Textbook of
Pediatric Dermatology

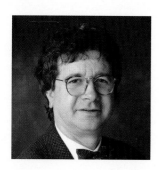

John Harper is Consultant in Paediatric Dermatology at Great Ormond Street Hospital for Children and Honorary Senior Lecturer at the Institute of Child Health, London. He trained at St Mary's Hospital, University of London, and his postgraduate thesis (MD) was on cutaneous manifestations of graft-versus-host disease. He was the founder Secretary of the British Society for Paediatric Dermatology and Chairman from 1988 to 1991, then President of the European Society for Pediatric Dermatology from 1993 to 1996. He is the author of *Handbook of Paediatric Dermatology* (Butterworth-Heinemann, London), and wrote the section of Genetics and Genodermatoses in the 'Rook' *Textbook of Dermatology* (Blackwell Science). Research interests include: atopic dermatitis, in particular genetics and new treatments; the inherited ichthyoses; developmental disorders of the skin and vitiligo. His work has established links worldwide in paediatric dermatology.

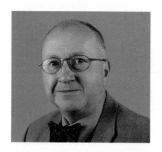

Arnold Oranje is Consultant in General and Paediatric Dermatology at the University Hospital Rotterdam, the Netherlands. He attended Erasmus University Rotterdam and completed his training in dermatology and venereology at the University Hospital Rotterdam. Dr Oranje was co-founder and Secretary of the Dutch Society for the Study of Sexually Transmitted Diseases. He was also founder and President of the Dutch–Belgian Society for Paediatric Dermatology. Dr Oranje was Secretary and President of the European Society for Pediatric Dermatology. He is co-editor of *Paediatric Dermatology*; a Dutch handbook and cd-rom (in English). He has written a thesis on gonococcal serology and numerous publications on different issues of dermatology and venereology. His current interests include atopic dermatitis, mastocytosis, and psychodermatology.

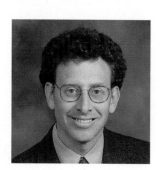

Neil Prose is Director of Pediatric Dermatology at Duke University Medical Center in Durham, North Carolina. He attended New York University School of Medicine and completed his training in dermatology and pediatrics at the State University of New York Health Science Center at Brooklyn. Dr Prose has served as President of the Society for Pediatric Dermatology, and on the board of directors of the Sulzberger Institute for Dermatologic Education. He is the co-author of the *Color Atlas of Pediatric Dermatology* (McGraw-Hill, New York), and has written numerous publications on the cutaneous manifestations of HIV infection in children. His current interests include the support of paediatric dermatology in developing countries, and the teaching of doctor–patient communication to medical students and physicians in training.

Textbook of Pediatric Dermatology

EDITED BY

JOHN HARPER MD, FRCP, FRCPCH
Consultant in Paediatric Dermatology
Great Ormond Street Hospital for Children
London, UK

ARNOLD ORANJE MD, PhD
Consultant in Paediatric and General Dermatology
University Hospital
Rotterdam, The Netherlands

NEIL PROSE MD
Director, Pediatric Dermatology
Duke University Medical Center, Durham
North Carolina, USA

IN TWO VOLUMES
VOLUME 2

FOREWORD BY
NANCY ESTERLY

b
**Blackwell
Science**

© 2000 by
Blackwell Science Ltd
Editorial Offices:
Osney Mead, Oxford OX2 0EL
25 John Street, London WC1N 2BL
23 Ainslie Place, Edinburgh EH3 6AJ
350 Main Street, Malden
  MA 02148 5018, USA
54 University Street, Carlton
  Victoria 3053, Australia
10, rue Casimir Delavigne
  75006 Paris, France

Other Editorial Offices:
Blackwell Wissenschafts-Verlag GmbH
Kurfürstendamm 57
10707 Berlin, Germany

Blackwell Science KK
MG Kodenmacho Building
7–10 Kodenmacho Nihombashi
Chuo-ku, Tokyo 104, Japan

First published 2000

Set by Excel Typesetters Co., Hong Kong
Printed and bound in Italy by G. Canale &
C. SpA, Turin

The Blackwell Science logo is a
trade mark of Blackwell Science Ltd,
registered at the United Kingdom
Trade Marks Registry

A catalogue record for this title
is available from the British Library

ISBN 0-86542-939-1

Library of Congress
Cataloging-in-publication Data

Textbook of pediatric dermatology / edited
  by John Harper, Arnold P. Oranje, Neil
  Prose.
      v. < 1– >   p.   cm.
    ISBN 0-86542-939-1
    1. Pediatric dermatology.   2. Skin—
  Diseases.   I. Harper, John I.   II. Oranje,
  Arnold P.   III. Prose, Neil S.
  RJ511. T492   1999
  618.92'5—dc21   99-38325
                                         CIP

DISTRIBUTORS

Marston Book Services Ltd
PO Box 269
Abingdon, Oxon OX14 4YN
(*Orders*: Tel: 01235 465500
          Fax: 01235 465555)

USA
  Blackwell Science, Inc.
  Commerce Place
  350 Main Street
  Malden, MA 02148 5018
  (*Orders*: Tel: 800 759 6102
                   781 388 8250
            Fax: 781 388 8255)

Canada
  Login Brothers Book Company
  324 Saulteaux Crescent
  Winnipeg, Manitoba R3J 3T2
  (*Orders*: Tel: 204 837 2987)

Australia
  Blackwell Science Pty Ltd
  54 University Street
  Carlton, Victoria 3053
  (*Orders*: Tel: 3 9347 0300
            Fax: 3 9347 5001)

For further information on
Blackwell Science, visit our website:
www.blackwell-science.com

Contents

vi   *Contents*

Contributors

ADRIAANS, Beverley
Consultant Dermatologist, Gloucester Royal Hospital, Great
West Road, Gloucester, GL1 3NN
Author of
Chapter 7.1: Tropical Ulcer

AL-ANARI, Huda
Fellow in Paediatric Infectious Diseases, Great Ormond Street
Hospital for Children NHS Trust, Great Ormond Street,
London, WC1 3JH
Co-author of
Chapter 5.10: Mycobacterial Infections of the Skin

ALBRECHT-NEBE, Helga
Department of Dermatology, Venereology and Allergology with
Asthma Outpatient Department, School of Medicine, Charité
Humboldt-University of Berlin, Schumannstrasse 20–21,
D-10117 Berlin, Germany
Author of
Chapter 25.11: Morphoea

ALONSO, Fausto Forin
Associate Professor of Dermatology, Santa Casa Medical School,
Sao Paulo, Brazil
Author of
Chapter 7.3: Cutaneous Larva Migrans

ANTAYA, Richard J
Assistant Professor, Dermatology and Pediatrics, Yale
University School of Medicine, CI501, 333 Cedar Street, New
Haven, CT 06520-8059, USA
Author of
Chapter 12.2: Infantile Acropustulosis
Chapter 19.18: Cutis Laxa
Co-author
Chapter 29.7: Hypereosinophilic Disorders

ANTON-LAMPRECHT, Ingrun
Professor, Formerly Director, Department of Dermatology,
Institute for Ultrastructure Research of the Skin, Ruprecht-
Karls University, Voss-Strasse 2, D-69115 Heidelberg,
Germany
Author of
Chapter 19.25: Prenatal Diagnosis of Inherited Skin Disorders

ARCHER, Clive B
Consultant Dermatologist and Honorary Clinical Senior
Lecturer, University of Bristol, Bristol Royal Infirmary,
Bristol, BS2 8HW
Author of
Chapter 3.4: Pharmacological Mechanisms in Atopic
Dermatitis

ATHERTON, David J
Consultant in Paediatric Dermatology, Great Ormond Street
Hospital for Children NHS Trust, Great Ormond Street,
London, WC1N 3JH
Author of
Chapter 19.4: Epidermolysis Bullosa

BAKER, Heidi B
Paediatric Dietitian, Leicester Royal Infirmary, Infirmary Square,
Leicester, LE1 5WW
Co-author of
Chapter 3.8: The Role of Diet in Atopic Dermatitis

BASELGA, Eulalia
Department of Dermatology, The Medical College of Wisconsin,
Milwaukee, WI 53226, USA
Co-author of
Chapter 13.3: Calcification and Ossification in the Skin

BAXBY, Derrick
Senior Lecturer in Microbiology, Department of Medical
Microbiology and Genitourinary Medicine, The University of
Liverpool, Duncan Building, Liverpool, L69 3BX
Co-author of
Chapter 5.5: Zoonotic Poxviruses

BECERRIL-CHIHU, Georgina
Attending Pediatric Dermatologist, National University of
Mexico, National Institute of Pediatrics, Mexico City, Mexico
Co-author of
Chapter 6.1: Skin Manifestations of Malnutrition

BENTON, E Claire
Department of Dermatology, Royal Infirmary of Edinburgh,
Edinburgh, EH3 9YW

Author of
> Chapter 5.1: Human Papillomavirus Infection and
> Molluscum Contagiosum

BETTENCOURT, Miriam S
Resident, Division of Dermatology, Duke University Medical
> Center, Durham, NC 27710, USA
Co-author of
> Chapter 4.7: Lichen Simplex Chronicus and Prurigo

BILO, Robert AC
Child Abuse Physician, Lindenhof Foundation (Office of the
> Confidential Doctor), University Hospital Rotterdam, The
> Netherlands
Co-author of
> Chapter 24.2: Sexually Transmitted Diseases in Children and
> Adolescents
> Chapter 26.2: Habit Disorders and Factitious Disease

BINGHAM, E Ann
Consultant Dermatologist, The Royal Hospitals Trust,
> Grosvenor Road, Belfast, BT12 6BA
Author of
> Chapter 3.7: Guidelines to Management of Atopic Dermatitis

BLACK, Carol M
Academic Rheumatology and Connective Tissue Diseases
> Unit, Royal Free Hospital, Rowland Hill Street, London,
> NW3 2PF
Author of
> Chapter 25.12: Systemic Sclerosis

BLACK, Martin M
St John's Institute of Dermatology, St Thomas' Hospital,
> Lambeth Palace Road, London, SE1 7EH
Author of
> Chapter 9.4: Erythema Nodosum and other forms of
> Panniculitis

BODEMER, Christine
Service de Dermatologie, Hôpital Necker-Enfants Malades, 149
> rue de Savres, 75015 Paris, France
Co-author of
> Chapter 29.1: Alopecia Areata

BOLOGNIA, Jean L
Professor of Dermatology, Department of Dermatology, Yale
> Medical School, 500 LCI, 333 Cedar Street, New Haven,
> CT 06520-3219, USA
Author of
> Chapter 14.1: Disorders of Hypopigmentation and
> Hyperpigmentation

BONIFAZI, Ernesto
Professore Associato di Dermatologia Pediatrica, Università di
> Bari, Policlinico, Piazza Giulio Cesare 11, 70124 Bari, Italy

Author of
> Chapter 2.2: Causative Factors (Napkin Dermatitis)
> Chapter 11.4: Pityriasis Lichenoides

BOS, Jan D
Academic Medical Center, University of Amsterdam,
> Meibergdreef 9, 1105 AZ, Amsterdam, The Netherlands
Author of
> Chapter 3.3: Immunology of Atopic Dermatitis

BROMBERG, Kenneth
Associate Professor of Pediatrics, Department of Pediatrics, State
> University of New York, Health Sciences Center at Brooklyn,
> 450 Clarkson Avenue, Brooklyn, NY 11203, USA
Co-author of
> Chapter 24.2: Sexually Transmitted Diseases in Children and
> Adolescents

BURGE, Susan
Consultant Dermatologist, The Churchill Hospital, Oxford,
> OX3 7LJ
Author of
> Chapter 19.9: Darier's Disease

BURNS, David A
Consultant Dermatologist, Leicester Royal Infirmary, Leicester,
> LE1 5WW
Author of
> Chapter 8.3: Other Noxious and Venomous Creatures

CAMBAZARD, Frederic
Service de Dermatologie, C.H.U. de Saint Etienne, Hôpital Nord,
> 42055 Saint Etienne Cedex 2, France
Author of
> Chapter 21.1: Langerhans' Cell and Non-Langerhans' Cell
> Histiocytosis
> Chapter 29.4: Striae

CLAYTON, Peter T
Professor of Paediatric Metabolic Disease and Hepatology,
> Institute of Child Health, London, WC1
Author of
> Chapter 29.10: Carotenaemia

CLAYTON, Yvonne M
Formerly of the Department of Medical Mycology, St John's
> Institute of Dermatology, St Thomas' Hospital, Lambeth
> Palace Road, London, SE1 7EH
Author of
> Chapter 5.15: Superficial Fungal Infections

CLIFF, Sandeep H
Department of Dermatology, St George's Hospital, Blackshaw
> Road, London, SW17 0QT
Co-author of
> Chapter 18.3: Disorders of Lymphatics

COHEN, Bernard
Associate Professor of Pediatrics and Dermatology, Johns
   Hopkins University School of Medicine
Director, Pediatric Dermatology, Johns Hopkins Children's
   Center, Division of Pediatric Dermatology, Brady 208, Johns
   Hopkins Hospital, 601 North Wolfe Street, Baltimore, MD
   21287, USA
Author of
   Chapter 1.13: Congenital Erosive and Vesicular Dermatosis

COLLIER, Paul M
Consultant Dermatologist
Royal Devon and Exeter Healthcare NHS Trust, Barrack Road,
   Exeter, EX2 5DW
Author of
   Chapter 12.3: Chronic Bullous Disease of Childhood

COLVEN, Roy
Division of Dermatology, University of Washington School of
   Medicine, Seattle, Washington, USA
Co-author of
   Chapter 1.5: Disorders of Subcutaneous Tissue in the
   Newborn

COOKSON, William OCM
Nuffield Department of Clinical Medicine, John Radcliffe
   Hospital, Headington, Oxford, OX3 9DU
Co-author of
   Chapter 3.2: Genetics of Atopic Dermatitis

COX, Helen
Department of Paediatric Dermatology, Great Ormond Street
   Hospital for Children NHS Trust, Great Ormond Street,
   London, WC1N 3JH
Co-author of
   Chapter 3.2: Genetics of Atopic Dermatitis

CUNLIFFE, William J
Professor of Dermatology, The General Infirmary at Leeds, Great
   George Street, Leeds, LS1 3EX
Author of
   Chapter 10.1: Acne

DANGOISSE Chantal
Service de Dermatologie, Hôpital Universitaire des Enfants
   Reine Fabiola, Avenue Crocq, 15, B-1020, Bruxelles, Belgium
Author of
   Chapter 29.5: Hyperhidrosis

DAVID, Timothy J
Professor of Child Health and Paediatrics, Booth Hall Children's
   Hospital, Charlestown Road, Blackley, Manchester, M9 7AA
Co-author of
   Chapter 3.8: The Role of Diet in Atopic Dermatitis

DENTON, Christopher P
Academic Rheumatology and Connective Tissues Diseases
   Unit, Royal Free Hospital, Rowland Hill Street, London,
   NW3 2PF
Co-author of
   Chapter 25.12: Systemic Sclerosis

DE MOOR, Anya
Snoekstraat 16, B-9300 Aalst, Belgium
Co-author of
   Chapter 13.1: Differential Diagnosis of Skin Nodules and
   Cysts

DE RAEVE, Linda E
Department of Paediatric Dermatology, Academic Hospital
   Free University of Brussels, Laabeeklaan 101, B-1090
   Brussels, Belgium
Author of
   Chapter 4.5: Nummular or Discoid Dermatitis
   Chapter 28.2: Treatment of Giant Congenital Melanocytic
   Naevi

DEVANEY, Kenneth
Associate Professor, Department of Pathology, University of
   Michigan Hospital, 1500 East Medical Center Drive, Ann
   Arbor, MI 48109, USA
Co-author of
   Chapter 13.4: Fibromatoses, Hyalinoses and Stiff Skin
   Syndrome

DILLON, Michael J
Professor of Paediatric Nephrology, Great Ormond Street
   Hospital for Children NHS Trust, Great Ormond Street,
   London, WC1N 3JH
Co-author of
   Chapter 25.8: Wegener's Granulomatosis, Polyarteritis
   Nodosa, Behçet's Disease and Relapsing Polychondritis

DONNAI, Dian
Department of Clinical Genetics, St Mary's Hospital, Hathersage
   Road, Manchester, M13 0JH
Author of
   Chapter 19.15: Incontinentia Pigmenti and Pigmentary
   Mosaicism

DUARTE, Ana M
Director, Division of Dermatology, Miami Children's Hospital,
   3100 SW 62 Avenue, Miami FL 33155-3009, USA
Author of
   Chapter 9.3: Annular Erythemas

EICHENFIELD, Lawrence F
Chief, Pediatric Dermatology and Laser Surgery, Children's
   Hospital and Health Center, University of California San
   Diego School of Medicine, California, USA
Author of
   Chapter 28.5: Sedation and Anaesthesia

ELEY, Brian
Department of Paediatrics and Child Health, University of Cape
  Town, Red Cross War Memorial Children's Hospital,
  Rondebosch, Cape 7700, South Africa
Co-author of
  Chapter 25.5: Purpura Fulminans

ENGELKENS, Herman Jan H
Department of Dermatology and Venereology, Ikazia
  Ziekenhuis, Montessoriweg 1, 3083 AN, Rotterdam, The
  Netherlands
Author of
  Chapter 5.13: Endemic Treponematoses: Yaws, Pinta and
  Endemic Syphilis

ENJOLRAS, Odile
Consultant, Paediatric Dermatology, hôpital Cochin pavillon
  Tarnier, 89 rue d'Assas, Paris 75006, and 'Consultation des
  Angiomes' hôpital Lariboisière, 2 rue Ambroise Paré, Paris
  75010, France
Co-author of
  Chapter 18.1: Vascular Malformations

ESTERLY, Nancy B
Professor of Pediatrics and Dermatology, The Medical College of
  Wisconsin, 9200 W. Wisconsin Avenue, Milwaukee, WI 53226,
  USA
Author of
  Chapter 18.2: Haemangiomas

EWING, Carol I
Consultant Paediatrician, Booth Hall Children's Hospital,
  Blackley, Manchester, M9 7AA
Co-author of
  Chapter 3.8: The Role of Diet in Atopic Dermatitis

FAIRLEY, Janet A
Department of Dermatology, The Medical College of Wisconsin,
  Milwaukee, WI 53226, USA
Co-author of
  Chapter 13.3: Calcification and Ossification in the Skin

FARNDON, Peter A
Professor of Clinical Genetics, University Department of Clinical
  Genetics, Birmingham Women's Hospital, Edgbaston,
  Birmingham, B15 2TG
Author of
  Chapter 19.16: The Gorlin (Naevoid Basal Cell Carcinoma)
  Syndrome

FERGUSON, James
Photodermatology Unit, Ninewells Hospital & Medical School,
  Dundee, DD1 9SY
Author of
  Chapter 15.1: The Idiopathic Photodermatoses

FRANCIS, Julie S
Associate Professor, Division of Dermatology, Department
  of Pediatrics, Children's Hospital and Medical Center,
  4800 Sand Point Way, NE, PO Box 537/CH-25, Seattle WA
  98105-0371, USA
Author of
  Chapter 19.11: Ectodermal Dysplasias

FRIEDEN, Ilona J
Clinical Professor, Department of Dermatology and
  Pediatrics, University of California San Francisco, Box 0316,
  San Francisco, CA 94143-0316, USA
Author of
  Chapter 4.3: Perioral Dermatitis

GARZON, Maria C
Director, Pediatric Dermatology, Assistant Professor of
  Dermatology and Pediatrics, College of Physicians and
  Surgeons of Columbia University, 161 Fort Washington
  Avenue, New York, NY 0032, USA
Author of
  Chapter 13.5: Lymphatoid Papulosis and Jessner's
  Lymphocytic Infiltrate

GELMETTI, Carlo
Dirigente Responsabile Servizio di Dermatologia Pediatrica,
  Instituto di Scienze Dermatologiche dell'Università di
  Milano, I.R.C.C.S. 'Ospedale Maggiore' di Milano, Via Pace 9,
  20122 Milano, Italy
Author of
  Chapter 4.4: Pompholyx
  Chapter 5.4: Gianotti–Crosti Syndrome

GLOVER, Mary T
Consultant Dermatologist, Newham Hospital, Glen Road,
  London, E13
Author of
  Chapter 3.11: Psychological Aspects of Atopic Dermatitis

GOLDSMITH, Portia C
Consultant Dermatologist, Whittington Hospital, Highgate Hill,
  London, N19 5NF
Co-author of
  Chapter 9.4: Erythema Nodosum and other forms of
  Panniculitis

GOODYEAR, Helen
Consultant Paediatrician, Birmingham Heartlands Hospital,
  Bordesley Green East, Birmingham, B9 5SS
Author of
  Chapter 3.10: Eczema Herpeticum
  Chapter 5.2: Herpes Simplex Virus Infections

GRIFFITHS, William Andrew David
Consultant Dermatologist, St John's Institute of Dermatology, St Thomas' Hospital, Lambeth Palace Road, London, SE1 7EH
Author of
Chapter 11.2: Pityriasis Rubra Pilaris

GROSSHANS, Edouard
Professor of Dermatology, University Louis Pasteur, Chief, Department of Dermatology, Hôpital Universitaire, Strasbourg, France
Co-author of
Chapter 11.6: Lichen Striatus

VAN GYSEL, Dirk
Department of Paediatrics, OLV Hospital, Aalst, Belgium
Co-author of
Chapter 1.7: Acquired Neonatal Infections
Chapter 9.2: Mastocytosis

HABIBI, Parviz
Senior Lecturer, Paediatric Intensive Care Unit, Department of Paediatrics, Imperial College School of Medicine at St Mary's, Norfolk Place, London W2 1PG
Co-author of
Chapter 5.8: Skin Manifestations of Meningococcal Infection

HALPERT, Evelyne
Professor of Paediatric Dermatology, Head, Paediatric Dermatology Department, Fundación Santa Fe de Bogata, Colombia
Author of
Chapter 7.2: Leishmaniasis

HAMM, Henning
Professor of Dermatology, Department of Dermatology, University of Würzburg, Josef-Schneider-Strasse 2, D-97080 Würzburg, Germany
Author of
Chapter 1.8: Developmental Abnormalities

HAMMERSCHLAG, Margaret
Department of Pediatrics, State University of New York, Health Sciences Center at Brooklyn, 450 Clarkson Avenue, Brooklyn, NY 11203, USA
Co-author of
Chapter 24.2: Sexually Transmitted Diseases in Children and Adolescents

HAPPLE, Rudolf
Department of Dermatology, Universität Marburg, Deutschhausstrasse 9, D-35033 Marburg, Germany
Author of
Chapter 19.1: Principles of Genetics, Mosaicism and Molecular Biology

HARPER, John Irwin
Consultant in Paediatric Dermatology, Great Ormond Street Hospital for Children NHS Trust, Great Ormond Street, London, WC1N 3JH
Author of
Chapter 3.2: Genetics of Atopic Dermatitis
Chapter 4.7: Lichen Simplex Chronicus and Prurigo
Chapter 13.1: Differential Diagnosis of Skin Nodules and Cysts
Chapter 19.24: Genetic Diseases which Predispose to Malignancy
Chapter 25.11: Morphoea
Chapter 25.15: Graft-Versus-Host Disease

HARVEY, David
Professor of Paediatrics, Department of Paediatrics, Imperial College School of Medicine, Hammersmith Hospital, DuCane Road, London, W12 0HS
Co-author of
Chapter 1.14: Iatrogenic Skin Disorders

HERNANDEZ, Carlos Arturo
Parasitology Laboratory, Instituto Nacional de Salud, Bogata, Colombia
Co-author of
Chapter 7.2: Leishmaniasis

HEYDERMAN, Robert S
Senior Lecturer, Department of Pathology and Microbiology, School of Medical Sciences, University of Bristol, University Walk, Bristol, BS8 1TD
Co-author of
Chapter 5.8: Skin Manifestations of Meningococcal Infection

HOEGER, Peter H
Department of Dermatology, University of Hamburg, Universitäts-Krankenhaus Eppendorf, Martinistr. 52, 20246 Hamburg, Germany
Author of
Chapter 1.6: Cutaneous Manifestations of Congenital Infections
Chapter 7.4: Myiasis
Co-author of
Chapter 13.1: Differential Diagnosis of Skin Nodules and Cysts

HOGAN, Peter A
Department of Dermatology, Royal Alexandria Hospital for Children, Sydney, Australia
Author of
Chapter 25.10: Cutaneous Manifestations of Endocrine Disease

HOLBROOK, Karen A
Senior Vice President for Academic Affairs and Provost, University of Georgia, 108 Old College, Athens, GA 30602, USA
Author of
 Chapter 1.1: Embryogenesis of the Skin

HONIG, Paul J
Professor of Pediatrics and Dermatology, University of Pennsylvania School of Medicine, Director of Pediatric Dermatology, Children's Hospital of Philadelphia, 34th and Civic Center Boulevard, Philadelphia, PA 19104, USA
Co-author of
 Chapter 2.3: Clinical Features and Differential Diagnosis (Napkin Dermatitis)

HORNUNG, Robin
Assistant Professor, Division of Dermatology, Department of Pediatrics, Children's Hospital & Regional Center, University of Washington School of Medicine, Seattle, WA 98105, USA
Author of
 Chapter 15.3: Photoprotection

HUSON, Susan M
Consultant Clinical Geneticist, Department of Clinical Genetics, Oxford Radcliffe Hospital, The Churchill, Old Road, Headington, Oxford, OX3 7LJ
Author of
 Chapter 19.13: The Neurofibromatoses

ILOWITE, Norman T
Chief, Pediatric Rheumatology and Professor of Pediatrics, Albert Einstein College of Medicine, Schneider Children's Hospital, Long Island Jewish Health System, New Hyde Park, NY 11040, USA
Author of
 Chapter 5.12: Lyme Disease

JORIZZO, Joseph L
Professor and Chairman, Department of Dermatology, Bowman Gray School of Medicine, Wake Forest University, Medical Center Boulevard, Winston-Salem, NC 27157-1071, USA
Author of
 Chapter 25.6: Urticarial Vasculitis
 Chapter 25.7: Erythema Elevatum Diutinum

JUDGE, Mary R
Consultant Dermatologist, Royal Bolton Hospital, Bolton, BL4 0JR
Author of
 Chapter 1.10: Collodion Baby and Harlequin Ichthyosis

KAHN, Teri A
Director, Pediatric Dermatology, The Cleveland Clinic Foundation, One Clinic Center, 9500 Euclid Avenue, Cleveland, OH 44195-5032, USA

Author of
 Chapter 29.9: Amyloidosis

KANGESU, Loshan
St Andrews Centre for Plastic Surgery, Broomfield Hospital, Court Road, Broomfield, Chelmsford, Essex, CM1 7ET
Author of
 Chapter 28.3: More Complex Skin Surgery

KAWASAKI, Tomisaku
Director, Japan Kawasaki Disease Research Center, Kubo Building, 1-1-1 Kandasuda-cho, Chiyoda-ku, Tokyo 101, Japan
Author of
 Chapter 25.9: Kawasaki's Disease

KENNEDY, Cameron
Consultant Dermatologist, Bristol Royal Infirmary, Bristol, BS2 8HW
Author of
 Chapter 29.2: Granuloma Annulare

DE KLERK, Johannis BC
Consultant Paediatrician, Sophia Kinderziekenhuis, Dr. Molewaterplein 60, 3015 GJ Rotterdam, The Netherlands
Co-author of
 Chapter 19.12: Inherited Metabolic Disorders and the Skin

KOBLENZER, Caroline Scott
Clinical Professor of Dermatology and Dermatology-in-Psychiatry, The University of Pennsylvania, 1812 Delancey Place, Philadelphia, PA 19103, USA
Author of
 Chapter 26.1: Coping with Chronic Skin Disease

KRAFCHIK, Bernice R
Professor, University of Toronto, Departments of Pediatrics and Medicine, Division of Dermatology, Hospital for Sick Children, 555 University Avenue, Toronto, Ontario, Canada
Author of
 Chapter 5.3: Viral Exanthems

KUNZ, Barbara
Department of Dermatology, University of Hamburg, Universitäts-Krankenhaus Eppendorf, Martinistrasse 52, 20246 Hamburg, Germany
Author of
 Chapter 3.6: Clinical Features and Diagnostic Criteria of Atopic Dermatitis

LACOUR, Marc
Hôpital de la Tour, 3 av. J-D Maillard, CH-1217, Meyrin, Switzerland
Author of
 Chapter 19.20: Buschke–Ollendorff Syndrome, Marfan's

Syndrome, Osteogenesis Imperfecta, Anetodermas and
Atrophodermas
Chapter 20.1: Disorders of Fat Tissue

FAT, Rudy FM Lai A
Department of Dermatology, Academic Hospital, PO Box 1884,
  Parimaribo-Suriname, Surinam
Author of
  Chapter 7.5: Leprosy

LAMERSON, Cindy
Department of Dermatology, University of Cincinnati, PO Box
  670592, Cincinnati, OH 45267-0592, USA
Co-author of
  Chapter 14.2: Vitiligo

LANDAU, Marina
Department of Dermatology, Sackler School of Medicine, Tel
  Aviv University, 6 Weizman Street, Tel Aviv 64239, Israel
Co-author of
  Chapter 27.2: Hypersensitivity Reactions to Drugs

LANGTRY, James AA
Consultant Dermatologist, Sunderland Royal Hospital,
  Sunderland, SR4 7TP
Author of
  Chapter 4.6: Seborrhoeic Dermatitis of Adolescence

LARCHER, Vic
Consultant Paediatrician, Queen Elizabeth Children's Services,
  Royal London Hospital, Whitechapel, London, E11 BB
Author of
  Chapter 24.3: Physical and Sexual Abuse

LEAUTE-LABREZE, Christine
Consultant Pediatric Dermatologist, Unité de Dermatologie
  Pédiatrique, Hôpital Pellegrin-Enfants, Place Amélie Raba
  Léon, 33076 Bordeaux, France
Co-author of
  Chapter 9.1: Urticaria

LEBWOHL, Mark
Professor and Chairman, Department of Dermatology, The
  Mount Sinai School of Medicine, 5 East 98th Street, New York,
  NY 10029-6574, USA
Author of
  Chapter 19.19: Pseudoxanthoma Elasticum

LEGRAIN, Valérie
Consultant Pediatric Dermatologist, Unité de Dermatologie
  Pédiatrique, Hôpital Pellegrin-Enfants, Place Amélie Raba
  Léon, 33076 Bordeaux cédex, France
Co-author of
  Chapter 25.4: Acute Haemorrhagic Oedema of the Skin in
  Infancy

LEONARD, Jonathan N
Consultant Dermatologist, St Mary's Hospital, Praed Street,
  London W2 1NY
Author of
  Chapter 12.4: Dermatitis Herpetiformis

LEVER, Rosemary
Consultant Dermatologist, Royal Hospital for Sick Children,
  Yorkhill, Glasgow, G3 8SJ
Author of
  Chapter 3.5: Microbiology of Atopic Dermatitis

LEVIN, Michael
Professor of Paediatrics, Imperial College School of Medicine at
  St Mary's, Norfolk Place, London, W2 1PG
Author of
  Chapter 25.5: Purpura Fulminans

LEVY, Moise L
Professor of Dermatology and Pediatrics, Baylor College of
  Medicine, Chief, Dermatology Service, Texas Children's
  Hospital, 6621 Fannin, MC 3-3315, Houston, TX 77030, USA
Author of
  Chapter 28.4: Lasers for Vascular and Pigmented Lesions
Co-author of
  Chapter 13.4: Fibromatoses, Hyalinoses and Stiff Skin
  Syndrome

LEWIS-JONES, M Susan
Consultant Dermatologist, Ninewells Hospital and Medical
  School, Dundee, DD1 9SY
Author of
  Chapter 5.5: Zoonotic Poxviruses

LIM, Henry W
Chairman, Department of Dermatology, Clarence S. Livingood
  Chair in Dermatology, Henry Ford Health System, 2799 West
  Grand Boulevard, Detroit, Michigan, USA
Co-author of
  Chapter 15.2: Porphyrias

LOVELL, Christopher R
Consultant Dermatologist, Royal United Hospital, Combe Park,
  Bath, BA1 3NG
Author of
  Chapter 4.10: Phytodermatoses

LUCKER, George PH
Department of Dermatology, Deventer Riekenhuis, PO Box 5001,
  7400 GC Deventer, The Netherlands
Co-author of
  Chapter 19.6: Palmoplantar Keratoses

LUKER, Jane
Department of Oral and Dental Science, Bristol Dental Hospital
  and School, Lower Maudlin Street, Bristol, BS1 2LY

Author of
> Chapter 22.1: Diseases of the Oral Mucosa and Tongue

LUNT, Peter W
Consultant Clinical Geneticist, Bristol Royal Hospital for Sick
    Children, St Michael's Hill, Bristol, BS2 8BJ
Author of
> Chapter 19.2: Chromosome Disorders

MAALOUF, Elia
Neonatal Research Fellow, Department of Paediatrics, Imperial
    College School of Medicine, Hammersmith Hospital,
    DuCane Road, London, W12 0HS
Author of
> Chapter 1.14: Iatrogenic Skin Disorders

MALLORY, Susan Bayliss
Professor of Medicine (Dermatology) and Pediatrics,
    Washington University School of Medicine, St Louis, MO
    63110, USA
Director of Pediatric Dermatology, St Louis Children's
    Hospital, 1 Children's Place, St Louis, MO 63110, USA
Author of
> Chapter 1.5: Disorders of Subcutaneous Tissue in the
> Newborn

MALONEY, Mary E
Professor of Medicine (Dermatology), University of
    Massachusetts, Division of Dermatology, University of
    Massachusetts Memorial Medical Center, 55 Lake Avenue
    North, Worcester, MA 01655, USA
Author of
> Chapter 28.1: Basic Skin Surgery Techniques

MASCARO, Jose M
Professor and Chairman of Dermatology, Hospital Clinic and
    Faculty of Medicine, University of Barcelona, Casanova 143,
    Barcelona 08036, Spain
Author of
> Chapter 15.2: Porphyrias

MAUNDER, John W
Director, Medical Entomology Centre, Cambridge Road,
    Fulbourn, Cambridge, CB1 5EL
Author of
> Chapter 8.1: Papular Urticaria

McCAULIFFE, Daniel P
Assistant Professor of Dermatology, University of North
    Carolina, Department of Dermatology, Room 3100,
    Thurston Building-CB#7287, Chapel Hill, NC 27599-7287,
    USA
Author of
> Chapter 1.11: Neonatal Lupus Erythematosus

McGRATH, John A
Department of Cell and Molecular Pathology, St John's Institute
    of Dermatology, St Thomas' Hospital, Lambeth Palace Road,
    London, SE1 7EH
Author of
> Chapter 19.26: DNA and Gene Analysis in Prenatal Diagnosis

McNALLY, Lisa
Infectious Diseases Unit, Great Ormond Street Hospital for
    Children NHS Trust, Great Ormond Street, London, WC1N
    3JH
Co-author of
> Chapter 5.10: Mycobacterial Infections of the Skin

METZKER, Aryeh
Consultant in Pediatric Dermatology, Department of
    Dermatology, Sourasky Medical Center, 6 Weizman Street,
    Tel Aviv 64239, Israel
Author of
> Chapter 11.3: Pityriasis Rosea

MICALI, Giuseppe
Associate Professor of Dermatology, Clinica Dermatologica,
    Universita di Catania, Piazza Sant' Agata la Vetere 5, 95100
    Catania, Italy
Co-author of
> Chapter 27.1: Principles of Paediatric Dermatological
> Therapy
> Chapter 27.3: Poisoning and Paediatric Skin

MICHEL, Jean-Loic
Service de Dermatologie, C.H.U. de Saint-Etienne, Hôpital
    Nord, 42055 Saint Etienne, Cedex 2, France
Co-author of
> Chapter 29.4: Striae

MORTIMER, Peter S
Physician to the Skin Department/Reader in Dermatology,
    St George's Hospital, Blackshaw Road, London,
    SW17 0QT
Co-author of
> Chapter 18.3: Disorders of Lymphatics

MORTUREUX, Patricia
Consultant Pediatric Dermatologist, Unité de Dermatologie
    Pédiatrique, Hôpital Pellegrin-Enfants, Place Amélie Raba
    Léon, 33076 Bordeaux, France
Co-author of
> Chapter 9.1: Urticaria

MOSS, Celia
Consultant Dermatologist, The Birmingham Children's
    Hospital, Steelhouse Lane, Birmingham, B4 6NL
Author of
> Chapter 19.23: Rothmund-Thomson Syndrome, Bloom's
> Syndrome, Dyskeratosis Congenita and Fanconi's Syndrome

MULLIKEN, John B
Director Craniofacial Center, Associate Professor of Surgery, Harvard Medical School, Children's Hospital, Boston, Massachusetts, USA
Co-author of
 Chapter 18.1: Vascular Malformations

MYERS, Sarah A
Box 3852, Duke University Medical Center, Durham, NC 27710, USA
Author of
 Chapter 5.11: *Bartonella* Infections: Bacillary Angiomatosis, Cat Scratch Disease and Bartonellosis

NEILL, Sallie M
Consultant Dermatologist, St Peter's Hospital, Guildford Road, Chertsey, Surrey, KT16 0PZ
Author of
 Chapter 24.1: Vulvovaginitis and Lichen Sclerosus

NEWTON BISHOP, Julia A
ICRF Cancer Medicine Research Unit, St James's University Hospital, Beckett Street, Leeds, LS9 7TF
Author of
 Chapter 16.1: Melanocytic Naevi and Melanoma

NORDLUND, James J
Professor and Chairman, Department of Dermatology, University of Cincinnati, PO Box 670592, Cincinnati, OH 45267-0592, USA
Author of
 Chapter 14.2: Vitiligo

NOVELLI, Vas
Consultant in Paediatric Infectious Diseases, Great Ormond Street Hospital for Children NHS Trust, Great Ormond Street, London, WC1N 3JH
Author of
 Chapter 5.10: Mycobacterial Infections of the Skin

OLSEN, Elise A
Professor of Medicine, Division of Dermatology, Box 3294, Duke University Medical Center, Durham, NC 27710, USA
Author of
 Chapter 23.1: Hair Disorders

ORANJE, Arnold P
Department of Dermato-venereology, University Hospital Rotterdam, Dr. Molewaterplein 60, 3015 GJ Rotterdam, The Netherlands
Author of
 Chapter 1.7: Acquired Neonatal Infections
 Chapter 2.1: General Aspects (Napkin Dermatitis)
 Chapter 2.4: Management (Napkin Dermatitis)
 Chapter 9.2: Mastocytosis

 Chapter 11.1: Psoriasis
 Chapter 13.4: Fibromatoses, Hyalinoses and Stiff Skin Syndrome
 Chapter 19.7: Keratosis Pilaris
 Chapter 19.12: Inherited Metabolic Disorders and the Skin
 Chapter 24.2: Sexually Transmitted Diseases in Children and Adolescents
 Chapter 26.2: Habit Disorders and Factitious Disease

OSBORNE, John P
Professor of Paediatrics and Child Health and Consultant Paediatrician, Royal United Hospital, Combe Park, Bath, BA1 3NG
Author of
 Chapter 19.14: Tuberous Sclerosis

PAIGE, David G
Consultant Dermatologist, The Royal Hospitals Trust, The Royal London Hospital, Whitechapel, London, E1 1BB
Author of
 Chapter 1.12: Restrictive Dermopathy
 Chapter 19.8: The Erythrokeratodermas

PALLER, Amy S
Professor of Pediatrics and Dermatology, Northwestern University Medical School, Head, Division of Dermatology, Children's Memorial Hospital, 2300 Children's Plaza, Chicago, IL 60614, USA
Author of
 Chapter 25.14: Immunodeficiency Syndromes

PATEL, Leena
Senior Lecturer in Child Health, Booth Hall Children's Hospital, Charlestown Road, Blackley, Manchester, M9 7AA
Co-author of
 Chapter 3.8: The Role of Diet in Atopic Dermatitis

PHILLIPS, Rod
Consultant in Paediatric Skin Disease, Royal Children's Hospital, Flemington Road, Parkville, Victoria 3052, Australia
Author of
 Chapter 25.2: Cystic Fibrosis

PIERINI, Adrián-Martín
Servicio de Dermatologia Pediatrica, Hospital de Pediatria 'Prof. Dr Juan P. Garrahan', Combate de los Pozos 1881, (1245) Buenos Aires, Argentina
Author of
 Chapter 5.16: Deep Mycoses and Opportunistic Infections
 Chapter 13.6: Skin Malignancies

PIERINI, Rita Garcia-Diaz de
Servicio de Dermatologia Pediatrica, Hospital de Pediatria 'Prof. Dr Juan P. Garrahan', Combate de los Pozos 1881, (1245) Buenos Aires, Argentina

Co-author of
   Chapter 13.6: Skin Malignancies

PIRACCINI, Bianca Maria
Department of Dermatology, University of Bologna, Bologna,
   Italy
Co-author of
   Chapter 23.2: Nail Disorders

VAN PRAAG, Marinus CG
Department of Dermatology, Sint Fanciscus Gasthuis, Rotterdam
   University Hospital, Leiden, Rotterdam, The Netherlands
Co-author of
   Chapter 1.7: Acquired Neonatal Infections

PRENDIVILLE, Julie S
Division of Pediatric Dermatology, University of British
   Columbia, British Columbia's Children's Hospital, 4480 Oak
   Street, Vancouver, BC V6H 3V4, Canada
Author of
   Chapter 8.2: Scabies and Lice

PROSE, Neil S
Director, Pediatric Dermatology, Duke University Medical
   Center, Box 3252 DUMC, Durham, NC 27710, USA
Author of
   Chapter 5.6: Cutaneous Manifestations of HIV Infection

DE PROST, Yves
Service de Dermatologie, Hôpital Necker-Enfants Malades, 149
   rue de Savres, 75015 Paris, France
Author of
   Chapter 29.1: Alopecia Areata

RABINOWITZ, Linda G
Associate Professor, Department of Pediatrics (Dermatology),
   Medical College of Wisconsin; Director, Vascular Birthmark
   Treatment Center, Children's Hospital of Wisconsin,
   Milwaukee, Wisconsin, USA
Author of
   Chapter 25.3: Henoch–Schönlein Purpura
   Chapter 29.6: Pigmented Purpuras
   Chapter 29.8: Angiolymphoid Hyperplasia with
   Eosinophilia

RAJKA, Georg
Frederik Stangsgt 44, 0264 Oslo, Norway
Author of
   Chapter 4.1: Infantile Seborrhoeic Dermatitis

RAWSTRON, Sarah A
Department of Pediatrics, State University of New York, Health
   Sciences Center at Brooklyn, 450 Clarkson Avenue, Brooklyn,
   NY 11203, USA

Co-author of
   Chapter 24.2: Sexually Transmitted Diseases in Children and
   Adolescents

RESNICK, Steven D
Chief, Division of Dermatology, Department of Adult and
   Pediatric Medicine, Bassett Healthcare, Cooperstown, NY
   13326; Associate Clinical Professor of Dermatology,
   Columbia University, College of Physicians and Surgeons,
   New York, NY, USA
Author of
   Chapter 5.7: Staphylococcal and Streptococcal Skin Diseases:
   Pyodermas and Toxin-mediated Syndromes

RICO, M Joyce
Chief, Dermatology Service, Dermatology-130, New York VA
   Medical Center, 423 East 23rd Street, New York, NY 10010,
   USA
Author of
   Chapter 12.1: Differential Diagnosis of Vesiculobullous
   Lesions

RING, Johannes
Department of Dermatology, Technische Universität, München,
   Biedersteiner Strasse 29, 80802 Munich, Germany
Co-author of
   Chapter 3.6: Clinical Features and Diagnostic Criteria of
   Atopic Dermatitis

ROBERTS, Nerys
Consultant Dermatologist, Chelsea and Westminster Hospital,
   Fulham Road, London, SW10 9NH
Author of
   Chapter 29.7: Hypereosinophilic Disorders

RODRIGUEZ, Gerzaín
Scientific Investigator, Instituto Nacional de Salud; Full
   Professor, Facultad de Medicina, Universidad Nacional de
   Colombia, Bogata, Colombia
Co-author of
   Chapter 7.2: Leishmaniasis

ROGERS, Maureen
Head, Department of Dermatology, The Children's Hospital
   Medical Centre, Hainsworth Street, Westmead, 2145,
   Australia
Author of
   Chapter 17.1: Epidermal Naevi

RUGGIERI, Martino
Division of Pediatric Neurology, Department of Pediatrics,
   University of Catania, Via S. Sofia, 78, Catania I-95125, Italy
Co-author of
   Chapter 19.13: The Neurofibromatoses

RUIZ-MALDONADO, Ramón
Professor of Dermatology and Pediatrics, National University of Mexico, National Institute of Pediatrics, Mexico City, Mexico
Author of
Chapter 6.1: Skin Manifestations of Malnutrition

RUTTER, Nicholas
Professor of Paediatric Medicine, University Hospital, Nottingham, NG7 2UH
Author of
Chapter 1.2: Physiology of the Newborn Skin

SANDLER, Boris
Professor of Paediatrics, University of Bordeaux II, Department of Neonatal Medicine, Hôpital Pellegrin-Enfants, Place Amélie Raba Léon, 33076 Bordeaux cédex, France
Co-author of
Chapter 1.4: Common Transient Neonatal Dermatoses

SEXTON, Daniel J
Professor of Medicine, Department of Medicine, Division of Infectious Diseases, Duke University Medical Center, Durham, NC 27710, USA
Author of
Chapter 5.14: Rocky Mountain Spotted Fever and Other Rickettsial Infections

SHAPIRO, Lori E
Division of Dermatology and Clinical Pharmacology, University of Toronto, Sunnybrook and Women's College Health Sciences Center, Room E-240, 2075 Bayview Avenue, Toronto, Ontario M4N 3M5, Canada
Co-author of
Chapter 27.2: Hypersensitivity Reactions to Drugs

SHEA, Christopher R
Associate Professor of Pathology and Medicine, Box 3712, Duke University Medical Center, Durham, NC 27710, USA
Author of
Chapter 13.2: Adnexal Disorders

SHEAR, Neil H
Professor of Medicine, Pharmacology and Pediatrics, University of Toronto, Sunnybrook and Women's College Health Sciences Center, Room E-240, 2075 Bayview Avenue, Toronto, Ontario, M4N 3M5, Canada
Author of
Chapter 27.2: Hypersensitivity Reactions to Drugs

SHETH, Anita P
Assistant Professor, University of Cincinnati College of Medicine and Children's Hospital Medical Center, Department of Dermatology, PO Box 670592, Cincinnati, OH 45267-0592, USA
Author of
Chapter 5.9: Pitted Keratolysis, Erythrasma and Erysipeloid

SIDHU-MALIK, Navjeet K
Assistant Professor of Dermatology, University of Virginia Health Sciences Center, Box 134 University Hospitals, Charlottesville, VA 22901, USA
Author of
Chapter 19.17: Ehlers–Danlos Syndromes

SIEGFRIED, Elaine C
Associate Professor of Pediatrics and Dermatology, St Louis University School of Medicine, St Louis, MO 63104, USA
Author of
Chapter 19.10: The Porokeratoses
Chapter 29.3: Knuckle Pads

SILLEVIS SMITT, J Henk
Department of Dermatology, Academisch Medisch Centrum, University of Amsterdam, Meibergdreef 9, 1105 AZ Amsterdam, The Netherlands
Author of
Chapter 12.5: Pemphigus, Pemphigoid and Epidermolysis Bullosa Acquisita

SMITH, Paul J
Consultant Plastic and Reconstructive Surgeon, Great Ormond Street Hospital for Children NHS Trust, Great Ormond Street, London, WC1N 3JH
Co-author of
Chapter 28.3: More Complex Skin Surgery

SOLOMON, Lawrence M
Head, Dermatology, Department of Pediatrics, Lutheran General Pediatric Hospital, 1775 Dempster Street, Park Ridge, IL 60068, USA
Author of
Chapter 11.5: Lichen Planus and Lichen Nitidus

SONG, Micheline
Service de Dermatologie, Hôpital Universitaire des Enfants Reine Fabiola, Avenue Crocq, 15, B-1020 Bruxelles, Belgium
Co-author of
Chapter 29.5: Hyperhidrosis

SONI, Bhavik P
Dermatology Associates of Tallahassee, 1707 Riggins Road, Tallahassee, FL 32308, USA
Co-author of
Chapter 25.6: Urticarial Vasculitis
Chapter 25.7: Erythema Elevatum Diutinum

SPRAKER, Mary K
Associate Professor of Dermatology and Pediatrics, Chief of Dermatology, Egleston Hospital, Emory University School of

Medicine, Department of Dermatology, 1639 Pierce Drive, Room 5001 WMB, Atlanta, Georgia 30322, USA
Author of
Chapter 1.9: Differential Diagnosis of Neonatal Erythroderma

STALDER, Jean-François
Clinique Dermatologique, CHU Hôtel Dieu, 44035 Nantes cédex, France
Author of
Chapter 1.3: Skin care of the Newborn

STAUGHTON, Richard
Consultant Dermatologist, Chelsea and Westminster Hospital, Fulham Road, London, SW10 9NH
Co-author of
Chapter 29.7: Hypereosinophilic Disorders

VAN STEENSEL, Maurice AM
MD Resident, Department of Dermatology, University Hospital Nijmegen, PO Box 9101, 6500 HB Nijmegen, The Netherlands
Co-author of
Chapter 19.3: Review of Keratin Disorders

STEIJLEN, Peter M
Associate Professor of Dermatology, Department of Dermatology, University Hospital Nijmegen, PO Box 9101, 6500 HB Nijmegen, The Netherlands
Author of
Chapter 19.3: Review of Keratin Disorders
Chapter 19.6: Palmoplantar Keratoses

STEPHAN, Jean-Louis
Unité d'Hematologie et Oncologie Pédiatrique, CHU de Saint Etienne, Hôpital Nord, 42055 Saint Etienne cedex 2, France
Co-author of
Chapter 21.1: Langerhans' Cell and Non-Langerhans' Cell Histiocytosis

TAÏEB, Alain
Professor of Dermatology, University Victor Segaleu Bordeaux II, Unité de Dermatologie Pédiatrique, Hôptial Pellegrin-Enfants, Place Amélie Raba Léon, 33076 Bordeaux cédex, France
Author of
Chapter 1.4: Common Transient Neonatal Dermatoses
Chapter 9.1: Urticaria
Chapter 11.6: Lichen Striatus
Chapter 25.4: Acute Haemorrhagic Oedema of the Skin in Infancy

TAMAYO-SANCHEZ, Lourdes
Head, Department of Paediatric Dermatology, Instituto Nacional de Pediatria, Secretaria de Salud Publica, Mexico, DF, Mexico

Co-author of
Chapter 4.7: Lichen Simplex Chronicus and Prurigo

TENNSTEDT, Dominique
Unité de Dermatologie, Université Catholique de Louvain, École de Santé Publique, Clos Chapelle-aux-Champs, 30-UCL 3033, 1200 Bruxelles, Belgium
Author of
Chapter 4.8: Juvenile Plantar Dermatosis

TIZARD, E Jane
Consultant Paediatrician and Nephrologist, Children's Renal Unit, Southmead Hospital, Westbury-on-Trym, Bristol, BS10 5NB
Author of
Chapter 25.8: Wegener's Granulomatosis, Polyarteritis Nodosa, Behçet's Disease and Relapsing Polychondritis

TORIELLO, Helga V
Director of Genetics Services, Devos Children's Hospital at Spectrum Health, 21 Michigan Street, Suite 465, Grand Rapids, MI 49503, USA
Author of
Chapter 19.21: Premature Ageing Syndromes

TOSTI, Antonella
Department of Dermatology, University of Bologna, Bologna, Italy
Author of
Chapter 23.2: Nail Disorders

TRAUPE, Heiko
Associate Professor of Dermatology, Universitäs-Hautklinik, Von-Esmarch-Strasse 56, 48149 Münster, Germany
Author of
Chapter 19.5: The Genetic Ichthyoses

VIEHMAN, Gregory E
Cary Skin Center, Apex NC 27502, USA
Co-author of
Chapter 13.2: Adnexal Disorders

DE WAARD-VAN DER SPEK, Flora B
Department of Dermato-venereology, University Hospital Rotterdam, Dr. Molewaterplein 60, 3015 GJ Rotterdam, The Netherlands
Co-author of
Chapter 11.1: Psoriasis

WAGNER, Annette
Assistant Professor of Pediatrics and Dermatology Northwestern University, School of Medicine, Division of Dermatology, #107, Children's Memorial Hospital, 2300 Children's Plaza, Chicago, Illinois 60614-3394, USA

Author of
> Chapter 19.22: Xeroderma Pigmentosum, Cockayne's Syndrome and Trichothiodystrophy

WAHRMAN, Julie E
Clinical Affiliate, Dermatology Division, Children's Hospital of Philadelphia, 34th and Civic Center Boulevard, Philadelphia, PA 19104, USA
Author of
> Chapter 2.3: Clinical Features and Differential Diagnosis (Napkin Dermatitis)

WARNER, John O
Professor of Child Health, University of Southampton, Child Health, Level G, Centre Block, Southampton General Hospital, Tremona Road, Southampton, SO16 6YD
Author of
> Chapter 3.9: Environmental Allergens in Atopic Dermatitis

WEST, Dennis P
Professor of Dermatology, Director, Dermatopharmacology Program, Department of Dermatology, Clinical Trials Unit/Suite 19–200, 675 North St Clair, Chicago, IL 60611-3008, USA
Author of
> Chapter 27.1: Principles of Paediatric Dermatological Therapy
> Chapter 27.3: Poisoning and Paediatric Skin

WESTON, William
Professor and Chairman of Dermatology, Box B 153, University of Colorado, School of Medicine, Denver, CO 80262, USA
Author of
> Chapter 9.5: Erythema Multiforme, Stevens–Johnson Syndrome and Toxic Epidermal Necrolysis

WHITE, Ian R
Consultant Dermatologist, St John's Institute of Dermatology, St Thomas' Hospital, Lambeth Palace Road, London, SE1 7EH
Author of
> Chapter 4.9: Allergic Contact Dermatitis

WILLIAMS, Hywel C
Professor of Dermato-Epidemiology, Department of Dermatology, Queen's Medical Centre, University Hospital NHS Trust, Nottingham, NG7 2UH
Author of
> Chapter 3.1: Epidemiology of Atopic Dermatitis

WISS, Karen
Associate Professor of Medicine (Dermatology) and Pediatrics, Director of Pediatric Dermatology, University of Massachusetts Medical School, 55 Lake Avenue North, Worcester, MA 01655, USA
Author of
> Chapter 25.1: Sarcoidosis, Pyoderma Gangrenosum, Crohn's Disease and Granulomatous Cheilitis

WOJNAROWSKA, Fenella
Professor of Dermatology, The Churchill Hospital, Old Road, Headington, Oxford, OX3 7LJ
Co-author of
> Chapter 12.3: Chronic Bullous Disease of Childhood

WOO, Patricia
Professor of Paediatric Rheumatology, University College London, Department of Paediatric Rheumatology, Great Ormond Street Hospital for Children NHS Trust, Great Ormond Street, London, WC1N 3JH
Author of
> Chapter 25.13: Juvenile Chronic Arthritis, Systemic Lupus Erythematosus and Dermatomyositis

YAMAMOTO, Kazuya
Department of Dermatology, National Children's Hospital, 3-35-31 Taishido Setagaya-ku, Tokyo 154, Japan
Author of
Chapter 4.2: Pityriasis Alba

ZUBKOV, Bella
Dermatology Associates of Glastonbury, 211 New London Turnpike, Glastonbury, CT 06033, USA
Co-author of
> Chapter 11.5: Lichen Planus and Lichen Nitidus

Preface

Paediatric dermatology is now recognized as a separate subspecialty in most countries, and societies devoted to our field are now established in Europe, the United States, South America and Asia.

The *Textbook of Pediatric Dermatology* is intended to be an authoritative and up-to-date text with 185 contributors from 18 different countries.

The book is formatted in sections which cover both the common diseases, such as atopic dermatitis and psoriasis, and the many rare disorders of the skin which occur in children. We have also included the latest advances in molecular genetics, and the newest and most promising modalities of treatment.

We wish to thank all of the many people who have been involved in the creation and production of this book. Special thanks go to Stuart Taylor and Alice Emmott at Blackwell Science, and to Rosemary Barton, Deborah Ladd, Hilly Versprille, Bhupendra Tank and the Medical Illustration Department at Great Ormond Street Hospital.

It has been an exciting challenge to bring together such a wealth of expert knowledge, from countries all over the world. We hope that this book will be a useful and user-friendly reference text for paediatricians, dermatologists, and all other individuals involved in the care of children.

John Harper
Arnold Oranje
Neil Prose

Please note: the spelling of the word 'Pediatric' in the title of this textbook was advised by the publishing company because of international marketing, but throughout the text we have maintained the traditional spelling of 'paediatric' according to its Greek derivation.

Foreword

During the past three decades pediatric dermatology has emerged as a specialty in its own right. Prior to that, interest in skin diseases of children was limited, except on the part of a few, mostly academic, physicians. Books on the subject were scarce and research in the field was in its infancy. In recent years, however, there has been a virtual explosion of medical knowledge resulting from efforts to understand the mechanisms of children's skin disease and to discover safe, effective modes of treatment. As interest in pediatric dermatology has increased exponentially, so has the need for accurate and up-to-date information. We now have regional, national and international societies as well as several journals devoted to physician education, but so too, is there a need for other resources.

To this end, Harper, Oranje and Prose have compiled an encyclopedic pediatric dermatology text authored by nearly 200 contributors from countries around the globe. The book is liberally illustrated with excellent quality color photographs and has some exceptional features. Important common diseases, for example, atopic dermatitis, have been divided into specific topics, each authored by an expert in that aspect of the disorder. This approach has permitted the editors to tap the expertise of the most knowledgeable investigators in the field, and has resulted in a truly international effort. There are chapters on modern genetic concepts including variations on mendelian inheritance, mosaicism and gene mapping, as well as the practical and ethical aspects of new molecular techniques and gene analysis used in prenatal diagnosis.

Factitious disease and coping mechanisms in the setting of chronic disease are discussed in their respective sections, and the effects of solar radiation and preventative measures are addressed in a lengthy chapter on photoprotection. Several chapters on surgery describe basic as well as complex techniques commonly used for pediatric patients such as tissue expansion, grafts of various sorts including cultured keratinocytes and the management of keloids, scars, and burn wounds. The use of lasers for treatment of vascular and pigmented lesions and sedation and anesthesia appropriate for children round out the offerings in the surgical arena. In the infectious diseases section, there are in-depth discussions of the *Bartonella* and zoonotic poxvirus diseases, the endemic treponematoses, leprosy, and leishmaniasis; infections that are often given short shrift in general dermatology textbooks. Written by contributors with firsthand knowledge in the diagnosis and care of patients with such disorders, these chapters broaden the scope of the book, and should better serve those practitioners caring for children in developing countries.

In short, this international effort has resulted in a beautifully organized, state-of-the-art textbook that has captured the excitement of new knowledge and well addresses the goal of launching pediatric dermatology into the new millennium.

Nancy B. Esterly, MD

Section 17
Epidermal Naevi/Epidermal Naevus Syndrome

17.1 Epidermal Naevi

MAUREEN ROGERS

Sebaceous naevus

Keratinocytic naevi

Inflammatory linear verrucous epidermal naevus

Follicular naevus

Porokeratotic eccrine ostial and dermal duct naevus

Syringocystadenoma papilliferum

Epidermal naevi with abnormalities in other organ systems

CHILD syndrome

Proteus syndrome

Sebaceous naevus syndrome

Naevus comedonicus syndrome

Widespread keratinocytic naevi with skeletal defects

Epidermal naevi with hypophosphataemic vitamin D-resistant osteomalacia and rickets

Epidermal naevi with endocrine abnormalities

Epidermal naevi with vascular malformations

Development of internal neoplasms

Epidermal naevi with pigmentary disorders

Conclusion

Definition

Epidermal naevi are hamartomas arising from the embryonic ectoderm whose pluripotential cells differentiate not only into keratinocytes but also into the cells forming the epidermal appendages. Although epidermal naevi may show an admixture of components either from area to area or within the same area at different times [1], these naevi are best classified according to their predominant component into sebaceous, keratinocytic, follicular and sweat

gland naevi. The general term epidermal naevus is often, however, still used for simplicity.

REFERENCE

1 Solomon LM, Esterly NB. Epidermal and other congenital organoid nevi. *Curr Prob Pediatr* 1975; 1: 3–56.

History

The polymorphic appearance of these lesions and the great variety in size and distribution has historically led to an extraordinary number of designations either descriptive or speculatively aetiological. In 1893 von Baerensprung [1] introduced the term naevus unius lateris to emphasize the unilateral distribution of the warty naevus he was describing. The speculative neural distribution led others to introduce such names as naevus nervosus and papilloma neuropathicum unilaterale, and the similarity to the lesions of ichthyosis was emphasized in the term ichthyosis hystrix. The term systematized naevus was employed for lesions which were bilateral and extensive. The fact that in lesions on the face and scalp a prominent sebaceous component can accompany epidermal hyperplasia was emphasized in the designation introduced by Robinson [2] of naevus sebaceous of Jadassohn; it is of interest, however, that what Jadassohn [3] originally described was an area of large well-formed sebaceous lobules in a naevus on the leg. Jadassohn [3] also initiated the term organ naevus to distinguish lesions with a congenitally determined excess of sebaceous glands and other constituents of the skin from pigmented naevus cell naevi. Mehregan and Pinkus [4] favoured the term organoid naevus. The comedo-like structures in naevi of follicular origin led to the descriptive terms such as naevus unilateralis comedonicus and naevus acneiformis while another designation given was naevus follicularis keratosis [5].

The recognition that these naevi could be associated with a wide variety of abnormalities in other organ systems and the description of these cases by a variety of authors led to a further plethora of descriptive or eponymous names including linear naevus

955

sebaceous syndrome, organoid naevus syndrome, Schim-melpenning–Feurstein–Mims syndrome, Jadassohn naevus phakomatosis and Solomon syndrome.

In an attempt at simplification and unification in this difficult area, Solomon and Esterly [6], noting that an admixture of histological features may occur in a single naevus and that the same abnormalities in other organ systems may occur with naevi of different type, suggested that the single term epidermal naevus be used and that the epidermal naevus syndrome be regarded as a single syndrome with considerable clinical variability. Recent understanding of the concepts of genetic mosaicism, however, has brought us back to an appreciation of the wide variety of separate entities within the still useful designations of epidermal naevus and epidermal naevus syndrome and led to a search for the genes involved in each of these entities.

REFERENCES

1 Von Baerensprung F. Naevus unius lateris. *Charite Ann* 1863; 2: 91.
2 Robinson SS. Naevus sebaceus (Jadassohn). *Arch Dermatol Syph* 1932; 26: 663–70.
3 Jadassohn J. Bermerkungen zur histologie der systematisierten naevi und uber 'talgdrusen-naevi'. *Ann Dermatol Syph (Paris)* 1895; 33: 335–94.
4 Mehregan AH, Pinkus H. Life history of organoid nevi. *Arch Dermatol* 1965; 91: 574–88.
5 Paige TN, Mendelson CG. Bilateral nevus comedonicus. *Arch Dermatol* 1967; 96: 172–5.
6 Solomon LM, Esterly NB. Epidermal and other congenital organoid nevi. *Curr Prob Pediatr* 1975; 1: 3–56.

Aetiology

Epidermal naevi follow the lines of Blaschko [1] which represent the migration tracks of clones of genetically identical cells. This observation led Happle [2,3] to propose that each type of epidermal naevus represents the cutaneous manifestation of a different mosaic phenotype. There are several different explanations for this mosaicism (Chapter 19.1). It may represent genetic mosaicism [2,3] which may be genomic, due to a non-lethal autosomal postzygotic mutation where the condition can occur in the next generation in a diffuse form (epidermolytic keratinocytic naevus) or a lethal autosomal postzygotic mutation which can survive only in the mosaic state (sebaceous naevus syndrome, Proteus syndrome) or it may result from functional X-chromosome mosaicism occurring as a result of lyonization (congenital hemidysplasia with ichthyosiform erythroderma and limb defects or CHILD syndrome). Alternatively, chromosomal mosaicism may be operating [4]. The very rare instances of apparently familial epidermal naevi [5–7] are difficult to explain but remain inconclusive in most cases because of lack of supporting biopsy evidence.

Confirmatory genetic studies are already available for some entities [8] and more can be expected over the next few years, clarifying the understanding of this presently very complicated group of conditions.

REFERENCES

1 Bolognia JL, Orlow SJ, Glick SA. Lines of Blaschko. *J Am Acad Dermatol* 1994; 31: 157–90.
2 Happle R. Lethal genes surviving by mosaicism: a possible explanation for sporadic birth defects involving the skin. *J Am Acad Dermatol* 1987; 16: 899–906.
3 Happle R. How many epidermal nevus syndromes exist? *J Am Acad Dermatol* 1991; 25: 550–6.
4 Stosiek N, Ulmer R, von den Driesch P, Claussen U, Hornstein OP, Rott H-D. Chromosomal mosaicism in two patients with epidermal verrucous nevus. *J Am Acad Dermatol* 1994; 30: 622–5.
5 Sahl WJ. Familial nevus sebaceus of Jadassohn: occurrence in three generations. *J Am Acad Dermatol* 1990; 22: 853–4.
6 Benedetto L, Blumenthal N, Sturman S. Familial nevus sebaceus. *J Am Acad Dermatol* 1990; 23: 130–2.
7 Meschia JF, Junkins E, Hofman KJ. Familial systematized epidermal nevus syndrome. *Am J Med Genet* 1992; 44: 664–7.
8 Paller AS, Syder AJ, Chan Y-M *et al*. Genetic and clinical mosaicism in a type of epidermal nevus. *N Engl J Med* 1994; 331: 1408–15.

Sebaceous naevus

Definition

This is a hamartoma in which the predominant component is sebaceous. The term organoid naevus is preferred by Mehregan and Pinkus [1] to emphasize that other 'organs' such as hair follicles, sweat glands and epidermis may also be involved.

Pathology

The histological appearance varies with the age of the lesion [2,3]. In the neonatal period and early infancy sebaceous glands are prominent, but throughout childhood they are underdeveloped. During childhood a typical finding is cords of undifferentiated cells resembling embryonic hair follicles [1]. At puberty epidermal proliferation with hyperkeratosis and papillomatosis occurs and prolific, large, mature sebaceous glands are a major feature. These are often in groups, abnormally high in the dermis and apparently unconnected with normal follicular canals [4]; some open on to the surface of the epidermis. The primordial follicular structures persist and remain small. Mature hair follicles are absent or extremely few in number [4] but ectopic apocrine glands are often seen.

The development of secondary tumours in sebaceous naevi is well recognized, usually presenting as a raised tumour but sometimes being found incidentally on histopathological examination of excised lesions. It may be more appropriate to regard many of these 'secondary tumours' as simply inherent components of these naevi which, as has been pointed out, may differentiate towards several different structures. The commonest secondary tumours are syringocystadenoma papilliferum [1,4] and areas of benign basaloid hyperplasia [4], the latter probably accounting for many of the reports of basal cell carcinoma [4]. The development of secondary tumours in epidermal naevi occurs usually in adult life but both benign and malignant tumours have rarely been reported in childhood [1,4,5–10]. These include keratoacanthoma [4], infundibuloma [9] basal cell carcinoma [5,8,9], syringocystadenoma papilliferum [1,10], sebaceous epithelioma [7], pilar leiomyoma [5] and squamous cell epithelioma [6]. It is postulated [4] that perhaps the lesions reported as squamous cell epithelioma [6] may have represented keratoacanthomas or pseudoepitheliomatous hyperplasia.

Clinical features

Sebaceous naevi occur particularly on the scalp and face as these are the areas where sebaceous glands are present in large numbers [11,12]. They are invariably present at birth and do not spread beyond their original distribution, growing in proportion to the patient [12]. The appearance changes with age [11]. At birth they are most characteristically oval or linear, flat or slightly raised plaques with a smooth, waxy surface, hairless on the scalp and varying in colour from pink to yellow (Fig. 17.1.1). Occasionally they are significantly raised from birth (Figs 17.1.2, 17.1.3), par-

ticularly in extensive lesions associated with neurological abnormalities. Rare lesions present as an erythematous papilloma (Fig. 17.1.4). They may occur in a centrofacial distribution, sometimes as a single line extending down the centre of the nose to the philtrum and even into the

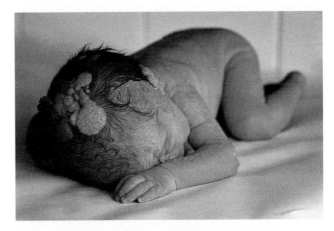

Fig. 17.1.2 Extensive sebaceous naevus, elevated from birth.

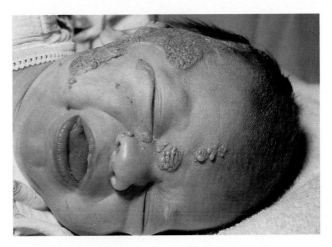

Fig. 17.1.3 Papillomatous sebaceous naevus, involving the centrofacial area.

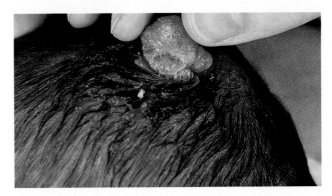

Fig. 17.1.4 Sebaceous naevus presenting as an erythematous, pedunculated nodule.

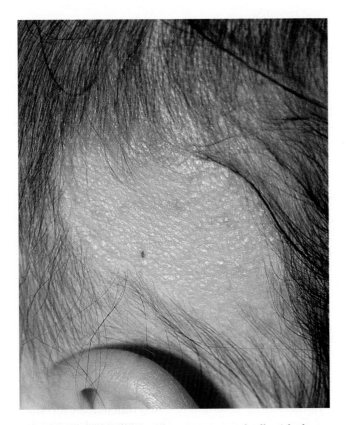

Fig. 17.1.1 Sebaceous naevus appearing as an oval yellowish plaque.

mouth (Fig. 17.1.5) and may involve the retroauricular area where a verrucous element is often prominent even in early life (Fig. 17.1.6). The centrofacial distribution also correlates with neurological involvement. Another rare presentation is as a solitary pedunculated lesion on the scalp [13]. At puberty sebaceous naevi, particularly on the scalp, often become more raised, warty and irritable (Fig. 17.1.7).

While sebaceous naevi almost always occur on the face and scalp they rarely involve other areas, with or without involvement of the head. Lentz *et al.* [14] describe a case with extensive linear plaques on the trunk and one arm, consisting of yellow waxy papules with a rather verrucous surface. Histology from an area on the back showed the typical appearance of a sebaceous naevus.

The majority of patients are otherwise normal but in some individuals, particularly those with large and/or centrofacial naevi, other abnormalities occur and this association is discussed below as the sebaceous naevus syndrome.

Management

The occasional early appearance of secondary tumours underlines the importance of emphasizing to the parents of a child with a sebaceous naevus that any alteration in the naevus should be reported. Any suspicious areas should be excised, and if possible the whole naevus removed. Removal is often indicated on cosmetic grounds, preferably before puberty when the lesions usually become raised and irritable. Because these are deep lesions involving a substantial part of the dermis, the treatment of choice, where feasible, is complete excision. A reduction in thickness with cosmetic improvement has been reported with carbon dioxide laser therapy [15]; it is important for the patient and family to appreciate that the risk of development of malignant secondary tumours is not removed by this procedure and that continued follow-up is required.

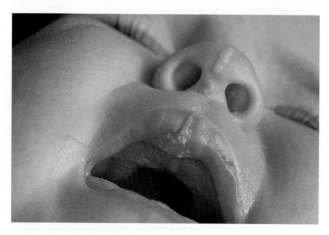

Fig. 17.1.5 Sebaceous naevus extending from the centre of the nose into the mouth.

REFERENCES

1 Mehregan AH, Pinkus H. Life history of organoid nevi. Special reference to nevus sebaceus of Jadassohn. *Arch Dermatol* 1965; 91; 574–88.
2 Lever WF, Lever GS. *Histopathology of the Skin*, 7th edn. Philadelphia: JB Lippincott, 1990: 594–6.
3 Poomeechaiwong S, Golitz LE. Hamartomas. *Adv Dermatol* 1990; 5: 257–88.
4 Wilson Jones E, Heyl T. Naevus sebaceus. A report of 140 cases with special

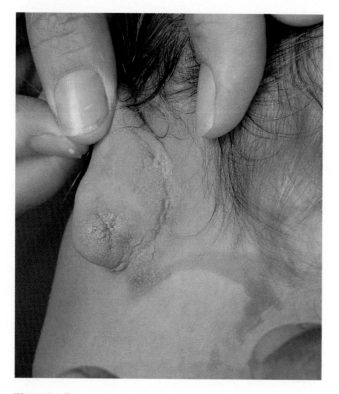

Fig. 17.1.6 Retroauricular sebaceous naevus, demonstrating a verrucous component.

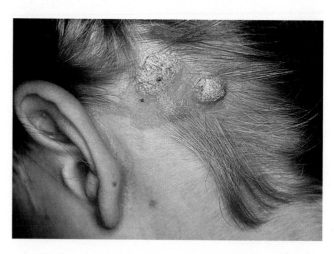

Fig. 17.1.7 Verrucous thickening of sebaceous naevus at puberty.

regard to the development of secondary malignant tumours. *Br J Dermatol* 1970; 82: 99–117.

5 Serpas De Lopez RME, Hernandez-Perez E. Jadassohn's sebaceous nevus. *J Dermatol Surg Oncol* 1985; 11: 68–72.

6 Parkin T. Naevus sebaceus (Jadassohn) with squamous cell epithelioma. *Br J Dermatol* 1950; 62: 167–70.

7 Ruiter M. Sebaceous epithelioma developing from a sebaceous naevus. *Dermatologica* 1964; 128: 403–5.

8 Goldstein GD, Whitaker DC, Argenyi ZB, Bardach J. Basal cell carcinoma arising in a sebaceous nevus during childhood. *J Am Acad Dermatol* 1988; 18: 429–30.

9 Piansay-Soriano EF, Pineda VB, Jimenez RI, Mungcal VC. Basal cell carcinoma and infundibuloma arising in separate sebaceous nevi during childhood. *J Dermatol Surg Oncol* 1989; 15: 1283–6.

10 Mostafa WZ, Satti MB. Epidermal nevus syndrome: a clinicopathologic study with 6-year follow-up. *Pediatr Dermatol* 1991; 8: 228–30.

11 Solomon LM, Esterly NB. Epidermal and other congenital organoid nevi. *Curr Prob Pediatr* 1975; 1: 3–56.

12 Rogers M, McCrossin I, Commens C. Epidermal nevi and the epidermal nevus syndrome. *J Am Acad Dermatol* 1989; 20: 476–88.

13 Pierini A-M, Lopez-Ramos N, Siminovich M, Garcia-Diaz R. Exophytic scalp tumor in a newborn. *Pediatr Dermatol* 1991; 8: 84–6.

14 Lentz CL, Altman J, Mopper C. Nevus sebaceus of Jadassohn. *Arch Dermatol* 1968; 97: 294–6.

15 Ashinoff R. Linear nevus sebaceus of Jadassohn treated with the carbon dioxide laser. *Pediatr Dermatol* 1993; 10: 189–91.

Keratinocytic naevi

Definition

These are epidermal naevi with differentiation exclusively or predominantly towards keratinocytes. Alternative names include naevus verrucosus and verrucous epidermal naevus.

Pathogenesis

The enormous clinical and histopathological [1] spectrum of keratinocytic naevi attests to the likelihood that this term encompasses a large number of different mosaic phenotypes, the separation of which will occur only as a result of definitive genetic studies. Some entities have, however, already been defined. One of the histopathological patterns is epidermolytic hyperkeratosis identical to that found in bullous ichthyosis, a condition found to be linked to point mutations in K1 or K10 genes [2]. Patients with epidermolytic epidermal naevi may have offspring with bullous ichthyosis [3]. It has been hypothesized that the naevus arises as a result of a postzygotic mutation producing a mosaic pattern of abnormality; the mutation could involve other organs including the gonads and affected offspring will carry the mutation in every cell producing a generalized abnormality. This hypothesis has now been proven with the demonstration, in patients with epidermolytic naevi, of mutations in one of the two K10 alleles in keratinocytes cultured from lesional but not non-lesional epidermis and the finding of the same mutation in their offspring with bullous ichthyosis [4]. In the epidermolytic naevus patients the mutation was absent or underrepresented in blood and fibroblasts indicating that genetic studies in these patients should be carried out on lesional epidermis rather than other tissues.

It is tempting to believe that the keratinocytic naevi showing acantholytic dyskeratotic histology represent mosaic forms of Darier's disease. Supporting this possibility are the facts that like the lesions in Darier's disease the condition appears as groups of brown keratotic papules, the onset may be delayed until at least later childhood and the condition may be photoaggravated [5,6]. There have been no definite reports of typical Darier's disease in the offspring of patients with this type of naevus but it is interesting to note [7] that in Cockayne's early review of the condition [8] zosteriform lesions were mentioned in members of families with Darier's disease, although the relationship of the individuals was not stated. Further evidence comes from reports of patients with acantholytic dyskeratotic naevi and ipsilateral typical nail and palmar changes of Darier's disease [6,7].

Chromosomal mosaicism has been demonstrated in skin cells from two patients with non-epidermolytic keratinocytic naevi, one with an extensive truncal lesion and another with a small lesion on the neck [9]. Variegated translocation mosaicism was found in skin cells from each, with an identical breakpoint on chromosome 1. Normal skin showed normal karyotypes.

Pathology

These naevi show a wide variety of histopathological appearances. In a study of 160 cases reviewed in detail by Su [1] the most common pattern was non-specific hyperkeratosis, papillomatosis and acanthosis with elongation of rete ridges. Others included pictures resembling the histopathology of seborrhoeic keratosis, acrokeratosis verruciformis, Darier's disease (acantholytic dyskeratosis), bullous ichthyosis (epidermolytic hyperkeratosis), verruca vulgaris, acanthosis nigricans and porokeratosis. A final pattern is psoriasiform which correlates with the clinical entity of inflammatory linear verrucous epidermal naevus (ILVEN) (see below). Other epidermal patterns have been reported elsewhere. One resembled the histopathology of Hailey–Hailey disease both on light and electron microscopy [10]. Two male patients showed naevi with histopathology showing many of the features of the verrucous stage of incontinentia pigmenti [11]. A unique pattern was described by Happle *et al.* [12] with acantholysis but no dyskeratosis; in view of the clinical appearance of filiform keratoses, cutaneous horns and lesions resembling large comedones, it was clinically designated naevus corniculatus. Brownstein *et al* [13] reported a case in which, beneath the common pattern of hyperkeratosis and acanthosis, there was a lichenoid tissue reaction. A pattern resembling that seen in the entity of verruciform xanthoma [14], with regular hyperkeratosis and acanthosis overlying collections of foamy histiocytes, has been reported, particularly in the CHILD syndrome [15,16] (see below). In patients with widespread lesions there may be different patterns in different areas. Secondary tumours occur rarely in epidermal naevi of keratinocytic type, but basal cell carcinoma [17], squamous cell carcinoma [18], trichoepithelioma [19] and keratoacanthoma [20] have all been reported.

Clinical features

Naevi with predominantly keratinocytic differentiation occur mainly on the trunk and limbs although occasionally the head is involved particularly as part of a very extensive lesion. They may be congenital but in over 50% of cases the onset is after birth, usually in the first year of life but occasionally as late as adolescence [21]. Unlike sebaceous naevi they may spread beyond their original distribution, usually for several months but occasionally for years [21–23]. They may be small and localized, extend from the trunk to an adjacent limb (Fig. 17.1.8) or be widespread, involving large areas of the trunk and limbs and occasionally the face. The colour may be light or dark grey (Fig. 17.1.9), brown (Fig. 17.1.10) or black. Most are darker than the surrounding normal skin but some are paler, particularly in dark-skinned individuals. Some lesions are very subtle and only slightly raised while others are very thick and warty or papillomatous. The colour and elevation may vary from area to area in an extensive naevus. Although many lesions remain unaltered after their initial appearance, they may become more elevated at puberty. Many different patterns occur [21,22] including single or multiple narrow or broad lines, an array of small papillomas (Fig. 17.1.11) or groups of plaques in a linear pattern (Fig. 17.1.12). On the limbs the lesions take a more or less straight longitudinal direction but on the trunk they form complicated curved and whorled configurations (Fig. 17.1.13). A midline cut off is seen in most areas of the trunk, but this is absent on the lower back where the lines of Blaschko cross the midline.

Woolly hair naevus (Fig. 17.1.14) had been reported in

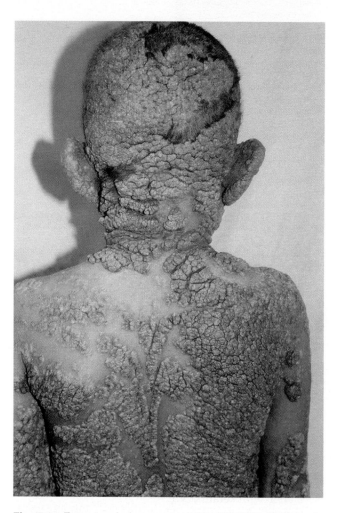

Fig. 17.1.9 Extensive, dark grey-coloured keratinocytic naevus. (Courtesy of Dr Y. Barakbah.)

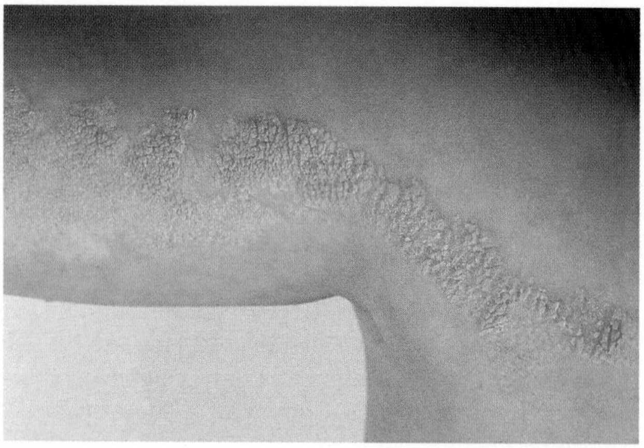

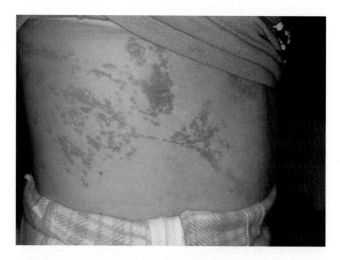

Fig. 17.1.10 Brown-coloured keratinocytic naevus.

Fig. 17.1.8 Keratinocytic naevus extending from the trunk to the arm.

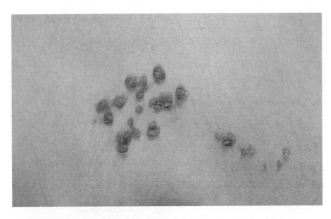

Fig. 17.1.11 Keratinocytic naevus, comprising an array of small papillomas.

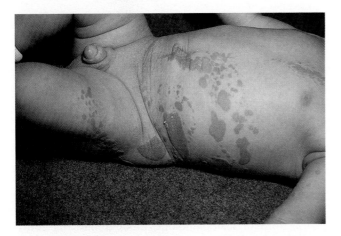

Fig. 17.1.12 Keratinocytic naevus on the trunk, comprising a linear array of plaques.

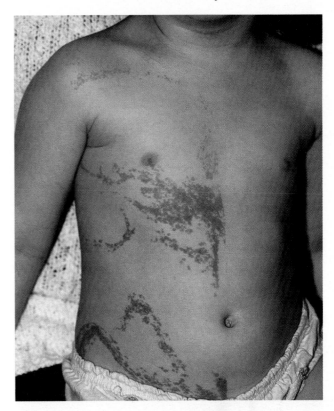

Fig. 17.1.13 Keratinocytic naevus on the trunk, comprising multiple curved lines and demonstrating a midline cut-off.

association with keratinocytic epidermal naevi [21,24–26]. The epidermal naevus usually involves the face and neck on the same side as the woolly hair naevus [24] but may be extensive and bilateral [25]. Very rarely the verrucous epidermal naevus and the woolly hair naevus occur in the same area [26].

Management

It seems that the dermis is involved in some way because recurrence is almost invariable following apparently successful removal with diathermy, cryosurgery or superficial dermabrasion. Deeper dermabrasion or partial thickness skin excision with a dermatome may be successful in ablating the lesion but only at the expense of scarring [27]. Excision is the treatment of choice for small plaques and narrow linear lesions and for areas of larger lesions which are particularly irritating or cosmetically troublesome. The use of argon or carbon dioxide laser treatment has achieved good results in some cases, particularly for the softer, more papillomatous type of lesion

[28,29]. Recurrence is always a potential problem and hypertrophic scarring a risk, particularly with the carbon dioxide laser. Flattening of thick lesions has been achieved on a temporary basis with topical retinoic acid, alone or combined with topical 5-fluorouracil [30]. Oral retinoids may produce significant improvement [31] but recurrence occurs quickly on their cessation and long-term use of these agents in a child is probably unjustified.

REFERENCES

1 Su WPD. Histopathologic varieties of epidermal nevus. *Am J Dermatopathol* 1982; 4: 161–70.
2 Syder AJ, Yu QC, Paller AS, Giudice G, Pearson R, Fuchs E. Genetic mutations in the K1 and K10 genes of patients with epidermolytic hyperkeratosis: correlation between location and disease severity. *J Clin Invest* 1994; 93: 1533–42.
3 Nazzaro V, Ermacora E, Santucci B, Caputo R. Epidermolytic hyperkeratosis: generalized form in children from parents with systematized linear form. *Br J Dermatol* 1990; 122: 417–22.
4 Paller AS, Syder AJ, Chan Y-M *et al.* Genetic and clinical mosaicism in a type of epidermal nevus. *N Engl J Med* 1994; 331: 1408–15.
5 Starink TM, Woerdeman MJ. Unilateral systematized keratosis follicularis. A variant of Darier's disease or an epidermal naevus (acantholytic dyskeratotic epidermal naevus)? *Br J Dermatol* 1981; 105: 207–14.
6 Cambiaghi S, Brusasco A, Grimalt R, Caputo R. Acantholytic dyskeratotic epidermal nevus as a mosaic form of Darier's disease. *J Am Acad Dermatol* 1995; 32: 284–6.
7 Munro CS, Cox NH. An acantholytic dyskeratotic epidermal naevus with other features of Darier's disease on the same side of the body. *Br J Dermatol* 1992; 127: 168–71.

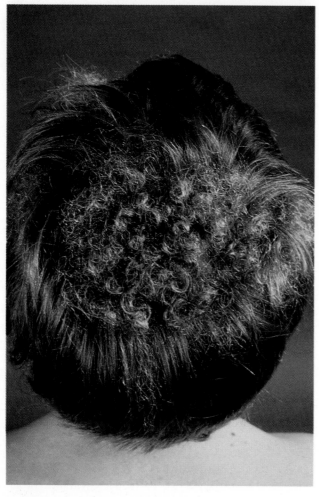

Fig. 17.1.14 Woolly hair naevus in a patient with a keratinocytic naevus on the neck.

8 Cockayne EA. Darier's disease. In: *Inherited Abnormalities of the Skin and its Appendages*. Oxford: Oxford University Press, 1933: 134–8.

9 Stosiek N, Ulmer R, von den Driesch P, Claussen U, Hornstein OP, Rott H-D. Chromosomal mosaicism in two patients with epidermal verrucous nevus. *J Am Acad Dermatol* 1994; 30: 622–5.

10 Vakilzadeh F, Kolde G. Relapsing linear acantholytic dermatosis. *Br J Dermatol* 1985; 112: 349–55.

11 Fletcher V, Williams ML, Lane AT. Histologic changes resembling the verrucous phase of incontinentia pigmenti within epidermal nevi: report of two cases. *Pediatr Dermatol* 1985; 3: 69–74.

12 Happle R, Steijlen PM, Kolde G. Naevus corniculatus: a new acantholytic disorder. *Br J Dermatol* 1990; 122: 107–12.

13 Brownstein MH, Silverstein L, Lefing W. Lichenoid epidermal nevus: 'linear lichen planus'. *J Am Acad Dermatol* 1989; 20: 913–15.

14 Chyu J, Medenica M, Whitney DH. Verruciform xanthoma of the lower extremity—report of a case. *J Am Acad Dermatol* 1987; 17: 695–8.

15 Palestine RF, Winklemann RK. Verruciform xanthoma in an epithelial nevus. *Arch Dermatol* 1982; 118: 686–91.

16 Zamora-Martinez E, Martin-Moreno L, Barat-Cascante A, Castro-Torres A. Another CHILD syndrome with xanthomatous pattern. *Dermatologica* 1990; 180: 263–6.

17 Horn MS, Sausker WF, Pierson DL. Basal cell epithelioma arising in a linear epidermal nevus. *Arch Dermatol* 1981; 117: 247.

18 Cramer SF, Mandel MA, Hauler R, Lever WF, Jensen AB. Squamous cell carcinoma arising in a linear epidermal nevus. *Arch Dermatol* 1981; 117: 222–4.

19 Lambert WC, Bilinski DL, Khan MY, Brodkin RH. Trichoepithelioma in a systematized epidermal nevus with acantholytic dyskeratosis. *Arch Dermatol* 1984; 120: 227–30.

20 Wilkinson SM, Tan CY, Smith AG. Keratoacanthoma arising within organoid naevi. *Clin Exp Dermatol* 1991; 16: 58–60.

21 Rogers M, McCrossin I, Commens C. Epidermal nevi and the epidermal nevus syndrome. *J Am Acad Dermatol* 1989; 20: 476–88.

22 Solomon LM, Esterly NB. Epidermal and other congenital organoid nevi. *Curr Prob Pediatr* 1975; 1: 3–56.

23 Submoke S, Piamphongsant T. Clinico-histopathological study of epidermal naevi. *Aust J Dermatol* 1983; 24: 130–6.

24 Lantis SD, Pepper MC. Woolly hair nevus. *Arch Dermatol* 1978; 114: 233–8.

25 Wright S, Lemoine NR, Leigh IM. Woolly hair naevi with systematized linear epidermal naevus. *Clin Exp Dermatol* 1986; 11: 179–82.

26 Peteiro C, Oliva NP, Zulaica A, Toribio J. Woolly-hair nevus: report of a case associated with a verrucous epidermal nevus in the same area. *Pediatr Dermatol* 1989; 6: 188–90.

27 Dellon AL, Luethke R, Wong L, Barnett N. Epidermal nevus: surgical treatment by partial-thickness skin excision. *Ann Plast Surg* 1992; 28: 292–6.

28 Ratz JL, Bailin PL, Wheeland RG. Carbon dioxide laser treatment of epidermal nevi. *J Dermatol Oncol Surg* 1986; 12: 567–70.

29 Hohenleutner U, Landthaler M. Laser therapy of verrucous epidermal naevi. *Clin Exp Dermatol* 1993; 18: 124–7.

30 Nelson BR, Kolansky G, Gillard M, Ratner D, Johnson TM. Management of linear verrucous epidermal nevus with topical 5-fluorouracil and tretinoin. *J Am Acad Dermatol* 1994; 30: 287–8.

31 Abdel-Aal MAM. Treatment of systematized verrucous epidermal naevus by aromatic retinoid (Ro. 10-9359). *Clin Exp Dermatol* 1983; 8: 647–50.

Inflammatory linear verrucous epidermal naevus

Definition

The term ILVEN was coined by Altman and Mehregan [1] to describe a distinct variety of keratinocytic epidermal naevus which was clinically inflammatory and which was psoriasiform on histopathology, although the same entity had been previously described as dermatitic epidermal naevus [2].

Pathogenesis

Adrian and Baden [3] found that the electrophoretic pattern of protein extracted from the scale in an ILVEN differed from that of normal stratum corneum and of psoriatic scale. A subsequent study showed that the epidermal protein pattern is not identical in each case of ILVEN [4]. Welch *et al.* [5] have demonstrated in ILVEN immunohistochemical features differing from those of non-inflammatory keratinocytic naevi, suggesting a distinctive pattern of clonal dysregulation of growth in these naevi; some of these changes resembled those seen in psoriasis. Ito *et al.* [6] found both similarities and differences in histopathogenesis of the parakeratotic epidermis between ILVEN and psoriasis. There is a report of a patient with ILVEN developing autoimmune thyroiditis, possibly coincidentally but raising the question of autoimmune involvement in the inflammatory component of ILVEN [7]. Familial cases have rarely been reported [8,9]; Hamm and Happle [8] suggest several possible explanations including X-linked inheritance with extreme lyonization.

Histopathology

The most distinctive histopathological finding is sharply demarcated alternating areas of hypergranulosis with overlying orthokeratotic hyperkeratosis and of hypogranulosis with overlying parakeratotic hyperkeratosis [10,11]. There is a psoriasiform epidermal hyperplasia with close-set elongation of the rete ridges and spongiosis, exocytosis and even microabscess formation may be seen. An upper dermal perivascular lymphohistiocytic inflammatory infiltrate is a regular feature. Sometimes the histopathology is less specific, mimicking a chronic eczema.

Clinical features

ILVEN presents as erythematous, extremely pruritic papules and plaques, with a raised scaly surface, occurring in narrow or, more often, wide linear patterns following the lines of Blaschko. The lower limb (Fig. 17.1.15), with or without extension to the buttock (Fig. 17.1.16) or inguinogenital area, is the commonest site of involvement [1,12,13] but lesions may involve the arm, the genital area and rarely other sites. It is almost always unilateral but widespread bilateral lesions have been reported [14,15]. Initially, a female predominance was reported [1] but further studies indicate that the sexes are affected equally [12,13]. In most cases the onset is in the first 5 years of life, often under 1 year and occasionally at birth [1,12,13]. Rarely, the onset is in later childhood or even adult life [1,14]. Once established, the lesions are persistent with no tendency to remission or improvement with time.

Patients with ILVEN are generally otherwise normal. The cases reported in association with severe skeletal abnormalities, in particular hypoplasia or aplasia of limb bones, may represent cases of CHILD syndrome [16–18].

Differential diagnosis

This includes naevoid psoriasis [19], lichen striatus, linear lichen planus, the erythematous scaly lesions which may occur in Goltz syndrome and a non-inflammatory epidermal naevus on which psoriasis has become superimposed as a Koebner phenomenon [13,20,21]. The differentiation of ILVEN from naevoid psoriasis is a difficult area; some lesions reported as ILVEN may have represented naevoid psoriasis and vice versa. Psoriatic lesions are in general less pruritic and may respond well to standard psoriasis therapy. Some indeed question the existence of linear or naevoid psoriasis as a distinct entity [21] and others [19] classify naevoid psoriasis as a separate form of ILVEN. Lichen striatus is usually less pruritic and less scaly than ILVEN, differs from it histologically and, unlike ILVEN, is self-limiting in several months to leave postinflammatory hypopigmentation.

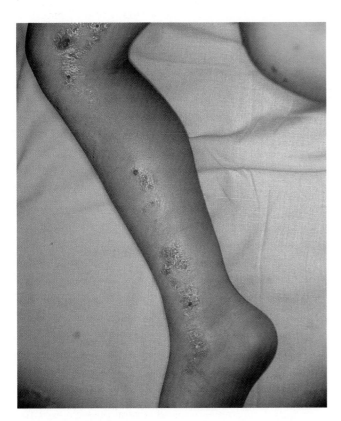

Fig. 17.1.15 Inflammatory linear verrucous naevus on the lower limb.

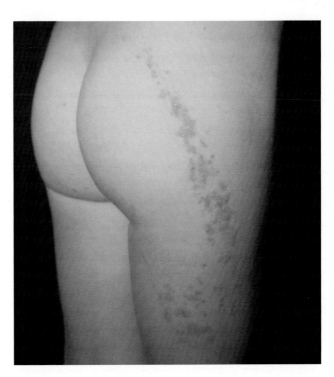

Fig. 17.1.16 Inflammatory linear verrucous naevus on the buttock and thigh.

Management

Treatment is in general quite unsatisfactory. Some relief from pruritis and lessening in thickness and degree of inflammation may be achieved with the use of strong topical [22] or intralesional corticosteroids [12]; however, this is usually short-lived on cessation of therapy. Similarly prompt recurrence is likely to follow electrodessication, cryotherapy, laser therapy and superficial dermabrasion. Long-lasting ablation is reported following cryotherapy [23] but the presence in this female patient of linear atrophic streaks raises the possibility that this may have been a case of Goltz syndrome. Topical calcipotriol, offers some hope [24], although this agent would have to be used with caution in children. For narrow lesions or parts of lesions surgical excision is the treatment of choice.

REFERENCES

1 Altman J, Mehregan AH. Inflammatory linear verrucous epidermal nevus. *Arch Dermatol* 1971; 104: 385–9.
2 Kaidbey KH, Kurban AK. Dermatitic epidermal nevus. *Arch Dermatol* 1971; 104: 166–71.
3 Adrian RM, Baden HP. Analysis of epidermal fibrous proteins in an inflammatory linear verrucous epidermal nevus. *Arch Dermatol* 1980; 116: 1179–80.
4 Bernhart JD, Owen WR, Steinman HK, Kaplan LA, Menkes AB, Baden HP. Inflammatory linear verrucous epidermal nevus. *Arch Dermatol* 1984; 120: 214–15.
5 Welch ML, Smith KJ, Skelton HG *et al.* Immunohistochemical features in inflammatory linear verrucous epidermal nevi suggest a distinctive pattern of clonal dysregulation of growth. *J Am Acad Dermatol* 1993; 29: 242–8.
6 Ito M, Shimuzi N, Fujiwara H, Maruyama T, Tezuka M. Histopathogenesis of inflammatory linear verrucose epidermal naevus: histochemistry, immunohistochemistry and ultrastructure. *Arch Dermatol Res* 1991; 283: 491–9.
7 Dereure O, Paillet C, Bonnel F, Guilhou J-J. Inflammatory linear verrucous epidermal naevus with autoimmune thyroiditis: coexistence of two autoimmune epithelial inflammations? *Acta Derm Venereol (Stockh)* 1994; 74: 208–9.
8 Hamm H, Happle R. Inflammatory linear verrucous epidermal nevus (ILVEN) in a mother and her daughter. *Am J Med Genet* 1986; 24: 685–90.
9 Alsaleh QA, Nanda A, Hassab-el-Naby HMM, Sakr MF. Familial inflammatory linear verrucous epidermal nevus (ILVEN). *Int J Dermatol* 1994; 33: 52–4.
10 Ackerman AB. *Histologic Diagnosis of Inflammatory Skin Disease.* Philadelphia: Lea & Febiger, 1978: 169–280.
11 Dupre A, Christol B. Inflammatory linear verrucose epidermal nevus. *Arch Dermatol* 1977; 113: 767–9.
12 Morag C, Metzker A. Inflammatory linear verrucous epidermal nevus: report of seven new cases and review of the literature. *Pediatr Dermatol* 1985; 3: 15–18.
13 Rogers M, McCrossin I, Commens C. Epidermal nevi and the epidermal nevus syndrome. *J Am Acad Dermatol* 1989; 20: 476–88.
14 Cheesbrough MJ, Kilby PE. The inflammatory linear verrucous epidermal naevus—a case report. *Clin Exp Dermatol* 1978; 3: 293–8.
15 Landwehr AJ, Starink TM. Inflammatory linear verrucous epidermal naevus. *Dermatologica* 1983; 166: 107–9.
16 Golitz LE, Weston WE. Inflammatory linear verrucous epidermal nevus. *Arch Dermatol* 1979; 115: 1208–9.
17 Barr RJ, Plank CJ. Verruciform xanthoma of the skin. *J Cutan Pathol* 1980; 7: 422–8.
18 Grosshans E, Laplanche G. Verruciform xanthoma or xanthomatous transformation of inflammatory epidermal nevus? *J Cutan Pathol* 1981; 8: 382–4.
19 Atherton DJ, Kahana M, Russell-Jones R. Naevoid psoriasis. *Br J Dermatol* 1989; 120: 837–41.
20 Bondi EE. Psoriasis overlying an epidermal nevus. *Arch Dermatol* 1979; 115: 624–5.
21 Thivolet J, Goujon C. Linear psoriasis and systematized epidermolytic nevus. *Arch Dermatol* 1982; 118: 285–6.
22 Cerio R, Wilson Jones E, Eady RAJ. ILVEN responding to occlusive potent topical steroid therapy. *Clin Exp Dermatol* 1992; 17: 279–81.
23 Fox BJ, Lapins MA. Comparison of treatment modalities for epidermal nevus: a case report and review. *J Dermatol Surg Oncol* 1983; 9: 879–85.
24 Gatti S, Carrozzo AM, Orlandi A, Nini G. Treatment of inflammatory linear verrucous epidermal naevus with calcipotriol. *Br J Dermatol* 1995; 132: 837–9.

Follicular naevus

(SYN. COMEDO NAEVUS, NAEVUS COMEDONICUS)

Pathogenesis

This naevus, which comprises numerous keratin-filled invaginations of the epidermis, appears to demonstrate a differentiation towards hair follicle structures, a concept supported by the occasional finding of small hair shafts and sebaceous lobules at their base.

One case of a localized naevus comedonicus showing otherwise typical histology demonstrated epidermolytic hyperkeratosis in the epidermal component at the base and on either side of the invagination [1]. Of particular interest was the fact that the patient had a child with bullous ichthyosis. In view of the discussion above regarding epidermolytic epidermal naevi, it seems likely that this case is an example of this condition with both keratinocytic and follicular differentiation.

There is a recent report of a naevus comedonicus in a patient with Alagille's syndrome, which has recently been assigned to chromosome 20, suggesting the possibility of genetic linkage of these two unusual conditions [2].

Histopathology [3,4]

This shows deep, wide invaginations of the epidermis filled with keratin. These represent dilated rudimentary follicular structures. The follicular wall may be atrophic or irregularly thickened. Small sebaceous gland lobules may be seen opening into the lower pole of the invagination. Hair is rarely formed by these rudimentary follicles but occasionally small hair shafts are seen at the base of the invaginations. A standard naevus verrucosus histopathology may be found between the groups of comedones [5]. Epidermolytic hyperkeratosis has been reported in the follicular wall in lesions which otherwise show the typical histopathology of naevus comedonicus [1,6]. A histological variant of naevus comedonicus, designated the dilated pore naevus, has been recently described [7]. The lesion was clinically typical of a naevus comedonicus and histologically showed multiple dilated pilar infundibula resembling aggregated dilated pores of Winer. Secondary tumours are rare in follicular naevi but tumours of hair follicle origin, including giant trichilem-mal cysts, and basal cell carcinoma have occurred in adult life [8,9].

Clinical features

Epidermal naevi with a predominantly follicular differen-tiation—the so-called naevus comedonicus—occur as a linear plaque on the scalp or as lines or wider bands on the face, trunk or limbs. They may be very extensive. They comprise groups of small or large dilated follicular open-ings and the contained comedones vary from small pin-head sized to large horny structures. The plugs may be extruded to produce a pitted or cribriform appearance [10]. These naevi are usually present at birth but rarely may appear in adolescence. After puberty, and occasion-ally even in younger patients [11], large nodules, equiva-lent to acne cysts, can occur and these can lead to deep and hypertrophic scarring. Small areas of follicular differentia-tion can occur in naevi of predominantly keratinocytic dif-ferentiation [12] and large naevi may show a verrucous change between the groups of comedones [5]. The rare development of a secondary tumour in a follicular naevus will usually be manifested by the development of a nodule [8,9].

Naevus comedonicus-like lesions occurring in areas which do not normally contain hair follicles, such as the soles or palms are probably in most cases examples of sweat duct naevi (see below) although there is a report of a patient with a classical extensive comedo naevus with extension onto the palmar skin, with similar histology in palmar and non-palmar areas [13].

Management

The treatment of choice for small lesions is excision with direct closure. Naevus comedonicus lesions are often extensive and complete excision is usually impossible without skin grafting. However, there is a report of the successful use of tissue expansion allowing complete removal of a large lesion [14]. Dealing with active infec-tion in cysts prior to definitive treatment and the use of prophylactic antibiotics at the time of surgery are essential [14]. More conservative surgical procedures such as der-mabrasion and shave excision are usually followed by recurrence because they do not remove the lesion to a sufficient depth. Comedones which are manually extracted quickly reform [15] and the use of topical retinoic acid has been disappointing [15,16]. Oral retinoids have reduced cyst formation with little effect on the comedones but recurrence has occurred swiftly on ces-sation [16] and their use in children is almost certainly unjustified. A surprisingly good response is reported to a once daily topical application of 12% ammonium lactate solution [10,16], with a decrease in the number of keratin

plugs and no new cyst formation. The use of long-term erythromycin completely controlled the development of abscesses in a 3-year-old child [11].

REFERENCES

1 Lookingbill DP, Ladda RL, Cohen C. Generalized epidermolytic hyperker-atosis in the child of a parent with nevus comedonicus. *Arch Dermatol* 1984; 120: 223–6.
2 Woods KA, Larcher VF, Harper JI. Extensive naevus comedonicus in a child with Alagille syndrome. *Clin Exp Dermatol* 1994; 19: 163–4.
3 Lever WF, Lever GS. *Histopathology of the Skin*, 7th edn. Philadelphia: JB Lip-pincott, 1990: 525.
4 Poomeechaiwong S, Golitz LE. Hamartomas. *Adv Dermatol* 1990; 5: 257–88.
5 Kim SC, Kang WH. Nevus comedonicus associated with epidermal nevus. *J Am Acad Dermatol* 1989; 21: 1085–8.
6 Barsky S, Doyle JA, Winkelmann RK. Nevus comedonicus with epider-molytic hyperkeratosis. *Arch Dermatol* 1981; 117: 86–8.
7 Resnik KS, Kantor GR, Howe NR, Ditre CM. Dilated pore nevus. *Am J Der-matopathol* 1993; 15: 169–71.
8 Leppard BJ. Trichilemmal cysts arising in an extensive comedo naevus. *Br J Dermatol* 1977; 96: 545–8.
9 Dudley K, Barr WG, Armin A, Massa MC. Nevus comedonicus in associa-tion with widespread, well-differentiated follicular tumours. *J Am Acad Dermatol* 1986; 15: 1123–7.
10 Cestari TF, Rubim M, Valentini BC. Nevus comedonicus: case report and brief review of the literature. *Pediatr Dermatol* 1991; 8: 300–5.
11 Glover MT, Ridley CM, Leigh IM. Extensive comedo nevus: benefit from long-term erythromycin. *Br J Dermatol* 1991; 125(suppl 38): 57–8.
12 Rogers M, McCrossin I, Commens C. Epidermal nevi and the epidermal nevus syndrome. *J Am Acad Dermatol* 1989; 20: 476–88.
13 Wood MG, Thew MA. Naevus comedonicus. *Arch Dermatol* 1968; 98: 111–16.
14 Marcus J, Esterly NB, Bauer BS. Tissue expansion in a patient with extensive nevus comedonicus. *Ann Plast Surg* 1992; 29: 362–6.
15 Beck MH, Dave VK. Extensive nevus comedonicus. *Arch Dermatol* 1980; 116: 1048–50.
16 Milton GP, DiGiovanna JJ, Peck GL. Treatment of nevus comedonicus with ammonium lactate solution. *J Am Acad Dermatol* 1989; 20: 324–8.

Porokeratotic eccrine ostial and dermal duct naevus

This term was coined by Abell and Read [1], describing a congenital linear lesion on the sole. It clinically resembled a verrucous epidermal naevus but on pathology showed large numbers of focal parakeratotic plugs resembling cornoid lamellae. These mainly arose from deep epider-mal invaginations which were identified as grossly dilated intraepidermal eccrine ducts but some arose more superficially, again related to sweat duct structures. The eccrine ducts below the level of origin of the cornoid lamellae often showed hyperplasia and a dilated lumen. The eccrine glands showed no abnormality. The keratotic plugs resembled those seen in naevus comedonicus but arose from eccrine ducts rather than hair follicles; also, the plugs in naevus comedonicus are rarely parakeratotic. In some cases of porokeratotic eccrine ostial and dermal duct naevus comedones are a major clinical feature particularly on the palmar skin, although other areas show a more non-specific verrucous appearance [2]. The condition occurs particularly on the limbs and may be very exten-sive [2]. The clinical absence of lesions with annular margins and atrophic centres and the origin of the cornoid lamellae in sweat ducts alone are believed to separate the condition from linear porokeratosis, in which the lamellae may originate from hair follicle infundibulum, sweat duct and interadnexal epidermis [1,3].

The cases reported as 'linear eccrine nevus with comedones' [4] and 'sweat duct naevus' [5] probably represent the same entity as porokeratotic eccrine ostial and dermal duct naevus. A case has been reported under the name of 'porokeratotic eccrine duct and hair follicle nevus' in which the parakeratotic plugs arose from both hair follicles and sweat ducts but not from the interadnexal epidermis [3]. In this case the lesion extended from the wrist onto palm and fingers; the plugs occurred in both hair follicles and sweat ducts on the wrist, but only in sweat ducts on palm and fingers.

REFERENCES

1 Abell E, Read SI. Porokeratotic eccrine ostial and dermal duct naevus. *Br J Dermatol* 1980; 103: 435–41.
2 Aloi FG, Pippione M. Porokeratotic eccrine ostial and dermal duct nevus. *Arch Dermatol* 1986; 122: 892–5.
3 Coskey RJ, Mehregan AH, Hashimoto K. Porokeratotic eccrine duct and hair follicle nevus. *J Am Acad Dermatol* 1982; 6: 940–3.
4 Blanchard L, Hodge S, Owen LG. Linear eccrine nevus with comedones. *Arch Dermatol* 1981; 117: 357–9.
5 Marsden RA, Fleming K, Dawber RPR. Comedo naevus of the palm—a sweat duct naevus. *Br J Dermatol* 1979; 101: 717–22.

Syringocystadenoma papilliferum

This is a hamartoma of disputed origin with a distinctive histopathology [1]. There is variable epidermal papillomatosis and cystic invaginations extend down from the epidermis, lined in their upper portion with squamous cells. Lower down many papillary projections, lined by glandular epithelium extend into the lumina of the invaginations. In most areas there are two rows of cells, the outer ones cuboidal with round nuclei and the inner ones high columnar cells which occasionally demonstrate decapitation secretion as seen in apocrine glands. Collections of tubular glands are often found deep to the invaginations and in some cases serial sections will identify connections between glands and invaginations. Lever and Lever [1] conclude that while most of these naevi are apocrine in differentiation, there is evidence that some appear to be eccrine.

Many cases occur within sebaceous naevi, with onset usually at or after puberty [2]. They may, however, be isolated lesions with onset birth or early infancy, occurring usually on the scalp or face [2] but also elsewhere, occurring on the neck [3], limbs [4] or trunk [5] and even in the inguinogenital area [2]. On the scalp they appear as a plaque or a linear arrangement of papules. Elsewhere they are usually linear lesions, clearly following the lines of Blaschko [3–5]. A rare clinical presentation is as a pedun-

culated nodule [2]. In early life they are pink or skin coloured and hairless on the scalp. Like sebaceous naevi they often become darker, raised and crusted at puberty because of epidermal hyperplasia.

These lesions are usually limited in extent, and excision with direct closure is often possible.

REFERENCES

1 Lever WF, Lever GS. *Histopathology of the Skin*, 7th edn. Philadelphia: JB Lippincott, 1990: 602–4.
2 Helwig EB, Hackney VC. Syringadenoma papilliferum. *Arch Dermatol* 1955; 71: 361–72.
3 Goldberg NS, Esterly NB. Linear papules on the neck of a child. *Arch Dermatol* 1985; 121: 1197.
4 Rostan SE, Waller JD. Syringocystadenoma papilliferum in an unusual location. *Arch Dermatol* 1976; 112: 835–6.
5 Premaltha S, Raghuveera Rao N, Yesudian P, Razack A, Zahra A. Segmental syringocystadenoma papilliferum in an unusual location. *Int J Dermatol* 1985; 24: 520–1.

Epidermal naevi with abnormalities in other organ systems

The term epidermal naevus syndrome has been used to describe the association of epidermal naevi with abnormalities in other organ systems but this term should now be abandoned [1]. Since the time of the comprehensive review of Solomon and Esterly [2] which added so much to the understanding of epidermal naevi and the abnormalities in other organ systems which may be associated with them, the concept of genetic mosaicism as an explanation for epidermal naevi has become better understood, elucidated in particular by Happle [1,3]. He proposes that each type of epidermal naevus represents the cutaneous manifestation of a different mosaic phenotype. It seems likely therefore that the initial concept of the epidermal naevus syndrome as a single syndrome with great clinical variability [2,4] is incorrect. Instead there are potentially many different 'epidermal naevus syndromes', or syndromes of which an epidermal naevus is a cutaneous feature [1,3,5]. It is likely that within the next few years genetic studies will conclusively separate many different phenotypes but until this time we can only postulate that certain collections of clinical features represent discrete entities.

REFERENCES

1 Happle R. How many epidermal nevus syndromes exist? *J Am Acad Dermatol* 1991; 25: 550–6.
2 Solomon LM, Esterly NB. Epidermal and other congenital organoid nevi. *Curr Prob Pediatr* 1975; 1: 3–56.
3 Happle R. Lethal genes surviving by mosaicism: a possible explanation for sporadic birth defects involving the skin. *J Am Acad Dermatol* 1987; 16: 899–906.
4 Rogers M, McCrossin I, Commens C. Epidermal nevi and the epidermal nevus syndrome. *J Am Acad Dermatol* 1989; 20: 476–88.
5 Rogers M. Epidermal nevi and the epidermal nevus syndromes: a review of 233 cases. *Pediatr Dermatol* 1992; 9: 342–4.

CHILD syndrome

Definition

The term CHILD syndrome was proposed by Happle *et al.* [1] as an acronym for the previously described constellation of findings of *c*ongenital *h*emidysplasia with *i*chthyosiform erythroderma and *l*imb *d*efects. Earlier cases had been described under various descriptions including unilateral ichthyosiform erythroderma [2,3]. Subsequently the skin lesion was perceived as a naevus and Happle [4] suggested the revised description congenital hemidysplasia with ichthyosiform naevus and limb defects.

Aetiology and pathogenesis

Happle believes that CHILD syndrome is a well-defined entity among the syndromes of which an epidermal naevus is a feature [5]. All except two of the reported cases have occurred in females [5] and the condition is believed to be inherited as an X-linked dominant trait, lethal in male embryos [1,5]. The male cases may have had an XXY phenotype or have resulted from a postzygotic mutation in an X chromosome. Happle [6] has pointed out the tendency for skin lesions, which show a striking lateralization, to have, in addition, an affinity for skin folds, a phenomenon he has labelled ptychotropism. The lesions may occur predominantly in these areas from the outset or may remain in these areas when, as often occurs, there has been resolution of significant areas of extensive lesions. He feels that the Lyon effect of functional X chromosome mosaicism results in a striking lateralization as well as in a patchy and linear pattern defining the lines of Blaschko; this distribution is modified by ptychotropism. So lyonization gives rise to areas prone to develop the naevus and ptychotropism seems to play a part in their manifestation. Others doubt whether lyonization could explain a condition with such striking lateralization [7].

Dale *et al.* [8] have demonstrated *in vivo* in lesional CHILD epidermis a failure of differentiation-specific protein markers to be properly expressed and a lack of downregulation of basal cell keratin expression; these changes are similar to those seen in other hyperproliferative states such as forms of harlequin ichthyosis and palmoplantar keratoderma. Cultured keratinocytes from lesional CHILD skin do not show these abnormalities, suggesting that dermal or systemic influences are important in the failure of expression of these markers [8]. A possible mechanism may relate to the finding of an increased synthesis of prostaglandin E_2 (PGE_2) by fibroblasts from lesional CHILD skin [9]. PGE_2 is known to stimulate keratinocyte growth and to induce bone resorption [10]. Peroxisomal deficiency has been demonstrated in fibroblasts from lesional skin in CHILD syndrome [11] and it is known that peroxisomes are involved in prostaglandin metabolism. More recent work, however, challenges this peroxisomal theory [10].

Pathology

On light microscopy there is marked hyperkeratosis and parakeratosis with an acanthotic epidermis. The granular layer is variably thickened or absent [1,7,10] and ghost granular cells may be seen [10]. A mixed inflammatory infiltrate occurs in the papillary dermis and may also infiltrate the epidermis. Collections of foam cells in the upper dermis have been noted in several cases producing the changes of verruciform xanthoma [12,13].

Clinical features

The condition presents at birth or soon after. The characteristic skin finding is a non-pruritic erythematous naevus with scaling which may be waxy and yellow occurring in a non-linear patter with a striking predominance on one side of the body and a midline cut-off [7]. There is often a nail dystrophy on affected limbs. Linear areas of spared skin may occur on the side of major involvement and linear areas of affected skin may be found on the opposite side; these linear areas follow the lines of Blaschko [1]. The other major finding is a skeletal aplasia or hypoplasia of variable, and sometimes extreme [12] degree, ipsilateral to the side of major skin involvement; there may be minimal changes on the other side. Punctate epiphyseal calcification may be seen on X-ray in infancy, disappearing after the early years of life. Scaly skin lesions, limb defects, chondrodysplasia punctata and peroxisomal deficiency are features shared by CHILD syndrome, Conradi–Hunermann syndrome and rhizomelic chondrodysplasia punctata, suggesting that these syndromes may be linked pathogenetically, although they differ in mode of inheritance and/or severity and distribution of cutaneous and bony defects [11].

Other associated findings in CHILD syndrome include ipsilateral structural renal and ureteric abnormalities. It is possible that skin involvement may sometimes be quite limited and that some cases described as inflammatory linear verrucous naevi with skeletal changes may have represented examples of CHILD syndrome.

REFERENCES

1 Happle R, Koch H, Lenz W. The CHILD syndrome. Congenital hemidysplasia with ichthyosiform erythroderma and limb defects. *Eur J Pediatr* 1980; 134: 27–33.
2 Rossman RE, Shapiro EM, Freeman RG. Unilateral ichthyosiform erythroderma. *Arch Dermatol* 1963; 88: 567–71.
3 Cullen SI, Harris DE, Carter CH, Reed WB. Congenital unilateral ichthyosiform erythroderma. *Arch Dermatol* 1969; 99: 725–9.

4 Happle R. The lines of Blaschko: a developmental pattern visualizing functional X-chromosome mosaicism. In: Wuepper KD, Gedde-Dahl T, eds. *Biology of Heritable Skin Diseases*.

5 Happle R. How many epidermal nevus syndromes exist? *J Am Acad Dermatol* 1991; 25: 550–6.

6 Happle R. Ptychotropism as a cutaneous feature of the CHILD syndrome. *J Am Acad Dermatol* 1990; 23: 763–6.

7 Hebert AA, Esterly NB, Holbrook KA, Hall JC. The CHILD syndrome. *Arch Dermatol* 1987; 123: 503–9.

8 Dale BA, Kimball JR, Fleckman P, Hebert AA, Holbrook KA. CHILD syndrome: lack of expression of epidermal differentiation markers in lesional ichthyotic skin. *J Invest Dermatol* 1992; 98: 442–9.

9 Goldyne ME, Williams ML. CHILD syndrome: phenotypic dichotomy in eicosanoid metabolism and proliferative rates among cultured dermal fibroblasts. *J Clin Invest* 1989; 84: 357–60.

10 Hashimoto K, Topper S, Sharata H, Edwards M. CHILD syndrome: an analysis of abnormal keratinization and ultrastructure. *Pediatr Dermatol* 1995; 12: 116–29.

11 Emami S, Rizzo WB, Hanley KP, Taylor JM, Goldyne ME, Williams ML. Peroxisomal abnormality in fibroblasts from involved skin of CHILD syndrome. *Arch Dermatol* 1992; 128: 1213–22.

12 Palestine RF, Winkelmann RK. Verruciform xanthoma in an epithelial nevus. *Arch Dermatol* 1982; 118: 686–91.

13 Zamora-Martinez E, Martin-Moreno L, Barat-Cascante A, Castro-Torres A. Another CHILD syndrome with xanthomatous pattern. *Dermatologica* 1990; 180: 263–6.

Proteus syndrome

An epidermal naevus is a frequent, although not universal feature of Proteus syndrome named after the Greek god Proteus, the polymorph [1]. It is a hamartomatous disorder characterized by bilateral, asymmetric, multifocal overgrowths of many tissues [2].

All cases are sporadic and the sexes are equally affected. The condition is best explained by the effect of a lethal autosomal mutation surviving by mosaicism [3,4]. The concept of a somatic mutation affecting production or regulation of tissue growth factors or their receptors could explain the sporadic occurrence, the random distribution of overgrowth, the wide range of findings within the phenotype and the cessation of asymmetrical growth and enlargement of hamartomas at puberty [5].

The naevus is of the keratinocytic type and is often flat, soft and papillomatous [6]. It is usually unilateral and often involves the neck. The trunk and limbs may also be involved but facial involvement is rare. Other features include subcutaneous hamartomatous masses containing combinations of adipose, collagenous, vascular and lymphatic tissue, pigmented and hypopigmented lesions and a characteristic cerebriform thickening of soles and sometimes palms, showing on histology an irregular proliferation of adipose and fibrous tissue [2].

The most characteristic non-cutaneous features are progressive, asymmetric macrodactyly, hemihypertrophy of any part of the skeleton, macrocephaly and exostoses especially of the skull. Visceral hamartomas may also occur including renal and lung cysts and pelvic lipomatosis [7]. Epibulbar choristomas are rarely reported [4,7,8]. Many patients are neurologically normal but developmental delay and seizures may be found [4,7,9].

Benign and malignant internal neoplasms, with onset in childhood have been encountered including parotid adenoma and papillary adenocarcinoma of the testis [8]. At a recent workshop at the National Institute of Health in the USA, diagnostic criteria and guidelines for patient evaluation were proposed [10].

REFERENCES

1 Wiedemann HR, Burgio GR, Aldenhoff P, Kuntze J, Kaufmann HJ, Schirg E. The Proteus syndrome. *Eur J Pediatr* 1983; 140: 5–12.

2 Nazzaro V, Cambiaghi S, Montagnani A, Brusasco A, Cerri A, Caputo R. Proteus syndrome. *J Am Acad Dermatol* 1991; 25: 377–83.

3 Happle R. Lethal genes surviving by mosaicism: a possible explanation for sporadic birth defects involving the skin. *J Am Acad Dermatol* 1987; 16: 899–906.

4 Cohen MM. Proteus syndrome: clinical evidence for somatic mosaicism and selective review. *Am J Med Genet* 1993; 47: 645–52.

5 Clark RD, Donnai D, Rogers J, Cooper J, Baraitser M. Proteus syndrome: an expanded phenotype. *Am J Med Genet* 1987; 27: 99–117.

6 Happle R. How many epidermal nevus syndromes exist? *J Am Acad Dermatol* 1991; 25: 550–6.

7 Costa T, Fitch N, Azouz EM. Proteus syndrome: report of two cases with pelvic lipomatosis. *Pediatrics* 1985; 76: 984–9.

8 Hornstein L, *et al.* Linear nevi, hemihypertrophy, connective tissue hamartomas and unusual neoplasms in children. *J Pediatr* 1987; 110: 404–8.

9 Malamitsi-Puchner A, Kitsiou S, Bartsocas CS. Severe Proteus syndrome in an 18-month-old boy. *Am J Med Genet* 1987; 27: 119–25.

10 Biesecker LG, Happle R, Mulliken JB *et al.* Proteus syndrome: diagnostic criteria, differential diagnosis, and patient evaluation. *Am J Med Genet* 1999; 84: 389–95.

Sebaceous naevus syndrome

This term refers to the association of a sebaceous naevus with neurological and/or ocular abnormalities. The sexes are equally affected and the condition always occurs sporadically and Happle [1] has postulated that it is caused by the action of a lethal autosomal mutation which survives by mosaicism. The naevus always involves the head [2] and may be of any size but large lesions and those extending to, or involving, the centrofacial area are well represented. There may be an associated epidermal naevus of the trunk which will usually demonstrate keratinocytic rather than sebaceous hyperplasia [3].

The major neurological features of the sebaceous naevus syndrome are mental retardation of varying degree, seizures (especially infantile spasms) and hemiparesis. Structural abnormalities demonstrated on neuroimaging include hemimegalencephaly, gyral malformations, grey matter heterotopia, enlarged ventricles, cortical hypoplasia, intracerebral calcification, intracranial vascular malformations, arachnoid cysts and intracranial tumours. These structural abnormalities are usually ipsilateral to the naevus [4].

The major ocular abnormalities are colobomas and choristomas (Fig. 17.1.17). Eyelid colobomas are most frequent but sometimes other ocular structures are involved. Choristomas represent congenital overgrowths of normal tissue in an abnormal location [5]. The varieties are

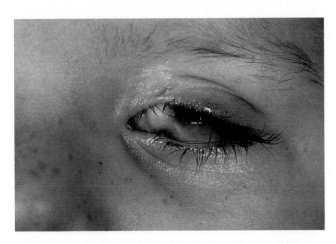

Fig. 17.1.17 Repaired coloboma of the upper eyelid and complex ocular choristoma in a patient with the sebaceous naevus syndrome.

dermoid, lipodermoid, single tissue choristoma and complex choristoma. Ocular choristomas occur in various parts of the eye. In the sebaceous naevus syndrome the choristomas are usually epibulbar and of the complex type and are sometimes bilateral and extensive.

It is likely that there is not one single sebaceous naevus syndrome with variable manifestations but several distinct phenotypes in which the cutaneous lesion is a naevus of the sebaceous type. These will eventually be confirmed by genetic studies but for the present certain constellations of findings stand out as distinct entities.

In one group there is a facial or scalp sebaceous naevus, often extensive and involving the centrofacial area, unilateral or bilateral ocular choristomas with or without colobomas, variable clinical neurological findings including seizures, motor and intellectual delay and demonstration of cerebral atrophy and/or intracranial vascular malformations on neuroimaging [2,3,6–8]. There are similarities to the encephalocraniocutaneous syndrome [9,10] in which epibulbar choristomas, facial papillomas and ipsilateral cerebral atrophy are features; however, there are also scalp lipomas with overlying alopecia and the histology of the facial papillomas shows angiofibroma or fibrolipoma. Epidermal naevi are not part of the phenotype.

In another group of patients the unifying feature is hemimegalencephaly [2,4,11–15]. There is an ipsilateral sebaceous naevus involving the face or scalp, seizures, mental retardation and contralateral hemiparesis. In most patients there is a facial hemihypertrophy involving soft tissue and/or bony structures on the same side as the naevus and in some hemihypertrophy involving the rest of the body [2,11]. There are some similarities to Proteus syndrome but the characteristic features of progressive hemihypertrophy, macrodactyly and gyriform plantar thickening are absent. Choristomas and colobomas are rarely reported in patients with hemimegalencephaly [11]. Imaging demonstrates pachygyria and

sometimes polygyria over the affected hemisphere and other changes include an ipsilateral enlarged lateral ventricle, irregularly thickened cortex, focal thickening of white matter, intracerebral calcification and hydrocephalus. The primary brain involvement is due to a neuronal migration disorder, resulting in aberrant cortical architecture and heterotopic grey matter [11,12]. Magnetic resonance imaging (MRI) is the best radiographic study for the demonstration of abnormalities related to neuronal migration defects as it provides better grey/white matter contrast than computed tomography (CT) scan [13].

Patients with sebaceous naevi and scalp aplasia cutis [16–19] may represent examples of a separate phenotype. The areas of aplasia cutis are often multiple. In most cases eyelid colobomas and ocular choristomas have also been present. Developmental delay, seizures and hemimegalencephaly have all been documented in individual cases in this group. Another recently described syndrome with overlapping features is the oculoectodermal or Toriello's syndrome [20–22] in which the major features are epibulbar dermoids and patchy scalp alopecia and/or aplasia cutis. Epidermal naevi have not been mentioned as part of the syndrome but descriptions have included a raised hyperkeratotic lesion on the face and hyperpigmented streaks on the trunk and limbs; arachnoid cyst and brainstem arteriovenous malformation have occurred in individual cases.

REFERENCES

1 Happle R. How many epidermal nevus syndromes exist? *J Am Acad Dermatol* 1991; 25: 550–6.
2 Clancy RR, Kurtz MB, Baker D, Sladky JT, Honig PJ, Younkin DP. Neurologic manifestations of the organoid nevus syndrome. *Arch Neurol* 1985; 42: 236–40.
3 David P, Elia M, Garcovich A, Colosimo C, Tagliaferri G, Macchi G. A case of epidermal nevus syndrome with carotid malformation. *Ital J Neurol Sci* 1990; 11: 293–6.
4 Baker RS, Ross PA, Baumann RJ. Neurologic complications of the epidermal nevus syndrome. *Arch Neurol* 1987; 44: 227–32.
5 Mansour AM, Barber JC, Reinecke RD, Wang FM. Ocular choristomas. *Surv Ophthalmol* 1989; 33: 339–58.
6 Lambert HM, Sipperley JO, Shore JW, Dieckert JP, Evans R, Lowd DK. Linear nevus sebaceous syndrome. *Ophthalmology* 1987; 94: 278–82.
7 Nuno K, Mihara M, Shimao S. Linear sebaceous nevus syndrome. *Dermatologica* 1990; 181: 221–3.
8 Kucukoduk S, Oznan H, Turanli AY, Dinc H, Selcuk M. A new neurocutaneous syndrome: nevus sebaceous syndrome. *Cutis* 1993; 51: 437–41.
9 Fishman MA. Encephalocraniocutaneous lipomatosis. *J Child Neurol* 1987; 2: 186–93.
10 Grimalt R, Ermacora E, Mistura L *et al*. Encephalocraniocutaneous lipomatosis: case report and review of the literature. *Pediatr Dermatol* 1993; 10: 164–8.
11 Pavone L, Curatolo P, Rizzo R *et al*. Epidermal nevus syndrome: a neurologic variant with hemimegalencephaly, gyral malformation, seizures and facial hemihypertrophy. *Neurology* 1991; 41: 266–71.
12 Hager BC, Dyme IZ, Guertin SR, Tyler RJ, Tryciecky EW, Fratkin JD. Linear nevus sebaceous syndrome: megalencephaly and heterotopic gray matter. *Pediatr Neurol* 1991; 7: 45–9.
13 El-Shanti H, Bell WE, Waziri MH. Epidermal nevus syndrome: subgroup with neuronal migration defects. *J Child Neurol* 1992; 7: 29–34.
14 Cavenagh EC, Hart BL, Rose D. Association of linear sebaceous

nevus syndrome and unilateral megalencephaly. *Am J Neuroradiol* 1993; 14: 405–8.

15 Demarel P, Wilms G, Casaer P. More association of linear sebaceous nevus syndrome and unilateral megalencephaly. *Am J Neuroradiol* 1994; 15: 196–7.

16 Frieden IJ. Aplasia cutis congenita: a clinical review and proposal for classification. *J Am Acad Dermatol* 1986; 14: 646–60.

17 Frieden I, Golabi M. Aplasia cutis congenita and the epidermal nevus syndrome: a previously unrecognized association. *Clin Res* 1985; 33: 130.

18 Lantis S, Leyden J, Thew M, Heaton C. Nevus sebaceus of Jadassohn: part of a new neurocutaneous syndrome. *Arch Dermatol* 1968; 98: 117–23.

19 Mimoumi F, Han BK, Barnes L *et al*. Multiple hamartomas associated with intracranial malformation. *Pediatr Dermatol* 1986; 3: 219–25.

20 Toriello HV, Lacassie Y, Droste P, Higgins JV. Provisionally unique syndrome of ocular and ectodermal defects in two unrelated boys. *Am J Med Genet* 1993; 45: 764–6.

21 Evers MEJW, Dijkman-Neerinex RHM, Hamel BCJ. Oculo-ectodermal syndrome: a new case. *Am J Med Genet* 1994; 53: 378–9.

22 Gardner J, Viljoen D. Aplasia cutis congenita with epibulbar dermoids: further evidence for syndromic identity of the ocular ectodermal syndrome. *Am J Med Genet* 1994; 53: 317–20.

Naevus comedonicus syndrome

Naevus comedonicus has been associated with a variety of abnormalities including unilateral and bilateral cataracts [1,2] and skeletal defects [2,3]. Spinal defects include congenital scoliosis, hemivertebrae, fused vertebrae and spina bifida occulta [3] and leg shortening, supernumary digit and hand and foot syndactyly are also reported [2]. Happle [4] postulates that this condition which always occurs sporadically and equally in both sexes is another example of the effect of a lethal autosomal mutation surviving by mosaicism.

REFERENCES

1 Whyte HJ. Unilateral comedo nevus and cataract. *Arch Dermatol* 1968; 97: 533–5.

2 Rogers M. Epidermal nevi and the epidermal nevus syndromes: a review of 233 cases. *Pediatr Dermatol* 1992; 9: 342–4.

3 Engber PB. The nevus comedonicus syndrome: a case report with emphasis on associated internal manifestations. *Int J Dermatol* 1978; 17: 745–9.

4 Happle R. How many epidermal nevus syndromes exist? *J Am Acad Dermatol* 1991; 25: 550–6.

Widespread keratinocytic naevi with skeletal defects

Series of patients with epidermal naevi contain individuals with widespread keratinocytic naevi and skeletal abnormalities of the spine, chest and in particular the limbs, especially the legs and feet [1–5]. Structural bony abnormalities demonstrated include deformity of the vertebral bodies, bifid ribs, limb reduction defects (usually more minor than in CHILD syndrome), duplication of fibula and accessory or bifid digits.

REFERENCES

1 Solomon LM, Fretzin DF, Dewald RL. The epidermal nevus syndrome. *Arch Dermatol* 1968; 97: 273–85.

2 Solomon LM, Esterly NB. Epidermal and other congenital organoid nevi. *Curr Prob Pediatr* 1975; 1: 3–56.

3 Rogers M, McCrossin I, Commens C. Epidermal nevi and the epidermal nevus syndrome. *J Am Acad Dermatol* 1989; 20: 476–88.

4 Rogers M. Epidermal nevi and the epidermal nevus syndromes: a review of 233 cases. *Pediatr Dermatol* 1992; 9: 342–4.

5 Grebe TA, Rimsza ME, Richter SF, Hansen RC, Hoyme HE. Further delineation of the epidermal naevus syndrome: two new cases with new findings and literature review. *Am J Med Genet* 1993; 47: 24–30.

Epidermal naevi with hypophosphataemic vitamin D-resistant osteomalacia and rickets

There have been several reports of hypophosphataemic vitamin D-resistant osteomalacia and rickets in association with epidermal naevi [1–8] both of sebaceous and keratinocytic type. The response to the combination of calcitriol and phosphorus in these patients is consistent with the entity of tumour-induced osteomalacia [9], which has been reported with a variety of ossifying and mesenchymal tumours and in which removal of the tumour may be associated with remission. It has been postulated that the epidermal naevus itself may be the cause of the condition. However, removal of the naevus does not result in resolution of the condition [7,8] and most patients with widespread epidermal naevi do not show this complication. Several of the reported patients have had vascular tumours in bones [4,5,7], lungs [5] or skin [1]. In the latter case [1] a homogenate of the vascular lesions but not of the sebaceous naevus induced phosphaturia when injected into a dog. In several other patients bone cysts have been found [1,2,6] but histopathological confirmation of their nature was not obtained. Widespread haemangiomatosis of the bone in the absence of an epidermal naevus has been reported to produce a similar rickets which recovered after irradiation of the bony lesions [10]. These findings suggest that the osteomalacia/rickets in patients with epidermal naevi may be explained by tumours other than the epidermal naevus. Most patients have had similar widespread, predominantly unilateral naevi, usually involving the head as well as the trunk and often with a papillomatous surface. It seems possible that this is a distinct mosaic phenotype [7]. One of the patients had in addition multiple, biopsy-proven, melanocytic naevi; most of these were standard compound or intradermal naevi but some were Spitz naevi [6].

Three patients with epidermal naevi and polyostotic fibrous dysplasia have been reported [11–13]. However, it has been pointed out [14] that none had precocious puberty and in all of the patients the predominant cutaneous lesion was a verrucous epidermal naevus rather than the usual macular hyperpigmentation. In one case hypophosphataemic rickets was present and Stosiek *et al.* [7] point out the clinical and radiological similarity of this case to their own in which intraosseous haemangiomas were found.

REFERENCES

1 Aschinberg LC, Solomon LM, Zeis PM, Justice P, Rosenthal IM. Vitamin D-resistant rickets associated with epidermal nevus syndrome: Demonstration of a phosphaturic substance in the dermal lesions. *J Pediatr* 1977; 91: 56–60.

2 Carey DE, Drenzer MK, Hamdan JA *et al.* Hypophosphatemic rickets/osteomalacia in linear sebaceous nevus syndrome: a variant of tumor-induced osteomalacia. *J Pediatr* 1986; 109: 994–1000.

3 Skovby F, Svejgaard E, Moller J. Hypophosphatemic rickets in linear sebaceous nevus sequence. *J Pediatr* 1987; 111: 855–7.

4 Becker W, Stosiek N, Peters K-P, Wolf F. Bone scan and red blood cell scan in a patient with epidermal naevus syndrome. *Eur J Nucl Med* 1990; 17: 369–71.

5 O'Neill EM. Linear sebaceous naevus syndrome with oncogenic rickets and diffuse pulmonary angiomatosis. *J Roy Soc Med* 1993; 86: 177–8.

6 Goldblum JR, Headington JT. Hypophosphatemic vitamin D-resistant rickets and multiple spindle and epithelioid nevi associated with linear nevus sebaceus syndrome. *J Am Acad Dermatol* 1993; 29: 109–11.

7 Stosiek N, Horstein OP, Hiller D, Peters K-P. Extensive linear epidermal nevus associated with haemangiomas of bones and vitamin D-resistant rickets. *Dermatology* 1994; 189: 278–82.

8 Oranje AP, Przyrembel H, Meradji M, Loonen MCB, de Klerk JBC. Solomon's epidermal nevus syndrome (type: linear nevus sebaceus) and hypophosphatemic vitamin D-resistant rickets. *Arch Dermatol* 1994; 130: 1167–71.

9 Fukumoto Y, Tarui S, Tsukuyama K *et al.* Tumor-induced vitamin D-resistant hypophosphatemic rickets/osteomalacia associated with proximal renal dysfunction and 1,25-dihydroxyvitamin D deficiency. *J Clin Endocrinol Metab* 1979; 49: 873–8.

10 Amir G, Boneh A, Tochner Z, Bar Ziv J. Widespread hemangiomatosis of bone associated with rickets: recovery after irradiation. *J Pediatr* 1993; 123: 269–72.

11 Grun G, Didier MF. Le syndrome d'Albright. Apropos de deux observations. *Bull Soc Franc Dermatol Syph* 1972; 79: 184–5.

12 Pierini AM, Ortonne JP, Floret D. Signes dermatologiques du syndrome de McCune–Albright. *Ann Dermatol Vénéréol* 1981; 108: 969–76.

13 Rustin MHA, Bunker CB, Gilkes JJH, Robinson TWE, Dowd PM. Polyostotic fibrous dysplasia associated with extensive linear epidermal naevi. *Clin Exp Dermatol* 1989; 14: 371–5.

14 Moss C, Parkin JM, Comaish JS. Precocious puberty in a boy with a widespread linear epidermal naevus. *Br J Dermatol* 1991; 125: 178–82.

Epidermal naevi with endocrine abnormalities

An adult male with a small keratinocytic naevus presented with hypogonadism and hypothyroidism and was found to have a pituitary tumour [1]. Precocious puberty has been twice reported in association with widespread keratinocytic naevi [2,3]. In neither was a cause demonstrated. In each case CT scan of the head was normal but a small hypothalamic hamartoma remains a possibility [2].

REFERENCES

1 Abou Zeid SA, Khalil SA, Meheesen AM, El-Beheiry AH, Salama MN. Epidermal nevus with cutaneous endocrinal associations. *Arch Dermatol* 1979; 115: 625–6.

2 Moss C, Parkin JM, Comaish JS. Precocious puberty in a boy with a widespread linear epidermal naevus. *Br J Dermatol* 1991; 125: 178–82.

3 Hogan P, Klingensmith G, Travers S, Weston W. Epidermal nevus with precocious puberty. *Pediatr Dermatol* 1992; 9: 221 (abstract).

Epidermal naevi with vascular malformations

As has been discussed, intracranial vascular malformations may occur in association with sebaceous naevi. There are reports of keratinocytic epidermal naevi in association with Klippel–Trenaunay syndrome [1,2]. Happle [2] suggests that the phenomenon of twin-spotting can be considered to explain this association but that another explanation is that these cases represent oligosymptomatic examples of Proteus syndrome.

REFERENCES

1 Wikler J, Starink TM. Acanthosis nigricans-like epidermal naevus and Klippel–Trenaunay syndrome. *Br J Dermatol* 1990; 123: 539.

2 Happle R. How many epidermal nevus syndromes exist? *J Am Acad Dermatol* 1991; 25: 550–6.

Development of internal neoplasms

Some patients with epidermal naevi appear to be at increased risk of the development of certain neoplasms of internal organs, often at a young age. Renal tumours are the most frequently encountered [1–5] and cases of nephroblastoma, rhabdomyosarcoma of the bladder and transitional cell carcinoma of the urinary tract have been reported in childhood, usually in patients with widespread keratinocytic naevi. Other reported neoplasms with onset in childhood include glioma [6] astrocytoma [6,7] parotid adenocarcinoma [8], odontoma [9] and ameloblastoma of the mandible [10].

REFERENCES

1 Solomon LM, Esterly NB. Epidermal and other congenital organoid nevi. *Curr Prob Pediatr* 1975; 1: 3–56.

2 Lansky LL, Funderburk S, Cuppage FE, Schimke RN, Diehl AM. Linear nevus sebaceous syndrome: hamartoma variant. *Am J Dis Child* 1972; 123: 587–90.

3 Dimond RL, Amon RB. Epidermal nevus and rhabdomyosarcoma. *Arch Dermatol* 1976; 112: 1424–6.

4 Rosenthal D, Fretzin DF. Epidermal nevus syndrome: report of association with transitional cell carcinoma of the bladder. *Pediatr Dermatol* 1986; 3: 455–8.

5 Rongioletti F, Rebora A. Epidermal nevus with transitional cell carcinomas of the urinary tract. *J Am Acad Dermatol* 1991; 25: 856–8.

6 Andriola M. Nevus unius lateralis and brain tumor. *Am J Dis Child* 1976; 130: 1259–61.

7 Meyerson LB. Nevus unius lateralis, brain tumor and diencephalic syndrome. *Arch Dermatol* 1967; 95: 501–4.

8 Berkeley WT. Nevus sebaceus (Jadassohn) complicated by bilateral salivary gland adenocarcinoma. *Plast Reconstr Surg* 1959; 23: 55–63.

9 Baghaei-Rad M, Doku HC, Ficarelli J. Epidermal nevus syndrome with maxillary involvement. *J Oral Maxillofac Surg* 1982; 40: 821–3.

10 Lovejoy FH, Boyle WE. Linear nevus sebaceus syndrome: report of two cases and review of the literature. *Pediatrics* 1973; 52: 382–7.

Epidermal naevi with pigmentary disorders

Epidermal naevi have been described in patients with the symptom complex designated as hypomelanosis of Ito [1], known now to represent a collection of different mosaic phenotypes. Solomon and Esterly [2] reported six patients with, in addition to pigmented verrucous epidermal naevi, large hypopigmented macules, large and small hyperpigmented macules, and multiple melanocytic naevi. There are also reports of patients with widespread epidermal naevi and naevus spilus-like lesions accompanied by skeletal [3,4] and neurological abnormalities [3].

REFERENCES

1 Rogers M. Epidermal nevi and the epidermal nevus syndromes: a review of 233 cases. *Pediatr Dermatol* 1992; 9: 342–4.
2 Solomon LM, Esterly NB. Epidermal and other congenital organoid nevi. *Curr Prob Pediatr* 1975; 1: 3–56.
3 Goldberg LH, Collins SAB, Siegel DM. The epidermal naevus syndrome: case report and review. *Pediatr Dermatol* 1987; 4: 27–33.
4 Mostafa WZ, Satti MB. Epidermal nevus syndrome: a clinicopathologic study with 6-year follow-up. *Pediatr Dermatol* 1991; 8: 228–30.

Conclusion

Much of the literature on epidermal naevi has concerned individuals or series [1] of patients with established abnormalities in other organ systems and it has been difficult to assess the risk of these abnormalities in the general population of patients with epidermal naevi. One large series attempting to look at unselected patients with these naevi and finding abnormalities in one-third of cases probably included as significant at least some abnormalities which were minor or coincidental [2]. Further, preferably multicentre, studies are required to address this issue. However, what is clear is that epidermal naevi are commonly encountered in paediatric dermatology practice and the majority of patients are free of other significant abnormalities. In view of the wide range of associated abnormalities that may occur it is essential that all of these patients have a detailed physical examination including neurological and ophthalmological assessment at presentation. If presentation is in the neonatal period, annual follow-up for several years is important. In general further investigation is indicated only in the presence of significant clinical abnormalities. However, it is recommended that even in the absence of clinical neurological abnormalities neuroimaging, preferably with MRI, be carried out in patients with sebaceous naevi which are extensive or which involve the centrofacial area, in patients with sebaceous naevi and ocular choristomas or colobomas and in patients with skull asymmetry. Skeletal radiology should ideally be undertaken in all patients with very widespread naevi involving trunk and limbs.

REFERENCES

1 Solomon LM, Esterly NB. Epidermal and other congenital organoid nevi. *Curr Prob Pediatr* 1975; 1: 3–56.
2 Rogers M, McCrossin I, Commens C. Epidermal nevi and the epidermal nevus syndrome. *J Am Acad Dermatol* 1989; 20: 476–88.

Section 18
Vascular and Lymphatic Anomalies

18.1 Vascular Malformations

ODILE ENJOLRAS AND JOHN B. MULLIKEN

Fast-flow vascular malformations
Arteriovenous malformation

Slow-flow vascular malformations
Venous malformation
Lymphatic malformation
Capillary malformation

The nomenclature and classification for superficial vascular anomalies have been debated in international workshops over 20 years. The nosology used in this chapter is that approved by the International Society for the Study of Vascular Anomalies (ISSVA), initiated in 1992. This system of classification is based on clinical, radiological, histopathological and haemodynamic characteristics. According to this system, there are two major categories of superficial vascular anomalies found in infancy and childhood: haemangiomas and vascular malformations [1–4]. Haemangiomas exhibit cellular proliferation; they grow during infancy, involute in childhood and never appear in an adolescent or an adult [5]. In contrast, vascular malformations are comprised of dysplastic vessels. These lesions do not exhibit endothelial cell proliferation and they never regress. Some vascular malformations are stable, whereas others expand.

Vascular malformations can be further divided into two categories, based on rheology and channel morphology (Table 18.1.1). Fast-flow vascular malformations may be either arterial and arteriovenous—arterial malformation (AM), arteriovenous fistula (AVF) or arterial venous malformation (AVM). Slow-flow vascular malformations may be venous malformations (VM), lymphatic malformations (LM) and capillary malformations (CM). There are also complex–combined vascular malformations—capillary–lymphatic malformations (CLM), capillary–venous malformations (CVM), lymphatic–venous malformations (LVM), arterial–capillary malformations (ACM), capillary–lymphatic–venous malformations (CLVM), capillary–arteriovenous malformations (CAVM) and capillary–arteriovenous–lymphatic malformations (CAVLM). Many eponymous syndromes fall into these categories. Vascular malformations can be either localized or diffuse (Table 18.1.2). Some lesions are inconsequential, while others may cause cosmetic problems, functional disability or even life-threatening complications. More than 90% of superficial vascular malformations in paediatric patients are easily diagnosed by clinical features. Radiological imaging is rarely necessary to make a correct diagnosis, but it is needed to delineate the vascular malformation, to detect an associated dysmorphogenetic anomaly and to determine therapy [6,7]. Interdisciplinary collaboration is necessary, not only for the diagnosis, but also for the treatment of vascular anomalies.

REFERENCES

1 Mulliken JB, Glowacki J. Hemangiomas and vascular malformations in infants and children: a classification based on endothelial characteristics. *Plast Reconstr Surg* 1982; 69: 412–20.
2 Mulliken JB, Young AE. *Vascular Birthmarks: Hemangiomas and Malformations.* Philadelphia: WB Saunders, 1988.
3 Enjolras O, Riché MC, Mulliken JB, Merland JJ. *Atlas des Hémangiomes et Malformations Vasculaires Superficielles.* Paris: McGraw Hill, 1990.
4 Takahashi K, Mulliken JB, Kozakewich HPW, Rogers RA, Folkman J, Ezekowitz RA. Cellular markers that distinguish the phases of hemangioma during infancy and childhood. *J Clin Invest* 1994; 9: 2357–64.
5 Esterly NB. Cutaneous hemangiomas, vascular stains and malformations, and associated syndromes. *Curr Prob Dermatol* 1995; 7: 65–108.
6 Enjolras O, Mulliken JB. The current management of vascular birthmarks. *Pediatr Dermatol* 1993; 10: 311–33.
7 Burrows PE, Paltiel H, Robertson RL. Diagnostic imaging in the evaluation of vascular birthmarks. *Dermatol Clin* 1998; 16: 455–88.

Fast-flow vascular malformations

Most fast-flow cutaneous vascular anomalies are AVMs. Pure AMs, i.e. arterial aneurysms, stenoses and ectasias, rarely occur alone in skin as symptomatic lesions. AMs can be associated with AVMs, and sometimes require surgical treatment. In skin, in contrast to the brain, a single, direct AVF is almost always the result of trauma.

Arteriovenous malformation

Localized or extensive arteriovenous malformations

Definition

An AVM is a fast-flow vascular malformation that is comprised of micro and macro AVFs. The epicentre, called the

Table 18.1.1 Classification of vascular anomalies according to the ISSVA 11th International Workshop, Rome, June 1996

Vascular tumours	Vascular malformations
Haemangioma	**Pure types**
Kaposiform	*Fast flow*
haemangioendothelioma	AM
(with or without KMP)	AVF (single direct AVF)
Tufted angioma (with or	AVM (with multiple AVFs)
without KMP)	
Others	*Slow flow*
	VM
	LM
	CM
	Complex–combined types
	CLM, CVM, CLVM, LVM, ACM, CAVM, CAVLM, etc. (concerning the eponymous syndromes with limb gigantism: KTS is CLVM, and Parkes–Weber syndrome is CAVM or CAVLM)

KMP, Kasabach–Merritt phenomenon; KTS, Klippel-Trenauney syndrome.

Table 18.1.2 Vascular malformations

Fast-flow vascular malformations
AVM
Localized or extensive AVM or syndromic AVM (Bonnet–Dechaume–Blanc or Wyburn-Mason syndrome, Brégeat's syndrome, Cobb's syndrome, Parkes–Weber syndrome)

Slow-flow vascular malformations
VM
Localized or extensive VM or syndromic VM (Maffucci's syndrome, glomangiomatosis, blue rubber bleb naevus syndrome or Bean's syndrome, familial VM, familial 'cavernous angiomatosis' of the brain)

LM

CM
• Localized or extensive PWS or syndromic PWS, (Sturger–Weber syndrome, PWS in complex–combined VMs = KTS and Parkes–Weber syndrome, Servelle–Martorell syndrome, Proteus syndrome, phacomatosis pigmentovascularis, OSD and midline CM)
• Localized or syndromic telangiectatic vascular malformations (cutis marmorata telangiectatica, Adams–Oliver syndrome, AT, Divry-Van Bogaert syndrome, Rendu–Osler–Weber disease)
• Localized or syndromic angiokeratomas (angiokeratoma corporis diffusum/Fabry's disease, etc.)

PWS, Port wine stain; VMs, vascular malformations; KTS, Klippel-Trenauney syndrome; OSD, occult spinal dysmorphism.

'nidus', consists of arterial feeders and enlarged veins that appear early on arteriography. AVMs are present at birth or they become evident in infancy or childhood. They never regress.

Pathology

An AVM is usually poorly delimited and consists of round or elongated arteries and veins with irregularly thickened fibromuscular walls, discontinuous elastic network and fibrosis in the stroma [1].

Clinical features

AVMs are very often misdiagnosed in childhood and mistaken for haemangiomas or port-wine stains (PWS). Puberty and trauma trigger growth, at which point the fast-flow nature becomes clinically evident. At this time, lesions may become infiltrated or develop a red or violaceous colour. A mass, either under normal skin or (more frequently) under a vascular stain may develop. Other signs include local warmth, a thrill or bruit and pulses of increased amplitude.

As an AVM worsens, draining veins become more evident, and are more tortuous and distended. Wherever the site of an AVM, the eventual consequences are alteration of skin colour, atrophy, recurrent ulceration [2], intractable pain and intermittent bleeding. All of these may occur in childhood, and haemorrhage can be life-threatening. A facial AVM, if localized to the skin and/or bones (ethmoid, maxillary or mandibular), leads to asymmetrical hypertrophy and gingival haemorrhage [3]. A nasal AVM can cause epistaxis. AVM in a digit may gradually narrow the distal phalanx and causes violaceous skin atrophy, due to ischaemia of the distal capillary bed and

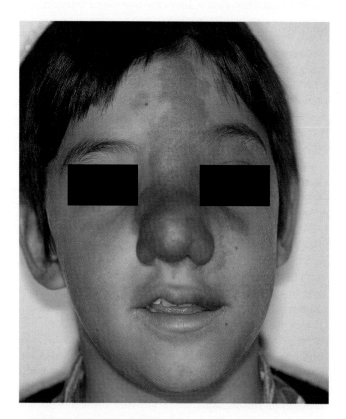

Fig. 18.1.1 Facial AVM mimicking CM in a boy with Bonnet–Dechaume–Blanc syndrome.

progressive shortening of the nailplate. The veins become prominent over the fingers and dorsum of the hand. Pseudokaposi sarcoma skin changes commonly occur in association with AVM in the lower limb [4–6], although they rarely develop before adolescence.

Radiological investigation is recommended as soon as AVM is suspected clinically. A number of techniques may be helpful in defining the extent and nature of the lesion as follows.

Ultrasonography combined with grey-scale and colour Doppler documents the arteriovenous (AV) shunting. An AVM is heterogeneously echogenic and exhibits numerous dilated arteries and veins with fast flow and low resistance. Vessels are tortuous.

Pulsed Doppler quantitates arterial output (e.g. from the carotid, axillary or femoral arteries) as compared with the uninvolved side. This technique allows the clinician to follow the progression of an AVM in a non-invasive fashion.

Computed tomography (CT) with contrast demonstrates the extent of an AVM but (unlike magnetic resonance imaging or MRI) cannot clearly differentiate between haemangioma, VM and AVM.

MRI of an AVM shows flow voids, corresponding to fast-flow vessels, in all sequences (spin–echo T1- and T2-weighted sequences) except gradient–echo (in which sequence increased signal is present in vascular spaces). There is no parenchymal staining.

Magnetic resonance angiography (MRA) portrays, without injection of contrast medium, the anomalous vascular network. It has replaced arteriography for follow-up of AVM.

Arteriography remains an indispensable tool in the work-up of AVMs and is used to depict the angioarchitecture clearly, especially prior to arterial embolization.

Prognosis

AVMs are the most unpredictable of all vascular malformations. They often enlarge, and cause local destruction and systemic effects. Once the initial diagnostic work-up is completed, the child should be carefully followed, both by frequent clinical evaluation, and by serial Doppler and/or MRI and MRA. An AVM usually remains quiescent in childhood, masquerading as a PWS or haemangioma. Failure to recognize its true nature can lead to dangerous mismanagement and result in severe complications. For example, partial excision or ligation of arterial feeders may trigger lesional growth, especially during

puberty. Mismanagement of a limb AVM can lead to gangrene and necessitate amputation [7]. Shunting through AVFs, particularly in large cephalic, pelvic or extremity AVMs, can cause congestive heart failure. This complication usually occurs after adolescence, but may rarely be seen in infancy and early childhood.

Differential diagnosis

AVM must be distinguished from haemangioma or PWS. With the aid of ultrasound and colour Doppler, haemangiomas are noted to have equatorial arterial feeders, peripheral veins and variable echogenicity. There may be evidence of fast flow, but there is no true AV shunting.

A few other dermatological lesions, all uncommon in the paediatric patient, mimic AVM. The epithelioid haemangioendothelioma, which usually occurs on the distal extremity, is a violaceous and locally aggressive infiltrative lesion [8]. Lupus erythematosus tumidus or sarcoidosis on the ear or nose and Melkersson–Rosenthal syndrome of the lip may rarely mimic AVM. In the latter, a bruit and thrill indicates the presence of an AVM. The pseudokaposi sarcoma changes which may develop uni-

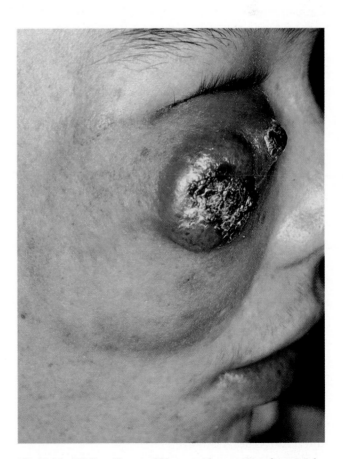

Fig. 18.1.2 AVM in a 15-year-old boy: rapid worsening after partial excision.

laterally in an evolving AVM of the limb are usually easily differentiated from true Kaposi's sarcoma. Dabska's tumour, a vascular tumour of childhood, can mimic an AVM of the ear. Dabska's tumour is firm and has no AV shunting. Biopsy shows endovascular papillary proliferation [9].

Treatment

Every AVM is potentially dangerous. In the paediatric age group, AV shunting is frequently latent and clinically inevident. An AVM is usually not treated in its quiescent stage. Early embolic/surgical treatment of a quiescent AVM in childhood is controversial, and should only be considered if surgical excision is easily achievable. The most useful guidelines for the management of an AVM are as follows: (a) employ a multidisciplinary approach; and (b) be modest about treatment outcomes and do not overestimate your therapeutic capabilities. The only acceptable surgical stratagem is complete resection [3,7,10]; partial excision may lead to transient clinical improvement, but the AVM inevitably re-expands over time, and may lead to severe disfigurement, limb amputation or death from visceral extension of a cephalic or truncal lesion. Ligation or proximal embolization of arterial feeding vessels is contraindicated. After a period of transient benefit, a vascular recruitment phenomenon occurs, as small arteries extend from the neighbouring arteries to supply the nidus. Furthermore, arterial ligation of large feeder vessels impedes access to the nidus at a time when therapeutic embolization becomes necessary. In a limb AVM, elastic stockings provide benefit and protect the skin from injury. Treatment of an AVM is always complex and difficult. However, intervention becomes necessary whenever local and/or cardiac complications occur. Therapies that have been used are as follows.

Transcatheter embolization of the AVM nidus, followed by flashlamp pulsed dye laser therapy for the residual skin component of the AVM. This technique improved the clinical outcome in one child with an ear AVM [11]; however, the long-term results are unknown so this procedure cannot be recommended.

Superselective arterial embolization. This can be an effective palliative treatment for some evolving AVMs, especially in those instances when surgical excision will be disfiguring or mutilating. In patients with maxillary or mandibular AVM, localized embolization should be performed prior to dental extraction, which can be perilous. Embolization of an AVM, unlike embolization of a single direct AVF, is never curative.

Microcatheter guide-wire systems, as used in intracra-

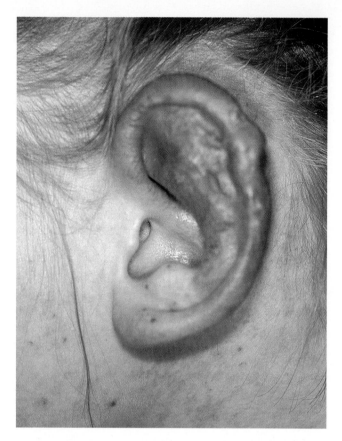

Fig. 18.1.3 Ear AVM, with adjacent neck and cheek involvement, in an 8-year-old girl.

nial neuroradiology, permit a superselective approach to the nidus. Direct puncture of the nidus, in association with local arterial and venous compression, is necessary when arteries are dysplastic and tortuous, or in children who have undergone previous arterial ligation. The embolic materials most commonly employed are liquid (ethanol, isobutylcyanoacrylate, Ethibloc), particles (Ivalon), or permanent implantable devices (microspheres) [12].

Surgical resection. In most cases, arterial embolization is performed prior to resection. This temporarily shrinks or occludes the nidus, and facilitates the surgical procedure that is performed 24–72 h later. Embolization minimizes intraoperative bleeding but does not affect the margins of the surgical resection; the AVM and the overlying skin must be widely excised [3]. Microsurgical free flap transfer is often necessary for reconstruction [13]. Cutaneous expansion, prior to embolization and resection, is an alternative surgical strategy. The overlying skin can be saved only if normal; vascular-stained skin that is left in place may lead to recurrence. After treatment, the patient should be followed carefully for many years by clinical examination, ultrasonography and/or MRA. Definitive cure is uncommon [14].

Syndromic arteriovenous malformation

Bonnet–Dechaume–Blanc (1937), Wyburn-Mason (1943) and Brégeat (1958) syndromes

These are sporadic, neuro-ocular anomalies associated with oculo-orbital, facial and brain (mesodiencephalon) AVMs [15–17]. These patients exhibit centrofacial and/or hemifacial fast-flow lesions, with ipsilateral retinal, optic nerve, optic chiasm, optic pathway, basal ganglia and cerebral AVMs. The patients present in childhood with multiple AVMs: the involved skin resembles a PWS, although it is warm and thick, and the lesions never follow a clear trigeminal distribution (as in Sturge–Weber syndrome or SWS). Retinal involvement is present in Bonnet–Dechaume–Blanc syndrome (also known as Wyburn-Mason syndrome). Brégeat syndrome has no retinal or choroidal AVM, but exhibits vascular anomalies in the conjunctiva. The jaws, nose and mouth are sometimes involved. All syndromic AVMs are present at birth and progressively worsen. Skin staining, infiltration, exophthalmos and hemianopia may develop, and some patients develop a variety of neurological symptoms. Wyburn-Mason also described mental changes. Modern ophthalmological and neuroradiological investigative procedures, including MRA, may be used to delineate the oculo-orbital and intracranial vascular anomalies. Because of the extent of the AVMs, therapeutic possibilities are usually limited. Mismanagement of the superficial lesions (namely arterial ligation, venous ligation, proximal embolization, partial excision and laser treatment) causes progressive expansion. Neurosurgical procedures are rarely curative.

Cobb's syndrome

This syndrome consists of cutaneous AVM, which may masquerade as PWS and spinal cord AVMs in the same metamere. These spinal cord AVMs are either (a) intramedullar or perimedullar and fed by spinal cord arteries; or (b) dural and fed by radicular meningeal arteries [18,19]. Vascular malformation in the vertebrae and paraspinal muscles can also occur in the same metamere. The syndrome is sporadic, and patients are at risk for local complications such as limb hypertrophy, ulceration and amputation. Neurological complications, including pain, sensory disturbance, neurogenic bladder and bowel, and motor symptoms (monoplegia, paraplegia or quadriplegia) depend on the location and extent of the lesion. These usually begin in childhood. MRI is the best test for screening, but intrathecal contrast myelography may be neces-

sary to delineate the lesion. Prior to surgery, the angioarchitecture of the lesion must be defined by selective arteriography. Neurosurgical treatment aims at complete removal of the spinal cord AVM nidus whenever possible, in order to minimize the risk for further neurological deterioration. Neuroendovascular treatment is an alternative to surgical extirpation.

Syndromic AVM in limb complex–combined vascular malformations

These include CAVM or CAVLM, with limb overgrowth (Parkes–Weber syndrome) (see below).

REFERENCES

1 Wassef M. Angiomes et malformations vasculaires cervico-céphaliques, aspects histopathologiques et classification. *J Mal Vasc* 1992; 17: 20–5.
2 Lee EB, Dubin HV. Ulcers associated with congenital arteriovenous fistulas. *Arch Dermatol* 1983; 119: 949–52.
3 Kohout MP, Hansen M, Pribaz JJ, Mulliken JB. Arteriovenous malformations of the head and neck: natural history and management. *Plast Reconstr Surg* 1998; 102: 643–54.
4 Bluefarb SM, Adams LA. Arteriovenous malformation with angiodermatitis: stasis dermatitis simulating Kaposi's disease. *Arch Dermatol* 1967; 96: 176–81.
5 Stewart W. Pseudoangiosarcomatose de Kaposi par fistules artérioveineuses. *Ann Dermatol Vénéréol* 1977; 104: 391–6.
6 Marshall E, Hartfield ST, Hartfield DR. Arteriovenous malformation simulating Kaposi's sarcoma. *Arch Dermatol* 1985; 121: 99–101.
7 McClinton MA. Tumors and aneurysms of the upper extremity. *Hand Clin* 1993; 9: 151–69.
8 Roudier-Pujol C, Enjolras O, Lacronique L *et al*. Hémangioendothéliome épithélioide multifocal en rémission partielle sous traitement par interféron alpha 2a. *Ann Dermatol Vénéréol* 1994; 121: 898–904.
9 Morgan J, Robinson M, Rosen L, Hunger H, Niven J. Malignant endovascular papillary angioendothelioma (Dabska tumor). *Am J Dermatopathol* 1989; 11: 64–8.
10 Enjolras O, Borsik M, Herbreteau D, Merland JJ. Prise en charge des malformations artérioveineuses. *Ann Dermatol Vénéréol* 1994; 121: 59–66.
11 Ashinoff R, Berenstein A, Geronemus R. Arteriovenous malformation treated with embolization and laser therapy. *Arch Dermatol* 1991; 127: 1642–4.
12 Burrows P, Fellows KE. Techniques for management of pediatric vascular anomalies. In: Cope C, ed. *Current Techniques in Interventional Radiology*, vol. 2. Philadelphia: Current Medicine, 1995: 12–27.
13 Dompmartin A, Labbe D, Barrelier MT, Theron J. Use of a regulating flap in the treatment of a large arteriovenous malformation of the scalp. *Br J Plast Surg* 1998; 51: 561–3.
14 Enjolras O, Deffrennes D, Borsik M, Diner P, Laurian C. Les 'tumeurs' vasculaires et les règles de prise en charge chirurgicale. *Ann Chir Plast Esthét* 1998; 43: 311–64.
15 Brégeat P. Brégeat syndrome. In: Vinken PJ, Bruyn GW, eds. *Handbook of Clinical Neurology: the Phakomatoses*, vol. 14. Amsterdam: North Holland Publishers, 1975: 474–9.
16 Théron J, Newton TH, Hoyt WF. Unilateral retinocephalic vascular malformations. *Neuroradiology* 1974; 7: 185–96.
17 Brodsky MC, Hoyt WF, Higashida RT, Hieshima G, Halbach VV. Bonnet–Dechaume–Blanc syndrome with large facial angioma. *Arch Ophthalmol* 1987; 105: 854–5.
18 Jessen RT, Thompson S, Smith EB. Cobb syndrome. *Arch Dermatol* 1977; 113: 1587–90.
19 Hodes JE, Merland JJ, Casasco A, Houdart E, Reizine D. Spinal vascular malformations: endovascular therapy. *Neurosurg Clin N Am* 1994; 5: 497–509.

Slow-flow vascular malformations

Venous malformation

Localized or extensive venous malformations

Definition and aetiology

VMs are slow-flow vascular malformations involving the collecting side of the vascular network. VMs may be localized or extensive, minor or distorting, single or multiple, and may be located on the head, extremities and/or trunk. The lesions are present at birth, but may become clinically evident later. Most VMs occur sporadically, although some are familial [1].

Pathology

VMs are comprised of ectatic, poorly defined, venous channels and lakes interconnected to form a complex network, which dissects normal tissues. Some lesions contain only dysplastic, enlarged venous channels (sometimes labelled as 'cavernous'). Other lesions consist of a spongy combination of ectatic venous channels and capillaries. The lining endothelium is flat. The walls are thin and irregular with islands of smooth muscle cells. Thrombosis and subsequent phleboliths are frequent. The dysplastic venous network drains to adjacent veins, many of which are varicose and lack valves.

Clinical features

Ectatic venous channels within the dermis give the lesions a characteristic blue colour. VMs swell with exertion or when the region is dependent. Skin temperature is normal, and there is no thrill or bruit. Depending on the size and site of the lesion, patients complain of either swelling, pain or a burning sensation. Increased stiffness and pain upon waking in the morning is also a frequent complaint. Distortion of anatomical structures worsens during childhood.

Head and neck VMs are usually unilateral, but bilateral involvement may rarely occur. Due to a mass effect, VMs can cause facial asymmetry and progressive distortion of facial features. Oral VMs typically cause dental malalignment and malocclusion. Intraorbital VMs vary in size depending on head position, and induce enlargement of the orbital cavity. Enophthalmia may occur when the patient is standing, but vision is not altered. A VM involving the orbit can communicate through the spheno-maxillary fissure with a lesion of the deep cheek and infratemporal fossa. Rarely optic nerve compression results from a VM lying near the orbital apex. Mucosal buccal VMs can involve the tongue, cheek, palate and oropharynx, but rarely impair speech. Pharyngeal and laryngeal VMs commonly cause obstructive sleep apnoea syndrome.

A pure VM involving the extremities is uncommon. Upper or lower limb VMs can be distal and may cause enlarged blue fingers or toes with sagging skin, in a segmental pattern. VMs can affect an entire upper or lower limb and adjacent trunk [2]. Many of these lesions are mislabelled in the literature as 'haemangioma' of the bone, intramuscular or synovial 'haemangioma' or 'cavernous haemangioma' [3–5]. These lesions progressively worsen in childhood and adolescence, and phleboliths are present. Because VMs frequently enlarge to involve skin, muscles, joints and bones, there may be increased limb girth. However, VMs rarely cause limb length discrepancy. A VM can be associated with slight limb length

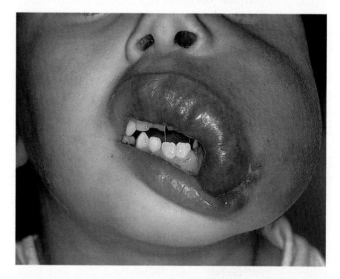

Fig. 18.1.4 VM of the cheek: distortion, swelling, blue colour and open bite.

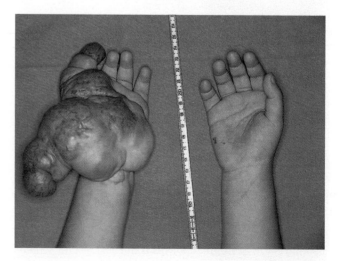

Fig. 18.1.5 Left hand VM involving the first and second fingers and adjacent palm.

undergrowth and affected children may limp; a pure VM does not cause limb overgrowth (as seen in the Klippel–Trenaunay syndrome or KTS). An extremity VM sometimes induces structural weakening of the bony shaft, and pathological fracture can occur with minimal trauma [2]. VM in the synovia of the knee joint causes episodic attacks of joint pain (due to effusion and bleeding) in the absence of an obvious history of trauma. These symptoms begin in childhood and result in intermittent stiffness and difficulty in walking and exercising. For a time, symptoms abate with bedrest. If not treated, synovial knee VMs result in amyotrophy, flexion of the knee and progressive ankylosis of the joint [2]. Upper limb VMs can also involve the joints, and may cause elbow swelling, pain and stiffness [5]. Haemarthrosis is particularly troublesome in children with VM-associated chronic disseminated intravascular coagulation (DIC). This disorder mimics the haemarthrosis seen in haemophiliacs, and leads to degenerative joint disease and destructive bone changes [2].

Blood coagulation profile (fibrinogen, D-dimers, soluble complexes, fibrin split degradation products and clotting factors) should always be obtained in the case of an extensive VM.

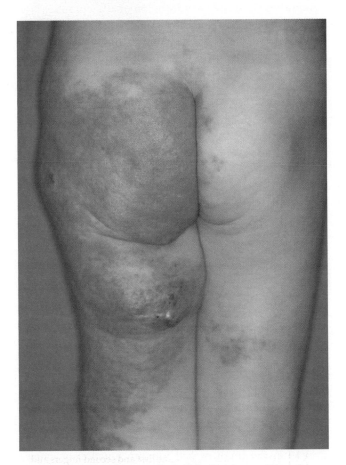

Fig. 18.1.6 Leg VM (skin, muscle and joint involvement) in a girl.

Because VMs are often much more extensive than clinically anticipated, radiological imaging is necessary as follows.

Plain radiography reveals phleboliths, often as early as at the age of 2 or 3 years. These round calcifications are pathognomonic of venous, slow-flow vascular lesions. Plain radiographs also portray bony distortion in facial VMs and bony thinning or periosteal reaction in limb VMs. These reactive periosteal and bony changes can mimic osteoid osteoma [4–6].

Ultrasonography, grey-scale and colour Doppler give information on the angioarchitecture. Most typically, a heterogeneous echogenicity and an ill-defined hypoechoic lacunar pattern are noted; arterial structures are not detected.

CT scans with iodinated contrast detect extension and display skeletal alteration.

MRI, with spin–echo T1- and T2-weighted sequences, is the best non-invasive imaging modality to delineate a VM. On spin–echo T2-weighted sequences, a VM gives a hypersignal brighter than fat. Selective sections in the three planes of space are particularly useful in demonstrating the involved structures. Gadolinium is not routinely used for contrast in the MRI study of a VM. In the case of a knee VM, MRI plus CT provides useful information, and eliminates the need for arthrography before treatment is undertaken.

Digital computed arteriography is not recommended as VMs are poorly visualized.

Phlebography shows the racemose complex of abnormal veins in limb VMs. However, this modality does not precisely demonstrate the anatomical location and size of the lesion, and therefore has limited usefulness in comparison to Doppler plus MRI.

Prognosis

VMs always expand, albeit slowly. They also may have a variety of associated anomalies as follows.

Cerebral developmental venous anomaly (DVA). DVA consists of dilated intramedullary veins converging into a large draining vein. This blood vessel enters either the superficial or the deep system in an area which lacks the normal cerebral draining veins. DVA is an uncommon trajectory of the brain venous drainage and it occurs in 0.05–0.5% of the general population. By contrast, patterns of DVA were found in 20% of 40 patients with extensive head and neck VMs [7]. In contrast to cerebral 'cavernoma' (previously known as 'cryptic' or 'angiographically occult' vascular malformation), opacification of DVA appears in the angiographic venous phase, as do normal veins. DVA, as well as 'cavernoma', can now be clearly imaged using CT and MRI with MRA. In patients with cephalic VMs, DVAs usually consist of ectatic and dilated veins which converge in the drainage system of the deep brain. Unlike true cerebral VMs ('cavernoma'), DVAs are symptom-free in most cases. Even though patients may develop headaches, they do not develop intracerebral haemorrhage, seizures or any neurological deficit. Therefore, DVA must be recognized but not treated. A true cerebral 'cavernoma' can occur in association with a superficial cervicofacial VM and in association with an intracerebral DVA, although very rarely.

Disseminated intravascular coagulopathy. In a child with an extensive VM, especially involving an extremity, a coagulation profile should be obtained [2]. Chronic DIC, characterized by low fibrinogen, elevated D-dimers, soluble complexes, split fibrin degradation products and normal or moderately low platelet count may be observed throughout life. This coagulopathy is completely different from Kasabach–Merritt syndrome (KMs) associated with aggressive vascular tumours of infancy (kaposiform haemangioendothelioma and tufted angioma) but not 'true' common haemangioma [8] (in KMs the platelet count is extremely low, i.e. 10 000/mm³ or less). Unfortunately, most of the DIC plus VM cases are mislabelled in the literature as 'haemangioma' and 'KMs' [9]. DIC worsens during surgical procedures, resulting in increased blood loss, multiple blood transfusions, and postoperative haematoma. A child with VM plus DIC should be treated with heparin during surgical procedures in order to minimize these haemorrhagic complications. This treatment has also proved to be useful in extensive VMs of the limb with recurrent spontaneous painful haematoma or joint bleeding. Slow flow in VM is more likely to cause DIC than thrombosis in the deep veins; pulmonary embolism in VM is extremely rare.

Differential diagnosis

A blue facial VM may be confused with the naevus of Ota. Also, Sinus pericranii, with abnormal cerebral venous drainage from the intracranial area mimics a VM of the middle of the forehead. CT scan of the frontal bone reveals the bony defect. Utilizing direct puncture of the venous lakes in the forehead and catheterization of the ostium, selective opacification of the communication between the sinus pericranii and the sagittal superior sinus is possible.

Dilated veins at the base of the nose are common in newborns. However, marked ectasia of the veins in the frontonasal area is occasionally due to collateral cerebral venous circulation through the cavernous sinus, superior ophthalmic vein, angular vein and facial vein, as a result of an AVM of the vein of Galen. This false VM deflates only after the intracranial lesion has been successfully treated.

In a deep cephalic or limb VM located under normal skin and within muscle, MRI indicates a slow-flow vascular lesion. Biopsy may be necessary to rule out a sarcoma (fibrosarcoma or rhabdomyosarcoma) or a neurofibroma.

In evaluating extremity lesions, it is important to differentiate clearly between a pure VM and a complex–combined vascular malformation such as CVM and CLVM also known as KTS.

Treatment

Selective catheterization of slow-flow lesions is difficult, and, therefore, arterial embolization is very seldom used. The best strategy for treatment of both cutaneous and intramuscular VMs is percutaneous intralesional sclerotherapy [10–14]. Various sclerosants have been used; the most effective are either Ethibloc (a mixture of zein, a corn protein, alcohol, contrast medium and additives) or 100% ethanol. Procedures are performed with real-time fluoroscopic control, and under general anaesthesia with careful monitoring [10–13]. Direct injection of ethanol into a VM can be dangerous, and local compression is used to prevent passage into the systemic circulation. Local complications include blistering, necrosis with scarring, and residual nerve deficit. Severe systemic complication such as renal toxicity, and even cardiac arrest, have been reported [10–13]. With the use of Ethibloc, local complications include inflammatory reaction, aseptic skin necrosis and chronic drainage with eventual scarring. Fever can occur but no severe systemic complications are reported [14]. Sodium tetradecyl or Aetoxisclerol injections are often effective for small VMs, and these are given with either local anaesthesia or without anaesthesia. There are few local side-effects [10].

For cephalic VMs, treatment must begin as soon as deformity and/or functional problems develop. Multiple sessions are required, combining sclerotherapy and surgical procedures. Open bite deformity requires orthodontic management and orthognathic surgical treatment after the secondary teeth have erupted.

Pure VMs involving the extremities often involve the skin, muscles and joints. For extensive VMs, it is impossible to sclerose or remove the entire lesion without damage to function, and marked scarring. Therefore, sclerotherapy and resection should be used to alleviate symptoms [2] rather than as an attempt to eradicate the lesion [3–5]. Elastic stockings provide comfort by reducing the venous pressure, and are indispensable. If an intramuscular VM in the thigh or calf impairs function or causes severe pain, the involved muscle can be excised. With intrasynovial knee VMs, recurrent episodes of haemarthrosis and restriction of joint motion are observed in active children as early as 6–10 years of age. Excision of the VM embedded in the synovia is possible and, after a 3-month period of physical therapy, the child often recovers painless joint mobility and normal function. Subtotal resection can be beneficial in VMs of the hands or feet, particularly in the digits.

Syndromic venous malformation

Maffucci's syndrome

Maffucci's syndrome, first described in 1881, is a combination of VMs and enchondromatosis. Lesions may be either diffuse or localized; some cases are unilateral and/or segmental. Maffucci's syndrome occurs sporadically, and without gender predilection. Lesions begin in infancy and develop throughout childhood and adulthood. Enchondromas, are both metaphyseal and diaphyseal, and are similar to those seen in Ollier's disease [15–17]. The tumours are easily demonstrated on plain radiograph as round or ovoid, well-demarcated radiolucent masses. They result from an abnormal development of cartilage in normal bone. Skeletal deformity and pathological fracture are common. Deformity of the hands is due to both cutaneous and skeletal lesions, but these usually do not occur in close proximity. Secondary dwarfism may develop due to shortening and deformity of long leg bones. The hands are involved in 89% of cases; fingers are involved in 88% of cases and toes in 61%, whereas the long bones of the limbs are involved in 30–40% of cases. Cranial and pelvic bones are rarely affected. Craniofacial lesions can be associated with various neurological defects and with ocular complications (e.g. proptosis secondary to tumours in the orbit). The incidence of malignant transformation in enchondromatosis may be as high as 30% [17]. Any painful enchondroma must be biopsied to rule out enchondrosarcoma.

VMs in Maffucci's syndrome consist of blue or red–blue, exophytic nodules, which can be emptied by manual compression. These lesions are similar to those seen in Bean's syndrome. Phleboliths are common. Cutaneous and bony lesions are both present at birth in 27% of cases [17]. The occurrence of a benign vascular tumour, a spindle cell haemangioendothelioma, was recently demonstrated in cutaneous blue nodules of Maffucci's syndrome [18]. A neural abnormality of the neuropeptidergic nervous system may be the cause of both the abnormal stimulation of growth and the tumour formation [19].

Familial glomangiomatosis

This relatively common syndrome, first described by Bailey is inherited in autosomal dominant fashion [20,21].

It consists of multiple, deep-blue, nodular dermal vascular lesions, isolated or grouped in a plaque-like distribution, occurring anywhere on the cutaneous surface. The lesions, which develop in childhood and adolescence, sometimes become tender, particularly with cold or manual compression. Within an affected family, some individuals have very few lesions and others exhibit hundreds [22–24]. Brachymetacarpia (of the fifth and fourth finger), also an autosomal dominant trait, can be an associated finding [24]. Arteriography in these lesions is always normal and therefore need not be performed. Venograms obtained by direct contrast injection indicate a well-demarcated dermal vascular anomaly; draining veins are not usually seen [24]. Histologically, these lesions differ from typical VMs by the presence of clusters of glomus cells lining endothelium-lined vascular spaces [23]. Ultrastructurally, these cells are smooth muscle cells; nonmyelinated nerve fibres are seen in close contact [22].

Blue rubber bleb naevus syndrome of Bean

Blue rubber bleb naevus syndrome was named by Bean in 1958. In this syndrome, VMs are both cutaneous and visceral. Familial examples (with autosomal dominant inheritance) are rare. Cutaneous lesions consist of blue soft nodules, which may or may not be painful. Occasionally, lesions aggregate in polylobular cutaneous blue masses (described as 'cavernous'). There are also small, colourless, dome-shaped, nipple-like lesions ('rubber bleb').

Visceral vascular anomalies predominantly affect the gastrointestinal (GI) system. They can be sessile (submucosal) or polypoid, and are best visualized by endoscopy. Vascular anomalies are found in the entire GI tract (oesophagus, stomach, small and large bowel), and also in the mesentery. These lesions may cause recurrent intestinal bleeding, and patients may require iron replacement therapy and blood transfusion to control anaemia. Other visceral locations include the oral cavity, nasopharynx, anus, genitalia, bladder, brain, spinal cord, liver, spleen, lungs, bones and skeletal muscles [25–40]. Clinically, in a given family, some individuals have only cutaneous lesions while others have both cutaneous and visceral anomalies. Histologically, in most specimens there is a network of large vascular lakes lined with a flat endothelium, and glomus cells are absent [39]. Vascular lesions in skin are treated using sclerotherapy, excision, cryosurgery or neodymium:yttrium–aluminium–garnet (Nd:YAG) laser photocoagulation, with scarring. Enteric lesions, when bleeding, require either endoscopic Nd:YAG laser photocoagulation or surgical resection [31–41].

Familial, multiple, cutaneous and mucosal venous malformations

This autosomal dominant syndrome is characterized by

multiple, small, dome-shaped VMs; larger anomalies also occur. The cutaneous lesions are similar to those seen in Bean's syndrome, but there is no GI involvement. The locus for this syndrome, in a three-generational family (15 out the 30 members examined were affected) maps to chromosome 9p [1].

Familial 'cavernous angiomatosis' of the brain

The disorder is characterized by multiple brain and occasional retinal VMs. Patients are at risk for intracranial haemorrhage. Other manifestations include VM in the skin and viscera, and a transverse limb defect. The gene for this familial autosomal dominant VM maps to the q11–q22 region of chromosome 7 [42,43].

REFERENCES

1 Vikkula M, Boon LM, Carraway KL *et al.* Vascular dysmorphogenesis caused by an activating mutation in the receptor tyrosine kinase TIE2. *Cell* 1996; 87: 1181–90.

2 Enjolras O, Ciabrini D, Mazoyer E *et al.* Extensive pure venous malformations in the upper and lower limbs. *J Am Acad Dermatol* 1997; 36: 219–25.

3 Loefgren EP, Loefgren KA. Surgical treatment of cavernous hemangioma. *Surgery* 1985; 97: 474–80.

4 Loxley SS, Thiemeyer JS, Ellsasser JC. Periosteal hemangioma. *Clin Orthop Rel Res* 1972; 85: 151–4.

5 Milner RH, Sykes PJ. Diffuse cavernous hemangiomas of the upper limb. *J Hand Surg* 1987; 12b: 199–202.

6 Schajowicz F, Rebecchini AC, Bosc-Mayol G. Intracortical hemangioma simulating osteoid osteoma. *J Bone Joint Surg (Br)* 1979; 61b: 94–5.

7 Boukobza M, Enjolras O, Guichard JP *et al.* Cerebral developmental venous anomalies associated with head-and-neck venous malformations. *Am J Neuroradiol* 1996; 17: 987–94.

8 Enjolras O, Wassef M, Mazoyer E *et al.* Infants with Kasabach–Merritt syndrome do not have 'true' hemangioma. *J Pediatr* 1997; 130: 631–40.

9 Hoeger PH, Helmke K, Winkler K. Chronic consumption coagulopathy due to occult splenic haemangioma: Kasabach–Merritt syndrome. *Eur J Pediatr* 1995; 154: 365–8.

10 Burrows PE, Fellows KE. Techniques for management of pediatric vascular anomalies. In: Cope C, ed. *Current Techniques in Interventional Radiology*, Vol. 2, 2nd edn. Philadelphia: Current Medicine, 1995: 12–27.

11 Riché MC, Hadjean E, Tran Ba Huy P, Merland JJ. The treatment of capillary–venous malformations using a new fibrosing agent. *Plast Reconstr Surg* 1983; 71: 607–12.

12 Dubois J, Sebag G, De Prost *et al.* Soft tissue venous malformations in children—percutaneous sclerotherapy with Ethibloc. *Radiology* 1991; 180: 195–8.

13 Yakes WF. Diagnosis and management of venous malformations. In: Salvader SJ, Trerotola SO, eds. *Venous Interventional Radiology with Clinical Perspectives*. New York: Thieme Medical, 1996: 139–50.

14 Herbreteau D, Riché MC, Enjolras O *et al.* Les malformations vasculaires veineuses et leur traitement par Ethibloc. *J Mal Vasc (Paris)* 1992; 17: 50–3.

15 Loewinger RJ, Liechtenstein JR, Dodson WE, Zeisen AZ. Maffucci's syndrome: a mesenchymal dysplasia and multiple tumour syndrome. *Br J Dermatol* 1981; 105: 331–6.

16 Johnson TE, Nasr AM, Nalbandian RM. Enchondromatosis and hemangioma (Maffucci's syndrome) with orbital involvement. *Am J Ophthalmol* 1990; 110: 153–9.

17 Kaplan RP, Wang JT, Amron DM, Kaplan L. Maffucci's syndrome: two case reports with a literature review. *J Am Acad Dermatol* 1993; 29: 894–9.

18 Enjolras O, Wassef M, Merland JJ. Syndrome de Maffucci: une fausse malformation veineuse? A propos d'un cas avec hémangioendothéliome à cellules fusiformes. *Ann Dermatol Vénéréol* 1998; 125: 512–15.

19 Robinson D, Tieder M, Halperin, Burshtein D, Nevo Z. Maffucci's syndrome, the result of neural abnormalitis. *Cancer* 1994; 74: 949–57.

20 André JM. La glomangiomatose de Bailey. In: *Les Dysplasies Vasculaires Systématisées*. Paris: Expansion Scientifique Française, 1973: 105–9.

21 Rudolph R. Familial multiple glomangiomatosis. *Ann Plast Surg* 1993; 30: 183–5.

22 Goodman TF, Abele DC. Multiple glomus tumours: a clinical and electron microscopy study. *Arch Dermatol* 1971; 103: 11–23.

23 Requena L, Sangueza OP. Cutaneous vascular proliferations. 2. Hyperplasias and benign neoplasms. *J Am Acad Dermatol* 1997; 37: 887–920.

24 Niechajev I. Multiple glomus tumors, special reference to radiological findings. *Scand J Plast Reconstr Surg* 1982; 16: 183–90.

25 Munkvad M. Blue rubber bleb nevus syndrome. *Dermatologica* 1983; 167: 307–9.

26 Wong SH, Lau WY. Blue rubber bleb nevus syndrome. *Dis Colon Rectum* 1982; 25: 371–4.

27 Freitzin DF, Potter B. Blue rubber bleb nevus. *Arch Dermatol* 1965; 116: 924–9.

28 Rice JS, Fischer DS. Blue rubber bleb nevus. *Arch Dermatol* 1962; 86: 503–11.

29 Belsheim MR, Sullivan SS. Blue rubber bleb nevus syndrome. *Canad J Surg* 1980; 23: 274–5.

30 Goraya JS, Marwaha KK, Vatve M *et al.* Blue rubber bleb nevus syndrome—a cause for recurrent episodic severe anemia. *Pediatr Hematol Oncol* 1998; 15: 261–4.

31 Morris L, Lynch PM, Gleason WA, Schauder C, Pinkel D, Duvic M. Blue rubber bleb nevus syndrome: laser photocoagulation of colonic hemangiomas in a child with microcytic anemia. *Pediatr Dermatol* 1992; 9: 91–4.

32 Sandhu KS, Cohen H, Radin R, Buck FS. Blue rubber bleb nevus syndrome presenting recurrences. *Dig Dis Sci* 1987; 32: 214–19.

33 Pasaboc LG, Gibbs PM, Kwan W. Blue rubber bleb nevus syndrome in the foot. *J Foot Ankle Surg* 1994; 33: 271–3.

34 Garen PD, Sahn EE. Spinal cord compression in blue rubber bleb nevus syndrome. *Arch Dermatol* 1994; 130: 934–5.

35 Radke M, Waldschmidt J, Stolpe HJ, Mix M, Richter I. Blue rubber bleb nevus syndrome with predominant urinary bladder hemangiomatosis. *Eur J Pediatr Surg* 1993; 3: 313–16.

36 Paules S, Baack B, Levisohn D. Tender bluish papules on the trunk and extremities, blue rubber bleb nevus syndrome. *Arch Dermatol* 1993; 129: 1505–9.

37 Busund B, Stray-Pedersen S, Iversen O, Austad J. Blue rubber bleb nevus syndrome with manifestations in the vulva. *Acta Obstet Gynecol Scand* 1993; 72: 310–3.

38 Radke M, Waldschmidt J, Stolpe HJ *et al.* Blue rubber bleb nevus syndrome with predominant urinary bladder hemangiomatosis. *Eur J Pediatr Surg* 1993; 3: 313–6.

39 Jumbou O, Bureau B, Fleischmann, Stalder JF. Blue rubber bleb naevus. *Ann Dermatol Vénéréol* 1993; 120: 241–3.

40 Olsen TG, Milroy SK, Goldman L, Fidler JP. Laser surgery for blue rubber bleb nevus. *Arch Dermatol* 1979; 115: 81–2.

41 Oranje AP. Blue rubber bleb nevus syndrome. *Pediatr Dermatol* 1986; 3: 304–10.

42 Filling-Katz M, Levin SW, Patronas NJ, Katz NNK. Terminal transverse limb defects associated with familial cavernous angiomatosis. *Am J Med Genet* 1992; 42: 346–51.

43 Dubovsky J, Zabramski JM, Kurth J *et al.* A gene responsible for cavernous malformations of the brain maps to chromosome 7q. *Hum Molec Genet* 1995; 4: 453–8.

Lymphatic malformation

Definition

LM consists of vesicles or pouches filled with lymphatic fluid. There are microcystic tissular LMs, macrocystic LMs and combined forms. LMs never regress. They can expand in the presence of inflammation or intralesional bleeding. Most LMs present during infancy or childhood. Ultrasonography detects intrauterine macrocystic LMs as early as the late first or second trimester of pregnancy [1].

Pathology

Microcystic LMs consist of dilated endothelium-lined, thin-walled and usually bloodless lymph capillaries and spaces. These vessels fill the dermis, and are sometimes intermingled with lymphocytes. Nodular collections of lymphocytes are often seen in the surrounding connective stroma. Occasionally, a dilated lymphatic vessel enlarges a dermal papilla, creating a vesicle. Blood within the anomalous spaces indicates either recent haemorrhage or a combined LVM. Mural thrombi may occur.

In macrocystic LMs, large cisterns do not communicate directly with the general lymphatic system, representing a sequestration phenomenon. The vessel walls are of variable thickness, with both striated and smooth muscle elements.

In combined macromicrocystic LMs, abnormal lymphatics connect deep muscular cisterns to the superficial dermis in a complex meandering network of anastomoses [2]. On electron microscopy, the basement membranes are found to be either fragmented or well formed [3].

Clinical features

Microcystic LM ('lymphangioma circumscriptum') is a plaque-like lesion involving skin and/or mucosal membranes. Clear and colourless, or blood-filled dark-red vesicles overlie an area of diffuse swelling; other lesions may present with intermittent red–brown dermal infiltration, flat-topped papules or slight hypertrichosis. Recurrent cellulitis and spontaneous ecchymoses are common.

Macrocystic LM ('cystic hygroma') is comprised of large cysts. These are visible as soft multilobular masses with slight blue discoloration of the skin. Macrocystic LMs can suddenly enlarge in response to nose, throat or dental infection, or to intracystic bleeding. When clinical diagnosis is equivocal, the following techniques may be employed: ultrasonography (cysts appear either anechoic or hypoechoic and homogeneous), CT (cysts are hypodense), MRI (cystic spaces are hypointense on T1-sequence, give hypersignal on T2 and show blood-filled levels if there is intracystic bleeding), direct puncture (clear liquid is recovered) and contrast injection.

Prognosis

An LM can be either a localized lesion, or it can involve a large area of skin, mucous membranes and viscera, causing significant complications [4–6]. LMs in the cheek, forehead and orbit are frequently both microcystic and macrocystic; they cause facial asymmetry and distortion of facial features. Bone overgrowth can occur, most commonly in the mandibular body, manifesting as class III malocclusion [7]. Eyelid and intraorbital LMs produce orbital enlargement, ocular dystopia, exophthalmia, occlusion of the visual axis and amblyopia [5,6]; sudden orbital proptosis and possible visual loss can result from bleeding within cysts. Bulky tongue LMs impair speech, and patients with such lesions develop swelling of the tongue with infection, bleeding and aggressive caries [7]. In the cervicofacial region, an extensive macromicrocystic LM can result in airway obstruction, sometimes necessitating tracheostomy. Cervical and axillary LM can invade the thorax, causing recurrent pleural and pericardial effu-

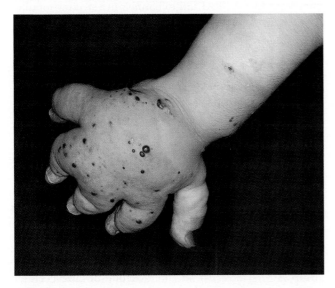

Fig. 18.1.7 Microcystic LM of the hand, with haemorrhagic lymphatic vesicles.

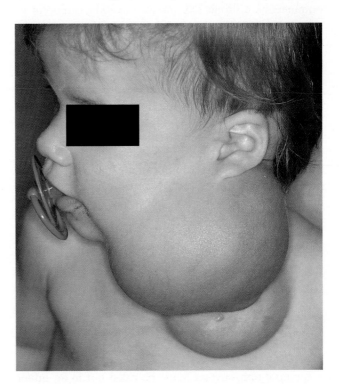

Fig. 18.1.8 Macrocystic cervical LM with acute inflammation.

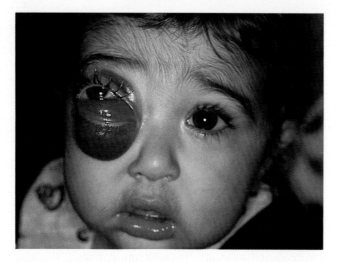

Fig. 18.1.9 Proptosis due to acute bleeding within an orbital LM.

sion. These may be lethal. Extensive limb LM is often associated with lymphoedema. The child experiences periodic cutaneous lymphorrhoea and chylous oozing. Very extensive forms may cause elephantiastic deformity of the limb. Skeletal changes, distortion and hypertrophy are common features in limb LM. The child with diffuse LM involving soft tissues and bones can present with sepsis unresponsive to antibiotics. Pelvic LM manifests with vulvar lymphangiectasias and vaginal chylous discharge, even before puberty. Abdominal LM with involvement of the gut may cause a protein-losing enteropathy and hypoalbuminaemia. Chronic DIC, as seen in VMs, can occur in some patients with extensive LMs.

Vanishing bone disease, also known as Gorham's syndrome or phantom bone syndrome, is an extensive progressive and spontaneous osteolytic process which is sometimes lethal. Capillaries and lymphatic clefts occupy the site of vanished bones and fibrosis replaces the bone. The disease demineralizes and destroys bones [8]. Radiographically, there is radiolucency of the affected bones and a 'licked stick of candy' appearance [9]. Depending on the location of lesions, complications may include bone pain, muscular atrophy, fractures, pleural effusion, ascites and cerebrospinal fluid rhinorrhoea. Gorham's syndrome causes death in 16% of cases. Phantom bone disorder in association with severe, chronic DIC and bleeding is reported [10].

Differential diagnosis

Any mass under normal skin in an infant can be an LM. The differential diagnosis includes deep haemangioma, teratoma, VM or, in the midline of the face, encephalocele.

Infantile fibrosarcoma must be ruled out in an infant with a bulky mass under normal skin, particularly in the chest, shoulder or cervical areas. These lesions of soft consistency, transillumination and multicystic appearance on CT or MRI, may mimic LM. One-third of these tumours are present at birth; they can grow to considerable size and metastasize [11].

Infantile rhabdomyosarcoma may present as an infiltrated pink or red plaque with firm pseudovesicles. These lesions, especially when on the face, may mimic microcystic LM, although different on palpation, and rapidly growing after birth.

Kimura's disease infiltrating the parotid and submaxillary gland under normal skin can be mistaken for macrocystic LM. These lesions can vary in volume, due to the high content of blood vessels and lymphatic clefts.

Microcystic lymphatic malformation, infiltrating large areas of skin with occasional bleeding, mimics the bruises of the Gardner–Diamond syndrome.

Benign lymphangioendothelioma is a rare benign vascular tumour occurring in the extremities or trunk. It sometimes appears in childhood, and may resemble lymphatic microcystic LM clinically, and low-grade angiosarcoma histologically [12].

Acral microcystic LM with haematic vesicles must be differentiated from APACHE syndrome (acral pseudolymphomatous angiokeratoma of children). This disorder is characterized by acquired, persistent painless, vascular papules. These lesions are unilateral and occur on distal regions of the foot or hand [13]. Histological findings are hyperkeratosis, dense dermal lymphohistiocystic infiltrate and prominent thick-walled blood vessels.

Sinusoidal 'haemangioma' is a misnomer for a dermal vascular anomaly occurring in childhood [14]. It presents clinically either as firm nodules or plaques mimicking LM. Histopathologically, it consists of interconnected, thin-lined, blood-filled, large channels in a striking lobular architecture, sometimes with pseudopapillary pattern.

Treatment

Sudden enlargement of an LM is usually the result of intralesional bleeding or cellulitis. Pain medication for the former, and antibiotics and anti-inflammatory drugs for the latter, are required. Bacterial infection within an LM may necessitate intravenous administration of antibiotics; rarely is incision and drainage of an abcess necessary.

Large cysts can be treated with aspiration of the lymphatic fluid, followed by percutaneous, image-guided, intralesional injection of sclerofibrosing agents. A number of substances have been used to shrink cysts, including Ethibloc, pure ethanol, bleomycin, dextrose, sodium morrhuate, sodium tetradecyl, OK-432 (a killed strain of group A *Streptococcus*) and tetracycline or doxycycline. Persistence is frequent [15–17].

Surgical resection of the LM offers potential cure.

Anatomical restrictions and difficulty in clearly separating normal from involved tissues can result in unsatisfactory outcome, with either incomplete excision or sacrifice of normal structures. The preferred surgical strategy is to extirpate the LM in a single region at one operation. Staged excisions or cutaneous expansion are necessary for extensive lesions.

Nd: YAG laser photocoagulation, with or without continuous ice-cube surface cooling, or interstitial Nd: YAG laser photocoagulation have been employed in the treatment of microcystic LM.

A favourable response to intravenous treatment with cyclophosphamide was reported in four children with life-threatening, unresectable, cervicofacial LM with airway and oesophageal compromise [18]. However, these results require confirmation.

In extensive LM with lymphoedema in the limbs, treatment with a pneumatic compression device, compressive bandaging and adapted elastic support stockings, may be helpful.

REFERENCES

1 Langer JC, Fitzgerald PG, Desa D *et al*. Cervicofacial cystic hygroma in the fetus, clinical spectrum and outcome. *J Pediatr Surg* 1990; 25: 58–62.
2 Whimster IW. The pathology of lymphangioma circumscriptum. *Br J Dermatol* 1976; 94: 473–86.
3 Kosek JC, Smolder BR, Egbert BM. Benign lymphangioendothelioma. *J Am Acad Dermatol* 1994; 31: 362–8.
4 Boyd JB, Mulliken JB, Kaban LB, Upton J, Murray JE. Skeletal changes associated with vascular malformations. *Plast Reconstr Surg* 1984; 74: 789–95.
5 Harris GJ, Sakol PJ, Bonavolonta G, De Concilis C. An analysis of 30 cases of orbital lymphangioma. *Ophthalmology* 1990; 97: 1583–92.
6 Gimeno-Aranguez M, Colomar Palmer P, Gonzalez Mediero I *et al*. Aspectos clinicos y morfologicos de los linfangiomas infantiles—revision de 145 casos. *An Esp Pediatr* 1996; 45: 25–8.
7 Padwa BL, Hayward PG, Ferraro NF, Mulliken JB. Cervicofacial lymphatic malformation: clinical course, surgical intervention, and pathogenesis of skeletal hypertrophy. *Plast Reconstr Surg* 1995; 95: 951–60.
8 Gorham LW, Stout AP. Massive osteolysis (acute spontaneous absorption of bone, phantom bone, disappearing bone). *J Bone Joint Surg* 1955; 37A: 985–1003.
9 Velez A, Ruiz-Maldonado R. Gorham's syndrome. *Int J Dermatol* 1993; 32: 884–7.
10 Lauret Ph, Monconduit M, Solnica J. Lymphangiomatose cutanée et osseuse disséminée avec coagulation intravasculaire disséminée. *Ann Dermatol Vénéréol* 1978; 105: 759–63.
11 Hayward PG, Orgill DP, Mulliken JB, Perez-Atayde AR. Congenital fibrosarcoma masquerading as lymphatic malformation: report of two cases. *J Pediatr Surg* 1995; 30: 84–8.
12 Wilson-Jones E, Winkelmann RK, Zachary CB, Reda AM. Benign lymphangioendothelioma. *J Am Acad Dermatol* 1990; 23: 229–35.
13 Kaddu S, Cerroni L, Pilatti A, Soyer HP, Kerl H. Acral pseudolymphomatous angiokeratoma. *Am J Dermatopathol* 1994; 16: 130–3.
14 Calonje E, Fletcher CDM. Sinusoidal hemangioma. *Am J Dermatopathol* 1991; 15: 1130–5.
15 Molitch HI, Unger EC, Witte CL, Van Sonnenberg E. Percutaneous sclerotherapy of lymphangiomas. *Radiology* 1995; 194: 343–7.
16 Ogita S, Tsuto T, Deguchi E, Tokiwa K, Nagashima M, Iwai N. OK-432 therapy for unresectable lymphangiomas in children. *J Pediatr Surg* 1991; 26: 263–70.
17 Dubois J, Garel L, Abela A *et al*. Lymphangiomas in children: percutaneous sclerotherapy with an alcoholic solution of zein. *Radiology* 1997; 204: 651–4.
18 Turner C, Gross S. Treatment of recurrent suprahyoid cervicofacial lymphangioma with intravenous cyclophosphamide. *Am J Pediatr Hematol Oncol* 1994; 16: 325–8.

Capillary malformation

Localized or extensive port-wine stain

Definition

A PWS is a macular CM that is present at birth and persists throughout life. In most cases, PWS is a cosmetic problem. However, it can also be an indicator of a more complex syndrome.

Pathology

PWS is comprised of regular, ectatic, thin-walled capillary to venular sized channels, located in the papillary and upper reticular dermis. In adults, fibrosis around vessels and progressive vascular dilatation develop.

Clinical features

PWS is a clinical diagnosis. It cannot be documented by arteriography or MRI. PWS may be localized or extensive, and may occur on the face, trunk or limbs. Facial PWS involves one or more of the three trigeminal areas (V1, V2, V3), and may be unilateral or bilateral. A PWS located on an extremity can remain unchanged and isolated throughout life, or it can be the first sign of a complex–combined vascular malformation. PWS can present in a scattered distribution over the entire body, or in a livedoid pattern. The lesions very rarely follow the lines of Blaschko. Areas of 'naevus anaemicus', comprised of vessels with dominant α-adrenergic tone, may be intermingled with PWS [1].

Prognosis

PWS usually grows in proportion to the rest of the body. The lesions are bright red at birth. During the first weeks they fade slightly, and then stabilize. Facial PWSs are prone to hyperplastic skin changes. Thickened skin, purple nodules and pyogenic granulomas begin to develop by adolescence. The hyperplastic lesions may sometimes mimic AVM. For unknown reasons, hyperplastic changes very rarely occur in extremity PWS. Facial PWSs are sometimes associated with progressive hyperplasia of soft and hard tissues. Lips and gums enlarge in areas of vascular staining. Peridontopathy, bleeding and dental hygiene problems are common. Overgrowth of the maxilla or mandible leads to skeletal asymmetry, occlusal tilt and open bite. Increased limb girth can present at birth in children with an extensive limb PWS; this asymmetry is stable and, unlike KTS, persists without progression until the child is fully grown. When the child has atopic dermatitis, psoriasis or acne, lesions may be worse in the area of PWS.

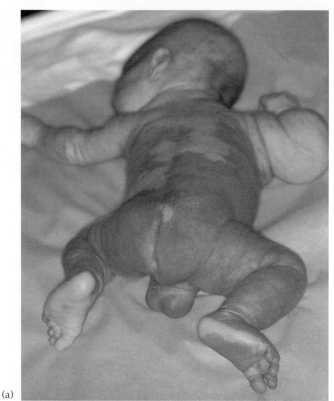

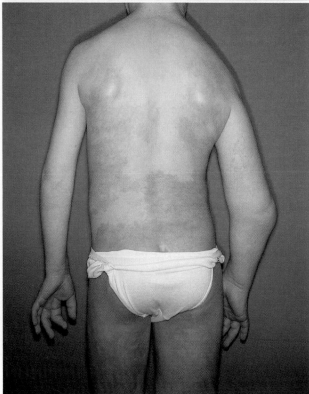

(a)

(b)

Fig. 18.1.10 (a,b) Same boy at birth and aged 8 years: the CM faded; the congenital right-sided hypertrophy (with CM in the leg, and without CM in the arm) did not worsen.

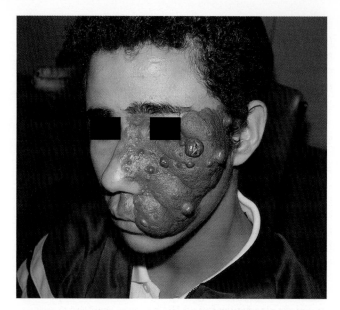

Fig. 18.1.11 V2 facial CM with hyperplastic skin changes mimicking AVM, in a 13-year-old boy.

Differential diagnosis

PWS must be differentiated in an infant from a salmon patch (also known as naevus flammeus neonatorum, naevus of Unna, 'stork bite' for the nuchal site and 'angel kiss' for the forehead). These occur in about half of neonates and may be seen in the nape of the neck, glabella, eyelid, nose and upper lip. These macules are usually more irregular and more discrete than PWS; they tend to fade completely in the facial region, and to persist in the occipital skin [2].

In childhood, AVM often mimics PWS. If there is concern about the possibility of AVM, Doppler evaluation is mandatory.

Tufted angioma (also known as angioblastoma of Nakagawa, or progressive capillary 'haemangioma') is an uncommon benign cutaneous vascular tumour [3–5] appearing most often during childhood. It is rarely present at birth [6]. This lesion grows slowly and then stabilizes. A wide area of skin may be involved. Tufted angiomas are tender, red, purple or brownish patches or indurated plaques, and are sometimes studded with red papules. The neck, upper chest and shoulders are the most frequent sites. Sclerosing tufted angioma on the lower limbs may exhibit a severe infiltrating course [6]. Histologically, this lesion is comprised of focal dermal collections of tightly packed capillaries, pericytes and endothelial cells, in a haphazard 'cannonball' distribution. There are glomerulus-like tufts and large irregular, blood-less endothelial-lined vascular clefts. A proliferation of eccrine glands is present in some of these lesions, and the overlying skin may sweat excessively when exposed to a warm environment [6]. These lesions must then be differentiated from eccrine angiomatous hamartomas, which present as erythematous plaques, or nodules under irregularly stained or hyperpigmented skin. These lesions may be associated with localized hypertrichosis and intermittent hyperhidrosis, and usually occur on the distal extremitiy [7].

Treatment

The preferred treatment of PWS in infancy and childhood is the pulsed dye laser. Because PWS enlarges in proportion to the growth of the child, laser therapy should be initiated as soon as possible. Younger children require fewer laser sessions, and may generally respond better to treatment [8]. Laser therapy is more effective in lesions on the face and trunk, than in those involving an extremity.

A successful result is defined as fading of the PWS, with little or no textural change. In a comparative study [9], the pulsed dye laser was found to be superior to the continuous wave dye laser with the Hexascan robotized device in 45% of patients (with less hyper- or hypopigmentation), whereas the continuous wave tunable dye laser was considered superior in 15%. There was no appreciable difference in the remaining 40% of patients.

Soft tissue hypertrophy does not respond to laser, and surgical correction may be necessary. Excision of the involved area must follow facial aesthetic units. Skin grafting rarely provides identical colour and texture of skin, and a border effect is frequently noticeable. Contour resection for labial hypertrophy may be helpful.

Orthodontic management for correction of the open bite is often required. Orthognathic surgical correction is performed at completion of skeletal growth. Careful dental care and mouth hygiene are important in cases of gingival involvement. If an epulis develops, electrodessication is curative.

Syndromic port-wine stain

Sturge–Weber syndrome

Definition, pathogenesis and aetiology. Sturge–Weber syndrome (SWS) is characterized by ocular anomalies, pial vascular malformations, and ipsilateral facial PWS. This constellation of findings reflects the common embryogenic origins, within the anterior neural primordium, of the frontopalpebronasal dermis (V1 area), the ocular choroid and the pia mater [10,11]. Recent studies of cranial morphogenesis indicate that any quantitative or qualitative anomaly in the phenotypic expression of cephalic neural crest derivatives, in a given facial region, can be a marker for an associated anomaly in the level of the brain from which they arise. Thus, a child with V1 PWS is at risk for SWS, the presumed cause being a somatic mutation in a common precursor cell on the anterior neural primordium [11].

Clinical features. Children with SWS may have extensive PWS, but always show clinical involvement of V1 [10]. A pial vascular anomaly, typical of SWS, can rarely occur in the absence of facial PWS.

In the presence of leptomeningeal involvement, patients may develop contralateral seizures, neurological deficits and hemiparesis or hemiplegia. These neurological complications are usually seen before the age of 2 years, and develop in about 20% of infants with V1 PWS. In addition, children with SWS often have delayed developmental milestones [12].

Patient with SWS may develop an increase in the ipsilateral choroidal vascularity, and glaucoma. Retinal detachment and blindness are additional complications.

SWS in an infant can be considered a near-medical emergency. Prompt pharmacological treatment of epilepsy prevents brain hypoxia and the resultant neuronal death and psychomotor deterioration.

Management. Ophthalmological examination (visual evaluation, fundoscopic examination and eye pressure measurement) must be done twice a year until puberty.

As soon as possible, the infant with V1 PWS must have a CT scan with iodinated contrast, or an MRI. MRI with T1-weighted sequences and gadolinium injection will detect a leptomeningeal vascular anomaly ipsilateral to the V1 PWS. Typically, but not in all cases, the leptomeningeal vascular anomaly is located in the occipital brain, and there is an asymmetrically enlarged ipsilateral choroid plexus. In infants younger than 6 months, accelerated myelination of the abnormal hemisphere may occur [13].

In advanced SWS, CT scan reveals focal cerebral atrophy and dense calcifications moulding the convolutions [14]. Single photon emission computed tomography (SPECT), which determines regional cerebral blood flow, and positron emission tomography (PET), which determines local cerebral glucose metabolism, are useful tools for monitoring the activity of central nervous system (CNS) disease. Local decreased cerebral blood flow and decreased cerebral glucose metabolism both correlate with anatomical involvement as seen on CT or MRI [15–17].

Treatment. Pharmacological treatment will minimize and prevent seizures and control glaucoma [17]. Pulsed dye laser therapy for the PWS is possible after control of seizure activity. Surgical treatment may be necessary for severe glaucoma. Hemispherectomy or callosotomy can stop progression of motor and psychomotor deterioration in children with seizures who are unresponsive to pharmacological treatment [18]. Management of labial and gingival hypertrophy and occlusal anomalies may be indicated.

Port-wine stains in complex–combined vascular malformations with progressive limb overgrowth

Definition, pathogenesis and aetiology. Eponyms have been used for many of the combined anomalies. These names should probably be abandoned because they are meaningless, misleading and do not indicate pathogenesis. A nosology based on flow characteristics and dysmorphic vascular channel types allows a more logical approach to diagnosis and management.

Slow-flow complex–combined type includes CVM and CLVM. These correspond to the popular eponym of Klippel-Trenauney syndrome (KTS). The multiple CMs that occur in this syndrome are most often located on the anterior-lateral aspect of the thigh, in a geographic pattern. Lymphatic vesicles, clear or haemorrhagic, may be present on the surface, and pulsations and bruit are absent. The involved vessels show evidence of inadequate venous return.

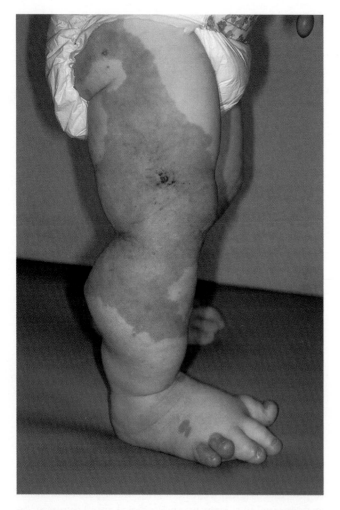

Fig. 18.1.12 Complex–combined vascular malformation (CLVM) of the lower limb.

Histologically, the anomalous veins have deformed, insufficient or absent valves. Venous fibromuscular dysplasia is the most consistent mural finding [19]. Limb bone overgrowth was originally suspected to be a consequence of venous stasis and venous hypertension, due to an anomalous deep venous system (e.g. agenesis, aplasia or duplication) [20,21]. However, in animal models, venous stasis does not affect longitudinal bone growth [22]. An alternate hypothesis suggests that an inborn mesodermal defect in early embryonic development causes the concomitant vascular anomalies and limb overgrowth [23]. Some of the veins (lateral marginal vein in the thigh) might represent persistent embryonic veins [24]. Based on family studies, multifactorial inheritance has been suggested [25]. In the case of monozygotic twins, only one twin in a pair is affected by either extensive CM, KTS or SWS. This observation is most consistent with a somatic mutation in early embryonic development.

High-flow complex–combined types include CAVM and CAVLM. These infrequent vascular anomalies probably correspond to the eponym Parkes–Weber syndrome. Cutaneous warmth, bruit and thrill are always present. There are usually numerous AV fistulas along the affected limb, particularly near the joints. In early childhood, however, arteriography may show only diffuse hypervascularity of the limb. In these patients, AV fistulas become obvious later in life. Bone overgrowth may result from the effect of AV shunting on the osteogenic function of osteoblasts [26].

Clinical features. Both slow-flow and fast-flow complex–combined vascular malformations occurring in limbs are characterized by CMs, dilated veins, occasional lymphangiectases and increased limb girth and limb length. All extremities may be involved, and truncal involvement also occurs.

Management. The child with either slow-flow or fast-flow complex–combined vascular malformations in a limb should be evaluated annually. Leg length should be evaluated clinically during infancy. After the age of 2 years, leg length is measured radiologically and, if abnormal, this study is repeated yearly. A shoe-lift is provided if a leg length discrepancy is over 1.5 cm. Ultrasonography, grey-scale and colour Doppler evaluation of limb arterial and venous vessels should be performed when the child is 3 or 4 years old. Simple radiographs will detect skeletal changes [27]. Arteriography is only necessary in cases where AVFs are suspected (Parkes–Weber syndrome). Phlebography may be indicated in the CVM or CLVM type (KTS). This study is used to define the incompetent venous system and document the deep venous system before embarking on surgical removal of superficial varicose veins (marginal vein) [26–28]. There are no indications for lymphography. In contrast to the findings in patients with pure extremity VMs, muscles and joints are rarely involved. However, MRI and MRA are sometimes useful to detect arterial feeders or draining veins penetrating muscles and bones.

Prognosis. The outlook in these syndromes depends on the type, extent and severity of the complex vascular anomalies, and on the bulk of the associated overgrowth. In teenagers with multiple AVFs (Parkes–Weber syndrome), the disorder may prevent normal function and may even be life-threatening. Complications include limb overgrowth, lytic bony lesions, pathological fractures, painful skin ulceration, distal pseudokaposi skin changes, high cardiac output and congestive heart failure. Children with extensive CVM and CLVM of the limbs and trunk (KTS) may have associated vascular abnormalities in the abdomen or chest, causing haematuria, intestinal bleeding, protein-losing enteropathy or haemothorax.

Differential diagnosis. These syndromes differ from pure limb VM, extensive CM with congenital limb hypertrophy and Maffucci's syndrome in the unilateral segmental form.

CVLM can be part of Proteus syndrome, or associated with SWS [21] or phacomatosis pigmentovascularis.

Treatment. Management is fundamentally conservative. Elastic compression stockings provide relief of pain due to venous engorgement. They are recommended only when grey-scale and colour Doppler evaluation have confirmed the adequate function of deep veins. Compressive bandaging and stockings and frequent massage minimize lymphoedema. Varicose veins, when severe, may be surgically treated during childhood. In correcting the haemodynamic disturbances, treatment must be individualized. Multiple procedures, performed properly by a skillful and experienced vascular surgeon, are needed in order to obtain satisfactory and lasting results [28].

In gross limb hypertrophy, staged surgical contour resection may be considered. However, these extensive procedures, albeit successful in the short term, often cause severe fibrosis and pedal lymphoedema [29]. In rare instances, amputation (digits, forefoot or distal limb) is needed to permit ambulation.

If there is leg length discrepancy and compensatory tilting of the pelvis, an adapted shoe-lift is provided to prevent scoliosis. However, in cases of significant leg length discrepancy (this may be as great as 6–8 cm), epiphysiodesis (surgical epiphyseal arrest) is indicated. This procedure is best performed when the child is approximately 11–13 years old, depending on his or her growth curve. If there is evidence of increased vascularization of the knee growth zone, embolization of the knee cartilage artery may retard the excess growth.

Bleeding from haemolymphatic vesicles on the thigh is a common problem. Treatment options include diathermal coagulation, YAG laser coagulation, limited excision or split thickness skin grafting for resurfacing. It is sometimes possible to excise the entire area and perform primary closure after tissue expansion of the normal adjacent skin.

Port-wine stain, venous malformations and limb hypotrophy (Servelle–Martorell syndrome)

Patients with this syndrome have PWS, venous anomalies and bone and soft tissue hypotrophy with weakening of the involved extremity [30,31]. Some patients with CVM and hypotrophy have documented arterial and/or deep venous hypoplasia. In a series of 109 patients with complex–combined vascular malformations of the extremities, hypotrophy was present in 6% of cases, and overgrowth in 32%; 62% had no growth alteration [26]. Some patients, classified in the literature as having Servelle–Martorell syndrome had lesions that were clearly pure, extensive limb VMs. This underscores the confusion caused by eponymous terminology.

Proteus syndrome

This is a sporadic, complex syndrome characterized by asymmetric growth and multiple hamartomatous tumours occurring in the trunk and/or extremities [32]. Proteus syndrome may result from a dominant lethal gene, surviving by mosaicism [33].

The tumour-like masses, cutaneous or visceral, represent the overgrowth of normal soft tissues (e.g. connective tissue, adipose tissue, Schwann cell structures), without any specific histological feature. Some deformities are congenital, others develop during childhood. Limb gigantism, overgrowth in hands and feet, cerebriform plantar thickening, and finger or toe macrodactyly are frequent findings. Severe scoliosis or kyphoscoliosis develop in cases with evolutive megaspondyly. Distortion of the facial features due to jugal lipoma is common. Verrucous linear epidermal naevi, following the lines of Blaschko are also present, and some consider Proteus syndrome to be part of the spectrum of epidermal naevus syndrome of Solomon. CMs, LMs (macrocystic) and complex–combined limb vascular malformations of the CVM and CLVM type frequently occur in Proteus syndrome; the incidence of this finding is underestimated in the literature. In most children with Proteus syndrome, intelligence is normal. Treatment focuses on the multiple disabilities; management may be orthopaedic, orthodontic or surgical [33–35]. The main differential diagnoses are von Recklinghausen type I neurofibromatosis and Bannayan–Zonana syndrome (multiple hamartomas, retardation of growth, macrocephaly). Patients with the latter syndrome do not develop acral gigantism, and rarely have extensive CMs.

Phacomatosis pigmentovascularis

The association between cutaneous vascular malformations and pigmented naevi, first reported by Ota, suggests a defect in the migration of neural crest cells. Happle hypothesized the genetic concept of 'twin spots' to explain this sporadic phenotype [36], which is more frequent in black and Japanese children. It is categorized into the following variants (Table 18.1.3): (a) type I is CM ('naevus flammeus') and naevus pigmentosus and verrucosus; (b) type II is CM and aberrant mongolian spots with or without naevus anaemicus; (c) type III is CM and naevus spilus (sometimes called giant speckled lentiginous naevus), with or without naevus anaemicus; and (d) type IV is CM, mongolian spots and naevus spilus, with or without naevus anaemicus. The authors have also observed the association of cutis marmorata telangiectatica congenita (CMTC) and aberrant mongolian spots. Each category is either cutaneous (type A), or cutaneous and syndromic (type B). Related syndromes in type B include SWS, KTS and/or naevus of Ota [37,38].

Occult spinal dysraphism and midline capillary malformations

Cutaneous hallmarks for occult spinal dysraphism (OSD) are most common in the lumbosacral area, but can also occur at the dorsal and cervical level [39]. They include lipoma, hairy patch, skin dimple, dermal sinus, faun tail and vascular birthmark (true haemangioma or CM). CM, occurring alone, is seldom a clue for OSD; most children with cutaneous indicators of OSD have two or more such markers.

Ultrasonography can be performed as a screening test in infants less than 6 months of age. However, in children with a midline CM and another axial sign, MRI is mandatory [40]. OSD must be detected early in life

Table 18.1.3 The various types of phacomatosis pigmentovascularis A and B

Cutaneous (A)	Type 1A	CM ('naevus flammeus') + naevus pigmentosus and verrucosus
	Type 2A	CM + aberrant mongolian spots ± naevus anaemicus
	Type 3A	CM + naevus spilus (or giant speckled lentiginous naevus) ± naevus anaemicus
	Type 4A	CM + aberrant mongolian spots + naevus spilus ± naevus anemicus
Syndromic (B)		Type 1b, 2b, 3b, 4b same as above plus either SWS or KTS, Ota naevus, etc.

because surgical correction may prevent neurological and orthopaedic impairment. Occipital CM can be associated with dysraphism in the skull (meningocele, encephalocele). The association of cephalic CM, scalp membranous aplasia cutis and neural tube closure defects is particularly significant [41].

Telangiectases

Localized telangiectatic vascular malformations

Definition and pathology. Telangiectases may present as fine irregular red or purple lines, punctate macules or minute papules. Stellate vessels may be noted. Individual telangiectasias may be surrounded by a white or 'anaemic' halo.

Unilateral naevoid telangiectasia (UNT) occurs in a systematized unilateral pattern. It predominantly affects females, and usually appears during puberty. Typically, it worsens with pregnancy. Elevated level of oestrogen and progesterone receptors have been demonstrated in areas of involved skin [42]. Hereditary benign telangiectasia is a familial disorder characterized by cutaneous and labial telangiectasias. In contrast to Rendu–Osler–Weber disease, visceral haemorrhage does not occur [43,44]. Generalized essential telangiectasia is another syndrome appearing sporadically in adult females.

Differential diagnosis. In an infant this includes the telangiectatic sequelae of neonatal lupus erythematosus (NLE), which are primarily located in sun-exposed areas. Anti-Ro (SSA) and/or anti-La (SSB) antibodies can be detected in the mothers and infants, and the mothers may have symptoms of connective tissue disease.

Telangiectasia macularis eruptiva perstans, a form of mastocytosis, is uncommon in childhood.

The vascular papules of 'glomeruloid hemangioma' in POEMS syndrome (polyneuropathy, organomegaly, endocrinopathy, M protein, skin changes), are histologically distinct [5].

Treatment. The pulsed dye laser is the treatment of choice.

Syndromic telangiectatic malformations

Cutis marmorata telangiectatica congenita (Van Lohuizen syndrome). CMTC is a congenital vascular anomaly which most often occurs sporadically; rare familial cases are reported [45]. The localized form is most common. CMTC consists of reticulated, violaceous bands, in a livedoid pattern, with areas of telangiectases and skin atrophy. Lesions of CMTC fade over a period of years, but rarely disappear completely. In long-standing CMTC, chronic ulcers may occur. Hypotrophy of the involved

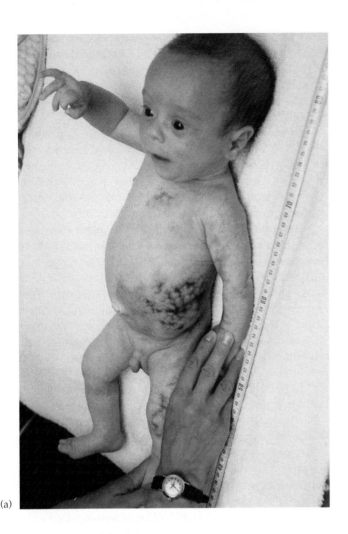

(a)

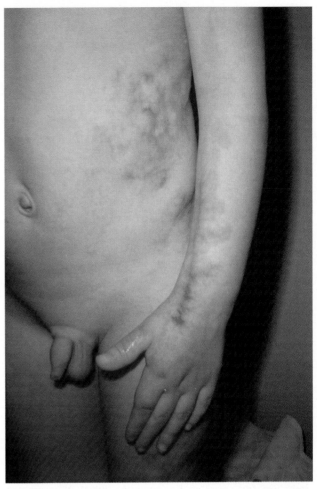

(b)

Fig. 18.1.13 (a, b) Same boy, 3-months old and 4 years old: he has a new type (V) of phacomatosis pigmentovascularis with aberrant mongolian spots (that faded) and cutis marmorata telangiectatica (that persisted).

limb is often present at birth, and usually becomes less prominent over time.

In a review of 152 cases, 23 involved only one or two limbs. Persistence into adulthood was noted in 20 patients; musculoskeletal ($n=53$), neurological ($n=29$) and vascular ($n=16$) anomalies were the most common associated features [45]. A constellation of other infrequent findings were also reported with CMTC [45,46]. In another study of 22 cases [47], six (27%) had associated anomalies (vascular malformations, glaucoma, limb atrophy); most of these cases were localized. Associated anomalies were also usually minor in another review of 35 patients [48].

Pulsed dye laser can be used to treat residual cutaneous lesions. CMTC must be differentiated from livedo reticularis, which is physiological in neonates. Persistent livedo is seen in primary antiphospholipid syndrome and

Sneddon's syndrome. 'Generalized phlebectasia' is a misnomer for CMTC: this term should be reserved for the extremely rare Bockenheimer's syndrome.

Adams–Oliver syndrome consists of CMTC, multiple lesions of aplasia cutis congenita in the scalp, with or without an underlying bone defect, and terminal transverse limb defects. This rare disorder is inherited as an autosomal dominant trait [49].

Ataxia telangiectasia (Louis–Bar syndrome). Ataxia telangiectasia (AT) is a complex neurovascular disorder of autosomal recessive inheritance. It occurs in approximately 1 in 40 000 live births. AT is the result of a mutation in the ATM gene, which has been localized to chromosome 11q22–23 [50].

Multiple telangiectases may begin to develop at 3 years of age, and are seen most commonly on the bulbar conjunctiva, near the canthus. Other locations include the face, neck and dorsum of the hand and foot. Premature photoageing, with associated freckling and loss of cutaneous fat, are seen. Premature greying of the hair may also occur.

Cerebellar ataxia typically begins during the second year of life. Dysarthric speech, choreoathetosis and myoclonic jerks also develop during early childhood, together with impaired intelligence.

MRI is useful in demonstrating cerebellar atrophy, a constant (although non-specific) finding. Recurrent sinobronchopulmonary infections occur in about 80% of patients. Granulomatous skin lesions, occurring in areas of ulceration and atrophy, have been reported [51]. Endocrinological dysfunction includes insulin-resistant diabetes, gonadal insufficiency and growth retardation.

Both humoral and cellular immunodeficiency occur in AT. Patients have decreased or absent serum immunoglobulin A (IgA), and decreased serum IgG-2. Lymphopenia and decreased counts of CD4+ lymphocytes may be noted. Patients with AT have high levels of α-fetoprotein and carcinoembryonic antigen.

AT is associated with an increased incidence of neoplasia. By adolescence, lymphoma and leukaemia are the main causes of death (10–15%). A variety of carcinomas, particularly breast cancer, occur in patients with AT.

Both affected homozygotes and carriers have an acute sensitivity to ionizing radiation and radiomimetic drugs, and experience unexpected severe reactions to these therapeutic regimens. AT heterozygotes are also at increased risk of cancer. Heterozygotes have been estimated to make up 0.5–1.5% of the population.

The discovery of ATM, the single gene responsible for AT, may eventually enable geneticists to offer carrier detection and prenatal diagnosis. Antibiotic therapy and physical therapy prevent bronchiectasis, but no treatment prevents progressive cerebellar ataxia.

Divry–Van Bogaert syndrome. This rare disease may be either sporadic or familial; most patients are male. Neurological manifestations result from non-calcifying leptomeningeal angiomatosis, and begin during adolescence. Multifocal ischaemic attacks and seizures lead to progressive dementia, and pseudobulbar and extrapyramidal symptoms.

Most patients develop livedo reticularis or cutis marmorata during childhood. At present, it is unclear whether the non-familial form of Divry–Van Bogaert syndrome, originally described in 1946, is identical to a subtype of the more recently described Sneddon's syndrome. In both conditions, MRI [52] and arteriogram of the brain reveal similar anomalies (stenosis, collateral circulation and, rarely, moya-moya pattern.)

Rendu–Osler–Weber disease (hereditary haemorrhagic telangiectasia or HHT) is an autosomal dominant disorder with a wide spectrum of serious complications. HHT can cause both recurrent bleeding from visceral telangiectasia, and life-threatening haemorrhage from visceral arteriovenous anomalies [53–57]. Various genotypes correspond to slightly different phenotypes of HHT. Endoglin, identified in 1994 as the gene for HHT type 1, maps to chromosome 9q3. HHT-1 is the first human disease defined by a mutation in a member of the transforming growth factor-β (TGF-β) receptor complex of endothelial cells [54].

Telangiectases are punctate, linear, stellate or nodular, and occur on the cheeks, nose, lips, oral mucosa and fingers. Recurrent epistaxis, the most frequent symptom of HHT, occurs in 80% of patients and usually develops during adolescence. GI bleeding, the second most common form of haemorrhage, begins in adulthood.

AVMs develop in the liver, brain or spinal cord, and lungs. Patients with lung disease may die from massive haemoptysis or haemothorax. AVMs in the lungs may also suppress pulmonary bacterial filtration: 41% of these patients have neurological complications from embolic cerebral abscesses. Due to pulmonary AVMs, a defect in the bacterial filtering function of the pulmonary circulation may allow bacteria to enter the systemic circulation; another mechanism may be the infection of a lung AVF, causing persistent bacteraemia [55]. CNS AVM in HHT can cause spinal cord or intracerebral haemorrhages.

Nasal, gastric or colonic endoscopy may be used to localize bleeding sites.

Electrodessication, laser (Nd : YAG, carbon dioxide or argon) and sclerotherapy have been used to stop bleeding. Patients who develop anaemia from GI haemorrhage may require iron replacement therapy and, occasionally, blood transfusion. In patients with HHT and pulmonary AVMs, antibacterial prophylaxis is recommended for dental, respiratory, GI or genitourinary procedures that place the patient at risk for bacteraemia.

Investigations in families with HHT can detect asymptomatic, unruptured intracranial AVMs; treatment guidelines must balance the lifetime risk for bleeding against surgical morbidity and mortality [56]. Familial CNS AVM has been reported [57].

Localized angiokeratomas

Angiokeratomas are small red to purple, keratotic papules. Lesions may be either localized, segmental or diffuse. Bleeding and irritation may occur. In the Fordyce form of angiokeratoma, multiple angiokeratomas develop on the scrotum. The Mibelli type, which begins during childhood, is characterized by multiple angiokeratomas on the fingers. Some occur in purple, hyperkeratotic plaques; lesions of this type may be present from birth, and may overly a CLVM.

The terms angiokeratoma corporis circumscriptum or Fabry type II disease have been used to describe patients with localized hyperkeratotic lesions present from birth. Angioma serpiginosum of Hutchinson refers to patients with multiple small lesions with mimimal hyperkeratosis; additional angiokeratomas develop over years. In angiokeratoma corporis diffusum, hundreds of small lesions develop over the entire skin surface.

Histologically, angiokeratomas consist of ectatic capillaries which fill the dermal papilla. Marked acanthosis and hyperkeratosis are present. Endothelial cells lining the abnormal capillaries stain for factor VIII related antigen.

Syndromic angiokeratomas (angiokeratoma corporis diffusum and lysosomal storage diseases)

Angiokeratomas may be an indicator of Fabry's disease, and other diseases of lysosomal storage. These are discussed in Chapter 19.12.

REFERENCES

1 Raff M. Die bedeutung adrenerger rezeptoren fur die enstelhung des naevus flammeus und des naevus anemicus. *Wiener Klin Wschr* 1981; 93(suppl 129): 3–14.

2 Leung AKC, Telmesani AMA. Salmon patches in Caucasian children. *Pediatr Dermatol* 1989; 6: 185–7.

3 Bernstein EF, Kantor G, Howe N, Savit RM, Koblenzer PJ, Uitto J. Tufted angioma of the thigh. *J Am Acad Dermatol* 1994; 31: 307–11.

4 Wilson-Jones E, Orkin M. Tufted angioma (angioblastoma). *J Am Acad Dermatol* 1989; 20: 214–25.

5 Tsang WYW, Chan JKC, Fletcher CDM. Newly characterized vascular tumors of skin and soft tissues. *Histopathology* 1991; 19: 489–501.

6 Catteau B, Enjolras O, Delaporte E *et al*. Angiome en touffes sclérosant. A propos de 4 observations aux membres inférieurs. *Ann Dermatol Vénéréol* 1998; 125: 682–7.

7 Sanmartin O, Botella R, Alegre V, Martinez A. Congenital eccrine angiomatous hamartoma. *Am J Dermatopathol* 1992; 14: 161–4.

8 Ashinoff R, Geronemus RG. Flashlamp-pumped pulsed dye laser for portwine stains in infancy: earlier versus later treatment. *J Am Acad Dermatol* 1991; 24: 467–72.

9 Dover JS, Geronemus R, Stern RS, O'Hare D, Arndt KA. Dye laser treatment of port-wine stains: comparison of the continuous-wave dye laser with a robotized scanning device and the pulsed dye laser. *J Am Acad Dermatol* 1995; 32: 237–40.

10 Enjolras O, Riché MC, Merland JJ. Facial port-wine stains and Sturge–Weber syndrome. *Pediatrics* 1985; 76: 48–51.

11 Couly G, Le Douarin NM. Mapping of the early primordium in quail-chick chimeras. II. *Dev Biol* 1987; 120: 198–214.

12 Pedailles S, Martin N, Launay V *et al*. Syndrome de Sturge–Weber–Krabbe, forme grave chez une jumelle monozygote. *Ann Dermatol Vénéréol* 1993; 120: 379–82.

13 Jacoby CG, Yuh WT. Accelerated myelination in early Sturge–Weber syndrome. *J Comput Assist Tomogr* 1987; 11: 26–31.

14 Adamsbaum C, Pinton F, Rolland Y *et al*. Accelerated myelination in early Sturge–Weber syndrome: MRI-SPECT correlation. *Pediatr Radiol* 1996; 26: 759–62.

15 Pinton F, Chiron C, Enjolras O *et al*. Early single photon emission computed tomography in Sturge–Weber syndrome. *J Neurol Neurosurg Psychiatr* 1997; 63: 616–21.

16 Chugani HT, Maziotta JC, Phelps MI. Sturge–Weber syndrome, a study of cerebral glucose utilization with positron emission tomography. *J Pediatr* 1989; 114: 244–53.

17 Arzimanoglou J, Aicardi J. The epilepsy of Strurge–Weber syndrome: clinical features and treatment in 23 patients. *Acta Neurol Scand* Suppl 1992; 140: 18–22.

18 Ito M, Sato K, Ohnuki A, Uto A. Sturge–Weber disease: operative indications and surgical results. *Brain Dev* 1990; 12: 473–7.

19 Lie JT. Pathology of angiodysplasias in Klippel–Trenaunay syndrome. *Pathol Res Pract* 1988; 183: 747–55.

20 Servelle M. Klippel and Trenaunay syndrome: 768 operated cases. *Ann Surg* 1985; 201: 365–73.

21 Stewart G, Farmer G. Sturge–Weber syndrome and Klippel–Trenaunay syndrome with absence of inferior vena cava. *Arch Dis Child* 1990; 65: 546–7.

22 Hansson LI, Strenström A, Thorngren KG. Effect of venous stasis on longitudinal bone growth in the rabbit. *Acta Othop Scand* 1975; 46: 177–84.

23 Baskerville PA, Ackroyd JS, Browse NL. The etiology of the Klippel–Trenaunay syndrome. *Ann Surg* 1985; 202: 624–7.

24 Ohashi I, Shibuya H, Ina H, Suzuki S. A study of venous anomalies of the lower extremities in patients manifesting Klippel–Trenaunay syndrome. *Fortschr Roentgenstr* 1993; 159: 205–7.

25 Alvoet GE, Jorens PG, Roelen LM. Genetic aspects of the Klippel–Trenaunay syndrome. *Br J Dermatol* 1992; 126: 603–7.

26 Matassi R. Differential diagnosis in congenital vascular–bone syndromes. *Semin Vascul Surg* 1993; 6: 233–44.

27 Boyd JB, Mulliken JB, Kaban LB, Upton J, Murray JE. Skeletal changes associated with vascular malformations. *Plast Reconstr Surg* 1984; 74: 789–95.

28 Loose DA. Surgical treatment of predominantly venous defects. *Semin Vasc Surg* 1993; 6: 252–9.

29 Rogalski R, Hensinger R, Loder R. Vascular abnormalities of the extremities, clinical findings and management. *J Pediatr Orthop* 1993; 13: 9–14.

30 Bircher AJ, Koo JYM, Frieden IJ, Berger TG. Angiodysplastic syndrome with capillary and venous malformation associated with soft tissue hypotrophy. *Dermatology* 1994; 189: 292–6.

31 Gibbon WW, Pooley J. Pathological fracture of the femoral shaft in a case of Servelle–Martorell syndrome (phleboectatic osteohypoplastic angiodysplasia with associated arteriovenous malformation). *Br J Radiol* 1990; 63: 574–6.

32 Wiedemann HR, Burgio GR, Aldendorff P *et al*. The Proteus syndrome. *Eur J Pediatr* 1983; 140: 5–12.

33 Lacombe D, Taïeb A, Vergnes P *et al*. Proteus syndrome in seven patients: clinical and genetic considerations. *Genet Couns* 1990; 2: 93–101.

34 Havard S, Enjolras O, Lessana-Leibowitch M, Escande JP. Syndrome Protée: 8 cas. *Ann Dermatol Vénéréol* 1994; 12: 303–8.

35 Darmstadt GL, Lane AT. Proteus syndrome. *Pediatr Dermatol* 1994; 11: 322–6.

36 Happle R, Steijlen PM. Phacomatosis pigmentovascularis gedeutet als ein phänomen der zwillingsflecken. *Hautarzt* 1989; 40: 721–4.

37 Ruiz-Maldonado R, Tamayo L, Laterza A, Brawn G, Lopez A. Phacomatosis pigmento vascularis: a new syndrome? Report of four cases. *Pediatr Dermatol* 1987; 4: 189–96.

38 Hagiwara K, Uezato H, Nonaka S. Phacomatosis pigmentovascularis type IIb associated with Sturge–Weber syndrome and pyogenic granuloma. *J Dermatol* 1998; 25: 721–9.

39 Enjolras O, Boukobza M, Jdid R. Cervical occult spinal dysraphism, MRI findings and the value of a vascular birthmark. *Pediatr Dermatol* 1995; 12: 256–9.

40 Tavafoghi V, Ghandchi A, Hambrick GW, Udverhelyi GB. Cutaneous signs of spinal dysraphism. Report of a patient with a tail-like lipoma and review of 200 cases in the literature. *Arch Dermatol* 1978; 114: 573–7.

41 Drolet B, Prendiville J, Golden J, Enjolras O, Esterly N. Membranous 'aplasia cutis' with hair collar. Congenital absence of the skin or neuroectodermal defect? *Arch Dermatol* 1995; 131: 1427–31.

42 Uhlin SR, McCarty KS. Unilateral nevoid telangiectatic syndrome, the role of estrogen and progesterone receptors. *Arch Dermatol* 1983; 119: 226–8.

43 Wells RS, Dowling GB. Hereditary benign telangiectasia. *Br J Dermatol* 1971; 84: 93–4.

44 Gold MH, Eramo L, Prendiville J. Hereditary benign telangiectasia. *Pediatr Dermatol* 1989; 6: 194–7.

45 Gelmetti C, Schianchi R, Ermacora E. Cutis marmorata telangiectatica congenita, 4 nouveaux cas et revue de la littérature. *Ann Dermatol Vénéréol* 1987; 114: 1517–28.

46 Pehr K, Moroz B. Cutis marmorata telangiectatica, long-term follow-up, review of the literature and report of a case in conjunction with congenital hypothyroidism. *Pediatr Dermatol* 1993; 10: 6–11.

47 Picascia DD, Esterly NB. Cutis marmorata telangiectatica congenita, report of 22 cases. *J Am Acad Dermatol* 1989; 20: 1098–104.

48 Devillers ACA, de Waard-van der Spek FB, Oranje AP. Cutis marmorata telangiectatica. Clinical features in 35 cases. *Arch Dermatol* 1999; 135: 34–8.

49 Bork K, Pfeifle J. Multifocal aplasia cutis congenita, distal limb hemimelia, and cutis marmorata telangiectatica in a patient with Adams–Oliver syndrome. *Br J Dermatol* 1992; 127: 160–3.

50 Savitsky K, Bar-Shira A, Gilad S *et al*. A single ataxia telangiectasia gene with a product similar to PI-3 kinase. *Science* 1995; 268: 1749–53.

51 Paller AS, Massey RB, Curtis MA. Cutaneous granulomatous lesions in patients with ataxia-telangiectasia. *J Pediatr* 1991; 119: 917–22.

52 Stockhammer G, Feller SR, Zelger B *et al*. Sneddon's syndrome diagnosis by skin biopsy and MRI in 17 patients. *Stroke* 1993; 24: 685–90.

53 Ference BA, Shannon TM, White RI, Zawin M, Burdge CM. Life-threatening pulmonary hemorrhage with pulmonary arteriovenous malformations and hereditary hemorrhagic telangiectasia. *Chest* 1994; 106: 1387–90.

54 McAllister KA, Grogg KM, Johnson DW *et al*. Endoglin, a TGF-β binding protein of endothelial cells, is the gene for hereditary haemorrhagic telangiectasia type 1. *Nat Genet* 1994; 8: 345–51.

55 Swanson DL, Dahl MV. Embolic abscesses in hereditary hemorrhagic telangiectasia. *J Am Acad Dermatol* 1991; 24: 580–3.

56 Ter Berg JW, Dippel DW, Habbema JD, Westermann CJ, Tulleken CA, Willemse J. Unruptured intracranial arteriovenous malformations with hereditary hemorrhagic telangiectasia. Neurosurgical treatment or not? *Acta Neurochir Wien* 1993; 121: 34–42.

57 Kadoya C, Momota Y, Ikegami Y, Urasaki E, Wada S, Yokota A. Central nervous system arteriovenous malformations with hereditary hemorrhagic telangiectasia: report of a family with three cases. *Surg Neurol* 1994; 42: 234–9.

Haemangiomas

NANCY B. ESTERLY

Disseminated cutaneous/visceral haemangiomatosis
Benign neonatal haemangiomatosis
Diffuse neonatal haemangiomatosis
Haemangiomatosis of the liver

Kasabach–Merritt syndrome

Haemangiomas are the most common benign tumours of infancy. Nevertheless, until recently, precise diagnosis has been confounded by the lack of a standardized nomenclature and confusion with other types of vascular lesions. In 1982, in a benchmark paper, Mulliken and Glowacki [1] proposed a classification system for the vascular birthmarks based on biological characteristics. They established two major categories: haemangiomas and vascular malformations. Haemangiomas are neoplasms that undergo a proliferative phase followed by stabilization and eventual spontaneous involution, whereas vascular malformations are structural anomalies representing morphogenetic errors of developing blood vessels and lymphatics. This classification system has become widely accepted as it allows for a more accurate diagnosis, predictable prognosis and rational choice of therapy.

Definition

The term haemangioma should be limited to vascular tumours that display a period of active growth followed by a period of inactivity and subsequent involution. These lesions may be present at birth but more often arise during the first few weeks of life. During the growth phase, endothelial cell proliferation has been substantiated by 3H-thymidine incorporation studies and the formation of multilaminated basement membranes [1,2].

Haemangiomas can be superficial, deep or mixed, but all three types of lesions undergo the same maturation sequence. Superficial haemangiomas (formerly called 'capillary' or 'strawberry' haemangiomas) are vivid red or scarlet, sharply circumscribed plaques or nodules, whereas deep haemangiomas (formerly called 'cavernous') are skin-coloured or bluish-purple and poorly circumscribed. These tumours can also be defined by their stage of maturation and referred to as proliferative or involuting [2].

REFERENCES

1 Mulliken JB, Glowacki J. Hemangiomas and vascular malformations in infants and children: a classification based on endothelial cell characteristics. *Plast Reconstr Surg* 1982; 12: 412–20.
2 Mulliken JB, Young AG. *Vascular Birthmarks. Hemangiomas and Malformations.* Philadelphia: WB Saunders, 1988.

Aetiology and pathogenesis

The pathogenesis of haemangiomas is not well understood. Embryological studies have demonstrated evidence of a simple dermal vasculature by the 35th day of gestation [1]. During subsequent weeks there is a gradual increase in the density and complexity of the cutaneous vessels with the formation of a superficial and a deep vascular plexus during the second trimester. Reorganization of the dermal vasculature continues throughout the remainder of gestation and into the first 3–4 postnatal months [2,3].

It seems reasonable to conclude that the process of angiogenesis is involved, not only in the construction of a definitive cutaneous vasculature, but also in the development of haemangiomas, most of which begin to proliferate while the dermal vasculature is still in a formative stage. Angiogenic molecules are known to stimulate the formation of capillary networks by their action on endothelial cells and pericytes. Marked expression of two such factors, vascular endothelial growth factor (VEGF) and basic fibroblast growth factor (bFGF), has been demonstrated in proliferating haemangiomas, providing circumstantial evidence in support of this concept [4]. Furthermore, high levels of bFGF have been detected in the urine of infants and children with haemangiomas [4]. It has been proposed that, during the rapid growth phase of these tumours, when proliferating cell nuclear antigen (PCNA) is strongly expressed, differentiation of the endothelial cells is induced, mediated in part by VEGF and bFGF. These cells in turn evoke an influx of mast cells, and there is prominent expression of tissue inhibitor of metalloproteinase type 1 (TIMP-1), a potent inhibitor of new blood vessel formation, thus inducing the involutional phase. It has been speculated that the mast cells play a role by secreting substances such as interferons and

997

transforming growth factors that downregulate angiogenesis and promote involution [4–7].

REFERENCES

1 Johnson CL, Holbrook KA. Development of human embryonic and fetal dermal vasculature. *J Invest Dermatol* 1989; 93: 10S–17S.
2 Perera P, Kurban AK, Ryan TJ. The development of the cutaneous microvascular system in the newborn. *Br J Dermatol* 1970; 83(suppl 5): 86–91.
3 Esterly NB. Cutaneous hemangiomas, vascular stains and malformations, and associated syndromes. *Curr Prob Dermatol* 1995; 7: 67–107.
4 Takahashi K, Mulliken JB, Kozakewich HPW, Rogers RA, Folkman J, Ezekowitz RAB. Cellular markers that distinguish the phases of hemangioma during infancy and childhood. *J Clin Invest* 1994; 93: 2357–64.
5 Gordon JR, Burd PR, Galli SJ. Mast cells as a source of multifunctional cytokines. *Immunol Today* 1990; 11: 458–64.
6 Arbiser JL. Angiogenesis and the skin. *J Am Acad Dermatol* 1996; 34: 486–97.
7 Folkman J. Clinical applications of research on angiogenesis. *N Engl J Med* 1995; 333: 1737–63.

Histopathology

Biopsies of both superficial (dermal) and deep (subcutaneous and deeper tissues) haemangiomas have a relatively uniform vessel morphology [1,2]. In the proliferative stage they are comprised of syncytial aggregates of plump endothelial cells and pericytes, some of which form lumina and others solid cords. These cells, like mature endothelial cells, express surface markers for alkaline phosphatase and factor VIII antigen [1]. Ultrastructurally, they contain microtubular Weibel–Palade bodies, another characteristic of mature endothelium. A thickened multilaminated basement membrane and elevated uptake of 3H-thymidine provide further evidence for a hyperproliferative state [3].

Pericytes, fibroblasts and, particularly, abundant mast cells are also characteristic of haemangiomas during their state of rapid growth [1]. In the late proliferative phase, the mast cells acquire finger-like processes and appear to interact with the adjacent connective tissue cells forming cytoplasmic bridges and membrane fusions [4].

During the involutional phase the endothelial cells flatten and the vascular channels become more ectatic producing large thin-walled vessels. Islands of fatty tissue and fibrous strands gradually replace the tumour cells. Tritiated thymidine studies no longer show evidence of proliferation and mast cells become less numerous, but there is persistence of the multilaminated basement membranes [1,2,4].

Immunohistochemical studies have demonstrated biological distinctions between haemangiomas and vascular malformations as well as differences in haemangiomas in various stages of evolution. The phase of rapid growth is characterized by large amounts of PCNA, type IV collagenase and VEGF. bFGF, CD31 and von Willebrand factor are also expressed in the proliferative phase. In contrast, elevated expression of TIMP-1, an inhibitor of new vessel formation, is a specific marker for the involutional phase

[5]. Identification of these markers in biopsy tissue could conceivably provide a means of staging haemangiomas.

REFERENCES

1 Mulliken JB, Glowacki J. Hemangiomas and vascular malformations in infants and children: a classification based on endothelial characteristics. *Plast Reconstr Surg* 1982; 69: 412–20.
2 Mulliken JB, Young AG. *Vascular Birthmarks. Hemangiomas and Malformations*. Philadelphia: WB Saunders, 1988.
3 Kojimahara M, Yamazaki K, Ooneda G. Ultrastructural study of hemangiomas. 1. Capillary hemangioma of the skin. *Acta Pathol Jpn* 1981; 31: 105–15.
4 Dethlefsen SM, Mulliken JB, Glowacki J. An ultrastructural study of mast cell interactions in hemangiomas. *Ultrastruct Pathol* 1986; 10: 175–83.
5 Takahashi K, Mulliken JB, Kosakewich HPW, Rogers RA, Folkman J, Ezekowitz AB. Cellular markers that distinguish the phases of hemangioma during infancy and childhood. *J Clin Invest* 1994; 93: 2357–64.

Clinical features

Haemangiomas show considerable variation in appearance depending on their size, anatomical location, depth and stage of evolution (Figs 18.2.1–18.2.3). Approximately one-third of haemangiomas are present at birth, and the remainder usually develop during the first month of life [1]. They are often preceded by a precursor lesion such as a blanched macule, an erythematous or telangiectatic patch with or without a pale halo, a closely packed cluster of bright red papules or a blue-tinged patch (Figs 18.2.4, 18.2.5) [2,3]. Precursor lesions are easily confused with

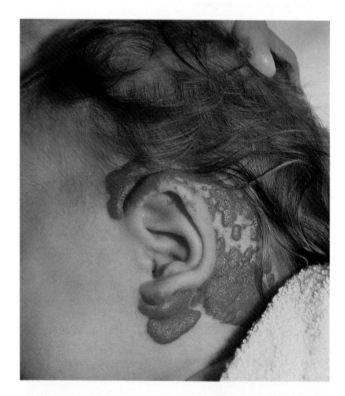

Fig. 18.2.1 Superficial haemangioma involving the ear and retroauricular skin.

port-wine stains and pigmentary abnormalities, or can simulate a scratch or bruise and mistakenly be attributed to traumatic injury.

Superficial haemangiomas evolve into vivid red, elevated, dome-shaped nodules or plaques of a rubbery consistency that can be partially blanched with pressure.

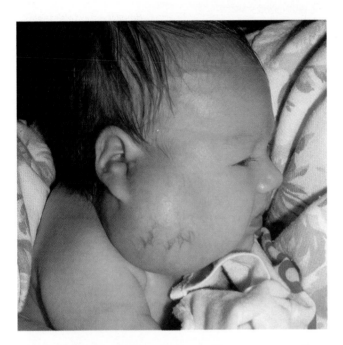

Fig. 18.2.2 Deep haemangioma in the parotid area, a common site.

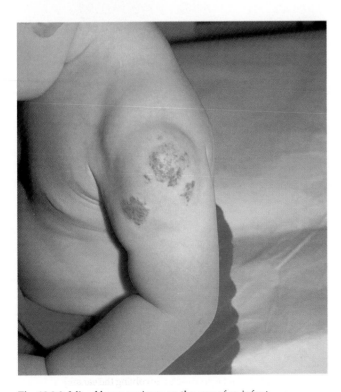

Fig. 18.2.3 Mixed haemangioma on the arm of an infant.

Deep haemangiomas are skin-coloured or bluish, somewhat more compressible and may have telangiectatic vessels on the surface as well as visible feeder vessels and draining veins. These haemangiomas characteristically fluctuate in size and deepen in colour with crying, activity or dependency of the affected part. Some deep lesions have a central superficial component and are called mixed haemangiomas.

Haemangiomas occur in 1.1–2.6% of white newborns and less frequently in black and Japanese (0.8%) neonates [3–6]. Prevalence figures for haemangiomas in white infants at 1 year of age are in the range of 10–12% [6,7]. These tumours occur with greater frequency in preterm infants with incidence figures in one retrospective survey of 22.9% in the 500–1000 g infants, 15.6% in the 1000–1500 g infants and 9.5% in the 1500–2000 g infants [8]. Girls are more frequently affected than boys with a sex ratio ranging from 5:1 to 2:1 [2,9–11], except in small preterm

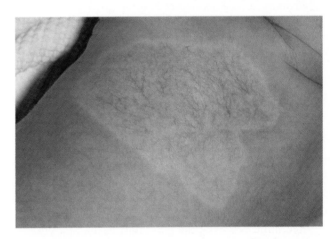

Fig. 18.2.4 Large precursor lesion on the back of a newborn infant, consisting of an area of pallor and telangiectases. Courtesy of Dr James Hogan.

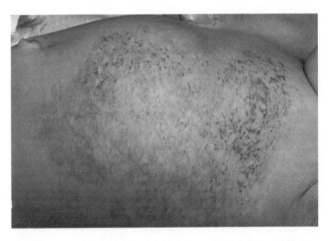

Fig. 18.2.5 Early, plaque-type haemangioma. Note the numerous cherry-red capillary tufts developing within the telangiectatic patch.

infants where the sex ratio is closer to 1:1 [8]. The recent observation that haemangiomas occur with increased frequency following chorionic villus sampling, which is performed between 10 and 12 weeks gestation, suggests that intrauterine factors play a role in the genesis of these lesions [9].

From 15 to 30% of infants with haemangiomas have multiple lesions; however, they are usually few in number [10–13]. Sites of predilection are the head and neck which, in some series, constitute as many as 50% of lesions [11,12,15]. Figures for prevalence of the various types of haemangiomas are not entirely reliable as many large series have included patients with vascular malformations erroneously labelled as haemangiomas. Nevertheless, superficial haemangiomas seem to be the most common type constituting approximately 50–60% of cases, whereas deep haemangiomas represent about 15% and combined superficial and deep lesions 25–35% [10,12].

Virtually all haemangiomas undergo a proliferative phase followed by a period of inactivity and then gradual involution. However, the timing of these phases varies considerably, even in different lesions in the same infant. In general, the growth phase persists for approximately 6–10 months, although an occasional deep haemangioma continues to enlarge slowly for another few months. Yet some have ceased proliferating as early as 3–4 months of age [12,14]. Maximum size is usually reached by the end of the first year. Rapidly proliferating tumours may ulcerate, particularly if large, and rarely a haemangioma may be disguised as an aggressively expanding ulcer with little evident vascular change, most often in the napkin area or on the lips [1,15].

Involution begins in the latter part of the first year or during the second year, although many haemangiomas start to regress earlier or later. The first perceptible change is loss of the brilliant red colour which, in the superficial haemangioma, is replaced by a dull purple hue. As the process of involution continues, the haemangioma becomes grey, first centrally, then peripherally, and begins to flatten and soften, gradually losing volume (Fig. 18.2.6). Unfortunately, the exact timetable for regression of a particular lesion cannot be predicted as time and rate of involution are unrelated to size, location, age of onset, sex of the child or type of haemangioma [16]. A notable exception is the lip where failure to regress or partial regression of a haemangioma is a predictably common outcome [15,17]. This has been attributed to direct continuous blood supply from the labial artery.

Another exception may be the congenital haemangioma which, in contrast to the nascent haemangioma, has completed its proliferative phase *in utero*. Intrauterine haemangiomas have been identified with high resolution ultrasonography as early as the second trimester of pregnancy [18–20]. These lesions have a predilection for the

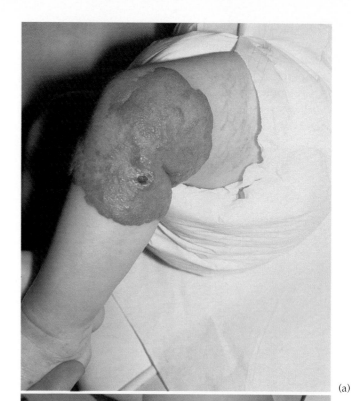
(a)

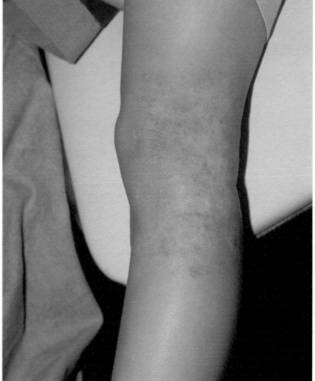
(b)

Fig. 18.2.6 (a) Large haemangioma on the knee of an infant. (b) The same child at 3 years of age. The haemangioma was allowed to involute spontaneously.

craniofacial area and lower limbs, and usually present as firm pink to violaceous nodules, sometimes with a central ulceration or scar. They occur with equal frequency in boys and girls [20]. Characteristically, these vascular tumours do not enlarge postnatally and have an accelerated natural involution, often beginning right after birth and finishing by the end of the first year. Striking dermal and subcutaneous atrophy is a frequent sequela of this rapid regression [20].

Diagnosis

Generally, the diagnosis of haemangioma is made on the basis of the clinical findings; however, some haemangiomas are easily confused with vascular malformations and other types of tumours. Arriving at the correct diagnosis is critical, particularly when complications arise or if surgery is contemplated. Radiological evaluation can help to delineate the type, size and extent of the lesion. Colour ultrasonography has been employed [21] but may be unsuccessful in distinguishing haemangiomas from arteriovenous malformations and will not define the extent of involvement or proximity to adjacent structures. More effective diagnostic studies include computed tomography (CT) scan with contrast and scintigraphy using radio-labelled red blood cells [22]. CT scans are particularly useful for detecting bone changes and radio-opaque structures such as phleboliths [23]. Radionuclide studies will distinguish haemangiomas from other vascular lesions and tumours but fail to localize the lesion accurately. Magnetic resonance imaging (MRI) is now considered the most informative radiological study as with this modality fast-flow and slow-flow lesions can be differentiated and the extent of involvement determined [24]. On MRI scan, haemangiomas appear as fast-flow lesions with flow voids and parenchymal tissue predominance; however, they must be distinguished from fast-flow arteriovenous malformations. Angiography is not often required for diagnostic purposes but is most useful for atypical lesions, or if surgery or embolization is contemplated. On angiograms, haemangiomas appear as well-circumscribed masses with intense persistent tissue staining, a well-organized lobular pattern and a recognizable pattern of feeder vessels and draining veins [25]. If radiological studies fail to clarify the diagnosis, a biopsy may provide more helpful information, particularly the exclusion of solid tumours.

Complications

Ulceration is the most common complication, occurring in 5–10% of haemangiomas [26] (Figs 18.2.7–18.2.10). This problem tends to develop during the phase of rapid proliferation and often causes considerable pain, particularly when the lips, genitalia, perirectal area or flexures are

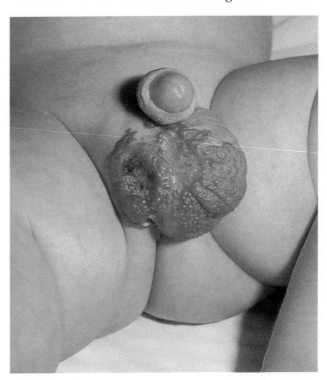

Fig. 18.2.7 Ulcerated haemangioma on the scrotum.

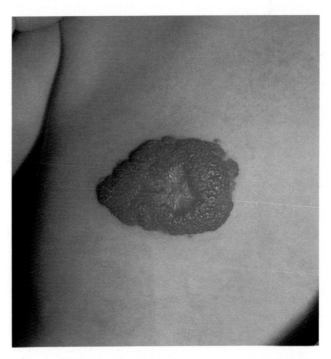

Fig. 18.2.8 Superficial haemangioma that has ulcerated and healed, leaving a small central scar.

involved [2,14,26]. Ulceration almost invariably results in scar formation and, if deep or extensive, can produce conspicuous scarring. Intervention is indicated, and local treatment with Burow solution compresses followed by

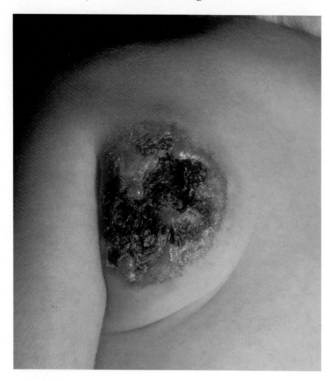

Fig. 18.2.9 Ulcerated, infected haemangioma on the back.

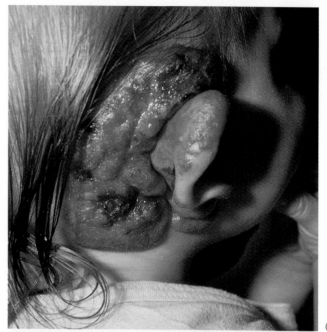

(a)

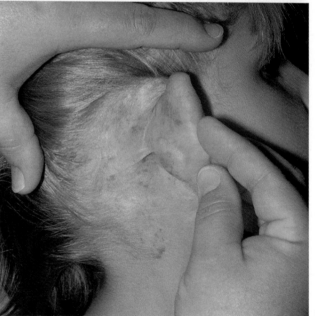

(b)

Fig. 18.2.10 (a) Ulcerated haemangioma in an infant several months of age. (b) The same child at 5 years of age. No treatment was given.

application of an antibiotic ointment and a non-adhesive biosynthetic dressing or an overlay of zinc oxide paste may suffice to induce healing [2]. Pain is promptly alleviated, and the ulcer protected from further trauma and entry of irritating substances. Alternatively, pulsed dye laser therapy is effective in causing rapid re-epithelialization, usually within 2 weeks. Large ulcers may require up to three treatments at 2-week intervals [26].

Infection secondary to ulceration of a haemangioma can be localized to the skin or can spread to the deeper tissues causing cellulitis or osteomyelitis. Suffusion of the skin surrounding the haemangioma, purulent drainage, warmth, tenderness, pain on motion of a limb and fever should alert the doctor to this possibility. Life-threatening septicaemia may supervene, particularly if infection is not detected early and treated promptly with systemic antibiotics. Group A β-haemolytic streptococci are frequently incriminated in these instances [27–29].

Bleeding from an eroded or traumatized haemangioma in the absence of a coagulopathy is usually insignificant and responsive to direct pressure. Nevertheless, it is distressing to parents who often need reassurance and specific instructions for handling this problem. The use of an enuresis blanket, which will detect even small amounts of bleeding during the night, may relieve parental anxiety [30]. Caretakers should be instructed to report evidence of bleeding in a timely fashion, and should be made aware of signs of blood loss such as pallor, bruising, petechiae, irritability and fatigue. These findings may signal bleeding from deep subcutaneous, intraoral or visceral haemangiomas as well. In the event of uncontrolled or persistent bleeding, the infant should be taken to an emergency room for a haematological evaluation and additional therapeutic measures.

Cardiac failure is a rare complication usually associated with large or numerous haemangiomas [31] (see disseminated haemangiomatosis below). High output congestive failure may respond to digitalis and diuretics but ultimately will require reduction of blood flow by drug-induced regression or extirpation of the haemangioma.

Impaired vision may be a consequence of periorbital haemangioma if there is obstruction of the visual axis, compression of the globe or expansion into the retrobulbar space. It is estimated that up to 80% of patients with periocular haemangiomas have these complications [32–34]. The risk is greatest with upper eyelid lesions which compromise vision more often than lower lid tumours and are also more common (approximately 75% of periocular haemangiomas). Iris haemangiomas, which may cause glaucoma, are associated only very rarely [35]. It is mandatory that patients with periorbital haemangiomas have an ophthalmological assessment early in their course and periodically thereafter in order to detect visual impairment. A CT or MRI scan is indicated if retrobulbar involvement is suspected because of displacement of the globe. The most frequent sequelae include astigmatic and myopic refractive errors, ptosis, strabismus, proptosis with keratitis and amblyopia due to stimulus deprivation. Prolonged obstruction of vision or compression of the optic nerve can eventuate in blindness. At times, simple patching of the normal eye will ensure use of the involved eye. If vision is in jeopardy, more aggressive measures such as intralesional or systemic corticosteroids [32–34] or excision [36], if feasible, may be required to preserve vision. However, none of these procedures are without risk [37].

Respiratory compromise is a consequence of obstruction of the airway by haemangioma in the nasal passages, oropharynx or laryngotracheal region. Inability to feed adequately may be a complicating factor. Infants with subglottic tumours experience difficulty before the age of 6 months and present with hoarseness, cough, inspiratory or biphasic stridor and cyanosis [38,39]. Approximately 50% of these infants have haemangiomas elsewhere on the body, most commonly involving the beard area [40]. Asymmetric narrowing of the subglottic airway in frontal radiographs of the neck is considered typical but cannot be relied upon as a consistent finding [41]. Definitive diagnosis must be made by endoscopy and/or biopsy. Some infants have required tracheostomy. Treatment modalities used to manage these haemangiomas include oral corticosteroids [38], intralesional corticosteroids [42], interferon-α [43], laser ablation [39] and surgical extirpation [44]. The risk of scarring and consequent subglottic stenosis must be taken into consideration [38].

Disfigurement, particularly from extensive and rapidly expanding haemangiomas of the head and neck, can be a serious problem and is an important reason for intervention. Some haemangiomas grow at an alarming rate and cause a host of complications depending on the sites of involvement. In two reported series of such children [45,46] problems included obstruction of the visual axis and of luminal structures, uncontrollable ulceration, infection, haemorrhage, coagulopathy and cardiopulmonary decompensation in addition to disfigurement. Multiple treatment modalities were required and were not always successful. More localized lesions can also be problematic, particularly from a psychosocial standpoint. Haemangiomas of the nasal tip (Cyrano nose; Fig. 18.2.11) are a case in point as they can significantly distort the nasal contour causing tremendous distress and embarrassment to the child and family alike. Some authors believe that early intervention is contraindicated as a more aesthetically pleasing result can be obtained by waiting for natural involution [47], whereas others feel that early intervention with systemic agents or surgery is the treatment of choice [1].

Skeletal changes such as overgrowth or hypoplasia of bone is often erroneously attributed to haemangiomas. In fact bony abnormalities are frequent concomitants of vascular malformations and only rarely result from proximate haemangiomas [48].

REFERENCES

1 Mulliken JB, Young AE. *Vascular Birthmarks: Hemangiomas and Vascular Malformations*. Philadelphia: WB Saunders, 1988.
2 Esterly NB. Cutaneous hemangiomas, vascular stains and malformations, and associated syndromes. *Curr Prob Dermatol* 1995; 7: 65–108.
3 Hidano A, Nakajima S. Earliest features of the strawberry mark in the newborn. *Br J Dermatol* 1972; 83: 138–44.
4 Pratt AG. Birthmarks in infants. *Arch Dermatol* 1953; 67: 302–5.
5 Jacobs AH, Walton RG. The incidence of birthmarks in the neonate. *Pediatrics* 1976; 58: 218–22.

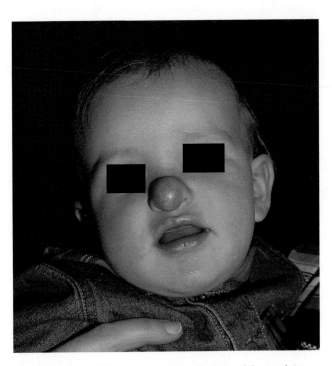

Fig. 18.2.11 Typical Cyrano nose, a haemangioma of the nasal tip.

6 Jacobs AH. Strawberry hemangioma: natural history of the untreated lesion. *Calif Med* 1957; 83: 8–10.

7 Holmdahl K. Cutaneous hemangiomas in premature and mature infants. *Acta Pediatr Scand* 1955; 44: 370–9.

8 Amir J, Krikler R, Metzker A *et al*. Strawberry hemangioma in preterm infants. *Pediatr Dermatol* 1986; 3: 331–2.

9 Burton BK, Schulz CJ, Angle B, Burd LI. An increased incidence of hemangiomas in infants born following chorionic villus sampling. *Prenat Diagn* 1995; 15: 209–14.

10 Lampe I, Latourette HB. Management of hemangiomas in infants. *Pediatr Clin N Am* 1959; 6: 511–28.

11 Margileth AM, Museles M. Current concepts in diagnosis and management of congenital cutaneous hemangiomas. *Pediatrics* 1965; 36: 410–16.

12 Moroz B. Long-term follow-up of hemangiomas in children. In: Williams HB, ed. *Symposium on Vascular Malformations and Melanotic Lesions*. St Louis: CV Mosby, 1983: 162–71.

13 Nakayama H. Clinical and histologic studies of the classification and natural course of the strawberry mark. *J Dermatol* 1981; 8: 277–91.

14 Bowers EA, Graham EA, Tomlinson EM. The natural history of the strawberry nevus. *Arch Dermatol* 1960; 82: 667–80.

15 Liang M, Frieden IJ. Perineal and lip ulcerations as the presenting manifestation of hemangioma of infancy. *Pediatrics* 1997; 99: 256–9.

16 Finn MC, Glowacki J, Mulliken JB. Congenital vascular lesions: clinical application of a new classification. *J Pediatr Surg* 1983; 18: 894–900.

17 Wisnicki JL. Hemangiomas and vascular malformations. *Ann Plast Surg* 1984; 12: 41–56.

18 Bronshtein M, Bar-Hava I, Blumenfelds Z. Early second trimester sonographic appearance of occipital hemangioma simulating encephalocele. *Prenat Diagn* 1992; 12: 695–8.

19 Treadwell MC, Sepulveda W, Leblanc LL, Romero R. Prenatal diagnosis of fetal hemangioma: case report and review of the literature. *J Ultrasound Med* 1993; 12: 683–7.

20 Boon LM, Enjolras O, Mulliken JB. Congenital hemangioma: evidence of accelerated involution. *J Pediatr* 1996; 128: 329–35.

21 Oates CP, Williams ED, Ward-Booth RP, Luyk NH. Doppler ultrasound: a valuable diagnostic aid in a patient with a facial hemangioma. *Oral Surg Oral Med Oral Pathol* 1985; 59: 458–9.

22 Front D, Groshar D, Weininger J. Technetium-99m labeled red blood cell imaging. *Semin Nucl Med* 1984; 14: 226–50.

23 Huston J III, Forbes JS, Ruefenacht DA *et al*. Magnetic resonance imaging of facial vascular lesions. *Mayo Clin Proc* 1992; 67: 739–47.

24 Meyer JS, Hoffer FA, Barnes PD *et al*. Biologic classification of soft-tissue vascular anomalies: MR correlation. *Am J Radiol* 1991; 157: 559–64.

25 Burrows PE, Mulliken JB, Fellows KE *et al*. Childhood hemangiomas and vascular malformations: angiographic differentiation. *Am J Roentgenol* 1983; 141: 483–8.

26 Morelli JG, Tan OT, Yohn JJ. Treatment of ulcerated hemangiomas in infancy. *Arch Pediatr Adolesc Med* 1994; 148: 1104–5.

27 Yagupsky P, Giladi Y. Group A beta-hemolytic streptococcal septicaemia complicating infected hemangioma in children. *Pediatr Dermaol* 1987; 4: 24–6.

28 Burech DL, Koranyi KI, Haynes RC. Serious group A streptococcal diseases in children. *J Pediatr* 1976; 88: 972–4.

29 Armstrong AL, Finch RG, Bailie FB. Serious group A streptococcal infections complicating cryotherapy to lip hemangiomas. *Clin Exp Dermatol* 1993; 18: 537–9.

30 Mallory SB, Morris P. Bleeding hemangioma detected by enuresis blanket. *Pediatr Dermatol* 1989; 6: 139–40.

31 Vaksman G, Rey C, Marache P *et al*. Severe congestive heart failure in newborns due to giant cutaneous hemangioma. *Am J Cardiol* 1987; 60: 392–4.

32 Kushner BJ. Infantile orbital hemangiomas. *Int Pediatr* 1990; 5: 249–57.

33 Haik BG, Jacobiec FA, Ellsworth RM *et al*. Capillary hemangioma of the lids and orbit: an analysis of the clinical features and therapeutic results in 101 cases. *Ophthalmology* 1979; 83: 760–89.

34 Nelson LB, Melick JE, Harley RD. Intralesional corticosteroid injections for infantile hemangiomas of the eyelid. *Pediatrics* 1984; 74: 241–5.

35 Ruttum MS, Mittelman D, Singh P. Iris hemangiomas in infants with periorbital capillary hemangiomas. *J Pediatr Ophthalmol Strabismus* 1993; 30: 331–3.

36 Deans RM, Harris GJ, Kivlin JD. Surgical dissection of capillary hemangiomas. An alternative to intralesional corticosteroids. *Arch Ophthalmol* 192; 110: 1743–7.

37 Ruttum MS, Abrams GW, Harris GJ, Ellis MK. Bilateral embolization associ-
ated with intralesional corticosteroid injection for capillary hemangioma of infancy. *J Pediatr Ophthalmol Strabismus* 1993; 30: 4–7.

38 Shikani AH, Marsh BR, Jones MM *et al*. Infantile subglottic hemangiomas: an update. *Ann Otol Rhinol Laryngol* 1986; 95: 336–47.

39 Riding K. Subglottic hemangioma: a practical approach. *J Otolaryngol* 1992; 21: 419–21.

40 Orlow SJ. Isakoff MS, Blei F. Increased risk of symptomatic hemangiomas of the airway in association with cutaneous hemangiomas in a 'beard' distribution. *J Pediatr* 1997; 131: 643–6.

41 Cooper M, Slovis TL, Madgy DN, Levitsky D. Congenital subglottic hemangioma: frequency of symmetric subglottic narrowing on frontal radiographs of the neck. *Am J Roentgenol* 1992; 159: 1269–71.

42 Meeuwis J, Bos EE, Hoeve LJ *et al*. Subglottic hemangiomas in infants: treatment with intralesional corticosteroid injection and intubation. *Int J Pediatr Otorhinolaryngol* 1990; 19: 145–50.

43 Ohlms LA, McGill TJI, Jones DT, Healy GB. Interferon alpha-2a therapy for airway hemangiomas. *Ann Rhinol Otolaryngol* 1994; 103: 1–8.

44 Gregg CM, Wistrak BJ, Koopmann CF. Management options for infantile subglottic hemangiomas. *Am J Otolaryngol* 1995; 16: 409–14.

45 Enjolras O, Riche MC, Merland JJ *et al*. Management of alarming hemangiomas in infancy: a review of 25 cases. *Pediatrics* 190; 85: 491–7.

46 Weber TR, Connors RH, Tracy TF Jr. Complex hemangiomas of infants and children. *Arch Surg* 1990; 125: 1017–21.

47 Thompson HG. Hemangiomas of the nose. In: Williams HB, ed. *Symposium on Vascular Malformations and Melanotic Lesions*. St Louis: CV Mosby, 1983: 109–14.

48 Boyd JB, Mulliken JB, Kaban LB. Skeletal changes associated with malformations. *Plast Reconstruct Surg* 1984; 74: 789–95.

Prognosis

The prognosis is excellent for most haemangiomas. Approximately 50–60% will have totally involuted by 5 years of age, 70–75% by 7 years of age and upwards of 90% by 9 years of age [1–3]. Occasionally the process is not completed for a few more years. At least 20% of children will have residual skin changes, most often pallor, alteration of skin texture, redundant skin, telangiectasia, atrophy and fibrofatty residuum. These changes seem to occur more frequently when the haemangioma has a prominent dermal component. Scarring is inevitable if ulceration has transpired. Patients with massive haemangiomas, particularly involving the face, or with pendulous lesions or areas of considerable textural change in any location should be referred to a plastic surgeon when natural regression is complete. In instances of severe disfigurement, if a good cosmetic result is achievable, corrective surgery should be considered prior to complete involution to prevent damage to the child's self-image [4,5]. Residual telangiectasia can be eradicated with the pulsed dye laser.

REFERENCES

1 Margileth AM, Museles M. Current concepts in diagnosis and management of congenital cutaneous hemangiomas. *Pediatrics* 1965; 36: 410–16.

2 Bowers RE, Graham EA, Tomlinson KM. The natural history of the strawberry nevus. *Arch Dermatol* 1960; 82: 667–80.

3 Lampe I, Latourette HB. Management of hemangiomas in infants. *Pediatr Clin N Am* 1959; 6: 511–28.

4 Dieterich-Miller C, Cohen B, Liggett J. Behavioral adjustment and self-concept of young children with hemangiomas. *Pediatr Dermatol* 1992; 9: 241–5.

5 Frieden IJ. Which hemangiomas to treat—and how? *Arch Dermatol* 1997; 133: 1593–5.

Differential diagnosis

Haemangiomas may be mistaken for other types of naevi or neoplasms depending on their stage of development. In the precursor stage they may be confused with naevus anaemicus or naevus depigmentosus, salmon patches and port-wine stains or a traumatic injury (scratch or bruise). Once developed, haemangiomas may resemble dermoid cysts, pyogenic granulomas, the nodules of infantile myofibromatosis, neuroblastomas, lipomas and plexiform neurofibromas. Perhaps the greatest difficulty lies in the distinction from lymphangiomas, venous malformations and blue rubber bleb naevus syndrome. The correct diagnosis may become obvious with time as rapid growth during the first month of life favours a diagnosis of haemangioma. However, ultrasound, CT or MRI scan and/or skin biopsy may be required in order to arrive at a definitive diagnosis.

Associations

Previously, the vascular lesions of several malformation syndromes have been mistakenly categorized as haemangiomas [1]. In fact, haemangiomas are rarely associated with structural abnormalities. Only a few such syndromes have true haemangiomas as a cardinal feature. The following associations appear to be genuine and are well documented in the literature.

Lumbosacral haemangiomas, tethered cord and multiple congenital anomalies

It is important to recognize this constellation of findings which, in some infants, may include defects in the skeletal system, nervous system and gastrointestinal and genitourinary tracts. The vascular component, which is present at birth, is initially flat and may consist of only a telangiectatic patch or small ulceration but gradually evolves into a more typical superficial plaque-like haemangioma. Although it may be asymmetrically placed, this lesion always spans the midline [2,3]. It may occasionally involve the legs as well as portions of the buttocks and genitalia [2]. Associated anomalies include imperforate anus, fistulae involving the gastrointestinal and/or the genitourinary tract, bony abnormalities of the sacrum, renal defects, skin tags in the genital or sacral area, and abnormalities of the genitalia. When a lipomeningomyelocele is present as well, it manifests as a paraspinal mass [2].

Infants with plaque-type haemangiomas in a lumbosacral distribution (Figs 18.2.12–18.2.14), even in the absence of other congenital defects or paraspinal masses, are at risk for tethered cord [3]. More often than not, affected infants initially appear normal neurologically. Despite the perceived absence of neurological deficit, appropriate radiological studies should be performed, as

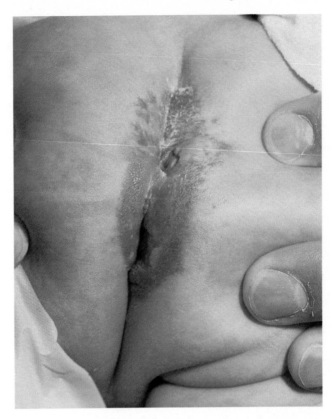

Fig. 18.2.12 Haemangioma of the perirectal area, necessitating temporary colostomy.

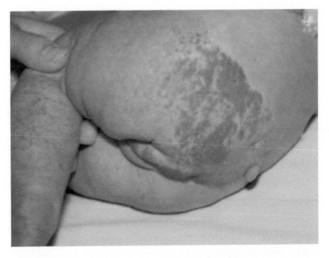

Fig. 18.2.13 Infant with lumbosacral haemangioma which extended down onto the legs. This infant had multiple congenital anomalies including imperforate anus, a rectovaginal fistula, renal abnormalities, a 1-cm skin tag in the sacral area and bony abnormalities of the sacrum.

failure to recognize tethered cord prior to onset of signs and symptoms can result in permanent neurological damage. For infants, plain spine films are not adequate to demonstrate spina bifida and tethered cord because the

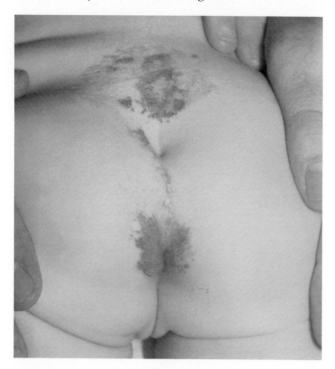

Fig. 18.2.14 Patchy plaque-type haemangioma involving the perineum and presacral skin. This infant had a deep sacral dimple, an anteriorly displaced anus and vertebral abnormalities. Note the grey patch within the haemangioma, a characteristic of these presacral, plaque-type haemangiomas.

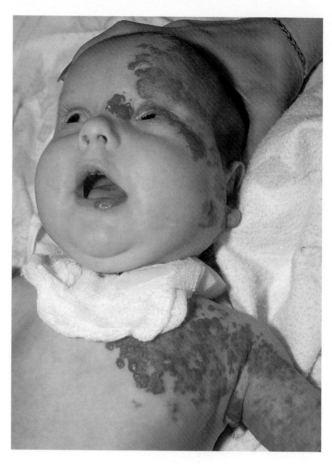

Fig. 18.2.15 This infant of 5 months had an emergency tracheostomy for respiratory compromise due to a subglottic haemangioma. Additional findings were a Dandy–Walker malformation and haemangioma involving the face, chest and right arm. She responded well to a course of oral corticosteroids.

vertebral lamina are poorly calcified. High resolution ultrasound may be useful in small infants, but MRI scan is the procedure of choice. Prompt surgical intervention is indicated for tethered cord, if possible prior to onset of neurological signs and symptoms [4]. These haemangiomas, like those elsewhere on the body, regress in early childhood eradicating the identifying cutaneous marker for the underlying defect(s).

PHACE syndrome (posterior fossa malformations, haemangiomas, arterial anomalies, coarctation of the aorta and cardiac defects, eye abnormalities)

In 1993 Reese *et al.* published a series of nine patients with this combination of congenital anomalies [5]. A second publication augmented the series, reviewed 41 cases collected from the literature, and proposed the acronym PHACE for this neurocutaneous syndrome [6]. Of the reported cases, 88% were female.

The haemangiomas in this syndrome are large and plaque-like, mainly localized to the face, unilateral or bilateral and often involve several dermatomes [5,6]. Severe cutaneous ulcerations, especially on the lips and ears are a frequent manifestation. Laryngotracheal haemangiomas also occur with some frequency. Posterior fossa abnormalities constitute the most common central

nervous system findings, particularly Dandy–Walker malformation (hypoplastic or absent cerebellar vermis and posterior fossa cyst; (Fig. 18.2.15). Structural vascular anomalies of the intracranial arteries, often involving the left carotid artery, as well as multiple defects of the heart and aorta have been documented [5–7]. Ocular abnormalities include congenital cataracts, microphthalmia and optic nerve hypoplasia. A few patients have also had sternal clefting and supra-abdominal raphe (see below).

This entity has been confused with Sturge–Weber syndrome. However, the ocular, cutaneous and central nervous system findings differ in the two syndromes. It has been suggested that PHACE syndrome represents a collection of malformations resulting from a common morphogenetic event *in utero*. The types of malformations characteristic of this syndrome would place the untoward event during the mid to late first trimester. The connection between the vascular dysplasia and the haemangiomas is as yet unexplained.

Infants with large and aggressive facial haemangiomas should be examined carefully for ocular and cardiac defects, signs of neurological dysfunction and respiratory signs and symptoms indicative of airway involvement. An MRI scan of the head should be obtained and cranial arteriography may also be indicated in selected cases. Cranial ultrasound can be used as a sceening procedure for structural defects in young infants with open fontanelles. A full cardiac evaluation including blood pressure in all four limbs is also required. These infants have been treated with a variety of modalities, most successfully with systemic corticosteroids and interferon-α [5,6].

Multiple cutaneous haemangiomas, right aortic arch and coarctation of the aorta

This unusual combination of defects has been reported in several infants [8]. The haemangiomas in these children are cervicofacial and associated with cardiovascular malformations of various types. The most peculiar feature is the right-sided aortic arch in association with a coarctation. It is unclear whether this triad represents a distinct syndrome.

Sternal malformation/vascular dysplasia syndrome

The salient features of this syndrome include a sternal cleft, an atrophic scar continuous with the median abdominal raphe, and haemangiomas of the face and anterior trunk [9]. It has been suggested that this constellation of abnormalities represents a primary disturbance in the ectodermal/mesodermal midline structures occurring at 8–10 weeks of gestation [10]. The haemangiomas involve the face, ears, neck and upper torso and proliferate in early infancy, at times causing necrosis and ulceration of the involved tissue. A few patients have had visceral hemangiomas as well [9]. Systemic corticosteroid [9], interferon-α and the pulsed dye laser [11] have been used to treat these patients.

Haemangiomatous branchial clefts, lip pseudoclefts and unusual facies

These patients have haemangiomatous branchial clefts in the retroauricular areas extending down along the sternocleidomastoid muscle. Associated defects include a peculiar facies with epicanthal folds, flat nasal bridge and blunted alae, nasolacrimal duct obstruction, pseudoclefts of the lips and retroverted auricles with uplifted lobules. Micro- or anophthalmia and conductive deafness may also occur [12].

REFERENCES

1 Burns AJ, Kaplan LC, Mulliken JB. Is there an association between hemangioma and syndromes with dysmorphic features? *Pediatrics* 1991; 88: 1257–67.
2 Goldberg NS, Hebert AA, Esterly NB. Sacral hemangiomas and multiple congenital anomalies. *Arch Dermatol* 1986; 122: 684–7.
3 Albright AL, Gartner JC, Weiner GS. Lumbar cutaneous hemangiomas as indicators of tethered spinal cords. *Pediatrics* 1989; 83: 977–80.
4 Merx JL, Niezen-Bakker SH, Thijssen HOM, Walder HAD. The tethered spinal cord syndrome: a correlation of radiologic features and preoperative findings in 30 patients. *Neuroradiology* 1989; 31: 63–70.
5 Reese V, Frieden IJ, Paller AS *et al.* The association of facial hemangiomas with Dandy–Walker and other posterior fossa malformations. *J Pediatr* 1993; 122: 379–84.
6 Frieden IJ, Reese V, Cohen D. The association of posterior fossa brain malformations, hemangiomas, arterial anomalies, coarctation of the aorta and cardiac defects, and eye abnormalities. *Arch Dermatol* 1996; 132: 307–11.
7 Pascual-Castroviejo I. The association of extracranial and intracranial vascular malformations in children. *Canad J Neurol Sci* 1985; 12: 139–48.
8 Vaillant L, Lorette G, Chantepic A *et al.* Multiple cutaneous hemangiomas and coarctation of the aorta with right aortic arch. *Pediatrics* 1988; 81: 707–9.
9 Hersh JH, Waterfill D, Rutledge J *et al.* Sternal malformation vascular dysplasia association. *Am J Hum Genet* 1985; 21: 177–86.
10 Opitz JM. Editorial comments on the papers by Hersh *et al.* and Kaplan *et al.* on sternal cleft. *Am J Hum Genet* 1985; 21: 201–2.
11 Blei F, Orlow SJ, Geronemus RG. Supraumbilical mid-abdominal raphe, sternal atresia, and hemangioma in an infant: response of hemangioma to laser and interferon alpha-2a. *Pediatr Dermatol* 1993; 10: 71–6.
12 Hall BD, deLorimier A, Foster LH. Brief clinical report: a new syndrome of hemangiomatous branchial clefts, lip pseudoclefts and unusual facial appearance. *Am J Med Genet* 1993; 14: 135–8.

Treatment

A course of non-intervention is usually followed because haemangiomas are benign and self-limited. Parents must be reassured that this choice is in the best interests of the child and will lead to the most satisfactory outcome. Most haemangiomas can be expected to involute spontaneously and, in many instances, a better cosmetic result is achieved than if there is active intervention. It is helpful to parents to establish visits at regular intervals to obtain measurements of the lesions as well as photographic documentation, particularly during the phase of involution. Often the changes associated with regression evolve slowly and the progress made over a fixed period of time is not easily appreciated without photographs. Parental anxiety may increase as the growing child becomes more aware of the skin lesion and of looking different [1]. Parents need guidance in responding to remarks and questions from family and friends as well as advice on how to handle their child's introduction to school. This may be an appropriate time for some children to have an evaluation by a plastic surgeon, particularly if it is obvious that cosmetic repair will be required because of incomplete regression of the haemangioma or the presence of redundant and texturally altered skin. Certain events require intervention: rapid growth of large facial haemangiomas causing disfigurement, haemangiomas involving the genital, anal, ocular, oropharyngeal and laryngeal structures, ulceration with or without secondary infection, Kasabach–Merritt syndrome, disseminated haemangiomatosis, cardiac failure and active bleeding from trauma. Options for treatment include surgical resection, cryotherapy, compression wraps or garments, embolization, laser ablation, ionizing radiation, corticosteroids and α-interferon [2].

Surgery

Resection or excision of a haemangioma may be the best or indeed the only option in an emergent situation such as Kasabach–Merritt syndrome or haemangiomatosis of the liver unresponsive to medical therapy [3]. It may also be the treatment of choice for carefully selected localized haemangiomas such as those on the upper eyelid [4] or for the deforming Cyrano nose [5]. It is important to convey to parents the attendant risks of these procedures and the fact that scarring is an inevitable outcome. In instances of severe disfigurement, carefully placed surgical scars may, nevertheless, represent an improvement in the child's appearance.

Cryotherapy

Cryotherapy is no longer in widespread use for the treatment of haemangiomas and is probably only minimally effective, particularly for large lesions. It may be performed repeatedly if necessary, however, atrophy, scarring and alteration of pigment are common sequelae [6–8].

Compression

Compression with an Ace bandage or Coban wrap is thought by some to facilitate involution of haemangiomas [9,10]. This modality is best utilized on the extremities; in other areas a pressure garment (Jobst garment) can be substituted. The true success of this strategy is unknown as it is impossible to evaluate this technique in a double-blind controlled fashion. Disadvantages are possible ulceration of the haemangioma, discomfort from the pressure and the cost of the garment.

Embolization

This technique, which requires special skill, is generally reserved for vascular lesions that are inoperable, inaccessible, actively haemorrhaging or require radical surgery [10–12]. It has also been employed prior to surgery to minimize intraoperative blood loss. An inert material is deposited in the vasculature with the aid of selective angiography causing blockage and shrinkage of the vascular mass. Risks include thrombosis and backflow of material, entry into the wrong vascular channel, inadvertent embolization of normal vessels, passage of material into the venous circulation, uncontrolled necrosis of involved tissue, loss of vision and sepsis [13]. Nevertheless, morbidity is relatively low if the procedure is performed by an experienced doctor. This approach to

haemangiomas has been used most often in hepatic haemangiomas and in Kasabach–Merritt syndrome.

Radiation

Ionizing radiation is no longer used for treatment of benign haemangiomas because of the risk of serious sequelae including late-onset radiation dermatitis [14], carcinoma or sarcoma [14,15] and cataracts [16] as well as adverse effects on the growing bones, cartilage, thyroid, gonads and breast tissue [17]. These sequelae are clearly dose-related [18]. Nevertheless, radiation therapy has been employed in emergent situations such as Kasabach–Merritt syndrome when the infant is unresponsive to other treatment modalities and is inoperable. In these instances, it is often difficult to judge efficacy as multiple therapies may be used simultaneously. Several studies have failed to document a clear-cut response to radiation therapy [18,19]; however, the use of this modality may be justifiable as a last resort, if careful attention is paid to the dose delivered.

Corticosteroids

Although there are a couple of reports of successful topical steroid therapy for haemangiomas, in general intralesional or systemic administration is required to produce an effect.

Intralesional corticosteroid has been used to halt proliferation and induce regression of problematic haemangiomas for many years. The largest experience has been with periocular tumours because they pose a great risk for serious sequelae and, therefore, require a rapid response. Furthermore, the focal nature of the tumour lends it to localized therapy. Intralesional injection usually requires light general anaesthesia but has several theoretical advantages: (a) ease and rapidity of administration; (b) alleged low frequency of complications; (c) rapid response; and (d) opportunity to employ additional treatment measures if it is ineffective. Generally triamcinolone (prolonged action) is combined with dexamethasone (rapid action) for injection which may be repeated in 4–8 weeks if response is inadequate [20–22].

Despite the impressive response of some children, enthusiasm for this modality is not shared universally. Complications have ranged from minor problems such as temporary discoloration of the skin due to deposits of injected material, haematomas, depigmentation of the injected site and reversible linear atrophy of the subcutaneous tissue [23] to more serious consequences including full thickness eyelid necrosis [24], central retinal artery occlusion from intravascular injection [25], and bilateral retinal and choroidal embolization with loss of vision [26]. Adrenal suppression from a single injection has also been reported [27]. Excessively rapid involution may also result in ulceration, scarring and damage to underlying structures.

Although haemangiomas elsewhere on the body are sometimes treated with intralesional injections, there is a paucity of reports on response rate. In one study 30 infants were treated without complications but the response rate was excellent in only 13% and good in 32% [28]; another series from Italy of 115 haemangiomas had only a 35% cure rate [28]. However, for carefully selected patients this modality has merit and may be especially useful for localized tumours of the lips, nasal tip, cheek and ears that cause significant obstruction or distortion [12].

Systemically administered corticosteroids have been an accepted treatment for problematic haemangiomas for 30 years [29]. The purpose of this therapy is to arrest the growth of the haemangioma and, if possible, to induce regression (Figs 18.2.16, 18.2.17). The most plausible time to initiate this treatment, therefore, is during the early rapid growth phase. Once this phase is completed corticosteroid therapy may no longer have any impact. This means that the doctor must anticipate imminent problems and use clinical judgement regarding choice of therapy. Prednisone is usually given in a dosage of 2–5 mg/kg/day in a single early morning dose; however, larger doses and alternate day, twice a day and even four times a day regimens have also been used successfully [5,11,12,29–31]. A response is usually apparent in 2–4 weeks. Once the tumour has stabilized or begun to regress, the medication should be tapered very slowly. A rapid taper often precipitates rebound growth, presumably because the lesion is still in its proliferative phase. In these circumstances, restoration of a higher dose for 2–4 weeks again followed by a slow taper will often avoid this problem.

Although it is sometimes difficult to distinguish steroid effect from spontaneous regression, rebound growth with reduction in steroid dose is evidence for a therapeutic response. Some studies suggest that about 30% of children with haemangiomas will have a dramatic response to systemic corticosteroids, 40% will have a minimal or equivocal response and 30% will fail this therapy [12]. Reasons for failure include poor patient selection, injudicious delay in initiating therapy and inadequate dosage. In support of this notion in a recently published series of 60 infants treated with an initial dose of 3 or 5 mg/kg/day (16 and 44 patients, respectively) 94% of infants experienced a good or excellent response [31]. Consideration of possible side-effects is important to the decision to use this therapy. In general, with careful patient selection and close monitoring of the infant while on the drug, the benefits outweigh the risks.

The mode of action of corticosteroid on haemangiomas is still unknown. Several theories such as increased sensitivity to vasoactive amines and interaction with other hormones have been postulated but never substantiated. The more recent study of Folkman and Ingber, demonstrating

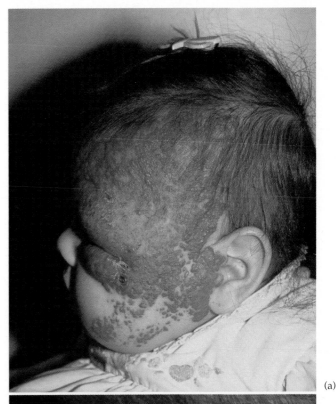
(a)

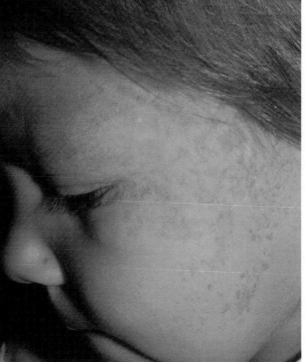
(b)

Fig. 18.2.16 (a) A 5-month-old child with a massive facial haemangioma closing the involved eyelid. (b) Same child at the age of 2 years following a course of oral prednisone.

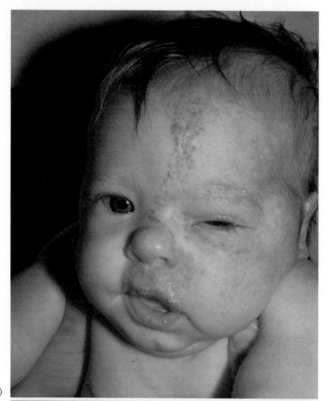

(a)

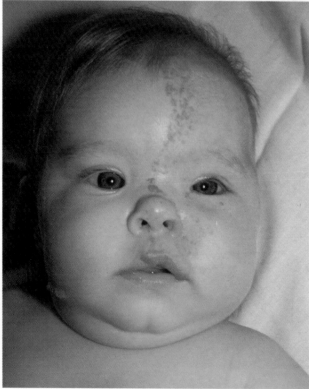

(b)

Fig. 18.2.17 (a) A 2-month-old infant with a large, superficial and deep haemangioma of the face, closing the left eye. (b) Same infant 2 months later following a course of oral prednisone.

that corticosteroids inhibit angiogenesis, suggest that steroids may act directly on the proliferating vessels [32].

Interferon-α

This agent represents a relatively new therapy for problematic haemangiomas. Developed initially as an antiviral agent, it was found to have a beneficial effect on rapidly proliferating, life-threatening haemangiomas [33], ulcerated haemangiomas [34] and in patients with Kasabach–Merritt syndrome [35]. The drug is administered by subcutaneous injection, usually in dosages of 3 million units/m²/day [12].

Response is slower than with corticosteroids but often occurs in steroid-insensitive lesions. In one prospective study [36], haemangiomas regressed by 50% or more in an average of 7.8 months. However, not all patients respond to interferon [37,38] indicating that this drug is also somewhat unpredictable in its effects. Toxic reactions are dose-related and include fever, chills, arthralgias, neutropenia, headaches and transient elevation of liver function tests, as well as a reversible retinal vasculopathy [12]. Spastic diplegia has also been reported [39]. The mechanism of action is unknown but may relate to interferon's ability to inhibit endothelial cell and fibroblast proliferation and to block response of muscle cells to platelet derived growth factors.

Laser therapy

The CO₂ laser has been in use for many years as a cutting instrument to minimize blood loss at surgery for problematic haemangiomas that require immediate intervention [40]. This laser is also employed in the management of subglottic haemangiomas [41,42] but has the attendant risk of subglottic stenosis from scarring.

More recently the flashlamp-pumped pulsed dye laser has been used to treat haemangiomas but, because its depth of penetration is limited to 1.2 mm, it is effective only for superficial lesions and surface telangiectases, including those remaining after involution [43–47]. As adverse effects are minimal with this laser, therapeutic trial is not unreasonable, particularly at sites of potential functional impairment, for ulcerations, or if disfigurement is likely from a large plaque-type haemangioma. Haemangiomas must be treated early while still relatively flat for an optimal response [43]. Treatments are performed every 3–4 weeks until the desired effect is obtained or it becomes clear that the lesion is not responding. Although it was hoped that early treatment of superficial haemangiomas would prevent development of a deep component, several studies have shown that this is not the case. Significant lightening may occur but there is no change in bulk [44,46,48]. Lasers that penetrate more deeply, such as the argon and neodymium:yttrium–aluminium–garnet

(Nd : YAG), unfortunately, have a greater risk for scarring. However, they may have a role in the treatment of deeper and more complicated haemangiomas [46,48,49].

With more widespread use of the pulsed dye laser, the need for anaesthesia for some patients has become more apparent. The use of topical eutectic mixture of local anaesthetics (EMLA) cream is effective in palliating the discomfort for most patients and does not adversely affect outcome.

REFERENCES

1 Tanner JL, Dechert MP, Frieden IJ. Growing up with a facial hemangioma: parent and child coping and adjustment. *Pediatrics* 1998; 101: 446–52.

2 Frieden IJ. Editor, special symposium: management of hemangiomas. *Pediatr Dermatol* 1997; 14: 57–83.

3 Weber TR, Connors RH, Tracy TF Jr. Complex hemangiomas of infants and children. *Arch Surg* 1990; 125: 1017–21.

4 Deans RM, Harris GJ, Kivlin JD. Surgical dissection of capillary hemangioma: an alternative to intralesional corticosteroids. *Arch Ophthalmol* 1992; 110: 1743–7.

5 Mulliken JB, Young AG. *Vascular Birthmarks. Hemangiomas and Malformations*. Philadelphia: WB Saunders, 1988.

6 Lampe I, Latourette HB. Management of hemangiomas in infants. *Pediatr Clin N Am* 1959; 6: 511–28.

7 Simpson JR. Natural history of cavernous hemangiomata. *Lancet* 1959; ii: 1057–9.

8 Wisnicki JL. Hemangiomas and vascular malformations. *Ann Plast Surg* 1984; 12: 41–56.

9 Miller SH, Smith RL, Shochat SJ. Compression treatment in hemangiomas. *Plast Reconstr Surg* 1976; 68: 573–9.

10 Larsen EC, Zinkham WH, Eggleston JC et al. Kasabach–Merritt syndrome: therapeutic considerations. *Pediatrics* 1987; 79: 971–80.

11 Enjolras O, Riche MC, Merland JJ et al. Management of alarming hemangiomas in infancy: a review of 25 cases. *Pediatrics* 1990; 85: 491–7.

12 Enjolras O, Mulliken JB. The current management of vascular birthmarks. *Pediatr Dermatol* 1993; 10: 311–33.

13 Denuth RJ, Miller SH, Keller F. Complication of embolization treatment for problem cavernous hemangiomas. *Ann Plast Surg* 1984; 13: 135–44.

14 Griffith BH. Management of the complications of radiation treatment of benign conditions. *Plast Reconstr Surg* 1965; 36: 207–17.

15 Goette DK, Detlefs RL. Postirradiation angiosarcoma. *J Am Acad Dermatol* 1985; 12: 922–6.

16 Bek V, Zahn K. Cataract as a late sequel of contact roentgen therapy of angiomas in children. *Acta Radiol* 1960; 54: 433–48.

17 Abdulkerin A, Boyd JA, Reeves RJ. Treatment of hemangioma of the skin in infancy and childhood by roentgen irradiation and radium. *Pediatrics* 1954; 14: 523–7.

18 Jung EG, Kohler V. Ruckbildung fruhkinlicher hamangioma nacht rontgen und pseudobestrahlung. *Arch Dermatol Res* 1977; 259: 21–8.

19 Walter J. On the treatment of cavernous hemangiomas with special reference to spontaneous regression. *J Fac Radiol (Lond)* 1953; 5: 134–40.

20 Nelson LB, Melick JE, Harley RD. Intralesional corticosteroid injections for infantile hemangiomas of the eyelid. *Pediatrics* 1984; 74: 241–5.

21 Kushner BJ. Infantile orbital hemangioma. *Int Pediatr* 1990; 5: 249–57.

22 Assaf A, Nasr A, Johnson T. Corticosteroids in the management of adnexal hemangiomas in infancy and childhood. *Ann Ophthalmol* 1992; 24: 12–18.

23 Vasquez-Botet R, Reyes BA, Vasquez-Botet M. Sclerodermiform linear atrophy after the use of intralesional steroids for periorbital hemangiomas: a review of complications. *J Pediatr Ophthalmol Strabismus* 1989; 26: 124–7.

24 Sutula FC, Gloves AT. Eyelid necrosis following intralesional corticosteroid injection for capillary hemangioma. *Ophthalm Surg* 1987; 18: 103–5.

25 Shorr N, Seiff SR. Central retinal occlusion associated with periocular corticosteroid injection for juvenile hemangioma. *Ophthalm Surg* 1986; 17: 229–31.

26 Ruttum MS, Abrams GW, Harris GJ et al. Bilateral retinal embolization associated with intralesional corticosteroid injection for capillary hemangioma of infancy. *J Pediatr Ophthalmol Strabismus* 1993; 30: 4–7.

27 Weiss AH. Adrenal suppression after corticosteroid injection of periocular hemangiomas. *Am J Ophthalmol* 1989; 107: 518–22.

28 Sloan GM, Reinisch JF, Nichter LS et al. Intralesional corticosteroid therapy for infantile hemangiomas. *Plast Reconstr Surg* 1989; 83: 459–66.

29 Fost NC, Esterly NB. Successful treatment of hemangiomas with prednisone. *J Pediatr* 1968; 73: 351–7.

30 Edgerton MT Jr. Steroid therapy of hemangiomas. In: Williams HB, ed. *Symposium on Vascular Malformations*. St Louis: CV Mosby, 1983: 74–83.

31 Sadan N, Wolach B. Treatment of hemangiomas of infants with high doses of prednisone. *J Pediatr* 1996; 128: 141–6.

32 Folkman J, Ingber DG. Angiostatic steroids: method of discovery and mechanism of action. *Ann Surg* 1987; 206: 374–83.

33 White CW, Wolf SJ, Korones DN et al. Treatment of childhood angiomatous diseases with recombinant interferon alfa-2a. *J Pediatr* 1991; 118: 59–66.

34 Blei F, Orlow SJ, Geronemus RG. Interferon alpha-2a therapy for extensive and lower extremity hemangioma. *J Am Acad Dermatol* 1993; 29: 98–9.

35 Orchard PJ, Smith CM III, Wood WG et al. Treatment of hemangioendotheliomas with alpha interferon. *Lancet* 1989; ii: 565–6.

36 Ezekowitz RAB, Mulliken JB, Folkman J. Interferon alpha-2a therapy for life-threatening hemangiomas of infancy. *N Engl J Med* 1992; 326: 1456–63.

37 Henley JD, Danielson CFM, Rothenberger SS et al. Kasabach–Merritt syndrome with profound platelet support. *Hematopathology* 1993; 99: 628–30.

38 Teillac-Hamel D, DeProst Y, Bodemer C et al. Serious childhood angiomas: unsuccessful alpha-2b interferon treatment. A report of four cases. *Br J Dermatol* 1993; 129: 473–6.

39 Folkman J. Clinical applications of research on angiogenesis. *N Engl J Med* 1995; 333: 1757–63.

40 Apfelberg DB, Maser MR, Lash H et al. Benefits of the CO_2 laser in oral hemangioma excision. *Plast Reconstr Surg* 1985; 75: 46–50.

41 Mizono G, Dedo HH. Subglottic hemangiomas in infants: treatment with the CO_2 laser. *Laryngoscope* 1984; 94: 638–41.

42 Healy G, McGill T, Friedman EM. Carbon dioxide laser in subglottic hemangioma: an update. *Ann Otol Rhinol Laryngol* 1984; 93: 370–3.

43 Ashinoff R, Geronemus RG. Capillary hemangioma treatment with the flashlamp-pumped pulsed dye laser. *Arch Dermatol* 1991; 127: 202–5.

44 Garden JM, Bakus AD, Paller AS. Treatment of cutaneous hemangiomas by the flashlamp-pumped pulsed dye laser: prospective analysis. *J Pediatr* 1992; 120: 555–60.

45 Maier H, Neumann R. Treatment of strawberry marks with flashlamp-pumped pulsed dye laser in infancy. *Lancet* 1996; 347: 131–2.

46 Landthaler M, Hohenleutner U, Abd El-Raheem T. Laser therapy of childhood hemangiomas. *Br J Dermatol* 1995; 133: 275–81.

47 Scheepers JH, Quaba AA. Does the pulsed dye laser have a role in the management of infantile hemangiomas? Observations based on 3 years' experience. *Plast Reconstr Surg* 1995; 95: 305–12.

48 Ashinoff R, Geronemus RG. Failure of the flashlamp-pumped pulsed dye laser to prevent progression to deep hemangioma. *Pediatr Dermatol* 1993; 10: 77–80.

49 Achauer BM, Chang C-J, Vander Kam VM. Management of hemangiomas in infancy: review of 245 patients. *Plast Reconstr Surg* 1997; 99: 1301–8.

Disseminated cutaneous/visceral haemangiomatosis

Rarely, an infant may develop numerous small cutaneous haemangiomas with or without accompanying visceral lesions. When the tumours are limited to the skin, this condition has been referred to as benign neonatal haemangiomatosis. When there is visceral involvement as well, it has been called diffuse, miliary, disseminated or multiple neonatal haemangiomatosis. In some infants, the haemangiomas occur predominantly in the liver and may be sparse or absent in the skin; in these instances, a diagnosis of haemangiomatosis of the liver or hepatic haemangioendothelioma is usually made. Although the terminology may vary, it should be appreciated that these entities form a continuum represented by varying degrees of involvement of the skin, liver and other viscera [1–20]. The histopathological features of these tumours are identical to those of solitary haemangiomas; likewise, they are also more common in female infants [2,3].

Benign neonatal haemangiomatosis

In this condition the haemangiomas remain localized to the skin and do not affect the viscera [1,2]. The lesions may be relatively sparse or number in the hundreds but are widely distributed and small and superficial in type (Fig. 18.2.18). These infants have an uncomplicated course and rarely require invasive studies or intervention. A careful history and thorough physical exam are critical and may obviate the need for expensive and anxiety-provoking tests. Choice of studies should be predicated on the clinical status of the infant. The haemangiomas may regress spontaneously as early as the first year of life and tend to involute completely.

Diffuse neonatal haemangiomatosis

This distinctive entity is manifest at birth or in early infancy by multiple haemangiomas involving at least three organ systems. Although not all infants reported under this rubric fulfil this criterion, the prototypic patient has myriads of bright red, blue or purple 2 mm to 2 cm, superficial papular haemangiomas covering the entire body surface (Fig. 18.2.19). These lesions may be present at birth or develop during the neonatal period. Haemangiomas also occur in the liver (64%), central nervous system (52%), gastrointestinal tract (52%), lungs (52%), eyes (32%), and mouth and tongue (44%) [3]. Less com-

monly the thyroid, spleen, pancreas, muscles, thymus, mesenteries, kidney, heart and genitourinary tract are affected. These tumours, like solitary haemangiomas, have a proliferative phase and a stationary phase and will usually regress, often as early as during the first year.

Ocular findings consist of haemangiomas of the lids, conjunctivae and irides, glaucoma secondary to new vessel formation, and ocular nerve palsies [4,5]. Infants with central nervous system involvement may develop neurological deficits, hydrocephalus or seizures. Large and/or numerous hepatic tumours may be manifest by hepatomegaly, a bruit, cardiac failure, obstructive jaundice and portal hypertension.

Depending on the history and physical findings, evaluation may include a complete blood count for anaemia or thrombocytopenia, urinalysis for haematuria, stool examination for fresh or occult blood, coagulation profile, ophthalmological examination, chest film, electrocardiogram and echocardiogram if there is cardiac failure, spinal tap for blood in the spinal fluid, ultrasound and CT or MRI scan of the head and abdomen to detect intracra-

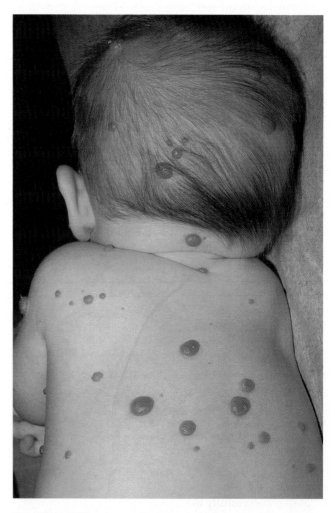

Fig. 18.2.19 Diffuse neonatal haemangiomatosis.

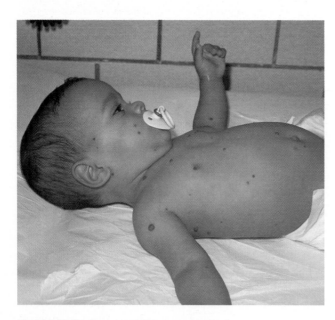

Fig. 18.2.18 Benign neonatal haemangiomatosis.

nial and abdominal haemangiomas, and radiolabelled red cell scans for delineation of hepatic lesions. Angiography may be indicated in special circumstances [6–10]. If the infant is jaundiced, liver function tests should be performed. Colour Doppler imaging represents a relatively new technique that has been found helpful in evaluating and monitoring response to treatment in these children [11]. Complications are frequent and, despite the histological benignity of this condition, only 40% of affected infants survive beyond the first few months [3]. Death can usually be attributed to massive gastrointestinal or intracranial bleeding or intractable cardiac failure due to arteriovenous shunting [3,12]. Kasabach–Merritt syndrome supervenes only rarely [3,12].

No definitive treatment has been identified. Medical modalities including high-dose prednisone (2–4 mg/kg/day), and oxygen, digitalis and diuretics for high output congestive failure have been successful in some instances [6,13,14]. Operative intervention, no longer considered the treatment of choice, may be necessary in those who do not respond to treatment and consists of hepatic artery ligation or lobectomy. If treatment is instituted early, tailored to the individual and carefully monitored, a successful outcome is possible with regression of the haemangiomas.

Haemangiomatosis of the liver

This entity is usually defined as a triad consisting of hepatomegaly, variable numbers of cutaneous haemangiomas and high-output cardiac failure (Fig. 18.2.20). The latter finding is felt to be due to unregulated shunting of blood through unduly large or numerous hepatic haemangiomas. These patients tend to be symptomatic early, usually presenting in the first few weeks of life [15,16]. Their subsequent course is dependent on the site, size, number and haemodynamic consequences of the lesions. Death, which occurs in up to 80–90% of infants in some reports, commonly results from intractable cardiac failure, haemorrhage or, rarely, obstructive jaundice, portal hypertension or a consumptive coagulopathy [16]. Evaluation should include abdominal ultrasound, and CT or MRI scan with contrast [7]. The technetium 99m red blood cell scan and colour Doppler imaging are two non-invasive modalities that provide excellent information regarding extent of involvement and response to therapy [8,9,11].

For many years, these patients were treated surgically by excision of the haemangiomas, lobectomy or hepatic artery ligation. More recently, medical therapy including systemic corticosteroids and supportive measures for cardiac failure has been shown to be efficacious in some but not all patients [8,9,11,16,17,19]. Radiation therapy, generally regarded as too risky or ineffective, has been employed successfully in rare cases [18,19] as has transarterial embolization [20]. As with diffuse cutaneous hae-

mangiomatosis, the tumours will regress spontaneously if the patient can be supported throughout the early months of life.

REFERENCES

1 Stern JK, Wolf Jr JE, Jarrett M. Benign neonatal hemangiomatosis. *J Am Acad Dermatol* 1981; 4: 442–5.
2 Held JL, Haber RS, Silvers DN, Grossman ME. Benign neonatal hemangiomatosis: review and description of a patient with unusually persistent lesions. *Pediatr Dermatol* 1990; 7: 63–6.
3 Golitz LE, Rudikoff J, O'Meara OP. Diffuse neonatal hemangiomatosis. *Pediatr Dermatol* 1986; 3: 145–52.
4 Haik BG, Clancy P, Ellsworth RM, Perina A, Zimmerman K. Ocular manifestations in diffuse neonatal hemangiomatosis. *J Pediatr Ophthalmol Strabismus* 1983; 20: 101–5.
5 Weiss MJ, Ernest JT. Diffuse congenital hemangiomatosis with infantile glaucoma. *Am J Ophthalmol* 1976; 81: 216–18.
6 Gozal D, Saad N, Bader D, Berger A, Jaffe M. Diffuse neonatal haemangiomatosis: successful management with high dose corticosteroids. *Eur J Pediatr* 1990; 149: 321–4.
7 Choi BI, Han MC, Park JH, Kim SH, Man MH, Kim C-W. Giant cavernous hemangioma of the liver: CT and MR imaging in 10 cases. *Am J Roentgenol* 1989; 152: 1221–6.

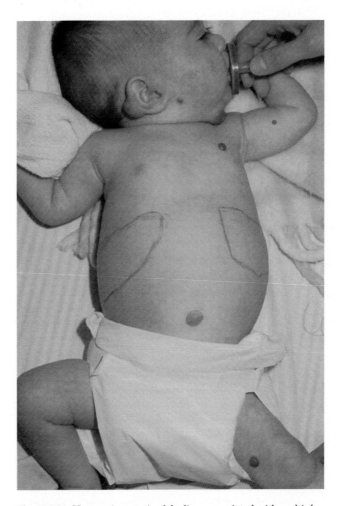

Fig. 18.2.20 Hemangiomatosis of the liver, associated with multiple, but not numerous, cutaneous haemangiomas. She responded promptly to a course of prednisone as well as digitalis and diuretics for congestive failure.

8 Stanley P, Geer GD, Miller JH, Gilsanz V, Landing BH, Boechat IM. Infantile hepatic hemangiomas. Clinical features, radiologic investigations, and treatment of 20 patients. *Cancer* 1989; 64: 936–9.

9 Kristidis P, De Silva M, Howman-Giles R, Gaskin KJ. Infantile hepatic haemangioma: investigation and treatment. *J Paediatr Child Health* 1991; 27: 57–61.

10 Esterly NB, Margileth AM, Kahn G *et al*. Special symposium. The management of disseminated eruptive hemangiomata. *Pediatr Dermatol* 1984; 1: 312–17.

11 Bruce S, Downe L, Devonald K, Ellwood D. Noninvasive investigation of infantile hepatic hemangioma: a case study. *Pediatrics* 1995; 95: 595–7.

12 Byard RW, Burrows PE, Izakawa T, Silver MM. Diffuse infantile haemangiomatosis: clinicopathological features and management problems in five fatal cases. *Eur J Pediatr* 1991; 150: 224–7.

13 Stenninger E, Schollin J. Diffuse neonatal hemangiomatosis in a newborn child. *Acta Pediatr* 1993; 82: 102–4.

14 Stillman AE, Hansen RC, Hallinan V, Strobel C. Diffuse neonatal hemangiomatosis with severe gastrointestinal involvement. *Clin Pediatr* 1983; 22: 589–91.

15 Nguyen L, Shandling B, Ein S, Stephens C. Hepatic hemangioma in childhood: medical management or surgical management? *J Pediatr Surg* 1982; 17: 576–9.

16 Cohen RC, Myers NA. Diagnosis and management of massive hepatic hemangiomas in childhood. *J Pediatr Surg* 1986; 21: 6–9.

17 Shannon K, Buchanan GR, Votteler TP. Multiple hepatic hemangiomas: failure of corticosteroid therapy and successful hepatic artery ligation. *Am J Dis Child* 1982; 136: 275–6.

18 Rotman M, John M, Stowe S, Inamdar S. Radiation treatment of pediatric hepatic hemangiomatosis and coexisting cardiac failure. *N Engl J Med* 1980; 302: 852.

19 Pereyra R, Andrassy RJ, Mahour GH. Management of massive hepatic hemangiomas in infants and children: a review of 13 cases. *Pediatrics* 1982; 70: 254–8.

20 Johnson DH, Vinson AM, Wirth FH *et al*. Management of hepatic hemangioendotheliomas of infancy by transarterial embolization: a report of two cases. *Pediatrics* 1984; 73: 546–9.

Kasabach–Merritt syndrome

This syndrome, as originally described in 1940, consists of thrombocytopenia, microangiopathic haemolytic anaemia and a localized consumption coagulopathy (disseminated intravascular coagulation or DIC) in association with a rapidly enlarging haemangioma. However, recent studies indicate that the vascular lesions in these patients have the features of a kaposiform haemangioendothelioma or tufted angioma, and may not represent classic haemangiomas [1,2]. Unlike classic haemangiomas there is no sexual predilection for these tumours. The prototypic patient is a young infant in the first few weeks of life with a large tumour of the head, trunk or limb [3,4]. Occasionally this syndrome complicates the course of a visceral or retroperitoneal tumour, disseminated haemangiomatosis or a vascular malformation [5–7].

Clinical features that should alert the clinician to the possibility of DIC, particularly in a young infant, include pallor, spontaneous petechiae and ecchymoses, prolonged bleeding from trauma or from the umbilicus or circumcision site, haematuria, epistaxis or haematochezia. The vascular lesion, which enlarges with remarkable rapidity, acquires a woody indurated consistency with discoloured haemorrhagic overlying skin suggesting cellulitis (Figs 18.2.21, 18.2.22). Initially the haemorrhagic lesions are

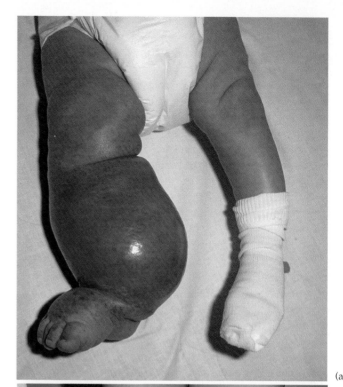

(a)

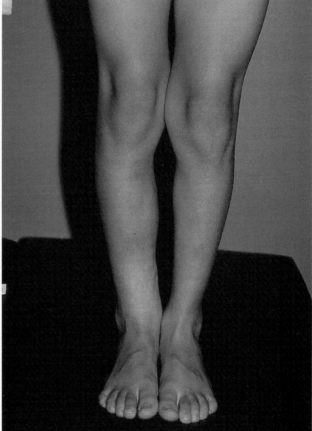

(b)

Fig. 18.2.21 (a) A 2.5-month-old infant with Kasabach–Merritt syndrome. Platelet count was 9000. (b) Same child at age 7 years old. He was treated with a course of prednisone and a Coban wrap.

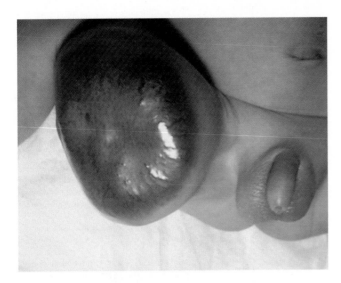

Fig. 18.2.22 A 6-week-old infant with massive congenital vascular lesions on the thigh. This infant failed a course of prednisone, aspirin and dipyridamole. The tumour was excised successfully with immediate return of the platelet count to normal.

restricted to the area of the haemangioma but subsequently they become more widespread.

It is important to obtain an immediate haematological evaluation if Kasabach–Merritt syndrome is suspected. Appropriate studies include a haematocrit and haemoglobin, a smear for fragmented red blood cells and a platelet count. If thrombocytopenia is identified then clotting studies including a prothrombin time, activated partial thromboplastin time, fibrinogen level and determination of fibrin split products at the least should be obtained. Because increased production of fibrinogen and other clotting factors may result in normal clotting in chronic DIC, fibrin split products should always be measured in these infants. Additional helpful tests include reptilase time, factor V and VIII levels, and identification of soluble fibrin and fibrinopeptide A in the plasma [8]. A haematologist should be consulted regarding interpretation of haematological studies and management.

The thrombocytopenia of Kasabach–Merritt syndrome has been attributed to sequestration and destruction of platelets within the expanding vascular mass. Normal to increased numbers of megakaryocytes are found in the bone marrow [8]. This explanation of pathogenesis is supported by studies demonstrating localization of platelets within the haemangioma by intravenous injection of Cr-labelled platelets [9]. Preferential accumulation of fibrinogen within the tumour has also been noted following administration of ^{131}I-labelled fibrinogen [10]. Both platelets and fibrinogen have a shortened survival time in these patients [9,10]. Although the pathophysiology is that of a localized consumption coagulopathy, the initiating factors have not been identified. It has been suggested that the endothelial cells may be

responsible or that enlargement of the tumour mass accompanied by stasis, accumulation of activated coagulation factors and increased local fibrinolysis, may produce an autocatalytic state resulting in depletion of platelets and coagulation factors when consumption exceeds production.

Mortality figures are as high as 20–30% of patients in some published reports. Nevertheless, as the disorder remits when the tumour begins to involute [4,7], treatment should be tailored to the individual depending on the severity of the condition and the age of the patient. Young infants, who are relatively inactive, tolerate mild to moderate thrombocytopenia without bleeding and may require only close observation until the haemangioma stabilizes and begins to regress. Precipitous changes in the clinical findings or haematological values mandate intervention. Restoration of platelets, coagulation factors and fibrinogen by administration of platelet concentrates, fresh frozen plasma and cryoprecipitate may be effective in controlling bleeding, but heparinization may be required as well [11,12]. Heparin is usually administered in a dose of 100 mg/kg every 4 h until bleeding stops and the patient is stabilized. Additional measures may be indicated for shock and high output cardiac failure.

Treatment should be directed at inducing involution of the tumour mass. Prednisone in doses of 2–5 mg/kg/day has been effective in restoring the platelet count to normal and shrinking the haemangioma in some patients [4,6,7,13,14]. Additional agents that have been variably successful include a combination of aspirin and dipyridamole [15], pentoxifylline [16], cyclophosphamide [17] and the antifibrinolytic agents tranexamic acid and ε-aminocaproic acid [5,7,18]. However, no single agent has been consistently effective in patients with this syndrome. Two other drug regimens that have been utilized more recently with success are high-dose intravenous methylprednisolone [19,20] and interferon-α [21–24]. Interferon may have to be administered for several months to induce permanent remission, and as with other modalities, not all patients have responded favourably [25].

Patients who have failed medical management have been successfully treated by surgical extirpation with or without prior embolization to control bleeding or by embolization alone [26,27]. Although this approach is fraught with serious risks, it may represent the only choice in emergent situations. Radiation therapy has also been advocated, but the attendant long-term sequelae make this modality a less acceptable choice [28–30].

REFERENCES

1 Enjolras O, Wassef M, Mazoyer E *et al*. Infants with Kasabach–Merritt syndrome do not have 'true' hemangiomas. *J Pediatr* 1997; 130: 631–40.
2 Vin-Christian K, McCalmont TH, Frieden IJ. Kaposiform hemangioendothelioma. An aggressive, locally invasive vascular tumor that can mimic hemangioma of infancy. *Arch Dermatol* 1997; 133: 1573–8.

3 Shim WKT. Hemangiomas of infancy complicated by thrombocytopenia. *Am J Surg* 1968; 116: 896–906.

4 Esterly NB. Kasabach–Merritt syndrome. *J Am Acad Dermatol* 1983; 8: 504–13.

5 Shulkin BL, Argenta LC, Kyung C *et al*. Kasabach–Merritt syndrome: treatment with epsilon-aminocaproic acid and assessment by indium 111 platelet scintigraphy. *J Pediatr* 1990; 117: 746–9.

6 Loh W, Miller JH, Gomperts ED. Imaging with technetium 99m-labelled erythrocytes in evaluation of the Kasabach–Merritt syndrome. *J Pediatr* 1988; 113: 856–9.

7 Larsen EC, Zinkham WH, Eggleston JC *et al*. Kasabach–Merritt syndrome: therapeutic considerations. *Pediatrics* 1987; 79: 971–80.

8 Bell R. Disseminated intravascular coagulation. *Johns Hopkins Med J* 1980; 146: 289–99.

9 Kontras SB, Green OC, King L *et al*. Giant hemangioma with thrombocytopenia: case report with survival and sequestration studies of platelets labeled with chromium 51. *Am J Dis Child* 1963; 105: 188–95.

10 Straub PW, Kessler SF, Schreiber A *et al*. Chronic intravascular coagulation in Kasabach–Merritt syndrome. *Arch Int Med* 1972; 129: 475–8.

11 Henley JD, Danielson CFM, Rothenberger SS *et al*. Kasabach–Merritt syndrome with profound platelet support. *Hematopathology* 1993; 99: 628–30.

12 deTerlizzi M, Bonifazi E, Toma MC *et al*. Kasabach–Merritt syndrome: successful management of coagulopathy with heparin and cryoprecipitate. *Pediatr Hematol Oncol* 1988; 5: 325–8.

13 Evans J, Batchelor ADR, Start G *et al*. Haemangioma with coagulopathy: sustained response to prednisone. *Arch Dis Child* 1975; 60: 809–12.

14 Enjolras O, Mulliken JB. The current management of vascular birthmarks. *Pediatr Dermatol* 1993; 10: 311–33.

15 Koerper MA, Addiego JE, deLorimio AA *et al*. Use of aspirin and dipyridamole in children with platelet trapping syndromes. *J Pediatr* 1983; 102: 311–14.

16 deProst Y, Teillac D, Bodemer C *et al*. Successful treatment of Kassabach–Merritt syndrome with pentoxifylline. *J Am Acad Dermatol* 1991; 25: 854–5.

17 Hurvits CH, Alkalay AL, Sloninsky L *et al*. Cyclophosphamide in life threatening vascular tumors. *J Pediatr* 1986; 109: 360–3.

18 Warrell RP Jr, Kempin SJ. Treatment of severe coagulopathy in the Kasabach–Merritt syndrome with amminocaproic acid and cryoprecipitate. *N Engl J Med* 1985; 313: 309–12.

19 Ozsoylu S, Ihren C, Gurgey A. High dose intravenous methylprednisolone for Kasabach–Merritt syndrome. *Eur J Pediatr* 1989; 148: 403–5.

20 Ozsoylu S. High dose of methylprednisolone for Kasabach–Merritt syndrome. *J Pediatr* 1991; 119: 676.

21 Klein C, Hauser M, Hadorn HB. Interferon alpha-2a therapy of consumptive coagulopathy in Kasabach–Merritt syndrome. *Eur J Pediatr* 1992; 152: 919.

22 White CW, Wolf SJ, Korones DN *et al*. Treatment of childhood angiomatous diseases with recombinant interferon alpha-2a. *J Pediatr* 1991; 118: 59–66.

23 Hatley RM, Sabio H, Howell CG *et al*. Successful management of an infant with a giant hemangioma of the retroperitoneum and Kasabach–Merritt syndrome with alpha-interferon. *J Pediatr Surg* 1993; 28: 1356–9.

24 Ezekowitz RAB, Mulliken JB, Folkman J. Interferon alpha-2a therapy for life-threatening hemangiomas of infancy. *N Engl J Med* 1992; 326: 1456–63.

25 Teillac-Hamel D, deProst Y, Bodemer C *et al*. Serious childhood angiomas: unsuccessful alpha-2b interferon treatment. A report of four cases. *Br J Dermatol* 1993; 129: 473–6.

26 El-Dessouky M, Azmy AF, Raine PAM *et al*. Kasabach–Merritt syndrome. *J Pediatr Surg* 1988; 23: 109.

27 Tanaka K, Shimao S, Okada T *et al*. Kasabach–Merritt syndrome with disseminated vascular coagulopathy treated by exchange transfusion and surgical excision. *Dermatologica* 1986; 173: 90.

28 Furst CJ, Silfversward C, Holm LE. Mortality in a cohort of radiation treated childhood skin hemangiomas. *Acta Oncol* 1989; 28: 789.

29 Griffeth BH. Management of the complications of radiation treatment of benign conditions. *Plast Reconstr Surg* 1965; 36: 207–17.

30 Goette DK, Detlefs RL. Postirradiation angiosarcoma. *J Am Acad Dermatol* 1985; 12: 922–6.

18.3 Disorders of Lymphatics

SANDEEP H. CLIFF AND PETER S. MORTIMER

The lymphatic system is composed of lymph, lymphatic vessels, lymph nodes and organs containing lymphoid tissue such as the spleen and bone marrow [1]. It is a vascular network consisting of channels through which lymph passes and ultimately ends up in the blood vascular system and should be considered as part of the peripheral cardiovascular system. The network ensures the maintenance of blood volume by returning to the general circulation fluid and protein that leaks from the blood vessels into the interstitial space [2]. The arrest of this circulation is incompatible with life and the obstruction or failure to develop components of this circulation *in utero* is associated with a significant morbidity [3].

The similarity of the development of the lymphatic system with the venous system is undisputed. However, our inability to identify immunohistochemically lymphatics from the venous system prevents us from reliably distinguishing the two vessels in most circumstances. Because of the limited reliable and sensitive investigative methods for highlighting the lymphatics, the significance of the lymphatics and the role played by the lymphatics both in the normal and diseased states remains largely unknown.

Role of lymphatics

The lymphatics serve two major roles: the regulation of homoeostasis (in conjunction with macrophages) and an immunological role.

Regulation of homoeostasis

Regulation of homoeostasis involves the following.
1 The return of macromolecules, in particular protein, leaked from blood vessels into the interstitium, to the blood stream.
2 The elimination from the tissues of unwanted cellular byproducts as well as dysfunctional cells.
3 The removal and processing of foreign organic (microbes) and inorganic material.
4 The draining of excess fluid from the interstitium thereby acting as a safety valve in case of fluid overload.
An understanding of the role of the lymphatics makes it possible to understand why the lymphatics parallel the veins so intimately.

Immunological function

1 The transport of antigens to the regional lymph nodes where an appropriate immune response may be elicited:

most antigens are presented to the central lymphoid system for the first time via the lymphatics.

2 Provides the major route from the skin for circulating cells such as T lymphocytes, macrophages and the dendritic cells.

3 Maintenance of the functioning lymph node [4].

Bacterial and other microorganism are channelled through lymphatics presumably as a protective mechanism to prevent noxious agents from directly entering the blood stream. Further support of this important role of lymphatics is the observation of recurrent erysipelas/cellulitis in patients with lymphoedema.

Components of lymph

Lymph is the main constituent of the lymphatics; it is clear and colourless in the skin. The protein composition of lymph is lower than that of plasma, although there is considerable variation between the lymphatic constituents depending upon the organ of origin. Lymph also contains all the coagulation factors, and therefore clots like plasma although less readily. There is a higher concentration of coagulation factors in lymph in hepatic lymphatics than in skin lymphatics simply because the factors are synthesized in the liver. The electrolyte concentration of lymph is the same as that found in plasma but the total cation concentration is slightly lower in the lymph whilst the chloride and bicarbonate levels tend to be higher.

Development of the lymphatics

Central lymphatic vessels develop in embryonic life as buds from the developing venous system and in the skin they develop from undifferentiated mesenchyme. The vessels are composed of a network of endothelial channels which are apparent initially from the sixth week of embryonic development.

The lymphatic system develops from four cystic spaces that appear on either side of the neck and in both groins. These large cisterns develop communications (lymphatic vessels) which allow most of the lymph from the lower limbs and abdomen to be channelled through the cisterns into the thoracic duct. This then ascends the left side of the thoracic vertebrae before entering the internal jugular vein in the left side of the neck. A separate lymphatic trunk drains lymph from the right upper limb and head, and enters the right internal jugular vein. Lymph nodes develop as condensations along the course of these lymphatic pathways.

Within the skin, lymphatics originate as blind-ending endothelial lined loops in the superficial dermis.

There are four main types of lymphatic vessels [5]: lymph capillaries, precollectors, collectors and lymphatic trunks. In the skin the network is constructed as a poly-

gonal mesh forming a two-dimensional grid located between the reticular and papillary dermis. This subpapillary plexus of lymphatics is overlaid by a horizontal meshwork of precapillary arterioles and postcapillary venules, and above this network lies the epidermis [5]. The precollectors drain the lymph from the capillary mesh vertically through the dermis and the subcutaneous layer to the large prefascial collectors. These larger collectors are demonstrable radiologically.

Structure of the lymphatics

The unidirectional flow of lymph is ensured in the healthy state by the presence of valves [6]. It is uncertain as to whether these valves are permanent or reactionary, being present under circumstances in which there is an increased lymph flow and depleted in areas in which flow is principally under the influence of gravity. This theory partly explains why fewer valves are seen in the upper limbs and the face. The structure of the lymphatics has been reviewed extensively [7]. Histologically, the initial lymphatics are large, with a lumen lined by an extremely attenuated endothelium. Under normal circumstances the vessel is collapsed and therefore not readily identifiable. The endothelium of the lymphatic has very few organ-specific characteristics: there are no fenestrae, pinocytotic vesicles or Weibel–Palade bodies, although some of these features have been reported [8]. Blood vessels have typically plump vascular endothelium and are rich in organ-specific characteristics.

Lymphatics possess gaps between the endothelial cells through which macromolecules may pass into their lumen. These gaps or open junctions are demonstrable ultrastructurally.

There is a degree of variability in the structure of the lymphatics in different tissues [9] reflecting possibly their varied and unique role. As the smaller vessels merge to form larger lymphatics, an external connective coat supports the endothelium. The lining of the larger lymphatics is similar to that of the veins: the tunica intima consists of endothelium and a surrounding layer of fibrous tissue, the tunica media consists of a few smooth muscle fibres and the tunica adventitia is composed mainly of fibrous tissue with some nerves present [10]. The basal lamina consists of a fine network of filaments embedded in a homogeneous matrix. This structure is replaced over time with an electron-dense lamina which is also present in lymphatics that have endured physical stress resulting from an increase in the intralymphatic pressure. Further studies have shown that these filaments are embedded into the outer sheath of the valves and into the coarse collagen bundles present in the dermis [11,12]. The filaments are thought to be paramount to the normal functioning of the vessels, they are believed to hold open the ports of entry into the lymphatics by being stretched when the interstitium swells due to an increase in interstitium fluid. Additionally, dermal elastic fibres [13,14] are now thought to act as a prelymphatic pathway by offering macromolecules a path of low resistance to the precollector lymphatics. They are ideally suited to this role since they are located perpendicularly in the upper dermis and in the mid dermis they are horizontally orientated.

Identification of the lymphatics

Identification of the dermal lymphatics in tissue sections is still not possible with a distinct marker. Attempts at identifying lymphatics involve the combination of stains for elastic fibres (orcein) and blood vessel endothelium (factor VIII related antigen). In the healthy skin, blood vessels stain positive with factor VIII related antigen and lymphatics negative; the addition of the elastic fibre stain allows the lymphatics to be distinguished. However, the negative factor VIII related antigen in lymphatic endothelium is thought to depend upon the fixative used and the type of lymphatic vessel being stained [15]. As yet there is no marker positive for lymphatics but negative for blood vessels.

REFERENCES

1 Olszewski WL. Lymphatics, lymph and lymphoid cells and integrated immune system. *Eur Surg Res* 1986; 18: 264–70.
2 Adair TH, Guyton AC. Physiology—lymph formation its control and lymph. In: Close M, Wallace S, eds. *Lymphatic Imaging*. Baltimore: Williams & Wilkins, 1985; 120–41.
3 Yoffey JM, Courtice FG. *Lymphatics, Lymph and Lymphomyeloid Complex*. New York: Academic Press, 1970.
4 Drayson MT, Ford WL. Afferent lymph and lymph borne cells: their influence on lymph node function. *Immunobiology* 1984; 168: 362–79.
5 Kubik S, Manestar M. Anatomy of the lymph capillaries and pre-collectors of the skin. In: Bollinger A, Partsch H, Wolfe JHN, eds. *The Initial Lymphatics*. Stuttgart: Georg Thieme Verlag, 1985: 66–75.
6 Daroczy J. New structural details of dermal lymphatics valves and their functional interpretation. *Lymphology* 1984; 17: 54–60.
7 Ryan TJ. Structure and function of lymphatics. *J Invest Dermatol* 1989; 93: 18S–24S.
8 Holden CA, Spaull J, Williams R, Spry CFF, Rusell-Jones R, Wilson-Jones E. The distribution of endothelial cell antigens in cutaneous tissue using methacarn and periodate lysine para formaldehyde fixation. *J Immunol Methods* 1986; 91: 45–52.
9 Leak LV, Burke JF. Ultrastructural studies on the lymphatic anchoring filaments. *J Cell Biol* 1986; 36: 129–49.
10 Boggan RP, Palfrey AJ. The microscope anatomy of human lymphatic trunks. *J Anat* 1973; 114: 389–405.
11 Pullinger BD, Florey HW. Some observations on the structure and function of lymphatics: their behaviour in local oedema. *Br J Exp Pathol* 1935; 16: 49–61.
12 Casely-Smith JR. The role of the endothelial intercellular junctions in the functioning of the initial lymphatics. *Angiologica* 1972; 9: 106–31.
13 Mortimer PS, Cherry GW, Jones RL, Barnhill RL, Ryan TJ. The importance of elastic fibres in skin lymphatics. *Br J Dermatol* 1983; 108: 561–6.
14 Mortimer PS, Jones RL, Ryan TJ. Human skin lymphatics; regional variation and relationship to elastin. Progress in lymphology; diagnostic, therapeutic and research approaches to lymphatic system structure and function. *Progress in Lymphology* 1985; 10: 59–64.
15 Witschi E. Teratogenic effects from overripeness of the egg. In: Fraser FC, McKessick VA eds. *Congenital Malformations, Proceedings of the Third International Conference*. Amsterdam: Excerta Medica, 1970.

Investigations

There are very few methods available to assess the lymphatics of the skin. *In vitro* studies using electron/light microscopy allow a structural assessment of the lymphatics but fail to give any functional information. *In vivo* assessment can be done using radiocontrast X-ray lymphangiography and isotope lymphography.

Contrast lymphangiography [1–4]

This test is indicated to confirm the diagnosis of a lymphatic abnormality and to determine, if possible, the type of lymphatic malfunction. The investigation requires the prior injection into the interstitial subcutaneous tissue of patent violet blue. This allows the visualization of the lymphatic network. Patients are usually admitted to hospital and a general anesthesia is normally required since patients can rarely remain still for long enough. This is particularly important in the presence of oedema where the technique may be technically difficult. The oily contrast medium lipiodol is then injected into a suitable peripheral lymphatic. The failure to opacify the collectors with this dye and its persistence in the tissues for several days confirms the diagnosis of lymphoedema. If there is an obstruction to the lymphatics then there is retrograde flow of dye into the dermal network, so called 'dermal backflow', which can also be visualized. Lymphangiography allows precise information on the presence of hypoplasia, megalymphatics and obstruction, and it still remains the 'gold standard' against which other techniques are assessed. Lymphangiography, however, is not without hazards; anaphylaxis to the contrast medium can occur and pulmonary oil embolism [5] has been reported. It is possible that the lipiodol may actually damage the lymphatics thereby exacerbating any lymphoedema present.

Indirect lymphangiography [6,7]

Indirect lymphangiography involves the intracutaneous injection of a water-soluble contrast medium via a pump over 10 min thereby creating a depot. Using the mammogram film method the intradermal and subcutaneous lymphatics may be visualized. The major advantage of this method is the single interstitial injection without the need for further cannulation of the vessels but the drawback is that the collectors are often not visualized.

Isotope lymphography [8,9]

Isotope lymphography has largely replaced contrast lymphangiography in most centres as the primary diagnostic technique. A radiolabelled protein or colloid is injected subcutaneously where it is specifically taken up by the lymphatics. This permits lymphoedma to be diagnosed as an outpatient investigation. Normally 0.3% of the injected dose will appear in the groin within 30 min and in venous disease this is increased to 3% over 1 h thereby allowing venous and lymphatic disease to be distinguished [9]. This technique allows quantitative analysis of lymph drainage. Gamma camera pictures will show the isotope reaching the groin and a delay to progress suggests either a proximal obstruction or hypoplasia of the lymphatics. The major disadvantage of this method is that unlike direct lymphangiography the subcutaneous collectors cannot be discriminated easily [10].

Fluorescence microlymphography [11]

This technique permits the visualization of the superficial dermal lymphatic network under the vital microscope by means of a fluorescent macromolecule—fluorescein isothiocynate (FITC)–dextran (molecular weight 150000). This is injected subepidermally and subsequently taken up by the dermal lymphatics. Recordings can then be made and both qualitative and quantitative interpretations made. It remains at present a research tool.

REFERENCES

1 Kinmonth JB. Lymphangiography in man. *Clin Sci* 1952; 11: 13–20.
2 Kinmonth JB. Lymphography in clinical surgery. *Ann Roy Coll Surg Engl* 1954; 15: 300–15.
3 Kinmonth JB. Lymphography 1977. A review of some technical points. *Lymphology* 1977; 10: 102–6.
4 Kinmonth JB, Harper RA, Taylor GW. Lymphangiography: a technique for its clinical use in the lower limb. *Br Med J* 1995; 1: 940–2.
5 Kinmonth JB. *The lymphatics—surgery, lymphography and diseases of the chyle and lymph systems*, 2nd edn. London: Edward Arnold, 1982.
6 Partsch H, Stoberl CH, Urbanek A, Wenzel-Hora BI. Clinical use of indirect lymphography in different forms of leg oedema. *Lymphology* 1988; 21: 152–60.
7 Partsch H, Wenzel-Hora B, Urbanek A. Differential diagnosis of lymphoedema after indirect lymphography with iotasol. *Lymphology* 1983; 16: 12–18.
8 Mostbeck A, Kahn P, Partsch H. Quantitative lymphography in lymphoedema. In: Bollinger A, Partsch H, Wolfe JH, eds. *The Initial Lymphatics*. Stuttgart: Georg Thieme Verlag, 1985: 123–30.
9 Stewart G, Gaunt J, Croft DN, Browse NL. Isotope lymphography: a new method of investigating the role of lymphatics. *Br J Surg*, 1985; 72: 906–9.
10 Proby C, Mortimer PS, Gaine J, Joseph A. Investigation of the swollen limb with isotope lymphography. *Br J Dermatol* 1988; 119: 44.
11 Bollinger A, Jager K, Sgier F, Seglias J. Fluorescence microlymphography. *Circulation* 1981; 64: 1195–9.

Developmental disorders of the lymphatic system

A number of human conceptuses are said to die prenatally, of which a number involve abnormalities of the lymphatic system. Chromosomal aneuploidy affects about 50% of human embryos [1] some of which involve lymphatic abnormalities.

Turner's syndrome

Turner's syndrome is defined as gonadal dysgenesis due to either an absent or a structurally defective X chromosome. It was originally described in seven girls by Turner in 1938 [2].

Aetiology

The frequency of Turner's syndrome is 1 per 2500 female births [3]. Typically about 80% of cases have 45 chromosomes with an XO sex complement which is thought to occur in as many as 4% of human conceptuses [4]. These cases are chromatin negative in buccal smears. The missing chromosome is considered lost either before or at fertilization. The remaining 15% are chromatin positive showing partial deletion [5] of the X-chromosome. These affected individuals are phenotypically similar to the XO but to a lesser extent.

It is postulated that the cardiac and pulmonary abnormalities noted in these patients are a direct consequence of encroachment on these structures from enlarged lymphatic sacs in the neighbouring area. The typical webbed neck is thought by some [6,7] to represent redundant skin which arose secondary to being stretched by a distended lymphatic in the neck region which then connected up with the venous system leaving the resultant web. Others [8] have felt that the hypoplastic lymphatics may be reflected in organs leading to altered haemodynamics and resulting in the congenital heart defects. The characteristic widely spaced nipples are thought to be possibly due to enlarged lymphatics *in utero* which are then relieved. All these theories are speculative based on the fact that Turner's syndrome is most often associated with congenital lymphatic malformations [9].

Pathology

Ovarian streaks are present instead of the normal gonads. These are composed of stroma-like cells without follicular activity or germ cells. A hormonal profile reveals an elevated follicle-stimulating hormone (FSH) and luteinizing hormone (LH) in the serum within the first few days of life due to the absence of the negative feedback mechanism [10].

A number of studies have shown that patients with Turner's syndrome have hypoplastic lymph vessels in the lower extremities and this explains why a significant finding in patients with Turner's syndrome is the presence of lymphoedema of the lower limbs at birth. This has been confirmed using lymphangiography [1] which has demonstrated impaired lymphatic drainage. Additionally, the vessels that do exist lack valves [11] thus inhibiting the forward propulsion of fluid. It has been hypothesized that the lymphatics distend as a result of a failure to drain into the jugular lymph sacs during embryonic life [11]. The hypoplastic lymph vessels may be considered as the cause of the oedema in Turner's syndrome. Some studies have shown that the abnormal vessels persist despite a resolution of the oedema [9] and others have found these abnormal vessels with no evidence of oedema, suggesting other factors may be involved in the pathogenesis of the oedema.

Clinical features

Turner's syndrome results in the early spontaneous loss of the fetus in over 95% of cases. Amongst the multiple malformations noted in this syndrome, congenital lymphatic disorders are frequently seen. The manifestations include cystic hygroma, hydrops fetalis and ascites which may be detected by ultrasound in the second trimester [6,12,13].

Characteristic clinical features of Turner's syndrome include a small stature, a broad-shaped chest and widely spaced nipples [8]. Other findings include a webbed neck, cubitus valgus, high arched palate, hypoplastic nails, abnormally shaped ears and multiple pigmented naevi. Often the lymphangiectatic oedema that is present in the acral sites at birth clears within the first few years. Other abnormalities include coarctation of the aorta—cardiac involvement occurring in up to 25% of cases. Eye involvement is also a feature with squints and ptosis. Intelligence is typically normal.

Endocrinologically, there is primary amenorrhoea and a failure to develop full secondary sexual characteristics.

Diagnosis

The clinical features may suggest the diagnosis in infancy and childhood but if they are subtle or absent then the diagnosis may be delayed until puberty when patients may present with primary amenorrhoea or absent secondary sexual characteristics. The diagnosis may be confirmed by examination of buccal smears which reveal the absence of the chromatin and presence of an increased urinary excretion of FSH.

REFERENCES

1 Alvin A, Diehl J, Lindsten J, Lodin A. Lymph vessel hypoplasia and chromosome aberrations in six patients with Turner's syndrome. *Acta Derm Venereol* 1967; 47: 25–33.
2 Turner H. A syndrome of infantilism, congenital webbed neck and cubitus valgus. *Endocrinology* 1938; 23: 566–74.
3 Maclean N, Harnden DG, Court Brown WM. Abnormalities of sex chromosome constitution in newborn babies. *Lancet* 1961; ii: 406–8.
4 DeAngelis CS, Feigin RD, Warshaw JB. *Principles and Practice of Paediatrics.* FA, Oski (ed), 1990: 259, 444.
5 Bowen P. Chromosomal abnormalites. *Clin Orthoped* 1964; 3: 40–58.
6 Clarke EB. Neck web and congenital heart defects: a pathogenic association in 45XO Turner syndrome? *Teratology* 1984; 29: 355–61.
7 Lacro R, Jones KL, Benirschke K. Coarctation of the aorta in Turner syn-
drome: a pathologic study of fetuses with nuchal cystic hygromas, hydrops fetalis, and female genitalia. *Pediatrics* 1988; 81: 445–51.
8 Noonan JA. Turner syndrome and partial anomalous pulmonary venous drainage. *Paediatrics* 1991; 87: 584–5.
9 Chervenak FA, Isaacson G, Blakemore KJ et al. Fetal cystic hygroma—cause and natural history. *N Engl J Med* 1983; 309: 822–5.
10 Conte FA, Grumbach MM, Kaplan SL et al. Correlation of LH releasing factor induced LH and FSH release from infancy to 19 years with the changing pattern of gonadotrophin secretion in a gonadal patients: relation to the restraint of puberty. *J Clin Endocrinol Metab* 1980; 50: 163–8.
11 Van der Putte SCJ. Lymphatic malformations in human fetuses. *Virchows Arch A Pathol Anat Histol* 1977; 376: 233–46.
12 Byrne J, Blanc WA, Warburton D et al. The significance of cystic hygromas in fetuses. *Hum Pathol* 1983; 15: 61–7.
13 Vitlay P, Bosze P, Gaad M et al. Lymph vessel defects in patients with ovarian dysgenesis. *Clin Genet* 1980; 18: 387–91.

Klippel–Trenaunay–Weber syndrome

The Klippel–Trenauany–Weber syndrome [1] is a widely used term to describe the condition of angio-osteohypertrophy.

Aetiology

The aetiology of this condition remains unknown and the severity of the phenotype is highly variable.

The combination of a port-wine stain on a limb with soft tissue swelling is termed the Klippel–Trenaunay–Weber syndrome which may sometimes by associated with bony overgrowth. The original description included a bony overgrowth of the affected limb [1] but that has since been modified.

Parkes-Weber subsequently described a syndrome which was associated with arteriovenous anastomosis in a limb [2] and differed from the Klippel–Trenaunay syndrome which principally involved the venous system; however, they were all given a single heading which has since been termed the Klippel–Trenaunay–Weber syndrome rather than distinguished from one another though they should be considered as separate entities. The distinction between these two entities may be complicated further since some unique features may not become apparent until the patient is older.

A variety of blood and lymph vascular malformations may be seen including haemangiomas, arteriovenous malformations, port-wine stains, lymphangiomas and lymphoedema [3].

Patients with this disorder may be designated into one of three broad groups depending upon the principal malformation: predominantly venous [1], predominantly arteriovenous fistulae [2] or mixed venous–lymphatic malformations.

Clinical features

The typical triad of clinical features seen are macromelia, varicosities and cutaneous angiomas. In the original description a naevus extending the full length of the lower limb, varices present from infancy on the affected limb and hypertrophy of all the tissues of the diseased side were reported. However, the exact combination of all these features are rarely seen. Other dermatological manifestations are now widely recognized and have been well reported [4]. They include aseptic cellulitis and cavernous haemangiomas seen in up to 50% of patients. Lymphoedema was seen in the majority of patients in Viljoen *et al.*'s study [4].

Diagnosis

This is made on the clinical features. Attempts to diagnose the condition antenatally via ultrasound have proved unreliable. Ultrasonic findings include polyhydramnios with a multiloculated mass on the anterior wall [5] and lower extremity hemihypertrophy [6].

Treatment

There is no effective treatment for this condition. The lymphoedema should be managed in the standard way as specified later. The vascular haemangioma is now amenable to treatment using the pulsed dye laser.

REFERENCES

1 Klippel M, Trenaunay P. Du naevus variqueux osteohypertrophique. *Arch Gen Med* 1900; 3: 641–72.
2 Parkes-Weber F. Angioma formation in connection with hypertrophy of limbs and hemi-hypertrophy. *Br J Dermatol* 1907; 19: 231–5.
3 Lewis BD, Doubilet PM, Heller VL *et al.* Cutaneous and visceral haemangiomata in the Klippel–Trenaunay–Weber syndrome: antenatal sonographic detection. *Am J Roentgenol* 1986; 147: 598–600.
4 Viljoen D, Saxe N, Pearn J, Beighton P. The cutaneous manifestations of the Klippel–Trenaunay–Weber syndrome. *Clin Exp Dermatol* 1987; 12: 12–17.
5 Hatjis CG, Philip AG, Anderson GG, Mann Li. The *in utero* ultrasonic appearance of Klippel–Trenaunay–Weber syndrome. *Am J Obstet Gynecol* 1981; 139: 972–4.
6 Warhit J, Goldman MA, Sacks L, Weiss LM, Pek H. Klippel–Trenaunay–Weber syndrome: appearance *in utero*. *J Ultrasound Med* 1983; 2: 515–18.

Noonan syndrome

This syndrome phenotypically resembles Turner's syndrome but the karyotype is normal (46XY or 46XX).

Aetiology

The syndrome may be familial [1] and various modes of inheritance have been proposed but direct transmission now favours an autosomal dominant inheritance pattern [2,3]; however, most reported cases are sporadic. Patients with Noonan syndrome may be male or female but because of the phenotypical similarity between Turner's and Noonan syndromes both have been confused in the female patient. The discovery by Ford *et al.* in 1959 [4] of the X-chromosomal abnormality in patients with Turner's syndrome has helped to differentiate these two conditions on chromosomal analysis.

Pathology

Skin biopsy specimens have not demonstrated any specific abnormality [3]. Biopsies of the pulmonary and femoral arteries have shown degeneration of the media with an excess of mucopolysaccharides and fragmentation of the elastic fibres [3]. From this it was proposed that there was a defect in the connective tissue; however, these results have not been reproduced.

Clinical features

Clinical features include a short stature and a short broad neck which may sometimes be webbed. The characteristic facies include hypertelorism, epicanthic folds and micronathia. Phenotypically very similar to Turner's syndrome, cardiovascular abnormalities are very common and in particular pulmonary stenosis. Other distinct features include a degree of mental retardation.

Congenital peripheral oedema occurs in Turner's syndrome but appears to be more common in Noonan syndrome. Some authors [5] have suggested the presence of lymphoedema persisting into adulthood as one of the differentiating features between the two syndromes. In Turner's syndrome the congenital oedema disappears in a few months or years in most cases, whilst in Noonan syndrome the lymphoedema is usually stationary or slowly progressive. In one study the incidence of lymphoedema in the over 16 year olds with Turner's syndrome was 3% compared to 15% in Noonan patients [6]. The aetiology of the lymphoedema in patients with Noonan syndrome remains unknown; it has been postulated that like Turner's syndrome the defect may result from an absence of the superficial lymphatic channels [7] or a valvular defect. Why some patients should improve and others not is not known but it is possible that the development of a collateral circulation may ensue after several years thereby reducing the lymphoedema. Prolonged lymphoedema will lead to inflammation and fibroblastic proliferation ultimately leading to irreversible brawny oedema with the concomitant risk of superinfection.

Studies of the lymphatics with lymphangiography have shown a variety of abnormalities in patients with Noonan syndrome including aplasia and hypoplasia of lymphatic vessels and lymphangiectasia [8,9]. The webbing of the neck (pterygium colli) may be explained by the regression of the cystic hygromas following the correction of lymphatic obstruction or the formation of collateral lymphatic channels.

Other abnormalities include a low posterior hairline,

scant pubic and axillary hair, poor beard growth in males and hirsutism in females.

Diagnosis

The combination of the above clinical features with a normal karyotype confirms the diagnosis. Investigations must exclude cardiovascular abnormalities in particular pulmonary stenosis which may shorten life expectancy.

Prenatal diagnosis can identify cystic hygromas with ultrasound in the second trimester [10] and even in the first trimester [11]. This evidence, coupled with the evidence that cystic hygromas are associated with an elevated α-fetoprotein level, have lead many to believe that prenatal diagnosis by serial detailed ultrasonography beginning in the late first trimester or early second trimester, and by the measurement of the maternal α-fetoprotein, should be offered to couples with a previous child with Noonan syndrome [12]. Based on some studies which have suggested the mode of inheritance is autosomal dominant [12] such prenatal tests should be offered to relatives of affected individuals.

Treatment

Treatment is aimed at correcting any cardiovascular abnormalities. Any cutaneous lesions such as the webbed neck are amenable to intervention but it should be remembered that these patients have an increased susceptibility to keloid formation.

REFERENCES

1 Goodman RM. Familial lymphoedema of the Meige's type. *Am J Med* 1965; 32: 651–4.
2 Nora JJ, Nora AH, Sinha AK *et al.* The Ullrich–Noonan syndrome (Turner phenotype). *Am J Dis Child* 1974; 27: 48–55.
3 Bolton MR, Pugh DM, Mattiolo LF *et al.* The Noonan syndrome: a family study. *Ann Intern Med* 1974; 80: 626–9.
4 Ford CE, Ford KW, Polani PE *et al.* A sex chromosome anomaly in a case of gonadal dysgenesis (Turner's syndrome). *Lancet* 1959; i: 711–13.
5 Summitt RL. Turner syndrome and Noonan's syndrome. *J Pediatr* 1969; 74: 155–6.
6 Char F, Rodriguez-Fernandez HL, Scott CI *et al. The Noonan Syndrome—a Clinical Study of 45 Cases. Birth Defects Original Article Series*, vol. 8. New York: the National Foundation, 1972.
7 Alvin A, Diehl J, Lindsten J, Lodin A. Lymph vessel hypoplasia and chromosome aberrations in six patients with Turner's syndrome. *Acta Derm Venereol* 1967; 47: 25–33.
8 Smith S, Schulman A, Weir EK, Beatty DW, Joffe HS. Lymphatic abnormalities in Noonan syndrome. *S Afr Med J* 1979; 56: 271–4.
9 Hoeffel JC, Juncker P, Remy J. Lymphatic vessel dysplasia in Noonan syndrome. *Am J Radiol* 1980; 134: 399–401.
10 Frigoletto FD, Birholtz JC, Driscoll SG, Finberg HJ. Ultrasound diagnosis of cystic hygroma. *Am J Obstet Gynecol* 1980; 136: 962–4.
11 Gustavii B, Edvall E. First trimester diagnosis of cystic nuchal hygroma. *Acta Obstet Gynaecol Scand* 1984; 63: 377–8.
12 Witt DR, Hoyme E, Zonana J *et al.* Lymphoedema in Noonan syndrome: clues to pathogenesis and prenatal diagnosis and review of the literature. *Am J Med Gen* 1987; 27: 841–56.

Lymphangiomas

Lymphangiomas are malformations characterized by anastomosing lymphatic channels with cystic spaces [1].

Aetiology

As with cystic hygromas 60% are present at birth and about 90% are apparent by the end of the second year [2] and spontaneous regression is rare. Their aetiology remains unknown. They do, however, possess the ability to extend and penetrate through tissues and surrounding structures [3].

They were originally grouped into three by Wegner 1877 [4] and the classification has since remained as follows.
1 Lymphangioma simplex—capillary-sized lymphatic channels.
2 Cavernous lymphangioma—dilated lymphatic channels with a fibrous surrounding.
3 Cystic hygromas.

Clinical features [5]

Patients usually present due to the cosmetically disfiguring lesion which is usually asymptomatic. Pain may be attributable to infection or haemorrhage. Since the lesion is composed of tiny vesicles, fluid occasionally weeps from them. Unlike cystic hygromas cavernous lymphangiomas are surrounded by a fibrous stroma and therefore do not transilluminate. The overlying skin occasionally shows some discoloration which is either due to hemorrhage or haemangiomatous elements (so-called haemangiolymphangiomas). The lesion, which is usually solitary, enlarges in proportion to the child. Cavernous lymphangiomas usually give rise to an ill-defined swelling sometimes involving a large area of a limb. The swelling is usually due to a combination of both lymphoedema and abnormally dilated lymphatic channels. Since the diffuse lymphangiomas involve the larger lymphatics, vesicles may not be apparent clinically, and therefore although this condition is present from birth, it may go unnoticed for many years and only manifest itself when disturbed either by accidental injury, surgery or infection.

Pathology

Lymphangiomas are firmer than cystic hygromas and are made up of tiny cysts with a dense stroma of connective and lymphoid tissue [6]. Occasionally, dilated blood capillaries are interspersed within the lymphangioma producing a very vascular lesion prone to haemorrhage (lymphangiohaemangioma).

Treatment

Because of the small cysts present, needle aspiration and the injection of sclerosing solution is usually without effect [7]. Surgical excision is the most effective treatment modality and is normally left until the patient is older to minimize the risk of damage to vital structures. Resection may either be a definitive procedure or staged depending upon the depth of the lesion. Residual lesions may be left behind resulting in recurrent growth. Hill and Briggs [7] concluded that complete surgical excision of the lymphangioma was rarely followed by recurrence whilst partial excision had a high recurrent rate [7]. Other treatment options include the carbon dioxide laser which has been effective in treating lymphangiomas of the head and neck.

REFERENCES

1 Bill AH, Sumner DS. A unified concept of lymphangioma and cystic hygroma. *Surg Gynecol Obstet* 1965; 120: 79–86.
2 Gross RE. *The Surgery of Infancy and Childhood*. Philadelphia: WB Saunders, 1953.
3 Fonkalsrud EW. Lymphangioma in infancy and childhood. *Pediatr Dig* 1969; 11: 29–36.
4 Wegner G. Uber Lymphangiome. *Arch Klin Chir* 1877; 20: 641.
5 Hill JT, Briggs JD. Lymphangioma. *West J Surg Obstet Gynecol* 1961; 48: 811–15.
6 Harkins GA, Briggs JD. Lymphangioma. *Surgery* 1960; 48: 811–15.
7 Fonkalsrud EW. Congenital malformations of the lymphatic system. *Semin Pediatric Surg* 1994; 3: 62–9.

Lymphangioma circumscriptum

Definition

Lymphangioma circumscriptum is characterized by a circumscribed area of vesicles present at or soon after birth.

Aetiology

The aetiology of this condition remains unknown. Since the lesions are frequently seen primarily in the newborn or soon after [1] it has been postulated that the lesions arise as a result of lymph sacs which have failed to connect to the lymphatic channels during embryological development. Under normal development it is well recognized that the lymph sacs usually develop independently of the blood vessels and that they become interconnected later. If this hypothesis is to be accepted then it is assumed that these defunct lymph sacs branch out producing lymphatic channels towards the skin surface. This occurs as a direct result of pressure produced from the compression of the muscular wall lining the sacs.

These structures are not part of the general lymphatic circulation and therefore do not function as a drainage system for the skin. To account for the lack of oedema noted in these structures it is felt that there must be a compensatory increase in the dermal lymphatics to drain lymph. The presence of this dual lymphatic network which are not connected to one another—one functional and one functionless—has been shown using the injection of dye intradermally [1].

Clinical features

Lymphangioma circumscriptum is characterized clinically by the presence of vesicles within a circumscribed area of skin, usually filled with a colourless fluid (Fig. 18.3.1). They range in size up to 5mm in diameter. Frequently haemorrhage may occur into the vesicles producing a pink or frankly red appearance. This may occur spontaneously or secondary to trivial trauma. Lesions are present most commonly at birth or soon afterwards. The commonest site of involvement is the proximal part of the limbs.

They may be subdivided into classical and localized lymphangioma circumscriptum [2] based on the degree of involvement of the skin. Classic cases involve an area of skin-bearing vesicles of $1\,cm^2$ or more; additionally, there is often more diffuse swelling of the subcutaneous tissue whilst localized lymphangioma circumscriptum involves an area of $1\,cm^2$ or less. As expected classical lymphangioma circumscriptum is associated with more complications than the localized variety which includes bleeding, infection, pain and localized erythema. The development of a squamous cell carcinoma within congenital lymphangioma circumscriptum has been reported in an 82-year-old female [3].

Investigations

Lymphangiography has been carried out on patients with

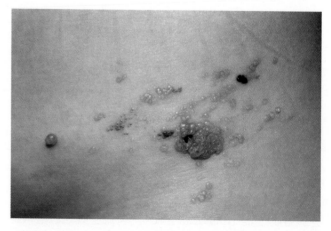

Fig. 18.3.1 Lymphangioma circumscriptum over the left flank in a young boy.

lymphangioma circumscriptum and shows the presence of a normal lymphatic network surrounding these sacs. No connection has been found between these individual lymph sacs and the normal lymphatics.

Treatment

There is no definitive treatment for this disorder and often it is best left untreated. Surgical excision is effective but incomplete excision is associated with a high relapse rate [2]. Other treatment modalities include CO_2, snow [4], liquid nitrogen, the use of sclerosants and local undercutting of the lesions [2] with mixed results.

REFERENCES

1 Whimster IW. The pathology of lymphangioma circumscriptum. *Br J Dermatol* 1976; 94: 473–86.
2 Peachey RDG, Lim CC, Whimster IW. Lymphangioma of skin. *Br J Dermatol* 1970; 83: 519–27.
3 Wilson GR, Cox NH, Mclean NR, Scott D. Squamous cell carcinoma arising within congenital lymphangioma circumscriptum. *Br J Dermatol* 1993; 129: 337–9.
4 Gant JQ Jr. Lymphangioma circumscriptum: successful treatment results with solid carbon dioxide. *Arch Dermatol* 1946; 54: 202–4.

Fetal cystic hygromas

Cystic hygromas (from the Greek term *hygros* meaning 'moist') develop from a defect in the formation of lymphatic vessels [1].

Aetiology

The fetal lymphatic vessels drain into two large sacs lateral to the jugular veins. These jugular lymph sacs eventually form communications with the venous system and become the terminal portion of the right lymphatic duct and thoracic duct [2]. If the lymphatic and venous structures fail to connect, the jugular lymph sacs enlarge and lymph accumulates in tissues forming cystic hygromas. These are typically located in the posterior triangle of the neck. If the jugular lymph sacs and the jugular veins ultimately connect then the cystic hygromas will regress and any peripheral oedema will resolve.

They are said to occur in approximately 1 in 12 000 births with an equal sex incidence. Around 60% are present at birth and 85% are detected before the end of the second year of life [3].

The combination of cystic hygromas, neck webbing and/or redundant posterior neck skin is frequently seen in fetuses with the 45XO karyotype (Turner's syndrome) [4]. Other chromosomal abnormalities have been reported with the same combination of lymphatic abnormalities including trisomy 18 [5], trisomy 21, fetal alcohol syndrome and trisomy 22 mosaicism. It remains unknown whether the redundant skin is a consequence of the hygroma or an independent finding.

Clinical features

These are uncommon tumours typically present at birth or in early infancy. They are typically located in the neck (Fig. 18.3.2) but have been reported in the popliteal fossa, retroperitoneal areas and in one case the groin, suggesting derivation from an embryonic iliac lymph sac. The present as single or multiloculated fluid-filled cavities, and present as soft, brilliantly translucent swellings. The cysts may vary from a few millimetres to a few centimetres. About one-third of cystic hygromas will enlarge as a result of infection or haemorrhage producing a tender swelling with a bluish hue. The enlargement of the cyst may produce compression of neighbouring structures such as the spinal accessory nerve leading to sudden shoulder drop. Its extension cephalically may occasionally result in stridor, cyanosis and apnoea although this is most uncommon.

Pathology

The wall of the cyst is lined by endothelial cells with occa-

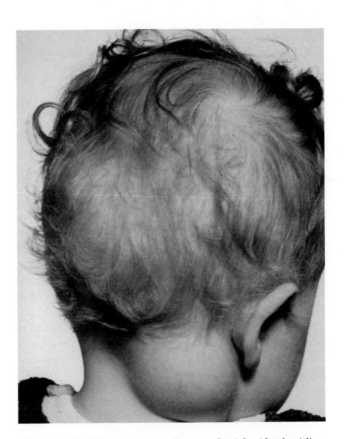

Fig. 18.3.2 Cystic hygroma presenting over the right side of a girl's neck. Courtesy of Professor Sir N Browse, St Thomas's Hospital, London.

sional lymphocytes and varying amounts of fibrous stroma. There may be focal areas of thrombosis and although rare internal haemorrhage may result from trauma such as birth.

Diagnosis

Cystic hygromas may be diagnosed reliably by ultrasound [6–8] with a characteristic posterolateral position and cystic appearance. The larger hygromas are often divided by fibrous septa and sometimes have a dense midline septum in the neck region. It is important to differentiate the cystic hygroma from other craniocervical masses including encephalocele, cystic teratoma and nuchal oedema. The diagnosis is confirmed by finding an intact skull and spinal column, the cystic nature of the lesion, the presence of septa and a relatively fixed position of the mass relative to the head. Other experimental tools include the measurement of α-feto protein levels prenatally in the amniotic fluid which in some series have been consistently elevated [7]. The cause for this elevation in α-fetoprotein remains unknown but one hypothesis includes the transudation of the protein through oedematous skin or bowel mucosa into the amniotic sac. However, whether the levels measured will enable clinicians to distinguish cystic hygromas from central nervous system abnormalities has yet to be determined.

Treatment

Once a diagnosis of cystic hygroma is made a detailed ultrasonic search should be made for evidence of pleural effusions and ascites [9]. Additional assessment of both renal and cardiac development is also needed. If cystic hygroma is associated with hydrops then the chance of survival is small. It is also necessary to determine the karyotype of the fetus for genetic counselling purposes. Treatment of the isolated cystic hygroma [2,10] is either by aspiration and injection of sclerosants such as bleomycin and OK-432 with the potential risk of recurrence and/or infection. Any subsequent surgical procedure is technically more difficult. Alternatively, careful excision may be the definitive procedure [11]. This is usually deferred until the patient is over 2 months old unless the lesion is compromising respiration. Due to their benign nature there is no indication to excise nerves or muscles. Recurrences tend to become evident within 3 months and are usually managed with sclerosing therapy.

Prognosis

Spontaneous remission is rare. There are no major sequelae to cystic hygromas.

REFERENCES

1 Young AE. Lymphatic malformations. In: Malliken JB, Young AE, eds. *Vascular Birthmarks. Haemangiomas and Malformations*. Philadelphia: WB Saunders, 1988.
2 Bill AH Jr, Sumner DS. A unified concept of lymphangioma and cystic hygroma. *Surg Gynecol Obstet*: 1965; 120: 79–86.
3 Chait D, Yonkers AJ, Beddoe M *et al.* Management of cystic hygromas. *Surg Gynecol Obstet* 1974; 139: 55–8.
4 Singh RP, Carr DH. The anatomy and histology of XO human embryos and fetuses. *Anat Rec* 1986; 155: 369–83.
5 Hodes ME, Cole J, Palmer CG *et al.* Clinical experience with trisomies 18 and 13. *J Med Genet* 1978; 15: 48–60.
6 Shaub M, Wilson R, Collea J. Fetal cystic lymphangioma (cystic hygroma): prepartum ultrasonic findings. *Radiology* 1976; 121: 449–50.
7 Adam AH, Robinson HP, Aust F *et al.* Prenatal diagnosis of fetal lymphatic abnormalities by ultrasound. *J Clin Ultrasound* 1979; 7: 361–4.
8 Young LW. Radiological case of the month. *Am J Dis Child* 1980; 134: 311–12.
9 Chervenak FA, Isaacson G, Blakemore KJ *et al.* Fetal cystic hygroma. *N Engl J Med* 1983; 309: 822–5.
10 Fonkalsrud EW. Surgical management of congenital malformations of the lymphatic system. *Am J Surg* 1974; 128: 152–9.
11 Gross RE. *The Surgery of Infancy and Childhood*. Philadelphia: WB Saunders, 1953.

Lymphoedema

Definition

Lymphoedema is the accumulation of lymph in the interstitial spaces caused by a fault in lymphatic drainage.

Aetiology

Lymphoedema results from a disturbance in the equilibrium between the load to be cleared from the interstitial space and the transport capacity of the clearing system, namely the lymphatic network. It is subdivided into primary and secondary causes, depending on the underlying aetiology.

Primary lymphoedema

The predominant defect in the primary lymphoedemas is in the lymphatic vessels as has been shown by lymphography [1,2]. No identifiable cause for this defect can be found. The lymphoedemas can be subdivided depending upon where the abnormality lies. Wolfe has classified the primary lymphoedemas by their lymphographic appearance [3]. His studies revealed four patterns as follows.
1 Distal hypoplasia in which the distal lymph vessels are too small and too few.
2 Proximal hypoplasia in which the proximal lymphatics are quantitatively or qualitatively abnormal with small fibrotic inguinal nodes.
3 Distal and proximal hypoplasia: a combination of the above.
4 Hyperplasia in which numerous tortuous lymphatics with large nodes present in the groin.

Approximately one-third of all cases are secondary to agenesis, hypoplasia or obstruction of the distal lymphatics with relatively normal proximal vessels [4]. The prognosis in this group is good. The degree of involvement is established early in the disease in about 40% of patients and therefore other parts of the body are rarely affected. However, the girth of the involved limb continues to increase over time.

In over half of the cases the primary defect involves the proximal lymphatics. In this group the extent and degree of the abnormality is more likely to progress and ultimately to require some surgical intervention.

Subtypes

Primary lymphoedema is most commonly seen in children. Clinical forms have been classified into three main groups depending upon the clinical presentation as follows.

1 Lymphoedema congenita [4] (Fig. 18.3.3) usually manifests at birth or shortly afterwards.

2 Lymphoedema praecox [5] (Fig. 18.3.4) presents with lymphoedema later in life usually at puberty although by definition before the age of 35 years.

3 Lymphoedema tarda presents after the age of 35 years.

Structural abnormality in the lymphatics

The severity of the underlying lymphatic abnormality is reflected in the age of onset of the lymphoedema [6].

1 The complete absence of lymphatic collectors usually presents with lymphoedema at birth (lymphoedema congenita).

2 Lymphatic hypoplasia refers to lymphatics which are fewer and smaller in number. These lymphatics under normal circumstances can clear a fluid load but under pathological conditions, such as following an infection, the lymphatics become overloaded and lymphoedema is manifest clinically. This is the cause seen most frequently in the commonest form of primary lymphoedema (praecox) and is confirmed on lymphography. Whether this reflects a poorly developed lymphatic network present from birth or a network that undergoes premature atrophy or ageing following injury or disruption such as that caused by infection remains undetermined.

3 Lymphatic varicosities are akin to venous varicosities and refer to a lymphatic network that is unaffected quantitatively but altered qualitatively resulting in dilated and tortuous vessels. These then probably lead to thrombosis in the vessels and lymphangitis. If the channels are grossly dilated as a result of incompetent valves then megalymphatics may ensue. This type is seen with lymphoedema tarda.

4 Obstruction to lymph flow along the subcutaneous lymphatics will result in a failure of forward flow of lymph. This will ultimately lead to retrograde filling of the subepidermal lymphatic plexus.

Incidence

Primary lymphoedema occurs in approximately 1 in

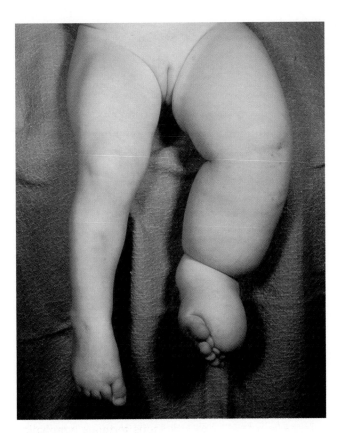

Fig. 18.3.3 Lymphoedema congenita affecting the lower leg of a young girl.

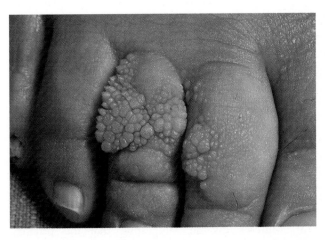

Fig. 18.3.4 Lymphoedema praecox: marked papillomatosis and skin thickening over the toes.

10000 people less than 20 years of age, with a female preponderance [7,8].

Investigations

A lack of sensitive methods of investigation makes it difficult to distinguish the exact cause of the lymphoedema. Investigations such as lymphangiograms are technically very difficult to perform in children and as a result are infrequently used for diagnostic purposes.

Clinical features

Congenital lymphoedema most often involves the dorsum of the foot, occasionally extending above the knee. Very occasionally it may occur in the upper extremities. In children who have involvement of the upper limbs there tends to be lymphoedema of other parts of the body such as their external genitalia [7]. The overlying skin can be normal and the hypertrophic changes seen in the later onset lymphoedemas may be absent.

The onset of the swelling in patients without congenital lymphoedema is usually insidious and fluctuant. Typically the swelling is more pronounced at the end of the day and does not decrease overnight.

Milroy's disease

Milroy, an American doctor, described a series of patients in 1892 in whom oedema was present from birth. The oedema was described as a non-tender chronic swelling of the lower extremities and typically did not affect the general health of the patients in any way [9]. This condition had been described previously by Nonne in 1891 [10] and Lettessier in 1865 [11] but it was Milroy who outlined the diagnostic criteria and studied the disease in the greatest detail.

Aetiology

Genetic studies suggest that it is inherited as an autosomal dominant trait with complete penetrance but variable expressivity [9] with an equal sex incidence. The aetiology of Milroy's disease remains unknown. Some authors have suggested that the lymphoedema may be a direct consequence of an increased arteriolar filtration [11]; however, this theory remains unproven and further studies suggest that the increased arteriolar blood flow is a secondary event to the oedema [12] from any cause. More recently, lymphography [13,14] to assess the lymphatics in patients has shown aplasia and hypoplasia in the affected limb of patients with Milroy's disease, suggesting that the primary defect is a congenital deficiency of viable lymphatics. Further studies with fluoresence microlymphography

have confirmed the complete absence of lymphatics [15].

Clinical features

The term Milroy's disease is often applied loosely to many different types of lymphoedema, but Milroy's disease as a cause of lymphoedema remains rare provided the correct criteria for diagnosis are adhered too. The incidence in one study was reported to be 3.4% of patients with lymphoedema, making it the smallest and rarest of the subgroups of primary lymphoedema [13]. The diagnostic criteria are as follows.
1 Chronic oedema, firm but pitting.
2 Affecting one or both of the lower extremities, the area involved is variable.
3 It must be present at birth or soon after.
4 It is permanent.
5 There is a positive family history.
6 There is no constitutional upset and it is compatible with life.
However, Milroy recognized three exceptions namely [16,17]:
1 A case where presentation occurred at puberty.
2 Additional involvement at age 20 following a fracture.
3 Scrotal involvement with spontaneous recovery of an affected foot.
In has been postulated that these 'exceptions' in fact represent lymphoedema praecox not true Milroy's disease.

Investigations

The diagnosis is made on clinical findings. Lymphography may additionally help in highlighting the principal defect, which in the vast majority of cases is hypoplasia of the distal lymphatics of the lower limbs and fibrosis of the lymph nodes as noted on inguinal node biopsy [7]. The degree of hypoplasia may range from aplasia to mild absence of the more proximal lymphatics which accounts for the variable prognosis of patients.

REFERENCES

1 Gough MH. Primary lymphodema: clinical and lymphangiographic studies. *Br J Surg* 1966; 53: 917–25.
2 Kinmonth JB, Eustace PW. Lymph nodes and lymph vessels in primary lymphoedema: their relative importance in aetiology. *Ann Roy Coll Surg Engl* 1976; 58: 278–84.
3 Wolfe JHN. The prognosis and possible cause of severe primary lymphoedema. *Ann Roy Coll Surg Engl* 1984; 66: 1172–4.
4 Allen EV. Lymphoedema of the extremities: classification, aetiology and differential diagnosis: a study of 300 cases. *Arch Intern Med* 1934; 54: 606–24.
5 Lewis JM, Wald ER. Lymphoedema preacox. *J Paediatr* 1984; 104: 641–8.
6 Kinmonth JB. Primary lymphoedema: clinical and lymphangiographic studies of 107 patients in which the lower limbs were affected. *Br J Surg* 1957; 45: 1–10.

7 Kinmonth JB, Wolfe JH. Fibrosis in the lymph nodes in primary lymphoedema. *Ann Roy Coll Surg Engl* 1980; 62: 344–54.

8 Browse NL. The diagnosis and management of primary lymphoedema. *Vasc Surg* 1986; 3: 181–4.

9 Esterly JR. Congenital hereditary lymphoedema. *J Med Genet* 1965; 2: 93–8.

10 Nonne M. Vier Falle von Elephantiasis Congentia Hereditaria. *Virchows Arch Pathol Anat* 1891; 125: 189.

11 Schroeder E, Helweg-Larsen HF. Chronic hereditary lymphoedema (Nonne–Milroy–Meige's disease). *Acta Med Scand* 1950; 137: 198–216.

12 Harrison TR, Pilcher C. Studies in congestive heart failure. *J Clin Invest* 1930; 8: 261–315.

13 Kinmonth JB. *The Lymphatics: Surgery, Lymphography and Diseases of the Chyle and Lymph Systems*, 2nd edn. London: Arnold, 1982.

14 Kinmonth JB, Taylor GW, Tracey GD, Marsh JD. Primary lymphoedema. *Br J Surg* 1957; 45: 1–10.

15 Bollinger A, Jaker K, Sgier J. Fluorescence microlymphography. *Circulation* 1981; 64: 1195–200.

16 Milroy WF. An undescribed variety of hereditary oedema. *N Y Med J* 1892; 56: 101–8.

17 Milroy WF. Chronic hereditary oedema: Milroy's Disase. *J Am Med Assoc* 1928; 91: 1172.

Secondary lymphoedema

Damage to the lymphatic channels may occur secondary to any number of causes. Typically secondary lymphoedema is uncommon in children but may occur as a result of surgical removal or radiation of lymph nodes for cancer treatment. Cancers that can result in lower limb swelling include melanoma, sarcoma and pelvic tumours. Lymphoproliferative tumours rarely cause lymphatic obstruction.

Trauma to the lymphatics may lead to lymphoedema. However, extensive trauma is needed to induce permanent lymphoedema due to the efficient regenerative powers of the lymphatics. This regeneration is impeded following scarring.

Filiarasis is considered to be the commonest cause of secondary lymphoedema worldwide. It occurs as a result of infection with the nematode worm (*Wucheria bancroftii*) which is transmitted by the mosquito through direct inoculation of the skin with microfilariae. These larvae migrate and mature in the lymphatics into adult worms leading to progressive damage to these vessels and ultimately causing lymphoedema.

Managing lymphoedema

Complications

Lymphoedema has three main consequences.

1 Swelling (oedema).

2 An increased susceptibility to infection of the involved area of skin.

3 A small but recognized risk of malignancy arising within the lymphoedematous skin.

The inadequate drainage of lymph from a limb produces oedema and characteristic changes in the skin. The swelling results in discomfort, limb heaviness and decreased mobility with a limitation in function. Ulti-mately patients may develop musculoskeletal problems due to an abnormally increased weight in the limbs [1]. Skin changes noted include thickening of the skin as shown by Stemmer's sign—a failure to pinch a fold of skin at the base of the second toe. Further changes include the development of exaggerated skin creases and hyperkeratosis [2]. Because of the lymphatic insufficiency there is dilatation of the upper dermal lymphatics giving rise to thin-walled blisters (lymphangiomas) which are prone to rupture and weep.

Cellulitis is a frequent complication of long-standing lymphoedema, recurrent episodes further impair lymph drainage and thereby exacerbate the lymphoedema. This can be very debilitating for the patient sometimes necessitating long-term prophylactic antibiotics. The aetiology of these recurrent infections are thought to be related to a failure of local immune mechanisms to respond to a bacterial organism [3]. Clinically patients may occasionally have a prodrome of a flu-like illness and within 24h they develop redness and tenderness in the lymphoedematous area. Often an organism cannot be isolated and some authors have questioned whether this is genuine cellulitis [4] or an inflammatory reaction.

Management

Successful treatment of lymphoedema requires close collaboration between the patient and the clinician. The patient should be informed of the diagnosis and the treatment programme and any psychological impact of the disease should be attended to though this is often neglected [5].

Prevention of inflammation

It is important to emphasize to the patient or parents the need for meticulous care of the skin; this is especially important in children, who commonly sustain abrasions and minor injuries to their limbs. Good hygiene, control of fungal infection between the digits and good antisepsis following trauma is vital. An emollient should be applied twice daily to avoid drying and fissuring of the skin. Trauma should be avoided as much as is feasible. The feet should be covered when ambulatory and a podiatrist should attend to nail care as needed. Prophylactic antibiotics have a role particularly in patients who encounter repeated inflammatory episodes.

Control and the reduction of the oedema can only be addressed if the physiology of the lymphoedema is understood: the movement of lymph from interstitial space into the non-contractile vessels and then along initial lymphatics relies upon changes in tissue pressure and can therefore be influenced by external massage [6,7], arterial pulsation [8] and passive movements [9]. The lymph then progresses into the contractile lymph vessels. Valves are present to ensure unidirectional flow. The contraction of the vessels is stimulated by the distension of the vessels in a manner similar to the heart. The propulsion of lymph through these collectors is influenced by exercise. Therefore application of measures known to enhance lymph drainage under normal conditions will help patients with congenital lymphoedemas by allowing an improved drainage through existing vessels and collaterals.

Massage

If performed correctly massage will encourage the movement of lymph through the intercommunicating network of skin and subcutaneous lymphatics to normally drained areas [10]. This is the principle of manual lymphatic drainage which is practised in many parts of Europe [11]. It is important that the patient is taught how to perform the technique since if it is too vigorous the resultant higher blood flow will lead to increased capillary filtration and exacerbate the condition. Other treatments employed to influence lymph return through the collateral circulation include the use of pneumatic compression therapy [11,12].

Exercise

Exercise is crucial to improve lymph drainage. Dynamic muscle contractions (isotonic exercises) have a dual function, both increasing absorption of lymph into the non-contractile vessels and increasing propulsion of lymph through the contractile vessels. Again as with massage this should be controlled to avoid an increase in capillary filtration and a deterioration in the oedema.

External support

It is vital to encourage the wearing of adequate hosiery. The principle of hosiery is (a) to create a counterforce to underlying muscle pumps; and (b) to normalize capillary function. The use of the highest compression strength (>40 mmHg) is recommended. Such garments last less than a few months in the young physically active person. This is the most effective means of controlling the acquired lymphangiomas seen at the sites of lymphoedema.

Drug therapy

Drug therapy is generally disappointing. The most commonly used drugs are the diuretics. However, these drugs have very little proven benefit in lymphoedema since their principle action is to reduce capillary filtration by reducing blood volume.

The Rutoside group of drugs has been advocated for lymphoedema. However, doses of Paroven up to 3 g daily for 6 months have shown little benefit in patients with postmastectomy lymphoedema [13]. Clinical trials using benzopyrones have shown benefit in certain forms of lymphodema [14]. More recently human work exploring the use of intra-arterial infusions of autologous lymphocytes have demonstrated promising results in oedema reduction [15].

Surgery

The use of surgical manoeuvres in treating lymphoedema has a limited role. They are considered as options if, despite all conservative measures, the limb remains so large or heavy that it interferes with the patient's mobility in an unacceptable way. It involves either the removal of excess tissue or the reconstruction of the lymphatics, bypassing the abnormality. Overall patient satisfaction with reduction surgery is good and only 20% report poor outcomes from surgery [16], although this is a selected group. Four types of excisional operation have been described [17] all aiming to reduce the size of the limb. Essentially the operations involve the excision of a large wedge of skin together with the subcutaneous tissue, which is either closed primarily or a skin flap or graft is used.

Lymphatic bypass

A number of methods have been tried to unite obstructed lymphatics with the venous system, thereby bypassing the obstruction [18,19]. These have a variable success rate in patients with secondary lymphoedemas where the obstruction can be identified. More recently, flaps of tissue rich in lymphatics have been implanted into the oedematous region [20]. The idea was that if the lymphatic vessels in the flaps remain functional they may eventually anastomose with the surrounding lymphatics and provide an alternative pathway for drainage from the oedematous region. The long-term success of this procedure has yet to be determined [21].

Malignancy

The patient should be alerted to report any changes noted in the limb because of the recognized risk of malignant transformation within the lymphoedematous limb [22]. Angiosarcoma and lymphangiosarcoma are potentially devastating but fortunately uncommon complications of long-standing lymphoedema occurring in less than 1% of cases [23–25]. Early detection and amputation can be life-saving, but recognition is often delayed. Other malignancies which have been reported in association with lymphoedema include squamous cell carcinoma and malignant melanoma [26–29].

REFERENCES

1 Mortimer PS, Regnard C. Lymphostatic disorders. *Br Med J* 1986; 1: 293.
2 Mortimer PS. Investigation and management of lymphoedema. *Vasc Med Rev* 1990; 1: 1–20.
3 Mortimer PS. Lymphoedema. *Surgery* 1996: 73–7.
4 Casley-Smith JR. Discussion of the definition, diagnosis and treatment of lymphoedema (lymphostatic disorder). In: Casley-Smith JR, Piller NB, eds. *Progress in Lymphology, Proceedings of the Xth International Congress of Lymphology*. South Australia: University of Adelaide Press, 1985: 1–16.
5 Smeltzer DM, Stickler GB, Schirger A. Primary lymphoedema in children and adolescents: a follow-up study and review. *Pediatrics* 1985; 76: 206–18.
6 Calnan JS, Pflug J, Reis ND, Taylor LM. Lymphatic pressures and the flow of lymph. *Br J Plast Surg* 1970; 23: 305–17.
7 Olszewski WL. *Peripheral Lymph: Formation and Immune Function*. Florida: CRC Press, 1985.
8 Parsons RJ, McMaster PD. The effect of the pulse upon the formation and flow of lymph. *J Exp Med* 1938; 68: 353–76.
9 Jacobsson S. Lymph flow from the lower leg in man. *Acta Chir Scand* 1967; 133: 79–81.
10 Hall JG, Morris B, Woolley G. Intrinsic rhythmic propulsion of lymph in unanesthetised sheep. *J Physiol* 1965; 180: 336–49.
11 Pohjola RT, Kolari PJ, Pekanhaki K. Intermittent pneumatic compression for lymphoedema. A comparison of two treatment modes. In: Partsch H, ed. *Progress in Lymphology*, vol XI. Amsterdam: Excerta Medica, 1988: 583–6.
12 Anonymous. Compression for lymphoedema. *Lancet* 1986; 1: 89.
13 Mortimer PS, Badger C, Clarke I, Pallett J. A double blind randomized, parallel group, placebo-controlled trial of *O*-(*b*-hydroxyethyl)-rutosides in chronic arm oedema resulting from breast cancer treatment. *Phlebology* 1995; 10: 51–5.
14 Casley-Smith JR, Morgan RG, Piller NB. Treatment of lymphoedema of the arms and legs with 5,6-benzo-(~)-pyrones. *N Engl J Med* 1993; 329: 1158–63.
15 Nagata Y, Murata R, Mitsumori M *et al*. Intra-arterial infusion of autologous lymphocytes for the treatment of refractory lymphoedema. *Eur J Surg* 1994; 160: 105–9.
16 Sakulsky SB. Lymphoedema: results of surgical treatment in 64 patients (1936–1984). *Lymphology* 1977; 10: 15–26.
17 Sistrunk WE. Further experiences with Kondoleon operation for elephantiasis. *J Am Med Assoc* 1918; 71: 800–6.
18 O'Brien BMcC, Schfiroff BB. Microlymphaticovenous and reconstructive surgery in obstructive lymphoedema. *World J Surg* 1979; 3: 3–15.
19 Nieuborg L. *The role of lymphaticovenous anastomosis in the treatment of postmastectomy oedema*. MD thesis, University of Amsterdam, 1982.
20 Savage RC. The surgical management of lymphoedema. *Surg Gynaecol Obstet* 1984; 160: 283–90.
21 Hurst PAE *et al*. Long-term results of the enteromesenteric bridge operation in the treatment of primary lymphoedema. *Br J Surg* 1985; 72: 272–4.
22 Alessi E, Sala F, Berti E. Angiosarcoma in lymphoedematous limbs. *Am J Dermatopathol* 1986; 8: 371–8.
23 Schmitz-Rixen T *et al*. Angiosarcoma in primary lymphoedema of the lower extremity—Stewart–Treves syndrome. *Lymphology* 1984; 17: 50–3.
24 Servelle M. Surgical treatment of lymphoedema: a report of 652 cases. *Surgery* 1987; 101: 485–95.
25 Woodward AH, Ivins JC, Soulf EH. Lymphangiosarcoma arising in chronic lymphoedematous extremities. *Cancer* 1972; 30: 562–8.
26 Tatnall FM, Mann BS. Non-Hodgkin's lymphoma of the skin associated with chronic limb lymphoedema. *Br J Dermatol* 1985; 113: 751–6.
27 Ruocco V *et al*. Kaposi's sarcoma in a lymphoedematous immunocompromised arm. *Int J Dermatol* 1984; 23: 56–60.
28 Epstein JL, Mendelsohn G. Squamous carcinoma of the foot arising in association with long-standing verrucous hyperplasia in a patient with congenital lymphoedema. *Cancer* 1984; 1: 943–7.
29 Bartal AH, Pinsky CM. Malignant melanoma appearing in post mastectomy lymphoedematous arm. A novel association of double primary tumours. *J Surg Oncol* 1985; 30: 316–18.

Lymphangitis

Acute lymphangitis

The role of the lymphatic network is to remove any noxious substances effectively, thereby preventing any further spread into the general circulation. Occasionally the lymphatics may be overloaded with a large infectious load leading to overt lymphangitis and even lymphadenitis. Lymphangitis represents inflammation of the lymphatic collectors and presents with tender red streaks passing up the limb which correspond to the inflamed vessels. Particularly on the medial side of the leg and thigh this presents as a diffuse erythema and distinction from an ascending cellulitis may be difficult. Usually any infection is limited by the lymph nodes which clinically manifest as painful swellings in the groin (lymphadenitis). Constitutional upset may be significant and is generally greater the more proximal the infection has extended.

Lymphatic tumours

Acquired progressive lymphangioma (benign lymphangioendothelioma)

This is a benign tumour which differs from simple acquired lymphangiomas clinically and histopathologically [1,2]. It presents as a reddish or bruise-like plaque which usually is located on the anterior abdominal wall, thigh or calf. Typically, the condition affects adolescents. It is usually localized, flat and grows slowly. It is thought to originate from lymphatic endothelium and therefore resembles a low-grade sarcoma or Kaposi's sarcoma histologically with anastomosing dilated channels which dissect collagen bundles and are lined by swollen endothelial cells but which are without cellular atypia.

Lymphangiomatosis

Diffuse lymphangiomas that slowly progress to an intrinsic proliferative process are termed lymphangiomatosis. They are indistinguishable from lymphangioma simplex histologically. The diagnosis is suggested by the slow progression and the infiltration of surrounding structures including bone. Typically it presents in children and in a large proportion of cases is confined to one limb [3]. Involvement of visceral organs is associated with a poor prognosis [4].

Maffucci's syndrome [5]

This is a diffuse haemolymphangiomatosis accompanied by severe widespread deformities of bone and cartilage. The lymphangiomas do not appear on lymphography to communicate with the main lymphatic pathways and often possess both blood vascular and lymphatic elements. As well as the vascular swellings patients develop firm nodules extending out from bones particularly the fingers and toes. These are enchondromas and are radiologically translucent. This disease has a high malignant potential including lymphangiosarcoma.

Chylous reflux

Chyle is a milky lymph which flows from the lacteals of the gut through the cisterna chyli and then through the thoracic duct. The appearance of chylous lymphangiomas is the commonest method of presentation in the lower limb, most commonly the thigh and perineum. Milky vesicles containing chyle may manifest in the skin at any point from toe to genitalia and are nearly always associated with lymphoedema.

Such forms of lymphoedema [6] develop early in life and subsequently chylous lymphangiomas appear. In most cases the condition tends to progress with increasing oedema and more chylous lymphangiomas. This may be because the downforce of lymph/chyle gradually undermines the function of more distal lymphatic valves. For chyle to appear in the leg it must reflux either from the point the cisterna chyli joins the retroperitoneal lymphatics or through fistulae adjoining the cisterna chyli with pelvic lymphatics. Lymphography usually shows incompetent megalymphatics, i.e. large, varicose main lymph trunks in which the valves are absent or totally incompetent. No obstruction is identified except in the thoracic duct in some cases.

The early age of onset, the association with congenital vascular anomalies such as cutaneous angiomas, and the demonstration of aberrant lymph pathways in the abdomen all suggest an embryological fault in development.

Treatment of chylous reflux into the lower limb is by surgery as no conservative/medical treatment offers any hope of cure. A low-fat diet will help to alleviate symptoms by reducing the volume of chyle. Surgical manoeuvres include (a) ligation of incompetent abdominal pathways; and (b) ligation of lymphatics in the groin or lumbar region. Once the reflux is controlled standard physical therapy measures should contain the lymphoedema.

REFERENCES

1 Wilson-Jones E, Winkelmann RK, Zachary CB et al. Benign lymphangioendothelioma. *J Am Acad Dermatol* 1990; 23: 229–34.
2 Meunier L, Barneon G, Meynadier J. Acquired progressive lymphangioma. *Br J Dermatol* 1996; 131: 706–8.
3 Sing H, Gomez C, Calonde E et al. Lymphangiomatosis of the limbs: clinicopathologic analysis of a series with a good prognosis. *Am J Surg Pathol* 1995; 19: 125–33.
4 Ramani P, Shah A. Lymphangiomatosis, histological and immunohistochemical analysis of four cases. *Am J Surg Pathol* 1992; 16: 764–71.
5 Carlton A, Elkington J StC, Greenfield JG et al. Maffucci's syndrome. *Q J Med* 1942; 11: 203–10.
6 Kinmonth JB. *Lymphatics, Lymphology and Diseases of the Chyle and Lymph Systems*, 2nd edn, London: Edward Arnold, 1982.

Cheilitis granulomatosa (orofacial granulomatosis)

Definition

Granulomatous cheilitis is a rare disorder characterized by the progressive and relentless enlargement of both lips.

Aetiology

Cheilitis granulomatosa was first described by Miescher [1] in 1945. He described six cases who presented with the sudden onset and subsequent chronic enlargement of the lips. The histology in these cases showed banal inflammation with granulomatous changes simulating sarcoidosis. Prior to this, such changes had been seen in a number of cases and were called a mixture of names including 'solid oedema' and 'cheilitis glandularis'. Melkersson [2] in 1928 had described a constellation of symptoms which had included chronic lip swelling present for up to 20 years previously, other features described included facial nerve palsy. Two years later Rosenthal [3] added scrotal tongue to the syndrome. This triad is now referred to as the Melkersson–Rosenthal syndrome. Some patients who present solely with granulomatous cheilitis are believed to represent an abortive or the early phase of this syndrome.

The exact aetiology remains unknown, an infectious cause has been proposed but no solid evidence has emerged to support this theory [4]. A genetic cause has not been excluded since siblings may be affected and solitary features such as the scrotal tongue may be present in other relatives. An association with Crohn's disease has been well documented in the literature [5]. In some cases the granulomatous cheilitis occurs as a localized form of Crohn's disease or is followed by ileal Crohn's disease many years later [6].

Pathology

Biopsy of a swollen lip reveals oedema and a perivascular lymphocytic infiltrate. Additional findings include noncaseating granuloma that are perivascular in distribution making them indistinguishable from Crohn's disease [6] or sarcoidosis [7]. Others have shown such granulomas in the lymphatic walls suggesting that the resulting lymphangitis [8] plays a role in the pathogenesis of the condition. Whether it is an infectious element or some other stimulant that provokes granuloma formation and leads to lymphatic damage remains undetermined. The lymphatic channels have not been studied extensively in this condition but it is felt by many that the persistent swelling and the limited response to treatment is a reflection of the lymphatic damage.

Clinical features

The early feature of this condition is the sudden onset of diffuse swelling of the lips, usually the upper lip is involved first (Fig. 18.3.5). Other sites distal to the lips including the forehead and eyelids have also been reported as early features of the disorder [9]. Generally the surrounding skin is of a normal colour although the mucous membranes may be intensely erythematous [10]. Initial signs may suggest angioneurotic oedema; however, the persistence over days with recurrent attacks which become more frequent makes this diagnosis unlikely. Gradually the lip takes on the consistency of rubber which may regress over a period of years. Other symptoms include scaling, fissuring and vesicles which are present over the vermillion border. Subjective symptoms are usually absent at the beginning although tenderness on pressure may be felt. Patients are typically afebrile and in good health although mild constitutional upset has been reported.

The scrotal tongue occurs in around 30% of cases and is associated with a loss of taste and reduced salivary secretion. Lower motor palsy of the seventh nerve may develop in about the same number of cases. It may occur at any stage of the cheilitis, but like the cheilitis it is intermittent and may sometimes be bilateral [11].

Diagnosis

The diagnosis of the Melkersson–Rosenthal syndrome is readily made in the presence of the triad of facial palsy, granulomatous cheilitis and scrotal tongue. The presence of the lip swelling alone may sometimes be difficult to dif-ferentiate from angioneurotic oedema; however, the persistence of oedema between attacks and the typical histology, if present, may help to confirm the diagnosis.

Treatment

Spontaneous recovery may occur but relapse can also occur many years after the condition has cleared [12]. There remains no effective treatment for this condition. Clofazimine, a phenazine iminoquinone derivative, at a dosage of 100 mg daily for 10 days followed by 200–400 mg weekly has been tried with reported benefit [13]. Neuhofer and Fritsch [13] in their study reported an excellent initial response after 2 weeks in patients with a fluctuant swelling. However, in those in whom the swelling was more persistent there was a slower response. There was a 50% relapse rate upon stopping treatment but these cases responded upon reintroduction of the clofazimine. The total duration of the treatment was 5–7 months. Its mode of action is unclear; however, it has been suggested that it may incite phagocytosis [13]. Further studies have confirmed the effectiveness of clofazimine in the treatment of cheilitis granulomatosa [14]. Other treatment modalities that have been tried include intralesional steroid injections with a variable response, often requiring repeated injections at regular intervals. The mix of combined intralesional injections with surgical reduction (cheiloplasty) has been effective in some studies [15–17], but the intralesional injections must be continued for sometime afterwards to prevent a rebound of the condition.

REFERENCES

1 Miescher G. Uber essentielle granulomatose Makrocheilie (cheilitis granulomatosa). *Dermatologica* 1945; 91: 57–85.
2 Melkersson E. Case of recurrent facial paralysis with angioneurotic oedema. *Hygiea* 1928; 90: 737–41.
3 Rosenthal C. Klinish-erbbiologischer Beitrag zur Konstitutionspathologie: Gemeinsame Auftreten von Facial isiahmung, Angioneurotischem Gesichtodem und Lingua plicata in Arthritismus-Familien. *Zentralbl Neurol Psychiatr* 1931; 131: 475–80.
4 Alpert B, Nelson R. Cheilitis granulomatosa: report of a case. *J Oral Surg* 1974; 32: 60–1.
5 Carr D. Granulomatous cheilitis in Crohn's disease. *Br Med J* 1974; 4: 636.
6 Talbot T, Jewell L, Schloss E *et al*. Cheilitis antedating Crohn's disease. Case report and literature review. *J Clin Gastroenterol* 1984; 6: 349–54.
7 Shedale SA, Foulds IS. Granulomatous cheilitis and a positive kveim test. *Br J Dermatol* 1986; 115: 619–22.
8 Nozicka Z. Endovasal granulomatous lymphangitis as a pathogenetic factor in cheilitis granulomatous. *J Oral Pathol* 1985; 14: 363–5.
9 Laymon CW. Cheilitis granulomatosa and Melkersson–Rosenthal syndrome. *Arch Dermatol* 1961; 83: 112–18.
10 Worsaae N, Christensen KC, Schiodt M. Melkersson–Rosenthal syndrome and cheilitis granulomatosa. *Oral Surg* 1982; 54: 404–13.
11 Graff-Radford SB. Melkersson–Rosenthal syndrome. *S Afr Med J* 1984; 60: 71–4.
12 Wadlington WB, Riley H, Lowbeer L. The Melkersson–Rosenthal syndrome. *Paedatrics* 1984; 73: 502–6.
13 Neuhofer J, Fritsch P. Cheilitis granulomatosa: therapy with clofazimine. *Hautarzt* 1984; 35: 459–63.

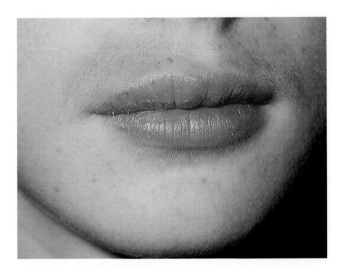

Fig. 18.3.5 Granulomatosis cheilitis affecting the upper lip.

14 Podmore P, Burrows D. Clofazimine—an effective treatment for Melkersson–Rosenthal syndrome or Meischer's cheilitis. *Clin Exp Dermatol* 1986; 11: 173–8.

15 Eisenbud L. Granulomatous cheilitis. *Oral Surg* 1971; 31: 384–9.

16 Krutchkoff D, James R. Cheilitis granulomatosa. Successful treatment with combined local triamcinolone injections and surgery. *Arch Dermatol* 1978; 114: 203–6.

17 Azaz B, Nitzan DW. Melkersson–Rosenthal syndrome. *Oral Surg* 1984; 57: 250–2.

Section 19
Genetic Disorders

19.1 Principles of Genetics, Mosaicism and Molecular Biology

RUDOLF HAPPLE

The impact of modern genetics on paediatric dermatology — and vice versa

The advances achieved recently in molecular genetics have revolutionized all fields of medicine including paediatric dermatology. A large number of inherited skin diseases has already been mapped at specific loci within the human genome [1] and the underlying structural or metabolic defects have been elucidated.

Paediatric dermatology has an important impact on this growing field of knowledge. In McKusick's catalogue of human genes and genetic disorders, the 12 most cited periodicals include one dermatological and four paediatric journals [1]. For paediatric dermatologists interested in clinical genetics an online version of McKusick's *Mendelian Inheritance in Man* is available.

In order to complete the huge task of human gene mapping, a close cooperation between clinicians and molecular geneticists is needed [2–4]. Absence of such cooperation has caused substantial mistakes such as the incorrect assignment of incontinentia pigmenti to Xp11 [5–7] or the erroneous mapping of focal dermal hypoplasia to Xp22.3 [8–10].

A good understanding of the large group of genodermatoses is not possible without a basic knowledge of modern genetic principles. Their relevance to paediatric dermatology is considered in this chapter. Some of these concepts, such as imprinting or anticipation, are so far of limited or no significance for paediatric dermatology because clinical examples are as yet lacking. Notwithstanding, such mechanisms are included because it is important that clinicians look with a prepared mind at genetically determined skin diseases.

What do we understand by the term 'genodermatosis'? It seems reasonable to give the following definition: a genodermatosis is a cutaneous phenotype caused by a single mutation that may be a point mutation, a deletion or a chromosomal aberration. Accordingly genodermatoses do not need to be inherited. In fact, many of them exclusively occur sporadically. Conversely, this definition excludes all phenotypes that are essentially caused by the action of more than one gene. Hence, psoriasis is not a genodermatosis, and the same is true for atopic dermatitis and for the familial occurrence of multiple dysplastic naevi [11].

A distinction between autosomal dominant and polygenic inheritance is important but often difficult. The penetrance and expression of a dominant phenotype may be influenced by modifying genes, and this is not far from polygenic inheritance with involvement of a major gene. From a heuristic point of view, however, it appears reasonable to assume polygenic inheritance rather than an unclear form of 'autosomal dominant inheritance'. It should be borne in mind that the terms linkage or genetic heterogeneity become meaningless when applied to a polygenic trait.

From the following overview it will become evident that the 'splitting' of similar phenotypes is a general trend enhanced by molecular genetics. Conversely, some interesting examples of 'lumping' of seemingly different phenotypes can be noted such as the unity of placental steroid sulphatase deficiency and X-linked recessive ichthyosis [12], or the common genetic origin of piebaldism and mast cell leukaemia [13].

Within the field of formal genetics, we shall first consider the classical rules of mendelian inheritance. Subsequently, the many exceptions and variations on this theme will be outlined. For the understanding of genetic mosaicism the study of cutaneous traits is especially suitable.

The future advances in gene mapping will have an important impact on prenatal diagnosis of inherited skin diseases, and the blurred outlines of gene therapy emerge above this field of research, although we are presently far from the stage of practical application.

REFERENCES

1 McKusick VA. *Mendelian Inheritance in Man. A Catalog of Human Genes and Genetic Disorders*, 12th edn. Baltimore: Johns Hopkins University Press, 1998.
2 De Bie L, de Paepe AM. Linkage analysis, a primer for dermatologists. *Eur J Dermatol* 1995; 5: 653–8.
3 Moss C, Savin J. *Dermatology and the New Genetics*. Oxford: Blackwell Science, 1995.
4 Harper JI. *Inherited Skin Disorders*. Oxford: Butterworth Heinemann, 1996.
5 Hodgson SV, Neville B, Jones RWA, Fear C, Bobrow M. Two cases of X/autosome translocation in females with incontinentia pigmenti. *Hum Genet* 1985; 71: 231–4.
6 Gorski JL, Burright EN, Harnden CE, Stein CK, Glover TW, Reyner EL. Localization of DNA sequences to a region within Xp11.21 between incontinentia pigmenti (IP1) X-chromosomal translocation breakpoints. *Am J Hum Genet* 1991; 48: 53–64.
7 Happle R. Mosaicism in human skin: understanding the patterns and mechanism. *Arch Dermatol* 1993; 129: 1460–70.
8 Friedmann PA, Rao KW, Teplin SW, Aylsworth AS. Provisional deletion mapping of the focal dermal hypoplasia (FDH) gene to Xp22.31. *Am J Hum Genet* 1988; 43 (suppl): A50.
9 Ballabio A, Andria G. Deletions and translocations involving the distal short arm of the human X chromosome: review and hypotheses. *Hum Mol Genet* 1992; 1: 221–7.
10 Happle R, Daniëls O, Koopman RJJ. MIDAS syndrome (microphthalmia, dermal aplasia, and sclerocornea): an X-linked phenotype distinct from Goltz syndrome. *Am J Med Genet* 1993; 47: 710–13.
11 Happle R. Dysplastic nevus 'syndrome': the emergence and decline of an erroneous concept. *J Eur Acad Dermatol* 1993; 2: 275–80.
12 Koppe JG, Marinkovic-Ilsen A, Rijken Y, De Groot WP, Jobsis AC. X-linked ichthyosis: a sulphatase deficiency. *Arch Dis Child* 1978; 53: 803–6.
13 Spritz RA, Holmes SA, Ramesar R, Greenberg J, Curtis D, Beighton P. Mutations of the KIT (mast/stem cell growth factor receptor) proto-oncogene account for a continuous range of phenotypes in human piebaldism. *Am J Hum Genet* 1992; 51: 1058–65.

Formal genetics

The mendelian rules of inheritance

Until recently human geneticists distinguished between autosomal dominant, autosomal recessive and X-linked inheritance. Today, Y-linked transmission and mitochondrial inheritance have been added.

Autosomal dominant inheritance

In the strict sense of Mendel's definition, the terms dominant and recessive should always refer to a phenotype and not to a genotype. Genetic traits are called dominant when

Table 19.1.1 Autosomal dominant traits explained by metabolic deficiencies

Disorder	Deficient gene product
Hereditary angio-oedema	C1-esterase inhibitor
Porphyria cutanea tarda	Uroporphyrinogen decarboxylase
Porphyria variegata	Protoporphyrinogen oxidase

they become manifest in a heterozygous state. Two different alleles are present at the underlying gene locus. For children of an affected individual the risk of recurrence is 50%.

It is important to realize that there are no 'dominant' or 'recessive' gene loci. For example, different alleles present at the locus of epidermolysis bullosa dystrophica may give rise to either autosomal dominant or autosomal recessive traits [1–3]. The same holds true for the phenotype of insulin-resistant diabetes with acanthosis nigricans [4,5].

A study of genodermatoses confirms the general rule that dominant traits usually involve defects of structural proteins. For example, neurofibromatosis type 1 has been explained by a defect of neurofibromin [6], whereas tuberous sclerosis type 2 is caused by a structural defect of tuberin [7,8]. However, exceptions from this rule may occur. Some autosomal dominant genodermatoses represent metabolic disorders (Table 19.1.1). For example, porphyria cutanea tarda is a rather common autosomal dominant trait characterized by a deficiency of the enzyme uroporphyrinogen decarboxylase [9]. Affected individuals have a 50% level of the enzyme. In hereditary angio-oedema, functional levels of activated C1-esterase inhibitor in the serum of patients range from 5 to 30% of normal rather than the expected 50% for the heterozygous state [10]. This has been tentatively explained by an increased catabolism of the protein [11].

In some classical autosomal dominant traits such as neurofibromatosis, tuberous sclerosis and naevoid basal cell carcinoma syndrome, molecular research has shown that benign hamartomas or malignant tumours of the skin or internal organs show homozygosity for the underlying gene. In other words, these lesions can be considered as circumscribed 'recessive' manifestations.

Variable expression and incomplete penetrance

As a characteristic feature of autosomal dominant inheritance, the degree of involvement may be rather variable. An impressive example is the mutation of adenomatous intestinal polyposis that may also give rise to the 'Gardner syndrome', a phenotype associated with multiple osteomas and cutaneous hamartomas such as sebaceous cysts, dermoid cysts, fibromas and leiomyomas [12]. The term 'incomplete penetrance' means that the trait is present but not detectable in some individuals. In fact, the terms 'variable expressivity' and 'reduced penetrance' are an academic paraphrasing of our ignorance.

Pleiotropism

A single gene defect may exert different effects on various tissues or organs. This phenomenon is called pleiotropism. For example, the gene of naevoid basal cell carcinoma syndrome gives rise to multiple palmar and plantar pits, maxillary cysts, fused ribs, calcification of the falx cerebri and reduced intelligence [13]. In fact, most of the human genes are pleiotropic.

Autosomal recessive inheritance

An autosomal recessive trait becomes manifest when the underlying allele is present in a homozygous state, i.e. two identical alleles are present at a given gene locus. For children of two heterozygous parents, the risk of recurrence is 25%. In general, only one generation is affected in a family.

The general rule that autosomal recessive traits are caused by an enzyme deficiency is confirmed when hereditary skin diseases are considered. For instance, tyrosinase is lacking in oculocutaneous albinism [14], and transglutaminase 1 is lacking in type 1 lamellar ichthyosis [15,16]. Further examples are given in Table 19.1.2.

When compared to autosomal dominant traits, individuals affected with autosomal recessive disorders show a rather constant degree of involvement and often resemble each other like sibs. Autosomal recessive traits are usually more severe than dominant traits.

X-linked inheritance

In X-linked skin diseases, the difference between dominant and recessive gene action is often blurred by the Lyon effect of X-inactivation [17,18]. For example, X-linked hypohidrotic ectodermal dysplasia is categorized, by scholastic convention, as an X-linked recessive trait although many heterozygous women show a more or less severe clinical involvement. For this reason it would also be justified to classify this phenotype as an X-linked

Table 19.1.2 Autosomal recessive traits explained by enzyme deficiencies

Disorder	Deficient enzyme
Lamellar ichthyosis type 1	Transglutaminase 1
Sjögren–Larsson syndrome	Fatty alcohol : NAD + oxidoreductase
Refsum's disease	Phytanic acid oxidase
Tyrosinaemia type II	Tyrosine aminotransferase
Oculocutaneous albinism	Tyrosinase
Congenital erythropoietic porphyria	Uroporphyrinogen III synthetase
Acrodermatitis acidaemica	Methylmalonic CoA mutase; Propionyl-CoA-Carboxylase

CoA, coenzyme A; NAD, nicotinamide adenine dinucleotide.

dominant trait. Some X-linked traits explained by enzyme deficiencies are listed in Table 19.1.3.

Sex-linkage versus X-linkage

The term sex-linked has previously been used as a synonym for X-linked but should be avoided because it is ambiguous: Y-linked traits are also sex-linked.

Hemizygosity

Because males possess only one X chromosome, most of the X-linked genes are present neither in a heterozygous nor in a homozygous state. This situation is called hemizygosity. As a consequence, X-linked gene defects are expressed in hemizygous males in a more severe degree than in heterozygous females. Presumably, the reduced life expectancy of men as compared to women can be explained by a hemizygous state of X-linked genes that account for about 5% of human genetic information.

X-inactivation

In female individuals, most X-linked genes are inactivated at an early stage of embryogenesis, a mechanism called Lyon effect or lyonization. In 1961, Lyon put forward her theory that dosage compensation is achieved by random X-inactivation [17]. The inactivated X chromosome can be either the maternal or the paternal one in different cells of the same individual, but the inactivated X remains the same in all daughter cells of a given cell line [19]. The resulting functional X-chromosome mosaicism may give rise to a characteristic pattern of skin lesions [20] (see below).

Escape from X-inactivation

There is increasing evidence that many genes located at different regions on either arm of the X chromosome escape inactivation, being interspersed among the inactivated genes [21]. From a clinical point of view, absence of any mosaic pattern in the skin of heterozygous women would indicate that the underlying gene escapes inactivation. For example, women heterozygous for the gene of

Table 19.1.3 X-linked traits explained by enzyme deficiencies

Disorder	Deficient enzyme
Fabry's disease	α-Galactosidase A
Menkes disease	Cu^{2+} transporting adenosine triphosphatase
X-linked recessive ichthyosis	Steroid sulphatase
	Sterol-Δ^8-isomerase
X-linked dominant chondrodysplasia punctata	3β-hydroxysteroid dehydrogenase
CHILD syndrome	

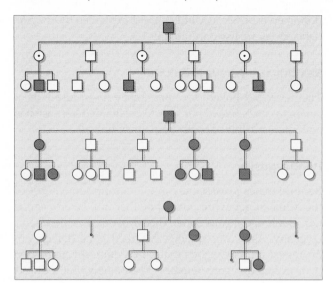

Fig. 19.1.1 Diagrammatic representation of three different forms of X-linked transmission. In X-linked recessive inheritance, one generation is skipped. In X-linked dominant inheritance with manifestation in both sexes, affected male individuals transmit the trait to all of their daughters but to none of their sons. In X-linked dominant, male-lethal inheritance, only female carriers are viable. They often have miscarriages.

X-linked recessive ichthyosis [22] do not display any skin changes. The same is true for epidermolysis bullosa of the Mendes da Costa type [22]. In keratosis follicularis spinulosa decalvans, women tend to be less severely affected than men but their skin lesions do not display any linear or otherwise mosaic arrangement, suggesting that the underlying X-linked gene escapes inactivation [22].

The three types of X-linked inheritance (Fig. 19.1.1)

X-linked recessive traits exclusively occur in male individuals. Characteristically, one generation is skipped because the disease is transmitted by clinically healthy female carriers. X-linked dominant non-lethal traits occur in both sexes. By contrast, X-linked dominant male-lethal traits are observed exclusively in female individuals because the underlying mutation has a lethal effect on hemizygous male embryos. Exceptionally such traits may also occur in male individuals with a normal XY constitution, and this can be explained by an early postzygotic mutation or by a gametic half chromatid mutation [23]. These men can transmit the trait to their daughters [24]. Conversely, a mother-to-son transmission of such phenotypes is not possible and has never been observed although this has been erroneously stated in the literature [25,26].

Y-linkage

In Y-linked traits two different modes of transmission should be distinguished. Firstly, there are pseudoautoso-

Table 19.1.4 Y-linked traits

Trait	MIM number
Stature/tooth size	475 000
Testes-determining factor (SRY)	480 000
Interleukin-3 receptor, Y-linked	430 000
Granulocyte–macrophage colony-stimulating factor receptor, α-subunit, Y-linked	425 000
Hairy pinnae of the ear (?)	425 500

SRY, sex-determining region

mal genes that have their counterpart on the X chromosome [27]. The pseudoautosomal region at the end of the short arm of the Y chromosome undergoes crossing-over with the telomeric part of the X chromosome. Traits determined by such genes show a transmission similar to autosomal traits. Secondly, the remaining Y-linked genes can be transmitted from father to son only [27].

Some examples of Y-linked traits are summarized in Table 19.1.4. A Y-linked gene relevant to paediatric dermatology is the SRY gene controlling the testis-determining factor localized at Yp11.3 [28]. Girls affected with MIDAS syndrome (microphthalmia–dermal aplasia–sclencornea) may show anomalies of external or internal genitalia and may display an SRY-positive status, indicating a translocation between the pseudoautosomal parts of Xp and Yp [29].

Hairy pinnae of the ear are another phenotype that may be Y-linked [30]. The trait is relevant to dermatology but certainly not to paediatric dermatology.

REFERENCES

1 Ryynänen M, Knowlton RG, Parente MG, Chung LC, Chu ML, Uitto J. Human type VII collagen: genetic linkage of the gene (COL7A1) on chromosome 3 to dominant dystrophic epidermolysis bullosa. *Am J Hum Genet* 1991; 49: 797–803.

2 Gruis NA, Bavinck JNB, Steijlen PM *et al*. Genetic linkage between the collagen VII (Co17A1) gene and the autosomal dominant form of dystrophic epidermolysis bullosa in two Dutch kindreds. *J Invest Dermatol* 1992; 99: 528–30.

3 Hovnanian A, Duquesnoy P, Blanchet-Bardon C *et al*. Genetic linkage of recessive dystrophic epidermolysis bullosa to the type VII collagen gene. *J Clin Invest* 1992; 90: 1032–6.

4 Kahn CR, Flier JS, Bar RS *et al*. The syndromes of insulin resistance and acanthosis nigricans: insulin receptor disorders in man. *N Engl J Med* 1976; 294: 739–45.

5 Yoshimasa Y, Seino S, Whittaker J *et al*. Insulin-resistant diabetes due to a point mutation that prevents insulin proreceptor processing. *Science* 1988; 240: 784–7.

6 Li Y, Bollag G, Clark R *et al*. Somatic mutations in the neurofibromatosis 1 gene in human tumors. *Cell* 1992; 69: 275–81.

7 The European Chromosome 16 Tuberous Sclerosis Consortium. Identification and characterization of the tuberous sclerosis gene on chromosome 16. *Cell* 1993; 75: 1305–15.

8 Wienecke R, König A, DeClue JE. Identification of tuberin, the tuberous sclerosis-2 product. *J Biol Chem* 1995; 270: 16409–14.

9 Sassa S, de Verneuil H, Anderson KE, Kappas A. Isolation and properties of human erythrocyte uroporphyrinogen decarboxylase: immunological demonstration of the enzyme defect in porphyria cutanea tarda. *Trans Assoc Am Phys* 1983; 96: 65–75.

10 Cicardi M, Igarashi T, Rosen FS, Davis AE III. Molecular basis for the deficiency of complement 1 inhibitor in type I hereditary angioneurotic edema. *J Clin Invest* 1987; 79: 698–702.

11 Quastel M, Harrison R, Cicardi M, Alper CA, Rosen FS. Behavior *in vivo* of normal and dysfunctional C1 inhibitor in normal subjects and patients with hereditary angio-neurotic edema. *J Clin Invest* 1983; 71: 1041–6.

12 Nishisho I, Nakamura Y, Miyoshi Y *et al*. Mutations of chromosome 5q21 genes in FAP and colorectal cancer patients. *Science* 1991; 253: 665–9.

13 Shanley S, Ratcliffe J, Hockey A *et al*. Nevoid basal cell carcinoma syndrome: review of 118 affected individuals. *Am J Med Genet* 1994; 50: 282–90.

14 Oetting WS, King RA. Molecular analysis of type I-A (tyrosine negative) oculo-cutaneous albinism. *Hum Genet* 1992; 90: 258–62.

15 Huber M, Rettler I, Bernasconi K *et al*. Mutations of keratinocytic transglutaminase in lamellar ichthyosis. *Science* 1995; 267: 525–8.

16 Parmentier L, Blanchet-Bardon C, Nguyen S, Prud' homme JF, Dubertret L, Weissenbach J. Autosomal recessive lamellar ichthyosis: identification of a new mutation in transglutaminase 1 and evidence for genetic heterogeneity. *Hum Mol Genet* 1995; 4: 1391–5.

17 Lyon MF. Gene action in the X-chromosome of the mouse (*Mus musculus* L.). *Nature* 1961; 190: 372–3.

18 Happle R. X-chromosomal vererbte Dermatosen. *Hautarzt* 1982; 33: 73–81.

19 Migeon BR. X-chromosome inactivation: molecular mechanisms and genetic consequences. *Trends Genet* 1994; 10: 230–5.

20 Happle R. Lyonization and the lines of Blaschko. *Hum Genet* 1985; 70: 200–6.

21 Disteche CM. Escape from X inactivation in human and mouse. *Trends Genet* 1995; 11: 17–22.

22 Happle R. Cutaneous manifestation of X-linked genes escaping inactivation. *Clin Exp Dermatol* 1992; 17: 69.

23 Lenz W. Half chromatid mutations may explain incontinentia pigmenti in males. *Am J Hum Genet* 1975; 27: 690.

24 Mahé A, Couturier J, Mathé C, Lebras F, Bruet A, Fendler JP. Minimal focal dermal hypoplasia in a man: a case of father-to-daughter transmission. *J Am Acad Dermatol* 1991; 25: 879–81.

25 Kurczynski TW, Berns JS, Johnson WE. Studies of a family with incontinentia pigmenti variably expressed in both sexes. *J Med Genet* 1982; 19: 447–51.

26 Hecht F, Hecht BK, Austin WJ. Incontinentia pigmenti in Arizona Indians including transmission from mother to son inconsistent with the half chromatid mutation model. *Clin Genet* 1982; 21: 293–6.

27 Burgoyne PS. Genetic homology and crossing over in the X and Y chromosomes of mammals. *Hum Genet* 1982; 61: 85–90.

28 Jäger RJ, Harley VR, Pfeiffer RA, Goodfellow PN, Scherer G. A familial mutation in the testis-determining gene SRY shared by both sexes. *Hum Genet* 1992; 90: 350–5.

29 Mücke J, Hepffner W, Thamm B, Theile H. MIDAS syndrome (microphthalmia, dermal aplasia and sclerocornea): an autonomous entity with linear skin defects within the spectrum of focal hypoplasias. *Eur J Dermatol* 1995; 5: 197–203.

30 Stern C, Centerwall WR, Sarkar SS. New data on the problem of Y-linkage of hairy pinnae. *Am J Hum Genet* 1964; 16: 455–71.

Exceptions and variations on mendelian inheritance

Today, so many exceptions from the rules of mendelian inheritance have been brought to light that it is an astonishing fact that Mendel was able to find the rules that have immortalized his name. Some of these modifying concepts and mechanisms are reviewed below.

Mitochondrial inheritance

The human mitochondrial genome contains 14 protein-coding regions that have been completely sequenced [1]. They are contained in a circular mitochondrial chromosome resembling that of a bacterium. There are no introns and there is very little flanking non-coding DNA. The mitochondrial mode of transmission is exclusively matrilineal. Remarkably, the presently known catalogue of mitochondrial disorders mainly contains muscular, neurological and ophthalmological diseases but so far no skin disorder [2].

Genomic imprinting

Some genes show the phenomenon of imprinting. When such a gene is derived from the mother it acts in a different way as compared to that derived from the father [3]. This different expression is apparently due to a different degree of methylation of DNA during gametogenesis [4]. Imprinting has been proposed to be present in neurofibromatosis I [5] and familial glomus tumours [6], and it may also play a role in the inheritance of atopy [7] and psoriasis [8].

Anticipation

A hundred years ago many doctors believed in anticipation. A genetic trait should worsen progressively from generation to generation. Until recently, modern geneticists have regarded this idea as a superstition. Remarkably, however, the concept of anticipation has now experienced a revival. In some traits such as fragile X syndrome, myotonic dystrophy or chorea Huntington, the number of trinucleotid repeats may increase from generation to generation, correlating with an increasing severity of the disease [9,10]. Although no example relevant to paediatric dermatology is so far known, clinicians should be aware of this concept.

Uniparental disomy

A child suffering from an autosomal recessive skin disorder may have only one heterozygous parent. Molecular research has shown that, by way of exception, both of the mutant chromosomes may be derived from one parent [11,12].

Compound heterozygosity

An individual may carry two different mutant alleles at the same locus. For example, compound heterozygosity for the alleles of Hurler's syndrome and Scheie's syndrome gives rise to an intermediate Hurler–Scheie phenotype [13]. Compound heterozygosity plays an important role in the autosomal recessive types of epidermolysis bullosa and other cutaneous traits [14,15]. It should not be confused with double heterozygosity which means heterozygosity at each of two separate loci on the same chromosome.

Pseudodominance

A seemingly dominant transmission of a recessive gene may occur when a clinically affected individual is mating with a heterozygous gene carrier. In this particular situation, the children have a 50% risk of recurrence. This may happen in a population with a high degree of inbreeding. Such pedigrees have been observed in mal de Meleda, a distinctive type of palmoplantar keratoderma occurring in the population of the island of Mljet (Meleda) off the Croatian coast [16].

Paradominance

Some mosaic phenotypes such as Becker naevus or Sturge–Weber–Klippel–Trenaunay syndrome usually occur sporadically but may affect, by way of exception, several members of a family. To explain this paradox, the concept of paradominant transmission has been proposed [17,18]. Heterozygous gene carriers would be, as a rule, phenotypically normal, and for this reason the mutant gene would be transmitted imperceptibly through many generations. The trait would become manifest only when a somatic event of allelic loss in an early stage of embryogenesis gave rise to a clone of cells that were either homozygous or hemizygous for the mutation (Fig. 19.1.2). In several other mosaic traits not fitting an established mode of mendelian inheritance, the concept of paradominant transmission may replace the terminological vagueness of 'incomplete penetrance' or 'reduced expression'.

Gonadal mosaicism

An autosomal dominant trait may occur in several siblings although both parents are healthy. The phenomenon has been conclusively explained by gonadal mosaicism [19]. Molecular proof for this concept has been provided in many hereditary disorders such as tuberous sclerosis [20], bullous congenital ichthyosiform erythroderma of Brocq

[21] and neurofibromatosis type 1 [22]. Gonadal mosaicism may be due either to an early postzygotic mutation affecting both germ cells and somatic tissues, or to a late postzygotic mutation affecting the germ cells alone. Such events should no longer be called 'somatic mutations'. Only those postzygotic mutations affecting somatic cells alone, without any germ line mosaicism, are true somatic mutations (Fig. 19.1.3).

Similarly, gonadal mosaicism for an X-linked trait, incontinentia pigmenti, has been documented in a healthy male [23].

The concept of gonadal mosaicism is important for genetic counselling. In a sporadic case of a severe autosomal dominant disorder, molecular analysis of the father's sperm may be a reasonable approach to exclude gonadal mosaicism, especially when the mutation rate of the involved gene is relatively high as in neurofibromatosis type 1 [22].

Founding effect

In an isolated population originating from a limited number of founding parents, some autosomal recessive disorders may be either absent or, conversely, particularly frequent due to the absence or presence of the mutation in the founding parents. For example, cartilage–hair hypoplasia is relatively common in the Finnish-speaking population of Finland, whereas phenylketonuria is virtually absent [16].

Point mutations versus deletions

Many traits showing a monogenic mode of inheritance are not due to a point mutation but to a deletion either present within a given gene or involving several neighbouring genes. It should be noted that the human genes have different sizes. For example, the insulin gene is relatively small [24], whereas the steroid sulphatase gene is rather large [25]. This may explain the rather high frequency of deletions found within the steroid sulphatase gene [26].

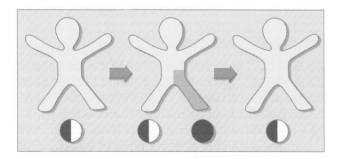

Fig. 19.1.2 Diagrammatic representation of paradominant inheritance. Heterozygotes are phenotypically normal. The trait is expressed only when loss of heterozygosity occurs in an early stage of embryogenesis and gives rise to a clonal population of cells either homozygous or hemizygous for the mutation.

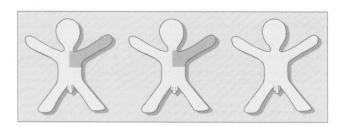

Fig. 19.1.3 A postzygotic mutation may involve both somatic and germinal tissues (left), somatic tissue only (middle) or germinal tissue only (right). The term 'somatic mutation' exclusively refers to a postzygotic event as shown in the middle.

Contiguous gene syndromes

Large deletions may involve several neighbouring genes, giving rise to a 'contiguous gene syndrome'. For example, a large deletion at Xp22.3 may result in a combination of X-linked recessive ichthyosis, chondrodysplasia punctata of the Maroteaux type and Kallmann's syndrome (hypogonadotrophic hypogonadism with anosmia) [27–29]. In such cases, the different entities are inherited together, simulating a monogenic multisystem birth defect.

Genetic heterogeneity

Molecular research has provided evidence that similar phenotypes are often genetically different. For example, there are two types of tuberous sclerosis that are so far indistinguishable at the clinical level. The underlying genes have been assigned to chromosomes 9q and 16p [30]. Analysis of keratins has provided proof that bullous ichthyosis of the Siemens type is genetically different from the Brocq type [31–33] as assumed earlier on the basis of clinical and histopathological criteria [34].

REFERENCES

1 Anderson S, Bankier AT, Barrell BG *et al*. Sequence and organization of the human mitochondrial genome. *Nature* 1981; 290: 457–65.
2 McKusick VA. *Mendelian Inheritance in Man. A Catalog of Human Genes and Genetic Disorders*, 12th edn. Baltimore: Johns Hopkins University Press.
3 Marx JL. A parent's sex may affect gene expression. *Science* 1988; 239: 352–3.
4 Hall JG. Genomic imprinting: review and relevance to human diseases. *Am J Hum Genet* 1990; 46: 857–73.
5 Miller M, Hall JG. Possible maternal effect on severity of neurofibromatosis. *Lancet* 1978; ii: 1071–3.
6 Van der Mey AGL, Maaswinkel-Mooy PD, Cornelisse CJ. Genomic imprinting in hereditary glomus tumours: evidence for new genetic theory. *Lancet* 1989; ii: 1291–4.
7 Cookson WOCM, Young RP, Sandford AJ *et al*. Maternal inheritance of atopic IgE responsiveness on chromosome 11q. *Lancet* 1992; 340: 381–4.
8 Traupe H, van Gurp PJM, Happle R *et al*. Psoriasis vulgaris, fetal growth, and genomic imprinting. *Am J Med Genet* 1992; 42: 649–54.
9 Sutherland GR, Richards RI. Invited editorial: anticipation legitimized: unstable DNA to the rescue. *Am J Hum Genet* 1992; 51: 7–9.
10 Harper PS, Harley HG, Reardon W *et al*. Anticipation in myotonic dystrophy: new light on an old problem. *Am J Hum Genet* 1992; 51: 10–16.
11 Engel E. A new genetic concept: uniparental disomy and its potential effect, isodisomy. *Am J Med Genet* 1980; 6: 137–43.
12 Spence JE, Perciaccante RG, Greig GM *et al*. Uniparental disomy as a mechanism for human genetic disease. *Am J Hum Genet* 1988; 42: 217–26.
13 McKusick VA, Howell RR, Hussels IE *et al*. Allelism, non-allelism, and genetic compounds among the mucopolysaccharidoses. *Lancet* 1972; I: 993–6.
14 Christiano AM, Anton-Lamprecht I, Amano S. Compound heterozygosity for COL7A1 mutations in twins with dystrophic epidermolysis bullosa: a recessive paternal deletion/insertion mutation and a dominant negative maternal glycine substitution result in a severe phenotype. *Am J Hum Genet* 1996; 58: 682–93.
15 Oshima J, Yu CE, Piussan C *et al*. Homozygous and compound heterozygous mutations at the Werner syndrome locus. *Hum Mol Genet* 1996; 12: 1909–13.
16 Vogel F, Motulsky AG. *Human Genetics. Problems and Approaches*, 2nd edn. Berlin: Springer Verlag, 1986: 509–11.
17 Happle R. Paradominant inheritance: a possible explanation for Becker's pigmented hairy nevus. *Eur J Dermatol* 1992; 2: 39–40.
18 Happle R. Klippel–Trenaunay syndrome: is it a paradominant trait? *Br J Dermatol* 1993; 128: 465.
19 Hall JG. Somatic mosaicism: observations related to clinical genetics. *Am J Hum Genet* 1988; 43: 355–63.
20 Verhoef S, Vrtel R, van Essen T *et al*. Somatic mosaicism and clinical variation in tuberous sclerosis complex. *Lancet* 1995; 345: 202.
21 Paller AS, Syder AJ, Chan YM *et al*. Genetic and clinical mosaicism in a type of epidermal nevus. *N Engl J Med* 1994; 331: 1408–15.
22 Lázaro C, Ravella A, Gaona A *et al*. Neurofibromatosis type I due to germ-line mosaicism in a clinically normal father. *N Engl J Med* 1994; 331: 1403–7.
23 Kirchman TTT, Levy ML, Lewis RA *et al*. Gonadal mosaicism for incontinentia pigmenti in a healthy male. *J Med Genet* 1995; 32: 887–90.
24 McKusick VA. *Mendelian Inheritance In Man. A Catalog of Human Genes and Genetic Disorders*, 12th ed. Baltimore: Johns Hopkins University, 1994: XLVII.
25 Bonifas JM, Morley BJ, Oakey RE *et al*. Cloning of a cDNA for steroid sulfatase: frequent occurrence of gene deletions in patients with recessive X chromosome-linked ichthyosis. *Proc Natl Acad Sci* 1987; 84: 9248–51.
26 Basler E, Grompe M, Parenti G *et al*. Identification of point mutations in the steroid sulfatase gene of three patients with X-linked ichthyosis. *Am J Hum Genet* 1992; 50: 483–91.
27 Bick D, Curry CJR, McGill JR *et al*. Male infant with ichthyosis, Kallmann syndrome, chondrodysplasia punctata, and an Xp chromosome deletion. *Am J Med Genet* 1989; 33: 100–7.
28 Meindl A, Hosenfeld D, Brückl W *et al*. Analysis of a terminal Xp22.3 deletion in a patient with six monogenic disorders: implications for the mapping of X linked ocular albinism. *J Med Genet* 1993; 30: 838–42.
29 Paige DG, Emilion GG, Bouloux PMG, Harper JI. A clinical and genetic study of X-linked ichthyosis and contiguous gene defects. *Br J Dermatol* 1994; 131: 622–9.
30 Povey S, Burley MW, Attwood J *et al*. Two loci for tuberous sclerosis: one on 9q35 and one on 16p13. *Ann Hum Genet* 1994; 58: 107–27.
31 Steijlen PM, Kremer H, Vakilzadeh F *et al*. Genetic linkage of the keratin type II gene cluster with ichthyosis bullosa of Siemens and with autosomal dominant ichthyosis exfoliativa. *J Invest Dermatol* 1994; 103: 282–5.
32 McLean WHI, Morley SM, Lane EB *et al*. Ichthyosis bullosa of Siemens—a disease involving keratin 2e. *J Invest Dermatol* 1994; 103: 277–81.
33 Kremer H, Zeeuwen P, McLean WHI *et al*. Ichthyosis bullosa of Siemens is caused by mutations in the keratin 2e gene. *J Invest Dermatol* 1994; 103: 286–9.
34 Steijlen PM, Perret CM, Schuurmans Stekhoven JH *et al*. Ichthyosis bullosa of Siemens: further delineation of the phenotype. *Arch Dermatol Res* 1990; 282: 1–5.

Polygenic inheritance

Many hereditary skin diseases are determined by more than one gene. Such polygenic traits are psoriasis [1], atopic dermatitis [2], and multiple melanocytic naevi including dysplastic naevi [3,4]. In polygenic traits, several scientific terms such as expression, penetrance, pleiotropism, linkage and genetic heterogeneity are meaningless and should be avoided. In all of these traits impressive pedigrees suggesting a dominant mode of inheritance have been documented but can be explained by a bias of ascertainment. Such phenotypes should no longer be taken as 'autosomal dominant traits with reduced penetrance and variable expression'.

Polygenic versus multifactorial traits

Both terms are often used synonymously, but the term 'polygenic' is preferred because a 'multifactorial trait' implies the influence of environmental factors too.

In polygenic traits, the risk of recurrence is not constant but increases with the number of affected individuals present in a given family. When compared to monogenic traits, it is rather difficult to elucidate the molecular basis of polygenic skin disorders [1,5]. However, important advances have been made in the genetic understanding of these common skin diseases by documenting a close association with major gene loci such as 11q13 in atopy [6–9] or chromosomes 1q21, 4q and 17q in psoriasis [10–13]. It should be noted, however, that 'linkage' of such major loci is only found in some families but absent in others [14–16].

In classical genetics, twin studies have been very useful to elucidate polygenic inheritance. The principle is to study unselected twin pairs and to compare monozygotic to dizygotic pairs. In polygenic traits, a concordant manifestation is found in both types of twin pairs but tends to be much higher (four- to fivefold) in monozygotic twins [2]. The Minnesota study [16] has yielded important information regarding the influence of the environment on atopic manifestations. The total immunoglobulin E (IgE) levels of monozygotic pairs showed a remarkable concordance even in those twins who had been separated at an early age and lived under different environmental conditions.

REFERENCES

1 Elder JT, Nair RP, Guo SW, Henseler T, Christophers E, Voorhees JJ. The genetics of psoriasis. *Arch Dermatol* 1994; 130: 216–24.
2 Schultz Larsen F, Holm NV, Henningsen K. Atopic dermatitis. A genetic epidemiologic study in a population-based twin sample. *J Am Acad Dermatol* 1986; 15: 487–94.
3 Happle R. Gregor Mendel und die dysplastischen Nävi. *Hautarzt* 1989; 40: 70–6.
4 Goldstein AM, Goldin LR, Dracopoli NC, Clark WH, Tucker MA. Two-locus linkage analysis of cutaneous malignant melanoma/dysplastic nevi. *Am J Hum Genet* 1996; 58: 1050–6.
5 Weeks DE, Lathrop GM. Polygenic disease: methods for mapping complex disease traits. *Trends Genet* 1995; 11: 513–20.
6 Cookson WOCM, Sharp PA, Faux JA, Hopkin JM. Linkage between immunoglobulin E responses underlying asthma and rhinitis and chromosome 11q. *Lancet* 1989; i: 1292–5.
7 Szepetowski P, Gaudray P. FCER1B, a candidate gene for atopy, is located in 11q13 between CD20 and TCN1. *Genomics* 1994; 19: 399–400.
8 Shirakawa T, Mao XQ, Sasaki S et al. Association of FcεRIβ in Japanese population. *Hum Mol Genet* 1996; 5: 1129–30.
9 Cox HE, Moffatt MF, Faux JA et al. Association of atopic dermatitis to the beta subunit of the high affinity immunoglobulin E receptor. *Br J Dermatol* 1998; 138: 182–7.
10 Tomfohrde JT, Silverman A, Barnes R et al. Gene for familial psoriasis susceptibility mapped to the distal end of human chromosome 17q. *Science* 1993; 264: 1141–5.
11 Tazi Ahnini R, Camp NJ, Cork MJ et al. Novel genetic association between the corneodesmosin (MHC S) gene and susceptibility to psoriasis. *Hum Mol Genet* 1999; 8: 1135–40.
12 Hardas BD, Zhao X, Zhang J, Longqing X, Stoll S, Elder JT. Assignment of psoriasis to human chromosomal band 1q21: coordinate overexpression of clustered genes in psoriasis. *J Invest Dermatol* 1996; 106: 753–7.
13 Matthews D, Fry L, Powles A et al. Evidence that a locus for familial psoriasis maps to chromosome 4q. *Nature Genet* 1996; 14: 231–3.
14 Matthews D, Fry L, Powles A, Weissenbach J, Williamson R. Confirmation of genetic heterogeneity in familial psoriasis. *J Med Genet* 1995; 32: 546–8.
15 Trembath R, Clough L, Frodsham A, Terwilliger J, Rosbotham J, Barker J. A complete genomic search for susceptibility loci in psoriasis. *J Invest Dermatol* 1996; 106: 901.
16 Hanson B, McGue M, Roitman-Johnson B, Segal NL, Bouchard TJ Jr, Blumenthal MN. Atopic disease and immunoglobulin E in twins reared apart and together. *Am J Hum Genet* 1991; 48: 873–9.

Mosaicism

Many genetic skin disorders reflect mosaicism. A mosaic is defined as an organism composed of two or more genetically different cell populations that are derived from a genetically homogeneous zygote. It has been proposed that all naevi reflect genetic mosaicism [1]. A classical archetypic pattern of cutaneus mosaicism is the system of Blaschko's lines (Figs 19.1.4, 19.1.5), but several other types have also been observed.

Archetypic patterns of pigmentary mosaicism

Mosaicism involving the melanocytes shows a particular diversity of cutaneous patterns. Four major types can be distinguished (Fig. 19.1.6) [4].

Type 1: lines of Blaschko

This is the commonest mosaic skin pattern and can be explained in the following way. At the time when the presence of a primitive streak confers a bilateral symmetry on the embryonic disc, precursor cells begin to proliferate in a transversal direction starting from the primitive streak (see Fig. 19.1.5a). This proliferation interferes with the longitudinal growth and increasing flexion of the embryo, resulting in a bizarre arrangement characterized by a V shape on the back (see Fig. 19.1.5b) and an S figure on the anterolateral aspects of the trunk [3]. This pattern can be subdivided into type 1a showing narrow bands and type 1b characterized by rather broad bands. A more thorough study may result in the description of additional intermediate subtypes of this archetypic pattern.

Type 1a: lines of Blaschko, narrow bands

This well-known pattern (see Fig. 19.1.6a) is observed in incontinentia pigmenti [5] (see Chapter 19.15). Furthermore, most cases of mosaic pigmentary disturbances previously categorized under the misleading term 'hypomelanosis of Ito' display this pattern (Fig. 19.1.7) [6].

Type 1b: lines of Blaschko, broad bands

This variation on the Blaschko theme (see Fig. 19.1.6b) is found in McCune–Albright syndrome, a phenotype characterized by polyostotic fibrous dysplasia, sexual precocity and rather broad linear lesions of hyperpigmentation [7].

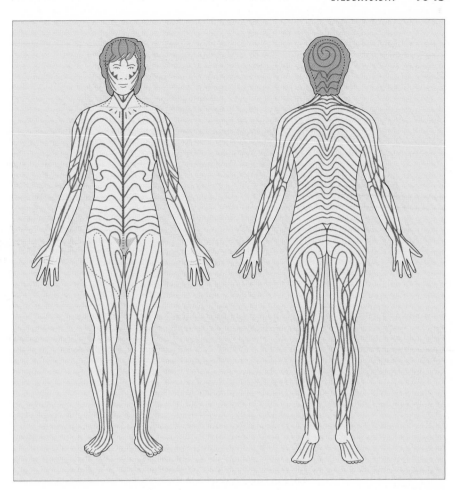

Fig. 19.1.4 Lines of Blaschko. This figure is adapted from Blaschko's original drawing (1901) and completed on the scalp according to more recent data [2].

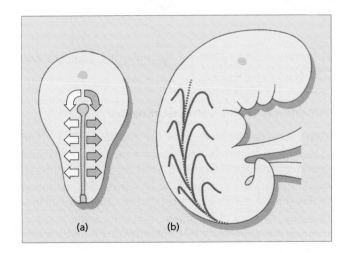

Fig. 19.1.5 Explanation of Blaschko's lines. (a) Precursor cells proliferate in a transversal direction starting from the primitive streak at the time when the presence of this streak confers a bilateral symmetry on the embryonic disk. (b) This transverse proliferation interferes with the longitudinal growth and the flexion of the embryo, resulting in a fountain-like pattern on the back [3].

Type 2: checkerboard pattern

This is a flag-like arrangement of alternating squares of pigmentary disturbance (see Fig. 19.1.6c) A typical example is systematized speckled lentiginous naevus, a disorder also known under the term naevus spilus [4,8]. A similar pattern has been observed in some cases of human chimerism [9,10].

Type 3: phylloid pattern

The Greek word *phylloid* means 'leaf-like'. The pattern is characterized by an arrangement of pigmentary disturbances similar to a floral ornament or Jugendstil painting (Fig. 19.1.6d). This pattern has been described only recently [4] and is therefore less well-known so far. However, its existence has been confirmed beyond doubt by demonstration of chromosomal mosaicism in several cases (Fig. 19.1.8) [11,12].

The phylloid pattern is composed of different elements such as oval leaf-like patches, lesions resembling the asymmetrical leaves of a begonia, large pear-shaped areas or areas showing a peculiar oblong configuration. Although this pattern may appear at first glance to be

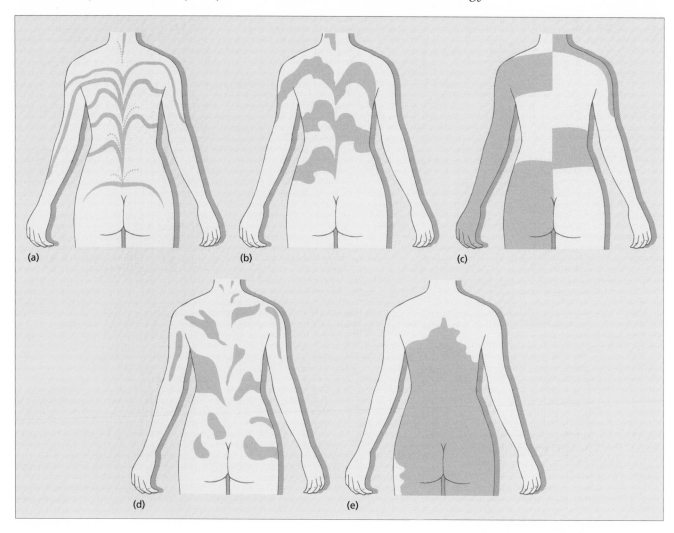

Fig. 19.1.6 Pigmentary patterns associated with human mosaicism. (a) Type 1a: lines of Blaschko, narrow bands; (b) type 1b: lines of Blaschko, broad bands; (c) type 2: checkerboard pattern; (d) type 3: phylloid pattern; and (e) type 4: patchy pattern without midline separation.

rather chaotic, it shows nevertheless a definitely non-random arrangement. For example, there is a strict dorsal and ventral midline separation of the lesions.

The number of cases displaying a phylloid pattern is so far limited. Possibly, a more thorough study will result in the delineation of different subtypes.

Type 4: patchy pattern without midline separation

The pattern displayed by giant melanocytic naevi as observed in neurocutaneous melanosis is unique because it does not respect the dorsal or ventral midline (see Fig. 19.1.6e). Because an involvement of the entire skin has never been observed, this phenotype can be best explained by a lethal mutation surviving by mosaicism

[13]. However, cytogenetic or molecular proof of this concept is so far lacking.

Functional versus genomic mosaics

Two major genetic categories are functional mosaicism resulting from the Lyon effect of X-inactivation and genomic mosaicism resulting from an autosomal mutation [11]. Functional mosaics can be inherited from mother to daughter, whereas genomic mosaics usually occur sporadically. By way of exception, however, some genomic mosaics can apparently be transmitted by paradominant inheritance [14].

Lethal versus non-lethal mutations

In functional X-chromosome mosaicism two different situations should be distinguished [11]. Firstly, the underlying gene may exert a lethal effect on male embryos which is why the trait occurs almost exclusively in female individuals (see Fig. 19.1.1). Secondly, the X-linked gene

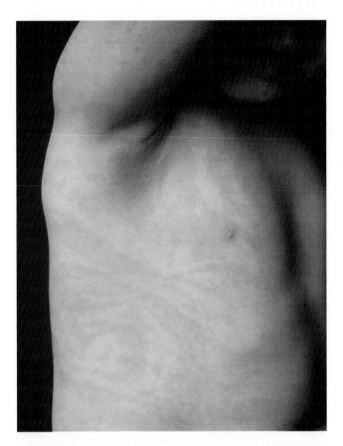

Fig. 19.1.7 Type 1a pattern in pigmentary mosaicism of the Ito type.

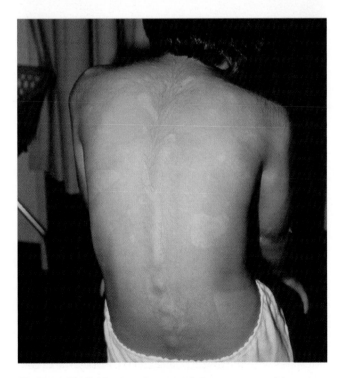

Fig. 19.1.8 Phylloid pattern in a case of pigmentary mosaicism. Courtesy of Dr K. Naritomi, Nishihara, Okinawa, Japan.

may be non-lethal. Affected male individuals are more severely involved and do not show a mosaic pattern of skin lesions, whereas affected female individuals do and are relatively mildly involved.

Similarly, autosomal gene defects resulting in genomic mosaicism may be either lethal or non-lethal. Most of the lethal autosomal mutations only occur sporadically although the paradominant traits represent an important exception from this rule [13]. Individuals affected with a mosaic phenotype originating from a non-lethal postzygotic mutation can transmit the underlying gene to their children who will show a diffuse involvement of the entire integument [11,15,16].

Functional mosaicism of X-linked male-lethal mutations

Some X-linked traits occur almost exclusively in girls because the underlying gene defect represents a lethal factor for hemizygous male embryos (Table 19.1.5). In female gene carriers the Lyon effect of X-inactivation accounts for survival (Fig. 19.1.9). Most of the affected girls show streaky skin lesions following a type 1a pattern of the lines of Blaschko.

By way of exception all of these phenotypes may be observed in male patients. Some of them have a gonosome constitution XXY, but others have a normal 46, XY karyotype. These cases can be explained either by an early postzygotic mutation or by a gametic half-chromatid mutation [11,17] (Fig. 19.1.10). Affected XY males can transmit the trait to their daughters. By contrast, a mother-to-son transmission is not possible and has so far never been convincingly documented.

It should be noted that incontinentia pigmenti maps to Xq28 and not elsewhere [18]. Until recently, molecular geneticists erroneously believed that a 'sporadic type' of incontinentia pigmenti had been regionally assigned to Xp11 [19,20]. However, all of the phenotypes assigned to Xp11 belong to the heterogeneous group of so-called 'hypomelanosis of Ito' characterized by genomic mosaicism involving the pigmentary system [11].

Similarly, many molecular geneticists so far adhere to the erroneous belief that focal dermal hypoplasia has been assigned to Xp22.3 [21]. What has been mapped to this

Table 19.1.5 X-linked male-lethal mutations giving rise to a mosaic cutaneous pattern

Incontinentia pigmenti
Focal dermal hypoplasia
MIDAS syndrome
X-linked dominant chondrodysplasia punctata
Oral-facial–digital syndrome, type 1
CHILD syndrome

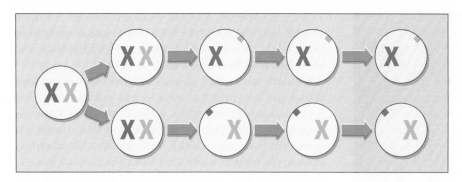

Fig. 19.1.9 Diagrammatic representation of random X-inactivation explaining the dorsoventral outgrowth of two functionally different populations of cells.

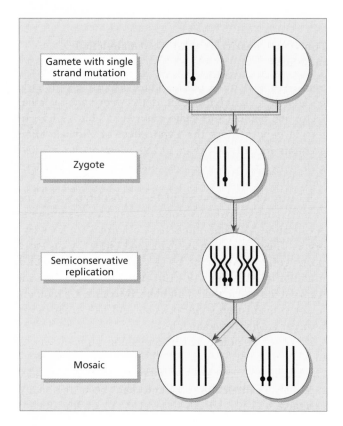

Fig. 19.1.10 A gametic half chromatid mutation may result in mosaicism already present at the two-cell stage.

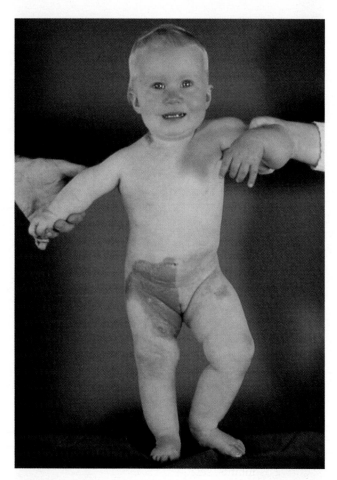

Fig. 19.1.11 CHILD syndrome.

locus, however, is MIDAS syndrome and not focal dermal hypoplasia [22].

A complex mosaic pattern: CHILD syndrome

A special case is the CHILD syndrome (congenital hemidysplasia with ichthyosiform erythroderma and limb defects) because the CHILD naevus associated with this X-linked dominant male-lethal trait is arranged in two different patterns that are often intermingled [23]. Characteristically, the CHILD naevus shows a marked lateralization diffusely affecting one half of the body with a strict midline demarcation (Fig. 19.1.11). Per contra,

the naevus may be arranged in streaks following the lines of Blaschko. Sometimes one half of the body is involved by a lateralization pattern whereas the opposite side shows some linear lesions. The striking lateralization pattern has been tentatively explained by the assumption that the event of X-inactivation coincides and interferes with the origin of a clone of organizer cells controlling a large developmental field that includes many internal organs as well as the skin of one side (Fig. 19.1.12) [3,11].

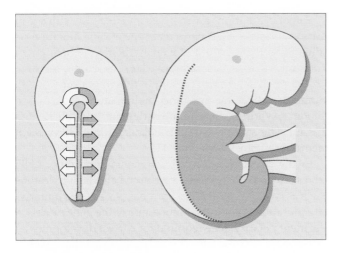

Fig. 19.1.12 Proposed explanation of the lateralization effect as observed in the CHILD syndrome. The event of X-inactivation would coincide and interfere with the origin of a clone of organizer cells controlling a large developmental field.

Table 19.1.6 X-linked non-lethal mutations giving rise to a mosaic cutaneous pattern

> X-linked hypohidrotic ectodermal dysplasia
> Menkes disease
> Dyskeratosis congenita, X-linked type
> Partington's syndrome
> Congenital generalized hypertrichosis, X-linked type

Functional mosaicism of X-linked non-lethal mutations

X-linked non-lethal mutations displaying a mosaic pattern in affected females are summarized in Table 19.1.6. Arrangements different from Blaschko's lines may be observed [24]. (It should be noted that in the strict sense of genetic nomenclature, Menkes disease would be a lethal trait because affected males do not reach the age of reproduction.)

A full-blown picture of Partington's syndrome is almost exclusively observed in males who show failure to thrive as infants, seizures, hemiplegia, gastroenteritis, recurrent pneumonia and a diffuse brown pigmentation of the skin [25]. Female individuals are only mildly affected and show a linear pattern of hyperpigmentation. Cutaneous amyloidosis is an epiphenomenon that may or may not be present which is why the syndrome should no longer be categorized as a particular type of amyloidosis [26].

In order to exclude or ascertain heterozygosity for X-linked hypohidrotic ectodermal dysplasia, sweat testing by use of a large skin area such as the back is a reliable method that has the advantage of being more simple and less expensive than a molecular analysis (Fig. 19.1.13) [27,28].

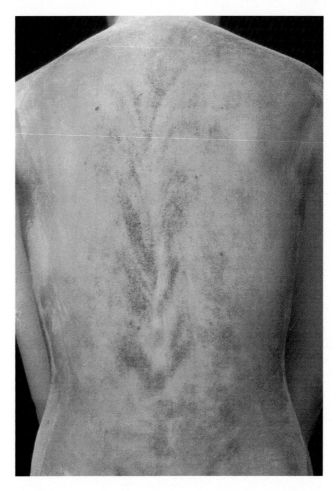

Fig. 19.1.13 Result of sweat testing in a woman heterozygous for X-linked hypohidrotic ectodermal dysplasia.

Table 19.1.7 Phenotypes that can be explained by autosomal lethal mutations surviving by mosaicism

> McCune–Albright syndrome
> Schimmelpenning syndrome
> Proteus syndrome
> Naevus comedonicus syndrome
> Encephalocraniocutaneous lipomatosis
> Delleman's syndrome
> Sturge–Weber–Klippel–Trenaunay syndrome
> Cutis marmorata telangiectatica congenita
> Pigmentary mosaicism of the Ito type
> Miliaria acantholytica
> Neurocutaneous melanosis

Genomic mosaicism of lethal mutations

Some mosaic phenotypes exclusively occur sporadically because the underlying autosomal gene exerts a lethal effect when present in a zygote [13]. The embryo can only survive when the mutant cells are growing in close proximity to normal tissue, i.e. in a mosaic state. Traits belonging to this category are summarized in Table 19.1.7.

Molecular proof of this concept has been provided in the McCune–Albright syndrome that is caused by mosaicism of a mutation in exon 8 of the $G_{s\alpha}$ gene [29,30]. Possibly, other mosaic phenotypes such as the Proteus syndrome may likewise represent defects of a G protein (guanine nucleotide-binding protein).

Most, if not all, cases of pigmentary mosaicism reported under the outdated term 'hypomelanosis of Ito' reflect mosaicism of a lethal mutation that may be a numeric chromosome aberration, translocation, ring chromosome, marker chromosome, pericentric inversion or point mutation [6,11]. Such cases do not always show the pattern of Blaschko's lines but may display a checkerboard or phylloid pattern [4].

Paradoxically, some phenotypes reflecting mosaicism of an autosomal lethal mutation may occur in several members of a family. This can be explained by the concept of paradominant inheritance [14] (see below).

Genomic mosaicism of non-lethal mutations

Some autosomal dominant traits may exceptionally occur in a quadrant or otherwise segmental distribution. Such cases can be explained by a postzygotic mutation that may have caused, simultaneously, gonadal mosaicism which is why these patients may transmit the trait to their children who will show a diffuse involvement of the entire integument (see Fig. 19.1.3) [11,15,31].

Other non-lethal autosomal mutations may manifest themselves in the following way. The entire integument is diffusely and rather mildly involved, reflecting a heterozygous state of the mutation. In addition, a circumscribed linear or otherwise segmental area of skin shows a severe involvement, reflecting a homozygous or hemizygous state due to allelic loss (see below).

Loss of heterozygosity (LOH)

Patients affected with disseminated superficial actinic porokeratosis may show, in addition, a circumscribed area of severe involvement in the form of linear porokeratosis. This can best be explained by loss of the normal allele through an early postzygotic mutational event [32,33].

A similar concept has been proposed to explain linear psoriasis [34]. Through somatic recombination occurring at an early stage of embryogenesis one of the daughter cells may become homozygous for a psoriasis gene, and the linear arrangement would reflect a clonal proliferation of this population of cells. In this way, a minor additive gene would act, in a homozygous state, as a major gene predisposing to the disease. The ultimate manifestation of linear psoriasis would depend on the influence of other predisposing genes as well as of environmental factors. This would explain why linear psoriasis usually develops later in life.

Somatic mutations are frequent and increase with age in various tissues [35]. A particular type of such mutations is allelic loss that accounts for many benign or malignant tumours such as neurofibroma [36], neurofibrosarcoma [37] or the hamartomas present in tuberous sclerosis [38]. Similarly, leukaemia and other malignancies occurring in Bloom's syndrome apparently originate from allelic loss [39,40]. The same is true for leukaemia in children with neurofibromatosis type 1 [41,42].

In the naevoid basal cell carcinoma syndrome, LOH gives rise to both basal cell carcinoma and benign lesions such as jaw cysts or ovarian fibromas [43,44]. The underlying mutation is a human homologue of the gene *patched*, a segment polarity gene required for correct developmental patterning of *Drosophila*. It has been shown that LOH at this locus is also an initial step in the development of sporadic basal cell carcinoma [45].

Two different segmental forms of autosomal dominant skin disorders

When an autosomal dominant skin disorder manifests itself in a quadrant, linear or otherwise segmental form, two different types of severity, reflecting different states of zygosity, can be distinguished (Fig. 19.1.14) [46]. Type 1 reflects heterozygosity and shows a degree of severity similar to that encountered in the non-mosaic phenotype. Type 2 involvement is more severe and originates from loss of heterozygosity for the underlying mutation. Such dichotomous types of segmental involvement have been described in various autosomal dominant traits (Table 19.1.8) [33,47].

Twin spotting

Loss of heterozygosity may give rise to twin spotting in the form of paired patches of mutant tissue that differ from each other and from the background tissue [48]. In an embryo heterozygous for two different recessive mutations localized on the same chromosome, an event of somatic recombination may result in two homozygous daughter cells that may constitute the stem cells of paired mutant patches (Fig. 19.1.15). Twin spotting has been extensively studied in plants and animals [49,50]. A similar mechanism has been proposed to explain some human skin disorders that occur close together.

Table 19.1.8 Autosomal dominant skin disorders exemplifying dichotomous types of segmental involvement

Neurofibromatosis type 1
Cutaneous leiomyomatosis
Multiple glomus tumours
Epidermolytic hyperkeratosis of Brocq
Darier's disease
Disseminated superficial actinic porokeratosis

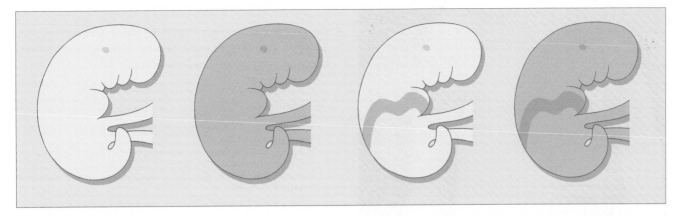

Fig. 19.1.14 Dichotomous types of segmental manifestation of autosomal dominant skin disorders. (a) Healthy phenotype; (b) diffuse manifestation in a heterozygous embryo; (c) segmental involvement of type 1, reflecting heterozygosity; (d) segmental involvement of type 2, reflecting loss of heterozygosity.

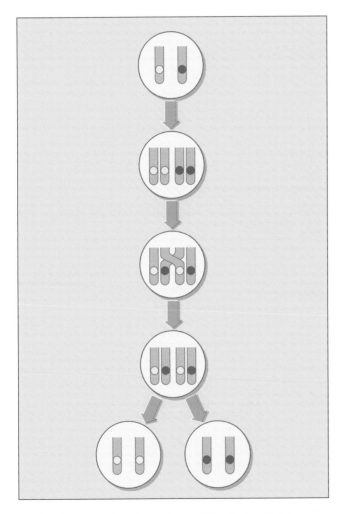

Fig. 19.1.15 Mechanism of somatic recombination in which two homozygous daughter cells give rise to allelic twin spotting.

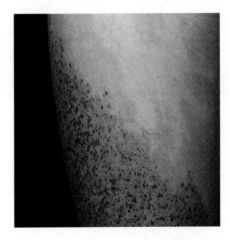

Fig. 19.1.16 Phacomatosis pigmentovascularis, a possible example of non-allelic twin spotting.

1 Vascular twin naevi. These are characterized by a cooccurrence of naevus telangiectaticus and naevus anaemicus [51]. This is presumably the most frequent form of twin spots occurring in human skin. There is circumstantial evidence in favour of the assumption that the underlying mutations are allelic [52].

2 Phacomatosis pigmentovascularis. A coexistence of teleangiectatic naevus and widespread pigmentary naevus is known under the term phacomatosis pigmentovascularis (Fig. 19.1.16). Most likely the underlying mutations are non-allelic [53].

3 Phacomatosis pigmentokeratotica. This phenotype is characterized by a simultaneous occurrence of speckled lentiginous naevus of a papular type and epidermal naevus of a non-epidermolytic, organoid type (Fig. 19.1.17) [54]. Nine cases have been found in the literature, and in most of these patients the two different types of naevi were found either in adjacent regions or in corresponding areas on either side of the body, suggesting a common origin from a somatic mutational event giving rise to a twin-spot phenomenon [55].

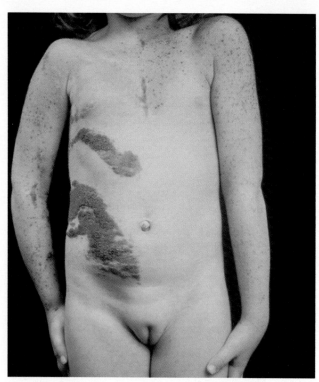

Fig. 19.1.17 Phacomatosis pigmentokeratotica. Courtesy of Dr Gianluca Tadini, Milan, Italy.

Table 19.1.9 Possible examples of twin spotting in human skin

Vascular twin naevi
Cutis tricolor
Phacomatosis pigmentovascularis
Phacomatosis pigmentokeratotica
Unilateral naevoid telangiectasia and Becker naevus

Table 19.1.10 Phenotypes that may be explained by paradominant inheritance

Becker naevus/Becker naevus syndrome
Sebaceous naevus/sebaceous naevus
  syndrome
Sturge–Weber–Klippel–Trenaunay syndrome
Naevus anaemicus
Unilateral naevoid telangiectasia

Other possible examples of twin spotting in human skin are summarized in Table 19.1.9. It should be noted, however, that molecular proof for the concept of twin spotting in human skin is so far lacking.

Paradominant inheritance

A particular mechanism giving rise to a mosaic phenotype is paradominant inheritance. This concept was first pro-

posed to explain the exceptional familial occurrence of Becker pigmented hairy naevus [14,33]. Cutaneous phenotypes that may be explained by paradominant inheritance are summarized in Table 19.1.10.

REFERENCES

1 Happle R. What is a nevus? A proposed definition of a common medical term. *Dermatology* 1995; 191: 1–5.
2 Happle R, Fuhrmann-Rieger A, Fuhrmann W. Wie verlaufen die Blaschko-Linien am behaarten Kopf? *Hautarzt* 1984; 35: 366–9.
3 Happle R. The lines of Blaschko: a developmental pattern visualizing functional X-chromosome mosaicism. *Curr Prob Dermatol* 1987; 17: 5–18.
4 Happle R. Pigmentary patterns associated with human mosaicism: a proposed classification. *Eur J Dermatol* 1993; 3: 170–4.
5 Bolognia JL, Orlow SJ, Glick SA. Lines of Blaschko. *J Am Acad Dermatol* 1994; 31: 157–90.
6 Read AP, Donnai D. Association of pigmentary anomalies with chromosomal and genetic mosaicism and chimerism. *Am J Hum Genet* 1990; 47: 166–7.
7 Happle R. The McCune–Albright syndrome: a lethal gene surviving by mosaicism. *Clin Genet* 1986; 29: 321–4.
8 Davis DG, Shaw MW. An unusual human mosaic for skin pigmentation. *N Engl J Med* 1964; 270: 1384–9.
9 Findlay GH, Moores PP. Pigment anomalies of the skin in the human chimaera: their relation to systematized naevi. *Br J Dermatol* 1980; 103: 489–98.
10 Fitzgerald PH, Donald RA, Kirk RL. A true hermaphrodite dispermid chimera with 46, XX and 46, XY karyotypes. *Clin Genet* 1979; 15: 89–96.
11 Happle R. Mosaicism in human skin: understanding the patterns and mechanisms. *Arch Dermatol* 1993; 129: 1460–70.
12 Horn D, Rommeck M, Sommer D, Körner H. Phylloid pigmentary pattern with mosaic trisomy 13. *Pediatr Dermatol* 1997; 14: 278–80.
13 Happle R. Lethal genes surviving by mosaicism: a possible explanation for sporadic birth defects involving the skin. *J Am Acad Dermatol* 1987; 16: 899–906.
14 Happle R. Paradominant inheritance: a possible explanation for Becker's pigmented hairy nevus. *Eur J Dermatol* 1992; 2: 39–40.
15 Hall JG. Somatic mosaicism: observations related to clinical genetics. *Am J Hum Genet* 1988; 43: 355–63.
16 Boltshauser B, Stocker H, Mächler M. Neurofibromatosis type 1 in a child of a parent with segmental neurofibromatosis (NF-5). *Neurofibromatosis* 1989; 2: 224–45.
17 Lenz W. Half chromatid mutations may explain incontinentia pigmenti in males. *Am J Hum Genet* 1975; 27: 690.
18 Sefiani A, Abel L, Heuertz S *et al*. The gene for incontinentia pigmenti is assigned to Xq28. *Genomics* 1989; 4: 427–9.
19 Gorski JL, Burright EN, Harnden CE, Stein CK, Glover TW, Reyner EL. Localization of DNA sequences to a region within Xp11.21 between incontinentia pigmenti (Ip1) X-chromosomal translocation breakpoints. *Am J Hum Genet* 1991; 48: 53–64.
20 Hodgson SV, Neville B, Jones RWA, Fear C, Bobrow M. Two cases of X/autosome translocation in females with incontinentia pigmenti. *Hum Genet* 1985; 71: 231–4.
21 Ballabio A, Andria G. Deletions and translocations involving the distal short arm of the human X-chromosome: review and hypotheses. *Hum Mol Genet* 1992; 1: 221–7.
22 Happle R, Daniëls O, Koopman RJJ. MIDAS syndrome (microphthalmia, dermal aplasia, and sclerocornea): an X-linked phenotype distinct from Goltz syndrome. *Am J Med Genet* 1993; 47: 710–13.
23 Happle R, Mittag H, Küster W. The CHILD nevus: a distinct skin disorder. *Dermatology* 1995; 191: 210–16.
24 Figuera LE, Pandolfo M, Dunne PW, Cantú JM, Patel PI. Mapping of the congenital generalized hypertrichosis locus to chromosome Xq24–q27.1. *Nature Genet* 1995; 10: 202–7.
25 Partington MW, Mariott PJ, Prentice RSA, Cavaglia A, Simpson NE. Familial cutaneous amyloidosis with systemic manifestation in males. *Am J Med Genet* 1981; 10: 65–75.
26 Gedeon AK, Mulley JC, Kosman H, Donnelly A, Partington MW. Localisation of the gene for X-linked reticulate pigmentary disorder with systemic manifestations (PDR), previously known as X-linked cutaneous amyloidosis. *Am J Med Genet* 1994; 52: 75–8.

27 Happle R, Frosch PJ. Manifestation of the lines of Blaschko in women heterozygous for X-linked hypohidrotic ectodermal dysplasia. *Clin Genet* 1985; 27: 468–71.

28 Bartstra HLJ, Hulsmans RFHJ, Steijlen PM, Ruige M, de Die-Smulders CEM, Cassiman JJ. Mosaic expression of hypohidrotic ectodermal dysplasia in an isolated affected female child. *Arch Dermatol* 1994; 130: 1421–4.

29 Weinstein LS, Shenker A, Gejman PV, Merino MJ, Friedman E, Spiegel AM. Activating mutations of the stimulatory G protein in the McCune–Albright syndrome. *N Engl J Med* 1991; 325: 1688–95.

30 Schwindinger WF, Francomano CA, Levine MA. Identification of a mutation in the gene encoding the α subunit of the stimulatory G protein of adenylyl cyclase in McCune–Albright syndrome. *Proc Natl Acad Sci USA* 1992; 89: 5152–6.

31 Happle R. Akanthokeratolytischer epidermaler Nävus: Vererbbar ist die Akanthokeratolyse, nicht der Nävus. *Hautarzt* 1990; 41: 117–18.

32 Happle R. Somatic recombination may explain linear porokeratosis associated with disseminated superficial actinic porokeratosis. *Am J Med Genet* 1991; 39: 237.

33 Happle R. Loss of heterozygosity in human skin. *J Am Acad Dermatol* 1999; 41: 143–61.

34 Happle R. Somatic recombination may explain linear psoriasis. *J Med Genet* 1991; 28: 337.

35 Martin GM, Ogburn CE, Colgin LM, Gown AM, Edland SD, Monnat RJ Jr. Somatic mutations are frequent and increase with age in human kidney epithelial cells. *Hum Mol Genet* 1996; 5: 215–21.

36 Colman SD, Williams CA, Wallace MR. Benign neurofibromas in type 1 neurofibromatosis (NF1) show somatic deletions of the NF1 gene. *Nature Genet* 1995; 11: 90–2.

37 Menon AG, Anderson KM, Riccardi VM *et al.* Chromosome 17p deletions and p53 gene mutations associated with the formation of malignant neurofibrosarcomas in von Recklinghausen neurofibromatosis. *Proc Natl Acad Sci USA* 1990; 87: 5435–9.

38 Green AJ, Smith M, Yates JRW. Loss of heterozygosity on chromosome 16p13.3 in hamartomas from tuberous sclerosis patients. *Nature Genet* 1994; 6: 193–6.

39 German J. Cytological evidence for crossing-over *in vitro* in human lymphoid cells. *Science* 1964; 144: 298–301.

40 Langlois RG, Bigbee WL, Jensen RH, German J. Evidence for increased *in vivo* mutation and somatic recombination in Bloom's syndrome. *Proc Natl Acad Sci USA* 1989; 86: 670–4.

41 Largaespada DA, Brannan CI, Jenkins NA, Copeland NG. *NF1* deficiency causes Ras-mediated granulocyte/macrophage colony stimulating factor hypersensitivity and chronic myeloid leukaemia. *Nature Genet* 1996; 12: 137–43.

42 Bollag G, Clapp DW, Shih S *et al.* Loss of *NF1* results in activation of the Ras signaling pathway and leads to aberrant growth in halmatopoietic cells. *Nature Genet* 1996; 12: 144–8.

43 Gailani MR, Bale SJ, Leffell DJ *et al.* Developmental defects in Gorlin syndrome related to a putative tumor suppressor gene on chromosome 9. *Cell* 1992; 69: 111–17.

44 Levanat S, Gorlin RJ, Fallet S, Johnson DR, Fantasia JE, Bale AE. A two-hit model for developmental defects in Gorlin syndrome. *Nature Genet* 1996; 12: 85–7.

45 Gailani MR, Ståhle-Bäckdahl M, Leffell DJ *et al.* The role of the human homologue of *Drosophila patched* in sporadic basal cell carcinomas. *Nature Genet* 1996; 14: 78–81.

46 Happle R. Segmental forms of autosomal dominant skin disorders: different types of severity reflect different states of zygosity. *Am J Med Genet* 1996; 66: 241–2.

47 Happle R. A rule concerning the segmental manifestation of autosomal dominant skin disorders: review of clinical examples providing evidence for dichotomous types of severity. *Arch Dermatol* 1997; 133: 1505–9.

48 Whitehouse HLK. *Genetic Recombination: Understanding the Mechanisms*. Chichester: John Wiley, 1982: 214–24.

49 Vig BK. Somatic crossing over in Glycine max (L.) Merrill: effect of some inhibitors of DNA synthesis on the induction of somatic crossing over and point mutations. *Genetics* 1973; 73: 583–96.

50 Ramel C, Magnusson J. Modulation of genotoxicity in *Drosophila*. *Mutation Res* 1992; 267: 221–7.

51 Happle R, Koopman R, Mier PD. Hypothesis: vascular twin naevi and somatic recombination in man. *Lancet* 1990; 335: 376–8.

52 Happle R. Allelic somatic mutations may explain vascular twin nevi. *Hum Genet* 1991; 86: 321–2.

53 Happle R, Steijlen PM. Phacomatosis pigmentovascularis gedeutet als ein Phänomen der Zwillingsflecken. *Hautarzt* 1989; 40: 721–4.

54 Happle R, Hoffmann R, Restano L, Caputo R, Tadini G. Phacomatosis pigmento-keratotica: a melanocytic-epidermal twin nevus syndrome. *Am J Med Genet* 1996; 65: 363–5.

55 Tadini G, Restano L, González-Pérez R *et al.* Phacomatosis pigmentokeratotica: report of new cases and further delineation of the syndrome. *Arch Dermatol* 1998; 134: 333–7.

Molecular biology and gene mapping

This is important for the purpose of genetic counselling including prenatal diagnosis [1–3] and for the endeavour to reach the ultimate goal of gene therapy, particularly for the most severe genetic disorders.

Methods of gene mapping

An initial step in the mapping of genes was the elucidation of X-linked inheritance implying the assignment of a trait to a specific chromosome [4]. Later, linkage of some diseases such as the nail–patella syndrome to the ABO locus on chromosone 9 was achieved. A further method was the study of translocations with the goal of localizing a given gene defect at the break point. During the 1970s, a major breakthrough was achieved by the technique of analysing rodent–human somatic cell hybrids. During the 1980s, *in situ* hybridization and the technique of cloning DNA sequences as yeast artificial chromosomes (YACs) has further accelerated the project of human gene mapping [5]. Important additional techniques are FISH (fluorescence *in situ* hybridization) as well as the use of restriction fragment length polymorphisms and variable number tandem repeats (VNTRs) for linkage analysis [1,6]. A frequently used term is the word LOD score ('logarithm of the odds'). Taken together with a specified recombination fraction (θ) the LOD score expresses the odds for and against linkage. A LOD score greater than 3 indicates that linkage is very likely. The frequency of recombination between two gene loci is indicated in terms of centimorgans (cM). One cM means that recombination occurs in one out of 100 meioses. One cM corresponds to a distance of about 1 million base pairs.

A list of regionally assigned phenotypes is given in Table 19.1.11.

Molecular analysis of mendelian disorders

For the molecular analysis of a monogenic trait, the following techniques and concepts have been itemized by McKusick [1].

1 Demonstration of a changed purine or pyrimidine base in the DNA of a cloned gene.

2 Absence, reduction or structural deviation of mRNA.

Table 19.1.11 Cutaneous traits mapped within the human genome

Location	Disorder	MIM Number	Gene or gene product
1p36.2–p34	Erythrokeratodermia variabilis	133 200	connexin 31
1p36–p34	Peutz–Jeghers syndrome	175 200	serine threonine kinase
1p34	Porphyria cutanea tarda	176 100	uroporphyrinogen III, decarboxylase
1p36.3–p36.2	Ehlers–Danlos syndrome type VI	225 400	lysylhydroxylase
1q13.2–q13.3	Bloom's syndrome	210 900	DNA helicase
1q21	Porphyria variegata	176 200	protoporphyrinogen oxydase
1q21	Ichthyosis vulgaris, autosomal dominant type	146 700	filaggrin
1q21	Vohwinkel's syndrome	124 500	loricrin
1q25–q31	Epidermolysis bullosa, Herlitz type	226 700	laminin 5
1q32	Van der Woude's syndrome	119 300	
1q32–q44	Ectodermal dysplasia/skin fragility syndrome	601 975	plakophilin
1q43	Chediak–Higashi syndrome	214 500	
1q44	Muckle–Wells syndrome	191 900	
2p16	Muir–Torre syndrome	158 320	DNA mismatch repair
2p16	NAME syndrome	160 980	
2q	Junctional epidermolysis bullosa with pylorus stenosis	226 730	α6 integrin
2q11–q13	Hypohidrotic ectodermal dysplasia, autosomal recessive type	224 900	
2q21	Xeroderma pigmentosum group B	278 710	nucleotide excision repair
2q31	Ehlers–Danlos syndrome type IV	130 050	COL3A1
2q31–q34.3	Ehlers–Danlos syndrome type I	130 000	COL5A2
2q31–q34.3	Ehlers–Danlos syndrome type II	130 000	COL5A2
2q33–q35	Lamellar ichthyosis type 2	601 277	
2q34	Ehlers–Danlos syndrome type X	225 310	fibronectin
2q34–q36	Bjørnstad's syndrome	262 000	
2q35	Waardenburg's syndrome type 1	193 500	PAX 3
3p25	Xeroderma pigmentosum group C	278 720	XPC excision repair
3p21.3	Dystrophic epidermolysis bullosa (8 separate types)	120 120	COL7A1
3q21–q24	Hailey–Hailey disease	169 600	
4q12	Piebaldism	172 800	c-KIT protooncogene
4q28–q31	Huriez's syndrome	181 600	
5q21–q22	Gardner's syndrome	175 100	
5q35.5	Lymphoedema, Nonne–Milroy type	136 352	vascular endothelial growth factor 5 receptor
6p21	Striated palmoplantar keratoderma	148 700	desmoplakin
7q11	Cutis laxa	123 700	elastin
7q21.1	Ehlers–Danlos syndrome tye VII	130 060	COL1A2
8p21.2	Atrichia, papular type	203 655	zink finger transcription factor protein, hairless gene
8p23–p22	Keratolytic winter erythema (Oudtshoorn disease)	148 370	
8p12–p11.2	Werner's syndrome	277 700	helicase
8q24	Tricho-rhino-phalangeal syndrome	190 350	
8q24	Epidermolysis bullosa simplex with muscular dstrophy	226 670	plectin 1
8q24.3	Rothmund–Thomson syndrome	268 400	DNA helicase RECQL4
8qter	Mal de Meleda	248 300	
9p21	Multiple trichoepithelioma	132 700	
9p21–p13	Cartilage-hair hypoplasia	250 250	
9q22	Naevoid basal cell carcinoma syndrome	109 400	PATCHED protein
9q34	Hereditary haemorrhagic teleangiectasia (Osler's disease)	187 300	endoglin
9q34.1	Tuberous sclerosis type 1	191 100	hamartin
9q34.1	Nail-patella syndrome	161 200	LIM homeodomain protein, LMX1B
9q34.1	Xeroderma pigmentosum group A	278 700	XPA excision repair
9q34.2–q34.3	Ehlers–Danlos syndrome type I	130 000	COL5A1
9q34.2–q34.3	Ehlers–Danlos syndrome type II	130 010	COL5A1
9q34.2–q34.3	Ehlers–Danlos syndrome type III	130 020	COL3A1
10pter	Refsum's disease	266 500	phytanic acid oxydase
10q11.2	Multiple endocrine neoplasia type 2b	162 300	RET protooncogene
10q11	Cockayne's syndrome	216 400	ERCC6 excision repair
10q22–q23	Cowden disease	158 350	PTEN
10q23.1–q23.2	Hermansky–Pudlak syndrome	203 300	transmembrane protein
10q24.3	Generalized atrophic benign epidermolysis bullosa	226 650	COL17A1
10q25.2–q26.3	Congenital erythropoietic porphyria (Günther's disease)	263 700	uroporphinogen III cosynthase
11p13	Omenn's syndrome	267 700	Rag-1
11q11–q13.1	Hereditary angio-oedema	106 100	C1 esterase inhibitor
11q13	Multiple endocrine neoplasia type 1	131 100	menin

Continued

Table 19.1.11 *Continued*

Location	Disorder	MIM Number	Gene or gene product
11q13.1	Multiple glomus tumors	138 000	
11q13.5–q14	Papillon–Lefèvre syndrome	245 000	
11q14–q21	Oculocutaneous albinism (OCA 1)	203 100	tyrosinase
11q23.3	Ataxia telangiectasia	208 900	phosphatidylinositol 3 kinase
12q11–q13	Epidermolytic hyperkeratosis of Brocq	113 800	keratin 1
	Ichthyosis bullosa of Siemens	146 800	keratin 2e
	Epidermolysis bullosa simplex (Köbner type, Weber–Cockayne type, Dowling–Meara type)	148 040	keratin 5
	Pachonychia congenita, Jadassohn–Lewandowsky type	167 200	keratin 6A
	Pachonychia congenita, Jackson–Lawler type	167 210	keratin 6B
	White sponge hyperplasia of the mucosa	193 900	keratin 4
	Monilethrix	158 000	hair cortex keratin 6
	Palmoplantar keratoderma, Norbotten type (keratin type II cluster)	144 200 148 030	
12q23–q24.1	Darier's disease	124 200	ATPA2 (SERCA 2)
12q24	Noonan syndrome	163 950	
13q.11–q12.1	Hidrotic ectodermal dysplasia of Clouston	129 500	
14q11	Lamellar ichthyosis type 1	242 100	transglutaminase 1
15q11.2–q12	Oculocutaneous albinism (OCA2)	203 200	P protein
15q21	Griscelli's syndrome	214 450	myosin Va
15q21.1	Marfan's syndrome type 1	134 797	fibrillin 1
15q22.1	Bloom's syndrome	210 900	DNA helicase
16p13.1	Pseudoxanthoma elasticum	264 800	
16p13.3	Tuberous sclerosis type 2	191 092	tuberin
16q12–q13	Cylindromatosis	123 850	
16q22.1–q22.3	Tyrosinaemia type II	276 600	
17p13	Onychohypoplasia of Hamm	no entry	
17p11.2	Sjögren–Larsson syndrome	270 200	fatty aldehyde, dehydroxygenase
17q11.2	Neurofibromatosis type I	162 200	neurofibromin
17q12–q21	Epidermolytic hyperkeratosis of Brocq	113 800	keratin 10
	Epidermolytic palmoplantar keratoderma	144 200	keratin 9
	Epidermolysis bullosa simplex (Köbner type, Weber–Cockayne type, Dowling–Meara type)	148 066	keratin 14
	Pachyonychia congenita, Jadassohn–Lewandowsky type	167 200	keratin 16
	Pachyonychia congenita, Jackson–Lawlor type	167 210	keratin 17
	Steatocystoma multiplex	148 069	keratin 17
	White sponge hyperplasia of the mucosa (keratin type I cluster)	193 900 148 040	keratin 13
17q21.2–q22	Tricho-dento-osseous syndrome	190 320	distal-less homoeo box 3, (DLX3)
17q21.31–q22.05	Ehlers–Danlos syndrome type VII	130 060	COL1A1, COL1A2
17q23–qter	Palmoplantar keratoderma with oesophageal cancer	148 500	envoplakin
17qter	Epidermodysplasia verruciformis	226 400	
18q12	Striated palmoplantar keratoderma	148 700	desmoglein
18q21.3	Erythropoietic protoporphyria	177 000	ferrocholestase
19q13.2–q13.3	Xeroderma pigmentosum group D	278 730	XPD helicase
20q13.2	McCune–Albright syndrome	139 320	$G_s\alpha$ protein (GNAS1)
Xp22.32	X-linked recessive ichthyosis	308 100	steroid sulphatase
Xp22.31	MIDAS syndrome	309 801	rho type GTPase activating protein
Xp22.2–p22.13	Keratosis follicularis spinulosa decalvans	308 800	
Xp22–p21	Partington's syndrome	301 220	
Xp11.3–p11.2	Wiskott–Aldrich syndrome	301 000	WAS protein
Xp11.23–p11.22	X-linked dominant chondrodysplasia punctata (Happle's syndrome)	302 960	sterol-Δ^8-isomerase
Xq12–q13.1	X-linked hypohidrotic ectodermal dysplasia	305 100	ectodysplasin A (tabby protein)
Xq13	Menkes disease	309 400	copper transporting protein, type ATPase 7A
Xq22.1	Angiokeratoma corporis diffusum	301 500	α-galactosidase A
Xq24–q27	Bazex–Dupré–Christol syndrome	301 845	
Xq24–q27.1	Congenital generalized hypertrichosis, X-linked type	307 150	
Xq26.3–q27	Albinism-deafness syndrome	300 700	
Xq27.3–qter	Hereditary bullous dystrophy, X-linked macular type	302 000	
Xq28	Incontinentia pigmenti	308 310	
Xq28	Dyskeratosis congenita, X-linked type	305 000	dyskerin (XAP 101)
Xq28	Goeminne's syndrome	314 300	
Xq28	CHILD syndrome	308 050	3β-hydroxysteroid dehydrogenase

3 Correction of a gene defect by transfection of the normal gene.

4 'Positional cloning': determination of the normal structure and function of a DNA segment where a given disease has been mapped [7].

5 Demonstration of an altered primary structure of a protein.

6 Failure of complementation in cell fusion experiments (e.g. XP).

7 Linkage of a trait to a restriction fragment length polymorphism (candidate gene approach).

8 Deficiency of enzymatic activity in a recessive trait (absence in homozygotes or intermediate levels in heterozygotes).

9 Mapping of a phenotype to a locus for a given molecule (candidate gene approach) [6,7].

10 Inference of enzyme deficiency from accumulation of a given substrate.

11 Correction by providing a substance not synthesized.

12 Delineation of an ultrastructural abnormality.

13 Homology between the human genome and that of other species, in particular the mouse [8,9].

An additional molecular method is somatic crossover point mapping in which cells are used from individuals having undergone intragenic recombination [10]. The regional assignment and subsequent cloning of genes has opened new ways of thinking for the clinical dermatologist and has in part transformed the rules of classification of diseases. New nosological categories are emerging. For example, antigen mapping has provided evidence for a striking analogy between acquired autoimmune bullous disorders and specific types of epidermolysis bullosa (see Chapter 19.4). The epidermal differentiation complex localized at 1q21 harbours genes responsible for various hyperkeratotic disorders such as Vohwinkel's syndrome and psoriasis [11,12]. Mutations within the KIT oncogen at chromosome 4q12 are responsible for both piebaldism and mast cell leukaemia. Mutations within the keratin clusters type I and II are responsible for epidermolytic ichthyosis, epidermolytic palmoplantar keratoderma, several types of epidermolysis bullosa simplex as well as for white sponge hyperplasia of the oral mucosa and pachyonychia congenita (Table 19.1.11) [13]. Conversely, molecular research has confirmed a fundamental difference between clinically related entities such as Darier's disease and Hailey–Hailey disease or between the various groups of xeroderma pigmentosum. In the McCune–Albright syndrome, the aetiological concept of a lethal mutation surviving by mosaicism was first proposed on the grounds of clinical features and subsequently confirmed by demonstrating mosaicism for an activating mutation in the GNAS-1 gene [14]. Hence, the disease belongs to the increasing group of G protein diseases. G

proteins (guanine nucleotide-binding proteins, alpha-stimulating polypeptide) have an important function in signal transduction such as visual transduction, olfactory transduction, hormone transduction or melanoma cell motility. Remarkably, Albright's hereditary osteodystrophy that should not be confused with McCune–Albright syndrome is caused by a mutation at the same locus, resulting in a decreased GNAS-1 activity [15]. McKusick [1] calls it poetic justice that two conditions described by Fuller Albright should have a defect in the same gene (MIM no. 139320), producing either deficiency or excess of a stimulatory G protein.

The homeobox (HOX) genes are probably of increasing significance for the understanding of the embryogenesis of human skin. HOX genes control the hierarchy of regulatory genes inducing embryonic development [16]. A clinical example is Waardenburg's syndrome that is caused by a mutation in the PAX-3 gene that belongs to a particular subgroup of homeobox genes.

REFERENCES

1 McKusick VA. *Mendelian Inheritance in Man. A Catalog of Human Genes and Genetic Disorders*, 12th ed. Baltimore: Johns Hopkins University Press, 1998.

2 Upadhyaya M, Fryer A, MacMillan J, Broadhead W, Huson SM, Harper PS. Prenatal diagnosis and presymptomatic detection of neurofibromatosis type 1. *J Med Genet* 1992; 29: 180–3.

3 Shimizu H, Niizeki H, Suzumori K *et al.* Prenatal diagnosis of oculocutaneous albinism by analysis of the fetal tyrosinase gene. *J Invest Dermatol* 1994; 103: 104–6.

4 Macias-Flores MA, Garcia-Cruz D, Rivera H *et al.* A new form of hypertrichosis inherited as an X-linked dominant trait. *Hum Genet* 1984; 66: 66–70.

5 Kere J, Grzeschik KH, Limon J, Gremaud M, Schlessinger D, de la Chapelle A. Anhidrotic ectodermal dysplasia gene region cloned in yeast artificial chromosomes. *Genomics* 1993; 16: 305–10.

6 De Bie SL, De Paepe AM. Linkage analysis, a primer for dermatologists. *Eur J Dermatol* 1995; 5: 653–8.

7 Uitto J. Genetic linkage mapping of heritable skin diseases: positional cloning versus the candidate gene approach. *J Invest Dermatol* 1994; 102: 825–6.

8 Searle AG, Edwards JH, Hall JG. Mouse homologues of human hereditary disease. *J Med Genet* 1994; 31: 1–19.

9 Kelly EJ, Palmiter RD. A murine model of Menkes disease reveals a physiological function of metallothionein. *Nature Genet* 1996; 13: 219–22.

10 Ellis NA, Groden J, Ye TZ *et al.* The Bloom's syndrome gene product is homologous to ReqQ helicases. *Cell* 1995; 83: 655–66.

11 Christiano AM, Maestrini E, Monaco A *et al.* Perturbations in the epidermal cornified cell envelope in Vohwinkel's syndrome: genetic linkage to the epidermal differentiation complex in 1q21 and identification of a mutation in the loricrin gene. *J Invest Dermatol* 1996; 106: 811.

12 Hardas BD, Zhao X, Zhang J, Longqing X, Stoll S, Elder JT. Assignment of psoriasis to human chromosomal band 1q21: coordinate overexpression of clustered genes in psoriasis. *J Invest Dermatol* 1996; 106: 753–8.

13 McLean WHI, Rugg EL, Lunny DP *et al.* Keratin 16 and keratin 17 mutations cause pachyonychia congenita. *Nature Genet* 1995; 9: 273–8.

14 Weinstein LS, Shenker A, Gejman PV, Merino MJ, Friedman E, Spiegel AM. Activating mutations of the stimulatory G protein in the McCune–Albright syndrome. *N Engl J Med* 1991; 325: 1688–95.

15 Levine MA, Ahn TG, Klupt SF *et al.* Genetic deficiency of the alpha subunit of the guanin nucleotide-binding protein G(s) as the molecular basis for Albright hereditary osteodystrophy. *Proc Natl Acad Sci* 1988; 85: 617–21.

16 Scott GA, Goldsmith LA. Homeobox genes and skin development: a review. *J Invest Dermatol* 1993; 101: 3–8.

Chromosome Disorders

PETER W. LUNT

Altered ploidy
Triploidy: 69,XXX or 69,XXY or 69,XYY

Autosomal anomalies
Aneuploidy
Structural anomalies
Microdeletions
Uniparental disomy

Sex chromosome anomaly
Turner's syndrome: 45,X0
Ring-X mosaic
Triple-X syndrome: 47,XXX
Klinefelter's syndrome: 47,XXY
XYY syndrome: 47,XYY
Sex reversal
XX males

Single gene conditions affecting chromosomes
Chromosome breakage syndromes
Fragile X syndrome
Robert's syndrome

The ever accelerating growth of genetic knowledge through or alongside the advance of the Human Genome Mapping Project (HGMP) is providing increasing insight into the diversity of ways in which the genetic material can be altered in mankind. Increasingly, many conditions are being found to be caused by alteration of whole sections of genetic material, but in only a few will this be sufficiently large to be seen under a microscope. The majority of such new 'chromosomal' conditions, which may speculatively include many yet to be discovered, exist as submicroscopic alterations only detectable by specific DNA hybridization. Efficient identification of these will be made possible through sophisticated chromosome painting techniques currently being developed. The completion of the descriptive part of HGMP (anticipated by 2002) will provide the greater challenge of coming to understand the organization of the DNA sequence and of chromosome structure. In particular one can anticipate that integrity of chromosome microstructure, and of any local pattern of DNA folding in a chromosome region, must be required both for normal regulatory control of gene expression and for enabling continual scrutiny for DNA mismatch repair. Thus, familiarity with chromosomal disorders can no longer be limited to the aneuploidies or structural rearrangements detectable microscopically, but increasingly in any field of medicine (and therefore also in dermatology), must include the more subtle deletions, duplications or other DNA rearrangements.

Chromosome anomalies can be classified as follows.

1 Altered ploidy:
  (a) triploid; or
  (b) tetraploid.
2 Autosomal anomaly:
  (a) aneuploidy;
  (b) structural anomaly:
      (i) balanced translocation or inversion;
      (ii) unbalanced duplication/deletion;
      (iii) ring or marker;
      (iv) mosaic anomaly;
  (c) microdeletion;
  (d) uniparental disomy.
3 Sex chromosome anomaly:
  (a) aneuploidy
      (i) full;
      (ii) mosaic;
      (iii) partial, or ring/marker chromosome;
  (b) sex reversal.
4 Other chromosome alteration due to single gene condition:
  (a) chromosome breakage;
  (b) fragile site;
  (c) centromere puffs.

History

Unbalanced autosomal anomalies are invariably associated with developmental delay/learning difficulty, and often cause severe mental retardation. Other typical manifestations include low birth weight, hypotonia, short stature/growth retardation, congenital anomalies which are often multiple and a dysmorphic appearance, often with microcephaly.

Aetiology

Aneuploidies and many other cases of chromosome disorder occur *de novo* with the affected child. Constitutional anomalies are present in sperm or egg; mosaic anomalies arise postzygotically. The exceptions are the structural rearrangements (balanced or unbalanced translocations or inversions) which can result from a familial balanced rearrangement. Autosomal microdeletions, if not *de novo*, can follow autosomal dominant inheritance. The inheritance of genetic faults affecting chromosome behaviour is that of the genetic syndrome concerned (mostly autosomal recessive or X-linked).

Altered ploidy

Triploidy: 69,XXX or 69,XXY or 69,XYY

Although triploidy (having three copies of each chromosome) is present in 2% of all conceptions, it accounts for 20% of first and second trimester miscarriages, and occurs in only 1 in 2500 births [1]. First week death is usual, but some do survive into early infancy. Triploid/diploid mosaicism may be as frequent in live births as full triploidy, and results in a specific retardation syndrome with some features of full triploidy but with asymmetry and with additional characteristic pigmentary and depigmentary signs on the skin [2].

A triploid pregnancy is often associated with hydatidiform changes in the placenta and with polyhydramnios. The newborn infant is usually severely growth retarded (often with bodily asymmetry), has hypotonia and a very large posterior fontanelle [3]. The majority have multiple congenital abnormalities including in the brain, heart, kidneys and genitalia. Skin syndactyly of the third and fourth fingers and variable syndactyly of the toes is characteristic. An increased proportion of digital whorls and a transverse palmar crease can often be noted [4].

Triploid/diploid mosaics are often recognized from their skin signs, and usually require skin biopsy for fibroblast culture for diagnostic confirmation. Typically the skin shows pigmentary and depigmentary changes following the lines of Blaschko which may initially have been classified as hypomelanosis of Ito [2], or erroneously as incontinentia pigmenti. Psychomotor retardation is usually severe although this may depend on the overall proportion of triploid cells and on brain malformation. Postnatal growth retardation and asymmetry can be expected, often with progressive scoliosis. Wide-spaced splayed toes of asymmetric disproportionate length, and skin syndactyly, particularly of the middle and ring fingers can also be diagnostic. Other malformations including iris or choroidal coloboma, cleft lip or palate, and asymmetrically missing teeth [3].

REFERENCES

1 Blackburn WR, Miller WP, Superneau DW, Cooley NR Jr, Zellweger H, Wertelecki W. Comparative studies of infants with mosaic and complete triploidy, an analysis of 55 cases. *Birth Defects* 1982; 18: 251–74.
2 Donnai D, Read AP, McKeown C, Andrews T. Hypomelanosis of Ito: a manifestation of mosaicism or chimaerism. *J Med Genet* 1988; 25: 809–18.
3 Gorlin RJ, Cohen MM, Levin LS. *Syndromes of the Head and Neck*, 3rd edn. New York: Oxford University Press, 1990.
4 Harris MJ, Poland BJ, Dill FJ *et al.* Triploidy in 40 human spontaneous abortuses: assessment of phenotype in embryos. *Obstet Gynaecol* 1981; 57: 600–6.

Autosomal anomalies

Aneuploidy

Trisomy 21

The growth, physical and dysmorphic features of children with Down's syndrome are well known [1]. Congenital malformation is frequent including a 40% incidence of congenital heart disease (particularly ventricular septal defect, atrioventricular septal defect or tetralogy of Fallot), and an 18% incidence of gastrointestinal (GI) anomalies (including duodenal atresia and Hirschprung's disease). The diagnosis in newborns, particularly if premature, may not be immediately obvious. Key features often include growth retardation, hypotonia, flat occiput, excess nuchal skin, epicanthic folds, transverse palmar creases, broad 'spade-like' hands, short incurved little finger due to a short middle phalanx and a wide 'sandle' gap between the first and second toes with deep longitudinal plantar crease. There is an increased risk in childhood of leukaemia, hypothyroidism and cataract.

Dermatoglyphic features typically include distally placed palmar axial triradii, an increased incidence of hallucal tibial arch (72% versus around 0.5% of controls), and all fingers having ulnar loops (31% versus 7% of controls) [2]. Skin infections, particularly around the genital area, buttocks and thighs are common, occurring in 50–60% of adolescents [3]. Usually these are follicular pustules, but may develop into abscesses. They may relate to an increased incidence of B- and T-cell dysfunction. Alopecia areata and vitiligo may reflect an increased prevalence of autoimmune disorders, while other skin problems which develop with age include patchy lichenification and acrocyanosis [4].

Trisomy 18

The median survival for babies born with trisomy 18 (Edward's syndrome) is only 5 days, although for those without cardiac defects the median is 40 days. Fewer than 10% survive beyond 1 year [5]. Characteristic features are a low birth weight, prominent occiput, low-set malformed ears, short palpebral fissures, small mouth and chin, thumb hypoplasia, rockerbottom feet with prominent heels and typical camptodactyly [1].

The most consistent dermatological features are nail hypoplasia and a dermatoglyphic pattern with arches on at least six fingertips. This will usually be associated with camptodactyly of the fingers and absence of distal flexion creases of the little finger, and often also of the third and fourth fingers. The hand is usually clenched with fixed overlapping of the index over the middle finger, and the fifth over the fourth finger [1]. Hypoplasia of subcutaneous and adipose tissue accompanying postnatal failure to thrive is common, while the multiple congenital anomalies (predominantly cardiac, genitourinary and central nervous system) can include a thyroglossal duct cyst [1].

Trisomy 13

Scalp defects, although also associated with 4p– or following dominant inheritance (including with toe aplasia in Adams–Oliver syndrome), are one of the hallmarks of trisomy 13 (Patau's syndrome). Survival beyond 3 years of the 14% who reach 1 year is exceptional, but recurrent chronic cellulitis affecting the parotid region and axilla, groin and abdominal wall is reported in at least two older children [6]. Capillary haemangioma, particularly in the glabellar region, can commonly be a prominent feature. Holoprosencephaly, a sloping forehead, bilateral or midline cleft lip and palate, and congenital heart and renal defects are frequent, as also is postaxial polydactyly, often with a rudimentary and flail postminimus sixth finger [1]. Hyperconvexity of the nails may be noted.

Trisomy 22

Preauricular tags or sinuses are a characteristic feature in infants who appear to have an extra chromosome 22 on banded karyotype [1]. Some of these cases in reality have trisomy for distal 11q as an unbalanced product of an 11/22 translocation [7], which may have a similar phenotype, and is only now becoming distinguishable from true trisomy 22 through *in situ* hybridization chromosome painting techniques. Microcephaly, large low-set ear pinnae, cleft palate, long philtrum, hypotonia, congenital heart defect, male hypogenitalism, long fingers and a finger-like thumb, are all features which may accompany the mental retardation [1].

Trisomy 8, trisomy 8 mosaic

Trisomy 8 is more commonly seen as a mosaic (85% of cases) than as complete trisomy (15% of cases), which may in part be due to a tendency for the abnormal cell line to be lost from the peripheral lymphocyte population with increasing age of the patient [1]. Diagnosis therefore often

requires skin biopsy and 'first pass' fibroblast culture analysis, as well as analysis of a more established fibroblast culture. A 'pure' trisomy 8 may be seen in fibroblasts, even if a standard karyotype from peripheral lymphocytes has been normal. The technique of chromosome painting by *in situ* hybridization may be about to revolutionize the approach to diagnosis of mosaic karyotypes through ability to detect low levels of mosaicism in interphase nuclei in many different tissue types.

Congenital distal joint contractures, which are usually progressive, with an accompanying absence of interphalangeal joint creases, illustrate one of the possible manifestations of chromosomal or other genetic mosaicism, and are frequently seen in trisomy 8. The feet can be characteristic, with between one and three deep plantar longitudinal furrows, again a feature of mosaicism. The other common diagnostic feature is absence or hypoplasia of the patella. Other dysmorphic features include a long face and high forehead, dysplastic ear pinnae, small mandible and everted lower lip, scoliosis and often a long slender trunk, congenital heart defect (in 25%) and hydronephrosis or ureteral obstruction (40%) [1]. Intelligence may depend on the proportion of normal cells in the brain, and varies from mild to moderate retardation, with some children able to function with support in an average school. The condition is not rare, with an incidence estimated at 1 in 25 000 to 50 000, but with a 5:1 male to female ratio [1]. Life expectancy is normal.

Trisomy 9

Trisomy 9, like trisomy 8, usually occurs only as a mosaic, and has the same requirement for fibroblast or other tissue cell culture to establish the diagnosis. Deep palmar or plantar creases are the characteristic dermatological feature. Low birth weight, failure to thrive, neurological impairment and psychomotor retardation are usual, leading to death in most cases by 4 months of age [1]. Dysmorphic features can include deep-set microphthalmic eyes, cleft lip or palate, dysplastic ears, short webbed neck and hypogenitalism. Congenital heart anomalies, hydronephrosis and joint contractures with talipes and dislocated hips are common.

REFERENCES

1 Gorlin RJ, Cohen MM, Levin LS. *Syndromes of the Head and Neck*, 3rd edn. New York: Oxford University Press, 1990.
2 Preus M, Fraser FC. Dermatoglyphics and syndromes. *Am J Dis Child* 1972; 124: 933–43.
3 Pueschel SM. Clinical aspects of Down syndrome from infancy to adulthood. *Am J Med Genet* 1990; suppl 7: 52–6.
4 Moss C, Savin J. *Dermatology and the New Genetics*. Oxford: Blackwell Science, 1995.
5 Carter PE, Pearn JH, Bell J, Martin N, Anderson NG. Survival in trisomy 18. *Clin Genet* 1985; 27: 59–61.
6 Redheendran R, Neu RL, Bannerman RM. Long survival in trisomy 13

syndrome: 21 cases including prolonged survival in two patients 11 and 19 years old. *Am J Med Genet* 1981; 8: 167–72.

7 Schinzel A. Mosaic-trisomy 22 and the problem of full trisomy 22. *Hum Genet* 1981; 56: 269–73.

Structural anomalies

Balanced rearrangements

Around 1 in 600 people in the general population carry a balanced chromosome rearrangement, usually as a translocation between two chromosomes, or as an inversion on one chromosome. If there is no loss or gain of genetic material this will usually have no discernible phenotypic effect, except where one of the breakpoints disrupts a gene, or otherwise interferes with the normal control of expression of a nearby gene. The clinical importance of a balanced translocation or inversion is the risk in offspring that the segregation products could result in an unbalanced karyotype with duplication or deletion of chromosomal material. If compatible with live birth, karyotypic imbalance will inevitably be associated with learning problems and often congenital abnormality; but may alternatively end in spontaneous miscarriage. Many translocations are familial, conferring consequent reproductive risk to several branches of a family.

The individual importance of balanced chromosome rearrangement is when the breakpoint does disrupt normal gene expression. In particular, the finding of a *de novo* balanced translocation in a single case of someone who has a dominant or X-linked disorder arising from a presumed new mutation, can provide not only the vital clue to chromosomal band location of the gene involved, but also the means for cloning the gene itself. In dermatology this approach has enabled cloning of the gene for X-linked hypohydrotic ectodermal dysplasia [1], and facilitated this for neurofibromatosis [2].

Unbalanced structural abnormalities

Genetic imbalance, particularly if resulting from a parental balanced translocation, will often be a combination of duplication and deletion of different chromosome material. The phenotype of any particular child may therefore represent a combination of the two components, which can only be described individually below.

2q37–

This has only recently been recognized as an entity, but may be relatively frequent. Many cases show overlap of features with pseudopseudohypoparathyroidism, although the latter is due to mutation in the Gs-α gene on chromosome 20 [3]. Thus short metacarpals, and short terminal phalanges (particularly of the thumb) are usual, but without biochemical evidence of parathyroid hormone resistance. A long neck with sloping shoulders, short palpebral fissures, high palate and joint laxity are typical. The skin may be abnormally dry, with troublesome dermatitis recorded in a majority of cases. Learning problems are usually mild to moderate, but many of the children have an unusually good visuospatial memory [4].

4p– (Wolf–Hirschhorn syndrome)

Midline scalp defects (found in 10% of cases), and preauricular dimples or skin tags are the most consistent dermatological feature from deletion of the tip of the short arm of chromosome 4 [5]. The phenotype is often distinctive, even in those cases requiring specific fluorescent *in situ* hybridization (FISH) study to detect submicroscopic microdeletion within band 4p16. Hypertelorism and wide nasal bridge give a characteristic 'Grecian helmet' appearence to the upper face. Iris coloboma, cleft lip or palate with micrognathia, narrowed external auditory meati, lobeless ear pinnae, congenital heart defect, sacral dimple and hypospadias are frequent. There is usually severe psychomotor and growth retardation, often with seizures, hypotonia and talipes. Around 35% die by the age of 2 years, but others survive to adulthood [5].

5p– (Cri-du-chat syndrome)

Characterized by microcephaly and a high-pitched 'mewing' cry in infancy, preauricular skin tags are the only noteable skin feature in deletion of the tip of the short arm of chromosome 5. The critical region is in bands 5p14 and 5p15, with some cases due to a cryptic microdeletion demonstrable only by FISH study. The degree of retardation which varies from mild to severe correlates with the size of the deletion. The facies is characterized by an increased inner canthal distance as well as true hypertelorism, micrognathia and maxillary overbite. Congenital heart defect is common [5].

9p trisomy

Duplication of the short arm of chromosome 9 is observed more frequently than either pure or mosaic full trisomy 9. Characteristic is hypoplasia of the finger nails, particularly symmetrically on the index and little fingers, due to hypoplasia of the terminal phalanx. Transverse palmar creases and contractures of some fingers may be present, with only a single flexion crease on the clinodactylous little finger. Mild syndactyly between the middle and ring fingers may also be found. There is moderate to severe retardation with IQ between 30 and 65. Facially there is a high, broad forehead, with large anterior fontanelle, open metopic suture, small deep-set eyes, large outstanding ears, large downturned mouth and everted lower lip [5,6].

11q duplication

This arises in most cases from an unbalanced product of a maternal 11q/22q translocation, which is relatively common. Preauricular tags or pits, often multiple, are seen in 85% of cases. A small mandible with retracted lower lip and cleft palate is characteristic. Psychomotor and growth retardation are expected, with congenital heart defect and hypogenitalism features in many cases [5].

12p tetrasomy mosaic (Pallister–Killian syndrome)

In Pallister–Killian syndrome there is an extra metacentric chromosome consisting of an isocentric duplication of the short arm of chromosome 12. This only occurs in mosaic form, and can often only be found in fibroblasts from skin biopsy or in dividing cells from a bone marrow aspirate. Cells with the abnormal karyotype may tend to be lost with increasing age [7]. The use of FISH with a specific 12p cosmid DNA probe may facilitate diagnosis from peripheral blood.

Multiple patches of skin depigmentation usually including the anterior scalp, are characteristic, and may include depigmentation along Blaschko's lines [8]. Scalp hair in infancy is sparse and fine, typically being absent from the frontal and temporal regions, although later it grows more normally. Eyebrows and eyelashes are sparse medially. Supernumerary nipples are frequently seen [5].

The facies is quite coarse, with a high forehead and puffy metopic skin and eyelids, and gives an overall look of a storage disorder. There is a long, prominent philtrum, and a thin upper lip which may have a sharp central V shape to the Cupid's bow; the lower lip is out-turned. The earlobes are thick. Other features include hypertelorism, ptosis, small mandible, short neck and macroglossia. Psychomotor retardation is severe, with infantile hypotonia, and deafness, absent speech and epilepsy apparent subsequently [5].

18q–

Skin dimples over the extensor surface of bony prominences characterize partial deletion of the long arm of chromosome 18 (involving band 18q21). The dimples can be on the cheek, subacromial, epitrochlear, over the knuckles or on the lateral aspect of the knee, and are usually bilateral [5]. A transverse palmar crease and excess of fingertip whorls with high total finger ridge count are usually noted.

The condition is recognized clinically by hypotonia, severe mental retardation (IQ rarely above 30), growth retardation, microcephaly, retruded midface, seizures, nystagmus, low-pitched voice, wide-spaced nipples, hypogenitalism, long thin tapered hands and proximally set

thumbs [5]. Congenital heart defects are common. Approximately 30% have immunoglobulin A (IgA) deficiency.

22p tetrasomy

An additional marker chromosome as a single extra copy (trisomy), or isoduplicate (tetrasomy) of the short arm of chromosome 22 (and including band 22q11 from the proximal long arm), results in cat-eye syndrome [9].This is characterized by the combination of iris or choroidal coloboma, and anal atresia. A majority of patients have bilateral preauricular ear tags or pits, 50% have renal anomalies and 40% have heart defects especially total anomalous pulmonary venous drainage (TAPVD) or tetralogy of Fallot [5]. The facies may show hypertelorism and downslant palpebral fissures. Although most children diagnosed have associated retardation, clinical expression can be variable, including the possibility of an asymptomatic carrier parent [10].

Ring chromosomes/marker chromosomes/mosaicism

Ring chromosomes, formed by terminal deletion of both ends of one chromosome and rejoining as a ring, tend to be unstable at mitosis [11]. With increasing age of a patient they can tend to disappear and hence often give rise to mosaic situations. Extra marker chromosomes similarly tend to default to a mosaic pattern. For both, the clinical presentation may predominantly be one of a mosaic abnormality, with asymmetry a prominent feature. Skin manifestation with depigmentation along the lines of Blaschko may be present [8]. Diagnosis may require skin biopsy for fibroblast culture, or bone marrow aspirate.

REFERENCES

1 Kere J, Srivastava AK, Montonen O *et al.* X-linked anhydrotic (hypohydrotic) ectodermal dysplasia is caused by a mutation in a novel transmembrane protein. *Nat Genet* 1996; 13: 409–16.

2 Schmidt MA, Michels VV, Dewald GW. Cases of neurofibromatosis with rearrangements of chromosome 17 involving band 17q11.2. *Am J Med Genet* 1987; 28: 771–7.

3 Wilson LC, Leverton K, Oude Luttikhuis ME *et al.* Brachydactyly and mental retardation: an Albright hereditary osteodystrophy-like syndrome localized to 2q37. *Am J Hum Genet* 1995; 56: 400–7.

4 Turnpenny PD, Lunt PW, Howell R *et al.* The phenotype of deletion 2q37 syndrome. *7th Manchester Birth Defects Conference*. Abstract, p. 48. Manchester: Regional Genetics Service, 1996.

5 Gorlin RJ, Cohen MM, Levin LS. *Syndromes of the Head and Neck*, 3rd edn. New York: Oxford University Press, 1990.

6 Young RS, Reed T, Hodes ME, Palmer CG. The dermatoglyphic and clinical features of the 9p trisomy and partial 9p monosomy syndromes. *Hum Genet* 1982; 62: 31–9.

7 Ward BE, Hayden MW, Robinson A. Isochromosome 12p mosaicism (Pallister–Killian syndrome): newborn diagnosis by direct bone marrow analysis. *Am J Med Genet* 1988; 31: 835–40.

8 Thomas IT, Frias JL, Cantu ES, Lafer CZ, Flannery DB, Graham JG Jr. Association of pigmentary anomalies with chromosomal and genetic mosaicism and chimaerism. *Am J Hum Genet* 1989; 45: 193–205.

9 Schinzel A, Schmid W, Fraccaro M *et al*. The 'cat eye syndrome': dicentric small marker chromosome probably derived from a no. 22 (tetrasomy pter→q11) associated with a characteristic phenotype. Report of 11 patients and delineation of the clinical picture. *Hum Genet* 1981; 57: 148–58.

10 Jones KL. *Smith's Recognisable Patterns of Human Malformation*, 4th edn. Philadelphia: WB Saunders, 1988.

11 Pezzolo A, Gimelli G, Cohen A *et al*. Presence of telomeric and subtelomeric sequences at the fusion points of ring chromosomes indicates that the ring syndrome is caused by ring instability. *Hum Genet* 1993; 92: 23–7.

Microdeletions

There are a number of genetic syndromes which are now recognized to be due to submicroscopic chromosomal microdeletion. Confirmation of diagnosis requires demonstration of microdeletion by *in situ* hybridization using a fluorescently tagged cosmid DNA probe (FISH), or by DNA restriction fragment hybridization. In addition, these techniques may be necessary to demonstrate deletion in patients with clinical features typical of a recognized chromosomal deletion syndrome (such as 4p− or 5p−), but in whom a standard karyotype appears to be normal [1].

Autosomal microdeletion syndromes follow dominant inheritance, and although most cases arise *de novo* there is a subsequent 50% risk to any offspring of affected subjects. The parents' karyotype should also in most cases be checked for similar microdeletion, or for chromosomal rearrangement predisposing to this. Even in *de novo* cases there remains a small sibling recurrence risk from the possibility of parental germinal mosaicism.

Williams syndrome: microdeletion 7q11

Williams syndrome [2,3] in children is characterized by a friendly personality and loquacious mimic speech ('cocktail party manner'), but with little understanding of the content. IQ can range from 40 to 85, but at least 40% of cases have only borderline retardation (IQ 70–85). The condition is often suspected initially from either the specific heart defect of supravalvular aortic stenosis, or from hypercalcaemia in early infancy. Pulmonary stenosis can also occur. Typically in early infancy there is hypotonia and feeding difficulty. Facial appearance is characteristic with a short nose, long philtrum with prominent philtral pillars, wide mouth with prominent lower lip, stellate iris and skin dimples lateral to the eyes. There is often clinodactyly of the little finger and hypoplastic, deeply set nails. Hypersensitivity to loud noise is another behavioural feature.

The microdeletion includes the elastin gene at 7q11 which is also involved in families with dominant inheritance for supravalvular aortic stenosis alone [4].

Langer–Giedion syndrome: deletion 8q24.1

Langer–Giedion syndrome (or trichorhinophalangeal syndrome type 2) [2] has several dermatological manifes-

tations. At birth and throughout infancy the baby has excess loose redundant skin. Scalp hair remains sparse, although eyebrows are full. The nails are brittle. A majority of patients develop multiple naevi on the face and extremities.

Typical facial features include a bulbous nasal tip, thin upper lip and prominent 'bat' ears, often with mild microcephaly. The nasal columella may extend onto the philtrum, often with a raised midline skin nodule below the lower lip. There is short stature and variable mild to moderate mental retardation, although intelligence can be normal. Multiple bony exostoses develop from around 2–3 years of age, and hand X-rays show cone-shaped phalangeal epiphyses [2].

WAGR: deletion or microdeletion 11p13

Wilms' tumour, aniridia, genital anomaly (hypospadias and cryptorchidism) and retardation (WAGR) can occur together in children deleted for chromosome band 11p13 [2]. The aniridia (PAX-6) and Wilms' tumour suppressor gene have now been cloned from this chromosome region, and are both deleted in the syndrome. There are no specific dermatological manifestations.

Angelman's syndrome and Prader–Willi syndrome: deletion/microdeletion or disomy 15q11

Angelman's syndrome (AS) is characterized by severe retardation, microbrachycephaly, epilepsy, frequent involuntary smiling or laughing and jerky ataxic movements. Prader–Willi syndrome (PWS) is characterized by infantile hypotonia, hypogenitalism, small hands and feet, and onset by 3–4 years of age of food craving and the development of gross truncal obesity. These syndromes are both due to disruption of normal gene expression at the chromosome 15q11 region. This can be through deletion of one copy of the 15q11 region from one parent, through uniparental disomy (where both copies of chromosome 15 originate in the same parent), or through mutation affecting a local 'imprinting centre' gene, thereby altering the normal local DNA methylation and hence imprinting pattern [5]. If the maternal copy is missing or extinguished the child has AS, whereas the same for the paternal copy results in PWS. In fact the expressed genes involved in the two conditions are different, but closely linked, and subject to the same imprinting centre regulation [5]. Although perhaps 99% of PWS cases can be accounted for by one of the above mechanisms, around 25% of cases of AS may be due to a postulated point mutation inherited from the mother and with high recurrence risk.

There is a skin pigment controlling gene in the same region, and both conditions are often associated with some degree of oculocutaneous albinism. Also in PWS a decreased pain sensitivity allows the children to pick at cuts or bruises on their skin, producing chronic sores and scars. Nasal picking can lead to troublesome nose bleeds [2].

Rubinstein–Taybi syndrome: microdeletion 16p13.3

This short-stature retardation syndrome [2] is recognized by the combination of microcephaly, typical facial features and broad thumbs and great toes which can in some cases be duplicated. The syndrome is caused by mutation in the cyclic AMP-responsive element-binding protein (CREB) gene, 11% of which are microdeletions [6]. Facial features include downslant palpebral fissures, and a beaked nose with nasal septum and columella giving a hook-like protrusion to the nasal tip. Hirsutism and a prominent naevus flammeus on the forehead, nape or back are often noted at birth. Supernumerary nipples may be present. Hypertrophic scarring and keloid formation is reported in several cases. Cardiac and renal abnormalities are quite common, and in males, testes are usually undescended [2].

Miller–Dieker syndrome: deletion/microdeletion 17p13

Lissencephaly presenting with intractable seizures from early infancy, together with a typical facies with high broad forehead and vertical glabellar furrows characterize Miller–Dieker syndrome due to microdeletion at 17p13 [2]. There are no other specific dermatological features.

Smith–Magenis syndrome: microdeletion 17p11.2

This behavioural and retardation microdeletion syndrome [7] may present to the dermatologist due to a tendency to self-mutilatory behaviour. Syndactyly between toes 2 and 4 may also be seen. Facial features are not striking, but the face tends to be broad with frontal bossing and a prominent chin. The hands tend to be small with short fingers and fifth finger clinodactyly. Conductive hearing loss is common, and speech is disproportionately delayed. There is impulsive aggression, but hugging behaviour is also characteristic.

Shprintzen/DiGeorge syndrome: microdeletion 22q11

After Down's syndrome, 22q11 microdeletion (Shprintzen or DiGeorge syndrome) which may have a birth incidence of at least 1 in 4000 is emerging as the single most common genetic cause of congenital heart defects [8]. Typically these involve outflow tract defects (i.e. truncus, transposition, Fallot's tetralogy, interrupted aortic arch), but also ventricular septal defect or other common defects; heart defects overall being present in over 75% of cases [9]. If not first diagnosed through paediatric cardiology, a child (or adult) with the condition may first present to diverse medical disciplines: to plastic surgery or ear, nose and throat (ENT) departments on account of a cleft or submucous cleft palate; to community paediatrics for speech and learning problems; to orthopaedics for joint laxity or distal arthrogryposis; to ophthalmology for retinal coloboma; to psychiatry for schizophrenic psychosis; to metabolic paediatrics for hypocalcaemia; and to haematology for myelodysplasia and thrombocytopoenia. Absence of the thymus occurs in around 14%, who will tend to be classified as DiGeorge syndrome. The consequent immunodeficiency, together with hypocalcaemia may predispose to *Candida* infection, and hence involvement of the dermatology department [2].

Facial features are characteristic and readily recognizable to those familiar with 22q11 syndrome. The nose is long and has a broad root, producing deep-set inner canthi due to thickened inner canthal skin. The alae nasi are narrowed and hypoplastic. There is a thin upper lip and the mouth may be small. The ear pinna is small and nearly circular. The fingers and toes are characteristically long and tapered, with an overall degree of hypotonia or joint laxity. Intelligence can be normal, but mild to moderate learning disability is usual, with particular speech and language delay [2].

X-linked recessive chondrodysplasia punctata: microdeletion Xp22

This condition [2] will often present to the dermatology department as a male infant or child with ichthyosis combined with mental retardation, sometimes microcephaly and neonatally stippled epiphyses. This combination arises from contiguous deletion of genes at the tip of the short arm of the X chromosome, which can be detected by FISH with an Xp22 probe.

The ichthyosis tends to be mild, affects the skin typically over the chest, back of legs, neck and axillae, and is associated with sparse hair. The ichthyosis arises since the deletion includes the steroid sulphatase gene, which can also be assayed biochemically from a fibroblast culture. On X-ray many epiphyseal centres, including paravertebral, larynx, trachea and long bones, show bilaterally symmetric punctate stippling, which tends to disappear with age. The relationship between this condition and X-linked dominant Conradi's disease (with male lethality) is not clear, although ichthyosis and stippled epiphyses are features of both [2]. A small nose and cataracts (which may also be seen in Conradi's disease) may also suggest some overlap with peroxisomal disorders, although without the rhizomelia and joint contractures of recessive rhizomelic chondrodysplasia punctata.

REFERENCES

1 Reid E, Morrison N, Barron L *et al.* Familial Wolf–Hirschhorn syndrome resulting from a cryptic translocation: a clinical and molecular study. *J Med Genet* 1996; 33: 197–202.
2 Gorlin RJ, Cohen MM, Levin LS. *Syndromes of the Head and Neck*, 3rd edn. New York: Oxford University Press, 1990.
3 Burn J. Williams syndrome. *J Med Genet* 1986; 23: 389–95.

4 Lowery MC, Morris CA, Ewart A *et al.* Strong correlation of elastin deletions, detected by FISH, with Williams syndrome: evaluation of 235 patients. *Am J Hum Genet* 1995; 57: 49–53.

5 Buiting K, Saitoh S, Gross S *et al.* Inherited microdeletions in the Angelman and Prader–Willi syndromes define an imprinting centre on human chromosome 15. *Nature Genet* 1995; 9: 395–400.

6 Wallerstein R, Anderson CE, Hay B *et al.* Submicroscopic deletions at 16p13.3 in Rubinstein–Taybi syndrome: frequency and clinical manifestations in a North America population. *J Med Genet* 1997; 34: 203–6.

7 Gorlin RJ, Toriello HV, Cohen MM. *Hereditary Hearing Loss and its Syndromes.* New York: Oxford University Press, 1995.

8 Wilson DI, Cross IE, Wren C *et al.* Minimum prevalence of chromosome 22q11 deletions. *Am J Hum Genet* 1994; 55(3): Suppl. A169, Abstract 975.

9 Goldberg R, Motzkin B, Marion R, Scambler PJ, Shprintzen RJ. Velo-cardio-facial syndrome: a review of 120 patients. *Am J Med Genet* 1993; 45: 313–19.

Uniparental disomy

Trisomy is not uncommon at conception, but is only compatable with fetal survival if the extra chromosome is chromosome 8, 9, 13, 18, 21 or 22, and in some of these cases only if the abnormal cell line is present as a mosaic. Other trisomic conceptuses can only survive if one of the chromosomes represented in three copies is lost [1]. This can result in a fetus having uniparental disomy (UPD), where both copies of one chromosome originate from the same parent [2]. This affects any gene on that chromosome whose expression is determined by imprinting with the sex of parental origin, usually through differential methylation of the two gene copies. Also, UPD could unmask a recessive condition for which the parent is a carrier, if that chromosome region is duplicated by its replication homologue (i.e. uniparental isodisomy) [3].

UPD for chromosome 15 is observed in a proportion of cases of PWS and AS (maternal or paternal UPD, respectively) [4,5], but is also reported with chromosome 7 in some cases of Russell–Silver syndrome [2], with chromosome 11 in some cases of Beckwith's syndrome [6] and with chromosomes 14 and 16 associated typically with growth retardation [1,7]. At least one case of Bloom's syndrome has occurred due to uniparental isodisomy for chromosome 15 [8]. UPD should be considered particularly where a prenatal chorion villous biopsy has identified confined placental mosaicism for a trisomic cell line [1].

REFERENCES

1 Kalousek DK, Langlois S, Barrett I *et al.* Uniparental disomy for chromosome 16 in humans. *Am J Hum Genet* 1993; 52: 8–16.

2 Kotzot D, Schmitt S, Bernasconi F *et al.* Uniparental disomy 7 in Silver–Russell syndrome and primordial growth retardation. *Hum Mol Genet* 1995; 4: 583–7.

3 Spence JE, Perciaccante RG, Greig GM *et al.* Uniparental disomy as a mechanism for human genetic disease. *Am J Hum Genet* 1988; 42: 217–26.

4 Nicholls RD, Knoll JHM, Butler MG, Karam S, Lalande M. Genetic imprinting suggested by maternal heterodisomy in non-deletion Prader–Willi syndrome. *Nature* 1989; 342: 281–5.

5 Malcolm S, Clayton-Smith J, Nichols M *et al.* Uniparental disomy in Angelman's syndrome. *Lancet* 1991; 337: 694–7.

6 Henry I, Puech A, Riesewijk A *et al.* Somatic mosaicism for partial paternal isodisomy in Wiedemann–Beckwith syndrome: a post-fertilization event. *Eur J Hum Genet* 1993; 1: 19–29.

7 Penman Splitt M, Cross I, Goodship J. Maternal uniparental isodisomy of chromosome 14 resulting from i (14q) formation. *J Med Genet* 1996; 33 (suppl. 1): S31 (abstract 5.027).

8 Woodage T, Prasad M, Dixon JW *et al.* Bloom syndrome and maternal uniparental disomy for chromosome 15. *Am J Hum Genet* 1994; 55: 74–80.

Sex chromosome anomaly

Turner's syndrome: 45,X0

Monosomy X (45,X0) may be the single most frequent chromosome abnormality at conception, but is associated with a fetal loss of over 95%. At least some live-born girls with Turner's syndrome are likely to be cryptic mosaics. Evidence for the presence of a Y chromosome (i.e. 45,X0/46,XY mosaic) should be sought using a Y-specific DNA probe to identify those girls at risk of gonadoblastoma.

The typical presentation of Turner's syndrome with short stature (mean adult height of 147 cm), webbed neck and low posterior hairline, neonatal pedal oedema and infertility due to gonadal dysgenesis, is well known [1]. Coarctation of the aorta or other cardiac malformation occurs in 10–16%, and renal malformation (particularly horseshoe kidney) in 38%. Typically the skin may show multiple pigmented naevi. Seborrhoea, xeroderma, hirsutism and keloid formation are increased in frequency, and small deep-set nails are common. The neck webbing probably results from resolution of nuchal oedema present *in utero*.

Intelligence levels in girls with Turner's syndrome are usually in the normal range, but may show specific visuospatial skill deficits, with a normal verbal IQ [2]. Gonadal dysgenesis is accompanied by infertility, but pregnancies using donor eggs have been sustained in some cases with appropriate hormone treatment following *in vitro* fertilization (IVF). Growth hormone is now well established as having a beneficial effect on height.

Mosaic Turner's syndrome is not uncommon and can be X0/XX, X0/XY or X0/XXX.

Ring-X mosaic

A ring-X is unstable and tends to be seen only as a mosaic. The abnormal cell line may have a terminal deletion of both Xp and Xq. Girls with this usually have significant mental retardation and coarse facial features, often with elongated palpebral fissures [3]. It may be that the normal X chromosome preferentially undergoes X-inactivation, thereby leading to a phenotypic effect of the abnormal X.

Triple-X syndrome: 47,XXX

Phenotypic effects of a 47,XXX karyotype are few, although they may include epicanthic folds and clinodactyly. Head circumference tends to be below the 50th centile, whereas height tends to be above this. Significant learning problems do occur, with a reduced IQ overall (Wechsler Intelligence Scale for Children mean of 85) [2]. There are no specific dermatological features.

Klinefelter's syndrome: 47,XXY

Klinefelter's syndrome [1] is characterized by boys with hypogonadism, tallish stature and infertility. Pubertal development is limited, and results in a female distribution of body hair. Gynaecomastia in young adults is common, but can be corrected surgically. There is a concomitant increased risk of male breast cancer. Congenital malformations occur with increased frequency (in up to 18% of boys), but without any specific associations. Schooling and emotional problems are frequent, with overall mean for IQ being around 88. The boys tend to have a shy immature personality, with low self-esteem, perhaps aggravated by peer response to their physical characteristics. Treatment with testosterone injections and locally applied testosterone cream may be helpful in some cases. Varicose veins and stasis ulcers are reported, but there are no other specific dermatological manifestations.

XYY syndrome: 47,XYY

Tall stature with excessive impulsive behaviour, lack of emotional control and temper tantrums together characterize XYY syndrome [1]. Antisocial behaviour with criminality is increased. IQ is reduced, with 38% scoring below 90, with verbal IQ affected more than performance IQ. Acne involving the face, chest and back, may be more frequent than in normal 46,XY males [4].

REFERENCES

1 Gorlin RJ, Cohen MM, Levin LS. *Syndromes of the Head and Neck*, 3rd edn. New York: Oxford University Press, 1990.
2 Ratcliffe SG, Butler GE, Jones M. Edinburgh study of growth and development of children with sex chromosome abnormalities. IV. *Birth Defects Orig Art Ser* 1990; 26(4): 1–44.
3 Dennis NR, Collins AL, Crolla JA, Cockwell AE, Fisher AM, Jacobs PA. Three patients with ring (X) chromosomes and a severe phenotype. *J Med Genet* 1993; 30: 482–6.
4 Voorhees JJ, Wilkins JW Jr, Hayes E, Harrell ER. Nodulocystic acne as a phenotypic feature of the XYY genotype. *Arch Dermatol* 1972; 105: 913–19.

Sex reversal

Women with a 46,XY karyotype and testicular feminization, may exhibit no obvious external abnormalities apart from a blind vagina and primary amenorrhoea. Partial or compete feminization of external genitalia can also occur in some XY infants with certain dysmorphic syndromes, such as Smith–Lemli–Opitz syndrome type 2 (SLO type 2), and campomelic dysplasia. SLO type 2 also typically includes microcephaly, hypotonia, cleft palate, congenital heart defect, proximal placement of a short thumb, postaxial polydactyly in the hands and 2, 3 toe syndactyly [1]. These babies often also have a prominent naevus flammeus over the forehead. This autosomal recessive condition is due to a block in the final step of cholesterol synthesis giving raised 7-dehydrocholesterol levels [2].

Campomelic dysplasia is a lethal skeletal dysplasia with short bowed lower limbs, small scapulae and cleft palate in addition to genital sex reversal in 46,XY infants. A dermatological feature is of pretibial skin dimples over the maximum bony convexity [1]. The condition is due to a *de novo* dominant mutation in the SOX-9 gene, but recurrence risk is not insignificant on account of parental germinal mosaicism [3].

XX males

Some XX males [1] do have Y chromosome sequences translocated into an X chromosome or inserted elsewhere in the genome, which can be detected using Y-specific DNA probes. Others may have genuine autosomal or X-chromosome gene mutations. There are no specifically associated dermatological features.

REFERENCES

1 Gorlin RJ, Cohen MM, Levin LS. *Syndromes of the Head and Neck*, 3rd edn. New York: Oxford University Press, 1990.
2 Seller MJ, Russell J, Tint GS. Unusual case of Smith–Lemli–Opitz syndrome 'type II'. *Am J Med Genet* 1995; 56: 265–8.
3 Cameron FJ, Hageman RM, Cooke-Yarborough C *et al.* A novel germ line mutation in SOX9 causes familial campomelic dysplasia and sex reversal. *Hum Molec Genet* 1996; 5: 1625–30.

Single gene conditions affecting chromosomes

Chromosome breakage syndromes

Fanconi's anaemia, Bloom's syndrome, Nijmegen breakage syndrome, Seemanova's syndrome, Rothmund–Thomson syndrome and ataxia telangiectasia, as detailed elsewhere (Chapters 19.23 and 19.24), may present with sun-sensitive dermatitis due to impaired repair of ultraviolet-induced DNA damage, or with patchy hypo- or hyper-pigmentation. Specific chromosomal breakage investigations may be required in each one.

Fragile X syndrome

This is the commonest single cause of retardation in males (and perhaps of mild retardation in females) after Down's syndrome, and should be considered in any boy with an IQ of 30–70, particularly if associated with large ears and head circumference above the 50th centile. Although originally recognized by the appearence of a fragile site at Xq27 with chromosomes cultured in a low-folate medium, diagnosis is now usually made from DNA analysis. The X-linked FRAXA gene contains a trinucleotide repeat which is expanded in fragile X syndrome. There can be marked joint laxity, and the skin can be lax with a velvety soft feel [1].

Robert's syndrome

Robert's syndrome [1] is diagnosed in the cytogenetic laboratory from centromeric puffing of chromosomes. The phenotype of this autosomal recessive condition is characterized by tetraphocomelia and bilateral cleft lip and palate. Death often occurs in early infancy, but others can survive, although 50% of these are mentally retarded. Superficial capillary haemangiomas on the forehead, midface, philtrum and ears can be a striking feature in the neonate.

REFERENCE

1 Gorlin RJ, Cohen MM, Levin LS. *Syndromes of the Head and Neck*, 3rd edn. New York: Oxford University Press, 1990.

19.3 Review of Keratin Disorders

MAURICE A.M. VAN STEENSEL AND
PETER M. STEIJLEN

In recent years, rapid progress has been made in our understanding of the molecular basis of many genetic skin diseases. Among these are a number of often distressing and sometimes even life-threatening disorders in which the process of keratinization is disturbed. Keratinization is a complex process and many molecules are involved in it. There are still many gaps in our knowledge of keratinization, but modern genetics has given us some insight into the function of keratins themselves, as well as in the effects of keratin mutations.

For a proper understanding of the effects of keratin mutation, some knowledge of keratin biology is necessary.

Keratin biology

There are at least 30 different keratins. They belong to the family of intermediate filament (IF) molecules [1]. These evolutionary conserved molecules are a major part of the cytoskeleton in many organisms and as such play an important role in maintaining the structural integrity of the cells and their surroundings.

Like all other IF molecules, keratins have a central α-helical 'rod' domain, flanked by end domains that are particular to the type of keratin in question (Fig. 19.3.1) [1–3]. This basic structure is strongly conserved throughout evolution, which suggests that it is essential to normal keratin function.

Keratins are subdivided on the basis of their end domains and their charge: acidic (keratins 10–21, type I) or basic/neutral (type II, keratins 1–9). The acidic keratins are coded for by a gene cluster on chromosome 17, the basic ones by genes on chromosome 12. The two forms also differ slightly in their basic structure: type I keratins lack H1 and H2 domains [1–3].

A peculiarity of keratin molecules is that they are never alone: they exist as obligate heterodimers of a type I and a type II chain [3]. The association between the chains is thought to take place through the rod domain that shows a motif of seven amino acids (the 'heptad motif') thought to mediate the association of the helices. Short, strongly conserved sequences at the beginning and the end of the rod domains, the helix initiation and helix termination motifs, respectively, are essential for the initiation and proper termination of the dimerization process [1,4]. Alterations in this motif should perturb keratin function and we will show that this is indeed the case. The keratin filaments aggregate into a network, the keratin IF (KIF) network, that interacts with adhesion structures in the keratinocytes: desmosomes and hemidesmosomes (reviewed in [5]). Thus the cytoskeleton of each cell is linked to its membrane and, via this membrane, to other cells.

During differentiation of the epidermal cells, the expression of keratins in the keratinocytes changes as the cells move upwards [6] (Table 19.3.1). Basal keratinocytes express K4 and K15 [6]. Upon their maturation to spinous layer cells, K5 and K14 are downregulated and K1, K2e and K10 are expressed. Nail and hair progenitor cells express mainly K6, K16 and K17 [2]. These keratins are also expressed in other regions in response to keratinocyte stress or injury [7]. Because of this, they can also be found in the palms and soles. K6 and K16 are also expressed in mucosal epithelia. K9 is expressed in the palms and soles only [8]. Non-epidermal keratins are expressed in mucous membranes and two of these, K4 and K13, have been implicated in a disorder of the mucosa (see below). As the keratinocytes reach the stratum granulosum, the expression of keratins ceases. The proteins produced in the upper layer are loricrin, involucrin, filaggrin and others [9,10]. The first three are a major part of the so-called cornified envelope (CE), an insoluble hydrophobic layer on the inner surface of the plasma membrane of the keratinocytes in the stratum corneum. This layer is made by cross-linking of the proteins mentioned, both to each other and to the KIF network [10]. A number of enzymes is

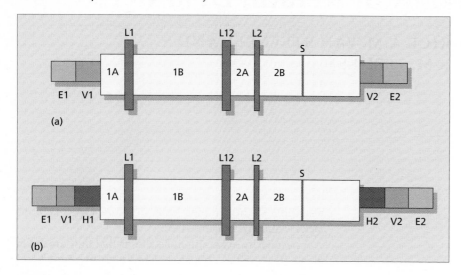

Fig. 19.3.1 Central α-helical rod domain: (a) type I; (b) type II.

Table 19.3.1 Differentiation-specific expression of keratins

Layer of epidermis	Expression of keratins
Stratum epinosum	
Upper	K2e
Lower	K1/K10, K6/K16, K4/K13, K9*
Stratum basale	K5/K14, K17

*Expression in palmoplantar skin only.

involved in this process, mainly transglutaminases [11]. In conclusion, keratins and other members of the IF family are responsible for the structural integrity of the epidermis. Disruption of the IF network will lead to abnormal keratinization and/or decreased resistance of the epidermis to mechanical stress. A number of disorders, characterized by abnormal keratinization and/or increased skin fragility, has in recent years been shown to be due to keratin mutations.

Disorders caused by keratin mutations

The diseases known to be caused by keratin mutations are listed in Table 19.3.2. These disorders are discussed below.

Epidermolysis bullosa simplex (EBS)

EBS [12] is caused by mutations in K5 and K14 (referenced in [13]). Both keratins are expressed in basal epidermal cells. Different mutations can give rise to different phenotypes depending upon their effect on keratin network formation. It has been shown that disturbed network formation is an essential component of the different forms of EBS [14].

The mildest form of EBS, Weber–Cockayne syndrome (MIM* no. 131 800), is characterized by blistering of the palms and soles only. Mutations have been found in the H1, 1A, L12 and 2B domains of K5 and K14 [13]. Though some of these mutations are located in conserved regions, they are probably not very disruptive to normal keratin function. The mild phenotype supports this.

*MIM numbers refer to Victor McKusick's *Mendelian Inheritance in Man*. This database can be found online at http://www.ncbi.nlm.nih.gov/omim/

Table 19.3.2 Keratin disorders

Disorder (and subtypes)	Keratins affected
Epidermolysis bullosa, simplex type	
Weber–Cockayne	K5/K14
Koebner	K5/K14
Dowling–Meara	K5/K14
Bullous congenital ichthyosiform erythroderma of Brocq	K1/K10
Epidermolytic epidermal nevus	K10, mosaic
Epidermolytic palmoplantar hyperkeratosis	K1/K9
Ichthyosis bullosa Siemens	K2e
Non-epidermolytic palmoplantar hyperkeratosis (NEPPK)	K1
Pachyonychia congenita	
Jadassohn–Lewandowsky	K6a/K16
Jackson–Lawler	K17
Focal NEPPK	K16
Steatocystoma multiplex	K17/K6b
White sponge nevus	K4/K13

This is different for the more severe forms of EBS, the Dowling–Meara (MIM no. 131760) and Koebner (MIM no. 131900) variants. The Koebner type of EBS is characterized by more generalized but still relatively mild blister formation. Mutations of K5 and K14 are located more inside the 1A or 2B segments of the rod domains. Interestingly, recessive forms of this variant have been found to represent human K14 'knockouts' [15,16]. The patients described were homozygous for a truncating mutation. Such a mutation introduces a 'STOP' codon in the DNA and, during the transcription process, mRNA. This codon stops translation of the mRNA, resulting in the absence of a protein product. The heterozygous parents were normal in both cases, indicating that one functional keratin allele is sufficient for normal IF formation. Moreover, it underlines the fact that disturbance of network formation (by dominant negative mutations) is the cause of the EBS phenotype. Another study has found patients homozygous for a mutation in the terminal half of the 1A domain of K14 [17]. They had a very mild EBS phenotype, which suggests

that the second half of the 1A domain is not as important for IF assembly as the first half. The heterozygous parents were normal.

In the most severe form of EBS, the Dowling–Meara variant, there is severe generalized herpetiform blistering. The mucous membranes are sometimes involved. Mutations in this subtype are located in the very beginning or the end of the rod domains. This interferes strongly with filament assembly. Thus a reasonable genotype–phenotype correlation has emerged, where mutations in the ends of the rod domains (the helix initiation and termination motifs) are associated with a severe phenotype and mutations elsewhere in the keratin genes are better tolerated and give rise to milder phenotypes. One problem in correlating genotype with phenotype still remains: it has emerged that keratins are 'promiscuous'. In some cases, a keratin chain that is not normally a partner for another chain can compensate partly for the absence of the obligate partner [4], thus ameliorating the mutant phenotype.

Bullous congenital ichthyosiform erythroderma of Brocq (BCIE) and ichthyosis bullosa of Siemens (IBS)

BCIE (MIM no. 113800) is a rare disorder, characterized by generalized blistering at birth accompanied by varying erythroderma and the development later in life of a generalized hyperkeratosis that is most pronounced on the large joints (Fig. 19.3.2). Inheritance is autosomal dominant. In this disorder, various mutations in K1 and K10 have been identified (referenced in [13]). These keratins are expressed mainly in the suprabasal layers of the epidermis, where the ultrastructural abnormalities of epidermolytic hyperkeratosis (EHK) are found: clumping of intermediate filaments, vacuolation and hyperkeratosis.

Mutations in K1 and K10 are located at the beginning or the end of the 1A rod domain, as in EBS. Milder forms of EHK have mutations in the H1 domain. It is interesting to note that in three different keratin disorders (BCIE, EBS and epidermolytic palmoplantar keratodermas (EPPK) see below) the same residues are mutated in three different keratins (asparagine 160, arginine 162, methionine 156). This indicates the functional importance of the conserved heptad motif. A most interesting finding was reported by Paller *et al.* [18]. They found that K10 mutations can also appear in a mosaic pattern in some individuals. Mosaicism means that cells carrying a mutation are intermingled with normal cells in the same individual. K10 mutations in a mosaic give rise to an epidermolytic epidermal naevus (MIM no. 600648), whereas presence of the mutation in all cells gives rise to BCIE.

IBS (MIM no. 146800) is a milder bullous ichthyosis without erythroderma (Fig. 19.3.3). Hyperkeratosis is mild and located on the flexural areas as well as on the umbilical skin and shins. Erosions are caused by minor trauma [19]. Ultrastructural features in this disorder again are indicative of keratin mutations: KIF clumping, vacuolation, this time in the upper layers of the stratum spinosum. One of the keratins expressed in this layer, K2e, was found to harbour mutations [20,21]. Again, the mutations cluster within the conserved domains.

Palmoplantar keratodermas

This is a very heterogeneous group of disorders, all characterized by abnormal keratinization of the skin of palms and soles. Their classification is based on morphology and associated features [22]. In recent years, the causative mutation of a number of palmoplantar keratodermas (PPKs) has been found.

The Vörner type (MIM no. 144200) shows diffuse thickening of the epidermis of palms and soles. Ultrastructural examination shows epidermolysis and clumping of keratin filaments [23]. The only keratin with expression limited to the skin of palms and soles is K9 and mutations have indeed been found in this keratin (referenced in [13]). Here again mutations cluster within the first few amino acids of the rod domain. Non-epidermolytic diffuse PPK has been associated with a mutation in K1 in one family, but linkage to the keratin cluster could not be found in others [24,25]. It is of interest that the mutation in this non-epidermolytic disease is located in the V1 domain of K1, which is expressed in the stratum spinosum. The V1 domain is probably not involved in cell–cell adherence; conversely, mutations in the rod domain certainly are, as they give rise to EHK (see above). Other PPKs have been mapped to different chromosomal regions [24,26]. One form of PPK, Vohwinkel's syndrome (or keratoderma hereditaria mutilans, MIM no. 124500), has been found to be caused by mutations in a keratin-associated molecule, loricrin [27]. Loricrin binds to K1, involucrin, filaggrins and other components of the CE and is thought to be required for the structural integrity of the CE [10]. How the mutation relates to the phenotype is presently unknown. Also, Vohwinkel's syndrome is heterogeneous, some cases being associated with deafness and probably due to a different mutation. Perhaps cross-linking of loricrin to the other components of the CE is impaired. The slight ichthyosis observed in some of the family members described in the article by Maestrini *et al.* [27] may be a consequence of fragility of the CE due to defective cross-linking.

Pachyonychia congenita (PC) is another group of PPKs. PC is characterized by dystrophic nail hypertrophy and hyperkeratosis of the nail bed, soles and palms. McKusick recognizes two basic variants, the Jadassohn–Lewandowsky (MIM no. 167200) and the Jackson–Lawler (MIM no. 167210) types. These are distinguished on the basis of associated symptoms [28]. Many other variants have been described, including PC with nail changes only [29] and PC with alopecia as the only associated symptom (personal communication, Van Steensel MAM and Steijlen PM, unpublished). Jadassohn-Lewandowsky PC has been found to be caused by mutations in K6a and K16 whereas K6b and K17 [30] mutations have been found in Jackson–Lawler PC [7,31]. In all cases, mutations were located in the 1A segment of the rod domain. The clinical differences between the two forms of PC can be well explained with the different expression patterns of K6, K16 and K17. A variant of Jadassohn–Lewandowsky PC, focal non-epidermolytic PPK (NEPPK, MIM no. 600962), has also been found to be due to K16 mutations [32]. This particular disease differs from Jadassohn–Lewandowsky PC in the degree of nail involvement. The mutation in focal NEPPK is in the same region as the mutation in PC. It is at present not clear why the phenotypes are different. In an interesting parallel to the situation with focal NEPPK and Jadassohn–Lewandowsky PC, it has turned out that keratin 17 mutations can cause both Jackson–Lawler PC

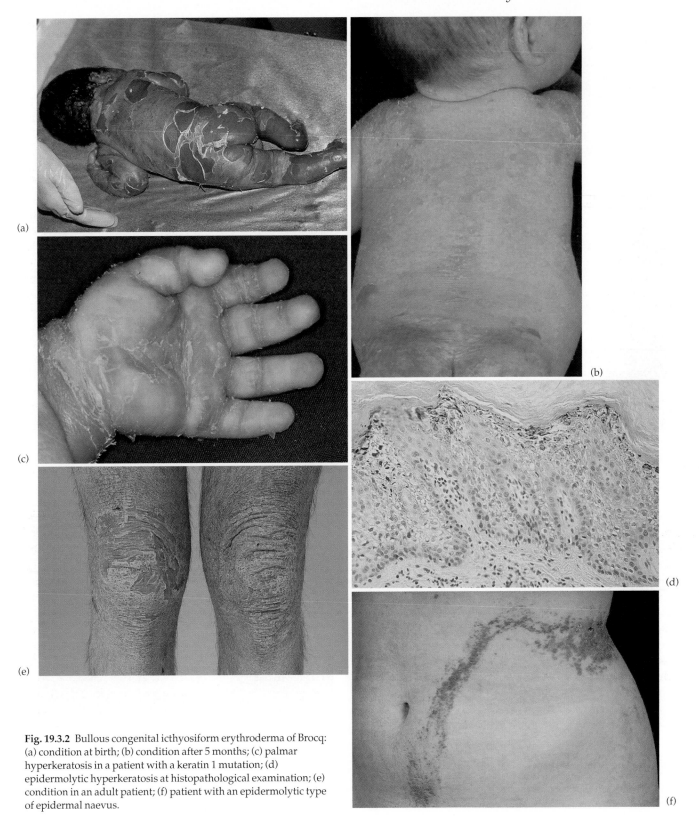

Fig. 19.3.2 Bullous icthyosiform erythroderma of Brocq: (a) condition at birth; (b) condition after 5 months; (c) palmar hyperkeratosis in a patient with a keratin 1 mutation; (d) epidermolytic hyperkeratosis at histopathological examination; (e) condition in an adult patient; (f) patient with an epidermolytic type of epidermal naevus.

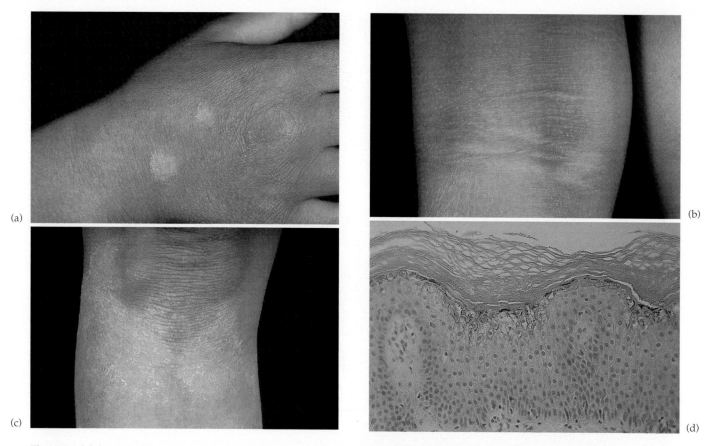

(a)

(b)

(c)

(d)

Fig. 19.3.3 Ichthyosis bullosa of Siemens: (a) mild scaling in a boy; (b) rimpled hyperkeratosis in flexural site of the knee; (c) condition in the mother of the boy; (d) epidermolytic hyperkeratosis limited to the upper layers of the stratum spinosum.

and steatocystoma multiplex without associated abnormalities [33]. Again, no association to specific mutations could be demonstrated. Since both phenotypes can occur within one family and be associated with one mutation only, the only logical explanation for this seems to be subtle differences in genetic background between individual family members. Theoretically, revertant mosaicism [34] could also explain this phenomenon, but this seems highly unlikely in view of the fact that reverting events are usually randomly distributed. Inheritance in all the above disorders is autosomal dominant. There is one report of autosomal recessive inheritance [35]. It is tempting to speculate that this case parallels the recessive K14 knockout mutations and that it is a K9 knockout.

White sponge 'naevus'

This is a rare autosomal dominant disorder (MIM no. 193900), characterized by the presence of thick white plaques in the mouth and occasionally on the mucosa of the oesophagus, nose, genitals and rectum (Fig. 19.3.4). Microscopically, plaques show vacuolization of suprabasal cells in a manner similar to epidermolytic hyperkeratosis. Linkage to the type I and II keratin clus-

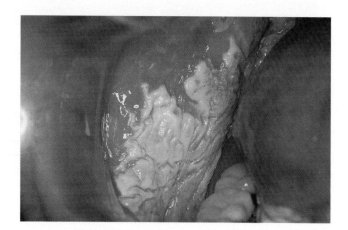

Fig. 19.3.4 White sponge naevus.

ters in two families and mutations in the K4 and K13 genes were subsequently found [36,37]. It will be no surprise that these mutations were located in the beginning of the 1A domains. It should be noted that this disorder is not a true naevus. Naevi are the result of genetic mosaicism [38], white sponge 'naevus' is not.

Other diseases possibly caused by keratin mutations

Keratins are expressed in a multitude of skin appendages. Hair and nails, especially, are composed of a distinct subset of keratins, the so-called 'hard' or trichocyte keratins [2]. Some disorders may be caused by mutations in one of these keratins.

One of these is monilethrix (MIM no. 158 000 and no. 252 200), which is characterized by beaded hair that breaks easily. This is most obvious on the occiput. Autosomal dominant and recessive modes of inheritance have been reported [39]. Linkage to the type II keratin gene cluster has been reported in a Scottish kindred [40]. Indeed, mutations in the hand keratins hHb1 and hHb6 have been found in this family [41,42]. In another family, however, linkage to 14q32–33 has been found [43]. It is likely that monilethrix is a heterogeneous disorder, at least at the molecular level. Another disorder that may be caused by keratin mutations is CHANDS (MIM no. 214 350). CHANDS is an acronym for curly hair, ankyloblepharon and nail dysplasia syndrome. The combination of abnormal hair and nail structure suggests the possibility of the involvement of keratins or associated molecules.

Finally, ankyloblepharon ectodermal dysplasia and clefting (of the palate) (AEC) or Hay–Wells syndrome (MIM no. 106 260) must be mentioned. One peculiar abnormality described in AEC syndrome is loss of scalp hair with subsequent inflammation of the epidermis [44]. Rothnagel *et al.* [45] described mice transgenic for a mutant human K6 gene. These mice showed a scarring alopecia and follicular keratosis. There was no cleft palate, but this is a variable feature in AEC syndrome [46]. Abnormalities of the teeth can also occur in Jadassohn–Lewandowsky PC, which is caused by a keratin mutation. The ectodermal dysplasia in AEC syndrome consists of dry skin [44,47]; abnormalities of the eccrine glands have not been reported. It would therefore be of interest to examine AEC syndrome patients for disorders of keratins or related molecules.

Conclusion

Given the present speed of progress in our understanding of the basic biology of the keratin disorders, it can be expected that the near future will bring many more revelations. Disease classification will be based on molecular data. Eponymous syndrome designations can be expected to disappear and it is reasonable to expect that disorders thought to be distinct will prove to have the same molecular basis, and vice versa. See for example the EBS variants. At present, the patient does not benefit very much from our increased understanding of the mechanisms underlying his or her disease. For some disorders, prenatal diagnosis is possible [48]. An accurate diagnosis is essential for reproductive counselling of patients and finding a mutation can confirm a clinical diagnosis. As far as therapy is concerned, nothing much can be offered at present.

However, increased knowledge will bring new avenues for therapeutic interventions. Recently, keratinocytes carrying a mutant transglutaminase were shown to express normal transglutaminase after transfection with a retrovirus carrying a normal gene [49]. This and other forms of gene therapy can be expected to become clinically feasible in the (possibly near) future. Pharmaceutical interventions, aimed at specific processes in keratinization that we are now learning to understand will also appear in clinical practice. Thus, an understanding of basic molecular processes will ultimately lead to better patient care.

REFERENCES

1 Fuchs E, Weber K. Intermediate filaments: structure, dynamics, functions and disease. *Ann Rev Biochem* 1994; 63: 345–82.
2 Bowden PE. Keratins and other epidermal proteins. In: Priestly GC, ed. *Molecular Aspects of Dermatology*. New York: Wiley, 1993: 19–54.
3 Steinert PM, Roop DR. Molecular and cellular biology of intermediate filaments. *Ann Rev Biochem* 1988; 57: 593–625.
4 Lu X, Lane EB. Retrovirus-mediated transgenic keratin expression in cultured fibroblasts: specific domain functions in keratin stabilization and filament formation. *Cell* 1990; 62: 681–96.
5 Garrod DR. Desmosomes and hemidesmosomes. *Curr Opin Cell Biol* 1993; 5: 30–40.
6 Fuchs E, Green H. Changes in keratin gene expression during terminal differentiation of the keratinocyte. *Cell* 1980; 19: 1033–42.
7 McLean WHI, Rugg EI, Lunny DP *et al.* Keratin 16 and keratin 17 mutations cause pachyonychia congenita. *Nature Genet* 1995; 9: 273–8.
8 Langbein L, Heid HW, Moll I *et al.* Molecular characterization of the body-site specific human cytokeratin 9: cDNA cloning, amino acid sequence and tissue specificty of gene expression. *Differentiation* 1993; 55: 57–72.
9 Mehrel T, Hohl D, Rothnagel JA *et al.* Identification of a major keratinocyte cell envelope protein, loricrin. *Cell* 1990; 61: 1103–12.
10 Rothnagel JA, Longley MA, Bundman DS *et al.* Characterization of the mouse loricrin gene: linkage with profilaggrin and the flaky tail and soft coat mutant loci on chromosome 3. *Genomics* 1994; 3: 450–6.
11 Folk JE. Transglutaminases. *Ann Rev Biochem* 1980; 49: 517–31.
12 Fine J-D, Bauer EA, Briggaman RA *et al.* Revised clinical and laboratory criteria for subtypes of inherited epidermolysis bullosa. *J Am Acad Dermatol* 1991; 24: 119–35.
13 Korge BP, Krieg T. The molecular basis for inherited bullous diseases. *J Mol Med* 1996; 74: 59–70.
14 Coulombe PA, Hutton ME, Letai A *et al.* Point mutations in human keratin 14 genes of epidermolysis bullosa simplex patients: genetic and functional analyses. *Cell* 1991; 66: 1301–11.
15 Chan Y-M, Anton-Lamprecht I, Yu Q-C *et al.* A human keratin 14 'knockout': the absence of K14 leads to severe epidermolysis bullosa simplex and a function for an intermediate filament protein. *Genes Dev* 1994; 8: 2574–87.
16 Rugg EL, McLean WHI, Lane EB *et al.* A functional 'knock-out' for human keratin 14. *Genes Dev* 1994; 8: 2563–73.
17 Hovnanian A, Pollack E, Hillal L *et al.* A missense mutation in the rod domain of keratin 14 associated with recessive epidermolysis bullosa simplex. *Nature Genet* 1993; 3: 327–32.
18 Paller AS, Syder AJ, Chan Y-M *et al.* Genetic and clinical mosaicism in a type of epidermal nevus. *N Engl J Med* 1994; 331: 1408–15.
19 Traupe H, Kolde G, Hamm H *et al.* Ichthyosis bullosa of Siemens: a unique type of epidermolytic hyperkeratosis. *J Am Acad Dermatol* 1986; 14: 1000–5.
20 Kremer H, Zeeuwen P, McLean WHI *et al.* Ichthyosis bullosa of Siemens is caused by mutations in the keratin 2e gene. *J Invest Dermatol* 1994; 103: 2886–9.

21 Rothnagel JA, Traupe H, Wojcik S *et al.* Mutations in the rod domain of keratin 2e in patients with ichthyosis bullosa of Siemens. *Nature Genet* 1994; 7: 485–90.

22 Lucker GPH. *Ichthyosis, Darier's disease and palmoplantar keratoderma. New insights in classification and therapy.* Thesis, Catholic University of Nijmegen, The Netherlands, 1996.

23 Hamm H, Happle R, Butterfass T *et al.* Epidermolytic palmoplantar keratoderma of Vörner: is it the most frequent type of hereditary palmoplantar keratoderma? *Dermatologica* 1988; 177: 138–45.

24 Kelsell DP, Stevens HP, Ratnavel R *et al.* Genetic linkage studies in non-epidermolytic palmoplantar keratoderma: evidence for heterogeneity. *Hum Mol Genet* 1995; 4: 1021–5.

25 Kimonis V, DiGiovanna JJ, Yang J-M *et al.* A mutation in the V1 end domain of keratin 1 in non-epidermolytic palmar-plantar keratoderma. *J Invest Dermatol* 1994; 103: 764–9.

26 Hennies H-C, Küster W, Mischke D *et al.* Localization of a gene for the striated form of palmoplantar keratoderma to chromosome 18q near the desmosomal cadherin gene. *Hum Mol Genet* 1995; 4: 1015–20.

27 Maestrini E, Monaco AP, McGrath JA *et al.* A molecular defect in loricrin, the major component of the cornified cell envelope, underlies Vohwinkel's syndrome. *Nature Genet* 1996; 13: 70–7.

28 Feinstein A, Friedman J, Schewach-Millet M. Pachyonychia congenita. *J Am Acad Dermatol* 1988; 19: 705–9.

29 Chang A, Lucker GPH, Van de Kerkhof PCM *et al.* Pachyonychia congenita in the absence of other syndrome abnormalities. *J Am Acad Dermatol* 1994; 30: 1017–18.

30 Smith FJ, Jonkman MF, van Goor H *et al.* A mutation in human keratin K6b produces a phenocopy of the K17 disorder pachyonychia congenita type 2. *Hum Mol Genet.* 1998; 7: 1143–8.

31 Bowden PE, Haley JL, Kansky A *et al.* Mutation of a type II keratin (k6a) in pachyonychia congenita. *Nature Genet* 1995; 10: 363–5.

32 Shamsher MK, Navsaria HA, Stevens HP *et al.* Novel mutations in keratin 16 gene underly focal non-epidermolytic palmoplantar keratoderma (NEPPK) in two families. *Hum Mol Genet*, 1995; 10: 1875–81.

33 Covello SP, Smith FJ, Sillevis Smitt JH *et al.* Keratin 17 mutations cause either steatocystoma multiplex or pachyonychia congenita type 2. *Br J Dermatol* 1998; 139: 475–80.

34 Jonkman MF, Scheffer H, Stulp R *et al.* Revertant mosaicism in epidermolysis bullosa caused by mitotic gene conversion. *Cell* 1997; 88: 543–51.

35 Alsaleh QA, Teebi AS. Autosomal recessive epidermolytic palmoplantar keratoderma. *J Med Genet* 1990; 27: 519–22.

36 Richard G, De Laurenzi V, Didona B *et al.* Keratin 13 point mutation underlies the hereditary mucosal epithelia disorder white sponge nevus. *Nature Genet* 1995; 11: 453–5.

37 Rugg EL, McLean WHI, Allison WE *et al.* A mutation in the mucosal keratin K4 is associated with oral white sponge nevus. *Nature Genet* 1995; 11: 450–3.

38 Happle R. What is a nevus? A proposed definition of a common term. *Dermatology* 1995; 191: 1–5.

39 Hamm H, Echternacht-Happle K, Happle R. Monilethrix: ausschlieslicher Befall der Körperbehaarung. *Z Hautler* 1984; 59: 1177–8.

40 Healy E, Holmes SC, Belgaid CE *et al.* A gene for monilethrix is closely linked to the type II keratin gene cluster at 12q13. *Hum Mol Genet* 1995; 4: 2399–402.

41 Winter H, Rogers MA, Langbein L *et al.* Mutations in the hair cortex keratin hHb6 cause the inherited hair disease monilethrix. *Nat Genet* 1997; 16: 372–4.

42 Winter H, Labreze C, Chapalain V *et al.* A variable monilethrix phenotype associated with a novel mutation, Glu402Lys, in the helix termination motif of the type II hair keratin hHb1. *J Invest Dermatol* 199; 111: 169–72.

43 Renwick JH, Izatt MM. Linkage data on monilethrix. *Cytogenet Cell Genet* 1988; 47: 108.

44 Fosko SW, Stenn KS, Bolognia JL. Ectodermal dysplasias associated with clefting: significance of scalp dermatitis. *J Am Acad Dermatol* 1992; 27: 249–56.

45 Rothnagel JA, Longley MA, Holder RA *et al.* Genetic disorders of keratins: are scarring alopecias a sub-set? *J Dermatol Sci* 1994; 7 (suppl): S164–9.

46 Cambiaghi S, Tadini G, Barbareschi M *et al.* Rapp–Hodgkin syndrome and AEC syndrome: are they the same entity? *Br J Dermatol* 1994; 130: 97–101.

47 Moss C, Savin J. *Dermatology and the New Genetics.* Oxford: Blackwell Science, 1995.

48 Rothnagel JA, Longley MA, Holder RA *et al.* Prenatal diagnosis of epidermolytic hyperkeratosis by direct gene sequencing. *J Invest Dermatol* 1994; 102: 13–16.

49 Choate KA, Medalie DA, Morgan JR *et al.* Corrective gene transfer in the human skin disorder lamellar ichthyosis. *Nature Med* 1996; 2: 1263–7.

Epidermolysis Bullosa

DAVID J. ATHERTON

Epidermolysis bullosa simplex
Rarer types of epidermolysis bullosa simplex

Dystrophic epidermolysis bullosa
Skin care
Topical antimicrobials
Other topical and systemic therapy
Prevention and treatment of complications
Prenatal diagnosis

Junctional epidermolysis bullosa

Epidermolysis bullosa (EB) is the name given to a group of genetically determined disorders characterized by excessive susceptibility of the skin and mucosae to separate from the underlying tissues following mechanical trauma (Fig. 19.4.1). The individual diseases vary in their impact from relatively minor disability (e.g. limitation of walking distance because of blistering of the feet) to death in infancy [1,2].

Some authors object to the use of the term for those diseases which fulfil the above criteria but which do not feature true epidermolysis, i.e. lysis of keratinocytes, and would prefer to call these conditions hereditary mechanobullous diseases, rather than EB. However, the term EB in the wider sense will be used in this chapter.

There are three broad categories of EB depending on the level of split within the skin (Fig. 19.4.2): EB simplex (EBS), dystrophic EB (DEB) and junctional EB (JEB). Within each of these categories, there are several subtypes which are clinically, and probably genetically distinct.

Epidermolysis bullosa simplex

Definition

This is a group of inherited disorders characterized by mechanically induced blistering occurring within the epidermis itself as a result of lysis of basal keratinocytes. Because of the characteristic level of cleavage, EBS is sometimes termed epidermolytic EB.

There are several established variants, of which the following are the most important.

1 EBS localized to hands and feet (Weber–Cockayne type).
2 Generalized EBS (Koebner type).
3 EBS herpetiformis (Dowling–Meara type).

There are, in addition, a number of rarer variants that are encountered from time to time.

1 Epidermolysis bullosa simplex with muscular dystrophy [3].
2 EBS superficialis [4]
3 Kallin's syndrome [5].
4 EBS with mottled pigmentation [6].
5 'Lethal' autosomal recessive EBS [7].

Aetiology and pathogenesis

The prevalence of the different forms of EBS has not been systematically studied, and can therefore only be estimated; it probably varies from country to country [8–10]. The prevalence of EBS localized to the hands and feet (Weber–Cockayne type) is about 10–20 per million. The generalized form is rarer, possibly about 2 per million. With increasing experience of clinical and pathological diagnosis of the Dowling–Meara variant, the impression is that the disease is commoner than previously believed, affected neonates being approximately as common as those with either dystrophic or junctional disease; prevalence is probably in the region of 5–10 per million. The superficial and autosomal recessive types are probably extremely rare, but some of the rare forms may be locally common, for example the Ogna variant, whose prevalence may be as high as 14 per million in Norway [10].

Almost all forms of EBS are inherited as autosomal dominant traits. There appear to be certain rare forms that are inherited as autosomal recessive traits, notably EBS with neuromuscular disease [11], 'lethal' EBS [7], and there is some evidence that at least occasionally, EBS localized to the hands and feet may be transmitted as an autosomal recessive trait [12].

Patients with the generalized and localized forms of EBS almost always have extensive family histories of the condition, and the occurrence of sporadic cases is r elatively unusual. As is generally the case with dominantly inherited diseases, severity may vary considerably

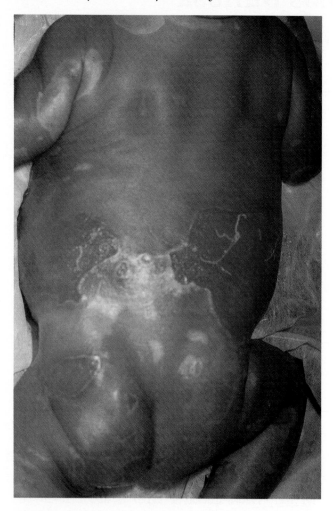

Fig. 19.4.1 The appearance of a 9-day-old child with EB showing erosions caused by lifting the child.

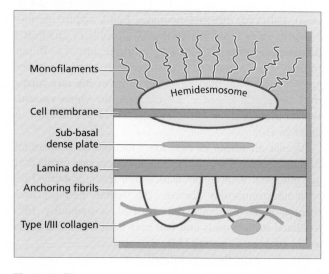

Fig. 19.4.2 Diagrammatic representation of the dermoepidermal junction.

between affected members of a single family. The majority of cases of EBS herpetiformis appear to be sporadic, but inheritance has been autosomal dominant in all reported familial cases to date [13].

Mutations can be found in about 50% of patients examined in the genes coding for keratins 5 or 14, which are, respectively, the predominant basic and acidic keratins in the skin [14,15]. These mutations have so far been clustered in six 'hot-spots' on the keratin molecules, and it is becoming clear that the site of each hot-spot will determine the clinical severity of the resulting disease. Thus the mutations so far identified in the more severe Dowling–Meara form of EBS have all been in the highly conserved regions at the beginning and end of the central rod domain, which are known to be important in the early stages of filament assembly. The mutations identified in the milder Weber–Cockayne and Koebner forms have been in the other four hot-spots. However, a proportion of EBS patients do not appear to have mutations in keratins 5 or 14, and their mutations are thought likely to be in the genes encoding other basal keratins, such as keratins 15 and 17, or a variety of keratin-associated proteins.

Pathology

The technique of taking biopsies in EB is of the greatest importance if the procedure is to provide useful tissue for the pathologist. The biopsy should be taken from clinically unaffected skin. Disruption of the skin should be induced by rubbing the area to be biopsied with a finger or an India rubber for about a minute. There should follow a delay of 5–10 min, after which the biopsy should be taken. In the author's view, a shave technique provides the best quality material, because artefact is minimal, fixation is rapid, orientation is easier and healing is good. A useful technique is to pass a hypodermic needle in a shallow tangential direction through the biopsy site after local anaesthesia has been achieved, and then to cut along the upper surface of the needle with a scalpel blade.

In all forms of EB, routine light microscopy may be misleading. For example, intraepidermal cleavage in EBS may appear to be subepidermal. EBS is characterized at the pathological level by true epidermolysis, i.e. intracellular keratinocyte lysis. At the ultrastructural level, this lysis occurs in the basal keratinocytes [16] in all forms. EBS of the generalized and localized types cannot currently be distinguished ultrastructurally. Conversely, EBS herpetiformis shows the distinctive feature of tonofibril clumping occurring within basal keratinocytes prior to their lysis [17], though this change cannot always be found easily, particularly in patients with clinical disease that is relatively mild. Prenatal diagnosis of EBS is discussed in Chapters 19.25 and 19.26.

Clinical features

Epidermolysis bullosa simplex localized to the hands and feet (Weber–Cockayne type)

This variant of EBS most characteristically has its onset in early childhood, but very often not until walking is established. In some cases, the condition is not revealed until adolescence or early adult life, when the subject is required to undertake unaccustomed activity, for example a forced march in the army. Those who have Weber–Cockayne EBS often do not consider themselves to have a medical problem, merely an exaggeration of the normal tendency to blister during or after hard walking or running, or after intensive use of the hands.

Rubbing of the feet by footwear is generally the major cause of blisters, and the commonest parts of the feet to be affected are the soles and the junctions between the sole and the sides of the toes or the main part of the foot. A particular feature of all types of EBS is a progressively increased tendency to blister as the environmental temperature rises. So great is this effect that some patients who have marked disability in hot summer weather may have little or none in the winter. Though it is sometimes implied that EBS of this type is a relatively trivial disease, some patients experience very substantial disability, mainly because of difficulty in walking. Some individuals may only be able to walk 100 or 200 m on a summer day before painful blistering occurs. Other patients may have problems with manual tasks, and may find it impossible to use hand tools for more than brief periods.

Blisters tend to be small, up to about 2 cm in diameter, and, despite their relatively superficial localization, they are generally tense (Fig. 19.4.3); they may even be haemorrhagic. A particular feature is an erythematous halo around blisters, a characteristic which, in the absence of secondary infection, is generally lacking in other types of EB. Nevertheless, secondary infection is common once blisters have ruptured. Though the blisters will heal rapidly in the absence of such secondary infection, the frequent recurrence of provocative trauma at affected sites tends to cause new blisters to occur underneath and at the margins of ones that are in the process of healing. A degree of hyperkeratosis often marks sites of recurrent blistering.

The nails are not usually affected unless subject to considerable trauma such as a heavy object being dropped on to toe nails or toe nails being trodden on. Areas of the body other than the hands and feet are rarely affected. The mouth is almost invariably spared.

Generalized epidermolysis bullosa simplex (Koebner type)

Generalized EBS tends to have an early onset, either

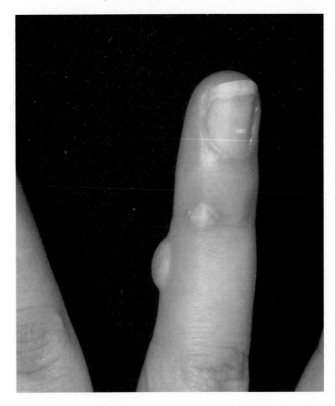

Fig. 19.4.3 Typical blisters in a 14-year-old with EBS.

during the perinatal period or during the first few months of life. It is not infrequently already present at birth.

In the perinatal period, blistering and erosions occur at sites determined by trauma during delivery and by handling in the nursery. Lesions heal quickly without scarring. Thereafter, the rate of new blister formation tends to slow down, with new lesions only appearing at sites of continuing friction, particularly in the napkin area.

Oral lesions do occur, but tend not to be prominent and only rarely interfere with feeding. Nail involvement is unusual, and when nails are occasionally shed following subungual blistering, they generally regrow without dystrophy.

Rubbing of the skin tends to be the main provocative factor. The blistering tendency is much more apparent in warm weather, to the extent that some patients' problems may be more or less confined to the summer months. As the child starts to crawl, lesions may occur on the knees, feet, elbows and hands. With the onset of walking, the principal problem localizes to the feet and ankles, with the hands being the next most frequently affected site. In adults, it is rare for lesions to occur elsewhere, though blisters can be provoked at any site under appropriate provocation.

The blisters are tense and occur at the same sites on the hands and feet as in the localized type of EBS. Likewise, secondary infection is perhaps the principal complication of the disorder. In the absence of such infection, the blisters heal fairly rapidly without blistering.

Epidermolysis bullosa simplex herpetiformis (Dowling–Meara type) [17–20]

Increasing recognition of this disorder is making it clear that this is a more common type of EBS than was previously believed. Clinically, it generally causes blistering with an onset in early infancy. There is a great range of severity in individual cases. Blistering may be exceptionally severe during the neonatal period, and these babies can present a devastating picture. Death in the neonatal period is probably not infrequent, and many of these severe cases were previously probably thought to have lethal JEB. In the severe case, blistering may appear to arise quite spontaneously, particularly in a hot environment. Blisters are perhaps even more often haemorrhagic than in other forms of EBS, and milia may be a transient feature after blisters have healed. It is important to be aware that milia are not pathognomonic of dystrophic forms of EB, and that they may occur, albeit rather fleetingly, in all the other forms, but perhaps particularly in Dowling–Meara EBS.

The hands and feet are the sites of predilection (Fig. 19.4.4), and blisters at these sites are similar to those seen in other forms of EBS. However, it is particularly characteristic for blistering on the palms and soles to be succeeded by focal keratoderma, though this is also seen, albeit usually to a lesser degree, in other types of EBS. On occasions, this keratoderma may be very prominent and associated with flexion deformity and loss of function.

A rather characteristic thickening of the nails is also commonly seen in Dowling–Meara EBS. Even in the neonatal period, involvement of the hands and feet is prominent, and is often already associated with nail thickening; this combination can be diagnostically helpful.

Blisters frequently occur at other sites on the face (Fig. 19.4.5), trunk and limbs, and tend to be disposed in groups with an erythematous border; hence the adjective herpetiformis. However, these groups are perhaps more often annular or arcuate than truly herpetiform. Of these other sites, the neck is particularly commonly affected. A major provocative factor appears to be friction from the seams of clothing. However, in this condition, groups of blisters may appear with remarkably little provocation. High environmental temperatures seem to be of great importance in reducing the threshold for blistering. Like other types of EBS, secondary infection is very common and is perhaps more of a problem in this than any other form of EB.

Oral involvement is usually not prominent. However, a proportion of severely affected neonates under the author's care have experienced extreme oropharyngeal blistering with potentially serious interference with feeding. These babies may demonstrate incoordination of swallowing with a tendency to aspirate feeds, and they frequently also demonstrate marked gastro-oesophageal reflux.

Hoarseness of the voice is quite often present, particularly in the more severely affected case; a weak cry may be noticeable in the neonatal period. Laryngeal involvement was previously considered virtually pathognomonic of the Herlitz type of JEB, but it is now clear that it also occurs regularly in Dowling–Meara EBS.

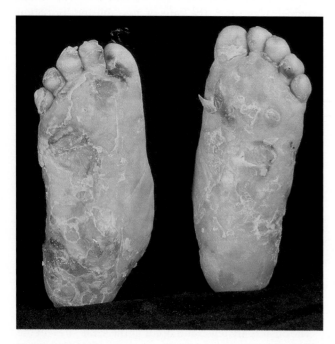

Fig. 19.4.4 The soles of a 5-year-old child with Dowling–Meara EBS.

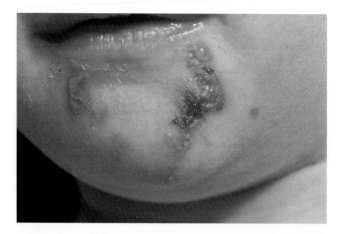

Fig. 19.4.5 Characteristic annular herpetiform blistering in Dowling–Meara EBS.

Prognosis

Generally, the prognosis in EBS is good, particularly in the common Weber–Cockayne type, the great majority of patients having a normal life expectancy. However, disability can be significant, patients' choices of career, housing, employment and leisure activity being constrained by limitations on the distance they can walk. While the Dowling–Meara type of EBS can undoubtedly be lethal in early infancy, the blistering tendency will probably improve with time, and some adults who had problems with the conditions as children later become more or less free from any evidence of the disease. However, other adults remain substantially disabled by Dowling–Meara EBS throughout their lives [21], particularly as a result of persisting blistering of the hands and feet, and palmar and plantar keratoderma.

Differential diagnosis

The principal problem in diagnosis of the commoner varieties of EBS is to distinguish them clinically from other forms of EB, though this is, in the main, only a problem in the neonatal period. Immunohistochemistry and electron microscopy of appropriate skin biopsies usually allow differentiation, but experience is required for reliable interpretation.

In the neonate, EB may be confused with any of the following: incontinentia pigmenti; miliaria crystallina; bullous ichthyosiform erythroderma; bullous impetigo or staphylococcal scalded skin syndrome; the EEC syndrome (ectodactyly–ectodermal dysplasia and clefting syndrome); AEC syndrome (ankyloblepharon ectodermal defects and cleft lip) and Rapp–Hodgkin forms of ectodermal dysplasia (which all feature lip and/or palatal clefting); neonatal or congenital varicella and herpes simplex; neonatal pemphigus or pemphigoid gestationis; infantile pemphigoid and cutis aplasia. In adults, pachyonychia congenita will need to be considered, particularly in Dowling–Meara EBS where palmar and plantar hyperkeratosis and nail thickening may both be prominent.

Treatment

In EBS localized to the hands and feet, and in generalized EBS, the long family association with the disease, combined with an awareness both of the provoking influences and the limitations of available therapy, make it fairly unusual for patients to seek medical assistance. When they do, the most useful contribution one can make is to provide advice about suitable footwear, general care of the feet and genetic counselling.

Fresh blisters should be drained after puncturing them with a sterile disposable needle, as they tend to extend if left alone. The blister roof should be left *in situ*. It is often useful to bathe blistered feet and hands in warm water containing potassium permanganate at a dilution of about 1:8000. The ideal dressing for erosions and blisters in patients with EBS has yet to be invented, and none of the currently available products seems very precisely to fit these patient's requirements. Patients and their parents generally make up their own minds about the dressing materials that most suit their own needs, and the dermatologist's priority is really to ensure, firstly that they are properly informed about the range of different types of dressing available, and secondly that they are able to secure a supply of their chosen dressings as economically as possible.

Patients often like to use topical antimicrobial applications because of the frequent occurrence of secondary bacterial infection. However, the ideal topical antimicrobial agent to protect these patients from secondary bacterial infections has yet to be developed, and the regular use of any particular preparation tends to be associated with the development of bacterial resistance to the antimicrobial employed. The author tends to prefer to concentrate on physical cleansing and the use of potassium permanganate soaks as described above. If anything is to be applied to individual lesions, an antiseptic is preferred to an antibiotic, although the author discourages patients from using either. Of those preparations that are currently available, the least unsuitable would include 1.5% hydrogen peroxide cream (Hioxyl, Quinoderm, Oldham, UK), 10% povidone-iodine aqueous solution or ointment (Betadine, Napp, Cambridge, UK) and 0.5% cetrimide cream (Cetavlex, Care, Wilmslow, UK).

It is important to provide children with EBS with footwear which allows them the maximum mobility while providing the best possible protection for their feet. Many children can wear 'off the peg' shoes if these incorporate appropriate design features. Ideally, these shoes are made of very soft leather, with the minimum number of internal seams. There should be plenty of room for the toes, in both the horizontal and vertical planes. Both the uppers and the insock should be made of permeable leather, in order to keep the foot as cool and dry as possible, and the inside of the sole should have a shape which is as anatomically appropriate as possible. Few 'off the peg' shoes fulfil these criteria, other than certain lines of Elephanten shoes (Intershoe Ltd, Stockton on Tees UK) which are more or less ideal. Socks should be absorbent and should therefore contain a high proportion of cotton. They should also provide additional cushioning; the towelling type of sport sock is ideal. It is sometimes useful for the patient to wear two pairs of socks as this helps to reduce friction.

A small proportion of babies and young children with generalized EBS, and a larger proportion with Dowling–Meara EBS may be very fragile, and they will need protective measures as described below under DEB (p. 1089). However, it is very important to avoid the use of heavy dressings which may increase the skin surface temperature and therefore the rate of blistering. In children with Dowling–Meara EBS it seems especially important to check that clothing does not have rough internal seams, and that it fits loosely, especially at the neck, wrists and ankles.

Avoidance of high environmental temperatures whenever possible is a helpful measure, and it is especially important to keep affected infants cool. The author's practice is to use an air-conditioned cubicle for these infants during any admission to hospital, and severely affected infants are provided with a portable air-conditioning unit for use at home in the early years. Topical application of 10% glutaraldehyde and 10% aluminium chloride hexahydrate have both been advocated for the soles of patients with Weber–Cockayne EBS [22,23], but neither have proven useful for the majority of patients.

A useful response of Dowling–Meara EBS to the oral 5-hydroxytryptamine (5-HT)-2 antagonists pipamperone and cyproheptadine has been reported [24], but the author's patients have had minimal benefit from cyproheptadine.

The author has occasionally used short courses of oral prednisolone to reduce blistering temporarily in Dowling–Meara EBS. The effectiveness of oral corticosteroid therapy in Weber–Cockayne EBS was documented many years ago [25]. The use of such treatment may be worth considering as a short-term measure when symptoms are particularly distressing in any form of EBS.

Neonates severely affected with Dowling–Meara EBS have required nasogastric feeding for a period which may last several months.

Rarer types of epidermolysis bullosa simplex

Epidermolysis bullosa simplex with muscular dystrophy

This is a rare form of EB which is now known to reflect mutations in the gene coding for plectin, a cytoskeleton-membrane anchoring protein [3,26,27]. Generalized blistering is of early onset, and the clinical features tend to be rather similar to those seen in junctional EB, with prominent periungual blistering, nail loss, atrophic scarring and dental enamel hypoplasia [28,29]. Progressive muscular dystrophy reflects the important role of plectin in muscle as well as in skin.

Epidermolysis bullosa simplex superficialis [4]

A group of patients has been described in which blistering occurs just below the stratum corneum; inheritance was autosomal dominant. Despite the superficial level of cleavage, peeling of the skin was not noted; the patients reported generalized blistering and, frequently, the development of superficial erosions and crusting without preceding blisters. Patients were also liable to a variable degree to milia, atrophic scarring, nail dystrophy, and oral and ocular involvement.

Kallin's syndrome [5]

This syndrome was described in two sisters, in whom it was thought likely to have been transmitted as an autosomal recessive trait. It featured blistering of the hands and feet, occasionally haemorrhagic, occurring mainly in the summer, essentially identical to those seen in patients with Weber–Cockayne EBS. However, these children also had hypodontia associated with a dental enamel dysplasia, increased curvature or thickening of the nails and diffuse alopecia without scarring. One of the sisters had been discovered to be totally deaf in one ear when she was 5 years old.

Epidermolysis bullosa simplex with mottled pigmentation [30–32]

This condition has now been described by several authors, and is likely to be transmitted by an autosomal dominant gene. Affected individuals have life-long, mechanically induced blistering, essentially indistinguishable from Koebner EBS, healing without scarring or atrophy. The mucosae are generally not affected. The blistering becomes less prominent with increasing age, and may even disappear. Pigmentary abnormalities are the main distinguishing feature of the disorder, and take the form of well-demarcated pigmented macules 2–5 mm in diameter, most profuse on the trunk and the proximal limbs, which may be present from very early in life and whose appearance does not seem to be a direct result of blistering. In several cases, there may be a mixture of hyper- and hypopigmented macules. Another fairly regular feature has been the development of small warty palmoplantar keratoses measuring 2–5 mm in diameter.

'Lethal' autosomal recessive epidermolysis bullosa simplex [7]

This disorder has been described in a single Sudanese family in which it appeared to be inherited as an autosomal recessive trait. Generalized blistering healed without scarring. Anaemia was common and most affected individuals died in early childhood. The cause of death was likely to have been laryngeal involvement resulting in upper airways obstruction.

Dystrophic epidermolysis bullosa

Definition

This is a group of inherited disorders characterized by mechanically induced blistering occurring immediately below the lamina densa of the basement membrane zone. Because of the characteristic level of cleavage, DEB is sometimes termed dermolytic EB. These disorders derive the name *dystrophic* from the tendency of the blisters to heal with atrophic scarring.

Aetiology and pathogenesis

DEB may be inherited as an autosomal dominant or an autosomal recessive trait. In general, it tends to be most severe when inherited as a recessive trait, and mildest when inherited as a dominant trait, but there is considerable clinical overlap. In sporadic cases, it is therefore imprudent to guess the mode of inheritance on clinical grounds alone. In the great majority of cases of dominant DEB, there is a clear family history, suggesting a low rate of new mutations. Most sporadic cases of DEB seem to be of recessive type, even where clinically mild.

There are few data to indicate the prevalence of DEB. In Norway the prevalence of dominant DEB has been estimated to be 1.4 per million [10]. In England an estimated prevalence for all recessive types of EB was 3 per million [33,34], of which most were probably cases of DEB. A more recent estimated prevalence from Scotland was 21.4 per million for all types of DEB [8].

Linkage and mutational analysis have demonstrated the likelihood that all types of DEB reflect mutations in the gene for type VII collagen (known as COL-7A1) [35,36], which has been localized to the short arm of chromosome 3 at the 3p21.1 locus [37]. Type VII collagen is a major component of anchoring fibrils [38,39]. It is a large molecule (approximately 1000 kDa), which is synthesized and secreted by keratinocytes. Structurally, it comprises a homotrimer of three α1 (VII) chains which associate to form a triple helix. The molecule has three domains: a central triple helical domain consisting of (Gly-X-Y) repeats and two non-helical globular domains termed NC-1 and NC-2. Type VII procollagen molecules associate via their carboxy-terminals, following which the NC-2 domains are cleaved off. The resulting type VII collagen molecules further condense to form anchoring fibrils.

It is becoming clear in DEB that the type of mutation or mutations present in the type VII collagen gene will be increasingly able to predict the clinical severity and prognosis of that individual's disease [40]. There is evidence that the most severe forms of recessive DEB reflect mutations that result in premature termination of translation and in truncated α1 (VII) chains [41–43], while alterations of the NC-2 domain cause milder recessively transmitted disease not manifest in heterozygotes [44]. Dominantly transmitted disease may generally reflect mutations affecting the triple helical domain [36].

Pathology

DEB is the clinical reflection of defective attachment of the basement membrane to the underlying dermis, manifest at the ultrastructural level by reduced numbers of morphologically abnormal anchoring fibrils [45]. The monoclonal antibody LH-7.2 binds to the basement membrane zone in normal skin, but not in severe recessive DEB. It is now clear that this antibody binds to the NC-1 domain of type VII collagen. While there is generally no binding at all in severe recessive DEB, binding is often weakly present in milder recessive DEB, but is normal in dominant DEB [46–50].

Clinical features

There is very wide variation in the severity of DEB in different patients, reflecting the many different mutations that may affect the type VII collagen gene. At its least severe, DEB can allow an almost normal quality and length of life, while at its most severe, it may cause major handicap and a relatively brief and painful life.

Skin

The clinical hallmark of DEB is the tendency for blistered areas to heal with atrophic scarring and the development of contractures. While the presence of milia in recently healed areas is highly characteristic of dystrophic forms of EB, milia may more transiently be seen in other types of EB.

Attempts have previously been made to subdivide DEB into a number of distinct subtypes. Such efforts were in practice hampered by the considerable degree of overlap observed between different subtypes, and it is the author's view that an obsession with precise categorization of the individual case is generally unnecessary and unhelpful. It is all too easy for an academic preoccupation with classification to distract from the more urgent and important matter of providing care and advice to the patient and their family. In the individual case it is sufficient for the purpose of clinical management to establish that the patient has a dystrophic form of the disease. Beyond this, the most important issue is whether it has been transmitted as an autosomal dominant or recessive trait, for the purposes of genetic counselling and prenatal diagnosis. However, apart from the wide variability in the severity of the different clinical manifestations of DEB in individual patients, it is possible to recognize a pattern of cutaneous disease in a minority of cases in which the trunk and proximal flexural areas are predominantly affected, in contrast to the more usual predilection for peripheral areas. In patients with this 'inverse' pattern [51,52], the hands tend to be less severely affected, but the non-cutaneous aspects of the disease are generally just as troublesome.

Blistering in DEB tends to be provoked predominantly by knocks and blows to the skin rather than by rubbing as is the case in EBS. Blisters in DEB therefore occur most frequently at skin sites where knocks and blows are common, such as the dorsa of the hands and feet, and the elbows and knees. However, persistent rubbing of the skin does also predispose to blistering, especially rubbing by clothing and bedding such as occurs around the neck, waist, groins, hips and lumbosacral area. Another prominent cause of blistering and ulceration is the attachment of anything adherent to the skin, such as adhesive tapes; this feature has great practical importance in the initial clinical recognition of the disease in the neonate and in the management of the patient. However, in the longer term, perhaps the most important provocative factor of all is excoriation by the patient of healing or recently healed areas of skin.

The blisters may vary considerably in size, and some patients may develop blisters that exceed 10 cm in diameter. The blisters tend to be rather flaccid, and are filled with either clear or blood-stained fluid. Healing of previously unblistered sites is generally fairly rapid. Crops of milia are common following initial re-epithelialization, but where an area is not subject to further blistering, the milia disappear after a few months. Discernible scarring is unusual following a single episode of blistering in a particular area, and generally only follows recurrent blistering. Blistering is much more easily provoked in areas that have previously been blistered, particularly when scarring has occurred. Healing areas tend to itch, and when the patient scratches, further blistering is likely to follow. This can establish a cycle of blistering, itching and reblistering, the situation being made worse by the decreasing quality of healing and the increasing ease with which reblistering therefore occurs. Scarring is often not apparent after a particular area of skin has only been blistered once, but becomes progressively more apparent the more often blistering occurs.

In the great majority of cases, blisters or, more often, erosions are present at or very shortly after birth. Rather commonly, an extensive eroded area is present at birth on one or both lower legs, usually on the dorsum and lateral aspect of the foot and on the medial and anterior aspect of the shin (Fig. 19.4.6). This type of lesion almost certainly evolves *in utero* as a result of the fetus rubbing one leg against the other. When unilateral and in the absence of other lesions suggestive of EB, the significance of this type of lesion may not be appreciated. Such congenital absence of the skin on the lower leg is not specific for any particular type of EB [53]. These areas usually heal fairly rapidly, though the resulting scarring frequently leads to some deformity, particularly to upward displacement of the great toe, and to diminished growth of the foot.

New blisters develop less frequently with increasing age. It is unclear whether this is because of a genuinely decreased tendency of the skin to blister or is simply a reflection of more effective avoidance of trauma by older patients. In patients who are more severely affected,

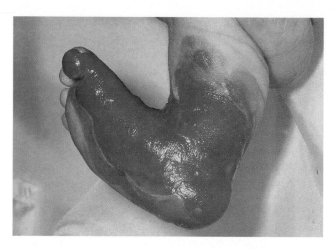

Fig. 19.4.6 Absence of skin at birth: a very characteristic presentation of EB.

this trend is often counterbalanced by the steadily increasing fragility of skin that has been repeatedly ulcerated in the past, and which becomes atrophic and as delicate as tissue paper. Whereas previously ulcerated areas would usually heal rapidly, these atrophic areas may now break down so frequently that they never seem to heal. The neck, axillae, elbows, hands, hips, knees and ankles seem to be among the most troublesome sites from this point of view. Nevertheless, most patients who survive into adult life may nevertheless enjoy a gradual improvement in the quality of scarred areas alongside a greater resistance of the skin to the development of new blisters. In those with mild DEB, scarring can almost disappear in adult life, leading to a remarkable improvement in the appearance, for example, of the hands. Patients with DEB quite frequently develop areas of dark macular pigmentation with rather characteristic irregular borders which may show histological features resembling malignant melanoma [54]. True malignant melanoma has been reported but is probably rare. [55].

The most sinister late complication of DEB is the tendency for epitheliomas, predominantly squamous carcinomas, to develop in recurrently ulcerated and scarred areas, particularly over bony prominences on the limbs [55–62]. The incidence of these tumours reaches its peak in the third and fourth decades. Tragically, patients are very often unaware of this danger and may therefore fail to bring such lesions to medical attention in good time. As a result, death from metastatic disease is frequent in some series [63]. Squamous carcinoma is a major cause of death in patients with severe DEB that survive into adult life.

Albopapuloid dystrophic epidermolysis bullosa

The term 'albopapuloid' was first used by Pasini [64] to describe the ivory-white papules he observed in two patients with DEB. These lesions are generally small and multiple, but may coalesce to form plaques up to about 4 cm in diameter. They are most often seen on the trunk, especially the lower back, but they have also occurred at other sites. Although it was initially believed that lesions of this type were specific to a particular autosomal dominant variant of DEB, it now seems more likely that they are non-specific though they tend to be seen most often in older children and adults with relatively mild DEB. They have been reported in otherwise unremarkable cases of recessively inherited DEB [65], and in both pretibial EB [66] and EB pruriginosa [67].

Epidermolysis bullosa pruriginosa

There appears to be a fairly distinctive clinical variant of DEB in which the predominant features are pruriginous papules or lichenified plaques, associated with scarring [67,68]. Lesions occur mostly on the limbs, particularly on the shins, but may also be seen on the trunk. Itching is often marked. Finger and toe nail dystrophy is very common, with thickening or loss of the nail plate. Because intact blisters are rarely seen, the fact that the patient has DEB can easily be overlooked. Mucosal lesions tend to be absent. Where familial cases have occurred, inheritance has generally been autosomal dominant.

Pretibial epidermolysis bullosa [66,69–71]

In this variant of DEB, blistering and scarring are predominantly located on the shins. There may be associated toe nail dystrophy.

Transient bullous dermolysis [72–75]

A subgroup of infants with DEB can be defined on the basis of abundant amounts of type VII collagen found intraepidermally on immunocytochemistry. These infants have a relatively good prognosis, with most enjoying virtual resolution of their disease by the end of the first year of life, though initially blistering may be severe, even fatal [76]. It appears likely that there is a transient abnormality of handling of type VII collagen in these cases. The intraepidermal type VII collagen may disappear within a few weeks of birth, so that it is important to take skin biopsies within the first 2 weeks of life if this variant of DEB is to be recognized.

It is important to be aware that sparse deposits of intraepidermal type VII collagen may be found quite commonly in all forms of DEB as long as the disease is active, if sufficiently sensitive methods are used, perhaps in up to a third of cases, but this finding probably has little significance [77].

Hands

Cutaneous scarring in DEB may lead to a variety of complications, particularly to joint contractures, and to fusion of the fingers and toes. Progressive hand deformity is common in patients who blister readily. When digital fusion is going to develop, one can usually detect the earliest signs of the process within the first year of life. By this age, it is possible to gauge some idea of the likely speed of its progression. The process of fusion seems to occur rather insidiously in the apices of the interdigital spaces, where careful examination will generally reveal small fissures. Occasionally, accidental trauma will lead to denudement of skin on the opposing aspects of more than one finger. If the fingers are opposed during healing, they may become fused within hours. Children with severe DEB are always at risk of acute loss of the entire skin cover of one or more fingers or of an entire hand, an injury known as 'degloving'. This is especially likely to happen when a small child stumbles whilst holding an adult's hand. The adult holds on tightly to prevent the child from falling only to remove the skin from much of the hand; it requires no imagination to realize how distressing such an event will be both to child and adult.

Surprisingly good hand function may be retained despite marked digital fusion, so long as opposition of index finger and thumb is retained. More disabling is the development of flexion contraction of the hand, due to fibrosis of the skin on the palmar aspects of the fingers and hand.

Nails

Subungual blisters are common, and are generally followed by partial or complete separation of the nail plate. The nail will usually regrow normally after this has occurred on one or two occasions, but repeated nail loss will lead to the development first of nail dystrophy and, then of permanent nail loss. In the very mildest cases of DEB, nail dystrophy may be an important diagnostic aid, particularly dystrophy of the great toe nails.

Upper gastrointestinal tract

Blistering of the oral (Fig. 19.4.7), pharyngeal and oesophageal mucosa is common in DEB, and may lead to a number of problems [78–81], of which the most important are as follows.
1 Pain, leading to reduced nutritional intake.
2 Progressive contraction of the mouth.
3 Progressive fixation of the tongue.
4 Dental caries due to oral infection and impaired dental hygiene.
5 Oesophageal dysmotility and strictures/webs [82–85].
6 Gastro-oesophageal reflux.

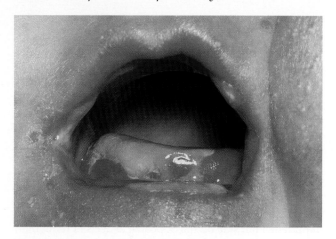

Fig. 19.4.7 The mouth of a 12-week-old baby with DEB.

Dysphagia is a rather common complication of DEB, particularly of severe recessively transmitted disease, but it can occasionally be seen in patients in whom skin involvement is relatively trivial. Many factors contribute to this dysphagia, and although great emphasis has been placed on the role of oesophageal strictures in causing dysphagia, these are not the only, nor perhaps even the most important cause. Major contributions are made by problems in the mouth, particularly by submucous fibrosis in the oral cavity, contraction of the oral and pharyngeal openings, and by fixation of the tongue. In addition, the teeth are often very poor and many may have been extracted. Extremely painful erosions are frequently present in the mouth and pharynx. Combinations of these problems cause patients great difficulties in chewing and swallowing normal food. Eating is often painful, slow and exhausting, so that only relatively small quantities of food can be coped with at any meal.

Gastro-oesophageal reflux, both symptomatic and asymptomatic, is exceedingly common in children with DEB from early infancy. It is probable that such reflux would contribute substantially to dysphagia by aggravating oral, pharyngeal and oesophageal ulceration, increasing dental decay and accelerating oesophageal stricture formation. Gastro-oesophageal reflux is an additional reason why children with DEB may restrict their nutritional intake. One of the author's patients has a laryngeal stricture which we believe is the consequence of recurrent aspiration of gastric acid; he now has a tracheostomy.

There is no evidence that the small intestine is affected and malabsorption is not a problem.

Constipation

Chronic constipation is a common complication of DEB. It is caused principally by anal fissuring, which leads to painful defaecation and therefore to faecal retention, faecal soiling and overflow, and to constipation [80,86]. The tendency to constipation is aggravated by a low dietary fibre intake [85, 87]. It seems probable that the tendency of these patients to take food in frequent small quantities, rather than in discrete meals of reasonable size, leads to a degree of disordered intestinal peristalsis, which will tend to aggravate the constipation still further. The tendency to chronic constipation is frequently compounded by suboptimal fluid intake, administration of oral iron supplements and generalized apathy.

These problems are frequently underestimated, but frequently have a major impact on the patient's quality of life. Besides causing great discomfort, they frequently exert a substantial adverse effect on the patient's nutritional status, principally because of secondary anorexia. Any decrease in appetite is critical in these patients since their dietary intake is already almost invariably low. A frequent and undesirable consequence of constipation is that its presence often discourages oral administration of iron.

Teeth

Rapidly progressive caries is a regular feature in patients with severe DEB. It results from chronic intraoral infection and gum disease, a high sucrose intake and the absence of the normal physical cleansing effect of food due to the diet being more or less liquid. The situation is made worse in severe DEB by the loss of the gingivobuccal sulci, causing residual food to remain applied to the buccal surfaces of the teeth for long periods, and by the loss of the normal cleansing of the teeth because of fixation and shrinkage of the tongue [88]. There is no evidence of a dental enamel defect [89].

Eyes [90–92]

Conjunctival bullae occur quite frequently in patients with severe DEB, and lead to conjunctival ulceration and painful corneal erosions. These may result in conjunctival and corneal scarring, and symblepharon, and may threaten vision in the longer term, both directly and indirectly by interfering with tear film stability and tear production.

Genitourinary tract

A few boys will develop phimosis, and scarring of the external genitalia in a girl led to diversion of the urine into a distended vagina and into the uterus [93]. Children of both sexes may very occasionally develop strictures of the urethral meatus, resulting in urinary retention [94]. The author has seen temporary but recurrent obstruction of the urethral meatus in boys leading to urine tracking under the epithelium of the glans.

Kidneys [95]

Chronic postinfectious glomerulonephritis, considered likely to be a complication of secondary streptococcal skin infection, has been reported in a 10-year-old child with severe DEB. Nephrotic syndrome secondary to renal amyloidosis has also been recorded in a 17-year-old patient.

Anaemia

Anaemia is a problem in most patients with severe DEB. Investigations demonstrate haematological features both of iron deficiency and of decreased red cell iron utilization ('anaemia of chronic disease'). The iron deficiency probably reflects both chronic blood loss from skin, mouth, oesophagus and anal canal, and poor iron intake.

Heart

There have been several reports of fatal dilated cardiomyopathy in children with severe DEB [96–98]. In one of these, the cause was suspected to have been secondary haemochromatosis following multiple blood transfusions [97]. A role for selenium deficiency has also been proposed [98].

Nutritional problems [87,89,100]

The malnutrition which occurs in severe DEB is a consequence of a combination of decreased nutritional intake and increased requirements. Intake is reduced for a variety of reasons, including oropharyngeal ulceration, fibrosis leading to restricted opening of the mouth, tethering of the tongue, oesophageal dysmotility and strictures, and secondary anorexia due to chronic constipation, resulting from anal fissures and faecal retention. Requirements are increased as a result of loss of blood and plasma from denuded epithelium, skin infection and continuous wound healing.

Children with severe DEB on unsupplemented diets tend to consume inadequate amounts of iron, zinc, magnesium, calcium, vitamins, protein, energy and fibre, and are shorter and thinner than normal controls.

Laboratory investigations indicate deficient levels of selected micronutrients, notably plasma iron and zinc, and vitamins A and B_6. The malnutrition that results exerts a major detrimental impact on growth, wound healing, resistance to infection, quality of life and mortality. Those who survive into adult life frequently demonstrate short stature, cachexia and delayed sexual maturation.

Growth

Children with more severe DEB tend to grow poorly.

A decrease in linear growth velocity is usually preceded by an inadequate rate of weight gain, implying that the growth effect is secondary to inadequate nutrition. Anaemia probably also makes a significant contribution.

Prognosis

There is an extraordinary variation in prognosis in DEB. Patients with the mildest clinical presentations will enjoy early cessation of blistering, occasionally even in the first year of life. Conversely, more severely affected individuals will experience increasing malnutrition, increasing anaemia and progressively increasing disability due to interference with joint mobility. While it is now relatively rare in good centres for children with DEB to die in infancy, death towards the end of the first decade remains a threat to the most severely affected. The final cause of death in these cases is very frequently overwhelming sepsis, probably mainly a reflection of deteriorating nutritional status. There is some correlation between the amount of type VII collagen seen immunohistochemically at the basement membrane and the prognosis, complete absence suggesting a worse outlook. The good prognostic significance of abundant intraepidermal type VII collagen has already been highlighted.

Differential diagnosis

Differential diagnosis is normally only a problem during the neonatal period. The principal conditions that require consideration at this time include 'sucking blisters', congenital herpes simplex, the various causes of cutis aplasia congenita, incontinentia pigmenti, focal dermal hypoplasia, bullous ichthyosiform erythroderma, transplacental herpes gestationis and pemphigus vulgaris, miliaria crystallina, bullous impetigo and staphylococcal scalded skin syndrome.

During the neonatal period, it is unwise to attempt to distinguish the various types of EB clinically. The later appearance of milia is indicative of DEB, though small numbers of milia can undoubtedly be seen from time to time in non-dystrophic types.

Early diagnostic biopsy is important, but considerable skill is required in interpretation of results, and such biopsies may be of limited value in centres unaccustomed to handling them. The technique of taking a biopsy in EB is discussed above. In the author's unit, all specimens are examined immunohistochemically with LH-7.2 antibody (for collagen VII) and GB3 antibody (for laminin 5), and ultrastructurally to identify the level of splitting and to examine the various structures normally present in the basement membrane zone.

Treatment [1,2,101,102]

It is advisable to keep new babies with EB in hospital until the clinical situation is stable and the parents feel confident enough to take over in their own home. There is a great deal to be done while the child is in hospital in addition to the basic skin care. Precise diagnosis has to be made, and much time needs to be spent with parents explaining the nature of their child's problems and its care. Feeding and nutritional problems have to be overcome. Before the child's departure from hospital, contact must be made with community nursing and medical staff, and local social services. The genetic implications need to be clarified with the parents, and the risks to further offspring must be delineated as far as possible at this stage. The availability of the means to prevent the birth of a similar child *must* be explained to parents; it is the clear responsibility of the child's doctors to do so whatever their personal views. It is advisable, lest the issue subsequently be neglected, to do this during the affected child's first admission.

Subsequently, in the author's unit the more mildly affected patients are generally reviewed in the outpatient clinic, but brief admissions are more appropriate for multidisciplinary review for the more severely affected.

Skin care

Skin care in patients with EB must incorporate the twin objectives of protection against trauma and provision of optimal conditions for healing of blisters and erosions, in such a way as to minimize disability. A third objective is surveillance for epidermal neoplasia in adult patients.

Neonates

The skin of neonates with EB may be extraordinarily sensitive, even to 'normal' handling. Infants transferred to the author's unit frequently have erosions on each side of the trunk where they have been picked up earlier. Sometimes there are five on each side, one for each of a nurse's or midwife's fingers. Therefore, special handling techniques are required.

Babies with EB should not be nursed naked. Such babies are usually uncomfortable, irritable and restless; they will therefore generally do themselves considerable harm, for example by rubbing their legs together, and their lesions heal relatively slowly. Babies wearing the correct dressings are usually more comfortable and are to some extent shielded from external mechanical trauma, particularly that which is self-induced. Young babies should be nursed on silk sheets to avoid trauma and to prevent any new lesions from sticking to the bedding during dressing changes. Once dressings are in place, the baby should be clothed in soft clothing, which provides added protection during handling. When picking up the baby, the hands should not be pushed underneath, but the baby should first be rolled away, and then allowed to roll back on to the hands and lifted. No child with EB of any age should ever be lifted under the arms. There is a danger that parents will be discouraged from handling their baby; however, it is important for them to do so, and handling should be encouraged once the correct techniques have been learnt.

Dressings should be changed as necessary. It is useful to drain new blisters after puncturing them with a sterile disposable needle, as they will often extend if left intact; the blister roof is left *in situ*. After bathing in warm water, the baby is patted, rather than rubbed, dry with a soft but nonfluffy sheet or towel. The author's unit currently employs the following dressing technique.

Method 1. This is currently the favoured method. Following bathing, erosions are covered with Mepitel (Mölnlycke). This dressing comprises a silicone mesh, which although 'sticky' to the touch, is easily removed from the wound, without pain or trauma. Aquacel, a hydrofibre dressing is applied under the Mepitel in very moist areas. A secondary dressing is applied over the Mepitel, e.g. Mesoft (Mölnlycke) or Release (Johnson and Johnson, Slough, UK). This combination is then secured by a suitable conforming bandage, e.g. J-Fast (Johnson and Johnson), and/or a tubular stretch bandage such as Tubifast (Seton, Oldham, UK). The great advantage of Mepitel is that it needs only to be changed once or twice a week, saving time for the carers and reducing pain for the child, whilst allowing healing to take place. The overlying absorbent secondary dressing can still be changed daily if there is any exudate.

Previous application of any cream or ointment appears to reduce the efficiency of Mepitel. However, creams or ointments may be applied over the Mepitel when this is necessary, e.g. topical corticosteroids to reduce pruritus (see below).

Mepitel has also proved invaluable for securing intravenous cannulae, as its adhesive properties hold the cannula in place, but, in contrast to adherent tapes, removal does not cause any damage to the skin.

The use of these dressings is generally associated with a good rate of re-epithelialization, probably reflecting both their occlusive and protective properties. However, they are not used solely to encourage healing of blistered areas; they are also useful for protection in any area, whether affected or not, which is liable to blistering. Parents should be encouraged to learn these techniques and to use them after they take the baby home.

Older infants and toddlers

Over the months that follow birth, dressing methods need to accommodate the child's increasing need for mobility and play. However, as the child becomes more mobile, the risk of external trauma from falls and knocks becomes a greater factor, at least initially. Later, as the child gradually learns to become more careful, the risk of mechanical trauma again diminishes. Sadly, toddlers are notoriously careless, and certain sites tend to become recurrently traumatized. In DEB, these sites become permanently scarred, which is a problem because such areas are less resistant to subsequent trauma than unscarred areas. The sites that are at special risk in the toddler are the elbows, wrists, hands, knees, shins, ankles and feet. Many parents elect to use protective dressings to cushion these sites. An appropriate technique is to use Lyofoam (Seton, Oldham, UK) (which can be used over Mepitel in an already eroded area or directly over the skin in healed areas), over which is applied Tubifast (Seton), an elasticated viscose tubular bandage. Tubipad (Seton), a foam-lined tubular bandage, on the areas that require protection. Alternatively, materials such as quilting can be sewn inside commercially bought clothing in order to protect at-risk areas.

The ideal dressing for erosions and blisters in patients with EB beyond infancy has yet to be invented. None of the currently available products seems very precisely to fit the requirements of these patients. Patients and their parents generally make up their own minds about the dressing materials that most suit their own needs, and the dermatologist's priority is to ensure that they are properly informed about the range of different types of dressing available and to secure a supply of the preferred dressings as economically as possible for the parents. There can be little question that relatively occlusive dressings are more effective in accelerating healing [103,104].

Clearly, avoidance of trauma is an important facet of treatment of these children. However, it is extremely difficult for parents to get the balance right between what could be regarded as appropriate avoidance of trauma and overprotection of the developing child. Children with EB should be brought up as normally as possible, in order to maximize their physical, manipulative and social skills. They gradually learn for themselves to take extra care, and to avoid situations in which trauma is likely to occur. Older children with EB learn to stand back when other children scuffle. However, during the toddler phase, they tend to be rather careless, and may need someone on hand to patch them up after tumbles. In order to give them the best chance of taking part in normal activities, the emphasis should be on the provision of protective dressings and clothing, rather than on the avoidance of all remotely physical activities.

It is particularly important to provide children with EB with footwear which allows them the maximum mobility while providing the best possible protection for their feet. Ideally, their shoes will be made of very soft leather, with the minimum number of internal seams. As outlined above, there should be plenty of room for the toes and per-

meable leather on the uppers and insock will keep the foot as cool and dry as possible. The inside of the sole should have a shape which is as anatomically appropriate as possible. In practice, few 'off the peg' shoes fulfil these criteria. However, certain lines of Elephanten shoes (UK Agents: Intershoe Ltd, Eveline House, Preston Farm Business Park, Stockton on Tees) appear to be more or less ideal. Some children will have mis-shapen feet due to early damage and subsequent scarring with contraction. They will require tailor-made shoes; Schein shoes have been recommended by some orthotists (Salt and Son, Birmingham, UK). In order to protect the toes from damage often caused by other children stepping on them, it is helpful to incorporate a protective toe-cap into tailor-made shoes, or to adapt 'off the peg' shoes.

Socks should be absorbent and contain a high proportion of cotton. Wearing two pairs of socks can help to reduce friction. Socks should provide additional cushioning for the foot; the towelling type of sport sock is ideal. Other clothing needs to be chosen carefully. Before purchase, all items should be inspected to check that they do not have rough internal seams, and that they fit loosely, especially at the neck, wrists and ankles. In the UK, a good range of suitable clothes is available from sources that specialize in clothing for those with skin diseases.

Older children and adults

The great majority of patients with EB find that new blisters develop less frequently with increasing age. It appears probable that there is a genuinely decreased tendency of the skin to blister, coupled with more effective avoidance of trauma by older patients. In the case of patients with severe DEB, this gradual improvement is sometimes counterbalanced by the steadily increasing fragility of skin which has previously been repeatedly ulcerated, and which may locally be atrophic and exceedingly delicate. These areas may break down so readily that they never heal for long. The neck, back, axillae, hips, knees and ankles seem to be among the most troublesome sites from this point of view. It is tempting to consider skin grafting such areas, but this has proved to be of limited value in ensuring permanent healing [55]. Similarly cultured keratinocytes from normal human skin have failed to produce lasting benefit [105].

Adults with DEB need to be aware of the need for constant surveillance of their skin for the development of squamous carcinoma. It is exceedingly unusual for such lesions to occur in the preadolescent. Sadly, it is not uncommon for patients with EB to become disenchanted with the medical profession; such patients may fail to ask for help with an unfamiliar skin lesion, and they are often not aware of the risk of malignancy. Even if they do seek medical advice, their doctor may also be ignorant of this important and potentially lethal complication. It is of the greatest importance that all patients with DEB be fully educated in relation to this risk and that they should report promptly any unusual skin lesion, particularly nodules, ulcers or crusted lesions which seem particularly unwilling to heal. They should be carefully examined at least once yearly, though this can be difficult to do in an outpatient setting because all dressings have to be removed; it may therefore be more convenient for patients to be admitted briefly for this purpose.

Topical antimicrobials

Secondary bacterial infection is a constant problem in blistered and eroded areas, and it frequently delays healing. Great caution must be exercised in the use of topical antibacterial agents in EB because of the twin risks of induction of bacterial resistance, and of adverse effects that may either be systemic as a result of their percutaneous absorption, or local, usually in the form of interference with healing.

One of the first reports of *Staphylococcus aureus* resistant to mupirocin related to a patient with EB [106]. Whereas at one time the use of this agent was advocated [107], it soon became clear that such an approach would inevitably be complicated by the induction of resistant *Staphylococcus aureus* [108].

The potentially serious hazards of systemic absorption of topical antibacterials should not be underestimated in patients with EB, particularly when they are used in children. The author has seen children with impaired hearing in whom previous ototoxicity was strongly suspected from ill-advised applications of bacitracin, polymyxin, neomycin or gentamicin, to extensive areas of deepithelialized skin under partially occlusive dressings. Chlorhexidine is potentially neurotoxic, and povidone-iodine may be thyrotoxic.

For these reasons, the use of topical antimicrobial agents should not be routine, and should generally be avoided wherever possible. The ideal topical antibacterial agent is unavailable which will protect these patients from the secondary bacterial infections that tend to be such a problem. Of those preparations that are currently available, the least unsuitable appear to be 1.5% hydrogen peroxide cream (Hioxyl) and 1% silver sulphadiazine cream (Flamazine).

Some patients apply various natural substances to ulcerated areas with the aim of accelerating healing. These include honey [109] and sucrose [110], which may discourage microorganisms by providing a hyperosmolar environment. Unfortunately, the beneficial or other effects of such agents have very rarely been the subject of scientific evaluation and it is therefore difficult to comment upon their value.

Other topical and systemic therapy

Over the years a number of systemic agents have been reported to have beneficial effects in DEB; the principal claims for such agents have been reduced blistering rates and accelerated healing.

Phenytoin, protease inhibitors, retinoids and tetracyclines

Early ultrastructural studies of recessive DEB suggested that collagen breakdown in the papillary dermis might contribute to the development of blisters. The subsequent observation that skin fibroblasts cultured from patients synthesize increased amounts of a structurally altered collagenase appeared to strengthen this view and provided the rationale for the therapeutic use of phenytoin, as this agent appeared able to reduce this collagenase production *in vitro*. After early reports of clinical benefit from oral phenytoin [111], a larger multicentre controlled trial failed to confirm this impression of therapeutic benefit [112], and phenytoin is no longer widely used. The author was always extremely anxious about its use in infants because of its significant adverse effects, which include megaloblastic anaemia, lymphoma, encephalopathy and choreoathetosis.

Following the demonstration that retinoids are able to inhibit collagenase activity *in vitro*, there was interest in their possible therapeutic value in recessive DEB. However, these drugs have not to date turned out to be helpful in practice [113], and if they are given in high dose may lead to increased skin fragility.

Tetracyclines have also been shown to inhibit collagenase, and minocycline has been reported to have decreased the rate of blistering in severe DEB [114]. Similarly topical protease inhibitors have been reported to have been helpful in reducing blistering rates [115].

Increased protease activity in DEB is currently regarded as a secondary phenomenon, and none of the above agents has proved to be of consistent therapeutic value in clinical practice.

Corticosteroids

Many patients with severe DEB were previously treated with oral corticosteroids [116], and this therapy did appear to lead to genuinely decreased blistering rates. However, the current consensus is that the longer term toxicity of this form of treatment outweighs any benefits, and it is generally avoided. Its use has been considered in specific situations, such as for a few months after restorative hand surgery, or after oesophageal dilatation for dysphagia, but there is no evidence that patients have enjoyed worthwhile degrees of benefit from this intervention.

Conversely, it appears that topical corticosteroids can be of great value in the treatment of pruritus in healing and healed areas. Dealing with the substantial pruritus experienced by many patients not only enhances patient comfort, but also has the important benefit of averting damaging excoriation and reblistering. This approach requires considerable judgement in terms of selection of an appropriate potency of topical corticosteroid for the individual patient depending on age, extent of the area to be treated and response to treatment. The author has used highly potent preparations intermittently without the development of worrying adverse effects. However, the optimum method of using topical corticosteroids in this situation has yet to be established.

Vitamin E

Over the years there has been interest in the possible value of vitamin E as a treatment for DEB, but little objective evidence of benefit.

Prevention and treatment of complications

Digital fusion and contracture

Corrective surgery should be undertaken as soon as the function of the hand is significantly impaired [117,118]. Function is mainly compromised by flexion and fusion of the first interdigital web. Ideally, only one hand should be operated upon at one time. The surgical procedure involves separating the fused digits, and then releasing any contractures as completely as possible. Split-skin grafts are then sewn into place in the resulting defects along the separated surfaces and on the palmar aspect of previously flexed joints. Where the hand is almost completely encased, the whole extremity may be more conveniently degloved before proceeding to separate the fingers completely and release the contractures.

Kirschner wires are sometimes used to maintain extension during the immediate postoperative period, and are particularly valuable in maintaining complete separation between thumb and index finger. However, it is of great importance to splint the hand in a flat position, with all joints extended as fully as possible between plaster of Paris slabs on the front and back of the hand. The dressings are changed under general anaesthesia at 1–2 weeks and again at about 4 weeks.

While this type of surgical procedure is technically relatively straightforward, the benefit may be limited by rapid recurrence of flexion deformity and digital fusion. For this reason, it is essential to use early postoperative hand splintage in an attempt to maintain extension and separation of the fingers. Traditionally, hard acrylic splints have been employed; these are generally made by taking an impression in dental alginate at the second dressing

change. The author prefers a new type of splint that is easier and cheaper to produce, more comfortable to wear and easier to replace when necessary. These splints are made of a thin and light thermoplastic material, with silicone rubber inserts between the digits [119]. After surgery, children initially wear the splints continuously for 3 months, then for decreasing periods during the day, until after 6 months they wear them only at night.

Unfortunately, these operations often need to be repeated from time to time. It may be necessary to relieve similar flexion contractures at other joints, especially in the feet, at the knees, the hips and in the axillae.

It is perhaps surprising that skin autografts can be so easily and successfully undertaken in patients with DEB. Attempts to grow therapeutically useful autologous keratinocyte sheets *in vitro* from patients with DEB have been frustrated by the tendency of the cells to separate from one another in culture.

Physiotherapy and maintenance of mobility

Physiotherapy probably has little part to play in the treatment of established flexion contractures, but is useful for the maintenance of mobility, which should have the effect of slowing down the progression of such contractures and, in children, the encouragement of normal motor development. Reasonable levels of physical activity should be encouraged, particularly in the case of children, who may mistakenly be immobilized by well-meaning parents or doctors. Patients should be reviewed regularly with full assessment of all joint ranges of movement, muscle power, gross and fine motor abilities and, in children, motor development [120]. Home exercises should be initiated for specific joints as soon as limitation of movement is detected at review. In addition, daily prone lying, and mouth and tongue exercises are recommended for all patients to delay soft tissue shortening and adherence. Patients with contractures may benefit from active exercises in a hydrotherapy pool, and, in some patients, passive 'stretches' may also be beneficial, though these need to be done with great care to avoid skin trauma. Splintage with suitable materials may be a useful additional approach.

Nail problems

Thickened, dystrophic finger and toe nails may be extremely unsightly; in the case of toe nails, they may interfere with wearing shoes. Such nails should be permanently removed surgically.

Dysphagia and nutrition [121,122]

Babies who are being bottle-fed require the softest available teats (generally those designed for premature infants). The opening can be enlarged by use of a hot needle to make feeding easier. The Haberman teat is particularly good and is long enough to ensure that the plastic neck of the bottle does not come into contact with the nose. This teat has the additional benefit of incorporating a valve that ensures easy delivery of feed without the need for the baby to suck hard; as a result babies with severe oral ulceration can often succeed in feeding with this teat rather than having to be fed by nasogastric tube. Some babies find it easier to take milk from a spoon than from a bottle.

Overcoming the combination of nutritional problems presented by many patients with DEB can prove exceedingly difficult. Some patients with dysphagia find it helpful to have their food liquidized, but others never accept this, unless they have been fed nothing else from infancy. However, apart from making it easier for the patient to eat, liquidizing the diet may help prevent further damage to the pharynx and oesophagus, and may reduce the frequency of the episodes of acute dysphagia they often experience. However, liquidizing food usually involves increasing its fluid content and therefore its bulk. If water or gravy is used for this purpose, the nutrient value of the food will be reduced, whereas this effect can be minimized by the use of milk or soup. The process may make food more bland and less appetising. Sieving food should be avoided as it removes fibre, which is retained if food is liquidized.

The diets of many patients are heavily dependent upon milk. This dependence should not be discouraged, but such a diet may be far from nutritionally complete, and will tend to be short on fibre and iron content. Although a high fibre intake is desirable, this is not practical using conventional foods in these patients because they tend to be difficult to eat and relatively low in nutrient value. Proprietary fibre-containing products are ideal, and are now widely available, e.g. Benefiber (Novartis, Frimley, UK) and Enrich (Abbott, Maidenhead, UK).

Though sucrose provides a highly effective means of increasing the patient's calorie intake, we like to restrict high sucrose foods, such as chocolate, to mealtimes, in order to minimize their harmful effect on the teeth. Though sucrose provides a highly effective means of increasing the patient's calorie intake, high sucrose foods, such as chocolate, should be restricted to meal-times in order to minimize their harmful effect on the teeth.

The author's own experience suggests that the best approach is to inform parents and patients of the nutritional properties of different foods, and to encourage them to focus on those that provide nutrition in its most concentrated and best balanced form. The aim is a well-balanced diet with a higher than normal content of protein, vitamins and minerals. The emphasis is on foods of soft, manageable consistency, with an attractive appearance and flavour.

Patients should be encouraged to take their food in discrete meals, rather than by eating small quantities continuously throughout the day. However, many children with EB will not be able to eat enough at only three meals, mainly because they find the process of eating both painful and tiring. A system of three or four main meals per day, plus two or three snacks, will often be more appropriate. It is often a good idea to put a limit on the time allowed for each meal or snack to prevent one meal from overlapping with the next.

The first 2 years of life are probably critical to the nutritional status of children with EB, and great efforts need to be directed towards improving nutrition during this period.

Since few patients do succeed in achieving even a normal nutritional intake, vitamin and mineral supplements are advisable. The author's practice is to give a complete vitamin supplement such as Ketovite (Paines and Byrne Ltd, Greenford, UK), a liquid iron supplement such as Sytron (Parke-Davis, Eastleigh, UK) and a zinc supplement such as Solvazinc (Cortecs, Deeside, UK).

Many children with severe DEB intermittently experience periods when they cannot eat at all, due either to pain in the mouth or throat, or to obstruction in the pharynx or oesophagus. If they are also unable to drink, it may be necessary to give fluid intravenously. A short admission for intravenous fluid administration allows for 'rest', and seems to accelerate recovery. Nasogastric feeding can be used to provide longer periods of rest with full nutritional support.

If swallowing difficulties become more constant, it may occasionally be beneficial to release the buccal mucosa, to allow fuller opening of the mouth. Dribbling can be improved at the same time by transplantation of the submandibular ducts back into the tonsillar fossa [55]. Improved access to the mouth is sometimes necessary for anaesthesia and dental work, but because these procedures also mobilize the tongue, they have the additional benefit of making it much easier for the patient to masticate, swallow and talk. Mouth opening can also be improved by exercises.

Improvements in dietary intake using conventional oral supplements are rarely sustained in patients with dysphagia and more invasive procedures such as nasogastric feeding frequently need to be considered [87,123]. Although insertion of a nasogastric tube does not require surgery, problems arise with tube placement, day-to-day management and disfigurement [121]. It is therefore best reserved for short-term use.

Oral verapamil administration has been advocated to alleviate oesophageal dysmotility and spasm [124]. The author's experience has been that any improvement is short-lived, and that verapamil will generally exacerbate the constipation which is already a major problem in most patients.

Surgical approaches which have been taken include balloon dilatation of the oesophagus [123] or endoscopy and oesophageal bougienage [124], but to date nutritional or anthropometric benefit following these procedures has never been documented. Patients themselves frequently report that improvement may be short-lived, with the intervals between subsequent dilatations tending to become progressively briefer. Intraoperative deaths due to rupture of the oesophagus have been reported, even from centres familiar with this type of intervention [124,125]. It is the author's view that the risks associated with these procedures make them highly undesirable. More radical procedures have included oesophageal reconstruction by reversed gastric tube [126], resection and end-to-end oesophageal anastomosis [127] and colon transplant [128]. Favourable results at 5-year follow-up have been reported [129], but the numbers of patients so treated has been small, and the associated risks are substantial.

Although the success of gastrostomy feeding in conditions such as cystic fibrosis and cerebral palsy has been well-documented, such intervention has not been reported in children with DEB, probably due to fears of poor healing and infection at the gastrostomy insertion site.

Gastrostomies have been inserted in over 40 children with DEB in the author's unit, some of whom have now been receiving feeding by gastrostomy for over 8 years [130]. It is preferable to insert a gastrostomy button device primarily, using an open operative technique. The Mic-Key device is particularly good (Medical Innovations, Utah, USA). Although it has generally been recommended that button devices be inserted only after a tract has formed from a previous gastrostomy, primary insertion offers certain advantages in DEB. It avoids an extra general anaesthetic; furthermore, button devices are small and unobtrusive, and therefore aesthetically much more acceptable, particularly to older children. Although percutaneous endoscopic gastrostomy insertion is now widely regarded as the procedure of choice in childhood, the author's experience has been that the endoscope causes substantial shearing damage in the oropharynx and oesophagus, therefore this technique is contraindicated in DEB. In most cases, it proves most convenient to deliver gastrostomy feeds overnight, over a period of about 8h, using a pump (e.g. Kangaroo, Sherwood Medical, Crawley, UK). The author favours a nutrient-dense, fibre-containing feed, for example, Jevity Plus (Abbott, Maidenhead, UK). With a gastrostomy, significant weight gains can be obtained. Additional benefits have been prevention of constipation, and the ease with which medicines and nutritional supplements such as iron can be given when the child has a gastrostomy.

Nutrient requirements increase markedly during adolescence because of rapid growth and the virtual doubling of body mass. Furthermore, if growth throughout childhood has been impaired, nutrition during adolescence should allow for catch-up growth. Since most adults with severe DEB demonstrate delayed sexual maturation and short stature, it is critical that the nutritional status of these patients is optimal at the onset of adolescence.

The author has found that younger children accept the procedure more readily than adolescents. Older children are more aware of their body image, and adolescent girls, in particular, may be alarmed by a sudden increase in weight. Psychological factors should be taken into account before surgery, with a psychologist and play specialist included in discussions.

Complications of gastrostomy are few, but include leakage around the device, enuresis because of nocturnal fluid administration and gastro-oesophageal reflux. The effect of long-term gastrostomy feeding on oral intakes in DEB is as yet unknown. It is the author's policy to encourage oral intake when possible, in the hope that at least some patients will be able to manage without a gastrostomy in adult life.

Gastrostomy insertion should be considered in preference to more invasive surgical procedures in children with DEB in whom dysphagia compromises nutritional intake.

Gastrostomy feeding can permit catch-up growth in children with growth failure, and offers further benefits which include amelioration of constipation and improved compliance with vitamin and mineral supplementation. Feeding by this route should not be considered exclusively for children who demonstrate growth failure. It can greatly alleviate the stresses associated with feeding children who are still just managing to maintain growth, but are not likely to continue to do so in the future, particularly at adolescence.

Gastro-oesophageal reflux

One needs to maintain a high level of vigilance for symptoms of gastro-oesophageal reflux in young children with DEB. If such symptoms appear, an early barium study should be undertaken; ideally evaluation will also include a cine swallow. If malrotation of the small intestine can be excluded, a combination of cisapride 0.1–0.3 mg/kg per dose three times daily (or domperidone 0.2–0.4 mg/kg per dose three to six times daily) and ranitidine 2–4 mg/kg per dose twice daily should be commenced. If gastro-oesophageal reflux is not confirmed, one option would be to undertake an isotopic milk scan but this may also fail to demonstrate reflux over the period of scanning, and it would be reasonable to start therapy if the level of suspicion on the basis of symptoms is high. In the author's experience, the normal practice of undertaking oesophageal pH monitoring is not feasible because it is not possible to secure the probe adequately. In practice, because gastro-oesophageal reflux is so common in infants with DEB, the author gives all of them rani-tidine from the time of referral and orders an early barium study.

Constipation

Low fibre intake is a contributory factor to constipation in DEB. Unfortunately, the oral and oesophageal problems of severely affected patients preclude the consumption of increased amounts of dietary fibre in the form of conventional foods (high-fibre cereals and breads, fruit and vegetables). Studies suggest that the fibre-containing liquid enteral formulas which have been commercially produced in recent years can improve gastrointestinal tolerance and function and reduce laxative use [131]. They have provided a new approach to the prevention and therapy of constipation in children with DEB, and one that should be preferred to the long-term use of laxatives. They have provided a new approach to the prevention and therapy of constipation in children with dystrophic EB, and one that should be preferred to the long-term use of laxatives [132].

Children with megarectum or faecal impaction, demonstrable on abdominal X-ray, should have their bowel emptied before the introduction of fibre-containing feed. This is not only humane, since it removes the necessity for the child to pass the accumulation of large, dry stools, but it also allows the increased fibre intake to take effect quickly and so encourages future compliance. If faecal impaction is present, commonly associated with faecal overflow, initial clearance can be achieved by administration of a polyethylene glycol–electrolyte solution (Klean-Prep, Norgine, Oxford, UK) [133]. Unfortunately, most children are defeated by the large volumes of solution that need to be drunk and a nasogastric tube often needs to be passed. The tube must be as soft and of as narrow a gauge as possible, and fixed with a non-adhesive dressing. The procedure also requires hospitalization of the patient for up to 2–3 days. A less invasive and faster method that can be employed in cases of less severe impaction, is the use of oral sodium picosulphate combined with magnesium sulphate, in the form of Picolax (Nordic, Middlesex, UK) or sodium picosulphate elixir. The prior application of topical local anaesthetic makes the procedure much less unpleasant for the patient.

Intractable constipation should be regarded in its own right as a reasonable indication for gastrostomy insertion because of the great improvements in constipation to be gained through gastrostomy feeding. Parents who were previously reluctant to give iron supplements, because of aggravation of constipation, are now happy to do so via the gastrostomy.

If children remain constipated despite taking adequate volumes of Enrich, it is important to check radiologically that faecal impaction is not present; its treatment is discussed above. If it is absent, the child can be prescribed a faecal softener such as docusate sodium (Dioctyl Paediatric Syrup, Medo Pharmaceuticals, Chesham, UK) or lactulose (Duphalac, Duphar Laboratories, Southampton, UK), which has the additional benefit of increasing bulk. It may in addition be worthwhile to encourage daily defaecation by the regular oral administration of senna for a period of a few months. The senna dose should then be progressively reduced. The routine administration of liquid paraffin is contraindicated because of the real risk of its entry into the respiratory tract in these patients. If constipation persists despite these measures, and where anal pain on attempted defaecation is marked, it may be worth considering an anal stretch under general anaesthesia.

Anaesthesia

Despite the delicacy of the oral and pharyngeal mucosa, and anxieties about acute laryngeal obstruction if blistering of the larynx were to occur following intubation, general anaesthesia has proved to be fairly straightforward in patients with EB, if certain precautions are taken [125,134,135].

All those involved in handling these children before, during and after surgery must be made aware of the extreme vulnerability of their skin. Patients must be moved about with great care. Trolleys and the operating table should be well padded so that pressure on the skin is kept to a minimum. No one should lean on the patient during the operation. Plenty of non-adherent soft gauze padding such as Melolin should separate blood pressure cuffs and tourniquets from the skin. Clingfilm is very useful to place under the child to reduce shearing forces and to prevent adherence; it is also valuable as a temporary covering for eroded areas when dressings are removed. Sticky tapes and other adhesive materials, such as those used to attach electrocardiogram (ECG) electrodes, must be avoided as the skin will come away when they are removed. Mepitel has proved very valuable for securing devices such as intravenous cannulae, as its adhesive properties hold the device securely, but, in contrast to adherent tapes, removal does not cause any damage to the skin. Non-adhesive elasticated netting, conforming bandages and sutures may also be useful. Heart rate is probably best monitored by the use of pulse oximetry. The eyes should be carefully closed and covered with Vaseline gauze or Geliperm.

General anaesthesia is preferred to extensive local anaesthesia, because the latter may cause blistering. To avoid undue facial manipulation, intubation is generally preferable, and an uncuffed tracheal tube should be selected, a size smaller than normally used. The tracheal tube and laryngoscope blade should be well lubricated. The tube should be fixed using ribbon gauze. All tubing should be padded, and where it touches the lips or skin, Vaseline gauze should be interposed. Occasionally, limitation of mouth opening or dental problems may make intubation difficult; in such cases, and for short procedures, inhalational anaesthesia can be maintained by means of a face mask, which should have a soft air cushion separated from the skin by Vaseline gauze. Vaseline gauze should also be placed against the patient's skin where the underside of the jaw is held by the anaesthetist. Oropharyngeal airways should not be used. The author is unaware of any reported cases in which laryngeal or tracheal obstruction has occurred following intubation in patients with DEB.

Pain

There can be no doubt that patients of all ages with EB experience a great deal of pain, predominantly from cutaneous ulceration, particularly at times of baths and dressing changes, from oropharyngeal ulceration and from anal fissures, particularly at the time of defaecation. Pain from the skin can be minimized by the use of the most appropriate dressings; Mepitel is extremely valuable from this point of view as daily changes are unnecessary. Similarly, pain from the oropharynx can be reduced by provision of a gastrostomy in selected cases, and pain on defaecation can be minimized by keeping the faeces soft.

Drugs like paracetamol (15 mg/kg), codeine (0.5–1 mg/kg), dihydrocodeine (0.5–1 mg/kg) and morphine (200–500 µg/kg) are often helpful if given orally in anticipation of the pain predictably associated with dressing changes. Amitriptyline has proved very helpful in the management of the chronic pain suffered by many children with severe DEB. Reduction of this pain can improve quality of life substantially, an improvement that can be manifest in enhanced mobility or better performance at school. The appropriate dose for this purpose is about 0.5 mg/kg at night.

Anaemia

Patients with more severe DEB almost invariably become anaemic within a few years of life. Investigations generally demonstrate haematological features both of iron deficiency and decreased red cell iron utilization ('anaemia of chronic disease') [136]. The iron deficiency probably reflects both chronic blood loss from the skin, mouth, oesophagus and anal canal, and poor iron intake.

Where there is evidence of iron deficiency, probably best indicated by a low mean cell volume (MCV), administration of iron supplements is appropriate, but it is generally found that oral iron therapy alone is of limited value in relieving the anaemia because of decreased red cell iron

utilization. It may therefore become necessary for some patients to have frequent blood transfusions in an attempt to control their profound anaemia, but this approach is both uncomfortable and associated with significant hazards which include infection and iron overload. In practice, transfusion is reserved for those patients who are substantially disabled by their anaemia and for patients undergoing surgical procedures. It has been our policy not to transfuse unless the anaemia is causing significant symptoms or handicap; in these relatively immobile individuals, transfusion is therefore rarely necessary until haemoglobin levels fall below 7 g/dl. It must be borne in mind that iron overload may become a problem if transfusions are given more often than every 6–8 weeks over prolonged periods. Every effort should be made to improve the patient's general condition, with particular attention paid to nutrition and care of the skin, as these measures may reduce the frequency at which transfusion is required.

In the past, the risk of anaphylaxis precluded the administration of parenteral iron preparations such as iron-dextran injection. However, more recently, a new intravenous iron preparation, iron (III) hydroxide-sucrose complex (Venofer) has become available, with the advantage of a much reduced risk of anaphylaxis. This can lead to a good rise in haemoglobin concentration in some patients [137], but administration is time-consuming and may need to be repeated rather frequently. It is possible that erythropoietin would allow higher haemoglobin levels to be achieved, with maintenance of these levels for longer periods between courses of parenteral iron, but there is a risk that this would merely have the effect of increasing iron demand without providing great improvements in haemoglobin concentration.

Teeth

While the teeth are usually structurally normal in DEB, they are prone to severe caries. Appropriate dental care includes improvements in the diet, improved cleaning of the teeth, the regular use of an antiseptic mouthwash after meals to clean away as much residual food as possible and oral fluoride supplements in areas where it is not adequately present in tap water [138]. It may be ueful to use an electric toothbrush such as the Braun Oral-B Plaque Remover.

In DEB, a conservative approach to dental therapy should be adopted, rather than wholesale extraction as has occasionally been recommended. Those who propose this approach argue that the patients do not require teeth as their diet is more or less liquid. The possession of teeth is helpful in giving the patients a more normal facial appearance, since dentures are not tolerated. Furthermore, shrinkage of the mouth may be accelerated by dental extractions.

Undoubtedly, extraction is sometimes the only practical option for severely carious teeth because of the difficulty of doing conservative dental work through the very restricted oral opening of these patients. Where extraction is necessary, healing is rapid. Patients may be unable to eat for 24–48 h after dental extraction because of unavoidable oropharyngeal trauma. For this reason, a nasogastric tube is useful in patients who do not already have a gastrostomy. The nasogastric tube is best secured by wrapping it around an elasticated bandage which is then passed around the head. Feeding should be provided via the tube until the patient is able to take drink and food comfortably.

Dribbling

Dribbling often occurs in children with severe DEB, mainly due to obliteration of the lingual and inferior gingivobuccal sulci. This has been successfully corrected by surgical relocation of the submandibular salivary ducts to the base of the tongue [78].

Eyes

The use of lubricants such as simple eye ointment BP (10% liquid paraffin, 10% wool fat in yellow soft paraffin) is valuable when patients have bullae or erosions, and in patients who experience recurrent lesions its use is recommended nightly on a prophylactic basis. Topical corticosteroids without preservative may be indicated in the acute phase of ulceration, but use should not be prolonged unless it is possible to monitor intraocular pressure.

Prenatal diagnosis

Prenatal diagnosis of DEB is discussed in Chapters 19.25 and 19.26.

Junctional epidermolysis bullosa

Definition

This is a group of inherited disorders characterized by mechanically induced blistering occurring within the basement membrane at the level of the lamina lucida.

Aetiology and pathogenesis

The incidence of JEB is particularly difficult to ascertain because most affected individuals die early in life. From the author's experience the incidence of new cases is estimated at approximately the same as for DEB, and is therefore likely to be around 20 per million births. A recent estimate of prevalence in Scotland—presumably exclusively of surviving patients—was 0.4 per million [8].

From the clinical and pathological point of view, it is helpful to divide JEB into two types: Herlitz (sometimes called 'lethal' junctional EB), and non-Herlitz.

It is now clear that all forms of JEB reflect mutations in the genes encoding components of the hemidesmosome-anchoring filament complex that appears to be of great importance in binding basal keratinocytes to the lamina densa.

It has been known for some time that basement membrane zone binding of the monoclonal antibody GB3 is absent or greatly reduced in all cases of Herlitz-type JEB. This antibody was found to recognise a lamina lucida protein originally designated as BM600 and subsequently renamed as nicein [139]. A basement membrane protein called kalinin was isolated at about the same time [140]; both proteins were subsequently shown to be identical [141]. It is now known that the anchoring filaments which complex with hemidesmosomes in the lamina lucida are comprised of this glycoprotein, now designated as laminin 5 [142].

Several variants of the laminin molecule have since been identified, all of which have been shown comprise 3 polypeptide chains, known as A, B1 and B2. All cases of Herlitz, and most cases of non-Herlitz junctional EB appear to reflect mutations in the genes encoding the α3, β3 and γ2 chains of laminin 5, which are designated LAMA3, LAMB3 and LAMC2 respectively [143,144, 145,146,147]. Other cases of non-Herlitz JEB have been caused by mutations in the genes coding for hemidesmosome components, namely β4 integrin and the 180-kDa bullous pemphigoid antigen (BPAG2), and it is likely that there will be others.

To date, all types of junctional epidermolysis bullosa have been transmitted as autosomal recessive traits [148,149].

Pathology

In JEB, separation of the epithelium occurs through the lamina lucida, between the lamina densa of the basement membrane and the basal keratinocytes. In most cases there is an abnormality of the structures known as hemidesmosomes, which appear to have a role in bonding these two structures; these tend to be absent, or reduced in number and hypoplastic, lacking sub-basal dense plates [150]. However, in some patients these structures appear to be normal both structurally and numerically [151]. Immunohistochemical staining with GB3 antibody is absent or reduced [152].

JEB with pyloric atresia appears to be a distinct subtype in which GB3 staining is normal or only slightly reduced despite typical ultrastructural findings of a lamina lucida split and absent or hypoplastic hemidesmosomes [153].

Exactly what is happening pathologically in the larynx is uncertain, but blistering on the edges of the cords is probably followed by the development of granulations, and eventually in at least some cases by squamous metaplasia and the development of mucous retention cysts [154]. The pathological basis for the profound failure to thrive observed in many babies remains unclear.

Clinical features

Previously JEB was more usually known as EB letalis. However, although JEB is undoubtedly more likely than the other categories of EB to result in death in infancy, a number of children do survive, some for a few years, and others into adult life, occasionally with relatively little handicap. Because of the regular occurrence of such survivors, the term EB 'letalis' is usually now avoided. Although not yet adequately differentiated, it seems clear that there are several distinct varieties of JEB. From the clinician's point of view there are three broad groups of patients.
1 Herlitz JEB (sometimes called 'lethal' JEB), the commonest form of JEB, in which death is probable within the first 2 years of life.
2 Benign JEB, in which many patients will survive into adult life.
3 JEB with pyloric atresia.
There are almost certainly intermediate types in addition.

Herlitz junctional epidermolysis bullosa [155]

In the great majority of cases, blistering is present at birth or develops within the first few days of life. Despite the likelihood of an early lethal outcome, the initial lesions may be deceptively mild. It is always a mistake to try to guess the type of EB or the prognosis on clinical grounds alone in the neonate, as there is little correlation between initial severity and outcome, either in terms of life expectancy or ultimate degree of handicap.

In the infant, the sites of blistering are essentially the same as in other types of EB. Subungual and mucosal blisters are equally typical and frequent in JEB as they are in DEB. Initially, healing is rapid, and milia are not infrequent though they are not as numerous or persistent as in DEB. Scarring is not a prominent feature as it is in DEB, but slightly atrophic areas are a not infrequent sequel to previous blistering. In the absence of profound scar formation, digital fusion and hand and foot deformity do not occur.

As time passes, healing tends to become more and more sluggish, and by the second year of life, if the child survives, the disease is often typified by the development of gradually extending areas of chronic ulceration. These are perhaps most characteristically seen around the mouth and nose. The development of exces-

sive granulation tissue in these non-healing areas is a peculiarity of JEB, and is perhaps most obvious in association with smaller ulcerations. Obstruction of the nares by granulation tissue is rather characteristic [156]. Whereas DEB is rarely associated with scalp lesions, the scalp is quite often affected in JEB. Chronic paronychia with nail loss is a frequent feature, with the nail being replaced by excessive granulation tissue, often leading to a drumstick appearance of the tips of the fingers and toes.

The mouth and pharynx are affected, often severely, causing substantial pain and difficulty with feeding, but erosive lesions at these sites are not complicated by oral submucous fibrosis, nor by pharyngeal and oesophageal strictures. However, the early appearance of profound failure to thrive is a regular and very distinctive feature of lethal JEB. The development of this complication of the disease has ominous significance for the infant as it tends to fail to respond to any attempt at correction, including the use of nasogastric hyperalimentation.

The disease is also serious because of its tendency to affect the larynx [154,157]. Many babies with JEB become hoarse very early in life; indeed the appearance of this symptom seems to be one of the few relatively reliable features that allow a clinical distinction to be made between JEB and DEB in the first weeks of life, though one needs to be aware that it is also frequently present in Dowling – Meara EB simplex. Hoarseness is usually followed by recurrent bouts of stridor, each of which carries a serious risk of fatal asphyxiation.

As in severe DEB, a degree of anaemia is common. In some cases this is severe. Also as in DEB, the pattern is a mixture of iron deficiency anaemia and anaemia of chronic disease. As in DEB anal fissuring, faecal retention and constipation are common. Ocular disease similar to that described in DEB may occur [158]. Involvement of the bladder and urethra appears to be an occasional complication of JEB in surviving children, almost certainly secondary to direct involvement of the epithelium by the disease. Rapid dental degeneration is the rule. Dental enamel hypoplasia appears to be common in JEB [159,160], and the resulting development of caries is accelerated by the dietary preference of affected children for foods and drinks with a high sucrose content.

Benign junctional epidermolysis bullosa [161,162]

The early clinical course of individuals with this type of EB seems to be rather similar to that of children with Herlitz JEB, though the development of excessive granulation tissue, growth failure and anaemia is less prominent. The patient survives through early childhood, with a gradually decreasing tendency to develop new blisters. Non-healing areas may remain a life-long problem for

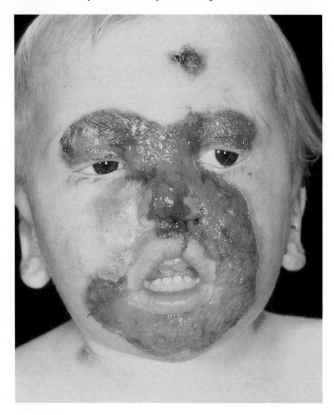

Fig. 19.4.8 Persistent and extending facial ulceration in a 1-year-old child with JEB.

such patients (Fig. 19.4.8). Areas of previous blistering show a variable degree of atrophy, and both nail dystrophy and scarring alopecia are prominent sequelae of previous blistering and ulceration. Clinical distinction of the Herlitz and 'benign' types of JEB is complicated by the reported death in early infancy of some of the siblings of patients with the clinically 'benign' type. Many of the noncutaneous features are qualitatively very similar, including involvement of the teeth, eyes, bladder and urethra [163,164].

Junctional epidermolysis bullosa with pyloric atresia [165]

Congenital pyloric atresia occurs in a small but significant number of infants with JEB, and the combination appears to indicate a distinct disorder, with a generally poor prognosis. Involvement of the genitourinary tract appears to be particularly frequent [166].

Prognosis

Death in the first 2 years of life is usual in the Herlitz form of JEB, but is not invariable. The cause of death is generally either acute respiratory obstruction due to laryngeal involvement or overwhelming sepsis consequent upon malnutrition. Conversely, survival into adult life is usual though not invariable in the benign form. Death in infancy is generally to be anticipated in the pyloric atresia-associated variant, but there have been occasional survivors [166,167]. There is a general tendency for the prognosis to be better the less reduced is immunohistochemical staining with GB3 antibody, except in the case of the JEB pyloric atresia variant in which the outlook is usually, but not invariably poor.

Differential diagnosis

The problem of differential diagnosis in the neonatal period is discussed under DEB above. The laryngo-onychocutaneous syndrome is a very rare condition that has certain clinical similarities with JEB [168].

Treatment

As in other forms of EB, specific treatment is not available, and there is no evidence that patients benefit from the administration of any systemic therapy other than nutritional supplements.

General skin care, pain control and the management of complications such as constipation, malnutrition, ocular disease and anaemia are essentially the same as in the case of DEB, though the author would hesitate to place a gastrostomy in a patient with JEB.

Patients with JEB usually tolerate a less liquid diet and, because there is much less mucosal scarring, the teeth are more accessible to the dentist. A normal conservative approach to dental treatment is therefore both more necessary and feasible.

Autologous epidermal grafts have been successfully used for the treatment of chronic facial ulceration in JEB [169].

The author has found that humidification of the inspired air is valuable in babies with subacute stridor. The onset of acute laryngeal obstruction in these cases is possibly more likely to reflect the development of granulations on the vocal cords than intact blisters, and therefore more intense stridor should be treated by inhalation of nebulized racemic adrenaline (racepinephrine, Vaponephrin, 0.5 ml in 2 ml normal saline; Fisons Pharmaceuticals, Loughborough, UK), and corticosteroids, such as beclomethasone dipropionate, 100 µg (Becotide suspension, Allen and Hanburys, Greenford, UK), both as often as 2-hourly. Although it is important to know the precise cause of the obstruction, laryngoscopy is not undertaken routinely because this would require the clinician to be prepared if necessary both to intubate the patient acutely and to undertake tracheostomy later. It is the author's view that tracheostomies are too difficult to maintain in babies with JEB because of the ulceration that occurs at the insertion of the tube and along the line of the ties used to hold it in place. Because some children will survive, surgical treatment of pyloric atresia in JEB pyloric atresia variant is justified.

REFERENCES

1 Priestley GC, Tidman MJ, Weiss JB, Eady RAJ, eds. *Epidermolysis Bullosa: a Comprehensive Review of Classification, Management and Laboratory studies.* Crowthorne: DEBRA, 1990.

2 Lin AN, Carter DM, eds. *Epidermolysis Bullosa: Basic and Clinical Aspects.* New York: Springer-Verlag, 1992.

3 Smith FJD, Eady RAJ, Leigh JM *et al.* Plectin deficiency results in muscular dystrophy with epidermolysis bullosa. *Nat Genet* 1996; 13: 450–7.

4 Fine J-D, Johnson L, Wright T. Epidermolysis bullosa simplex superficialis. *Arch Dermatol* 1989; 125: 633–8.

5 Nielsen PG, Sjolund E. Epidermolysis bullosa simplex localisata associated with anodontia, hair loss and nail disorders: a new syndrome. *Acta Derm Venereol (Stockh)* 1985; 65: 526–30.

6 Fischer T, Gedde-Dahl T. Epidermolysis bullosa simplex and mottled pigmentation: a new dominant syndrome. *Clin Genet* 1979; 15: 228–38.

7 Salih MAM, Lake BD, El Hag MA, Atherton DJ. Lethal epidermolytic epidermolysis bullosa: a new autosomal recessive type of epidermolysis bullosa. *Br J Dermatol* 1985; 113: 135–43.

8 Horn HM, Priestley GC, Tidman MJ. Epidemiology of epidermolysis bullosa in Scotland. *Br J Dermatol* 1995; 133: 1005.

9 Kero M. Occurrence of EB in Finland. *Acta Derm Venereol (Stockh)* 1984; 64: 57–62.

10 Gedde-Dahl T. EB. *A Clinical, Genetic and Epidemiological Study.* Baltimore: Johns Hopkins Press, 1971.

11 Fine J-D, Stenn J, Johnson L *et al.* Autosomal recessive epidermolysis bullosa simplex: generalized phenotypic features suggestive of junctional or dystrophic EB, and association with neuromuscular disease. *Arch Dermatol* 1989; 125: 931–8.

12 Fine J-D, Johnson L, Wright T, Horiguchi Y. Epidermolysis bullosa simplex: identification of a kindred with autosomal recessive transmission of the Weber–Cockayne type. *Pediatr Dermatol* 1989; 6: 1–5.

13 Gedde-Dahl T. Epidermolysis bullosa simplex (intra-epidermal epidermolysis bullosa) and allied conditions. In: Wojnarowska F, Briggaman RA, eds. *Management of Blistering Diseases.* London: Chapman & Hall, 1990: 196–204.

14 Leigh IM, Lane EB. Mutations in the genes for epidermal keratins in epidermolysis bullosa and epidermolytic hyperkeratosis. *Arch Dermatol* 1993; 129: 1571–7.

15 Lane EB. Keratin diseases. *Curr Opp Genet Dev* 1994; 4: 412–18.

16 Haneke E, Anton-Lamprecht I. Ultrastructure of blister formation in epidermolysis bullosa hereditaria. V. Epidermolysis bullosa simplex localisata type Weber–Cockayne. *J Invest Dermatol* 1982; 164: 219–23.

17 McGrath JA, Ishida-Yamamoto A, Tidman MJ, Heagerty AHM, Schofield OMV, Eady RAJ. Epidermolysis bullosa simplex (Dowling–Meara): a clinicopathological review. *Br J Dermatol* 1992; 126: 421–30.

18 Buchbinder LH, Lucky AW, Ballard E *et al.* Severe infantile epidermolysis bullosa simplex Dowling–Meara type. *Arch Dermatol* 1986; 122: 190–8.

19 Hachem-Zadeh S, Rappersberger K, Livshin R, Konrad K. Epidermolysis bullosa herpetiformis Dowling–Meara in a large family. *J Am Acad Dermatol* 1988; 18: 702–6.

20 Furumura M, Imayama S, Hori Y. Three neonatal cases of epidermolysis bullosa herpetiformis (Dowling–Meara type) with severe erosive skin lesions. *J Am Acad Dermatol* 1993; 28: 859–61.

21 McGrath JA, Burrows NP, Russell-Jones R, Eady RAJ. Epidermolysis bullosa simplex Dowling–Meara: troublesome blistering in an adult patient. *Dermatology* 1993; 186: 68–71.

22 DesGroseilliers J-P, Brisson P. Localized epidermolysis bullosa: report of two cases and evaluation of therapy with glutaraldehyde. *Arch Dermatol* 1974; 109: 70–2.

23 Tkach JR. Treatment of recurrent bullous eruption of the hands and feet (Weber–Cockayne disease) with topical aluminium chloride. *J Am Acad Dermatol* 1982; 6: 1095–6.

24 Tadini G, Ermacora E, Cambiaghi S, Brusasco A, Cavalli R. Positive response to 5HT-2 antagonists in a family affected by epidermolysis bullosa Dowling–Meara type. *Dermatology* 1993; 186: 80.

25 Readett MD. Localized epidermolysis bullosa. *Br Med J* 1961; 1: 1510–11.

26 McLean WHI, Pulkinnen L, Smith FJD *et al.* Loss of plectin causes epidermolysis bullosa with muscular dystrophy: cDNA cloning and genomic organisation. *Genes & Dev* 1996; 10: 1724–35.

27 Gache Y, Chavanas S, Lacour JP *et al.* Defective expression of plectin/HD1 in epidermolysis bullosa simplex with muscular dystrophy. *J Clin Invest* 1996; 97: 2299–307.

28 Fine J-D, Stenn J, Johnson L *et al.* Autosomal recessive epidermolysis bullosa simplex. *Arch Dermatol* 1989; 125: 931–8.

29 Niemi K-M, Sommer H, Kero M *et al.* Epidermolyis bullosa simplex associated with muscular dystrophy with recessive inheritance. *Arch Dermatol* 1988; 124: 551–4.

30 Bruckner-Tuderman L, Vogel A, Ruegger S *et al.* EB simplex with mottled pigmentation. *J Am Acad Dermatol* 1989; 21: 425–32.

31 Coleman R, Harper JI, Lake BD. Epidermolysis bullosa with mottled pigmentation. *Br J Dermatol* 1993; 128: 679–85.

32 Combemale P, Kanitakis J. Epidermolysis bullosa simplex with mottled pigmentation. *Dermatology* 1994; 189: 173–8.

33 Davison BCC. Epidermolysis bullosa. *J Med Genet* 1965; 2: 233–42.

34 Horn HM, Priestley GC, Tidman MJ. Epidemiology of epidermolysis bullosa in Scotland. *Br J Dermatol* 1995; 133: 1005.

35 Uitto J, Christiano AM. Molecular basis for the dystrophic forms of EB: mutations in the type VII collagen gene. *Arch Dermatol Res* 1994; 287: 16–22.

36 Uitto J, Pulkinnen L, Christiano AM. Molecular basis of dystrophic and junctional forms of EB: mutations in the type VII collagen and kalinin (laminin 5) genes. *J Invest Dermatol* 1994; 103: 39S–46S.

37 Parente MG, Chung LC, Ryynanen J *et al.* Human type VII collagen: C-DNA cloning and chromosomal mapping of the gene (COL7A1) on chromosome 3 to dominant dystrophic epidermolysis bullosa. *Am J Hum Genet* 1991; 24: 119–35.

38 Sakai L, Keene DR, Morris NP, Burgeson RE. Type VII collagen is a major structural component of anchoring fibrils. *J Cell Biol* 1986; 103: 1577–86.

39 Burgeson RE. Type VII collagen, anchoring fibrils and epidermolysis bullosa. *J Invest Dermatol* 1993; 101: 252–5.

40 Christiano AM, Ryynanen M, Uitto J. Dominant dystrophic epidermolysis bullosa: identification of a Gly-to-Ser substitution in the triple-helical domain of type VII collagen. *Proc Natl Acad Sci USA* 1994; 91: 3549–53.

41 Christiano AM, Anhalt G, Gibbons S, Bauer EA, Uitto J. Premature termination codons in the type VII collagen gene (COL7A1) underlie severe mutilating recessive dystrophic epidermolysis bullosa. *Genomics* 1994; 21: 160–8.

42 Hilal L, Rochat A, Duquesnoy P *et al.* A homozygous insertion-deletion in the type VII collagen gene (COL7A1) in Hallopeau–Siemens dystrophic epidermolysis bullosa. *Nature Genet* 1993; 5: 287–93.

43 Hovnanian A, Hilal L, Blanchet-Bardon C *et al.* Recurrent nonsense mutations within the type VII collagen gene in patients with severe recessive dystrophic epidermolysis bullosa. *Am J Hum Genet* 1994; 55: 289–96.

44 Christiano AM, Greenspan DS, Hoffman GG *et al.* A missense mutation in type VII collagen in two affected siblings with recessive dystrophic epidermolysis bullosa. *Nature Genet* 1993; 4: 62–6.

45 Bruckner-Tuderman L, Mituhashi Y, Schnyder UW, Bruckner P. Anchoring fibrils and type VII collagen are absent from skin in severe recessive dystrophic epidermolysis bullosa. *J Invest Dermatol* 1989; 93: 3–9.

46 Heagerty AHM *et al.* Identification of an epidermal basement membrane defect in recessive forms of dystrophic epidermolysis bullosa by LH 7.2 monoclonal antibody: use in diagnosis. *Br J Dermatol* 1986; 115: 125–31.

47 Bruckner-Tudeman L, Niemi KM, Kero M, Schnyder UW, Reunala T. Type VII collagen is expressed but anchoring fibrils are defective in dystrophic epidermolysis bullosa inversa. *Br J Dermatol* 1990; 122: 383–90.

48 Leigh IM, Eady RAJ, Heagerty AH, Purkis PE, Whitehead PA, Burgeson RE. Type VII collagen is a normal component of epidermal basement membrane, which shows altered expression in recessive dystrophic epidermolysis bullosa. *J Invest Dermatol* 1988; 90: 639–42.

49 McGrath JA, Ishida-Yamamoto A, O'Grady A, Leigh IM, Eady RAJ. Structural variations in anchoring fibrils in dystrophic epidermolysis bullosa: correlation with type VII collagen expression. *J Invest Dermatol* 1993; 100: 366–72.

50 McGrath JA, Leigh IM, Eady RAJ. Intracellular expression of type VII col-

lagen during wound healing in severe recessive dystrophic epidermolysis bullosa and normal human skin. *Br J Dermatol* 1992; 127: 312–17.

51 Hashimoto I, Anton-Lamprecht I, Hofbauer M. Epidermolysis bullosa dystrophica inversa: report on two sisters. *Hautarzt* 1976; 27: 532–7.

52 Pearson R, Paller A. Dermolytic (dystrophic) epidermolysis bullosa inversa. *Arch Dermatol* 1988; 124: 544–7.

53 Wojnarowska FT, Eady RAJ, Wells RS. Dystrophic epidermolysis bullosa presenting with congenital absence of skin: report of four cases. *Br J Dermatol* 1983; 108: 477–83.

54 Hoss DM, McNutt NS, Carter DM *et al*. Atypical melanocytic lesions in epidermolysis bullosa. *J Cutan Pathol* 1994; 21: 164–9.

55 Terrill PJ, Mayou BJ, McKee P, Eady RAJ. The surgical treatment of dystrophic epidermolysis bullosa. *Br J Plast Surg* 1992; 45: 426–34.

56 Reed WB, College J, Francis MJO *et al*. Epidermolysis bullosa dystrophic with epidermal neoplasms. *Arch Dermatol* 1974; 110: 894–902.

57 Didolkar M, Gerner R, Moore G. Epidermolysis bullosa dystrophica and epithelioma of the skin. *Cancer* 1974; 33: 198–202.

58 Carapeto FJ, Pastor JA, Martin J, Agurruza J. Recessive dystrophic epidermolysis bullosa and mutiple squamous cell carcinoma. *Dermatologica* 1982; 165: 39–46.

59 Song IC, Dicksheet S. Management of squamous cell carcinoma in a patient with dominant-type epidermolysis bullosa dystrophica: a surgical challenge. *Plast Reconstr Surg* 1985; 75: 732–6.

60 Lentz SR, Raish RJ, Orlowski EP, Marion JM. Squamous cell carcinoma in epidermolysis bullosa: treatment with systemic chemotherapy. *Cancer* 1990; 66: 1276–8.

61 McGrath JA, Schofield OMV, Mayou BJ, McKee PH, Eady RAJ. Epidermolysis bullosa complicated by squamous carcinoma: report of 10 cases. *J Cutan Pathol* 1992; 19: 116–23.

62 Carlesimo M, Giustini S, Richetta A, Calvieri S. Multiple squamous cell carcinomas developing in dystrophic epidermolysis bullosa. *Eur J Dermatol* 1993; 3: 564–7.

63 Keefe M, Wakeel RA, Dick DC. Death from metastatic cutaneous squamous cell carcinoma in autosomal recessive dystrophic epidermolysis bullosa despite permanent inpatient care. *Dermatologica* 1988; 177: 180–4.

64 Pasini A. Dystrophie cutanee bulleuse atrophiante et albo-papuloide. *Ann Dermatol Syph* 1928; 9: 1044–66.

65 Ramelet A-A, Boillat C. Epidermolyse bulleuse dystrophique albopapuloide autosomique recessive. *Dermatologica* 1985; 171: 397–406.

66 Garcia-Perez A, Carapeto FJ. Pretibial epidermolysis bullosa: report of two families and review of the literature. *Dermatologica* 1975; 150: 122–8.

67 McGrath JA, Schofield OMV, Eady RAJ. Epidermolysis bullosa pruriginosa: dystrophic epidermolysis bullosa with distinctive clinicopathological features. *Br J Dermatol* 1994: 130; 617–25.

68 Russell-Jones R. Epidermolysis bullosa: report of a family and discussion of the dominant dystrophic types. *Clin Exp Dermatol* 1979; 4: 303–8.

69 Furue M, Ando I, Inoue Y *et al*. Pretibial epidermolysis bullosa. *Arch Dermatol* 1986; 122: 310–13.

70 Lichtenwald DJ, Hanna W, Sauder DN, Jacubovic HR, Rosenthal D. Pretibial epidermolysis bullosa: report of a case. *J Am Acad Dermatol* 1990; 22: 346–50.

71 Gassia V, Basex J, Ortonne J-P. Pretibial epidermolysis bullosa. *J Am Acad Dermatol* 1990; 22: 663–4.

72 Hashimoto K, Matsumoto M, Jacobelli D. Transient bullous dermolysis of the newborn. *Arch Dermatol* 1985; 121: 1429–38.

73 Hashimoto K, Burk JD, Bale GF *et al*. Transient bullous dermolysis of the newborn: two additional cases. *J Am Acad Dermatol* 1989; 21: 708–13.

74 Fine JD, Horiguchi Y, Stein DH *et al*. Intraepidermal type VII collagen. *J Am Acad Dermatol* 1990; 22: 188–95.

75 Hatta N, Takata M, Shimuzu H. Spontaneous disappearance of intraepidermal type VII collagen in a patient with dystrophic epidermolysis bullosa. *Br J Dermatol* 1995; 133: 619–24.

76 Smith LT, Sybert VP. Intraepidermal retention of type VII collagen in a patient with recessive dystrophic epidermolysis bullosa. *J Invest Dermatol* 1990; 94: 261–4.

77 Phillips RJ, Harper JI, Lake BD. Intraepidermal collagen type VII in dystrophic epidermolysis bullosa: report of five new cases. *Br J Dermatol* 1992; 26: 222–30.

78 Travis SPL, McGrath JA, Turnbull AJ *et al*. Oral and gastrointestinal manifestations of epidermolysis bullosa. *Lancet* 1992; 340: 1505–6.

79 Ergun GA, Lin AN, Danneberg AJ, Carter DM. Gastrointestinal manifesta-

tions of epidermolysis bullosa: a study of 100 patients. *Medicine* 1992; 71: 121–7.

80 Orlando RC, Bozymski EM, Briggaman RA, Bream CA. Epidermolysis bullosa: gastrointestinal manifestations. *Ann Int Med* 1974; 81: 203–6.

81 Fortier-Beaulieu M, Teillac D, De Prost Y. Atteinte digestive au cours de l' epiderolyse bulleuse dystrophique receesive. *Ann Dermatol Vénéréol* 1987; 114: 963–71.

82 Mauro MA, Parker LA, Hartley WS *et al*. Epidermolysis bullosa: radiographic findings in 16 cases. *Am J Radiol* 1987; 149: 925–7.

83 Hillemeier C, Touloukian R, McCallum R, Gryboski J. Esophageal web: a previously unrecognized complication of epidermolysis bullosa. *Pediatrics* 1981; 67: 678–82.

84 Tishler JM, Han SY, Helman CA. Esophageal involvement in epidermolysis bullosa dystrophica. *Am J Radiol* 1983; 141: 1283–6.

85 Gryboski JD, Touloukian R, Campanella RA. Gastrointestinal manifestations of epidermolysis bullosa in children *Arch Dermatol* 1988; 124: 746–52.

86 Clayden GS. Dysphagia and constipation in epidermolysis bullosa. In: *Epidermolysis Bullosa: a Comprehensive Review of Classification, Management and Laboratory Studies*. Crowthorne: DEBRA, 1990: 67–71.

87 Allman SA, Haynes L, Mackinnon P, Atherton DJ. Nutrition in dystrophic epidermolysis bullosa. *Pediatr Dermatol* 1992; 9: 231–8.

88 Crawford EG, Burkes EJ, Briggaman RA. Hereditary epidermolysis bullosa: oral manifestations and dental therapy. *Oral Surg* 1976; 42: 490–500.

89 Wright JT, Fine J-D, Johnson L. Hereditary epidermolysis bullosa: oral manifestations and dental management. *Pediatr Dent* 1993; 15: 242–7.

90 McDonnell PJ, Spalton DJ. The ocular signs and complictions of epidermolysis bullosa. *J Roy Soc Med* 1988; 81: 576–8.

91 Gans LA. Eye lesions of epidermolysis bullosa. *Arch Dermatol* 1988; 124: 762–4.

92 Iwamoto M, Haik BG, Iwamoto T *et al*. The ultrastructural defect in conjunctiva from a case of recessive dystrophic epidermolysis bullosa. *Arch Ophthalmol* 1991; 109: 1382–6.

93 Shackelford GD, Bauer EA, Graviss ER, McAlister WH. Upper airway and external genital involvement in epidermolysis bullosa dystrophica. *Pediatr Radiol* 1982; 143: 429–32.

94 Kretkowski RC. Urinary tract involvement in epidermolysis bullosa. *Pediatrics* 1973; 51: 938–41.

95 Mann JFE, Zeier M, Zilow E *et al*. The spectrum of renal involvement in epidermolysis bullosa dystrophica hereditaria: report of two cases. *Am J Kidney Dis* 1988; 11: 437–41.

96 Sharratt GP, Lacson AL, Cornel G, Virmani S. Echocardiography of intracardiac filling defects in infants and children. *Pediatr Cardiol* 1986; 7: 189–94.

97 Brook MM, Weinhouse E, Jarenwattananon M, Nudel DB. Dilated cardiomyopathy complicating a case of epidermolysis bullosa dystrophica. *Pediatr Dermatol* 1989; 6: 21–3.

98 Melville C, Atherton D, Burch M, Cohn A, Sullivan I. Fatal cardiomyopathy in dystrophic epidermolysis bullosa. *Br J Dermatol* (in press).

99 Lechner-Gruskay D, Honig PJ, Pereira G *et al*. Nutritional and metabolic profile of children with epidermolysis bullosa. *Pediatr Dermatol* 1988; 5: 22–7.

100 Fine J-D, Tamura T, Johnson L. Blood vitamin and trace metal levels in epidermolysis bullosa. *Arch Dermatol* 1989; 125: 374–9.

101 Pessar A, Verdicchio JF, Caldwell D. Epidermolysis bullosa: the paediatric dermatological management and therapeutic update. *Adv Dermatol* 1988; 3: 99–120.

102 Dunnill MGS, Eady RAJ. The management of dystrophic epidermolysis bullosa. *Clin Exp Dermatol* 1995; 20: 179–88.

103 Eisenberg M. The effect of occlusive dressings on re-epithelialization of wounds in children with epidermolysis bullosa. *J Pediatr Surg* 1986; 10: 892–4.

104 Mallory SB. Adjunctive therapy for epidermolysis bullosa. *J Am Acad Dermatol* 1982; 6: 951–2.

105 McGrath JA, Schofield OMV, Ishida-Yamaoto A *et al*. Cultured keratinocyte allografts and wound healing in severe recessive dystrophic epidermolysis bullosa. *J Am Acad Dermatol* 1993; 29: 407–19.

106 Rahman M, Noble WC, Cookson B. Mupirocin-resistant *Staphylococcus aureus*. *Lancet* 1987; ii: 387.

107 Lin AN, Caldwell D, Varghese M *et al*. Efficacy of long-term mupirocin therapy in epidermolysis bullosa and its effect on growth and lifespan of cultured fibroblasts. *J Invest Dermatol* 1986; 87: 152.

108 Moy JA, Caldwell-Brown D, Lin AN, Pappa KA, Carter DM. Mupirocin-resistant *Staphylococcus aureus* after long-term treatment of patients with epidermolysis bullosa. *J Am Acad Dermatol* 1990; 22: 893–5.

109 Zumla A, Lulat A. Honey—a remedy rediscovered. *J Roy Soc Med* 1989; 82: 384–5.

110 Chirife J, Scarmato G, Herszage L. Scientific basis for use of granulated sugar in treatment of infected wounds. *Lancet* 1982; i: 560.

111 Cooper TW, Bauer EA. Therapeutic efficacy of phenytoin in recessive dystrophic epidermolysis. *Arch Dermatol* 1984; 120: 490–5.

112 Caldwell-Brown D, Stern RS, Lin AN *et al.* Lack of efficacy of phenytoin in recessive dystrophic epidermolysis bullosa. *N Engl J Med* 1992; 327: 163–7.

113 Fritsch P, Klein G, Aubock J, Hintner H. Retinoid therapy of recessive dystrophic epidermolysis bullosa. *J Am Acad Dermatol* 1983; 9: 766.

114 White JE. Minocycline for dystrophic epidermolysis bullosa. *Lancet* 1989; i: 966.

115 Ikeda S, Manabe M, Muramatsu T, Takamori K, Ogawa H. Protease inhibitor therapy for recessive dystrophic epidermolysis bullosa. *J Am Acad Dermatol* 1988; 18: 1246–52.

116 Moynahan EJ. The treatment and management of epidermolysis bullosa. *Clin Exp Dermatol* 1982; 7: 665–72.

117 Grieder JL, Flatt AE. Surgical restoration of the hand in epidermolysis bullosa. *Arch Dermatol* 1988; 124: 765–7.

118 Terrill PJ, Mayou BJ, Pemberton J. Experience in the surgical management of the hand in dystrophic epidermolysis bullosa. *Br J Plast Surg* 1992; 45: 435–42.

119 Mullett FLH, Smith PJ. Hand splintage for dystrophic epidermolysis bullosa. *Br J Plast Surg* 1993; 46: 192–3.

120 Mullett FLH, Atherton DJ. Physiotherapy for epidermolysis bullosa: a starting point. *Physiotherapy* 1990; 76: 660–2.

121 Haynes L. Epidermolysis bullosa. In: Shaw V, Lawsib M, eds. *Clinical Paediatric Dietetics*. Oxford: Blackwell Scientific Publications, 1994: 295–302.

122 Birge K. Nutrition management of patients with epidermolysis bullosa. *J Am Diet Assoc* 1995; 95: 575–9.

123 Feurle G, Weidauer H, Baldauf G *et al.* Management of esophageal stenosis in recessive dystrophic epidermolysis bullosa. *Gastroenterology* 1984; 87: 1376–80.

124 Kern IB, Eisenberg M, Willis S. Management of eosophageal stenosis in epidermolysis bullosa dystrophica. *Arch Dis Child* 1989; 64: 551–6.

125 Griffin R, Mayou B. The anaesthetic management of patients with dystrophic epidermolysis bullosa. *Anaesthesia* 1993; 48: 810–15.

126 Harmel RP. Esophageal replacement in two siblings with epidermolysis bullosa. *J Pediatr Surg* 1986; 21: 175–6.

127 Sehhat S, Amirie SA. Oesophageal reconstruction for complete stenosis due to dystrophic epidermolysis bullosa. *Thorax* 1977; 32: 697–9.

128 Absolon KB, Finney LA, Waddill GM *et al.* Esophageal reconstruction—colon transplant in two brothers with epidermolysis bullosa. *Surgery* 1969; 65: 832–6.

129 De Leon R, Mispireta LA, Absolon KB. Five-year follow-up of colonic transplants in patients with epidermolysis bullosa producing esophageal obstruction. *Med Ann Dist Columbia* 1974; 43: 241–4.

130 Haynes L, Atherton DJ, Ade-Ajayi N, Wheeler R, Kiely EM. Gastrostomy and growth in dystrophic epidermolysis bullosa. *Br J Dermatol* 1996; 134: 872–9.

131 Shankardass K, Chuchmach S, Chelswick K *et al.* Bowel function of long-term tube-fed patients consuming formulae with and without dietary fiber. *J Parent Ent Nutr* 1990; 14: 508–12.

132 Haynes L, Atherton D, Clayden G. Constipation in epidermolysis bullosa: successful treatment with a liquid fiber-containing formula. *Pediatr Dermatol* 1997; 14: 393–6.

133 Ingebo KB, Heyman MB. Polyethylene glycol–electrolyte solution for intestinal clearance in children with refractory encopresis. *Am J Dis Child* 1988; 142: 340–2.

134 James I, Wark H. Airway management during anaesthesia in patients with epidermolysis bullosa dystrophica. *Anesthesiology* 1982; 56: 323–6.

135 Tomlinson AA. Recessive dystrophic epidermolysis bullosa: the anaesthetic management of a case for major surgery. *Anaesthesia* 1983; 38: 485–91.

136 Hruby MA, Esterly NB. Anaemia in epidermolysis bullosa letalis. *Am J Dis Child* 1973; 125: 696–9.

137 Atherton DJ, Cox I, Hann I. Intravenous iron (III)-hydroxide sucrose complex for anaemia in epidermolysis bullosa. *Brit J Dermatol* 1999; 140: 773.

138 Nowak AJ. Oropharyngeal lesions and their management in epidermolysis bullosa. *Arch Dermatol* 1988; 124: 742–5.

139 Verrando P, Pisani A, Ortonne J-P. The new basement membrane antigen recognized by the monoclonal antibody GB3 is a large size glycoprotein: modulation of its expression by retinoic acid. *Biochim Biophys Acta* 1988; 942: 45–6.

140 Marinkovich MP, Lunstrum GP, Keene DR, Burgeson RE. The dermo-epidermal junction of human skin contains a novel laminin variant. *J Cell Biol* 1992; 119: 695–703.

141 Marinkovich MP, Verrando, Keene DR *et al.* The basement membrane proteins kalinin and nicein are structurally and immunologically identical. *Lab Invest* 1993; 69: 295–9.

142 Burgeson RE, Chiquett M, Deutzmann R *et al.* A new nomenclature for laminins. *Matrix Biol* 1994; 14: 209–11.

143 Pulkkinen L, Christiano AM, Gerecke D *et al.* A homozygous nonsense mutation in the beta 3 chain gene of laminin 5 (LAMB3) in Herlitz junctional epidermolysis bullosa. *Genomics* 1994; 24: 357–60.

144 Aberdam D, Galliano MF, Vailly J *et al.* Herlitz's junctional epidermolysis bullosa is linked to mutations in the gene (LAMC2) for the gamma 2 subunit of nicein/kalinin (LAMININ-5). *Nat Genet* 1994; 6: 299–304.

145 Kivirikko S, McGrath JA, Baudoin C *et al.* A homozygous nonsense mutation in the alpha 3 chain gene of laminin 5 (LAMA3) in lethal (Herlitz) junctional epidermolysis bullosa. *Hum Mol Genet* 1995; 4: 959–62.

146 McGrath JA, Pulkkinen L, Christiano AM *et al.* Altered laminin 5 expression due to mutations in the gene encoding the beta 3 chain (LAMB3) in generalized atrophic benign epidermolysis bullosa. *J Invest Dermatol* 1995; 104: 467–74.

147 Mellerio JE, Eady RA, Atherton DJ, Lake BD, McGrath JA. E210K mutation in the gene encoding the beta3 chain of laminin-5 (LAMB3) is predictive of a phenotype of generalized atrophic benign epidermolysis bullosa. *Br J Dermatol* 1998; 139: 325–31.

148 Cross HE, Wells RS, Esterly JR. Inheritance in epidermolysis bullosa letalis. *J Med Genet* 1968; 5: 189–96.

149 Cross HE, Wells RS, Esterly JR. Inheritance in epidermolysis bullosa letalis. *J Med Genet* 1968; 5: 189–96.

150 Hashimoto I, Gedde-Dahl T, Schnyder UW, Anton-Lamprecht I. Ultrastructural studies in epidermolysis bullosa. IV. Recessive dystrophic types with junctional blistering. *Arch Dermatol Res* 1976; 257: 17–32.

151 Tidman M, Eady R. Hemidesmosome heterogeneity in junctional epidermolysis bullosa revealed by morphometric analysis. *J Invest Dermatol* 1986; 86: 51–6.

152 Schofield O, Fine JD, Verrando P, Heagerty AHM, Ortonne JP, Eady RAJ. GB3 monoclonal antibody for the diagnosis of junctional epidermolysis bullosa: results of a multicenter study. *J Am Acad Dermatol* 1990; 23: 1078–83.

153 Lacour J, Hoffman P, Bastiani-Griffet F *et al.* Lethal junctional epidermolysis bullosa with normal expression of BM600 and pyloric atresia: a new variant of junctional epidermolysis bullosa. *Eur J Pediatr* 1992; 151: 252–7.

154 Davies H, Atherton DJ. Acute laryngeal obstruction in junctional epidermolysis bullosa. *Pediatr Dermatol* 1987; 4: 98–101.

155 Pearson RW, Potter B, Strauss F. Epidermolysis bullosa hereditaria letalis. *Arch Dermatol* 1974; 109: 349–55.

156 Oakley CA, Wilson N, Ross JA, Barnetson RStC. Junctional epidermolysis bullosa in two siblings. *Br J Dermatol* 1984; 111: 533–43.

157 Kenna MA, Stool SE, Mallory SB. Junctional epidermolysis bullosa of the larynx. *Pediatrics* 1986; 78: 172–4.

158 Hammerton ME, Turner TW, Pyne RJ. A case of junctional epidermolysis bullosa (Herlitz–Pearson) with corneal bullae. *Aust J Ophthalmol* 1984; 12: 45–8.

159 Brain EB, Wigglesworth JS. Developing teeth in epidermolysis bullosa hereditaria letalis. *Br Dent J* 1968; 124: 255–60.

160 Gardner DG, Hudson CD. The disturbances in odontogenesis in epidermolysis bullosa hereditaria letalis. *Oral Surg* 1975; 40: 483–93.

161 Hintner H, Wolff K. Generalised atrophic benign epidermolysis bullosa. *Arch Dermatol* 1982; 118: 375–84.

162 Paller AS, Fine J-D, Kaplan S, Pearson RW. The generalised atrophic benign form of junctional epidermolysis bullosa. *Arch Dermatol* 1986; 12: 704–10.

163 Turner TW. Two cases of junctional epidermolysis bullosa (Herlitz–Pearson). *Br J Dermatol* 1980; 102: 97–107.

164 Ichiki M, Kasada M, Hachisuka H, Sasai Y. Junctional epidermolysis bullosa with urethral stricture. *Dermatological* 1987; 175: 244–8.

165 Valari MD, Phillips RJ, Lake BD, Harper JI. Junctional epidermolysis bullosa and pyloric atresia: a distinct entity. Clinical and pathological studies in five patients. *Br J Dermatol* 1995; 133: 732–6.

166 Berger T, Detlefs R, Donatucci C. Junctional epidermolysis bullosa, pyloric atresia and genitourinary disease. *Pediatr Dermatol* 1986; 3: 130–4.

167 Hayashi AH, Galliani CA, Gillis DA. Congenital pyloric atresia and junctional epidermolysis bullosa: a report of long-term survival and a review of the literature. *J Pediatr Surg* 1991; 28: 1341–5.

168 Phillips RJ, Atherton DJ, Gibbs ML, Strobel S, Lake BD. Laryngo-onycho-cutaneous syndrome: an inherited epithelial defect. *Arch Dis Child* 1994; 70: 319–26.

169 Carter DM, Lin AN, Varghese MC, Caldwell D, Pratt LA, Eisinger M. Treatment of junctional epidermolysis bullosa with epidermal autografts. *J Am Acad Dermatol* 1987; 17: 246–50.

19.5   The Genetic Ichthyoses

HEIKO TRAUPE

Isolated vulgar ichthyoses
Autosomal dominant ichthyosis vulgaris (ADI)
X-linked recessive ichthyosis

Associated ichthyoses of the vulgaris type
Refsum's syndrome (heredopathia atactica polyneuritiformis)
Associated steroid sulphatase deficiency
Multiple sulphatase deficiency

Isolated congenital ichthyoses
Harlequin ichthyosis

The lamellar ichthyoses
Autosomal dominant lamellar ichthyosis
Autosomal recessive lamellar ichthyosis

The epidermolytic ichthyoses
Bullous ichthyotic erythroderma of Brocq
Annular epidermolytic ichthyosis
Ichthyosis bullosa of Siemens
Ichthyosis hystrix of Curth–Macklin
Genetic counselling of the epidermolytic ichthyoses

Associated congenital ichthyoses
Sjögren–Larsson syndrome
Trichothiodystrophy syndromes
Comèl–Netherton syndrome
Happle's syndrome
Dorfman's syndrome
Hystrix-like ichthyosis with deafness (HID) syndrome
KID syndrome
Ichthyosis follicularis with atrichia and photophobia (IFAP)
 syndrome

Recently recognized ichthyoses

Definition

The term 'ichthyosis' is loosely applied to a broad number of scaling diseases. These disorders are grouped together because they have in common a conspicuous scaling which is generalized and affects the entire skin [1].

By tradition ichthyoses are considered universal scaling disorders and separated from those which involve only parts of the body such as palmoplantar keratosis or erythrokeratodermias. However, the distinction between erythrokeratodermias and ichthyoses is a bit arbitrary. The same applies to the distinction between ichthyosis and ichthyosiform dermatosis. In the author's understanding the proper adjective for ichthyosis is 'ichthyotic' and not ichthyosiform which actually means ichthyosis-like. Though the author prefers to use the term ichthyosis only in the context of a genetic keratinization disorder, many colleagues also include acquired disorders of keratinization under the label of 'ichthyotic'. The causes of acquired disturbances of cornification include malignancies, such as lymphoproliferative diseases, drug interactions, especially those interfering with epidermal lipid metabolism, or renal failure to name but a few [2]. In this chapter acquired causes of disorders of keratinization will not be addressed. They do not play a major role in paediatric dermatology and are seen mainly in adults.

Historical aspects and classification

The genetic ichthyoses are a perfect example of a group of diseases in which first clinical and later genetic heterogeneity was appreciated. The first ichthyosis described in detail was a peculiar type of ichthyosis hystrix referred to as porcupine man (Fig. 19.5.1). Robert Willan devoted a whole chapter of his textbook of dermatology written in 1808 to the description of members of the Lambert family who were affected by a very severe type of ichthyosis hystrix. These family members were regarded by their contemporaries as porcupine men and as a new species of man. They attracted considerable interest in their spectacular disease.

Willan [3] introduced the term ichthyosis for their skin disease. In the beginning of the 20th century further clinical heterogeneity of the ichthyoses was recognized and it was suggested to separate ichthyosis vulgaris from congenital ichthyosis [4]. In 1902 the French dermatologist Brocq [5] even distinguished between a bullous and a nonbullous type of congenital ichthyotic erythroderma. In the 1930s Hermann Werner Siemens advanced a genetic understanding of the various ichthyoses and proposed to use pedigree analysis and formal modes of transmission such as autosomal recessive transmission versus autosomal dominant transmission as a means of distinguishing between various types of ichthyosis [6]. The rediscovery of X-linked recessive ichthyosis (XRI) by Wells and Kerr

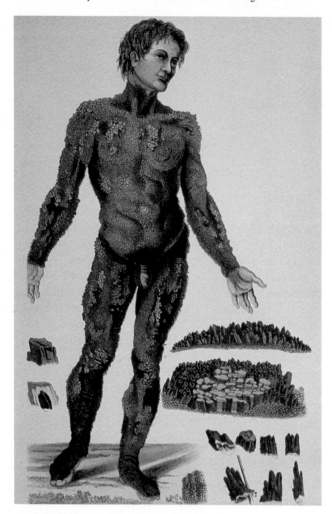

Fig. 19.5.1 Ichthyosis hystrix; drawing of a 'porcupine man' by Tilesius 1802. This man belonged to the Lambert family.

[7] stimulated the interest of the general dermatologists and paediatricians in ichthyosis and paved the way for a molecular understanding of this disorder as a consequence of steroid sulphatase deficiency [8,9].

Recently molecular genetic research has unravelled the basis of several other ichthyoses. Thus bullous ichthyotic erythroderma (BIE) and ichthyosis bullosa of Siemens (IBS) have been identified as keratin disorders and one particular type of lamellar ichthyosis has been shown to be due to a mutation in transglutaminase 1 [10,11]. These advances in the molecular understanding of ichthyosis also provide new insights about the normal function of the epidermis. In particular they reaffirm the two-compartment model ('bricks and mortar' model) of the stratum corneum as proposed by Elias [12]. In this model the stratum corneum is viewed as a structure consisting of protein-rich corneocytes, i.e. 'bricks' filled with keratins forming the cytoskeleton, and intercellular multilamellar lipidsheets, i.e. 'mortar' representing the water permeability barriers. Disorders of cornification can arise either

by defects in the mortar, that is a disturbed composition of epidermal lipids, or by defects within the protein-rich corneocytes.

However, when confronted with an individual patient the doctor does not see a keratin mutation or a deficiency of steroid sulphatase or transglutaminase K, but he or she sees a patient with a scaly skin and perhaps further symptoms. To arrive at the definite diagnosis it is useful to ask two questions as follows.

1 Has the ichthyosis been present at birth or at least within the first 4 weeks of life and may thus be regarded as being congenital or was the onset of major scaling noticed only after the age of 3 months? This question allows the differentiation between congenital ichthyoses and non-congenital ichthyoses. The latter are usually referred to as ichthyosis of the vulgaris type. In practice this information often has to be obtained from the parents and sometimes may not be reliable. Then it can help to ascertain whether the clinical features are suggestive of ichthyosis vulgaris or congenital ichthyosis. Thus severe scaling, marked involvement of the flexural folds and definite involvement of palms and soles are suggestive of congenital ichthyosis, while the sparing of flexural folds or partial sparing of these folds as well as absent palmar and plantar involvement or the presence of accentuated creases are suggestive of an ichthyosis belonging to the vulgaris group.

2 Is the ichthyosis the only manifestation of the underlying gene defect or does the patient have further signs and symptoms in the sense of a syndrome or associated ichthyosis? If only dry skin is present then the underlying gene defect apparently is restricted in its expression to the epidermis as is the case in lamellar ichthyosis, while a pleiotropic gene action involves several tissues and thus results in a syndromic or associated ichthyosis.

By combining these two questions we can categorize a given case of ichthyosis into four different major groups: isolated vulgar ichthyoses, associated vulgar ichthyoses, isolated congenital ichthyoses and associated congenital ichthyoses.

After having made a selection within one of these four groups a number of differential diagnoses can then be considered, and in many instances a specific diagnosis, such as Sjögren–Larsson syndrome of XRI, can be made.

REFERENCES

1 Traupe H. *The Ichthyoses. A Guide to Clinical Diagnosis. Genetic Counseling, and Theory.* Berlin: Springer-Verlag, 1989: 3–14.
2 Kütting B, Traupe H. Der erworbene Ichthyosis-ähnliche Hautzustand. Eine Herausforderung zur diagnostischen Abklärung. *Hautarzt* 1995; 46: 836–40.
3 Willan R. *On Cutaneous Diseases*, vol. 1. London: Barnard, 1808.
4 Riecke R. Über Ichthyosis Congenita. *Arch Dermatol Syph (Wien)* 1900; 54: 289–340.
5 Brocq L. Erythrodermie congénitale ichthyosiforme avec hyper epidermotrophie. *Ann Dermatol Syph* 1902; 3: 1–31.
6 Siemens HW. Die Vererbung in der Ätiologie der Hautkrankheiten. In:

Jadassohn J, ed. *Handbuch der Haut- und Geschlechtskrankheiten*, vol. 3 Berlin: Springer-Verlag, 1929: 1–165.

7 Wells RS, Kerr CB. Clinical features of autosomal dominant and sex-linked ichthyosis in an English population. *Br Med J* 1966; 1: 947–50.

8 Koppe JG, Marinkovic-Ilsen A, Rijken Y, De Groot WP, Jöbis AC. X-linked ichthyosis. A sulphatase deficiency. *Arch Dis Child* 1978; 53: 803–6.

9 Shapiro LJ, Weiss R, Webster D, France JT. X-linked ichthyosis due to steroid sulphatase deficiency. *Lancet* 1978; 1: 70–2.

10 Huber M, Rettler I, Bernasconi K *et al*. Mutations of keratinocyte transglutaminase in lamellar ichthyosis. *Science* 1995; 267: 525–8.

11 Russel LJ, Di Giovanna JJ, Rogers GR *et al*. Mutations in the gene for transglutaminase 1 in autosomal recessive lamellar ichthyosis. *Nature Genet* 1995; 9: 279–83.

12 Elias PM. Plastic wrap revisited. The stratum corneum two-compartment model and its clinical implications. *Arch Dermatol* 1987; 123: 1405–6.

Isolated vulgar ichthyoses

Autosomal dominant ichthyosis vulgaris (ADI)

ADI can range in expression from very mild to considerable hyperkeratosis and in its mild form may be present in 1 in 250 individuals in the general population [1]. Autosomal dominant inheritance of this condition was used as a main argument by Siemens to separate ADI from lamellar ichthyosis which mostly follows an autosomal recessive mode of inheritance. The clinical and genetic features of ADI could be fully appreciated only after XRI had been delineated by Wells and Kerr [1]. Though the vast majority of cases with ichthyosis vulgaris do not start before the age of 6 months, it has been claimed that occasionally ichthyosis vulgaris can already be present at birth and begin even as collodion baby [2]. However, it is not clear whether these exceptional cases perhaps represent autosomal dominant lamellar ichthyosis instead of ADI.

Clinical features

Typical cutaneous features of ADI include light grey scales covering mainly the extensor surfaces of the extremities and the trunk (Fig. 19.5.2). The groin and the big flexures are always spared. Prominent follicular keratosis (keratosis pilaris) is usually seen especially in younger patients and occurs in 75% of all ADI patients, but only in about 12.7% of the general population [3]. On palms and soles accentuated creases can be seen. This has been designated the ichthyosis hand, but it should be borne in mind that such accentuated palmoplantar markings can be found also in atopic dermatitis and in several other ichthyoses such as Refsum's syndrome and sometimes in lamellar ichthyoses. There has been a long-standing debate on the relationship between atopic dermatitis and ichthyosis vulgaris. In the author's experience quite a number of patients suffering from ichthyosis vulgaris come to the attention of the dermatologist because of an accompanying atopic dermatitis which is itchy and may constitute a major problem for the child, while the ichthyosis may be overlooked and dismissed as 'dry skin' only. From a clinical point of view about a third of all children with atopic

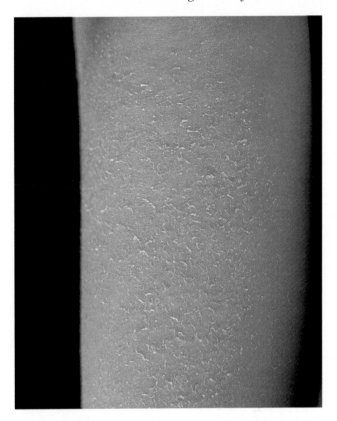

Fig. 19.5.2 Autosomal dominant ichthyosis vulgaris: fine translucent scaling.

dermatitis also suffer from ichthyosis vulgaris. Keratosis pilaris is particularly frequent and may reach up to 90% in this subgroup of patients.

A three-generation family in which ADI was associated in several family members with keratosis punctata of the palmar creases has been reported [4].

Histopathology and ultrastructure

Histological examination reveals an increased stratum corneum with orthohyperkeratosis and a reduced or in part lacking granular layer, while the remaining epidermis can be normal or sometimes even atrophic. Perivascular infiltrates, if present at all, are slight. At the ultrastructural level the diminished granular layer is reflected by reduced and abnormal keratohyalin granules which have a crumbly or spongy appearance [5]. The major protein component of keratohyalin is filaggrin. Filaggrin and its precursor profilaggrin are absent in severely affected ADI patients and reduced in intensity in less severely affected patients [6]. This reflects a defect in post-transcriptional control of profilaggrin expression [7].

X-linked recessive ichthyosis

Having an incidence of 1 in 2000 males XRI is the second

most common type of ichthyosis [8]. An X-linked recessive mode of inheritance in a family suffering from ichthyosis was first noted by Lundborg in 1927 [9]. However, this disease became forgotten for many years until it was rediscovered by Wells and Kerr in 1966 [1]. In particular they correlated clinical features of XRI with the histological aspect and thus made possible a clear-cut differential diagnosis from autosomal dominant ichthyosis vulgaris.

Clinical features

The clinical spectrum of XRI was only fully appreciated after it had been recognized that the disease is due to a deficiency of steroid sulphatase and includes ichthyosis, birth complications and cryptorchidism [10]. Corneal opacities which, however, do not affect the visual acuity can be a further ophthalmological manifestation in up to 50% of patients. Cutaneous findings in XRI include a fine scaling directly after birth which then diminishes and returns at the age of 3–4 months with a marked (in most cases) dark brown scaling with rhombic firmly adherent hyperkeratosis covering the arms, legs and trunk (Fig. 19.5.3). Therefore this type of ichthyosis has often also been called ichthyosis nigricans or 'ichthyose noire' in the French literature. However, in about one-third of patients the hyperkeratoses have a light grey colour and they may show phenotypic variability even within the same family. Very often the neck is involved with dark grey hyperkeratosis and this may give the children 'a dirty look' which is not found in ADI. Many children suffer from this because their peers at school assume that they do not wash properly.

Because the enzyme deficiency is expressed in placental tissue (placental sulphatase deficiency), insufficient cervical dilatation is sometimes found in pregnant women and can cause weakness of labour and prolonged delivery. A history of birth complications is thus sometimes obtained. In a series of 33 patients diagnosed postnatally with XRI there was a history of forceps delivery in three and caesarean section in one, while in another six pregnancies infusions with oxytocin because of weakness in labour had been given [11].

Several studies have independently found that testicular maldescent is present in about 20% of patients [11]. This figure is far above the prevalence of cryptorchidism to be expected in the male population after the first year of life, which is about 1%. Since uncorrected cryptorchidism can affect normal gonadal and sexual development and can be the cause of hypogenitalism, all boys in whom XRI is diagnosed should be systematically investigated for the presence of testicular maldescent and proper treatment should be given. The reason for this association may be that in more than 80% of cases steroid sulphatase deficiency is caused by a deletion of the steroid sulphatase gene [12] and more importantly XRI may be due to a contiguous gene defect. A study showed that nine out of 33 investigated patients had evidence of such a contiguous gene defect [13] which means that not only the steroid sulphatase gene but also adjacent genes are deleted. Congenital defects of the abdominal wall have also been reported in a unique case of XRI and could also be due to a contiguous gene defect [14].

Histopathology

In most books it can be found that XRI is characterized by an epidermal hyperplasia and an increased granular layer. While this is so in the majority of the cases sometimes a reduced granular layer and an almost atrophic epidermis can be found especially if the biopsy is taken from a site of extreme scaling. Since in other types of ichthyosis this has to be done in order to appreciate the complete histological features—a good example of this is epidermolytic hyperkeratosis—histological findings are only of additional value when making a diagnosis of XRI.

Biochemical aspects

The best means of confirming the diagnosis is to perform an enzyme test to demonstrate steroid sulphatase deficiency. However, this enzyme test is done only in a few laboratories in Europe. A DNA diagnosis by demonstrating absence of the steroid sulphatase gene or neighbouring DNA probes can be done in many molecular genetic institutes, but fails to identify point mutations. In practice the doctor will often be faced with the situation where a molecular or biochemical confirmation of the clinical diagnosis is not available. In this situation it may be useful to employ lipoprotein electrophoresis which is a test that can be done in any biochemistry laboratory and typically shows an increased electromobility of β-lipoprotein

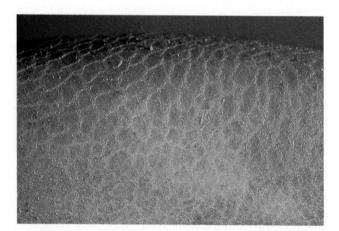

Fig. 19.5.3 XRI: dark-brown rhombic scales.

(Fig. 19.5.4) [15]. The reason for this increased electromobility of β-lipoprotein particles is that cholesterol sulphate is accumulated within this fraction and alters the electric charge and thus the electrophoretic mobility of lipoprotein. When ordering such a test it is useful to provide a stored blood sample from a previous patient as a positive control and from patients who are normal and the biochemist should be informed of the special interest in the electrophoretic mobility, otherwise he or she will report normal results.

Somewhat surprisingly, the skin barrier properties in patients with XRI have been shown to be superior to those of normal controls [16]. In particular, the response to sodium lauryl sulphate was less marked when evaluated by transepidermal water loss.

Genetic aspects

The genetics of XRI are very intriguing because the gene is located in the Xp22.3 region immediately below the pseudoautosomal region and has non-functional sequences on the long arm of the Y chromosome. In mice the steroid sulphatase gene behaves as a pseudoautosomal trait and there are frequent crossovers between the X and Y chromosome [17]. Pseudoautosomal genes do not undergo the X-inactivation which is typical of most genes on the X chromosome. It is of interest that the steroid sulphatase gene—although it no longer resides in the

pseudoautosomal region in humans—also escapes the common X-inactivation, which means that normal women have a considerably higher steroid sulphatase activity than normal males, while women who are heterozygous gene carriers have a steroid sulphatase activity in the range of normal males [18]. Thus steroid sulphatase testing allows even recognition of female gene carriers who cannot be deduced from pedigree data because they have no affected offspring.

A Sardinian family with ichthyosis has been reported in whom the transmission pattern was consistent with XRI, while biochemical studies showed normal levels of steroid sulphatase and molecular investigations ruled out the Xp22.3 region where the steroid sulphatase locus has been mapped [19].

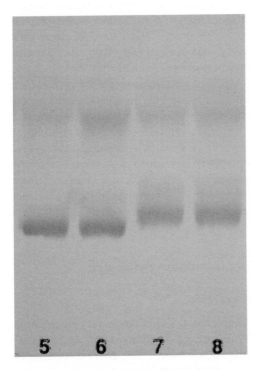

Fig. 19.5.4 Lipoprotein electrophoresis in XRI: note increased electromobility of β-lipoprotein in the XRI patients (lanes 7 and 8) compared to normal controls (lanes 5 and 6).

REFERENCES

1 Wells RS, Kerr CB. Clinical features of autosomal dominant and sex-linked ichthyosis in an English population. *Br Med J* 1966; 1: 947–50.
2 Larrègue M, Ottavy N, Bressieux JM, Lorette J. Bébé collodion. Trente-deux nouvelles observations. *Ann Dermatol Vénéréol* 1986; 113: 773–85.
3 Mevorah B, Maruzzi A, Frenk E. The prevalence of accentuated palmoplantar markings and keratosis pilaris in atopic dermatitis, autosomal ichthyosis, and control dermatological patients. *Br J Dermatol* 1985; 112: 679–85.
4 Del-Rio E, Vazquez-Veiga H, Aguilar A, Velez A, Sanchez-Yus E. Keratosis punctata of the palmar creases. A report on three generations, demonstrating an association with ichthyosis vulgaris and evidence of involvement of the acrosyringium. *Clin Exp Dermatol* 1994; 19: 165–7.
5 Anton-Lamprecht I, Hofbauer U. Ultrastructural distinction of autosomal dominant ichthyosis vulgaris and X-linked recessive ichthyosis. *Hum Genet* 1972; 15: 261–4.
6 Sybert VP, Dale BA, Holbrook KA. Ichthyosis vulgaris: identification of a defect in synthesis of filaggrin correlated with an absence of keratohyalin granules. *J Invest Dermatol* 1985; 84: 191–4.
7 Nirunsukiri W, Presland RB, Brumbaugh SG, Dale BA, Fleckman P. Decreased profilaggrin expression in ichthyosis vulgaris is a result of selectively impaired post-transcriptional control. *J Biol Chem* 1995; 270: 871–6.
8 Lykkesfeldt G, Hoyer H, Ibsen HH, Brandrup F. Steroid sulphatase deficiency. *Clin Genet* 1985; 28: 231–7.
9 Lundborg H. Geschlechtsverbundene Vererbung von Ichthyosis simplex (vulgaris) in einer schwedischen Bauernsippe. *Hereditas* 1927; 8: 45–8.
10 Traupe H, Happle R. Clinical spectrum of steroid sulfatase deficiency: X-linked recessive ichthyosis, birth complications, and cryptorchidism. *Eur J Pediatr* 1983; 140: 19–21.
11 Traupe H. *The Ichthyoses. A Guide to Clinical Diagnosis. Genetic Counseling and Therapy.* Berlin: Springer-Verlag, 1989: 54–78.
12 Yen P, Allen E, Marsh E *et al.* Cloning and expression of steroid sulfatase cDNA and the frequent occurrence of deletions in steroid sulfatase deficiency: implications for X-Y interchange. *Cell* 1987; 49: 443–53.
13 Paige DG, Emilion GG, Bouloux PM, Harper JI. A clinical and genetic study of X-linked recessive ichthyosis and contiguous gene defects. *Br J Dermatol* 1994; 131: 622–9.
14 Bousema MT, Oranje AP, van Diggelen OP. X-linked ichthyosis and congenital abdominal wall defects. *Int J Dermatol* 1991; 30: 53.
15 Epstein EH, Krauss RM, Shackleton CHL. X-linked ichthyosis: increased blood cholesterol sulfate and electrophoretic mobility of low-density lipoprotein. *Science* 1981; 214: 659–60.
16 Johansen JD, Ramsing D, Vejlsgaard G, Agner T. Skin barrier properties in patients with recessive X-linked ichthyosis. *Acta Derm Venereol* 1995; 75: 202–4.
17 Keitges E, Rivest M, Siniscalco M, Gartler SM. X-linkage of steroid sulphatase in the mouse is evidence for a functional Y-linked allele. *Nature* 1985; 315: 226–7.
18 Müller CR, Migl B, Traupe H, Ropers HH. X-linked steroid sulphatase:

evidence for different gene-dosage in males and females. *Hum Genet* 1980; 54: 197–9.

19 Robledo R, Melis P, Schillinger E *et al.* X-linked ichthyosis without STS deficiency: clinical, genetical, molecular studies. *Am J Med Genet* 1995; 59: 143–8.

Associated ichthyoses of the vulgaris type

Refsum's syndrome (heredopathia atactica polyneuritiformis)

Refsum's syndrome is due to an accumulation of phytanic acid because of a defective phytanic acid oxydase [1]. The disease was first described under the name of heredopathia atactica polyneuritiformis by Sigvald Refsum in the years 1944–1946 [2].

Clinical features

Refsum's syndrome is an autosomal recessive disorder that features failing night vision, retinitis pigmentosa, constriction of visual fields, anosmia, neurosensory deafness, peripheral neuropathy, diminished deep tendon reflexes, an impaired arterioventricula (AV) conduction and a scaly skin resembling a mild form of ichthyosis vulgaris. An infantile form of Refsum's syndrome has been described and is due to deficiency of catalase-containing particles (peroxisomes) [3]. To date infantile Refsum's syndrome has not been associated with skin symptoms and therefore is not discussed in more detail. Only in a few patients does the condition begin in the first year of life. In most patients there is slow but continual evolution of the disease with an onset well after puberty and the presenting sign may be failing night vision. Because Refsum's syndrome is uncommon, its diagnosis is often delayed for many years. Cutaneous features of Refsum's syndrome include a light, fair scaling with a wrinkled appearance of the skin and accentuated palmar creases strikingly similar to those seen in ADI vulgaris. Disseminated naevi which may have a yellow appearance can be of diagnostic value [4] especially if biopsied. Routine histology usually fails to make a clear-cut differential diagnosis from ADI because as in ADI the granular layer can be reduced. The correct diagnosis should be suspected on clinical grounds and special lipid stains, for example with Sudan red which will show marked lipid droplets in the keratinocytes as well as in melanocytes.

An exceptional case of adult Refsum's disease with only very mild retinal changes, normal visual fields and normal dark adaptation has been reported [5].

Therapeutic aspects

A diet low in phytol should be prescribed in all patients. In practice this means that dairy products and green vegeta-bles must be avoided because phytol is a side chain of the chlorophyll molecule and accumulates in dairy products. When this diet is initiated the patient may lose weight initially and the clinical situation could even become worse. Due to the weight loss there can be a mobilization of lipids stored in the subcutaneous tissue and therefore an increase in serum levels of phytanic acid often occurs. Plasmapheresis should then be considered.

Associated steroid sulphatase deficiency

Clinical features

XRI can be associated with a number of other conditions such as Kallman's syndrome, hypertrophic pyloric stenosis [6], unilateral renal aplasia, chondrodysplasia punctata, mental retardation and even hypergonadotropic hypogonadism [7]. The clinical consequences of such associations can be dramatic as far as normal sexual development is concerned. The association of ichthyosis and hypogonadism should prompt the question whether the ichthyosis could represent XRI. Previously such cases have been reported under the misnomer of Rud's syndrome [8].

As discussed above, this is due to contiguous gene defects involving the steroid sulphatase gene and genes in the vicinity of the steroid sulphatase locus. Not only has the gene for Kallman's syndrome been cloned and assigned to the Xp22.3 region [9], but also a gene for chondrodysplasia punctata has been recognized by molecular techniques to represent a further arylsulphatase designated arylsulphatase E. These advances were achieved by extensively analysing DNA from overlapping yeast artificial chromosome clones that included the critical Xp22.3 region. Moreover, two further genes that encode previously unrecognized sulphatases have been identified and these arylsulphatases have been named 'D' and 'F' [10]. Arylsulphatase E is probably inhibited by warfarin and may be the link between exposition to warfarin and its embryopathy which is also characterized by chondrodysplasia punctata. Previously it had been shown that X-linked recessive chondrodysplasia punctata can be due to deletion of the terminal short arm of the X chromosome [11].

Multiple sulphatase deficiency

Clinical features

Multiple sulphatase deficiency is a severe neuropaediatric disorder featuring psychomotor retardation usually starting in the second year of life. Mental regression, speech deterioration and development of severe motor deficits are typical for this condition [12]. Affected children who already may have learned to walk become unsteady and require support to stand or walk. During the third year of life the condition of the children usually rapidly deteriorates. Eventually patients need to be fed via a gastric tube and death usually occurs between 4 and 12 years of age. The neurological findings correspond to those found in the late-onset type of infantile metachromatic leucodystrophy and can be related to arylsulphatase A deficiency. This is thought to be due to a post-translational modification common to all sulphatases. In addition, patients display typical features of mucopolysaccharidosis such as a coarse facial appearance, growth retardation, lumbar kyphosis and hepatosplenomegaly. These symptoms can also be seen in arylsulphatase B deficiency. As a clinical correlate of steroid sulphatase deficiency the children usually present with mild ichthyosis. It should be noted, however, that multiple sulphatase deficiency is also present in girls and the reason for steroid sulphatase deficiency is quite different from that in XRI. Recently a Saudi variant of multiple sulphatase deficiency has been described which takes a more benign course.

Biochemical and genetic aspects

Biochemical evidence supports the notion that in multiple sulphatase deficiency the initial synthesis of sulphatase polypeptides is normal, but the half-life of these sulphatases is much reduced to 4–6h compared to 6 days in normal cells [13]. From a biochemical point of view, multiple sulphatase deficiency is quite unique since seven known sulphatases become deficient. Multiple sulphatase deficiency should be suspected in children with a neurodegenerative disorder also featuring ichthyosis. Because multiple sulphatase deficiency is very uncommon the dermatologist is not very likely to be confronted with these children, who are usually taken care of by paediatricians and neurologists, since ichthyosis is only a minor complaint.

REFERENCES

1 Dykes PJ, Marks R, Davies MG, Reynold DJ. Epidermal metabolism in heredopathia atactica polyneuritiformis (Refsum's disease). *J Invest Dermatol* 1978; 70: 126–9.
2 Refsum S. Heredopathia atactica polyneuritiformis. *Acta Psychiatr Scand* 1946; 38(suppl): 1–303.
3 Wanders RJ, Schutgens RB, Schrakanp G *et al*. Infantile Refsum disease: deficiency of catalase-containing particles (peroxisomes), alkyldihydroxyacetone phosphate synthase and peroxisomal beta-oxidation enzyme proteins. *Eur J Pediatr* 1986; 145: 172–5.
4 Puissant A, Dry J, Noury JY, Laudat P, Noury-Duperrat G. Syndrome de Refsum-Thiebaut avec naevi xanthomateuse disséminés. *Bull Soc Franc Dermatol Syph* 1972; 79: 462–4.
5 Yamamoto S, Onozu H, Yamada N, Hayasaka S, Watanabe A. Mild retinal changes in a 47-year-old patient with phytanic acid storage disease. *Ophthalmologica* 1995; 209: 251–5.
6 Stoll C, Grosshans E, Binder P, Roth M. Hypertrophic pyloric stenosis associated with X-linked ichthyosis in two brothers. *Clin Exp Dermatol* 1983; 8: 61–4.
7 Paige DG, Emillion GG, Bouloux PMG, Harper JI. A Clinical and genetic study of X-linked recessive ichthyosis and contiguous gene defects. *Br J Dermatol* 1994; 131: 622–9.
8 Traupe H. *The Ichthyoses. A Guide to Clinical Diagnosis, Genetic Counseling and Therapy*. Berlin: Springer-Verlag, 1984; 91–7.
9 Franco B, Guioli S, Pragliola A *et al*. A gene deleted in Kallmann's syndrome shares homology with neural cell adhesion and axonal path-finding molecules. *Nature* 1991; 353: 529–36.
10 Franco B, Meroni G, Parenti G *et al*. A cluster of sulfatase genes on Xp22.3: mutations in chondrodysplasia punctata (CDPX) and implications for warfarin embryopathy. *Cell* 1995; 81: 15–25.
11 Curry CJR, Magenis RE, Brown M *et al*. Inherited chondrodysplasia punctata due to a deletion of the terminal short arm of an X-chromosome. *N Engl J Med* 1984; 311: 1010–15.
12 Rampini S, Isler W, Baerlocher K, Bischoff A, Ulrich J, Plüss HJ. Die Kombination von metachromatischer Leukodystrophie und Mucopolysaccharidose als selbständiges Krankheitsbild (Mukosulfatose). *Helv Pediatr Acta* 1970; 25: 436–61.
13 Horwitz AL, Warshawsky L, King J, Burns G. Rapid degradation of steroid sulfatase in multiple sulfatase deficiency. *Biochem Biophys Res Commun* 1986; 135: 389–96.

Isolated congenital ichthyoses

Harlequin ichthyosis

An extensive discussion of harlequin ichthyosis as well as its differential diagnosis from collodion baby and other types of congenital ichthyoses is given in Chapter 1.10.

The lamellar ichthyoses

Biochemical studies and molecular genetics

Lamellar ichthyosis comprises several genetic entities but it has been extremely difficult to appreciate these different types by clinical, histological or ultrastructural means. Many, but not all children with lamellar ichthyosis are born as a collodion baby (Fig. 19.5.5), i.e. they are encased in a membrane which covers the skin. Most of these collodion babies later develop into lamellar ichthyosis, but a self-healing type of collodion baby is recognized [1].

The term lamellar ichthyosis is usually used as a synonym with non-bullous congenital ichthyosis. For a

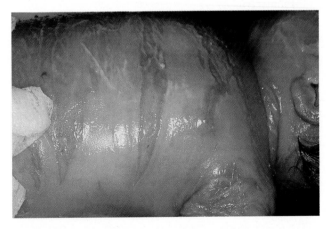

Fig. 19.5.5 Collodion baby. Courtesy of Professor Happle, Marburg.

long time it was believed to represent a single entity, but in 1984 a distinct autosomal dominant subtype of lamellar ichthyosis was delineated [2].

In the following years ultrastructural investigations [3,4] and lipid biochemical studies [5] suggested further heterogeneity of autosomal recessive lamellar ichthyosis (ARLI). In particular Williams and Elias claimed to distinguish between an erythrodermic subtype of lamellar ichthyosis characterized by elevated *N*-alkanes in scales and a non-erythrodermic subtype in which normal *N*-alkanes but increased free steroids were found in the scales. While it cannot be disputed that some patients show very high *N*-alkane levels in their scales, these lipids probably have an exogeneous origin [6]. Other groups tried to attack the problem of ARLI by employing enzymatic methods based on scale analysis and this seemed to support the essential dichotomy of lamellar ichthyosis into an erythrodermic versus a non-erythrodermic type [7]. However, from a clinical point of view it has to be stated that even within the same family, and that means within the same mutation, the phenotype of lamellar ichthyosis can vary considerably and be both erythrodermic and non-erythrodermic [8,9].

Ultrastructural examination may provide better markers than the analysis of scale lipids or scale enzymes and Kanerva *et al.* [3] described a type characterized by massive cholesterol depositions within the stratum corneum. A further type characterized by vacuolated membrane structures within the keratinocytes of the granular and spinous layer and abnormal vesicular keratinosomes (lamellar bodies) has been described [4]. These two types can then be distinguished from a type that has no such features. In individual patients further subtypes have been postulated on the grounds of subtle changes when examined by electron microscopy.

Because electron microscopy is not available in many departments of dermatology and because the above-mentioned changes are quite subtle it remains to be seen how useful an ultrastructural approach to classification is in the long term.

More recently Hohl *et al.* performed an analysis of the cornified cell envelope in lamellar ichthyosis and pointed out the disturbed membrane anchorage of transglutaminase 1 [10]. It was assumed that this disturbed membrane anchorage could alter the cross-linking of loricrin and involucrin when forming the cornified cell envelope. This line of work has continued and the same group have shown that some, but not all, patients have point mutations in transglutaminase 1 [11]. In contrast, in a previous study using scale as a material, membrane-bound transglutaminase was found to be either normal in patients with lamellar ichthyosis or even to be three-fold elevated in patients with a non-erythrodermic phenotype [12].

Molecular studies have shown that many, but not all, families with ARLI show linkage with the 14q region,

where the gene for transglutaminase K resides [13]. Moreover, in a few patients point mutations affecting the transglutaminase gene have been found [14]. However, many patients apparently seem to have compound mutations and the functional relevance of the mutations is not yet clear. Because the epidermis contains several different types of transglutaminase, such as tissue transglutaminase, epidermal transglutaminase and transglutaminase K, it is conceivable that a defect in one of these can be partly compensated by the others. Histochemical investigation by the author's own group on a series of six probands from four families showed a marked reduction of transglutaminase 1 when assayed by incorporation of biotinylated monodansylcadaverin in two out of six patients [15]. Direct histochemical analysis has shown that also self-healing collodion baby is often associated with transglutaminase 1 deficiency (M Raghunath, personal communication, 1999).

Autosomal dominant lamellar ichthyosis

Autosomal dominant lamellar ichthyosis was first described in 1984 [2] and is characterized by large dark grey scales covering the entire body and a very pronounced plantar keratosis with yellowish scales. The palms are less severely involved, but can exhibit accentuated creases. On the back of the hands, feet, wrists and knees there can be prominent lichenification.

Histological investigations show a hyperplastic epidermis and an increased granular layer. Ultrastructural investigations have revealed an increased transforming zone of up to six cell layers between the granular and the horny cell layer. Normally this zone measures only one cell layer [16]. Further cases of autosomal dominant lamellar ichthyosis have been reported from Spain and France [17,18].

Autosomal recessive lamellar ichthyosis

Patients suffering from ARLI can be born with a clinical phenotype of a collodion baby. When the collodion membrane peels off some of the patients suffer at birth from marked ichthyotic erythroderma, which means that the entire skin is highly inflamed. This erythroderma should not be mixed up with the rather subtle erythema which can be seen in almost all types of lamellar ichthyosis. It should be noted that even those types of lamellar ichthyosis which traditionally have been regarded as belonging to the classical lamellar type and being non-erythrodermic also show some residual erythema below the scales. Patients with the erythrodermic phenotype of lamellar ichthyosis tend to have very marked involvement of the palms and soles and, often, in later life, the scales in these patients are translucent and scaling can be mild. In contrast there are patients with a non-erythrodermic course of lamellar ichthyosis who often exhibit plate-like dark grey scales and usually show only slight involvement of the palms and soles. In the author's experience, these patients often show transglutaminase 1 deficiency. As stated above, some patients cannot be classified along the lines of erythrodermic or non-erythrodermic lamellar ichthyosis, and it should be borne in mind that apparently even transglutaminase 1 deficiency features a broad clinical spectrum.

From a genetic point of view, it can be stated that lamellar ichthyosis (non-bullous congenital ichthyosis) is heterogeneous because autosomal dominant lamellar ichthyosis could be excluded from the long arm of chromosome 14 (A. Reis, personal communication, 1996) and because even in ARLI linkage studies have firmly established genetic heterogeneity [19].

The epidermolytic ichthyoses

Epidermolytic ichthyoses are those types of ichthyoses which can be bullous and at the histological level are characterized by the features of epidermolytic hyperkeratosis. From a clinical point of view, at least three different types can be distinguished; BIE, annular epidermolytic ichthyosis (AEI) and IBS. The former two entities are caused either by mutations in keratin 1 or 10 [20,21] while IBS is due to a different keratin, keratin 2e, which is expressed only in the upper layer of the stratum granulosum [22,23]. The assumption that ichthyosis hystrix of Curth–Macklin also constitutes an epidermolytic ichthyosis [9] was based on the very similiar histological appearance of this disease. However, linkage analysis done in one family with ichthyosis hystrix Curth–Macklin excluded the gene from the common keratin gene loci [24].

Bullous ichthyotic erythroderma of Brocq

This autosomal dominant disease is characterized by marked erythroderma and severe blistering at birth (Fig. 19.5.6). During the first year of life the blistering and erythema usually become less and hystrix-like keratoses develop instead. Predilection sites are the axilla, the elbows and flexural aspects. In some families patients have severe involvement of the palms and soles and harbour mutations in keratin 1, while keratin 10 mutations appear to be unassociated with the presence of palmoplantar involvement.

Histological features

Histological examination of BIE reveals a basket-weave orthohyperkeratosis, a huge stratum corneum and strong periodic acid–Schiff (PAS)-positive deposits in the horny layer. The granular layer as well as the spinous layer is degenerated (Fig. 19.5.7). Coarse keratohyalin granules can be seen. The keratinocytes of the granular layer and the spinous cell layer show cytoplasmic oedema and a perinuclear vacuolization, whereas the basal and suprabasal keratinocytes usually appear normal.

Genetic aspects

As discussed above, the disease is due to mutations either in keratin 1 or 10. It should be noted that sometimes this mutation can occur *de novo* and may manifest itself in the parent generation only in the form of an epidermal naevus showing on histological examination epidermolytic hyperkeratosis [25,26]. This constellation is indicative of germ-line mosaicism and the presence of an epidermal naevus showing the histological features of epidermolytic hyperkeratosis should alert the doctor to discuss with the patient the possibility of the development of full-blown BIE in his or her children.

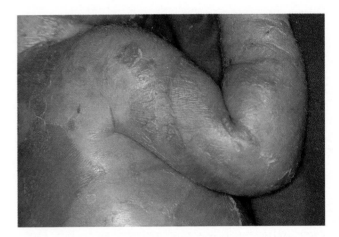

Fig. 19.5.6 BIE in a neonate with 'enfant brûlé'. Courtesy of Dr Peter Steijlen, Nijmegen.

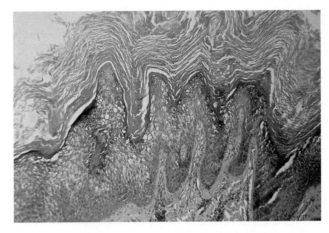

Fig. 19.5.7 Histopathological features of epidermolytic hyperkeratosis in BIE.

Annular epidermolytic ichthyosis

AEI represents a distinct clinical phenotype characterized by the development of numerous annular polycyclic erythematous hyperkeratotic plaques on the trunk and the proximal extremities [27]. The disease is much milder than classical BIE and the probands suffer from bouts of disease activity.

Histological examination shows the typical pathology of epidermolytic hyperkeratosis and an abnormal keratin filament network. However, one has to take the biopsy from a site with maximal clinical involvement. Molecular analysis of one family revealed a CG to GA two base pair mutation in the same allele of keratin 10 in the affected individuals, resulting in an arginine to glutamate substitution at residue 83 of the 2B helical segment [28]. The mild phenotype of AEI may thus be due to a position effect of the mutation which affects the centre of the rod domain and not the ends of the rod domain.

Ichthyosis bullosa of Siemens

Ichthyosis of Siemens was first described by Siemens in 1937 [29], who compared the blistering in this disease to that of epidermolysis bullosa simplex and stressed that the blisters occurred after minor mechanical trauma. The absence of erythroderma and a different distribution of involved skin areas, namely the sparing of the trunk except for a small region around the navel, prompted Siemens to separate the entity from the BIE of Brocq. In 1986 the author reported a second family and recognized the histological features of this disease as being those of epidermolytic hyperkeratosis. However, in contrast to BIE epidermolytic hyperkeratosis affects only the granular layer and is much less pronounced than in BIE. From a clinical point of view very often large superficially denuded areas can be seen in this phenomenon which were called 'Mauserung' by Siemens (Fig. 19.5.8). Hyperkeratoses are rather prominent on flexural sites as well as over the knees and elbows and on the back of the hands and feet. In contrast, palms and soles are always spared from the hyperkeratotic process.

As is the case in IBS, it is very important to choose a site of maximal scaling for the biopsy in order to appreciate the typical features of epidermolytic hyperkeratosis in this disease [30]. It is of interest that mutations in keratin 2e underlying this disease tend to cluster in the highly conserved carboxy-terminal of the rod domain of keratin 2e revealing a mutational hot-spot [22].

Ichthyosis hystrix of Curth–Macklin

In 1954 Ollendorff-Curth and Macklin [31] reported on a family with an ichthyosis hystrix-like cornification disorder. Despite many clinical resemblances to BIE and many

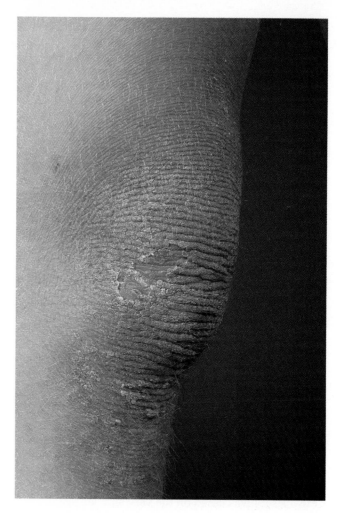

Fig. 19.5.8 IBS: Mauserung phenomenon (denudation) on a knee.

histological resemblances to epidermolytic hyperkeratosis, Anton-Lamprecht *et al.* were able to detect subtle ultrastructural differences between BIE and ichthyosis hystrix of Curth–Macklin [32]. Molecular analyses excluded a keratin gene in at least one family, which seems to support this distinction. From a clinical point of view some family members suffer from ichthyotic erythrodermas while others do not. In typical cases the entire trunk as well as the flexural surfaces of the extremities and the palms and soles are covered by very heavy, papillomatous dark hyperkeratosis. Blisters generally do not occur in this disease.

Genetic counselling of the epidermolytic ichthyoses

The epidermolytic ichthyoses can be very severe and some parents may want a prenatal diagnosis. In those cases, in which a molecular work-up of keratin mutations has been done, this will be possible, for example with a chorion biopsy and subsequent DNA analysis. Even in cases with no previous genetic work-up a prenatal diagnosis can be tried because the mutations in these diseases tend to cluster in mutational hot-spots. Moreover, fetoscopy and ultrastructural analysis of the specimen obtained could be performed in centres specialized in these procedures. In any case, one should discuss the question of possible prenatal diagnosis well in advance and contact either the molecular or the ultrastructural centre in due time. Also it is meaningful to discuss with the parents whether they are sure that they want an abortion if the child is affected. For a mother it may be difficult to follow through with the pregnancy when she is aware that her child will have a severe skin disease. Sometimes, it may be easier not to know the outcome of the pregnancy in advance.

REFERENCES

1 Frenk E, de Techtermann F. Self-healing collodion baby: evidence for autosomal recessive inheritance. *Pediatr Dermatol* 1992; 9: 95–7.

2 Traupe H, Kolde G, Happle R. Autosomal dominant lamellar ichthyosis: a new skin disorder. *Clin Genet* 1984; 26: 457–61.

3 Kanerva L, Niemi K-M, Lauharanta J, Lassus A. New observations on the fine structure of lamellar ichthyosis and the effect of treatment with etretinate. *Am J Dermatopathol* 1983; 5: 555–67.

4 Arnold ML, Anton-Lamprecht I, Melz-Rothfuss B, Hartschuh W. Ichthyosis congenita type III. Clinical and ultrastructural characteristics and distinction within the heterogenerous ichthyosis congenita group. *Arch Dermatol Res* 1988; 280: 268–78.

5 Williams ML, Elias PM. Heterogeneity in autosomal recessive ichthyosis. Clinical and biochemical differentiation of lamellar ichthyosis and nonbullous congenital ichthyosiform erythroderma. *Arch Dermatol* 1985; 121: 477–88.

6 Williams ML, Vogel JS, Ghadially R, Brown BE, Elias PM. Exogenous origin of N-alkanes in pathologic scale. *Arch Dermatol* 1992; 128: 1065–71.

7 Bergers M, Traupe H, Dunnwald SC et al. Enzymatic distinction between two subgroups of autosomal recessive lamellar ichthyosis. *J Invest Dermatol* 1990; 94: 407–12.

8 Bernhardt M, Baden HP. Report of a family with an unusual expression of recessive ichthyosis. Review of 42 cases. *Arch Dermatol* 1986; 122: 428–33.

9 Traupe H. *The Ichthyoses. A Guide to Clinical Diagnosis, Genetic Counseling and Therapy.* Berlin: Springer-Verlag, 1989: 111–34.

10 Hohl D, Huber M, Frenk E. Analysis of the cornified cell envelope in lamellar ichthyosis. *Arch Dermatol* 1993; 129: 618–24.

11 Huber M, Rettler I, Bernasconi K et al. Mutations of keratinocyte transglutaminase in lamellar ichthyosis. *Science* 1995; 267: 525–8.

12 van Hooijdonk CAEM, Steijlen PM, Bergers M, Mier PD, Traupe H, Happle R. Epidermal transglutaminase in the ichthyoses. *Acta Derm Venerol* 1991; 71: 173–5.

13 Russell LJ, DiGiovanna JJ, Hashem N, Compton JG, Bale SJ. Linkage of autosomal recessive lamellar ichthyosis to chromosome 14q. *Am J Hum Genet* 1994; 55: 1146–52.

14 Russell LJ, DiGiovanna JJ, Rogers GR et al. Mutations in the gene for transglutaminase 1 in autosomal recessive lamellar ichthyosis. *Nat Genet* 1995; 9: 279–83.

15 Ragunath M, Hennies HC, Velten F, Wiebe V, Steinert PM, Reis A, Traupe H. A novel in situ method for the detection of deficient transglutaminase activity in the skin. *Arch Dermatol Res* 1998; 290: 621–7.

16 Kolde G, Happle R, Traupe H. Autososmal dominant lamellar ichthyosis: ultrastructural characteristics of a new type of congenital ichthyosis. *Arch Dermatol Res* 1985; 278: 1–5.

17 Toribo J, Redondo VF, Peteiro C, Zulaica A, Fabeiro JM. Autosomal dominant lamellar ichthyosis. *Clin Genet* 1986; 30: 122–6.

18 Larrègue M, Ottavy N, Bressieux JM, Lorette J. Bébé collidion. Trente-deux nouvelles observations. *Ann Dermatol Vénéréol* 1986; 113: 773–85.

19 Parmentier L, Blanchet-Bardon C, Nguyen S, Prud'homme JF, Dubertret L, Weissenbach J. Autosomal recessive lamellar ichthyosis: identification of a new mutation in transglutaminase 1 and evidence for genetic hetrogeneity. *Hum Mol Genet* 1995; 4: 1391–5.

20 Rothnagel JA, Dominey AM, Dempsey LP et al. Mutations in the rod domain of keratins 1 and 10 in epidermolytic hyperkeratosis. *Science* 1992; 257: 1128–30.

21 Chipev CC, Korge BP, Markova N et al. A leucine–proline mutation in the H1 subdomain of keratin 1 causes epidermolytic hyperkeratosis. *Cell* 1992; 70: 821–8.

22 Rothnagel JA, Traupe H, Wojcik S et al. Mutations in the rod domain of keratin 2e in patients with ichthyosis bullosa of Siemens. *Nat Genet* 1994; 7: 485–90.

23 Kremer H, Zeeuwen P, McLean WH et al. Ichthyosis bullosa of Siemens is caused by mutations in the keratin 2e gene. *J Invest Dermatol* 1994; 103: 286–9.

24 Bonifas JM, Bare JW, Chen MA, Ranki A, Neimi KM, Epstein EH Jr. Evidence against keratin gene mutations in a family with ichthyosis hystrix Curth–Macklin. *J Invest Dermatol* 1993; 101: 890–1.

25 Lookingbill DP, Laddu RL, Cohen C. Generalized epidermolytic hyperkeratosis in a child of a parent with nevus comedonicus. *Arch Dermatol* 1984; 120: 223–6.

26 Nazzzaro V, Ermacora E, Santucci B, Caputo R. Epidermolytic hyperkeratosis: generalized form in children from parents with systematized linear form. *Br J Dermatol* 1990; 122: 417–22.

27 Sahn EE, Weimer CE Jr, Garen PD. Annular epidermolytic ichthyosis: a unique phenotype. *J Am Acad Dermatol* 1992; 27: 348–55.

28 Joh G-Y, Traupe H, Rothnagel JA et al. A novel dinucleotide mutation in keratin 10 in the annular epidermolytic ichthyosis variant of bullous congenital ichthyosiform erythroderma. *J Invest Dermatol* 1997; 108: 357–61.

29 Siemens HW. Dichtung und Wahrheit über die Ichthyosis bullosa mit Bemerkungen zur Systematik der Epidermolysen. *Arch Dermatol* 1937; 175: 590–608.

30 Traupe H, Kolde G, Hamm H, Happle R. Ichthyosis bullosa of Siemens: a unique type of epidermolytic hyperkeratosis. *J Am Acad Dermatol* 1986; 14: 1000–5.

31 Ollendorf-Curth H, Allen FH Jr, Schnyder UW, Anton-Lamprecht I. Follow-up of a family group suffering from ichthyosis hystrix type Curth–Macklin. *Hum Genet* 1972; 17: 37–48.

32 Anton-Lamprecht I, Curth HO, Schnyder UW. Zur Ultrastruktur hereditärer Verhornungsstörungen. II. Ichthyosis hystrix Typ Curth–Macklin. *Arch Dermatol Forsch* 1973; 246: 77–91.

Associated congenital ichthyoses

Sjögren–Larsson syndrome

Clinical features

This syndrome was delineated by Sjögren and Larsson in 1957, who reported on 28 patients belonging to 13 families and concluded that these patients who exhibited pronounced congenital ichthyosis, severe mental retardation, symmetric spastic paralysis and an ocular involvement characterized by glistening spots, suffered from a distinct genetic disease [1]. In the North Swedish province of Västerbotten the incidence of this disease is 10.2 per 100 000 inhabitants, while it is very rare outside Sweden [2]. Most cases in Germany can be related to a Swedish source of the gene and in particular to movements of the Swedish army during the Thirty Years War in Germany. Onset of the neurological manifestations—pathological reflexes, muscular hypertonus, paralysis of legs and mental retardation—is usually between 4 and 13 months of age [3]. The cutaneous findings are rather typical and characterized by yellowish or dark-brown papillomatous keratoses, giving the skin a lichenified appearance

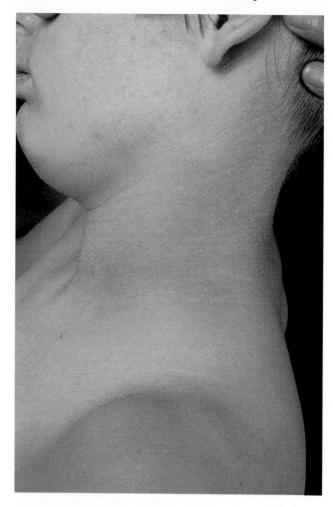

Fig. 19.5.9 Sjögren–Larsson syndrome: keratotic lichenification.

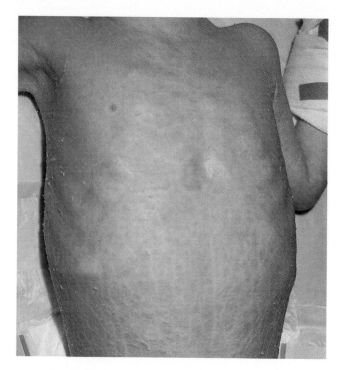

Fig. 19.5.10 Ichthyosis in Tay's syndrome.

(Fig. 19.5.9). These typical changes can be noted at the age of a few months, so that the correct diagnosis can be suspected in the neonatal period while the neurological and more florid dermatological symptoms become manifest later.

Histological features

The histology of the Sjögren–Larsson syndrome is non-specific and shows the features of a hyperplastic epidermis.

Biochemical aspects

A defect of fatty alcohol oxidation has been recognized in fibroblasts in the epidermis and jejunal mucosa from Sjögren–Larsson syndrome patients as the main biochemical alteration underlying this disease [4]. Linkage studies show that the locus for Sjögren–Larsson syndrome is between the locus D17S805 on the centromeric part of chromosome 17 and D17S783 and D17S959 on the telomeric side of this chromosome [5].

The human gene for fatty aldehyde dehydrogenase (FALDH) has been shown to map to the Sjögren–Larsson syndrome region on chromosome 17 on the short arm (p11.2) [6]. Moreover, sequence analysis of FALDH amplified from fibroblast mRNA and genomic DNA from three unrelated patients revealed distinct mutations including deletions and insertions and a point mutation in this gene which plays a role in fatty alcohol oxydation. These findings suggest that Sjögren–Larsson syndrome is actually caused by mutations in the FALDH gene. However, it should be noted that a few patients with striking similarities to the Sjögren–Larsson syndrome—also showing ichthyosis, mental retardation and asymptomatic spasticity—have been described who exhibit a normal fatty alcohol aldehyde dehydrogenase activity and thus may have a neurocutaneous disorder distinct from Sjögren–Larsson syndrome [7].

Trichothiodystrophy syndromes

Clinical features

Trichothiodystrophy, or sulphur-deficient brittle hair, is an autosomal recessive disorder characterized by reduced sulphur content and mental and physical retardation. Numerous additional clinical features may be present, producing a range of heterogeneous syndromes. Many cases exhibit ichthyosis (Fig. 19.5.10) and are referred to as Tay syndrome [8,9]. In fact Tay first pointed out the peculiar association of ichthyotic erythroderma, hair shaft abnormalities and mental and growth retardation as a new recessive disorder.

Using polarization microscopy it was found that the hair shafts in Tay's syndrome exhibit a zebra-like pattern of dark and light bands (Fig. 19.5.11) identical to that seen in the brittle hair, intellectual impairment, decreased fertility and short stature (BIDS) syndrome [10]. Later, it was found that some patients regarded as having Tay's syndrome also exhibit severe photosensitivity and that in these patients a facial dysmorphism different from that seen in most patients with Tay's syndrome is present. These differences prompted Rebora and Crovoto to regard this group of patients as suffering from the PIBIDS syndrome [11].

Since then it has been established that patients with the PIBIDS syndrome suffer from a DNA defect and that this DNA repair defect is due to mutations in the gene for xeroderma pigmentosum type D [12]. This is quite surprising since patients with trichothiodystrophy whether they represent the BIDS syndrome, the Tay syndrome or the PIBIDS syndrome do not suffer from skin cancer. Nevertheless, several independent investigations have established that the gene product of the xeroderma pigmentosum type D (XPD) gene, which is a DNA helicase, shows mutations in a number of patients with trichothiodystrophy. It is of interest that mutations in the same gene can also give rise to Cockayne's syndrome, which is a multisystem disorder with profound growth retardation, progressive pigmentary retinopathy, optic disc atrophy, cataracts and a characteristic facies with large sunken eyes, temporal wasting and a thin prominent nose. Further symptoms of Cockayne's syndrome include neurological abnormalities such as delayed psychomotor development, mental retardation, microcephaly, spasticity, ataxia and sensorineural deafness.

It is difficult to understand how it is possible that the same gene accounts for three rather distinct groups of diseases—xeroderma pigmentosum (a disease characterized by skin cancer), Cockayne's syndrome and the spectrum of trichothiodystrophy syndromes. The possible explanation could be that the *XPD* gene product is not only involved in nucleotide excision repair but is also part of a complex of proteins that serves as a transcription factor, i.e. transcription-factor IIh (TFIIH), and that thus genes involved in trichothiodystrophy syndromes have essential roles in transcription. Chu and Mayne have advanced the hypotheses that the XPD gene product in its function as a transcription factor can affect the methylation status of nearby genes and that a possible role of the gene product in demethylation could consequently influence developmental regulation of gene expression and underlie the decrease of sulphur-rich hair proteins in these disorders [13].

In summary, only two of the many syndromes caused by mutations in the XPD gene exhibit ichthyosis—Tay's and PIBIDS syndrome. Clinically, Tay's syndrome is characterized by severe congenital ichthyosis, brittle hair, dysplastic nails, mild mental retardation, growth retardation and a proneness to infections and hypergonadism, whereas PIBIDS syndrome is characterized by a mild ichthyosis, marked photosensitivity, an unusual facies that is not progeroid, a proneness to infections, short stature, mental retardation, dysplastic nails and the same hair abnormalities, such as trichoschisis and the typical tiger-tail pattern on polarizing microscopy.

Prenatal diagnosis of the trichothiodystrophy syndromes is possible if they exhibit a DNA repair defect [14] and in the future it should be possible to obtain a prenatal diagnosis by demonstration of the underlying mutations in the XPD gene.

Comèl–Netherton syndrome

Clinical features

The Comèl–Netherton syndrome is an autosomal recessive disease of unknown cause. Severe congenital generalized exfoliative erythroderma in newborns and infants can be a possible first sign of this disease (Fig. 19.5.12), which has previously been misdiagnosed as generalized seborrhoeic dermatitis (Leiner's disease) [15,16]. In many cases the eczema-like changes disappear during the first year of life and ichthyosis linearis circumflexa [17] develops. According to the literature this particular phenotype with typical annular and serpiginous lesions, often bordered by distinctive double-edged scales, is the predominant phenotype seen in patients (Fig. 19.5.13). However, Traupe and others have argued that the more severe involvement in which the entire integument remains inflamed even in adult life may be underdiagnosed [18]. This latter phenotype corresponds to severe congenital ichthyotic erythroderma. Both ends of the spectrum of the

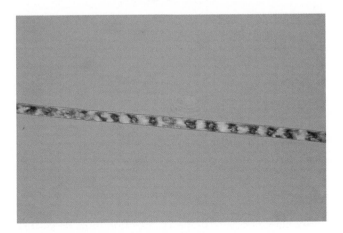

Fig. 19.5.11 Zebra pattern of dark and light bands of a hair using polarizing microscopy in Tay's syndrome.

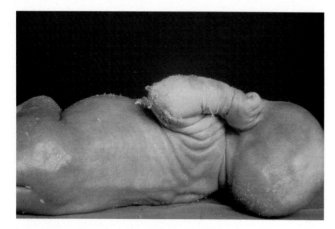

Fig. 19.5.12 Comèl–Netherton syndrome showing congenital generalized exfoliative erythroderma in a neonate. This girl died from pseudomonas sepis at 10 months.

Comèl–Netherton syndrome have in common a peculiar hair abnormality, which is referred to as trichorrhexis invaginata (Fig. 19.5.14). In order to make a definite diagnosis, it is important to shave hair from the scalp and perhaps even to investigate hairs from the eyebrows. The Comèl–Netherton syndrome is often associated with atopy, and failure to thrive in infancy is a feature in many severely affected patients. This failure to thrive can be life-threatening and recurrent infections can form part of the clinical syndrome [15,18]. In severely affected patients the disease often has a lethal outcome.

Histological features

Histological examination reveals pronounced dermal inflammatory processes as well as exocytosis of the lymphocytes, macrophages and neutrophils. In severely affected cases the upper prickle cell layer often shows degenerative and necrolytic changes with blurred cell boundaries, contrasting with the hyperplastic lower most portion of the epidermis. In patients with the ichthyosis linearis circumflexa similar eczematous but less pronounced changes are found. The granular layer is usually diminished and may be lacking completely in those parts of the biopsy which correspond to the active border of the specimen. On electron microscopy inclusion bodies can be seen in keratinocytes of the granular and prickle cell layer, but similar inclusion bodies are found in other diseases with the histology of an acute eczema. The typical hair abnormality, trichorrhexis invaginata, may be caused by periodic inflammatory changes in deep follicular areas during eczematous episodes. Such an incomplete cornification within the keratogenous zone of the growing hair shaft would lead to circumscribed segments with weak cortical keratin and subsequent intussusception of the distal shaft into the proximal portion could cause the hair abnormality.

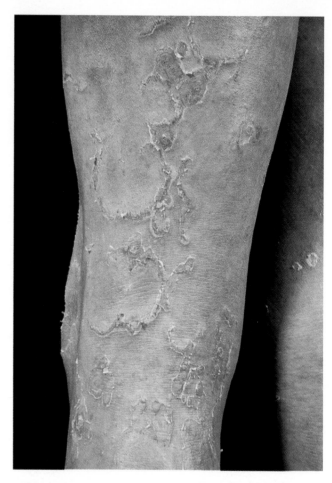

Fig. 19.5.13 Ichthyosis linearis circumflexa as a cutaneous mild manifestation of Comèl–Netherton syndrome.

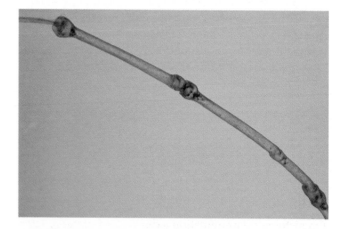

Fig. 19.5.14 Trichorrhexis invaginata in the Comèl–Netherton syndrome.

Treatment

In the newborn period special attention must be paid to the problems of hypernatraemic dehydration and because of a failure to thrive some infants can be prone to develop serious and life-threatening infections, which may require hospitalization in the intensive care unit.

Happle's syndrome

Clinical features

Happle's syndrome is an X-linked dominant type of ichthyosis that was defined in 1977–1979 by Rudolph Happle as an X-linked dominant variant of chondrodysplasia punctata characterized by a mosaic pattern of skin lesions [19,20]. For historic reasons, this type is also sometimes referred to as Conradi–Hünermann type which shows autosomal dominant inheritance. Since then, the existence of the so-called autosomal dominant Conradi–Hünermann type has become disputed because a number of cases published many years ago showing no skin involvement and referred to as Conradi–Hünermann type have now been recognized as examples of warfarin embryopathy [21].

The main features of Happle's syndrome are chondrodysplasia punctata, severe erythrodermic ichthyosis at birth evolving into streaky hyperkeratosis in later life, patchy cicatricial alopecia, cataracts, which are often sectorial, and short stature [19,22]. In older children systemized atrophoderma mainly involving the hair follicles (Fig. 19.5.15), pigmentory disturbances and ichthyosis are noted. The hyperkeratoses are arranged in a mosaic-like pattern following the lines of Blaschko and are more pronounced in atrophic areas.

Non-cutaneous findings include stippled calcifications of the area of enchondral bone formation, which is a characteristic skeletal manifestion of all chondrodysplasia punctata types, a short stature and asymmetric shortening of legs giving rise to moderate or severe kyphoscoliosis in later life. However, a symmetrical shortening of the tubular bones has also been reported in a girl with typical cutaneous involvement [23]. Unilateral hexadactyly and severe dysplasia of the hip joints can also be noted in some cases. Many patients show an asymmetric facial appearance and frontal bossing. Cataracts can be seen in up to two-thirds of cases. They can be sectorial and confined to a quadrant of the eye [22].

Histological and ultrastructural features

On histological examination a diminished granular layer, slight acanthosis and perivascular infiltrates in the upper dermis can be seen. Follicular hyperkeratosis can be striking. Special stains for calcium may reveal calcifications in the epidermis especially in areas displaying follicular hyperkeratosis. On electron microscopy a large number of electron-lucent vacuoles containing electron-dense stellate bodies can be seen in the keratinocytes of the granular layer. These bodies probably represent calcium crystals.

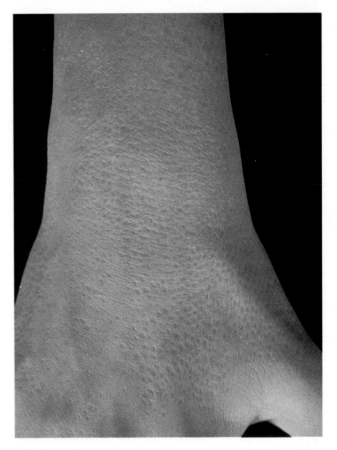

Fig. 19.5.15 Happle syndrome: note the follicular atrophoderma in an older child.

Moreover, degeneration of Langerhans' cells is a further typical finding [24].

Newborn babies suffering from Happle's syndrome exhibit thick and spiky adherent hyperkeratosis on their whole body. The histopathological examination of thick scales from such hyperkeratotic lesions often display calcium in the centre of these keratotic plaques. Histopathological examination of such thick scales is easy and the scales can be collected without pain so that the examination of such scales is helpful in making the diagnosis of Happle's syndrome [25].

Genetic aspects

Because of a homologous mouse mutant which shares the major clinical findings of Happle's syndrome and which also behaves as an X-linked dominant trait that is lethal for male embryos [26], it was expected that the gene for Happle's syndrome should be located in humans on the X chromosome Xq28 region. However, multiple recombinations in a linkage study of three families excluded the Xq28 region as a site of the gene [27]. Surprisingly, multiple crossovers were found with 26 other markers spread along the rest of the X chromosome and two point linkage analysis seems to exclude the gene from the entire X chromosome. To account for the paradox of an X-linked gene which is excluded from the X chromosome the hypothesis of an unstable premutation that can become silent in males has been advanced [28]. This last explanation would also account for the unexpected sex ratio of males to females of 1.2 to 1 among surviving siblings and for the striking clinical variability of the phenotype, including stepwise increases in disease expression in sucessive generations. So far, Happle's syndrome has been observed in four boys [29]. It is of interest that one of these cases concerns an XXY male, i.e. a patient with Klinefelter's syndrome [30]. A similar situation has been found among males with incontinentia pigmenti who also show a mosaic disease expression, and in four of 12 cases studied cytogenetically had an XXY karyotype. Very recently mutations in the emopamil binding protein that acts as a δ 8–δ 7 sterol isomerase have been identified in several patients with Happle's syndrome [31]. Apparently these mutations are stable.

Dorfman's syndrome

Clinical features

In 1974 Maurice Dorfman *et al.* [32] delineated this entity which is characterized by congenital ichthyosis, severe fatty changes of the liver and variable neurological and ocular involvement. At birth, mild ichthyotic erythroderma is often present and the scaling is generalized and fine. Due to the hyperkeratosis, the skin may have a lichenified appearance [33]. Non-cutaneous findings include involvement of the eye, muscles, nerves, liver and possibly also the gastrointestinal tract. Bilateral cataracts can be present in infancy or develop during adult life. Elevated serum muscle enzymes reflect mild muscular weakness. The neurological impairment includes ataxia, bilateral neurosensory hearing loss and a fine horizontal nystagmus. Liver biopsies often disclose a severe fatty degeneration.

The typical diagnostic features are multiple lipid vacuoles in virtually every granulocyte and monocyte but not in small lymphocytes when blood cells are stained in a Wright stained buffy coat preparation. This phenomenon is also called Jordon's anomaly and is due to the accumulation of neutral lipids in this storage disease [34]. Patients often have a Mediterranean descent and cases in Sicily could be attributed to the Arab domination of Sicily during the seventh century [35]. Two siblings with the typical clinical features of this multisystem triglyceride storage disorder have been described who lacked congenital ichthyosis.

Hystrix-like ichthyosis with deafness (HID) syndrome

Clinical features

HID syndrome is characterized shortly after birth by red patches developing on the skin and evolving into ichthyotic erythroderma accompanied by hystrix-like hyperkeratosis (Fig. 19.5.16). There is a bilateral inner hearing loss, which is severe and borders on total deafness. A superficial, punctate keratitis may be present in some cases [36–39]. Alopecia ichthyotica and the absence of eyebrows, dystrophic eyelashes and dystrophic nails can be further findings. Interestingly, a severe mycotic infection beneath the hyperkeratosis can often be found. Retinoid treatment may be helpful in controlling the mycotic infections [40]. The disease is frequently mistaken for ichthyosis hystrix of Curth–Macklin. Another diagnosis that has to be considered is the keratosis, ichthyosis and deafness (KID) syndrome, which shows more localized lesions and has the typical facial involvement with bizarre sharply outlined hyperkeratotic plaques. Histological examination shows altered keratinocytes in which the cell nucleus is surrounded by an empty halo. These changes are often clustered in the upper prickle cell and granular layers, while the remaining epidermis may look normal.

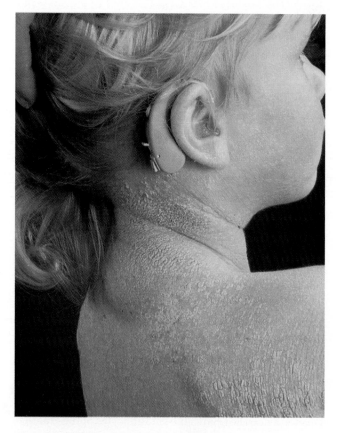

Fig. 19.5.16 HID syndrome. Reproduced from Traupe [18].

On electron microscopy a marked reduction in tonofibrils, few keratohyalin granules and an abnormal production of membrane-bound granules containing mucous substances can be seen [41].

KID syndrome

The term KID syndrome denotes a disease that features localized erythematous, scaly skin lesions, usually severe keratitis and bilateral deafness [42]. There has been a long-standing debate over whether KID syndrome actually represents an ichthyosis or should rather be regarded as an erythrokeratoderma. Since most cases of KID syndrome show rather localized involvement of the skin, the latter classification might be more appropiate [43,44], but the term KID syndrome has become firmly entrenched in the medical literature. The syndrome is characterized by sharply outlined verrucous hyperkeratotic plaques on the face [33] (Fig. 19.5.17) and on the extremities. If involved the trunk has only slight scaling. Further features may include scarring alopecia (80%) ophthalmological defects (95%), especially vascularizing keratitis and neurosensory deafness (90%). Very typical for the cutaneous involvement is the palmoplantar hyperkeratosis, which has a typical reticulated pattern, and which is often described as leather-like. An increased susceptibility to viral bacterial and mycotic skin infections has been observed [44]. Dentition can also be abnormal. Squamous cell carcinoma has been described in seven of 71 cases which accounts for 11% of patients [45]. This may be the most severe manifestation of the disease.

Histological features are those of a non-specific hyperplastic epidermis, but follicular plugging can be striking.

In most cases, KID syndrome appears to be sporadic [46], but in three reports an autosomal dominant transmission has been reported.

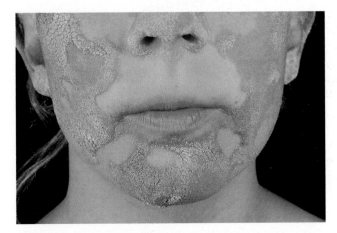

Fig. 19.5.17 KID syndrome: note sharply outlined verrucous, hyperkeratotic plaques on the face. Courtesy of Professor W. Küster, Marburg.

Ichthyosis follicularis with atrichia and photophobia (IFAP) syndrome

This syndrome is characterized by the presence of marked ichthyosis with prominent follicular keratosis, atrichia and marked photophobia in affected boys, and was first reported by MacLeod in 1909 [47]. The absence of hair (congenital atrichia) is the most striking clinical feature of IFAP syndrome. Follicular involvement can result in thorn-like projections, giving the skin the feeling of a nutmeg grater [48]. Photophobia refers to a marked sensitivity to light; however this does not imply a tendency for sunburn. The children avoid bright light, but are at risk of true photosensitivity as would be the case in PIBIDS syndrome. Torticollis was a problem in some cases. The mode of transmission is unclear and both X-linked as well as autosomal dominant inheritance patterns have been proposed [49,50].

REFERENCES

1 Sjögren T, Larsson T. Oligophrenia in combination with congenital ichthyosis and spastic disorders. *Acta Psychiatr Scand* 1957; 32 (suppl. 113): 1–113.
2 Jagell S, Gustarson KH, Holmyren G. Sjögren–Larsson syndrome in Sweden. A clinical, genetic and epidemiological study. *Clin Genet* 1981; 19: 233–56.
3 Liden S, Jagell S. The Sjögren–Larsson syndrome. *Int J Dermatol* 1984; 23: 247–53.
4 Judge MR, Lake BD, Smith VV, Besley GT, Harper JI. Depletion of alcohol (hexanol) dehydrogenase activity in the epidermis and jejunal inucosa in Sjögren–Larsson syndrome. *J Invest Dermatol* 1990; 95: 632–4.
5 Pigg M, Jagell S, Sillén A, Weissenbach J, Gustavson KH, Wadelius C. The Sjögren–Larsson syndrome gene is close to D17S805 as determined by linkage analysis and allelic association. *Nat Genet* 1994; 8: 361–4.
6 De Laurenzi V, Rogers GR, Hamrock DJ *et al.* Sjögren–Larsson is caused by mutations in the fatty aldehyde dehydrogenase gene. *Nat Genet* 1996; 12: 52–7.
7 Koone MD, Rizzo WB, Elias PM, Williams ML, Lightner V, Pinnell SR. Ichthyosis, mental retardation, and asymptomatic spasticity. A neurocutaneous syndrome with normal fatty alcohol. *Arch Dermatol* 1990; 126: 1485–90.
8 Tay CH. Ichthyosiform erythroderma, hair shaft abnormalities, and mental and growth retardation. A new recessive disorder. *Arch Dermatol* 1971; 104: 4–13.
9 Happle R, Traupe H, Gröbe H, Bonsmann G. The Tay syndrome (congenital ichthyosis with trichothiodystrophy). *Eur J Pediatr* 1984; 141: 147–52.
10 Brown AL, Belser RB, Crounse RG, Wehr BF. A congenital hair defect. Trichoschisis with alternating birefringence and low sulfur content. *J Invest Dermatol* 1970; 54: 496–509.
11 Rebora A, Crovoto F. PIBIDS syndrome—trichothiodystrophy with xeroderma pigmentosum (group D) mutation. *J Am Acad Dermatol* 1987; 16: 940–7.
12 Broughton BC, Steingrimsdottir H, Weber CA, Lehmann AR. Mutations in the xeroderma pigmentosum group D DNA repair/transcription gene in patients with trichothiodystrophy. *Nat Genet* 1994; 7: 189–94.
13 Chu G, Mayne L. Xeroderma pigmentosum, Cockayne syndrome and trichothiodystrophy: do the genes explain the diseases? *Trends Genet* 1996; 12: 187–92.
14 Sarasin A, Blancet-Bardon C, Renault G, Lehmann A, Arlett C, Dumez Y. Prenatal diagnosis in a subset of trichothiodystrophy patient defective in DNA repair. *Br J Dermatol* 1992; 127: 485–91.
15 Judge MR, Morgan G, Harper JI. A clinical and immunological study of Netherton's syndrome. *Br J Dermatol* 1994; 131: 615–21.
16 Hausser I, Anton-Lamprecht I. Severe congenital generalized exfoliate

erythroderma in newborns and infants: a possible sign of Netherton syndrome. *Pediatr Dermatol* 1996; 13: 183–99.

17 Comèl M. Ichthyosis linearis circumflexa. *Dermatologica* 1949; 98: 112–36.

18 Traupe H. *The Ichthyoses. A Guide to Clinical Diagnosis, Genetic Counseling and Therapy.* Berlin: Springer-Verlag, 1984: 168–78.

19 Happle R, Matthias HH, Macher E. Sex-linked chondrodysplasia punctata? *Clin Genet* 1977; 11: 73–6.

20 Happle R. X-linked dominant ichthyosis. *Clin Genet* 1979; 15: 239–40.

21 Hosenfeld D, Wiedemann HR. *Chondrodysplasia Punctata im Erwachsenenalter als Cumarinembroyopathie Erkannt. 6. Symposium Klinische Genetik in der Pädiatrie,* 3–5 July 1987, Bad Homburg.

22 Happle R. Cataracts as a marker of genetic heterogeneity in chondrodysplasia punctata. *Clin Genet* 1981; 19: 64–6.

23 Gobello T, Mazzanti C, Fileccia P et al. X-linked dominant chondrodysplasia punctata (Happle syndrome) with uncommon symmetrical shortening of the tubular bones. *Dermatology* 1995; 191: 323–7.

24 Kolde G, Happle R. Histologic and ultrastructural features of the ichthyototic skin in X-linked dominant chondrodysplasia punctata. *Acta Derm Venereol* 1984; 64: 389–94.

25 Yanagihara M, Ueda K, Asano N, Ozawa T, Nakatani A, Hirose M. Usefulness of histopathologic examination of thick scales in the diagnosis of X-linked dominant chondrodysplasia punctata (Happle). *Pediatr Dermatol* 1996; 11: 1–4.

26 Happle R, Phillips RJS, Roessner A, Jünemann G. Homologous genes for X-linked chondrodysplasia punctata in man and mouse. *Hum Genet* 1983; 63: 24–7.

27 Traupe H, Vetter U, Happle R et al. Exclusion of the biglycan (BGN) gene as a candidate gene for the Happle syndrome, employing an intragenic single strand conformational polymorphism. *Hum Genet* 1993; 91: 89–90.

28 Traupe H, Müller D, Atherton D et al. Exclusion mapping of the X-linked dominant chondrodysplasia punctata/ichthyosis/cataract/short stature (Happle) syndrome: possible involvement of an unstable premutation. *Hum Genet* 1992; 89: 659–65.

29 Happle R. X-linked dominant chondrodysplasia punctata/ichthyosis/cataract syndrome in males. *Am J Med Genet* 1995; 57: 493.

30 Sutphen R, Amar MJ, Kousseff BG, Toomey KE. XXY with X-linked dominant chondrodysplasia punctata (Happle syndrome). *Am J Med Genet* 1995; 489–92.

31 Derry JMJ, Gormally E, Means GD et al. Mutations in a delta 8–delta 7 sterol isomerase in the tattered mouse and x-linked dominant chondrodysplasia punctata. *Nat Genet* 1999, 22: 286–90.

32 Dorfman ML, Hershko C, Eisenberg S, Sagher F. Ichthyosiform dermatosis with systemic linidosis. *Arch Dermatol* 1974; 110: 261–6.

33 Venencie PY, Armengaud D, Foldès C, Vieillefond A, Coulombel L, Hadchonael M. Ichthyosis and neutral lipid storage disease (Dorfman–Chanarin syndrome). *Pediatr Dermatol* 1988; 5: 173–7.

34 Williams ML, Koch TK, O'Donell JJ et al. Ichthyosis and neutral lipid storage disease. *Am J Med Genet* 1985; 20: 711–26.

35 Musumecis DI, Agata A, Romano C, Patané C, Cutrone D. Ichthyosis and neutral lipid storage disease. *Am J Med Genet* 1988; 29: 377–82.

36 Wesalowski R, Schroten H, Neuen-Jacob E et al. Multisystem triglyceride storage disorder without ichthyosis in two siblings. *Acta Paediatr* 1994; 83: 93–8.

37 Gülzow J, Anton-Lamprecht I. Ichthyosis hystrix gravior Typus Rheydt: ein otologisch—dermatologisches Syndrom. *Laryng Rhinol Otol* 1977; 56: 949–55.

38 Schnyder UW. Ichthyosis hystrix Typus Rheydt (Ichthyosis hystrix gravior mit praktischer Taubheit). *Z Hautkr* 1977; 52: 763–6.

39 Traupe H. *The Ichthyoses. A Guide to Clinical Diagnosis, Genetic Counseling, and Therapy.* Berlin: Springer-Verlag, 1989: 191–7.

40 Badillet C, Blanchet-Bardon C, Cabral O, Puissant A. Etude mycologique de trois cas d'erythrodermie avec keratite et surdité (ichthyose de Rheydt). *Bull Soc Mycol Med* 1982; 11: 197–8.

41 Anton-Lamprecht I. Ultrastructural criteria for the distinction of different types of inherited ichthyoses. In: Marks R, Dykes PJ, eds. *The Ichthyoses.* Lancaster: MTP Press, 1978: 71–8.

42 Skinner BA, Greist MC, Norins AL. The keratitis ichthyosis, and deafness (KID) syndrome. *Arch Dermatol* 1981; 117: 285–9.

43 Traupe H. *The Ichthyoses. A Guide to Clinical Diagnosis, Genetic Counseling and Therapy.* Berlin: Springer-Verlag, 1989: 198–202.

44 Caceres-Rios H, Tamayo-Sanchez L, Duran-Mckinster C, Orozco ML, Ruiz-Maldonado R. Keratitis, ichthyosis, and deafness (KID syndrome): review

of the literature and proposal of a new terminology. *Pediatr Dermatol* 1996; 13: 105–13.

45 Hazen PG, Carney P, Lynch WS. Keratitis, ichthyosis, and deafness syndrome with development of multiple cutaneous neoplasms. *Cameo* 1989; 28: 190–1.

46 Langer K, Konrad K, Wolff K. Keratitis, ichthyosis and deafness (KID) syndrome: report of three cases and a review of the literature. *Br J Dermatol* 1990; 122: 689–97.

47 MacLeod JMH. Three cases of ichthyosis follicularis associated with baldness. *Br J Dermatol* 1909; 21: 165–89.

48 Eramo LR, Esterly NB, Zieserl EJ, Stock EL, Hermann J. Ichthyosis follicularis with alopecia and photophobia. *Arch Dermatol* 1985; 121: 1167–74.

49 Hamm H, Meinecke P, Traupe H. Further delineation of the ichthyosis follicularis, atrichia, and photophobia (IFAP) syndrome. *Eur J Pediatr* 1991; 150: 627–9.

50 Rothe MJ, Weiss DS, Dubner BH, Weitzner JM, Lucky AW, Schachner L. Ichthyosis follicularis in two girls: an autosomal dominant disorder. *Pediatr Dermatol* 1990; 7: 287–92.

Recently recognized ichthyoses

When a given case of ichthyosis does not fit with any of the entities discussed so far, a number of further, uncommon entities should be considered, including the following.

Ichthyosis en confetti is characterized by congenital reticular ichthyotic erythroderma with erythematous ichthyotic skin in reticular arrangement on the trunk [1]. Patients are born with the features of erythodermic lamellar ichthyosis, but during puberty patches of normal skin enclosed by erythematous ichthyotic skin appear in a reticular arrangement on the trunk. This disease was first described by Marghescu *et al.* under the designation congenital reticular ichthyosiform erythroderma [2].

Vohwinkel's disease. Congenital ichthyosis can be associated with keratoderma hereditaria mutilans of Vohwinkel [3,4]. Ichthyosis in this association is mild and may be overlooked. Vohwinkel's disease is characterized by a palmoplantar keratosis with a 'honey-combed' appearance and often severe keratotic constricting bands around the distal fingers and toe joints. This can even result in loss of fingers and toes especially on the fourth and fifth digit. Patients with Vohwinkwel's disease have been found to have mutations in loricrin.

Zunich's syndrome. In congenital migratory ichthyosis with neurological and ophthalmological abnormalities (Zunich's syndrome), the skin phenotype resembles the peeling skin syndrome, and is associated with migratory scaling, facial dysmorphism, retinal colobomas and abnormalities in spacing, size and number of teeth as well as a conductive hearing loss, psychomotor delay and autistic mannerism [5].

Schwachmann's syndrome. The association of ichthyosis, growth retardation and scanty hair on the scalp is suggestive of Schwachmann's syndrome, which comprises exocrine pancreatic insufficiency, growth retardation and bone marrow hypoplasia resulting in neutropenia [6]. These children show changes resembling that of lamellar ichthyosis, especially on the legs. Moreover, they often also exhibit dystrophic nails and teeth and are prone to severe infections.

Stormorken's syndrome. A syndrome that has been discussed in a number of articles concerns a family in which three generations of affected members have suffered from thrombocytopathia, muscle fatigue, asplenia, miosis, migraine, dyslexia and ichthyosis [7] (Stormorken's syndrome). Headache is also a prominent sign present in the family in all four generations in which the syndrome has been observed. Nasal and conjunctival bleeding are part of the headache picture in some of the inviduals exhibiting the haemorrhagic symptoms. The thrombocytopathia in this disorder may be due to abnormal serotonin storage, uptake and release [8].

Congenital ichthyosis with hypogonadism and growth retardation may constitute a distinct syndrome that is clinically characterized by generalized erythroderma, fine scaling on the trunk, palmoplantar keratoderma, severely affected nails and hepatosplenomegaly [9].

Cardiofacio cutaneous (CFC) syndrome. Mild ichthyosis can also be found in the CFC syndrome which in addition features curly hair, low-set ears with thickened outer helix, broad depressed bridge of nose, epicanthic folds, sparse eyebrows and eyelashes, thick focal yellowish palmar hyperkeratosis and extensive keratosis pilaris on extensor and flexor surfaces of the arms [10]. Moreover, these patients suffer from psychomotor and growth retardation, brain atrophy, hydrocephalus, nystagmus and cardiac abnormalities, such as pulmonary stenosis and atrial septal defects.

Miscellaneous. Ichthyosis has also been found in patients suffering from restrictive dermopathy and Gaucher's disease [11] and more recently, a congenital sensory neuropathy associated with ichthyosis and anterior chamber cleavage syndrome has been delineated as a possible unique entity, featuring ichthyosis and absence of sensation for light touch, vibration, position and temperature. Nerve action potentials are small or absent and sural nerve biopsies show almost complete absence of myelinated nerve fibres with multiple bundles of abnormally arranged axons [12].

REFERENCES

1 Brusasco A, Tadini G, Cambiaghi S, Ermacora E, Grimalt R, Caputo R. A case of congenital reticular ichthyiosiform erythroderma—ichthyosis 'en confettis'. *Dermatology* 1994; 188: 40–5.

2 Marghescu PO, Anton-Lamprecht I, Rudolph PO, Kaste R. Kongenitale retikuläre ichthyosiforme Erythrodermie. *Hautarzt* 1984; 35: 522–9.

3 Camisa C, Hesel A, Rossana C, Parks A. Autosomal dominant keratoderma, ichthyosi-form dermatosis and elevated serum beta-glucuronidase. *Dermatologica* 1988; 177: 341–7.

4 Traupe, H. *The Ichthyoses. A Guide to Clinical Diagnosis, Genetic Counseling and Therapy.* Berlin: Springer-Verlag, 1989: 211–13.

5 Zunich J, Esterly NB, Holbrook KA, Kaya CI. Congenital migratory ichthyosiform dermatosis with neurologic and ophthalmologic abnormalities. *Arch Dermatol* 1985; 121: 1149–56.

6 Goeteyn M, Oranje A, Vuzevski VD, de Groot R, Suijlekom LWA. Ichthyosis, exocrine pancreatic insufficiency, impaired neutrophil chemotaxis, growth retardation, and metaphyseal dysplasia (Shwachman syndrome). *Arch Dermatol* 1991; 127: 225–30.

7 Stormorken H, Sjaastad O, Langslet A, Suly I, Egge K, Diderichsen J. A new syndrome. Thrombocytopenia, muscle fatigue, asplenia, miosis, migraine, dyslexia and ichthyosis. *Clin Genet* 1985; 28: 367–74.

8 Sjaastad O. The hereditary syndrome of thromobocytopathia, bleeding tendency, extreme miosis, muscular fatigue, asplenia, headache, etc. ('Stormorken's syndrome'). I. The headache. *Headache* 1994; 34: 221–5.

9 Arnold ML, Anton-Lamprecht I, Albrecht-Nebe H. Congenital ichthyosis with hypogonadism and growth retardation—a new syndrome with peculiar ultrastructural features. *Arch Dermatol* 1992; 284: 198–208.

10 Borradori L, Blancet-Bardon C. Skin manifestations of cardio-facio-cutaneous syndrome. *J Am Acad Dermatol* 1993; 28: 815–19.

11 Sherer DM, Metlay LA, Sinkin RA, Mongeon C, Lee RE, Woods JR Jr. Congenital ichthyosis with restrictive dermopathy and Gaucher disease: a new syndrome with associated prenatal diagnostic and pathologic findings. *Obstet Gynecol* 1993; 81: 842–4.

12 Quinlivan R, Robb S, Hughes RA, Hall SM, Calver D. Congenital sensory neuropathy in association with ichthyosis and anterior chamber cleavage syndrome. *Neuromusc Disord* 1993; 3: 217–21.

Therapy

Topical therapy

Therapy is bound to be symptomatic because the many different causes of ichthyosis cannot be cured. In many cases with only mild involvement topical therapy aimed at hydration of the epidermis will be sufficient. Commonly used active substances include sodium chloride, urea, lactic acid and propylene glycol. Sodium chloride in a concentration of 5–10% in aqueous cream is especially effective if applied directly after a bath or shower when the skin is still a little wet. In the author's experience it is very difficult for pharmacists to make good creams containing sodium chloride, which often tends to crystallize in a cream. However, in Germany, topical creams including sodium chloride and urea are available from the pharmaceutical company Galderma.

Vitamin A acid (0.1% tretinoin) has been used for a long time for topical therapy of ichthyosis and is effective [1]. However, many patients experience unpleasant itching. A possible way to avoid this may be to apply topical vitamin A acid only every other day, or to combine lower concentrations of tretinoin with urea. Also, the 13-*cis*-isomeric form is better tolerated and 0.1% 13-*cis*-retinoic acid was found to be superior to its base cream when applied over 4 weeks. However, only four out of 10 patients treated were regarded as good responders [2]. New topical retinoids such as tazarotene may soon prove to be useful—as they are in psoriasis. Urea treatment was initially introduced by Swanbeck in 1968 [3] who demonstrated that urea strongly increased the water-binding capacity of scales from psoriatic patients. It has become very popular in German speaking and Scandinavian countries [4]. The clinical efficacy of urea can be further increased if it is combined with lactic acid, sodium chloride or vitamin A. Urea is used in concentrations between 5 and 10%.

Similar to urea, lactic acid is a moisturizer related to the α-hydroxy acids [5] and is rather effective in controlling dry and hyperkeratotic skin. Van Scott and Yu [6] were able to show that lactic acid reduces the hyperkeratotic states by weakening the intercellular bonding and corneocyte cohesion.

Goldsmith and Baden [7] observed that an occlusive treatment with 60% propylene glycol is also effective in scale removal. However, propylene glycol without occlusion gives less optimal results. In the author's experience, many creams containing some water, for example Eucerin cum aqua or Unguentum emulsificans aquosum, produce good results if applied under occlusion overnight.

For practical reasons, the author prefers to treat patients with ichthyosis with ointments containing urea in concentrations of 5–10%. In Germany, a product called Unguentum Cordes, is commercially available and can be used as a base. It is possible to combine for example 10% urea with 5% lactic acid as is done in a number of commercially available products, e.g. Eucerin (Beiersdorf). Salicylic acid should not be used because intoxications have repeatedly been reported after the use of this topical ointment in children with ichthyosis [8]. Also, urea should not be used in children under the age of 1 year because in very small children high plasma urea concentrations have been reported, for example in collodion babies.

More recently, topical calcipotriol therapy has been tried in a number of patients with ichthyosis including children [9]. Whilst this vitamin D derivative seems to be effective in many patients with ichthyosis, it is not clear whether it is safe. In contrast to psoriasis almost the entire skin surface has to be treated in children with ichthyosis, which could result in hypercalcaemia and possible ectopic calcification as a side-effect, e.g. in the urogenital tract. There is one report of a hypercalcaemic crisis after excessive topical use of a vitamin D derivative [10]. If a whole body treatment is done at all, blood calcium levels must be monitored at regular intervals. Calcipotriol therapy is therefore not very attractive for children, and topical treatment modalities which require less monitoring are preferable in this age group. A drawback inherent to topical therapy is that many children and their parents become weary of applying the ointments twice a day and tend to treat only once daily, or even less. Therefore, the skin condition usually improves markedly when the children are treated as inpatients, but often deteriorates when treatment is continued on an outpatient basis.

Systemic therapy

Children with very severe ichthyosis, such as lamellar ichthyosis, can be treated with retinoids [11]. The response to retinoids is in part dependent on the underlying disease, thus children with Sjögren–Larsson syndrome respond to a very low dosage of retinoids, and in bullous types of ichthyosis the dosage of retinoids should not exceed 0.3 mg/kg body weight because otherwise the blistering tendency can be increased. Conversely, typical lamellar ichthyosis usually requires acitretin in a dosage of 0.5–1 mg/kg body weight. Care must also be taken when treating children with the Comèl–Netherton syndrome because patients with severe expression of the disease—Netherton phenotype—can actually become worse. It is now generally accepted that retinoids should not replace but supplement topical therapy. The aim is to find the necessary (low) dose for maintenance therapy. In children with severe XRI it may be best to try treating only during the winter (Fig. 19.5.18) as the skin condition improves in the summer (so-called interval therapy). Patients with ichthyosis vulgaris usually do not require systemic retinoid therapy. One has to be keep in mind that

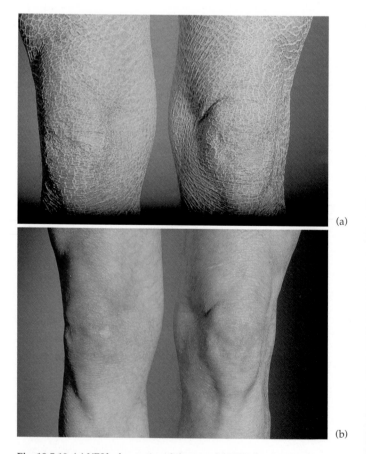

(a)

(b)

Fig. 19.5.18 (a) XRI before retinoid therapy. (b) XRI after 'interval' therapy with acitretin in the winter. Courtesy of Professor L. Bruckner-Tudermann, Münster.

systemic retinoids may be prescribed for many years. Before beginning this long-term therapy X-rays of the knees, hip, hands, feet and elbows should be taken. At the beginning of the retinoid era most dermatologists were afraid of possible side-effects on the bones and regular monitoring at yearly intervals was advised. It is now acceptable for children to have further radiological studies if complaints relating to the musculoskeletal system are noted. However, keeping a growth chart is suggested since retinoids can induce premature closing of the epiphyseal line. This side-effect occurred despite monitoring in one of our young patients and resulted in a shortened (3 cm) leg (asymmetrical shortening). Disseminated retinoid-induced skeletal hyperostosis (DISH) syndrome is a side-effect observed in older patients but not in children. The usual laboratory studies (blood cell counts, lipids, liver enzymes, creatinine, etc.) should be done after 4 weeks and later every 2 months. If newborns are treated the tablets may have to be dissolved and care must be taken that this procedure is performed in the dark in order to prevent an inactivation of the active substance by day light. Gene therapy may become available in some ichthyoses, for example in the form of an ointment containing 'good' DNA. In dominantly transmitted diseases the aim may be to achieve silencing of the mutant gene because it is the gene product of the mutant gene that interferes with the normal function of, for example, keratin molecules. However, it will take several years before gene therapy turns into a realistic option for ichthyosis patients.

REFERENCES

1 Stüttgen G. Zur Lokalbehandlung von Keratosen mit Vitamin-A-Säure. *Dermatologica* 1962; 124: 65–80.
2 Steijlen PM, Reifenschweiler DOH, Ramaekers FCS *et al*. Topical treatment of ichthyoses and Darier's disease with 13-*cis*-retinoic acid. *Arch Dermatol Res* 1993; 285: 221–6.
3 Swanbeck G. A new treatment of ichthyosis and other hyperkeratotic conditions. *Acta Derm Venereol* 1966; 48: 123–7.
4 Grice K, Sattar H, Baker H. Urea and retinoic acid in ichthyosis and their effect on transepidermal water loss and water holding capacity of stratum corneum. *Acta Derm Venereol* 1973; 53: 114–18.
5 Rubin MG. The clinical use of alpha hydroxy acids. *Australas J Dermatol* 1994; 35: 29–33.
6 van Scott EF, Yu RJ. Control of keratinization with α hydroxy acids and related compounds. I. Topical treatment of ichthyotic disorders. *Arch Dermatol* 1974; 110: 586–90.
7 Goldsmith LA, Baden HP. Management and treatment of ichthyosis. *N Engl J Med* 1972; 286: 821–3.
8 Germann R, Schindera I, Kuch M, Seitz U, Altmeyer S, Schindera F. Lebensbedrohliche Salicylatintoxikation durch perkutane Resorption bei einer schweren Ichthyosis vulgaris. *Hautarzt* 1996; 47: 624–7.
9 Lucker GPH, van de Kerkhof PCM, van Dijk MR, Steijlen PM. Effect of topical calcipotriol on congenital ichthyosis. *Br J Dermatol* 1994; 131: 546–50.
10 Hoeck HC, Laurberg G, Laurberg P. Hypercalcaemic crisis after excessive topical use of a vitamin D derivative. *J Intern Med* 1994; 235: 281–2.
11 Lacour M, Mehta-Nikhar B, Atherton DJ, Harper JI. An appraisal of acitretin therapy in children with inherited disorders of keratinization. *Br J Dermatol* 1996; 134: 1023–9.

19.6 Palmoplantar Keratoses

PETER M. STEIJLEN AND GEORGES P.H. LUCKER

Diffuse hereditary palmoplantar keratoderma without associated features

Palmoplantar keratoderma diffusa circumscripta Unna
Palmoplantar keratoderma transgrediens et progrediens Greither
Palmoplantar keratoderma cum degeneratione granulosa Vörner
Palmoplantar keratoderma of Sybert
Mal de Meleda
Palmoplantar keratoderma Gamborg Nielsen
Acral keratoderma

Diffuse hereditary palmoplantar keratodermas with associated features

Palmoplantar keratodermas mutilans Vohwinkel
Carcinoma of the oesophagus with keratosis palmaris et plantaris (Howel-Evans)
Palmoplantar keratoderma with scleroatrophy (Huriez syndrome)
Hidrotic ectodermal dysplasia (Clouston's syndrome)
Palmoplantar keratoderma and sensorineural deafness
Mutilating palmoplantar keratoderma with periorificial keratotic plaques (Olmsted's syndrome)
Palmoplantar keratoderma with periodontitis
Palmoplantar keratoderma with clubbing of the fingers and toes and skeletal deformity (Bureau–Barrière–Thomas)

Focal hereditary palmoplantar keratodermas without associated features

Keratosis palmoplantaris areata et striata
Keratosis palmoplantaris nummularis

Focal hereditary palmoplantar keratodermas with associated features

Tyrosinaemia type II
Pachyonychia congenita
Focal palmoplantar and oral mucosa hyperkeratosis syndrome
Keratosis palmoplantaris papillomatosa et verrucosa

Papular hereditary palmoplantar keratodermas without associated features

Keratosis palmoplantaris punctata (Davies–Colley, Buschke, Fischer, Brauer)
Acrokeratoelastoidosis (AKE)
Focal acral hyperkeratosis

Papular hereditary palmoplantar keratodermas with associated features

Syndrome of cystic eyelids, palmoplantar keratosis, hypodotia and hypotrichosis (Schöpf–Schulz–Passarge syndrome)

The palmoplantar keratodermas (PPKs) comprise a large and heterogeneous group of disorders of keratinization which are characterized by gross thickening of the palmoplantar skin. There are both hereditary and acquired forms.

Hereditary forms of PPK may occur as a symptom of more generalized disorders of keratinization, such as autosomal dominant ichthyosis vulgaris, bullous ichthyosiform erythroderma, lamellar ichthyosis, erythrokeratoderma and Darier's disease. This chapter deals with the monogenic PPKs which are without associated features, and the PPKs which have associated features. In the latter group the PPK is one of the major findings and sometimes the hallmark of a congenital syndrome. Classification of the monogenic PPKs is often difficult, because of inter- and intrafamiliar variations, difference in nomenclature and the large number of reported cases. Many authors have attempted to classify the hereditary forms [1–7]. In recent years, a large number of new entities have been described, and manifestations which were previously considered to be distinct entities have been shown to be variants of the same type of keratoderma. Furthermore, the application of molecular biological techniques, such as linkage studies and mutational analysis, has led to the reclassification of some of these diseases. Since the clinical findings provide the first indication for a possible diagnosis the classification according to Greither still forms a good starting point [3]. Based on the new available data, this classification has been adapted and updated (Table 19.6.1) [6]. Most important features in the classification of PPKs are the specific morphology and distribution of the hyperkeratosis (diffuse, focal, punctate), presence or absence of associated features and pattern of inheritance. It should always be kept in mind that for most of the diseases the clinical features are often not fully expressed in early childhood (life of lesions). Additional criteria are the age of onset of the keratoderma, severity of the disease process and histopathological findings. In some cases the ultimate diagnosis can be made by the demonstration of mutations in specific genes. An integrated approach is necessary for giving a correct diagnosis. The classification in this chapter is necessarily provisional and must be modified continually as new information becomes available.

The MIM numbers accompanying several of the

Table 19.6.1 Hereditary palmoplantar keratoses

	Inheritance	No associated features	Associated features
Diffuse	AD	Unna–Norrbotten Greither Vörner–Thost Sybert	Vohwinkel Howel–Evans Huriez Clouston PPK and sensorineural deafness Olmsted
	AR	Mal de Meleda Gamborg Nielsen Acral keratoderma	Papillon–Lefèvre Bureau–Barrière–Thomas
Nummular/Linear	AD	Wachters PPK nummularis	Richner–Hanhart Pachyonychia congenita Focal palmoplantar and oral mucosa hyperkeratosis syndrome
	AR		Pachyonychia congenita Jakac–Wolf
Papular	AD	Punctate PPK* Acrokeratoelastoidosis* Focal acral hyperkeratosis	
	AR		Schöpf–Schulz-Passarge

*A few rare cases with associated features have been reported.

diseases refer to McKusick's *Mendelian Inheritance in Man, a Catalog of Human Genes and Genetic Disorders* [8]. An updated on-line version is also available (OMIM) [9].

REFERENCES

1 Franceschetti A, Schnyder UW. Versuch einer klinisch-genetischen Klassifikation der hereditären Palmoplantarkeratosen unter Berücksichtigung assoziierter Symptome. *Dermatologica* 1960; 120: 154–78.
2 Schnyder UW, Klunker W. Erbliche verhornungsstörungen der Haut. In: Gottron HA, Schnyder UW, eds. *Handbuch der Haut- und Geschlechtskrankheiten.* Berlin: Springer, 1966: 861–961.
3 Greither A. Erbliche Palmoplantarkeratosen. *Hautarzt* 1977; 28: 395–403.
4 Voigtländer V, Schnyder UW. Palmoplantarkeratosen. In: Korting GW, ed. *Dermatologie in Praxis und Klinik.* Stuttgart: Thieme Verlag, 1980: 26–36.
5 Salamon T. An attempt at classification of inherited disorders of keratinization localized mainly, not exclusively on the palms and soles. *Dermatol Monatsschr* 1986; 172: 601–5.
6 Lucker GPH, Kerkhof van de PCM, Steijlen PM. The hereditary palmoplantar keratoses: an updated review and classification. *Br J Dermatol* 1994; 131: 1–14.
7 Stevens HP, Kelsell DP, Bryant SP *et al.* Linkage of an American pedigree with palmoplantar keratoderma and malignancy (palmoplantar ectodermal dysplasia type III) to 17q24. Literature survey and proposed updated classification of the keratodermas. *Arch Dermatol* 1996; 132: 640–51.
8 McKusick VA. *Mendelian Inheritance in Man. A Catalog of Human Genes and Genetic Disorders,* 12th edn. Baltimore: Johns Hopkins University Press, 1998.
9 OMIM (on-line *Mendelian Inheritance in Man*) available via www.ncbi.nlm.nih.gov/omim/

Diffuse hereditary palmoplantar keratoderma without associated features

Palmoplantar keratoderma diffusa circumscripta Unna (MIM no. 148 400)
(SYN. TYLOSIS, PALMOPLANTAR KERATODERMA TYPE NORRBOTTEN)

History

In his thesis of 1880, Thost described a family with an autosomal dominant diffuse non-transgredient PPK [1]. 110 years after the publication of Thost, Küster and Becker re-examined Thost's family clinically and histologically and found the histopathological features of epidermolytic hyperkeratosis which are characteristic of PPK type Vörner. They concluded that this proved that the PPK type Thost is identical with PPK type Vörner [2]. In 1883 Unna published a clinically identical PPK in two families [3]. Since he did not mention any histological findings it is not known if epidermolytic hyperkeratosis was present. When examining skin biopsies from patients with clinically suspected PPK of Unna–Thost several authors found invariably the histological features of epidermolytic hyperkeratosis as found in Vörner's PPK [4]. The usually reported high frequency of PPK type Unna–Thost should therefore be questioned since it appears that PPK type Vörner is far more frequent when histological examination is performed routinely [4]. As long as the patients from the families described by Unna are not examined histologically even the existence of a PPK type Unna–Thost should be questioned. Between 1985 and 1994 Swedish patients with a diffuse PPK were reported [5–7]. They were examined using light and electron microscopy. No signs of epidermolytic hyperkeratosis were found. This PPK has a very high frequency of 1 in 180 and may be a unique type of diffuse PPK.

Aetiology

This PPK is determined by an autosomal dominant gene with a high penetrance. The gene for the Norrbotten type, which is clinically and histologically identical to the original description of the Thost type, is localized to chromosome 12q11–q13 [8]. In another family with a more or less diffuse PPK histologically without epidermolytic hyperkeratosis, mutations were found in the V1 end domain of keratin 1 [9]. On the basis of the molecular biological findings it now appears that the diffuse PPK is heterogeneous.

Pathology

PPK type Thost is said to show non-specific changes with orthohyperkeratosis, acanthosis and thickening of the granular layer [1]. Histological re-examination of some members of the Thost family, however, showed epidermolytic hyperkeratosis consistent with PPK type Vörner [2]. This discrepancy can be best explained by the variable expression of the epidermolytic hyperkeratosis in the biopsy. Unless one or more biopsies are performed and carefully examined the diagnosis of PPK of Vörner can be missed [2]. The Norrbotten type did not differ histologically from the description made by Thost [6].

Clinical features

Diffuse PPK type Unna mostly presents in the first month of life and is usually evident by the age of 2 years. An even, very thick hyperkeratosis covers diffusely the palms and soles, starting periferally and extending to the centre. At the beginning the margins show a violaceous border, which usually subsides after several years. A tendency to spread towards the extensor surfaces is lacking (not 'transgrediens'). Aberrant keratotic lesions may appear on the dorsa of the hands and feet as well as the knees and elbows. Marked hyperhidrosis is usual and dermatophyte infections are frequently found. The nails may be thickened.

Differential diagnosis

Diffuse PPK type Unna should be differentiated from PPK type Vörner by careful histological examination and from the other autosomal dominant and autosomal recessive diffuse PPKs (see Table 19.6.1 and below).

Treatment

Patients can be helped by the application of keratolytics like salicylic acid (contraindicated in very young children), urea, lactic acid and propylene glycol in white soft paraffin, a gel or an ointment. Occlusion under polyethylene often has a better effect. Topical retinoids have some effect but systemic retinoids like acitretin are more effective. Because of possible side-effects systemic retinoids should be prescribed after serious consideration. Fungal and bacterial superinfections should be treated adequately, if necessary using systemic therapy.

REFERENCES

1 Thost A. *Über Erbliche Ichthyosis Palmaris et Plantaris Cornea*. Inaugural dissertation. Heidelberg, 1880.
2 Küster W, Becker A. Indication for the identity of palmoplantar keratoderma type Unna–Thost with type Vörner. Thost's family revisited 110 years later. *Acta Derm Venereol (Stockh)* 1992; 72: 120–2.
3 Unna PG. Uber das Keratoma palmare et plantare hereditarium. Eine Studie zur Kerato-Nosologie. *Arch Dermatol Syph (Berlin)* 1883; 15: 231–70.
4 Hamm H, Happle R, Buterfass T, Traupe H. Epidermolytic palmoplantar keratoderma of Vörner: is it the most frequent type of hereditary palmoplantar keratoderma? *Dermatologica* 1988; 177: 138–45.
5 Gamborg Nielsen P. Hereditary palmoplantar keratoderma in the northernmost county of Sweden. *Acta Derm Venereol* 1985; 65: 224–9.
6 Gamborg Nielsen P, Hofer PA, Lagerholm B. The dominant form of hereditary palmoplantar keratoderma in the northern most county of Sweden (Norrbotten). *Dermatology* 1994; 188: 188–93.
7 Gamborg Nielsen P, Brändström A. Adoption of a demographic database for family studies of hereditary palmoplantar keratoderma type Gamborg Nielsen. *Dermatology* 1994; 188: 194–9.
8 Lind L, Lundström A, Hofer P-A, Holmgren G. The gene for diffuse palmoplantar keratoderma of the type found in northern Sweden is localized to chromosome 12q11–q13. *Hum Mol Genet* 1994; 3: 1789–93.
9 Kimonis V, DiGiovanni JJ, Yang J-M, Doyle SZ, Bale SJ, Compton JG. A mutation in the V1 end domain of keratin 1 in non-epidermolytic palmarplantar keratoderma. *J Invest Dermatol* 1994; 103: 764–9.

Palmoplantar keratoderma transgrediens et progrediens Greither (MIM no. 148400)

(SYN. PROGRESSIVE DIFFUSE PALMOPLANTAR KERATODERMA, GREITHER'S SYNDROME)

History

In 1952 Greither described a diffuse PPK with hyperhidrosis. His observation was confirmed in 1960 by Salamon, in 1962 by Grin *et al.*, in 1967 by Rook and in 1969 by Hübner and Ziegenbalg [1–5].

Aetiology

This disorder is determined by an autosomal dominant trait. PPK type Greither has been linked to 1p36.2–34, the same locus as erythrokeratodermia variabilis [6]. Richard *et al.* excluded linkage to chromosome 1p32–34 in another family with Greither's PPK indicating that this disease might be heterogeneous [7].

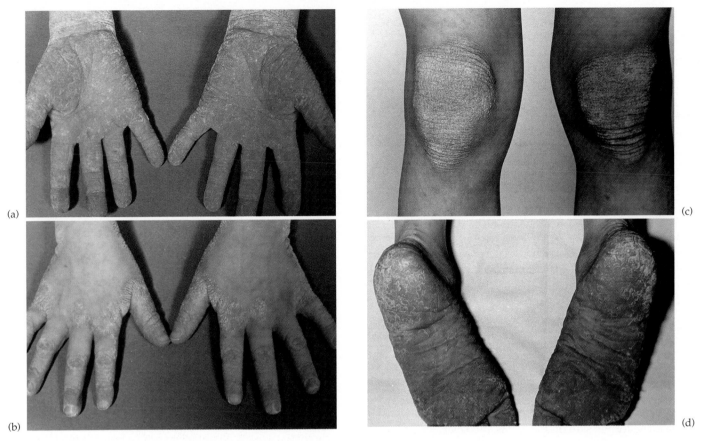

Fig. 19.6.1 (a–d) PPK transgrediens et progrediens Greither. Courtesy of Dr Colin S. Munro, Southern General Hospital, Glasgow, UK.

Pathology

Histological examination shows orthohyperkeratosis, acanthosis and a slight perivascular infiltrate [1].

Clinical features (Fig. 19.6.1)

PPK Greither presents in infancy and is characterized by a diffuse hyperkeratosis which progresses and spreads to the dorsal aspects of the hands and feet (transgrediens) often with a violaceous border and hyperhidrosis. Additional hyperkeratotic lesions can be seen on the knees, elbows and in the region of the Achilles tendon. Worsening of the keratosis is seen in childhood, followed by a stationary course after puberty and finally a tendency to improve is noted in the fifth decade.

Differential diagnosis

It differs from the Unna–Thost variety by showing extension to the dorsal aspects of the hands, knees, elbows and Achilles tendons. Furthermore, PPK type Greither improves in the fifth decade. It differs from mal de Meleda because of the dominant inheritance and the variable intrafamiliar expression. PPK type Greither must be discriminated from the erythrokeratodermas.

Treatment

Therapy in children consists of the application of topical keratolytics. Systemic retinoids can be effective but are usually reserved for adults because of possible side-effects.

REFERENCES

1 Greither A. Keratosis extremitatum hereditaria progrediens mit dominantem Erbgang. *Hautarzt* 1952; 3: 198–203.
2 Salamon T. Uber einige Fälle von Keratosis extremitatum hereditaria progrediens mit dominantum Erbgang (Greither). *Z Haut Geschl Krankh* 1960; 29: 289–98.
3 Grin E, Salamon T, Milicevic M. Keratosis palmo-plantaris progrediens hereditaria mit dominantem Erbgang. *Arch Klin Exp Dermatol* 1962; 214: 378–93.
4 Rook AJ. Progressive palmoplantar keratodermia. Greither's syndrome. *Br J Dermatol* 1967; 79: 302.
5 Hübner U, Ziegenbalg W. Keratosis extremitatum hereditaria transgrediens et progrediens dominans. *Derm Mschr* 1969; 155: 340–3.
6 Gedde-Dahl TJ, Rodge S, Helsing P et al. Greither's disease and erythrokeratoderma variabilis (EKV) caused by the same mutation on chromosome 1. *Human Genome Mapping Workshop*, 1993; 1 (abstract).
7 Richard G, Whyte YM, Smith L et al. Linkage studies in erythrokeratodermias: fine mapping, genetic heterogeneity, and analysis of candidate genes. *J Invest Dermatol* 1996; 107: 481.

Palmoplantar keratoderma cum degeneratione granulosa Vörner (MIM no. 144200)

(SYN. EPIDERMOLYTIC PALMOPLANTAR KERATODERMA, PALMOPLANTAR KERATODERMA TYPE THOST)

History

In 1909 Vörner described a diffuse PPK which was histologically characterized by epidermolytic hyperkeratosis (granular degeneration or acanthokeratolysis) [1]. Küster and Becker re-examined the family described by Thost clinically and histologically and demonstrated that the PPK in this family was identical to that described by Vörner [2]. In fact Vörner described the PPK of Thost. In 1994 Reis *et al.* elucidated the cause of this disease by identifying mutations in the gene coding for keratin 9 [3]. PPK type Vörner is probably the most frequent and the most investigated and elucidated form of PPK.

Aetiology

This PPK is an autosomal dominant disease and is caused by point mutations in the gene coding for keratin 9 which lies on chromosome 17q12–21 [4–9]. Keratin 9 is expressed in the suprabasal compartment of the epidermis and is specific for the skin on the palms and soles. Mutations in the gene coding for keratin 9 leads to disruption of the keratin–filament network and cytolysis. Alsaleh and Teebi described two children with PPK type Vörner of consanguinous unaffected parents [10]. An explanation for this observation might be the presence of the mutation only in the gonads of one of the parents (gonadal mosaicism). Another explanation might be that the parents are both heterozygous for a mutation that leads to a complete loss (knock-out) of keratin 9 expression. As carriers they produce only a normal keratin 9 by the non-mutated allele and show no symptoms. Their children, however, might become homozygous for the mutation and as such represent total knock-outs for keratin 9 leading to severe palmoplantar keratoderma. Torchard *et al.* demonstrated cosegregation of the PPK type Vörner with breast and ovarian cancer [8].

Pathology

This PPK is characterized histologically (light and electron microscopy) by the features of epidermolytic hyperkeratosis including perinuclear vacuolization, large keratohyaline granules, clumping of tonofilaments, cellular degeneration in spinous and granular cells and sometimes blister formation [7,9,11–16]. The features of epidermolytic hyperkeratosis are mostly clearly present in the biopsy but sometimes the abnormalities are subtle and careful light and electron microscopical examination in several biopsies is necessary [17]. Epidermolytic hyperk-

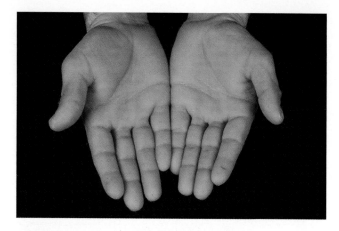

Fig. 19.6.2 PPK cum degeneratione granolosa Vörner.

eratosis also occurs in several other skin conditions as well, such as bullous congenital ichthyosiform erythroderma of Brocq, ichthyosis bullosa of Siemens and some linear epidermal naevi. PPK nummularis is another PPK characterized by epidermolytic hyperkeratosis [18].

Clinical features (Fig. 19.6.2)

The symptoms and the mode of transmission of PPK Vörner do not differ much from those of PPK Unna except that these patients do not always have hyperhidrosis and they may develop blisters [11–16]. Knuckle pad lesions have been reported [19]. To date at least 33 family observations and 11 sporadic cases have been published [16]. In this disorder the hyperkeratosis may be more extreme on the pressure points. A correct classification of diffuse PPKs is impossible without histological examination. PPK type Vörner appears to be the most frequent type of hereditary PPK [20].

Differential diagnosis

PPK type Vörner can be differentiated from the other diffuse types of PPK by the histopathological characteristics of epidermolytic hyperkeratosis.

Treatment

The treatment is the same as for the type Unna. However, systemic retinoids may cause excessive peeling and even blistering.

REFERENCES

1 Vörner H. Zur Kenntnis des Keratoma hereditarium palmare et plantare. *Arch Dermatol Syph (Berlin)* 1901; 56: 3–31.
2 Küster W, Becker A. Indication for the identity of Palmoplantar Keratoderma Type Unna–Thost with Type Vörner. Thost's family revisited 110 years later. *Acta Derm Venereol (Stockh)* 1992; 72: 120–2.
3 Reis A, Hennies HC, Langbein *et al.* Keratin 9 gene mutations in epidermolytic palmoplantar keratoderma (EPPK). *Nat Genet* 1994; 6: 174–9.

4 Reis A, Hennies H-C, Langbein L et al. Nat Genet 1994; 6: 174–9.

5 Bonifas JM, Matsumura K, Chen MA et al. Mutations of keratin 9 in two families with palmoplantar epidermolytic hyperkeratosis. J Invest Dermatol 1994; 103: 474–7.

6 Hennies H-C, Zehender D, Kunze J, Küster W, Reis A. Keratin 9 gene mutational heterogeneity in patients with epidermolytic palmoplantar keratoderma. Hum Genet 1994; 93: 649–54.

7 Navsaria HA, Swensson O, Ratnavel RC et al. Ultrastructural changes resulting from keratin-9 gene mutations in two families with epidermolytic palmoplantar keratoderma. J Invest Dermatol 1995; 104: 425–9.

8 Torchard D, Blanchet-Bardon C, Serova O et al. Epidermolytic palmoplantar keratoderma congregates with a keratin 9 mutation in a pedigree with breast and ovarian cancer. Nat Genet 1994; 6: 106–10.

9 Kobayashi S, Tanaka T, Matsuyoshi N, Imamura S. Keratin 9 point mutation in the pedigree of epidermolytic hereditary palmoplantar keratoderma perturbs keratin intermediate filament network formation. FEBS Lett 1996; 386: 149–55.

10 Alsaleh QA, Teebi AS. Autosomal recessive epidermolytic palmoplantar keratoderma. J Med Genet 1990; 27: 519–22.

11 Klaus S, Weinstein GD, Frost P. Localized epidermolytic hyperkeratosis. A form of keratoderma of the palms and soles. Arch Dermatol 1970; 101: 272–5.

12 Fritsch P, Hönigsman H, Jaschke E. Epidermolytic hereditary palmoplantar keratoderma. Report of a family and treatment with an oral aromatic retinoid. Br J Dermatol 1978; 99: 561–8.

13 Kanitakis J, Tsoitis G, Kanitakis C. Hereditary epidermolytic palmoplantar keratoderma (Vörner type). Report of a familial case and review of the literature. J Am Acad Dermatol 1987; 17: 414–22.

14 Moriwaki S, Tanaka T, Horiguchi Y, Danno K, Imamura S. Epidermolytic hereditary palmoplantar keratoderma. Histologic, ultrastructural, protein–chemical, and DNA analyses in two patients. Arch Dermatol 1988; 104: 555–9.

15 Berth-Jones J, Hutchinson PE. A family with palmoplantar epidermolytic hyperkeratosis. Clin Exp Dermatol 1989; 14: 313–16.

16 Requena L, Schoendorff, Sanchez Yus E. Hereditary epidermolytic palmoplantar keratoderma (Vörner type)—report of a family and review of the literature. Clin Exp Dermatol 1991; 16: 383–8.

17 Küster W, Zehender D, Mensing H, Hennies HC, Reis A. Keratosis palmoplantaris diffusa Vörner Klinische, formalgenetische und molekularbiologische untersuchungen bei 22 families. Hautarzt 1995; 46: 705–10.

18 Wachters DHJ, Frensdorf EL, Hausman R et al. Keratosis palmoplantaris nummularis ('hereditary painful callosities'). Clinical and histopathologic aspects. J Am Acad Dermatol 1983; 9: 204–9.

19 Nogita T, Nakagawa H, Ishibashi Y. Hereditary epidermolytic palmoplantar keratoderma with knuckle pad-like lesions over the finger joints. Br J Dermatol 1991; 125: 496.

20 Hamm H, Happle R, Buterfass T, Traupe H. Epidermolytic palmoplantar keratoderma of Vörner: is it the most frequent type of hereditary palmoplantar keratoderma. Dermatologica 1988; 177: 138–45.

Palmoplantar keratoderma of Sybert

Sybert *et al.* described a family in 1988 with a PPK, starting with erythema and scaling of both palms and soles in the first year of life [1]. The palmoplantar lesions eventually progressed to a severe diffuse hyperkeratosis causing deformities and spontaneous amputations of the digits. In childhood additional lesions developed in the natal cleft and groins. With increasing age, hyperkeratoses developed on the elbows, knees, dorsa of the hands and feet, posterior aspects of the forearms and anterior aspects of the legs. The pedigree was consistent with an autosomal dominant mode of inheritance.

Differential diagnosis

This diffuse, transgreding and mutilating PPK has to be differentiated from mal de Meleda, PPK of Gamborg–Nielsen and PPK of Greither. The clinical features resemble those found in mal de Meleda which, however, is an autosomal recessive disorder. PPK of Gamborg Nielsen shows less extension onto the dorsal surfaces, fewer additional hyperkeratoses and is recessively inherited. The severity and extent of involvement are much greater than in PPK of Greither.

REFERENCE

1 Sybert VP, Dale BA, Holbrook KA. Palmar-plantar keratoderma. A clinical, ultrastructural and biochemical study. J Am Acad Dermatol 1988; 18: 75–86.

Mal de Meleda (MIM no. 248 300)

(SYN. MELEDA DISEASE, KERATOSIS EXTREMITATUM HEREDITARIA TRANSGREDIENS ET PROGREDIENS, KERATODERMA PALMOPLANTARIS TRANSGREDIENS)

History

This rare PPK was first described by Hovarka and Ehlers in 1897 and further delineated amongst others by Brunner and Fuhrman in 1950 and Francechetti *et al.* in 1972 [1–8].

Aetiology

The inheritance is autosomal recessive. This very rare disorder has, as a result of inbreeding, an endemic prevalance on the adriatic island Mljet (Meleda). The causative gene has been mapped on chromosome 8q [9].

Pathology

The histological findings consist of hyperkeratosis with some parakeratosis and a marked acanthosis. A prominent perivascular mononuclear infiltrate is often present.

Clinical features (Fig. 19.6.3)

It is characterized by a diffuse, thick hyperkeratosis with a prominent erythematous border. The thick hyperkeratosis may lead to flexure contractures. The disease has its onset in early infancy and follows a progressive course and extension onto the dorsal surfaces. Constricting bands surrounding the digits are typical [7], rarely resulting in spontaneous amputation of the digits [6]. Concomitant lesions can be found at other sites, especially the elbows and knees [4]. Perioral erythema and hyperkeratosis may be present [8,10], resembling the clinical features of Olmsted syndrome. Hyperhidrosis of the affected parts with maceration of the hyperkeratotic masses and consequent production of a rancid odour is pronounced. Bacterial and fungal superinfection is common. Nail changes (koilonychia, nail thickening, subungual hyperkeratosis) are usually present.

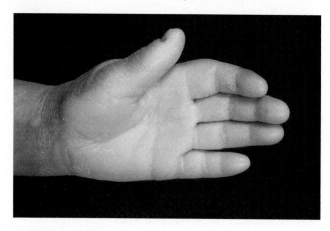

Fig. 19.6.3 Mal de Meleda.

Differential diagnosis

The disease has to be differentiated from PPK transgrediens et progrediens Greither and PPK of Sybert which both have a dominant mode of inheritance. PPK of Gamborg Nielsen displays less severe hyperkeratosis, no nail deformities and no distant keratoses, except for the knuckle pads.

Treatment

A good response to retinoids has been reported [10–12], especially a reduction of the hyperkeratosis, but the erythema may become more prominent [12].

REFERENCES

1 Hovorka O, Ehlers E. Meledakrankheit. *Arch Dermatol Syph* 1896; 34: 51.
2 Kogoj F. Die Krankheit von Mljet (mal de Meleda). *Acta Derm Venereol (Stockh)* 1934; 15: 264–9.
3 Bosnjakovic S. Vererbungsverhältnisse bei der sog. Krankheit von Mljet (mal de Meleda). *Acta Derm Venereol (Stockh)* 1938; 19: 88.
4 Niles HD, Klumpp MM. Mal de Meleda. Review of the literature and report of four cases. *Arch Dermatol Syph* 1939; 39: 409–21.
5 Brunner MJ, Fuhrman DL. Mal de Meleda. Report of a case and results of treatment with vitamin A. *Arch Dermatol Syph* 1950; 61: 820–3.
6 Miani G, Rasdoni L. Strozzamenti anulari e amputazioni spontanee della dita nelle keratodermie. *Arch Ital Derm Vener* 1952; 25: 23–30.
7 Degos MMR, Delort J, Charlas J. Ainhum avec kératodermie palmoplantaire. *Bull Soc Fr Derm Syph* 1963; 70: 136–8.
8 Franchetti AT, Reinhart V, Schnyder UW. La maladie de Meleda. *J Génét Hum* 1972; 20: 267–96.
9 Fisher J, Bouadjar B, Heilig R, Fizames C, Prud'homme J-F, Weissenbach J. Genetic linkage of Meleda disease to chromosome 8qter. *Eur J Hum Genet* 1998; 6: 542–7.
10 Brambilla L, Pigatto PD, Boneschi V, Altomare GF, Finzi AF. Unusual cases of Meleda keratoderma treated with aromatic retinoid etretinate. *Dermatologica* 1984; 168: 283–6.
11 Blanchet-Bardon C, Nazzaro V, Rognin C, Geiger JM, Puissant A. Acitretin in the treatment of severe disorders of keratinization. Results of an open study. *J Am Acad Dermatol* 1991; 24: 982–6.
12 van de Kerkhof PCM, van Dooren-Greebe RJ, Steijlen PM. Acitretin in the treatment of mal de Meleda. *Br J Dermatol* 1992; 127: 191–2.

Palmoplantar keratoderma Gamborg Nielsen (MIM no. 244 850)

History

In 1983 Gamborg Nielsen recognized a severe form of diffuse PPK which he distinguished from the autosomal dominant diffuse PPK Unna-Norrbotten type and mal de Meleda [1,2].

Aetiology

This disorder has an autosomal recessive inheritance of an until now unknown gene.

Pathology

Considerable hyperkeratosis and hypergranulosis is found. On electron microscopy abnormal keratin hyaline granules are observed [3].

Clinical features

Gamborg Nielsen delineated a severe form of PPK represented by six patients in two families, both living in the northernmost county of Sweden [1,2]. This type was characterized by a very thick hyperkeratosis, distinctly demarcated from normal skin. The dorsal aspects of the finger joints showed knuckle pads. A bluish-red zone was observed in four patients. One patient demonstrated transgression of the keratoderma to the dorsal surfaces of the hands. Another featured mutilating symptoms due to constricting bands surrounding the fingers [1]. Except for the knuckle pads on the dorsa of the fingers, no additional hyperkeratoses were observed.

Differential diagnosis

The type Unna-Norrbotten is less severe and has an autosomal dominant manner of inheritance. PPK type Sybert exhibits more transgression and distant keratoses and is inherited as an autosomal dominant trait. Compared to mal de Meleda, the Gamborg Nielsen type differs only in the extension of the keratoderma. It displays less severe hyperkeratoses, no nail deformities and no distant keratoses except for the knuckle pads. It might be possible that in Sweden an incomplete form of mal de Meleda exists [2]. Similar, though less severe cases have been described in the Japanese literature as the 'Nagashima type'.

REFERENCES

1 Gamborg Nielsen P. Mutilating palmoplantar keratoderma. *Acta Derm Venereol (Stockh)* 1983; 63: 365–7.

2 Gamborg Nielsen P. Two different clinical and genetic forms of hereditary palmoplantar keratoderma in the northernmost county of Sweden. *Clin Genet* 1985; 28: 361–6.

3 Kastl L, Anton-Lamprecht I, Gamborg Nielsen P. Hereditary palmoplantar keratosis of the Gamborg Nielsen type. Clinical and ultrastructural characteristics of a new type of autosomal recessive palmoplantar keratosis. *Arch Dermatol Res* 1990; 282: 363–70.

Acral keratoderma

Nesbitt *et al.* described three siblings with a keratoderma characterized by diffuse and striate hyperkeratosis of the palms and soles, hyperkeratotic plaques over the dorsum of the hands and toes and linear hyperkeratotic lesions over the Achilles tendon, ankles, elbows and knees. In one subject the right fifth toe was missing while a constricting band completely encircled the left fifth toe at the base. Histopathologically dyskeratotic changes without epidermolytic hyperkeratosis were observed.

Differential diagnosis

The keratoderma is clinically dissimilar from PPK mutilans by the presence of striate hyperkeratosis on the palmar surface of the fingers, the absence of starfish-shaped hyperkeratosis and the lack of a violaceous border surrounding the PPK. In addition the pedigree suggests an autosomal recessive inheritance pattern which also justifies discriminating this disease from PPK varians. The typical clinical features enable a distinction between acral keratoderma and mal de Meleda [1].

REFERENCE

1 Nesbitt LT, Rotschild H, Ichinose H, Stein W, Levy L. Acral keratoderma. *Arch Dermatol* 1975; 111: 763–8.

Diffuse hereditary palmoplantar keratodermas with associated features

Palmoplantar keratodermas mutilans Vohwinkel (MIM no. 124 500)

(SYN. VOHWINKEL'S SYNDROME, KERATODERMIA HEREDITARIA MUTILANS)

History

In 1929 Vohwinkel described a mutilating keratoderma [1]. After the first publication about 30 cases have been reported [2].

Aetiology

Vohwinkel is an autosomal dominant disease. Maestrini *et al.* mapped the disease to the epidermal differentiation complex (EDC) at chromosome 1q21 and identified a mutation in the major cornified envelope protein loricrin [3]. This family showed in addition to the typical symptoms ichthyosis. Korge *et al.* could exclude linkage to the EDC complex in a family without ichthyosis. They concluded that Vohwinkel's disease might be heterogeneous [4].

Pathology

Orthohyperkeratosis and hypergranulosis and a sparse perivascular lymphocytic infiltrate in the dermis can be observed.

Clinical features (Fig. 19.6.4)

PPK Vohwinkel is a diffuse PPK characterized by honey-combed hyperkeratosis, a violaceous border and hyperhidrosis [1–14]. It presents in infancy and is characterized by strangulating fibrous bands leading to progressive constriction and eventually spontaneous amputation of the digits (pseudoainhum). In addition, patients may present distinctive keratotic lesions on the elbows and knees and the dorsa of hands and feet, with a peculiar, linear and starfish-shaped configuration. In one patient, grossly mutilating keratoderma was accompanied by keratosis of the groins and perianal skin [12]. A number of associated findings have been noted to occur sporadically: alopecia [9,12], high-tone acoustic impairment [9,11], deafness [7,13], spastic paraplegia, myopathy [11], ichthyosiform dermatoses [2,3,5,6] and nail anomalies.

Differential diagnosis

The presence of constricted digits (pseudoainhum) can occasionally be seen in other PPKs, among them mal de Meleda, pachyonychia congenita (PC), acral keratoderma and Olmsted's syndrome.

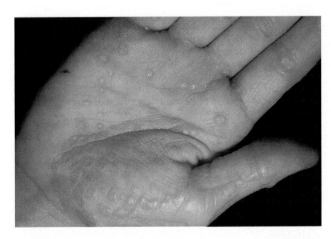

Fig. 19.6.4 PPK mutilans Vohwinkel. Courtesy of Dr Colin S. Munro, Southern General Hospital, Glasgow, UK.

Treatment

Oral retinoids are effective and can be used after good consideration of the risk–benefit ratio [2,11,14].

REFERENCES

1 Vohwinkel KH. Keratoderma hereditarium mutilans. *Arch Dermatol Syphil* 1929; 158: 354–64.
2 Camisa C, Rossana C. Variant of keratoderma hereditaria mutilans (Vohwinkel's syndrome). Treatment with orally administered isotretinoin. *Arch Dermatol* 1984; 120: 1323–8.
3 Maestrini E, Monaco AP, McGrath JA *et al*. A molecular defect in loricrin, the major component of the cornified cell envelope, underlies Vohwinkel's syndrome. *Nature Genet* 1996; 13: 70–7.
4 Korge BP, Pünter C, Stephenson A, Munro CS. Evidence of genetic heterogeneity in Vohwinkel's keratoderma. *J Invest Dermatol* 1996; 107: 481.
5 Wirz F. Keratoma hereditaria mutilans: Zu dem gleichnämigen Aufsatz von Dr KH Vohwinkel. *Arch Dermatol Syph* 1930; 159: 311–12.
6 Greschebin S. Observations on ainhum: does it exist as an independent disease? *Urol Cutan Rev* 1936; 40: 98–102.
7 Drummond A. A case of unusual skin lesions. *Ir J Med Sci* 1939; Feb: 85–9.
8 Piers F. Hereditary keratodermia and ainhum. *Br J Dermatol* 1967; 79: 693–8.
9 Gibbs RC, Frank SB. Keratoma hereditaria mutilans (Vohwinkel): differentiating features of conditions with constriction of digits. *Arch Dermatol* 1966; 94: 619–25.
10 Sierra JO, Blesa G, Montero E. Syndrome de Vohwinkel: etude de quatre cas. *Ann Dermatol Syph* 1975; 102: 41–5.
11 Chang Sing Pang AFI, Oranje AP, Vuzevki VD, Stolz E. Successful treatment of keratoderma hereditaria mutilans with an aromatic retinoid. *Arch Dermatol* 1981; 117: 225–8.
12 Ruiz-Maldonado R, Larano-Ferral N. Mutilating palmoplantar hyperkeratosis with alopecia and erythematous inguinal and perianal lesions. *Int J Dermatol* 1972; 11: 31.
13 Fitzgerald DA, Verbov JL. Hereditary palmoplantar keratoderma with deafness. *Br J Dermatol* 1996; 134: 939–42.
14 Rivers JK, Duke EE, Justus DW. Etretinate: management of keratoma hereditaria mutilans in four family members. *J Am Acad Dermatol* 1985; 13: 43–9.

Carcinoma of the oesophagus with keratosis palmaris et plantaris (Howel-Evans) (MIM no. 148 500)

(SYN. TYLOSIS)

History

A family in whom six members developed an oesophagal carcinoma in two generations was reported in 1954 by Clarke and McConell [1]. At that time the authors did not recognize that these cases also showed PPK. After the discovery of another family with the association of PPK and oesophagal carcinoma, PPK was found in the patients of the first family [2]. In 1958 Howel-Evans *et al*. further delineated the phenotype in both the families from Liverpool [3]. The largest of these two families has recently been reviewed by Ellis *et al*. [4]. Additionally, many families and sporadic individuals were described [5–10].

Aetiology

The disease is inherited in an autosomal dominant way, with complete penetrance. Risk *et al*. mapped the disease in the 17q23 region telomeric to the keratin gene cluster [11]. This finding was confirmed by other groups [10,12].

Pathology

Histopathological examination of biopsies of the hyperkeratotic lesions show marked orthohyperkeratosis and acanthosis but no signs of epidermolytic hyperkeratosis.

Clinical features

In the study by Howel-Evans *et al*. the incidence of oesophageal carcinoma was 18 out of 48 tylotic members and only one out of 87 non-tylotic members. In this paper the average age of onset of the palmoplantar hyperkeratosis was 5–15 years and of the oesophageal carcinoma 43 years. In the paper by Yesudian *et al*. [8] of those affected, three of the fourth-generation tylotics developed squamous carcinoma of the tylotic skin and only one of these died of carcinoma of the oesophagus. Palmoplantar keratosis presented at birth. Skin cancer developed in the second decade of life. This family probably suffered from Huriez's disease instead of Howel-Evans syndrome.

In one American pedigree Stevens *et al*. described 125 affected individuals in seven generations [10]. Eight had squamous cell cancer of the oesophagus. Hyperkeratosis showed a focal distribution and was most prominent on the pressure sites of the soles. They disappeared completely with prolonged bedrest or inactivity. The palms were mostly not involved except in manual workers. Hyperkeratoses developed on other places after friction and recurrent trauma. Oral hyperkeratosis preceded the plantar lesions in children [10]. (Peri)follicular hyperkeratosis, keratosis pilaris and multiple epithelial cysts were other features [10].

Acquired PPK, beginning late in life and apparently not genetically determined, has also been described in association with internal malignancy [13–17].

Differential diagnosis

The oral hyperkeratosis as described in the family of Stevens *et al*. [10] should be distinguished from the oral hyperkeratosis as can be observed in pachyonychia congenita Jadassohn–Lewandowsky which is due to a mutation in keratin 16 or 6a (see below). The thickened nails in pachyonychia congenita are an important distinguishing feature [10]. The patients in the study of Stevens *et al*. [10] showed a more localized plantar keratoderma which also makes the distinction to 'focal palmoplantar and oral mucosa hyperkeratosis syndrome' as described by Laskaris *et al*. necessary (see below) [18].

REFERENCES

1 Clarke CA, McConell RB. Six cases of carcinoma of the oesophagus occurring in one family. *Br Med J* 1954; 2: 1137–8.

2 Clarke CA, Howel-Evans AW, McConnell RB. Carcinoma of the oesophagus associated with tylosis. *Br Med J* 1957; 1: 945.

3 Howel-Evans W, McConnell RB, Clarke CA *et al*. Carcinoma of the oesophagus with keratosis palmaris et plantaris (tylosis): a study of two families. *Quart J Med* 1958; 27: 413–29.

4 Ellis A, Field JK, Field EA *et al*. Tylosis associated with carcinoma of the oesophagus and oral leukoplakia in a large Liverpool family—a review of six generations. *Eur J Cancer Oral Oncol* 1994; 30b: 102–12.

5 Shine I, Allison PR. Carcinoma of the oesophagus and tylosis. *Lancet* 1996; i: 951–3.

6 Tyldesly WR. Oral leukoplakia associated with tylosis and esophageal carcinoma. *J Oral Pathol* 1974; 3: 62–70.

7 Ritter SB, Petersen G. Esophageal cancer, hyperkeratosis, and oral leukoplakia: occurrence in a 25-year-old woman. *J Am Med Assoc* 1976; 235: 1723.

8 Yesudian P, Premalatha S, Thambiah AS. Genetic tylosis with malignancy: a study of a South Indian pedigree. *Br J Dermatol* 1980; 102: 597–600.

9 Marger RS, Marger D. Carcinoma of the oesophagus and tylosis: a lethal genetic combination. *Cancer* 1993; 72: 17–19.

10 Stevens HP, Kelsell DP, Bryant SP *et al*. Linkage of an american pedigree with palmoplantar keratoderma and malignancy (palmoplantar ectodermal dysplasia type III) to 17q24. Literature survey and proposed updated classification of the keratodermas. *Arch Dermatol* 1996; 132: 640–51.

11 Risk JM, Field EA, Field JK *et al*. Tylosis oesophageal cancer mapped. *Nature Genet* 1994; 8: 319–21.

12 Hennies H-C, Hagedorn M, Reis A. Palmoplantar keratoderma in association with carcinoma of the esophagus maps to chromosome 17q distal to the keratin gene cluster. *Genomics* 1995; 29: 537–40.

13 Parnell DD, Johnson SAM. Tylosis palmaris et plantaris. Its occurrence with internal malignancy. *Arch Dermatol* 1969; 100: 7–9.

14 Riddick L, Brodkin RH, Gibbs RC. Palmar and plantar keratoderma with hyperpigmentation and gynaecomastia. Report of a case associated with primary adenocarcinoma of the lung. *Acta Derm Venereol (Stockh)* 1971; 51: 69–72.

15 Kerdel FA, MacDonald DM. Palmo-plantar keratoderma associated with carcinoma of the bronchus. *Acta Derm Venereol (Stockh)* 1981; 62: 178–80.

16 Votion V, Mineur P, Mirgaux M, Aupaix M. Hyperkératose palmoplantaire associée a un adénocarcinome gastrique. *Dermatologica* 1982; 165: 660–3.

17 Hillion B, Le Bozec P, Moulonguet-Michau I *et al*. Hyperkératose palmoplantaire filiforme et cancer du sein. *Ann Dermatol Vénéréol* 1990; 117: 834–6.

18 Laskaris G, Vareltzidis A, Augerinou G. Focal palmoplantar and oral mucosa hyperkeratosis syndrome: a report concerning five members of a family. *Oral Surg* 1980; 50: 250–3.

Palmoplantar keratoderma with scleroatrophy (Huriez syndrome) (MIM no. 181600)

Definition

This is an inherited disorder of keratinization, characterized by diffuse scleroatrophic keratoderma of the palms and soles, sclerodactyly, nail anomalies (aplasia, ridging and clubbing) and possible malignant degeneration of the affected skin.

History

The syndrome was first described by Huriez *et al.* in two families resident in the North of France [1–3]. So far, nine families [1–10] and one case report [11] have been published.

Aetiology

The condition is autosomal dominantly inherited.

Pathology

The epidermal Langerhans' cells are virtually absent in the involved skin only [8]. The resulting diminution of recognition and presentation of tumour-associated antigens, might contribute to the proneness to malignant degeneration. Histopathological changes are aspecific.

Clinical features (Fig. 19.6.5)

The disease usually starts at birth or during early childhood and persists unchanged throughout adult life. The PPK consists of a discrete, sometimes lamellated hyperkeratosis with atrophy, diffusely covering especially the palmar skin. The plantar skin usually displays less severe involvement. Atrophic plaques may be found

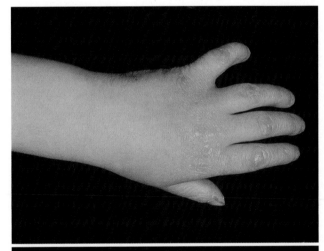

(a)

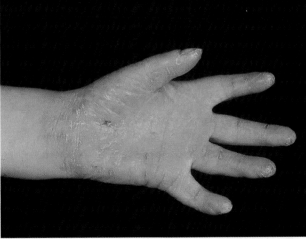

(b)

Fig. 19.6.5 (a,b) PPK with scleroatrophy (Huriez syndrome).

on the dorsa of the hands and fingers. Obligatorily associated features are sclerodactyly and nail changes. The sclerodactyly strongly resembles scleroderma, although the genetic inheritance, absence of systemic symptoms, lack of vasomotor phenomena, appearance of the initial symptoms at birth or in early childhood, and absence of progression during adulthood, enable a differentiation. Nail changes consist of aplasia, ridging and clubbing. Hypohidrosis is associated in half of the cases. The distinctive feature of this syndrome is the risk of the development of squamous cell carcinoma on the affected skin, which may occur as early as the third or fourth decade. These have been observed in 15 of 100 affected family members (average 13%). Four of them had died from metastasis of their cutaneous malignancy and one had died from squamous cell carcinoma of the oesophagus. This unusually high mortality rate might be explained by the frequently low grade of differentiation. As several affected family members described were often young, the life-time risk is probably even higher.

Treatment

Until now, only one patient with the Huriez syndrome has been treated with retinoids for 5 years. This patient did not develop any further squamous cell carcinomas in this period [12].

REFERENCES

1 Huriez CL, Agache P, Bombart M *et al.* Epitheliomas spinocellulaires sur atrophie cutanée congénitale dans deux familles à morbidité cancéreuse élevée. *Bull Soc Fr Derm Syph* 1963; 70: 24–8.
2 Huriez CL, Agache P, Souillart F *et al.* Scléroatrophie familiale des extrémités avec dégénérescence cellulaires multiples. *Bull Soc Fr Derm Syph* 1963; 70: 743–4.
3 Huriez CL, Deminati M, Agache P *et al.* Génodermatose scléro-atrophique et kératodermique des extrémités. *Ann Dermatol Syphiligr* 1969; 96: 135–46.
4 Lambert D, Planche H, Chapuis JL. La génodermatose scléro-atrophiante et kératodermique des extrémités. *Ann Dermatol Vénéréol* 1977; 104: 654–7.
5 Fischer S. La génodermatose scléro-atrophianta et kératodermique des extrémités. *Ann Dermatol Venereol* 1978; 105: 1079–82.
6 Shaw M, Formentini E, de Kaminski AR. Genodermatosis escleroatrofiante y queratodermica de las extremidades frecuentemente degenerativa. *Med Cut Ibero Lat Am* 1978; 5: 291–6.
7 Kavanagh GM, de Berker D, Jardine P, Peachey RD. The scleroatrophic syndrome of Huriez. *Br J Dermatol* 1993; 129 (suppl. 42): 21 (abstract).
8 Hamm H, Traupe H, Bröcker E, Schubert H, Kolde G. The scleroatrophic syndrome of Huriez: a cancer-prone genodermatosis. *Br J Dermatol* 1996; 134: 512–18.
9 Yesudian P, Premalatha S, Thambiah AS. Genetic tylosis with malignancy: a study of a South Indian pedigree. *Br J Dermatol* 1980; 102: 597–600.
10 Lucker GPH, Zeedijk N, Steijlen PM. The Huriez syndrome. Scleroatrophic palmoplantar keratoderma. *Eur J Dermatol* 1997; 7: 155–7.
11 Patrizi A, Lernia VD, Patrone P. Palmoplantar keratoderma with sclerodactyly (Huriez syndrome). *J Am Acad Dermatol* 1992; 26: 855–7.
12 Delaporte E, Guyen-Mailfer CN, Janin A *et al.* Keratoderma with scleroatrophy of the extremities or sclerotylosis (Huriez syndrome): a reappraisal. *Br J Dermatol* 1995; 133: 409–16.

Hidrotic ectodermal dysplasia (Clouston's syndrome) (MIM no. 129 500)

History

Hidrotic ectodermal dysplasia was first described by Nicolle and Hallipré in a French-Canadian family in 1859 [1]. In 1929 Clouston described the disease in five generations of a large French-Canadian family [2]. Later familial cases from other countries were reported [3–7].

Aetiology

The disease is inherited in an autosomal dominant manner. The gene locus has recently been mapped to the pericentromeric region of chromosome 13q [8].

Clinical features

It is characterized by dystrophy of the nails, defects of the hair and palmoplantar keratosis [2,9–11]. Sparsity of the hair of the scalp, face, eyebrows, eyelashes, axillae and genitalia, varies in severity from mild thinning to complete baldness [3]. In some, alopecia appears maximally soon after birth, though in the majority, hair loss is gradual, less severe and occurs only after puberty. Hyperkeratosis of the palms and soles has a papillomatous aspect with multiple small fissures and increases generally with age. Skin thickening has also been reported on the finger knuckles, knees and elbows [3]. Biochemically, a depletion of hair matrix protein related to a disruption of disulphide bond formation in the keratin of the integumentary system, may account for the clinical features in the hair and skin [4]. Sensorineural deafness [5,6], polydactylism, syndactylism, clubbing of the fingers, mental retardation, dwarfism [7], photophobia [4] and strabismus [12], may be associated.

REFERENCES

1 George DI, Escobar VH. Oral findings of Clouston's syndrome (hidrotic ectodermal dysplasia). *Oral Surg* 1984; 57: 258–62.
2 Clouston HR. A hereditary ectodermal dystrophy. *Canad Med Assoc J* 1929; 21: 18–31.
3 Rajagopalan K, Hai Tay C. Hidrotic ectodermal dysplasia. *Arch Dermatol* 1977; 113: 481–5.
4 Patel R-RA, Bixler D, Norins AL. Clouston syndrome: a rare autosomal dominant trait with palmoplantar hyperkeratosis and alopecia. *J Craniofac Gen Dev Biol* 1991; 11: 176–9.
5 Feinmesser M, Zelig S. Congenital deafness associated with onychodystrophy. *Arch Otolaryngol* 1961; 74: 507–8.
6 Robinson GC, Miller JR, Bensimon JR. Familial ectodermal dysplasia with sensorineural deafness and other anomalies. *Pediatrics* 1962; 30: 797–802.
7 Schinzel A. A case of multiple skeletal anomalies, ectodermal dysplasia and severe growth and mental retardation. *Helv Paediatr Acta* 1980; 35: 243–51.
8 Kibar Z, Der Kaloustian VM, Brais B, Hani V, Fraser FK, Rouleau GA. The gene responsible for Clouston hidrotic ectodermal dysplasis maps to the pericentromeric region of chromosome 13q. *Hum Mol Genet* 1996; 5: 543–7.

9 Clouston HR. Hereditary ectodermal dystrophy. *Canad Med Assoc J* 1939; 40: 1–7.
10 Wilkey WD, Stevenson GH. A family with inherited ectodermal dystrophy. *Canad Med Assoc J* 1945; 53: 226–30.
11 Williams M, Fraser FC. Hidrotic ectodermal dysplasia: Clouston's family revisited. *Canad Med Assoc J* 1967; 96: 36–9.
12 McKusick VA. *Mendelian Inheritance in Man. A Catalog of Human Genes and Genetic Disorders*, 11th edn, Baltimore: Johns Hopkins University Press, 1994.

Palmoplantar keratoderma and sensorineural deafness

History

In 1992 Sharland *et al.* [1] described a new syndrome of diffuse PPK invariably associated with a slowly progressive, bilateral, high frequency, cochlear hearing loss.

Clinical features

The onset of deafness in infancy and early childhood precedes the PPK, after which both progress slowly with age. The two abnormalities never appear as isolated defects in the family described. Combination of sensorineural hearing loss and palmoplantar keratosis has been recognized previously [2,3].

Differential diagnosis

A variable relationship between the inheritance of skin lesions and acoustic impairment has been reported in Olmsted's syndrome [4] and PPK mutilans Vohwinkel [5]. Clouston's syndrome also includes other ectodermal defects [6].

REFERENCES

1 Sharland M, Bleach NR, Goberdhan PD, Patton MA. Autosomal dominant palmoplantar hyperkeratosis and sensorineural deafness in three generations. *J Med Genet* 1992; 29: 50–2.
2 Bititci OO. Familial hereditary progressive sensorineural hearing loss with keratosis palmaris et plantaris. *J Laryngol* 1975; 89: 1143–6.
3 Konigsmark BW. Hereditary deafness in man. *N Engl J Med* 1969; 281: 713–20.
4 Olmsted HC. Keratoderma palmaris et plantaris congenitalis. *Am J Dis Child* 1927; 33: 757–64.
5 Gibbs RC, Frank SB. Keratoma hereditaria mutilans (Vohwinkel): differentiating features of conditions with constriction of digits. *Arch Dermatol* 1966; 94: 619–25.
6 Clouston HR. A hereditary ectodermal dystrophy. *Canad Med Assoc J* 1929; 21: 18–31.

Mutilating palmoplantar keratoderma with periorificial keratotic plaques (Olmsted's syndrome)

History

In 1927 Olmsted described a congenital PPK, leading to flexural deformities and spontaneous amputation of two distal phalanges [1]; 11 further cases have been reported [2–10].

Aetiology

The disease has an autosomal dominant pattern of inheritance.

Clinical features

The syndrome consists of congenital diffuse, sharply marginated keratoderma of the palms and soles with flexion deformities of the digits, leading to constriction or spontaneous amputation, periorificial keratoses and onychodystrophy. Perianal involvement has been reported in four cases [1,3,4]. Leucokeratosis was present in two cases [4]. In one patient, additionally, groins and inner thighs, ears and anterior neck, were all involved by the age of 2 years. This patient also featured universal alopecia, absence of a premolar tooth, joint hypermobility, and at the age of 20 years, linear hyperkeratotic streaks in the anticubital fossae as well as the flexor surfaces of the forearms [4]. A case has been reported with a congenital non-mutilating PPK and nail dystrophy who developed progressive perioral and perineal keratoderma and, additionally, bilateral corneal epithelial dysplasia leading to severe corneal scarring and impairment of vision [8].

Differential diagnosis

The principal genetic syndromes to be excluded in the differential diagnosis include hidrotic ectodermal dysplasia of the Clouston type, PC, mal de Meleda and PPK of Vohwinkel. The condition mimics acrodermatitis enteropatica, which has to be excluded by determination of the plasma zinc level. In retrospect, it is possible that other cases of Olmsted's syndrome may have been misdiagnosed as such.

Treatment

Mechanical removal, full thickness excision of affected skin, followed by grafting as well as systemic etretinate have been reported to be effective in single cases [1,6–7,11].

REFERENCES

1 Olmsted HC. Keratoderma palmaris et plantaris congenitalis. *Am J Dis Child* 1927; 33: 757–64.
2 Keir M. Keratodermia palmaris et plantaris. *J Roy Soc Med* 1967; 79: 419–21.
3 Ruiz-Maldonado R, Lozano-Ferral N. Hiperqueratosis palmoplantar mutilante con hipotriquia y con lesiones eritematoescamosas inguinales y perianales. *Int J Dermatol* 1972; 11: 31–5.

4 Poulin Y, Perry HO, Muller SA. Olmsted syndrome-congenital palmoplantar and periorificial keratoderma. *J Am Acad Dermatol* 1984; 10: 600–10.

5 Harms M, Bergues JP, Saurat JH. Syndrome de Olmsted (kératodermie palmoplantaire et périorificielle congénitale). *Ann Derm Vénéréol* 1985; 112: 479.

6 Atherton DJ, Sutton C, Jones BM. Mutilating palmoplantar keratoderma with periorificial keratotic plaques (Olmsted syndrome). *Br J Dermatol* 1990; 122: 245–52.

7 Judge MR, Misch K, Wright P, Harper J. Palmoplantar and periorofacial keratoderma with corneal epithelial dysplasia: a new syndrome. *Br J Dermatol* 1991; 125: 186–8.

8 Lucker GPH, Steijlen PM. The Olmsted syndrome: mutilating palmoplantar and periorificial keratoderma. *J Am Acad Dermatol* 1994; 31: 508–9.

9 Cambiaghi S, Tadini G. Olmsted syndrome in twins. *Arch Dermatol* 1995; 131: 738–9.

10 Kress DW, Seraly MP, Falo L. Kim B, Jegasothy BV, Cohen B. Olmsted syndrome. Case report and identification of a keratin abnormality. *Arch Dermatol* 1996; 132: 797–800.

11 Rivers JK, Duke EE, Justus DW. Etretinate: management of keratoderma hereditaria mutilans in four family members. *J Am Acad Dermatol* 1985; 13: 43–9.

Palmoplantar keratoderma with periodontitis (MIM no. 245 000)

(SYN. PAPILLON–LEFÈVRE SYNDROME OR PLS)

History

In 1924 Papillon and Lefèvre reported the coexistence of a PPK and severe dental anomalies in a brother and sister [1].

Aetiology

This condition is inherited as an autosomal recessive trait. Disorders of leucocyte functions might account for the prominent gingival and cutaneous infections. Some investigators have demonstrated disturbances in both polymorphonuclear leucocyte motility and bactericidal functions [2–4] or in bactericidal functions only [5–7], whereas others have not found any defects in leucocyte function [8,9]. The precise underlying mechanism for susceptibility to infections in PLS patients, however, remains to be determined. The causative gene has been mapped on chromosome 11q14 [10].

Pathology

Histopathological changes are non-specific. Electron microscopic features include lipid-like vacuoles in the corneocytes and granulocytes, reductions in tonofilaments and irregular keratohyalin granules.

Clinical features (Fig. 19.6.6)

PLS is characterized by a diffuse transgreding palmoplantar keratosis and premature loss of both the deciduous and permanent teeth [1]. In addition to the well-known palmoplantar hyperkeratosis, numerous PLS patients show scaly erythematous lesions over the knees, elbows and interphalangeal joints, commonly misdiagnosed as psoriasis [11]. Redness and thickening of the palms and soles usually appear in the first years of life, together with the breakthrough of the deciduous teeth. A spontaneous improvement parallels the subsiding of the gingiva inflammation after the loss of the permanent teeth. Associated hyperhidrosis causes an unpleasant odour [12]. An increased susceptibility to infections has been observed in about 20% of PLS patients [13]. The skin is reported to be the most common site affected by infections. Internal organs are less frequently involved [14].

Differential diagnosis

An analogue syndrome combining the features of PLS with flat feet, onychogryphosis, arachnodactyly and acro-osteolysis has been described in one family by several authors [15–17]. The Schopf–Schultz–Passarge syndrome can be distinguished by the presence of cysts on the eyelids and hypotrichosis as additional symptoms [18].

Treatment

Etretinate [14] and acitretin [19] appeared to be effective in the treatment of the hyperkeratosis and has been associated with remission of the pyodermas [14]. It was suggested that if the treatment is started at an early age normal adult dentition might be possible [19]. Other authors advise professional oral hygiene [20].

REFERENCES

1 Papillon MM, Lefèvre P. Deux cas de keratodermie palmaris et plantire symetrique familiale (Maladie de Meleda) chez le frere et la soer. Coexistance dans le deux cas d'alterations dentaires graves. *Soc Franc Dermatol Syph* 1924; 31: 82.

2 Van Dyke TE, Taubman MA, Ebersole JL *et al*. The Papillon–Lefèvre syndrome: neutrophil dysfunction with severe periodontal disease. *Clin Immunol Immunopathol* 1984; 31: 419–29.

3 Levo Y, Wollner S, Hacham-Zadeh S. Immunological study of patients with the Papillon–Lefèvre syndrome. *Clin Exp Immunol* 1980; 40: 407–10.

4 Stadler JF, Torres M, Taraud D *et al*. Anomalies fonctionelles des polynucléairs dans la maladie de Papillon–Lefèvre: trois observations. *Nouv Presse Med* 1982; 11: 2135–8.

5 Shams el Din A, Benton FR, Bottomley WK *et al*. Hyperkeratosis, periodontosis and chronic pyogenic infections in a 15-year-old boy. 1. *Ann Allergy* 1984; 53: 11–14.

6 Shams el Din A, Benton FR, Bottomley WK *et al*. Hyperkeratosis, periodontosis and chronic pyogenic infections in a 15-year-old boy. 2. *Ann Allergy* 1984; 53: 55–6.

7 Borroni G, Pagani A, Carcaterra A *et al*. Immunological alterations in a case of Papillon–Lefèvre syndrome with recurrent cutaneous infections. *Dermatologica* 1985; 170: 27–30.

8 Lyberg T. Immunological and metabolic studies in two siblings with Papillon–Lefèvre syndrome. *J Periodont Res* 1982; 17: 563–8.

9 Schroeder HE, Segar RA, Keller HU, Rateitschalk-Plüss EM. Behaviour of neutrophilic granulocytes in a case of Papillon–Lefèvre syndrome. *J Clin Periodontol* 1983; 10: 618–35.

10 Laass MW, Hennies HC, Preis S *et al*. Localisation of a gene for Papillon-Lefèvre syndrome to chromosome 11q14-q21 by homozygosity mapping. *Hum Genet* 1997; 101: 376–82.

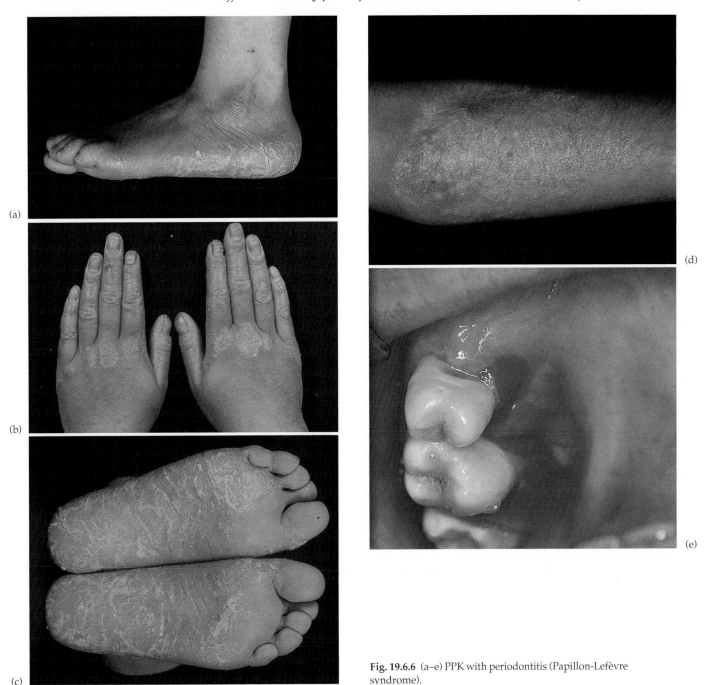

Fig. 19.6.6 (a–e) PPK with periodontitis (Papillon-Lefèvre syndrome).

11 Bork K, Löst C. Extrapalmoplantare Hautsymptome und weitere klinische und ätiologische, insbesondere immunologische Gesichtspunkte beim Papillon–Lefèvre-Syndrom. *Hautarzt* 1980; 31: 179–83.

12 Bach JN, Levan NE. Papillon–Lefèvre syndrome. *Arch Dermatol* 1968; 97: 154–8.

13 Haneke E. The Papillon–Lefèvre syndrome: keratosis palmoplantaris with periodontopathy: report of a case and review of the cases in the literature. *Hum Genet* 1979; 51: 1–35.

14 Bergman R, Friedman-Birnbaum R. Papillon–Lefèvre syndrome: a study of the long-term clinical course of recurrent pyogenic infections and the effects of etretinate treatment. *Br J Dermatol* 1988; 119: 731–6.

15 Haim S, Munk J. Keratosis palmo-plantaris congenita, with periodontosis, arachnodactyly and peculiar deformity of the terminal phalanges. *Br J Dermatol* 1965; 77: 42.

16 Smith P, Rosenzweig KA. Seven cases of Papillon–Lefèvre syndrome. *Periodontics* 1967; 5: 52.

17 Puliyel JM, Sridharan Iyer KS. A syndrome of keratosis palmo-plantaris congenita, pes planus, onychogryphosis, periodontosis, arachnodactyly and a peculiar acro-osteolysis. *Br J Dermatol* 1986; 115: 243–8.

18 Schöpf E, Schulz H-J, Passarge E. Syndrome of cystic eyelids, palmo-plantar keratosis, hypodontia and hypotrichosis as a possible autosomal recessive trait. *Birth Defects* 1971; 8: 219–21.

19 Nazzaro V. Blanchet-Bardon C, Mimoz C, Revuz J, Puissant A. Papillon-Lefèvre syndrome. Ultrastructural study and successful treatment with acitretin. *Arch Dermatol* 1988; 124: 533–9.

20 D'Angelo M, Margiotta V, Ammatuna P, Sammartano F. Treatment of pre-pubertal periodontitis. A case report and discussion. *J Clin Periodontol* 1992; 19: 214–19.

Palmoplantar keratoderma with clubbing of the fingers and toes and skeletal deformity (Bureau–Barrière–Thomas)

In 1959 Bureau, Barrière and Thomas described four members of one family, presenting with a diffuse, symmetrical, non-transgredient palmoplantar keratosis, clubbing of the fingers and toes and skeletal changes consisting of bone hypertrophy and thinning of the cortex of long bones [1,2]. Hedstrand *et al.* [3] reported on two sisters of consanguineous parents, presenting with PPK, starting in childhood, clubbing of fingers and toes together with unusual skeletal changes in the terminal phalanges. X-ray investigation revealed a peculiar deformity of the terminal phalanges. The distal end seemed splayed out and showed marginal effects suggesting atrophy [3]. In both families the PPK was accompanied by a marked hyperhidrosis. A patient was described with PPK, drumstick finger, hypotrichosis, hypohidrosis and dental dysplasia [4].

REFERENCES

1 Bureau Y, Horeau M, Barrière H, Dufaye C. Deux observations de doigts en baguettes de tambors avec hyperkératose palmoplantaire et lésions osseuses. *Bull Soc Fr Dermatol Syph* 1958; 65: 328–30.
2 Bureau Y, Barrière H, Thomas M. Hippocratisme digital congénital avec hyperkératose palmo-plantaire et troubles osseux. *Ann Derm Syph* 1959; 86: 611–22.
3 Hedstrand H, Berglund G, Werner I. Keratodermia palmaris et plantaris with cubbing and skeletal deformity of the terminal phalanges of the hands and feet. *Acta Derm Venereol (Stockh)* 1972; 52: 278–80.
4 Koch HJ, Hübner U, Schaarschmidt, Thiel W. Keratosis palmoplantaris mit Trommelschlegelfingern, Hypotrichose, Hypohidrose und Zahndysplasie. *Hautarzt* 1991; 42: 399–401.

Focal hereditary palmoplantar keratodermas without associated features

Keratosis palmoplantaris areata et striata (MIM no. 148 700)

(SYN. KERATOSIS PALMOPLANTARIS VARIANS WACHTERS)

History

Originally, striata and arata types of PPK were described: in 1924 by Fuchs [1], in 1925 by Brünauer [2] and in 1929 by Siemens [3]. In 1963 in his thesis Wachters [4] demonstrated that both arata and striata types of keratosis occurred in one family. He considered both types as manifestations of the same disorder and proposed the term keratosis palmoplantaris varians [4]. It is, however, possible to find only one subtype occurring in a family. In 1996 a case was reported presenting both keratosis palmoplantaris varians and keratosis palmoplantaris punctata [5].

Aetiology

This form of PPK is inherited in an autosomal dominant manner. The locus of this disorder occurring in a well-documented family was appointed to chromo-some 18q near the desmosomal cadherin gene cluster [6,7].

Pathology

Hyperkeratosis, hypergranulosis, acanthosis and papillomatosis. No signs of epidermolytic hyperkeratosis are observed.

Clinical features (Fig. 19.6.7)

Characteristic is the great inter- and intrafamilial variability. The palmar keratoses have either a nummular, linear, membranaceous, fissured or periungual configuration. The keratoses on the soles always have a nummular aspect and are localized on the pressure points [3,4,8,9]. The lesions become manifest at the soles mostly in the first or second year of life. The palms are affected later in life [6].

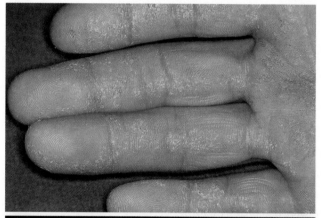
(a)

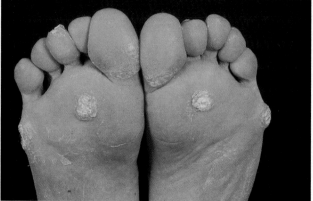
(b)

Fig. 19.6.7 (a,b) Keratosis palmoplantaris areata et striata. (b) is from Lucker GPH, Van de Kerkhof PCM, Steijlen PM. The hereditary palmoplantar keratoses: an updated review and classification. *Br J Dermatol* 1994; 131: 1–14.

Differential diagnosis

Keratosis palmoplantaris areata et striata should be differentiated from Howel-Evans syndrome in which plantar keratoderma can also have a more focal aspect, from keratosis palmoplantaris nummularis which is characterized histologically by epidermolytic hyperkeratosis and from the focal PPKs with associated features (see below).

REFERENCES

1 Fuchs H. Zur Kenntniss der herdweisen Keratosen an Händen und Füssen. *Acta Derm Venereol (Stockh)* 1924; 5: 11–58.
2 Brünauer SR. Zur Symptomatologie und Histologie der kongenitalen Dyskeratosen. *Dermatol Ztschr* 1925; 42: 6–26.
3 Siemens HW. Keratosis palmo-plantaris striata. *Arch Derm Syph (Berlin)* 1929; 157: 392–408.
4 Wachters DHJ. *Over de verschillende morphologische vormen van de keratosis palmoplantaris, in het bijzonder over de 'keratosis palmoplantaris varians'.* Thesis, State University Leiden, The Netherlands, 1963: 49–67.
5 Lucker GPH, Steijlen PM. Keratosis palmoplantaris varians et punctata. Klinische Variabilität eines einzigen gentischen Defectes? *Hautarzt* 1996; 47: 858–9.
6 Küster W, Hennies H-C, Reis A. Keratosis palmoplantaris striata Brünauer–Fuhs–Siemens. Klinische, lipidbiochemische und molekularbiologische Untersuchungen. *Z Hautkr* 1995; 70: 263–8.
7 Hennies H-C, Küster W, Mischke D, Reis A. Localization of a locus for the striated form of palmoplantar keratoderma to chromosome 18q near the desmosomal cadherin gene cluster. *Hum Molec Genet* 1995; 4: 1015–20.
8 Baes H, de Beukelaar L, Wachters D. Kératodermie palmoplantaire variante. *Ann Dermatol Syph* 1969; 96: 45–50.
9 Bologa EI. Ein Fall van plantarer, inselförmiger Keratose in 5 Generatiuonen mit dominanten Erbgang. *Hautarzt* 1965; 16: 231.

Keratosis palmoplantaris nummularis (MIM no. 114 140)
(SYN. HEREDITARY PAINFUL CALLOSITIES)

Nummular keratotic lesions, nearly exclusively located on the plantar pressure points, with pain as the major complaint, are characteristic for the disease and have been reported in 34 patients out of 14 families [1–6]. The lesions usually appear when the child begins to walk. They progress slowly and are often accompanied by pain. The palms may be involved after a period of mechanical traumatization. Extrapalmoplantar lesions have been observed in only two patients [4,5]. The major histological feature found in nearly all patients, is local epidermolytic hyperkeratosis [5].

Differential diagnosis

It differs from the PPK Vörner in that the Vörner type of palmoplantar keratosis displays diffuse palmoplantar epidermolytic hyperkeratosis. The disease can be differentiated from other focal PPKs by the presence of epidermolytic hyperkeratosis on histology.

REFERENCES

1 Samberger F. Zur Pathologie der Hyperkeratosen. *Arch Derm Syph (Berlin)* 1905; 77: 173–90.
2 Bloom D. Keratosis palmaris et plantaris hereditaria (occurring in four generations). *Arch Dermatol* 1932; 25: 1123.
3 Gasser I. Über atypische Palmo-Plantar-Keratosen. *Dermatol Wchnschr* 1950; 121: 289–96.
4 Roth W, Penneys NS, Fawcett N. Hereditary painful callosities. *Arch Dermatol* 1978; 114: 591–2.
5 Wachters DHJ, Frensdorf EL, Hausman R, van Dijk E. Keratosis palmoplantaris nummularis (hereditary painful callosities). *J Am Acad Dermatol* 1983; 9: 204–9.
6 Nogita T, Furue M, Nakagawa H, Ishibashi Y. Keratosis palmoplantaris nummularis. *J Am Acad Dermatol* 1991; 25: 113–14.

Focal hereditary palmoplantar keratodermas with associated features

Tyrosinaemia type II (MIM no. 276 600)
(SYN. RICHNER–HANHART SYNDROME, TYROSINE TRANSAMINASE DEFICIENCY)

History

This syndrome was first described by Richner in 1938 [1] and later by Hanhart in 1947 [2].

Aetiology

Tyrosinaemia type II is a rare disorder of tyrosine metabolism. Deficiency of the enzyme tyrosine aminotransferase (TAT), leading to increased serum levels of tyrosine and phenolic acid metabolites of tyrosine, is the biochemical basis for tyrosinaemia type II [3–5]. The TAT gene was mapped to the long arm of chromososome 16 (16q22.1–q22.3) [6]

Pathology

Histologically eosinophilic cytoplasmic inclusions are present in the Malpighian layer of a thickened epidermis [7].

Clinical features

This syndrome is characterized clinically by focal painful palmoplantar keratoses, bilateral pseudoherpetic corneal ulcerations and mental retardation [1,2,8,9]. The typical cutaneous changes of tyrosinaemia type II consist of painful circumscribed hyperkeratotic plaques on the palms and soles. Occasionally aberrant hyperkeratotic lesions are present in areas such as the elbows, knees or even the tongue [3]. Hyperhidrosis of the palms and soles is frequently associated [6,10,11]. Mild herpetiform corneal erosions and dendritic ulcers develop within the first months of life and may lead to corneal scarring and glaucoma [12]. Skin lesions usually occur when eye lesions have developed, although the skin lesions may exist without eye lesions [13].

REFERENCES

1 Richner H. Hornhautaffektionen bei Keratoma palmare et plantare hereditarium. *Klin Monatsbl Augenheilkd* 1938; 100: 580–8.
2 Hanhart E. Neue Sonderformen von Keratosis palmo-plantaris, u a eine regelmässig-dominante Form mit systematisierten Lipomen, ferner zwei einfach rezessive, mit Schwachsinn und z. T. mit Hornhautveränderungen des Auges (Ektodermalsyndrom). *Dermatologica* 1947; 94: 286–308.
3 Larrègue M, de Giacomoni PH, Bressieux JM, Odievre M. Syndrome de Richner–Hanhart ou tyrosinose oculo-cutanee. *Ann Dermatol Vénéréol* 1979; 106: 53–62.
4 Fellman JH, Vanbellinghen PJ, Jones RT, Koler RD. Soluble and mitochondrial forms of tyrosine aminotransferase. Relationship to human tyrosinaemia. *Biochemistry* 1969; 8: 615–22.
5 Goldsmith LA, Thorpe J, Roe CR. Hepatic enzymes of tyrosine metabolism in tyrosinaemia II. *J Invest Dermatol* 1979; 73: 530–2.
6 Natt E, Westphal E, Toth-Fejel SE *et al.* Inherited and *de novo* deletion of the tyrosine aminotransferase genelocus at 16q22.1–22.3 in a patient with tyrosinemia type II. *Hum Genet* 1987; 77: 352–8.
7 Goldsmith LA, Kang E, Bienfang DC, Jimbow K, Gerald R, Baden HP. Tyrosinaemia with plantar and palmar keratosis and keratitis. *J Paediatr* 1973; 83: 798–805.
8 Goldsmith LA. Tyrosine-induced skin disease. *Br J Dermatol* 1978; 98: 119–23.
9 Goldsmith LA. Tyrosinaemia II. *Arch Int Med* 1985; 145: 1697–700.
10 Hunziker N. Richner–Hanhart syndrome and tyrosinaemia type II. *Dermatologica* 1980; 160: 180–9.
11 Rehak A, Selim MM, Yadav G. Richner–Hanhart syndrome (tyrosinaemia II). *Br J Dermatol* 1981; 104: 469–75.
12 Bienfang DC, Kuwabara T, Pueschel SM. The Richner–Hanhart syndrome: report of a case associated with tyrosinaemia. *Arch Ophthalmol* 1976; 94: 1133–7.
13 Fraser NG, MacDonald J, Griffths WAD, McPhie JL. Tyrosinaemia type II (Richner–Hanhart syndrome)—report of two cases treated with etretinate. *Clin Exp Dermatol* 1987; 12: 440–3.

Pachyonychia congenita (subtypes: Jadassohn–Lewandowsky (MIM no. 167 200), Jackson–Lawler (MIM no. 167 210))

Definition

PC is a heterogeneous group of diseases characterized by hypertrophic nail dystrophy with nail bed keratosis.

History

PC was originally described by Muller in 1904 [1] and Wilson in 1905 [2]. Jadassohn and Lewandowsky [3] reported in 1906 on the association with PPK and other ectodermal defects.

Aetiology

PC is inherited in an autosomal dominant manner. An autosomal recessively inherited form of the disorder has been described [4]. PC Jadassohn–Lewandowsky is caused by a heterozygous mutation in the gene coding either for keratin 6 or 16. The keratins 6 and 16 are present in the nail bed around nail progenitor cells; they are abundant in the suprabasal layers of palmoplantar skin, in mucosal epithelia, especially in the oral region and in hair follicles. In PC Jackson–Lawler a mutation in the gene coding for keratin 17 has been found. Keratin 17 has a slightly different reaction pattern as compared to keratin 6 and 16. It is less present in palmoplantar skin and undocumented in oral epithelium. Traumatic damage due to a compromised keratin cytoskeleton leads to the distinct clinical features [5,6].

Pathology

Light microscopical examination of lesional plantar skin in PC Jadassohn–Lewandowsky showed many darkly stained perinuclear inclusions in spinous and granular cells. Electron microscopical examination showed perinuclear arranged keratin aggregates [5]. Histopathology of a blister did not reveal the features of epidermolytic hyperkeratosis [7].

Clinical features (Fig. 19.6.8)

PC is characterized by discoloration and thickening of the nails, usually beginning within the first month of life. The thickening results from subungual hyperkeratosis, with an upward angulation of the distal nail tip, whereas the lateral borders often curve towards the centre. Several subdivisions have been proposed [7–9]. A retrospective study of PC performed by Feinstein *et al.* in 1988 [10] disclosed 168 cases. Based on the main pathological symptoms found in this survey, the following classification was proposed:

1 Type I: Jadassohn–Lewandowsky type (56% of cases) hyperkeratosis of nails, palmoplantar keratosis, follicular keratosis and oral leucokeratosis.
2 Type II: Jackson–Lawler type (25% of cases) clinical findings of type I plus bullae of palms and soles, palmar

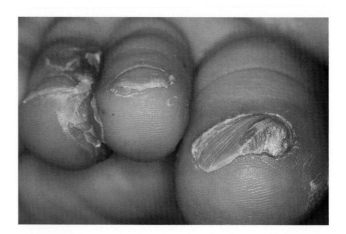

Fig. 19.6.8 PC.

and plantar hyperhidrosis, natal or natal teeth and steatocystoma multiplex.

3 Type III. (12% of cases) clinical findings of types I and II plus angular cheilosis, corneal dyskeratosis and cataracts.

4 Type IV (7% of cases) clinical findings of types I, II and III plus laryngeal lesions, hoarseness, mental retardation, hair anomalies and alopecia [10].

Chang *et al.* demonstrated that the coexistence of associated symptoms, however, is not an absolute prerequisite for the diagnosis [11]. A late-onset form of the disease has also been reported [12,13].

Differential diagnosis

PC should be differentiated from other PPKs associated with oral leucokeratosis like the Howel-Evans syndrome and the 'focal palmoplantar and oral mucosa hyperkeratosis syndrome'.

Treatment

Local keratolytic measures appeared to be useful in reducing hyperkeratosis [13]. Systemic retinoids can be effective in severe cases [14].

REFERENCES

1 Muller C. On the causes of congenital onychogryphosis. *München Med Wchnschr* 1904; 49: 2180–2.
2 Wilson AG. Three cases of hereditary hyperkeratosis of the nail bed. *Br J Dermatol* 1905; 17: 13–4.
3 Jadassohn J, Lewandowsky F. Pachyonychia congenita. In: *Jacobs Ikonographia Dermatologica*. Berlin: Urban and Schwarzenberg, 1906: 29–31.
4 Haber RM, Rose TH. Autosomal recessive pachyonychia congenita. *J Am Acad Dermatol* 1988; 19: 705–11.
5 McLean WHI, Rugg EL, Lunny DP *et al*. Keratin 16 and keratin 17 mutations cause pachyonychia congenita. *Nat Genet* 1995; 9: 273–8.
6 Bowden PE, Haley JL, Kansky A, Rothnagel JA, Jones DO, Turner RJ. Mutation of a type II keratin gene (K6a) in pachyonychia congenita. *Nat Genet* 1995; 10: 363–5.
7 Schönfeld PHIR. The pachyonychia congenita syndrome. *Acta Derm Venereol (Stockh)* 1980; 60: 45–9.
8 Kumer L, Loos HO. Congenital pachyonychia (Riehl type). *Wien Klin Wochenschr* 1935; 48: 174–8.
9 Sivasundram A, Rajagopalan K, Sarojini T. Pachyonychia congenita. *Int J Dermatol* 1985; 24: 179–80.
10 Feinstein A, Friedman J, Schewach-Millet M. Pachyonychia congenita. *J Am Acad Dermatol* 1988; 19: 705–11.
11 Chang A, Lucker GPH, Kerkhof van de PCM, Steijlen PM. Pachyonychia congenita in the absence of other syndrome abnormalities. *J Am Acad Dermatol* 1994; 30: 1017–18.
12 Paller AS, Moore JA, Scher R. Pachyonychia congenita tarda. A late-onset form of pachyonychia congenita. *Arch Dermatol* 1991; 127: 701–3.
13 Lucker GPH, Steijlen PM. Pachyonychia congenita tarda. *Clin Exp Dermatol* 1995; 20: 226–9.
14 Dupré A, Christol B, Bonafé JL, Touron P. Pachonychia congénitale. Descriptions de 3 cas familiaux. Traitement par le rétinoïde aromatique (RO 10.9359). *Ann Dermatol Vénéréol* 1981; 108: 145–9.

Focal palmoplantar and oral mucosa hyperkeratosis syndrome (MIM no. 148 730)

(SYN. FOCAL PALMOPLANTAR AND GINGIVAL KERATOSIS, FOCAL NON-EPIDERMOLYTIC PPK OR NEPPK)

History

In 1964 Fred *et al.* described the combination of PPK and hyperkeratosis of the oral mucosa in one patient [1]. Raphael *et al.* described this combination of clinical features in a family with four affected relatives [2]. Subsequently, the syndrome has been reported in families involving several generations [3–6].

Aetiology

Shamser *et al.* demonstrated two different heterozygous mutations in the keratin 16 gene in two families [6].

Pathology

Histological examination of biopsies taken from the labial gingiva and the soles revealed severe hyperkeratosis and acanthosis [5]. In the family described by Shamser *et al.* no signs of epidermolytic hyperkeratosis could be observed [6].

Clinical features

The syndrome is characterized by hyperkeratosis of the palms, soles and oral mucosa. The hyperkeratosis is especially marked on the weight-bearing areas of the soles, the pressure-related areas of the palms and the attached gingiva. Besides the attached gingiva, hyperkeratotic lesions develop in areas of the oral mucosa subjected to friction and irritation. The hyperkeratosis, which has a symmetrical distribution, appears in early childhood or around puberty. The hyperkeratotic lesions increase in severity with age and vary among patients, even in the same family. Subungual and circumungual hyperkeratosis of the nails may be an associated feature [5]. In 1995 Shamser *et al.* described two families with focal PPK, follicular and orogenital hyperkeratosis. Subtle nail changes with widening of the onychocorneal band was observed in affected members.

Differential diagnosis

This disease can be differentiated from pachyonychia congenita Jadassohn–Lewandowsky by the absence of thickened nails and from the Howel-Evans syndrome by the absence of oesophageal carcinoma. Furthermore, in the Howel-Evans syndrome linkage to the keratin clusters has been excluded.

REFERENCES

1 Fred HL, Gieser RG, Berry WR, Eiband JM. Keratosis palmaris et plantaris. *Arch Int Med* 1964; 113: 866–71.
2 Raphael AL, Baer PN, Lee WB. Hyperkeratosis of gingival and plantar surface. *Periodontics* 1968; 6: 118–20.
3 James P, Beggs D. Tylosis: a case report. *Br J Oral Surg* 1973; 11: 143–5.
4 Gorlin RJ. Focal palmoplantar and marginal gingival hyperkeratosis—a syndrome. *Birth Defects* 1976; 12: 239–42.
5 Laskaris G, Vareltzidis A, Avgerinou G. Focal palmoplantar and oral mucosa hyperkeratosis syndrome: a report concerning five members of a family. *Oral Surg* 1980; 50: 250–3.
6 Shamser MK, Havsaria HA, Stevens HP *et al.* Novel mutations in keratin 16 gene underly focal non-epidermolytic palmoplantar keratoderma (NEPPK) in two families. *Hum Molec Genet* 1995; 4: 1875–81.

Keratosis palmoplantaris papillomatosa et verrucosa

In 1975, Jakac and Wolf described a clinically distinct keratoderma in four relatives of one family, which has its onset between 2 and 6 years of age and is characterized by a verrucous–papillomatous aspect [1]. The PPK, accompanied by a violaceous red border, is nummular at onset and progresses to cover the entire surface of the palms and soles. The keratosis is sharply confined to the palms and soles. Fingers and toes have an atrophic skin and are contracted in flexion. Aberrant keratotic lesions may be present at the knees, lower arms and buttocks. Because of a profuse hyperhidrosis, which is a constant accompanying feature of the disease, and the pronounced papillomatosis, secondary infections may lead to periostitis and osteomyelitis. In one of the patients, gingivitis and periodontitis, leading to preliminary loss of teeth, was observed.

REFERENCE

1 Jakac D, Wolf A. Papillomatös-verruköse Form der palmo-plantaren Keratodermie kombiniert mit anderen Anomalien der Verhornung sowie dysplastischen Zahnveränderungen. *Hautarzt* 1975; 26: 25–9.

Papular hereditary palmoplantar keratodermas without associated features

Keratosis palmoplantaris punctata (Davies–Colley, Buschke, Fischer, Brauer) (MIM no. 148 600)

(SYN. KERATOSIS PALMOPLANTARIS PAPULOSA, PUNCTATE POROKERATOSIS, POROKERATOSIS PUNCTATA PALMARIS ET PLANTARIS, PALMOPLANTAR KERATOSIS ACUMINATA, PUNCTATE POROKERATOTIC KERATODERMA)

Pathology

Histological examination reveals a compact column of parakeratosis resembling that of a cornoid lamella, without evidence of dyskeratosis or hydropic degeneration in the epidermis, differentiating the condition from porokeratosis [1–3,11].

Clinical features (Fig. 19.6.9)

The clinical presentation of numerous tiny keratotic papules, strictly limited to the volar aspects of the hands and feet, has been designated by numerous terms, causing much confusion [2–6]. Lesions generally develop between the second and fourth decade, with the age of onset ranging from 12 to 70 years. The papular keratoses progress slowly and remain asymptomatic. Despite a great interfamilial clinical variation, a uniform expression exists within an individual family. Localized forms limited to the palmar creases have been described [1]. Most of the patients exhibit no associated features. Nevertheless, spastic paralysis [7], morbus Bechterew [8] and facial sebaceous hyperplasia [5] have been reported in associated with PPK punctata. Additionally, a coincidental [9] and a possible familial [10] association with gastrointestinal malignancy have been discussed. Stevens *et al.* [12] found an association between punctate PPK and malignancy in a four-generation family. They speculated about the possibility that both the PPK and the malignancies may be caused by a defect in the same gene or that two tightly linked genetic mutations cosegregate through the family [12]. Kelsell *et al.* excluded linkage with the keratin clusters on chromosome 12 and 17 [13].

REFERENCES

1 Weiss RM, Rasmussen JE. Keratosis punctata of the palmar creases. *Arch Dermatol* 1980; 116: 669–71.
2 Friedman SJ, Herman PS, Pittelkow MR, Daniel WP. Punctate porokeratotic keratoderma. *Arch Dermatol* 1988; 124: 1678–82.
3 Lestringant GG, Berge T. Porokeratosis punctata palmaris et plantaris. A new entity? *Arch Dermatol* 1989; 125: 816–20.
4 Herman PS. Punctate porokeratotic keratoderma. *Dermatologica* 1973; 147: 206–13.
5 Schiff BL, Pawtucket RI, Hughes D. Palmoplantar keratosis acuminata with facial sebaceous hyperplasia. *Arch Dermatol* 1974; 109: 86–7.
6 Sakas EL, Gentry RH. Porokeratosis punctata palmaris et plantaris (punctate porokeratosis). Case report and literature review. *J Am Acad Dermatol* 1985; 13: 908–12.
7 Powell FC, Venencie PY, Gordon H, Winkelmann RK. Keratoderma and spastic paralysis. *Br J Dermatol* 1983; 109: 589–96.
8 Nielsen PG. Punctate palmoplantar keratoderma associated with morbus Bechterew and HLA-B-27. *Acta Derm Venereol (Stockh)* 1988; 68: 346–50.
9 Fegueux S, Crickx B, Perron J, Grossin M, Belaïch S. Hyperkératose palmoplantaire filiforme et cancer recto-sïgmoidien. *Ann Dermatol Vénéréol* 1988; 115: 1145–6.
10 Bennion SD, Patterson JW. Keratosis punctata palmaris et plantaris and adenocarcinoma of the colon. *J Am Acad Dermatol* 1984; 10: 587–91.
11 Osman Y, Daly TJ, Don PC. Spiny keratoderma of the palms and soles. *J Am Acad Dermatol* 1992; 26: 879–81.
12 Stevens HP, Kelsell DP, Leigh IM, Ostlere LS, MacDermot KD, Rustin MHA. Punctate palmoplantar keratoderma and malignancy in a four-generation family. *Br J Dermatol* 1996; 134: 720–6.
13 Kelsell DP, Stevens HP, Ratnavel R *et al.* Genetic linkage studies in non-epidermolytic palmoplantar keratoderma: evidence for heterogeneity. *Hum Molec Genet* 1995; 4: 1021–5.

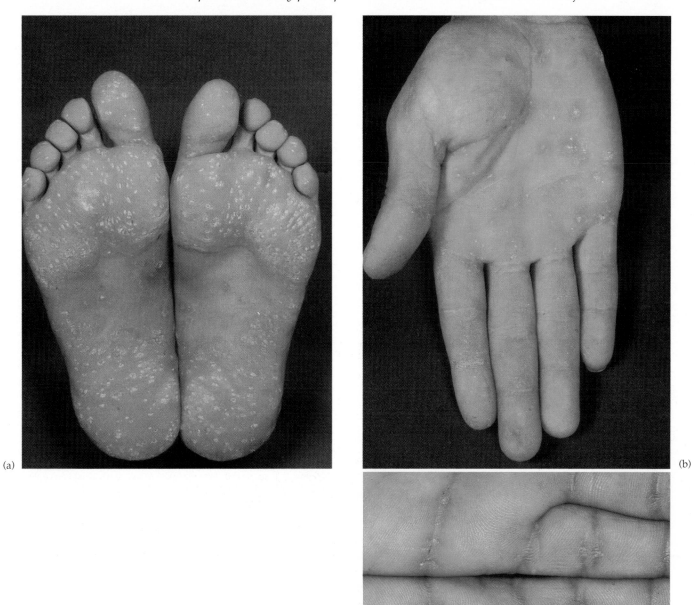

(a)

(b)

(c)

Fig. 19.6.9 (a–c) Keratosis palmoplantaris punctata.

Acrokeratoelastoidosis (AKE) (MIM no. 101850)

Costa described in 1953 a clinical entity which he called AKE [1,2]. Clinically, the disease is characterized by small yellowish, round to oval keratotic papules, extending the marginal and dorsal surfaces of palms and soles. Centrally, the keratotic papules may confluence to a diffuse keratoderma of the palms and soles. The process begins in childhood or adolescence. The number of papules gradually increases over several years. Local hyperhidrosis is present. Histologically, the disease is characterized by elastorrhexis [1,2]. In 1995 Lossos *et al.* described a family with four members suffering from leucoencephalopathy and a PPK resembling AKE [3]. The disease must be differentiated histologically from focal acral hyperkeratosis and clinically from degenerative collagenous plaques of the hands [4], which is an entirely separate acquired condition, occurring in an older age group on the sun-exposed parts of the hands.

REFERENCES

1 Costa OG. Acrokeratoelastoidosis: a hitherto undescribed skin disease. *Dermatologica* 1953; 107: 164.
2 Jung EG, Beil FU, Anton-Lamprecht I, Greten H, Nemetschek T. Akrokeratoelastoidosis. *Hautarzt* 1974; 25: 127–33.
3 Lossos A, Cooperman H, Soffer D *et al.* Hereditary leukoencephalopathy and palmoplantar keratoderma: a new disorder with increased skin collagen content. *Neurology* 1995; 45: 331–7.
4 Ritchie EB, Williams HM. Degenerative collagenous plaques of the hands. *Arch Dermatol* 1966; 93: 202–3.

Focal acral hyperkeratosis

This dermatosis is clinically similar but histologically dissimilar to AKE [1]. It appears to be a focal disorder of keratinization with insidious onset in childhood, reaching a maximum in early life and causing only cosmetic embarrassment. With the exception of one Arab patient, all patients are of black African descent. In addition to the typical papules along the borders of the hands and feet, hyperkeratotic papules may be present over the interphalangeal joints of the fingers and toes as well as the heels. On histological examination, elastorrhexis is lacking, differentiating the disease from AKE.

REFERENCE

1 Dowd PM, Harman RRM, Black MM. Focal acral hyperkeratosis. *Br J Dermatol* 1983; 109: 97–103.

Papular hereditary palmoplantar keratodermas with associated features

Syndrome of cystic eyelids, palmoplantar keratosis, hypodontia and hypotrichosis (Schöpf–Schulz–Passarge syndrome) (MIM no. 224 750)

Schöpf *et al.* reported two sisters with a syndrome of cystic eyelids, hypodontia, hypotrichosis and palmoplantar keratosis [1]. A similar grouping of ectodermal defects was reported by Burket *et al.* in a man who presented as a sporadic case [2]. Unique in his report were multiple facial tumours of the follicular infundibulum (Mehregan and Butler) [3]. Happle and Rampen described the development of squamous cell carcinoma in association with this syndrome [4]. PLS can be differentiated easily. Periodontitis, which is an integral part of PLS, was absent in the cases of Schöpf's syndrome. Eyelid cysts have not been described in PLS.

REFERENCES

1 Schöpf E, Schulz H-J, Passarge E. Syndrome of cystic eyelids, palmo-plantar keratosis, hypodontia and hypotrichosis as a possible autosomal recessive trait. *Birth Defects* 1971; 8: 219–21.
2 Burket JM, Burket BJ, Burket DA. Eyelid cysts, hypodontia and hypotrichosis. *J Am Acad Dermatol* 1984; 10: 922–5.
3 Mehregan AH, Butler JD. A tumor of follicular infundibulum. *Arch Dermatol* 1961; 83: 78–81.
4 Happle R, Rampen FHJ. Multiple eyelid hidrocystoma syndrome: a new cancer syndrome? In: Wilkinson DS, Mascaró JM, Orfanos CE, Albers J, eds. *Clinical Dermatology—the CMD Case Collection. World Congress of Dermatology*, Berlin, 24–29 May 1987. Stuttgart: Schattauer, 1987: 290–1.

Keratosis Pilaris

ARNOLD P. ORANJE

Definition

Keratosis pilaris is a cutaneous finding associated with a variety of diseases. It is defined by the presence of keratotic plugging of hair follicles, surrounded by varying degrees of erythema. When keratosis pilaris is accompanied by atrophy, it is referred to as keratosis pilaris atrophicus [1,2].

History

The clinical entities of keratosis pilaris and keratosis pilaris atrophicus are the source of historical confusion. This is the result of overlap among syndromes, the presence of intermediate forms and the existence of numerous synonyms in the dermatology and genetics literature [3].

Particularly confusing is the entity 'ichthyosis follicularis', a term coined by Lesser in 1885 [4,5]. Another disorder that, historically, has received much attention is keratosis follicularis spinulosa decalvans (also initially described as ichthyosis follicularis). This entity was first described in the Dutch literature by Lameris in 1905 and Rochat in 1906 in a Dutch-German family [6,7]. In 1925, Siemens investigated this same family [8].

REFERENCES

1 McKusick VA. *Mendelian Inheritance in Man*, 13th edn. Baltimore: Johns Hopkins University Press, 1995.
2 Rand RE, Arndt KA. Follicular syndromes with inflammation and atrophy. In: Fitzpatrick TB, Eisen AZ, Wolff K, Freedberg IM, Austen KF, eds. *Dermatology in General Medicine*, 3rd edn. McGraw Hill, 1979: 717–21.
3 Touraine A. Essai de classification des keratoses congenitales. *Ann Dermatol* 1958; 85: 257–66.
4 Eramo LR, Burton Esterly N, Zieserl EJ, Stock EL, Herrmann J. Ichthyosis follicularis with alopecia and photophobia. *Arch Dermatol* 1985; 121: 1167–74.
5 Lesser E. Ichthyosis follicularis. In: Eiemssen N, ed. *Handbook of Skin Diseases*. New York: William Wood, 1885.
6 Lameris HJ. Ichthyosis follicularis. *Ned Tijdschr Geneeskd (Dutch J Med)* 1905; 41: 1524.
7 Rochat GF. Familiaire cornea degeneratie. *Ned Tijdschr Geneeskd (Dutch J Med)* 1906; 42: 515–18.
8 Siemens HW. Keratosis follicularis spinulosa decalvans. *Arch Dermatol Syph* 1926; 151: 384–7.

Aetiology and pathogenesis

In the isolated form, keratosis pilaris is essentially physiological. About 40% of children suffer from mild keratosis pilaris. In a questionnaire study undertaken by Poskitt and Wilkinson, the mean age of improvement was 16 years [1]. Keratosis pilaris may also be seen in relation to malnutrition/nutritional deficiency, xerosis and ichthyosis vulgaris [2,3].

Keratosis pilaris atrophicans occurs in a number of syndromes with different inheritance patterns: (a) keratosis pilaris atrophicans faciei; (b) atrophoderma vermiculata; (c) keratosis follicularis spinulosa decalvans; and (d) folliculitis spinulosa decalvans [4].

Keratosis pilaris atrophicans faciei, or ulerythema ophryogenes, is inherited in autosomal dominant fashion. Physical findings occur predominantly in the eyebrows. Genetic linkage studies have not yet been performed.

Atrophoderma vermiculata, also known as atrophoderma reticulata, acne vermoulante, folliculitis ulerythema reticulata, folliculitis ulerythematosa and honeycomb atrophy, is characterized by reticulate scarring on the cheeks. The disease is inherited as an autosomal recessive trait, and genetic linkage has not yet been performed.

Keratosis follicularis spinulosa decalvans has been extensively studied. Families have been described in Finland, Switzerland and The Netherlands. In all three family studies, pedigree analysis shows X-linked inheritance [5–7]. Nearly complete expression in women can be explained by skewed lyonization. Harth *et al.* have described fully expressed keratosis follicularis spinulosa decalvans in a woman [8].

In a large Dutch family which descends from the cohort originally investigated by Lameris and Siemens, Oosterwijk *et al.* located the gene to Xp21.2–p22.2 [5,9]. In 54 individuals (including 21 affected males), DNA linkage analysis was performed using DNA probes of the X chromosome. Multipoint analysis placed the gene defect between DXS16 and DXS269. The gene locus has since been narrowed to Xp22.13–p22.2 [10], but in another German family the same research team could not confirm these results and suggested the possibility of genetic heterogeneity [11].

Pathology

The histopathology is non-specific and is generally not useful in diagnosis. The follicular orifice is distended by a keratin plug. In keratosis pilaris, mild inflammation is present. In keratosis pilaris atrophicans, severe inflammation may occur in the early stages. In late stages of keratosis pilaris atrophicans, atrophy of the epidermis is noted [5,12].

REFERENCES

1 Poskitt L, Wilkinson JD. Natural history of keratosis pilaris. *Br J Dermatol* 1994; 130: 711–13.
2 Guillet G, Sanciaume C, Hennunestre JP *et al.* Keratose pilaire generalisée. *Ann Dermatol Vénéréol* 1982; 109: 1061–6.
3 Mevorah B, Marazzi A, Frenk E. The prevalence of accentuated palmoplantar marking and keratosis pilaris in atopic dermatitis, autosomal dominant ichthyosis and control dermatological patients. *Br J Dermatol* 1985; 112: 679–85.
4 Oranje AP, Osch van LDM, Oosterwijk JC. Keratosis pilaris atrophicans. *Arch Dermatol* 1994; 130: 500–2.
5 Van Osch LDM, Oranje AP, Keukens FM *et al.* Keratosis follicularis spinulosa decalvans. *J Med Genet* 1992; 29: 36–40.
6 Franceschetti A, Jaccottet M, Jadassohn W. Manifestations cornéennes dans la keratosis follicularis spinulosa decalvans (Siemens). *Ophthalmologica* 1957; 133: 259–63.
7 Kuokkanen K. Keratosis follicularis spinulosa decalvans in a family from northern Finland. *Acta Derm Venereol (Stockh)* 1971; 51: 146–50.
8 Richard G, Harth W. Keratosis follicularis spinulosa decalvans. Therapie mit Isotretinoin und Etretinat im entzundlichen Stadium. *Hautarzt* 1993; 44: 529–34.
9 Oosterwijk JC, Nelen M, van Zandvoort PM *et al.* Linkage analysis of keratosis follicularis spinulosa decalvans, and regional assignment to human chromosome Xp21.2–p22.2. *Am J Hum Genet* 1992; 50: 801–7.
10 Oosterwijk JC, van der Wielen MJ, van de Vosse E *et al.* Refinement of the localisation of the X linked keratosis follicularis spinulosa decalvans (KFSD) gene in Xp22.13–p22.2. *J Med Genet* 1995; 32: 736–9.
11 Oosterwijk JC, Richard G, van der Wielen MJ *et al.* Molecular genetic analysis of two families with keratosis follicularis spinulosa decalvans: refinement of gene localisation and evidence for genetic heterogeneity. *Hum Genet* 1997; 100: 520–4.
12 Sallakachart P, Nakjang Y. Keratosis pilaris: a clinicohistopathologic study. *J Med Assoc Thai* 1987; 70: 386–9.

Clinical features

Keratosis pilaris

Lesions occur predominantly on the extensor surfaces of the arms (Fig. 19.7.1) and legs, but may also involve the face, buttocks and trunk. Keratosis pilaris often improves in the summer months, and flares in the winter. Clinical signs of atopy are observed in at least one-third of patients [1,2].

Keratosis pilaris is characterized by the presence of rough, follicular papules, and varying degrees of erythema. Erythema may be particularly severe in children with extensive facial involvement (keratosis pilaris rubra faciei). A number of diseases are associated with keratosis pilaris (Table 19.7.1) [3–9].

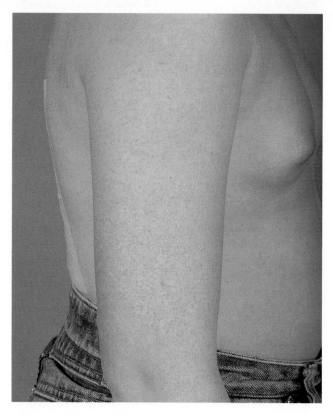

Fig. 19.7.1 Keratosis pilaris on the arms.

Table 19.7.1 Keratosis pilaris and keratosis pilaris atrophicans associated disorders and syndromes in childhood

Keratosis pilaris	Physiological
	Atopic dermatitis
	Lichen spinulosa
	Ichthyosis vulgaris
	Other ichthyoses (Mevorah *et al.* [3])
	Renal insufficiency (Guillet *et al.* [4])
	Prolidase deficiency (Larrègue *et al.* [5])
	Down's syndrome (Finn *et al.* [6])
	Monilethrix
	Fairbank's syndrome (Marks [7])
	Keratosis pilaris follicularis non-atrophicans
Keratosis pilaris atrophicans	Keratosis pilaris atropicans faciei (ulerythema oophryogenes)
	Atrophoderma vermiculata
	Keratosis follicularis spinulosa decalvans
	Folliculitis spinulosa [8]
	Noonan's syndrome (now called cardiofaciocutaneous syndrome (Ward *et al.* [9])
	Woolly hair

Monilethrix is characterized by beaded hair shafts that break easily (see Chapter 23.1). The hair is often unremarkable at birth, and becomes abnormal during the first year of life. Follicular hyperkeratosis is seen on the neck and occipital scalp. The eyebrows may also be affected [10].

Lichen spinulosa or keratosis spinulosa is characterized by grouped follicular papules with keratotic spines in nummular patches, on the trunk and extremities. Boys are most often affected, and the disorder usually disappears at puberty [11]. There are no known associations with syndromes or systemic diseases.

Keratosis pilaris atrophicans

Keratosis pilaris atrophicans faciei is characterised by redness and atrophic scarring of the eyebrows (Fig. 19.7.2). The symptoms are present at birth or begin during infancy. Typical keratosis pilaris is observed at other sites. Combinations of keratosis pilaris atrophicans faciei and Noonan's syndrome or woolly hair have been described [12–14]. The association with Noonan's syndrome has been designated as cardiofaciocutaneous syndrome [9].

Atrophoderma vermiculata is characterized by symmetrical reticulate atrophy and scarring of the cheeks. Small pits with sharp edges give the skin a 'worm-eaten' appearance. Lesions are always limited to the face, and begin after the age of 5 years. Asymmetric forms limited to one cheek have been described [15].

Keratosis follicularis spinulosa decalvans is a rare X-linked disease that affects both the skin (Fig. 19.7.3) and the eyes (Fig. 19.7.4). It is characterized by follicular hyperkeratosis of the skin and corneal dystrophy. Several families have been described, the largest one of German-Dutch origin [16–18].

The follicular papules are associated with loss of hair, especially of the scalp, eyebrows and eyelashes. Marked photophobia may result from the corneal dystrophy. Other prominent findings are scarring alopecia of the scalp and absence of the eyebrows and eyelashes. X-linked keratosis follicularis spinulosa decalvans lacks

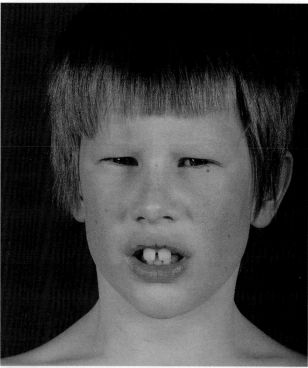

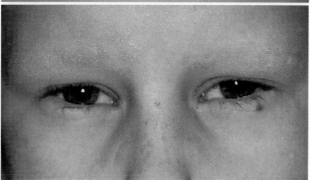

Fig. 19.7.3 Keratosis follicularis spinulosa decalvans in the face.

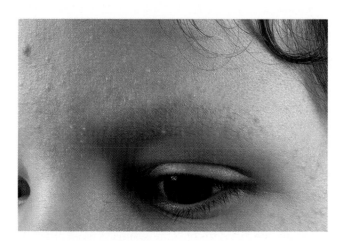

Fig. 19.7.2 Keratosis pilaris atrophicans faciei.

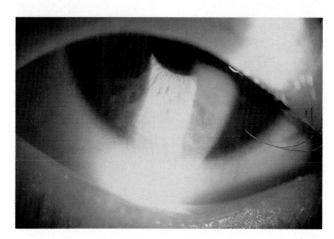

Fig. 19.7.4 Patchy corneal dystrophy in keratosis follicularis spinulosa decalvans.

severe inflammation. In the author's study of the largest known pedigree, hyperkeratosis of the knees (Fig. 19.7.5) and calcaneal region of the soles was noted, together with a high cuticle on the nails (Fig. 19.7.6) [16].

Symptoms are never present at birth, and generally develop in early childhood. Complete spontaneous improvement often occurs at puberty [16].

Of female carriers 50% are asymptomatic [16–18]. Symptomatic female carriers develop dry skin, minimal follicular hyperkeratosis and mild hyperkeratosis of the soles, but have no eye findings. Fully expressed keratosis follicularis spinulosa decalvans has been described once in a female [19].

Phrynoderma. Nicholls observed hyperkeratotic folliculitis in some African labourers who suffered from vitamin A deficiency [20]. More recently, the same physi-

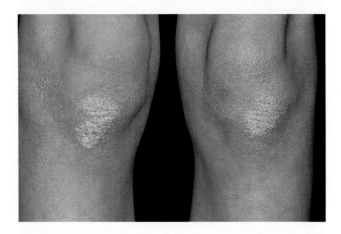

Fig. 19.7.5 Hyperkeratosis on the knees in keratosis follicularis spinulosa decalvans.

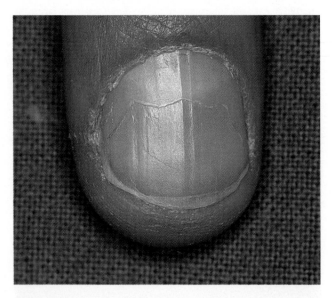

Fig. 19.7.6 A prominent cuticle of the nails in keratosis follicularis spinulosa decalvans (aspecific sign).

cal finding has been noted to occur after intestinal bypass [21]. Phrynoderma has not been described extensively in children.

REFERENCES

1 Rand RE, Arndt KA. Follicular syndromes with inflammation and atrophy. In: Fitzpatrick TB, Eisen AZ, Wolff K, Freedberg IM, Austen KF, eds. *Dermatology in General Medicine*, 3rd edn. McGraw 1979: 717–21.
2 Poskitt L, Wilkinson JD. Natural history of keratosis pilaris. *Br J Dermatol* 1994; 130: 711–13.
3 Mevorah B, Marazzi A, Frenck E. The prevalence of accentuated palmoplantar markings and keratosis pilaris in atopic dermatitis, autosomal dominant ichthyosis and control dermatological patients. *Br J Dermatol* 1985; 112: 679–85.
4 Guillet C, Sanciaume C, Hehunestre JP *et al.* Keratose pilaire generalisée et hypervitaminose à chez une enfant insuffisante renale. *Ann Dermatol Vénéréol* 1982; 109: 1061–6.
5 Larrègue M, Charpentier C, Laidet B *et al.* Déficit en prolidase et en manganese. *Ann Dermatol Vénéréol* 1982; 109: 667–8.
6 Finn OA, Grant PW, McCallum DI *et al.* A singular dermatosis of Mongols. *Arch Dermatol* 1978; 114: 1493–4.
7 Marks R. Follicular hyperkeratosis and ocular abnormalities associated with Fairbank's syndrome. *Br J Dermatol* 1967; 79: 118–19.
8 Oranje AP, van Osch LDM, Oosterwijk JC. Keratosis pilaris atrophicans. *Arch Dermatol* 1994; 130: 500–2.
9 Ward KA, Moss C, McKeown C. The cardio-facio-cutaneous syndrome: a manifestation of the Noonan syndrome? *Br J Dermatol* 1994; 131: 270–4.
10 Despontin K, Krafchik B. What syndrome is this? Monilethrix. *Pediatr Dermatol* 1993; 10: 192–4.
11 Boyd AS. Lichen spinulosus: case report and overview. *Cutis* 1989; 43: 557–60.
12 McKusick VA. *Mendelian Inheritance in Man*, 10th edn. Baltimore: Johns Hopkins University Press, 1992.
13 Pierini DO, Pierini AM. Keratosis pilaris atrophicans faciei (ulerythema oophryogenes): a cutaneous marker of Noonan's syndrome. *Br J Dermatol* 1979; 100: 409–16.
14 Neild VS, Pegum JS, Wells RS. The association of keratosis pilaris atrophicans and woolly hair, with and without Noonan's syndrome. *Br J Dermatol* 1984; 110: 357–62.
15 Arrieta E, Milgram-Sternberg Y. Honeycomb atrophy on the right cheek. *Arch Dermatol* 1994; 130: 481–2.
16 Osch van LDM, Oranje AP, Keukens FM *et al.* Keratosis follicularis spinulosa decalvans. *J Med Genet* 1992; 29: 36–40.
17 Franceschetti A, Jaccottet M, Jadassohn W. Manifestations cornéennes dans la keratosis follicularis spinulosa decalvans (Siemens). *Ophthalmologica* 1957; 133: 259–63.
18 Kuokkanen K. Keratosis follicularis spinulosa decalvans in a family from northern Finland. *Acta Derm Venereol (Stockh)* 1971; 51: 146–50.
19 Harth W, Richard G, Schubert H. Keratosis follicularis spinulosa decalvans: the complete syndrome in a female (German language). *Z Hautkr* 1992; 67: 1080–4.
20 Nicholls L. Phrynoderma: a condition due to vitamin deficiency. *Ind Med Gazette* 1933; 68: 681–7.
21 Barr RJ, Riley RJ. Bypass phynoderma. *Arch Dermatol* 1984; 120: 919–21.

Prognosis

Keratosis pilaris resolves completely in at least one-third of the cases. Lesions involving the arms and legs are more likely to persist into adulthood than facial lesions. Most cases of keratosis pilaris atrophicans eventuate in atrophy, without persistent inflammation [1–3].

Differential diagnosis

Normally, the diagnosis of keratosis pilaris is not difficult.

Keratosis pilaris involving the face may mimic milia, miliaria and acne vulgaris. Other childhood causes of follicular keratoses include pityriasis rubra pilaris and Darier's disease. Early cases of keratosis pilaris atrophicans faciei may be confused with the common form of keratosis pilaris, and late forms with seborrhoeic dermatitis. Atrophoderma vermiculata may be misdiagnosed as acne vulgaris or lupoid sycosis.

Treatment

There is no effective therapy for keratosis pilaris. Emollients are rarely effective. Mild, temporary relief can be obtained with keratolytic agents, such as 10% urea. Topical corticosteroids may also temporarily reduce the keratotic and inflammatory components [4].

Similar results with topical therapy are seen in keratosis pilaris atrophicans. Dermabrasion is helpful in selected cases [5]. End-stage atrophy can be treated only by grafting [6]. Isotretinoin or etretinate are not useful in the treatment of keratosis pilaris atrophicans [4,7]. Response to all therapies (keratolytics, antibiotics, corticosteroids and retinoids) is limited.

REFERENCES

1 Poskitt L, Wilkinson JD. Natural history of keratosis pilaris. *Br J Dermatol* 1994; 130: 711–13.
2 Arrieta E, Milgram-Stenberg Y. Honeycomb atrophy on the right cheek. *Arch Dermatol* 1994; 130: 481–2.
3 Oranje AP, van Osch LDM, Oosterwijk JC. Keratosis pilaris atrophicans. *Arch Dermatol* 1994; 130: 500–2.
4 Baden HP, Byers R. Clinical findings, cutaneous pathology and response to therapy in 21 patients with keratosis pilaris atrophicans. *Arch Dermatol* 1994; 130: 469–75.
5 Rand RE, Arndt KA. Follicular syndromes with inflammation and atrophy. In: Fitzpatrick TB, Eisen AZ, Wolff K, Freedberg IM, Austen KF, eds. *Dermatology in General Medicine*, 3rd edn. New York: McGraw Hill, 1987: 717–21.
6 van Osch LDM, Oranje AP, Keukens FM *et al*. Keratosis follicularis spinulosa decalvans. *J Med Genet* 1992; 29: 36–40.
7 Arrieta E, Milgram-Sternberg Y. Honeycomb atrophy on the right cheek. *Arch Dermatol* 1994; 130: 481–2.

19.8   The Erythrokeratodermas

DAVID G. PAIGE

Erythrokeratoderma variabilis

Erythrokeratoderma en cocardes

Erythrokeratoderma progressiva symmetrica

Syndromes associated with erythrokeratoderma

Definition

The erythrokeratodermas are a group of rare genodermatoses characterized by well-demarcated, hyperkeratotic, erythematous plaques. Three types have been delineated based solely on clinical features: erythrokeratoderma variabilis (EKV), erythrokeratoderma en cocardes (EKC) and erythrokeratoderma progressiva symmetrica (EPS). Recent genetic advances are beginning to allow a better understanding of the true nosological status of these three variants.

Erythrokeratoderma variabilis

(SYN. KERATOSIS RUBRA FIGURATA,
ERYTHROKERATODERMIA FIGURATA VARIABILIS,
MENDES DA COSTA'S SYNDROME)

History

In 1907 DeBuy Wenniger described a girl with an erythrokeratodermia of variable configuration [1]. Two further cases were described in 1922 by Rille (keratosis rubra figurata) [2] and Jeanselme [3]. In 1925 Mendes da Costa described the same condition in a mother and daughter naming the disorder EKV [4]. He described the rash as being characterized by erythematous, hyperkeratotic plaques which showed 'outlines like the boundary lines of seacoasts on maps'. He also noted the other typical feature of this condition describing erythematous areas which moved hour by hour. Noordhoeck [5] and Schnyder and Sommacal-Schopf [6] subsequently reported large family studies, thus establishing the autosomal dominant pattern of inheritance.

Pathogenesis

Van der Schroeff reported linkage data on two large dutch kindreds showing close linkage with the Rh locus on chromosome 1 (located at 1p36.2-p34) [7,8]. More recent studies have shown that EKV is due to a mutation in the GJB3 gene which codes for a gap junction protein called connexin 31 [9,10].

Pathology

The histological changes within the skin are non-specific; the diagnosis depends on the clinical features and family history [11–13]. Light microscopy reveals non-specific compact hyperkeratosis with a varying degree of basket-weave hyperkeratosis and parakeratosis. There is underlying acanthosis and papillomatosis. A sparse, mononuclear perivascular infiltrate is seen in the upper dermis. Electron microscopy has shown a decrease in keratinosomes (membrane coating granules) in the granular layer [12,13] in some patients but this has not been found in other reports [14,15]. A dense perinuclear tonofilament and keratohyaline granule complex has been described [15] but this finding is not consistent. Immunohistochemical studies have revealed abnormal basal cytokeratin staining [16] and an increase in suprabasal involucrin [17]. Autoradiographic studies have shown that the epidermal proliferation rate is normal [18].

Clinical features

The characteristic skin lesions of EKV usually present before the age of 1 year but may rarely occur later in childhood or early adulthood [5,19–23]. The sex incidence is equal. Irregularly shaped, macular patches of erythema occur at any site and appear to migrate slowly over the body (Fig. 19.8.1). They normally last from hours to days and may be accompanied by some fine scaling. Changes in ambient temperature, emotional upsets or external pressure may induce new lesions. Patients may also develop more fixed geographic, hyperkeratotic plaques most commonly on the extensor surfaces, buttocks and face. These are well demarcated and range from red to yel-

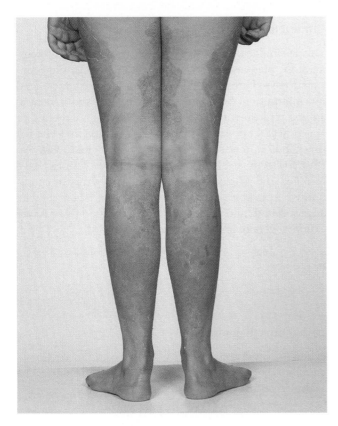

Fig. 19.8.1 Irregularly outlined patches of erythema accompanied by scaling in a 14-year-old girl with EKV.

lowish brown in colour. Palmoplantar keratoderma is rarely associated [20,21,24]. The clinical features are variable both within a single family and an individual patient. The condition may flare during use of the oral contraceptive pill or pregnancy and it may improve after the menopause [12].

Prognosis

EKV normally continues into adult life [11,21]. There is a tendency for the hyperkeratotic plaques to appear or extend up until puberty and then remain stationary. The erythematous lesions may decrease in intensity or even disappear after puberty [21,25].

Differential diagnosis

The transient nature of the erythematous lesions distinguishes EKV from other erythrokeratodermas and pityriasis rubra pilaris.

Treatment

Before the development of the retinoids a variety of therapies were tried such as oral vitamin A, X-rays and intralesional steroids [26–29]. Etretinate [30–32], acitretin [33]

and isotretinoin [12] have all been shown to be effective treatments for both types of skin lesion of EKV. Emollients, topical retinoic acid and 5% lactic acid may be of some use in those intolerant of retinoids [12].

REFERENCES

1 DeBuy Wenniger LM. Erythrodermie congénitale ichthyosiforme avec hyperépidermotrophie. *Ned Tijdschr Geneesk* 1907; 1A: 510–15.
2 Rille JH. Krankenvorstellungen. *Zentbl Haut Geschl Krankh* 1922; 7: 161.
3 Jeanselme E. Un cas d'erythrokératodermie symétrique, en placards à extension géographique. *Bull Soc Fr Dermatol Syph* 1922; 29: 150–6.
4 Mendes da Costa S. Erythro- et keratodermia variabilis in a mother and daughter. *Acta Derm Venereol (Stockh)* 1925; 6: 225–61.
5 Noordhoeck FJ. *Over Erythro- et Keratodermia variabilis*. Utrecht thesis, 1950. Cited in: Gottron HA, Schnyder UW, eds. *Vererbung von Hautkrankheiten*. Berlin: Springer-Verlag, 1966: 923.
6 Schnyder UW, Sommacal-Schopf D. Fourteen cases of erythrokeratodermia figurata variabilis within one family. *Acta Genet Statist Med* 1957; 7: 204–6.
7 Van der Schroeff JG, Nijenhuis LE, Meera Khan P *et al*. Genetic linkage between erythrokeratodermia variabilis and Rh locus. *Hum Genet* 1984; 68: 165–8.
8 Van der Schroeff JG, Van Leeuwen-Cornelisse I, Van Haeringen A, Went LN. Further evidence for localization of the gene of erythrokeratoderma variabilis. *Hum Genet* 1988; 80: 97–8.
9 Richard G, Smith LE, Bailey RA *et al*. Mutations in the human connexin gene GJB3 cause erythrokeratoderma variabilis. *Nature Genet* 1998; 20: 366–9.
10 Richard G, Lin J–P, Smith L *et al*. Linkage studies in erythrokeratodermias: fine mapping, genetic heterogeneity, and analysis of candidate genes. *J Invest Dermatol* 1997; 109: 666–71.
11 Gewirtzman GB, Winkler NW, Dobson RL. Erythrokeratoderma variabilis. A family study. *Arch Dermatol* 1978; 114: 259–61.
12 Rappaport IP, Goldes GA, Goltz RW. Erythrokeratoderma variabilis treated with isotretinoin—a clinical, histological and ultrastructural study. *Arch Dermatol* 1986; 122: 441–5.
13 Vandersteen PR, Muller SA. Erythrokeratoderma variabilis. An enzyme histochemical and ultrastructural study. *Arch Dermatol* 1971; 103: 362–70.
14 Jurecka W. Erythrokeratodermia variabilis. *Arch Dermatol* 1986; 122: 1356.
15 Macfarlane AW, Chapman SJ, Verbov JL. Is erythrokeratoderma one disorder? A clinical and ultrastructural study of two siblings. *Br J Dermatol* 1991; 124: 487–91.
16 Mcfadden N, Oppedal BR, Ree K, Brandtzaeg P. Erythrokeratoderma variabilis: immunohistochemical and ultrastructural studies of the epidermis. *Acta Derm Venereol* 1987; 67: 284–8.
17 Kanitakis J, Zambruno G, Viac J, Thivolet J. Involucrin expression in keratinization disorders of the skin—a preliminary study. *Br J Dermatol* 1987; 117: 479–86.
18 Schellander FG, Fritsch PO. Variable erythrokeratodermien: enzymhistochemische und autoradiographische untersuchungen an 2 Fällen. *Arch Klin Exp Derm* 1969; 235: 241–51.
19 Cram D. Erythrokeratodermia variabilis and variable circinate erythrokeratodermias. *Arch Dermatol* 1970; 101: 68–73.
20 Schellander FG, Fritsch PO. Variable erythrokeratoderma: an unusual case. *Arch Dermatol* 1969; 100: 744–8.
21 Brown J, Kierland RR. Erythrokeratodermia variabilis. Report of three cases and review of the literature. *Arch Dermatol* 1966; 93: 194–201.
22 Hacham-Zadeh S, Even-Paz Z. Erythrokeratodermia variabilis in a Jewish Kurdish family. *Clin Genet* 1978; 13: 404–8.
23 Luy JT, Jacobs AH, Nickoloff BJ. A child with erythematous and hyperkeratotic patches. Erythrokeratodermia variabilis. *Arch Dermatol* 1988; 124: 1271–2, 1274.
24 Wollina U, Knopf B, Schaaschmidt H, Frille I. Familial coexistence of erythrokeratodermia variabilis and keratosis palmoplantaris transgrediens et progrediens. *Hautarzt* 1989; 40: 169–72.
25 Itin P, Levy CA, Sommacal-Schopf D, Schnyder UW. Family study of erythrokeratodermia figurata variabilis. *Hautarzt* 1992; 43: 500–4.
26 Budlovsky G. Kerato- et erythrodermia variabilis. *Zbl Haut Geschlechtskr* 1935; 51: 32–3.
27 Carteaud A, Dorfman L. Erythrokératodermie variable de Mendes da Costa. *Presse Méd* 1963; 71: 2685–7.

28 Kanaar P. Zur histochemie und symptomatischen therapie der erythro- et keratodermia variabilis (Mendes da Costa). *Hautarzt* 1965; 16: 126–9.

29 Wulf K, Koch H, Schlutz KH. Erythrokeratodermia figurata variabilis vom typ Mendes da Costa eine durch Vitamin A beeinflussbare dermatose. *Derm Wochenschr* 1960; 142: 1012–16.

30 Marks R, Finlay AY, Holt PJA. Severe disorders of keratinization: effects of treatment with Tigason (etretinate). *Br J Dermatol* 1981; 104: 667–73.

31 Magyarlaki M, Drobnitsch I, Zombai E, Schneider I. A case of erythrokeratodermia figurata variabilis successfully treated with tigason. *Z Hautkr* 1989; 64: 881–2, 885–7.

32 Larregue M, Bressieux JM, Titi A *et al.* Mendes da Costa erythrokeratoderma variabilis. Effect of RO 10-9359 (Tigason). *Ann Dermatol Vénéréol* 1988; 115: 1123–5.

33 Van de Kerkhof PCM, Steijlen PM, Van Dooren-Greebe RJ, Happle R. Acitretin in the treatment of erythrokeratodermia variabilis. *Dermatologica* 1990; 181: 330–3.

Erythrokeratoderma en cocardes

(SYN. GÉNODERMATOSE EN COCARDES, GÉNODERMATOSE ERYTHÈMATOSQUAMEUSE CIRCINÉE VARIABLE, MALADIE DE DEGOS, DEGOS DISEASE)

History

In 1947 Degos and colleagues described a possible new genodermatosis in a 13-year-old girl, her father and her paternal uncle, which was characterized by erythematous plaques and intermittent erythematous lesions with an annular or 'en cocarde' appearance [1]. During the following decade four more reports of the same condition appeared in the French literature [2–5]. More recently, further families have been described with almost certainly the same condition under the names 'congenital ichthyosis with erythema centrifugum' [6], 'familial annular erythema' [7] and erythrokeratodermia anularis migrans [8].

Pathogenesis

The aetiology of erythrokeratoderma en cocardes (EKC) is unknown. Both Degos *et al.*'s original family [1] and Barrière's sibship [3] suggest an autosomal dominant inheritance. This inheritance pattern was further supported by Kelly's study of a family of 31 members spanning five generations with 12 affected members. Many authors regard EKC as a variant of EKV and Cram reported a 9-year-old Dutch boy with features of both [9]. The relationship to EKV remains uncertain but linkage studies of EKC families and analysis of their connexin genes on chromosome 1p should help this.

Pathology

Light microscopy changes are non-specific and the same for the erythematous plaques and annular lesions. They show hyperkeratosis, occasional parakeratosis, acanthosis and a mild perivascular monocytic infiltrate in the upper dermis [3].

Clinical features

This is similar to EKV in that fixed erythematous hyperkeratotic plaques appear in infancy, commonly on extensor surfaces. However, this condition is also characterized by intermittent annular lesions which show central scaling with surrounding erythema, giving a targetoid or 'en cocardes' appearance [1–6]. The eruption may clear at times but it tends to progress during childhood. An ichthyosiform scaling may remain after lesions have resolved. Intercurrent infection may exacerbate the condition whereas sunlight tends to improve it. There may be an associated mild peeling of the palmar skin [1] or rarely a more severe palmoplantar keratoderma [6].

Prognosis

The condition normally progresses into adult life.

Differential diagnosis

Erythema gyratum perstans, tinea corporis, erythema annulare centrifuguum and Netherton's syndrome can be excluded on clinical and histological grounds.

Treatment

Treatment is as for EKV.

REFERENCES

1 Degos R, Delzant O, Morival H. Erythème desquamatif en plaques congénital et familiar (génodermatose nouvelle?). *Bull Soc Fr Dermatol Syph* 1947; 54: 442.

2 Gougerot H, Grupper C. Génodermatose erythèmato-squameuse circinée, variable: 'Maladie de Degos' (Variable circinate erythematosquamous genodermatosis: 'Degos disease'). *Bull Soc Fr Dermatol Syph* 1948; 55: 396.

3 Barrière H. Eruption congénital, erythèmato-squameuse, variable. Génodermatose de Degos. *Bull Soc Fr Dermatol Syph* 1950; 57: 547–8.

4 Bazex A, Dupré A. Génodermatose à erythèmes circinés variables. *Ann Dermatol Syph* 1956; 83: 612–17.

5 Bureau Y, Jarry H, Barrière H. Génodermatose à type d'erythème desquamatif récidivant par poussées depuis l'enfance. *Bull Soc Fr Dermatol Syph* 1955; 62: 25.

6 Kelly LJ, Koscard E. Congenital ichthyosis with erythema annulare centrifugum. A new form of ichthyosis affecting 12 members of a family of 31 in five generations. *Dermatologica* 1970; 140: 75–83.

7 Beare JM, Froggatt P, Jones JH, Neill DW. Familial annular erythema. An apparently new dominant mutation. *Br J Dermatol* 1966; 78: 59–68.

8 Vakilzadeh F, Rose I. Erythrokeratodermia anularis migrans—a new genetic dermatosis? *Hautarzt* 1991; 42: 634–7.

9 Cram DL. Erythrokeratoderma variabilis and variable circinate erythrokeratodermas. *Arch Dermatol* 1970; 101: 68–73.

Erythrokeratoderma progressiva symmetrica (SYN. GOTTRON'S SYNDROME, DARIER–GOTTRON'S SYNDROME)

History

In February, 1922 Gottron presented a patient at a Berlin dermatology society meeting with symmetrical erythematous plaques over extensor surfaces calling the condition 'symmetrical progressive erythrokeratoderma' [1,2]. However, the first case reported was probably by Brocq and Dubreuilh in 1908 although this patient had previously been reported by Darier in 1886 [3]. Darier published a further case in 1911 under the name of 'progressive and symmetrical verrucous erythrokeratodermia' [4] but Gottron's name remains the most commonly associated with this rare dermatosis. More recently numerous isolated cases and affected families have been described [5–12].

Pathogenesis

The aetiology is unknown. The inheritance is probably autosomal dominant with variable penetrance. Ruiz-Maldonado *et al.* reported two sporadic cases of EPS from consanguineous parents but six other cases came from three families (in which 16 relatives were affected) suggesting an autosomal dominant inheritance pattern [5]. Rodriguez-Pichardo *et al.* reported one sporadic case and a kindred with seven affected members spanning five generations that followed an autosomal dominant pattern [8]. Reviewing all the reported cases the inheritance appears autosomal dominant although 30–40% of these were sporadic cases and presumably new mutations. Recently, Macfarlane *et al.* described two sisters born to non-consanguineous, unaffected parents [13]. The younger sister developed EKV at the age of 17 months whereas the elder sister developed the clinical signs of EPS at the age of 6 years. The skin ultrastructural findings were identical and they conjecture that EKV and EPS may be different phenotypic expressions of a single genetic disorder. However, the epidermal proliferation rate, which is increased in EPS [7] and normal in EKV [14], was not measured. Linkage and mutation studies to the connexin genes on chromosome 1p should help clarify the relationship of these disorders.

Pathology

Light microscopy is non-specific and shows hyperkeratosis, patchy parakeratosis overlying an acanthotic epidermis with preservation of the granular layer. Vacuolation around the nuclei has been reported in the granular layer. A sparse, lymphohistiocytic, perivascular infiltrate is seen in the upper dermis [5,6]. Electron microscopy shows markedly swollen mitochondria in the granular cells and vacuolation in the cells of the lower stratum corneum. Desmosomes, keratohyaline granules and tonofilament bundles appear normal [6].

Clinical features

EPS usually appears in early childhood, often in the first year of life, and shows an equal sex incidence. It is characterized by fixed, large, well-defined, hyperkeratotic plaques [5–12]. They are normally symmetrical with a somewhat reddish-orange or brownish colour. Lesions are commonly on the limbs, buttocks, shoulders and fingers and also may involve the face. The chest and abdomen are usually spared, unlike the involvement of EKV. An erythematous, palmoplantar keratoderma is seen in about 50% of cases. The plaques tend to extend during the first decade of life and then remain static. They may improve during summer. The clinical severity shows a marked variation even within individual families [5].

Prognosis

There is some tendency to improvement after puberty but lesions persist into adult life [5,8,10].

Differential diagnosis

EKV and pityriasis rubra pilaris can be distinguished by the clinical features and psoriasis by histological differences.

Treatment

Topical therapies are of limited benefit but oral etretinate therapy produces a good response [5,6,8,10].

REFERENCES

1 Gottron HA. Congenital angelegte symmetrische progressive Erythrokeratodermie. *Zentbl Haut Geschl Krankh* 1922; 4: 493–4.
2 Gottron HA. Congenital symmetrical progressive erythrokeratoderma. *Arch Dermatol Syph* 1923; 7: 416.
3 Brocq M, Dubreuilh W. Erythrokératodermie symétrique en placards. *Bull Soc Fr Dermatol Syph* 1908; 19: 327–32.
4 Darier J. Erythrokératodermie verruceuse en nappe symétrique et progressive. *Bull Soc Fr Dermatol Syph* 1911; 22: 252–64.
5 Ruiz-Maldonado R, Tamayo L, Del Castillo V *et al.* Erythrokeratodermia progressiva symmetrica. Report of 10 cases. *Dermatologica* 1982; 164: 133–41.
6 Nazzaro V, Blanchet-Bardon C. Progressive symmetric erythrokeratoderma. Histological and ultrastructural study of patient before and after treatment with etretinate. *Arch Dermatol* 1986; 122: 434–40.
7 Hopsu-Havu VK, Tuohimaa P. Erythrokeratodermia congenitalis progressiva symmetrica (Gottron). An analysis of kinetics of epidermal cell proliferation. *Dermatologica* 1971; 142: 137–44.
8 Rodriguez-Pichardo A, Garcia-Bravo B, Sanchez-Pdreno P, Camacho-Martinez F. Progressive symmetric erythrokeratodermia. *J Am Acad Dermatol* 1988; 19: 129–30.
9 Hopsu-Havu UK, Peltonen L. Erythrokeratodermia congenitalis progressiva symmetrica (Gottron). *Dermatologica* 1970; 141: 321–8.

10 Nir M, Tanzer F. Progressive symmetric erythrokeratoderma. *Dermatologica* 1978; 156: 268–73.

11 Kudsi S, Naeyaert JM. Progressive symmetric erythrokeratodermia of Darier Gottron. *Dermatologica* 1990; 180: 196–7.

12 Dupertuis MC, Laroche L, Huault MC, Blanchet-Bardon C. Progressive and symmetrical erythrokeratoderma of Darier-Gottron. *Ann Dermatol Vénéréol* 1991; 118: 775–8.

13 Macfarlane AW, Chapman SJ, Verbov JL. Is erythrokeratoderma one disorder? A clinical and ultrastructural study of two siblings. *Br J Dermatol* 1991; 124: 487–91.

14 Schellander FG, Fritsch PO. Variable erythrokeratoderminen: enzymhistochemische und autoradiographische untersuchungen an 2 Fällen. *Arch Klin Exp Derm* 1969; 235: 241–51.

Syndromes associated with erythrokeratoderma

A number of reports exist in the literature describing 'erythrokeratoderma' associated with other abnormalities. Giroux described a large French-Canadian family over five generations with a distinct autosomal dominant, neurocutaneous syndrome [1]. This was characterized by a symmetrical erythrokeratoderma appearing in infancy on extensor surfaces with a tendency for improvement in summer. The eruption usually cleared spontaneously by middle-age but showed occasional relapses later in life. A progressive neurological disease was seen from the age of 40 years characterized by ataxia, spasticity and decreased tendon reflexes.

In the 1960s, Schnyder described a possible new neurocutaneous syndrome characterized by a partial EPS, neurosensory deafness, myopathy and peripheral neuropathy [2,3]. Similar cases have been described by Beare *et al.* and Kiesewetter *et al.* [4,5]. The EPS-like skin changes appear in the first few years of life and progress until puberty but unlike EPS they tend to be asymmetrical. The histological changes are non-specific and similar to those of EPS. However, the possible association of keratitis, nail dystrophy and recurrent skin infections with this disorder suggest it is most likely a variant of the KID syndrome (keratitis, ichthyosis and deafness), which is also characterized by asymmetrical erythrokeratoderma [6,7].

Recent genetic advances have shown that mutations in different gap junction protein (connexin) genes may be responsible for deafness [8,9], deafness and mutilating keratoderma (Vohwinkel's syndrome) [10] and Charcot-Marie Tooth disease (ataxia and deafness) [11]. As Connexin 31 mutations cause EKV it seems likely that further connexin gene mutations may explain some of the above disorders. Families with EKV and ataxia have already shown linkage to 1p34-35; a region with a number of connexin genes [12].

REFERENCES

1 Giroux JM, Barbeau A. Erythrokeratodermia with ataxia. *Arch Dermatol* 1972; 106: 183–8.

2 Schnyder UW. Erythrokeratodermia progressiva (krankendemonstration). *Arch Klin Exp Dermatol* 1964; 219: 973–6.

3 Schnyder VW, Wissler H, Wendt G. Eine weitere form von atypischer erythrokeratodermie mit schwerbörigkeit und cerebraler schädigung. *Helv Paediatr Acta* 1968; 23: 220–30.

4 Kiesewetter F, Simon M Jr, Fartasch M, Gevatter M. Progressive partially symmetric erythrokeratodermia with deafness: histological and ultrastructural evidence for a subtype distinct from Schnyder's syndrome. *Dermatology* 1993; 186: 222–5.

5 Beare JM, Nevin NC, Frogatt P *et al.* Atypical erythrokeratoderma with deafness, physical retardation and peripheral neuropathy. *Br J Dermatol* 1972; 87: 308–14.

6 Skinner BA, Greist MC, Norins AL. The keratitis ichthyosis and deafness syndrome. *Arch Dermatol* 1981; 117: 285–9.

7 Burns FS. A case of generalised congenital keratoderma with unusual involvement of the eyes, ears and nasal and buccous membranes. *J Cutan Dis* 1915; 33: 255–60.

8 Xia JH, Liu CY, Tang BS *et al.* Mutations in the gene encoding gap junction protein beta-3 associated with autosomal dominant hearing impairment. *Nature Genet* 1998; 20: 370–3.

9 Kelsell DP, Dunlop J, Stevens HP *et al.* Connexin 26 mutations in hereditary non-syndromic sensorineural deafness. *Nature* 1997; 387: 80–3.

10. Maestrini E, Korge BP, Ocaña-Sierra J *et al.* A missense mutation in connexin 26, D66H, causes mutilating keratoderma with sensorineural deafness (Vohwinkel's syndrome) in three unrelated families. *Hum Mol Genet* 1999; 8: 1237–43.

11. Bergoffen J, Scherer SS, Wang S *et al.* Connexin mutations in X-linked Charcot-Marie-Tooth disease. *Science* 1993; 267: 2039–42.

12. Richard G, Lin J-P, Smith L *et al.* Linkage studies in eryhtrokeratodermias: fine mapping, genetic heterogeneity, and analysis of candidate genes. *J Invest Dermatol* 1997: 109: 666–71.

19.9   Darier's Disease

SUSAN BURGE

Definition

Darier's disease (Darier–White disease, keratosis follicularis) is a dominantly inherited dermatosis which is characterized by warty papules and a nail dystrophy. The histopathological changes include focal acantholysis, dyskeratosis and hyperkeratosis.

History

The disease was described in 1889 by White in the USA and Darier in France [1,2]. Estimates of prevalence range from 1 in 100 000 in Denmark [3] to 1 in 36 000 in the northeast of England [4].

Aetiology and pathogenesis

Inheritance is autosomal dominant with complete penetrance but variable expression [4–6]. The gene has been mapped to a single locus on chromosome 12q23–q24.1 [7–8]. The gene product, SERCA2, is a sarco-endoplasmic reticulum calcium pump. It seems likely that the mutation interferes with the normal internal calcium 'signalling' that regulates processes such as cell proliferation, differentiation and adhesion.

Localized, linear 'naevoid' lesions of Darier's disease probably reflect genetic mosaicism arising from a mutation in early embryogenesis. The genetic defect may be the same as in patients with generalized disease. Theoretically, patients with linear lesions have a small chance of bearing a child with generalized disease if the somatic mutation has also affected the gametes [10,11].

Although the genetic defect is known the pathogenesis of Darier's disease is unclear. The pathological changes in the epidermis include acantholysis, dyskeratosis and hyperkeratosis (see below). The earliest event appears to be disruption of adhesion between the suprabasal keratinocytes. Lesions are triggered by ultraviolet light in the sunburn range [12,13], but physical forces such as suction do not breakdown the adhesion junctions [14].

Although perilesional skin looks normal both clinically and ultrastructurally, the abnormality in Darier's disease is present in all the keratinocytes in affected individuals. When normal looking skin from patients with Darier's disease is grown in explant cultures, the keratinocytes dissociate from each other and the pattern of growth is disorganized. Epidermal cells from unaffected individuals grown in the presence of these diseased cells or in the medium in which they were cultured also dissociate and lose desmosomes. The acantholytic cells may release a protease activator into the medium [15–18].

Intercellular adhesion between keratinocytes is mediated predominantly by transmembrane glycoproteins of the cadherin family which are present in specialized adhesion junctions, the desmosomes. Desmosomal cadherins interact with the cytokeratin filaments in the cytoskeleton either directly or indirectly via linking proteins. Keratinocytes round-up and separate from each other when adhesion is disrupted and the cytokeratin filaments collect around the cell nucleus, when they are no longer linked to the desmosomes.

Immunohistology has shown that epidermal cytokeratins and desmosomal components are expressed normally in intact epidermis. Non-specific changes are apparent after acantholysis. The desmosomal cadherins are internalized in the acantholytic cells. Some of the acantholytic suprabasal cells express cytokeratins typical of basal cells, probably because the epitopes are unmasked when the cytokeratin filaments are redistributed around the nucleus [19,20].

Pathology [21]

Foci of suprabasal cell acantholysis, hyperkeratosis and dyskeratosis are present in the epidermis (Fig. 19.9.1). Narrow intraepidermal clefts or lacunae containing acantholytic cells form above the basal cells. Epidermal villi project into the lacunae and sometimes the epidermis proliferates down into the dermis below the lesions. Desmosomes are reduced in number in the lesions and the acantholytic cells contain intracytoplasmic desmosomes [22,23].

The dyskeratotic keratinocytes are known as corps ronds and grains. Both contain clumped cytokeratin

1153

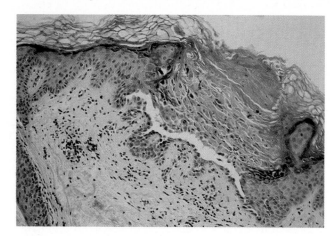

Fig. 19.9.1 The hyperkeratotic papule in this biopsy shows typical features of Darier's disease. The suprabasal cleft contains acantholytic cells. Dyskeratotic cells are present in the granular layer and the horny plug (×200; stain H & E).

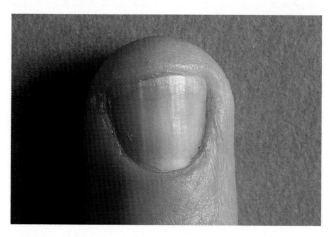

Fig. 19.9.2 Longitudinal white line in the nail is an early sign of Darier's disease which may be associated with nail fragility, notching and splitting. Courtesy of Dr John Harper.

filaments and cytoplasmic vacuoles [24,25]. Corps ronds, which are in the spinous and granular layers, have a central homogeneous nucleus surrounded by a clear halo. Grains, which have elongated pyknotic nuclei surrounded by homogeneous dyskeratotic material, are usually seen in or just below the horny layer.

Clinical features [4,5]

Expression of the disease varies. Males and females are affected with equal frequency. More than 60% of patients develop signs between the ages of 6 and 20 years, but onset peaks between the ages of 11 and 15 years. The disease has not been observed in infants.

More than 95% of patients have acral involvement and children may have hand involvement before any other signs of the disease. In one study, seven of 13 children had nail involvement, eight had palmar pits and 10 had acrokeratosis verruciformis. Only three of these children had the typical rash of Darier's disease [4].

The most specific acral sign of Darier's disease is a combination of longitudinal red and white lines extending from the base to the free edge of the nail plate (Fig. 19.9.2). These may be associated with V-shaped notching of the free edge, subungual hyperkeratosis or splinter haemorrhages. The nails are fragile so they break and split, but initially these changes may be blamed on biting or trauma. Most patients have pits or punctate keratotic papules on palms and soles. The fine palmar pits are easier to detect in children on prints of the palms [4]. Children may develop haemorrhagic macules or blisters on the hands and feet, but these are rare and have only been observed in 6% of patients [5,26,27].

Acrokeratosis verruciformis may be an early sign of the disease on the backs of the hands and feet (Fig. 19.9.3). The

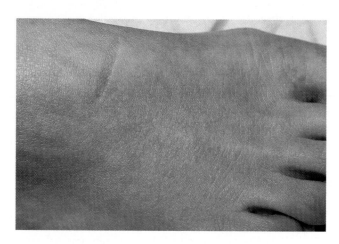

Fig. 19.9.3 Small flesh-coloured papules of acrokeratosis verruciformis scattered over the dorsum of both feet in this patient with Darier's disease.

flat-topped papules are skin-coloured and are always bilateral.

The greasy, crusted papules in Darier's disease are flesh-coloured, yellow or brown (Fig. 19.9.4), but children with pigmented skin may present with hypopigmented macules or papules (Fig. 19.9.5) [28–30]. Papules appear on seborrhoeic areas of the trunk, the supraclavicular fossae, the sides of the neck, the forehead, ears and scalp (Figs 19.9.6, 19.9.7). At first the lesions are discrete but later may coalesce into crusted, malodorous plaques. Most patients have some flexural involvement, occasionally this is severe. The condition is usually mild in children so the rash is often overlooked until summer when symptoms and signs are exacerbated by heat and sweating. Sun, particularly sunburn, may provoke lesions 1 or 2 weeks after the exposure. Itching is common, but not invariable. Pain is unusual in uncomplicated disease.

Mucosal involvement has been described in some

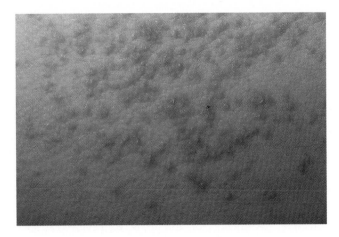

Fig. 19.9.4 The crusted papules are yellowish-brown and rather greasy. Collections of papules coalesce into plaques.

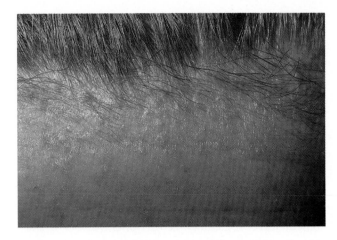

Fig. 19.9.7 The forehead, particularly along the hair line, is often involved in Darier's disease. The keratotic papules may be misdiagnosed as acne vulgaris.

Fig. 19.9.5 Darier's disease may present with hypopigmented lesions in children with pigmented skin. This child had typical hyperpigmented papules in addition to hypopigmented macules and papules.

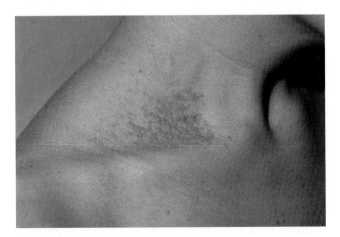

Fig. 19.9.6 It is common for the supraclavicular fossae to be involved in Darier's disease.

patients. Papules or verrucous plaques develop on the palate, alveolar ridges, buccal mucosa or tongue.

Zosteriform, linear disease has been described in children and adults [11]. Keratotic papules appear on one side of the body in streaks or whorls following Blaschko's lines. Palmar pits and nail changes may be present on the same side of the body [10]. These naevoid lesions are also aggravated by heat, sweating or sun. The histopathological changes are identical to those in generalized disease. This pattern of disease may reflect genetic mosaicism (see above) [10,11].

Complications [5]

Patients are prone to widespread cutaneous infections, particularly with herpes simplex virus. Immune function has been investigated, but no specific or consistent abnormality has been demonstrated [31]. Herpes infection causes erythema, crusting and pain. Vesicles may not be seen. The possibility of infection with herpes simplex should be considered in any patient with a painful exacerbation of the rash. Secondary bacterial overgrowth is common in the keratotic debris and may account for malodour. Infection with *Staphylococcus aureus* may cause blisters. Rarely involvement of the salivary ducts causes salivary gland obstruction in adults.

Associated conditions

Neuropsychiatric problems such as mental impairment and epilepsy have been described in some families, but the incidence of these conditions in Darier's disease is probably low [14].

Prognosis

Darier's disease is chronic and life long, but severity is unpredictable and fluctuates. Some patients always have relatively mild disease; however, the condition slowly gets worse in others. A few patients do seem to improve in old age [5].

Differential diagnosis

Crusted plaques on the trunk, flexural lesions and scaling in the scalp may suggest seborrhoeic dermatitis, but discrete warty papules are not a feature of this disease. Large comedones are sometimes seen in Darier's disease in association with the keratotic papules on the face or chest and initially the disease may be misdiagnosed as acne.

Acrokeratosis verruciformis simulates plane warts.

Patients with Hailey–Hailey disease sometimes have longitudinal white lines in the nails but do not have nail fragility [32]. Palmar pits have been described in Hailey–Hailey disease, but are rare. Solitary red or white lines in the nails may occur in association with subungual tumours. Flexural skin is pigmented, thickened and papillomatous in the benign forms of acanthosis nigricans, but the soft tags are different from the warty papules of Darier's disease. Confluent and reticulate papillomatosis begins around puberty usually in girls. The flat, brown papules appear between the breasts and in the middle of the back, and gradually spread across the trunk. The distribution and pigmentation may suggest Darier's disease.

The diagnosis of Darier's disease is confirmed by a biopsy which shows the characteristic histopathological changes. Intraepidermal splits with acantholysis and dyskeratosis are also seen in Hailey–Hailey disease, which usually presents in young adults, and in transient or persistent acantholytic dermatosis (Grover's disease), but this condition affects adults not children.

Treatment

Treatment must be tailored to the individual. Children who have mild disease and are asymptomatic need no treatment. Some children, even those with mild disease, may be so embarrassed by their appearance, that they refuse to wear clothes which reveal the affected skin or take part in activities such as swimming. These children may need emotional support some of which can be provided by a trained dermatology nurse. The disease must be explained to the family and discussed with school teachers. Teenagers should be advised about their choice of career as it may be wise not to work in hot or sweaty conditions. Cosmetic camouflage may be appreciated by older children. Genetic counselling may be appropriate for some teenagers.

Itching is the most troublesome symptom. Cool cotton clothing, sun avoidance and sun-block creams will reduce exacerbations in the summer. Simple emollients such as aqueous cream used as a soap substitute, may be helpful. Some patients prefer emollients containing urea or lactic acid (Aquadrate, Calmurid) but sometimes these sting. A mild or moderately potent topical steroid (e.g. clobetasone butyrate) may reduce irritation but unfortunately steroids have little effect on the progress of the disease. Topical steroids may be prescribed in combination with an antibiotic to reduce secondary infection in crusted plaques or malodorous flexural disease. Antiseptics may also be helpful. Retinoids, the vitamin A derivatives, are the most effective treatments for moderate to severe Darier's disease, but are rarely needed in children.

Topical retinoids (isotretinoin gel; tretinoin cream; tazarotene gel) reduce hyperkeratosis, but irritate the skin. The retinoid can be applied on alternate days until the patient tolerates more frequent applications. Emollients such as aqueous cream or mild topical steroids may reduce irritation [14,33]. The oral retinoids, etretinate, acitretin and isotretinoin, are of great value in Darier's disease. Acitretin has supplanted the older retinoid, etretinate [34]. Oral retinoids are toxic so they should only be prescribed for children with severe disease. All oral retinoids are teratogenic. Pregnancy must be avoided during treatment and for 2 years after stopping acitretin (or etretinate) or for 1 month after stopping isotretinoin. Dose-related side-effects include mucosal dryness, nose bleeds, skin fragility, itching and elevated triglycerides, cholesterol and liver enzymes. Retinoids may cause skeletal hyperostosis and extraosseous calcification, but the risk is low and the significance of these changes is not known. Acitretin, in a dose of no more than 0.5 mg/kg/day, has been recommended as an effective long-term treatment for inherited disorders of keratinization in children, but side-effects must be monitored carefully, particularly liver function [35]. Isotretinoin, 0.5–1 mg/kg/day, is not as effective in disorders of keratinization, but may be a more suitable choice in teenage girls because of the short half-life [36].

REFERENCES

1 White J. A case of keratosis (ichthyosis) follicularis. *J Cutan Genito-Urin Dis* 1889; 7: 201–9.
2 Darier J. Psorospermose folliculaire végètant. *Ann Dermatol Syph* 1889; 10: 597–612.
3 Svendsen I, Albrectsen B. The prevalence of dyskeratosis follicularis (Darier's disease) in Denmark. *Acta Derm Venereol (Stockh)* 1959; 39: 256–69.
4 Munro CS. The phenotype of Darier's disease: penetrance and expressivity in adults and children. *Br J Dermatol* 1992; 127: 126–30.
5 Burge SM, Wilkinson JD. Darier–White disease: a review of the clinical features in 163 patients. *J Am Acad Dermatol* 1992; 27: 40–50.
6 Beck A, Finocchio A, White J. Darier's disease: a kindred with a large number of cases. *Br J Dermatol* 1977; 97: 335–9.
7 Parfitt E, Burge S, Craddock N *et al.* The gene for Darier's disease maps between D12S78 and D12S79. *Hum Molec Genet* 1994; 3: 35–8.

8 Carter SA, Bryce SD, Munro CS *et al.* Linkage analyses in British pedigrees suggest a single locus for Darier disease and narrow the location to the interval between D12S105 and D12S129. *Genomics* 1994; 24: 378–82.

9 Sakuntabhai A, Ruiz-Perez V, Carter S *et al.* Mutations in ATP2A2, encoding a Ca^{2+} pump, cause Darier disease. *Nat Genet* 1999; 21: 271–7.

10 Munro CS, Cox NH. An acantholytic dyskeratotic epidermal naevus with other features of Darier's disease on the same side of the body. *Br J Dermatol* 1992; 127: 168–71.

11 Starink T, Woerdeman MJ. Unilateral systematized keratosis follicularis. A variant of Darier's disease or an epidermal naevus (acantholytic dyskeratotic epidermal naevus)? *Br J Dermatol* 1981; 105: 207–14.

12 Baba T, Yaoita H. UV radiation and keratosis follicularis. *Arch Dermatol* 1984; 120: 1484–7.

13 Hedblad MA, Nakatani T, Beitner H. Ultrastructural changes in Darier's disease induced by ultraviolet irradiation. *Acta Derm Venereol* 1991; 71: 108–12.

14 Burge S. Darier's disease—the clinical features and pathogenesis. *Clin Exp Dermatol* 1994; 19: 193–205.

15 Ishibashi Y, Kukita A. Influence of cell dissociation on normal epidermal cells in Hailey–Hailey's disease and Darier's disease. *Curr Prob Dermatol* 1983; 11: 59–68.

16 Ishibashi Y, Kajiwara Y, Andoh I *et al.* The nature and pathogenesis of dyskeratosis in Hailey–Hailey's disease and Darier's disease. *J Dermatol* 1984; 11: 335–53.

17 Burge SM, Ryan TJ, Cederholm-Williams SA. Darier's disease: an immunohistochemical study using antibodies to proteases. *Br J Dermatol* 1989; 121: 613–21.

18 Burge SM, Cederholm-Williams SA, Garrod DR, Ryan TJ. Cell adhesion in Hailey–Hailey disease and Darier's disease: immunocytological and explant-tissue-culture studies. *Br J Dermatol* 1991; 125: 426–35.

19 Burge SM, Fenton DA, Dawber RPR, Leigh IM. Darier's disease: an immunohistochemical study using monoclonal antibodies to human cytokeratins. *Br J Dermatol* 1988; 118: 629–40.

20 Burge SM, Garrod DR. An immunohistological study of desmosomes in Darier's disease and Hailey–Hailey disease. *Br J Dermatol* 1991; 124: 242–51.

21 Weedon D. Darier's disease. In: Symmers WSC, ed. *The Skin*, 3rd edn, vol. 9. London: Churchill Livingstone, 1992: 280–1.

22 El-Gothamy Z, Kamel MM. Ultrastructural observations in Darier's disease. *Am J Dermatopathol* 1988; 10: 306–10.

23 Arai H, Hori Y. An ultrastructural observation of intracytoplasmic desmosomes in Darier's disease. *J Dermatol* 1977; 4: 223–34.

24 Gottlieb S, Lutzner M. Darier's disease. An electron microscopic study. *Arch Dermatol* 1973; 107: 225–30.

25 Mesquita-Guimaräes J, Mesquita-Guimaräes I. Cellular differentiation in Darier's disease. Ultrastructural aspects. *J Submicrosc Cytol* 1984; 16: 387–94.

26 Jones W, Nix T, Clark W. Hemorrhagic Darier's disease. *Arch Dermatol* 1964; 89: 523–7.

27 Coulson IH, Misch KJ. Haemorrhagic Darier's disease. *J Roy Soc Med* 1989; 82: 365–6.

28 Berth-Jones J, Hutchinson PE. Darier's disease with peri-follicular depigmentation. *Br J Dermatol* 1989; 120: 827–30.

29 Singal R, Honig B, Morison W, Farmer E. Hypopigmented, hyperkeratotic papules in two siblings. *Arch Dermatol* 1992; 128: 397–402.

30 Jacyk WK, Visser AJ. Leukodermic macules in keratosis follicularis (Darier's disease). *Int J Dermatol* 1992; 31: 715–17.

31 Patrizi A, Ricci G, Neri I, Specchia F, Varotti C, Masi M. Immunological parameters in Darier's disease. *Dermatologica* 1989; 178: 138–40.

32 Burge S. Hailey–Hailey disease: a clinical study. *Br J Dermatol* 1991; 125(suppl 38): 13–14.

33 Burge SM, Buxton PK. Topical isotretinoin in Darier's disease. *Br J Dermatol* 1995; 133: 924–8.

34 Christophersen J, Geiger JM, Danneskiold Samsoe P *et al.* A double-blind comparison of acitretin and etretinate in the treatment of Darier's disease. *Acta Derm Venereol* 1992; 72: 150–2.

35 Lacour M, Mehta-Nikhar B, Atherton DJ, Harper JI. An appraisal of acitretin therapy in children with inherited disorders of keratinization. *Br J Dermatol* 1996; 134: 1023–9.

36 Dicken CH, Bauer EA, Hazen PG *et al.* Isotretinoin treatment of Darier's disease. *J Am Acad Dermatol* 1982; 6: 721–6.

19.10   The Porokeratoses

ELAINE C. SIEGFRIED

Definition

The porokeratoses are a group of cutaneous lesions that share characteristic histological features. Several clinically distinct subtypes have been identified. The five most well-described variants are porokeratosis of Mibelli, linear porokeratosis, porokeratosis palmaris et plantaris disseminata, disseminated superficial porokeratosis (DSP) and disseminated superficial actinic porokeratosis (DSAP). Malignant epithelial neoplasms, arising in adulthood, have been reported in association with all five subtypes; the risk may be as high as 7–11% [1–3]. Many forms of altered immune response have been documented in association with onset or exacerbation of porokeratosis (most often DSP and DSAP), and subsequent development of skin cancers. These include organ transplantation, lymphoreticular malignancy acquired immune deficiency syndrome (AIDS), treatment with immunosuppressive drugs, ionizing radiation psoralens and ultraviolet A (PUVA) and combined UVA/UVB exposure [4–13]. Recent data supports the concept that porokeratoses represent a focal abnormal clone of keratinocytes.

History

The condition was originally recognized by Mibelli in 1889 [14]. He described a familial condition with onset in childhood, and coined the term 'porokeratosis' to emphasize what he believed to be representative features of the lesion: abnormal keratinization and origination within the pores of sweat ducts. Four years later, Respighi described the disseminated superficial variant [15]. In 1966, Chernosky defined DSAP (also known as porokeratosis of Chernosky) as a distinct clinical entity characterized by small, inconspicuous lesions occurring in adults, on sun-exposed areas [16]. A subsequent detailed light microscopic analysis of 35 clinically varied cases was published by Reed and Leone in 1970. They observed that the majority of lesions were not associated with ostia of eccrine or pilosebaceous ducts, and asserted that the well-accepted term 'porokeratosis' is a misnomer [17]. A more precise term was not proposed. The rare subtypes were subsequently described, porokeratosis palmaris et plantaris

disseminata in 1971 [18,19], and linear porokeratosis in 1974 [20].

Aetiology and pathogenesis

Clinical and laboratory observations support a common pathogenesis for all subtypes of porokeratosis. Multiple clinical variants have been reported in the same patient [21–24]. Comparative histological and cytochemical studies have included several subtypes of porokeratosis, and have not identified significant differences [3,4,19,25–27].

The histological features of porokeratosis seem to hold a clue to epidermal differentiation. Beginning with Mibelli's original description, this has inspired many detailed observations and hypotheses about their pathogenesis. Reed and Leone first proposed the theory that porokeratoses arise from a precarious mutant clone of keratinocytes, and enlarge by centripetal migration [17]. Since then, an array of additional and supportive data has been generated. Microfluorometry has been used to demonstrate increases in abnormal DNA ploidy from lesional keratinocytes of several types of porokeratosis, compared to controls [3,19,27]. Cultured keratinocytes from lesional, but not adjacent normal skin exhibit an increased number of non-specific chromosomal aberrations. Immunohistochemical analyses of a variety of markers of keratinocyte differentiation (involucrin, filaggrin, loricrin, cytokeratins) reveal a pattern similar to that of other premalignant and malignant keratinocytic lesions [8,28–30]. Scattered keratinocytes within the majority of lesions of porokeratosis of Mibelli and DSAP exhibit immunostaining with monoclonal antibodies directed against p53, a tumour suppressor nucleoprotein [1,8,26]. This suggests an increase in p53 mutation, a finding that has been observed in a variety of premalignant and malignant neoplasms. Immunohistochemical analysis for proliferating cell nuclear antigen (PCNA) revealed expression of the protein in less than half of the cases indicating that increased cellular proliferation is not a uniform feature of these porokeratoses [26]. Abnormalities of the underlying dermal fibroblasts have also been suspected [31]. Chromosome analyses of cultured lesional

1158

dermal fibroblasts did not reveal an increased number of mutations [3]. However, these cells are hypersensitive to the lethal effects of X-irradiation [3,4].

Pathology

The diagnosis of porokeratosis is confirmed histologically, with a biopsy of the keratotic border of the lesion that reveals a classic cornoid lamella. The cornoid lamella was first described in association with porokeratosis, and is characteristic but not pathognomonic [31]. Although the name 'porokeratosis' implies an association with ostia of the eccrine sweat ducts, this is an uncommon finding. More often, cornoid lamellae project from hair follicles [17]. This easily recognized 'horny plate' consists of a sloping column of parakeratotic cells nestled within an invagination of the epidermis. The apex of the invagination points away from the centre of the lesion, while the superficial parakeratotic column leans towards it (Fig. 19.10.1). The cornoid lamella marks an abnormal, often atrophic segment of epidermis. The granular layer is absent; keratinocytes are vacuolated, dyskeratotic or frankly necrotic; the basal layer may show liquefactive degeneration; and there may be exocytosis of lymphocytes [25,32]. The majority of lesions have an associated inflammatory cellular infiltrate within the papillary dermis, consisting primarily of T-lymphocytes expressing UCHL-1, Leu-3a and MB-2 monoclonal markers with an admixture of CD1 and Leu-6 positive Langerhans cells.

Histological changes within the centre of the lesion have been less well studied, and are variable. The epidermis is atrophic within DSAP, and may be atrophic or show psoriasiform hyperplasia in porokeratosis of Mibelli. The centre of both subtypes show increased immunostaining with p53 [26]. The epidermis peripheral to the cornoid lamella may be atrophic or unremarkable.

Clinical features

Of the well-described subtypes of porokeratosis, only the classic Mibelli type and linear porokeratosis present in childhood; DSAP and disseminated palmoplantar porokeratosis are autosomal dominant conditions that remain clinically inapparent until adulthood.

Descriptions of other rare clinical variants have been published. Classical and localized [2,3,27], hyperkeratotic [33], reticulate [34] and ulcerated [35] forms probably fit the Mibelli subtype. Punctate porokeratoses [22,36] are probably variants of disseminated palmoplantar porokeratosis.

Porokeratosis of Mibelli is an autosomal dominant condition, with a high incidence of new mutation. The male to female ratio is 2–3:1. Lesions may appear in early childhood or beyond, starting as verrucous papules that slowly enlarge into annular or gyrate plaques with a prominent

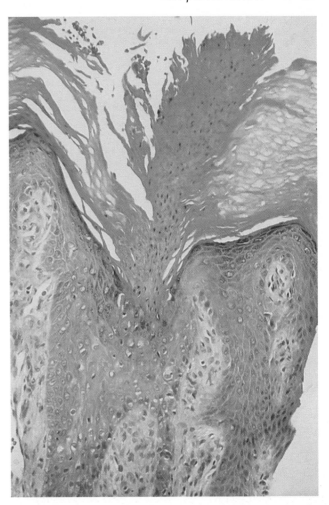

Fig. 19.10.1 A prominent cornoid lamella marks a focus of dyskeratotic keratinocytes in this biopsy specimen from the border of a porokeratosis of Mibelli (40× magnification).

double-edged, keratotic border (Fig. 19.10.2). The centre may be hyperkeratotic or atrophic [17,33]. Lesions are usually acral. Involvement limited to the face [9] and genitalia [10] has been described.

Linear porokeratosis was initially described as a variant of porokeratosis of Mibelli. It usually presents at birth or in childhood with localized or extensive lesions distributed along the lines of Blaschko [20,37–39] (Fig. 19.10.3). A clinically ambiguous presentation was reported in a neonate, with linear erosions and crusts rather than the characteristic double-edged border, subverting the correct biopsy specimen and diagnosis for several months [35].

A Blaschko's distribution strongly supports the theory that linear porokeratosis represents a mosaic genetic mutation. A genetic mosaic is an organism composed of two or more genetically different populations of cells that originate from one zygote. When the skin is involved, unique patterning is seen, reflecting the cellular hetero-

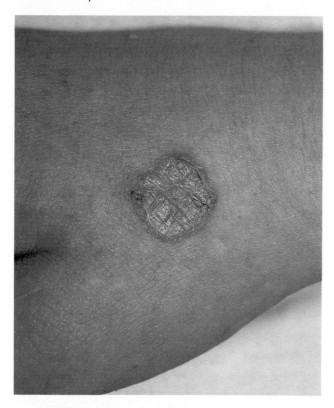

Fig. 19.10.2 A solitary porokeratosis of Mibelli on the hand of a 7-year-old girl.

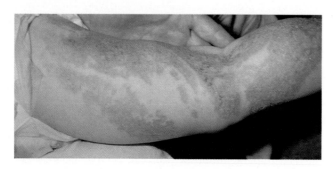

Fig. 19.10.3 Extensive lesions of linear porokeratosis in a 10 month-old boy. Courtesy of Dr Ilona Frieden.

geneity. The distribution is known as Blaschko's lines. The pattern is linear and whorled, and may be bilaterally symmetric, with a midline demarcation (see Chapter 19.1). Autosomal mosaicism is only heritable if the germ cells are affected [40].

Onset or exacerbation of Mibelli's porokeratosis has been reported in immunosuppressed individuals following organ or bone marrow transplantation [6,41–43]. Less profound alterations of immune surveillance have been associated with the porokeratoses of adulthood; an exhaustive search for immune system dysfunction in otherwise healthy children with porokeratosis is not warranted.

Prognosis

The porokeratoses are generally chronic and progressive. Discomfort is rare, but intense pruritus has been reported [11]. Lesions that are large, multiple or on cosmetically important areas may be disfiguring.

The risk of malignant transformation is 7% in Caucasians and 11.6% in Japanese people with Mibelli lesions [12]. Malignancy does not occur in childhood, but increases over time. The average latency period before tumour development is between two and seven decades [3]. Squamous cell carcinoma is the most commonly associated tumour; Bowen's disease and basal cell carcinoma have also been reported [3]. Malignant tumours may occur in a higher proportion of linear porokeratosis, or variants with large lesions [3,27].

Spontaneous resolution of lesions has been reported in an adult with linear and annular lesions [44], and remission was reported in an adult with DSP and paraneoplastic dermatomyositis after excision of her tumour [45]. The decision to treat versus monitor must be tailored to each patient. A wide variety of therapeutic modalities have been utilized, with suboptimal results.

Differential diagnosis

The porokeratoses have such distinct clinical features that the diagnosis is often made clinically. Occasionally 'confirmatory' skin biopsy will instead reveal the histological features of other disorders. The sharp keratotic margin and clinical morphology of DSP and DSAP has been described in a case of cutaneous T-cell lymphoma [46]. Cutaneous phaeohyphomycosis [47,48] and dermatophytosis [48] have been superimposed on lesions of superficial porokeratosis. Porokeratosis of Mibelli has a more distinct clinical appearance but cutaneous T-cell lymphoma has also mimicked its features [49]. Polycyclic lesions may suggest other conditions: tinea corporis, granuloma annulare, elastosis perforans serpiginosa or ichthyosis linearis circumflexa. Linear porokeratosis may be clinically confused with a number of dermatoses that follow the lines of Blaschko: epidermal naevus, naevus sebaceous and linear psoriasis. Eroded lesions in a neonate may be suggestive of intrauterine varicella zoster, herpes simplex or Goltz syndrome [35]. In all cases, skin biopsy from the border will support the diagnosis and rule out the other conditions. The biopsy specimen should be oriented for sectioning perpendicular to the long axis of the border.

Treatment

As with any genodermatosis, a genetic history should be obtained and counselling should be provided. Parents of a child with porokeratosis of Mibelli should be examined for skin lesions. There is a 50% risk of disease in each child born to an affected individual. The inheritance pattern of linear porokeratosis is unclear. An autosomal pattern of transmission has been reported for other genodermatoses that present as somatic mosaics [50].

A treatment of choice has not been defined for the porokeratoses; many alternatives have been published, usually as single case reports in adults or small, uncontrolled series. Therapeutic categories include active non-intervention, surgical removal or ablation, topical therapy and systemic therapy (Table 19.10.1). Only a few of these options are appropriate for the initial treatment of children.

The decision to treat must be tailored to each family, by carefully weighing of the risks and benefits. Active non-intervention should always be accompanied by anticipatory guidance for patients and care-givers along with regular follow-up to monitor for significant changes. High-quality, close-up photographic images can be of value in this effort.

Aggressive therapy should be reserved for problematic lesions, i.e. those that are symptomatic, large, rapidly growing or disfiguring. In general, non-painful options should be selected. For example, intralesional corticosteroids do not provide significant advantages for children over potent topical (or occluded) preparations. If a painful surgical approach is indicated, age-appropriate recommendations for control of pain and anxiety should be followed [51–53].

Excision can be curative with a single treatment for limited lesions. Full thickness excision is required to prevent recurrence; primary closure may not be possible. Ablative techniques are generally less costly, and less time-consuming than excision, but have some disadvantages. CO_2 laser and cryotherapy have been used most often; there is little data on cosmetic outcome in children following dermabrasion, curettage or electrodesiccation. Ablated tissue is not available for histological examination. Rapid recurrence has been reported following CO_2 laser vaporization to the upper to middle dermis [12].

Table 19.10.1 Treatment options for porokeratosis in children*

Surgical excision[12,58]
Surgical ablation
Co_2 laser vaporization [12,34,36,59]
dermabrasion† [59]
cryosurgery [60]
Topical
corticosteroids
anthralin [36]
5-FU†[61]
calcipotriol [62]

*Limited data on efficacy for all treatment modalities in children.
†Limited data on safety in children.

Postoperative pain may be poorly tolerated, and traditional wound care, with frequent dressing changes is not easily accomplished in young children.

Topical therapy is the most acceptable route for the majority of patients. However, long-term therapy is often required. Poor compliance will result in suboptimal results, and prolonged use of some medications (potent topical corticosteroids, calcipotriol) requires close follow-up, paying special attention to problems associated with systemic absorbtion [53]. There is no data on the efficacy of topical 5-fluorouracil (5-FU) for the treatment of paediatric porokeratoses. Case reports have documented the relative safety of extensively applied topical 5% 5-FU cream for up to 10 years in children with other problems [53–55]. A potential adverse effect is injury from inadvertent transfer to other sensitive tissues, such as the cornea. Systemic absorption in adults is estimated to be 6 mg following a daily application of 2 g, far below the 12 mg/kg/day for cancer chemotherapy, and toxic effects have not been reported. However, enhanced absorption is expected from eroded areas, and the increased ratio of body surface area to weight in small children puts them at higher risk for systemic toxicity. Although X-irradiation has been successfully used it is contraindicated because of an associated high risk of carcinogenesis [4].

Systemic therapies, including dexamethasone pulse [56], oral vitamin A, isotretinoin [57] and etretinate [37], have been utilized for adults with extensive involvement, with unclear benefit. The risks of these treatments outweigh their benefits for children.

REFERENCES

1 Puig L, Alerge M, Costa I, Matias-Guiu X, de Moragas JM. Overexpression of p53 in disseminated superficial actinic porokeratosis with and without malignant degeneration. *Arch Dermatol* 1995; 131: 353–4.
2 Goerttler E, Jung E. Porokeratosis of Mibelli and skin cancer. *Humangenetik* 1975; 26: 291–6.
3 Otsuka F, Iwata M, Watanabe R, Chi H, Ishibashi Y. Porokeratosis: clinical and cellular characterization of its cancer-prone nature. *J Dermatol* 1992; 19: 702–6.
4 Watanabe R, Otsuka F. Cultured skin fibroblasts derived from three patients with disseminated superficial actinic porokeratosis (DSAP) are hypersensitive to the lethal effects of x-radiation but not to those of ultraviolet (UV) light. *Exp Dermatol* 1993; 2: 175–8.
5 Morton CA, Shuttleworth D, Douglas WS. Porokeratosis and Crohn's disease. *J Am Acad Dermatol* 1995; 32: 894–7.
6 Ghigliotti G, Nigro A, Gambini C, Farris A, Burroni A, de Marchi R. Mibelli's porokeratosis after bone marrow transplantation. *Ann Dermatol Vénéréol* 1992; 119: 968–70.
7 Rothman IL, Wirth PB, Klaus MV. Porokeratosis of Mibelli following heart transplant. *Int J Dermatol* 1992; 31: 52–4.
8 Kanitakis J, Misery L, Nicolas JF et al. Disseminated superficial porokeratosis in a patient with AIDS. *Br J Dermatol* 1994; 131: 284–9.
9 Levell NJ, Bewley AP, Levene GM. Porokeratosis of Mibelli on the penis, scrotum and natal cleft. *Clin Exp Dermatol* 1994; 19: 77–8.
10 Enk A, Bork K, Hoede N, Knop J. Atypical facial porokeratosis of Mibelli. *Br J Dermatol* 1991; 125: 596–8.
11 Kanzaki T, Miwa N, Kobayashi T, Ogawa S. Eruptive pruritic papular porokeratosis. *J Dermatol* 1992; 19: 109–12.

12 McCullough TL, Lesher JL Jr. Porokeratosis of Mibelli: rapid recurrence of a large lesion after carbon dioxide laser treatment. *Pediatr Dermatol* 1994; 11: 267–70.

13 Fleischer AB, Donahue MJ, Feldman SR. Tanning salon porokeratosis. *J Am Acad Dermatol* 1993; 29: 787–8.

14 Mibelli V. Porokeratosis. In: Morris MA, ed. *International Atlas of Rare Skin Diseases*. Hamburg: Leopold Voss, 1889: 8–10.

15 Respighi E. Di una ipercheraosi non ancora descritta. *G Ital Mal Ven Pell* 1893; 28: 356–86.

16 Chernosky MD. Porokeratosis: report of 12 patients with multiple superficial lesions. *South Med J* 1966; 59: 289–94.

17 Pinkus H. Porokeratosis. *Arch Dermatol* 1970; 102: 235–6.

18 Guss SB, Osbourn RA, Lutzner MA. Porokeratosis plantaris, palmaris, et disseminata: a third type of porokeratosis. *Arch Dermatol* 1971; 104: 366–73.

19 Beers B, Jaszcz W, Sheetz K, Hogan DJ, Lynch PJ. Porokeratosis palmaris et plantaris disseminata. *Arch Dermatol* 1992; 128: 236–9.

20 Rahbari H, Cordero AA, Mehregan AH. Linear porokeratosis—a distinctive clinical variant of porokeratosis of Mibelli. *Arch Dermatol* 1974; 109: 526–8.

21 Feldman SR, Crosby DL, Tomsick RS. Scaly atrophic lesions both scattered and in linear arrays. Disseminated superficial actinic porokeratosis in a patient with linear porokeratosis. *Arch Dermatol* 1991; 127: 1219–22.

22 Gautam RK, Bedi GK, Schgal VN, Singh N. Simultaneous occurrence of disseminated superficial actinic porokeratosis (DSAP), linear, and punctate porokeratosis. *Int J Dermatol* 1995; 34: 71–2.

23 Lucker GP, Steijlen PM. The coexistence of linear and giant porokeratosis associated with Bowen's disease. *Dermatology* 1994; 189: 78–80.

24 Happle R. Somatic recombination may explain linear porokeratosis associated with disseminated superficial actinic porokeratosis. *Am J Med Genet* 1991; 39: 237.

25 Jurecka W, Neumann A, Knobler RM. Porokeratoses: immunohistochemical, light and electron microscopic evaluation. *J Am Acad Dermatol* 1991; 24: 96–101.

26 Magee JW, McCalmont TH, LeBoit PE. Overexpression of p53 tumor suppressor protein in porokeratosis. *Arch Dermatol* 1994; 130: 187–90.

27 Otsuka F, Umebayashi Y, Watanabe S, Kawashima M, Hamanaka S. Porokeratosis large skin lesions are susceptible to skin cancer development: histological and cytological explanation for the susceptibility. *J Cancer Res Clin Oncol* 1993; 119: 395–400.

28 Gray MH, Smoller BS, McNutt NS. Carcinogenesis in porokeratosis. Evidence for a role relating to chronic growth activation of keratinocytes. *Am J Dermatopathol* 1991; 14: 61–2.

29 Hohl D. Expression patterns of loricrin in dermatological disorders. *Am J Dermatopathol* 1993; 15: 20–7.

30 Ito M, Fujiwara H, Maruyama T, Oguro K, Ishihara O, Sato Y. Morphogenesis of the cornoid lamella: histochemical, immunohistochemical, and ultrastructural study of porokeratosis. *J Cutan Pathol* 1991; 18: 247–56.

31 Otsuka F, Wantanabe R, Kawashima M, Tomita Y, Ohahr K, Ishibashi Y. Porokeratosis with large skin lesions. Histologic, cytologic and cytogenetic study of three cases. *Acta Derm Venerol* 1991; 71: 437–40.

32 Shumack S, Commens C, Kossard S. Disseminated superficial actinic porokeratosis. *Am J Dermatopathol* 1991; 13: 26–31.

33 Jacyk WK, Esplin L. Hyperkeratotic form of porokeratosis of Mibelli. *Int J Dermatol* 1993; 32: 902–3.

34 Merkle T, Hohenleutner U, Braun-Falco O, Landthaler M. Reticulate porokeratosis—successful treatment with CO_2 laser vaporization. *Clin Exp Dermatol* 1992; 17: 178–81.

35 Fisher CA, LeBoit PE, Frieden IJ. Linear porokeratosis presenting as erosions in the newborn period. *Pediatr Dermatol* 1995; 12: 318–22.

36 Kosogabe M, Tada J, Arata J. Punctate porokeratotic keratoderma. *Jap J Dermatol* 1991; 101: 553–60.

37 Guillot P, Taieb A, Fontan I, Bilhou-Nabera C, Viard E. Linear porokeratotis of Mibelli in monozygotic twin girls. *Ann Dermatol Vénéréol* 1991; 118: 519–24.

38 Goldman GD, Milstone LM. Generalized linear porokeratotis treated with etretinate. *Arch Dermatol* 1995; 131: 496–7.

39 Taniguchi Y, Yuasa T, Shimizu M. Linear porokeratosis. *J Dermatol* 1993; 20: 489–92.

40 Happle R. Mosaicism in human skin. *Arch Dermatol* 1993; 129: 1460–70.

41 Rothman IL, Wirth PB, Klaus MV. Porokeratosis of Mibelli following heart transplant. *Int J Dermatol* 1992; 31: 52–4.

42 Wilkinson SM, Cartwright PH, English JSC. Porokeratosis of Mibelli and immunosuppression. *Clin Exp Dermatol* 1991; 16: 61–2.

43 Kormorowski RA, Clowry LJ. Porokeratosis of Mibelli in transplant recipients. *Am J Clin Pathol* 1989; 91: 71–4.

44 Adriaans B, Salisbury JR. Recurrent porokeratosis. *Br J Dermatol* 1991; 124: 383–6.

45 Tsambaos D, Spiliopoulos T. Disseminated superficial porokeratosis: complete remission subsequent to discontinuation of immunosuppression. *J Am Acad Dermatol* 1993; 28: 651–2.

46 Hsu WT, Toporcer MB, Kantor GR, Vonderheid EC, Kadin ME. Cutaneous T-cell lymphoma with porokeratosis-like lesions. *J Am Acad Dermatol* 1992; 27: 327–30.

47 Hsu MM, Lee JY. Cutaneous and subcutaneous phaeyphomycosis caused by exserohilum rostratum. *J Am Acad Dermatol* 1993; 28: 340–4.

48 Chu P, LeBoit PE. Dermatophytosis in lesions of disseminated superficial actinic porokeratosis. *J Am Acad Dermatol* 1994; 30: 146–7.

49 Breneman DL, Breneman JC. Cutaneous T-cell lymphoma mimicking porokeratosis of Mibelli. *J Am Acad Dermatol* 1993; 29: 1046–8.

50 Paller AS, Syder AJ, Yiu-Mo Chan BS, Hutton E, Tadini G, Fuchs E. Genetic and clinical mosaicism in a type of epidermal nevus. *New Engl J Med* 1994; 331: 1408–15.

51 Siegfried EC. Diagnostic and therapeutic surgical interventions in pediatric dermatology. *Curr Opin Dermatol* 1995; 2: 142–54.

52 Siegfried EC. Diagnostic and therapeutic surgical interventions in pediatric dermatology. *Curr Opin Dermatol* 1995; 3: 169–75.

53 Siegfried EC. Principles of treatment. In: Schachner LA, Hansen RC, eds. *Peditric Dermatology*. New York: Churchill Livingstone, 1996.

54 Nelson BR, Kolansky G, Gillard M, Ratner D, Johnson TM. Management of linear verrucous epidermal nevus with topical 5-fluorouracil and tretinoin. *J Am Acad Dermatol* 1994; 30: 287–8.

55 Strange PR, Lang PG Jr. Long-term management of basal cell nevus syndrome with topical tretinoin and 5-fluorouracil. *J Am Acad Dermatol* 1995; 27: 842–5.

56 Verma KK, Singh OP. Dexamethasone pulse treatment in disseminated porokeratosis of Mibelli. *J Dermatol Sci* 1994; 7: 71–2.

57 McCallister RE, Estes SA, Yarbrough CL. Porokeratosis plantaris, palmaris et disseminata. Report of a case and treatment with isotretinoin. *J Am Acad Dermatol* 1985; 13: 598–603.

58 Rabbin PE, Baldwin HE. Treatment of porokeratosis of Mibelli with CO_2 laser vaporization versus surgical excision with split-thickness skin graft. *J Dermatol Surg Oncol* 1993; 19: 199–202.

59 Spencer JM, Katz BE. Successful treatment of porokeratosis of Mibelli with diamond fraise dermabrasion. *Arch Dermatol* 1992; 128: 1187–8.

60 Limmer BL. Cryosurgery of porokeratosis plantaris, palmaris et discreta. *Arch Dermatol* 1979; 115: 582–3.

61 McDonald SG, Peterka ES. Porokeratosis (Mibelli): treatment with topical 5-fluorouracil. *J Am Acad Dermatol* 1983; 8: 107–10.

62 Harrison PV, Stollery N. Disseminated superficial actinic porokeratosis responding to calcitriol. *Clin Exp Dermatol* 1994; 19: 95.

19.11 Ectodermal Dysplasias

JULIE S. FRANCIS

The original ectodermal dysplasias
X-linked hypohidrotic ectodermal dysplasia
Autosomal recessive hypohidrotic ectodermal dysplasia
Hidrotic ectodermal dysplasia

Ectodermal dysplasias with involvement primarily of appendages of the epidermis and oral ectoderm (hair, teeth, nails and sweat glands)
Tooth and nail syndrome
Trichodentosseus syndrome
Ectodermal dysplasias with cleft lip/palate
Rapp–Hodgkin syndrome
Ankyloblepharon, ectodermal dysplasia, cleft lip/palate syndrome
Ectrodactyly, ectodermal dysplasia, clefting syndrome

Ectodermal dysplasias with eye abnormalities
Schöpf–Schulz–Passarge syndrome
Oculodentodigital dysplasia

Ectodermal dysplasias with pigmentary abnormalities
Naegeli–Franceschetti–Jadassohn syndrome

Ectodermal dysplasias with abnormal dermatoglyphics
Absence of dermal ridge patterns, onychodystrophy and palmoplantar anhidrosis

The ectodermal dysplasias are a large, diverse group of inherited disorders that share in common developmental abnormalities of two or more of the following: (a) hair; (b) teeth; (c) nails; (d) sweat glands; and (e) other ectodermal structures. An extensive review of the ectodermal dysplasias and a classification system was proposed by Freire-Maia and Pinheiro in 1984 in an effort to impose order on a poorly defined group of disorders [1]. Involvement of the appendages of the epidermis and oral ectoderm (hair, teeth, nails and sweat glands) is the primary basis of their classification system even though many ectodermal dysplasias also involve abnormalities of other ectoder-mal structures including keratinocytes, melanocytes, the mammary gland, thymus, thyroid, anterior pituitary, adrenal medulla, oral, nasal, rectal and genital mucosa, external ear, central nervous system, lens, cornea, conjunctiva, lacrimal gland and lacrimal duct. Clinical abnormalities of these structures must be sufficiently prominent for the disorder to be classified as

an ectodermal dysplasia [1]. Solomon *et al.* suggest that a disorder must also be congenital, diffuse and nonprogressive in order to be considered an ectodermal dysplasia [2,3]. Many conditions that involve abnormalities of ectodermal structures are not considered ectodermal dysplasias because these features are neither major nor sufficiently prominent.

From over 150 ectodermal dysplasias [4], the conditions arbitrarily chosen for discussion in this chapter include the most common ectodermal dysplasias, those most likely to present to the dermatologist for diagnosis and those that are of particular interest to the author. Those ectodermal dysplasias defined by single case reports or by a few affected individuals in a single family are, in general, not included. Those ectodermal dysplasias that exhibit prominent features unrelated to ectodermal structures such as dwarfism, cardiac defects, neutropenia, hypogonadism and severe mental retardation are not discussed as they are unlikely to present to the dermatologist for diagnosis. Incontinenti pigmenti, focal dermal hypoplasia of Goltz and hypomelanosis of Ito also exhibit many features that warrant their discussion outside the category of ectodermal dysplasias, even though ectodermal structures may be affected. The reader is referred to Freire-Maia's book for a review of those ectodermal dysplasias not discussed in this chapter [1].

Classification of the ectodermal dysplasias is phenotypically based as little is known about the pathogenesis or the biochemical and molecular defects of these disorders. The appendages of the epidermis and oral ectoderm (hair, nails, sweat glands and teeth) all develop at different time periods during development as downward epithelial projections from the epidermis, guided along their developmental path by underlying collections of mesenchymal cells. Other structures of ectodermal origin affected in many of the ectodermal dysplasias (certain bones of the head and face, mammary gland, lacrimal gland, thymus, thyroid, palate, etc.) also develop dependent on a relationship between the surface epithelium and underlying mesenchyme [5,6]. In this region of the epithelial–mesenchymal interface, complex and poorly understood events occur which may be disrupted during development leading to the formation of abnormal ectodermal structures [5]. A unifying concept that defines the developmental errors seen in the various ectodermal dysplasias, must explain how a single mutant gene exerts affects on a number of ectodermal derivatives over a broad time period in development.

Doctors treating patients with any of the ectodermal dysplasias, should inform these individuals of an international patient advocacy and support group, the National Foundation for Ectodermal Dysplasias (NFED) (Mascoutah, Illinois, USA, Email nfed1@aol.com). The NFED serves people with ectodermal dysplasia and their families through support networks, publications on treatment and care, treatment funds, dental implant programmes, scholarships, regional diagnostic centres and the funding of research programmes.

REFERENCES

1 Freire-Maia N, Pinheiro M. *Ectodermal Dysplasias: a Clinical and Genetic Study.* New York: Alan R. Liss, 1984.
2 Solomon LM, Keuer EJ. The ectodermal dysplasias. Problems of classification and some newer syndromes. *Arch Dermatol* 1980; 116: 1295–9.
3 Solomon LM, Cook B, Klipfel W. The ectodermal dysplasias. *Dermatol Clin* 1987; 5: 231–7.
4 Pinheiro M, Freire-Maia N. Ectodermal dysplasias: a clinical classification and a causal review. *Am J Med Genet* 1994; 53: 153–62.
5 Holbrook KA. Structural abnormalities of the epidermally derived appendages in skin from patients with ectodermal dysplasia: insight into developmental errors. In: Salinas CF, Opitz JM, Paul NW, eds. *Recent Advances in Ectodermal Dysplasias.* New York: Alan R. Liss, 1988: 15–44.
6 Cohen RL. Clinical perspectives on premature tooth eruption and cyst formation in neonates. *Pediatr Dermatol* 1984; 1: 301–6.

The original ectodermal dysplasias

Even though there are scattered reports of individuals affected with ectodermal dysplasia prior, the term 'hereditary ectodermal dysplasia' was first coined by Weech in 1929 to describe those individuals with congenital anomalies of structures that arise from embryonic ectoderm [1]. In his detailed report of two individuals affected with X-linked anhidrotic ectodermal dysplasia (now termed 'hypohidrotic'), Weech proposed a subclassification of anhidrotic ectodermal dysplasia for those individuals with deficient sweating [1]. In the same year, Clouston reported a large kindred with hereditary abnormalities of the hair and nails, palmoplantar hyperkeratosis, localized areas of hyperpigmentation and normal sweating. He used the term 'hereditary ectodermal dystrophy' to describe this disorder which later became known as hidrotic ectodermal dysplasia [2,3]. This initial subclassification of the group of ectodermal dysplasias into anhidrotic and hidrotic has been superseded by more recent classification systems but these two ectodermal dysplasias, X-linked hypohidrotic ectodermal dysplasia (HED) and hidrotic ectodermal dysplasia, are considered the original ectodermal dysplasias and are discussed in

detail in this section. Autosomal recessive HED is included for convenience even though its genetic heterogeneity to X-linked HED was not recognized for almost 40 years after Weech's and Clouston's respective reports [4].

REFERENCES

1 Weech AA. Hereditary ectodermal dysplasia (congenital ectodermal defect). A report of two cases. *Am J Dis Child* 1929; 37: 766–90.
2 Clouston HR. A hereditary ectodermal dystrophy. *Canad Med Assoc J* 1929; 21: 18–31.
3 Clouston HR. The major forms of hereditary ectodermal dysplasia (with an autopsy and biopsies on the anhydrotic type). *Canad Med Assoc J* 1939; 40: 1–7.
4 Passarge E, Nuzum CT, Schubert WK. Anhidrotic ectodermal dysplasia as autosomal recessive trait in an inbred kindred. *Humangenetik* 1966; 3: 181–5.

X-linked hypohidrotic ectodermal dysplasia
(SYN. CHRIST–SIEMENS–TOURAINE SYNDROME, ANHIDROTIC ECTODERMAL DYSPLASIA)

Definition

X-linked HED is the most common of the ectodermal dysplasias and is characterized by hypotrichosis, hypodontia, hypohidrosis and distinctive facial features.

History

X-linked HED was first described in 1848 by Thurnam [1]. In 1921, Thadini determined it was an X-linked disorder and later reported that female carriers manifest varying signs of the condition [2]. The prevalence is assessed at approximately 1 in 100 000 live male births [3].

Aetiology

The disorder is X-linked recessive and the gene has been mapped to the q12–q13.1 region of the X chromosome [4,5]. A patient has been reported with a deletion at locus DXS732, within the Xq12–13 region; this is considered a candidate locus for the X-linked HED gene [6]. The gene has not yet been identified and the basic defect is unknown, but a homologous animal, the tabby mouse, allows for developmental studies in X-linked HED [6,7]. Injections of epidermal growth factor (EGF) for 7 days after birth resulted in the development of sweat glands in the tabby mouse [8], suggesting that the precursors for the eccrine glands are present in the newborn tabby but have not received the proper inductive signals for their development. The action of EGF on the developing eccrine glands may be non-specific, as the genes for EGF and its receptor are autosomal and not localized to the X chromosome. Immunolabelling studies with antibodies to EGF and its receptor in tabby skin at different stages of development showed no difference with normal controls [9], suggesting the basis for the EGF response is unrelated to the primary gene defect.

Pathology

The epidermis is thin with effacement of rete ridges. The striking finding is absent or sparse eccrine glands and ducts in affected males (Fig. 19.11.1) [10–12]. Hair follicles and sebaceous glands are variably reduced in number and may appear rudimentary [10,11,13]. Apocrine glands may be absent, sparse or even normal [12]. The nasal mucosa demonstrates almost complete loss of ciliated cells [14]. Mucous glands of the upper respiratory tract may be sparse or absent [10]. Mucous-secreting glands in the duodenum may also be absent [11]. Light and scanning electron microscope findings of hair shaft abnormalities are variable and include longitudinal clefts or grooves and transverse fissuring. The bulb of the hair shaft is dystrophic in some individuals [15]. Radiographs of the mandible reveal dental hypoplasia or aplasia [10,16].

Clinical features

Hair

The scalp hair is sparse, fine, lightly pigmented and grows slowly (Fig. 19.11.2). Eyebrows are scanty or absent; sometimes just the outer two-thirds are missing. The eyelashes may be normal, sparse or completely absent. Secondary sexual hair in the beard, pubic and axillary regions is variably present and may be normal. Hair on the torso and extremities is usually absent [10,13,17,18]. Approximately 70% of obligate female carriers describe their hair as being sparse or fine [17].

Teeth

Dental abnormalities vary from complete absence of teeth to sparse, abnormally shaped teeth. Studies reveal a mean of 24 missing teeth, out of a total of 28, in affected males [17,19]. Dentition is delayed and the erupted teeth tend to be small, widely spaced, and are frequently conical or peg-shaped (Fig. 19.11.3). Both deciduous and permanent teeth are affected. The alveolar ridges are hypoplastic (Fig. 19.11.4) which gives rise to full, everted lips [16,20]. About 80% of obligate female carriers have distinct dental abnormalities including absent permanent teeth and small or peg-shaped teeth (Fig. 19.11.5) [17].

Nails

The nails are normal in most individuals. Thin, brittle nail plates with longitudinal ridges have been described in some individuals.

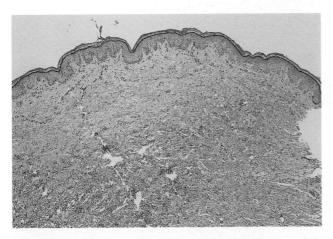

Fig. 19.11.1 Skin biopsy from the trunk of an affected male with X-linked HED. Note the absence of hair follicles, sebaceous glands and eccrine glands (haematoxylin and eosin; 10× original magnification).

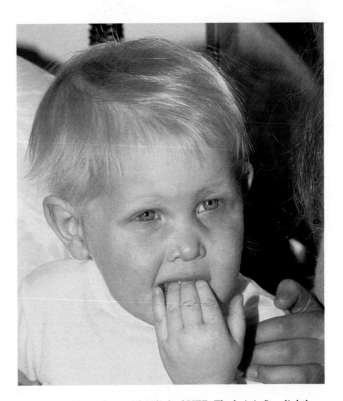

Fig. 19.11.2 Young boy with X-linked HED. The hair is fine, lightly pigmented and sparse.

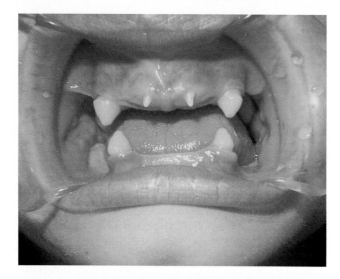

Fig. 19.11.3 This individual with X-linked HED exhibits absent, hypoplastic and peg-shaped teeth.

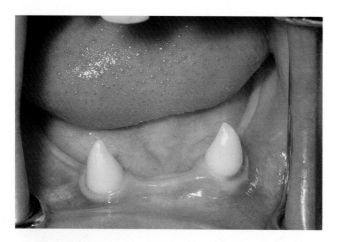

Fig. 19.11.4 Hypoplastic aveolar ridges and peg-shaped teeth in an affected male with X-linked HED.

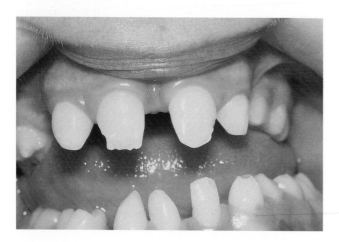

Fig. 19.11.5 This heterozygous female for X-linked HED exhibits abnormally shaped and absent permanent teeth.

Sweat glands

Sweating is severely diminished or absent due to a paucity or absence of eccrine glands. The ability to thermoregulate by evaporative cooling is inadequate and hyperthermia can occur with physical exertion or in a warm environment. This is particularly problematic in infants and young children who may experience recurrent bouts of fever as high as 42°C. Heat intolerance does occur in older children and adults, but they learn to control their body temperature by drinking cold liquids, wetting their skin or clothing and seeking out cool surroundings [17]. About 25% of heterozygote females experience heat intolerance and almost half notice their ability to sweat is reduced [17]. The hypohidrotic areas of skin in carrier females occur in defined linear patterns corresponding to the lines of Blaschko [21]. Diminished apocrine sweating in affected individuals is not problematic.

Skin

At birth, affected males may demonstrate marked scaling or peeling of their skin which may be mistaken for a collodion membrane [22]. In children and adults, the skin is fine, smooth and dry. Periorbital hyperpigmentation and fine wrinkling around the eyes are characteristic features of the disorder (Fig. 19.11.6). Eczema is common and is

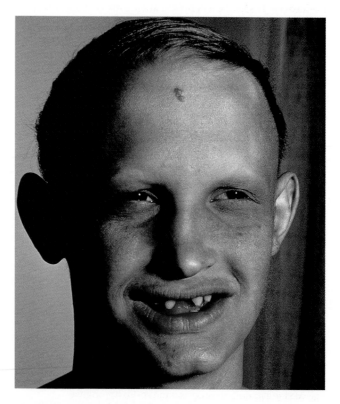

Fig. 19.11.6 Periorbital hyperpigmentation and fine wrinkling in an affected male with X-linked HED.

prominent in flexural areas [18,23]. Small milia-like papules may be found on the face [12,13].

Other ectodermal structures

Diminished or absent salivary glands and mucous glands of the nose, mouth and ears cause numerous otolaryngological complications including nasal obstruction caused by thick, fetid nasal discharge and adherent nasal crusts, sinusitis, recurrent upper respiratory tract infections, feeding problems in infancy, xerostomia, hoarse voice and impacted cerumen [13,17,24]. Diminished production of tear film from the lacrimal glands may cause dry eyes, photophobia and corneal damage [12,25].

A third of affected males have abnormalities of the nipples including absent, simple or accessory nipples [17,26]. Female carriers may also be affected with marked breast asymmetry, inadequate breast milk production or athelia. Pituitary and adrenal insufficiency have been reported [12].

Craniofacial features

The facies are distinctive with relative frontal bossing, concave midface, saddle nose and everted lips (Fig. 19.11.6) [10,13,16]. A third of affected males have ears that are described as simple or satyr [17]. The distinctive facial features may not be obvious at birth, but become more noticeable with age (Fig. 19.11.7). Carrier females may exhibit similar facial features (Fig. 19.11.8).

Other clinical features

Diminished or absent mucous glands of the tracheal, bronchial, oesophageal, gastric and colonic mucosa cause problems with recurrent bronchitis, pneumonia, dysphagia and gastro-oesophageal reflux and constipation [12,17,27]. Reactive airways with wheezing is a common problem [17]. There is no convincing evidence for thyroid or parathyroid abnormalities, nor for a primary immune deficiency associated with X-linked HED [17].

Prognosis

Failure to thrive occurs in up to 40% of affected males [17]. Height and weight are compromised in early childhood but appear to normalize with time. Mortality in infancy and early childhood is historically 25%, primarily due to hyperthermia, failure to thrive and respiratory infections [17]. Febrile seizures can occur with hyperpyrexia [17,23]. Speech problems may exist due to hypodontia, nasal obstruction and impacted cerumen [23,24].

Differential diagnosis

Affected infants with scaling skin may be misdiagnosed as collodion babies with lamellar ichthyosis. The saddle nose and abnormal teeth have caused diagnostic confusion with congenital syphilis [12,13]. Once the characteristic facies and lack of sweating are evident, there are very few disorders to consider in the differential diagnosis. HED with hypothyroidism displays hypohidrosis with hyperthermia and hypotrichosis but the teeth are normal, the nails are significantly dystrophic and the skin has

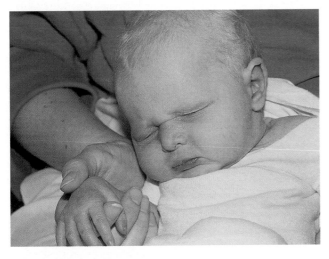

Fig. 19.11.7 The facial features of X-linked HED may not be obvious at birth, but become more pronounced over time. This 2-week-old infant is also seen in Fig. 19.11.2 at the age of 2 years.

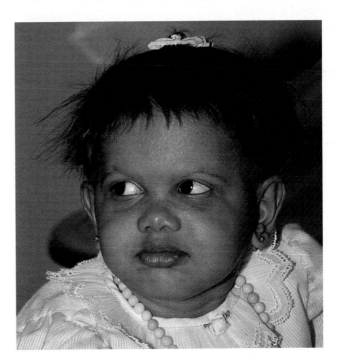

Fig. 19.11.8 This heterozygous female for X-linked HED exhibits a concave midface, saddle nose and everted lips.

mottled-brown areas of pigmentation [28]. Fried's tooth and nail syndrome manifests hypotrichosis, hypodontia and prominent everted lips but the sweating is normal [28]. Basan's syndrome is characterized by hypotrichosis, hypodontia and hypohidrosis but also by severe nail dystrophy and congenital absence of dermatoglyphics [23]. Genetic heterogeneity for HED is probable and it is important to try to distinguish the more common X-linked form from the autosomal recessive form (see below) for the purposes of genetic counselling and reproductive planning.

Treatment

A multidisciplinary approach to the management of these individuals is advocated [29]. Early diagnosis is crucial to avoid life-threatening complications in infancy, for planning long-term management and to define recurrent risks for families [30]. Female carriers may be detected in most cases by careful clinical examination for patchy distribution of scalp and body hair, sweat pores and hypodontia [23]. The use of restriction fragment length polymorphism linkage analysis on affected families can detect female carriers with considerable accuracy. Prenatal diagnosis is also possible in a majority of families at risk for the disorder [31].

Prevention of hyperthermia is critical. This is done by avoiding heat and physical overexertion, cooling the body with wet clothing and cool drinks and by air-conditioning home and school environments. Early dental restoration with bonding, overdentures or implants is imperative [25,32,33]. Nasal crusting and discharge can be managed with saline nose drops and a home humidifier. Consumption of large amounts of liquids, or artificial saliva preparations minimize dry mouth and swallowing difficulties [34]. Dry eyes may be treated with artificial tears. The daily use of lubricating drops facilitates the removal of impacted ear wax. Pulmonary difficulties are managed by avoidance of smoky, dusty environments, adequate humidification and the use of chest physiotherapy and antibiotics when appropriate [35].

REFERENCES

1 Thurnam J. Two cases in which the skin, hair and teeth were very imperfectly developed. *Med Chir Trans* 1848; 31: 71–82.
2 Thadini KI. A toothless type of man. The 'Bhudas' of India—a case of sex-linked inheritance. *J Hered* 1921; 12: 87–8.
3 Kerr CB, Wells RS, Cooper KE. Gene effect in carriers of anhidrotic ectodermal dysplasia. *J Med Genet* 1966; 3: 169–76.
4 Zonana J, Jones M, Clarke A et al. Detection of *de novo* mutations and analysis of their origin in families with X linked hypohidrotic ectodermal dysplasia. *J Med Genet* 1994; 31: 287–92.
5 Thomas NS, Chelly J, Zonana J et al. Characterisation of molecular DNA rearrangements within the Xq12–q13.1 region, in three patients with X-linked hypohidrotic ectodermal dysplasia (EDA). *Hum Mol Genet* 1993; 2: 1679–85.
6 Zonana J, Gault J, Davies KJ et al. Detection of a molecular deletion at the

DXS732 locus in a patient with X-linked hypohidrotic ectodermal dysplasia. *Am J Hum Genet* 1993; 52: 78–84.
7 Blecher SR. Anhidrosis and absence of sweat glands in mice hemizygous for the tabby gene: supportive evidence for the hypothesis of homology between tabby and human anhidrotic (hypohidrotic) ectodermal dysplasia (Christ–Siemens–Touraine syndrome). *J Invest Dermatol* 1986; 87: 720–2.
8 Blecher SR, Kapalanga J, Lalonde D. Induction of sweat glands by epidermal growth factor in murine X-linked anhidrotic ectodermal dysplasia. *Nature* 1990; 345: 542–4.
9 Kim S, Francis JS, Holbrook KA. The presence of epidermal growth factor and epidermal growth factor receptor in skin of fetal tabby mice. *Clin Res* 1993; 41: 38A.
10 Clouston HR. The major forms of hereditary ectodermal dysplasia (with an autopsy and biopsies on the anhydrotic type). *Canad Med Assoc J* 1939; 40: 1–7.
11 Arnold ML, Anton-Lamprecht I, Rauskolb R. Prenatal diagnosis of ectodermal dysplasias. *Semin Dermatol* 1984; 3: 247–52.
12 Butterworth T, Ladda RL. *Clinical Genodermatology*, vol. I. New York: Praeger, 1981: 208–17.
13 Weech AA. Hereditary ectodermal dysplasia (congenital ectodermal defect). A report of two cases. *Am J Dis Child* 1929; 37: 766–90.
14 Baer ST, Coulson IH, Elliman D. Anhidrotic ectodermal dysplasia: an ENT presentation in infancy. *J Laryngol Otol* 1988; 102: 458–9.
15 Micali G, Cook B, Blekys I, Solomon LM. Structural hair abnormalities in ectodermal dysplasia. *Pediatr Dermatol* 1990; 7: 27–32.
16 Vierucci S, Baccetti T, Tollaro I. Dental and craniofacial findings in hypohidrotic ectodermal dysplasia during the primary dentition phase. *J Clin Pediatr Dent* 1994; 18: 291–7.
17 Clarke A, Phillips DIM, Brown R, Harper PS. Clinical aspects of X-linked hypohidrotic ectodermal dysplasia. *Arch Dis Child* 1987; 62: 989–96.
18 Reed WB, Lopez DA, Landing B. Clinical spectrum of anhidrotic ectodermal dysplasia. *Arch Dermatol* 1970; 102: 134–43.
19 Crawford PJM, Aldred MJ, Clarke A. Clinical and radiographic dental findings in X-linked hypohidrotic ectodermal dysplasia. *J Med Genet* 1991; 28: 181–5.
20 Levin LS. Dental and oral abnormalities in selected ectodermal dysplasia syndromes. In: Salinas CF, Opitz JM, Paul NW, eds. *Recent Advances in Ectodermal Dysplasias*. New York: Alan R. Liss, 1988: 205–27.
21 Happle R, Frosch PJ. Manifestation of the lines of Blaschko in women heterozygous for X-linked hypohidrotic ectodermal dysplasia. *Clin Genet* 1985; 27: 468–71.
22 The Executive and Scientific Advisory Boards of the National Foundation for Ectodermal Dysplasias, Mascoutah, Illinois. Scaling skin in the neonate: a clue to the early diagnosis of X-linked hypohidrotic ectodermal dysplasia (Christ–Siemens–Touraine syndrome). *J Pediatr* 1989; 114: 600–2.
23 Clarke A. Hypohidrotic ectodermal dysplasia. *J Med Genet* 1987; 24: 659–63.
24 Coston GN, Salinas CF. Speech characteristics in patients with hypohidrotic ectodermal dysplasia. In: Salinas CF, Opitz JM, Paul NW, eds. *Recent Advances in Ectodermal Dysplasias*. New York: Alan R. Liss, 1988: 229–34.
25 Wright JT, Finley WH. X-linked recessive hypohidrotic ectodermal dysplasia. Manifestations and management. *Ala J Med Sci* 1986; 23: 84–7.
26 Söderholm AL, Kaitila I. Expression of X-linked hypohidrotic ectodermal dysplasia in six males and in their mothers. *Clin Genet* 1985; 28: 136–44.
27 The Executive and Scientific Advisory Boards of the National Foundation for Ectodermal Dysplasias, Mascoutah, Illinois. Gastrointestinal complaints in individuals with hypohidrotic ectodermal dysplasia (Christ–Siemens–Touraine syndrome). *Pediatr Dermaol* 1995; 12: 288–9.
28 Freire-Maia N, Pinheiro M. *Ectodermal Dysplasias: A Clinical and Genetic Study*. New York: Alan R. Liss, 1984.
29 Farrington FH. The team approach to the management of ectodermal dysplasias. In: Salinas CF, Opitz JM, Paul NW, eds. *Recent Advances in Ectodermal Dysplasias*. New York: Alan R. Liss, 1988: 237–42.
30 Sybert VP. Early diagnosis in the ectodermal dysplasias. In: Salinas CF, Opitz JM, Paul NW, eds. *Recent Advances in Ectodermal Dysplasias*. New York: Alan R. Liss, 1988: 277–8.
31 Zonana J. Hypohidrotic (anhidrotic) ectodermal dysplasia: molecular genetic research and its clinical applications. *Semin Dermatol* 1993; 12: 241–6.
32 Nowak AJ. Dental treatment for patients with ectodermal dysplasia. In:

Salinas CF, Opitz JM, Paul NW, eds. *Recent Advances in Ectodermal Dysplasias*. New York: Alan R. Liss, 1988: 243–52.

33 Guckes AD, Brahim JS, McCarthy GR, Rudy SF, Cooper LF. Using endosseous dental implants for patients with ectodermal dysplasia. *J Am Dent Assoc* 1991; 122: 59–62.

34 Myer CM. The role of an otolaryngologist in the care of ectodermal dysplasia. *Pediatr Dermatol* 1987; 4: 34–5.

35 Myer CM. Otolaryngologic manifestations of the ectodermal dysplasias. In: Salinas CF, Opitz JM, Paul NW, eds. *Recent Advances in Ectodermal Dysplasias*. New York: Alan R. Liss, 1988: 253–6.

Autosomal recessive hypohidrotic ectodermal dysplasia

An autosomal recessive form of X-linked HED has been described which is clinically indistinguishable from the X-linked form and females appear to be as severely affected as males (Fig. 19.11.9) [1–4]. Autosomal recessive mode of inheritance has been inferred from pedigrees in which females are severely affected or inbreeding is present. A number of these pedigrees are more consistent with X-linked inheritance when carefully reviewed and the clinical evidence to support an autosomal recessive form of classic X-linked HED has been minimal [5]. Recently, four families with possible autosomal recessive HED were identified and genotyped using markers closely flanking the X-linked hypohidrotic locus [6]. In three families, the disorder did not segregate with the X-linked locus, supporting the existence of autosomal recessive inheritance in these few families although gonadal mosaicism could not be ruled out in one family. To date, in over 95% of families evaluated with HED, linkage to the q12–q13.1 region of the X chromosome has been demonstrated, suggesting the proportion of individuals with autosomal recessive inheritance is small [7]. Genetic counselling for families of affected females should stress the likelihood of X-linked recessive inheritance [5].

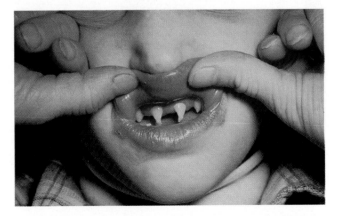

Fig. 19.11.9 This female with autosomal recessive HED exhibits clinical features indistinguishable from males affected with X-linked HED. Note the severely affected teeth and the periorbital hyperpigmentation just visible at the top of the photograph.

REFERENCES

1 Freire-Maia N, Pinheiro M. *Ectodermal Dysplasias: a Clinical and Genetic Study*. New York: Alan R. Liss, 1984.

2 Crump IA, Danks DM. Hypohidrotic ectodermal dysplasia. A study of sweat pores in the X-linked form and in a family with probable autosomal recessive inheritance. *J Pediatr* 1971; 78: 466–73.

3 Gorlin RJ. Hypohidrotic ectodermal dysplasia in females. A critical analysis and argument for genetic heterogeneity. *Z Kinderheilk* 1970; 108: 1–11.

4 Anton-Lamprecht I, Schleiermacher E, Wolf M. Autosomal recessive anhidrotic ectodermal dysplasia: report of a case and discrimination of diagnostic features. In: Salinas CF, Opitz JM, Paul NW, eds. *Recent Advances in Ectodermal Dysplasias*. New York: Alan R. Liss, 1988: 183–95.

5 Sybert VP. Hypohidrotic ectodermal dysplasia: argument against an autosomal recessive form clinically indistinguishable from X-linked hypohidrotic ectodermal dysplasia (Christ–Siemens–Touraine syndrome). *Pediatr Dermatol* 1989; 6: 76–81.

6 Munoz F, Jorgenson R, Sybert VP *et al.* Evidence for a rare autosomal recessive form of hypohidrotic ectodermal dysplasia (ARHED) clinically indistinguishable from the X-linked disorder at the EDA locus. *Am J Hum Genet* 1995; 57: A221.

7 Zonana J. Hypohidrotic (anhidrotic) ectodermal dysplasia: molecular genetic research and its clinical applications. *Semin Dermatol* 1993; 12: 241–6.

Hidrotic ectodermal dysplasia

(SYN. CLOUSTON'S SYNDROME, FISCHER–JACOBSEN–CLOUSTON SYNDROME, WALDEYER–FISCHER SYNDROME, JACOBSEN'S SYNDROME)

Definition

Hidrotic ectodermal dysplasia is an autosomal dominant ectodermal dysplasia defined by generalized hypotrichosis, dystrophic nails and hyperkeratosis of the palms and soles.

History

This distinct ectodermal dysplasia is named after Clouston, a doctor in Quebec, Canada, who defined much of what we know about the disorder [1,2]. Several reports describe a large kindred originally from France, who then migrated to Canada, the USA and Scotland [1–5]. Five generations of a large Malaysian-Chinese kindred have also been reported [6].

Aetiology

The disorder is inherited as an autosomal dominant trait; expression is mildly variable [5]. The basic defect is unknown. A structural hair keratin defect has been postulated [7] but linkage analyses to any of the keratin genes has not been accomplished in affected families.

Pathology

Various abnormal physical properties of the hair shaft

have been found including low disulphide-bonded protein content, increased water content, altered birefringence in polarized light, reduced elastic modulus and reduced tensile strength [7]. The hair shaft is abnormally shaped; it may be twisted, small, have longitudinal grooves and be square in cross section. The pigment may be absent [8]. Cells of the cuticle are atrophic or even absent near the tips of the hair shafts though relatively normal near the base. The cortex of the hair shaft is more fibrillar, coarse and disorganized compared with normal hair shafts [8]. Hair follicles in skin biopsies are reduced in number and when present may appear dystrophic, with thickened connective tissue sheaths surrounding them [9]. Sebaceous glands are sparse and apocrine glands are sparse or absent. Eccrine glands are normal in number; in one affected individual, a single, rather than a double, layer of eccrine ductal cells was present [9]. Skin biopsy of the palmoplantar thickening shows acanthosis, orthohyperkeratosis and hypergranulosis [9].

Clinical features [1–4,6,10]

Hair

Scalp hair is sparse, fine, brittle, pale in colour and slow growing (Fig. 19.11.10). Hair loss may become more pronounced over time and total alopecia can occur. The eyebrows and eyelashes are thin or absent. Body, pubic and axillary hairs are also affected.

Teeth

The teeth are normal but caries are common.

Nails

Nail dystrophy is characteristic of HED but can be variable. Generally, the nail plate is short, thick, slow growing and discolored (Fig. 19.11.11). The nail plate may be completely absent. Frequent infections of the nail folds can occur.

Sweat glands

Sweating is normal in affected individuals.

Skin

The skin tends to be dry and rough; it is unclear how this is related to the paucity of sebaceous glands described in some affected individuals. Diffuse palmar and plantar hyperkeratosis is a frequent finding (Fig. 19.11.12), and can be severe. It may extend onto the dorsum of the hands and feet, and fissuring can occur. Malignant degeneration of the palmoplantar hyperkeratosis has been reported.

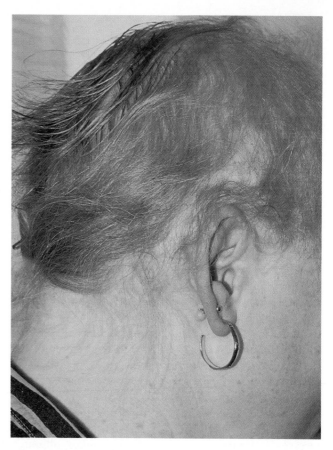

Fig. 19.11.10 The scalp hair is sparse, fine and brittle in this female with hidrotic ectodermal dysplasia.

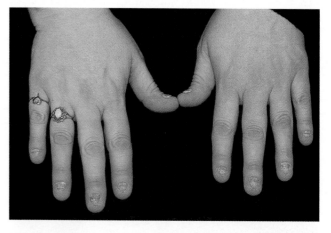

Fig. 19.11.11 The nail plates are thick, short and discolored in this individual with hidrotic ectodermal dysplasia.

The skin may also be thickened over the knees, elbows, joints of the fingers and knuckles. Localized hyperpigmentation of the skin is a striking finding and may be found over the knuckles, elbows, axillae, areolae and bony prominences.

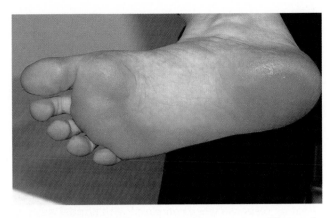

Fig. 19.11.12 Diffuse palmoplantar hyperkeratosis is seen frequently in hidrotic ectodermal dysplasia. This individual exhibits mild plantar hyperkeratosis.

Other ectodermal structures

Various eye abnormalities have been described including conjunctivitis, strabismus and congenital cataract. In one family with HED, five affected individuals developed bilateral premature cataracts [11]. Oral leucoplakia has been described in a number of families [10,12]. Diffuse eccrine poromatosis was reported in one patient [13].

Craniofacial features

There are no characteristic craniofacial features. Thickened skull bones have been described.

Other features

Tufting of the terminal phalanges was described in Clouston's original report [1].

Prognosis

The nail and skin dystrophies can become more pronounced over time. Physical development and life span are unaffected.

Differential diagnosis

Pachyonychia congenita shares the features of palmoplantar hyperkeratosis, oral leucoplakia and thickened, discolored nails but the hair is usually normal and the teeth erupt prematurely [10,14]. Individuals with Coffin–Siris syndrome have sparse hair and absent or hypoplastic nails, most notably the fifth fingernail and toenail. They lack the palmoplantar hyperkeratosis, their facial features are characteristic and they have associated mental retardation [14].

Treatment

Nail ablation may sometimes be necessary, emollients for hyperkeratosis sometimes helpful and artificial hair pieces useful in some individuals.

REFERENCES

1 Clouston HR. A hereditary ectodermal dystrophy. *Canad Med Assoc J* 1929; 21: 18–31.
2 Clouston HR. The major forms of hereditary ectodermal dysplasia (with an autopsy and biopsies on the anhydrotic type). *Canad Med Assoc J* 1939; 40: 1–7.
3 Joachim H. Hereditary dystrophy of the hair and nails in six generations. *Ann Intern Med* 1936; 10: 400–2.
4 Wilkey WD, Stevenson GH. A family with inherited ectodermal dystrophy. *Canad Med Assoc J* 1945; 53: 226–30.
5 Williams M, Fraser FC. Hydrotic ectodermal dysplasia—Clouston's family revisited. *Canad Med Assoc J* 1967; 96: 36–8.
6 Rajagopalan K, Tay CH. Hidrotic ectodermal dysplasia. Study of a large Chinese pedigree. *Arch Dermatol* 1977; 113: 481–5.
7 Gold RJM, Scriver CR. The characterization of hereditary abnormalities of keratin: Clouston's ectodermal dysplasia. *Birth Defects* 1971; 7: 91–5.
8 Escobar V, Goldblatt LI, Bixler D, Weaver D. Clouston syndrome: an ultrastructural study. *Clin Genet* 1983; 24: 140–6.
9 Pierard GE, Van Neste D, Letot B. Hidrotic ectodermal dysplasia. *Dermatologica* 1979; 158: 168–74.
10 Levin LS. Dental and oral abnormalities in selected ectodermal dysplasia syndromes. In: Salinas CF, Opitz JM, Paul NW, eds. *Recent Advances in Ectodermal Dysplasias*. New York: Alan R. Liss, 1988: 205–27.
11 Hazen PG, Zamora I, Bruner WE, Muir WA. Premature cataracts in a family with hidrotic ectodermal dysplasia. *Arch Dermatol* 1980; 116: 1385–7.
12 George DI, Escobar VH. Oral findings of Clouston's syndrome (hidrotic ectodermal dysplasia). *Oral Surg Oral Med Oral Pathol* 1984; 57: 258–62.
13 Wilkinson RD, Schopflocher P, Rozenfeld M. Hidrotic ectodermal dysplasia with diffuse eccrine poromatosis. *Arch Dermatol* 1977; 113: 472–6.
14 Freire-Maia N, Pinheiro M. *Ectodermal Dysplasias: a Clinical and Genetic Study*. New York: Alan R. Liss, 1984.

Ectodermal dysplasias with involvement primarily of appendages of the epidermis and oral ectoderm (hair, teeth, nails and sweat glands)

The ectodermal dysplasias in this section exhibit abnormalities primarily of the appendages of the epidermis and oral ectoderm (hair, teeth, nails and sweat glands) without prominent involvement of other ectodermal structures. The two major ectodermal dysplasias in this category are the tooth and nail syndrome and trichodentosseous (TDO) syndrome. A sufficient number of families and individuals have been reported with these disorders that a thorough discussion is warranted. The tooth and nail syndrome is probably underreported because the clinical manifestations may be subtle. Though individuals with TDO syndrome have characteristic facies, the features are not marked and the hair and nail abnormalities are prominent. A number of other ectodermal dysplasias affect primarily just the hair, teeth, nails and sweat glands including dermodontodysplasia [1,2], trichoonychodental dysplasia [3], trichodermodysplasia with dental alterations [4], tricho-odonto-onychial dysplasia [5], odonto-onychodermal dysplasia [6], odonto-onychodysplasia with alopecia [7], hair–nail dysplasia [8], Fried's tooth and nail syndrome [9], hypoplastic enamel, onycholysis, hypohidrosis [10] and pili torti and onychodysplasia [11,12]. These specific ectodermal dysplasias are not discussed in this chapter because they are extremely rare. Most are described on the basis of one kindred with as few as two affected individuals.

REFERENCES

1 Pinheiro M, Freire-Maia N. Dermo-odontodysplasia: an 11-member, four-generation pedigree with an apparently hitherto undescribed pure ectodermal dysplasia. *Clin Genet* 1983; 24: 58–68.
2 Pinheiro M, Gomes-de-Sá-Filho FP, Freire-Maia N. New cases of dermo-odontodysplasia? *Am J Med Genet* 1990; 36: 161–6.
3 Koshiba H, Kimura O, Nakata M, Witkop CJ. Clinical, genetic, and histologic features of the trichoonychodental (TOD) syndrome. *Oral Surg Oral Med Oral Pathol* 1978; 46: 376–85.
4 Pinheiro M, Freire-Maia DV, Miranda E, Silva-Filho OG, Freire-Maia N. Trichodermodysplasia with dental alterations: an apparently new genetic ectodermal dysplasia of the tricho-odonto-onychial subgroup. *Clin Genet* 1986; 29: 332–6.
5 Pinheiro M, Freire-Maia N, Roth AJ. Tricho-odontoonychial dysplasia—a new mesoectodermal dysplasia. *Am J Med Genet* 1983; 15: 67–70.
6 Fadhil M, Ghabra TA, Deeb M, Der Kaloustian VM. Odonto-onychodermal dysplasia: a previously apparently undescribed ectodermal dysplasia. *Am J Med Genet* 1983; 14: 335–46.
7 Pinheiro M, Freire-Maia N, Gollop TR. Odonto-onychodysplasia with alopecia: a new pure ectodermal dysplasia with probable autosomal recessive inheritance. *Am J Med Genet* 1985; 20: 197–202.
8 Pinheiro M, Freire-Maia N. Hair–nail dysplasia—a new pure autosomal dominant ectodermal dysplasia. *Clin Genet* 1992; 41: 296–8.
9 Fried K. Autosomal recessive hydrotic ectodermal dysplasia. *J Med Genet* 1977; 14: 137–9.
10 Witkop CJ, Brearley LJ, Gentry WC. Hypoplastic enamel, onycholysis, and hypohidrosis inherited as an autosomal dominant trait. A review of ectodermal dysplasia syndromes. *Oral Surg Oral Med Oral Pathol* 1975; 39: 71–86.
11 Calzavara-Pinton P, Carlino A, Benetti A, De Panfilis G. Pili torti and onychodysplasia. Report of a previously undescribed hidrotic ectodermal dysplasia. *Dermatologica* 1991; 182: 184–7.
12 Traupe H. A new syndrome is born. *Dermatologica* 1991; 182: 139–40.

Tooth and nail syndrome

(SYN. HYPODONTIA AND NAIL DYSGENESIS, WITKOP'S SYNDROME; AUTOSOMAL DOMINANT DYSPLASIA OF NAILS AND HYPODONTIA)

Definition

Tooth and nail syndrome is an ectodermal dysplasia with severe hypodontia of permanent teeth and distinctive congenital nail defects.

History

This syndrome was first described by Witkop in 1965 who subsequently reported multiple affected individuals in a number of families [1,2].

Aetiology

The mode of inheritances is autosomal dominant with variable expressivity.

Pathology

Examination of the hair shaft by light microscope does not reveal specific abnormalities [2]. None of 29 affected individuals reported by Hudson and Witkop described heat intolerance, yet of the four individuals who underwent sweat testing, two had reduced or slightly reduced sweating response when compared with normal controls [2].

Clinical features [1–4]

Hair

The scalp hair may be fine, thin and brittle. Eyebrows and eyelashes are usually normal. Axillary, pubic and body hair are normal.

Teeth

Hypodontia of the permanent teeth is a characteristic feature of this disorder. The primary teeth are frequently normal in appearance though they may be small. The disorder is usually not diagnosed until the permanent teeth fail to erupt. There may be partial or total absence of permanent teeth; mandibular incisors, second molars and maxillary canines are most frequently missing.

Nails

The nails are small, thin, brittle and spoon-shaped. Longitudinal ridging is common. The toenails are often more severely involved than the fingernails and may be absent at birth. Nail abnormalities may improve with time.

Sweat glands

Sweating abnormalities are not considered a prominent feature of this disorder. Individuals do not report heat intolerance or difficulty sweating, but sweat tests have been performed in a limited number of affected individuals.

Skin

The skin is essentially normal.

Other ectodermal structures

No other ectodermal structures are reported to be affected.

Craniofacial features

The facies are normal though full, everted lips are described in a number of affected families.

Other abnormalities

There are no other abnormalities.

Prognosis

Affected individuals are healthy.

Differential diagnosis

The nail and teeth abnormalities are subtle in some individuals and may be missed. The presence of well-formed aveolar ridges, normal sweating and facies help distinguish this disorder from X-linked HED. Hypodontia, taurodontia and sparse hair is a rare ectodermal dysplasia reported in a few individuals [5]. Taurodontia, defined as an increased size of the tooth pulp chamber, appears to be the only feature which distinguishes it from the tooth and nail syndrome and it is unclear if these disorders are distinct.

Treatment

This consists of appropriate dental restoration.

REFERENCES

1 Witkop CJ Jr. Genetic diseases of the oral cavity. In: Tiecke RW, ed. *Oral Pathology*. New York: McGraw-Hill, 1965; 812–13.
2 Hudson CD, Witkop CJ Jr. Autosomal dominant hypodontia with nail dysgenesis. Report of 29 cases in six families. *Oral Surg Oral Med Oral Pathol* 1975; 39: 409–23.
3 Giansanti JS, Long SM, Rankin JL. The 'tooth and nail' type of autosomal dominant ectodermal dysplasia. *Oral Surg Oral Med Oral Pathol* 1974; 37: 576–82.
4 Murdoch-Kinch CA, Miles DA, Poon CK. Hypodontia and nail dysplasia syndrome. *Oral Surg Oral Med Oral Pathol* 1993; 75: 403–6.
5 Levin LS. Dental and oral abnormalities in selected ectodermal dysplasia syndromes. In: Salinas CF, Opitz JM, Paul NW, eds. *Recent Advances in Ectodermal Dysplasias*. New York: Alan R. Liss, 1988: 205–27.

Trichodentosseus syndrome

Definition

TDO syndrome is a well-defined ectodermal dysplasia with kinky hair, hypoplasia of tooth enamel and asymptomatic sclerotic bone changes.

History

Lichtenstein *et al.* defined the features of this disorder in 107 individuals and proposed the name TDO syndrome [1]. Robinson *et al.* were the first authors to describe this syndrome, but did not detect bone involvement as part of the disorder [2]. Some authors argue that the clinical manifestations observed in some families are varied enough to suggest genetic heterogeneity and they classify TDO syndrome into three subtypes differing from each other primarily by the degree of bone involvement [3,4]. Variable expression of a single gene seems a more plausible explanation for other authors [5].

Aetiology

The mode of inheritance for all types is autosomal dominant. The basic defect is unknown.

Pathology

On dental radiographs, unerupted teeth and taurodontia (increased size of the tooth pulp chamber) are found [6]. Scanning electron microscopic analysis of affected teeth show pits and depressions in the tooth enamel, uniformly thin tooth enamel and an abnormal collagenous membrane around the open apices [7]. Radiographs of the skull reveal sclerosis and sometimes thickening of the calvarium. The long bones may also be sclerotic [5].

Clinical features [1,2,4,5,7]

Hair

At birth, the scalp hair is thick and kinky or curly; it may straighten in later life. The eyelashes may also be curly.

Teeth

Teeth abnormalities are present in all patients and include pitted, hypoplastic enamel with brownish-yellow discoloration of both primary and permanent teeth, and taurodontia. Tooth eruption may be delayed and abscesses are common. Multiple dental caries occur and lead to early loss of teeth.

Nails

Fingernails are thin, brittle and peel readily. Toenails may be thickened or normal.

Sweat glands

Sweating abnormalities are not found in this disorder.

Skin

The skin is normal and other ectodermal structures are normal.

Craniofacial features

There is frontal bossing, the jaw is square and the head is elongated. Partial premature fusion of the cranial sutures occurs in three-quarters of affected individuals. The bones of the skull are radiographically dense and may be thick. This is not problematic for the patient and may be found incidentally when radiographs of the skull are obtained for unrelated reasons.

Other abnormalities

Clinodactyly is rarely seen.

Prognosis

Affected individuals are healthy, but lose most of their teeth by the age of 30 years [1].

Differential diagnosis

Curly hair and nail dysplasia is also seen in CHANDS syndrome (curly hair, ankyloblepharon and nail dysplasia) but ankyloblepharon makes this disorder distinct. Tooth and nail syndrome lacks kinky or curly hair.

Treatment

This includes appropriate dental restoration.

REFERENCES

1 Lichtenstein J, Warson R, Jorgenson R, Dorst JP, McKusick VA. The tricho-dento-osseous (TDO) syndrome. *Am J Hum Genet* 1972; 24: 569–82.
2 Robinson GC, Miller JR, Worth HM. Hereditary enamel hypoplasia: its association with characteristic hair structure. *Pediatrics* 1966; 37: 498–502.
3 Freire-Maia N, Pinheiro M. *Ectodermal Dysplasias: a Clinical and Genetic Study.* New York: Alan R. Liss, 1984.
4 Shapiro SD, Quattromani FL, Jorgenson RJ, Young RS. Tricho-dento-osseous syndrome: heterogeneity or clinical variability. *Am J Med Genet* 1983; 16: 225–36.
5 Quattromani F, Shapiro SD, Young RS *et al.* Clinical heterogeneity in the tricho-dento-osseous syndrome. *Hum Genet* 1983; 64: 116–21.
6 Levin LS. Dental and oral abnormalities in selected ectodermal dysplasia syndromes. In: Salinas CF, Opitz JM, Paul NW, eds. *Recent Advances in Ectodermal Dysplasias.* New York: Alan R. Liss, 1988: 205–27.
7 Melnick M, Shields ED, El-Kafrawy AH. Tricho-dento-osseous syndrome: a scanning electron microscopic analysis. *Clin Genet* 1977; 12: 17–27.

Ectodermal dysplasias with cleft lip/palate

A number of ectodermal dysplasias exhibit cleft lip/palate as a characteristic feature (Table 19.11.1). Individuals with Rapp–Hodgkin syndrome exhibit abnormalities of all four epidermal appendages, distinctive mid facial hypoplasia and cleft lip/palate. The AEC syndrome (ankyloblepharon, ectodermal dysplasia and cleft lip/palate) exhibits the defining feature of ankyloblepharon in addition to cleft lip/palate and dysplasia of

Table 19.11.1 Ectodermal dysplasias with cleft lip/palate*

ED with cleft lip/palate
Rapp–Hodgkin syndrome†
Rare syndromes with ED and cleft lip/palate
  Regional ED–cleft lip/palate syndrome [1]
  Allanson–McGillivray syndrome [2]

ED with cleft lip/palate and ankyloblepharon
AEC syndrome†
Rare syndromes with ED, cleft lip/palate and ankyloblepharon
  ED–cleft lip/palate–mental retardation (syn: Bowen–Armstrong syndrome) [3]
  ED–cleft palate–ankyloblepharon–alveolar synechiae with autosomal recessive inheritance [4]

ED with cleft lip/palate and acral limb defects
EEC syndrome†
Rare syndromes with ED, cleft lip/palate and acral limb defects
  ED–cleft lip/palate–popliteal pterygium syndrome (syn: Rosselli–Gulienetti syndrome) [5]
  ED–cleft lip/palate–oligodontia–syndactyly–hair alterations (syn: Martinez syndrome) [6]
  ED–cleft lip/palate–abnormal ears–syndactyly–mental retardation (syn: Zlotogora–Ogur syndrome) [7–10]
  odentotrichomelic syndrome (syn: ED with extensive tetramelic deficiencies syndrome) [11,12]
  autosomal recessive ED with corkscrew hair [13,14]

ED, ectodermal dysplasia
*See cleft lip/palate section for references.
†See text for full discussion of syndrome.

four epidermal appendages. EEC syndrome (ectrodactyly, ectodermal dysplasia and clefting) is the most common of those ectodermal dysplasias with cleft lip/palate and acral limb defects. Dermatologists should be aware of the distinctive scalp dermatitis and erosions seen in this group of disorders that is most severe and characteristic of the AEC syndrome. Other ectodermal dysplasias with cleft lip/palate are listed in Table 19.11.1 and references provided below. Most are classified based on a few case reports and are extremely rare.

REFERENCES

1 Fara M. Regional ectodermal dysplasia with total bilateral cleft. *Acta Chir Plast* 1971; 13: 100–5.
2 Allanson JE, McGillivray BC. Familial clefting syndrome with ectropion and dental anomaly—without limb anomalies. *Clin Genet* 1985; 27: 426–9.
3 Bowen P, Armstrong HB. Ectodermal dysplasia, mental retardation, cleft lip/palate and other anomalies in three sibs. *Clin Genet* 1976; 9: 35–42.
4 Seres-Santamaria A, Arimany JL, Muñiz F. Two sibs with cleft palate, ankyloblepharon, alveolar synechiae, and ectodermal defects: a new recessive syndrome? *J Med Genet* 1993; 30: 793–5.
5 Rosselli D, Gulienetti R. Ectodermal dysplasia. *Br J Plast Surg* 1961; 14: 190–204.
6 Martinez BR, Monasterio LA, Pinheiro M, Freire-Maia N. Cleft lip/palate–oligodontia–syndactyly–hair alterations, a new syndrome: review of the conditions combining ectodermal dysplasia and cleft lip/palate. *Am J Med Genet* 1987; 27: 23–31.
7 Ogur G, Yuksel M. Association of syndactyly, ectodermal dysplasia and

cleft lip and palate: report of two sibs from Turkey. *J Med Genet* 1988; 25: 37–40.

8 Zlotogora J, Zilberman Y, Tenenbaum A, Wexler MR. Cleft lip and palate, pili torti, malformed ears, partial syndactyly of fingers and toes, and mental retardation: a new syndrome. *J Med Genet* 1987; 24: 291–3.

9 Zlotogora J. Syndactyly, ectodermal dysplasia, and cleft lip/palate. *J Med Genet* 1994; 31: 957–9.

10 Rodini ESO, Richieri-Costa A. Autosomal recessive ectodermal dysplasia, cleft lip/palate, mental retardation, and syndactyly: the Zlotogora–Ogur syndrome. *Am J Med Genet* 1990; 36: 473–6.

11 Freire-Maia N. A newly recognized genetic syndrome of tetramelic deficiencies, ectodermal dysplasia, deformed ears, and other abnormalities. *Am J Hum Genet* 1970; 22: 370–7.

12 Pavone L, Rizzo R, Tiné A *et al.* A case of the Freire-Maia odontotrichomelic syndrome: nosology with EEC syndrome. *Am J Med Genet* 1989; 33: 190–3.

13 Bustos T, Simosa V, Pinto-Cisternas J *et al.* Autosomal recessive ectodermal dysplasia. I. An undescribed dysplasia/malformation syndrome. *Am J Med Genet* 1991; 41: 398–404.

14 Abramovits-Ackerman W, Bustos T, Simosa-Leon V, Fernandez L, Ramella M. Cutaneous findings in a new syndrome of autosomal recessive ectodermal dysplasia with corkscrew hairs. *J Am Acad Dermatol* 1992; 27: 917–21.

Rapp–Hodgkin syndrome

(SYN. HYPOHIDROTIC ECTODERMAL DYSPLASIA WITH CLEFT LIP AND CLEFT PALATE; ANHIDROTIC ECTODERMAL DYSPLASIA WITH CLEFT LIP AND CLEFT PALATE)

Definition

Rapp–Hodgkin syndrome is characterized by hypotrichosis, teeth abnormalities, nail dysplasia and hypohidrosis. Cleft palate, with or without cleft lip and distinctive mid-facial hypoplasia, are characteristic features of the disorder.

History

Rapp–Hodgkin syndrome was first described by Rapp and Hodgkin in 1968, who reported a family with three affected members [1]. In 1971, Summitt and Hiatt described a sporadic case with similar findings [2]. Wannarachue *et al.* re-evaluated the original family described by Rapp and Hodgkin, noted the similarity to Summitt and Hiatt's patient, and defined the distinct clinical syndrome [3].

Aetiology

The mode of inheritance is autosomal dominant. Spontaneous mutations have been reported. The basic defect is unknown.

Pathology

Hypoplasia or absence of the follicles and sebaceous glands from skin biopsies have been reported, with a decrease in number, size and degree of maturation in those follicles present. The eccrine glands are also hypoplastic and may be absent [1,2,4]. Hair shaft abnormalities include fine twists along the length of the hair shaft, longitudinal grooves and varying shapes on cross-sectional view. The pattern of the cuticular cells is abnormal and the hairs show alternating bands of birefringence under polarizing light. Salinas and Montes suggest that the morphological changes of the hair shaft should be termed 'pili canaliculi' rather than 'pili torti' [5].

Clinical features

Hair

The scalp hair is coarse, wiry and slow growing (Fig. 19.11.13). In children it may be sparse and can progress to total alopecia in adults. The eyelashes are coarse and sparse and the lateral third of the eyebrows is frequently absent. Body, pubic and axillary hair may also be involved [1,5–7].

Teeth

Teeth are decreased in number, small, conically shaped and prone to extensive caries (Fig. 19.11.14) [1,8]. Congenitally absent teeth have been reported.

Nails

The nails are typically short, thickened proximally and slow growing (Fig. 19.11.15). They are variably dystrophic and discolored [1,8].

Sweat glands

Affected individuals describe heat intolerance and decreased sweating but hyperpyrexia is not a striking feature [6,7]. Sweat pore openings on the palms may be small and sparse. There may be a disproportionate amount of sweating on the scalp in some individuals [5].

Skin

The skin tends to be dry.

Other ectodermal structures

Aplasia of the lacrimal duct is a notable ocular finding—with resultant epiphora (tearing) and recurrent conjunctivitis—which occurs in about a third of patients. Other less common ocular manifestations include corneal opacities, corneal vasularization, ectropion and corneal scarring [2,3,6,8].

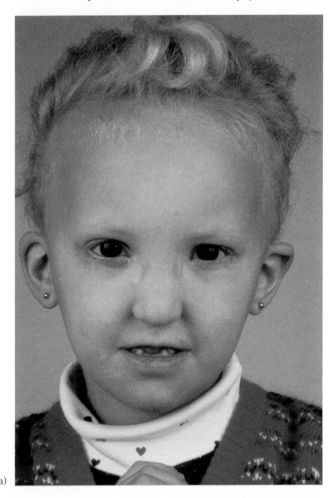
(a)

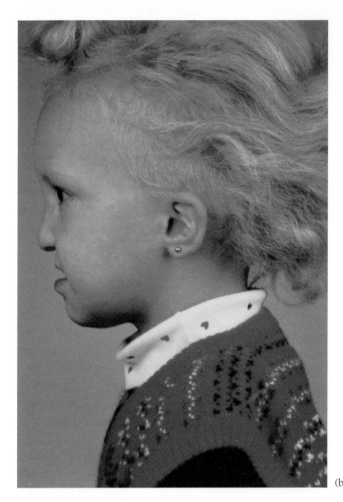
(b)

Fig. 19.11.13 (a) Front and (b) side profiles of a young girl with Rapp–Hodgkin syndrome. Note the coarse, wiry scalp hair, sparse eyebrows, high, broad forehead and midfacial hypoplasia. Reproduced with permission from Schroeder and Sybert [7].

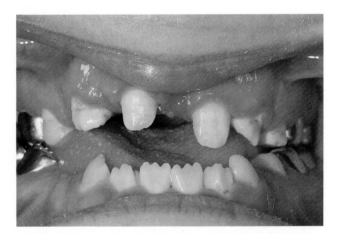

Fig. 19.11.14 Small, absent, and abnormally shaped teeth in an individual with Rapp–Hodgkin syndrome. She has extensive caries.

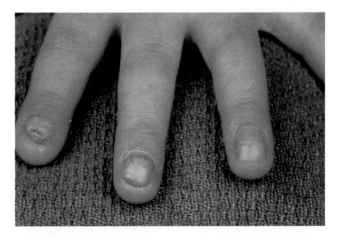

Fig. 19.11.15 The nails in this individual with Rapp–Hodgkin syndrome are short, thickened and discolored. Reproduced with permission from Schroeder and Sybert [7].

Craniofacial features

The facies are characterized by a high broad forehead, a narrow pinched nose with a short columella, a small mouth and pronounced mid-facial hypoplasia (Fig. 19.11.13) [9,10]. Hypoplasia of the mid-facial tissue as well as displacement of the maxilla contribute to the mid-facial hypoplasia [10]. The external ear may have various anomalies and the external auditory canal may be stenotic [2,6]. Cleft palate with or without cleft lip are characteristic features of the disorder. Submucous clefts and a bifid or absent uvula may be overlooked when cleft lip is absent [9].

Other abnormalities

Hypospadias is a distinctive feature and is found in up to half of affected males [9]. Hypoplasia and fusion of the labia have been described in one female [9]. Short stature is a common but variable feature [3,7]. Syndactyly of the second and third toe have been reported [6,9].

Prognosis

Undiagnosed palatal defects may cause feeding difficulty, nasal regurgitation and poor weight gain in infancy [9]. The combination of stenotic external ear canals, palatal abnormalities and eustachian tube abnormalities contribute to significant problems with recurrent otitis media and secondary hearing impairment [6]. Speech abnormalities also occur for similar reasons. Life expectancy is not compromised.

Differential diagnosis

Several ectodermal dysplasia syndromes are associated with cleft lip and palate, and significant overlap may occur. It may be difficult to distinguish AEC syndrome (Hay–Wells syndrome) from Rapp–Hodgkin in the absence of ankyloblepharon. Some authors question the concept that Rapp–Hodgkin and AEC syndromes are separate entities [11]. Though scalp dermatitis and erosions are reported in Rapp–Hodgkin syndrome, they are more characteristic and severe in the AEC syndrome [12]. EEC syndrome shares many features with Rapp–Hodgkin but the presence of ectodactyly is unique to the EEC syndrome [12]. A number of other rare ectodermal dysplasias also exhibit cleft palate and lip but other features such as mental retardation, hypoplasia of the thumbs, mottled hyperpigmentation and hypertelorism distinguish them [12].

Treatment

A number of defects associated with Rapp–Hodgkin

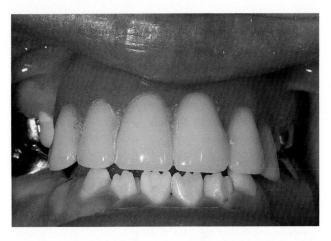

Fig. 19.11.16 Placement of overdentures improves the dental appearance of the same individual with Rapp–Hodgkin syndrome seen in Fig. 19.11.14.

syndrome such as hypospadias, labial abnormalities, syndactyly and dysmorphic craniofacial features can be minimized with appropriate surgical intervention. Routine otolaryngology and audiology examinations can minimize the complications associated with ear canal and palatal abnormalities. Speech therapy may be required. Individuals with lacrimal duct abnormalities require routine ophthalmological examinations to minimize secondary complications. The lacrimal duct abnormalities may be surgically correctable [13]. Frequent dental examination and restorative measures can minimize caries (Fig. 19.11.16) [6].

REFERENCES

1 Rapp RS, Hodgkin WE. Anhidrotic ectodermal dysplasia: autosomal dominant inheritance with palate and lip anomalies. *J Med Genet* 1968; 5: 269–72.
2 Summitt RL, Hiatt RL. Hypohidrotic ectodermal dysplasia with multiple associated anomalies. *Birth Defects* 1971; 7: 121–4.
3 Wannarachue N, Hall BD, Smith DW. Ectodermal dysplasia and multiple defects (Rapp–Hodgkins type). *J Pediatr* 1972; 81: 1217–18.
4 Viljoen DL, Winship WS. A new form of hypohidrotic ectodermal dysplasia. *Am J Med Genet* 1988; 31: 25–32.
5 Salinas CF, Montes GM. Rapp–Hodgkin syndrome: observations on 10 cases and characteristic hair changes (pili canaliculi). In: Salinas CF, Opitz JM, Paul NW, eds. *Recent Advances in Ectodermal Dysplasias*. New York: Alan R. Liss, 1988: 149–68.
6 O'Donnell BP, James WD. Rapp–Hodgkin ectodermal dysplasia. *J Am Acad Dermatol* 1992; 27: 323–6.
7 Schroeder HW, Sybert VP. Rapp–Hodgkin ectodermal dysplasia. *J Pediatr* 1987; 110: 72–5.
8 Crawford PJM, Aldred MJ, Clarke A. Rapp–Hodgkin syndrome: an ectodermal dysplasia involving the teeth, hair, nails, and palate. Report of a case and review of the literature. *Oral Surg Oral Med Oral Pathol* 1989; 67: 50–62.
9 Walpole IR, Goldblatt J. Rapp–Hodgkin hypohidrotic ectodermal dysplasia syndrome. *Clin Genet* 1991; 39: 114–20.
10 Hart TC, Kyrkanides S. Cephalometric analysis of Rapp–Hodgkin syndrome. *J Med Genet* 1994; 31: 758–60.
11 Cambiaghi S, Tadini G, Barbareschi M, Menni S, Caputo R. Rapp–Hodgkin syndrome and AEC syndrome: are they the same entity? *Br J Dermatol* 1994; 130: 97–101.

12 Fosko SW, Stenn KS, Bolognia JL. Ectodermal dysplasias associated with clefting: significance of scalp dermatitis. *J Am Acad Dermatol* 1992; 27: 249–56.
13 Hicks C, Pitts J, Rose GE. Lacrimal surgery in patients with congenital cranial or facial anomalies. *Eye* 1994; 8: 583–91.

Ankyloblepharon, ectodermal dysplasia, cleft lip/palate syndrome

(SYN. AEC SYNDROME, HAY–WELLS SYNDROME)

Definition

AEC syndrome is characterized by cleft lip/palate, severe scalp erosions and abnormalities of the epidermal appendages including hypotrichosis, hypodontia, absent or dystrophic nails and mild hypohidrosis. The distinctive feature is ankyloblepharon filiforme adnatum, partial thickness fusion of the eyelid margins.

History

In 1976, Hay and Wells described seven patients from four families with an inherited disorder characterized by congenital filiform fusion of the eyelids, dysplasia of the epidermal appendages and cleft lip/palate. Five of these original seven patients had ankyloblepharon filiforme adnatum and one had small nodules removed from her eyelids as a child, presumably remnants of spontaneously lysed ankyloblepharon [1].

Aetiology

The mode of inheritance is autosomal dominant with variable expression. The basic defect is unknown.

Pathology

Scanning electron microscopy of the affected hair shaft shows various defects including fractures of the cuticle and pili torti, none of which are specific for the disorder [2]. Skin biopsy of involved scalp tissue shows a thin granular layer and stratum corneum. Hair follicles are reduced in size and arrector pili muscles appear hypertrophic [3]. Sweat stimulation tests reveal a patchy loss of sweat glands over most of the body [1].

Clinical features

Hair

Scalp hair is wiry, coarse and sparse; alopecia is common. The eyebrows and eyelashes are short, brittle and sparse. Body, pubic and axillary hair may be sparse or absent [1,2,4].

Teeth

Hypodontia is common. Those teeth that are present are frequently small, conical and discolored [1,2,4,5].

Nails

Nail abnormalities are variable even within an individual and include distal hypoplasia and thickened, hyperconvex plates. Complete absence of nails is a frequent finding [1]. Chromic paronychia has been reported [2].

Sweat glands

Heat intolerance is described by a significant number of individuals but hyperpyrexia is not a problem [4]. Sweat pores are reduced in number in affected individuals [1].

Skin

At birth, over three-quarters of affected newborns have red, eroded, peeling skin like a collodion membrane (Fig. 19.11.17) [4]. This resolves over the first few weeks and the underlying skin is dry (Fig. 19.11.18). Over two-thirds of individuals have chronic problems with severe recurrent scalp erosions and scalp infections which are a major feature of AEC syndrome (Fig. 19.11.19) [4].

Plamoplantar keratoderma was reported in four of the original seven patients described by Hays and Wells [1]. It is not a common finding in affected children but may be more pronounced in adults.

Other ectodermal structures

Ankyloblepharon filiforme adnatum (strands of epithelial tissue between the eyelids) are a cardinal feature of the disorder but are noted in only 70% of patients

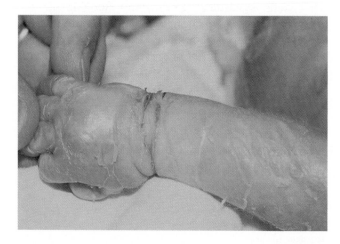

Fig. 19.11.17 Peeling, red, parchment-like skin in a newborn with AEC syndrome.

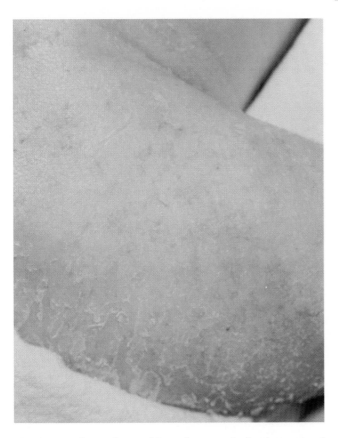

Fig. 19.11.18 The parchment skin resolves over the first few weeks of life and the underlying skin is dry as seen in this 1-month-old baby with AEC syndrome.

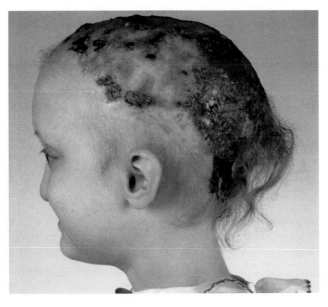

Fig. 19.11.19 Severe scalp erosions and extensive granulation tissue in a 5-year-old girl with AEC syndrome.

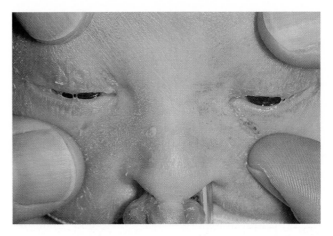

Fig. 19.11.20 Ankyloblepharon filiforme adnaturm (strands of epithelial tissue between the eyelids) in a newborn with AEC syndrome.

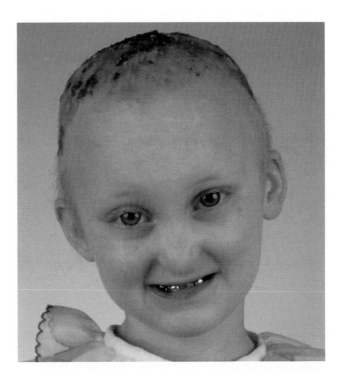

Fig. 19.11.21 The characteristic craniofacial features of a broad nasal bridge and maxillary hypoplasia are seen in this young girl with AEC syndrome.

(Fig. 19.11.20) [1,2,4]. The strands may lyse spontaneously and may be difficult to detect. Lacrimal duct atresia or obstruction occurs in over half of affected individuals [4]. Supernumerary nipples may be present [2,4].

Craniofacial features

Typical craniofacial features include a broadened nasal bridge and maxillary hypoplasia (Fig. 19.11.21) [6]. The ears may be small and low-set with deformities of the auricle [4]. The ear canals may be webbed and abnormally shaped [2]. Cleft lip is a variable feature but cleft palate is seen in most individuals [1,2,4].

Other abnormalities

Other features seen occasionally in AEC syndrome include cutaneous syndactyly of the second and third toes, hypospadias and vaginal dryness and erosions [4].

Prognosis

Abnormalities of the external ear canals and palate frequently cause problems with chronic otitis media and secondary hearing loss. Atresia of the lacrimal duct can lead to excessive lacrimation, chronic conjunctivitis and photophobia. Scalp erosions and chronic scalp infections may be severe enough to warrant surgical intervention with skin engraftment [4]. Prenatal diagnosis may be possible in affected families by ultrasound of cleft palate/lip [7].

Differential diagnosis

It may be difficult to distinguish AEC syndrome from Rapp–Hodgkin syndrome particularly if ankyloblepharon are absent. Though reported in Rapp–Hodgkin syndrome, scalp erosions and infections are more characteristic for AEC syndrome. CHANDS is a rare autosomal recessive ectodermal dysplasia with curly, kinky hair, hypoplastic nails and the defining feature of ankyloblepharon. It can be distinguished from AEC by absence of cleft palate and lack of typical craniofacial features [8,9]. In the newborn period, the eroded, peeling skin seen in AEC syndrome may be mistaken for epidermolysis bullosa [10].

Treatment

Emollients are appropriate for the collodion-like membrane in the newborn. The ankyloblepharon filliforme adnatum may require surgical correction or may lyse spontaneously. The lacrimal duct atresia may be surgically correctable [11]. The scalp requires aggressive wound care and treatment with topical or systemic antibiotics as warranted [4]. Other abnormalities such as cleft lip/palate, hypospadias and the maxillary hypoplasia may be surgically corrected [6]. Teeth preservation and restoration is imperative [5].

REFERENCES

1 Hay RJ, Wells RS. The syndrome of ankyloblepharon, ectodermal defects and cleft lip and palate: an autosomal dominant condition. *Br J Dermatol* 1976; 94: 277–89.
2 Greene SL, Michels VV, Doyle JA. Variable expression in ankyloblepharon–ectodermal defects–cleft lip and palate syndrome. *Am J Med Genet* 1987; 27: 207–12.
3 Fosko SW, Stenn KS, Bolognia JL. Ectodermal dysplasias associated with clefting: significance of scalp dermatitis. *J Am Acad Dermatol* 1992; 27: 249–56.
4 Vanderhooft SL, Stephan MJ, Sybert VP. Severe skin erosions and scalp infections in AEC syndrome. *Pediatr Dermatol* 1993; 10: 334–40.
5 Rule DC, Shaw MJ. The dental management of patients with ankyloblepharon (AEC) syndrome. *Br Dent J* 1988; 164: 215–18.
6 Satoh K, Tosa Y, Ohtsuka S, Onizuka T. Ankyloblepharon, ectodermal dysplasia, cleft lip and palate (AEC) syndrome: surgical corrections with an 18-year follow-up including maxillary osteotomy. *Plast Reconstr Surg* 1994; 93: 590–4.
7 Bronshtein M, Gershoni-Baruch R. Prenatal transvaginal diagnosis of the ectrodactyly, ectodermal dysplasia, cleft palate (EEC) syndrome. *Prenat Diagn* 1993; 13: 519–22.
8 Baughman FA. CHANDS: the curly hair–ankyloblepharon–nail dysplasia syndrome. *Birth Defects* 1971; 7: 100–2.
9 Toriello HV, Lindstrom JA, Waterman DF, Baughman FA. Re-evaluation of CHANDS. *J Med Genet* 1979; 16: 316–17.
10 Taïeb A, Legrain V, Surlève-Bazeille JE, Sarlangue J, Maleville J. Generalized epidermolysis bullosa with congenital synechiae, associated malformations and unusual ultrastructure: a new entity? *Dermatologica* 1988; 176: 76–82.
11 Hicks C, Pitts J, Rose GE. Lacrimal surgery in patients with congenital cranial or facial anomalies. *Eye* 1994; 8: 583–91.

Ectrodactyly, ectodermal dysplasia, clefting syndrome

Definition

The main features of the EEC syndrome are ectrodactyly (spilt hand or foot deformity), cleft lip/palate, tear duct anomalies and abnormalities of the epidermal appendages including hypotrichosis, hypodontia, dystrophic nails and occasional hypohidrosis.

History

The association of ectrodactyly, cleft lip/palate and ectodermal dysplasia was initially described by Rüdiger *et al.* who recognized this combination of defects represents a specific syndrome termed EEC syndrome [1]. Over 150 cases have subsequently been described [2].

Aetiology

The mode of inheritance is autosomal dominant with marked variability in expression and evidence for reduced penetrance [3–7]. The basic defect is unknown. Deletions or translocations in the chromosomal region 7q11.2–q21.3 as well as a balanced inversion of chromosome 7(q22.1; q36.3) have been reported in some affected individuals [8–10].

Pathology

Radiographs of hand or foot deformities show missing or hypoplastic metacarpals and metatarsals [11]. Scanning electron microscopic studies of hair shafts of affected individuals show longitudinal grooves, distorted bulbs and cuticular defects [12,13]. These findings can be seen in a number of other ectodermal dysplasias and are not specific to this disorder.

Clinical features

Hair

The scalp hair is fine and sparse, light-coloured and may be wiry in texture. Eyebrows and eyelashes are short, thin and sparse. Axillary, pubic and body hair may also be affected [1,4,11,12].

Teeth

Teeth may be small, abnormally shaped or missing [1,4,11,12]. Premature loss of secondary teeth is common presumably due to multiple caries from enamel hypoplasia.

Nails

The nail plates may be dystrophic, hypoplastic or completely absent even when there are no bony defects of the involved digit [3,4].

Sweat glands

Sweating is usually normal but heat intolerance is noted by a few individuals [4,11,14].

Skin

Dry skin and hyperkeratosis, particularly of the lower extremities, are reported in some individuals [14,15]. Scalp dermatitis is seen rarely [12,16].

Other ectodermal structures

Atresia or hypoplasia of the lacrimal duct are seen in over 90% of affected individuals [2,15,17]. Secretions from the lacrimal gland may be diminished [17]. Nipple anomalies are reported in a few individuals [15].

Craniofacial features

The nose may be broad, the chin pointed, and there may be minor variable ear anomalies, but the facies are not distinct. Cleft palate with or without cleft lip occurs in three-quarters of affected individuals and is a major feature of this disorder [15]. Choanal atresia has been reported [18].

Other abnormalities

Ectrodactyly (lobster claw deformity) is a major feature of this disorder and occurs in over 90% of affected individuals (Fig. 19.11.22). About three-quarters of individuals with ectrodactyly have both hand and foot involvement [15]. Structural abnormalities of the genitourinary tract occur in about one-third of individuals; the most common structural finding is megaureter [19,20]. Abnormalities of the external genitalia have also been described [20]. Mental retardation is a variable and uncommon feature of the disorder occurring in less than 10% of affected individuals [15] and may be limited to those with chromosomal deletions as part of a contiguous gene syndrome. Hearing loss occurs in about 15% of individuals [15]. It is uncertain whether this is primary or secondary to recurrent otitis media. Isolated growth hormone deficiency has been reported in one individual [21].

Prognosis

A significant number of affected individuals experience excessive tearing, conjunctivitis and blepharitis as a result of lacrimal duct hypoplasia. Photophobia, corneal ulcers as well as corneal scarring and perforation may occur as a result of lacrimal gland hypoplasia [17]. Recurrent urinary tract infections, both symptomatic and asymptomatic, may be a problem in individuals with genitourinary anomalies [19]. Prenatal diagnosis may be possible with ultrasonography for limb and palatal defects in affected families [22].

Differential diagnosis

A few other ectodermal dysplasias involve limb abnormalities and cleft palate/lip. Though clefting is not a constant feature, odentotrichomelic syndrome may be

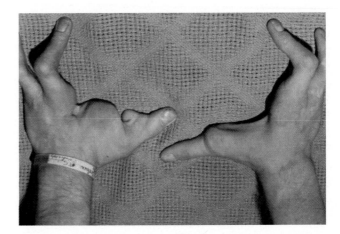

Fig. 19.11.22 Ectrodactyly of the hands in a young man with EEC syndrome.

differentiated by severe tetramelic reductions and autosomal recessive mode of inheritance [2]. Other rare syndromes such as Martinez syndrome, Zlotogora–Ogur syndrome and Rosselli–Gulienetti syndrome can be differentiated from EEC by specific limb abnormalities and mode of inheritance (see Table 19.11.1).

Treatment

Treatment involves surgical correction of the cleft lip/palate, lacrimal duct, limb defects and genitourinary abnormalities as indicated.

REFERENCES

1 Rüdiger RA, Haase W, Passarge E. Association of ectrodactyly, ectodermal dysplasia and cleft lip-palate. The EEC syndrome. *Am J Dis Child* 1970; 120: 160–3.
2 Fosko SW, Stenn KS, Bolognia JL. Ectodermal dysplasias associated with clefting: significance of scalp dermatitis. *J Am Acad Dermatol* 1992; 27: 249–56.
3 Rosenmann A, Shapira T, Cohen MM. Ectrodactyly, ectodermal dysplasia and cleft palate (EEC syndrome). Report of a family and review of the literature. *Clin Genet* 1976; 9: 347–53.
4 Küster W, Majewski F, Meinecke P. EEC syndrome without ectrodactyly? Report of eight cases. *Clin Genet* 1985; 28: 130–5.
5 Majewski F, Küster W. EEC syndrome sine sine? Report of a family with oligosymptomatic EEC syndrome. *Clin Genet* 1988; 33: 69–72.
6 Tse K, Temple IK, Baraitser M. Dilemmas in counselling: the EEC syndrome. *J Med Genet* 1990; 27: 752–5.
7 Anneren G, Anderson T, Lindgren PG, Kjartansson S. Ectrodactyly–ectodermal dysplasia–clefting syndrome (EEC): the clinical variation and prenatal diagnosis. *Clin Genet* 1991; 40: 257–62.
8 Qumsiyeh MB. EEC syndrome (ectrodactyly, ectodermal dysplasia and cleft lip/palate) is on 7q11.2–q21.3. *Clin Genet* 1992; 42: 101.
9 Hasegawa T, Hasegawa Y, Asamura S et al. EEC syndrome (ectrodactyly, ectodermal dysplasia and cleft lip/palate) with a balanced reciprocal translocation between 7q11.21 and 9q12 (or 7q11.2 and 9q12) in three generations. *Clin Genet* 1991; 40: 202–6.
10 Akita S, Kuratomi H, Abe K et al. EEC syndrome in a girl with paracentric inversion. *Clin Dysmorphol* 1993; 2: 62–7.
11 Bixler D, Spivack J, Bennett J, Christian JC. The ectrodactyly–ectodermal dysplasia–clefting (EEC) syndrome. Report of two cases and review of the literature. *Clin Genet* 1971; 3: 43–51.
12 Trüeb RM, Bruckner-Tuderman L, Wyss M et al. Scalp dermatitis, distinctive hair abnormalities and atopic disease in the ectrodactyly–ectodermal dysplasia–clefting syndrome. *Br J Dermatol* 1995; 132: 621–5.
13 Micali G, Cook B, Blekys I, Solomon LM. Structural hair abnormalities in ectodermal dysplasia. *Pediatr Dermatol* 1990; 7: 27–32.
14 Richieri-Costa A, de Vilhena-Moraes SA, Ferrareto I, Masiero D. Ectodermal dysplasia/ectrodactyly in monozygotic female twins. Report of a case—review and comments on the ectodermal dysplasia/ectrodactyly (cleft lip/palate) syndromes. *Rev Bras Genet* 1986; 9: 349–74.
15 Rodini ESO, Richieri-Costa A. EEC syndrome: report on 20 new patients, clinical and genetic considerations. *Am J Med Genet* 1990; 37: 42–53.
16 Trüeb RM, Bruckner-Tuderman L, Burg G. Ectrodactyly–ectodermal dysplasia–clefting syndrome with scalp dermatitis. *J Am Acad Dermatol* 1993; 29: 505.
17 McNab AA, Potts MJ, Welham RAN. The EEC syndrome and its ocular manifestations. *Br J Ophthalmol* 1989; 73: 261–4.
18 Christodoulou J, McDougall PN, Sheffield LJ. Choanal atresia as a feature of ectrodactyly–ectodermal dysplasia–clefting (EEC) syndrome. *J Med Genet* 1989; 26: 586–9.
19 Nardi AC, Ferreira U, Netto NR et al. Urinary tract involvement in EEC syndrome: a clinical study in 25 Brazilian patients. *Am J Med Genet* 1992; 44: 803–6.
20 Rollnick BR, Hoo JJ. Genitourinary anomalies are a component manifestation in the ectodermal dysplasia, ectrodactyly, cleft lip/palate (EEC) syndrome. *Am J Med Genet* 1988; 29: 131–6.
21 Knudtzon J, Aarskog D. Growth hormone deficiency associated with the ectrodactyly–ectodermal dysplasia–clefting syndrome and isolated absent septum pellucidum. *Pediatrics* 1987; 79; 410–12.
22 Köhler R, Sousa P, Jorge CS. Prenatal diagnosis of the ectrodactyly, ectodermal dysplasia, cleft palate (EEC) syndrome. *J Ultrasound Med* 1989; 8: 337–9.

Ectodermal dysplasias with eye abnormalities

The lens, cornea, conjunctiva, lacrimal gland, nasolacrimal duct, tarsal gland and eyelashes are all ectodermal derivatives and are involved in a significant number of the ectodermal dysplasias. Dysplasia of the lacrimal duct is the most common abnormality and may lead to excessive tearing and chronic conjunctivitis. Dysplasia of the lacrimal gland causes decreased production or absence of tears which may lead to dry eye, photophobia and corneal erosion or ulceration. Hypoplasia or aplasia of the lacrimal duct may be found in Rapp–Hodgkin syndrome and AEC syndrome, and is found in over 90% of individuals with EEC syndrome. Hypoplasia of the lacrimal glands is reported in X-linked hypohidrotic ectodermal dysplasia and in EEC syndrome. The two ectodermal dysplasias reviewed in this section, Schöpf–Schulz–Passarge syndrome, and oculodentodigital dysplasia are rare but their eye findings are specific and distinct. Small cysts along the eyelid margins in addition to hair, teeth and nail abnormalities distinguish the Schöpf–Schulz–Passarge syndrome. Oculodentodigital dysplasia is characterized by small eyes and microcornea in addition to sparse hair, abnormal teeth and camptodactyly of the fourth and fifth fingers.

Schöpf–Schulz–Passarge syndrome

Definition

This rare, unique ectodermal dysplasia is characterized by bilateral cysts of the eyelid margins, hypodontia, hypotrichosis, nail dystrophy and palmoplantar hyperkeratosis.

History

In 1971, Schöpf et al. reported two sisters with a unique form of ectodermal dysplasia that later became known as Schöpf–Schulz–Passarge syndrome [1]. It has been reported in only seven individuals.

Aetiology

The mode of inheritance is autosomal recessive. The basic defect is unknown.

Pathology

Histopathology of the eyelid cysts shows features of benign apocrine hidrocystomas, thought to arise from the glands of Moll [1–3].

Clinical features [1–4]

Hair

Scalp hair, eyebrows and eyelashes are thin and scanty. Body hair may also be affected.

Teeth

Primary teeth may be small and widely spaced. Most secondary teeth fail to erupt; those that do are lost prematurely. Most of the few reported individuals with this disorder are edentulous by young adulthood.

Nails

Nail plates are frequently narrow with longitudinal ridges. They may be thickened or completely absent.

Sweat glands

Sweating is normal.

Skin

Diffuse palmoplantar keratoderma is a characteristic feature of the disorder. The severity varies among individuals and may not be obvious until late childhood or early adult life. Numerous facial telangiectasias with or without fine scattered milia have been described in several affected individuals.

Other ectodermal structures

The eyelid cysts are a distinctive feature. They are 1 to 2 mm in size and appear as pearly beads along the lid margins. They usually become clinically apparent in late childhood or early adult life.

Craniofacial features

The facies are normal appearing. There are no other abnormalities.

Prognosis

The eyelid cysts are asymptomatic. The palmoplantar hyperkeratosis may be severe with cracks and fissures.

Differential diagnosis

The teeth abnormalities and eyelid cysts distinguish this disorder from hidrotic ectodermal dysplasia. This disorder is differentiated from Papillon–Lefèvre syndrome by the presence of eyelid cysts and the lack of periodontitis which is a major feature of the later [5].

Treatment

Emollients for the palmoplantar hyperkeratosis may minimize fissures.

REFERENCES

1 Schöpf E, Schulz HJ, Passarge E. Syndrome of cystic eyelids, palmo-plantar keratosis, hypodontia and hypotrichosis as a possible autosomal recessive trait. *Birth Defects* 1971; 7: 219–21.
2 Burket JM, Burket BJ, Burket DA. Eyelid cysts, hypodontia, and hypotrichosis. *J Am Acad Dermatol* 1984; 10: 922–5.
3 Font RL, Stone MS, Schanzer C, Lewis RA. Apocrine hidrocystomas of the lids, hypodontia, palmar-plantar hyperkeratosis, and onychodystrophy. A new variant of ectodermal dysplasia. *Arch Ophthalmol* 1986; 104: 1811–13.
4 Monk BE, Pieris S, Soni V. Schöpf–Schulz–Passarge syndrome. *Br J Dermatol* 1992; 127: 33–5.
5 Freire-Maia N, Pinheiro M. *Ectodermal Dysplasias: a Clinical and Genetic Study*. New York: Alan R. Liss, 1984.

Oculodentodigital dysplasia
(SYN. OCULODENTO-OSSEOUS DYSPLASIA)

Definition

Oculodentodigital dysplasia is characterized by sparse hair, enamel hypoplasia, camptodactyly and characteristic facies with small eyes.

History

The syndrome was originally described by Lohmann in 1920 and more fully defined by Gorlin *et al.* in 1963 [1].

Aetiology

Mode of inheritance is autosomal dominant with variable expressivity. New mutations are common. The basic defect is unknown.

Pathology

Radiographs show shortening of the fifth finger with a cube-shaped hypoplastic middle phalanx. Despite a normal clinical appearance, radiographs of the feet show hypoplasia or absence of the middle phalanx of one or more toes. Radiographs of the teeth show generalized enamel hypoplasia.

Clinical features [1–5]

Hair

The scalp hair is dry, lustreless, slow growing and can be sparse. The eyebrows and eyelashes may be sparse or absent.

Teeth

All teeth exhibit severe hypoplasia of the enamel. The teeth are friable, small, prone to caries and yellowish in colour. Both primary and secondary teeth are affected.

Nails are normal as are the *sweat glands* and skin.

Other ectodermal structures

Individuals may have microcornea, microphthalmia or both. Variable iris abnormalities have been described.

Craniofacial features

The facies are distinctive with small palpebral fissures, a long slender nose, hypoplastic alae nasi and prominent columella. Occular hypertelorism and epicanthal folds are seen in some individuals. The mandible may be large and broad. Minor ear anomalies have been described such as thin pinnae and bifid ear lobes. Cleft palate has been described in several individuals.

Other abnormalities

Bony anomalies are seen in almost every individual and include hyperostoses of the calvarium, small paranasal sinuses, broad, thick clavicles and ribs, and abnormal trabeculation of the long bones. The most frequent skeletal abnormality is absence of the middle phalynx of the fifth finger. Camptodactyly of the fourth and fifth fingers occurs in over 80% of individuals and syndactyly of the fourth and fifth fingers and toes may be present but is not a constant feature.

Prognosis

Rare neurological abnormalities have been described due to spinal cord compression from severe cranial hyperostosis [6]. Despite the associated eye abnormalities, vision is usually normal. Glaucoma is reported in 10–15% of affected individuals [5]. Conductive hearing loss may occur possibly due to deformity of the bony ossicles.

Differential diagnosis

Microphthalmos is described in a number of other syndromes but none with the characteristic facies, and hair and teeth abnormalities seen in oculodentodigital dysplasia.

Treatment

Syndactyly may require surgical correction.

REFERENCES

1 Gorlin RJ, Meskin LH, St Geme JW. Oculodentodigital dysplasia. *J Pediatr* 1963; 63: 69–75.
2 Reisner SH, Kott E, Bornstein B *et al*. Oculodentodigital dysplasia. *Am J Dis Child* 1969; 118: 600–7.
3 Eidelman E, Chosack A, Wagner ML. Orodigitofacial dysostosis and oculodentodigital dysplasia. Two distinct syndromes with some similarities. *Oral Surg Oral Med Oral Pathol* 1967; 23: 311–19.
4 Gillespie FD. A hereditary syndrome: 'dysplasia oculodentodigitalis'. *Arch Ophthalmol* 1964; 71: 187–92.
5 Judisch GF, Martin-Casals A, Hanson JW, Olin WH. Oculodentodigital dysplasia. Four new reports and a literature review. *Arch Ophthalmol* 1979; 97: 878–84.
6 Beighton P, Hamersma H, Raad M. Oculodento-osseous dysplasia: heterogeneity or variable expression? *Clin Genet* 1979; 16: 169–77.

Ectodermal dysplasias with pigmentary abnormalities

A number of the ectodermal dysplasias exhibit pigmentary abnormalities of the skin. Individuals with X-linked HED and autosomal recessive HED exhibit characteristic periorbital hyperpigmentation. Localized hyperpigmentation of flexural regions and over bony prominences is a striking feature in individuals with hidrotic ectodermal dysplasia. Reticulate hyperpigmentation of the arms and axilla was described in one of the original seven patients with AEC syndrome reported by Hay and Wells [1]. Reticulate hyperpigmentation also occurs as a prominent feature in Naegeli–Franceschetti–Jadassohn syndrome which is discussed in this section. Other ectodermal dysplasias with prominent pigmentary abnormalities include autosomal dominant anonychia with bizarre flexural pigmentation described in one family by Verbov [2], and an autosomal recessive disorder with mottled hypo- and hyperpigmentation described in four siblings by Berlin [3]. Individuals with Berlin's syndrome also exhibit palmoplantar hyperkeratosis, hypotrichosis, abnormal teeth, mental retardation and stunted growth [3].

REFERENCES

1 Hay RJ, Wells RS. The syndrome of ankyloblepharon, ectodermal defects and cleft lip and palate: an autosomal dominant condition. *Br J Dermatol* 1976; 94: 277–89.
2 Verbov J. Anonychia with bizarre flexural pigmentation—an autosomal dominant dermatosis. *Br J Dermatol* 1975; 92: 469–74.
3 Berlin C. Congenital generalized melanoleucoderma associated with hypodontia, hypotrichosis, stunted growth and mental retardation occurring in two brothers and two sisters. *Dermatologica* 1961; 123: 227–43.

Naegeli–Franceschetti–Jadassohn syndrome

(SYN. NAEGELI'S SYNDROME)

Definition

This syndrome is defined by reticulate hyperpigmentation, palmoplantar keratoderma, hypohidrosis, enamel defects and absence of dermatoglyphics.

History

In 1927, Naegeli first described the disorder in a father and two daughters. In 1954 Franceschetti and Jadassohn re-examined the original family and determined the inheritance pattern to be autosomal dominant [1].

Aetiology

Mode of inheritance is autosomal dominant. The basic defect is unknown.

Pathology

Skin biopsies from affected individuals show diminished or absent eccrine glands [2]. In areas of hyperpigmentation, the epidermis and melanocytes are normal appearing. The melanin content of basal keratinocytes is variable and numerous pigment-laden macrophages are present in the superficial dermis. Numerous eosinophilic colloid–amyloid bodies are present in the superficial dermis of affected individuals and are occasionally localized around eccrine glands and ducts [3]. Sweat stimulation with pilocarpine may be negative or weakly positive [2].

Clinical features [2,4]

Teeth

Teeth are yellow and prone to severe caries. Most affected individuals lose all of their teeth in their thirties or forties.

Hair is normal.

Nails

Nails may be brittle; the distal nail plate may be thick with subungual hyperkeratosis. Malalignment of the great toenails can be present in one-third to one-half of individuals. Some affected individuals have normal nails.

Sweat glands

Hypohidrosis is a significant feature of the disorder and varies in severity. Flushing, dizziness and hyperthermia can occur during physical exercise or in a hot environment. Hypohidrosis does not improve with age.

Skin

Grey–brown reticulate pigmentation begins as early as 3 months of age but is universally present by the sixth year of life. All patients exhibit reticulate pigmentation of their abdomen. The neck is frequently involved and pigment changes may also be seen on the trunk and flexures. Some individuals may show marked pigmentation around their eyes and mouth. The pigmentation begins to fade in the teenage years and may disappear entirely with age.

Diffuse keratoderma of the palms and soles is a cardinal feature of Naegeli–Franceschetti–Jadassohn syndrome. Some individuals may exhibit a punctate keratoderma and others exhibit accentuation of the keratoderma in their palmar creases. Onset of the keratoderma usually begins in late childhood and does not improve with age.

The normal dermatoglyphic ridge pattern of the fingertips is absent in all affected individuals. A few newborns have been described with transient blisters of the soles.

Other ectodermal structures are normal as are *craniofacial features*. The are no *other abnormalities*.

Prognosis

Affected individuals are healthy.

Differential diagnosis

Incontinentia pigmenti shares some features with Naegeli–Franceschetti–Jadassohn syndrome, but the hyperpigmentation is preceded by vesicular and verrucous stages, palmoplantar hyperkeratosis is absent and the inheritance is X-linked. Pachyonychia congenita shares several features with Naegeli–Franceschetti–Jadassohn syndrome but hyperpigmentation is unusual. Dermatopathia pigmentosa reticularis may be confused with this syndrome but there is scarring alopecia of the scalp and eyebrows, the teeth are normal and the reticulate pigmentation does not fade with time.

Treatment

Environmental temperature control is necessary in those individuals with significant hypohidrosis.

REFERENCES

1 Franceschetti A, Jadassohn W. A propos de l''incontinentia pigmenti', délimitation de deux syndromes différents figurant sous le même terme. *Dermatologica* 1954; 108: 1–28.

2 Itin PH, Lautenschlager S, Meyer R, Mevorah B, Rufli T. Natural history of the Naegeli–Franceschetti–Jadassohn syndrome and further delineation of its clinical manifestations. *J Am Acad Dermatol* 1993; 28: 942–50.
3 Frenk E, Mevorah B, Hohl D. The Naegeli–Franceschetti–Jadassohn syndrome: a hereditary ectodermal defect leading to colloid–amyloid formation in the dermis. *Dermatology* 1993; 187: 169–73.
4 Sparrow GP, Samman PD, Wells RS. Hyperpigmentation and hypohidrosis. The Naegeli–Franceschetti–Jadassohn syndrome: report of a family and review of the literature. *Clin Exp Dermatol* 1976; i: 127–40.

Ectodermal dysplasias with abnormal dermatoglyphics

Abnormalities or congenital absence of dermatoglyphics are rare and can be found in several ectodermal dysplasias. The formation of dermatoglyphics begins in the second month of gestation with the appearance of the volar pads which are mounds of tissue found over the terminal and ventral tips of each digit. The volar pads stimulate development of the primary and secondary epidermal ridges which promote formation of the sweat ducts and glands, and dermatoglyphic patterns [1]. These developmental events explain how abnormalities of dermatoglyphics (also known as dermal ridge patterns or epidermal ridge patterns) are found in association with abnormalities of sweat ducts and glands. An absence or decrease of dermatoglyphics is found in affected males with X-linked hypohidrotic ectodermal dysplasia (Fig. 19.11.23), in affected individuals with Naegeli–Franceschetti–Jadassohn syndrome, Rapp–Hodgkin syndrome, AEC syndrome and have been described as prominent features in two other ectodermal dysplasias. One of these, Jorgenson's syndrome, has been reported in only one kindred as an autosomal dominant disorder characterized by unusual fine, sparse dermatoglyphics and hypohidrosis. Coarse, scanty scalp hair, sparse eyelashes, short, thick nails and defective teeth are also fea-

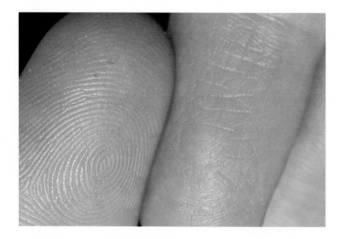

Fig. 19.11.23 Fingertips of an unaffected individual (left) and affected individual (right) with X-linked hypohidrotic ectodermal dysplasia. Note the absence of dermatoglyphics in the affected individual.

tures of the syndrome [2]. The other ectodermal dysplasia defined by congenital absence of dermatoglyphics, has been described in several kindreds and is called, absence of dermal ridge patterns, onychodystrophy and palmoplantar anhidrosis [3]. This disorder is discussed in detail below.

REFERENCES

1 Holbrook KA. Structural abnormalities of the epidermally derived appendages in skin from patients with ectodermal dysplasia: insight into developmental errors. In: Salinas CF, Opitz JM, Paul NW, eds. *Recent Advances in Ectodermal Dysplasias*. New York: Alan R. Liss, 1988: 15–44.
2 Jorgenson RJ. Ectodermal dysplasia with hypotrichosis, hypohidrosis, defective teeth, and unusual dermatoglyphics (Basan syndrome?). *Birth Defects* 1974; 10: 323–5.
3 Freire-Maia N, Pinheiro M. *Ectodermal Dysplasias: a Clinical and Genetic Study*. New York: Alan R. Liss, 1984.

Absence of dermal ridge patterns, onychodystrophy and palmoplantar anhidrosis
(SYN. BASAN'S SYNDROME)

Definition

This is a rare ectodermal dysplasia characterized by congenital absence of dermatoglyphics, nail dystrophy, transient congenital facial milia and absence of sweating on the palms and soles. Blistering in the neonatal period is also a prominent feature of the disorder.

History

This disorder was first reported by Baird who described 16 affected individuals in a kindred of 28 members over four generations [1,2]. Similar cases have since been reported by Basan, Reed and Schreiner and Límová, but it was unclear that these were the same disorder until Cirillo-Hyland *et al.* reported a fourth-generation male subject of Baird's kindred with features of all the previously described kindreds [3–6].

Aetiology

The mode of inheritance is autosomal dominant with variable expressivity.

Pathology

Microscopic examination of material obtained from the facial milia reveal fragments of cornified debris. Skin biopsies from the affected areas of the palms show a flat epidermis with sparse or absent eccrine ducts and glands [1,4]. Thickened collagen bundles have been described in the skin involved with flexion contractures [1].

Clinical features [1,2,4–6]

Hair and *teeth* are normal.

Nails

The nails are short, wide and rough in texture. Single transverse grooves as well as longitudinal ridges are reported. The distal free edge of the nail plate may be attached to the underlying hyponychium. This feature along with the tendency of the fingertips to taper distally can give the appearance of clubbing.

Sweat glands

No sweat gland openings are visible on the palms and soles and sweating is absent in these areas.

Skin

Complete congenital absence of dermatoglyphics is a defining feature of the disorder. At birth the palms and soles are smooth and thin and the palmar creases are frequently underdeveloped. Numerous facial milia are present at birth and are described in all affected individuals. They gradually disappear during the first 6 months of life. Discrete bullae may be present on the hands and feet at birth, rupture easily and resolve. Individuals may develop occasional blisters on the hands and feet in hot weather. Calluses develop on the palms and soles with age and fissures are problematic, especially around the nails.

Other ectodermal structures

Diminished tear production has been described in some individuals.

Craniofacial features are normal.

Other abnormalities

Flexion contractures of the fingers and/or toes are a major feature of the disorder and are found in about three-quarters of affected individuals. Webbing of toes is found less frequently.

Prognosis

Heat intolerance is usually not a problem and affected individuals are healthy.

Differential diagnosis

X-linked HED is differentiated by its mode of inheritance, characteristic facial features and involvement of teeth and hair. Jorgenson's syndrome also exhibits abnormal dermatoglyphics and hypohidrosis but in addition, involves the hair and teeth [7]. Epidermolysis bullosa progressiva is distinguished by onset of acral blistering in childhood, eventual loss of nails, and loss of dermatoglyphics that occurs over years [8].

Treatment

The flexion contractures and toe webbing may require surgical release.

REFERENCES

1 Baird HW. Kindred showing congenital absence of the dermal ridges (fingerprints) and associated anomalies. *J Pediatr* 1964; 64: 621–31.
2 Baird HW. Absence of fingerprints in four generations. *Lancet* 1968; ii: 1250.
3 Freire-Maia N, Pinheiro M. *Ectodermal Dysplasias: a Clinical and Genetic Study*. New York: Alan R. Liss, 1984.
4 Reed T, Schreiner RL. Absence of dermal ridge patterns: genetic heterogeneity. *Am J Med Genet* 1983; 16: 81–8.
5 Límová M, Blacker KL, LeBoit PE. Congenital absence of dermatoglyphs. *J Am Acad Dermatol* 1993; 29: 355–8.
6 Cirillo-Hyland VA, Zackai EH, Honig PJ, Grace KR, Schnur RE. Re-evaluation of a kindred with congenital absence of dermal ridges, syndactyly, and facial milia. *J Am Acad Dermatol* 1995; 32: 315–18.
7 Jorgenson RJ. Ectodermal dysplasia with hypotrichosis, hypohidrosis, defective teeth, and unusual dermatoglyphics (Basan syndrome?). *Birth Defects* 1974; 10: 323–5.
8 Haber RM, Hanna W. Epidermolysis bullosa progressiva. *J Am Acad Dermatol* 1987; 16: 195–200.

Acknowledgements

I wish to thank Drs Sybert, and Vanderhooft for contributing photographs for use in this chapter, and Chris Neely-Jones for her secretarial assistance.

19.12 Inherited Metabolic Disorders and the Skin

JOHANNIS B.C. DE KLERK AND ARNOLD P. ORANJE

Aminoacidopathies
Phenylketonuria (PKU)/hyperphenylalaninaemia (HPA)
Tyrosinaemia
Homocystinuria

Organic acidurias
Alkaptonuria
Propionic acidaemia
Methylmalonic acidaemia
Biotinidase deficiency

Transport defects
Hartnup's disease

Lysosomal storage diseases
Alpha-N-acetylgalactosaminidase deficiency
Fabry's disease
Fucosidosis
Mucopolysaccharidoses
GM_1 gangliosidosis
Farber lipogranulomatosis: ceramidase deficiency

Hyperlipoproteinaemias

Acrodermatitis enteropathica

So far more than 300 human diseases due to inborn errors of metabolism have been recognized [1,2]. This number is still increasing as new techniques become available (mass spectrometry of urinary and plasma metabolites, molecular biology). Many of these disorders, however, remain undetected or are misdiagnosed. Many practitioners and paediatricians think of inborn errors of metabolism only in relation to clinical features such as psychomotor retardation, seizures or in case of unexplained hypoglycaemia [3].

Most inborn errors of metabolism are autosomal recessive disorders. Many patients develop symptoms only later in infancy, or even in adolescence or adulthood. This chapter mainly describes the key symptoms of inborn errors of metabolism related to the skin and hair (Tables 19.12.1, 19.12.2). Porphyrias, hyperlipidaemias and the ichthyoses are detailed elsewhere.

REFERENCES

1 Saudubray JM, Charpentier C. Clinical approach to inherited metabolic diseases. In: Scriver CR, Beaudet AL, Sly WS, Valle D, eds. *The Metabolic and Molecular Bases of Inherited Disease. Clinical Phenotypes: Diagnosis/Algorithms*, 7th edn. New York: McGraw-Hill, 1995: 327–400.
2 Saudubray JM, Ogier de Baulny H, Charpentier C. Clinical approach to inherited metabolic diseases. In: Fernandes J, Saudubray JM, van den Berghe G, eds. *Inborn Metabolic Diseases: Diagnosis and Treatment*, 2nd edn. Berlin: Springer Verlag, 1995: 3–39.
3 Saudubray JM, Ogier H, Bonnefont JP *et al.* Clinical approach to inherited metabolic disease in the neonatal period: a 20-year survey. *J Inher Metab Dis* 1989; 12 (suppl 1): 25–41.

Aminoacidopathies

Phenylketonuria (PKU)/hyperphenylalaninaemia (HPA)

Definition

PKU is an autosomal recessively inherited aminoacidopathy, caused by deficiency of L-phenylalanine hydroxylase in the liver [1].

History

In 1934, Fölling [2] described 10 patients with oligophrenia with a typical dermatitis on air-exposed skin, muscle hypotonia and with a green coloration of the urine after addition of ferrichloride. He named this condition imbecillitas phenylpyruvica, because of the abnormal amount of phenylpyruvic acid in the urine.

In 1937, this condition was named oligophrenia phenylpyruvica by Jervis [3], indicating the different clinical stages of this disease. In 1953, treatment with a phenylalanine-restricted diet by using casein-hydrolysate was described by Bickel *et al.* [4].

Pathogenesis

PKU is a genetically determined disease with an autosomal recessive inheritance. A small group of patients (1–2%) with HPA have defects of biopterin synthesis metabolism which may result in a deficiency of neuro-

Table 19.12.1 Skin abnormalities in metabolic diseases

Skin abnormalities	Type, location	Disease/first symptoms (FS)
Yellow papules on the buttocks	Eruptive xanthomas	Type I, IV and V hyperlipidaemia FS: after childhood
Yellow–red papulonodular lesions on extensor aspect of the knees, elbows	Tuberous xanthomas	Type II and III hyperlipidaemia FS: possible in childhood
Soft yellow plaques	Plane xanthomas (striatum palmare)	Hyperlipidaemia in 50% of cases FS: possible in childhood
Decreased pigmentation, erythema/scaling, fair skin	Eczema, hypopigmentation	Phenylketonuria FS: infancy
Dark urine, bluish pigmentation	Dark-grey/blue nappies	Alkaptonuria FS: infancy
Hyperpigmentation	Diffuse hyperpigmentation on face, neck and hands	Gaucher's disease FS: childhood
Yellow plaques; yellowish indurated skin; coarse facial features	Xanthomas in axillae, waxy induration of the trunk and legs	Niemann–Pick disease FS: childhood
Palmoplantar hyperkeratosis and erosions	Keratoderma	Tyrosinaemia II FS: childhood
Red cheeks	Malar flush, livido reticularis, ulceration	Homocystinuria FS: childhood
Red pinpoint lesions around the navel and legs; pain in extremities and abdomen	Angiokeratomas	Fabry's disease FS: late childhood, or adulthood
Red pinpoint lesions; coarse facial features	Angiokeratomas	Fucosidosis FS: infancy
Red pinpoint lesions, coarse facial features	Angiokeratomas	Galactosialidosis FS: childhood
Pink urine; skin erosions and poikiloderma (face, hands)	Pink nappies	Congenital erythropoietic porphyria FS: infancy
Symmetrical circumorificial and acral vesicular erythematous lesions; alopecia	Acral located eczema	Acrodermatitis enteropathica, (secondary) zinc deficiency FS: neonate
Neonatal erythroderma; erythema, sharply demarcated in the napkin and intertriginous areas	Erythroderma or seborrhoeic dermatitis-like	Holocarboxylase synthetase deficiency, (biotin-responsive) FS: neonate
Alopecia, and same skin abnormalities as above	Acrodermatitis enteropathica-like	Biotinidase deficiency FS: neonate
Erythematosquamous eruption in napkin, acral and periorificial areas; scalded skin	Seborrhoeic dermatitis or staphylococcal scalded skin-like eruption	Propionic acidaemia FS: neonate
		Methylmalonic acidaemia FS: neonate
Scaly skin; small stature; hypogonadism; mental retardation; short stature	Ichthyosis, X-linked	Steroid sulphatase deficiency FS: neonate to early childhood
Scaly skin at birth	Ichthyosis	Sjögren–Larsson syndrome; fatty alcohol oxidation defect FS: neonate
Areas of scaling, circumscribed in lines or bands	Ichthyosis	Chondrodysplasia punctata; multiple peroxisomal enzyme deficiency FS: neonate
Erythema; ecchymoses; purpura; telangiectasia; ulceration	Erythematous purpuric partly ulcerative dermatosis	Prolidase deficiency FS: neonate
Nodular swellings on ankle, wrist, elbow and friction sites	Granulomatous tumours	Farber lipogranulomatosis (ceramidase deficiency) FS: early childhood
Fat pads on buttocks, thickened skin; lipoatrophy (linear) on legs	Lipoatrophy, lipomatosis	Carbohydrate-deficient glycoprotein syndrome type I FS: infancy
Brittle hair; pili torti	Hair shaft abnormality	Menkes disease; copper deficiency FS: infancy
Ivory-coloured papules on the back; coarse face, thick nose, broad hands, short fingers	Skin infiltrations	Mucopolysaccharidosis

Table 19.12.2 Classification of inborn errors of metabolism

Amino acidopathies
PKU, HPA
Tyrosinaemia type II (Richner–Hanhart syndrome)
Homocystinuria

Organic acidurias
Alkaptonuria
Propionic acidaemia
Methylmalonic acidaemia
Biotinidase deficiency

Transport defects
Hartnup's disease

Lysosomal storage diseases
α-NAGA deficiency/Schindler's disease
Fabry's disease
Fucosidosis
Mucopolysaccharidoses
GM$_1$ type I gangliosidosis
Farber lipogranulomatosis: ceramidase deficiency

transmitters. Due to the neurological sequelae the name of 'malignant PKU' is used for this group [5].

The genetic incidence of PKU varies in various countries; over 100 mutations in the phenylalanine hydroxylase gene have already been described. In Ireland its frequency is high (1 in 400 births), in Finland very low (1 in 40 000 births).

Clinical features

In the more severe classical untreated or late detected forms of PKU (plasma phenylalanine concentrations ≥1200 μmol/l, (normal values 60 mmol/l)) retarded development, seizures, microcephaly and mental retardation are constant clinical features.

The skin is characterized by decreased pigmentation, photosensitivity, eczema, lightly pigmented eyes, fair hair and sclerodermoid changes. Synthesis of brain neurotransmitters is reduced due to competitive inhibition of tyrosine and tryptophan hydroxylation. In mild PKU or non-PKU HPA (plasma phenylalanine levels ≥240 μmol/l but not over 480) reflects a less severe clinical phenotype.

Untreated pregnant women with HPA/PKU have a high risk to spontaneous miscarriages (maternal PKU syndrome); their offspring often shows low birth weight, microcephaly, retarded development and cardiac malformations [6,7].

Prognosis

In classical PKU early dietary treatment with a phenylalanine-restricted diet can prevent psychomotor delay and mental retardation.

Patients with defective biopterin biosynthesis should be carefully monitored for neurological symptoms. Some patients with these defects have a rather benign course; however, some of them show severe neurological sequela even if well treated. The long-term prognosis of these disorders is still unknown. Prevention of the maternal PKU syndrome will be a main issue in the near future, as the generation of early detected patients by newborn screening has now reached adulthood.

Differential diagnosis

In the neonatal period, premature infants and patients with liver disease, plasma levels of phenylalanine can be abnormally high. This can lead to a false-positive PKU screening test due to other metabolic defects, such as classical galactosaemia or tyrosinaemia (see below). The dermatological manifestations in PKU can mimic eczema and scleroderma-like lesions with pigment changes.

Screening and treatment

In the USA and most Western countries, PKU screening is included in the national neonatal screening programme, either by a semi-quantitative microbiological procedure (Guthrie card) or by a quantitative chemical reaction (Quantase test) [8].

A low phenylalanine–tyrosine supplemented diet should be introduced as soon as possible if plasma phenylalanine concentrations exceed 360 μmol/l. Vitamins, minerals and calcium should be added according to need and age. The diet should be adhered to for life by all patients, or at least during school age and especially by women to prevent maternal PKU syndrome. Some centres change to a protein-restricted diet in adulthood. During treatment the hair colour may darken due to tyrosine supplementation in the diet (Fig. 19.12.1).

In patients with defects in biopterin metabolism, administration of tetrahydrobiopterin (BH4) and precursors of neurotransmitters (L-dopa, carbidopa and 5-hydroxytryptophan) is the treatment of choice, depending on the enzymatic defect.

REFERENCES

1 Güttler F. Hyperphenylalaninaemia: diagnosis and classification of the various types of phenylalanine hydroxylase deficiency in childhood. *Acta Pediatr Scand* 1980; 280 (suppl): 1–80.
2 Fölling A. Uber Ausscheidung von Phenylbrenztraubensaüre in den Harn als Stoffwechselanomalie in Verbindung mit Imbezillität. *Höppe-Seylers Z. Physiol Chem* 1934; 227: 169.
3 Jervis GA. Phenylpyruvic oligophrenia. *Arch Neurol Psychiatr* 1937; 38: 944.
4 Bickel H, Gerrad I, Hickmans EM. Influence of phenylalanine intake on phenulketonuria. *Lancet* 1953; ii: 812.
5 Blau N, Thony B, Heizmann CW *et al.* Tetrahydrobiopterin deficiency: from phenotype to genotype. *Pteridines* 1993; 4: 1–10.
6 Lenke RL, Levy HL. Maternal phenylketonuria and hyperphenylalaninaemia. *N Engl J Med* 1980; 303: 1202–8.
7 Klerk JBC de, Wadman SK, Dijkhuis HJ *et al.* Maternal PKU syndrome in

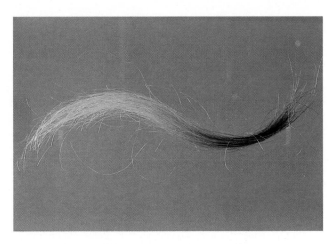

Fig. 19.12.1 Change of hair pigmentation after the start of a phenylalanine-restricted, tyrosine-supplemented diet in a lately detected classical phenylketonuria patient. Courtesy of Professor F.J. van Sprang.

an exceptional family with unexpected PKU. *J Inher Metab Dis* 1987; 10: 162–70.
8 Smith I, Cook B, Beasley M. Review of neonatal screening programme for phenylketonuria. *Br Med J* 1991; 303: 333–5.

Tyrosinaemia

Definition

Tyrosinaemia type I is the hepatorenal type due to fumarylacetoacetase deficiency [1]. No skin abnormalities are present.

Tyrosinaemia type II (Richner–Hanhart syndrome) is the oculocutaneous form of tyrosine catabolism due to a defect of hepatic cytosol aminotransferase [2]. Tyrosinaemia type II is an autosomal recessive disorder.

History

Richner (in 1938) and Hanhart (in 1947) recognized a distinctive oculocutaneous syndrome. Its association with tyrosinaemia was suggested 35 years after the original clinical description. Many patients have probands of Italian ancestry, although other patients have been described from all over the world.

Pathogenesis

Oculocutaneous tyrosinaemia or Richner–Hanhart syndrome is one of the known inborn errors of tyrosine catabolism, and is due to a defect of hepatic cytosol aminotransferase. This results in increased plasma tyrosine levels as well as in abnormal urinary tyrosine metabolites.

Alkaptonuria, another tyrosine-related disorder, characterized by dark-stained urine and cerumen, and arthri-

tis and ochronosis in the fourth decade of life, is discussed below.

Intracellular crystallization is proposed as the mechanism for tissue damage. The levels of amino acids in the epidermis may exceed those in plasma, as tyrosine levels in plasma exceed saturation. The skin lesions are limited to volar surfaces and are associated with polymorphonuclear infiltrates.

Clinical features

Tyroxinaemia type I presents in the neonatal period as an acute disease with severe liver failure or as a more chronic form later in life with rickets, failure to thrive, porphyria-like attacks and liver failure [1]. No skin abnormalities are present.

Oculocutaneous tyrosinaemia or Richner–Hanhart syndrome is characterized by skin abnormalities showing painful palmar and sole erosions and hyperkeratosis. These symptoms often begin as painful blisters.

The eye lesions are often observed within the first year (but usually within the first decade) as bilateral erosions with photophobia or therapy-resistant keratitis. As a result, visual impairment can occur if correct diagnosis and treatment are delayed. Tyrosine crystals in the eye can also be observed on slit-lamp examination.

The basis for the neurological symptoms, often seen in this disease, is not known.

Prognosis

Dietary restriction of phenylalanine and tyrosine can resolve the ophthalmological abnormalities within a week. The skin lesions will recover within a few months. Pregnancy in patients with tyrosinaemia type II has been described [3].

Differential diagnosis

Painful blisters in oculocutaneous tyrosinaemia should be considered as a differential diagnosis of various blistering diseases, such as different forms of epidermolysis bullosa.

Treatment

Oculocutaneous tyrosinaemia with eye crystals is treated with a phenylalanine- and tyrosine-restricted diet (the diet should also be low in phenylalanine because the conversion from the amino acid phenylalanine to tyrosine by L-phenylalanine hydroxylase is not hampered). Dietary intervention is often successful. On dietary treatment, neurological symptoms generally disappear [4].

REFERENCES

1 Kvittingen EA. Tyrosinaemia type I—an update. *J Inher Metab Dis* 1991; 14: 554–62.
2 Paige DG, Clayton P, Bowron A *et al*. Richner–Hanhart syndrome (oculocutaneous tyrosinaemia type II). *J Roy Soc Med* 1992; 85: 759–60.
3 Francis DEM, Kirby DM, Thompson GN. Maternal tyrosinaemia type II: management and successful outcome. *Eur J Pediatr* 1992; 151: 196–9.
4 Barr DGD, Kirk JM, Laing SC. Outcome of tyrosinaemia type II. *Arch Dis Child* 1991; 66: 1249–50.

Homocystinuria

Definition

Cystathionine β-synthase (CBS) deficiency is a genetic disorder of trans-sulphuration [1].

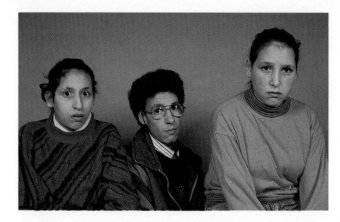

Fig. 19.12.2 Three Moroccan siblings with CBS-deficient pyridoxine responsive homocystinuria before treatment. The boy's lenses have been extracted, the elder girl showing the facial malar flush.

History

The enzyme defect was identified in 1964 by Mudd *et al.*, after the first clinical description in 1963 by both Carson and Neill in Northern Ireland and Gerritsen *et al.* in the USA [1].

Pathogenesis

CBS deficiency is a disorder of trans-sulphuration resulting in elevated plasma levels of homocyst(e)ine and methionine and a decreased level of cysteine [1]. CBS deficiency is inherited as an autosomal recessive trait; pyridoxine responsiveness is probably related to mutations of specific regions of the protein.

Clinical features

Affected patients have a multisystem involvement, including eyes (ectopis lentis), skeleton (marfanoid habitus, premature osteoporosis, bone deformities: pectus carinatum, pectus excavatum), central nervous system (mental retardation), vascular system (thromboembolic events), skin (malar flush) and hair.

Reversible hypopigmentation in some treated homocystinuric patients has been reported, the mechanism is undefined, although some data suggest tyrosinase inhibition by homocyst(e)ine caused by interaction of homocyst(e)ine with copper at the active site of tyrosinase [2]. Malar flush in untreated patients is a roughening, red colouring of the skin of the cheeks, as seen in farmers (Fig. 19.12.2).

Prognosis

Clinical variability is present and mild cases may not be recognized until severe complications, like thromboembolic accidents, develop. Even mild hyperhomocyst(e)inaemia has been related to higher risk of occlusive vascular disease, partly related to methylenetetrahydrofolate metabolism.

Differential diagnosis

The classical phenotype is often confused with Marfan's syndrome, an autosomal dominantly inherited disease, and with eye lens dislocation, skeletal involvement and vascular complications (aneurysma of the aorta). Homocystinuria and Marfan's syndrome are both systemic diseases with (different) collagen abnormalities. Mental retardation is not associated with Marfan's syndrome in contrast to homocystinuria.

Treatment

About half of the patients with homocystinuria due to CBS deficiency, respond to pharmacological doses of pyridoxine (3 doses at 100–250mg daily orally). Pyridoxal-5-phosphate is a co-factor for CBS and pyridoxine treatment (vitamin B$_6$) will increase the conversion of pyridoxine non-responsive homocysteine to cysteine in patients with CBS deficiency. Betaine (di-methylglycine, as a methyl donor) is also used in the treatment of homocystinuria to stimulate the remethylation of homocysteine to methionine [3,4].

REFERENCES

1 Mudd SH, Skovby F, Levy HL *et al*. The natural history of homocystinuria due to cystathionine β-synthase deficiency. *Am J Hum Genet* 1985; 94: 1–31.
2 Rish O, Townsend D, Berry SA *et al*. Tyrosine inhibition due to interaction of homocysteine with copper: the mechanism for reversible hypopigmentation in homocystinuria due to cystathionine β-synthase deficiency. *Am J Hum Genet* 1995; 57: 127–32.
3 Mudd SH, Levy HL, Skovby F. Disorders of trans-sulfuration. In: Scriver CR, Beaudet AL, Sly WS, Valle D, eds. *The Metabolic and Molecular Bases of Inherited Disease*, 7th edn. New York: McGraw-Hill 1995: 1279–327.
4 Wilcken DEN, Wilcken B, Dudman NPD, Tyrell PA. Homocystinuria—the

effect of betaine in the treatment of patients not responsive to pyridoxine. *N Engl J Med* 1983; 309: 448–53.

Organic acidurias

Alkaptonuria

Definition

Alkaptonuria is an autosomal recessive hereditary disease in which the enzyme homogentisic acid oxidase is absent. Due to this effect homogentisic acid accumulates and is excreted in urine.

History

Studies on alkaptonuria have been of great importance in the development of ideas about inherited metabolic diseases. In 1908, Sir Archibald Garrod discussed alkaptonuria in one of the Croonian lectures [1].

Pathogenesis

Due to homogentisic acid oxidase enzyme deficiency, homogentisic acid accumulates and is excreted in urine. Homogentisic acid is an intermediary product in the metabolism of the aromatic amino acids, phenylalanine and tyrosine.

Clinical features

If urine contains homogentisic acid, the acid is gradually oxidized to a melanin-like product, resulting in dark-stained urine. This may lead to early recognition of the disease (black–brown darkening of used napkins). The main features of alkaptonuria are signs due to the presence of homogentisic acid in urine, darkened cerumen of the ears, pigmentation of cartilage, generalized pigmentation in connective tissues (ochronosis) and, later in life, arthritis and bluish pigmentation of the sclera. The skin manifestations are the first diagnostic signs.

Prognosis

Arthropathy occurs in the major joints and spine in the third and fourth decade. Calcification in the heart valves has been described. In comparison with the general population a higher incidence of cardiovascular disease due to arteriosclerosis is described.

Differential diagnosis

A familial and specific intestinal malabsorption of tryptophan, known as 'blue napkin syndrome', has been described [2]. Unabsorbed tryptophan is converted to indican by intestinal bacteria (which can also mimic Hartnup's disease).

The bluish pigmentation is suggestive of haemochromatosis or naevus of Ito. The same pigmentation can be observed after local treatment with phenolic solutions.

The ochronic arthritis as manifestation of long-standing alkaptonuria, resembles gouty arthritis or rheumatoid arthritis.

Treatment

Several attempts to treat alkaptonuria have been studied (vitamin C, vitamin B_{12}, cortisone) without any clinical effect. Dietary restriction of phenylalanine and tyrosine (or general protein restriction) seems to be logical in order to reduce the production of homogentisic acid. The final outcome, however, is unclear. The symptomatic prevention of complications (joints, heart) seems to be the primary therapeutic goal.

REFERENCES

1 Garrod AE. The Croonian Lectures on inborn errors of metabolisms. Lecture II: Alkaptonuria. *Lancet* 1908; ii: 73.
2 Drummond KN, Michael AF, Ulstrom RA, Good RA. The blue diaper syndrome: familial hypercalcemia with nephrocalcinosis and indicausia. *Am J Med* 1964; 37: 928.

Propionic acidaemia

Definition

Propionic acidaemia, as well as methylmalonic acidaemia, are autosomal recessively inherited inborn errors of branched-chain amino acid metabolism.

History

In 1961 Childs described an infant with episodic metabolic ketoacidosis, protein intolerance and elevated plasma glycine concentrations. Many children with similar clinical and biochemical findings have since been described. Propionic acidaemia due to a deficiency of propionyl coenzyme A (CoA) carboxylase deficiency and different forms of methylmalonic acidaemia, all with remarkably elevated plasma glycine concentrations, fit in this description.

Pathogenesis

The essential amino acids – isoleucine, valine, methionine and threonine – are metabolized into propionyl CoA. Propionyl CoA is converted into methylmalonyl CoA by the enzyme propionyl CoA carboxylase. Deficiency of this enzyme causes propionic acidaemia [1].

Clinical features

The clinical characteristics of propionic acidaemia and methylmalonic acidaemia are similar. Patients are commonly seen in the first weeks of life with vomiting, metabolic acidosis, failure to thrive, hypotonia and mental retardation: neonatal death occurs.

Propionic acidaemia is one of the so-called ketotic hyperglycinaemia syndromes, and is characterized by increased concentrations of free propionate in blood and urine. 1-Methylcitrate and 3-hydroxypropionate are major diagnostic urinary metabolites. During decompensation plasma odd-numbered fatty acids, ammonia and glycine levels are elevated.

In the course of propionic acidaemia (even under treatment), patients can develop large superficial desquamation of the skin with epidermolysis that resembles staphylococcal scalded skin syndrome. This complication, potentially due to nutrient or essential amino acid deficiency, has recently been described as acrodermatitis enteropathica-like syndrome (Figs 19.12.3, 19.12.4). Generalized candidiasis often occurs. Alopecia often appears at the end of a period of decompensation and is reversible (Fig. 19.12.5).

Pancytopenia, due to bone marrow depression caused by the abnormal organic acids, is a common feature.

Prognosis

The acute neonatal form of propionic acidaemia has a poor prognosis. Symptomatic treatment with bicarbonate to correct the ketoacidosis and peritoneal dialysis to remove the accumulated toxic metabolites can lead to survival in the neonatal period. However, at any age, each metabolic derangement is potentially life-threatening and often severe psychomotor retardation is a common feature.

Patients affected with the late-onset form will often be on a life-long dietary restriction of one or more essential amino acids, which in excess are the precursors of toxic metabolites. (Semi)-synthetic formulas can provide the required daily intake of protein.

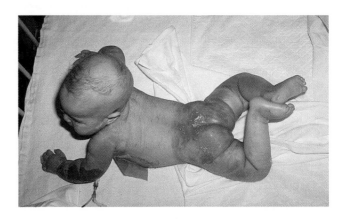

Fig. 19.12.4 Note the sparse scalp hair in the same patient as in Fig. 19.12.3.

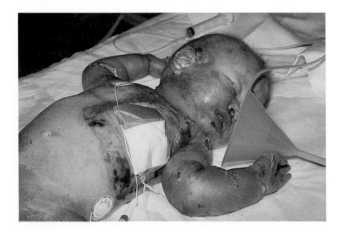

Fig. 19.12.3 Acrodermatitis-like lesions after metabolic decompensation in a non-biotin responsive propionic acidaemia patient.

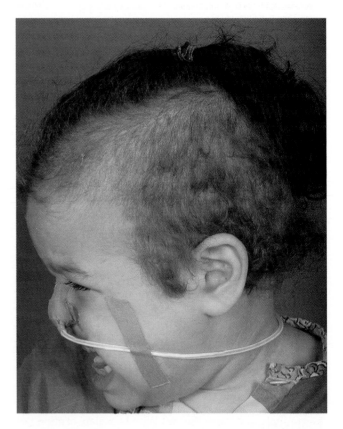

Fig. 19.12.5 Alopecia after metabolic decompensation with pancytopenia in a 6-year-old patient with propionic acidaemia. The girl died at the age of 7 years.

Differential diagnosis

The different forms of ketotic hyperglycinaemia syndromes, such as methylmalonic acidaemia and other organic acidaemias, should be ruled out by proper diagnosis by gas chromatographic mass spectrometric techniques.

Treatment

Propionyl CoA carboxylase requires biotin (10 mg daily) as a co-factor. Dietary treatment with special amino acid mixtures are available. Metronidazole, an antibiotic which inhibits colonic flora, has been found specifically effective in reducing urinary excretion of propionate metabolites. Supportive treatment with multivitamins, calcium is necessary. L-carnitine supplementation 100 mg/kg/day (secondary deficiency caused by urinary loss of esterified propionyl CoA) is indicated.

Some severe neonatal cases have been treated with liver transplantation; the outcome of this treatment is not yet clear.

REFERENCES

1 Fenton WA, Rosenberg LE. Disorders of propionate and methylmalonate metabolism. In: Scriver CR, Beaudet AL, Sly WS, Valle D, eds. *The Metabolic and Molecular Bases of Inherited Disease*, 7th edn. New York: McGraw-Hill: 1423–49.
2 De Raeve I, De Meirleir L, Ramet J *et al*. Acrodermatitis enteropathica-like cutaneous lesions in organic acidurias. *J Pediatr* 1994; 124: 416–20.

Methylmalonic acidaemia

Definition

Inherited deficiency of methylmalonyl CoA mutase activity in humans is caused by mutations at many different loci. Methylmalonic acidaemia is one of the most common organic acidurias.

History

In 1967 critically ill infants with metabolic ketoacidosis and developmental delay, with accumulated huge amounts of methylmalonate in blood and urine, were first described.

The early description, combined with new knowledge, has demonstrated that many different biochemical bases for inherited forms of methylmalonic acidaemia are present: among them defects of the mutase apoenzyme and defects of synthesis of adenosylcobalamine only.

Pathogenesis

Cobalamin (vitamin B_{12}) transport, or biosynthesis defects affecting the synthesis of both adenosylcobalamin and methylcobalamin, are the main causes of this disease. Some children with distinct mutations designated as type C, D and F also show homocystinuria as a result of methyltetrahydrofolate involvement.

Clinical features

Presenting symptoms are similar to propionic acidaemia: vomiting, failure to thrive, lethargy, hypotonia, and attacks of ketoacidosis and dehydration. Propionyl CoA metabolites, like 1-methylcitrate, 3-hydroxypropionate and 3-hydroxyisovalerate, are usually found in urine with gas chromatographic analysis techniques. Vitamin B_{12} deficiency must be excluded.

As in propionic acidaemia, skin disorders can appear during decompensation periods [2,3]. Erythematosquamous eruptions around the orificia and acra with lamellar desquamation, often with alopecia and candidiasis, can occur during metabolic decompensation (Figs 19.12.6, 19.12.7).

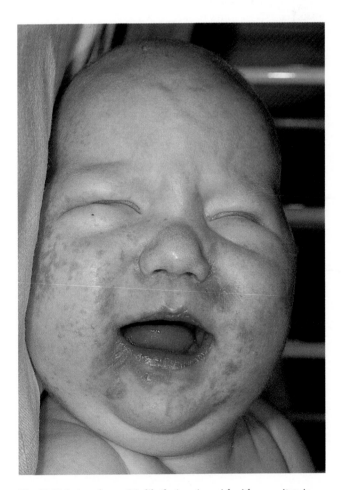

Fig. 19.12.6 Acrodermatitis-like lesions in a girl with non-vitamin responsive methylmalonic acidaemia.

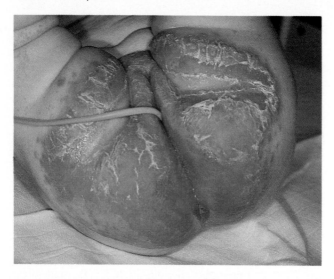

Fig. 19.12.7 Perineal region of the same patient as in Fig 19.12.6. The girl died at the age of 11 months with severe metabolic decompensation.

Prognosis

Early diagnosis and dietary treatment influence the prognosis [1].

Treatment

A tentative treatment with pharmacological doses of vitamin B_{12}, a protein-restricted diet or a restriction of branched-chain amino acids (the precursors), in combination with supportive treatment with L-carnitine, is the therapy of choice. Fasting should be avoided to prevent ketoacidosis.

REFERENCES

1 Saudubray JM, Ogier H, Bonnefont JP *et al*. Clinical approach to inherited diseases in the neonatal period: a 20-year-survey. *J Inher Met Dis* 1989; 12 (suppl 1): 1–17.
2 Koopman RJJ, Happle R. Cutaneous manifestations of methylmalonic acidemia. *Arch Dermatol Res* 1990; 282: 272–3.
3 Bodemer C, de Prost Y, Bachollot B *et al*. Cutaneous manifestations of methylmalonic and propionic acidemia: a description of 38 cases. *Br J Dermatol* 1994; 131: 93–9.

Biotinidase deficiency

Definition

Biotinidase deficiency is an autosomal recessive rare disease and is diagnosed by demonstrating deficient enzyme activity in serum (less than 10% of normal serum activity) [1].

Clinical features

Most symptoms present between 1 week and 2 years, averaging 6 months, with seizures, hypotonia, ataxia, developmental delay, skin rash and alopecia. Other symptoms include optic atrophy, hearing loss, conjunctivitis and fungal infections, which are probably due to abnormalities in immunoregulation.

Most symptomatic children show lactic acidosis and organic aciduria revealing elevated concentrations of β-hydroxyisovalerate, β-methylcrotonylglycine, lactate, β-hydroxyproprionate and methylcitrate.

Alopecia or skin eruption is the initial symptom in about 20% of the patients and is present during the clinical course in at least 60% of the patients. The alopecia is non-scarring.

Perioral erosions, crusts and conjuctival erosions and crusts are frequent findings.

Prognosis

Not all children with biotinidase deficiency respond to biotin therapy. Despite therapy some of the patients still develop ataxia or other neurological symptoms.

Differential diagnosis

Holocarboxylase deficiency and biotidinase deficiency can present with the same clinical features like vomiting, hypotonia, skin rash, alopecia, seizures, ataxia and metabolic ketoacidosis.

Treatment

Biotin, a member of the water-soluble B-complex group, 10 mg daily orally is the treatment of choice and can change the clinical picture dramatically.

REFERENCE

1 Nyhan WL. Inborn errors of biotin metabolism. *Arch Dermatol* 1987; 123: 1696–8.

Transport defects

Hartnup's disease

Definition

Hartnup's disease is an autosomal recessively inherited disorder, leading to an impaired transport of neutral amino acids, limited to kidneys and small intestine.

Pathogenesis

Urinary amino acid analysis shows a typical neutral hyperaminoaciduria. The increased urinary loss of tryptophan and reduced absorption of tryptophan leads to a reduced synthesis of niacin due to an impaired availability of tryptophan [1].

Clinical features

Most affected individuals remain asymptomatic. Photosensitivity is usually the first sign with a pellagra-like appearance and starts in childhood. The rash has been described predominantly on the sun-exposed areas of the body. Exposure to sunlight can form blisters, appearing as sunburn blisters. Neurological signs, like intermittent cerebellar ataxia (even in the neonatal period; the authors' personal observation, 1993), pyramidal signs and psychotic behaviour, have been described. Some affected patients are mildly mentally retarded.

Prognosis

From prospective and retrospective studies of Hartnup's disease patients identified by neonatal screening and with a long-term follow-up, even without therapy, it has become clear that very few become symptomatic.

The most recent hypothesis is that the cause of disease in the Hartnup's disorder is multifactorial [1].

It seems likely that Hartnup's disease does not adversely affect pregnancy and is not damaging to the fetus.

Differential diagnosis

Photosensitivity in early childhood is seen in Bloom's syndrome, Cockayne's syndrome, xeroderma pigmentosum, lupus erythematosus and some forms of porphyria.

Treatment

Treatment with nicotinamide four to six times at 100–250 mg daily leads to clearing of the rash and may lead to disappearance of the ataxia.

REFERENCE

1 Scriver ER, Mahon B, Levy HL *et al.* The Hartnup phenotype: mendelian transport disorder, multifactorial disease. *Am J Hum Genet* 1987; 40: 401.

Lysosomal storage diseases

Alpha-*N*-acetylgalactosaminidase deficiency

Definition

Schindler's disease (α-*N*-acetylgalactosaminidase or α-NAGA deficiency) is a recently recognized lysosomal storage disease with a clinically heterogeneous picture [1].

History

In 1985, this neurodegenerative disease was first described by Schindler as being a lysosomal storage disease in two affected brothers with primary neurological involvement.

Pathogenesis

In 1986, Van Diggelen found the marked deficiency of α-NAGA in blood and cultured fibroblasts.

The deficient enzyme activity causes neuroaxonal pathology, presumably involving neuroaxonal transport leading to dystrophy.

Clinical features

Two phenotypes have been identified. Type I disease is an infantile-onset neuroaxonal dystrophy with a rapid neurodegenerative course with severe psychomotor retardation, blindness and myoclonic seizures. Type II disease was identified in an adult Japanese woman with mild mental retardation and angiokeratoma corporis diffusum [2]. Both forms of this disease have identical patterns of urinary glycopeptide accumulation due to almost no detectable α-NAGA activity. Both types have an autosomal recessive inheritance.

Differential diagnosis

Similar structural lesions have been observed in Seitelberger's disease, Hallervorden–Spatz disease and other forms of inherited neuroaxonal dystrophy.

Type II form of the disease should be differentiated from other diseases with angiokeratoma like Fabry's disease, sialidosis, GM_1, gangliosidosis and fucosidosis.

Prognosis and treatment

Psychomotor retardation and seizures have been described. Appropriate supportive care as needed is the only treatment of choice.

REFERENCES

1 Diggelen OP van, Schindler D, Kleijer WJ *et al*. Lysosomal α-*N*-acetylgalactosaminidase deficiency: a new inherited metabolic disease. *Lancet* 1987; ii: 804.
2 Kanzaki T, Wang AM, Desnick RJ. Lysosomal α-*N*-acetylgalactosaminidase deficiency, the enzymatic defect in angiokeratoma corporis diffusum with glycopeptiduria. *J Clin Invest* 1991; 88: 707.

Fabry's disease

Definition

Fabry's disease results from the defective activity of the lysosomal enzyme, α-galactosidase A and is an inborn error of glycosphingolipid metabolism.

History

The first patients with angiokeratoma corporis diffusum were described by Anderson in England and Fabry in Germany in 1898 [1,2].

Pathogenesis

The enzymatic defect, transmitted by an X-linked recessive gene, leads to deposition of these glycosphingolipid substrates in body fluids and in many cell types in the heart, kidneys, eyes and other tissues [3].

Clinical features

Clinical manifestations during childhood or adolescence are the onset of pain and paraesthesias in the extremities and angiokeratoma (teleangiectases in the skin). Angiectases as an early manifestation may lead to diagnosis in childhood. With age, there is a progressive increase in size and number of these cutaneous vascular lesions. The lesions may be flat and there is slight hyperkeratosis. The localization of the lesions is usually between the knees and the umbilicus. Hips, back, buttocks and scrotum are mostly involved. Hypohidrosis is reported in atypical variants; corneal and lenticular opacities are early findings.

Prognosis

Renal failure and cardiac or cerebrovascular disease is the main cause of death.

Differential diagnosis

Patients with Fabry's disease should be distinguished from other patients with angiokeratoma corporis diffusum, like Schindler's disease, considering the X-linked inheritance.

Treatment

Prophylactic administration of low-maintenance dosages of diphenylhydantoin have been found to provide relief from the periodic invalidating crises of pain and constant discomfort [4]. Angiokeratoma can be removed for cosmetic appearance by laser treatment with little scarring [5]. Up to now, enzyme replacement therapy has not been successful.

REFERENCES

1 Anderson W. A case of angiokeratoma. *Br J Dermatol* 1898; 10: 113.
2 Fabry J. Ein Beitrag zur Kenntnis der Purpura haemorrhagica nodularis. *Arch Dermatol Syph* 1898; 43: 187.
3 Kint JA. Fabry's disease, α-galactosidase deficiency. *Science* 1970; 167: 1268.
4 Lockman LA, Hunninghake DB, Krivit W, Desnick RJ. Relief of pain of Fabry's disease by diphenylhydantoin. *Neurology* 1973; 23: 871.
5 Newton JA, McGibbon HD. The treatment of multiple angiokeratoma with the argon laser. *Clin Exp Dermatol* 1987; 12: 23.

Fucosidosis

Definition

Fucosidosis is a lysosomal storage disease due to a deficiency of α-fucosidase.

History

Patients resembling the phenotype of mucopolysaccharidoses were characterized in the late 1960s as having aspartylglucosaminuria, mannosidosis, mucolipidosis and fucosidosis, depending on the specific metabolites found by metabolic investigations of the urine.

Pathogenesis

The deficiency of α-fucosidase results in accumulation of glycoproteins, glycolipids and oligosaccharides.

Clinical features

The severity of the disease is variable. The more severely affected patients present in infancy with growth retardation, psychomotor retardation, dysostosis multiplex and coarse facies. The more mildly affected patients show angiokeratoma and anhidrosis.

Prognosis

In one study, over 40% of the patients had died before the age of 10 years [1]. A more normal sweat sodium chloride value is indicative of the milder phenotype. A review of 77 patients indicates a death percentage of 41% after the age of 20 years.

Differential diagnosis

The angiokeratoma that occur in fucosidosis cannot be distinguished from those seen in Fabry's disease and adult type α-NAGA deficiency. In one-third of fucosidosis patients under 10 years of age, and in 75% between 10 and 20 years of age angiokeratomas were found.

Other rare but similar disorders of glycoprotein degradation are α-mannosidosis, β-mannosidosis, sialidosis and aspartylglucosaminuria. Dysostosis multiplex should be distinguished from those seen in mucopolysaccharidoses. Sialidosis was not reported until the late 1970s.

Treatment

No treatment is available for these autosomal recessive disorders. Prenatal diagnosis by biochemical analysis is reliable and has been demonstrated by analysis of chorionic villus biopsy samples or cultured amniotic fluid cells [2].

REFERENCES

1 Willems PJ, Gatt R, Darby JK *et al*. Fucosidosis revisited: a review of 77 patients. *Am J Med Genet* 1991; 38: 111.
2 Butterworth J, Guy GJ. α-L-fucosidase of human skin fibroblasts and amniotic fluid cells in tissue culture. *Clin Genet* 1977; 12: 297.

Mucopolysaccharidoses

Definition

The mucopolysaccharidoses (MPS) are a group of lysosomal storage disorders caused by a deficiency of enzymes catalysing the stepwise degradation of mucopolysaccharides (glycosaminoglycans) (Table 19.12.3).

Depending on the enzymatic block, the catabolism of dermatan sulphate (DS), heparan sulphate (HS) or keratan sulphate (KS), singly or in combination, may be hampered; chondroitin sulphate (CS) may be involved.

Depending on the enzymatic deficiency, a different clinical picture exists.

Table 19.12.3 Classification of MPS

Type	Name	MPS product in urinary excretion
I H	Hurler	DS/HS
I S	Scheie	DS/HS
I H/S	Hurler/Scheie	DS/HS
II	Hunter	DS/HS
III A, B, C, D	Sanfilippo	HS
IV	Morquio	KS/CS
VI	Maroteaux–Lamy	DS
VII	Sly	DS/HS/CS

History

The MPSs are a group of disorders caused by a deficiency of lysosomal enzymes needed for the stepwise degradation of glucosaminoglycans (mucopolysaccharides).

Hurler's disease (MPS type I) and Hunter's disease (MPS type II) were originally described as congenital dysostosis multiplex (and gargoylismus).

Understanding about classification of lysosomal storage diseases with mucopolysacchariduria in MPS came only later.

Pathogenesis

Accumulation of undegraded glycosaminoglycan molecules stored in lysosomes eventually results in tissue and organ dysfunction. Depending on the enzyme deficiency a corresponding syndrome or syndrome subtype will develop.

Clinical features

The MPSs share many clinical features with multisystem involvement, hepatosplenomegaly, dysostosis multiplex and coarse facies. Severe mental retardation is characteristic of Hurler's syndrome, the severe form of Hunter's syndrome, and later in infancy in Sanfilippo's syndrome (MPS type III). Morquio's syndrome (MPS type IV) is predominantly related to the skeleton. Short trunk, dwarfism, kyphosis and scoliosis are typical skeletal anomalies of Morquio's syndrome.

Prognosis

The disease takes a chronic and progressive course with multisystem involvement. Mental retardation is a common feature, except in Morquio's disease. Supportive management with attention to respiratory and cardiovascular complications can improve the quality of life of these patients.

Differential diagnosis

Analysis of urinary glycosaminoglycans can discriminate between the classes of glycosaminoglycans, but not distinguish subgroups.

The easy spot test is inexpensive and useful for screening but can be both false positive and false negative. Definite diagnosis of MPS can only be established by enzyme assays. Mucoliposis and sialidosis should be considered if MPS investigations are negative.

Treatment

Enzyme replacement therapy is studied in animal models.

Bone marrow transplantation in MPS I and IV suggests that sufficient enzyme can be provided by haematopoietic cells. This approach needs to be evaluated in the long term [2].

REFERENCES

1 Neufeld EF, Muenzer J. The mucopolysaccharidoses. In: Scriver CR, Beaudet AL, Sly WS, Valle D, eds. *The Metabolic and Molecular Bases of Inherited Disease*, 7th edn. New York: McGraw-Hill, 1995: 2465–94.
2 Hoogerbrugge PM, Brouwer OF, Fischer A. Allogeneic bone marrow transplantation in metabolic diseases. *Blood* 1993; 82: 344.

GM$_1$ gangliosidosis

Definition

GM$_1$ gangliosidosis is a disorder involving the sphingolipids. There are two recognized types of this disorder in the paediatric age group. Type I is characterized by onset in early infancy, leading to death within 2 years of age. Type II occurs later in infancy leading to death usually at 3–10 years of age.

History

GM$_1$ gangliosidosis was the second ganglioside storage disease described, the first one was Tay–Sachs disease. Originally, it was described as Landing's disease: generalized neurovisceral lipidosis.

Pathogenesis

Accumulation of ganglioside GM$_1$ was documented by O'Brien *et al.* [2]. The primary defect is a severe deficiency of acid β-galactosidase. Intraneural storage is localized primarily to neurones of the basal ganglia.

Clinical features

The psychomotor development of an infant with GM$_1$ gangliosidosis is retarded in the first year of life. Many patients have facial abnormalities, including frontal bossing, large low-set ears, mild macroglossia and gum hypertropy. Cherry-red spots, identical to those in Tay–Sachs disease, are present in about 50% of patients. Hepatomegaly is usually present after 6 months of life and splenomegaly occurs in the majority of patients. The skin is often thick, hirsute and rough. Hyperpigmented macules and patches on the trunk and extremities are reported. Cutaneous manifestations are not common in GM$_1$ gangliosidosis [1].

Prognosis

Infantile GM$_1$ gangliosidosis presents with bone changes and neurological deterioration leading to early death. Progressive psychomotor deterioration with bony abnormalities is seen in juvenile GM$_1$ gangliosidosis.

Differential diagnosis

This includes lysosomal storage diseases with neurological symptoms.

Treatment

As far as is known, treatment can only be symptomatic.

REFERENCES

1 Calsur Selsor L, Lesher JL. Hyperpigmented macules and patches in a patient with GM$_1$ type I gangliosidosis. *J Am Acad Dermatol* 1989; 20: 878–82.
2 O'Brien JS, Stern MB, Landing BH *et al.* Generalized gangliosidosis. *Am J Dis Child* 1965; 109: 388.

Farber lipogranulomatosis: ceramidase deficiency

Definition

Farber's disease is an autosomal recessively inherited disorder of lipid metabolism, associated with a deficiency of a lysosomal acid ceramidase and tissue accumulation of ceramide.

History

So far the phenotype has been divided into six subtypes. It is likely that the diagnosis has been frequently missed because of the variability of the clinical picture.

Pathogenesis

Accumulation of ceramide has been reported in all well-documented cases. The granuloma formation and histiocytic response appear to be a consequence of ceramide accumulation.

Clinical features

Subcutaneous nodules near the joints and over pressure points, and progressively painful and deformed joints are the main clinical manifestations. Hoarseness due to laryngeal involvement can lead to aphonia, feeding and respiratory difficulties, failure to thrive and intermittent fever. Symptoms usually appear between the age of 2 weeks and 4 months. Different subtypes have been described.

The diagnosis can be demonstrated by a deficiency of acid ceramidase in cultured skin fibroblasts or in white blood cells. Prenatal diagnosis by measuring enzyme activity in cultured amniocytes has been proved useful.

Prognosis

The disease often leads to death within the first few years; according to the subtype, a more prolonged life-span can be observed.

Differential diagnosis

Juvenile rheumatoid arthritis and fibromatosis hyalinica multiplex can resemble the clinical picture of Farber's disease [3].

Histopathological and enzymatic investigations are necessary to confirm the final diagnosis.

Treatment

No specific treatment is available. Systemic corticosteroids may provide some relief. Tracheostomy may be needed to prevent respiratory insufficiency. Bone marrow transplantation may be an ultimate therapy in the future.

REFERENCES

1 Moser HW, Moser AB, Chen WW. Ceramidase deficiency: Farber lipogranulomatosis. In: Scriver CR, Beaudet AL, Sly WS, Valle D, eds. *The Metabolic and Molecular Bases of Inherited Disease*, 6th edn. New York: McGraw-Hill, 1989: 1645–53.
2 Fensom AH, Benson PI, Neville BRG *et al.* Prenatal diagnosis of Farber's disease. *Lancet* 1979; ii: 990.
3 Mancini GMS, Stojanov L, Willemsen R *et al.* Juvenile Hyaline Fibromatosis. *Dermatology* 1999; 198: 18–25.

Hyperlipoproteinaemias

Definition

Genetic hyperlipoproteinaemias are caused by defects of structural components of lipoproteins, or receptors which affect the formation or removal of lipoproteins [1]. They consist of a group of disorders characterized by elevated serum cholesterol levels and/or elevated triglyceride levels.

History

Hyperlipoproteinaemias are usually grouped according to the classification of Frederickson. They are all inherited disorders. Hyperlipoproteinaemias are classified into five groups, numbered I–V [2] (Table 19.12.4).

Aetiology

Lipoproteins are complexes that transport lipids within the blood: triglycerides, cholesterol (esterified and unesterified), phospholipids and fat-soluble vitamins. The major lipoprotein particles are chylomicrons, very low density lipoproteins (VLDL), low density lipoproteins (LDL) and high density lipoproteins (HDL).

The major consequences of lipoprotein disorders are premature arteriosclerosis and atherosclerosis in heterozygous or homozygous familial hypercholesterolaemia (FH). Life-threatening acute pancreatitis is the cause of death in untreated hypertriglyceridaemia and hyperchylomicronaemia caused by lipoprotein-lipase deficiency (LPL) or apolipoprotein CII deficiency [3].

Pathology

Histopathological features consist of upper dermal infiltrates of non-xanthomized histiocytes, varying in appearance corresponding with clinical features such as plane or more papular or nodular presentations. Based on the age of the lesion and differentiation, the infiltrate contains histiocytes, fully matured foam cells and Touton giant cells [4]. In all forms of xanthomas, the lipid within the foam cells stains positively with fat stains such as oil red O, scarlet or Sudan red [4]. These foam cells are characteristic of xanthomas. Depending upon the kind of xanthomas, the infiltrate is mixtured with lymphocytes and neutrophils [4,5]. In tendinous xanthomas older lesions

Table 19.12.4 Hyperlipoproteinaemias according to Frederickson type I–V

	I	II	III	IV	V
Inheritance	AR	AD	AR	AD	AR
Dermatology symptoms	Eruptive xanthomas	Tendinous, tuberous, plane xanthomas xanthelasma	Plane, tendinous, tuberous xanthomas	Eruptive, tuberous xanthomas	Eruptive, tuberous xanthomas,
Age	Infants, teenagers	Children	Adults	Adults (obesity)	Adults (obesity)
Laboratory	VLDL, TG, CM raised	C, LDL raised	C, TG raised; LDL, HDL low or N	VLDL, TG raised	VLDL, TG, CM raised

AD, autosomal dominant; AR, autosomal recessive; C, cholesterol; CM, chylomicrons; TG, triglycerides.

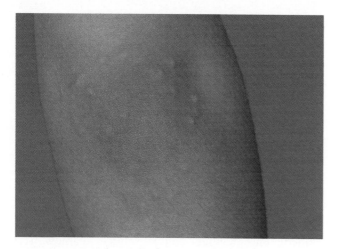

Fig. 19.12.8 Xanthomas in a boy with homozygous FH.

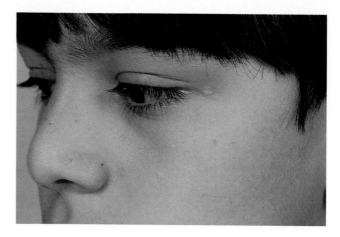

Fig. 19.12.9 Xanthelasma in a boy with homozygous FH, an extremely rare manifestation.

are associated with fibrosis, while in plane xanthomas it is rare [4]. Xanthomas, especially relevant in disseminated xanthomatosis, consist of non-Langerhans' cell histiocytes, that are S100 protein negative [6,7].

Clinical features

The most important clinical features of FH are premature arteriosclerosis and xanthomatosis. Xanthomas tuberosa can occur in the Achilles tendon and the tendons around the elbows, knees and the back of the hand. The age of appearance depends on the heterozygous or homozygous state of the disease. Xanthelasma, which is lipid accumulation of the soft connective tissue on the eyelids is also a recognizable clinical feature.

Xanthoma and xanthelasma appear between the third and fourth decade of life in heterozygous FH, while they already can be seen in early childhood in the homozygous FH patients (incidence 1 in 10^6 in the Caucasian population).

LPL deficiency (Fredrickson type I) is characterized by attacks of acute abdominal pain caused by pancreatitis in untreated patients; the mortality rate is high.

Xanthomas consist of papules, nodules or tumours that contain lipid. There are several types: plane xanthomas, eruptive xanthomas, tendinous xanthomas (Fig. 19.12.8), tuberous xanthomas and xantholasma (Fig. 19.12.9). A plane xanthoma is a flat or only slightly elevated plaque, commonly located in palmar and digital creases. An eruptive xanthoma is reddish-yellow and appears in crops. These xanthomas are mostly seen on the buttocks or extremities. A tendinous xanthoma is nodular and located on tendons especially of the elbows, hands, knees and feet. The tumour is skin coloured or yellow. A tuberous xanthoma is a nodule located on the extensor sites of the elbows, hands, buttocks or knees, which is skin coloured or yellow.

Prognosis

Untreated homozygous FH leads to early death in the second decade by coronary heart disease (CHD) or cerebral vascular accidents (CVA).

Heterozygous FH leads to CHD and CVA between the third and fourth decade of life.

Differential diagnosis

Secondary causes of hyperlipidaemias, including hepatic disease, diabetes mellitus and drug-induced causes, must be excluded.

Treatment

In FH a fat-restricted, linoleic-enriched diet should be advised by an experienced dietitian, combined with a fibre-rich diet. Physical exercise, an active non-smoking attitude and prevention of obesity should encouraged.

In homozygous FH, cholestyramine and hydroxymethyl-glutaryl CoA reductase (HMG CoA reductase) inhibitors, including lovostatin, pravastatin an simvastatin, are the drugs of choice, even at an early age [8]. Lipoapheresis and orthotopic liver transplantation are recent experimental therapies now evaluated to prevent early death of CHD in homozygous FH [9].

In LPL deficiency a fat-restricted, medium chain triglyceride (MCT) enriched diet is the treatment of choice.

REFERENCES

1 Brown MS, Goldstein JC. A receptor mediated pathway of cholesterol homeostatis. *Science* 1986; 232: 34–47.
2 Fredricksen DS, Lees RS. A system for phenotyping hyperlipoproteinaemia. *Circulation* 1965; 31: 321–7.
3 Santamarina-Fojo S. Genetic dyslipoproteinemias: role of lipoprotein lipase and apolipoprotein C-II. *Curr Opin Lipidol* 1992; 3: 186–95.

4 McKee P. *Pathology of the Skin*, 2nd edn. London: Mosby Wolfe, 1996: 7, 1–7, 10.

5 Crowe MJ, Gross DJ. Eruptive xanthoma. *Cutis* 1992; 50: 31–2.

6 Winkelmann RK. Cutaneous syndromes of non-X histiocytosis. A review of the macrophage–histiocyte diseases of the skin. *Arch Dermatol* 1981; 117: 667–72.

7 Soong VY, Rabkin MS, Thomas JM. Nodular lesions on the face and trunk: xanthoma disseminatum. *Arch Dermatol* 1991; 1127: 1717–22.

8 Stein EA. Treatment of familial hypercholesterolemie with drugs in children. *Arteriosclerosis* 1989; 9: 1146–51.

9 Gordon BR, Saal S. Advances in LPL apheresis for the treatment of severe hypercholesterolemia. *Curr Opin Lipidol* 1994; 5: 69–73.

Acrodermatitis enteropathica

Definition

Acrodermatitis enteropathica is a biochemical disease of metal metabolism by zinc deficiency. There is an inability to absorb sufficient zinc from the diet.

History

Acrodermatitis enteropathica was recognized in 1936 by a Swedish dermatologist [1].

Aetiology and pathophysiology

Acrodermatitis enteropathica is an autosomal recessively inherited disease. Deficiency of zinc-dependent enzymes leads to the typical clinical features of hair, muscle and bone. A large number of enzymes with zinc as a co-factor is probably the basis of the heterogeneity of the symptoms.

Serum alkaline phosphatase is a zinc-containing enzyme and is decreased at all ages in acrodermatitis enteropathica, but is not an early indicator of the disease. The disturbance of zinc homoeostasis results from a partial block in the intestinal absorption [2].

Clinical features

Clinical symptoms of acrodermatitis enteropathica are those of zinc deficiency. They represent general symptoms like failure to thrive, anorexia, tremor, diarrhoea and apathy, as well as local hair and skin symptoms. The classical triad is acral dermatitis, alopecia and diarrhoea. The skin presents with skin rash, alopecia, fine brittle hair, perioral and perianal vesiculobullous, pustular and hyperkeratotic dermatitis. Nail dystrophy may also occur [3]. Symptoms develop after the neonatal period (mostly after weaning).

Laboratory findings show low plasma or serum zinc levels.

Prognosis

If the diagnosis is made correctly and in time, the prognosis in general is good.

Differential diagnosis

Biotinidase deficiency, malnutrition and several types of epidermolysis bullosa and severe seborrhoeic dermatitis must be considered. A skin biopsy is not always diagnostic. Essential fatty acid deficiency is one of the most common differential diagnoses. Some types of organoacidaemias due to aberrant degration of branched-chain amino acids like propionic acidaemia and methylmalonic acidaemia [4,5] have acrodermatitis-like lesions. It should be noted that severe hypoalbuminaemia is associated with low serum zinc values.

Treatment

Zinc supplementation, usually leads to a rapid improvement of the clinical features. At least twice the normal daily requirements must be given initially. The therapy will need to be continued life long.

REFERENCES

1 Brandt T. Dermatitis in children with disturbances of general condition and absence of food. *Acta Derm Venereol* 1936; 17: 513–46.

2 Atherton DJ, Muller DPR, Aggett PJ *et al*. A defect in zinc uptake by jejunal biopsies in acrodermatitis enteropathica. *Clin Sci* 1970; 56: 505–7.

3 Neldner KH, Hambridge KM, Walravens PA. Acrodermatitis enteropathica. *Int J Dermatol* 1978; 17: 380–7.

4 Koopman RJJ, Happle R. Cutaneous manifestations of methylmalonic acidemia. *Arch Dermatol Res* 1990; 282: 272–7.

5 Bodemer C, de Prost Y, Bachollet B *et al*. Cutaneous manifestations of methylmalonic acidemia and propionic acidemia: a description of 38 cases. *Br J Dermatol* 1994; 131: 93–8.

The Neurofibromatoses

SUSAN M. HUSON AND MARTINO RUGGIERI

Neurofibromatosis type 1

Neurofibromatosis type 2

Other neurofibromatoses
Segmental or mosaic neurofibromatosis type 1
Autosomal dominant café-au-lait spots alone
Watson's syndrome
Schwannomatosis

In the earlier medical literature, the term neurofibromatosis or von Recklinghausen's disease was used to describe all patients with various combinations of café-au-lait spots and tumours of the peripheral and/or central nervous system (CNS). It is now clear that there are several distinct forms of neurofibromatosis, the differentiation of these disorders clinically is important—their natural history and management is quite different. Another problem in older literature is the use of the term 'forme fruste' to describe patients with limited disease features when the phenotype simply reflects one stage in the natural history of a progressive disease. Thus children with multiple café-au-lait spots do not have a forme fruste of neurofibromatosis type 1 (NF1), they have these lesions alone because neurofibromas do not appear until adulthood in the majority of cases.

Riccardi [1,2] has proposed a classification of neurofibromatosis that includes seven different types and an eighth category for cases 'not otherwise specified'. The definition of the different forms depends on the occurrence, number and distribution of the major features of neurofibromatosis—café-au-lait spots, tumours of the nervous system (neurofibromas and schwannomas) and Lisch nodules. The classification has not come into widespread use partly because the type 3 mixed, type 6 variant and type 7 late-onset forms are not defined sufficiently to permit their general use. Viskochil and Carey [3] have proposed an alternative classification which provides the basis for relating phenotype to genotype which may well prove the most satisfactory approach in the long term. However, at present the authors prefer to follow the National Institutes of Health (NIH) consensus conference classification [4]. The panel recommended a numerical

classification and felt that in 1987 only NF1 (formerly von Recklinghausen's disease or peripheral neurofibromatosis) and NF2 (formerly bilateral acoustic or central neurofibromatosis) could be clearly defined. The phenotypic overlap between these two disorders is small in the majority of cases and they are caused by mutations in different genes that do not have obvious overlap in function. Other forms of neurofibromatosis do exist but apart from mosaic or segmental NF1 they are all extremely rare. In this chapter NF1 is reviewed in detail, other forms of neurofibromatosis are mentioned briefly with emphasis on how they may present in paediatric dermatological practice.

Neurofibromatosis type 1

NF1 is one of the commonest autosomal dominant disorders in man. The gene has a high rate of mutation and approximately half of the people with NF1 have no family history. NF1 has a prevalence of around 1/5000 in most populations studies and an estimated birth frequency of 1/2500 [5].

Definition

The diagnosis is a clinical one using the NIH consensus development conference statement [4] diagnostic criteria for NF1. The criteria are met in an individual who has two or more of the following.
1 Six or more café-au-lait macules of over 5 mm in greatest diameter in prepubertal individuals and over 15 mm in greatest diameter in postpubertal individuals.
2 Two or more neurofibromas of any type or one plexiform neurofibroma.
3 Freckling in the axillary or inguinal regions.
4 Optic glioma.
5 Two or more Lisch nodules (iris hamartomas).
6 A distinct osseous lesion such as sphenoid dysplasia or thinning of the long bone cortex with or without pseudarthrosis.
7 A first-degree relative (parent, sibling or offspring) with NF1 by the above criteria.

History

Illustrations of patients with probable NF1 can be found dating back to the second century [6,7], the first clinical reports date from the 18th century [8]. By 1849, Smith [9] was able to cite 75 references; he reported two further cases and postulated but was unable to prove, that the tumours had a neural origin. In 1882 von Recklinghausen [10] confirmed their origin and named the tumours neurofibromas. In 1896, the other major dermatological feature, café-au-lait spots, were recognized as being part of the disease by three French doctors [11,12]. The first half of the 20th century saw reports of other disease features and numerous complications, but it was only with the first large cohort studies of Borberg [13] and Crowe *et al.* [14] in the 1950s that the natural history and very variable phenotypic spectrum began to emerge. In the last two decades there has been a marked increase in clinical and scientific research in the field of neurofibromatosis, with the distinct clinical phenotypes and different molecular pathogenesis of the two major forms being determined [15].

Pathogenesis

Genetics

NF1 is an autosomal dominant condition with very variable expression even within families. It has virtually 100% penetrance by the age of 5 years [5], the majority of patients develop six or more café-au-lait spots in the first 2 years of life. Approximately 50% of cases represent new mutations, the mutation rate is one of the highest recorded in humans.

The NF1 gene

Before the application of molecular genetic techniques there had been no major advances in our understanding of the pathogenesis of NF1. The gene was mapped to chromosome 17 by linkage analysis in 1987 [16,17] and cloned in 1990 [18–20]. Von Deimling *et al.* [21] and [22] have recently reviewed developments since the cloning of the gene.

The gene spans over 350 kb of genomic DNA, encoding an RNA of 11–13 kb with at least 59 exons. Its protein product has been named *neurofibromin* and contains 2818 amino acids with an estimated molecular mass of 220 kDa. The *NF1* gene has four alternatively spliced transcripts, three of which have been studied in detail and show, to some extent, differential expression in various tissues. A portion of the coding sequence of the *NF1* gene (about 13%) shows close homology to the guanosine triphosphatase (GTPase) activating protein (GAP) family. The region is known as the GAP-related domain (NF1—GRD). GAP proteins are involved in the regulation of *ras* and the presence of this domain supports a tumour suppressor function for the *NF1* gene. Some but not all tumours associated with NF1 that have been studied show loss of heterozygosity at the *NF1* gene locus providing further evidence for a tumour suppressor action. *Neurofibromin* is involved in the control of cell growth and differentiation by at least three possible mechanisms: (a) as an upstream downregulator of p21 *ras*; (b) as a downstream effector of p21 *ras*; and (c) as a link between tubulin and p21 *ras*.

The mouse *NF1* gene shows strong homology to the human locus. Mice that have been created that are homozygous for a mutation in the *NF1* gene lack *neurofibrominin* in all tissues and do not survive beyond the day 14 embryo stage. They show widespread developmental anomalies and embryonic death is attributable to a severe heart malformation. Heterozygote mice do not show classical NF1 disease features but appear to have an increased susceptibility to some of the tumours that are seen in the human disease, such as phaeochromocytoma and myeloid leukaemias [23,24].

Genotype/phenotype correlation

The large size of the gene has made mutation analysis difficult. No hot-spot for mutation has emerged, the identified changes being spread throughout the gene [25]. No obvious genotype/phenotype correlation has emerged except in the small minority of patients who have been shown to have a deletion of the whole gene [26,27]. Distinctive features of these patients are that they have more severe intellectual handicap than normally seen in NF1, facial dysmorphism (although a specific phenotype has not yet emerged), large hands and the development of cutaneous neurofibromas at a much earlier age than normal.

Easton *et al.* [28] have studied the basis for the phenotypic variation of NF1 and concluded that it is largely determined by the action of modifying genes, which may vary from one disease feature to another. Thus the pathogenesis of NF1 is likely to be a complex process. Research is now concentrating on the identification of the function of the other domains of the *NF1* gene and the genes which modify its action.

Pathology

Only the pathology of the major features of NF1 and plexiform neurofibromas, a complication relatively specific to the disorder, are discussed here. For other tumours which occur, the underlying pathology is usually the same as when they occur in isolation [29].

Café-au-lait spots

Microscopically, café-au-lait spots present as focal hyperpigmentation in the basal area of an otherwise normal epidermis, axillary freckles show a similar appearance. There is an increase in dopa-positive melanocytes [30] which show an increased number of melanin macroglobules. Melanocytes with melanin macroglobules are also found though in much lower numbers throughout the skin of NF1 patients. However, these lesions are not specific to NF1 being an occasional finding in normal individuals and being seen in other disorders including Albright's syndrome, LEOPARD syndrome (lentigines, electrocardiogram abnormalities, ocular hypertelorism, pulmonary stenosis, abnormalities of genitalia, retardation of growth and deafness), and xeroderma pigmentosum [31].

Neurofibromas

These can develop anywhere in the body in NF1, arising from sensory and autonomic nerves. Histologically, they are indistinguishable from neurofibromas occurring as isolated lesions in the general population. The clinical features of neurofibromas depend on their site of development, as discussed below; there is also some site-dependent histological variation. Dermal neurofibromas are well circumscribed but not encapsulated, and although they arise from the terminal branches of cutaneous nerves, the nerve of origin is not usually obvious. Conversely, nodular neurofibromas develop on nerve roots or major peripheral nerves, are more sharply demarcated and have an apparent capsule of perineural cells. The fibres of the nerve of origin pass through nodular neurofibromas and are not stretched over their surface as is seen in schwannomas [32].

Microscopically, both dermal and nodular neurofibromas are spindle cell tumours originating from peripheral nerve sheaths [32]. The primary cell of origin is still uncertain as neurofibromas contain a mixture of Schwann cells and perineural fibroblasts. Common features include the formation of collagen fibres and myxoid degeneration. Mitotic activity is low. The tumour is not locally invasive. Mast cells are seen scattered throughout the tumour tissue. Dermal neurofibromas are not thought to have the potential for sarcomatous degeneration.

Plexiform neurofibromas

These lesions are classically thought always to occur in association with NF1. However, they can occasionally be seen as isolated lesions in otherwise healthy individuals and presumably they then represent some form of somatic mosaicism (see section on segmental neurofibromatosis for further discussion). Plexiform neurofibromas can be discrete nodular tumours developing on a nerve or nerve root, or diffuse tumours associated with diffuse hypertrophy of surrounding connective tissue and other structures [33]. Microscopically they are moderately cellular spindle

cell neoplasms. The tumour cells are embedded in an abundant extracellular myxoid matrix, which often contains numerous mast cells. Plexiform neurofibromas are locally invasive, growing within and along the nerve, enlarging the nerve fascicles and elongating each fascicle; this growth causes the fascicles to twist on themselves, eventually creating a lesion resembling a tangle of worms. In the early stages of the lesion, hypercellular fascicles are found. As the lesion develops, there is an increase in the number of Schwann cells and/or perineural cells. A few residual axons that have not been destroyed by the tumour can be found. As the lesion grows, the fascicle can either become hypocellular and myxomatous or even more cellular; the two pathologies can be found side by side in a single lesion. Plexiform neurofibromas have the potential for malignant degeneration into sarcomas [32,33].

Lisch nodules

These lesions are melanocytic hamartomas [34] which on light microscopy are shown to be composed of a haphazard population of spindle-shaped cells with slender dendritic processes intermixed with round, plumper cells. On electron microscopy, these cells are shown to be melanocytes with many interwoven cytoplasmic processes and there is a mixture of immature and mature cells.

Clinical features

The clinical features of NF1 are diverse and can affect almost any organ system. Clinically, it is useful to consider them in three groups.

1 The major defining features. These are café-au-lait spots, freckling in specific areas, dermal neurofibromas and Lisch nodules. They are distinct disease features which are present in the vast majority of affected individuals and form the basis for the diagnostic criteria.

2 Minor disease features. These are short stature and macrocephaly. They are present in a significant proportion of patients but are not so specific that they are used as part of the diagnostic criteria.

3 Complications. These are defined as any condition that occurs at an increased frequency in patients with NF1 compared with the general population. Some of the complications are relatively specific to NF1 such as sphenoid wing dysplasia. Others are seen as isolated problems in the general population (e.g. scoliosis, the malignancies related to NF1), and here the question is whether there is actually an increased frequency in NF1 patients and if so how great is the increase. Purists may argue that some of the things that are described as disease complications would be better classified as disease associations (e.g. juvenile xanthogranulomas), but such a distinction complicates the issues unnecessarily.

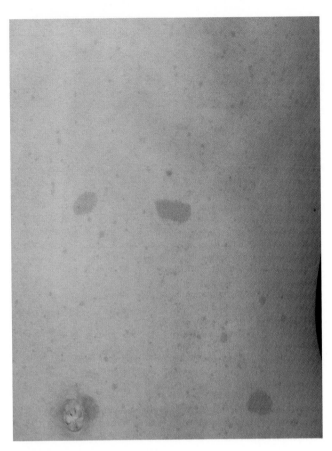

Fig. 19.13.1 Multiple café-au-lait macules in a 9-year-old boy. Courtesy of Dr John Harper.

Major defining features

Café-au-lait spots and skin fold freckling. Café-au-lait spots and freckling are not unique to NF1, at least 10% of the general population having one or two spots [35,36]. What is important in NF1 is the number of café-au-lait spots, the majority of affected patients having six or more (Fig. 19.13.1). Six was the number of café-au-lait spots that Crowe *et al.* [14] suggested after their large study of NF1 as being useful in the diagnosis to distinguish clearly the NF1 population from individuals with one or two café-au-lait spots as a variant of normal. There are very few other conditions associated with six or more café-au-lait spots and as discussed in the section below on differential diagnosis they have other specific disease features. However, clinical judgement has to be used and whilst the authors are usually happy to reassure parents of children (providing they are aged 2 years or more) who have three or less café-au-lait spots and no other features that there is nothing to worry about, follow-up is usually suggested for those with four or more because of the possibility of other forms of neurofibromatosis, particularly NF2. In practice these cases are rare, and as seen in Table 19.13.1 all the children in the Welsh NF1 study had six or more café-au-lait spots [37].

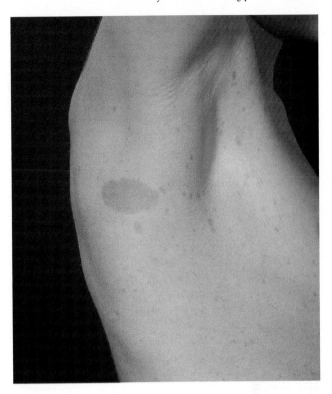

Fig. 19.13.2 Axillary freckling. Courtesy of Dr John Harper.

The café-au-lait spots are the first disease manifestation to appear and one or two may be present at birth. In the Welsh study [37] 82% of parents had noticed the spots for the first time within the first year of life. They continue to develop in number throughout childhood, but appear to stop developing or even disappear in adulthood (Table 19.13.1). The spots vary in diameter from 0.5 to 50 cm or more, but are usually less than 10 cm. They increase in size as the child grows and for the diagnostic criteria spots greater than 0.5 cm are counted in prepubertal individuals but only those greater than 1.5 cm in postpubertal individuals. The spots usually have smooth contours, but some, particularly the larger ones, have irregular outlines. Their colour intensity varies with background skin pigmentation and in children with very pale complexions they are best seen under ultraviolet light.

Freckling in the axillae (Fig. 19.13.2) and other specific areas (around the base of the neck, the groins and submammary regions in females) is the other characteristic pigmentary change in NF1. In obese people freckles can sometimes be seen between skinfolds. Occasionally patients have no demarcation between the zones of freckling, with freckles all over the trunk and proximal extremities. The freckles resemble café-au-lait spots but are only 1–3 mm in diameter. They appear after the spots; the youngest patient with axillary freckling in the Welsh study was 3 years [37]. Table 19.13.1 shows the percentage

Table 19.13.1 Percentage of patients with the cutaneous features of NF1 by age in the Welsh study (data derived from references 37,40)

Age (years)	No of cases	Feature				
		Café-au-lait spots (%)	Axillary freckling (%)	Inguinal freckling (%)	Submammary freckling (% females)	Dermal neurofibromas (%)
0–5	7	100	14	0	0 (0/5)	0
6–10	14	100	50	14	0 (0/6)	14
11–15	21	100	62	38	0 (0/14)	33
16–20	14	93	86	57	33 (1/3)	93
21–30	28	93	75	46	31 (5/16)	100
31–40	26	89	92	62	53 (9/17)	100
41–50	13	62	77	46	36 (4/11)	100
51–60	13	77	69	23	20 (1/5)	100
61–70	13	62	62	23	0 (0/4)	100
71–85	6	0	67	17	0 (0/6)	100

of patients in each age group with the different cutaneous features of NF1.

Peripheral neurofibromas. Clinically, there are two forms of peripheral neurofibroma depending on where in the peripheral nervous system they develop. Dermal neurofibromas develop on the cutaneous nerve endings and are present in nearly all adults with NF1. Nodular neurofibromas, arise on the major peripheral nerve trunks and occur in only a small proportion of patients (no one has recorded the exact number systematically, but it is perhaps in the region of 5%).

Dermal neurofibromas. These develop after the café-au-lait spots, usually in the teens or twenties. It is unusual to see children under 10 years with a large number of lesions. The number of neurofibromas which develop is extremely variable even within families, ranging from lesions that are hardly obvious at first glance on clinical examination to very occasional patients who are covered with neurofibromas all over their body (Fig. 19.13.3). At the present time there are no obvious childhood predictors as to which patients will develop a lot of neurofibromas.

Dermal neurofibromas lie within the dermis and epidermis and move passively with the skin. The majority are discrete nodules with a characteristic violaceous colour; they feel soft, almost gelatinous and vary from 0.1 cm to several centimetres in diameter. When pressed, the tumours tend to evaginate into the subcutaneous tissue, a sign first referred to by Crowe *et al.* [14] and called button-holing. Some neurofibromas become pedunculated as they grow. They develop mainly on the trunk and are only present in large numbers on exposed areas of the body in more severe cases, even then they rarely develop on the shins, palms or soles. Only 18% of patients in the Welsh study had obvious lesions on the head and neck. Women with NF1 often comment on an increase in size and number of neurofibromas during pregnancy sometimes

with partial regression after delivery. To our knowledge there have been no reports of women developing more neurofibromas when using oral contraceptives.

Dermal neurofibromas are the only major defining feature associated with significant morbidity. Although some patients complain of pruritus, they are rarely painful. Dermal neurofibromas are not thought to undergo sarcomatous change, but it is sensible to remove rapidly enlarging painful lesions. Haemorrhage into a neurofibroma can be a cause of sudden painful enlargement. The distressing aspect of these lesions to the patient is their appearance, some patients never coming to terms with this.

Nodular neurofibromas. These arise from the major peripheral nerve trunks and have a much firmer consistency and more defined margins than dermal neurofibromas. When present, they may give rise to neurological symptoms, which are not a feature of dermal lesions. Pressure on nodular neurofibromas may give rise to paraesthesiae. Removal of these lesions is more difficult than for dermal neurofibromas because of their position in relation to major nerve trunks.

Lisch nodules. Lisch nodules are harmless iris hamartomas. They cause no symptoms. They can occasionally be detected on general examination as yellow–brown lesions but are much more readily seen, and more definitely distinguished from common iris naevi, by slit-lamp examination. The nodules appear as smooth dome-shaped lesions up to 2 mm in diameter. They vary from clear to lightly pigmented and they usually have very distinct borders. It is their elevation and shape which distinguishes them from the common flat naevi, which can be a similar colour. Lisch nodules develop during childhood, after the café-au-lait spots but before the neurofibromas and are therefore useful for confirming the diagnosis in children with no family history and only multiple café-au-lait spots. Flueler and Boltshauser [38] found 33% of children under

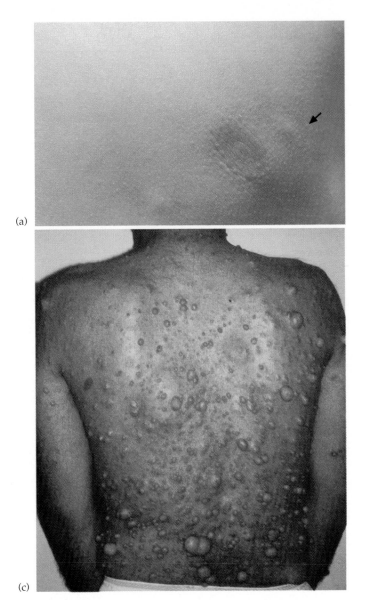

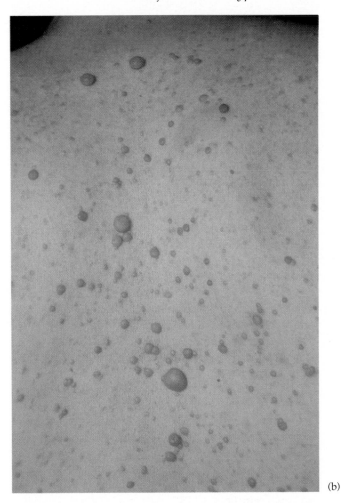

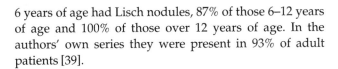

Fig. 19.13.3 Dermal neurofibromas at different stages of development. (a) Early subtle lesions which are best viewed with tangential lighting. Courtesy of Dr John Harper. (b) More obvious and florid lesions. Courtesy of Dr John Harper. (c) Extremely severely affected for his age. With permission from Chapman & Hall [15].

6 years of age had Lisch nodules, 87% of those 6–12 years of age and 100% of those over 12 years of age. In the authors' own series they were present in 93% of adult patients [39].

Minor disease features

Macrocephaly. Just under half of the patients in most large studies have had macrocephaly, the cause of which is unknown [37]. A child with NF1 does not therefore need to be investigated unless there are other features suggestive of intracranial pathology or serial head circumferences are showing progressive enlargement.

Short stature. Approximately one-third of patients are at or below the third centile in height [37]. When compared with data from their normal siblings the children with

NF1 were found to be approximately 7–8 cm shorter than expected. One should be aware, however, that very occasionally children with NF1 have a disturbance of growth because of pituitary/hypothalamic involvement by an optic chiasm glioma. The cause of short stature in the majority of NF1 cases is not known; those patients who have had investigation of short stature have not shown any causative factor.

The complications of NF1

If the NF1 phenotype consisted only of the features already discussed, the disease would be considered a dermatological problem which only occasionally causes significant morbidity in individuals with very many neurofibromas. It is the disease complications which make NF1 a disease with significant morbidity and mortality. As they can involve almost any body system, it also means that during their life-time individuals with NF1 may need to see any one of a number of specialists including dermatologists, clinical geneticists, neurologists, ophthalmologists, orthopaedic surgeons, paediatricians, and so on. Furthermore, the complications only occur in a proportion of patients and their occurrence cannot be predicted, even within families. Patients and their families find this uncertainty and the large number of different events that could happen, one of the most difficult aspects of the disease to come to terms with. From a doctor's viewpoint the challenge is to offer appropriate disease monitoring without causing unnecessary anxiety.

The exact frequency of complications in NF1 is difficult to determine because of underdiagnosis in mildly affected individuals and because of the failure to distinguish between the different forms of neurofibromatosis in some older studies (e.g. [14]). The Welsh study attempted to overcome this by performing a population-based study of only NF1 [37,40,41]. Even then, the data suggested that mildly affected individuals had been underascertained. The most accurate study of disease complications would come from following a large cohort of NF1 patients from birth and this has not been done.

Table 19.13.2 lists the NF1 disease complications, their frequency based on the Welsh study and their age of presentation. For detailed discussion of the different complications the reader is referred to one of the textbooks on neurofibromatosis [2,15,42]. Only those which may present in dermatological practice and learning difficulties (because of their frequency) are reviewed here. As can be seen in Table 19.13.2, the actual chance of patients developing many of the complications is small, only 1 or 2%; it is the relative risk of these conditions developing in NF1 when compared with the general population that is large.

Plexiform neurofibromas. In the older literature the terms elephantiasis neuromatosa or fibroma pendulum were often used to describe plexiform neurofibromas. These lesions take two forms clinically, diffuse and nodular, the former being the most frequent (present in 30% of cases in the Welsh study) [37]. None of the 135 patients in that study had a nodular plexiform neurofibroma.

Diffuse plexiform neurofibromas present as large subcutaneous swellings with ill-defined margins varying from a few centimetres in diameter to those which involve a whole area of the body (Fig. 19.13.4). Their consistency is usually soft, although within the mass hypertrophied nerve fibres can sometimes be palpated. The skin overlying them is often abnormal owing to a combination of hypertrophy, café-au-lait pigmentation or hypertrichosis. Diffuse plexiform neurofibromas develop in early childhood and are probably all obvious on careful examination within the first year or two of life.

They can occur anywhere on the body; in the Welsh

Table 19.13.2 The complications of NF1 (data derived from references 37,41)

Complications	Frequency (%)	Age of presentation
Plexiform neurofibromas		
All lesions	26.7	0–18
Large lesions of head and neck	1.2	0–1
Limb/trunk lesions associated with significant skin/bone hypertrophy	5.8	0–5
Intellectual Handicap		
Severe	0.8	
Moderate	2.4	
Minimal/learning difficulties	29.8	
Epilepsy		
No known cause	4.4	
Secondary to disease complications	2.2	Life long*
Hypsarrhythmia	1.5	0–5
CNS tumours		
Optic glioma†‡	1.5	0–20
Other CNS tumours	1.5	Life long
Spinal neurofibromas	1.5	Life long
Malignancy		
Peripheral nerve sarcoma	1.5	Life long
Pelvic rhabdomyosarcoma	1.5	0–5
Orthopaedic complications		
Scoliosis (requiring surgery)	4.4	0–18
Scoliosis (less severe)	5.2	
Pseudarthrosis of tibia and fibula	3.7	0–5
Vertebral scalloping‡§	10.0	
Other complications		
Aqueduct stenosis	1.5	0–30
Gastrointestinal neurofibromas	2.2	Life long
Renal artery stenosis	1.5	Life long
Phaeochromocytoma	0.7	From 10 years onwards
Duodenal carcinoid	1.5	
Congenital glaucoma	0.7	0–1
Juvenile xanthogranuloma	0.7	0–5
Complications not seen in Welsh study but definitely associated with NF1	Presumed frequency ≤1	
Sphenoid wing dysplasia§		Congenital
Lateral thoracic meningocele§		Life long
Atypical forms of childhood leukaemia		0–18
Cerebrovascular disease		Usually in childhood

* 'Life long' indicates cases have been reported presenting in all age groups.
† If cranial MRI scanning performed, found in 15% of cases.
‡ Feaures which are often asymptomatic and found on examination or imaging of appropriate body area.
§ Frequency from Riccardi [2].

study they were most frequent on the trunk (44% of lesions) followed by the limbs (38%) and the head and neck (18%). Plexiform neurofibromas in certain positions are associated with a characteristic appearance and associ-

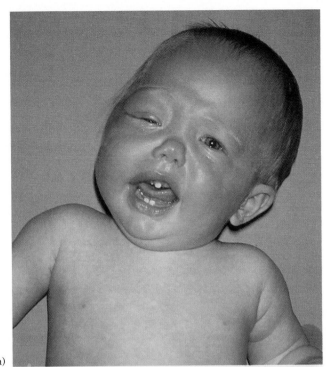

(a)

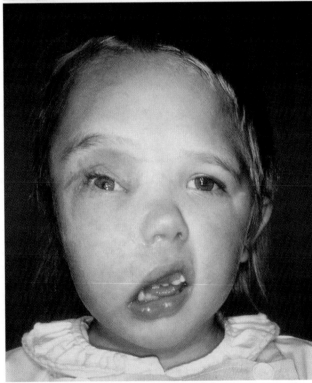

(b)

Fig. 19.13.4 Severe facial plexiform neurofibroma at 2 months (a) and 4 years of age (b), by which stage she had no useful sight in the right eye and several debulking operations. With permission from Chapman & Hall [15].

ated problems. For example on the face, when they involve the orbital area, they are often associated with sphenoid wing dysplasia. The most severe facial lesions involve all the branches of the trigeminal nerve and the resulting cosmetic disfigurement is significant [43,44]. Plexiform neurofibromas on the limbs may be associated with hypertrophy of underlying bones, giving rise to problems such as leg length discrepancy. Plexiform neurofibromas involving the perineal region in girls can be a cause of sexual ambiguity [45]. When assessing these lesions, the superficial area of involvement may be misleading in terms of the extent of the underlying lesion. Lesions in the pelvis can be associated with ureteric obstruction; those near the spinal column can erode the vertebrae and cause spinal collapse; and those in the region of the trachea can give rise to respiratory obstruction. Fortunately plexiform neurofibromas associated with these severe secondary problems are extremely rare. The majority of lesions are just associated with cosmetic problems and are rarely painful.

Nodular plexiform neurofibromas are lesions in which one or more nerves in an area develop multiple nodular neurofibromas almost continuously along their length. The age of onset of development of these lesions is uncertain. In our experience patients have presented during adolescence or early adulthood. The lesions have either presented as nodular subcutaneous masses (which have been misdiagnosed as lymph nodes in several patients) or because of pain.

Surgery for both types of plexiform neurofibromas is difficult because of their diffuse nature and ill-defined margins. They are often very vascular and definitive removal of those lesions involving major nerve trunks would obviously result in significant neurological deficit.

Plexiform neurofibromas harbour potential for sarcomatous degeneration, although the risk is probably small. This possibility should be considered in any plexiform lesion which begins to enlarge rapidly or becomes painful [46].

Juvenile xanthogranulomas. These lesions appear to be more common in NF1 than in the general population; 1 of 135 patients (0.7%) in the Welsh population had them. Their appearance and natural history seems to be similar in NF1 than when they occur in the general population. There have been several reports of the triple association of NF1, juvenile xanthogranuloma and juvenile myeloid leukaemia [47]. It is difficult to know whether this is a true association or simply a reflection of reporting bias a prospective follow-up study of children presenting with NF1 and juvenile xanthogranuloma is needed.

Learning difficulties. Aside from plexiform neurofibromas, learning difficulties are the most frequent NF1 complication. The learning difficulties in NF1 are relatively mild when compared with those seen in other pha-comatoses such as tuberous sclerosis. Indeed they are often not obvious in the preschool child. All the population-based studies of NF1 have shown that 25–30% of patients require some form of educational assistance, usually in the form of extra help in a normal school [48]. Several groups have looked at the neuropsychological profile of children with NF1 in detail [49–52]. All the studies showed an overall slight left shift of the IQ of the NF1 children compared with age-matched or sibling controls. Some of the studies showed that the children performed better on verbal than performance testing and had particular difficulties with visuospatial orientation, attention span and short-term memory. These problems are found in as many as 60% of NF1 children. The situation is further compounded with the frequency of co-ordination problems in NF1 children. In one study, 43% of the patients had co-ordination problems [52] and in another [49] all the NF1 individuals performed far worse than their unaffected siblings in a standardized examination for subtle neurological signs.

Intellectual handicap severe enough to present as developmental delay in preschool children is unusual in NF1. If a child with NF1 has significant developmental delay then a search should be made for underlying NF1 neurological problems and if none are found, then other unrelated causes of developmental delay should be investigated.

Natural history and prognosis

The morbidity and mortality of NF1 are largely dictated by the occurrence of its complications. Of the major defining features only the neurofibromas consistently cause the patients problems (usually from a cosmetic viewpoint), although children with very obvious café-au-lait spots are occasionally teased by their peer group. NF1 has only recently been the subject of systematic clinical research and so there are relatively few published long-term studies of patient cohorts [2,53,54]. Although cross-sectional studies like the Welsh one give some insight into the disease-related mortality. Of 25 deceased affected relatives, the cause of death was definitely attributable to NF1 in six cases (24%). The causes of death were pelvic rhabdomyosarcoma in two children aged 6 months and 2 years; a frontal astrocytoma in a 32-year-old patient; neurofibrosarcoma in a 24-year-old patient; obstructive hydrocephalus following removal of a neurofibroma at C1–2 in a 51-year-old patient; and acute left ventricular failure and haemorrhage into an undiagnosed phaeochromocytoma in a 54-year-old patient.

The best follow-up data available on NF1 patients are those from the 39-year follow-up of cases identified by Borberg in 1951 [13], undertaken by Sorenson *et al.* [53]. Survival rates to June 1983 of patients who were alive on 1 January 1944 were lower than the year, age and sex specific death rates of the general population. Mortality

was increased among probands, especially females, compared with affected relatives; female relatives had a survival rate just below that of the general population. Borberg's probands were originally identified through hospital inpatient records and the authors concluded that patients requiring admission to hospital had a poor prognosis, whereas incidentally diagnosed relatives had a considerably better outcome. This study also showed that NF1 patients with one malignancy (including CNS tumours and phaeochromocytoma) had an increased risk of developing a second malignancy, which occurred in 16 out of 70 patients (23%); this was compared with an expected rate of 4% in the general Danish population.

Thirty-nine of the 947 patients evaluated as part of Riccardi's neurofibromatosis research programme [2] had died during the follow-up period; in 28 cases the cause was related to NF1. The marked difference between this and the proportion of deaths related to NF1 in the Welsh study was probably due to ascertainment bias in a specialist neurofibromatosis clinic population. Neurofibrosarcoma was the cause of death in 17 of Riccardi's patients, with a mean age at death of 31.12 years. In 14 of the 17 patients, the malignancy arose in a pre-existing plexiform neurofibroma. Of the remaining 11 patients, five died of complications related to paraspinal neurofibromas; three from complications of diffuse plexiform neurofibromas; and single patients from an astrocytoma, metastatic carcinoid tumour and complications of childhood onset renovascular hypertension.

Zoller *et al.* [54] in 1995, reported a 12-year follow-up of the cohort originally described by Samuelsson and Axelson [55]. Twenty-two deaths occurred in the NF1 group, whereas 5.1 deaths were expected in the general Swedish population ($P < 0.001$). Of the listed causes of death they were clearly NF1 related in 10 out of 22 patients.

In terms of clinical practice, the question most frequently asked by parents of newly diagnosed children is 'How many neurofibromas will develop and what complications will arise?' Both questions are almost impossible to answer accurately from available data. None of the long-term studies have looked at neurofibroma development, cross-sectional studies [37] show the number of neurofibromas is roughly proportional to age, although the numbers within a given age group are very variable from patient to patient. With regard to complications, it seems reasonable that patients reaching adulthood with no serious complications have a relatively low risk of serious disease-related problems (see Table 19.13.2).

Differential diagnosis

The commonest conditions misdiagnosed as NF1 are other forms of neurofibromatosis, particularly segmental neurofibromatosis and NF2. The distribution of clinical features in the former are distinct and are discussed below.

NF2 should be considered in assessing children or teenagers with a few café-au-lait spots (usually six or less) in association with multiple nodular peripheral nerve lesions—the clinical appearance of peripheral schwannomas in NF2 is identical to that of peripheral nodular neurofibromas in NF1.

Young children who have six or more café-au-lait spots and no family history should be followed up. They usually have NF1, and other disease features usually appear [56]. Families with only autosomal dominant café-au-lait spots (see below) are extremely rare. Café-au-lait spots are recorded as a feature of many dysmorphic syndromes—presumably they simply reflect the one or two café-au-lait spots seen in the general population. The conditions other than NF1 that can result in more than six café-au-lait spots, are extremely rare. The authors have seen them in individuals with various ring chromosome syndromes (usually being investigated because of developmental delay and short stature), DNA repair syndromes such as ataxia telangiectasia and Schimke immuno-osseous dysplasia syndrome [57] where the individuals presented with a combination of extreme short stature, immunological and nephrological problems.

Other conditions that are confused with NF1 largely fall into two groups: (a) those associated with abnormal skin pigmentation confused with Café-au-lait spots; and (b) those associated with cutaneous or subcutaneous tumours. The former group include McCune–Albright syndrome, multiple lentigenes (LEOPARD) syndrome, Bannayan–Riley–Ruvalcaba syndrome, and urticaria pigmentosa. In the latter group multiple lipomatosis is by far the most common and adults presenting with multiple lipomas are often misdiagnosed as having NF1 in primary care. Rarer conditions include Proteus syndrome, congenital generalized fibromatosis and steatocystoma multiplex.

Management

It is recommended that individuals with NF1 have an annual clinical review [4,58,59,60]. The purpose of the assessment is to monitor disease progression, particularly with respect to the development of complications. The age of presentation of the various complications (see Table 19.13.2) must be appreciated. Thus, in the first 2 years of life one is particularly monitoring for plexiform neurofibromas, glaucoma, sphenoid wing dysplasia and pseudarthrosis. Psychological assessments become important in preschool children. Apart from learning difficulties and plexiform neurofibromas, most other complications of NF1 present with symptoms—the exception to this is hypertension due to renal artery stenosis or phaeochromocytoma, therefore the annual review of all ages must include blood pressure measurement. In the authors' opinion, there is no necessity for routine screening investigations, such as cranial magnetic resonance imaging (MRI) scans in the follow-up of asymptomatic patients.

There are no specific treatments for NF1 available that prevent any of the disease manifestations developing. Treatment of the different complications should be carried out by the appropriate specialist. Of the major defining features only the neurofibromas cause symptoms. Some patients complain of pruritus in relation to their neurofibromas (21% of the adult patients in the Welsh study complained that they had had pruritus in relation to their neurofibromas at some time) [37]. However, the principle problem is their cosmetic burden and the uncertainty as to how many will appear during a patient's life time. In the Welsh study, 20% of 94 adults were persistently distressed by the appearance of their neurofibromas. To offer the patients the chance to have each neurofibroma removed as it develops is unrealistic. It is more practical to encourage a patient to come to terms with the variation in NF1 and its natural history, and through this to accept the appearance of their cutaneous neurofibromas. Patients should be offered removal of particularly large or unsightly lesions on exposed parts of the body or those that are a problem because of rubbing on clothing. There seems to be no particular advantage in undertaking removal of neurofibromas by laser treatment as opposed to a standard surgical approach. Patients are helped by having access to a plastic or dermatological surgeon who is sympathetic to their problem and conscious of the importance of the cosmetic outcome of surgery.

Given the frequency of mast cells in neurofibromas, Riccardi [58,61] proposed that the itching was caused by release of compounds such as histamine and that mast cells play an important part in neurofibroma growth control. Riccardi has shown that the mast cell stabilizer ketotifen is effective in controlling neurofibroma-associated pruritus [2,62,63]. There was also some suggestion of a subjective control of growth rate. Another observation was that patients who underwent surgery whilst on treatment were noted to have a decreased amount of blood loss from tumours during the operation. In the authors' experience, very few of the patients have found their pruritus severe enough to want to take regular medication. Experience with ketotifen in other centres has been less conclusive. Rubinstein A. (personal communication, 1992) embarked on a trial of its use in controlling pruritus, alternating the drug with a placebo for 2-month periods during an 8-month trial. From a clinic population of 400 NF1 patients, only 12 (3%) had persistent and generalized pruritus. In view of the small numbers the trial was not completed. Assessment of 12 patients suggested an effect on pruritus but not on growth.

Many tertiary referral centres now have a specialized neurofibromatosis clinic. In this setting, patients are offered co-ordinated care and follow-up by a group of health professionals, including a paediatrician, ophthalmologist, dermatologist, neurologist, neurosurgeon, orthopaedic surgeon, otolaryngologist, plastic surgeon, clinic geneticist, specialist genetic nurse/genetic counseller, social worker and psychologist. Usually one of the group acts as the overall co-ordinator of patient care and involves the others at certain times in the patient's life or because of specific symptoms. As most patients with NF1 will never develop major complications not all patients need to attend a specialist clinic on a regular basis. After initial assessment in the Oxford clinic, many of the patients are discharged to follow-up with paediatricians in childhood and with their general practitioners in adulthood. The clinic is used for family support when NF1 is newly diagnosed, specialist genetic counselling and assessment of unusual symptoms or complications.

With regard to genetic counselling, the 50% risk to offspring of an affected individual is straightforward; more difficult to share with families is the varied and unpredictable nature of the disease. If one presumes that the concerns of prospective parents will include moderate to severe mental retardation, the complications that develop in childhood and cause life-long morbidity and the risk of developing a brain tumour or malignant tumour elsewhere, then the combined risk to offspring of an affected parent of developing one of these complications is 8% [41].

If children at risk of NF1 have not developed multiple café-au-lait spots by the end of their second year of life, then it is unlikely that they have inherited the NF1 gene. The Oxford clinic offers the children annual review until the age of 5 years to ensure disease status. In the 50% of cases with no family history, examination of the skin and eyes of the parents is important, as children with NF1 have been born to parents with segmental neurofibromatosis or Lisch nodules as their only disease feature—these parents would have a higher risk of recurrence than parents with no disease features, where the chance of having another child with NF1 is probably only a little above that of the general population risk [41,64,65].

Neurofibromatosis type 2

NF2 was not established as a separate entity until 1970 [66]. It is now clear that NF1 and NF2 are distinct both at a clinical and molecular level. The clinical overlap arises because café-au-lait spots and peripheral nerve tumours occur in both conditions. In NF2, however, the nerve tumours are schwannomas and not neurofibromas. NF2 is much less variable than NF1 with the symptomatic disease features being limited to the nervous system (including the eye). The majority of patients develop bilateral acoustic neuromas, usually in early adulthood. NF2 is much less common than NF1 with a prevalence of 1 in 210 000 and an estimated birth incidence of 1 in 33 000–40 562 [67].

Detailed discussion of the presentation and management of the neurological features of NF2 is inappropriate here (see references 68–70 for detailed reviews).

Definition

The initial NIH diagnostic criteria for NF2 [4] proved too narrow for routine clinical use. The original NIH Consensus Development Conference criteria proved too narrow for routine clinical use. A number of authors have suggested expansion of the criteria [67,68,69]. The most recent by Gutman *et al.* [60] recommend two categories of patients, those with definite NF2 and those with presumptive or probable NF2. The purpose of having the latter grouping is to identify individuals who need to be kept under long-term surveillance for the development of other disease features. The criteria proposed by Gutman *et al.*, which are widely accepted, are as follows.

1 Individuals with the following clinical features have confirmed (definite) NF2.
- Bilateral vestibular Schwannomas (VS).
- A family history of NF2 [first-degree relatives] *plus* a unilateral VS diagnosed less than 30 years or any two of: meningioma, glioma, Schwannoma, juvenile posterior subcapsular lenticular opacities/juvenile cortical cataracts.

2 Individuals with the following clinical features should be evaluated for NF2 (presumptive or probable NF2).
- Unilateral VS less than 30 years *plus* at least one of the following: meningioma, glioma, Schwannoma, juvenile posterior subcapsular lenticular opacities/juvenile cortical cataracts.
- Multiple meningiomas (two or more) plus unilateral VS diagnosed less than 30 years or one of the following: glioma, schwannoma, juvenile posterior subcapsular lenticular opacities/juvenile cortical cataracts.

Pathogenesis

NF2 is an autosomal dominant condition. About half the patients presenting will have no family history. The *NF2* gene was provisionally localized to chromosome 22 through studies of loss of heterozygosity of chromosome 22 DNA markers in acoustic neuromas in 1986 [71]. This was confirmed by linkage studies the following year [72]. The identification of germ-line deletions in NF2 patients in the critical area of chromosome 22 facilitated the cloning of the diseased gene in 1993 [73,74]. The *NF2* gene is a tumour suppressor gene which spans 110 kb and comprises 16 constitutive exons and one alternatively spliced exon. The *NF2* gene sequence shows strong harmology to the highly conserved protein 4.1 family. The *NF2* encoded protein is most similar to moezin, ezrin and radixin and it was named Merlin (moezin–ezrin–radixin-like protein) [74]. The primary role of the protein 4.1 family appears to be in mediating communication between the extracellular milieu and the cytoskeleton.

Pathology

Of the tumours that can occur in NF2, only the schwannoma is likely to present to the dermatologist for diagnosis and hence is the only one discussed here. Schwannomas are histologically distinct from neurofibromas although terminology can be confusing as schwannomas are sometimes referred to as neurinomas, neurilemmomas or neuromas. In addition, occasional tumours from patients with both NF1 and NF2 can have mixed histology with schwannomatous and neurofibromatous components [33]. Clinically, it is impossible to distinguish schwannomas and neurofibromas when they occur on major peripheral nerves, the cutaneous lesions seen in NF2 are more easily distinguishable as discussed below.

Macroscopically, the surface of the schwannoma is usually firm and the tissue has a white or yellowish colour. The nerve of origin can often be identified in the capsule of the tumour [33,75]. Microscopically, fusiform cells predominate within a fibrous capsule [76]. Many schwannomas show a biphasic histopathological growth pattern. One architecture, designated Antoni type A, consists of interwoven fascicles of elongated cells with conspicuous spindle-shaped nuclei that often exhibit palisading and contribute to the formation of Verocay bodies. Occasionally, the spindle cells form whirls resembling those found in meningiomas or isolated wavy fascicles similar to those occurring in neurofibromas [75]. The other architecture (Antoni type B) consists of a reticular, microcystic appearance, lower cellularity and regressive changes including fatty degeneration and accumulation of macrophages. Immunochemical reactivity can be useful in distinguishing schwannomas from other spindle cell neoplasms [33]. The calcium-binding protein S100 is strongly expressed in both normal and neoplastic Schwann cells.

Clinical features

The major features of NF2 are bilateral acoustic neuromas. Histologically, these lesions are schwannomas which develop on the vestibular branch of the acoustic nerve and some authors now refer to them as vestibular schwannomas. They develop in 85–92% of NF2 patients [68,69], a further 6% of cases in both these series had unilateral lesions. The first symptoms of NF2 that the patient experiences are usually related to their acoustic neuromas and consist of deafness, with or without associated vertigo and/or tinnitus. The lesions usually become symptomatic in early adult life (average age 22.6 years, range 2–52 years in the study of Evans *et al.* [68]). Other neurological tumours that may develop are meningiomas (45% of cases), spinal root schwannomas (26%), astrocytomas (4%) and ependymomas (2.5%). These lesions present with symptoms relating to their site or origin.

Dermatological features of NF2

A small but significant number of NF2 patients seek a dermatological consultation prior to the onset of symptoms from their neurological tumours because of the development of cutaneous or subcutaneous disease-related lesions. Those with more florid skin involvement are occasionally misdiagnosed as having NF1 prior to the development of the more characteristic NF2 tumours.

Dermatological involvement in NF2, is much more marked in those patients with the severe form of NF2 who present at a younger age—hence the importance of the awareness of paediatric dermatologists of this form of neurofibromatosis. NF2 patients fall into two broad categories clinically. There is quite marked intrafamily similarity in disease course, but marked interfamilial variation. Those patients presenting with what has been designated as mild NF2, tend to have principally bilateral acoustic neuromas as their only symptomatic lesions presenting after the age of 25 years. Those with the severe form of NF2 often present in childhood with a meningioma or spinal schwannoma. The patients with the severe form of NF2 tend to have multiple nervous system tumours and their acoustic neuromas become symptomatic before the age of 25 years. Cutaneous involvement is much more likely than in the mild form of the disease.

Café-au-lait spots. These are present in more NF2 patients than in the general population; 43% of patients in the study of Evans *et al.* [68] had between one and six spots. Thirty-nine per cent of cases had three or less spots, 3% had four spots and only 1% six spots. It is therefore only very occasional NF2 cases that have sufficient café-au-lait spots to satisfy the NF1 diagnostic criteria and therefore should not be easily confused. The other point is that NF2 patients do not develop the other pigmentary anomalies seen in NF1 such as axillary freckling.

Peripheral nerve tumours. These occur less consistently and in much smaller numbers than in NF1. In the study of Evans *et al.* [68], 68% of patients had peripheral nerve tumours, which varied in number from one to 27. Clinically, there are three types of peripheral nerve tumour in NF2, although histologically they are usually schwannomas. However, as discussed above some may be mislabelled as neurofibromas and others may have a mixed appearance histologically. In cases where the diagnostic debate is between NF1 and NF2 it is worth a review of tumour histology by an experienced neuropathologist; a diagnosis of schwannoma makes NF2 the likely diagnosis. The three types of peripheral nerve tumours that are distinguishable clinically in NF2 are as follows.

NF2 plaques. These are the most frequent cutaneous lesions in NF2 and occurred in 48% of patients in the

Evans *et al.* study [68]. They are discrete, well-circum-scribed, slightly raised cutaneous lesions usually less than 2 cm in diameter. Their surface is roughened, may be slightly pigmented and often contains excess hair. The age at which these lesions develop has not been formally studied, but they probably develop in early childhood (Fig. 19.13.5).

Peripheral nerve schwannomas. These appear clinically like the nodular tumours in NF1. They are subcutaneous, often spherical lesions that develop on the larger periph-eral nerves. The nerve is often thickened at either end of the tumour and a number of nodular tumours may develop in one particular part of the same nerve. Forty-three per cent of patients in the Evans *et al.* study had these lesions [68].

NF1-like cutaneous lesions. The least common type of peripheral tumour is similar to the dermal neurofibromas seen in NF1 and have a violaceous colour. They occurred in 27% of patients in the Evans *et al.* study [68], but were much fewer in number than would normally be seen in an adult with NF1.

Ophthalmological features. These are usually asympto-matic but are useful in diagnostic confirmation. However, a minority of NF2 patients will initially present in early childhood with visual problems due to their disease, e.g. a cataract causing symptoms or an optic nerve sheath meningioma or a particularly large retinal hamartoma developing in an area critical for vision.

Cataracts were present in 81% of the patients in the series of Parry *et al.* [69], 72.4% had posterior capsular cataracts, 41.4% had cortical cataracts and 32.8% had both types. The lesions only caused significant visual distur-bance in two of 47 individuals. The exact frequency of the other ocular features in NF2 is uncertain; they occur much less frequently than the lens changes. They include retinal hamartomas (either combined pigment epithelium and retinal hamartomas, congenital hypertrophy of retinal pigment epithelium or astrocytic hamartomas), epiretinal membranes and optic discs gliomas.

Differential diagnosis

As discussed above, the main differential diagnosis is from NF1 in those cases with more marked peripheral manifestations. There may also be some families who are just predisposed to the development of multiple schwan-nomas (often referred to as schwannomatosis) and this entity is discussed below.

Other neurofibromatoses

Only those conditions which present to a dermatologist are discussed here. For a review of all possible forms of neurofibromatosis see Riccardi [2] and Viskochil and Carey [77].

Segmental or mosaic neurofibromatosis type 1

Definition, prevalence and history

The term segmental NF1 is used to describe patients with one or more NF1 disease features limited to specific body segments. Segmental NF1 has been reported with increas-ing frequency. In a review of the literature up to 1995 we identified 140 cases. In terms of frequency of cases referred to the Oxford Neurofibromatosis Clinic segmental NF1 appears to be at least as common as NF2 and a clinical study is on-going in our region; the cases ascertained to date give a prevalence for segmental NF1 of 1 in 70–80 000 of the population (on 0.0013%).

The first case was reported by Gammel in 1931 [78]. He described a 60-year-old man with multiple neurofibromas confined to a limited area of the abdomen and referred to it as localized neurofibromatosis. Crowe *et al.* [14] in their large study of neurofibromatosis identified four cases with café-au-lait spots and/or neurofibromas in restricted areas of the body. They termed the disease sectorial neurofibromatosis and postulated somatic mosaicism of the NF1 gene as the likely cause. In 1977 Miller and Sparkes [79] suggested the term segmental neurofi-bromatosis which has become widely used. Roth *et al.* [80] reported four new cases and reviewed the literature up to 1987. They suggested that even within segmental neurofibromatosis different clinical subtypes were emerg-ing which they divided as follows [80].
1 True segmental neurofibromatosis or unilateral seg-mental—disease features limited to a unilateral segment of the body.
2 Bilateral segmental—where segments of the body are involved on both sides of the midline which can either be symmetrical or asymmetrical.
3 Segmental cases with deep involvement—those with segmental skin changes associated with underlying NF1 complications such as deep neurofibromas or bony dys-plastic changes.
4 Hereditary segmental—to describe cases where parents with segmental neurofibromatosis had transmitted the full-blown disorder to their offspring.

The above authors simply refer to segmental neuro-fibromatosis. With the very clear distinction between NF1 and NF2 it is important to use the term segmental NF1, particularly as cases with unilateral features of NF2 have been reported [68]. A further possible change in terminology would be to use the term *mosaic NF1* to reflect the probable disease pathogenesis and to enable the inclu-sion of cases who clinically have mild generalized NF1 but have been shown to be mosaic at the molecular level [81].

Pathogenesis

The assumed pathogenesis of segmental NF1 is somatic mosaicism of a mutation in the NF1 gene, although this is as yet unproven at the molecular level in a case with segmental involvement. Colman *et al.* [81] and Ainsworth *et al.* [82] have described individuals with generalized NF1 clinically but who were mosaic for an NF1 mutation on molecular analysis. Presumably the phenotype of somatic mutation of the NF1 gene depends upon the timing of the mutation. Viskochil and Carey [77] have proposed that cases of segmental NF1 should be classified according to the somatic mutation hypothesis determined by (a) the timing of the mutation (early versus late embryonic development); and (b) the source of tissue affected by the mutation. Taken to its extremes this hypothesis would mean that the reported cases of generalized NF1 who are mosaic at the molecular level, represent mutations occurring very early in embryonic development, the extreme of which would be mutation in the zygote. At the other end of the spectrum would be the individuals with isolated café-au-lait spots or neurofibromas and no other disease features, the lesions representing somatic mutation in terminally differentiated cells.

The somatic mutation scheme of Viskochil and Carey has four categories.
1 Single site/single manifestation, i.e. late neural crest mutation leading to a single disease manifestation.
2 Single site/multiple manifestations, e.g. early neural crest mutation leading to café-au-lait spots and neurofibromas in a distinct location.
3 Multiple site/single manifestation, i.e. bilateral dermatomal neurofibromas arising from a midline mutation early in somite development.
4 Multiple site/multiple manifestations, i.e. the full NF1 phenotype in patients with zygotic or very early postzygotic mutation.

Genetics

The majority of reported cases of segmental NF1 have no affected relatives with the disease. There are, however, a handful of cases [64,83–86] (reviewed in [64]) where parents with segmental NF1 have children with full-blown disease; it is assumed these cases represent gonosomal mosaics with involvement of both somatic and gonadal tissue. A further family reported by Uhlin [87], in which a patient with segmental NF1 had an aunt and cousins with generalized disease might be explained by the dominant inheritance of an NF1 premutation in all cells. From the clinical viewpoint these cases emphasize the importance of examining both the skin and irides of parents of apparently isolated cases of NF1. It is of note that Riccardi and Lewis [84] reported a family where a mother had more than 100 Lisch nodules bilaterally as the only manifestation of NF1, and her two sons both had generalized NF1; a similar family has been reported (R. Tenconi, personal communication, 1996) where a mother had only unilateral Lisch nodules and a son with full-blown NF1. It is important to realize that even though the segment of the body affected is distant from the gonads, there can be gonadal involvement. Therefore, it is difficult to reassure individuals fully with apparent segmental NF1 that there is no risk of NF1 occurring in their offspring (the issue of genetic counselling is discussed in the section on management). More difficult to explain pathogenetically are the cases of vertical transmission of segmental NF1 reported by Rubinstein *et al.* [83] and Segal *et al.* [88,89]. In the family of Rubinstein *et al.* a 59-year-old father had multiple dermal neurofibromas over the left trunk, and his 21-year-old daughter a recurrent surgically excised plexiform neurofibroma of the left side of the face. The case of Segal *et al.* was a 62-year-old father with a 39-year history of 30 operations for removal of painful nodular neurofibromas from the left leg who had a 32-year-old daughter with two neurofibromas removed from the left flank. A chromosome 1:5 balanced translocation (p32;q31) was found on cytogenetic studies in the skin biopsies taken from the father's affected region but not from the right leg or lymphocyte culture. No analysis was available on the daughter [88]. Among the cases referred to the Oxford Neurofibromatosis Clinic the authors identified two further families with apparent vertical transmission of segmental NF1: a father with multiple localized dermal and nodular neurofibromas had a daughter with a segmental ('checkerboard') [90,91] pattern of distribution of café-au-lait spots and freckling, and a mother with freckling in a dermatomal distribution had a son with localized NF1 pigmentary changes. The apparent occurrence of segmental NF1 in successive generations is difficult to explain on the basis of gonosomal mosaicism. One must speculate that in these families an NF1 gene is segregating which has variable expression within the same individual. One possibility is an inherited premutation which has become a full mutation only in certain body areas. Another mechanism could be that the NF1 gene in these families, for some reason is expressed normally and abnormally in different parts of the body. This might be explained genetically by inactivation caused by positional-effect variegation [92].

Clinical features

Patients with segmental NF1 usually seek a medical opinion because of the unusual appearance of the affected area. Some of the cases the authors have seen have been initially diagnosed as generalized NF1. The clinical features of segmental NF1, as predicted by the somatic mutation hypothesis, reflect the timing of the mutation in relation to embryonic development and the tissues

Table 19.13.3 Clinical features of segmental NF1 in 140 reported cases (data derived from references 14,64,78–80,83–89,93–162) and 45 cases seen in the Oxford Neurofibromatosis Clinic

	Literature (1931–95)	Oxford (1990–96)
Total no. of patients	140	45
Unilateral		
No. of patients	106	25
Sex	42 M; 53 F; 11 unknown	11 M; 14 F
Age (mean; range)	43 years; 10 months to 83 years	29 years; 7–55 years
Age at presentation (mean; range)	23 years; birth to 74 years	4 years; birth to 45 years
No. of patients with CAL+freckles	20	14 (14 with 'HB')
No. of patients with multiple NFs only	57 (3 with PNF+NFs)	6 (none with 'HB')
No. of patients with CAL (freckles)+NFs	29 (4 with PNF+CAL)	5 (5 with 'HB')
No. of patients with NF1 complications	12 (PNFs (2), MH (2), STH+VD (1), epilepsy (3), scoliosis (3), FH (1))	13 [PNFs (4), LD (2), scoliosis (3), PDA (2), OPG (1), tongue NFs (1)]
Extent of lesions		
entire hemibody	4	1
one body segment	20	9
dermatomal distribution	82	15
Lish nodules		
present	6	1
not examined	21	0
Inherited segmental NF1 (no. of families)		
segmental to full-blown NF1 transmission	7	2
segmental to segmental transmission	2	0
Bilateral		
symmetrical		
No. of patients	14	7
Sex	5 M; 9 F	2 M; 5 F
Age (mean range)	51; 7–70 years	36; 14–60 years
Age at presentation (mean; range)	15; 7–68 years	16; birth to 30 years
No. of patients with CAL+freckles	1 (only Lisch nodules)	0
No. of patients with multiple NFs only	8 (1 with NFs+PNF)	6 (none with 'HB')
No. of patients with CAL (freckles)+NFs	5 (1 with PNF+CAL)	1 (1 with 'HB')
No. of patients with NF1 complications	3 [PNFs (2), clitoral hypertrophy (1)]	0
Extent of lesions		
entire hemibody	0	0
one body segment	3	3
dermatomal distribution	13	4
Lisch nodules		
present	1	0
not examined	2	0
Inherited segmental NF (no. of families)		
segmental NF1 to full-blown NF1 transmission	1	0
segmental to segmental transmission	0	0
asymmetrical		
No. of patients	13	12
Sex	4 M; 9 F;	8 M; 4 F
Age (mean; range)	29; 11–58 years	22; 9–70 years
Age at presentation (mean; range)	29; 6–47 years	4.5; birth to 44 years
No. of patients with CAL+freckles	3 (1 with only multiple CAL)	9 (9 with 'HB')
No. of patients with multiple NFs only	3	1 (none with 'HB')
No. of patients with CAL (freckles)+NFs	7 (1 with only PNF+CAL)	2 (1 with 'HB')
No. of patients with NF1 complications	2 [scoliosis (1), epilepsy (1)]	4 LD (2), PDA (1), scoliosis (1)
Extent of lesions		
entire hemibody	0	0
one body segment	0	0
dermatomal distribution	13	12
Lisch nodules		
present	0	2
not examined	5	0
Inherited segmental NF (no. of families)		
segmental NF1 to full-blown NF1 transmission	0	0
segmental to segmental NF1 transmission	0	2

Continued

Table 19.13.3 *Continued*

	Literature (1931–95)	Oxford (1990–96)
Plexiform neurofibromas only		
No. of patients	7	1
Sex	0 M; 7 F	1 M; 0 F
Age (mean; range)	22.5 years; 23–30 years	14
Age at presentation (mean; range)	13.8 years; birth to 24 years	12 months
Extent of lesion		
unilateral	5	1
bilateral	2	0
Café-au-lait spots	—	—
Freckling	—	—
Dermal/nodular NFs	—	—
Lisch nodules	—	—
Other NF1 complications	—	—
Inherited segmental NF (no. of families)		
segmental NF1 to full-blown NF1 transmission	0	0
segmental to segmental NF1 transmission	0	0

CAL, café-au-lait spots; F, female; FH, face hemihypertrophy; 'HB', hyperpigmented background; LD, learning difficulties; M, male; MH, mental handicap; NFs, neurofibromas; OPG, optic pathways glioma; PDA, pseudarthrosis; PNF, plexiform neurofibromas; STH, soft tissue hypertrophy; VD, vascular dilatation.

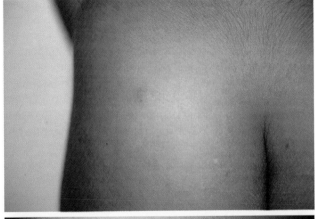

(a)

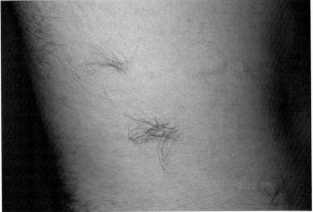

(b)

Fig. 19.13.5 (a) NF2 plaque in a ten-year-old girl who was referred to the Oxford Neurofibromatosis Clinic because of an unusual combination of skin features. These included a vulval plexiform neurofibroma (clinical diagnosis, no biopsy taken) and a variety of hypo- and hyper-pigmented skin lesions. On review some of these were NF2 plaques. Neuroaxis scanning was undertaken and it showed bilateral acoustic neuromas and several other lesions compatible with the diagnosis of NF2. (b) NF2 plaques made more obvious by their hair growth in a 16-year-old patient with NF2.

involved. This is reflected clinically in a very varying phenotype. The area of involvement has varied from one segment to one half of the body or more than one involved segment of the body on both sides of the midline either in a symmetrical or asymmetrical arrangement. Unilateral involvement has been generally ascribed to patients with involvement of one segment or one half of the body. Within the affected area there may be café-au-lait spots plus or minus freckling or neurofibromas alone; these features together; or one of these combinations plus an associated NF1 complication (Fig. 19.13.5). Table 19.13.3 summarizes the clinical findings in the 140 cases reported to 1995 [14,64,78–80,83–89,93–162] and the 45 patients assessed in the Oxford Neurofibromatosis Clinic.

The authors are at present undertaking a more detailed clinical and molecular study of segmental NF1. What is not clear is whether the segment involved has a dermatomal distribution or follows Blaschko's lines as suggested by Moss and Green [64]. Our preliminary impression is that some of the cases with neurofibromas alone appear to have a dermatomal distribution, whereas those with pigmentary changes alone have a distribution suggesting that they developed along Blaschko's lines. When looking at age of presentation of skin lesions it seems clear that patients with an earlier onset of symptoms are those with pigmentary changes, and those with neurofibromas alone develop lesions at older ages. Nonetheless, it is of note that not all of those with pigmentary changes develop neurofibromas when they grow older.

The appearance of the individual neurofibromas is exactly the same as when they occur in the generalized disease. However, at least in some patients, the segment involved seems to be more severely affected even if it lies in parts of the body not usually associated with dense neurofibromas in the generalized disease. This accords with Happle [163] who has reported severe involvement of the affected area in other mosaic skin disorders. Happle suggests that in segmental forms of autosomal dominant skin disorders, two different types of manifestations, reflecting different states of zygosity, can be distinguished: (a) a mild type of involvement, corresponding to that encountered in the non-mosaic phenotype, which reflects a heterozygous state of the underlying postzygotic mutation; and (b) a severe type of manifestation which would reflect a loss of heterozygosity for the same allele. Due to reduced penetrance, the heterozygous state may go unnoticed, whereas allelic loss will result in a severe type of mosaic manifestation.

In cases with pigmentary changes, and in those with pigmentary changes and associated neurofibromas, often the whole segment of skin is darker than the unaffected parts of the body (see Table 19.13.3), suggesting that the NF1 gene affects the pigment of the whole skin and not just the area within café-au-lait spots or freckles. Within the affected segment of skin there are multiple café-au-lait spots and/or freckling (and/or neurofibromas). Several of the authors' patients have had intense freckling within the affected segment, regardless of where this segment is situated on the body. Moss and Green [64] have suggested that some cases of naevus spilus represent segmental NF1 and the authors would agree with this.

Patients with solitary plexiform neurofibromas presumably also have a form of segmental NF1. We found eight such patients reported as segmental NF1 in the literature reviewed and we have observed one further case at the Oxford Neurofibromatosis Clinic (see Table 19.13.3). The clinical features and natural history of such lesions appear to be the same as when the occur as a complication of the generalized disease.

Management

These is no management specific to segmental NF1. Patients need to be advised they do not have generalized NF1 and are at a low risk of developing any disease-associated complications (see Table 19.13.3). Those considering children need to be aware of the small risk of having a child with generalized NF1. The exact level of risk is not definable with present knowledge. Studies of pigmentary anomalies in chimeric mice suggest the degree of gonadal involvement is proportional to the area of skin involved [164]. In clinical practice, the authors emphasize the low risk compared with generalized NF1 and if the patient is helped by an estimate of risk we use an empiric figure depending on the size of the segment involved.

Autosomal dominant café-au-lait spots alone

There have been a handful of families reported worldwide with multiple café-au-lait spots as the only disease feature segregating as an autosomal dominant [2,165–167]. The segregation of DNA markers in the region of the NF1 gene has been studied in three of these families. Two showed evidence of non-linkage [165,166] and the other appeared to be linked to the NF1 locus [167]. When assessing children with multiple café-au-lait spots as the only feature and no family history, NF1 is by far the most likely diagnosis [56], although the diagnosis cannot be confirmed until other disease features appear.

Watson's syndrome

In 1967, Watson [168] described three families with the combined features of pulmonary stenosis, multiple café-au-lait spots and intelligence at the lower end of the normal range, segregating as an autosomal dominant. The features which distinguished the condition from NF1 were pulmonary stenosis and the fact that intellectual problems were found in all members of the family which is unusual in NF1. A few similar families have since been reported. Allanson *et al.* [169] followed up the original Watson patients and confirmed that their phenotype had remained distinct from typical NF1. Although a few individuals have had Lisch nodules on slit lamp examination, and some had developed neurofibromas, both of these features were present at a very much lower frequency than is usually seen in NF1. The same group demonstrated linkage with markers for the NF1 gene in two families. Subsequently Tassabehji *et al.* [170] have identified an NF1 mutation in a separate Watson's syndrome family. The pathogenesis of this very distinctive phenotype is unclear.

Schwannomatosis

This term is used to describe patients with a predisposition to developing multiple schwannomas but without other features of NF2. As is the case with other forms of neurofibromatosis, the older literature on the subject tends to be confusing. One reason is because of different terminology, some authors preferring the term neurilemmomatosis [171]. Further confusion arises from the fact that some reports include cases who would now be considered to have definite NF2 or who were too young for this diagnosis to be excluded at the time of reporting [171,172].

Despite this, it is the experience of those who have assessed large numbers of NF2 cases [173,174] that within their cohort are patients with only peripheral and spinal nerve schwannomas. MacCollin *et al.* [173] have reported on 14 patients with multiple schwannomas but without acoustic nerve involvement seen at the neurofibromatosis clinic at the Massachusetts General Hospital. Of these three had lesions localized on one limb suggesting somatic mosaicism. Of the other 11 patients, two had only peripheral nerve schwannomas, six had peripheral and spinal schwannomas, one had peripheral and cranial nerve schwannomas, one had spinal and cranial nerve schwannomas and one had only spinal involvement. Only one patient had a positive family history. They conclude the most likely pathogenetic mechanism is an autosomal dominant tumour suppressor gene, which may be allelic to the NF2 gene; they commented, however, that the absence of family history in so many cases would be unusual for this model.

Evans *et al.* [174] report on their experience of schwannomatosis in the UK. There were 21 familial cases from five families and seven isolated cases. They emphasize the overlap between schwannomatosis and NF2, in their familial cases the majority of affected members only had multiple schwannomas, but one or two members in each case had either a unilateral acoustic neuroma or a meningioma. In one of their families a brother and sister were considered to have the classical phenotype of schwannomatosis for many years, until one of them developed bilateral acoustic neurofibromas at the age of 44 years; this patient's son had a more typical course of classical NF2 with bilateral acoustic neurofibromas diagnosed on scan at the age of 22 years. The majority of their cases, however, only had peripheral and spinal schwannomas. DNA markers for the NF2 gene segregated with the disease in their two largest families. They conclude that schwannomatosis is likely allelic to NF2 with particular mutations predisposing to this relatively specific phenotype.

Presentation of schwannomatosis in dermatology clinics

As many of the reported cases have presented because of their peripheral nerve lesions, initial presentation to a dermatology clinic is not unusual. Patients must be carefully screened for other signs of NF2 and offered long-term follow-up for monitoring for the development of further lesions. They should also be referred for genetic counselling. It is hoped with further understanding of the pathogenesis of the condition at the molecular level that diagnostic DNA tests will be developed.

Acknowledgements

Dr M. Ruggieri has been funded by Consiglio Nazionale delle Ricerche (CNR), Rome, Italy, grant no. Al96.00176.04, and is a recipient of a PhD in Paediatrics by MURST, from the Division of Paediatric Neurology, Paediatric Clinic, University of Catania, Italy. He also acknowledges the IBFSNC, CNR, Catania, Italy and the Oxfordshire Health Services Research Committee for research support. We thank Jennifer Wright for her tireless secretarial assistance.

REFERENCES

1 Riccardi VM. Neurofibromatosis: clinical heterogeneity. *Curr Prob Cancer* 1982; 7: 1–34.

2 Riccardi VM. *Neurofibromatosis: Phenotype, Natural History and Pathogenesis*, 2nd edn. Baltimore: Johns Hopkins University Press, 1992.

3 Viskochil D, Carey JC. Nosological considerations of the neurofibromatoses. *J Dermatol* 1992; 19: 873–80.

4 National Institutes of Health Consensus Development Conference Statement: Neurofibromatosis. *Arch Neurol* 1988; 45: 575–8.

5 Huson SM, Clark P, Compston DAS, Harper PS. A genetic study of von Recklinghausen neurofibromatosis in south east Wales I: Prevalence, fitness, mutation rate, and effect of parental transmission on severity. *J Med Genet* 1989; 26: 704–11.

6 Zanca A, Zanca A. Antique illustrations of neurofibromatosis. *Int J Dermatol* 1980; 19: 55–8.

7 Hecht F. Recognition of neurofibromatosis before von Recklinghausen. *Neurofibromatosis* 1989; 2: 180–4.

8 Huson SM. Neurofibromatosis: historical perspective, classification and diagnostic criteria. In: Huson SM, Hughes RAC, eds. *The Neurofibromatoses: a Pathogenetic and Clinical Overview*. London: Chapman & Hall, 1994: 1–22.

9 Smith RW. *A Treatise on the Pathology, Diagnosis and Treatment of Neurofibroma*. Dublin: Hodges & Smith, 1849.

10 von Recklinghausen FD. *Ueber die Multiplen Fibrome der Haut und ihre Beziehung zu den Multiplen Neuromen*. Berlin: Hirschwald, 1882.

11 Marie P, Bernard A. Neurofibromatose généralisée. *Soc Med Hop Paris* 1896; 13: 777.

12 Chauffard MA. Dermato-fibromatose pigmentaire (ou neurofibromatose généralisée). *Soc Med Hop Paris* 1896; 13: 200.

13 Borberg A. Clinical and Genetic Investigations into Tuberous Sclerosis and Recklinghausen's Neurofibromatosis. Acta Psychiat Neurol, 1951 (suppl); 71: 1–239.

14 Crowe FW, Schull WJ, Neel JV. *A Clinical, Pathological and Genetic Study of Multiple Neurofibromatosis*. Springfield, Illinois: C. Thomas, 1956.

15 Huson SM, Hughes RAC. *The Neurofibromatoses: a Pathogenetic and Clinical Overview*. London: Chapman & Hall, 1994.

16 Barker D, Wright E, Nguyen K *et al.* Gene for von Recklinghausen's neurofibromatosis is in the pericentromeric region of chromosome 17. *Science* 1987; 236: 1100–2.

17 Seizinger BR, Rouleau GA, Ozelius LG *et al.* Genetic linkage of von Recklinghausen neurofibromatosis to the nerve growth factor receptor gene. *Cell* 1987; 49: 589–94.

18 Cawthon RM, Weiss R, Xu G *et al.* A major segment of the neurofibromatosis type 1 gene: cDNA sequence, genomic structure and point mutations. *Cell* 1990; 62: 193–201.

19 Viskochil D, Buchberg AM, Xu G *et al.* Deletions and a translocation interrupt a cloned gene at the neurofibromatosis type 1 locus. *Cell* 1990; 62: 187–92.

20 Wallace MR, Marchuk DA, Anderson LB *et al.* Type 1 neurofibromatosis gene: identification of a large transcript disrupted in three NF1 patients. *Science* 1990; 249: 181–6.

21 Von Deimling A, Krone W, Menon AG. Neurofibromatosis type 1: pathology, clinical features and molecular genetics. *Brain Pathol* 1995; 5: 153–62.

22 Upadhyaya M, Cooper DN. *Neurofibromatosis type 1 from genotype to phenotype*. Oxford: Bios Scientific Publishers Ltd, 1998.

23 Jacks T, Shih TS, Schmitt EM, Brionson RT, Bernards A, Weinberg RA. Tumour predisposition in mice heterozygous for a targeted mutation in NF1. *Nature Genet* 1994; 7: 353–61.

24 Brannan CI, Perkins AS, Vogel KS *et al.* Targeted disruption of the neurofibromatosis type 1 gene leads to developmental abnormalities in heart and various neural crest-derived tissues. *Genes Devel* 1994; 8: 1019–29.

25 Upadhyaya M, Shaw DJ, Harper PS. Molecular basis of neurofibromatosis type 1 (NF): mutation analysis and polymorphisms in the NF1 gene. *Hum Mut* 1994; 4: 83–101.

26 Kayes LM, Burke W, Riccardi VM *et al.* Deletions spanning the neurofibromatosis 1 gene: identification and phenotype of five patients. *Am J Hum Genet* 1994; 52: 424–36.

27 Wu B-L, Austin MA, Schneider GH, Boles RG, Korf BR. Deletion of the entire NF1 gene detected by FISH: four deletion patients associated with severe manifestations. *Am J Med Genet* 1995; 59: 528–35.

28 Easton DF, Ponder MA, Huson SM, Ponder BAJ. An analysis of variation in expression of NF1: evidence for modifying genes. *Am J Hum Genet* 1993; 53: 305–13.

29 Enzinger FM, Weiss SW. *Soft Tissue tumours*, 2nd edn. St Louis: CV Mosby, 1998.

30 Benedict PH, Szabo G, Fitzpatrick TB, Sinesi SJ. Melanotic macules in Albright's syndrome and in neurofibromatosis. *J Am Med Assoc* 1968; 205: 72–80.

31 Fitzpatrick TB, Martuza RL. Clinical diagnosis of von Recklinghausen's neurofibromatosis. *Ann NY Acad Sci* 1986; 486: 383–5.

32 Harkin JC, Reed RJ. *Tumours of the peripheral nervous system. Atlas for Tumour Pathology*, second series fascicle 3. Washington DC: Armed Forces, Institute of Pathology, 1969: 67–106.

33 Wiestler OD, Radner H. Pathology of neurofibromatosis 1 and 2. In: Huson SM, Hughes RAC, eds. *The Neurofibromatoses, a Pathogenetic and Clinical Overview*. London: Chapman & Hall 1994; 135–59.

34 Perry HD, Font RL. Iris nodules in von Recklinghausen's neurofibromatosis. Electron microscopic confirmation of their melanocytic origin. *Arch Ophthalmol* 1982; 100: 1635–40.

35 Johnson BL, Charneco DL. Café au lait spots in neurofibromatosis and in normal individuals. *Arch Dermatol* 1970; 102: 442–6.

36 Kopf AW, Levine LJ, Rigel DS, Friedman RJ, Levenstein M. Prevalence of congenital nevus like nevi, nevi spili and café au lait spots. *Arch Dermatol* 1985; 121: 766–9.

37 Huson SM, Harper PS, Compston DAS. Von Recklinghausen neurofibromatosis: a clinical and population study in South East Wales. *Brain* 1988; 111: 1355–81.

38 Flueler U, Boltshauser E. Iris hamartoma as diagnostic criterion in neurofibromatosis. *Neuropaediatrics* 1986; 17: 183–5.

39 Huson SM, Jones D, Beck L. Ophthalmic manifestations of neurofibromatosis. *Br J Ophthalmol* 1987; 71: 235–8.

40 Huson SM. *Clinical and genetic studies of von Recklinghausen neurofibromatosis*. MD thesis, University of Edinburgh. 1986.

41 Huson SM, Compston DAS, Harper PS. A genetic study of von Recklinghausen neurofibromatosis in South East Wales. II. Guidelines for genetic counselling. *J Med Genet* 1989; 26: 712–21.

42 Rubenstein AE, Korfe BR. *Neurofibromatosis: a Handbook for Patients, Families and Health Care Professionals*. New York: Thieme, 1990.

43 Poole MD. Experiences in the surgical treatment of cranio-orbital neurofibromatosis. *Br J Plast Surg* 1989; 42: 155–62.

44 Angel MF, Persing JA, Edgerton MT. Reconstructive surgery for neurofibromatosis. In: Huson SM, Hughes RAC, eds. *The Neurofibromatoses A Pathogenetic and Clinical Overview*. London: Chapman & Hall, 1994: 70–97.

45 Griebel ML, Redman JF, Kemp SF, Elders MJ. Hypertrophy of clitoral hood: presenting signs of neurofibromatosis in female child. *Urology* 1991; 37: 337–9.

46 Huson SM. Neurofibromatosis 1 and 2. In: Eeles RA, Ponder BAJ, Easton DF, Horwich A, eds. *Genetic Predisposition to Cancer*. London: Chapman & Hall, 1996: 70–97.

47 Morier P, Mérot Y, Paccaud D *et al.* Juvenile chronic granulocytic leukaemia juvenile xanthogranulomas and neurofibromatosis. Case report and review of the literature. *J Am Acad Dermatol* 1990; 22: 962–5.

48 Ferner RE. Intellect in neurofibromatosis. In: Huson SM, Hughes RAC, eds. *The Neurofibromatoses. A Pathogenetic and Clinical Overview*. London: Chapman & Hall, 1994: 233–52.

49 Hofman KJ, Harris EL, Bryan RN, Denckla MB. Neurofibromatosis type 1: the cognitive phenotype. *J Paediatr* 1994; 124: 51–8.

50 Legius E, Descheemaeker MJ, Spaepen A *et al.* Neurofibromatosis type 1 in childhood: a study of the neuropsychological profile in 45 children. *Genet Couns* 1994; 5: 51–60.

51 North K, Joy P, Yidille D *et al.* Specific learning disability in children with neurofibromatosis type 1: significance of MRI abnormalities. *Neurology* 1994; 44: 878–83.

52 Ferner RE, Hughes RAC, Weinman J. Intellectual impairment in neurofibromatosis 1. *J Neurol Sci* 1996; 138: 125–33.

53 Sorensen SA, Mulvihill JT, Nielsen A. Long-term follow-up of von Recklinghausen neurofibromatosis: survival and malignant neoplasms. *N Engl J Med* 1986; 314: 1010–15.

54 Zoller M, Rembeck B, Akesson HO, Angervall L. Life expectancy, mortality and prognostic factors in neurofibromatosis type I. *Acta Derm Venereol (Stockh)* 1995; 73: 136–40.

55 Samuelsson B. Axelsson R. Neurofibromatosis: a clinical and genetic study of 96 cases in Gothenburg, Sweden. *Acta Derm Venereol (Stockh)* 1981; 95 (suppl): 67–71.

56 Korf BR. Diagnostic outcome in children presenting with multiple café au lait spots. *Pediatrics* 1992; 90: 924–7.

57 Ludman MD, Cole DEC, Crocker JFS, Cohen MM. Schimake immunoosseous dysplasia: case report and review. *Am J Med Genet* 1993; 47: 793–6.

58 Riccardi VM. Von Recklinghausen neurofibromatosis. *N Engl J Med* 1981; 305: 1617–27.

59 Huson SM, Upadhyaya M. Neurofibromatosis 1: clinical management and genetic counselling. In: Huson SM, Hughes RAC, eds. *The Neurofibromatoses. A Pathogenetic and Clinical Overview*. London: Chapman & Hall, 1994: 354–81.

60 Gutman DH, Aylsworth A, Carey JC *et al.* The diagnostic evaluation and multidisciplinary management of neurofibromatosis and neurofibromatosis 2. *JAMA* 1997; 278: 51–7.

61 Riccardi VM. The pathophysiology of neurofibromatosis. Dermatologic insights into heterogeneity and pathogenesis. *J Am Acad Dermatol* 1980; 3: 157–66.

62 Riccardi VM. Mast-cell stabilization to decrease neurofibroma growth. *Arch Dermatol* 1987; 123: 1011–16.

63 Riccardi VM. A controlled multiphase trial of ketotifen to minimise neurofibroma associated pain and itching. *Arch Dermatol* 1993; 129: 577–81.

64 Moss C, Green SH. What is segmental neurofibromatosis? *Br J Dermatol* 1994; 130: 106–10.

65 Riccardi VM, Lewis RA. Penetrance of von Recklinghausen neurofibromatosis: a distinction between predecessors and descendants. *Am J Hum Genet* 1988; 42: 284–9.

66 Young DF, Eldridge R, Gardner WJ. Bilateral acoustic neuromas in a large kindred. *J Am Med Assoc* 1970; 214: 347–53.

67 Evans DGR, Huson SM, Donnai D *et al.* A genetic study of type 2 neurofibromatosis in the United Kingdom: prevalence, mutation rate, fitness and confirmation of maternal transmission effect on severity. *J Med Genet* 1992; 29: 841–6.

68 Evans DGR, Huson SM, Neary W *et al.* A clinical study of type 2 neurofibromatosis. *Q J Med* 1992; 304: 603–18.

69 Parry DM, Eldridge R, Kaiser-Kupfer MI, Bouzas EA, Pikus A, Patronas N. Neurofibromatosis (NF2): clinical characteristics of 63 affected individuals and clinical evidence for heterogenicity. *Am J Med Genet* 1994; 52: 450–61.

70 Short PM, Martuza RL, Huson SM. Neurofibromatosis 2: clinical features, genetic counselling and management issues. In: Huson SM, Hughes RAC, eds. *The Neurofibromatoses: a Pathogenetic and Clinical Overview*. London: Chapman & Hall, 1994: 414–44.

71 Seizinger BR, Martuza RL, Gusella JF. Loss of genes on chromosome 22 in tumorigenesis of human acoustic neuroma. *Nature* 1986; 322: 644–7.

72 Rouleau GA, Seizinger BR, Ozelius LG *et al.* Genetic linkage analysis of bilateral acoustic neurofibromatosis to a DNA marker on chromosome 22. *Nature* 1987; 329: 246–8.

73 Rouleau GA, Merel P, Lutchman M *et al.* Alteration in a new gene encoding a putative membrane organising protein causes neurofibromatosis type 2. *Nature* 1993; 363: 515–21.

74 Trofatter JA, MacCollin MM, Rutter JL *et al.* A novel moesin-, ezrin-, radixin-like gene is a candidate for the neurofibromatosis 2 tumor suppressor. *Cell* 1993; 72: 826.

75 Bouldin TW. Nerve biopsy. In: Garcia J *et al.* eds. *Diagnostic Neuropathology*, vol. II. New York: Macmillan, 1990: 175–92.

76 Kleihues P, Burger PC, Scheithauer BW. *Histological Typing of Tumours of the Central Nervous System*, 2nd edn. Berlin: Springer-Verlag, 1993.

77 Viskochil D, Carey JC. Alternate and related forms of the neurofibromatoses. In: Huson SM, Hughes RAC, eds. *The Neurofibromatoses: a Clinical and Pathogenetic Overview*. London: Chapman & Hall, 1994: 445–574.

78 Gammel JA. Localised neurofibromatosis. *Arch Dermatol* 1931; 113: 837–8.

79 Miller RM, Sparkes RS. Segmental neurofibromatosis. *Arch Dermatol* 1977; 113: 837–8.

80 Roth R, Martines M, James W. Segmental neurofibromatosis. *Arch Dermatol* 1987; 123: 917–20.

81 Colman S, Rasmussen SA, Ho VT, Abernathy CR, Wallace M. Somatic mosaicism in a patient with neurofibromatosis type 1. *Am J Hum Gen* 1995; 58: 484–90.

82 Ainsworth PJ, Weksberg R, Shuman C. Somatic mosaicism in a case of sporadic neurofibromatosis. *Am J Hum Gen* 1995; 57 (suppl): A81–A440.

83 Rubenstein A, Bader JL, Aron AA, Wallace S. Familial transmission of segmental neurofibromatosis. *Neurology* 1983; 33 (suppl 2): 76.

84 Riccardi VM, Lewis RA. Penetrance of von Recklingausen neurofibromatosis: a distinction between predecessors and descendants. *Am J Hum Genet* 1988; 42: 284–9.

85 Boltshauer E, Stocker H, Machler M. Neurofibromatosis type 1 in a child of a parent with segmental neurofibromatosis (NF-5). *Neurofibromatosis* 1989; 2: 244–5.

86 Theiler R, Stocker H, Boltshauer E. Zur Klassierung atypischer Neurofibromatosis-Formen. *Schweiz Med Vschr* 1991; 121: 446–55.

87 Uhlin SR. Segmental neurofibromatosis. *South Med J* 1980; 73: 526–7.

88 Segal R, Wenger SL, Pollack I. *Chromosome translocation and familial transmission in segmental neurofibromatosis.* Presented at the Joint Section on Disorders of the Spine and Peripheral Nerves, AANS/CNS, California, 13–17 February 1991: 40 (abstract).

89 Segal R. Segmental neurofibromatosis of the sciatic nerve. Case report. *Neurosurgery* 1993; 33: 948.

90 Happle R. Pigmentary patterns associated with human mosaicism: a proposed classification. *Eur J Dermatol* 1993; 3: 170–4.

91 Happle R. Mosaicism in human skin. *Arch Dermatol* 1993; 129: 1460–70.

92 Dreesen TD, Henikoff S, Loughney K. A pairing-sensitive element that mediates trans-inactivation is associated with the *Drosophila* brown gene. *Genes Devel* 1991; 5: 331–40.

93 Streitmann von B. Neurofibromatosis localizata. *Z Haut Geschlkr* 1955; 19: 324–9.

94 Winkelmann RK, Johnson LA. Cholinesterases in neurofibromas. *Arch Dermatol* 1962; 85: 106–14.

95 Korting GW, Tupath-Barniske R. Neurofibromatosis disseminata und Herpes Zoster in selben Segmenbereich. *Dermat Wochensch B* 1965; 151: 33–7.

96 Diekmann, Huther W, Pfeiffer RA. Ungewohnilche Erscheinungsformen der Neurofibromatose (von Recklinghausensche Krankeit) in Kindesalter. *Zeit Kinderheilk* 1967; 101: 191–222.

97 Nicholls EM. Somatic variation and multiple neurofibromatosis. *Hum Hered* 1969; 19: 473–9.

98 Sava P, Mourot M, Carbillet JP, Gille P. A propos d'un cas de neurofibromatose avec hyertrophie segmentaire d'un membre. *Ann Pediatr* 1975; 22: 353–61.

99 Biemer E, Muhlbauer WD. Ein fall einer lokalisierten Neurofibromatosis der rechten Gesichtshalfte. In: Hohler H, ed. *Plastiche und Wiendessherstellmas Chirurie.* Stuttgart: Schattauer, 1975: 357–67.

100 Riccardi VM. Neurofibromatosis: clinical heteogenicity. *Curr Prob Cancer* 1982; 7: 16 (1–34).

101 Zonana J, Weleber G. Segmental neurofibromatosis and iris hamartomata (Lisch nodules). *Smith Workshop* 1983: 140–1 (abstract).

102 Weleber G, Zonana J. Iris hamartomas (Lish nodules) in a case of segmental neurofibromatosis. *Am J Ophthal* 1983; 96: 740–4.

103 Saul RA, Stevenson RE. Segmental neurofibromatosis: a distinct type of neurofibromatosis? *Proc Greenwood Genet Center* 1984; 3: 3–6.

104 Dawson TAJ. Regional eruptive neurofibromatosis. *Br J Dermatol* 1984; 111 (suppl 26): 65.

105 Takiguchi PS, Ratz JL. Bilateral dermal neurofibromatosis. *J Am Acad Dermatol* 1984; 10: 451–3.

106 Oranje AP, Vuzevski VD, Kalis TJ, Marts WFM, van Joost TH, Stolz E. Segmental neurofibromatosis. *Br J Dermatol* 1985; 112: 107–12.

107 Gelain A, Formica C, Segantini L. Von Recklinghausen neurofibromatosis. Case report with extensive involvement of the sciatic nerve. *Ital J Orthop Traumatol* 1988; 14: 529–32.

108 Pullara TJ, Greeson JD, Stoker GL, Fenske NA. Cutaneous segmental neurofibromatosis. *J Am Acad Dermatol* 1985; 13: 999–1003.

109 Guisasola L, Alonso M, Vives R, Moreno R, Ledo A. Neurofibromatosis segmentaria. *Actas Dermo-Sif* 1977; 77: 143–6.

110 Diaz F, Gallo S, Chaume A, Martinez A, Alliaga A. *Neurofibromatosis segmentria.* Presented at the XIth Congreso Hispano-Portugues de Dermatologia, Mayo, 1986: 4.

111 Monk BE, Salisbury JR, Pembroke AC. Segmental neurofibromatosis. *Clin Exp Dermatol* 1986; 2: 653–5.

112 Carey JC, Baty BJ, Johnson JP, Morrison T, Skolnick M, Kivlin J. The genetic aspects of neurofibromatosis. *Ann NY Acad Sci* 1986; 486: 45–56.

113 Rawlings CE, Wilkins RH, Cook WA, Burger PC. Segmental neurofibromatosis. *Neurosurgery* 1987; 20: 946–9.

114 Pujol RM, Tuneu A, De Morgas JM, Moreno A. Neurofibromatosis segmentaria. *Med Cut ILA* 1987; 15: 425–8.

115 Koedijk FHJ. Segmental neurofibromatosis. *Br J Dermatol* 1987; 117: 790–1.

116 Stotts JS, Steinman HK. Congenital, segmental pigmented lesions. *Arch Dermatol* 1987; 123: 251–6.

117 Gretzula JC, Weber PJ, McGregor JM, Weber M. Multiple papules in a localized area. *Arch Dermatol* 1988, 124: 1101–6.

118 McFadden JP, Logan R, Griffiths WAD. Segmental neurofibromatosis and pruritus. *Clin Exp Dermatol* 1988; 13: 265–8.

119 Calzavara PG, Carlino A, Anzola GP, Pasolini MP. Segmental neurofibromatosis. Case report and review of the literature. *Neurofibromatosis* 1988; 1: 318–22.

120 Archer CB, Glover M, Atherton DJ. Segmental neurofibromatosis with generalized cafè au lait spots. *Br J Dermatol* 1988; 119 (suppl 33): 96–7.

121 Jung EG. Segmental neurofibromatosis (NF-5). *Neurofibromatosis* 1988; 1: 306–11.

122 Zulaica A, Peteiro C, Pereiro M Jr, Pereiro Ferreiros M, Quintas C, Toribio J. Neurofibromatosis segmentaria. *Med Cut ILA* 1989; 17: 41–3.

123 Calzavara Pinton PG, Carlino A, Marini D. Neurofibromatosi segmentale. Descrizione di un caso clinico e revisione della letteratura. *Giorn Ital Dermatol Venereol* 1989; 124: 231–4.

124 Kaplan DL, Pestana A. Cutaneous segmental neurofibromatosis. *South Med J* 1989; 82: 516–17.

125 Sharma SC, Ray RC. Segmental neurofibromatosis. *Indian J Pathol Microbiol* 1989; 32: 229–31.

126 Allegue F, Espana A, Fernandez-Garcia JM, Ledo A. Segmental neurofibromatosis with contralateral lentiginosis. *Clin Exp Dermatol* 1989; 14: 448–50.

127 Sanchez Conejo-Mir J, Herrera Saval A, Camacho Martinez F. Segmental neurofibromatosis. *J Am Acad Dermatol* 1989; 20: 681–2.

128 Gersell DJ, Fulling KH. Localized neurofibromatosis of the female genitourinary tract. *Am J Surg Pathol* 1989; 13: 873–8.

129 Bousema MT, Vuzevszki VD, Oranje AP, Heule F, Stolz E, van Joost T. Non-von Recklinghausen neurofibromatosis resembliing a giant pigmented nevus. *J Am Acad Dermatol* 1989; 20: 358–62.

130 Bembibre MC, Musitani V, Levy T, Gandini O. Segmental neurofibromatosis. *Rev Assoc Odontol Argent* 1989; 77: 76–7.

131 Samuelsson B, Akesson HO. Neurofibromatosis in Gothemburg, Sweden. IV. Genetic analysis. *Neurofibromatosis* 1989; 2: 107–15.

132 Pizarro Redondo A, Borbujo Martinez J, Gonzàlez Hermosa MR, Casado Jimènez M. Neurofibromatosis segmentaria. *Riv Clin Esp* 1990; 187: 82–3.

133 Angelo C, Paradisi M, Celano G, Ferranti G, Ruatti P. Neurofibromatosi segmentale: a proposito di un caso clinico. *Chron Derm* 1990; 2: 183–7.

134 Sloan J, Fretzin D, Bovenmyer D. Genetic counselling in segmental neurofibromatosis. *J Am Acad Dermatol* 1990; 22: 461–7.

135 Smith S, Heymann WR. Segmental neurofibromatosis in an octuagenarian. *J Am Geriatr Soc* 1990; 308: 807–8.

136 Jaakkola S, Muona P, James WD *et al.* Segmental neurofibromatosis: immunocytochemical analysis of cutaneous lesions. *J Am Acad Dermatol* 1990; 22: 617–21.

137 Trattner A, David M, Hodak E, Ben-David E, Sandbank M. Segmental neurofibromatosis. *J Am Acad Dermatol* 1990; 23: 866–9.

138 Rossi A, Manzo R, Villano PA. Su di un caso di neurofibromatosi segmentale. *Dermatol Oggi* 1991; 5: 28–31.

139 Friedman DP. Segmental neurofibromatosis (NF-5): a rare form of neurofibromatosis. *Am J Neuroradiol* 1991; 12: 971–2.

140 Paoletti S, Celano G, Atzori F. Neurofibromatosi segmentale. decsrizione di un caso. *Chron Derm* 1991; 1: 135–7.

141 Rose I, Vakilzadeh F. Bilaterale segmentale Neurofibromatose. *Hautarzt* 1991; 42: 770–3.

142 Sieb JP, Schultheiss R. Segmental neurofibromatosis of the sciatic nerve: case report. *Neurosurgery* 1992; 31: 1122–5.

143 Cecchi R, Giomi A, Tuci F, Brunetti L, Seghieri G. Bilateral segmental neurofibromatosis. *Dermatology* 1992; 185: 59–61.

144 Gerhard G, Hamm H. Die unilaterale Lentiginose—eine segmentale Neurofibromatose ohne Neurofibrome. *Hautarzt* 1992; 43: 491–5.

145 Mohri S, Atsusaka K, Sasaki T. Localized multiple neurofibromatosis. *Clin Exp Dermatol* 1992; 17: 195–6.

146 Goldberg NS. What is segmental neurofibromatosis? *J Am Acad Dermatol* 1992; 26: 638–40.

147 Nicoletti A, Puccini S, Marelli MA, Crippa D. Neurofibromatosi bilaterale segmentaria (NF-S). A proposito di un casi clinico. *G Ital Dermatol Venereol* 1992; 127: 563–5.

148 Monfrecola G, Perrelli P, Nappa P, Brunetti B. Su di un caso di neurofibromatosi segmentale. *Ann It Derm Clin Sper* 1992; 46: 115–17.

149 Korf B. Diagnostic outcome in children with multiple cafè au lait spots. *Pediatrics* 1992; 90: 924–7.

150 Micali G, Lembo D, Verano C. Neurofibromatosi segmentale: descrizione di un caso clinico e revisione della letteratura. *Gior Int Derm Ped* 1992; 4: 63–70.

151 Zimmermann-Schroeder J. Bilateral segmental form of neurofibromatosis von Recklinghausen. *Aktuel Dermatol* 1992; 18: 277–9.

152 Micali G, Lembo D, Giustini S. Segmental neurofibromatosis with only macular lesions. *Pediatr Dermatol* 1993; 10: 43–5.

153 Finley EM, Kolbusz RV. Segmental neurofibromatosis clinically appearing as a nevus spilus. *Int Dermatol* 1993; 5: 358–60.

154 Huet P, Dandurand M, Joujoux M, Guillot B. Neurofibromatose segmentaire. *Ann Dermatol Vénéréol* 1993; 120: 450–4.

155 Filosa G, Bugatti L, Coccia I, Ciattaglia G. Neurofibromatosi segmentale: due casi. *G Ital Dermatol Venereol* 1993; 128: 373–6.

156 Ruxin TA, Pierson JC, Helm TN, Bergfield WF. Stump the expert. *J Dermatol Surg Oncol* 1994; 20: 304, 351–2.

157 Selvaag E, Thune P, Larsen TE. Segmental neurofibromatosis presenting as a giant nevus spilus. *Acta Derm Venereol* 1994; 74: 327–34.

158 Sawanda S, Honda M, Niimura M. Molecular genetic analysis of the von recklinghausen neurofibromatosis (NF1) gene using polymerase chain reaction-single strand conformation polymorphism (PCR-SSCP) method. *J Dermatol* 1994; 21: 294–300.

159 Menni S, Cavicchini S, Brezzi A, Piccinino R. A case of segmental macular neurofibromatosis. *Acta Derm Venereol (Stockh)* 1994; 74: 329.

160 Westenend PJ, Smedts F, de Jong MC, Lommers EJ, Assmann KJ. A 4-year-old boy with neurofibromatosis and severe renovascular hypertension due to renal artery dysplasia. *Am J Surg Pathol* 1994; 18: 512–16.

161 Ingordo V, D'Andria G, Mendicini S, Grecucci M, Baglivo A. Segmental neurofibromatosis: is it uncommon or underdiagnosed? *Arch Dermatol* 1995; 131: 959–60.

162 Wolkenstein P, Mahmoudi A, Zeller J, Revuz J. More on the frequency of segmental neurofibromatosis. *Arch Dermatol* 1995; 131: 1465.

163 Happle RH. Segmental forms of autosomal dominant skin disorders: different types reflect different states of zygosity. *Am J Med Genet* 1996; 66: 241–2.

164 Gardner RL. Cell lineage and cell commitment in the early mammalian embryo. In: Warshaw TB, ed. *The Biological Basis of Reproductive and Developmental Medicine.* Amsterdam: Elsevier Science, 1983: 31–41.

165 Brunner HG, Hulsebos T, Steijlen PM *et al.* Exclusion of the Neurofibromatosis 1 locus in a family with inherited café au lait spots. *Am J Med Genet* 1994; 46: 472–4.

166 Charrow J, Listernick R, Ward K. Autosomal dominant multiple café au lait spots and neurofibromatosis 1: evidence of non-linkage. *Am J Med Genet* 1993; 45: 606–8.

167 Abeliovich D, Gelman-Kohan Z, Silverstein S *et al.* Familial café au lait spots: a variant of neurofibromatosis type 1. *J Med Genet* 1995; 32: 985–6.

168 Watson GH. Pulmonary stenosis, café au lait spots and dull intelligence. *Arch Dis Child* 1967; 42: 303–7.

169 Allanson JE, Upadhyaya M, Watson G *et al.* Watson syndrome: is it a subtype of type 1 neurofibromatosis? *J Med Genet* 1991; 28: 752–6.

170 Tassabehji M, Strachan T, Sharland M *et al.* Tandem duplication within a neurofibromatosis type 1 (Nf1) gene exon in a family with features of Watson syndrome and Noonan syndrome. *Am J Hum Genet* 1993; 53: 90–5.

171 Shishiba T, Niimura M, Ohtsuka F, Tsura N. Multiple cutaneous neurofibromas as a skin manifestation of neurilemmomatosis. *J Am Acad Dermatol* 1984; 10: 744–54.

172 Purcell SM, Dixon SL. Schwannomatosis. An unusual variant of Neurofibromatosis or a Distinct Clinical Entity? *Arch Dermatol* 1989; 125: 390–3.

173 MacCollin M, Woodfinn W, Kronn D, Short MP. Schwannomatosis: a clinical and pathological study. *Neurology* 1996; 46: 1072–9.

174 Evans DGR, Mason S, Huson SM, Ponder M, Harding AE, Strachan T. Spinal and cutaneous schwannomatosis is a variant form of type 2 neurofibromatosis. A clinical and molecular study. *J Neurol Neurosurg Psychiatr* 1997; 62: 361–6.

19.14 Tuberous Sclerosis

JOHN P. OSBORNE

Definition

The tuberous sclerosis complex (TSC) (syn. Bourneville's disease, Pringle's disease, epiloia) is a serious genetic condition inherited as an autosomal dominant trait but with a high spontaneous mutation rate. It is best known for its association with seizures, learning disorder and skin manifestations. Initially thought to be uncommon and always associated with learning difficulties, it is now known that it is much more common and that only half of those affected have learning difficulties, a further quarter have seizures but not learning difficulty while the remainder have neither, being asymptomatic neurologically but having skin or visceral lesions.

History

It was first clearly described in 1880 by Bourneville [1] who recognized the pathological features of tubers with areas of sclerosis at postmortem in patients with epilepsy and mental retardation (Fig. 19.14.1). In 1908 Vogt [2] reported the classical triad of tuberous sclerosis (TS) consisting of learning difficulties, seizures and the facial skin rash, then called adenoma sebaceum. This rash is now correctly described as angiofibromatosis since histologically there is no primary involvement of the sebaceous glands (Figs 19.14.2, 19.14.3). Vogt also noted that cardiac and renal tumours can be present and in 1920 Van Der Hoeve [3] described the retinal tumours which he called retinal phacomas (the Greek word *phakos* means spot): he also noted that 'phacomas' can also occur in the intestine, bone and thyroid. For a long time the diagnosis was only considered in those with learning difficulties and the first attempts at an estimate of prevalence, in 1935, extrapolated the prevalence from the number of affected individuals in mental institutions [4] and suggested a figure of 1 in 30 000. A number of prevalence studies [5–8] have been undertaken since then, most of which suggest an overall prevalence of around 1 in 27 000 but with a much higher prevalence in children of nearer 1 in 10 000. This is supported by a long-term study in Minnesota, USA [9], suggesting a figure of 1 in 10 000 for a whole population. Because we are not good at detecting intellectually normal

children with TSC, the birth incidence may be as high as 1 in 7000 [10].

Aetiology and pathology

Although TSC is an extremely variable condition, all variations of the disease would appear to occur within families except where there is a deletion of the autosomal dominant polycystic kidney disease (ADPKD) gene in addition. The first gene locus to be identified (TSC1) showed linkage to the ABO blood group on chromosome 9q3.4 [11] but subsequent studies have confirmed the existence of a second gene on chromosome 16 [12]. This gene (TSC2) has been identified [13] and it is extremely close to the gene for ADPKD. The protein product for TSC2, tuberin, has been isolated. It has some areas of homology with *RAP-1* proteins suggesting that tuberin may mediate its activity in the same way. There is evidence to suggest that tuberin exhibits a weak but specific guanosine triphosphatase (GTPase) activating activity *in vitro* towards *RAP-1*. This would be compatible with the hypothesis that tuberin may function as a negative regulator for GTPase. Tissue analysis of human tissue has shown that tuberin localizes to the Golgi stacks and that pharmacological destruction of the Golgi apparatus coincidently abolishes antituberin immunofluorescence. Double-indirect immunofluorescence demonstrates colocalization of the two proteins in cultured cell lines. Additional evidence suggesting that tuberin is a tumour suppressor gene has been produced by using a tetracycline responsive promoter to cause an overproduction of tuberin: these cells suffer from significantly inhibited cell growth.

So far it has proved extremely difficult to identify small deletions in TSC2 but techniques for the detection of abnormalities of tuberin will be easier to develop and may prove more useful in some families. At the moment, unless a gene deletion has been identified, there is no molecular test for TSC and therefore for the majority, antenatal diagnosis by chorionic villus sampling is not available. These molecular studies remain predominantly research techniques. Whilst a few families remain who do not clearly link to chromosome 9 or 16, there is no convincing proof for a third or further locus but the existence of only two loci

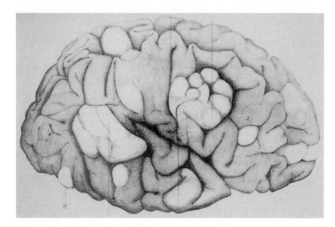

Fig. 19.14.1 A copy of one of the original illustrations from Bourneville's paper in 1880 showing 'tuber-like' growths with areas of sclerosis—hence the term TS.

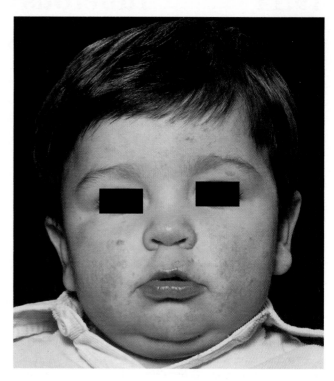

Fig. 19.14.3 Early facial erythema in a boy of 18 months who presented with infantile spasms in the first year of life. Facial erythema can precede the development of angiofibromatosis.

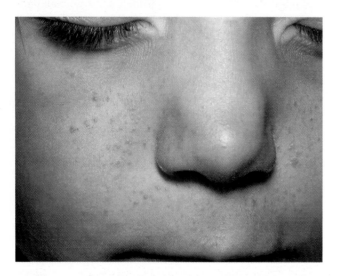

Fig. 19.14.2 A close-up view of early facial angiofibromatosis in a girl of 8 years.

cannot be guaranteed. Previously, chromosome 11 was thought to be a possible locus but these families are now predominately linked to the gene on chromosome 16. The suggestion of a locus on chromosome 12 was never very convincing. There is perhaps surprisingly no evidence of a significant difference in the phenotype of TSC between those families linking to TSC1 compared to TSC2 (unless the ADPKD gene is also affected) [14].

Truncation of the protein tuberin has been detected in some individuals with a non-inactivating deletion of the TSC2 gene. This may turn out to be an easier test for abnormalities in individuals where the tuberin protein product is shortened but it will not detect inactivating deletions. Such abnormalities could include deletions, insertions and substitutions causing a stop codon to be formed. The abnormally short tuberin protein product can then be detected.

The TSC1 gene has been identified on 9q34 and the protein product, termed harmartin, identified [15]. Harmartin has homology to a putative yeast protein of unknown function and since it is also a tumour suppressor protein, it must participate in a novel pathway of cell control. No large genomic deletions have yet been found at TSC1.

The knowledge that the two TSC genes are tumour suppressor genes [16,17] has been shown to explain the clinical features of the disease. An affected individual starts life as an embryo with a single defective gene which was either an inherited or a spontaneous mutation. During the normal growth and development of the fetus, and later in life, a second defect occurring during meiosis leaves the cell with no functioning gene. This then gives rise to the benign hamartomas that are the hallmark of the disease. It remains to be seen whether disease-modifying agents affect the growth rate of these hamartomas: since cell division does not normally occur within the central nervous system (CNS), cerebral tubers will not be affected by such treatment.

The Eker rat is an excellent example of a mendelian dominant predisposition to a specific cancer (renal carcinoma). It has been reported that it is a germ-line insertion in the rat homologue of the human tuberous sclerosis (TSC2) gene which gives rise to this abnormality in the Eker rat [18]. A tumour suppressor function of the TSC2 gene in the Eker rat has been demonstrated. Although the phenotype of TS in humans differs from that in the Eker rat, renal carcinoma does occur infrequently in humans with TS. Late in life Eker rats may additionally develop haemangioscarcomas of the spleen, leiomyosarcomas of the uterus and adenomas of the pituitary. Neurological abnormalities have not yet been shown but have not been studied in detail. The rat TSC2 gene shares more than 90% identical amino acid pattern when compared to the human gene. In the rat it has been shown that a C-terminal truncated TSC2 protein was localized in the nucleus but the full length protein was found predominantly in the perinuclear region of the cytoplasm. It has also been shown that the introduction of the wild-type TSC2 gene can rescue the Eker rat from carcinogenesis. It seems likely that this Eker rat model will be invaluable in studying molecular mechanisms of the TSC2 gene.

Clinical genetics

TS is an autosomal dominant condition with a high mutation rate of approximately 65%. Since we do not yet know that screening for complications of TSC is worthwhile, the main reason for examining the parents is for genetic counselling. If the parents wish to have further children, they should have a detailed dermatological and ophthalmic clinical examination followed by cranial imaging and a renal ultrasound scan. Cranial imaging for diagnosis is probably best done with a computed tomography (CT) scan to look for calcified subependymal nodules (Fig. 19.14.4): cranial magnetic resonance imaging (MRI) scanning is more likely to show tubers but the appearances are not always diagnostic and calcified subependymal nodules, which are diagnostic, can be missed on cranial MRI scanning (Figs 19.14.5, 19.14.6).

MRI scanning shows cortical tubers most clearly on T2-weighted images except in the fetus and newborn (perhaps for up to 3 months) when because of the relative lack of myelination, T1-weighted images are best. T1 images are most likely to show areas of calcification. Recent evidence suggests that flare sequences may be shown to be superior in due course. Gadolinium enhancement can be used to show the vascularity of a giant cell astrocytoma. Not all enhancing lesions are giant cell astrocytomas requiring treatment.

A renal ultrasound scan can be confusing if a single cyst is seen since this occurs in otherwise normal individuals: it should be done to look for polycystic kidney disease or angiomyolipomas (AML). If AML are the only evidence of TSC, confirmation by CT scan is advisable. However, if all investigations are normal there still remains a risk of recurrence of approximately 2% which may be due to germinal mosaicism rather than non-penetrance which is rare [6,8]. Echocardiography in adults causes confusion when possible calcified areas of myocardium are detected (e.g.

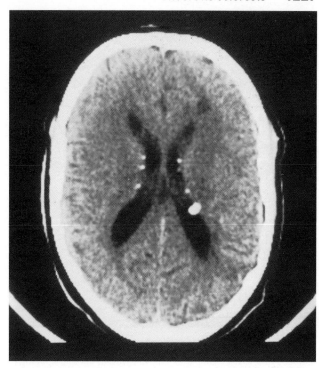

Fig. 19.14.4 This cranial CT scan shows multiple calcified subependymal nodules. In the left frontal region there is an area of reduced opacification which represents a subcortical tuber: these are sometimes visible on CT scans.

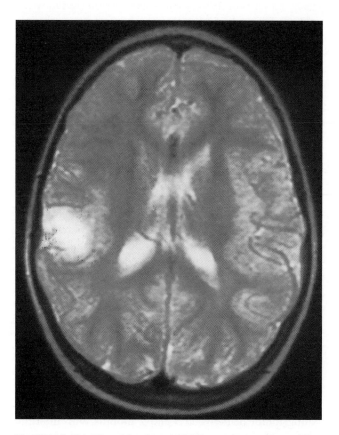

Fig. 19.14.5 This T2-weighted cranial MRI scan shows a large white area in the cortex of the left hemisphere which is a cortical tuber.

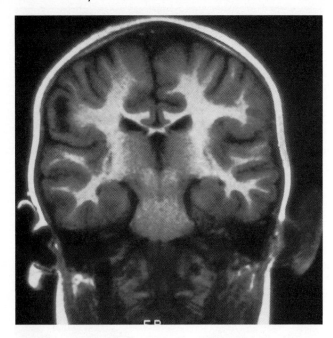

Fig. 19.14.6 This T1-weighted coronal cranial MRI scan shows an 'empty gyms' in the right parietal region which is another imaging feature of a cortical tuber.

papillary muscle) and is not recommended. As an autosomal dominant condition each fetus of an affected individual has a 50% risk of inheriting TS, the severity of which is random (with the exception of polycystic renal disease) and cannot be predicted.

Siblings of an affected individual should also be offered screening when they are old enough to request it themselves for potential genetic counselling. Earlier investigation is only justified to exclude polycystic renal disease or in the neonatal period when echocardiography may be contributory and where this evidence of TSC may subsequently disappear, or if the sibling has symptoms requiring investigation. Asymptomatic siblings should be offered a full screen (including cranial imaging) if their parents have not been examined but a full dermatological and eye examination may be sufficient if the parents were found to be unaffected after full investigations (see below).

Clinical features

Neurological

Almost any organ in the body can be affected with the possible exception of skeletal muscle and spinal cord but it is the serious neurological sequelae that dominate the paediatric presentation. The most common scenario is of a young infant of between 3 and 7 months with infantile spasms. However, partial seizures, absence seizures and tonic–clonic seizures are also found even in infancy. Not all affected individuals have seizures which only occur in between two-thirds and three-quarters of patients. Of those with seizures, two-thirds will start their seizures in the first year but 10% will occur for the first time in schoolage children and in 4% seizure onset is in adult life [8].

Learning disorder due to TSC is not thought to occur in the absence of seizures. The distribution of learning ability in individuals with TSC is thought to be bimodal with the vast majority of individuals with learning difficulties requiring supervision for daily living: often these patients have little or no language and despite needing help with feeding, dressing and toileting, they are usually fully mobile. Little is known about the detailed neuropsychology of TSC. Clinically, there are sometimes areas of extraordinary ability in individuals with otherwise severe deficits and occasional severe localized deficits in individuals functioning normally. The possibility of a specific defect (using a test of visual discrimination and attentional set-shifting, the ID/ED shift) was recently reported in about half of individuals with TSC who have a normal IQ. The significance of this is not yet known. There is a slight excess of males with learning difficulty and this is not thought to be due to an increased number of cerebral tubers but to the more frequent occurrence of early onset, severe and more intractable seizures in males.

Between 10 and 20% of infants presenting with infantile spasms will have TS as the cause: all children with infantile spasms should have their skin examined.

Focal neurological deficits also occur in TSC with a hemiparesis, usually mild, being most common. The cause of the hemiparesis can be due to an episode of status epilepticus or neurosurgery but in others is uncertain. Third nerve palsies have been seen. The head circumference is often slightly large and microcephaly should make one question the diagnosis, or consider two diagnoses.

Behaviour problems are one of the most distressing features of the disease. The combination of hyperactivity and autism is particularly difficult. While these difficulties are more common in those with learning difficulties, they can occur in those with normal intellect who have had seizures. Improvement in behaviour is sometimes seen when better seizure control is achieved but it takes time to appear. In contrast to children with idiopathic autism, children with TS and autism can still often learn from straightforward behavioural modification. Treatment of the hyperactivity is problematic since drug treatment is thought to be contraindicated by the presence of seizures. Some of the drugs used for the treatment of the seizures may cause behavioural problems, usually aggression, especially clonazepam and clobazam: withdrawal of these drugs can produce dramatic improvements. Self-injury is often due to drugs or to frustration and poor communication which can be relieved by attention to the detail of day-to-day life at home and at school. This can also result in some improvement of both behaviour and hyperactivity, occasionally dramatically so.

Skin manifestations

The earliest skin manifestations of TSC [19] include forehead plaques and shagreen patches as well as the more commonly recognized hypomelanic macules. Forehead plaques may be present at birth (Fig. 19.14.7) or appear shortly afterwards and can initially look like a capillary haemangioma. They can occur anywhere over the scalp at the front of the face and neck. When fully developed they are a firm, fleshy, slightly raised lesion which is commonly red but can be yellow or brown.

Shagreen patches when first developing may also look like a capillary haemangioma but there is usually some palpable thickening of the dermis. The typical site is posteriorly in the lumbar region (Fig. 19.14.8), occasionally at the top of the thigh, is a useful clue. The shagreen patch is a roughened area of usually red but occasionally pale or slightly pigmented skin. Sometimes the appearance is similar to orange peel and the consistency is that of soft rubber. The patches may be only a few millimetres in size or extremely large being 10–15 cm in diameter. Large lesions sometimes have a crop of smaller lesions around them and occasionally only the smaller lesions are seen when they may be scattered over the back or localized in the more common area around the loin. Only a large classic shagreen patch should be considered a diagnostic

feature. Histologically, again these are angiofibromas. They are rarely present in infancy but usually appear by adolescence. They are asymptomatic apart from their cosmetic appearance and are found in about 25% of individuals with TS.

Facial angiofibromas (see Fig. 19.14.3) are often heralded by excessive facial flushing in infancy but are rarely obvious before the age of 2 years. They gradually become more prominent with time and will persist throughout life. Typical lesions are erythematous papules or nodules occurring bilaterally, symmetrically, particularly over the nasolabial folds and cheeks, sometimes in a butterfly distribution. They rarely affect the forehead or scalp and curiously tend to spare the upper lip but appear again over the chin. They are present in about 85% of patients over the age of 5 years and can occasionally arise for the first time in adult life. In difficult cases biopsy is required to establish a firm diagnosis. The finding of angiofibromatous tissue is characteristic but the large giant cells are the diagnostic feature: forehead plaques, shagreen patches and ungual fibromas have similar histology.

Hypomelanotic macules also occur in normal individuals and are not always present in TS. The greater the number, the greater the chance that TSC is the cause. They are found most frequently on the trunk and the limbs and can be any shape (Figs 19.14.9, 19.14.10): the description ash leaf patch should be avoided since it is not particularly helpful. In younger adults a confetti pattern of small discrete hypomelanotic macules on the arms and legs is not uncommon. All these hypomelanotic areas reflect light 365 nm in wavelength because of the absence of melanin and the use of an ultraviolet lamp is therefore helpful in their detection (Fig. 19.14.11). New lesions can appear with time and old lesions can disappear. Histologically, these lesions have normal numbers of melanocytes

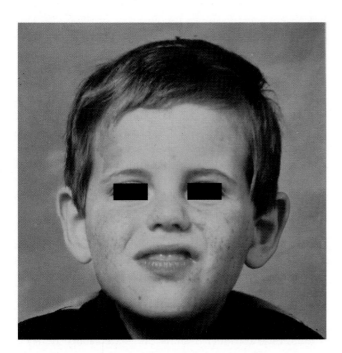

Fig. 19.14.7 This large facial forehead plaque was noted when this boy developed infantile spasms: it was the earliest skin sign of TS.

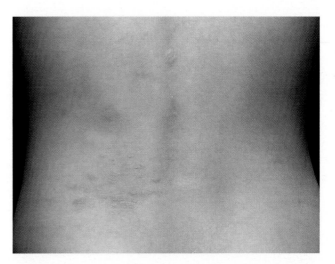

Fig. 19.14.8 This shagreen patch is at a typical site but is made up of multiple small areas of affected skin. The few small lesions distant from the main area are sometimes called satellite lesions.

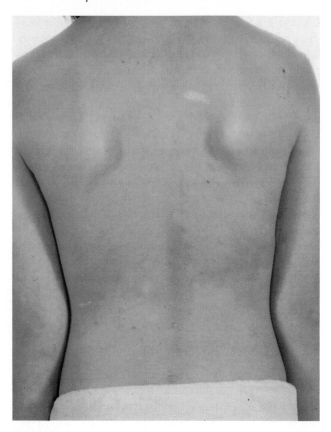

Fig. 19.14.9 A single ovate hypomelanotic macule in a girl of 8 years. She also shows two small circular patches in the midline just above her pants: these are very small shagreen patches and are sometimes referred to as satellite patches.

Fig. 19.14.11 Ultraviolet light makes hypomelanotic maules of TS easier to see.

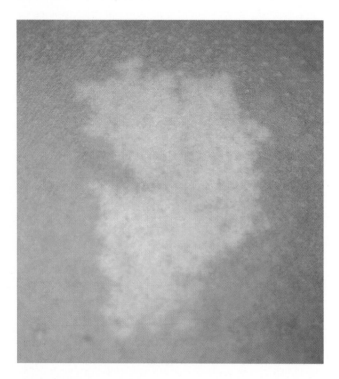

Fig. 19.14.10 An irregular hypomelanotic macule—these are not infrequent in TS.

but absent melanosomes. Involvement of the scalp (Fig. 19.14.12) by hypomelanotic lesions results in poliosis (hypopigmented hairs) which also occur at the eyebrows, eyelashes and pubic and body hair. Café-au-lait patches are not found in TSC in greater numbers than in the normal population [20].

Periungual fibromas usually lie on top of the nail or in a groove in the nail (Fig. 19.14.13) but are occasionally seen underneath the nail. Their presence can sometimes be presumed when longitudinal grooving is apparent but this can arise through other causes. They are much more common on the toes (Fig. 19.14.14) than on the hands. Histologically they are angiofibromas. They are uncommon in the first decade but become more common with time: they can even appear for the first time in middle-age. A single lesion is suggestive of the diagnosis of TSC if the histology is confirmed: two fibromas are essential for a certain diagnosis.

Unusual lesions include larger hamartomas. Occipital angiofibromas in the subcutaneous tissues can be quite troublesome but such lesions can occasionally be seen anywhere. Skin tags, also called molluscum fibrosum pendulum, are common especially around the neck.

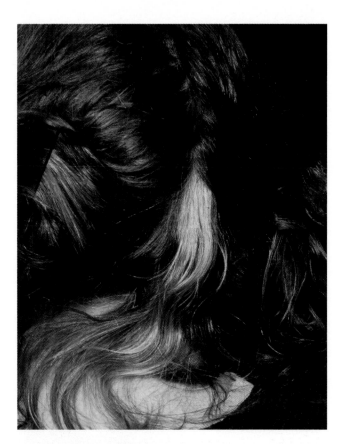

Fig. 19.14.12 Poliosis of the scalp in TS.

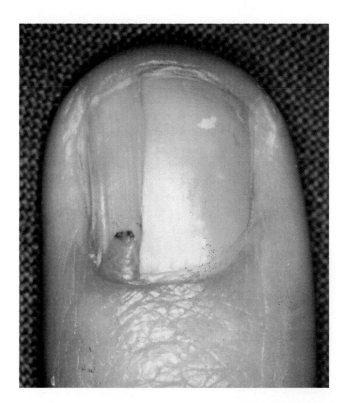

Fig. 19.14.13 This ungual fibroma in a teenage girl has caused a groove to develop in the nail.

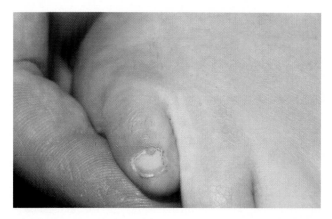

Fig. 19.14.14 This ungual fibroma was found in a boy of 3.5 years.

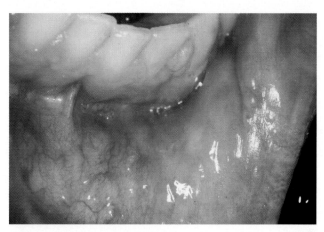

Fig. 19.14.15 A gum fibroma is visible next to the canine tooth.

Examination of the mouth can reveal fibromas around the teeth (Fig. 19.14.15) or even on the tongue. These are not usually sufficiently distinctive to be diagnostic and the picture can be confused by gum overgrowth particularly from phenytoin. Dental pits are thought to be more common in individuals with TS particularly affecting adult teeth. The pits may be more common in TSC but can occur in individuals without TSC and are not thought to be diagnostic.

Retinal lesions

The retinal phacomas are astrocytomas and are present in about 25% of affected individuals [8]. An astrocytoma affecting the macula will cause amblyopia but otherwise visual acuity is unaffected. The retinal phacomas are most frequently seen close to the optic disc (Fig. 19.14.16) and unlike retinoblastomas do not appear to increase in size with time. New retinal phacomas are not thought to appear but non-calcified retinal hamartomas are more difficult to see and can calcify with time, making the distinction problematic.

Cardiac lesions

Cardiac rhabdomyomas can be detected on echocardiography as echogenic lesions. On echo they are predominately seen in the ventricles or intraventricular septum but at postmortem are also seen in the atria. In young children they are more easily visible than in adults where papillary muscles in particular cause increasing echogenicity with age. Echocardiography is also technically more troublesome in adults with a thicker sternum and more intervening lung. Rhabdomyomas can be seen as early as the second trimester of pregnancy and are found with increasing frequency so that at birth it is thought that at least 60% of affected individuals may have rhabdomyomas. They may rapidly decrease in size following birth, possibly because of reduction in the glycogen content within the rhabdomyoma (Fig. 19.14.17). They can be associated with obstruction to outflow and with replacement of myocardial tissue or intraventricular volume resulting in poor cardiac output.

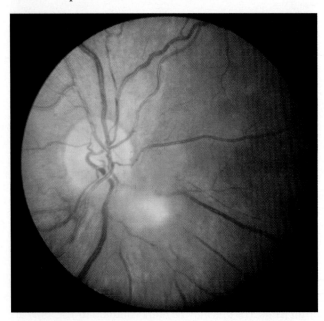

Fig. 19.14.16 This retinal photograph shows a calcified retinal phacoma: histologically these are astrocytomas.

Arrhythmias can occur including the Wolff–Parkinson–White (WPW) syndrome and this can also cause heart failure. It is possible that WPW syndrome may resolve more frequently in TSC than in other conditions possibly due to the resolution of the rhabdomyomas. If the electrocardiogram (ECG) is normal and the infant does not have cardiac compromise from rhabdomyomas then cardiac problems should not arise as the child grows. Rhabdomyomas are thought to get smaller as age increases as cross-sectional studies show smaller lesions with increasing age. It is thought that 80% of infants with cardiac rhabdomyomas will have TSC, the chances increasing with an increasing number of rhabdomyomas.

Renal disease

The kidney is often affected in TSC but the natural history is not well documented [21]. Cystic disease, clinically indistinguishable from ADPKD can occur from infancy causing hypertension and renal failure [22]: these individuals usually have a deletion of both the TSC2 gene and the gene for ADPKD (see above). However, polycystic kidney disease can occur without such a dual deletion and cysts are found in families with linkage to the TSC1 gene. Histologically, the cysts are lined with a hyperplastic eosinophilic epithelium which is thought to be pathognomonic. AMLs are a more common lesion and are often thought to arise in a previously normal kidney during or after puberty. They give a very hyperintense echo on ultrasound and are frequently bilateral but may be associated with cysts. CT will, in the majority of patients, show evidence of lipomatous tissue confirming the diagnosis of AML. Renal carcinoma is rare and may be more slow growing than renal carcinoma in the absence of TSC. On ultrasound these lesions are not echogenic but of mixed echogenicity or are even poorly echogenic, whilst still being clearly solid tissue. CT scanning may show an absence of lipomatous elements. Biopsy is often difficult to interpret since AMLs may contain areas of tissue which look remarkably like renal carcinoma. Staining with HMB-45 helps since renal carcinoma does not seem to

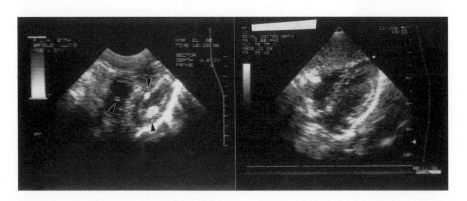

Fig. 19.14.17 These two echocardiograms were taken 6 weeks apart. At birth (on the left) three rhabdomyomas were present but they are no longer visible at 6 weeks of age.

stain while AML does. Some kidneys at postmortem are completely riddled with multiple small AMLs and cysts causing gross distortion of normal renal architecture, suggesting that the second hit (a defect in the previously normal gene pair to the abnormal gene—see above) occurred early in renal development. Haemorrhage is the most common complication of AML causing pain and frank haematuria. Haemorrhage into the collecting system can cause clot colic whereas haemorrhage into the kidney causes fever and localized renal pain. Haemorrhage rupturing through the kidney occurs infrequently but leads to fairly catastrophic blood loss. Haemorrhage occurs more frequently in females who may also be more likely to have AML. The most sensible treatment is that which is most conservative [23] since the risk of further haemorrhage from other lesions on the same or alternate sides remains and cannot be accurately predicted. Selective embolization of the feeding artery is the treatment of choice and nephrectomy should be avoided whenever possible. Renal failure occurs in approximately 1% of individuals with TS most frequently due to polycystic kidney disease but also due to small dysplastic kidneys and from nephrectomy for haemorrhage from AML or for the treatment of renal carcinoma. Renal transplantation does not seem to cause unexpected problems. AMLs also occur in the liver where they rarely cause symptoms, possibly because of the lower blood pressure and flow. AMLs are also occasionally seen in the spleen. Cysts can also be seen in liver and spleen.

Bony changes on X-ray include cysts, periosteal new bone formation and areas of sclerosis but symptomatic bone disease is rare. Rectal polyps are common and are benign: they are asymptomatic.

Pneumothorax, haemoptysis and respiratory insufficiency can occur due to pulmonary lymphangioleiomyomatosis. This occurs almost exclusively in females and can run a more protracted course than the same disease in individuals without TSC. It is thought that progesterone may have a beneficial effect on the course of the disease. Most females with lung disease also have renal disease.

Course and prognosis

Life expectancy has previously been reduced [24] by intercurrent infections and poorly controlled epilepsy in particular, but with modern medical management, life expectancy is thought to have improved. The occasional patient will succumb to a giant cell astrocytoma or to renal failure and even more infrequently to lung disease. Sudden unexpected death can also occur in any individual with epilepsy but the mechanism is not known. Some patients will succumb because of intractable epilepsy including non-convulsive status epilepticus. The disease

itself, however, is not a dementia and affected individuals should therefore be treated vigorously.

Diagnosis

The diagnosis of TS still largely rests on clinical judgement. This can lead to difficulties. Whilst the diagnosis is usually clear-cut in severely affected individuals, in others it may be quite difficult to confirm or refute. For this reason diagnostic criteria are still required. Multiple lesions, implying multiple second hits to the gene are always more convincing of the diagnosis. Gomez suggested the use of diagnostic criteria which have been refined with time [25] (Table 19.14.1). Primary diagnostic criteria are those features which, on their own, almost guarantee the diagnosis of TSC. These include facial angiofibromas and more than one ungual fibroma or calcified retinal hamartoma or cortical tubers or subependymal glial nodule. It is likely that a shagreen patch, if typical in site and appearance, is diagnostic. There have been reports of individuals with shagreen patches and no other clinical evidence of TSC but not since full evaluation through imaging has been available. A similar likelihood of diagnosis would occur with a typical forehead fibrous plaque. Individuals with multiple bilateral renal AML are not thought to have TSC but this has never been proven by follow-up of their offspring to show the risk of children with TSC.

In the presence of an affected first-degree relative, a single lesion suggesting a second hit, because these are

Table 19.14.1 Diagnostic features of TS

Primary diagnostic criteria
Facial angiofibromas
Ungual fibromas
Calcified retinal hamartomas
Multiple cortical tubers
Multiple subependymal glial nodules

Possible additional primary diagnostic criteria
Multiple bilateral renal AMLs
Forehead fibrous plaque
Shagreen patch

Diagnostic criteria with an affected first-degree relative
Histologically proven giant cell astrocytoma
Histologically proven cardiac rhabdomyomas or echocardiographic evidence of more than one lesion in children
Single cortical tuber
Single retinal hamartoma

Secondary diagnostic criteria (two or more needed for diagnosis)
Typical hypomelanic macules
Bilateral polycystic kidneys
Radiographic honeycomb lung (due to pulmonary lymphangiomyomastosis)
Single cardiac rhabdomyoma
Single renal angiomyolipoma
Multiple subcortical hypomyelinated lesions or wedge-shaped cortical-subcortical calcification

rare in the general population, would suggest a diagnosis of TSC. This would include a histologically proven giant cell astrocytoma, cardiac rhabdomyoma or cortical tuber as well as clinical evidence of a single retinal hamartoma and echocardiographic evidence of more than one rhabdomyoma in a child (in adults because of the possible confusion with papillary muscles such a lesion would need to be very large to be diagnostic in the absence of other evidence). Secondary diagnostic criteria are conditions which ideally suggest the need for further investigation: in the absence of supportive diagnostic evidence on imaging, it will remain difficult to make a confident diagnosis of TSC. At least two secondary criteria are therefore required and in many situations it will remain difficult to decide whether or not the individual is affected. All these lesions can occur in isolation in unaffected individuals.

The investigation of the fetus during pregnancy where either the mother or father is affected may help anticipate problems during or before delivery. Fetal echocardiography can be used to monitor for cardiac rhabdomyomas but their detection will be too late to consider termination of pregnancy. More recently cranial fetal MRI imaging has been shown to detect TSC lesions. In the fetus, the lesions are best shown on T1-weighted images rather than the T2-weighted images which are best used after about 3 months of age. It may therefore be possible to show evidence of intracranial disease but again this will be too late to consider a termination of pregnancy. Once the fetus is born, it is possible to examine the skin and multiple hypomelanotic macules would be suggestive but not diagnostic. Echocardiography is best repeated on the newborn infant since it provides better pictures than fetal echocardiography. Ideally echocardiography should be done within 48 h of birth since the normal infant rapidly resorbs glycogen from the heart within 48 h of birth: rhabdomyomas are full of glycogen and the resorption of this glycogen may account for the rapid diminution in size of some cardiac rhabdomyomas after birth. Reduction in size, however, cannot be guaranteed and symptomatic infants may require surgical removal of lesions if these are strategically sited. Fundoscopy through dilated pupils is worthwhile at birth. In the absence of any signs, cranial imaging is problematic. It usually requires a general anaesthetic which makes it a less than ideal investigation. In addition the calcification seen on cranial CT scanning are not always present at birth as the calcification progresses during the course of the first year of life. It may therefore be better to image the infant at the age of 1 or 2 years by which time the parents frequently have decided that they may as well let the child, if remaining asymptomatic, decide on the need for imaging when older. Siblings of individuals affected with TSC should at least be examined dermatologically and ophthalmologically for evidence of TSC. In the author's view, even if the parents are clinically unaffected, it would be wise to offer cranial CT and renal ultrasound scanning to siblings because of the risk that more than one affected child can be born to apparently unaffected parents.

Treatment

Management of the seizures has been greatly aided in recent years by the discovery that vigabatrin is remarkably effective in infantile spasms due to TS [26]. Vigabatrin is probably the treatment of choice (50 mg/kg for 2–3 days, increasing to 100 mg/kg for 2–3 days and then to 150 mg/kg for 2–3 days if necessary). If vigabatrin fails, then treatment of infantile spasms with steroids is advised. The author prefers oral prednisolone 20 mg three times a day regardless of age or weight but some paediatric neurologists still use adrenocorticotrophic hormone (ACTH), usually 40 or 50 international units daily. Other drugs which help with infantile spasms include nitrazepam, sodium valproate and lamotrigine. However, in many cases treatment fails and in many others seizures recur despite initial success. Partial seizures in infancy and other types of generalized seizures are probably best treated with vigabatrin first, followed by sodium valproate or carbamazepine. As children get older, vigabatrin seems to have less effect, but it is still worth trying. Sodium valproate and carbamazepine remain the best alternatives. However, due to the persistence of seizures in many children, all anticonvulsants need to be considered. Clonazepam and clobazam can be effective but cause behavioural problems in a high proportion of children so treated and the older anticonvulsants such as phenytoin and phenobarbitone can be of great help. Lamotrigine has not been particularly effective in older children with tuberous sclerosis and whilst gabapentin would be suitable on theoretical grounds, little is known about its efficacy in TS. Myoclonic seizures and drop attacks are particularly troublesome and respond to the same anticonvulsants if they respond at all. In intractable cases a course of steroids occasionally helps at any age and acetazolamide or a ketogenic diet (which may be impossible in those with behavioural difficulties) can reduce seizures.

Neurosurgery for intractable epilepsy, until recently, has been thought to be contraindicated in TS because of the presence of multiple intracranial lesions any of which might be epileptogenic. However, a few patients have been so treated with remarkable initial success [27] suggesting that not all the lesions are epileptogenic. Clearly the presence of multiple epileptogenic sites on an electroencephalogram (EEG) or clinical evidence of multiple focality, would not suggest that surgery would be successful but in an individual with a single active lesion, surgery could be considered.

Management of the giant cell astrocytomas which occur

in about 5% of individuals with TSC is neurosurgical. In individuals with normal intellect who report the symptoms of raised intracranial pressure (predominantly drowsiness, vomiting, double vision, unsteadiness and headaches) rapid cranial imaging allows a early diagnosis and neurosurgery can be extremely effective. Recurrences are rare and neither chemotherapy nor radiotherapy are thought to be of value in preventing recurrence. Indeed since we now know this condition to be a defect of a tumour suppressor gene, it is probably wise to avoid radiotherapy. It is in individuals with intellectual deficits that delayed diagnosis causes greater problems. The tumours grow very slowly and erode into adjacent tissues if not treated. Because of this screening for giant cell astrocytomas has been suggested but it can not yet be recommended. Giant cell astrocytomas virtually always arise around the foramen of Monro and thereby cause the symptoms of raised intracranial pressure due to obstruction of drainage of cerebrospinal fluid (CSF). Symptoms do therefore usually arise early. Giant cell astrocytomas enhance on cranial CT or MRI scanning. Some subependymal nodules may also enhance without necessarily representing giant cell astrocytomas: certainly they may enhance without necessarily subsequently enlarging. The presence therefore of an enlarging lesion causing obstructive hydrocephalus is suggestive of the diagnosis of a giant cell astrocytoma. Before screening can be recommended it is also useful to know how frequently to recommend imaging. Since some individuals can present with symptoms of a giant cell astrocytoma only weeks after a normal cranial CT or MRI, annual scans are probably not adequate and yet more frequent imaging is hardly realistic particularly in those who would require a general anaesthetic in order to accomplish the procedure. Best practice therefore is to arrange promptly for cranial imaging in an individual with symptoms suggestive of raised intracranial pressure. An increase in seizure activity is not an indication for repeat scanning in the absence of other suggestive symptoms or signs.

Screening for renal disease is undoubtedly worthwhile in order to exclude polycystic kidney disease. However, the management of AML is hampered by a lack of understanding of the natural history of these lesions. We know that individuals who develop symptomatic renal disease, pain and haemorrhage, usually have lesions of more than 3.5 or 4 cm in size. To suggest, however, that all lesions of that size are therefore best treated before symptoms arise, is not appropriate since there are individuals with even larger lesions who have never had symptoms. Screening for renal disease is therefore premature but is carried out by centres trying to understand the natural history of the disorder.

Paediatricians are frequently asked for advice about immunization in children with TS. While there is no proof that immunization is harmful, the need to avoid fits in the first year of life is so important that the risk of provoking such fits should be minimized. The Medical Advisors to the Tuberous Sclerosis Association in the UK, do not agree on the advice to be offered but many feel that immunization with pertussis and measles should be avoided. This advice does leave the child susceptible to wild infection, which would be more serious, and is not appropriate in countries where measles and pertussis are still endemic and common.

Patients with facial angiofibromatosis are most likely to complain of the cosmetic appearance as they reach puberty and during adult life. Individuals with severe learning difficulties will not themselves complain but the appearance can undoubtedly upset those who care for them. This does not necessarily mean that treatment is appropriate for cosmetic reasons, but it is sometimes necessary to prevent recurrent bleeding through shaving in males or through self-inflicted trauma in both sexes. Dermabrasion, curettage, cryosurgery and electrocautery were previously most commonly used, with the occasional surgical removal of large papillomatous lesions. However, recurrence was usually apparent within weeks or months of the initial treatment and was not usually seen as successful either by the patients or their carers. Since laser therapy became available, it has rapidly become the treatment of choice. Initially, argon lasers were used but this has been superseded by the flash lamp pulsed dye laser. Most patients are treated under general anaesthesia and several sessions may be required. The difficulty in attending for a number of treatments and the problems for caring for an individual with learning difficulties following laser treatment, reduce the take up by patients of what would otherwise be much more successful treatment. The result, however, can be very effective for angiomatous lesions, particularly with the flash lamp pulsed dye laser. More nodular lesions with a more fibrous component, are better treated with a CO_2 laser despite the relatively high risk of hypertrophic scarring: this may be reduced by new scanning systems for CO_2 lasers. These lasers may also effect melanin pigmentation leading to hypopigmentation post-treatment. Forehead fibrous plaques can also be treated by laser in the same way as facial angiofibromatous lesions are treated. Shagreen patches are usually hidden and do not therefore require treatment but ungual fibromas can be quite troublesome. These lesions can cause cosmetic disfigurement or bleeding. In manual workers, bleeding can be quite problematic. The best treatment for these lesions has not yet been determined but excision followed by laser treatment may turn out to be more effective than surgery alone.

Treatment of the hypomelanotic lesions is usually not necessary apart from advice to use sun block agents to prevent sunburn during periods of exposure.

The Tuberous Sclerosis International organization exists to support national TS associations. Their aim is to increase the knowledge of TSC throughout the world and to co-ordinate research. They can be contacted through the Tuberous Sclerosis Association of Great Britain in Bromsgrove, Worcestershire, UK.

REFERENCES

1 Bourneville DM. Sclerose tubereuse des circonvolutions cerebrales: idiote et epilepsie hemiplegique. *Arch Neurol (Paris)* 1880; 1: 81–91.

2 Vogt H. Zur diagnostik der tuberosen skelrose. *Z Erforsch Behandl Jugendl Schwachsinns* 1908; 2: 1–12.

3 Van der Hoeve J. Eye symptoms in tuberous sclerosis of the brain. *Trans Ophthalmol Soc UK* 1920; 40: 329–34.

4 Gunther M, Penrose LS. The genetics of epiloia. *J Genet* 1935; 31: 413–30.

5 Hunt A. Tuberous sclerosis; a new estimate of prevalence within the Oxford region. *J Med Genet* 1983; 21: 272–7.

6 Sampson JR, Scahill SJ, Stephenson JBP *et al.* Genetic aspects of tuberous sclerosis in the West of Scotland. *J Med Genet* 1989; 26: 28–31.

7 Umpathy D, Johnston AW. Tuberous sclerosis: prevalence in the Grampian Region of Scotland. *J Ment Def Res* 1989; 33: 349–55.

8 Webb DW, Fryer AE, Osborne JP. Morbidity associated with tuberous sclerosis: a population study. *Dev Med Child Neurol* 1996; 38: 146–55.

9 Wiederhold TW, Gomez MR, Rurland LT. Incidence and prevalence of tuberous sclerosis in Rochester, Minnesota, 1950 through 1982. *Neurology* 1985; 35: 600–3.

10 Webb DW, Fryer AE, Osborne JP. On the incidence of fits and mental retardation in tuberous sclerosis. *J Med Genet* 1991; 28: 395–7.

11 Fryer AE, Chalmers A, Connor JM *et al.* Evidence that the gene for tuberous sclerosis is on chromosome 9. *Lancet* 1987; i: 659–61.

12 Kandt RS, Haines JL, Smith M *et al.* Linkage of an important gene locus for tuberous sclerosis to a chromosome 16 marker for polycystic kidney disease. *Nature Genet* 1992; 2: 37–41.

13 The European Chromosome 16 Tuberous Sclerosis Consortium. Identification and characterisation of the tuberous sclerosis gene on chromosome 16. *Cell* 1993; 75: 1305–15.

14 Povey S, Burley MW, Attwood J *et al.* Two loci for tuberous sclerosis; one on 9q34 and one on 16p13. *Ann Hum Genet* 1994; 58: 107–27.

15 van Slegtenhorst M, de Hoogt R, Hermans C *et al.* Identification of the tuberous sclerosis gene TSC1 on chromosome 9q34. *Science* 1997; 277 (5327): 805–8.

16 Kobayashi T, Hirayama Y, Kobayashi E, Kubo Y, Hino O. A germ line insertion in the tuberous sclerosis (Tsc2) gene give rise to the Eker rat model of dominantly inherited cancer. *Nat Genet* 1995; 9: 70–4.

17 Green AJ, Smith M, Yates JRW. Loss of heterozygosity on chromosome 16p13.3 in hamartomas from tuberous sclerosis patients. *Nature Genet* 1994; 6: 193–6.

18 Green AJ, Johnson P, Yates JRW. The tuberous sclerosis gene on chromosome 9q34 acts as a growth suppressor. *Hum Mol Genet* 1994; 3: 1833–4.

19 Webb DW, Clarke A, Fryer A, Osborne JP. The cutaneous features of tuberous sclerosis: a population study. *Br J Dermatol* 1996; 135: 1–5.

20 Bell SD, MacDonald DM. The prevalence of café au lait patches in tuberous sclerosis. *Clin Exp Dermatol* 1985; 10: 562–5.

21 Webb DW, Kabala J, Osborne JP. A population study of renal disease in patients with tuberous sclerosis. *Br J Urol* 1994; 74: 151–4.

22 Webb DW, Super M, Normand ICS, Osborne JP. Tuberous sclerosis and polycystic kidney diease. *Br Med J* 1993; 306: 1258–9.

23 Oesterling JE, Fishman EK, Goldman SM, Marshall FF. The management of renal angiomyolipoma. *J Urol* 1986; 135: 1121–4.

24 Shepperd CW, Gomez MR, Lie JT, Crowson C. Causes of death of patients with tuberous sclerosis. *Mayo Clin Proc* 1991; 66: 792–6.

25 Osborne JP. Diagnosis of tuberous sclerosis. *Arch Dis Child* 1988; 63: 1423–5.

26 Chiron C, Dumas C, Jambaqué I, Mumford J, Dulac O. Randomized trial comparing vigabatrin and hydrocortisone in infantile spasms due to tuberous sclerosis. *Epilepsy Res* 1997; 26: 389–95.

27 Bebin EM, Kelly PJ, Gomez MR. Surgical treatment for epilepsy in cerebral tuberous sclerosis. *Epilepsia* 1993; 34: 651–7.

Incontinentia Pigmenti and Pigmentary Mosaicism

DIAN DONNAI

Blaschko's lines

Incontinentia pigmenti

Pigmentary mosaicism

Incontinentia pigmenti (IP) and hypomelanosis of Ito are often confused in the older literature but it is most important that they are distinguished from each other since they have different aetiologies and implications for genetic counselling and different clinical effects and natural histories. IP, sometimes known as Bloch–Sulzberger syndrome, is an X-linked dominant single gene disorder. A similar, but clinically distinct, disorder has been observed in several females with X-autosome translocations involving a possible locus at Xp11. At first this was thought to indicate the genetic locus for familial IP but that has been mapped elsewhere on the X chromosome. The disorder associated with X-autosome translocations is sometimes referred to as IP1 and the familial form as IP2. Hypomelanosis of Ito (incontinentia pigmenti achromians) is the dermatological phenotype associated with various types of genetic mosaicism. Since skin manifestations may be hypo- or hyperpigmentation the terms IP achromians and hypomelanosis of Ito are inappropriate. Happle has proposed that a better term would be pigmentary mosaicism.

Blaschko's lines

The clinical similarities of IP2, IP1 and pigmentary mosaicism are due to the distribution of skin lesions in Blaschko's lines. These were first described in 1901 by Blaschko [1], a dermatologist, who noted the occurrence of several skin disorders in a constant pattern in over 100 patients. Interest in these lines was revived by Jackson [2]. Curth and Warburton [3] suggested that the pigmentation following Blaschko's lines in IP2 reflected functional X chromosome mosaicism due to lyonization (X inactivation). Happle [4] widened the debate, suggesting that any disorder which manifested in Blaschko's lines reflected genetic mosaicism, either due to functional mosaicism such as that resulting from lyonization, or due to a somatic gene mutation or to chromosomal non-

disjunction. Blaschko's lines do not correspond to embryological body segments, to the territory supplied by individual nerves or blood vessels, or to Langer's lines. The pattern of Blaschko's lines is circumferential around the trunk, forming a V pattern over the spine, and stopping in the midline anteriorly. The pattern is linear over the shoulders and hips and down the limbs. It is thought that the lines represent the clonal boundaries of cells migrating from the neural crest via the dorsal route.

REFERENCES

1 Blaschko A. *Die Nervenverteilung in der Haut in ihrer Beziehung zu den Erkrankungen der Haut*. Wien-Leipzig: Braumüller, 1901.
2 Jackson R. The lines of Blaschko: a review and reconsideration. *Br J Dermatol* 1976; 95: 349–60.
3 Curth HO, Warburton D. The genetics of incontinentia pigmenti. *Arch Dermatol* 1965; 92: 229–35.
4 Happle R. Mosaicism in human skin. *Arch Dermatol* 1993; 129: 1460–70.

Incontinentia pigmenti

Definition

IP is a multisystem disorder predominantly affecting females. The cutaneous manifestations are diagnostic and classically occur in four stages: vesicular, verrucous, hyperpigmented and atrophic. Not all individuals have all of the cutaneous manifestations which may variably be accompanied by a variety of dental, ocular, neurological and developmental anomalies. It has been suggested that all of the observed findings could be explained by defects in cells of neural crest origin. Classical IP is a familial disorder; pedigree analysis supports X-linked dominant inheritance with male lethality. Familial IP is sometimes referred to as IP2 (MIM no. 308300) and should be distinguished from IP1, the disorder observed in females with X-autosome translocations involving Xp11, and from hypomelanosis of Ito (pigmentary mosaicism) which are discussed below.

History

IP2 was probably first described in 1906 by Garrod [1],

although Bardach [2], Bloch [3], Siemens [4] and Sulzberger [5] defined the condition further. Since then there have been a large number of small series and individual case reports. In 1976 Carney [6] reviewed the literature and, from published reports and his personal series, derived risk figures for cutaneous and non-cutaneous features. However, this analysis is of a group of patients which have been ascertained in a biased way (by publication) and may also be aetiologically heterogeneous. Not all the published reports contained sufficient information to be sure the individuals reported had classical IP2 and some may be examples of pigmentary mosaicism. The gene in familial cases was mapped in 1989 to Xq28 [7].

Aetiology

Review of pedigrees with familial IP suggests that the condition is due to an X-linked dominant gene with lethality in affected males. This mode of inheritance is supported by the high female to male ratio, female to female transmission, and by the increased incidence of miscarriage. In the study of familial IP [8], out of 111 patients, 53 were adult females who had been pregnant at least once. They had a total of 158 pregnancies. Forty (25%) ended in miscarriage, 32 in normal males, 56 in affected females and 30 in normal females. IP has also been reported in males with Klinefelter's syndrome [9,10]. The half chromatid mutation model and postzygotic mutation have been suggested to explain the survival of occasional sporadic males with IP [11]. Father to daughter transmission has been reported [12,13], in each case the father was the first affected member of the family and assumed to be a somatic mosaic. Migeon *et al.* [14] studied five heterozygous females from three kindreds segregating IP and found that cells expressing the mutation were eliminated from skin fibroblast cultures and, to varying degrees, from haematopoietic tissues. Other authors, including Curtis *et al.* [15], have reported skewed X inactivation with preferential inactivation of the IP X chromosome. Two affected half-sisters linked through their unaffected father were both shown to have preferentially inactivated their paternal X chromosome, implying that he was the source of the mutation and likely to be a gonadal mosaic [16].

The most convincing evidence of X-linkage has come from close linkage of IP2 to markers in subchromosomal band Xq28 [7]. Genetic studies have been conducted resulting in maximum LOD scores of up to 13 for markers in the distal portion of Xq28 [17].

Pathology

In the early vesicular cutaneous stage there is massive infiltration of eosinophils into the epidermis, with marked peripheral blood leucocytosis with up to 65% eosinophils. The pathogenesis of the inflammation is unknown and is not directed specifically at the melanocytes. The pigmentary incontinence which gives the condition its name is postinflammatory hyperpigmentation. In time the hyperpigmentation fades. In the so-called atrophic phase, Moss and Ince [18] observed that although the lesions are described as hypopigmented, the contrast with normal skin was probably because of the lack of hair follicles and reduced vascularity. These authors also demonstrated a linear arrangement of sweating and non-sweating skin similar to that described in X-linked hypohidrotic ectodermal dysplasia.

Clinical features

Skin

The cutaneous manifestations of IP are diagnostic; however, their absence does not entirely exclude the diagnosis, especially in first-degree female relatives of classical cases who have several non-cutaneous features. Classically, the dermatological features are described in four stages, but all stages do not necessarily occur and several stages may overlap. There may be a stage which precedes stage 1, the vesicular stage. This author has observed so-called erythema toxicum neonatorum distributed in Blaschko's lines which lasted 24 h before the occurrence of typical vesicles at the age of 48 h in an affected daughter of an affected mother.

Stage 1. The first stage is characterized by blisters, often preceded by localized erythema, which occur anywhere on the body but usually spare the face. The lesions of the first stage develop within the first few weeks after birth, often within the first week. A linear distribution along the limbs and circumferentially around the trunk is classical, although not always so well defined (Fig. 19.15.1). Crops

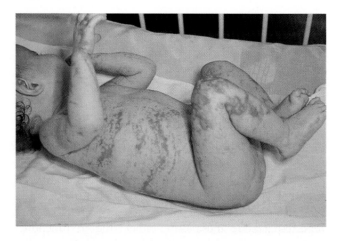

Fig. 19.15.1 Female aged 2 weeks demonstrating vesicular phase of IP in the distribution of Blaschko's lines.

of blisters may occur in the groin and axillary regions and on the vertex of the scalp. Each crop of blisters clears within weeks and may be replaced by new crops at the same or different sites. In general, the vesicles clear within the first 6 months of life although they may recur during acute febrile illness in childhood. These later eruptions are less severe and more short-lived than those which appear in the neonatal period.

Stage 2. The so-called verrucous lesions were observed in just over one-third of the 111 patients reported by Landy and Donnai [8]. These lesions were often short-lived and trivial compared to the initial vesicular eruption and therefore might have been under-reported. In the cases where there was a positive history the lesions had appeared by 2 months and all had cleared by 3 years. The lesions were predominantly seen on the distal limbs, especially the digits and ankles (Fig. 19.15.2). They did not necessarily appear in the same areas as the vesicles. The crusting lesions which develop at the vertex following blistering at that site may be similar to the verrucous lesions but these tended to persist and to be followed by an area of alopecia.

Stage 3. This is the stage which gives its name to the condition but its presence and extent are very variable. It can range from small streaks of pigmentation in the groin (Fig. 19.15.3) to more extensive lesions, especially following Blaschko's lines around the trunk (Fig. 19.15.4). The nipples are frequently involved in the increased pigmentation, and the axillae and groins are invariably affected in patients with pigmentation elsewhere. The pigmentation usually has appeared by 6 months but occasionally not until 2–3 years. By 10 years the lesions have faded in about 25% of cases and the majority of pigmented lesions disappear by the age of 16 years.

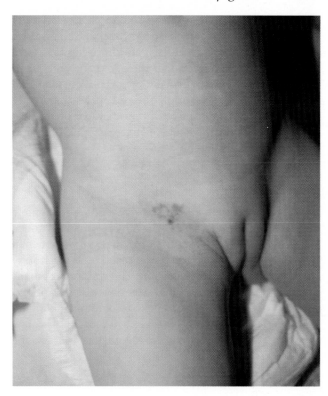

Fig. 19.15.3 Female aged 1 year with small area of increased pigmentation in right groin region.

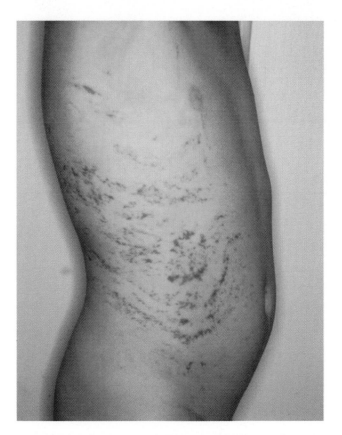

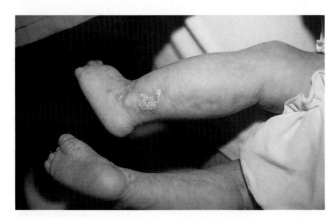

Fig. 19.15.2 Female aged 6 months demonstrating verrucous phase of IP.

Fig. 19.15.4 Female aged 4 years demonstrating widespread pigmentation in the distribution of Blaschko's lines.

Stage 4. This is the so-called atrophic phase classically seen in affected adult females. However, in the series of Landy and Donnai [8] these pale linear lesions were observed in many girls under the age of 10 years, concurrent with hyperpigmented or even vesicular and verrucous lesions. The atrophic lesions are less frequently observed on the trunk and are more often seen on the posterior aspect of the upper and lower legs (Fig. 19.15.5) and over the shoulders and upper arms.

Nails

Nail dystrophy is frequent, occurring in approximately 40% of affected individuals. The range of manifestations is wide, from mild ridging or pitting to severe nail dystrophy resembling onychomycosis. Nail dystrophy may be a transient phenomenon. The child whose nails are illustrated in Fig. 19.15.6 was affected for approximately 6 months before complete resolution. Subungual keratotic lesions have been described [19–21]. The histology of these lesions correspond to that seen in the verrucous cutaneous lesions of stage 2 showing hyperkeratosis, acanthosis, papillomatosis and focal dermal dyskeratosis.

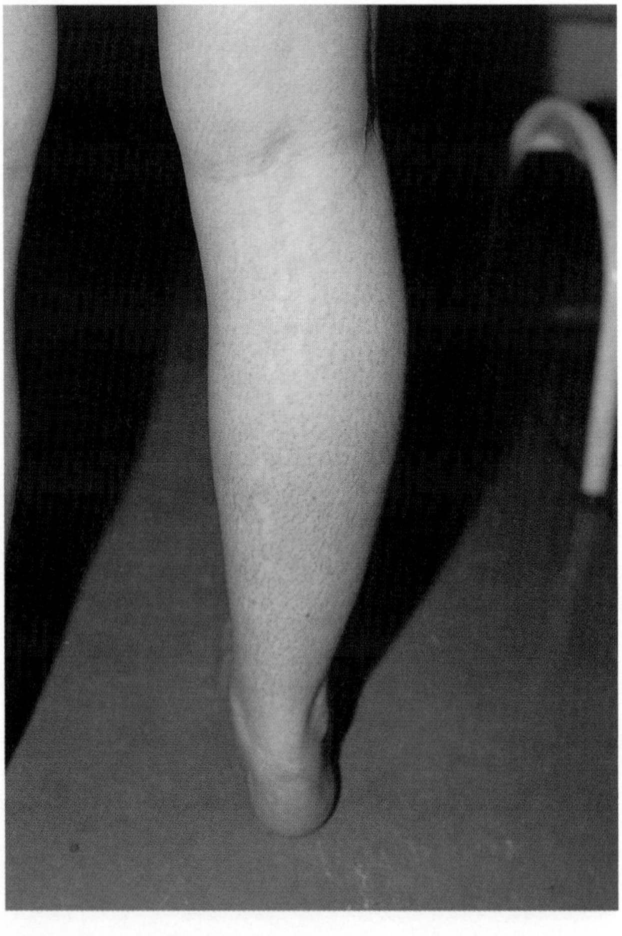

Hair

Whilst hair abnormalities are common it is rare for affected females to have major cosmetic problems. Alopecia, especially at the vertex and usually after blistering or verrucous lesions at this site, is common. Hair is often described as sparse early in childhood, and later in life as lustreless, wiry and coarse. Wiklund *et al.* [22] described the hair in later life as 'woolly hair naevus'.

Teeth

Dental abnormalities are common, occurring in over 80% of cases. Either, or both, deciduous and permanent dentition may be affected, and abnormalities include hypodontia, delayed eruption, impaction and malformation of the crowns, especially conical forms and accessory cusps [21]. Deciduous teeth may be retained into adult life (Fig. 19.15.7). Dental features can be of diagnostic value in adult females, and if present in adult first-degree

Fig. 19.15.5 Adult female demonstrating so-called atrophic phase of IP in a linear lesion over right calf.

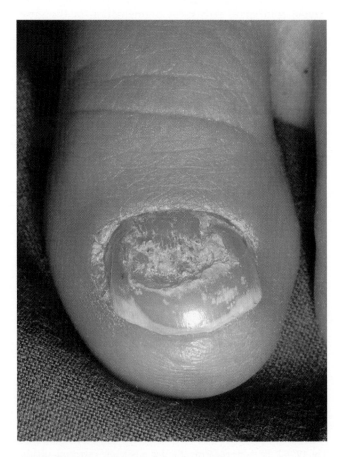

Fig. 19.15.6 Nails of child aged 3 years with IP.

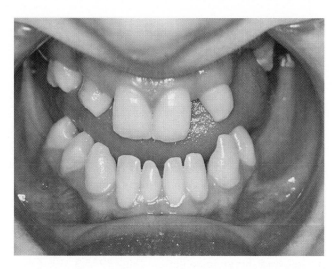

Fig. 19.15.7 Teeth of adult female with IP demonstrating hypodontia and missing upper incisors.

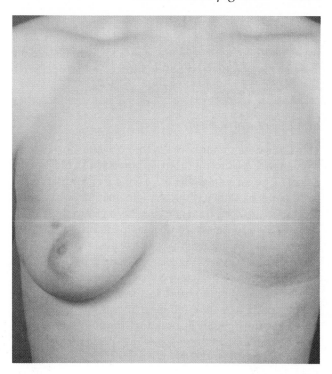

Fig. 19.15.8 Same adult female as in Fig. 19.15.7 demonstrating unilateral aplasia of breast and nipple.

female relatives of an affected case should stimulate a search for other signs such as atrophic skin lesions or hair anomalies.

Breasts

Breast anomalies have rarely been reported in patients with IP but in the series of Landy and Donnai [8], breast anomalies occurred in 10% of cases. One woman had unilateral breast and nipple aplasia (Fig. 19.15.8) whilst 10 others had supernumerary nipples.

Eyes

The incidence of ocular abnormalities in IP is high and may approach 40%. Strabismus occurs in almost one-third of patients, often in association with refractive errors. Occasionally microphthalmos, cataract and optic atrophy are seen. The characteristic lesion, however, of ocular IP involves anomalies of the developing retinal vessels and the underlying pigmented cells [23,24]. Areas of retinal ischaemia promote new vessel proliferation with subsequent bleeding and fibrosis, a somewhat similar process to that found in retinopathy of prematurity. Signs of this process are present in many IP patients but the process is generally limited and only in 10% of patients may it progress to gross intraocular scarring with severe visual loss. When this occurs it is usually only in one eye. Retinal detachment has occasionally been described [25]. Despite the high frequency of ophthalmic complications over 90% of patients have normal vision.

Neurological signs

Although Carney's review [6] found a high frequency of neurological abnormalities the group of patients reviewed may well have been biased and aetiologically heterogeneous. More recent figures from the study of Landy and Donnai [8], where strict diagnostic criteria were applied, suggest a considerably lower incidence of central nervous system (CNS) abnormalities. Whilst 14% of patients had seizures, these were transient and not associated with mental retardation in 8%. Only 6% of patients had persistent seizures. In this group the seizures developed before 12 weeks of age, often in the first week of life, and were associated with a degree of mental retardation. Just under 10% of the 111 patients studied had mental retardation, although in only one-third of these could it be classed as severe. The incidence of retardation in familial cases is 3% compared to 15% in the sporadic cases studied.

Other signs

Although there have been reports of IP patients with recurrent infections, suggesting that immunodeficiency might be a factor, and patients with malignancy, these do not seem to be reported in the larger series of strictly diagnosed familial cases. Similarly, skeletal abnormalities other than those associated with severe neurological deficits have not been described other than in clinical anecdotes.

Differential diagnosis

Any condition with skin manifestations in Blaschko's lines may be confused with IP and strict diagnostic criteria are crucial.

Incontinentia pigmenti 1

This is the designation given to the condition observed in women with X-autosome translocations with a breakpoint at Xp11. The early stage 1 and 2 lesions are not observed in these patients, rather whorled pigmentation or hypopigmentation are seen from early on. As a group these individuals have more severe developmental problems and Sybert [26] has argued that such cases should not be called true IP. Recent molecular studies by Hatchwell have demonstrated random X inactivation in uncultured fibroblasts, lending support to the hypothesis that the phenotype is a manifestation of mosaicism with some cells being functionally disomic for a portion of the X chromosome rather than the effects being due to disruption of a single genetic locus [27].

Hypomelanosis of Ito (*pigmentary mosaicism, incontinentia pigmenti achromians*)

This heterogeneous group of mosaic conditions should be considered in any 'atypical' or severely affected sporadic case of IP.

Goltz focal dermal hypoplasia

This condition with lesions in Blaschko's lines is sometimes confused with IP and it is likely to have the same X-linked dominant mode of inheritance. However, the skin lesions are quite distinct, consisting of focal absence of the dermis in the distribution of Blaschko's lines, with multiple papillomas of mucous membranes as well as linear hyper- and hypopigmentation (Fig. 19.15.9, 19.15.10). Skeletal abnormalities, including limb reduction defects, and major eye abnormalities, including microphthalmia and anophthalmia, are common.

X-linked dominant chondrodysplasia punctata

The early phases of skin manifestations in this condition are ichthyosiform erythroderma and these can sometimes

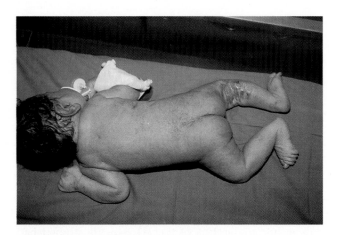

Fig. 19.15.9 Differential diagnosis: newborn female with Goltz focal dermal hypoplasia. Note skin deficiencies on back of right leg and lobster claw deformity of right foot.

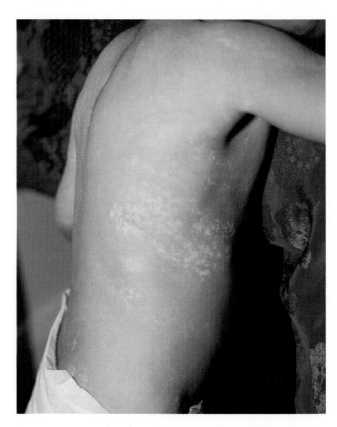

Fig. 19.15.10 Same female as in Fig. 19.15.9. Shown at 3 years. Note atrophic skin with fat herniation in distribution of Blaschko's lines.

be mistaken for the verrucous phase of IP. The hyperkeratotic phase is followed by linear scarring with follicular pitting. Alopecia is sometimes a major problem as are skeletal abnormalities and cataracts.

Treatment

During the neonatal period and when blisters are present it is important to guard against infection and keep the lesions as dry as possible. These is no effective treatment to hasten resolution of any of the phases of IP. It has been suggested that there should be regular screening for retinal abnormalities and that photocoagulation or cryotherapy might be helpful in promoting regression of neovascular changes. Genetic counselling and examination of first-degree female relatives should be offered.

REFERENCES

1 Garrod AE. Peculiar pigmentation of the skin of an infant. *Trans Clin Soc Lond* 1906; 39: 216.
2 Bardach M. Systematisierte Naevusbildungen bei einem eineiigen Zwillingspaar. *Z Kinderheilkd* 1925; 39: 542–50.
3 Bloch B. Eigentumliche, bisher nicht beschriebene Pigmentaffektion (Incontinentia Pigmenti). *Schweiz Med Wochenschr* 1926; 7: 404–5.
4 Siemens HW. Die Melanosis corii degenerative eine neue Pigmentdermatose. *Arch Dermatol Syph (Berl)* 1929; 157: 382–91.
5 Sulzberger MB. Uber eine bisher nicht beschriebene congenitale Pigmentanomalie (IP). *Arch Dermatol Syph (Berl)* 1928; 154: 19–32.
6 Carney RG. Incontinentia pigmenti: a world statistical analysis. *Arch Dermatol* 1976; 112: 535–42.
7 Sefiani A, Abel L, Heuertz S *et al.* The gene for incontinentia pigmenti is assigned to Xq28. *Genomics* 1989; 4: 427–9.
8 Landy SJ, Donnai D. Incontinentia pigmenti (Bloch–Sulzberger syndrome). *J Med Genet* 1993; 30: 53–9.
9 Ormerod AD, White MI, McKay E, Johnston AW. Incontinentia pigmenti in a boy with Klinefelter's syndrome. *J Med Genet* 1987; 24: 439–41.
10 Garcia-Dorado J, De Unamo P, Fernandez-Lopez E *et al.* Incontinentia pigmenti: XXY male with family history. *Clin Genet* 1990; 38: 128–38.
11 Lenz W. Half chromatid mutations may explain incontinentia pigmenti in males. *Am J Hum Genet* 1975; 27: 690–1.
12 Sommer AM, Liu PH. Incontinentia pigmenti in a father and his daughter. *Am Med Genet* 1984; 17: 655–9.
13 Emery MM, Siegfried EC, Stone MS *et al.* Incontinentia pigmenti: transmission from father to daughter. *J Am Acad Dermatol* 1993; 29: 368–72.
14 Migeon BR, Axelman J, De Beur SJ *et al.* Selection against lethal alleles in females heterozygous for incontinentia pigmenti. *Am J Hum Genet* 1989; 44: 100–6.
15 Curtis ARJ, Lindsay S, Boye E *et al.* A study of X chromosome activity in two incontinentia pigmenti families with probable linkage to Xq28. *Eur J Hum Genet* 1994; 2: 51–8.
16 Kirchman TTT, Levy ML, Lewis RA *et al.* Gonadal mosaicism for incontinentia pigmenti in a healthy male. *J Med Genet* 1995; 32: 887–90.
17 Smahi A, Hyden-Granskog C, Peterlin B *et al.* The gene for the familial form of incontinentia pigmenti (IP2) maps to the distal part of Xq28. *Hum Mol Gen* 1994; 3: 273–8.
18 Moss C, Ince P. Anhydrotic and achromians lesions in incontinentia pigmenti. *Br J Dermatol* 1987; 116: 839–50.
19 Hartman DL. Incontinentia pigmenti associated with subungual tumours. *Arch Dermatol* 1966; 94: 632–5.
20 Mascaro JM, Palon J, Vires P *et al.* Painful subungual keratotic tumours in incontinentia pigmenti. *J Am Acad Dermatol* 1985; 13: 913–18.
21 Simmons DA, Kegel MF, Scher RK, Hines YC. Subungual tumours in incontinentia pigmenti. *Arch Dermatol* 1986; 122: 1431–4.
22 Wiklund DA. Incontinentia pigmenti. A four-generation study. *Arch Dermatol* 1980; 116: 701–3.
23 Goldberg MF, Custis PH. Retinal and other manifestations of incontinentia pigmenti (Bloch–Sulzberger syndrome). *Ophthalmology* 1993; 100: 1645–54.
24 Francois J. Incontinentia pigmenti and retinal changes. *Br J Ophthal* 1984; 68: 19–25.
25 Wald KJ, Mehta MC, Katsumi O *et al.* Retinal detachments in incontinentia pigmenti. *Arch Ophthalmol* 1993; 111: 614–17.
26 Sybert VP. Incontinentia pigmenti nomenclature. *Am J Hum Genet* 1995; 55: 209–11.
27 Hatchwell E, Robinson D, Crolla JA, Cockwel AE. X-inactivation analysis in a female with hypomelanosis of Ito associated with a balanced X;17 translocation: evidence for functional disomy of Xp. *J Med Genet* 1996; 33: 216–20.

Pigmentary mosaicism

Definition

Pigmentary mosaicism is a group of multisystem disorders affecting males and females. The condition is named after the cutaneous manifestations which are flat hypo- or hyperpigmented lesions in the distribution of Blaschko's lines.

History

Ito [1] described a woman with hypopigmented lesions in a zig-zag pattern around her trunk and in a linear pattern down her arms. No other physical abnormality was reported apart from asymmetry of breast size and he named the condition IP achromians. The condition was later renamed hypomelanosis of Ito. Takematsu *et al.* [2] identified over 70 published cases with similar skin pigmentary abnormalities. Of the reviewed patients three-quarters had one or more abnormalities of the CNS, hair, teeth, eyes or skeletal system. Flannery *et al.* [3] first proposed the hypothesis that the pigmentary abnormalities might be a non-specific sign of chromosomal mosaicism based on his observations of a girl with 45,X/46,Xr(Y) mosaicism in skin fibroblasts who had pigmentary lesions. Donnai *et al.* [4], Thomas *et al.* [5] and Sybert *et al.* [6] described further series of patients with hypomelanosis of Ito and chromosomal mosaicism detected on skin biopsy, confirming Flannery's hypothesis. More recently, Happle, recognizing that the skin changes in hypomelanosis of Ito might be hypo- or hyperpigmentation, has proposed a better term would be pigmentary mosaicism.

Aetiology

The recognition that chromosomal mosaicism was the basis of many cases of hypomelanosis of Ito explained the varied clinical manifestations of the disorder and their asymmetrical expression. Chromosomal mosaicism is rarely demonstrated in cultured blood lymphocytes and the abnormal cell line is usually only found in cultured fibroblasts. A wide variety of aneuploid cell lines have been described, including (a) triploidy; (b) trisomies, monosomies and structural abnormalities of autosomes including rings, inversions and deletions; (c) monosomies and structural abnormalities of sex chromosomes; and (d) X autosome translocations. The only consistent feature is that at least two chromosomally different cell lines are present. More recently, females have been described with skin pigmentary abnormalities in Blaschko's lines where there was only one cell line present with a structural abnormality involving an X chromosome. In some of these cases it has been demonstrated that there is functional mosaicism due to abnormal X-inactivation [7].

In some series and in this author's experience, chromosomal mosaicism is only found in about one-third of the cases of patients diagnosed clinically as having pigmentary mosaicism. There are a number of possible explanations for this: the aneuploid cell line may not be present in the tissue examined, a microdeletion may be responsible or the abnormality may be a point mutation of a single gene present in a mosaic form. Moss *et al.* [8], recognizing that the skin pigmentary pattern may reflect epidermal rather than dermal mosaicism, studied cells of neural crest origin. Keratinocyte cultures were performed in four patients with pigmentary mosaicism, three had previously yielded normal chromosomal results on blood and fibroblast culture, in one a single cell out of 70 fibroblasts analysed showed an abnormal chromosome pattern. The keratinocyte culture confirmed this abnormal finding in this patient, and in a further patient whose fibroblast culture was negative a trisomy 7 cell line was demonstrated in keratinocytes.

There have been a number of reports claiming familial occurrence. Groshans *et al.* [9] reported a mother and three daughters. The daughters were severely retarded and had depigmented lesions on their trunks, the mother had only a single depigmented lesion. This family history is consistent with an X-linked disorder and the histology reported was not characteristic of pigmentary mosaicism and rather suggested X-linked dominant chondrodysplasia punctata. Rubin [10] described a female case of hypomelanosis of Ito, her father was reported to have had similar skin problems which were no longer present but no further clinical details were given. The proband's older brothers were reported as having depigmented areas but the distribution is more like that seen in vitiligo than pigmentary mosaicism. The third report of familial hypomelanosis of Ito in the literature is by Jelinek *et al.* [11]. The proband was a 4-year-old girl whose dead paternal great aunt was said to have had similar skin findings. None of these published reports are convincing.

Pathology

Histological features are relatively non-specific and include decreased numbers of melanocytes and melanosomes in the basal layer of the epidermis in the light areas of skin.

Clinical features

Skin

There can be hypo- or hyperpigmentation (Fig. 19.14.11–19.14.13). In some individuals pigmentary disturbance is recognized at birth or soon after, but in racially light-skinned individuals the pigmentary abnormalities may not be apparent unless sought, and may only be

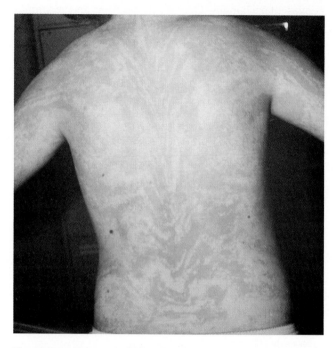

Fig. 19.15.11 Four-year-old female with pigmentary mosaicism. Note increased pigmentation in distribution of Blaschko's lines.

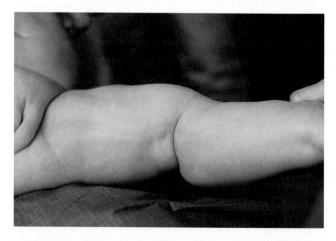

Fig. 19.15.12 Six-month-female with pigmentary mosaicism. Note linear depigmented lesions on back of left leg.

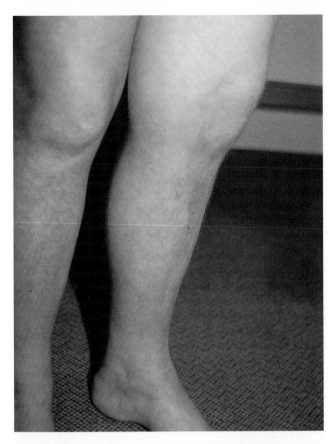

Fig. 19.15.13 Eight-year-old female. Note linear areas of increased pigmentation on legs.

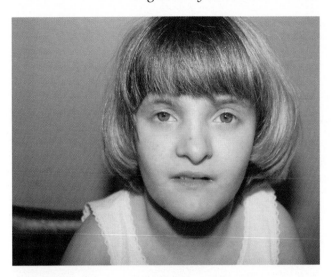

Fig. 19.15.14 Female with pigmentary mosaicism due to diploid/triploid mosaicism. Note heterochromia of irides.

commonly have hypodontia, absent teeth, irregularities of teeth spacing and size and unusual dental cusps [12].

Eye abnormalities

Eye abnormalities are frequently reported in patients with pigmentary mosaicism. These include microphthalmia, iris coloboma, heterochromia of the irides (Fig. 19.15.14) and pinpoint pupils [4]. Abnormal variations in the retinal pigmentary pattern are often observed, occasional patients have optic atrophy.

Limb and skeletal abnormalities

Joint contractures, particularly talipes [5], and camptodactyly of the fingers are particularly common, as is asymmetry of size of limbs and body parts. Kyphoscoliosis is frequently seen and may result from structural abnormalities of the vertebrae or from differential growth of the two sides of the body. Digital abnormalities are particularly common in patients who have diploid/triploid mosaicism (Fig. 19.15.15) [4]. Polydactyly, ectrodactyly, syndactyly and triphalangeal thumbs have also been reported.

Central nervous system abnormalities

In contrast to IP where mental retardation is rare, severe, moderate or mild mental retardation is commonly found in patients with pigmentary mosaicism. In some series more than 60% of patients had an IQ below 70 [13]. Early onset seizures are common and may be difficult to control. The association of severe epilepsy with mental retardation is thought to result from abnormal neuronal migration. In some patients magnetic resonance imaging (MRI) has

visualized under ultraviolet (UV) light. In at least two personally observed patients pigmentary patterns were looked for in the first year of life including with UV light, and not found, but developed over the course of the next 2 years. Unlike IP, no preceding vesicular or verrucous phase is seen. The edges of the hypo- or hyperpigmented areas are indistinct and close inspection reveals variations in pigment within the broader, generally hyper- or hypopigmented lines. There are few longitudinal reports of individual patients. In 15 personally observed cases there has been a general increase in hypo- or hyperpigmentation in infancy but after that, in follow-up, extending in some cases to 7 years, the skin pigmentary abnormalities have remained constant.

Hair, nails and teeth

Hair abnormalities are common, Sybert *et al.* [6] reported variations in colour and texture of hair. Occasional patients have areas of alopecia. Commonly, patients have slight variations in colour of the hair, often termed 'pepper and salt' colouring. Nail abnormalities are not so common as in IP but ridging and occasional hypoplasia or absence of nails is observed. Patients with pigmentary mosaicism

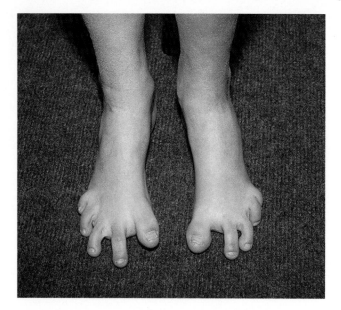

Fig. 19.15.15 Feet of same female as in Fig. 19.15.14. Note widespaced toes with expanded ends and flexion deformities.

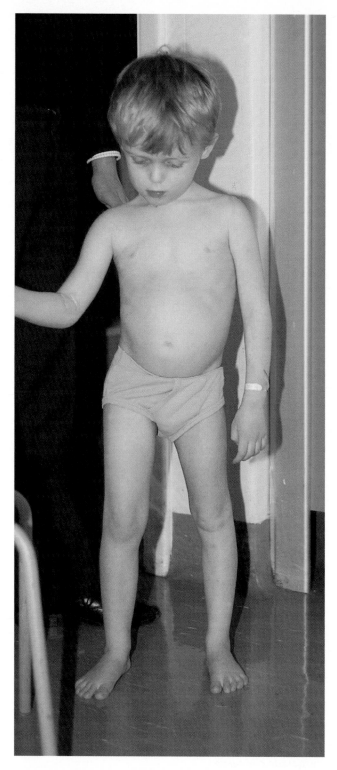

Fig. 19.15.16 Four-year-old male with pigmentary mosaicism. Note hypertrophy of right leg and left side of chest.

confirmed neuronal migration defects, and histological examination has revealed pachygyria, heterotopias as well as structural abnormalities of the brain. Autistic behaviour is a complication present in about 10% of patients [13].

Other abnormalities

Numerous abnormalities have been reported in individual patients. These include cardiac defects [6], ventricular septal defects (VSD), kidney anomalies including unilateral renal agenesis and horsehoe kidneys [5] and genital abnormalities such as hypospadias and vaginal skin tags.

Growth

Macrocephaly has been reported in a number of individuals with pigmentary mosaicism, and in older individuals truncal obesity has been a feature. Hemihypertrophy is observed and is not necessarily limited to one side of the body but may involve, for example, one arm and the contralateral leg (Fig. 19.15.16).

Differential diagnosis

The differential diagnosis of pigmentary mosaicism is similar to that for IP considered above.

Treatment

Treatment is symptomatic. Seizures should be fully investigated and treated. Asymmetry of growth and specific abnormalities may require orthopaedic treatment and educational support is frequently necessary.

REFERENCES

1 Ito M. Studies on melanin. IX. Incontinentia pigmenti achromians—a singular case of nevus depigmentosus systematicus bilateralis. *Tohoku J Exp Med* 1952; 55(suppl): 57–9.

2 Takematsu H, Sato S, Igarashi M, Seiji M. Incontinentia pigmenti achromians (Ito). *Arch Dermatol* 1983; 119: 391–5.

3 Flannery DB, Byrd JR, Freeman WE, Perlman SA. Hypomelanosis of Ito; a cutaneous marker of chromosomal mosaicism. *Am J Hum Genet* 1985; 37: A93.

4 Donnai D, Read AP, McKeown C, Andrew T. Hypomelanosis of Ito: a manifestation of mosaicism or chimerism. *J Med Genet* 1988; 25: 809–18.

5 Thomas IT, Frias JL, Cantu ES, Lafer CZ, Flannery DB, Graham JG. Association of pigmentary anomalies with chromosomal and genetic mosaicism and chimerism. *Am J Hum Genet* 1989; 45: 193–205.

6 Sybert VP, Pagon RA, Donlan M, Bradley CM. Pigmentary abnormalities and mosaicism for chromosomal aberration. Association with clinical features similar to hypomelanosis of Ito. *J Pediatr* 1990; 116: 581–6.

7 Hatchwell E, Robinson D, Crolla JA, Cockwel AE. X-inactivation analysis in a female with hypomelanosis of Ito associated with a balanced X;17 translocation: evidence for functional disomy of Xp. *J Med Genet* 1996; 33: 216–20.

8 Moss C, Larkins S, Stacey M, Blight A, Farndon PA, Davison EV. Epidermal mosaicism and Blaschko's lines. *J Med Genet* 1993; 30: 752–5.

9 Groshans EM, Stoebner P, Bergoend J, Stoll C. Incontinentia pigmenti achromians (Ito)—etude clinique et histopathologique. *Dermatologica* 1971; 142: 65–78.

10 Rubin MB. Incontinentia pigmenti achromians—multiple cases within a family. *Arch Dermatol* 1972; 105: 424–5.

11 Jelinek JE, Bart RS, Sciff GM. Hypomelanosis of Ito (incontinentia pigmenti achromians—report of three cases and review of the literature). *Arch Dermatol* 1973; 107: 596–601.

12 Happle R, Vakilzadeh F. Harmartomatous dental cusps in hypomelanosis of Ito. *Clin Genet* 1982; 21: 65–8.

13 Anon. Hypomelanosis of Ito. *Lancet* 1992; 339: 65–652.

19.16   The Gorlin (Naevoid Basal Cell Carcinoma) Syndrome

PETER A. FARNDON

Definition

The three main components of the Gorlin syndrome (naevoid basal cell carcinoma or NBCC) are multiple basal cell carcinomas (BCC), recurrent jaw cysts and non-progressive skeletal anomalies. Other hallmarks are palmar and plantar pits, ectopic calcification and an increased incidence of congenital malformations.

It is a fully penetrant autosomal dominant disorder with extremely variable expression, both within and between families. Not only does the variability manifest itself in the presence or absence of a particular feature, but also in its severity.

Adult patients with the Gorlin syndrome may present to any speciality as there are over 100 recognized features. In the absence of a family history, most children are diagnosed because of jaw cysts, a (usually unexpected) histological diagnosis of BCC in a biopsied skin lesion or skeletal anomalies found on X-rays taken for other reasons. Occasionally a child may present with hundreds of 'naevi' but it is unusual for aggressive BCCs to be the presenting feature in childhood.

Another common name for the syndrome is basal cell naevus syndrome but this name is inappropriate because histologically the naevi are BCCs, although not all behave aggressively. It has also been suggested that it be known as the NBCC syndrome, although 10% of adults do not develop BCCs. Rather than focus on one feature of the condition, it may be better to use the eponymous title of Gorlin syndrome, in recognition of Professor Robert Gorlin's contributions, especially as parents and patients prefer not to have a condition which contains the word 'carcinoma'.

History

Skeletal signs of the syndrome have been found in Egyptian mummies, presumed to be father and son [1]. The first reported cases appear to be those of Jarisch and White in 1894 [2,3].

The term basal cell naevus was coined by Nomland [4] when he reported an unusual case of invasive BCC of the face that occurred in adult life from congenital pigmented basal cell tumours. Clinically, the tumours resembled pigmented moles (naevi); microscopically the cells were 'like dark staining basal cells'. Thus the name 'nevus of basal cells' was used.

Gorlin and Goltz's description of two patients and review of the literature in 1960 [5] drew the condition to wide attention. However, Howell and Caro in the dermatological literature in 1959 [6] had attempted to correlate the clinical features of the unusual tumours in the syndrome with the interpretations which then prevailed, and introduced the term 'basal cell naevus syndrome'. For many years, clinicians had puzzled over rare cases of multiple tumours that, histologically, seemed to be epithelioma adenoides cysticum (EAC), but clinically behaved like rodent ulcers. Some believed that the tumours were unique, whilst others believed that the tumours were EAC transformed into rodent ulcers. Howell and Caro proposed that the tumours were a unique type of BCC which was capable of aggressive behaviour in adults, and were associated with developmental anomalies. They pointed out that the harmless clinical appearance of the tumours, especially in childhood, contrasted strikingly with the microscopic appearance and destructive behaviour of tumours in adulthood. They also felt that although ionizing radiation was curative, its use was not prudent because of the multiplicity of tumours and the concern over new ones erupting in the irradiated area.

Mason et al. [7] proposed the term naevoid basal cell carcinoma syndrome because of the confusion over the term 'naevus'.

Gorlin presented extensive reviews of the syndrome in 1987 [8] and 1995 [9], combining information from a personal series of patients and a review of 216 papers.

Aetiology and pathogenesis

A population-based study in north-west England gave a minimum prevalence of 1 in 55 600 [10].

Rahbari and Mehregan [11] reported a group of 59 children under the age of 19 years with a histologically proven BCC. Ten had a BCC which had developed in a pre-existing naevus sebaceous. Of the others, 13 (26%) had features of the Gorlin syndrome. Two other children were developing a second BCC but they had no signs of the syndrome on X-ray or examination.

The syndrome is an autosomal dominant condition, giving a 1 in 2 risk that a child of an affected parent will inherit the disorder. The gene is located at 9q22.3 and there is no evidence for genetic heterogeneity.

A new mutation rate of up to 40% has been suggested [12], and a paternal age effect reported [13]. The new mutation rate obtained from the literature may be an overestimate because not all parents were thoroughly investigated. The author knows of several families whose child was considered to have a new mutation until careful examination confirmed that one of the parents had the syndrome, albeit with very mild features.

Most, if not all, features of the Gorlin syndrome suggest that the gene is primarily involved in the control of cell growth and active in all three germ layers of the embryo.

The clinical behaviour of the naevi and BCCs fits the paradigm of Knudson's two-hit hypothesis [14] and suggests that the gene also acts as a tumour suppressor. A naevus may result when function of the normal allele is lost in a cell which already has an inherited or acquired mutation in the other copy of the gene. As only a proportion of naevi behave aggressively, it seems likely that at least one further event altering cellular control is required for a naevus to become locally invasive. Treatment by radiation appears to provide this stimulus in some patients with the Gorlin syndrome.

Following the localization of the gene to chromosome 9q22.3–31 [15–17], evidence that the gene is indeed a tumour suppressor gene came from studies of loss of heterozygosity in BCCs [18] and jaw cysts [19]. The alleles lost at 9q22.3–31 were those inherited from the unaffected parent, as expected from Knudson's hypothesis.

Other features of the Gorlin syndrome, especially the congenital malformations, do not fit easily into a loss of function model, and require further explanation. A gene dosage effect could explain the congenital malformations and the variation in expression.

The gene was isolated by positional cloning in 1996 [20,21] and was shown to have strong homology with the *Drosophila* patched gene, *Drosophila* patched is involved in establishing segment polarity in embryos, an integral part of the highly conserved *hedgehog* signalling pathway. *Patched* (ptc) and *smoothened* (smo) proteins form a membrane receptor complex, in which ptc represses the function of smo. When the secreted protein *hedgehog* binds to ptc, the repression is released, allowing smo to signal intracellularly, affecting several pathways and transcription factors. Phenotypic variability (presence/absence and severity of features) within families with Gorlin syndrome may therefore be due to fluctuations between levels of several proteins in an extremely dosage-sensitive pathway, whilst the jaw cysts and BCCs occur when the wild-type allele is lost releasing the cell from the control exerted by that allele. Indeed, the majority of mutations characterized in the author's laboratory appear to cause truncation of the protein giving further support to the postulated mechanisms.

Pathology

Histology of basal cell carcinomas

The naevi and NBCCs are histologically identical to BCCs. About one-third of patients have two or more types of NBCCs, including superficial, multicentric, solid, cystic, adenoid and lattice-like [22]. NBCCs are more commonly associated with melanin pigmentation and foci of calcification than non-syndromic BCCs, but otherwise cannot be distinguished.

Histology of jaw cysts

The histological features are characteristic [23]. The cysts are lined by a parakeratotic stratified squamous epithelium which is usually about five to eight cell layers thick and without rete ridges. Rarely the form of keratinization is orthokeratotic. The basal layer is well defined with regularly orientated palisaded cells. Satellite cysts, epithelial rests and proliferating dental lamina are sometimes seen in the cyst capsules.

Palmar and plantar pits

The pits appear to be caused by premature desquamation of horny cells along the intercellular spaces, but are not due to degeneration of the horny cells themselves. Light microscopy reveals a lack of keratinization of pit tissue and a proliferation of basaloid cells in irregular rete ridges [24].

Electron microscopy [25] showed that the epithelium at the base of the pits consists of keratinocytes containing poorly developed tonofibrils. Discharge of cementsomes from the horny cells was incomplete, perhaps due to a shortened transit time of keratinocytes, so failing to provide enough intercellular cement.

Scanning electron microscopy [24] showed the stratum corneum overlying the epithelium at the bases of the pits to be thin, irregular and containing large defects. The stratum corneum at the margins of the pits was thicker, more compact and more adherent. The pit walls descended from a gently rounded top to a point of sharp transition between pit epithelium and normal epithelium.

Response to radiation

As some patients respond to therapeutic irradiation by later developing crops of BCCs in the treated area, *in vitro* studies of cellular radiation hypersensitivity have been undertaken. They have given conflicting results. It appears, however, that the cancer susceptibility is not caused by nor manifested as chromosome instability, nor that increased cell killing is a major effect of the gene.

Little *et al.* [26] demonstrated a moderate degree of radiation hypersensitivity in one family member whereas the remaining affected and non-affected individuals from the same family responded normally. They suggested that isolated cases of *in vitro* radiation hypersensitivity may not relate to the underlying genetic disorder. It seems likely that the response to radiation may be affected by other genes of major effect, and their delineation by comparing family members with the syndrome will be helpful.

Ultraviolet radiation

Circumstantial evidence that exposure to sunlight may be deleterious comes from population studies: 14% of cases in a north-west England study [10] developed a BCC before the age of 20 years, compared with 47% in Australia (G. Trench, personal communication).

Laboratory experiments with ultraviolet radiation, however, have been inconclusive. Fibroblasts have been found to have no differences in sensitivity [27] following ultraviolet C (UVC) whilst others were more sensitive to UVC [28].

The majority of experiments have been conducted with UVC radiation (254 nm), but epidemiological and clinical studies indicate that UVB radiation (280–320 nm) in sunlight is responsible for the induction of most skin cancers in humans.

Gorlin syndrome fibroblasts have been shown to be hypersensitive to killing by UVB but not UVC radiation [29,30] compared with skin fibroblasts from normal individuals. This was not due to a defect in the excision repair of pyrimidine dimers [30].

Response to parathormone

It was considered that there may be a relationship between Gorlin syndrome and pseudohypoparathyroidism because ectopic calcification and short metacarpals are features of both. Later studies [31] using cyclic adenosine monophosphate (cAMP) failed to confirm initial reports of an absence of phosphorus diuresis following intravenous injection of parathormone. No biochemical abnormalities have been detected in the author's series.

Clinical features and natural history

The major features of the syndrome which present in childhood are shown in Table 19.16.1, compiled from a

Table 19.16.1 Summary of frequency of features in childhood in Gorlin's syndrome by organ system

	%
Skin	
Milia	42
Meibomian cysts	6
Epidermal cysts	44
Skin tags	6
Palmar pits	
<10 years	65
<15 years	80
Plantar pits	49
Naevi <20 years	53
Basal cell carcinomas	
<20 years	14
>20 years	73
>40 years	92
Jaw cysts	
10 years	13
20 years	51
>40 years	79–90
Misshapen/missing teeth	30
Skeletal	
High arched palate	6
Sloping shoulders	61
Sprengel shoulder	46
Pectus excavatum	20
Thoracic scoliosis	47
Short fourth metacarpal	26
Short terminal phalanx thumbs	9
Stiff thumbs	6
Polydactyly	8
OFC	97
Operative delivery	62
Facial features	
Bossing	79
'Typical face'	70
Prognathism	46
Eyebrows arched	28
Palpebral fissures	
downslanting	30
upslanting	13
Eye anomalies	30
Strabismus	19
Cataracts	4
Cleft lip and palate	7
Other features	
Mental retardation	?3
Epilepsy	6
Medulloblastoma	5
Ovarian fibroma	24 adult females
Undescended testes	6 males
Inguinal hernia	17 males
Cardiac fibroma	2.5
X-ray findings	
Cervical/thoracic vertebral anomalies	60
Rib anomalies	70
Calcification: Falx <15 years	40
: diaphragm sella (20 years)	100

OCP, occipito-frontal head circumference.

review of the literature and the author's own observations of over 140 patients many of whom have been followed for more than 10 years. Some features are described in more detail below.

Developmental history

Of children in the author's series 62% had an operative delivery. The average birth weight was 4.1 kg, and head circumference 38 cm, both greatly increased when compared with siblings. Walking was delayed until an average of 18 months; siblings walked at 12–13 months. Several children had investigations for hydrocephalus because of striking macrocephaly—the head circumference was grossly above the 97th centile but growth continued parallel with the centile lines. Many children initially have a motor delay, but appear to catch up. All children known to the author have attended mainstream school, a few needing additional help.

In the literature 'mental retardation' has been reported in about 3%. In the population study in the north-west of England there were no cases of moderate or severe mental retardation in 84 cases [10] apart from treated cases of medulloblastoma. About 6% of patients in that study required prolonged anticonvulsant therapy for grand mal seizures.

Build

Patients tend to be tall. Their heights are usually above the 97th centile, often in marked contrast to unaffected siblings. Some patients exhibit a marfanoid build.

Shape and size of cranium

One of the most striking features is the increased head size present from birth. All children and adults in the author's series had a head circumference on or above the 97th centile and above the corresponding centile line for height. The head gives the appearance of being long in the anteroposterior (AP) plane, with a prominent and low occiput.

Facial appearance

About 70% of patients have the characteristic facies but there is intrafamilial variation. Figures 19.16.1 and 19.16.2 show children and an adult with the syndrome.

Frontal, temporal and biparietal bossing in 80% give a prominent appearance to the upper part of the face, and patients often adopt hairstyles which disguise the bossing. There is often facial asymmetry. Some patients have well-developed supraorbital ridges, giving the eyes a sunken appearance. The eyebrows are often heavy, fused and arched. There is a broad nasal root and hyper-

telorism. The inner canthal, interpupillary and outer canthal distances are all generally above the 97th centile, but appear to be in proportion with the head circumference. The mandible is long and often prominent with the lower lip protruding in front of the upper. There is a well-established association with cleft lip/palate which occurs in 5–6%.

It can be very helpful to compare a person's facial appearance with siblings because there is usually a striking difference in the facial gestalt between unaffected and affected siblings.

In a personally examined series, 26% of cases had ophthalmic problems, 56% having a convergent strabismus. Of patients reported in the literature 10–15% have ophthalmic abnormalities including congenital blindness due to corneal opacity, congenital glaucoma, coloboma of the iris, choroid or optic nerve, convergent or divergent strabismus, nystagmus, cataracts and microphthalmia, ptosis, proptosis, medullated nerve fibres and retinal hamartomas.

Small keratin-filled cysts (milia) are found on the face in 30%, most commonly in the infraorbital areas, but they can also occur on the forehead. Meibomian cysts on the corneal surface of the eyelids can cause great distress as they repeatedly discharge material.

Skin tags are especially common around the neck; like the naevi, histology reveals the typical features of a BCC, but the skin tags do not generally change in size or shape.

Jaw cysts

Some 13% of cases develop a jaw cyst by the age of 10 years and 51% by the age of 20 years. The majority occur after the seventh year. The youngest affected case known to the author presented with jaw swelling at 5 years old. The peak incidence is in the third decade—about 10 years earlier than isolated odontogenic keratocysts. Around 26% of cases over the age of 40 years in the author's series had not developed signs or symptoms of cysts; Gorlin gave a figure of 10% [8].

The mandible is involved far more frequently than the maxilla, with keratocysts occurring most usually at the angle of the mandible (Fig. 19.16.3).

Patients can be remarkably free of symptoms until cysts reach a large size, especially when the ascending ramus is involved. Presentation can be with swelling and/or pain of the jaw, pus discharging into the oral cavity or displaced, impacted or loose teeth.

Misshapen teeth, missing teeth and a susceptibility to caries are more common in patients than in unaffected relatives.

Chest and trunk

Epidermoid cysts occur on the limbs and trunk in over

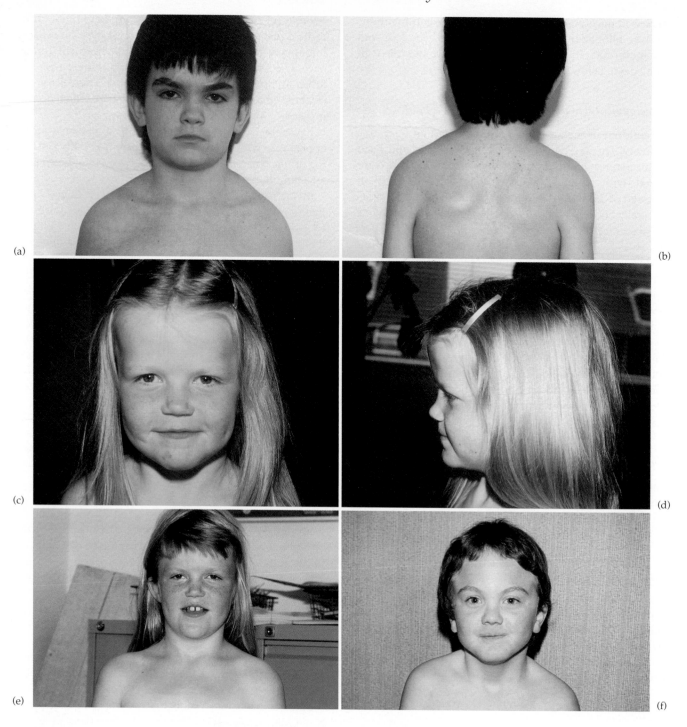

Fig. 19.16.1 (a–f) Four children with Gorlin syndrome showing the degree of variation in facial appearance, frontal bossing and sloping of the shoulders. Sprengel shoulder is also shown.

50% of cases. They are usually 1–2 cm in diameter, and are particularly common around the knee.

Rib anomalies may give an unusual shape to the chest, including a characteristic downward sloping of the shoul-ders (see Fig. 19.16.1). The rib anomalies, together with kyphoscoliosis may cause pectus excavatum or carinatum in about 30–40% of patients. Sprengel deformity has been found in some surveys to be as common as 25%. Of males 17% have inguinal herniae.

Hands and feet

The distinctive pits found on the palms and soles appear

to be pathognomonic [32]. They increase in number with age, are permanent and when found in a child are a strong diagnostic indicator. They may vary from only a few to over a hundred. BCCs have very rarely arisen in the base of the pits.

In the author's series, 65% had palmar pits by the age of 10 years rising to 80% by the age of 15 years. They were present in 85% cases over the age of 20 years.

The pits are small (1–2 mm), often asymmetric, shallow depressions, with the colour of the base being white, flesh coloured or pale pink (Fig. 19.16.4). They are found more commonly on the palms (77%) than on the soles (50%). Pits can also appear independently on the sides of the fingers, when they are tiny bright red pin-pricks.

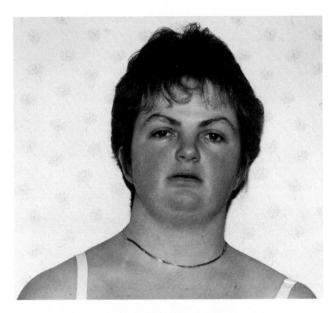

Fig. 19.16.2 An adult patient with Gorlin syndrome showing many of the facial features associated with the syndrome—arched eyebrows, downslanting palpebral fissures and sloping shoulders. Frontal bossing is disguised by the cut of the hair.

Although the pits will be easier to see in children who have been playing in a dirty environment, they should be differentiated from palmar lesions caused by excoriation of dirt under the skin. In most patients the pits can be better visualized if the hands are soaked in warm water for about 10 min.

Thumb anomalies (short terminal phalanges and/or small stiff thumbs) occur in about 10%. Pre- or postaxial polydactyly of hands or feet is found in 8%. The fourth metacarpal is short in 15–45% of patients, but is not a good diagnostic sign as it is found in about 10% of the normal population.

Hallux valgus can be severe, requiring operation.

Naevi and basal cell carcinomas

As 'naevi' and the BCCs found in the syndrome are histologically identical, they can both be classified as NBCCs. Clinically, however, the 'naevi' often develop first and behave differently from the BCCs which can appear to arise from naevi. For the purposes of the clinical description which follows, it is helpful to treat 'naevi' and 'NBCCs' as though they were separate entities.

Naevi. Naevi affect 53% of patients less than 20 years old, rising to 74% over the age of 20 years. Ordinary naevus cell naevi occur in about 4% of unaffected relatives but are present from birth, whilst affected family members report that the naevi tend to occur multiply in crops, their numbers increasing with time. Naevi also appear as individual lesions. A patient may develop no naevi, a few or many hundreds. The naevi are flesh coloured, reddish brown or pearly, the groups resembling moles, skin tags, ordinary naevus cell naevi or haemangiomas (Fig. 19.16.5). Some grow rapidly for a few days to a few weeks, but then most remain static.

Although 53% of cases under the age of 20 years have naevi, only 14% present clinically in this age group with a

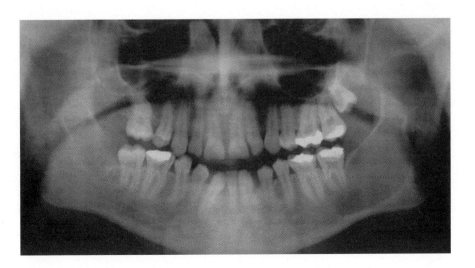

Fig. 19.16.3 An orthopantogram of a 17-year-old male showing a large cyst in the angle and ramus of the left mandible.

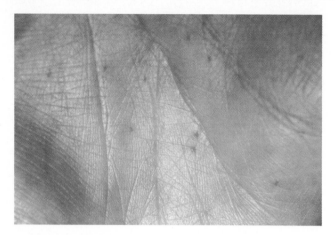

Fig. 19.16.4 Palmar pits.

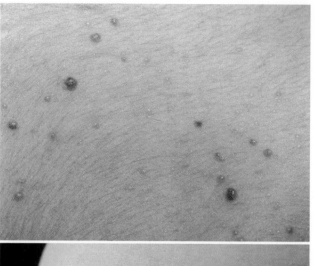
(a)

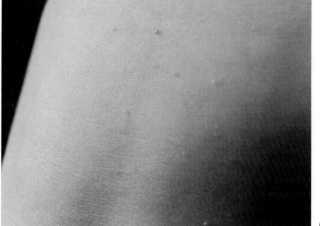
(b)

Fig. 19.16.5 (a,b) Naevi: note variation in size and appearance, some being reddish-brown, skin coloured or translucent.

rapidly growing BCC. It is unusual to develop aggressive BCCs before puberty.

Naevoid basal cell carcinomas. BCCs can arise in any area of the skin, affecting the face, neck and upper trunk in preference to the abdomen, lower trunk and extremities. The areas around the eyes, nose, malar regions and upper lip are the most frequently affected sites on the face. Usually only a few become aggressive, when they are locally invasive and behave like ordinary BCCs. Evidence of aggressive transformation of an individual lesion includes, as expected, an increase in size, ulceration, bleeding or crusting. Some patients can develop aggressive BCCs without first developing naevi. It is rare for metastasis to occur: only two cases have been cited [8].

In the author's series, no children under the age of 10 years developed an NBCC requiring treatment. Of those aged 15 20% had received treatment for one or more NBCC, 45% aged 20 years, 70% of those aged 25 years, 80% of those aged 40 years, and 92% of those aged 45 years.

Skeletal X-rays

Musculoskeletal features may be readily apparent on clinical examination, but X-ray investigation should always be undertaken when the syndrome is suspected.

Bifid, anteriorly splayed, fused, partially missing or hypoplastic ribs are found in 70% (Fig. 19.16.6). The third and fourth ribs are most frequently involved. Bifid ribs are found in about 6% of the normal population.

Abnormalities of the cervical or thoracic vertebrae are helpful diagnostic signs, being found in about 60% (Fig. 19.16.7). C6, C7, T2 and T1 are most frequently involved. Spina bifida occulta of the cervical vertebrae, or malfor-

mations at the occipitovertebral junction, are common. In addition to lack of fusion of the cervical or upper thoracic vertebrae, fusion or lack of segmentation has been documented in about 40%. A defective medial portion of the scapula is occasionally found.

As rib and spine anomalies are present at birth they are helpful diagnostic signs, but 14% of cases do not have anomalies of cervicothoracic spine and/or ribs.

Small pseudocystic lytic bone lesions, most often in the phalanges, metapodial and carpal and tarsal bones may be found in about 35% patients. There may be just one or two lesions, or they may involve almost the entire bone. The long bones, pelvis and calvarium may also be affected. Histologically, these bone radiolucencies are hamartomas composed of fibrous connective tissue, nerves and vessels.

Ectopic calcification

Calcification of the falx cerebri is a very useful diagnostic

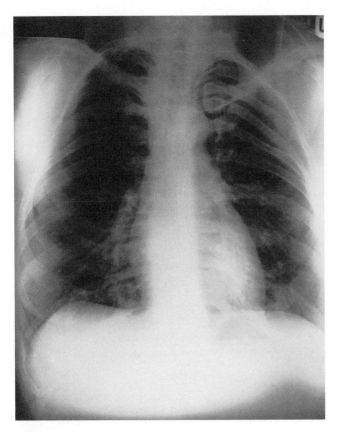

Fig. 19.16.6 Chest X-ray showing upper vertebral anomalies, variation in thickness of ribs and bifid ribs. The sloping left shoulder is due to the rib anomalies.

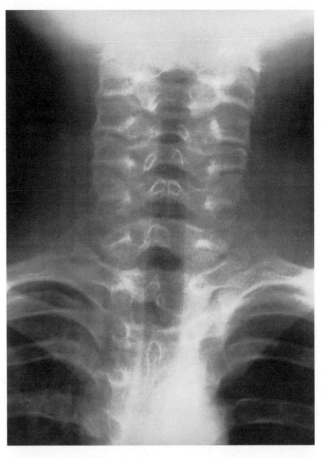

Fig. 19.16.7 Cervical and upper thoracic spine X-ray of a 10-year-old girl showing spina bifida occulta of C2–T3. The spinous processes of T1 and T2 are fused.

sign. It can appear very early in life, is often strikingly apparent from late childhood and its degree progresses with age. In the author's series it was present in 40% less than 15 years and 95% by age 25 years. Falx calcification first appears as a faint line in the upper falx (Fig. 19.16.8), the faint line becoming more prominent and giving the appearance of several individual sheets of calcification (Fig. 19.16.9). In some patients it can be very florid, up to 1 cm wide. It has a characteristic lamellar appearance (Fig. 19.16.10), in comparison with the single sheet of calcification found in 7% of the normal older population.

Calcification of the falx in a child should strongly raise Gorlin's syndrome as a diagnosis. A normal variant of the skull, a prominent frontal crest, can simulate falx calcification on the AP skull film, and should be considered if the calcification appears to be a single line beginning inferiorly.

Ectopic calcification also occurs in other membranes — the tentorium cerebelli (40%), petroclinoid ligaments (20%), dura, pia and choroid plexus.

Calcification of the diaphragma sellae causing the appearance of bridging of the sella turcica (Fig. 19.16.11) is another useful early diagnostic sign, found in 84% of cases, compared with 4% of the normal population in later life. It is present in almost 100% cases by the age of 20 years.

Calcification may also occur subcutaneously in apparently otherwise normal skin of the fingers and scalp.

Central nervous system

Medulloblastoma is a well-recognized complication, with an incidence of about 5%. Gorlin syndrome is found in 1–2% of children with medulloblastoma [33], presenting at an average age of about 2 years. This is about 5 years before the average age of presentation in children with isolated medulloblastoma. Meningioma, glioblastoma multiforme and craniopharyngioma have also been described in adults.

Cardiovascular system

In the north-west England population study, cardiac

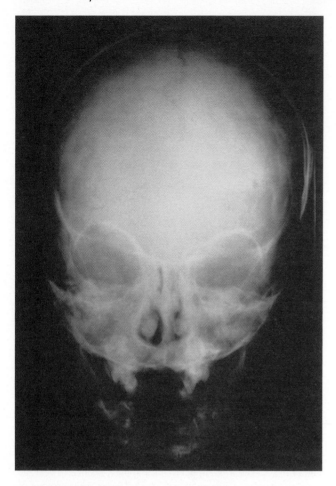

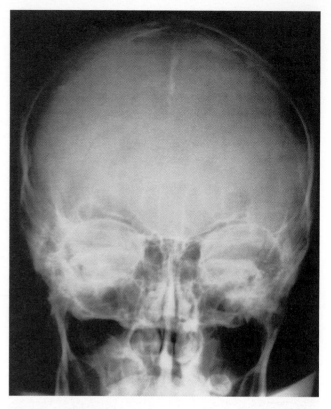

Fig. 19.16.9 Skull X-ray of an 18-year-old male showing upper falx calcification in plaques.

Fig. 19.16.8 Falx calcification. Skull X-ray of 2-year-old boy: a fine line of calcification is just visible in the upper falx.

fibroma was found in 2.5% [10]. One child died at 3 months of age from multiple cardiac fibromas, whilst another case has been followed for over 20 years with a single 2 cm cardiac fibroma in the interventricular septum, which has remained unchanged. Long-term prognosis is generally good, but resection may be necessary. The incidence in childhood of an isolated cardiac fibroma is between 0.027 and 0.08%, affecting most frequently the interventricular septum.

Mesentery

Just as cysts of the skin and jaws are integral parts of the syndrome so are chylous or lymphatic cysts of the mesentery, but these are rare. They may present, if large, as painless movable masses in the upper abdomen, or rarely may cause symptoms of obstruction. In most cases, however, they are discovered at laparotomy or on X-ray if calcified.

Genitourinary system

Calcified ovarian fibromas have been reported in 25–50%

of women with the syndrome [10] and may be mistaken for calcified uterine fibroids, especially if they overlap medially. They do not seem to reduce fertility but may undergo torsion. There is no evidence to suggest that they should be removed prophylactically.

Kidney malformations (horseshoe kidney, unilateral renal agenesis, renal cysts) have been described in isolated case reports but it is not known if their frequency is increased.

Neoplasia in other organs

Tumours in many other organs have been reported but rarely affect children. They include renal fibroma, melanoma, leiomyoma, rhabdomyosarcoma, adrenal cortical adenoma, seminoma, fibroadenoma of the breast, thyroid adenoma, carcinoma of the bladder, Hodgkin's disease and chronic leukaemia. There does not appear to be a particular neoplasm occurring at a frequency which would warrant selective screening.

Diagnosis and prognosis

Diagnosis

Diagnosis in a child at 50% risk of having inherited the

condition may not be easy because of the extreme variation in expression, both within and between families. Some children may have only rib anomalies whilst others have the 'typical face' without other signs. Gene tracking and mutation analysis may be helpful for presymptomatic diagnosis.

For apparently isolated cases, detailed examination and X-ray investigation of the parents should be undertaken before concluding that a child's condition is the result of a new mutation. If an adult has no physical signs, no pertinent history and normal radiology, it is unlikely that he or she has Gorlin syndrome. Direct mutation analysis of the gene may be helpful.

Confident diagnosis is obviously vital for subsequent surveillance for complications such as BCCs and jaw cysts, and for giving genetic information. Clinically, it relies on a detailed family history, and physical and X-ray examinations.

Family history

The family history may help to confirm the diagnosis in cases of doubt, although the variability of the condition may give seemingly disparate features in family members.

Physical examination

Particularly helpful are skeletal anomalies, typical facies, naevi and palmar and plantar pits. The most valuable measurement is the head circumference. Measurements should also include height, inner and outer canthal and interpupillary distances. The head circumference should be plotted on a chart which takes height into account [34].

X-ray and imaging investigations

X-ray signs may aid diagnosis in those who have equivocal physical signs. X-rays should include the following.
1 Skull: AP.
2 Skull: lateral.
3 Panoramic views of the jaws (plain films may miss lesions).
4 Chest X-ray.
5 Cervical and thoracic spine: AP and lateral.
6 Hands (for pseudocysts).
Ultrasound examinations for ovarian and cardiac fibromas may be helpful according to age.

Diagnostic criteria

Diagnostic criteria are given in Table 19.16.2 based on the most frequent and/or specific features of the syndrome [10]. These criteria were based on examination of family

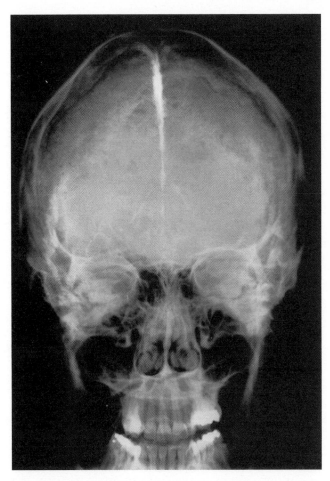

Fig. 19.16.10 Falx calcification. Skull X-ray of a 24-year-old woman showing florid falx calcification, extending inferiorly.

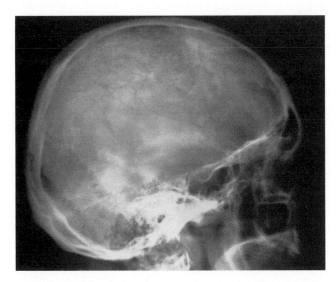

Fig. 19.16.11 Skull X-ray of a 44-year-old man showing bridged sella and characteristic 'low' occiput.

Table 19.16.2 Diagnostic criteria for NBBC syndrome. A diagnosis can be made when two major *or* one major and two minor criteria are fulfilled. If a first-degree relative is affected, the presence of one major or two minor criteria is diagnostic

Major criteria

1 Multiple (>2*) BCCs or one under the age of 30 years or >10 basal cell naevi

2 Odontogenic keratocyst (proven on histology) or polyostotic bone cyst

3 Palmar or plantar pits (3 or more)

4 Ectopic calcification: lamellar or early (<20 years) falx calcification

Minor criteria

1 Congenital skeletal anomaly: bifid, fused, splayed or missing rib or fused vertebrae

2 OFC >97th centile with bossing

3 Cardiac or ovarian fibroma

4 Medulloblastoma

5 Lymphomesenteric cysts

6 Congenital malformation: cleft lip and/or palate, polydactyly, eye anomaly (cataract, coloboma, microphthalmia).

*Note that the numbers of BCC given were based on a study carried out in England; the numbers of BCC for diagnosis will be inappropriate for sunnier climes.
OFC, occipito-frontal head circumference.

cases in England, a land not noted for excessive sunlight. The numbers of BCCs acceptable as a major criterion will vary according to the climate, and will need adaptation for countries such as Australia.

Prediction of disease status by gene tracking

As locus heterogenity has not been reported, presymptomatic and prenatal diagnosis is possible by gene tracking using DNA markers from 9q22.3–q31. For an individual family this will depend on the availability of DNA samples from appropriate family members.

There are several highly informative DNA markers which flank the gene, including D9S196/D9S197 and D9S180 [35] which have an intermarker distance of about 3.6 cM. As there is complete positive genetic interference over 9q22.3–31 [35,36] the error due to double recombinants when using flanking DNA markers for diagnosis will be extremely low. The closest flanking markers are D9S280 and D9S287 with a recombination rate of less than 1%.

Confirmation of diagnosis by mutation analysis

The definitive diagnostic test is to demonstrate a mutation in the patched gene, although this may be labour intensive as there are 24 exons. Detailed genotype/phenotype correlations are awaited, especially for the effects of missense mutations.

Prognosis

Because of the variability, presumably due to the other genes in a dosage-sensitive pathway, members of a sibship may be affected to different degrees. There is no evidence in the author's series that children are more severely affected than their parents, although jaw cysts and BCCs may be detected earlier through surveillance and may give the impression that these features have occurred at an earlier age. The skeletal signs are non-progressive and are not consistent between family members. Of adults with the syndrome 10% develop neither jaw cysts nor BCCs. It is unusual for new jaw cysts to appear from about the mid-30s. A child where the diagnosis is made on histological examination of an isolated lesion will not necessarily develop a large number of BCCs later.

The author has the clinical impression that some families seem especially prone to develop BCCs—occurring at a younger age and in greater number—than other families, in which members develop relatively few BCCs, and perhaps much later in life. The congenital malformations, however, generally do not follow a family-specific pattern: usually only one member is affected.

In the author's series, two patients had unexpected problems during general anaesthesia. There was difficulty in intubation in an adult female because muscle relaxation of the jaw did not occur following induction with thiopentone and suxamethonium, and in a child who was subsequently shown to have a laryngeal web. Southwick and Schwartz [37] also reported three patients who developed severe bradycardia and hypotension during induction of general anaesthesia.

Differential diagnosis

Differential diagnosis of the palmar pitting is porokeratosis of Mantoux [32] which is a rare form of non-hereditary papular keratosis of the hands and feet, with a few lesions occasionally sprinkled over the ankles. The lesions are changeable and usually disappear with time. The depressions are always found on the summit of the papillary excrescences, resembling an enlarged sudoriferous pore. Older lesions show a blackish vegetation with a finely lobulated or mulberry-like surface at the bottom of the depression which is eventually shed, leaving a small depression with a slightly raised margin and a red base. The material resembles a cornified comedone. The characteristic lesion is a translucent papule which erupts in recurring crops over months or years.

A family with trichoepitheliomas, milia and cylindromas presenting in the second and third decades and inherited as an autosomal dominant was reported by Rasmussen [38]. The milia were miniature trichoepitheliomas and appeared only in sun-exposed areas. Cylindromatosis

[39] (turban tumour syndrome) demonstrates considerable variation in the extent of distribution and age of onset within families, and may be the same condition.

Multiple BCCs, follicular atrophoderma on the dorsum of hands and feet, decreased sweating and hypotrichosis are features of Bazex's syndrome [40]. The pitting on the backs of the hands is reminiscent of orange peel and quite unlike the pits of Gorlin syndrome. The inheritance pattern is either autosomal or X-linked dominant.

A dominantly inherited condition similiar to Bazex syndrome was reported in a single family [41]. Rombo syndrome is characterized by vermiculate atrophoderma, milia, hypotrichosis, trichoepitheliomas, BCCs and peripheral vasodilation with cyanosis. The skin is normal until later childhood, BCCs develop later and there is no reduction in sweating.

A single family with another autosomal or X-linked dominant syndrome of hypotrichosis, BCCs, milia and excessive sweating was reported by Oley *et al.* [42].

In Cowden syndrome (multiple hamartoma syndrome) [43] mucocutaneous changes develop in the second decade, consisting of multiple facial papules, both smooth and keratotic, concentrated around the orifices, and generally associated with hair follicles. Numerous small hyperkeratotic and verrucous growths are found on the dorsal aspect of the hands and feet, and round translucent palmoplantar keratoses are also common. Similar lesions, including verrucous papules, occur on the oral mucosa. Multiple skin tags are also frequent. Most patients have a broad forehead and a large head circumference. Adenomas occur in the thyroid; gastrointestinal polyps occur in 60% and there is an increased incidence of breast cancer.

Arsenic exposure may cause multiple BCCs.

Multiple self-healing squamous epitheliomas (ESS1) [44], an autosomal dominant disorder, has also been mapped to the same area of chromosome 9q [45]; the majority of patients have been of Scottish origin. The skin tumours are invasive but then undergo spontaneous resolution over a period of months; there does not appear to be an increase in developmental anomalies as in Gorlin syndrome (D.R. Goudie, personal communication, 1997).

Patients with Gorlin syndrome may have café-au-lait patches but they number less than the six required for the diagnosis of neurofibromatosis type 1 (NF1), nor is axillary freckling present. In fact, physical appearances of some patients with NF1 and Gorlin syndrome are very similar.

Pseudohypoparathyroidism may be considered because of ectopic calcification and short fourth metacarpals.

Cardiac fibromas are also found in tuberous sclerosis and Beckwith–Wiedemann syndrome.

Surveillance

It is recommended that families are offered regular screening and that one clinician monitors and co-ordinates the overall programme [10]. Predictive testing by DNA analysis may be justified to identify family members for surveillance.

During pregnancy

Ultrasound scans may be offered during pregnancy to detect cardiac tumours and developmental malformations, which may require early decisions about neonatal surgery, and to detect an extremely enlarged head which may necessitate operative delivery.

Neonatal

A detailed neonatal examination may confirm the physical signs of a large head, cleft palate or eye anomaly. X-rays may confirm bifid ribs or vertebral abnormalities. An echocardiogram is best performed early as at least two cases have presented before 3 months of age with fibromas.

Childhood

Six-monthly neurological examination may detect a deficit indicative of a medulloblastoma. Routine scanning with computed tomography (CT) or excessive use of X-rays is not recommended because of concerns about inducing skin malignancies. At 3 years the examinations could be reduced to annually until 7 years after which a medulloblastoma is very unlikely. Although these examinations are of low sensitivity and specificity a parent will have contact with a specialist department should suspicious symptoms develop.

Annual dental screening should commence from about 8 years, usually including a panoramic X-ray of the jaw. Orthopantograms are justified because of complications of untreated jaw cysts.

At least annual examination of the skin from puberty is recommended but as a lesion may suddenly become aggressive, the patient needs open access to the specialist taking responsibility for treatment of the skin. It is especially important to offer early treatment for lesions of the eyelids, nose, ears and scalp. Patients must be warned to inspect all areas of the body—BCCs have been reported on the vulva, and the mucosa of the anal sphincter.

Exposure to sunlight

As sunlight may be one of the environmental agents promoting the appearance of BCCs [46], it is sensible to recommend basic sunscreening precautions, including the wearing of a wide-brimmed hat to offer some protection to the areas around the eyes.

Treatment

Skin

Local treatment. Alarm can be generated particularly in childhood when a skin tag or naevus is shown on histology to be a BCC. This may result in a feeling that immediate treatment is required for all other skin lesions present, and indeed, some authors do urge treatment for all such lesions. Other authors reserve treatment for lesions which show signs that they are active. As many naevi remain quiescent for long periods, they may not need to be removed but kept under frequent review. The author's practice is to have a lower threshold for local treatment for individual lesions occurring around the eyes, nose, mouth and ears.

The most suitable form of treatment may vary depending on the type, size and site of the NBCC. Surgical excision, cryotherapy, curettage and diathermy, topical 5-fluorouracil and Moh's microsurgery [47] have all been used. The priorities are to ensure complete eradication of aggressive BCCs, and to preserve normal tissue to prevent disfigurement. Topical 5-fluorouracil appears effective for superficial multicentric BCCs without follicular involvement but should not be used for deeply invasive BCCs.

The management of a girl who had inherited Gorlin syndrome from her father was reported after being treated for 10 years with a combination of topical tretinoin and 5-fluorouracil [48]. At 25 months of age, she had several red papules and numerous naevocellular and milia-like lesions confirmed on biopsy to be BCCs. After invasive BCCs had been removed, the other lesions were treated with twice daily total body application of 0.1% tretinoin cream followed by 5% 5-fluorouracil cream. Lesions around the eyes were treated with 5-fluorouracil alone twice daily. The hundreds of tumours disappeared after initiation of the combined therapy; most of the remaining tumours did not grow. The patient was examined every 3 months and lesions that demonstrated signs of growth or appeared to be deeply invasive were managed by shave excision and curettage. Development appeared normal and she showed neither clinical nor laboratory evidence of toxicity.

A few patients (usually adults) have hundreds of aggressive BCCs and treatment may seem overwhelming and hopeless. A great deal of support may therefore be required, not least to encourage attendance at follow-up clinics and to accept early treatment. There is a patient support group in the UK.

Treatment by radiation. Radiotherapy should be avoided because of clinical evidence that new lesions can appear in the irradiated field [37,49]. Children who received craniospinal irradiation as part of the treatment for a medulloblastoma have developed thousands of BCCs in the irradiated area (Fig. 19.16.12). The BCCs often develop within an extremely short latent period of 6 months to 3 years. This is earlier than, and in a distribution different from, other affected family members [49]. It may be that some families are not as radiosensitive as others, but until laboratory tests can detect these, radiotherapy should be avoided for all families.

Systemic retinoids. There are a few reports of oral synthetic retinoids (etretinate, isotretinoin and 13-*cis*-retinoic acid) preventing the development of new tumours, inhibiting the growth of existing tumours, and causing the regression of superficially invasive BCCs.

In two reports [50,51], etretinate at a dose of 1 mg/kg/day resulted in regression of 76% and 83% of lesions for 5 months, respectively, but new lesions appeared in both adult patients within 3 months of treatment being discontinued. Less aggressive surgery was required in a 63-year-old female patient, who received

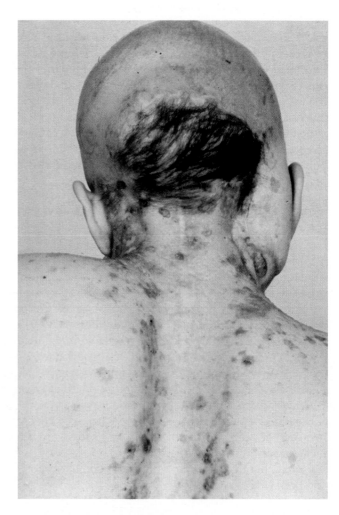

Fig. 19.16.12 Multiple BCCs arising in the field irradiated some years previously as part of treatment for a medulloblastoma.

treatment with oral etretinate, initially at 1 mg/kg/day [52].

Isoretinoin at 0.4 mg/kg/day prevented the formation of the majority of new BCCs and reduced the rate of growth of existing lesions in twin 26-year-old males who had hundreds of lesions [53]. The protective effect was lost following dose reduction to 0.2 mg/kg/day.

In a series of reports, Peck *et al.* [54] followed the progress of 12 adult patients with multiple BCCs, five of whom had Gorlin syndrome. Oral isotretinoin was given at 1 mg/kg/day increasing to an average maximum dose of 4.6 mg/kg/day for an average of 8 months. Approximately 8% of 270 selected BCC underwent complete clinical and histological remission. Twenty per cent of tumours showed partial and a further 44% minimal regression. Five patients withdrew because of the side-effects associated with retinoids. The dose of isotretinion was reduced to 0.25–1.5 mg/kg/day in the seven remaining patients. Partial regression of tumours was shown in only one patient. New tumours started to develop in a patient with Gorlin syndrome when on a chemopreventative dose of isotretinoin of 0.25 mg/kg/day. He developed 29 new BCCs in the 13 months following discontinuation of treatment [54].

A study of the chemopreventive potential of retinoids gave disappointing results in 981 adult patients with a previous history of two or more BCCs. Low dose isotretinoin (10 mg/day) adminstered for 36 months did not significantly reduce the rate of development of new tumours [55].

There is significant toxicity associated with prolonged retinoid use. As well as potential teratogenicity there are side-effects such as chelitis, pruritis, peeling of the palms and soles, eczema and diffuse idiopathic skeletal hyperostosis [56], dictating that retinoids should be used in carefully controlled circumstances. Their long-term role in the management of Gorlin syndrome is uncertain until synthetic retinoids become available which demonstrate reduced toxicity whilst maintaining an antineoplastic effect.

Photodynamic therapy. Photodynamic therapy (PDT) involves systemic or topical administration of a photosensitizer followed by exposure of the target area to light. In 1984, Tse *et al.* [57] treated 40 BCCs in three adult patients in whom conventional treatments had failed or were no longer possible, with 82.5% complete and 17.5% partial clinical response. There was a 10.8% recurrence rate.

This approach is also being evaluated in Gorlin syndrome by the Roswell Park Cancer Institute in Buffalo, New York (A.R. Roseroff, personal communication, 1997). Although complete clinical BCC response rate was high (93%) in 796 nodular and superficial lesions in 20 adults with 1 mg/kg systemic Photofrin, the results in three children were less satisfactory with a poorer response and scarring. Systemic PDT is therefore not recommended for prepubertal children. A major disadvantage of Photofrin is that it can produce a generalized photosensitivity for 4–8 weeks and so new generation photosensitizers are being developed. Topical treatment with δ-aminolevlinic acid (ALA) has given a 95% initial clinical response rate on treatment of 150 BCCs in two children with Gorlin syndrome who developed multiple lesions in fields irradiated for Hodgkin's disease and medulloblastoma. The healing response was better than with systemic administration of photosensitizer and left no scarring. This approach may prove to be especially useful in such cases where there are thousands of superficial BCCs.

Jaw cysts

As proliferating dental lamina and satellite cysts may occur in the fibrous wall of the primary cyst cavity, marsupialization may be successful only if no satellite cysts are left behind. Small single lesions with regular spherical outlines can usually be completely enucleated provided access is good. For the large multilocular lesions, excision and immediate bone grafting is the treatment of choice at the first operation [58].

The odontogenic keratocyst has a tendency to recur after surgical treatment, with reported rates varying up to 62%. New cysts may form from satellite cysts associated with the original, or from the dental lamina.

REFERENCES

1 Satinoff MI, Wells C. Multiple basal cell naevus syndrome in ancient Egypt. *Med Hist* 1969; 13: 294–6.
2 Jarisch W. Zur Lehre con den Hautgeschwulsten. *Arch Dermatol Syph* 1894; 28: 162–222.
3 White JC. Multiple benign cystic epitheliomas. *J Cutan Genitourin Dis* 1894; 12: 477–84.
4 Nomland R. Multiple basal cell epitheliomas originating from congenital pigmented basal cell nevi. *Arch Dermatol Syph* 1932; 25: 1002–8.
5 Gorlin RJ, Goltz RW. Multiple nevoid basal-cell epithelioma, jaw cysts and bifid rib: a syndrome. *N Engl J Med* 1960; 262: 908–12.
6 Howell JB, Caro MR. The basal cell nevus: its relationship to multiple cutaneous cancers and associated anomalies of development. *Arch Dermatol* 1959; 79: 67–80.
7 Mason JK, Helwig EB, Graham JH. Pathology of the nevoid basal cell carcinoma syndrome. *Arch Pathol* 1965; 79: 401–8.
8 Gorlin RJ. Nevoid basal-cell carcinoma syndrome. *Medicine* 1987; 66: 96–113.
9 Gorlin RJ. Nevoid basal cell carcinoma syndrome. *Dermatol Clin* 1995; 13: 113–25.
10 Evans DGR, Ladusans EJ, Rimmer S, Burnell LD, Thakker N, Farndon PA. Complications of the naevoid basal cell carcinoma syndrome: results of a population based study. *J Med Genet* 1993; 30: 460–4.
11 Rahbari H, Mehregan AH. Basal cell epithelioma (carcinoma) in children and teenagers. *Cancer* 1982; 49: 350–3.
12 Jones KL, Smith DW, Harvey MA, Hall BD, Quan L. Older paternal age and fresh gene mutation: data on additional disorders. *J Pediatr* 1975; 86: 84–8.
13 Gorlin RJ. Multiple nevoid basal cell carcinoma syndrome. In: Gorlin RJ, Cohen MM, Levin LS, eds. *Syndromes of the Head and Neck*, 3rd edn. Oxford: Oxford University Press, 1990: 372–80.
14 Knudson AG. Mutation and cancer: statistical study of retinoblastoma. *Proc Natl Acad Sci USA* 1971; 68: 820–3.

15 Farndon PA, Del Mastro RD, Evans DGR, Kilpatrick MW. Location of gene for Gorlin syndrome. *Lancet* 1992; 339: 581–2.

16 Reis A, Kuster W, Gebel E *et al.* Localisation of the gene for the naevoid basal cell carcinoma syndrome. *Lancet* 1992; 339: 617.

17 Gailani MR, Bale SJ, Leffell DJ *et al.* Developmental defects in Gorlin syndrome related to a putative tumor suppressor gene on chromosome 9. *Cell* 1992; 69: 111–17.

18 Bonifas JM, Bare JW, Kerschmann RL, Master SP, Epstein EH. Parental origin of chromosome 9q22.3–q31 lost in basal cell carcinomas from basal cell nevus syndrome patients. *Hum Molec Genet* 1994; 3: 447–8.

19 Levanat S, Gorlin RJ, Fallet S *et al.* A two-hit model for developmental defects in Gorlin syndrome. *Nature Genet* 1996; 12: 85–7.

20 Hahn H, Wicking C, Zaphiropoulos PG *et al.* Mutations of the human homolog of *Drosophila* patched in the nevoid basal cell carcinoma syndrome. *Cell* 1996; 85: 841–51.

21 Johnson RL, Rothman AL, Xie J *et al.* Human homolog of patched, a candidate gene for the basal cell nevus syndrome. *Science* 1996; 272: 1668–71.

22 Gorlin RJ, Vickers RA, Klein E, Williamson JJ. The multiple basal cell nevi syndrome. *Cancer* 1965; 18: 89–104.

23 Ahlfors E, Larsson A, Sjogren S. The odontogenic keratocyst: a benign cystic tumor? *J Oral Maxillofac Sur* 1984; 42: 10–19.

24 Howell JB, Freeman RG. Structure and significance of the pits with their tumors in the nevoid basal cell carcinoma syndrome. *J Am Acad Dermatol* 1980; 2: 224–38.

25 Hashimoto K, Howell JB, Yamanishi Y, Holubar K, Berhard R. Electron microscope studies of palmar and plantar pits of nevoid basal cell epithelioma. *J Invest Dermatol* 1972; 59: 380–93.

26 Little JB, Nichols WW, Troilo P, Nagasawa H, Strong LC. Radiation sensitivity of cell strains from families with genetic disorders predisposing to radiation-induced cancer. *Cancer Res* 1989; 49: 4705–14.

27 Lehmann AR, Kirk-Bell S, Arlett CF *et al.* Repair of UV light damage in a variety of human fibroblast cell strains. *Cancer Res* 1977; 37: 904–10.

28 Nagawaswa F, Little FF, Burke MJ *et al.* Study of basal cell nevus fibroblasts after treatment with DNA damaging agents. *Basic Life Sci* 1984; 29B: 775–85.

29 Ananthaswamy HN, Applegate LA, Goldberg LH *et al.* Skin fibroblasts from basal cell nevus patients are hypersensitive to killing by solar UVB radiation. *Photochem Photobiol* 1989; 49: 60S.

30 Applegate LA, Goldberg LH, Ley RD, Ananthaswamy HN. Hypersensitivity of skin fibroblasts from basal cell nevus syndrome patients to killing by ultraviolet B but not by ultraviolet C radiation. *Cancer Res* 1990; 50: 637–41.

31 Murphy KJ. Subcutaneous calcification in basal cell carcinoma syndrome: response to parathyroid hormone and relationship to pseudohypoparathyroidism. *Clin Radiol* 1969; 20: 287–93.

32 Howell JB, Mehregan AH. Pursuit of the pits in the nevoid basal cell carcinoma syndrome. *Arch Dermatol* 1970; 102: 586–97.

33 Evans DGR, Farndon PA, Burnell LD, Rao Gattamaneni H, Birch JM. The incidence of Gorlin syndrome in 173 consecutive cases of medulloblastoma. *Br J Cancer* 1991; 64: 959–61.

34 Bushby KMD, Cole T, Matthews JNS, Goodship JA. Centiles for adult head circumference. *Arch Dis Child* 1992; 67: 1286–7.

35 Povey S, Armour J, Farndon P *et al.* Report on the third international workshop on human chromosome 9. *Ann Hum Genet* 1994; 58: 177–250.

36 Kwiatkowski DJ, Dib C, Slaugenhaupt S, Povey S, Gusella JF, Haines JL. An index marker map of chromosome 9 provides strong evidence for positive interference. *Am J Hum Genet* 1993; 53: 1279–88.

37 Southwick GJ, Schwartz RA. The basal cell nevus syndrome: disasters occurring among a series of 36 patients. *Cancer* 1979; 44: 2294–305.

38 Rasmussen JE. A syndrome of trichoepitheliomas, milia and cylindromas. *Arch Dermatol* 1975; 111: 610–14.

39 Welch JP, Wells RS, Kerr CB. Ancell–Spiegler cylindromas (turban tumours) and Brooke–Fordyce trichoepitheliomas: evidence for a single genetic entity. *J Med Genet* 1968; 5: 29–35.

40 Viksnins P, Berlin A. Follicular atrophoderma and basal cell carcinomas: the Basex syndrome. *Arch Dermatol* 1977; 113: 948–51.

41 Michaelsson G, Olsson E, Westermark P. The Rombo syndrome. *Acta Derm Venereol* 1981; 61: 497–503.

42 Oley CA, Sharpe H, Chenevix-Trench G. Basal cell carcinomas, coarse sparse hair, and milia. *Am J Med Genet* 1992; 43: 799–804.

43 Starink TM, van der Veen JPW, Arwert F *et al.* The Cowden syndrome: a clinical and genetic study in 21 patients. *Clin Genet* 1986; 29: 222–33.

44 Ferguson-Smith MA, Wallace DC, James ZH, Renwick JH. Multiple self-healing squamous epithelioma. *Birth Defects Original Article Series* 1971; VII: 157–63.

45 Goudie DR, Yuille MAR, Leversha MA, Furlong RA, Carter N. Multiple self-healing squamous epitheliomata (ESS1) mapped to chromosome 9q22–q31 in families with common ancestry. *Nature Genet* 1993; 3: 165–9.

46 Goldstein AM, Bale SJ, Peck GL, DiGiovanna JJ. Sun exposure and basal cell carcinomas in the nevoid basal cell carcinoma syndrome. *J Am Acad Dermatol* 1993; 29: 34–41.

47 Mohs FE, Jones DL, Koranda FC. Microscopically controlled surgery for carcinomas in patients with nevoid basal cell carcinoma syndrome. *Arch Dermatol* 1980; 116: 777–9.

48 Strange PR, Lang PG Jr. Long-term management of basal cell nevus syndrome with topical tretinoin and 5-fluorouracil. *J Am Acad Dermatol* 1992; 27: 842–5.

49 Strong LC. Genetic and environmental interactions. *Cancer* 1977; 40: 1861–6.

50 Cristofolini M, Zumiani G, Scappni P *et al.* Aromatic retinoid in chemoprevention of the progression of nevoid basal cell carcinoma syndrome. *J Dermatol Surg Oncol* 1984; 10: 778–81.

51 Hodak E, Ginzburg A, David M *et al.* Etretinate treatment of the nevoid basal cell carcinoma syndrome. *Int J Dermatol* 1987; 26: 606–9.

52 Sanchez-Conejo-Mir J, Camacho F. Nevoid basal cell carcinoma syndrome: combined etretinate and surgical treatment. *J Dermatol Surg Oncol* 1989; 15: 868–71.

53 Goldberg LH, Hsu SH, Alcalay J. Effectiveness of isotretinoin in preventing the appearance of basal cell carcinomas in basal cell nevus syndrome. *J Am Acad Dermatol* 1989; 21: 144–5.

54 Peck GL, DiGiovanna JJ, Sarnoff DS *et al.* Treatment and prevention of basal cell carcinoma with oral isotretinoin. *J Am Acad Dermatol* 1988; 19: 176–85.

55 Tangrea JA, Edwards BK, Taylor PR *et al.* Long-term therapy with low-dose isotretinoin for prevention of basal cell carcinoma: a multicenter clinical trial. *J Natl Cancer Inst* 1992; 84: 328–32.

56 Theiler R, Hubscher E, Wagenhauser FJ, Panizzon R, Michel B. Diffuse idiopathic skeletal hyperostosis (DISH) and pseudocoxarthritis following long-term etretinate therapy. *Schweizer Med Wochenschr* 1993; 123: 649–53.

57 Tse DT, Kersten RC, Anderson RL. Hematoporphyrin derivative photoradiation therapy in managing nevoid basal cell carcinoma syndrome. A preliminary report. *Arch Ophthalmol* 1984; 102: 990–4.

58 Posnick JC, Clokie CML, Goldstein JA. Maxillofacial considerations for diagnosis and treatment in Gorlin's syndrome: access osteotomies for cyst removal and orthognathic surgery. *Ann Plast Surg* 1994; 35: 512–18.

19.17 Ehlers–Danlos Syndromes

NAVJEET K. SIDHU-MALIK

Definition

The Ehlers–Danlos syndromes (EDS) are a heterogeneous group of connective tissue diseases consisting of 10 different subtypes. In 1986, the Seventh International Congress of Human Genetics standardized the growing and confusing list of EDS subcategories [1]. The cardinal features, which are shared to varying degrees by most of the subtypes, include hyperextensible skin with a soft, doughy or velvety texture, dystrophic scarring, easy bruising, joint hypermobility and connective tissue fragility [1]. The genetic pattern of inheritance differs for the subtypes and additional systemic involvement may occur in some of the EDS syndromes. The diagnosis is based on the history, inheritance pattern, clinical examination and possible biochemical or genetic testing (which is available for some of the subtypes). Some EDS variants are relatively benign entities and have no significant associated morbidity; other variants, however, have systemic complications. There are no established figures for the incidence of EDS. McKusick [2] in 1972 estimated EDS to be one of the most common inherited diseases of connective tissue. As symptoms are often unnoticed, especially in the milder subtypes, EDS may be underdiagnosed, and a more recent estimate of incidence is 1 in 5000 [3]. Some of the cardinal features such as soft skin, easy scarring and bruising are difficult to assess during infancy and only become evident during childhood; whereas, other features such as joint hypermobility may present at birth with congenital hip dislocation, kyphoscoliosis and muscle hypotonia.

EDS IX, originally called X-linked cutis laxa and later reclassified as occipital horn syndrome, was excluded from the EDS subcategories when it was found to be a copper transport defect. EDS IX was thus left vacant in the numbering, as was EDS XI which has been renamed the familial articular hypermobility syndrome. Nonetheless, occipital horn syndrome is often still listed with the EDS syndromes and will also be reviewed in this chapter.

History

Although there are references to EDS-like diseases in ancient literature [4], the first reported case dates to 1682 when van Meek'ren [5], a Dutch surgeon, described a patient with hyperextensible skin. The features of EDS were undoubtedly present in the contortionists exhibited at fairs and curiosity shows that were popular in the 19th century. Various reports of these performers appeared in the medical literature [6]. The first extensive clinical description of a patient with EDS should be credited to Tschernogobow [7], a Russian dermatologist, who in 1891 described two patients with hyperextensible skin with scarring and fragility, joint hyperextensibility and molluscoid pseudotumours. He also conjectured that this may represent a disorder of underlying connective tissue. Ehlers [8] in 1901 reported a case of a patient with hyperextensible skin, joint laxity and easy bruisibility, and in 1908 Danlos [9] described a second patient with the additional features of pseudotumours at sites of trauma. In 1936, Weber [10] reviewed the numerous case reports describing various conditions with loose skin and joints, and suggested the name EDS for the disorder encompassing skin fragility and hyperextensibility, joint laxity and molluscoid pseudotumours. McKusick in 1960 [11] recognized that EDS encompasses a genetically heterogeneous group of diseases. Subsequently, additional subtypes have been described, and at present there are 10 EDS subtypes.

Aetiology and/or pathogenesis

As EDS is comprised of a heterogeneous group of diseases, distinct abnormalities involving abnormal collagen synthesis or processing have been described for the characterized subtypes (EDS IV, VI and VII). EDS IX results from abnormal copper utilization without a primary collagen defect and has been reclassified as a disorder of metal transport. No abnormality has thus far been described for EDS I, II, III, V, VIII and X and additional genetic and biochemical research is necessary to identify the underlying defect.

EDS I. No biochemical defect has been determined [12]. Genetic linkage studies have thus far been unable to identify a candidate gene, although several collagen genes have been excluded [13].

EDS II. No biochemical defect in collagen has been determined and linkage studies, thus far, have not localized the gene [14].

EDS III. No biochemical or genetic abnormality has been identified.

EDS IV. EDS IV results from a type III collagen defect with heterogeneous mutations in the COL3A1 gene [14]. These mutations lead to abnormal type III procollagen structure, synthesis or secretion, resulting in a thin dermis with abnormal collagen fibrils [15]. Fibroblast cultures demonstrate decreased synthesis or secretion of procollagen III [16]. Skin extracts also have decreased collagen III levels, and serum levels of procollagen III aminopeptide are decreased.

EDS V. No biochemical or genetic abnormality has been described for this subtype.

EDS VI. EDS VI was the first of the inherited disorders of collagen to be biochemically characterized [17]. The defect consists of a deficiency of lysyl hydroxylase, an important enzyme involved in collagen cross-linking. The lysyl hydroxylase gene has been identified and studies of families suggest that a heterogeneous group of mutations are responsible for the abnormal enzyme activity [18]. The diagnosis is confirmed by decreased levels of lysyl hydroxylase enzyme activity in fibroblast culture.

EDS VII. EDS VII consists of three subgroups A, B and C. EDS VIIA and VIIB are caused by type I collagen gene defects which result in a precursor procollagen molecule with an abnormal aminoterminal cleavage site that cannot be processed to mature collagen. EDS VIIA and VIIB are distinguished by mutations in COL1A1 and COL1A2 genes, respectively, which disrupt or delete the *N*-proteinase cleavage site of proα1(I) and proα2(I) collagen chains [19,20]. EDS VIIC results from deficiency of procollagen I *N*-proteinase enzyme activity with improper processing of both α1(I) and α2(I) collagen chains [21]. These mutations lead to alterations in crosslink formation in the type I collagen molecule with resulting decreased tissue strength.

EDS VIII. No biochemical defect has been reported for this disorder.

EDS IX. Abnormal copper utilization, similar to that found in Menkes syndrome, has been identified as the biochemical abnormality which results in defective activity of the copper-dependent enzyme lysyl oxidase. Lysyl oxidase is important for the formation of cross-links in collagen and elastin molecules. With the characterization of the gene for Menkes syndrome, it was found that EDS IX results from mutations in the some gene [22]; thus, EDS IX has been reclassified as a disorder of metal (copper) transport and has been excluded from the EDS group [1].

EDS X. No biochemical defect has been reported for this disorder.

Pathology

Routine light microscopic examination of the skin is unrevealing. Electron microscopy of the dermis has demonstrated abnormal collagen fibrils in some of the EDS subtypes including EDS I, II, IV and VIIC [15,23,24].

Clinical features

The clinical features associated with EDS are present to differing degrees in the individual subtypes and are summarized in Table 19.17.1. An overview of the clinical features is presented below and the specific features associated with each subtype will be reviewed as the individual subtypes are discussed.

Cutaneous aspects

Cutaneous features of EDS include skin hyperextensibility and fragility [3,4,25]. The skin is soft, and is often described as velvety and doughy with a chamois leather texture. The skin is easily extended and, upon release, recoils back to its original shape (Fig. 19.17.1). This finding differs from the lax skin of cutis laxa which, after stretching, does not recoil. Hyperextensibility and skin softness can be difficult to assess in infants because of subcutaneous fat and is more easily evaluated in slightly older children.

Skin fragility (dermatorrhexis) is manifested by tearing of the skin after minor trauma. Sites commonly involved include knees, shins, elbows and the face, especially the forehead and chin (Fig. 19.17.2). Scarring occurs most commonly during childhood as infants begin to crawl and walk and experience minor trauma and improves with increasing age. Cutaneous fragility also results in easy bruising, delayed wound healing and poor healing after suturing with a higher incidence of wound dehiscence. Prominent bruising has at times led to concerns about child abuse in affected children. Scars characteristically widen and develop fine 'cigarette paper' or 'papyraceous' wrinkling in addition to a shiny surface with overlying telangiectasias.

Table 19.17.1 Summary of clinical, genetic and biochemical features of the EDS subtypes

Subtype	Inheritance	Clinical features	Biochemical defect
I Gravis	AD	Skin: soft, markedly hyperextensible with easy bruising, fragility; heals poorly with scarring, and 'cigarette paper' wrinkling—especially during childhood. Joints: hypermobility. Other: history of premature birth, varicose veins, mitral valve prolapse	Unknown
II Mitis	AD	Skin: soft, hyperextensible, but with less frequent bruising and scarring than EDS I. Joints: hypermobility less than with EDS I. Other: mitral valve prolapse, rare prematurity	Unknown
III Benign familial hypermobility	AD	Skin: soft, no hyperextensibility, normal scar formation. Joints: marked hypermobility	Unknown
IV Arterial, vascular, ecchymotic	AD (AR)	Skin: thin, translucent, veins visible, marked bruising with normal scarring and rare hyperextensibility; hands and feet prematurely aged. Joints: rare hypermobility. Other: bowel, arterial, and uterine rupture with risk of death; premature or low birth weight infants	Type III collagen defect with abnormal collagen synthesis, secretion, and structure
V X-linked	XLR	Similar to EDS II	Unknown
VI Ocular	AR	Skin: hyperextensible, fragile, with easy bruising. Joints: marked hypermobility. Other: hypotonia at birth, delayed development, and kyphoscoliosis; possible ocular fragility	Lysyl hydroxylase deficiency
VII Arthrochalasis multiplex	AD	Skin: soft, mild hyperextensibility and bruising, no increased fragility. Joints: extreme laxity with dislocations. Other: hypotonia	Type I collagen gene defect: A: COL1AI mutation B: COLA2I mutation C: deficiency of procollagen *N*-proteinase
VIIC Human dermatospraxis	AR	Skin: marked fragility, easy tearing and bruising. Joint: mild hypermobility. Other: growth retardation, umbilical hernias, blue sclerae	
VIII Periodontal	AD	Skin: soft, mild hyperextensibility, easy bruising, scars on shins with purple discoloration. Joints: hypermobility. Other: early onset peridontal disease	Unknown
IX X-Linked	XLR	Skin: soft with laxity at birth. Joints: not hyperextensible. Other: bladder diverticuli, skeletal abnormalities with occipital horns, short humeri, broad clavicles	Lysyl oxidase defect with abnormal copper utilization
X	AR	Skin and joints: like EDS II. Other: clotting defect with abnormal platelet adhesion	Fibronectin defect

AD, autosomal dominant; XLR, X-linked recessive.

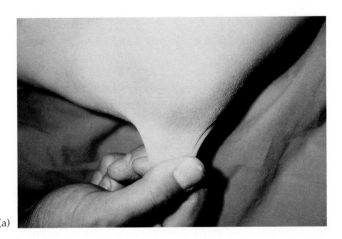 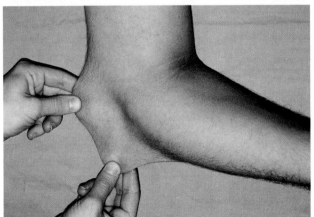

(a) (b)

Fig. 19.17.1 (a,b) Hyperextensibility of the skin is present with marked stretching upon gentle pulling.

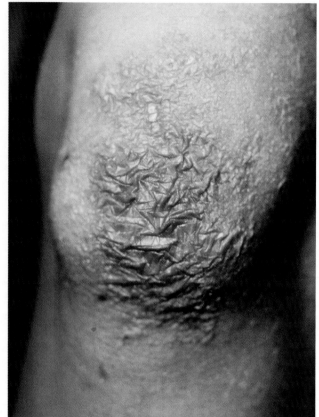

(a)

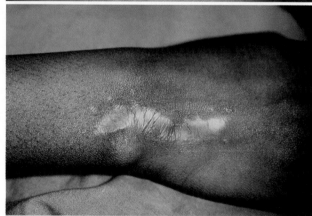

(b)

Fig. 19.17.2 Skin fragility with abnormal scarring. (a) knee with cigarette paper or papyraceous wrinkling after trauma. (b) Scar widening after healing.

EDS IV typically lacks significant hyperextensibility of skin, but is associated with pale skin with readily visible veins on the torso.

Unique cutaneous findings in some patients with EDS are molluscoid pseudotumours and spheroids (Fig. 19.17.3). Molluscoid pseudotumours are fleshy areas of redundant skin that present in early childhood and occur over areas of recurrent trauma such as the elbows, knees and heels. Spheroids are small subcutaneous, cyst-like nodules that occur over bony prominences of the legs and

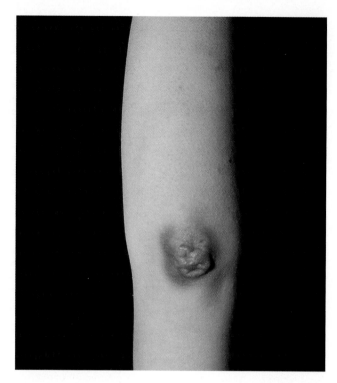

Fig. 19.17.3 Molluscoid pseudotumours present on the elbow with redundant skin and bruising.

arms. These are calcified on X-ray examination and result from trauma induced fibrosis and calcification of the subcutaneous fat lobules [26,27].

Additional cutaneous features include looseness of palmar skin, and an increased number of palmar creases (Fig. 19.17.4). Elastosis peforans serpigenosa has been reported in some affected individuals [28]. Peizogenic papules, herniations of fat lobules through fascia at the medial and lateral aspects of the feet, may also be present. Pregnancy-associated striae gravidum do not occur in patients with EDS.

Musculoskeletal aspects

Joint hypermobility is a cardinal feature of EDS (except EDS IV) and involves both large and small joints (Fig. 19.17.5) [29]. Generally this is first noticed when a child exhibits a delay in beginning to walk and remains unsteady with a greater number of falls and it improves with increasing age. At any age, females display greater mobility than males. Clinical evaluation of joint hyperextensibility includes examination of small joints such as fingers assessing the ability to dorsiflex the fifth finger beyond 90° and the ability to appose thumb to flexor forearm. Large joint hyperextensibility is evaluated by the presence of knee and elbow hyperextension and the ability to bend and touch palms of hands flat to the floor. Severe hypermobility as seen with EDS VI and VII can

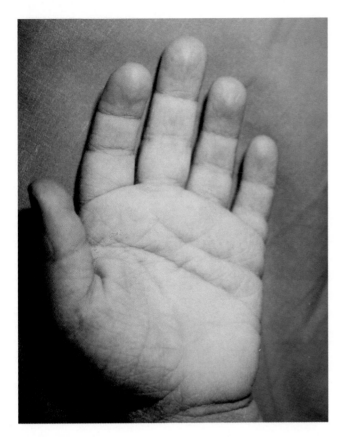

Fig. 19.17.4 Palmar aspect of hands with increased wrinkling and loose appearance of the skin.

present at birth with hypotonia, kyphoscoliosis and congenital hip dislocations.

Early onset osteoarthritis is a significant complication and commonly involves weight-bearing joints such as the knees and ankles. Other musculoskeletal complications include recurrent joint effusions, which occur most commonly in knees, ankles and elbows, pes planus (flat-footedness) and kyphoscoliosis [30]. Haemarthrosis may occur in EDS IV. Joint instability results in delayed walking in childhood and joint subluxation.

Cardiovascular aspects

Structural cardiac abnormalities are not specifically associated with EDS and may be present due to random association [31,32]. Mitral valve prolapse has been reported most often with EDS III and IV and results from redundant chordae tendinae and valve cusps. EDS IV is also associated with spontaneous and life-threatening rupture of large arteries, especially the descending aorta [33]. Intracranial aneurysm and arteriovenous fistulae rupture may occur with EDS IV, but have also been reported with other EDS types [34].

Genitourinary aspects

Urinary bladder diverticulae are found in most EDS types, but are specifically associated with EDS IX. These may result in vesicoureteral reflex and have an associated risk of recurrent urinary tract infections.

Neurological aspects

The central nervous system is not primarily involved and intelligence is generally normal [35]. Significant neurological complications include muscle hypotonia in EDS VI and haemorrhage from intracranial arterial aneurysm in EDS IV.

Ocular aspects

Minor ocular findings include epicanthal folds, ease in everting upper eyelid (Metenier's sign), redundant upper eyelid skin and strabismus that is secondary to the laxity of tendons supporting the extrinsic muscles of the eyes {36]. EDS VI (ocular variant) has been associated with more significant ocular complications of retinal detatchment and scleral perforation which may occur during childhood [37], although a more recent review of patients suggests that these serious ocular complications have been overestimated and that myopia is the most common finding in this EDS subgroup [38].

Dental and oral aspects

Gorlin's sign, the ability to touch the tip of the nose with the tongue, has sometimes been associated with EDS; nonetheless, this finding is not specific as it occurs in 10% of unaffected individuals [39]. EDS VIII is associated with early onset periodontal disease [40].

Obstetric complications

Complications of pregnancy occur in both mother and infants with EDS and are related to the specific type [41]. These include maternal joint subluxation, cervical insufficiency with risk of miscarriage and preterm labour. EDS IV is associated with the greatest risks, including uterine rupture which has an estimated maternal mortality of 25%. Fetuses affected with EDS have a higher incidence of prematurity resulting from maternal premature rupture of membranes.

Ehlers–Danlos syndrome subtypes

Ehlers–Danlos syndrome type I, II and III—the classic subtypes

EDS I, II and III, often described as the classic subtypes,

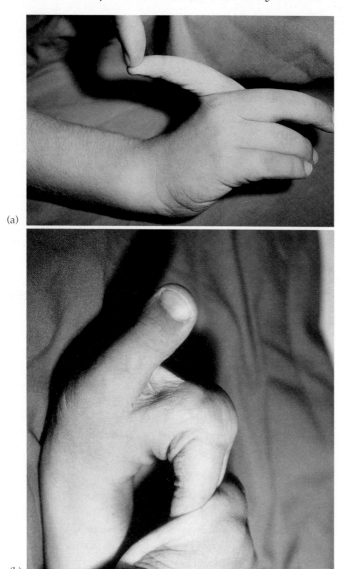

(a)

(b)

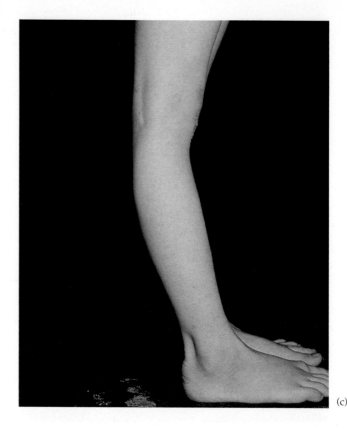

(c)

Fig. 19.17.5 (a–c) Joint hypermobility: (a) and (b) demonstrate small joint hypermobility with extension of fingers beyond 90°; (c) large joint hypermobility is evidenced by hyperextension of the knees.

are clinically similar with varying severity of involvement. They have autosomal dominant inheritance, and together comprise an estimated 80% of all EDS cases [4]. These may present in early childhood with delayed motor development including delay in walking, skin fragility with easy tearing after minor trauma, severe bruising and scarring at sites of frequent trauma such as forehead, chin, knees and shins.

EDS I

EDS I, also called the gravis variant, is the most severe of the three classic subtypes and comprises 40% of all EDS subtypes [4]. It is characterized by moderate to severe involvement with skin hyperextensibility, poor wound healing and marked joint hypermobility. The skin is soft with a velvety texture and can easily be streched with

recoil to its original form upon release. Increased fragility of the skin results in large wounds following minor trauma, and poor wound healing leads to widened scars with characteristic 'cigarette paper' wrinkling and atrophy. Large scars with hyperpigmentation develop during childhood in areas of repeated trauma such as knees, elbows, and shins. Molluscoid pseudotumours and subcutaneous spheroids may also develop on areas of trauma. Other findings include a history of premature rupture of fetal membranes in 50% of affected infants, scoliosis and pes planus, and lower extremity venous varicosities. Cardiac features include mitral valve prolapse in up to half of patients and the rare occurrence of arterial rupture. A common complication is early onset osteoarthritis secondary to the joint hyperextensibility.

EDS II

EDS II, the mitis form, is a milder variant of EDS I. It is inherited as an autosomal dominant trait and comprises 40% of all EDS subtypes [4]. The skin is soft, velvety and hyperextensible, but there is less skin fragility than with EDS I and scar formation is generally normal. The joints are less hypermobile than with EDS I and history of prematurity is rare. Mitral valve prolapse is still present in many patients. This EDS subtype may often be undiagnosed because of the mild degree of skin and joint involvement and associated complications.

EDS III

EDS III, benign familial hypermobility syndrome, is characterized primarily by joint hypermobility. It is inherited as an autosomal dominant trait and comprises 10% of all cases of EDS [4]. The skin is soft, but hyperextensibility and exaggerated scarring only occur in a minority of patients. Complications of joint dislocation and early onset osteoarthritis may be present.

EDS IV

EDS IV is also called the arterial–ecchymotic type of Sack–Barabas, in addition to vascular, arterial or ecchymotic EDS. This EDS subtype is quite distinct in that it lacks skin and joint hyperextensibility and is associated with life-threatening complications [42]. It is an uncommon subtype and exhibits autosomal dominant inheritance pattern, although there are a few reported cases of autosomal recessive transmission.

The skin of patients is thin and translucent with easily visible veins on the abdomen, trunk and extremities. A minority of patients have soft skin with mild hyperextensibility. Marked bruising of the skin after minor trauma often occurs. The skin of the hands and feet is thin and wrinkled with a resulting aged and acrogeric appearance. A characteristic facies with thin nose, thin lips, hollow cheeks, prominent eyes and thin hair has been described [43].

Life-threatening complications include rupture of the bowel and medium-sized arteries. Bowel rupture frequently involves the ascending colon. Arterial rupture most often occurs in abdominal mesenchymal, splenic and renal arteries, and in the descending aorta. Pregnancy may be complicated by uterine rupture.

EDS IV can present in infancy and childhood with low birth weight, prematurity, congenital hip dislocations, increased bruising and the facies described above; although, without a family history it is most often not suspected until vascular, bowel or pregnancy complication have occurred later in life. Treatment of this EDS type con-

sists of supportive care for management of vessel or bowel rupture. Pregnancy requires close monitoring.

EDS V

EDS V, or X-linked type, has X-linked recessive inheritance and is clinically similar to EDS type II with findings of soft skin and mild joint and skin hyperextensibility. This extremely rare disorder has been described in only two families with a total of eight affected persons [44,45]. Without a clear family history to confirm X-linked inheritance, the diagnosis of EDS type II should be considered. Some controversy exists as to whether this is a distinct subtype rather than variable expression of EDS II [3].

EDS VI

EDS VI, ocular scoliotic type, is a rare autosomal recessive disorder exhibiting joint laxity, kyphoscoliosis and muscle hypotonia. Skin findings include fragility with easy bruising, hyperextensibility and abnormal scarring. Major complications can include severe thoracic deformity with respiratory insufficiency [46], in addition to vascular and gastrointestinal ruptures [47].

Newborns generally present wth muscular hypotonia with poor cry, problems with sucking and delayed motor development. Kyphoscoliosis may be present at birth and is thought to be due to muscular hypotonia with resulting ligamentous laxity. Vertebral bodies are normal. There is marked joint laxity which may result in joint dislocations.

Ocular fragility complicated by retinal detatchment and globe rupture was initially reported as a major feature [47, 48], leading to the description 'ocular form' of EDS. A subsequent review [38] of the clinical features in patients biochemically confirmed to have EDS VI suggests that this may be less common than initially thought. Blue sclerae may also be present.

EDS VII

EDS VII consists of three subgroups. EDS VIIA and VIIB, also known as arthrochalasis multiplex congenita, and EDS VIIC, also referred to as human dermatospraxis.

EDS VIIA and VIIB are autosomal dominant disorders. They exhibit severe joint laxity with bilateral congenital hip dislocations and dislocation of other joints throughout life. Muscular hypotonia may be present at birth and is associated with delayed gross motor development. Skin features include softness, mild increase in bruising and mild hyperextensiblity without significantly increased fragility.

A disorder with extreme skin fragility, called dermatospraxis, was first identified in cattle in 1971; only recently has the human counterpart, EDS VIIC, been described [21,24,49]. It is characterized by autosomal recessive inheritance with marked skin fragility with easy tearing of the skin, skin laxity, increased bruisibility, growth retardation, umbilical hernias and blue sclerae.

EDS VIII

EDS VIII, periodontal form, displays autosomal dominant inheritance and is a rare variant with generalized periodontal disease [50,51]. There is early loss of teeth in the second to third decades due to gingival inflammation and alveolar bone loss. Other features include easy bruisability that presents in early childhood, and a characteristic purplish discoloration of scars limited to the shins (Fig. 19.17.6). Joint hypermobility and cutaneous hyperextensibility may be present to a minor degree.

EDS IX

EDS IX, Occipital horn syndrome, is a rare disorder with X-linked recesive inheritance [52–54]. Characteristic features, which are present at birth, include soft, lax and redundant skin. The skin, however, is not hyperelastic and

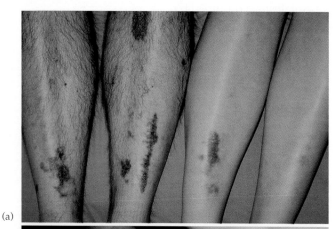

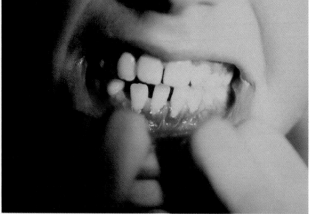

Fig. 19.17.6 EDS VIII. (a) Parent (left) and child (right) with characteristic scarring on anterior shins with bruising and purple discoloration. (b) Periodontal disease is present in this child with gingival fragility and retraction of tissue surrounding the gums.

does not demonstrate easy bruising or abnormal scarring. During childhood, formation of bladder diverticuli may occur with complications of bladder rupture, ureteral obstruction and hydronephrosis. Skeletal changes such as exostoses at sites of tendon insertion, also called occipital horns, osteoporosis, short humeri and short, broad clavicles are characteristic. A mild, chronic diarrhoea of unclear aetiology and orthostatic hypotension are also found in affected males. Female carriers are asymptomatic.

EDS X

EDS X, an autosomal recessive disorder, has been reported in a single family [55]. It is characterized by mild skin hyperextensibility, poor wound healing, easy bruising and mild joint hypermobility. Excessive bleeding was noted and a platelet adhesion defect which improved with the addition of fibronectin was identified.

Prognosis

The prognosis of the various EDS subtypes is based upon the specific associated features and their complications and has been reviewed above.

Differential diagnosis

The differential diagnosis of EDS includes syndromes specifically associated with joint hypermobility or cutaneous laxity. Familial articular hypermobility syndrome was initially classified as EDS XI, but displays joint laxity alone, without skin laxity and must be considered in patients with joint hypermobility without other stigmata of EDS. Cutis laxa has increased cutaneous laxity with acrogeric appearance but is distinguished by lack of recoil after stretching of the skin. Increased cutaneous fragility is found in osteogenesis imperfecta and this diagnosis may be considered in patients with EDS VI.

The diagnosis of EDS is based primarily on clinical history, family history to clarify inheritance, and careful physical examination to evaluate involvement of the various systems. Biochemical or genetic testing may be undertaken to confirm diagnosis in the EDS subtypes that have a characterized defect. In EDS IV, fibroblast cultures demonstrate decreased synthesis or secretion of procollagen III, in addition to decreased collagen III levels in skin extracts and decreased serum levels of prcollagen III aminopeptide [16]. Decreased lysyl hydroxylase enzyme activity in fibroblast culture confirms diagnosis of EDS VI [18]. The clinical diagnosis of the EDS VII subtypes can be confirmed through evaluation of type I collagen processing which shows abnormalities in α1, α2 or both peptides [19–21]. Electron microscopic studies of skin in EDS VIIC shows markedly irregular collagen fibres.

Treatment

The management of an EDS patient is dependent upon which system is involved. Joint laxity may result in early onset osteoarthritis or joint dislocations and may require orthopaedic or rheumatological follow-up. Physical therapy to strengthen supporting muscles and stabilize loose joints may be necessary in children who are experiencing delay in motor development. Bracing may be required to support unstable joints and assist with walking. Sports with joint impact such as gymnastics or long distance running are best avoided in children with significant joint hyperextensibility. Repeated hyperextension of joints to perform 'joint tricks' should also be discouraged as this stresses an unstable joint increasing the risk of joint dislocation and early onset osteoarthritis.

In children with severe skin fragility, protective pads over knees, shins and elbows may be helpful in preventing lacerations. Poor wound healing and scar formation has implications for any surgical procedure to be performed and the surgeon must be aware of the potential problems.

Because of the risk of sudden and potentially fatal vascular or bowel haemorrhage in EDS IV, patients should be advised to wear medical alert tags or bracelet with their diagnosis. EDS type IV females must be made aware of the complications associated with pregnancy.

Most importantly, counselling, reviewing the inheritance and the specific features of the subtype involved is essential for all families. The clinical and genetic heterogeneity of the EDS subtypes must be stressed with careful explanation of the expected risks and complications associated with the specific diagnosis. Clearly, the diagnosis of EDS II in a family has minimal impact on family planning or activity level of an affected individual; whereas, the diagnosis of EDS IV, VI or VII has significant life-long sequelae. The dramatic vascular complications of EDS IV have often been stressed in the older literature on EDS and it is essential to clarify that these are not associated with all the EDS subtypes. Patient support groups exist in the UK and the USA and are a valuable referral source for patients.

REFERENCES

1 Beighton P, de Paepe A, Danks D *et al.* International Nosology of heritable disorders of connective tissue, Berlin, 1986. *Am J Med Genet* 1988; 29: 585–94.
2 McKusick VA. The Ehlers–Danlos syndrome. In: *Heritable Disorders of Connective Tissue*, 4th ed. St Louis: CV Mosby, 1972: 292–371.
3 Steinmann B, Royce PM, Superti-Furga A. The Ehlers–Danlos Syndrome. In: Royce PM, Steinmann B, eds. *Connective Tissue and its Heritable Disorders.* New York: Wiley-Liss, 1993: 351–407.
4 Beighton P. The Ehlers–Danlos syndromes. In: Beighton, ed. *McKusick's Hertiable Disorders of Connective Tissue*, 5th edn. St Louis: CV Mosby, 1993: 189–251.
5 van Meek'ren JA. De dilatabilitate extraordinaria cutis. In: *Observations Medicochirugicae. Ger Fil Medicinae Studioso.* Amsterdam: Ex Officina Henrici & Viduae Theodori Boom, 1862: 134–6.
6 Beighton P. *The Ehlers–Danlos Syndrome.* London: Heinemann Medical, 1970.
7 Tschernogobow A. Cutis laxa (presentation at first meeting of Moscow Dermatologic and Venereologic Society, 13 November 1891). *Mhft Prakt Derm* 1892; 14: 76.
8 Ehlers E. Cutis Laxa, Neigung zu hemorrhagien in der Haut, Loekerung mehrerer artikulationen. *Dermatal Zeitschr* 1901; 8: 173.
9 Danlos M. Un cas de cutis laxa avec tumeurs par contusion chronique des coudes et des Mace De Lepinay. *Bull Soc Franc Dermatol* 1908; 19: 70.
10 Weber FP. The Ehlers–Danlos syndrome. *Br J Dermatol Syph* 1936; 48: 609.
11 McKusick VA. The Ehlers–Danlos syndrome. In: *Heritable Disorders of Connective Tissue*, 2nd edn. St Louis: CV Mosby, 1960.
12 Vogel A, Holbrook KA, Steinmann B, Gitzelmann R, Byers PH. Abnormal collagen fibril structure in the gravis form (type I) of the Ehlers–Danlos syndrome. *Lab Invest* 1979; 40: 201–6.
13 Sokolov BP, Prytkov AN, Tromp G, Knowlton RG, Prockop DJ. Exclusion of COL1A1, COL1A2, and COL3A1 genes as candidate genes for Ehlers–Danlos syndrome type I in one large family. *Hum Genet* 1991; 88: 125–9.
14 Byers PH. Ehlers–Danlos syndrome: recent advances and current understanding of the clinical and genetic heterogeneity. *J Invest Dermatol* 1994; 103: 47S–52S.
15 Byers PH, Holbrook KA, Mcgillivray. Clinical and ultrastructural heterogeneity of type IV Ehlers–Danlos syndrome. *Hum Genet* 1979; 47: 141–50.
16 De Paepe A. Ehlers–Danlos syndrome type IV. Clinical and molecular aspects and guidelines for diagnosis and management. *Dermatology* 1994; 189 (suppl 2): 21–5.
17 Pinnell SR, Krane SM, Kenzora JE, Glimcher MJ. A heritable disorder of connective tissue: hydroxylysine-deficient collagen disease. *N Engl J Med* 1972; 286: 1013–20.
18 Yeowell HR, Pinnell SR. The Ehlers–Danlos syndromes. *Semin Dermatol* 1993; 12: 229–40.
19 Cole WG, Chan D, Chambers GW, Walker ID, Bateman JF. Deletion of 24 amino acids from the proα1(I) chain of type I procollagen in a patient with the Ehlers–Danlos syndrome type VII. *J Biol Chem* 1986; 261: 5496–503.
20 Wirtz MK, Glanville RW, Steinmann B, Rao VH, Hollister DW. Ehlers–Danlos syndrome type VIIB. Deletion of 18 amino acids comprising the N-telopeptide region of a proα2(I) chain. *J Biol Chem* 1987; 262: 16376–85.
21 Smith LT, Wertelecki W, Milstone LM *et al.* Human dermatospraxis: a form of Ehlers–Danlos syndrome that results from failure to remove the amino-terminal peptide of type I procollagen. *Am J Hum Genet* 1992; 51: 235–44.
22 Levinson B, Gitschier J, Bulpe D, Whitney S, Yang S, Packman S. Are X-linked cutis laxa and Menkes disease allelic? *Nature Genet* 1993; 3: 6.
23 Rizzo R, Contri MB, Micali G *et al.* Familial Ehlers–Danlos syndrome type II: abnormal fibrillogenesis of dermal collagen. *Pediatr Dermatol* 1987; 4: 197–204.
24 Wertelecki W, Smith LT, Byers PH. Initial observations of Human dermatospraxis: Ehlers–Danlos syndrome type VIIC. *J Pediatr* 1992; 121: 558–64.
25 Byers PH, Holbrook KA. Ehlers–Danlos syndrome. In: Emery AEH, Rimoin DL, eds. *Principles and Practice of Medical Genetics*, 2nd edn. New York: Churchill Livingstone, 1990: 1065–81.
26 Beighton P, Thomas ML. The radiology of the Ehlers–Danlos syndrome. *Clin Radiol* 1969; 20: 354–61.
27 Weber FP, Aitken JK. Nature of the subcutaneous spherules in some cases of the Ehlers–Danlos syndrome. *Lancet* 1938; i: 198–9.
28 Mehregan AH. Elastosis perforans serpiginosa. *Arch Dematol* 1968; 97: 381–93.
29 Beighton P. Articular manifestations of the Ehlers–Danlos syndrome. *Semin Arthr Rheum* 1971; 1: 246–61.
30 Beighton P, Horan F. Orthopaedic aspects of the Ehlers–Danlos syndrome. *Semin Arthr Rheum* 1971; 1: 246–61.
31 Beighton P. Cardiac abnormalities in the Ehlers–Danlos syndrome. *Br Heart J* 1969; 31: 227–32.
32 Pyeritz RE. Cardiovascular manifestations of heritable disorders of connective tissue. *Prog Med Genet* 1983; 5: 191–301.
33 McFarland W, Fuller DE. Mortality in Ehlers–Danlos syndrome due to spontaneous rupture of large arteries. *N Engl J Med* 1964; 271: 1309–10.
34 Shohet I, Rosenbaum I, Frand M *et al.* Cardiovascular complications in the Ehlers–Danlos syndrome with minimal external findings. *Clin Genet* 1964; 31: 148–52.
35 Pretorious ME, Butler IJ. Neurologic manifestations of Ehlers–Danlos syndrome. *Neurology* 1983; 33: 1087–9.

36 Pemberton JW, Freeman HM, Schepens CL. Familial retinal detachment and the Ehlers–Danlos syndrome. *Arch Ophthalmol* 1966; 76: 817–24.

37 Beighton P. Serious ophthalmological complications in the Ehlers–Danlos syndrome. *Br J Ophthalmol* 1970; 54: 263–8.

38 Wenstrup RJ, Murad S, Pinnell SR. Ehlers–Danlos syndrome type VI: clinical manifestations of lysyl hydroxylase deficiency. *J Pediatrics* 1989; 115: 405–9.

39 Gorlin RJ, Cohen MM, Levin LS. Ehlers–Danlos syndromes. In: *Syndromes of the Head and Neck*, 4th edn. New York: Oxford University Press, 1990: 429–41.

40 Stewart RE, Hollister DW, Rimoin DL. A new variant of Ehlers–Danlos syndrome: an autosomal dominant disorder of fragile skin, abnormal scarring, and generalized periodontitis. *Birth Defects* 1977; 13(3B): 85–93.

41 Hordnes K. Ehlers–Danlos syndrome and delivery. *Acta Obstet Gynecol Scand* 1994; 73: 671–3.

42 Pepin MG, Superti-Furga A, Byers PH. Natural history of Ehlers–Danlos syndrome type IV (EDS IV): review of 137 cases. *Am J Hum Genet* 1992; 51: A44 (abstract).

43 Pope FM, Narcisi P, Nicholls AC, Liberman M, Oorthuys JWE. Clinical presentations of Ehlers–Danlos syndrome type IV. *Arch Dis Child* 1988; 63: 1016–25.

44 Beighton P. X-linked recessive inheritance of the Ehlers–Danlos syndrome. *B Med J* 1968; 2: 409–11.

45 Beighton P, Curtis D. X-linked Ehlers–Danlos syndrome type V; the next generation. *Clin Genet* 1985; 27: 472–8.

46 Chamson A, Berbis P, Fabre JE, Privat Y, Frey J. Collagen biosynthesis and isomorphism in a case of Ehlers–Danlos syndrome type VI. *Arch Dermatol Res* 1987; 279: 303–7.

47 Sussman M, Lichtenstein JR, Nigra TP, Martin GR, Mckusick VA. Hydroxylysine-deficient skin collagen in a patient with a form of Ehlers–Danlos syndrome. *J Bone Joint Surg* 1974; 56: 1228–34.

48 Pinnell SR, Krane SM, Kenzora JE, Glincher MJ. A heritable disorder of connective tissue: hydroxylysine-deficient collagen disease. *N Engl J Med* 1972; 286: 1013–20.

49 Petty EM, Seashore MR, Braverman IM, Spiesel SZ, Smith LT, Milstone LM. Dermatospraxis in children: a case report and review of the newly recognized phenotype. *Arch Dermatol* 1993; 129: 1310–15.

50 Stewart RE, Hollister DW, Rimoin DL. A new variant of Ehlers–Danlos syndrome: an autosomal dominant disorder of fragile skin, abnormal scarring, and generalized periodontitis. *Birth Defects* 1977; 13(3B): 85–93.

51 Nelson DL, King RA. Ehlers–Danlos syndrome type VIII. *J Am Acad Dermatol* 1981; 5: 297–303.

52 Kuivaniemi H, Peltonen L, Palotie A, Kaitila I, Kivirikko KI. Abnormal copper metabolism and deficient lysyl oxidase activity in a heritable connective tissue disorder. *J Clin Invest* 1982; 69: 730–3.

53 Peltonen L, Kuivaniemi H, Palotie A, Horn N, Kaitila I, Kivirikko KI. Alterations in copper and collagen metabolism in the Menkes syndrome and a new subtype of the Ehlers–Danlos syndrome. *Biochemistry* 1983; 22: 6156–63.

54 Kuivaniemi H, Peltonen L, Kivirikko KI. Type IX Ehlers–Danlos syndrome and Menkes syndrome: the decrease in lysyl oxidase activity is associated with a corresponding deficiency in the enzyme protein. *Am J Hum Genet* 1985; 37: 798–808.

55 Arneson MA, Hammerschmidt DE, Furcht LT, King RA. A new form of Ehlers–Danlos syndrome: fibronectin corrects defective platelet function. *J Am Med Assoc* 1980; 244: 144–7.

19.18 Cutis Laxa

RICHARD J. ANTAYA

Definition

The term cutis laxa (dermatochalasis, dermatomegaly) denotes the clinical expression of several extremely rare, heterogeneous disorders of elastic tissue characterized by loose, inelastic skin which is pendulous and hangs in folds, giving a prematurely aged or bloodhound-like appearance. Some forms with significant systemic involvement are better termed generalized elastolysis.

Aetiology and/or pathogenesis

Cutis laxa may be inherited or acquired, and both may manifest in childhood. The mechanisms leading to cutis laxa are not well understood. There may be defects in the synthesis or degradation of the elastic fibres, or the structure of elastic fibres may be defective. Some patients with congenital cutis laxa have diminished levels of elastin production as well as its mitochondrial RNA (mRNA), suggesting a defect at the molecular level in production of elastin [1]. Elevated serum elastase (neutral protease) activity has been demonstrated in a patient with recessively inherited cutis laxa and suggests a possible role for this enzyme; however, elevated activity has been shown in normals as well [2]. A deficiency of the copper-dependent elastase inhibitor has been postulated also, but this has not been proven [3]. In some forms there may be a defect in the normal relationship between serum copper, ceruloplasmin and copper-dependent elastase inhibitor activity [3,4].

An immunological basis is suggested for the acquired forms that have been reported following ill-defined febrile illnesses or surgery [5–8]. It has been associated with apparent hypersensitivity reactions to penicillin [9], isoniazid [7] or Calmette–Guèrin bacillus inoculation (in one adult only). Drugs such as D-penicillamine may produce cutis laxa by chelating copper, which is required for the function of enzymes responsible for the cross-linking of elastin and collagen [10].

Pathology

Haematoxylin and eosin stained tissue is generally un-remarkable. With elastic stains (Verhoeff) there may be diminished elastic fibres either throughout the dermis or primarily in the upper or lower dermis. Elastic fibres that are seen may be short, fragmented, clumped and often display thickening centrally with tapering to a point at the ends. In advanced cases elastic fibres may be completely absent, with only dust-like granules staining positive for elastic tissue [11]. The findings vary with the stage of the disease and location on the body, but even clinically uninvolved skin may display the characteristic changes [12]. Some cases exhibit moderate non-specific chronic inflammation with lymphocytes, histiocytes [12] and neutrophils [13]. There may be a mucinous stroma in areas of abnormal elastic tissue [3,12].

Ultrastructurally, there are various patterns of abnormal elastic fibres, of which the most significant is the presence of electron-dense amorphous or granular deposits associated with bundles of microfibrils [12,14,15]. A deficiency of elastin with normal microfibril formation has been observed in some cases [14]. Both acquired and congenital types display similar ultrastructural findings [14]. Internal organs such as lung [15], aorta and gastrointestinal (GI) tract may display similar changes in elastic fibres [3,5].

Clinical features and prognosis

Patients with cutis laxa demonstrate striking features with notably loose, redundant skin that sags and hangs in pendulous folds, giving the appearance that the skin is too large for the body (Fig. 19.18.1). Inelasticity is best demonstrated by lack of recoil when stretched from its resting position. This is in contrast to that observed in Ehlers–Danlos syndrome. The highly characteristic facial features are likened to that of a bloodhound, with marked sagging of the skin, accentuation of the nasolabial and other facial folds, ectropion and blepharochalasis. Because the corners of the mouth sag, individuals often appear mournful. Despite the senescent appearance in early ages, children may 'grow into' their abnormal skin and have a more normal appearance in adulthood. The cutaneous manifestations amongst the various types of cutis laxa are fairly similar, although there

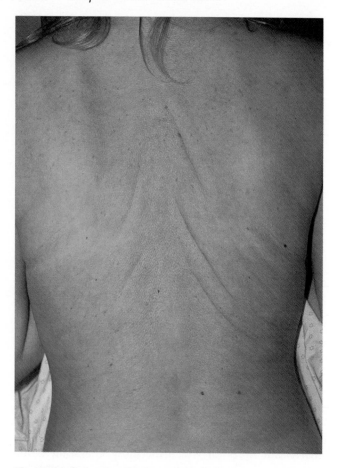

Fig. 19.18.1 Redundant skin in an adolescent girl with cutis laxa.

exists great variability in the internal manifestations and prognoses.

Cutis laxa can be inherited or acquired and there are subclassifications of each type. A self-limited congenital form has also been described.

Inherited types

One autosomal dominant and two autosomal recessive forms have been well described. An X-linked recessive form, characterized by a defect in the enzyme lysyl oxidase, which functions in cross-linking both collagen and elastin, has been reclassified as Ehlers–Danlos syndrome type IX, and is only mentioned here for historical perspective. Facial dysmorphism with hooked nose, short columella, everted nostrils and long upper lip is quite characteristic of the inherited forms of cutis laxa.

The exceedingly rare autosomal dominant form has primarily cutaneous involvement, with few systemic manifestations, a relatively benign course and a normal life expectancy [16–18]. It may appear at any age from birth to adulthood, but generally has a later onset than the recessive forms. It most likely displays incomplete penetrance [17]. Bronchiectasis, emphysema, diverticuli, hernias, uterine prolapse [16], hoarseness, mitral valve prolapse, dilatation of the sinuses of Valsalva [18], pulmonary artery stenosis [17], coarctation of the aorta [19] and dilatation and tortuosity of the carotid artery, presenting as a pulsating mass in the lateral neck [17] have been associated with this form [16]. Facial involvement is universal and cosmesis is usually the main concern, as most affected lack systemic involvement.

The more severe form of autosomal recessive cutis laxa is associated with emphysema, which may develop in the first months of life [16]. Cutis laxa is present at birth, involves nearly all of the body surface and, unlike other forms, can worsen over time. A hoarse, low-pitched voice is thought to result from lax, redundant vocal chords. Diaphragmatic hernia may cause respiratory distress in the neonatal period [3]. Diverticuli of the oesophagus, stomach, small intestine and rectosigmoid as well as inguinal, obturator and umbilical hernias are common. Bladder diverticuli present with symptoms of enuresis and frequency but are largely asymptomatic. Emphysema is associated with recurrent pulmonary infections, resulting in cor pulmonale and death in the first few years of life.

The other autosomal recessive form of cutis laxa is associated with delayed development and ligamentous laxity. Pre- and postnatal growth retardation seem to be defining criteria of this disorder [20]. Cutis laxa, nearly always present at birth, involves the face, trunk and extremities, and is especially severe over the hands, feet and abdomen [20,21]. Congenital dislocation of the hip is common and usually bilateral [20,21]. All joints exhibit generalized laxity, especially those of the hands, which leads to unusual positioning [20,21]. Affected infants exhibit wide sutures and a large anterior fontanelle with delayed closure. Other craniofacial abnormalities include broadening of the nasal bridge with apparent hypertelorism, prominent nasal tip, long philtrum, downslanting palpebral fissures, epicanthal folds, frontal bossing, low-set ears and a high-arched palate. Other inconstant findings are macular coloboma, myopia, iris hypoplasia, simian crease, cleft lip [22], ureteropelvic junction obstruction with hydronephrosis [20], osteoporosis [23] and Dandy–Walker malformation associated with minor heart and osseous defects [24]. The prognosis for intellectual and motor development is unpredictable, but there appears to be a tendency for improved performance with age [20]. There have been no reported deaths so far. Some patients have been products of consanguineous marriages, suggesting an autosomal recessive inheritance. However, because of the disproportionate number of affected females and miscarriages involving male siblings, an X-linked dominant mode of inheritance is possible.

Acquired types

Acquired elastolysis presents as a generalized insidious disease, typically associated with internal manifestations in all adults and infrequently in children. It usually begins in adulthood but has been reported in children [4,5,7,9,25,26]. Laxity varies in distribution and is progressive over several years. Only the facial and ear involvement has been reported in patients less than 10 years of age [5,7,26], with more generalized, adult presentation in older children [4,9]. Most reported cases have been males. Inflammatory skin lesions such as generalized vesicular eruptions [5], erythema multiforme, urticaria and dermatitis herpetiformis-like eruptions [9] occur before or concurrent with cutaneous laxity. Associated internal disorders include emphysema, GI and genitourinary diverticuli, inguinal hernias and rectal prolapse. The GI manifestations are most common and often asymptomatic.

Death from emphysema and aortic rupture has been reported. Increased serum immunoglobulin A (IgA) was reported in two children, but its significance is unknown [9,26]. Of the few cases reported in children only one had systemic involvement (tracheobronchiomegaly) and one death resulted. This suggests a better prognosis for those developing this type of acquired cutis laxa in childhood. However, there have been no reports of spontaneous resolution. Its association with recent drug therapy, particularly penicillin [9] and isoniazid [7], and evidence of tuberculosis in two children [7,25] suggest a hypersensitivity reaction as a possible aetiology.

Another type of acquired cutis laxa was first described by Marshall *et al.* [27] as postinflammatory elastolysis and cutis laxa (PECL). Almost all cases have occurred in previously healthy black females 4 years of age or younger, living in tropical climates [6,8,27–29]. A relapsing acute inflammatory phase lasting several months or years exhibits crops of recurrent inflammatory skin lesions resembling Sweet's syndrome. The primary lesion is a non-pruritic, bright red papule. The papules expand to well-circumscribed, erythematous oval plaques measuring 2–10 cm. As they extend peripherally, they leave a hypopigmented centre. Some lesions consist of erythema and swelling in geographic patterns while others resemble papular urticaria. Malaise, fever and peripheral eosinophilia typify the acute phase [27]. The chronic phase is characterized by localized or, less commonly, extensive areas of cutis laxa and dermal atrophy occurring in foci of prior inflammation [6]. There is no consistent systemic involvement. However, fatal aortitis [28] and coronary involvement [29] have been reported and the cutaneous manifestations do not always parallel internal organ involvement [29]. The aetiology is unknown. It seems to have features intermediate between anetoderma and acquired cutis laxa. Hypersensitivity, possibly to arthropod bites, has been proposed [6].

Transient neonatal cutis laxa

Transient neonatal cutis laxa presents in infants born to mothers treated with penicillamine for Wilson's disease [10,30], rheumatoid arthritis [31] or cystinuria [32] during gestation. Generalized cutis laxa associated with inguinal hernias are characteristic, and as its name implies, cutaneous changes resolve during the first year of life in all but the most severe cases [7,10,18,30,31]. Joint mobility is usually normal. Pulmonary complications [21], joint hyperflexibility, severe fragility of veins, varicosities, micrognathia, low-set ears [30] and impaired wound healing [32] have been reported associations in the severely affected. Low serum zinc but normal serum copper suggests a possible role for low zinc levels in the development of this form of cutis laxa [30]. Most have normal postnatal levels of serum copper and ceruloplasmin, and it was postulated that intermittently low serum copper levels [33] *in utero* had induced both collagen and elastic tissue defects, which self-corrected postnatally [10]. This is supported by similar findings in animal studies [34]. The effects of penicillamine are more severe in infants of mothers treated for rheumatoid arthritis and cystinuria than for Wilson's disease [31]. This may be explained on the basis that in Wilson's disease there is a high proportion of unbound copper, which is chelated by penicillamine and excreted, thus effectively reducing the penicillamine level and resultant toxicity.

Differential diagnosis

Cutis laxa may be differentiated from Ehlers–Danlos syndrome because in the latter the skin is extensible but exhibits brisk recoil. This is due to normal elastic fibres in association with abnormal collagen in Ehlers–Danlos syndrome. Pseudoxanthoma elasticum (PXE) usually spares the face and presents with yellowish confluent papules especially in flexural skin. Histologically, PXE demonstrates abnormal elastic fibres in the deeper portions of the dermis, with relative sparing of the papillary dermis. There is also calcification, which is not present in cutis laxa. Granulomatous slack skin, an atrophic patch stage of cutaneous T-cell lymphoma, is characterized by pendulous folds that hang from the axillae and groin. Anetoderma also exhibits cutaneous laxity, but it is usually a localized, macular type, and has not been associated with systemic elastolysis. Costello's syndrome should be considered in the differential diagnosis of the recessive form of cutis laxa with developmental delay. Children with Costello's syndrome usually have high birth weights and, despite clinically lax skin, display normal elastic tissue histologically [35].

De Barsy's syndrome, comprised of intrauterine growth retardation, wrinkled atrophic skin, open sutures, somatic and mental retardation and hypermobility of small joints can be differentiated from the recessive form of cutis laxa with delayed development by the presence of muscular hypotonia, athetoid posturing and brisk tendon reflexes [21].

Other conditions such as neurofibromatosis, trisomy 18, Patterson's syndrome (pseudoleprechaunism), 'wrinkly skin syndrome', gerodermia osteodysplastica, SCARF (skeletal abnormalities, cutis laxa, craniosynostosis, ambiguous genitalia, retardation and facial abnormalities) syndrome [36] and leprechaunism display abnormally lax skin folds and are distinguished by their associated characteristics.

Treatment

Therapy is limited. Surgical repair of associated internal defects such as hernias, diverticuli and rectal prolapse is sometimes necessary. Plastic surgery is effective for removal of excess skin folds, thereby improving the appearance and limiting the emotional trauma from severe disfigurement [37]. Repeated surgeries are often required as the redundant skin recurs over time. Unlike the collagen diseases, no problems with wound healing have been reported. Treatment with systemic steroids controlled the eruption of PECL well in one case, partially in another [27] and a blood transfusion along with dicloxacillin prompted regression of the inflammatory response but not the elastolysis in another patient. Dapsone controlled the inflammatory lesions in the systemic acquired form; however, methaemoglobinaemia complicated the treatment [9]. Penicillamine is not helpful [12]. Pulmonary function tests are useful for early detection of emphysema. Family members should be examined for signs of cutis laxa, and for those families with inherited forms, genetic counselling should be performed.

REFERENCES

1 Olsen DR, Fazio MJ, Shamban AT *et al.* Cutis laxa: reduced elastin gene expression in skin fibroblast cultures as determined by hybridizations with a homologous cDNA and an exon 1-specific oligonucleotide. *J Biol Chem* 1988; 263: 6465–7.

2 Anderson LL, Oikarinen AI, Ryhanen L, Anderson CE, Uitto J. Characterization and partial purification of a neutral protease from the serum of a patient with autosomal recessive pulmonary emphysema and cutis laxa. *J Lab Clin Med* 1985; 105: 537–46.

3 Goltz RW, Hult AM, Goldfarb M, Gorlin RJ. Cutis laxa. *Arch Dermatol* 1965; 92: 373–87.

4 Ferreira MC, Spina V. A case of cutis laxa with abnormal copper metabolism. *Br J Plast Surg* 1973; 26: 283–6.

5 Reed WB, Horowitz RE, Beighton P. Acquired cutis laxa. *Arch Dermatol* 1971; 103: 661–9.

6 Verhagen AR, Woerdeman MJ. Postinflammatory elastolysis and cutis laxa. *Br J Dermatol* 1975; 92: 183–90.

7 Koch SE, Williams MD. Acquired cutis laxa: case report and review of disorders of elastolysis. *Pediatr Dermatol* 1985; 2: 282–8.

8 Saxe N, Gordon W. Acute febrile neutrophilic dermatosis (Sweet's syndrome). *S Afr Med J* 1978; 52: 253–6.

9 Kerl H, Burg G, Hashimoto K. Fatal, penicillin-induced generalized post-inflammatory elastolysis (cutis laxa). *Am J Dermatopathol* 1983; 5: 267–76.

10 Linares A, Zarranz JJ, Rodriguez-Alarcon J, Diaz-Perez JL. Reversible cutis laxa due to maternal D-penicillamine treatment. *Lancet* 1979; ii: 43.

11 Mehregan AH, Lee SC, Nabai H. Cutis laxa (generalized elastolysis). *J Cutan Pathol* 1978; 5: 116–26.

12 Nanko H, Jepsen LV, Zachariae H, Sogaard H. Acquired cutis laxa (generalized elastolysis). *Acta Derm Venereol (Stockh)* 1979; 59: 315–24.

13 Jablonska S. Inflammatorische Hautveranderungen, die einer erworbenen Cutis laxa vorausgehen. *Hautarzt* 1966; 17: 341–6.

14 Hashimoto K, Kanzaki T. Cutis laxa. *Arch Dermatol* 1975; 111: 861–73.

15 Sayers CP, Goltz RW, Mottaz J. Pulmonary elastic tissue in generalized elastolysis (cutis laxa) and Marfan's syndrome. *J Invest Dermatol* 1975; 65: 451–7.

16 Beighton P. The dominant and recessive forms of cutis laxa. *J Med Genet* 1972; 9: 216–21.

17 Hayden JG, Talner NS, Klaus SN. Cutis laxa associated with pulmonary artery stenosis. *J Pediatr* 1986; 72: 506–9.

18 Brown FR, Holbrook KA, Byers PH *et al.* Cutis laxa. *Johns Hopkins Med J* 1982; 150: 148–53.

19 Balboni FA. Cutis laxa and multiple vascular anomalies, including coarctation of the aorta. *Bull St Francis Hosp (Roslyn)* 1963; 19: 26–34.

20 Sakati NO, Nyhan WL, Shear CS *et al.* Syndrome of cutis laxa, ligamentous laxity, and delayed development. *Pediatrics* 1983; 72: 850–6.

21 Gorlin RJ, Cohen MM. Craniofacial manifestations of Ehlers–Danlos syndromes, cutis laxa syndromes, and cutis laxa-like syndromes. *Birth Defects: Orig Art Ser* 1990; 25 (4): 39–71.

22 Patton MA, Tolmie J, Ruthnum P, Bamford S, Baraister M, Pembrey M. Congenital cutis laxa with retardation of growth and development. *J Med Genet* 1987; 24: 556–61.

23 Sakati NO, Nyhan WL. Congenital cutis laxa and osteoporosis. *Am J Dis Child* 1983; 137: 452–4.

24 Biver A, De Rijcke S, Toppet V *et al.* Congenital cutis laxa with ligamentous laxity and delayed development, Dandy–Walker malformation and minor heart and osseous defects. *Clin Genet* 1994; 42: 318–22.

25 Bernstein BA, Sorbera RS, Maloney PL, Doku HC. Cutis laxa: report of a case. *J Oral Surg* 1971; 29: 201–4.

26 Wanderer AA, Ellis EF, Goltz RW, Cotton EK. Tracheobronchiomegaly and acquired cutis laxa in a child. *Pediatrics* 1969; 44: 709–15.

27 Marshall J, Heyl T, Weber HW. Post-inflammatory elastolysis and cutis laxa. *S Afr Med J* 1966; 40: 1016–22.

28 Heyl T, Simson IW, Cronje RE. Post-inflammatory cutis laxa and aortitis (acquired systemic elastolysis). *Br J Dermatol* 1971; 85 (suppl 7): 37–43.

29 Muster AJ, Bharati S, Herman JJ *et al.* Fatal cardiovascular disease and cutis laxa following acute febrile neutrophilic dermastosis. *J Pediatr* 1983; 102: 243–8.

30 Harpey JP, Jaudon MC, Clavel JP, Galli A, Darbois Y. Cutis laxa and low serum zinc after antenatal exposure to penicillamine. *Lancet* 1983; ii: 858.

31 Solomon L, Abrams G, Dinner M, Berman L. Neonatal abnormalities associated with D-penicillamine treatment during pregnancy. *N Engl J Med* 1977; 296: 54–5.

32 Mjolnerod OK, Rasmussen K, Dommerud SA, Gjeruldsen ST. Congenital connective-tissue defect probably due to D-penicillamine treatment in pregnancy. *Lancet* 1971; i: 673–5.

33 Rosa FW. Teratogen update: penicillamine. *Teratology* 1986; 33: 127–31.

34 Keen CL, Cohen NL, Lonnerdal B, Hurley LS. Teratogenesis and low copper status resulting from triethylenetetramine in rats. *Proc Soc Exp Biol Med* 1983; 173: 598–605.

35 Davies SJ, Hughes HE. Costello syndrome: natural history and differential diagnosis of cutis laxa. *J Med Genet* 1994; 31: 486–9.

36 Koppe R, Kaplan P, Hunter A, MacMurray. Ambiguous genitalia associated with skeletal abnormalities, cutis laxa, craniostenosis, psychomotor retardation, and facial abnormalities (SCARF syndrome). *Am J Med Genet* 1989; 34: 305–12.

37 Thomas WO, Moses MH, Craver RD, Galen WK. Congenital cutis laxa: a case report and review of loose skin syndromes. *Ann Plast Surg* 1993; 30: 252–6.

19.19 Pseudoxanthoma Elasticum

MARK LEBWOHL

Definition

Pseudoxanthoma elasticum is an inherited disease of connective tissue which results in a wide array of cutaneous, ocular and systemic manifestation. Calcification of elastic tissue results in characteristic changes in the skin, eyes and cardiovascular systems. The resulting clinical picture can be quite variable, but in its most severe form, is a model for accelerated ageing. The clinical presentation of pseudoxanthoma elasticum in the paediatric age group has been well described [1].

History

Felix Balzer first reported a patient with yellow xanthomatous flexural skin lesions in 1884. On histopathological examination he observed thickened and broken elastic fibres in the skin and heart [2]. In 1896, Jean Darier differentiated the skin lesions and xanthomas and called the disease 'pseudo-xanthome elastique' [3]. Angioid streaks were also first described at the end of the 19th century [4,5] but it was not until 1929 that the ophthalmologist Gronblad and the dermatologist Strandberg firmly established a link with the skin lesions of pseudoxanthoma elasticum and attributed both to an underlying elastic tissue defect [6,7]. The cardiovascular calcification that occurs in pseudoxanthoma elasticum was definitively described in 1944 in a group of 29 Swedish patients with the disorder [8]. Since that time reviews of large numbers of patients have been conducted by Connor et al. at the Mayo Clinic [9], by McKusick [10], by Pope [11] and by Neldner [12]. A review of the history of pseudoxanthoma elasticum would not be complete without mention of the detailed description of this disorder's light microscopic and ultrastructural findings published by Danielsen in her doctoral thesis in 1979 [13].

Aetiology and pathogenesis

Pseudoxanthoma elasticum has been reported in most countries and racial groups around the world [10,12]. Several published studies have reported a female to male ratio of approximately 2:1 [10,12]. Both autosomal dominant and autosomal recessive inheritance patterns, however, should result in an equal number of male and female cases. The discrepancy may be explained by a tendency of males to ignore cutaneous lesions or by hormonal or environmental effects that cause the disease to become more noticeable in females.

The exact prevalence of the disorder is not known because we do not have a simple serological test for the diagnosis of pseudoxanthoma elasticum. In one of the earliest reviews of this disease, McKusick estimated that pseudoxanthoma elasticum occurs in at least 1 in 160 000 people [10]. In a study by Altman et al. in the Seattle area the prevalence of pseudoxanthoma elasticum was estimated at 1 in 70 000 [14]. In Denver Neldner found a prevalence of 1 in 90 000 to 1 in 100 000 [12]. He published his data in the most comprehensive review of pseudoxanthoma elasticum in a systematic 10-year study of 100 patients with the disease.

A key flaw exists in all attempts to estimate the prevalence of this disease. There are patients who have skin lesions which are mild or even undetectable except on biopsy. Patients have been reported who have accelerated cardiovascular disease and angioid streaks without the skin lesions of pseudoxanthoma elasticum. On biopsy of normal-appearing flexural skin, however, these patients have been found to have histological evidence of the disease [15]. There have also been reports of patients with angioid streaks and histological evidence of pseudoxanthoma elasticum on biopsy of scars despite the absence of characteristic skin lesions [16]. Are these patients heterozygote carriers for an autosomal recessive form of pseudoxanthoma elasticum? Or do they have a mild form of autosomal dominantly inherited pseudoxanthoma elasticum? Does the diagnosis of pseudoxanthoma elasticum require the presence of skin lesions? In an attempt to standardize the diagnosis of pseudoxanthoma elasticum for investigators and clinicians reporting their findings, a consensus conference was held in 1992. The conference was attended by almost all of the investigators working in pseudoxanthoma elasticum and resulted in publication of a classification system that was agreed upon by the participants [17].

According to that classification, major and minor criteria were established for the diagnosis of pseudoxanthoma elasticum, and patients who meet all major criteria are unequivocally identified as having the disease (Table 19.19.1). In patients who do not have characteristic skin lesions but have other features of the disease such as angioid streaks, histological evidence of pseudoxanthoma elasticum or a family history of the disease, a provisional classification of category II pseudoxanthoma elasticum can be established. If patients subsequently develop skin lesions, they can be reclassified as having category I disease as they would then meet all of the major criteria for the diagnosis of pseudoxanthoma elasticum. Category II patients have one major criterion, angioid streaks and either histological evidence of pseudoxanthoma elasticum or a family history of the disease or both (Table 19.19.2). Once a primary defect responsible for pseudoxanthoma elasticum is discovered, the above classification will undoubtedly be replaced by a more accurate classification system.

Studies of the genetics of pseudoxanthoma elasticum suffer from the same difficulty that plagues epidemiological studies. For many years pseudoxanthoma elasticum was presumed to be an exclusively autosomal recessive disease and many authors of textbooks of dermatology still consider autosomal recessive transmission to be the most common form of inheritance despite isolated reports of two or three generations of pseudoxanthoma elasticum. However, in 1966 20 instances of inheritance from parent to child were reported [18]. More instances of autosomal dominant inheritance were presented by Pope [19] who also reported autosomal recessive inheritance [20].

In 1975, Pope classified 121 pseudoxanthoma elasticum patients from England and Wales according to a system that recognized the genetic heterogeneity of the disease and included two autosomal dominant and two autosomal recessive forms [11]. According to Pope's classification patients with autosomal dominant inheritance comprised 53% of the group studied. Twelve of the 64 patients with this inheritance pattern had severe systemic manifestations including angina, claudication and hypertension. This group, characterized as autosomal dominant type 1, all had the classical flexural rash of pseudoxanthoma elasticum. The 52 remaining patients with autosomal dominant inheritance had milder cutaneous and systemic symptoms but had myopia, high arched palates, loose jointedness and blue sclerae. Of the two recessive types of pseudoxanthoma elasticum, one included 54 patients with typical flexural lesions but few systemic complications. The recessive type 2 group included only three patients with 'generalized cutaneous pseudoxanthoma elasticum'.

A critique of this classification was published by Neldner who disagreed with many of its aspects [12]. Specifically, Neldner suggested that the patients with autosomal recessive type 2 generalized cutaneous lesions might actually have a form of cutis laxa. In Neldner's survey of 100 patients, only three (3%) had autosomal dominant inheritance.

How can two investigators examining patients with the same disease find such great discrepancies in the inheritance patterns? At least in part, these discrepancies can be explained by differences in the definition of pseudoxanthoma elasticum. Clinically apparent skin lesions are required for a diagnosis of pseudoxanthoma elasticum according to Neldner, whereas some of Pope's patients did not have skin lesions. How then does one classify a patient with angioid streaks, cardiovascular complica-

Table 19.19.1 Criteria for the diagnosis of pseudoxanthoma elasticum

Major criteria
Characteristic skin involvement (yellow cobblestone lesions in flexural locations)
Characteristic histopathological features of lesional skin (elastic tissue and calcium or von Kossa stains)
Characteristic ocular disease (angioid streaks, peau d'orange, or maculopathy) in adults older than 20 years of age

Minor criteria
Characteristic histopathological features of non-lesional skin (elastic tissue and calcium or von Kossa stains)
Family history of PXE in first-degree relatives

Table 19.19.2 Classification of pseudoxanthoma elasticum

Category I* (3 major criteria)	Category IIa (1 major criterion and 2 minor criteria)	Category IIb (1 major criterion and 1 minor criterion)	Category IIc (1 major criterion and 1 minor criterion)	Category IId (2 minor criteria)
Characteristic yellow skin lesions in flexural sites	Angioid streaks	Angioid streaks	Angioid streaks	Family history of PXE in first-degree relatives
Elastic fibre calcification — lesional skin	Elastic fibre calcification — non-lesional skin	Elastic fibre calcification non-lesional skin	Family history of PXE in first-degree relatives	Elastic fibre calcification non-lesional skin
Ocular disease in adults	Family history of PXE in first-degree relatives			

*Subtypes: recessive, dominant, sporadic.

tions, a family history of pseudoxanthoma elasticum and histological evidence of the disease without apparent skin lesions? Some would consider this patient to be heterozygous for autosomal recessively inherited pseudoxanthoma elasticum. Others would consider the disease to be autosomal dominantly inherited with variable expressivity. Both autosomal dominant and autosomal recessive forms of the disease have been described and until more definitive tests exist, the classification showed in Table 19.19.2 adequately describes patients with different features of pseudoxanthoma elasticum. The locus for pseudoxanthoma elasticum has now been mapped to chromosome 16p13.1 [21]. Discovery of the responsible gene should enable us to answer many of the questions raised above.

The overwhelming preponderance of evidence suggests a genetic abnormality of either elastic tissue or another substance intimately associated with elastic tissue in pseudoxanthoma elasticum. All of the complications of pseudoxanthoma elasticum occur in elastic tissue-containing organs such as the skin, Bruch's membrane of the eye and the internal elastic lamina of arteries. Histological and ultrastructural studies certainly corroborate the profound involvement of elastic tissue in this disease.

While it has been difficult to demonstrate a primary genetic abnormality in elastic tissue in patients with pseudoxanthoma elasticum, fibroblasts of patients with pseudoxanthoma elasticum produce dramatically reduced amounts of fibrillin 2, an elastin-associated fetal protein that forms the scaffolding upon which elastic tissue is formed [22]. This protein contains many calcium-binding epidermal growth factor-like amino acid sequences, and a solitary change in these sequences could result in a dramatic increase in calcification. Thus, fibrillin 2 is certainly a candidate gene for the primary defect in pseudoxanthoma elasticum.

Other possible candidate genes that have been suggested include lysyl oxidase and reduced lysyl oxidase activity has been demonstrated in some patients [23].

Pathology

On light microscopy there is an increase in elastic tissue. Much of the elastic tissue is clumped and fragmented particularly in the middle and deep dermis.

On staining with haematoxylin and eosin, calcification of dermal components is visible as clumped, faintly basophilic material. The Von Kossa stain, a calcium stain that demonstrates the negatively charged ions that bind to calcium, is useful for demonstrating the calcification that occurs in pseudoxanthoma elasticum, and a diagnosis of pseudoxanthoma elasticum should be questioned if dermal calcification cannot be demonstrated with this stain (Fig. 19.19.1). The Verhoeff–Van Gieson stain is an elastic tissue stain that demonstrates the fragmentation of

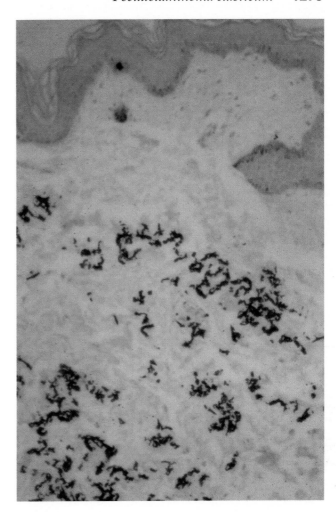

Fig. 19.19.1 Von Kossa stain to demonstrate calcification in pseudoxanthoma elasticum.

elastic fibres that occurs in pseudoxanthoma elasticum (Fig. 19.19.2a). Figure 19.19.2b shows normal elastic tissue in an unaffected individual for comparison.

On staining with Alcian blue, there is a marked increase in mucopolysaccharides. Upon digestion with hyaluronidase, it can be shown that much of this Alcian blue positive material is hyaluronic acid. A number of studies have demonstrated marked increases in dermal mucopolysaccharides in lesional skin of patients with pseudoxanthoma elasticum. Both dermatan sulphate and hyaluronic acid are increased [24–26]. Of great interest, the increase in mucopolysaccharides is also demonstrable in clinically unaffected skin of patients with pseudoxanthoma elasticum. This has been clearly shown in non-lesional buttock skin. The authors suggested that deposition of mucopolysaccharides precedes the calcification of elastic tissue, and the negatively charged mucopolysaccharides may contribute to elastic tissue calcification by electrostatic forces [24]. This leads to the intriguing possibility that by preventing this increase in mucopolysaccharides, we may one day be able to

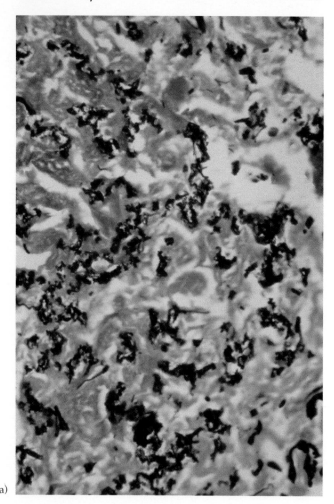

(a)

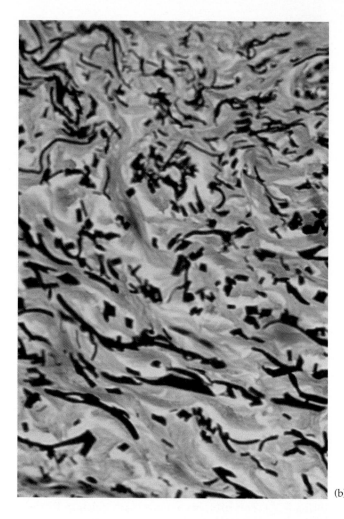

(b)

Fig. 19.19.2 Van Gieson stain: (a) showing fragmentation of elastic fibres in pseudoxanthoma elasticum; (b) in normal skin for comparison.

prevent the calcification that occurs in pseudoxanthoma elasticum.

On electron microscopy, profound changes in both elastic tissue and collagen have been described. Elastic fibres contain irregularly shaped holes and electron-dense bodies. Some elastic fibres contain holes surrounded by a striking discrete electron-dense borderline [13,27].

Numerous abnormalities of collagen have also been described including collagen fibrils that are thin, thick, laterally fused and twisted as well as decreased in number and broken down to particles [13,27–30].

Clinical features

The skin lesions of pseudoxanthoma elasticum are said to resemble cobblestones or plucked chicken skin. They have also been called 'xanthoma-like' because of their yellowish colour. The skin lesions typically begin on the neck

(Fig. 19.19.3). The next most commonly involved sites are the axillae (Fig. 19.19.4) but any flexural area can be affected, including the skin superior to the umbilicus (Fig. 19.19.5). Wrists are less commonly affected. Skin lesions begin as yellow macules that can develop into yellow papules. In more severe cases, papules become confluent to form yellow plaques that simulate plane xanthomas. In very severe cases patients develop redundant folds of skin in flexural areas (Fig. 19.19.6) and skin can be strikingly hyperextensible. In patients who are severely affected, the sagging of facial skin can be striking. This results in a 'hound dog'-like appearance that has been seen in patients with cutis laxa. The skin lesions of pseudoxanthoma elasticum exhibit a Koebner phenomenon, having a tendency to develop within scars. This has been used diagnostically in that biopsy of scars may aid in the diagnosis of pseudoxanthoma elasticum in patients without clinically apparent skin lesions [16]. Similarly, in patients with angioid streaks and accelerated cardiovascular disease who do not have skin lesions, biopsy of intertriginous areas such as the neck or axillae can establish a diagnosis of pseudoxanthoma elasticum [15].

Skin lesions can occasionally be quite subtle. In one

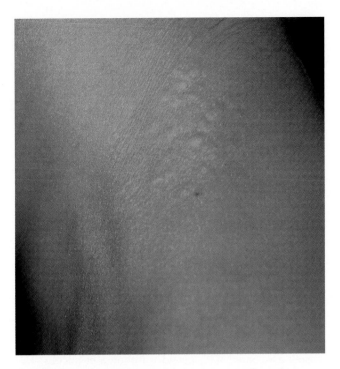

Fig. 19.19.3 Typical 'xanthoma-like' skin lesions on the neck.

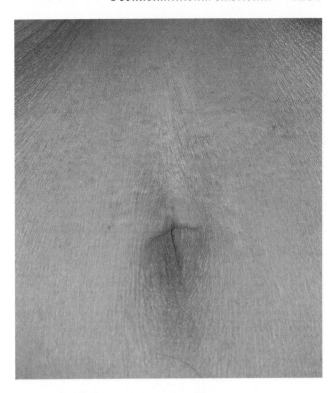

Fig. 19.19.5 Affected skin above the umbilicus.

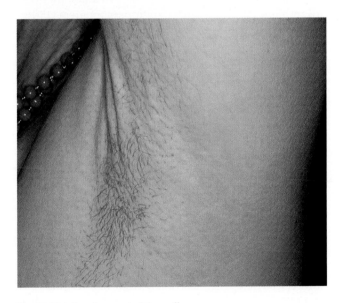

Fig. 19.19.4 Involvement of the axilla.

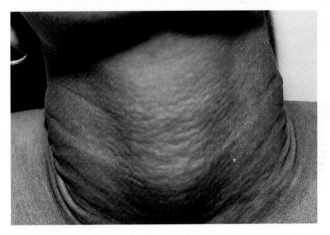

Fig. 19.19.6 Severe involvement with redundant folds of skin around the neck.

patient examined at the Mount Sinai Medical Center in New York City, pseudoxanthoma elasticum was found incidentally in normal-appearing skin around an excised naevus. The patient was subsequently found to have asymptomatic angioid streaks and mild skin lesions on the neck and in the axillae, groin and periumbilical area.

Mucosal lesions develop in many patients. They are easily seen on the mucosal aspect of the lower lip (Fig. 19.19.7) and under the tongue. Histological evidence of pseudoxanthoma elasticum has been found in rectal mucosa [31], and a patient has been reported with lesions of pseudoxanthoma elasticum on the dorsal aspect of the penis [12].

Variants

Perforation of calcified elastic fibres through the epidermis in patients with pseudoxanthoma elasticum has been called 'perforating pseudoxanthoma elasticum' [32]. There have been many reports of elastosis perforans ser-

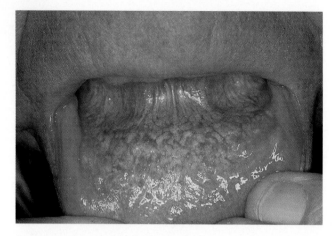

Fig. 19.19.7 Mucosal lesions on the lower lip.

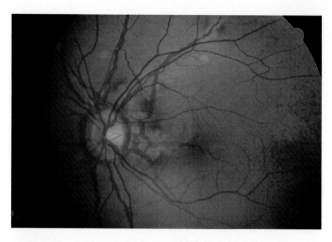

Fig. 19.19.8 Angioid streaks on the retina.

piginosa occurring in patients with pseudoxanthoma elasticum, and it is likely that many of these patients in fact had perforating pseudoxanthoma elasticum [33–35]. While extrusion of dermal material is common to all of the perforating disorders, perforating pseudoxanthoma elasticum is clearly distinct from the other disorders in that the extruded material consists of calcified elastic fibres.

Another unusual form of pseudoxanthoma elasticum has been called 'localized acquired cutaneous pseudoxanthoma elasticum'[36]. This condition appears to be more common in obese, multiparous, black females several of whom have had hypertension. Skin lesions usually occur on the abdomen, particularly in the periumbilical area. In several instances perforation of the epidermis with dermal extrusion of calcified elastic fibres has been reported [37]. The reported cases have been sporadic without any family history of pseudoxanthoma elasticum, and the patients do not generally have other stigmata of pseudoxanthoma elasticum, although there has been a solitary report of a black woman with chronic renal failure who developed perforating pseudoxanthoma elasticum and was found to have angioid streaks [38]. Neldner and Martinez-Hernandez have also reported a multiparous black woman with cirrhosis who was thought to have localized acquired pseudoxanthoma elasticum with skin lesions on the breasts as well as the abdomen [36].

Ocular manifestations

Angioid streaks, the ocular hallmark of pseudoxanthoma elasticum, represent breaks in Bruch's membrane, an elastic tissue-containing membrane of the retina that can become calcified and crack. Angioid streaks appear as blood vessel-like lines that are grey or brown in darkly pigmented individuals (Fig. 19.19.8) and red in fair-skinned patients. They often encircle the optic disc in a peripapillary distribution or radiate out from the optic disc. Their size is often similar to that of retinal vessels but they can occasionally be much wider than retinal vessels.

Although they have been reported in patients with many different conditions, angioid streaks are most closely associated with pseudoxanthoma elasticum. The large majority of adults with pseudoxanthoma elasticum have angioid streaks [12]. Because the skin lesions of pseudoxanthoma elasticum can be subtle or inapparent [15,16], it is possible that many of the patients reported with angioid streaks may have occult pseudoxanthoma elasticum. Angioid streaks have also been reported in several patients with Paget's disease and sickle cell anaemia [39,40].

In patients with pseudoxanthoma elasticum, angioid streaks often develop in teenage years. Other ocular features of pseudoxanthoma elasticum included mottled 'p'eau d'orange' which consists of mottled pigmentation of the retinal pigment epithelium, and drusen which appear as small hypopigmented holes in Bruch's membrane. The development of subretinal neovascularization in these patients can lead to haemorrhage, scarring and loss of vision. If haemorrhage involves the macular area, patients may develop loss of central vision and can become legally blind. Peripheral vision is maintained, however, so that patients do not become totally blind.

Cardiovascular manifestations

Just like other elastin-containing tissues, the internal elastic lamina of arteries can become calcified. Calcification of arteries can be seen on simple X-rays in up to one-third of patients [12]. Reduced peripheral pulses commonly result from arterial calcification in patients with pseudoxanthoma elasticum. Intermittent claudication, presumably due to reduced circulation, has been reported in up to 30% of patients [12]. Claudication has been reported as early as the age of 9 years in a patient with pseudoxanthoma elasticum [12]. Intermittent claudication of the arms can also occur and may present as aching, weakness or fatigue on upper extremity exertion. Occlusion of vessels has been demonstrated in arteriograms of the arms [31].

Calcification of the coronary arteries can lead to accelerated cardiovascular disease with symptoms and complications simulating arteriosclerosis. There have been patients with angina or myocardial infarctions in teenage years. A patient was reported who developed angina pectoris at the age of 11 years and underwent three vessel coronary artery bypass graft surgery at the age of 18 years [10]. An Australian journal reported three teenage patients with pseudoxanthoma elasticum who died of myocardial infarctions, leading the authors to call this disease the 'sudden death syndrome' [41].

The severity of skin lesions does not correlate with the development of cardiovascular disease. At the Mount Sinai Medical Center, the author has seen four patients who developed cardiovascular disease at early ages in the absence of other risk factors for atherosclerosis. All had angioid streaks and histological evidence of pseudoxanthoma elasticum but no skin lesions [15]. This has led to the suggestion that any patient with unexplained accelerated heart disease be examined for pseudoxanthoma elasticum. Examination for angioid streaks by a retina specialist and skin biopsy of normal-appearing axillary skin or scars may reveal the diagnosis in patients without skin lesions [16].

Other cardiovascular complications of pseudoxanthoma elasticum that have occurred include a restrictive cardiomyopathy reported in one patient [42] and cardiac valvular abnormalities that are common. Heart valves contain elastic tissue so it is not surprising that they are affected in patients with this disease. A number of cardiac valvular abnormalities can occur including fibrous thickening of the atrioventricular valves and mitral valve prolapse. The latter abnormality occurs in approximately two-thirds of patients [43].

Hypertension has been reported in the region of 9–48% of patients, depending on the series of patients studied [31,44]. It is clear that hypertension increases with age. There are, however, two sisters with pseudoxanthoma elasticum reported, one of whom died at the age of 10 years of complications of hypertension and a second who had elevated blood pressure at the age of 6 years [45]. Several additional reports of hypertension occurring in the teenage years or earlier have been published [46,47]. Elevation of blood pressure has been attributed to narrowing of the renal artery in at least some cases [48,49].

Other systemic manifestations

In some patients, calcification of the arteries will lead to cracking of the blood vessel and haemorrhage. Bleeding

has been reported in many sites including the uterus, nose, joints, gastrointestinal tract and others. Gastrointestinal bleeding develops in almost 10% of patients [12,44]. In some women, gastrointestinal bleeding occurs during pregnancy [50]. When radiographic and endoscopic examinations are undertaken, the source of bleeding is rarely found [12]. Fortunately, bleeding is often minor and self-limited, but occasionally partial gastrectomy is required.

Other consequences of arterial calcification include central nervous system complications such as stroke and dementia. These are attributed to calcification of cerebral arteries and reduced circulation or intracranial haemorrhage [51,52].

Pulmonary calcification has been noted in isolated foci on chest X-rays in a few patients with pseudoxanthoma elasticum [53,54]. It is quite interesting that pulmonary calcification is minor and not associated with clinical sequelae in patients with pseudoxanthoma elasticum even though the lungs contain elastic tissue.

Differential diagnosis

The clinical differential diagnosis of pseudoxanthoma elasticum includes actinic elastosis. This is most easily seen on the posterior neck of elderly light-skinned patients where skin takes on a yellowish hue similar to that seen in pseudoxanthoma elasticum. Plane xanthomas can also simulate the skin lesions of confluent plaques of pseudoxanthoma elasticum. Exposure of the skin to calcium salts such as calcium chloride can lead to cutaneous ulceration followed by the development of yellow papules that may resemble pseudoxanthoma elasticum. Farmers have been reported with persistent yellow lesions resembling pseudoxanthoma elasticum following a solitary exposure to saltpetre which they were using to fertilize their fields [55,56]. Histologically there is calcification of elastic fibres indistinguishable from that seen in pseudoxanthoma elasticum. Von Kossa stains show calcification of elastic fibres in the dermis.

Patients treated with penicillamine also can develop skin lesions that may resemble pseudoxanthoma elasticum clinically [57]. Some of these patients develop widespread redundant yellow folds of skin that are not accentuated in the typical flexural sites characteristically affected in pseudoxanthoma elasticum. Histologically, elastic tissues are not calcified in patients treated with penicillamine, distinguishing this phenomenon from true pseudoxanthoma elasticum. More commonly, patients treated with penicillamine develop elastosis perforans serpiginosa [58–60].

Finally, calcification of the dermis can occur in several circumstances such as electrical burns or other damaged tissue, conditions associated with hypercalcaemia or hyperphosphataemia, or idiopathic calcinosis cutis.

These conditions are usually easily distinguished both histologically and clinically from pseudoxanthoma elasticum.

Treatment

Several steps can be taken to minimize the complications of pseudoxanthoma elasticum. Because of the tendency to bleeding, use of anticoagulants such as warfarin or heparin should be minimized, and patients should avoid platelet inhibitors such as aspirin.

Echocardiograms can be performed to look for mitral valve prolapse or other cardiac valvular abnormalities. If heart valve abnormalities exist, it has been suggested that prophylactic antibiotics be prescribed at the time of dental work to prevent valvular infection. To prevent accelerated cardiovascular disease, a low-fat, low-cholesterol diet, avoidance of cigarette smoking, control of blood pressure and aerobic exercises have been advised.

Checking the stool for blood, particularly during pregnancies, has been advocated by some authors. Regular use of an Amsler grid and consultation with a retina specialist may help prevent ocular bleeding and visual loss. Similarly, avoidance of exercises that cause trauma to the head must be stressed.

Cosmetically deforming redundant folds of skin can be removed surgically with excellent results [61]. Despite the elastic tissue defect in pseudoxanthoma elasticum, patients generally heal very well following surgery.

It has also been suggested that oestrogens make pseudoxanthoma elasticum worse and should therefore be avoided. The role of dietary calcium in the development of pseudoxanthoma elasticum remains controversial. Patients with significant calcium intake early in life may have a worse prognosis and this has led to the suggestion that high calcium-containing foods such as milk or calcium supplements be avoided [62].

With the era of gene therapy on the horizon, it is likely that pseudoxanthoma elasticum patients will be treated in much more sophisticated ways in the future. For the time being, however, many of the therapeutic measures described are preventive in nature. It is therefore imperative that family members of patients with pseudoxanthoma elasticum be examined so that a diagnosis can be established as early as possible in life.

REFERENCES

1 Hacker SM, Ramos-Caro FA, Beers BB, Flowers FP. Juvenile pseudoxanthoma elasticum: recognition and management. *Pediatr Dermatol* 1993; 10: 19–25.
2 Balzer F. Recherches sur les caracteres anatomiques due xanthelasma. *Arch Physiol* (Series 3) 1884; 4: 65–80.
3 Darier J. *Pseudo-Xanthome Elastique. IIIe Congres Intern de Dermat de Londres*, 5 August 1896.
4 Doyne RW. Choroidal and retinal changes; the result of blows on the eyes. *Trans Ophthalmol Soc UK* 1889; 9: 129.
5 Knapp H. On the formation of dark angioid streaks as an unusual metamorphosis of retinal hemorrhage. *Arch Ophthalmol* 1892; 21: 289–94.
6 Gronblad E. Angioid streaks—pseudoxanthoma elasticum. Vorlaufige Mitteilung. *Acta Ophthalmol* 1929; 7: 329.
7 Strandberg J. Pseudoxanthoma elasticum. *Z Haut Geschlechtskr* 1929; 31: 689–94.
8 Carlbourg U. Study of circulatory disturbances, pulse wave velocity and pressure pulses in larger arteries in cases of pseudoxanthoma elasticum and angioid streaks: a contribution to the knowledge of the function of the elastic tissue and the smooth muscles in larger arteries. *Acta Med Scand* 1944; 151: 1–209.
9 Connor PJ, Juergens JL, Perry HO *et al.* Pseudoxanthoma elasticum and angioid streaks: a review of 106 cases. *Am J Med* 1961; 30: 537–43.
10 McKusick VA. *Heritable Disorders of Connective Tissue*, 4th edn. St Louis: CV Mosby, 1972; 475–520.
11 Pope FM. Pseudoxanthoma elasticum: an historical survey. *Trans St John's Hosp Dermatol Soc* 1972; 58: 235–50.
12 Neldner KH. Pseudoxanthoma elasticum. *Clin Dermatol* 1988; 6: 1–155.
13 Danielsen L. Morphological changes in pseudoxanthoma elasticum and senile skin. *Acta Derm Venereol (Stockh)* 1979; 83 (suppl): 1–79.
14 Altman LK, Fialkow PJ, Parker F *et al.* Pseudoxanthoma elasticum: an underdiagnosed genetically heterogenous disorder with protean manifestations. *Arch Intern Med* 1974; 134: 1048–54.
15 Lebwohl M, Halperin J, Phelps RG. Occult pseudoxanthoma elasticum in patients with premature cardiovascular disease. *N Engl J Med* 1993; 329: 1237–9.
16 Lebwohl M, Phelps RG, Yannuzzi L *et al.* Diagnosis of pseudoxanthoma elasticm by scar biopsy in patients without characteristic skin lesions. *N Engl J Med* 1987; 317: 347–50.
17 Lebwohl M, Neldner K, Pope FM *et al.* Classification of pseudoxanthoma elasticum: report of a consensus conference. *Am Acad Dermatol* 1994; 30: 103–7.
18 Wise D. Hereditary disorders of connective tissue. In: Galtron HA, Schnyder UW, eds. *Vererbung vo Hautkrankherten.* Berlin: Julius Springer Verlag, 1966; 30: 201–12.
19 Pope FM. Autosomal dominant pseudoxanthoma elasticum. *J Med Genet* 1974A; 11: 152–7.
20 Pope FM. Two types of autosomal recessive pseudoxanthoma elasticum. *Arch Dermatol* 1974B; 110: 209–12.
21 Struk B, Neldner KH, Rao V, St John P, Lindpaintner K. Mapping of both autosomal recessive and dominant variants of pseudoxanthoma elasticum to chromosome 16p13.1. *Human Mol Genet* 1977; 6: 1823–8.
22 Sapadin A, Schwartz E, Lebwohl M. Fibrillin synthesis in cultured pseudoxanthoma elasticum fibroblasts. *J Invest Dermatol* 1994; 102: 603.
23 Christiano AM, Lebwohl MG, Boyd CD, Uitto U. Workshop on Pseudoxanthoma Elasticum: Molecular Biology and Pathology of the Elastic Fibers. *J Invest Dermatol* 1992; 99: 660–3.
24 Lebwohl, M, Longas MO, Konstadt J *et al.* Hyaluronic acid and dermatan sulfate in nonlesional pseudoxanthoma elasticum skin. *Clinica Chimica Acta* 1995; 238: 101–7.
25 Smith JG Jr, Davidson EA, Clark RD. Dermal elastin in actinic elastosis and pseudoxanthoma elasticum. *Nature* 1962; 195: 716–17.
26 Fisher ER, Rodnan GP, Lansing AI. Identification of the anatomic defect in pseudoxanthoma elasticum. *Am J Pathol* 1958; 34: 977–91.
27 Lebwohl M, Schwartz E, Lemlich G, Lovelace O, Shaikh-Bahai F, Fleischmajer R. Abnormalities of connective tissue components in lesional and nonlesional tissue of patients with pseudoxanthoma elasticum. *Arch Dermatol Res* 1993; 285: 121–6.
28 Teller H, Vester G. Elektronmikroskopische Untersuchungsergebnisse an der kollagenen Intercellularsubstanz des Koriums beim *Pseudoxanthoma elasticum. Dermatol Wochenschr* 1957; 36: 1373.
29 Pasquali-Ronchetti I, Volpin D, Baccarani-Contri M, Castellani I, Peserico A. Pseudoxanthoma elasticum. Biochemical and ultrastructural studies. *Dermatologica* 1981; 163: 307–25.
30 Ross R, Fialkow PS, Altman LK. Fine structure alterations of elastic fibers in pseudoxanthoma elasticum. *Clin Genet* 1978; 13: 213–23.
31 Goodman RM, Smith EW, Paton D *et al.* Pseudoxanthoma elasticum: a clinical and histopathological study. *Medicine* 1963; 42: 297–334.
32 Graham JH, Hunter GA. Perforating pseudoxanthoma elasticum. *Arch Dermatol* 1976; 112: 1781.
33 Bos WH. Pseudoxanthoma elasticum associated with perforating elastoma. *Dermatologica* 1968; 136: 296–7.

34 Schutt DA. Pseudoxanthoma elasticum and elastosis perforans serpiginosa. *Arch Dermatol* 1965; 91: 151–2.

35 Takahashi H, Nagao S, Iijima S *et al.* A case of elastosis perforans serpiginosa associated with pseudoxanthoma elaticum. *Nippon Hifuka Gakkai Zasshi* 1982; 92: 91–101.

36 Neldner KH, Martinez-Hernandez A. Localized acquired cutaneous pseudoxanthoma elasticum. *Arch Dermatol* 1979; 1: 523–30.

37 Hicks J, Carpenter CL, Reed RJ. Periumbilical perforating pseudoxanthoma elasticum. *Arch Dermaol* 1979; 115: 300–3.

38 Nickoloff BJ, Noodleman FR, Abel EA. Perforating pseudoxanthoma elasticum associated with chronic renal failure and hemodialysis. *Arch Dermatol* 1985; 121: 1321–2.

39 Gass JDM, Clarkson JG. Angioid streaks and disciform macular detachment in Paget's disease. *Am J Ophthalmol* 1973; 75: 576–86.

40 Nagpal KC, Asdourian G, Goldbaum M *et al.* Angioid streaks and sickle haemoglobinopathies. *Br J Ophthalmol* 1976; 60: 31–4.

41 Wiehelm K, Paver K. Sudden death in pseudoxanthoma elasticum. *Med J Aust* 1972; 2: 1363–5.

42 Navarro-Lopez F, Llorian A, Ferrer-Roca O *et al.* Restrictive cardiomyopathy in pseudoxanthoma elasticum. *Chest* 1980; 78: 113–15.

43 Lebwohl MG, DiStefano D, Prioleau PG *et al.* Pseudoxanthoma elasticum and mitral-valve prolapse. *N Engl J Med* 1982; 307: 228–31.

44 Eddy DD, Farber EM. Pseudoxanthoma elasticum. Internal manifestations: a report of cases and a statistical review of the literature. *Arch Dermatol* 1962; 86: 729–40.

45 Parker JC, Friedman-Kien AE, Sien S *et al.* Pseudoxanthoma elasticum and hypertension. *N Engl J Med* 1964; 271: 1204–6.

46 Kansy J, Osiecka Z, Biernat A *et al.* Pseudoxanthoma elasticum with hypertension in a 13-year-old girl. *Pediatr Pol* 1980; 55: 633–7.

47 Irani C, Dagonet Y, Cassasoprana A *et al.* Pseudoxanthoma elasticum with aortic insufficiency and arterial hypertension in a 12-year-old boy. *Arch Fr Pediatr* 1984; 41: 337–9.

48 Farreras-Valenti P, Rozman C, Jurado-Grau J *et al.* Gronblad–Strandberg–Touraine syndrome with systemic hypertension due to unilateral renal angioma: cure of hypertension after nephrectomy. *Am J Med* 1965; 39: 355–60.

49 Dymock RB. Pseudoxanthoma elasticum: report of a case with renovascular hypertension. *Aust J Dermatol* 1979; 20: 82–4.

50 McCaughey RS, Alexander LC, Morrish JA. The Gronblad–Strandberg syndrome: a report of three cases presenting with massive gastrointestinal hemorrhage during pregnancy. *Gastroenterol* 1956; 31: 156–68.

51 Galle G, Galle K, Huk W *et al.* Stenoses of the cerebral arteries in pseudoxanthoma elasticum. *Arch Psychiatr Nervenkr* 1981; 231: 61–70.

52 Messis CP, Budzilovich GN. Pseudoxanthoma elasticum: report of an autopsied case with cerebral involvement. *Neurology* (NY) 1970; 20: 703–9.

53 Mamtora H, Cope V. Pulmonary opacities in pseudoxanthoma elasticum: report of two cases *Br J Radiol* 1981; 54: 65–7.

54 Jackson A, Loh CL. Pulmonary calcification and elastic tissue damage in pseudoxanthoma elasticum. *Histopathology* 1980; 4: 607–11.

55 Christensen OB. An exogenous variety of pseudoxanthoma elasticum in old farmers. *Acta Derm Venereol* (Stockh) 1978; 58: 319–21.

56 Otkjaer-Nielsen AO, Christensen OB, Hentzer B *et al.* Salpeter induced dermal changes electron microscopically indistinguishable from pseudoxanthoma. *Acta Derm Venereol* (Stockh) 1978; 58: 323–7.

57 Light N, Meyrick Thomas RH, Stephens A *et al.* Collagen and elastin changes in D-penicillamine-induced pseudoxanthoma elasticum-like skin. *Br J Dermatol* 1986; 114: 381–8.

58 Kirsch N, Hukill PB. Elastosis perforans serpiginosa induced by penicillamine. Electron microscopic observations. *Arch Dermatol* 1977; 113: 630–5.

59 Abel M, Town B. Elastosis perforans serpiginosa associated with penicillamine. *Arch Dermatol* 1977; 113: 1303.

60 Pass F, Goldfischer S, Sternlieb I *et al.* Elastosis perforans serpiginosa during penicillamine therapy for Wilson disease. *Arch Dermatol* 1973; 108: 713–5.

61 Kaplan EN, Henjyoji EY, Pseudoxanthoma elasticum: a dermal elastosis with surgical implications. *Plast Reconstr Surg* 1976; 58: 595–600.

62 Renie WA, Pyeritz RE, Combs J *et al.* Pseudoxanthoma elasticum: high calcium intake in early life correlates with severity. *Am J Med Genet* 1984; 19: 235–44.

Buschke–Ollendorff Syndrome, Marfan's Syndrome, Osteogenesis Imperfecta, Anetodermas and Atrophodermas

MARC LACOUR

Buschke–Ollendorff syndrome
Papular elastorrhexis

Marfan's syndrome

Osteogenesis imperfecta

Anetodermas
Postinflammatory elastolysis and cutis laxa

Atrophodermas
Atrophoderma of Pasini and Pierini
Familial follicular atrophoderma and basal cell carcinoma
Atrophoderma vermiculate
Linear atrophoderma of Moulin
Focal facial dermal dysplasias

Buschke–Ollendorff syndrome

(SYN. FAMILIAL JUVENILE ELASTOMA, DERMATOFIBROSIS LENTICULARIS DISSEMINATA WITH OSTEOPOIKILOSIS, DISSEMINATA DERMATOFIBROSIS ORTHOPOIKILOSIS, NAEVUS ELASTICUS)

Definition

Buschke–Ollendorff syndrome (BOS) is an autosomal dominant disorder clinically characterized by the appearance of disseminated connective tissue naevi of the elastic type and osteopoikilosis.

History

In 1928, Buschke and Ollendorff described a 41-year-old woman with pea-sized papules symmetrically distributed over the upper part of the back and arms, lumbar region, buttocks and thighs [1]. These skin changes, histologically compatible with connective tissue naevi, were reported as dermatofibrosis lenticularis disseminata and were associated with osteopoikilosis. Osteopoikilosis is an uncommon cause of multiple osteosclerotic bone lesions (syn: osteopathia condensans disseminata, spotted bones, familial disseminated osteosclerosis). It was first described by Stieda in 1905 [2] and subsequently by Albers-Schoenberg (in 1915) [3]. From the many further

reports [4–10], it became clear that BOS could be transmitted in an autosomal dominant pattern and that, in the same family, affected individuals would usually present with both skin and bone changes, but could also have only one of these two sites involved [11]. In 1977, Morrisson *et al.* [12] reported 16 patients from different families in whom the skin lesions of disseminated dermatofibrosis showed the characteristic histological changes of juvenile elastoma. This confirmed earlier findings by Cairns [5] and indicated that the specific dermatological abnormality of BOS is consistent with connective tissue naevi of the elastic type (naevus elasticus). Juvenile elastoma was first described by Weidman *et al.* in 1933 [13]. The disorder, a hamartomatous malformation of elastic tissue, may be sporadic or inherited as an autosomal dominant trait. In the many cases reported, radiological investigations for osteopoikilosis have either not been mentioned [14–16] or were negative [17]. Familial juvenile elastoma should, however, be considered as a 'forme fruste' of BOS on the basis of the similar histology and the intrafamilial variation in penetration of the bone and/or skin changes [12,18]. More recent reports of BOS have been published [18–24].

Aetiology and pathogenesis

The basic defect in BOS remains unknown but certainly involves a focal alteration of elastin, a fundamental component of the extracellular matrix. Structural abnormalities of the elastic fibres have been described [12,25] and Uitto *et al.* demonstrated elevated elastin accumulation in involved skin relative to uninvolved skin and to skin of controls [26]. This is in keeping with more recent *in vitro* data showing increased production of tropoelastin and elastin messenger RNA from both lesional and non-lesional skin fibroblasts from BOS patients [27].

The similarity of the oval-shaped, well-circumscribed lesions of the skin (disseminated dermatofibrosis) and the bone (osteopoikilosis) led Buschke and Ollendorff to suggest that these abnormalities were related. Changes in microfibrils of both tissues have been proposed as a common link [25]. However, it is also possible that disseminated dermatofibrosis and/or osteopoikilosis in the same patient/family are related to the variable expression of two unrelated but closely located genes.

Pathology

Histologically and ultrastructurally, the skin lesions of BOS consist of hypertrophic, broad interlacing elastic fibres surrounding normal collagen bundles. These changes are usually present in the mid and lower dermis, sparing the papillary dermis [5,12]. Variation in the amount of both elastic and collagen fibres, as well as peculiar branching of the elastin, have been described [9,24,25,27–29]. The adjacent uninvolved skin is morphologically normal but is not sharply demarcated from lesional skin.

The lesions of BOS are therefore histologically distinct from familial cutaneous collagenoma (increased collagen and decreased, thin and fragmented elastic fibres), from the shagreen patch of tuberous sclerosis (increased collagen and paucity of elastic fibres) and from pseudoxanthoma elasticum (elastic fibres fragmentation and calcification).

Osteopoikilosis histologically consists of thickened trabeculae of lamellar bone [30,31]. Changes in microfibrils have been described [25].

Clinical findings

The cutaneous lesions in BOS may be present at birth but usually develop in the first or second decade. Their appearance later in adulthood is rarer. They consist of multiple, pea-sized, flesh-, yellow- or white-coloured papules symmetrically distributed on the buttocks, upper thighs and lumbar region [11,12,19,29,32]. More frequently, lesions comprise larger yellowish nodules, often grouped and sometimes coalescing into plaques [12,28], or can be asymmetrically distributed [9,10,18,33]. Confluence of the lesions is frequent but only exceptionally affects the whole tegument [27]. Once established, the lesions usually stay unchanged and remain asymptomatic (Fig. 19.20.1).

The radiological findings of osteopoikilosis consist of multiple, well-circumscribed round or oval opacities, each 1–10 mm in diameter. They are usually found in the epiphyses and metaphyses of long bones and the pelvis, but are also frequent in the spongiosa of the phalanges, carpal and tarsal bones. The ribs, skull and spine are very rarely affected, which is helpful to exclude other osteocondensing conditions such as metastases, mastocytosis and tuberous sclerosis [21]. Osteopoikilosis is of no pathological significance and is usually an incidental finding, found in 12 of 211 000 radiographs in one series [34]. It can occur in the fetus but usually takes many years to develop and may not be detectable before the late adolescent or adult

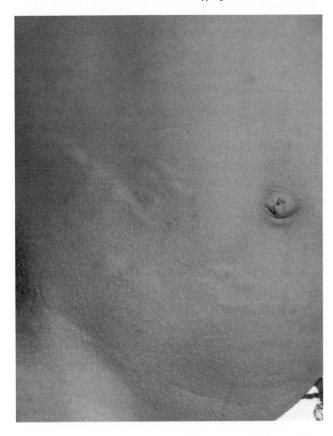

Fig. 19.20.1 Juvenile elastoma on the abdomen of a child with BOS.

period. Familial osteopoikilosis in the absence of skin changes has been described [35].

BOS usually remains an asymptomatic and benign disorder throughout life. However, muscle fibrosis and contractures may complicate the disorder [36] and several associations have been described [11], most of which are likely to be purely coincidental. One exception to this is the association with otosclerosis [5,22,37,38], possibly as a consequence of a generalized connective tissue disorder.

Differential diagnosis and treatment

History, careful clinical examination and appropriate radiological investigations of the patient and whole family are essential to identify BOS. Indeed, the differential diagnosis of the cutaneous findings is quite large (Table 19.20.1). In the absence of bone changes in any member of the family, a biopsy will differentiate BOS from other connective tissue naevi.

The lesions of BOS remain asymptomatic and rarely cause a cosmetic problem, thus no treatment is necessary. Informing close relatives of the diagnosis is advisable to avoid misinterpretation of incidental radiographs and allow genetic counselling of this autosomal dominant syndrome.

Table 19.20.1 Differential diagnosis of cutaneous elastoma in the Buschke–Ollendorff syndrome

Shagreen patch (tuberous sclerosis)
Collagenoma
Pseudoxanthoma elasticum
Lichen myxoedematous
Dermal nodules of Hunter syndrome
Smooth muscle hamartoma
Leiomyoma
Neurofibroma
Lipoma

REFERENCES

1 Buschke A, Ollendorff H. Ein Fall von Dermatofibrosis disseminata und Osteopathia condensans disseminata. *Dermatol Wochenschr* 1928; 86: 257–62.

2 Stieda A. Ueber umschriebene Knochenverdichtungen im Bereich des Substantia spongiosa im Röntgenbilde. *Bruns Beitr Klin Chir* 1905; 45: 700–3.

3 Albers-Schoenberg HE. Eine seltene, bisher nicht bekannte Strukturanomalie des Skelettes. *Fortschr Roentgenstr* 1915; 23: 174–5.

4 Berlin R, Hedensiö B, Lilja B et al. Osteopoikilosis—a clinical and genetic study. *Acta Med Scand* 1967; 181: 305–14.

5 Cairns RJ. Familial juvenile elastoma: osteopoikilosis (two cases). *Proc Roy Soc Med* 1967; 60: 1267.

6 Grupper C, Cardinne A. Disseminated lenticular dermatofibrosis with osteopecila (father and son). Buschke–Ollendorff syndrome. *Ann Dermatol Syph Paris* 1974; 101: 405–7.

7 Marshall J. Osteopoikilosis and connective tissue naevi: a syndrome of hereditary polyfibromatosis. *S Afr Med J* 1970; 44: 775–7.

8 Pastinszky J, Csato Z. On skin variations in osteopoikilia (Buschke–Ollendorff syndrome). *Z Haut Geschlechtskr* 1968; 43: 313–23.

9 Schorr WF, Opitz JM, Reyes CN. The connective tissue naevus—osteopoikilosis syndrome. *Arch Dermatol* 1972; 81: 249–52.

10 Smith AD, Waisman M. Connective tissue naevi: familial occurrence and association with osteopoikilosis. *Arch Dermatol* 1960; 81: 249–52.

11 Verbov J, Graham R. Buschke–Ollendorff syndrome—disseminated dermatofibrosis with osteopoikilosis. *Clin Exp Dermatol* 1986; 11: 17–26.

12 Morrison JG, Jones EW, MacDonald DM. Juvenile elastoma and osteopoikilosis (the Buschke–Ollendorff syndrome). *Br J Dermatol* 1977; 97: 417–22.

13 Weidman FD, Anderson NP, Ayres S. Juvenile elastoma. *Arch Dermatol Syph* 1933; 28: 182–9.

14 Staricco RG, Mehregan AH. Naevus elasticus and naevus elasticus vasularis. *Arch Dermatol* 1961; 84: 943–7.

15 de Graciansky P, Leclerc R. Le 'naevus elasticus' en tumeurs disséminées. *Ann Dermatol Syph* 1960; 87: 5–25.

16 Dammert K, Niemi KM. Naevus elasticus (elastoma juvenile Weidman) and naevus collagenicus lumbosacralis in Pringle's disease. *Dermatologica* 1968; 137: 36–45.

17 Marguery MC, Samalens G, Pieraggi MT et al. Conjunctive nevus of the disseminated elastic type without osteopoikilosis or Weidman juvenile elastoma. *Ann Dermatol Vénéréol* 1991; 118: 465–8.

18 Huilgol SC, Griffiths WA, Black MM. Familial juvenile elastoma. *Australas J Dermatol* 1994; 35: 87–90.

19 Dahan S, Bonafe JL, Laroche M et al. Iconography of Buschke–Ollendorff syndrome: X-ray computed tomography and nuclear magnetic resonance of osteopoikilosis. *Ann Dermatol Vénéréol* 1989; 116: 225–30.

20 Ramme K, Kolde G, Stadler R. Dermatofibrosis lenticularis disseminata with osteopoikilosis. Buschke–Olldendorff syndrome. *Hautarzt* 1993; 44: 312–14.

21 Roberts NM, Langtry JA, Branfoot AC et al. Case report: osteopoikilosis and the Buschke–Ollendorff syndrome. *Br J Radiol* 1993; 66: 468–70.

22 Schnur RE, Grace K, Herzberg A. Buschke–Ollendorff syndrome, otosclerosis, and congenital spinal stenosis. *Pediatr Dermatol* 1994; 11: 31–4.

23 Thieberg MD, Stone MS, Siegfried EC. What syndrome is this? Buschke–Ollendorff syndrome. *Pediatr Dermatol* 1993; 10: 85–7.

24 Trattner A, David M, Rothem A et al. Buschke–Ollendorff syndrome of the scalp: histologic and ultrastructural findings. *J Am Acad Dermatol* 1991; 24: 822–4.

25 Reymond JL, Stoebner P, Beani JC et al. Buschke–Ollendorf syndrome. An electron microscopic study. *Dermatologica* 1983; 166: 64–8.

26 Uitto J, Santa Cruz DJ, Starcher BC et al. Biochemical and ultrastructural demonstration of elastin accumulation in the skin lesions of the Buschke–Ollendorff syndrome. *J Invest Dermatol* 1981; 76: 284–7.

27 Giro MG, Duvic M, Smith LT et al. Buschke–Ollendorff syndrome associated with elevated elastin production by affected skin fibroblasts in culture. *J Invest Dermatol* 1992; 99: 129–37.

28 Ehlers G, Mayerhausen W. Buschke–Ollendorff syndrome. *Z Hautkr* 1989; 64: 869–74.

29 Raque CJ, Wood MG. Connective tissue naevus. Dermatofibrosis lenticularis disseminata with osteopoikilosis. *Arch Dermatol* 1970; 102: 390–6.

30 Schmorl G. Anatomische befunde bei einem Falle von Osteopoikilie. *Fortschr Geb Roentgenstr* 1931; 44: 1–8.

31 Hess W. Roentgenologische und pathologisch-anatomische Beobachtungen bei einem Fall von Osteopoikilie. *Fortschr Geb Roentgenstr* 1940; 62: 252–8.

32 Verbov J. Buschke–Ollendorff syndrome (disseminated dermatofibrosis with osteopoikilosis). *Br J Dermatol* 1977; 96: 87–90.

33 Atherton DJ, Wells RS. Juvenile elastoma and osteopoikilosis (the Buschke–Ollendorff syndrome). *Clin Exp Dermatol* 1982; 7: 109–13.

34 Jonasch E. 12 Faelle von Osteopoikilie. *Fortrschr Roentgenstr* 1955; 82: 344–53.

35 Sarralde A, Garcia Cruz D, Nazara Z et al. Osteopoikilosis: report of a familial case. *Genet Couns* 1994; 5: 373–5.

36 Walpole IR, Manners PJ. Clinical considerations in Buschke–Ollendorff syndrome. *Clin Genet* 1990; 37: 59–63.

37 Strosberg JM, Adler RG. Otosclerosis associated with osteopoikilosis. *J Am Med Assoc* 1981; 246: 2030–1.

38 Piette Brion B, Lowy Motulsky M, Ledoux Corbusier M et al. Dermatofibromas, elastomas and deafness: a new case of the Buschke–Ollendorff syndrome. *Dermatologica* 1984; 168: 255–8.

Papular elastorrhexis

Papular elastorrhexis is a rare variant of connective tissue naevus in which there is normal collagen and a decreased amount of elastic fibres. The disorder, appearing in adolescence, has recently been described in three single patients [1,2]. In these non-familial cases, the cutaneous findings were distinct from papular acne scars and not associated with extracutaneous abnormalities. Schirren *et al.* described three members of one family presenting with non-follicular, distributed, white papules on the trunk and extremities [3]. The clinical appearance with absence of osteopoikilosis and the histological findings (decreased, fragmented elastic fibres and normal collagen) were compatible with papular elastorrhexis. However, on the basis of the genetic background, the authors believed that papular elastorrhexis was an abortive form of the Buschke–Ollendorff syndrome and suggested that connective tissue naevi with the most prominent alterations in the elastic tissue should be classified under the term elastic tissue naevi. Others, however, believe that most connective tissue naevi-like lesions, including papular elastorrhexis, in adults are papular acne scars [4].

REFERENCES

1 Bordas X, Ferrandis C, Ribera M et al. Papular elastorrhexis: a variety of nevus anelasticus? *Arch Dermatol* 1987; 123: 433–4.

2 Sears JK, Seabury Stone M, Argenyi Z. Papular elastorrhexis: a variant of connective tissue nevus. *J Am Acad Dermatol* 1988; 19: 409–14.

3 Schirren H, Schirren CG, Stolz W *et al.* Papular elastorrhexis: a variant of dermatofibrosis lenticularis disseminata (Buschke–Ollendorff syndrome)? *Dermatology* 1994; 189: 368–72.
4 Wilson BB, Dent CH, Cooper PH. Papular acne scars. A common cutaneous finding. *Arch Dermatol* 1990; 126: 797–800.

Marfan's syndrome

Definition

Marfan's syndrome (MFS) is an autosomal dominant disorder of connective tissue due to the abnormal expression of fibrillin 1 and characterized by manifestations in the cardiovascular, musculoskeletal and ophthalmic systems (Table 19.20.2).

History

In 1896, the French paediatrician, Marfan, described a 5-year-old girl with tall stature, disproportionately long limbs and fingers [1]. He used the term 'dolichostenomelia' which is now often referred to as the marfanoid habitus. A few years later, Marfan's patient developed scoliosis [2] and another very similar patient was described by Achard, who introduced the word arachnodactyly for the spider fingers [3]. Following reports of associated dislocation of the lens (ectopia lentis) and mitral valve regurgitation with the disorder, Weve, in 1931, proposed the name 'dystrophica mesodermalis congenita, typus Marfanis' [4]. This was condensed to Marfan's syndrome in 1938 by Apert [5]. In 1956, McKusick, a major contributor to the characterization of MFS [6], already suggested that elastic fibre or a component intimately associated with elastic fibre was defective in MFS. Many studies (on collagens, elastin, etc.) failed and it was only in the late 1980s that fibrillin was described as a molecule tightly linked with elastic fibres [7,8]. In a very short time, both the positional cloning approach and the candidate gene strategy resulted in the cloning and localization of two fibrillin genes [9–13]. As seen on Table 19.20.2, mutations of the fibrillin 1 gene (FBN1, located on chromosome 15) were shown in MFS

and autosomal dominant ectopia lentis [14]; mutations on the fibrillin 2 gene (FBN2, on chromosome 5) are linked to the MFS-related disorder called congenital contractural arachnodactyly (CCA) [15].

Finally, two anecdotes in the MFS saga are worth mentioning: it is likely that Marfan's original patient did not have MFS but rather CCA [16], and there is quite an interest in knowing whether Abraham Lincoln was affected by MFS [17,18].

Aetiology

Fibrillin, an acidic glycoprotein with an estimated molecular mass of 350 kDa, is a major constituent of the 10-nm microfibrils of the extracellular matrix. Its primary structure is characterized by several cysteine-rich motives, reminiscent of the epidermal growth factor (EGF) peptide module including six similarly spaced cysteinyl residues [7,19,20]. The role of fibrillin as the underlying cause of MFS is supported by three independent lines of experimental evidence: (a) antisera to fibrillin showed a decreased amount of microfibrils in MFS tissue samples [21,22]; (b) defective synthesis and secretion of fibrillin by dermal fibroblasts was demonstrated in 26 probands with MFS [23]; and (c) linkage and mutational analysis of several affected kindred confirmed a genetic homogeneity between MFS and the fibrillin gene [24]. It should, however, be noted that the question of homogeneity in MFS has been disputed [25,26].

Functionally, the 10-nm microfibrils, including fibrillin serve at least three functions: (a) as a link between elastin and other matrix structures (i.e. the basement membrane at the dermoepidermal junction); (b) as a scaffolding on which elastin is deposited (i.e. in the tunica media of the aorta); and (c) as a structural component in tissues that do not contain elastin (i.e. the ciliary zonule) [27]. The genetic analysis provided precise insights into the structural/functional features of fibrillin. However, such studies failed to define predictable genotype/phenotype correlations. This is highly in keeping with the variable expression of MFS features in affected individuals of the

Table 19.20.2 Fibrillin gene disorders

	Marfan	Congenital contractural arachnodactyly	Autosomal dominant ectopia lentis	Marfan-craniosynostosis syndrome
Habitus	Marfanoid	Marfanoid	—	Marfanoid
Cardio-vascular manifestations	+	—	—	+
Ectopia lentis	+	—	+	(+)
Joints	Looseness	Contractures	—	Looseness
Cranial abnormality	—	—	—	+
Gene defect	Fbn-1	Fbn-2	Fbn-1	Fbn-1

same family. This implies that other factors are involved in the development of the clinical phenotype. Indeed, the same mutation (P1148A) was shown in individuals with MFS, isolated ectopia lentis (EL) and the MFS-related but clinically distinct Shprintzen–Goldberg syndrome [28].

Clinical features

Musculoskeletal features

Dolichostenomelia is the characteristic skeletal abnormality in MFS [29]. It encompasses tall stature, decreased upper to lower segment ratio (US/LS, a value <0.85 in adults is significant), dolichocephaly and arachnodactyly of fingers and toes (Fig. 19.20.2). Pectus excavatum/carinatum can be present at birth or develop as a result of excessive longitudinal growth. Scoliosis or kyphoscoliosis occur in 30–60% of MFS individuals [6]. Ligamentous laxity and generalized hypermobility are common and can cause spinal pain, arthralgia, ligament injury or other musculoskeletal symptoms in up to three-quarters of children and in nearly all adults with MFS [30].

Cardiovascular manifestations

These are responsible for the shorter lifespan of MFS individuals. Multivalvular incompetence predominates in childhood whereas most adults suffer from degenerative complications of the aorta. Dilatation of the aorta is due to the fragmentation of elastic fibres in the tunica media. This leads to the typical cystic medial necrolysis and provokes aortic aneurysms, often before the age of 40 years. Aortic regurgitation, which correlates with the aortic root diameter, is the most common valvular complication (as high as 70% in adults). Mitral valve prolapse is the next most frequent finding [6,29].

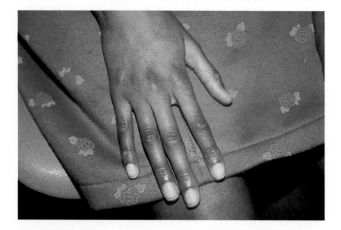

Fig. 19.20.2 MFS: macrodactyly of fingers and toes. Courtesy of Professor R. Winter.

Ocular manifestations

EL is usually bilateral and occurs in 50–80% of MFS individuals. The lens displacement is usually upward. Although EL is the most frequent ocular manifestation in MFS, visual loss more often results from secondary myopia, retinal detachment, glaucoma or iritis [31–33].

Cutaneous manifestations

These are minor findings in MFS. Striae atrophicae are the most common dermal manifestations of MFS and are usually found on the deltoid, pectoral and lumbar regions [34–36]. They can be found in two-thirds of MFS individuals and their number increases with age [30]. Histologically, they do not differ from striae in the normal population [37].

Skin hyperextensibility is also found in two-thirds of MFS patients, regardless of their age, and significantly correlates with joint laxity [30]. The combination of a marfanoid habitus and skin hyperextensibility, but apparently without MFS, has been described [38].

Papyraceous scars can occur but are not a typical feature of MFS patients whose cutaneous incisions or lacerations usually heal promptly [30].

Finally, isolated reports include the association of MFS with poliosis [39], LEOPARD syndrome (lentigines, electrocardiogram abnormalities, ocular hypertelorism, pulmonary stenosis, abnormalities of genitalia, retardation growth and deafness) [40], Ehlers–Danlos syndrome [41], neurofibromatosis [42] and elastosis perforans serpiginosa [43].

Diagnosis

The diagnosis of MFS is mainly clinical [44] and relies on the presence of cardinal manifestations (Table 19.20.3). Helpful and simple screening tests include the thumb sign (Fig. 19.20.3), the wrist sign (positive if the thumb and little finger overlap when wrapped around the opposite wrist) and the US/LS ratio. A severe infantile form of the disorder is recognized [45]. A marfanoid habitus is found in two rarer fibrillin disorders (see Table 19.20.2). CCA presents with joint contractures and abnormalities of the external ears but without cardiovascular or ocular manifestations [15,16]. The marfanoid–craniosynostosis syndrome (Shprintzen–Goldberg) is a clinically distinct variant of MFS, reported in only 11 individuals and characterized by additional findings such as craniofacial abnormalities, mental retardation, hypotonia and congenital abdominal wall weakness [28,46].

Other differential diagnoses include homocystinuria, Stickler's syndrome (hereditary arthrophthalmopathy), annuloaortic ectasia (Erdheim's disease) and mitral valve prolapse syndrome [47,48].

Table 19.20.3 Minimum criteria for the diagnosis of Marfan syndrome

Sporadic case	Involvement of the skeleton and at least two other systems, with at least one major manifestation (below in bold)
Familial case	Involvement of at least two systems, with at least one major manifestation

With the following diagnostic manifestations:

Skeletal
   Anterior chest deformity (asymmetric pectus excavatum/ carinatum), dolichostenomelia, arachnodactyly, scoliosis, thoracic lordosis or reduced thoracic kyphosis, tall stature (compared to unaffected relatives), high narrowly arched palate and dental crowding, protrusio acetabulae, abnormal appendicular joint mobility
Ocular
   Ectopia lentis, flat cornea, elongated globe, retinal detachment, myopia
Cardiovascular
   Dilatation of the ascending aorta, aortic dissection, aortic regurgitation, mitral regurgitation due to mitral valve prolapse, calcification of the mitral annulus, mitral valve prolapse, abdominal aortic aneurysm, dysrythmia, endocarditis
Pulmonary
   Spontaneous pneumothorax, apical web
Skin and integument
   Striae distensae, inguinal hernia, other hernia
Central nervous system
   Dural ectasia (lumbosacral meningocele, dilated cisterna magna), learning disability (verbal-performance discrepancy), hyperactivity with or without attention deficit disorder

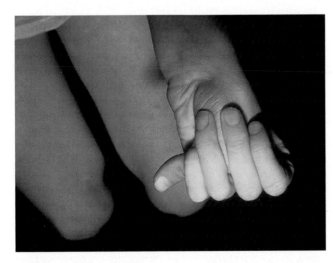

Fig. 19.20.3 MFS: the 'thumb sign'. Courtesy of Professor R. Winter.

Management

The dermatologist will rarely need to be involved in multidisciplinary teams managing MFS. In recent years, the increased lifespan and decreased morbidity in MFS have mainly been achieved through the improvement of cardiovascular, orthopaedic and ocular surgery [33,49–51].

Beta-blockers are useful to reduce/delay aortic dilatation [52,53]. Pregnancy remains a problem, due to the high risk of ruptured aneurysms, but can be managed in women with minimal cardiovascular findings [54–56].

REFERENCES

1 Marfan AB. Un cas de déformation congénitale des quatre membres plus prononcée aux extrémités, caractérisée par l'allongement des os avec un certain degré d'amincissement. *Bull Mem Soc Méd Hôp Paris* 1896; 13: 220.
2 Méry H, Babonneix L. Un cas de déformation congénitale des quatre membres: hyperchondroplasie. *Bull Mem Soc Méd Hôp Paris* 1902; 19: 671.
3 Achard C. Arachnodactylie. *Bull Mem Soc Méd Hôp Paris* 1902; 19: 834.
4 Weve H. Veber Arachnodactylie (Dystrophia mesodermalis congenita, typus Marfanis). *Arch Augenheilk* 1931; 104: 1.
5 Apert E. Les formes frustes du syndrome dolichosténomélique de Marfan. *Nourisson* 1938; 26: 1.
6 McKusick VA. The Marfan syndrome. In: McKusick VA, ed. *Heritable Disorders of Connective Tissue*. St Louis: CV Mosby, 1972: 61–201.
7 Sakai LY, Keene DR, Engvall E. Fibrillin, a new 35-kD glycoprotein, is a component of extracellular microfibrils. *J Cell Biol* 1986; 103: 2499.
8 Sakai LY, Keene DR. Fibrillin: monomers and microfibrils. *Methods Enzymol* 1994; 245: 29–52.
9 Blanton SH, Sarfarazi M, Eiberg H *et al*. An exclusion map of Marfan syndrome. *J Med Genet* 1990; 27: 73–7.
10 Dietz HC, Pyeritz RE, Hall BD *et al*. The Marfan syndrome locus: confirmation of assignment to chromosome 15 and identification of tightly linked markers at 15q15–q21.3. *Genomics* 1991; 9: 355–61.
11 Dietz HC, Cutting GR, Pyeritz RE *et al*. Marfan syndrome caused by a recurrent *de novo* missense mutation in the fibrillin gene see comments. *Nature* 1991; 352: 337–9.
12 Lee B, Godfrey M, Vitale E *et al*. Linkage of Marfan syndrome and a phenotypically related disorder to two different fibrillin genes see comments. *Nature* 1991; 352: 330–4.
13 Maslen CL, Corson GM, Maddox BK *et al*. Partial sequence of a candidate gene for the Marfan syndrome see comments. *Nature* 1991; 352: 334–7.
14 Kainulainen K, Karttunen L, Puhakka L *et al*. Mutations in the fibrillin gene responsible for dominant ectopia lentis and neonatal Marfan syndrome. *Nat Genet* 1994; 6: 64–9.
15 Putnam EA, Zhang H, Ramirez F *et al*. Fibrillin-2 (FBN2) mutations result in the Marfan-like disorder, congenital contractural arachnodactyly. *Nature Genet* 1995; 11: 456–8.
16 Beals RK, Hecht F. Congenital contractural arachnodactyly. A heritable disorder of connective tissue. *J Bone Joint Surg Am* 1971; 53: 987–93.
17 Gordon AM. Abraham Lincoln, the famous case of Marfan's syndrome. *Dtsch Med J* 1967; 18: 256–60.
18 McKusick VA. The defect in Marfan syndrome. *Nature* 1991; 352: 279–81.
19 Pereira L, D'Alessio M, Ramirez F *et al*. Genomic organization of the sequence coding for fibrillin, the defective gene product in Marfan syndrome. *Hum Mol Genet* 1993; 2: 1762.
20 Handford P, Downing AK, Rao Z *et al*. The calcium binding properties and molecular organization of epidermal growth factor-like domains in human fibrillin-1. *J Biol Chem* 1995; 270: 6751–6.
21 Hollister DW, Godfrey M, Sakai LY *et al*. Immunohistologic abnormalities of the microfibrillar-fiber system in the Marfan syndrome. *N Engl J Med* 1990; 323: 152–9.
22 Godfrey M, Menashe V, Weleber RG *et al*. Cosegregation of elastin-associated microfibrillar abnormalities with the Marfan phenotype in families. *Am J Hum Genet* 1990; 46: 652–60.
23 Milewicz DM, Pyeritz RE, Crawford ES *et al*. Marfan syndrome: defective synthesis, secretion, and extracellular matrix formation of fibrillin by cultured dermal fibroblasts. *J Clin Invest* 1992; 89: 79–86.
24 Tsipouras P, Del Mastro R, Sarfarazi M *et al*. Genetic linkage of the Marfan syndrome, ectopia lentis, and congenital contractural arachnodactyly to the fibrillin genes on chromosomes 15 and 5. The International Marfan Syndrome Collaborative Study. *N Engl J Med* 1992; 326: 905–9.
25 Boileau C, Junien C, Collod G *et al*. The question of heterogeneity in Marfan syndrome. *Nature Genet* 1995; 9: 230–1 (letter).

26 Dietz H, Francke U, Furthmayr H *et al*. The question of heterogeneity in Marfan syndrome. *Nat Genet* 1995; 9: 228–31 (letter).

27 Godfrey M. From fluorescence to the gene: the skin in the Marfan syndrome. *J Invest Dermatol* 1994; 103: 58S–62S.

28 Sood S, Eldadah ZA, Krause WL *et al*. Mutation in fibrillin-1 and the Marfanoid–craniosynostosis (Shprintzen–Goldberg) syndrome. *Nature Genet* 1996; 12: 209–11.

29 Pyeritz RE, McKusick VA. The Marfan syndrome: diagnosis and management. *N Engl J Med* 1979; 300: 772–7.

30 Grahame R, Pyeritz RE. The Marfan syndrome: joint and skin manifestations are prevalent and correlated. *Br J Rheumatol* 1995; 34: 126–31.

31 Maumenee IH. The eye in the Marfan syndrome. *Trans Am Ophthalmol Soc* 1981; 79: 684–733.

32 Nelson LB, Maumenee IH. Ectopia lentis. *Surv Ophthalmol* 1982; 27: 143–60.

33 Roussat B, Chiou AG, Quesnot S *et al*. Surgery of ectopia lentis in Marfan disease in children and young adults. *J Fr Ophtalmol* 1995; 18: 170–7.

34 Fazekas A, Szego L, Vigvary L. Striae distensae elasticae in Marfan's syndrome. *Orv Hetil* 1973; 114: 2290–2.

35 McKusick VA. Transverse striae distensae in the lumbar area in father and two sons. *Birth Defects* 1971; 7: 260–1.

36 Shuster S. The cause of striae distensae. *Acta Derm Venereol (Stockh)* 1979; 59 (suppl): 161–9.

37 Pinkus H, Keech MK, Mehregan AH. Histopathology of striae distensae, with special reference to striae and wound healing in the Marfan syndrome. *J Invest Dermatol* 1966; 46: 283–92.

38 Sakatsume Y, Saito M, Hara Y *et al*. A case of marfanoid body habitus associated with an excessive hyperextensibility of the skin—an unclassified case in inherited connective tissue diseases. *Nippon Naika Gakkai Zasshi* 1988; 77: 499–505.

39 Herman KL, Salman K, Rose LI. White forelock in Marfan's syndrome: an unusual association, with review of the literature. *Cutis* 1991; 48: 82–4.

40 Torok L, Szentendrei L, Szili M *et al*. Progressive cardiomyopathic lentiginosis (LEOPARD syndrome) in three patients, combined with Marfan syndrome. *Z Hautkr* 1990; 65: 197–201.

41 Fazekas A. Simultaneous occurrence of Ehlers–Danlos syndrome and Marfan's syndrome. *Orv Hetil* 1976; 117: 154–8.

42 Copeland T, Tiwary CM, Coker S. Coexistence of neurofibromatosis and Marfan's syndrome. *South Med J* 1986; 79: 489–92.

43 Mehregan AH. Elastosis perforans serpiginosa: a review of the literature and report of 11 cases. *Arch Dermatol* 1968; 97: 381–93.

44 Beighton P, de Paepe A, Danks D *et al*. International nosology of heritable disorders of connective tissue, Berlin, 1986. *Am J Med Genet* 1988; 29: 581–94.

45 Morse RP, Rockenmacher S, Pyeritz RE *et al*. Diagnosis and management of infantile Marfan syndrome. *Pediatrics* 1990; 86: 888–95.

46 Shprintzen RJ, Goldberg RB. A recurrent pattern syndrome of craniosynostosis associated with arachnodactyly and abdominal hernias. *J Craniofac Genet Dev Biol* 1982; 2: 65–74.

47 Devereux RB, Brown WT. Genetics of mitral valve prolapse. *Prog Med Genet* 1983; 5: 139–61.

48 Glesby MJ, Pyeritz RE. Association of mitral valve prolapse and systemic abnormalities of connective tissue. A phenotypic continuum see comments. *J Am Med Assoc* 1989; 262: 523–8.

49 Sponseller PD, Hobbs W, Riley LH *et al*. The thoracolumbar spine in Marfan syndrome. *J Bone Joint Surg Am* 1995; 77: 867–76.

50 Gott VL, Gillinov AM, Pyeritz RE *et al*. Aortic root replacement. Risk factor analysis of a 17-year experience with 270 patients. *J Thorac Cardiovasc Surg* 1995; 109: 536–44.

51 David TE, Feindel CM, Bos J. Repair of the aortic valve in patients with aortic insufficiency and aortic root aneurysm. *J Thorac Cardiovasc Surg* 1995; 109: 345–51 (discussion 351–2).

52 Shores J, Berger KR, Murphy EA *et al*. Progression of aortic dilatation and the benefit of long-term beta-adrenergic blockade in Marfan's syndrome. *N Engl J Med* 1994; 330: 1335–41.

53 Pyeritz RE, Francke U. The Second International Symposium on the Marfan Syndrome. *Am J Med Genet* 1993; 47: 127–35.

54 Beighton P. Pregnancy in the marfan syndrome. *Br Med J Clin Res Ed* 1982; 285: 464.

55 Farhi J, Orvieto R, Ben Rafael Z. Pregnancy in Marfan's syndrome. *Harefuah* 1993; 125: 396–8, 448.

56 Maruyama T, Totsuka N, Akahane K *et al*. Two cases of Marfan syndrome complicated with aortic dissection during pregnancy. *Kokyu To Junkan* 1993; 41: 85–8.

Osteogenesis imperfecta
(SYN. LA MALADIE DE LOBSTEIN)

Definition and overview

Osteogenesis imperfecta (OI) is a heterogeneous group of disorders characterized by bone fragility that is accompanied by other evidence of connective tissue malfunction, including abnormalities in teeth (dentinogenesis imperfecta), hearing loss, alterations in scleral hue and evidence of soft tissue dysplasia [1].

Historic cases may include an Egyptian mummy and Ivar the Boneless, the Scandinavian conqueror of England in the ninth century. The first accurate descriptions date back to the late 18th and early 19th centuries and the term osteogenesis imperfecta was introduced in 1906 [2].

OI is part of a group of heterogeneic disorders due to alterations in collagen biosynthesis (Table 19.20.4). It should be noted that this list is likely to expand rapidly over the next few years, as further characterization of the more than 25 different genes of collagens is achieved.

The 19 types of collagens share common structural properties such as a triple-helical domain characterized by the repetition of three amino acids $(Gly-X-Y)_n$, an abundance of hydroxyproline and hydroxylysine residues and a trimeric association (homo- or heterotrimers depending on the collagen type). The distribution of the different types of collagens varies both in location and quantity. For example, collagen type VII forms the anchoring fibrils at the dermoepidermal junction, type II is present in the cartilage and vitreous humour and type IV is found in basement membranes. Alterations in the biosynthesis of type I collagen, which is ubiquitous and represents the vast majority of collagen in the body, are found both in OI and Ehlers–Danlos syndromes (type II and VIIb). The clinical heterogeneity of OI phenotypes (from mild to lethal) is clearly reflected by the numerous point mutations, insertions and deletions found in the COL1A1 and COL1A2 genes [1,3,4].

OI is usually divided into four major types which are

Table 19.20.4 Disorders due to collagen genes defects

Collagen	Disorder	Gene
Type I	Osteogenesis imperfecta type I–IV	COL1A1, COL1A2
	Ehlers–Danlos type VIIA	COL1A1
	Ehlers–Danlos type II and VIIB	COL1A2
Type II	Chondrodysplasias	COL2A1
Type III	Ehlers–Danlos type IV	COL3A1
Type IV	Alport syndrome	COL4A5
Type VII	Epidermolysis bullosa Recessive dystrophic Dominant dystrophic	COL7A1

briefly described in Table 19.20.5. Prenatal diagnosis is possible with ultrasonography and/or genetic analysis from chorionic villous samples in appropriate families [1,5].

Cutaneous features

The skin in OI is characteristically thin and translucent [6].

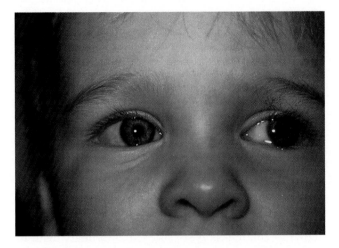

Fig. 19.20.4 OI: blue sclerae in OI type I. Courtesy of Professor R. Winter.

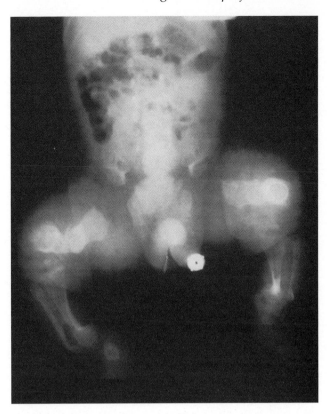

Fig. 19.20.5 OI: skeletal abnormalities in OI type II. Courtesy of Professor R. Winter.

Table 19.20.5 Characteristics of osteogenesis imperfecta types I–IV

	Type I	Type II	Type III	Type IV
Synonym	Dominant inheritance with blue sclerae	Perinatal lethal	Progressive deforming	Autosomal dominant with normal sclerae
Frequency	1/15 000–20 000	1/20 000–60 000	AR type frequent in South-African blacks	Undetermined
Clinical features	Blue sclerae; fractures in childhood and adolescence healing without deformity; normal stature; hearing loss in 50% of cases; rare DI (Fig. 19.20.4)	Dark sclerae; soft calvarium; short bowed legs; platyspondyly; early death from respiratory failure; characteristic radiological picture; common hearing loss	Faint blue sclerae lightening with age; osteopenic skeleton at birth; fractures from first year of life with marked deformity; very short stature; frequent DI	Normal sclerae; variable short stature; mild to moderate bone deformity; common DI; hearing loss in <50% of cases
Inheritance	AD	AD (new); AR (rare)	AD; AR	AD
Biochemical basis	Decreased production of type I procollagen; substitution for residue other than glycine in triple helix of α1 (I)	COL1A1 and COL1A2 genes rearrangements; substitutions for glycyl residues in the triple helical domain of the α1 (I) or α2 (I) chain; small deletion in α2 (I) on the background of a null allele	AD: point mutation in the α1 (I) or α2 (I) chain. AR frameshift mutation preventing incorporation of pro-α2 (I) into molecules	Point mutations in the α2(I) chain and (rarely) in the α1(I) chain; small deletions in α2(I) chain
Differential diagnosis	Child abuse	Thanatophoric dysplasia Achondrogenesis AR hypophosphatasia	Child abuse	Child abuse

AD, autosomal dominant; AR, autosomal recessive; DI, dentinogenesis imperfecta. Modified from [1]

Occasional cutaneous findings include elastosis perforans serpiginosa [7–11], and possibly wider scars than usual, as well as subcutaneous haemorrhages after minor trauma [6]. Macular atrophy (anetoderma) was reported by Blegvad and Haxthausen [12].

REFERENCES

1 Byers PH. Disorders of collagen biosynthesis and structure. In: Scriver CR, Beaudet AL, Sly WS, Valle D, eds. *The Biochemical and Molecular Bases of Inherited Disease*. New York: McGraw-Hill, 1995: 4029–77.
2 Tsipouras P. Osteogenesis imperfecta. In: Beighton P, ed. *McKusick's Heritable Disorders of Connective Tissue*. St Louis: CV Mosby, 1993: 281–314.
3 Zhuang J, Tromp G, Kuivaniami H *et al*. Direct sequencing of PCR products derived from cDNAs for the Proa1 and Proa2 chains of type 1 procollagen as a screening method to detect mutations in patients with osteogenesis imperfecta. *Hum Mutat* 1996; 7: 89–99.
4 Prockop DJ. Collagens: molecular biology, diseases, and potentials for therapy. *Ann Rev Biochem* 1995; 64: 403–34.
5 Chamson A, Bertheas MF, Frey J. Collagen biosynthesis in cell culture from chorionic villi. *Prenat Diagn* 1995; 15: 165–70.
6 McKusick VA. Osteogenesis imperfecta. In: Mckusick VA, ed. *Disorders of Connective Tissue*. St Louis: CV Mosby, 1972: 390–454.
7 Reed WB, Pidgeaon JW. Elastosis perforans serpiginosa with osteogenesis imperfecta. *Arch Dermatol (Chicago)* 1964: 89: 342.
8 Relias A, Sakellariou G, Tsoitis G *et al*. Lutz–Miescher elastosis perforans serpiginosa and osteogenesis imperfecta. *Ann Dermatol Syph Paris* 1968; 95: 491–504.
9 Carey TD. Elastosis perforans serpiginosa. *Arch Dermatol* 1977; 113: 1444–5.
10 Kingsley HJ. Peculiarities in dermatology. Case reports. II. Elastosis perforans serpignosa associated with osteogenesis imperfecta. *Cent Afr J Med* 1968; 14: 176.
11 Mehregan AH. Elastosis perforans serpiginosa: a review of the literature and report of 11 cases. *Arch Dermatol* 1968; 97: 381–93.
12 Blegvad O, Haxthausen H. Blue sclerotics and brittle bones, with macular atrophy of the skin and zonular cataracts. *Br Med J* 1921; 2: 1071.

Anetodermas

(SYN. MACULAR ATROPHY, DERMATITE ATROPHIANTE MACULEUSE)

Definition and history

Anetoderma is a clinicohistological entity characterized by a focal loss of dermal elastic tissue. Derived from *anetos*, the Greek word for 'relaxed', the term 'anetodermia' was introduced in 1891 by Jadassohn, who described a 23-year-old woman with a 5-year history of erythematous macules on the arms, progressing into slightly depressed lesions, with an atrophic, wrinkled epidermis and a feeling of lack of substance on finger palpation [1]. Larger, irregular and violaceous macules forming loose, soft and depressible sac-like lesions were also present on the elbows. A similar inflammatory onset was reported in 1884 by Pelizzari [2], who described a 45-year-old man with papular, round or oval lesions evoking superficial scars. The characteristic depression of the final stage was preceded by erythematous papular lesions, clinically distinct from urticaria by the absence of pruritus and by the chronicity of the lesions. In 1891, Schweninger and Buzzi [3] described a 29-year-old woman with multiple protrud-

ing white lesions which appeared over an 8-year period over the upper back and later involving the chest, the neck, the chin and the upper part of the arms. This eruption, at times pruriginous, included both depressed and protruding elements in which the atrophic epidermis did not oppose to the finger the resistance of the normal skin. The pseudotumoral lesions, surrounded by a rigid ring, could be temporarily reduced by pressure. No inflammatory process preceded the eruption [3].

In 1954, around 200 cases of anetoderma had already been reported under the names of 'macular atrophy of the skin', 'dermatitis atrophicans maculosa' or its French equivalent 'dermatite atrophiante maculeuse' [4]. The term '(macular) anetoderma' later became more widespread. Classically, primary or 'idiopathic' cases with an inflammatory onset were usually reported as of the Jadassohn type and non-inflammatory ones as of the Schweninger–Buzzi type. Many associations were also described, as well as cases where anetoderma developed on the same site of a pre-existing localized dermatosis. Several classifications have been proposed to group the many forms of this clinicohistological syndrome [4–6]. However, until the mechanisms leading to the disappearance of elastin in the dermis are better understood, anetoderma in children is best classified as primary, with or without associated morphological abnormalities, and secondary (Table 19.20.6).

Aetiology

Primary anetoderma

The mechanism leading to the focal loss of elastin fibres in primary anetoderma remains unknown. The normal appearance of the elastin fibres in the surrounding skin makes a genetic defect of the elastin gene unlikely. Furthermore, mutations of the elastin gene have now been associated with two other syndromes, namely supravalvular aortic stenosis [7] and Williams' syndrome [8]. The presence of inflammatory cells in early lesions of both inflammatory and non-inflammatory anetoderma suggests that the process may be secondary to the release of elastase and related proteases from polymorphonuclear cells, fibroblasts and macrophages [9,10]. This would indicate that the basic abnormality is focal elastolysis [11,12].

Table 19.20.6 Classification of anetoderma in children

Primary
Isolated (±familial)
In association with morphological abnormalities (±familial)

Secondary
To a disorder with systemic expression (Anti-phospholipid syndrome, syphilis, chicken pox, HIV)
To a localized pre-existing dermatosis (Mastocytosis, pilomatrixomas)

Phagocytosis of elastin by macrophages has been demonstrated [13]. The exact role of decay-accelerating factor, which is thought to protect elastin fibres against damage [14], and the significance of complement activation, C3 being deposited on the remaining fibres [15,16], are unclear. Of interest is the similarity between severe anetoderma with confluent lesions and acquired cutis laxa [12], this would suggest a similar abnormal function of the lysyl oxidase.

The occurrence of familial cases of anetoderma suggest that abnormalities leading to the focal absence of elastin may be genetically transmitted. In these cases, anetoderma was an isolated finding [17] or associated with systemic abnormalities [18–22]. Consanguinity was present in some families [18,19,21,22]. Modes of inheritance were autosomal recessive [18], autosomal dominant [19] or undefined [17,20–22].

Finally, many morphological abnormalities have been described in association with primary anetoderma (Table 19.20.7). The heterogeneity of these associations as well as the heterogeneity of the clinical presentations of primary anetoderma (very few cases, if any, are identical to the cases of Jadassohn or Schweninger-Buzzi [4]) indicate the fact that anetoderma is a clinicohistological entity which is likely to be the end result of not one, but several aetiologies.

Table 19.20.7 Morphological abnormalities described with anetoderma

Eye abnormalities
Cataract
Keratoconus
Corneal opacities
Optic atrophy (secondary to bony changes)
Osteoarticular abnormalities
Abnormal calcifications
Kyphoscoliosis
Shortening of a limb
Congenital fusion of cervical vertebrae
Spina bifida
Osteopetrosis
Metaphyseal dysplasia
Hip dislocation
Cardiovascular abnormalities
Mitral valve prolapse
Aortic insufficiency
Wolff–Parkinson–White
Miscellaneous
Emphysema
Protrusion of teeth
Pyramidal syndrome
Myotonic dystrophy
Diverticulum of mid-oesophagus
Blegvad–Haxthausen syndrome
(Anetoderma, osteogenesis-imperfecta)

Modified from [12].

Secondary anetoderma

In secondary anetoderma, typical lesions are either associated with an underlying systemic disease or occur in a site previously occupied by a specific dermatosis. Several causes are recognized as follows.

Infections. Syphilis was historically the most common infectious dermatosis associated with anetoderma [4]. Anetodermic lesions have been described as a consequence of secondary, tertiary and congenital syphilis. Since penicillin, this aetiology is rare [23]. It is interesting to note that in such cases, anetodermic lesions could occur both on previously healthy skin [23] and lesional skin [24]. Furthermore, both depressed and bulging lesions could coexist in the same patient. These findings are characteristic of secondary anetoderma and have been described with most of the following systemic conditions listed below.

Varicella is certainly the most common cause of anetoderma in children. In most cases, only few lesions develop on the trunk or upper limbs in the months following chicken pox. They can occur in association with typical varicella scars [12,25]. As such, anetoderma is a limited and benign condition that often goes unnoticed. When new lesions of anetoderma keep appearing several years after chicken pox, the link between varicella and anetoderma is less clear [25,26]. Some authors consider chicken pox as the causative factor [25] whereas others think that the two events are coincidental and unrelated [12]. One possibility is that lesions preceding anetoderma, being varicella or any other cutaneous disease, are simply revelatory of a cutaneous tendency to atrophy [4,27].

Other reported infectious triggers include upper respiratory tract infections [28], lepromatous leprosy [29], pityriasis versicolor, Lyme disease [30,31] and human immunodeficiency virus (HIV) [32]. The association with tuberculosis has never been convincing [4].

A distinction should be made for perifollicular anetodermic lesions in middle-aged women, possibly following infection with elastase-positive strains of *Staphylococcus epidermidis*. This has been proposed as a separate entity called perifollicular macular atrophy [33]. Whether the latter represents a variant of anetoderma or misdiagnosed papular acne scars [34] is still disputable.

Autoimmune disorders. The association between anetoderma and systemic or discoid lupus erythematosus (LE) was discussed at the beginning of the 20th century [35]. Despite many further reports [36–41], a clear relationship between LE and anetoderma was never established. In these cases anetoderma usually develops in adulthood either before or after clinical signs of LE. Patients often have positive direct immunofluorescence and serological abnormalities similar to those of LE [12,42,43]. However, criteria are often lacking for the diagnosis of true LE [16]. It recently became clear that anetoderma occurs more often in patients with the lupus anticoagulant antibodies than in patients with LE and no lupus anticoagulant [40]. It therefore appears that anetoderma is more a feature of the antiphospholipid syndrome than of LE [40,44]. Many such cases harbour microthromboses, which could correspond to the 'capillarites' already described in 1941 [6].

Localized dermatoses. Several dermatological afflictions may occasionally be complicated by anetoderma. In such cases, local infiltration by inflammatory cells is responsible for the elastolysis. Disorders thus associated with secondary anetoderma include urticaria pigmentosa [27,45–47], vesicular Langerhans' cell histiocytosis (Hashimoto–Pritzker form) [48], pilomatricomas [49–52], prurigo nodularis with Pautrier's neuromas [53], plasmacytoma or lymphoid hyperplasia [54,55] and surgical scars [56].

Histopathology

A focal complete loss of normal diameter elastin fibres in the dermis is the major histological characteristic of anetoderma and is necessary for defining the disease process [4,57,58]. The overlying epidermis is conserved. Fine elastic fibres or abnormal, irregular, granular, twisted fibres may remain, as a probable consequence of the elastolysis [58]. Immunoreactivity to microfibrils closely related to elastin, such as vibronectin and amyloid P component, is also decreased in anetoderma [59]. The fibrillin network remains, however, conserved throughout the dermis [11,59].

A perivascular and periadnexal inflammatory infiltrate is present in all cases of anetoderma, whether with or without an inflammatory presentation. This infiltrate is mainly composed of T-helper lymphocytes [60]. Plasma cells can be present. They were originally described as a frequent finding in syphilis [4], but were more recently found not to correlate with the age, type or location of the lesions or associated diseases [58]. Histiocytes and macrophages can be present, with or without granuloma formation [13,58]. Eosinophils are less frequent. Finally, as mentioned above, microthromboses should prompt research of an associated antiphospholipid syndrome [44].

Clinical features

Anetoderma in children is rare. The most common form is limited to a few lesions occurring in the months following chicken pox (Fig. 19.20.6). Primary anetoderma, as a widespread and progressive disease, usually starts in adulthood but may present in children. In a series of 16 patients, anetoderma began in the first decade in five patients and in the second decade in three [12]. Anetoderma was the

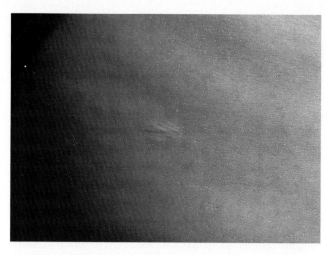

Fig. 19.20.6 Anetodermic chicken pox scar in a 5-year-old child.

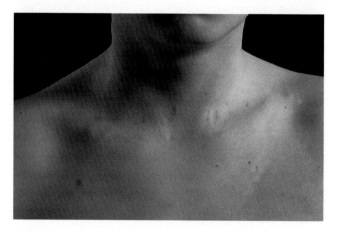

Fig. 19.20.7 Primary anetoderma around the neck of a 15-year-old boy.

only finding in all patients, except one with an associated hypothyroidism at presentation and with hip dislocation, mitral valve prolapse and vitiligo, 50 years later. Hence in children, anetoderma can be considered as a benign condition [25].

The sites most commonly involved are the chest, arms, upper back and neck (Fig. 19.20.7). Less frequently the face [12], abdomen and lower limbs are affected [4]. The palms and soles are spared. The number of lesions may vary from only a few to several hundred.

Initial lesions are usually pink macules, either isolated or in crops, with a diameter of 0.5–1 cm. These progressively evolve into atrophy. Other presentations include urticarial wheals, larger plaques of erythema or solid pseudotumoral lesions. Whatever the initial presentation, the lesions leave a localized area of wrinkled skin which is slightly depressed and, on pressure, admits the fingertip through a ring of normal surrounding skin. Ballooned, sac-like, easily depressible lesions are also often present. Both depressed and bulging pseudotumoral lesions

Table 19.20.8 Differential diagnosis of anetodermic lesions

Chicken pox scars
Papular acne scars
Lichen sclerosus et atrophicus (LSA)
Atrophoderma of Pasini and Pierini
Perifollicular macular atrophy
Atrophoderma vermiculare
Acquired cutis laxa
Striae distensae
Connective tissue naevus
Neurofibromas
Piezogenic papules
Focal dermal hypoplasia (Goltz)

usually coexist in most patients, but it is possible to observe only one type of lesion. The coalescence of sac-like lesions can occur, giving an aspect very similar to acquired cutis laxa (see Chapter 19.18). The atrophic lesions of anetoderma never heal and remain unchanged throughout life. Sensitivity over the lesions is always conserved.

The disease process may be self-limited over a few months but often progresses for years, either continuously or as a succession of exacerbations and remissions.

Differential diagnosis

The diagnosis of anetoderma in children can be made on clinical grounds only. A biopsy to confirm the absence of dermal elastic fibres may be helpful in atypical [61] or in progressive cases. The histological differential diagnosis mainly consists of mid-dermal elastolysis with wrinkling, a disorder of middle-aged women [62], and postinflammatory elastolysis and cutis laxa, a disorder of African children (see below).

Once concomitant morphological abnormalities have been excluded, further investigations are usually not warranted in this age group [25]. Only in late adolescence and adulthood is screening for the various associated systemic disorders and prolonged follow-up indicated [12,40]. A list of the clinical differential diagnoses is shown on Table 19.20.8.

Treatment

Many treatment modalities have been advocated in anetoderma. These include penicillin, aspirin, phenytoin, dapsone, vitamin E, nicotinate and intralesional steroids. Unfortunately, none of these seem to be effective [12] and so far anetoderma, once present, remains throughout life.

REFERENCES

1 Jadassohn J. Ueber eine eigenartige Form von 'Atrophia maculosa cutis'. *Arch Dermatol Syph* 1891; (suppl 1): 342–58.
2 Pelizzari C. Eritema orticato atrofizzante: atrofia parziale idiopathica delle pelle. *G Ital Mal Ven* 1884; 19: 230–43.
3 Schweninger E, Buzzi F. Multiple benign tumour-like new growths on the skin. In: Unna PG, Morris M, Besner E, ed. *International Atlas of Rare Skin Diseases*. Hamburg, Germany: Leopold Voss, 1889–1899: 4–5.
4 Deluzenne RL. Les anétodermies maculeuses. *Ann Dermatol Vénéréol* 1956; 83: 618–30.
5 Chargrin L, Silver H. Macular atrophy of the skin. *Arch Dermatol* 1931; 24: 614–43.
6 Touraine A. Anétodermie urticarienne de type Pelizzari. *Bull Soc Fr Dermatol Syphiligr* 1941; 48: 602–8.
7 Curran ME, Atkinson DL, Ewart AK et al. The elastin gene is disrupted by a translocation associated with supravalvular aortic stenosis. *Cell* 1993; 73: 159–68.
8 Ewart AK, Morris CA, Atkinson D et al. Hemizygozity at the elastin locus in a developmental disorder, Williams' syndrome. *Nature Genet* 1993; 5: 11–16.
9 Werb Z, Gordon S. Elastase secretion by stimulated macrophages. Characterization and regulation. *J Exp Med* 1975; 142: 361–77.
10 Ohlsson K, Ohlsson I. The neutral proteases of human granulocytes. Isolation and partial characterization of granulocyte elastases. *Eur J Biochem* 1974; 42: 519–27.
11 Venencie PY, Winkelmann RK, Moore BA. Ultrastructural findings in the skin lesions of patients with anetoderma. *Acta Derm Venereol (Stockh)* 1984; 64: 112–20.
12 Venencie PY, Winkelmann RK, Moore BA. Anetoderma. Clinical findings, associations, and long-term follow-up evaluations. *Arch Dermatol* 1984; 120: 1032–9.
13 Zaki I, Scerri L, Nelson H. Primary anetoderma: phagocytosis of elastic fibres by macrophages. *Clin Exp Dermatol* 1994; 19: 388–90.
14 Werth VP, Ivanov IE, Nussenzweig V. Decay-accelerating factor in human skin is associated with elastic fibers. *J Invest Dermatol* 1988; 91: 511–16.
15 Kossard S, Kronman KR, Dicken CH et al. Inflammatory macular atrophy: immunofluorescent and ultrastructural findings. *J Am Acad Dermatol* 1979; 1: 325–34.
16 Bergman R, Friedman Birnbaum R, Hazaz B et al. An immunofluorescence study of primary anetoderma. *Clin Exp Dermatol* 1990; 15: 124–30.
17 Friedman SJ, Venencie PY, Bradley RR et al. Familial anetoderma. *J Am Acad Dermatol* 1987; 16: 341–5.
18 Temtamy SA, El Meligh MR, Badrawy HS et al. Metaphyseal dysplasia, anetoderma and optic atrophy: an autosomal recessive syndrome. *Birth Defects* 1974; 10: 61–71.
19 Mollica F, Li Volti S, Guarneri B. New syndrome: exostoses, anetodermia, brachydactyly. *Am J Med Genet* 1984; 19: 665–7.
20 Grimalt MF, Korting GW. Anetodermie und Osteopsathyrose. *Z Hautkr Geschl* 1957; 22: 361–5.
21 Field CE. Albers–Schönberg disease: an atypical case. *Proc Roy Soc Med* 1939; 32: 320–4.
22 Ellis RWB. Osteopetrosis. *Proc Roy Soc Med* 1934; 27: 1563–71.
23 Clement M, du Vivier A. Anetoderma secondary to syphilis. *J Roy Soc Med* 1983; 76: 223–4.
24 Duperrat B, De Sablet M, Fontaine A. Anétodermie syphilitique incipiens. *Bull Soc Fr Dermatol Syph* 1958; 65: 22–3.
25 Tousignant J, Crickx B, Grossin M et al. Anétodermie post-varicelleuse: 3 observations. *Ann Dermatol Vénéréol* 1990; 117: 355–7.
26 Degos R, Larrègue M. Anétodermie de type Schweninger–Buzzi ayant débuté après une varicelle. *Bull Soc Fr Dermatol Syph* 1971; 78: 218.
27 Thivolet J, Cambazard F, Souteyrand P et al. Les mastocytoses à évolution anétodermique (revue de la literature). *Ann Dermatol Vénéréol* 1981; 108: 259–66.
28 Ferrara RJ. Macular atrophy following infection: report of a case. *Arch Dermatol* 1959; 79: 516–18.
29 Bechelli LM, Valeri V, Pimenta WP et al. Anétodermie de Schweninger–Buzzi chez des femmes atteintes de lèpre lépromateuse et chez des femmes non-atteintes. *Dermatologica* 1967; 135: 329–36.
30 Pautrier L-M. Les rapports de la dermatite chronique atrophiante, de l'anétodermie et de la sclérodermie: l'étude des troubles du métabolisme du tissu conjonctif. *Bull Soc Fr Dermatol Syph* 1929; 36: 973–8.
31 Malane MS, Grant Kels JM, Feder HM Jr et al. Diagnosis of Lyme disease based on dermatologic manifestations. *Ann Intern Med* 1991; 114: 490–8.
32 Ruiz Rodriguez R, Longaker M, Berger TG. Anetoderma and human immunodeficiency virus infection. *Arch Dermatol* 1992; 128: 661–2.
33 Varadi DP, Saqueton AC. Perifollicular elastolysis. *Br J Dermatol* 1970; 83: 143–50.

34 Wilson BB, Dent CH, Cooper PH. Papular acne scars. A common cutaneous finding. *Arch Dermatol* 1990; 126: 797–800.

35 Thibierge MG. Le lupus érythémateux à forme d'atrophodermie en plaques. *Ann Dermatol Syph* 1905; 6: 913–26.

36 Candio P, Lembo G, Saggiorato F *et al.* A case of anetoderma associated with discoid type lupus erythematosus. Clinico-histologic and pathogenetic observations. *G Ital Dermatol Venereol* 1986; 121: 269–72.

37 Edelson Y, Grupper C. Maculate anetoderma and lupus erythematosus. *Bull Soc Fr Dermatol Syph* 1970; 77: 753–6.

38 Hassan ML, Schroh RG, Konopka H. Anetoderma and lupus erythematosus. Study of two cases. *Med Cutan Ibero Lat Am* 1987; 15: 341–9.

39 Schnitzler L, Abimelech PH, Naveau B. Pseudotumoral lupus anetoderma. Child chorea. Development over 28 years. *Ann Dermatol Vénéréol* 1988; 115: 679–84.

40 Stephansson EA, Niemi KM, Jouhikainen T *et al.* Lupus anticoagulant and the skin. A long-term follow-up study of SLE patients with special reference to histopathological findings. *Acta Derm Venereol* 1991; 71: 416–22.

41 Temime P, Baran LR, Friedmann E. Pseudotumoral anetoderma and chronic lupus erythematosus. *Ann Dermatol Syph Paris* 1971; 98: 141–6.

42 Hodak E, Shamai Lubovitz O, David M *et al.* Primary anetoderma associated with a wide spectrum of autoimmune abnormalities. *J Am Acad Dermatol* 1991; 25: 415–18.

43 Hodak E, Shamai Lubovitz O, David M *et al.* Immunologic abnormalities associated with primary anetoderma. *Arch Dermatol* 1992; 128: 799–803.

44 Disdier P, Harle JR, Andrac L *et al.* Primary anetoderma associated with the antiphospholipid syndrome. *J Am Acad Dermatol* 1994; 30: 133–4.

45 Carr RD. Urticaria pigmentosa associated with anetoderma. *Acta Derm Venereol (Stockh)* 1971; 51: 120–2.

46 Gebauer KA, Navaratnam TE, Holgate C. Pruritic pigmented papules posing permanent problems. Urticaria pigmentosa (UP) with secondary anetoderma. *Arch Dermatol* 1992; 128: 107, 110.

47 Thivolet J, Pierini AM, Cambazard F *et al.* Mastocytose cutanée avec anétodermie secondaire et alopécie cicatricielle associée à une valvulopathie. *Ann Dermatol Vénéréol* 1981; 108: 269–75.

48 Higgins CR, Tatnall FM, Leigh IM. Vesicular Langerhans' cell histiocytosis—an uncommon variant. *Clin Exp Dermatol* 1994; 19: 350–2.

49 Balus L, Cristiani R, Amantea A *et al.* Tumeur de Malherbe anetodermique. *Ann Dermatol Vénéréol* 1990; 117: 641–3.

50 Shames BS, Nassif A, Bailey CS *et al.* Secondary anetoderma involving a pilomatricoma. *Am J Dermatopathol* 1994; 16: 557–60.

51 Kelly SE, Humphreys F, Aldridge RD. The phenomenon of anetoderma occurring over pilomatricomas letter; comment. *J Am Acad Dermatol* 1993; 28: 511.

52 Moulin G, Bouchet B, Dos Santos G. Les modifications anétodermiques de tégument au-dessus des tumeur de Malherbe. *Ann Dermatol Vénéréol* 1978; 105: 43–7.

53 Hirschel Scholz S, Salomon D, Merot Y *et al.* Anetodermic prurigo nodularis (with Pautrier's neuroma) responsive to arotinoid acid. *J Am Acad Dermatol* 1991; 25: 437–42.

54 Jubert C, Cosnes A, Wechsler J *et al.* Anetoderma may reveal cutaneous plasmacytoma and benign cutaneous lymphoid hyperplasia letter. *Arch Dermatol* 1995; 131: 365–6.

55 Jubert C, Cosnes A, Clerici T *et al.* Sjögren's syndrome and cutaneous B cell lymphoma revealed by anetoderma. *Arthr Rheum* 1993; 36: 133–4.

56 Dupre A. Dermatoses in scar tissue: necrobiosis lipodica diabeticorum, erythema elevatum diutinum, pretibial myxedema, anetoderma, etc. *Ann Dermatol Vénéréol* 1979; 106: 383.

57 Oikarinen AI, Palatsi R, Adomian GE *et al.* Anetoderma: biochemical and ultrastructural demonstration of an elastin defect in the skin of three patients. *J Am Acad Dermatol* 1984; 11: 64–72.

58 Venencie PY, Winkelmann RK. Histopathologic findings in anetoderma. *Arch Dermatol* 1984; 120: 1040–4.

59 Dahlback K, Ljungquist A, Lofberg H *et al.* Fibrillin immunoreactive fibers constitute a unique network in the human dermis: immunohistochemical comparison of the distributions of fibrillin, vitronectin, amyloid P component, and orcein stainable structures in normal skin and elastosis. *J Invest Dermatol* 1990; 94: 284–91.

60 Venencie PY, Winkelmann RK. Monoclonal antibody studies in the skin lesions of patients with anetoderma. *Arch Dermatol* 1985; 121: 747–9.

61 Taieb A, Dufillot D, Pellegrin Carloz B *et al.* Postgranulomatous anetoderma associated with Takayasu's arteritis in a child. *Arch Dermatol* 1987; 123: 796–800.

62 Kim JM, Daniel Su WP. Mid dermal elastolysis with wrinkling. *J Am Acad Dermatol* 1992; 26: 169–73.

Postinflammatory elastolysis and cutis laxa

This disorder may be regarded as a severe variant of anetoderma [1–4]. It typically occurs in African or Afro-Caucasian children. An acute onset with inflammatory plaques or urticarial lesions precedes a prolonged course of similar exacerbations which lead to atrophy and sometimes severe disfigurement. Most of the body can be involved with diffuse anetodermic changes. It is thought to be a reaction to arthropod bites, possibly aggravated by sun exposure, and is histologically characterized by the destruction of elastic fibres in the upper and mid-dermis.

REFERENCES

1 O'Brien JP. Is actinic damage the provoking cause of post-inflammatory elastolysis and cutis laxa? *Br J Dermatol* 1976; 95: 105–6.

2 Lewis PG, Hood AF, Barnett NK *et al.* Post-inflammatory elastolysis and cutis laxa. A case report. *J Am Acad Dermatol* 1990; 22: 40–8.

3 Verhagen AR, Woerdeman MJ. Post-inflammatory elastolysis and cutis laxa. *Br J Dermatol* 1975; 92: 183–90.

4 Marshall J, Heyl T, Weber HW. Post-inflammatory elastolysis and cutis laxa: a report on a new variety of this phenomenon and a discussion of some syndromes characterized by elastolysis. *S Afr Med J* 1966; 40: 1016–22.

Atrophodermas

Atrophoderma of Pasini and Pierini

(SYN. SLERODERMIE ATROPHIQUE D'EMBLEE, DYSCHROMIC AND ATROPHIC VARIATION OF SCLERODERMA, MORPHOEA PLANA ATROPHICA, ATROPHOSCLERODERMA SUPERFICIALIS, SCLERODERMIE ATYPIQUE LILACEE NON INDUREE (GOUGEROT))

Definition

Atrophoderma of Pasini and Pierini (APP) is a distinctive form of dermal atrophy, appearing as one or more sharply demarcated, depressed areas. Whether APP is a distinct entity or a variation of localized scleroderma (morphoea) has been disputed since its original description [1–5]. However, most authors would now regard APP as an atrophic non-indurated, possibly abortive, variant of localized scleroderma [6–8].

History

Described in 1923 by Pasini [9] and in more detail by Pierini [10], the condition had been reported earlier under various names [11,12]. The name idiopathic atrophoderma of Pasini and Pierini was introduced in 1958 by Canizares *et al.* [13] and many reports have followed [14–20].

Aetiology

The label 'idiopathic' has been well preserved in the literature [21,22] and the disorder remains of an uncertain origin. The occasional reports of the concomitant occurrence of APP and morphoea [2,22–24] and of APP and lichen sclerosus et atrophicus (LSA) [4,25] just rendered the distinction of APP more difficult and did not provide any significant insights into its pathogenesis. The only recent progress is the finding of serological evidence of *Borrelia burgdorferi* infection in a proportion of patients with APP [8] and morphoea [20,26,27]. Culture of *B. burgdorferi* [28] or polymerase chain reaction (PCR) obtained evidence of spirochaetes from active lesions furthermore suggest a pathogenic role, but this remains controversial [29]. For those who consider that APP, as morphoea, is the result of an intrinsic susceptibility which can be triggered by various environmental factors, *B. burgdorferi* should be accepted as a relevant aetiology in endemic areas. The few reports of a clinical response of APP to antibiotics may also argue for a role of a bacterial trigger. However, as mentioned above, the origin of APP still remains unknown in a large majority of cases.

Pathology

In early lesions of APP, there is focal homogenization and minimal thickening of collagen bundles in association with a mild perivascular infiltrate. In a series of 17 biopsies, Buechner and Kufli [8] also found a slight atrophy of the epidermis in six specimens and an increased pigmentation of basal cell layer in 16. The perivascular infiltrate mainly consists of T lymphocytes and histiocytes/macrophages. Deposition of immunoglobulin M (IgM), IgA and C3 have been described [30,31]. In most cases there is no alteration of the elastic fibres and the eccrine sweat glands, hair follicles and sebaceous glands remain intact. Slight sclerosis of collagen in the reticular dermis can be found as the lesions age. Histological differentiation of APP and residual pigmented lesions after involution of morphoea is not possible [4].

Clinical features

APP has a female to male ratio of 2:1 [1]. APP can occur at any age between 7 and 66 years, but usually develops in the teens or the 20s. Childhood presentation is not uncommon.

The lesions, single or multiple, are round or oval, sharply demarcated, grey or violet–brown areas that are slightly depressed below the normal surrounding skin (Fig. 19.20.8). Size ranges from 2 to several centimetres in diameter. Classic lesions present as 'cliff-drop' inverted plateaux lacking the lilac border of morphoea. They are usually bilateral, involving the back in the great majority of cases (85%) and less frequently the trunk, groin and proximal limbs, but never the face and distal extremities.

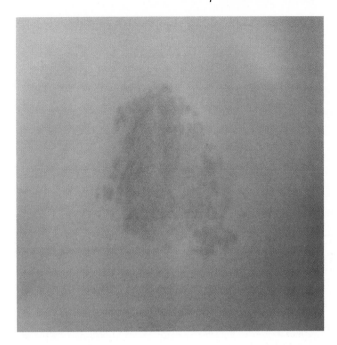

Fig. 19.20.8 APP.

Table 19.20.9 Distinct features of atrophoderma of Pasini-Pierini (APP) and morphea

	APP	Morphea
Age of onset	Teens to 20s	Teens to 40s
Colour	Grey, bluish, violet-brown	Lilac ring
Course	Protracted, 10–20 years	Shorter, 3–5 years
Initial finding	Atrophy	Induration, inflammation
progressing to:	Possible induration	Atrophy
Appendageal structures	Preserved	Destroyed

Confluence of lesions can occur as well as unilateral presentations [22,32,33]. APP is known to follow a long protracted course but remains a benign disorder in which morbidity is mainly cosmetic. Progression to systemic scleroderma is exceptional [34].

Clinical features that have been used to make APP a distinct variant of morphoea are listed in Table 19.20.9.

Diagnosis and treatment

APP is primarily a clinical diagnosis (see Table 19.20.9) and, in most cases, its differentiation with morphoea is mostly semantic. However, the recognition of this entity is helpful to avoid aggressive immunosuppressant therapy now widely given for early, rapidly progressive morphoea.

Lipoatrophic and panatrophic (Gower's) disorders both

involve the thinning and disappearance of the subcutaneous fat, this not being a feature of APP [35].

Antibiotic therapy of early APP has long been debated [4,8,36,37] and may be relevant in patients with positive serology to *B. burgdorferi*. Many authors, however, regard antibiotic therapy in APP as useless.

REFERENCES

1 Pierini LE, Abulafia J, Mosto SJ. Atrophodermie idiopathique progressive et états voisins. *Ann Dermatol Syph* 1970; 97: 391–416.

2 Quiroga MI, Woscoff A. L'atrophodermie idiopathique progressive (Pasini–Pierini) et la sclérodermie atypique lilacée non indurée (Gougerot). *Ann Dermatol* 1961; 88: 507–20.

3 Kogoj FR. Qu'est-ce que la maladie de Pasini–Pierini? *Ann Dermatol* 1961; 88: 247–56.

4 Jablonska S, Szczepanski A. Atrophoderma Pasini–Pierini: is it an entity? *Dermatologica* 1962; 125: 226–42.

5 Brunauer SR. Zur Terminologie der sogenannten 'idiopatischen progressiven Atrophodermie von Pasini und Pierini' sowie ueber die Stellung dieser Affektion im System des Dermatosen. *Hautarzt* 1964; 15: 108–12.

6 Kencka D, Blaszczyk M, Jablonska S. Atrophoderma Pasini–Pierini is a primary atrophic abortive morphea. *Dermatology* 1995; 190: 203–6.

7 Altmeyer P, Adam B, Bacharach-Buhles M. Zur Klassifikation des zirkumscripten Sklerodermie. *Hautarzt* 1990; 41: 16–21.

8 Buechner SA, Rufli T. Atrophoderma of Pasini and Pierini. Clinical and histopathologic findings and antibodies to *Borrelia burgdorferi* in 34 patients. *J Am Acad Dermatol* 1994; 30: 441–6.

9 Pasini A. Atrofodermia idiopathica progressiva. *G Ital Dermatol* 1923; 58: 785–809.

10 Pierini LE, Vivoli D. Atrofodermia idiopathica progressiva (Pasini). *G Ital Dermatol* 1936; 77: 403–9.

11 Brocq F. Sclérodermie en plaques superficielles sans infiltrations à foyers multiples, fait de passage vers les atrophies cutanées. *Ann Dermatol Syph* 1909; 189.

12 Gougerot H. Sclerodermies atypiques: la forme lilacée non indurée en plaques ou en bandes. *Bull Soc Fr Dermatol Syph* 1932; 39: 1667–9.

13 Canizares D, Sachs PA, Jaimovich L *et al.* Idiopathic atrophoderma of Pasini and Pierini. *Arch Dermatol* 1958; 79: 42–60.

14 Abrahams I. Atrophoderma of Pasini–Pierini. *Arch Dermatol* 1968; 98: 103.

15 Bourgeois Spinasse J, Grupper C. Unilateral Pasini–Pierini atrophoderma in bands. *Bull Soc Fr Dermatol Syph* 1969; 76: 494–6.

16 Duperrat B, de Sablet M. Atypical liliaceous scleroderma of Gougerot (Pasini and Pierini atrophoderma). *Bull Soc Fr Dermatol Syph* 1969; 76: 296.

17 Flegel H, Reink H. Pasini-Pierini syndrome, idiopathic atrophoderma. *Z Haut Geschlechtskr* 1965; 39: 268–72.

18 Haldar B. Case of atrophoderma of Pasini and Pierini. *Indian J Dermatol* 1974; 19: 71.

19 Labouche F, Balouet G, Cherif Cheikh JL *et al.* A propos of 2 cases of Pasini–Pierini atrophoderma. *Bull Soc Fr Dermatol Syph* 1967; 74: 670–2.

20 Rimbaud P, Meynadier J, Peraldi R. Atrophoderma of Pasini and Pierini. *Bull Soc Fr Dermatol Syph* 1969; 76: 573–5.

21 Goncharova LI, Kharitonova NI. Idiopathic Pasini–Pierini atrophoderma associated with guttate scleroderma. *Vestn Dermatol Venerol* 1988; 7: 68–9.

22 Murphy PK, Hymes SR, Fenske NA. Concomitant unilateral idiopathic atrophoderma of Pasini and Pierini (IAPP) and morphea. Observations supporting IAPP as a variant of morphea. *Int J Dermatol* 1990; 29: 281–3.

23 Szczepanski A. Pasini–Pierini atrophoderma coexisting with circumscribed scleroderma in the light of clinical observations and function tests. *Przegl Dermatol* 1970; 57: 631–6.

24 Kee CE, Brothers WS, New W. Idiopathic atrophoderma of Pasini and Pierini with coexistent morphea. *Arch Dermatol* 1960; 82: 154–7.

25 Heymann WR. Coexistent lichen sclerosus et atrophicus and atrophoderma of Pasini and Pierini. *Int J Dermatol* 1994; 33: 133–4.

26 Aberer E, Neumann R, Stanek G. Is localized scleroderma a *Borrelia* infection? *Lancet* 1985; ii: 278.

27 Rufli T, Lehner S, Aeschlimann A *et al.* Zum erweiterten Spektrum zeckenübertragener Spirochätosen. *Hautarzt* 1986; 37: 597–602.

28 Aberer E, Stanek G, Ertl M *et al.* Evidence for spirochetal origin of circumscribed scleroderma (morphea). *Acta Derm Venereol (Stockh)* 1987; 67: 225–31.

29 Hoesly JM, Mertz LE, Winkelmann RK. Localized scleroderma (morphea) and antibody to *Borrelia burgdorferi*. *J Am Acad Dermatol* 1987; 17: 455–8.

30 Berman A, Berman GD, Winkelmann RK. Atrophoderma (Pasini–Pierini). Findings on direct immunofluorescent, monoclonal antibody, and ultrastructural studies. *Int J Dermatol* 1988; 27: 487–90.

31 Kernohan NM, Stankler L, Sewell HF. Atrophoderma of Pasini and Pierini. An immunopathologic case study. *Am J Clin Pathol* 1992; 97: 63–8.

32 Wokalek H, Schmidt HG, Niedner R *et al.* Idiopathic progressive atrophoderma of Pasini–Pierini with the presence of antinuclear antibodies. *Hautarzt* 1985; 36: 154–60.

33 Iriondo M, Bloom RF, Neldner KH. Unilateral atrophoderma of Pasini and Pierini. *Cutis* 1987; 39: 69–70.

34 Bisaccia EP, Scarborough DA, Lowney ED. Atrophoderma of Pasini and Pierini and systemic scleroderma. *Arch Dermatol* 1982; 118: 1–2 (letter).

35 Franck JM, MacFarlane D, Silvers DN *et al.* Atrophoderma of Pasini and Pierini: atrophy of dermis or subcutis? *J Am Acad Dermatol* 1995; 32: 122–3.

36 Salamon T, Milicevic M. Concerning four cases of idiopathic atrophoderma of Pasini and Pierini. *Dermatologica* 1968; 136: 479–88.

37 Lohrer R, Barran L, Kellnar S *et al.* Pasini and Pierini idiopathic and progressive atrophoderma in childhood. *Monatsschr Kinderheilkd* 1986; 134: 878–80.

Familial follicular atrophoderma and basal cell carcinoma

(SYN. BAZEX–DUPRÉ–CHRISTOL SYNDROME)
(see Chapter 19.24)

The Bazex–Dupré–Christol syndrome represents a familial premalignant genodermatosis whose fundamental feature is an anomaly of the hair follicle. It is characterized by follicular atrophoderma, congenital hypotrichosis and basocellular neoformations that include basal cell naevi and basal cell carcinoma.

Atrophoderma vermiculate

(SYN. ULERYTHEMA ACNEIFORME, ACNE VERMOULANTE, ATROPHODERMA RETICULATA SYMMETRICA FACIEI, ATROPHODERMA RETICULATUM, HONEYCOMB ATROPHY)

Atrophoderma vermiculate (AV) is a rare disorder characterized by the bilateral occurrence on the cheeks of fine atrophic pits, representing widely dilated follicles and producing a honeycomb reticulate appearance. AV usually begins in the first decade and follows a slow progressive course over many years. It is fairly asymptomatic, but erythema, follicular plugs or papules with a perifolliculitis may precede the atrophic depressions. An autosomal dominant inheritance has been reported.

The disorder is clearly distinct from acne scars and should be considered as part of a group of closely related syndromes characterized by keratosis pilaris succeeded by atrophy. Apart from AV, this group includes keratosis pilaris atrophicans (ulerythema ophryogenes) and keratosis pilaris decalvans (keratosis follicularis spinulosa decalvans).

Variants of AV include unilateral presentation, presence of milia and association with Rombo's syndrome [1–8].

REFERENCES

1 Arrieta E, Milgram Sternberg Y. Honeycomb atrophy on the right cheek. Folliculitis ulerythematosa reticulata (atrophoderma vermiculatum). *Arch Dermatol* 1988; 124: 1101, 1104.

2 Brazzelli V, Borroni G. Early and late histologic aspects of atrophodermia vermiculata. A case study. *G Ital Dermatol Venereol* 1990; 125: 285–9.

3 Degos R, Touraine R, Belaich S *et al.* Lutz–Miescher verruciform perforating elastoma associated with vermiculated atrophoderma. *Ann Dermatol Syph Paris* 1967; 94: 406–7.

4 Dupre A, Carrere S, Bonafe JL *et al.* Syringomes éruptifs généralisés, milium et atrophodermie vermiculée. Syndrome de Nicolau et Balus. *Dermatologica* 1981; 162: 281–6.

5 Frosch PJ, Brumage MR, Schuster Pavlovic C *et al.* Atrophoderma vermiculatum. Case reports and review. *J Am Acad Dermatol* 1988; 18: 538–42.

6 Michaelsson G, Olsson E, Westermark P. The Rombo syndrome: a familial disorder with vermiculate atrophoderma, milia, hypotrichosis, trichoepitheliomas, basal cell carcinomas and peripheral vasodilation with cyanosis. *Acta Derm Venereol (Stockh)* 1981; 61: 497–503.

7 Savatard L. Honeycomb atrophy. *Br J Dermatol* 1943; 55: 259–66.

8 McKee GM, Parounagian MB. Folliculitis ulerythematosa reticulata. *J Cutan Dis* 1918; 36: 337.

Linear atrophoderma of Moulin

In 1992, Moulin *et al.* [1] reported five patients affected by a new clinical entity. The cutaneous lesions were characterized by multiple, acquired, hyperpigmented, depressed, unilateral large bands, closely following Blaschko's lines. All patients presented with lesions in the first or second decade, with a rapid (< 1 year) and asymptomatic onset. The absence of peripheral inflammation ('lilac ring'), induration or sclerodermic changes was confirmed by a follow-up of 2–30 years. The histological features in three patients did not show any inflammation in the dermis nor alterations of the connective tissue. The elastic fibres remained normal. Except for hyperpigmentation, the epidermis showed no alterations. In these patients, as well as in a further report [2], the topography of the lesions, the absence of inflammation or sclerodermiform changes and the absence of associated findings allowed a clear distinction from morphoea, scleroderma, APP or from other disorders following Blaschko's lines, such as incontinentia pigmenti, Goltz's syndrome and linear and whorled naevoid hypermelanosis (reticulate hyperpigmentation Iijima).

The aetiology of the disorder is unknown. These dysembriologic lesions of a late onset are part of the group of dermatoses whose expression follows Blaschko's lines as a consequence of a somatic mutation, a functional mosaicism or a hemi-chromatidic mutation in a gamete.

REFERENCES

1 Moulin G, Hill MP, Guillaud V *et al.* Bandes pigmentées atrophiques acquises suivant les lignes de Blaschko. *Ann Dermatol Vénéréol* 1992; 119: 729–36.

2 Baumann L, Happle R, Plewig G *et al.* Atrophodermia linearis Moulin. Ein neues Krankheitsbild, das den Blaschko-Linien folgt. *Hautarzt* 1994; 45: 231–6.

Focal facial dermal dysplasias

(SYN. BRAUER'S SYNDROME, SETLEIS SYNDROME, CONGENITAL ECTODERMAL DYSPLASIA OF THE FACE, BITEMPORAL SCARS WITH ABNORMAL EYELASHES, HEREDITARY SYMMETRICAL SYSTEMIC APLASTIC NAEVI, BITEMPORAL APLASIA CUTIS CONGENITA, BITEMPORAL FORCEPS MARKS SYNDROME)

The focal facial dermal dysplasias (FFDD) are all characterized by congenital bilateral temporal atrophic lesions. Since the first description by Brauer in 1929 [1], other reports described over 100 affected individuals in 12 families [2–10]. Although all patients exhibited bitemporal atrophic lesions, differences in the mode of inheritance and associated clinical features suggested that not one but several related entities could present with FFDD. Whether these entities represent a spectrum of facial abnormalities with genetic homogeneity or two, or more, separate disorders is debatable [2,11]. A classification, proposed by Kowalski *et al.* [6] and based on the clinical features and mode of inheritance, is retained here since it has the advantage of grouping several related entities with a common presenting feature (temporal atrophic marks) under the same heading. This classification is, however, not entirely satisfactory, as sporadic cases may be difficult to fit into any group, and may require modification with the genetic characterization of the disorder(s).

The atrophic lesions are usually present at birth and are histologically characterized by an atrophic epidermis overlying a thinned dermis with scarcity or absence of adnexae.

Type I autosomal dominant focal facial dermal dysplasia [1,5,8]

In three large pedigrees, all affected individuals had scar-like pigmented atrophic lesions, up to 1 cm in diameter, bilaterally appearing on the temporal areas of the face. A few variations were noted: (a) occasional unilateral involvement; (b) lines radiating out from between the eyebrows and across the forehead; (c) finger-point depressions on the mid forehead or on the chin; and (d) clefting of the chin. An autosomal dominant inheritance characterizes this group. In one pedigree, the association with mental disturbance and abdominal carcinoma is questioned [8].

Type II autosomal recessive focal facial dermal dysplasia [5,6]

This type is characterized by the same bitemporal scar-like facial lesions at birth, but with an autosomal recessive inheritance. The three affected children described by Jensen [5] also exhibited double rows of upper eyelashes. In the other family, a rim of fine lanugo hair surrounded some lesions, which were hypopigmented [6].

Type III focal facial dermal dysplasia with other facial features (Setleis syndrome) [3,4,7,9,10,12]

Setleis described five children of Puerto-Rican origin who presented the following features: (a) scar-like temporal defects; (b) sharply slanted eyebrows; (c) abnormalities of the eyelashes (absent or multiple rows); (d) an aged leonine appearance with a low-set frontal hairline; (e) puckered skin around the eyes; (f) a median cleft on the chin; and (g) 'rubbery' nose and jaw. Other 'carbon copy' patients originated from the same Puerto-Rican area [4,7,9,12], and from other parts of the world [3]. The inheritance of FFDD with other facial features is apparently variable, being autosomal recessive [3,7,10] or autosomal dominant with variable expression [4].

REFERENCES

1 Brauer A. Hereditaerer symmetrischer systematisierter Naevus aplasticus bei 38 Personen. *Dermatol Wochenschr* 1929; 89: 1163–8.
2 Magid M, Prendiveille J, Esterly N. Focal facial dermal dysplasia: bitemporal lesions resembling aplasia cutis congenita. *J Am Acad Dermatol* 1988; 18: 1203–7.
3 Clark R, Golabi M, Lacassie Y. Expanded phenotype and ethnicity in Setleis syndrome. *Am J Med Genet* 1989; 34: 354–7.
4 Di Lernia V, Neri I, Patrizi I. Focal facial dermal dysplasia: two familial cases. *J Am Acad Dermatol* 1991; 25: 389–91.
5 Jensen N. Congenital ectodermal dysplasia of the face. *Br J Dermatol* 1971; 84: 410–16.
6 Kowalski D, Fenske N. The focal facial dermal dysplasia: report of a kindred and a proposed new classification. *J Am Acad Dermatol* 1992; 27: 575–82.
7 Marion R, Chitayat D, Hutcheon G. Autosomal recessive inheritance in the Setleis bitemporal 'forceps mark' syndrome. *Am J Dis Child* 1987; 141: 895–7.
8 McGeoch A, Reed W. Familial focal facial dermal dysplasia. *Arch Dermatol* 1973; 107: 591–5.
9 Rudolph R, Schwartz W, Leyden J. Bitemporal aplasia cutis congenita: occurrence with other cutaneous anomalies. *Arch Dermatol* 1974; 110: 615–18.
10 Setleis H, Kramer B, Valcarel M. Congenital ectodermal dysplasia of the face. *Pediatrics* 1963; 32: 540–8.
11 Freire-Maia N, Pinheiro M. *Ectodermal Dysplasias: a Clinical and Genetic Study.* New York: Alan R. Liss, 1986.
12 Rudolph R, Schwartz W, Leyden J. Emendation to 'bitemporal aplasia cutis congenita'. *Arch Dermatol* 1974; 110: 636.

Premature Ageing Syndromes

HELGA V. TORIELLO

Conditions with true premature ageing
Hutchinson–Gilford syndrome
Werner syndrome
Cockayne's syndrome
Rothmund–Thomson syndrome

Conditions with skin atrophy/lipoatrophy
Wiedemann–Rautenstrauch syndrome
DeBarsy syndrome
Acrometageria
Mandibuloacral dysplasia
Lenz–Majewski syndrome
Mulvihill–Smith syndrome
Lenaert syndrome

Conditions with skin laxity
Cutis laxa
Cutis laxa–mental retardation syndrome
Wrinkly skin syndrome
Gerodermia osteodysplastica
Costello syndrome
Hernandez (Ehlers–Danlos-like) syndrome
Kresse syndrome

Conditions in which individuals appear aged
Marfanoid ageing syndrome
Lee syndrome
Berlin syndrome

The causes of a prematurely aged phenotype can be heterogeneous. In general, true premature ageing, thin skin with local or generalized lipoatrophy, cutis laxa or skin hyperextensibility, or simply an older appearance than would be expected for the person's age all can lead to what is considered a prematurely aged phenotype. This chapter is arranged so that phenotypically similar conditions are grouped together. There will be some overlap, in that some conditions have elements of more than one group.

Conditions with true premature ageing

Hutchinson–Gilford syndrome

(SYN. PROGERIA)

Definition

Hutchinson–Gilford syndrome (HGS) is a rare condition characterized by premature ageing, short stature and recognizable skin and hair manifestations. Early death is the rule.

History

Hutchinson [1] first described this condition in 1886; 11 years later Gilford [2] reported a similar patient. Since then, over 70 cases have been reported [3].

Aetiology and pathogenesis

Most cases have been sporadic, but eight reports of affected siblings have been published, thus suggesting heterogeneity exists, with typical HGS probably caused by an autosomal dominant mutation, and a second form caused by homozygosity for an autosomal recessive gene. Several studies examining the various properties of cultured fibroblasts have been done in an attempt to elucidate the basic genetic defect. Clark and Weiss [4] observed the presence of elevated levels of a glycoprotein 200 in HGS fibroblasts. Colige et al. [5] noted an increase of elastin and α_1 and α_2 type IV procollagen messenger RNA (mRNA) in HGS fibroblasts. Giro and Davidson [6] also noted increased elastin and procollagen IV production in HGS fibroblasts, but had similar findings in one of the unaffected parents as well. However, differences with respect to response to various growth factors in HGS cells was believed to be important to the development of the HGS phenotype. Briata et al. [7] described reduced insulin receptor gene expression in HGS cells. Sugita et al. [8] described reduced unscheduled DNA synthesis and plasminogen activator-like protease activity in HGS fibroblasts.

Pathology

Various skin biopsy analyses have been published, with abnormal findings including a superabundant network of thick and irregular elastin fibres in reticular dermis [5], epidermal atrophy and hyaline fibrosis of the dermis with loss of appendages [9] and capillary dilatation in the dermis [10].

Clinical features (Figs 19.21.1, 19.21.2)

In general, HGS is characterized by effects on several systems. Most affected individuals have low birth weight, with further diminution of growth near the end of the first year of life. The resultant growth rate is approximately half the normal rate [11]. The skin shows changes within the first 6 months, characteristic with tautness and a scleroderma-like appearance. Superficial veins are prominent, and sweating diminished. Over time, areas of hyperpigmentation appear [12,13]. Alopecia also begins during the first year of life, and tends to be generalized, but particularly affects the scalp and eyebrows. Eyelashes may be spared [11].

The facial manifestations include the appearance of macrocephaly, with frontal bossing. The eyes appear prominent, and the nasal tip is grooved. Lips are thin, and micrognathia is common. Ears may protrude, and lobes are small or absent. Other findings include a pyriform chest, the development of joint stiffness, short terminal phalanges and osteoporosis. Following fractures, bone healing may be depressed [11,14]. X-rays demonstrate resorption of distal clavicles and phalanges. The voice is described as highly pitched.

Prognosis

Most individuals succumb to cardiovascular disease, with diffuse atherosclerosis noted on autopsy [15]. Mean age at death is 13.4 years [16], with range between 7 and 27 years [17]. Ogihara *et al.* [18] described a 45-year-old man with a diagnosis of HGS, but since alopecia did not occur until the age of 20 years, it is likely he had a distinct disorder. Intellectual functioning is at or above the normal range.

Differential diagnosis

It is possible that there is an autosomal recessive form of progeria which closely resembles HGS. Distinct manifes-

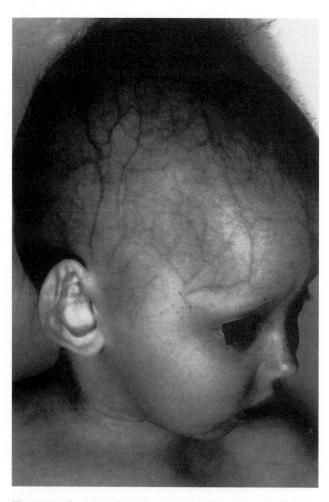

Fig. 19.21.1 Progeria: there is loss of hair with prominent scalp veins, micrognathia and abnormal ears. Reproduced from Harper [29] courtesy of Dr D.J. Gawkrodger and Butterworth Heinemann.

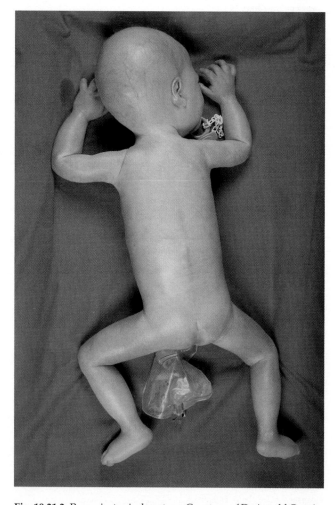

Fig. 19.21.2 Progeria: typical posture. Courtesy of Dr Arnold Oranje.

tations in the recessive form include complete resorption of clavicles and distal phalanges by 5 years of age and facial differences, including sparing of eyebrows, no groove on the nasal tip, full cheeks and more pronounced micrognathia. Possible examples of this condition include the children reported by Mostafa and Gabr [19], Rava [20], Franklyn [21], Maciel [22], Khalifa [23], Monu *et al.* [24], Hou and Wang [25] and LeMerrer *et al.* [26].

Other patients with the diagnosis of HGS [27] may actually have mandibuloacral dysplasia, thus this condition should also be considered in the differential diagnosis.

Treatment

Brown [28] described the results of treating HGS patients with nutritional supplementation and growth hormones. They observed a tripling in linear growth rate and reduction of basal metabolic rate. Long-term effects of such treatment is unknown.

REFERENCES

1 Hutchinson J. Congenital absence of hair and mammary glands with atrophic condition of skin and its appendages. *Med Chirur Trans* 1886; 69: 473–7.
2 Gilford H. On a condition of mixed premature and immature development. *Med Chirur Trans* 1897; 80: 17–45.
3 Yu QX, Zeng LH. Progeria: report of a case and a review of the literature. *J Oral Pathol Med* 1991; 20: 860–88.
4 Clark MA, Weiss AS. Elevated levels of glycoprotein gp200 in progeria fibroblasts. *Mol Cell Biochem* 1993; 120: 51–60.
5 Colige A, Roujeau JC, De La Rocque F, Nusgens B, Lapiere ChM. Abnormal gene expression in skin fibroblasts from a Hutchinson–Gilford patient. *Lab Invest* 1991; 64: 799–806.
6 Giro M, Davidson JM. Familial co-segregation of the elastin phenotype in skin fibroblasts from Hutchinson–Gilford progeria. *Mech Ageing Devel* 1993; 70: 163–76.
7 Briata P, Bellini C, Vignolo M, Gherzi R. Insulin receptor gene expression is reduced in cells from a progeric patient. *Mol Cell Endocrinol* 1991; 75: 9–14.
8 Sugita K, Suzuki N, Fujii K, Niimi H. Reduction of unscheduled DNA synthesis and plasminogen activator activity in Hutchinson–Gilford fibroblasts during passageing *in vitro*: partial correction by interferon-beta. *Mutat Res* 1995; 316: 133–8.
9 Beauregard S, Gilchrest BA. Syndromes of premature ageing. *Dermatol Clin* 1987; 5: 109–21.
10 Erdem N, Gunes AT, Avci O, Osma E. A case of Hutchinson–Gilford progeria syndrome mimicking scleredema in early infancy. *Dermatology* 1994; 188: 318–21.
11 DeBusk FL. The Hutchinson–Gilford progeria syndrome. *J Pediatr* 1972; 80: 697–724.
12 Mallory SB, Krafchik BR. Hutchinson–Gilford syndrome. *Pediatr Dermatol* 1990; 7: 317–19.
13 Gillar PJ, Kaye CI, McCourt JW. Progressive early dermatologic changes in Hutchinson–Gilford progeria syndrome. *Pediatr Dermatol* 1991; 8: 199–206.
14 Moen C. Orthopedic aspects of progeria. *J Bone Joint Surg* 1982; 64A: 542–6.
15 Baker PB, Baba N, Boesel CP. Cardiovascular abnormalities in progeria. *Arch Pathol Lab Med* 1981; 105: 384–6.
16 Dyck JD, David TE, Burke B, Webb GD, Henderson MA, Fowler RS. Management of coronary artery disease in Hutchinson–Gilford syndrome. *J Pediatr* 1987; 111: 407–10.
17 Badame AJ. Progeria. *Arch Dermatol* 1989; 125: 540–4.
18 Ogihara T, Hata T, Tanaka K, Fukuchi K, Tabuchi Y, Kumahara Y. Hutchinson–Gilford progeria syndrome in a 45-year-old man. *Am J Med* 1986; 81: 135–8.
19 Mostafa AH, Gabr M. Heredity in progeria. *Arch Pediatr* 1954; 71: 163–72.
20 Rava G. Su un nucleo familiare di progeria. *Minerv Med* 1967; 180: 1502–9.
21 Franklyn PP. Progeria in siblings. *Clin Radiol* 1976; 27: 327–33.
22 Maciel AT. Brief clinical report: evidence of autosomal recessive inheritance of progeria (Hutchinson–Gilford). *Am J Med Genet* 1988; 31: 483–7.
23 Khalifa MM. Hutchinson–Gilford progeria syndrome: report of a Libyan family and evidence of autosomal recessive inheritance. *Clin Genet* 1989; 35: 125–32.
24 Monu JUV, Benka-Coker LBO, Fatunde Y. Hutchinson–Gilford progeria syndrome in siblings. *Skel Radiol* 1990; 19: 585–90.
25 Hou J-W, Wang T-R. Clinical variability in neonatal progeroid syndrome. *Am J Med Genet* 1995; 58: 195–6.
26 Le Merrer M, Guillot M, Briard M-L, Maroteaux P. Lethal progeroid syndrome with osteolysis. *Ann Genet* 1991; 34: 82–4.
27 Ramesh V, Jain RK. Progeria in two brothers. *Aust J Derm* 1987; 28: 33–5.
28 Brown WT. Progeria: a human-disease model of accelerated ageing. *Am J Clin Nutr* 1992; 55: 1222S–4S.
29 Harper J, ed. *Inherited Skin Disorders*. Oxford: Butterworth Heineman, 1996.

Werner syndrome

Definition

This condition is perhaps the best example of a premature ageing syndrome, characterized by the combination of short stature, sclerodermatous skin, hypogonadism, proneness to diabetes, increased incidence of malignancy and early-onset greying, baldness, cataracts, atherosclerosis and osteoporosis.

History

Werner, in a 1904 doctoral thesis, first described this condition in four siblings [1]. Since then there have been over 200 patients reported, with recent emphasis on molecular mechanisms.

Aetiology and pathogenesis

The condition is clearly inherited as an autosomal recessive trait [2]. The gene maps to 8p12 [3,4] although a candidate gene has not yet been identified. As mentioned above, much work has been done to identify the genetic defect responsible for Werner syndrome (WS) [5–10]. In general, this work is based on reduced growth potential in cultured fibroblasts, as well as increased chromosome breaks and mutations in the cells of WS patients. The characterization of the spontaneous mutations has shown that deletions are primarily responsible [10]. One line of research has attempted to characterize gene function [8,9] and includes the findings of excessive fibronectin secretion and premature expression of DNA synthesis inhibitors. Another group has investigated the DNA ligation mechanism, and determined that in WS cells, the DNA ligation process was hypermutable and prone to error [10].

Pathology

Gawkrodger *et al.* [11] described skin biopsy findings in

one patient. The significant findings included hyalinization of dermal collagen, but no epidermal atrophy or loss of appendages. Electron microscopic evaluation demonstrated accumulation of amorphous material between normal collagen bundles.

Clinical features

Tannhauser [12] published 12 principle characteristics of WS. These are: (a) short stature, which is unusual in that the trunk is stocky but the extremities are thin—age of onset is in the second decade; (b) premature greying of the hair, with age of onset in the early 20s; (c) premature baldness, with onset in the 20s; (d) scleropoikiloderma-like skin; (e) trophic leg ulcers; (f) juvenile cataracts; (g) hypogonadism which is associated with reduced fertility; (h) tendency to develop diabetes; (i) calcification of blood vessels; (j) osteoporosis; (k) metastatic calcification; and (l) tendency to occur in families. Since that publication, which was in 1945, it has become clear that individuals with WS are at high risk of developing cancer [13,14], with the incidence over 10% [2]. The average age of diagnosis of WS is 38.7 years, with a range of 21–58 [15].

Prognosis

Average age of death is 47 years, with a range of 31–63 years. The most common causes of death are cardiovascular disease and malignancies [8]. Intellect is not impaired.

Differential diagnosis

Rothmund–Thomson syndrome closely resembles WS, but may be distinguished by its earlier age of onset. Acrometageria and mandibuloacral dysplasia may also be confused with WS.

Treatment

Rubin *et al.* [16] described the results of daily treatment with human insulin-like growth factor 1, and the resultant increase in bone density in a 43-year-old woman with WS. However no other symptoms were ameliorated.

REFERENCES

1 Werner CWO. *Uber Katarakt in Verbindung mit Sklerodermie.* Thesis, Kiel, Germany; Schmidt and Klauning; 1904.
2 Goto M, Tanimoto K, Horiuchi Y, Sasazuki T. Family analysis of Werner's syndrome: a survey of 42 Japanese families with a review of the literature. *Clin Genet* 1981; 19: 8–15.
3 Thomas W, Rubenstein M, Goto M, Drayna D. A genetic analysis of the Werner syndrome region on human chromosome 8p. *Genomics* 1993; 16: 685–90.
4 Goto M, Rubenstein M, Weber J, Woods K, Drayna D. Genetic linkage of Werner's syndrome to five markers on chromosome 8. *Nature* 1992; 355: 735–8.
5 Monnat RJ. Werner syndrome: molecular genetics and mechanistic hypotheses. *Exp Gerontol* 1992; 27: 447–53.
6 Poot M, Hoehn H, Runger TM, Martin GM. Impaired S-phase transit of Werner syndrome cells expressed in lymphoblastoid cell lines. *Exp Cell Res* 1992; 202: 267–73.
7 Faragher RGA, Kill IR, Hunter JAA, Pope M, Tannock C, Shall S. The gene responsible for Werner syndrome may be a cell division 'counting' gene. *Proc Natl Acad Sci* 1993; 90: 12030–4.
8 Thweatt R, Goldstein S. Werner syndrome and biological ageing: a molecular genetic hypothesis. *BioEssays* 1993; 15: 421–6.
9 Rasoamanantena P, Thweatt R, Labat-Robert J, Goldstein S. Altered regulation of fibronectin gene expression in Werner syndrome fibroblasts. *Exp Cell Res* 1994; 213: 121–7.
10 Runger TM, Bauer C, Dekant B *et al.* Hypermutable ligation of plasmid DNA ends in cells from patients with Werner syndrome. *J Invest Dermatol* 1994; 102: 45–8.
11 Gawkrodger DJ, Priestley GC, Vijayalaxmi, Ross JA, Narcisi P, Hunter JAA. Werner's syndrome. Biochemical and cytogenetic studies. *Arch Dermatol* 1985; 121: 636–41.
12 Thannhauser SJ. Werner's syndrome (progeria of the adult) and Rothmund's syndrome: two types of closely related heredofamilial atrophic dermatoses with juvenile cataracts and endocrine features: a critical study of five new cases. *Ann Intern Med* 1945; 23: 559–626.
13 Rosen RS, Cimini R, Coblenz D. Werner's syndrome. *Br J Radiol* 1970; 43: 193–8.
14 Bjornberg A. Werner's syndrome and malignancy. *Acta Derm Venereol (Stockh)* 1976; 56: 149–50.
15 Epstein CJ, Martin MG, Schultz AL, Motulsky AG. Werner's syndrome: a review of its symptomology, natural history, pathologic features, genetics, and relationship to the natural ageing process. *Medicine* 1966; 45: 177–221.
16 Rubin CD, Reed B, Sakhaee K, Pak CYC. Treating a patient with the Werner syndrome and osteoporosis using recombinant human insulin-like growth factor. *Ann Intern Med* 1994; 121: 665–8.

Cockayne's syndrome (see Chapter 19.22)

Cockayne's syndrome is a heterogeneous condition. The classic form is characterized by postnatal growth deficiency, cataracts, pigmentary retinopathy, skin photosensitivity, hearing loss and mental retardation. A severe form has been described, and includes prenatal growth deficiency and earlier onset of symptoms. A mild form has also been described, and includes normal growth and intelligence.

Rothmund–Thomson syndrome (see Chapter 19.23)

Rothmund–Thomson syndrome is an inherited disorder whose phenotype includes early childhood onset poikiloderma, with occasional occurrence of cataracts and skeletal anomalies. An increased risk of malignancy is one of the manifestations.

Conditions with skin atrophy/lipoatrophy

Wiedemann–Rautenstrauch syndrome
(SYN. NEONATAL PROGEROID SYNDROME)

Definition

Wiedemann–Rautenstrauch syndrome (WRS) is a premature ageing syndrome characterized by intrauterine growth retardation, short stature, typical facial appearance, natal teeth, lipoatrophy and paradoxical caudal fat accumulation. Fewer than 15 patients have been described.

History

Rautenstrauch and Snigula [1] first described two sisters with a progeria-like syndrome in 1977. Wiedemann [2] described two additional patients 2 years later; Devos *et al.* [3] suggested the eponym WRS.

Aetiology

This is almost certainly an autosomal recessive trait in that both affected siblings and parental consanguinity have been described [1,3,4]. The basic genetic defect is unknown, although Beavan *et al.* [5] described deficient decorin expression in one patient originally described by Rautenstrauch and Snigula. Decorin is a small proteoglycan which may interact with collagen I and II to influence the rate of fibril formation. However, the authors did not consider a decorin deficiency to be the primary defect, because decorin expression returned to normal levels in adolescence in that patient. Mazzarello *et al.* [6] described reduced thymidine kinase activity in skin fibroblasts, suggesting a DNA metabolism defect.

Pathology

Brain examination by Martin *et al.* [7] on the patient described by Devos *et al.* [3] showed a sudanophilic leucodystrophy with tigroid streaks. Hagadorn *et al.* [8] did not find this in their patient, and suggested heterogeneity may exist. Skin biopsy done on one patient only demonstrated marked hypoplasia of corium [9]. Proliferation rate of fibroblasts was half that of normal controls.

Clinical features

Affected individuals have intrauterine growth retardation with failure to thrive and short stature. The progeroid appearance is apparent at birth, with the phenotype consisting of a pseudohydrocephaloid appearance (although the occipitofrontal circumference is within normal limits), sparse hair, prominent scalp veins, widened anterior fontanelles and malar hypoplasia. One to four natal teeth are almost always present, with these teeth lost and subsequent dentition delayed. Skin is dry, thin and wrinkled. Hands and feet appear large. Generalized lipoatrophy is present, although paradoxical caudal fat accumulation occurs during childhood. One child also had fat accumulation in the axillae and on the proximal portion of the digits [9]. Feeding difficulties are common. Over time, the nose appears beaked. Mental retardation is invariably present with mild to severe levels reported. Joint contractures, cardiac defects, hydronephrosis and congenital hearing loss are occasional manifestations.

Prognosis

Longevity is unknown, with the oldest patients 16 years at the time of the report. One child died at the age of 5 years of bronchopneumonia. As noted above, mental retardation is present, with levels between mild and severe. One 16-year-old had developed ataxia [10].

Differential diagnosis

Natal teeth are present in Hallerman–Streiff, Ellis–van Creveld and Ullrich Fremerez–Dohna syndromes. Progeroid facial appearance at birth occurs in Hallermann–Streiff, Berardinelli–Seip, van Lohuizen's, Bamatter's and deBarsy's syndromes. The syndrome described by Petty *et al.* [11] should be distinguished from WRS.

REFERENCES

1 Rautenstrauch T, Snigula F. Progeria: a cell culture study and clinical report of familial inheritance. *Eur J Pediatr* 1977; 124: 101–11.
2 Wiedemann HR. An unidentified neonatal progeroid syndrome: follow up report. *Eur J Pediatr* 1979; 130: 65–70.
3 Devos EA, Leroy JG, Fryns JP, Van Den Berghe H. The Wiedemann–Rautenstrauch or neonatal progeroid syndrome: report of a patient with consanguineous parents. *Eur J Pediatr* 1981; 136: 245–8.
4 Castincyra G, Panal M, Presas HL, Goldschmidt E, Sanchez JM. Two sibs with Wiedemann–Rautenstrauch syndrome: possibilities of prenatal diagnosis by ultrasound. *J Med Genet* 1992; 29: 434–6.
5 Beavan LA, Quentin-Hoffmann E, Schonherr E, Snigula F, Leroy JG, Kresse H. Deficient expression of decorin in infantile progeroid patients. *J Biol Chem* 1993; 268: 9856–62.
6 Mazzarello P, Verri A, Mondello C *et al.* Enzymes of DNA metabolism in a patient with Wiedemann–Rautenstrauch progeroid syndrome. *Ann NY Acad Sci* 1992; 663: 440–1.
7 Martin JJ, Ceuterick CM, Leroy JG, Devos EA, Roelens JG. The Wiedemann–Rautenstrauch or neonatal progeroid syndrome. Neuropathological study of a case. *Neuropediatrics* 1984; 15: 43–8.
8 Hagadorn JI, Wilson WG, Hogge WA, Callicott JH, Beale EF. Neonatal progeroid syndrome: more than one disease? *Am J Med Genet* 1990; 35: 91–4.
9 Rudin C, Thommen L, Fliegel C, Steinmann B, Buhler U. The neonatal pseudohydrocephalic progeroid syndrome (Wiedemann–Rautenstrauch). *Eur J Pediatr* 1988; 147: 433–8.
10 Rautenstrauch T, Snigula F, Wiedemann HR. Neonatales progeroides syndrom (Wiedemann–Rautenstrauch). Eine follow-up studie. *Klin Padiatr* 1994; 206: 440–3.
11 Petty EM, Laxova R, Wiedemann HR. Previously unrecognized congenital progeroid disorder. *Am J Med Genet* 1990; 35: 383–7.

DeBarsy syndrome

Definition

DeBarsy syndrome phenotype consists of progeroid appearance, growth and mental retardation, cutis laxa, corneal clouding and athetoid movements.

History

DeBarsy *et al.* [1] described the combination of prenatal growth retardation, skin laxity, minor craniofacial anomalies, cloudy corneas, large anterior fontanelle with delayed closure and athetoid movements in a single girl in 1968. Since then several patients have been described, including three as unknown cases [2–11].

Aetiology and pathogenesis

This is clearly inherited as an autosomal recessive trait based on several examples of affected siblings. The basic genetic defect is unknown, although Karnes *et al.* [11] found that fibroblasts contained reduced levels of elastin messenger RNA (mRNA), which in turn could be attributable to decreased transcription or increased degradation of mRNA.

Pathology

Skin biopsy done by DeBarsy *et al.* [1] demonstrated normal epidermis, but thinner than normal dermis. The collagen fibres were described as having few fasciculations and elastic fibres were thin, short and decreased in number. Kunze *et al.* [3] described marked degeneration of the elastic and collagen fibres. Karnes *et al.* [11] also described decreased elastic fibres, as well as skin biopsy changes over time. In the neonatal period, their patient had hyperkeratosis and papillomatosis of the epidermis, with a deficiency of elastic fibres. At 10 months, the epidermis was normal and the dermis thin. The adnexal structures were located at the dermoepidermal junction instead of their usual location. Elastic fibres remained decreased in number and size.

Electron microscopy demonstrated variability in the collagen bundle size, as well as increased microfibrillar component of elastin and thinning of the amorphous component of elastin.

Clinical features

Children with DeBarsy syndrome generally have intrauterine growth retardation and subsequent slow growth. Corneal clouding or cataracts are virtually constant; and the facial phenotype is described as progeroid. Although few authors have delineated the specific features which contribute to this progeroid appearance, comparison of photographs of published patients suggests that the prominent forehead, prominent nasal bridge and thin lips are highly characteristic. The eyes usually appear deeply set. The ears are described as large and dysplastic, with a relatively unfolded helix. Hypotonia is a virtually constant findings, as is mild cutis laxa and thin wrinkled skin, particularly of the extremities. Small joints are often

hyperflexible, and hip dislocation or clubfoot occur frequently. Athetoid movements are common, but it is unclear whether it is present in all affected individuals. Mental retardation affects most, but not all.

Prognosis

Lifespan is unknown, because the oldest reported individual was 20 years old at the time of the report and did not have any life-threatening health problems.

Differential diagnosis

Apparently some children with DeBarsy syndrome are initially diagnosed as having WRS, but the presence of natal teeth and caudal fat accumulation in WRS should distinguish between the two. The other premature ageing syndromes should also be considered in the differential diagnosis.

Treatment

None is known.

REFERENCES

1 DeBarsy AM, Moens E, Dierckx L. Dwarfisms, oligophrenia and degeneration of the elastic tissue in skin and cornea: a new syndrome? *Helv Paediatr Acta* 1968; 23: 305–13.
2 Schierenberg M, Donne W, Schiafone P *et al*. De Barsy–Moens–Dierckx-Syndrom: ein ungewohnlicher Verlauf bei einem Fruhgeborenen. *Klin Padiatr* 1994; 206: 444–6.
3 Kunze J, Majewski F, Montgomery P, Hockey A, Karkut I, Riebel T. De Barsy syndrome—an autosomal recessive, progeroid syndrome. *Eur J Pediatr* 1985; 144: 348–54.
4 Stanton RP, Rao N, Scott CI. Orthopaedic manifestations in de Barsy syndrome. *J Pediatr Orthop* 1994; 14: 60–2.
5 Harrod MJ, Keele D, Stevenson RE. The De Barsy syndrome. *Proc Greenwood Genet Cent* 1984; 3: 134.
6 Hoefnagel D, Pomeroy J, Wurster D, Saxon A. Congenital athetosis, mental deficiency, dwarfism, and laxity of skin and ligaments. *Helv Paediatr Acta* 1971; 26: 397–402.
7 Burck U. De Barsy-Syndrom—eine weitere Beobachtung. *Klin Padiatr* 1974; 186: 441–4.
8 Riebel T. DeBarsy–Moens–Dierckx-Syndrom: Beobachtung bei Geschwistern. *Mschr Kinderheilk* 1976; 124: 96–8.
9 Siedel H, Stengel-Rutkowski S, Schimanek P, Miller K, Mertin B. Non-chromosomal dysmorphic syndromes (MCA/MR syndromes). 1. Similar abnormal phenotype in two mentally retarded brothers. *Dysmorph Clin Genet* 1987; 1: 101–8.
10 Saul R, ed. Unknown case (R.F.W.). *Proc Greenwood Genet Cent* 1983; 2: 70–1.
11 Karnes PS, Shamban AT, Olsen DR, Fazio MJ, Falk RE. De Barsy syndrome: report of a case, literature review, and elastic gene expression studies of the skin. *Am J Med Genet* 1992; 42: 29–34.

Acrometageria

Definition

This is a presumed spectrum of phenotypes which encompasses acrogeria, which primarily affects the hands and feet, and metageria, which involves the limbs as well as other structures.

History

Gottron [1] first described a progeroid syndrome which primarily affected the skin of the hands and feet. Since then, over 40 cases have been described. In 1974, Gilkes *et al.* [2] described two patients with phenotypes similar to but believed to be distinct from acrogeria and HGS or WS. Greally *et al.* [3] described in 1992 a boy with manifestations that overlapped between acrogeria and metageria, and hypothesized that there was a single entity which included acrogeria and metageria in the phenotypic spectrum. They suggested acrogeria as the name for this condition.

Aetiology and pathogenesis

Although most affected individuals are the only such family members affected, Kaufman *et al.* [4] described a pedigree consistent with autosomal dominant inheritance, in which one individual clinically had metageria and two others had acrogeria. The other cases therefore could represent fresh mutations. Although a defect in collagen III synthesis was suggested by Pope *et al.* [5] and Bouillie *et al.* [6], Bruckner-Tuderman *et al.* [7] did not find abnormal collagen III levels. It is possible that acrometageria is heterogeneous, or that patients with collagen III deficiency actually have a distinct connective tissue disorder, such as Ehlers–Danlos syndrome type IV.

Pathology

Meurer *et al.* [8] examined the skin in a man diagnosed with acrogeria. Subcutaneous fat was diminished. Dermal papillae were flattened, and there was orthokeratotic hyperkeratosis. Collagen fibre number was decreased, whereas elastin fibres were increased, although they were fragmented in appearance. The granular endoplasmic reticulum was dilated so cells appeared vacuolized. In the vacuoles as well as extracellular area, pseudoelastin was present. Bruckner-Tuderman *et al.* [7] also examined the skin from a patient with acrogeria, but noted differences between biopsy sites. These differences included reduced thickness of the dermis and more collagen bundle abnormalities in the foot specimen as compared to the axilla specimen. A third report of skin biopsy results did not note any abnormalities in a specimen taken from the buttock [3].

Clinical features

Clinical manifestations in patients with acrogeria were reviewed by Meurer *et al.* [8] and Greally *et al.* [3] and are essentially limited to the skin and skeleton. Cutaneous findings include skin atrophy of the extremities, particularly the hands and feet; atrophic nose tip; hyperpigmentation; dystrophic and thickened nails; hypertrophic scars; and in rare cases other cutaneous manifestations (e.g. psoriasis, scleroderma). Skeletal changes are minor, and are most often limited to short limbs. Other described changes include osteoporosis, acro-osteolysis and hypermobile joints [9].

The described cutaneous changes in metageria are more severe, and the phenotype also includes metabolic and cardiovascular changes. Skin manifestations include more severe atrophy affecting the limbs, thin scalp hair and generalized limb lipoatrophy. Metabolic disturbances are primarily limited to early-onset diabetes; cardiovascular changes consist of premature atherosclerosis. The facial phenotype includes beaked nose and prominent eyes.

Prognosis

In general, the lifespan is dependent on the severity of the diabetes and atherosclerosis, if present. Intellect appears unimpaired, although the patient of Greally *et al.* [3] was moderately mentally retarded.

Differential diagnosis

WS and DeBarsy's syndrome must be included in the differential diagnosis, but can be distinguished by age of onset in the case of WS, and phenotypic differences in the case of DeBarsy's syndrome.

Treatment

Diabetes and atherosclerosis should be treated.

REFERENCES

1 Gottron H. Famiare akrogerie. *Arch Derm Syph* 1941; 181: 571–83.
2 Gilkes JJH, Sharvill DE, Wells RS. The premature ageing syndromes. Reports of eight cases and description of a new entity named metageria. *Br J Dermatol* 1974; 91: 243–62.
3 Greally JM, Boon LY, Lenkey SG, Wenger SL, Steele MW. Acrometageria: a spectrum of 'premature ageing' syndromes. *Am J Med Genet* 1992; 44: 334–9.
4 Kauffman I, Thiele B, Mahrle G. Simultaneous occurrence of metageria and Gottron's acrogeria in one family. *Z Hautkr* 1985; 60: 975–84.
5 Pope FM, Nicholls AC, Jones PM, Wells RS, Lawrence D. EDS IV (acrogeria): new autosomal dominant and recessive types. *J Roy Soc Med* 1980; 73: 180–6.
6 Bouillie MC, Venencie PY, Thomine E, Ogier H, Puissant A, Lauret P. Syndrome d'Ehlers–Danlos type IV a type d'Acrogerie. *Ann Dermatol Vénéréol* 1986; 113: 1077–85.
7 Bruckner-Tuderman L, Vogel A, Schnyder UW. Fibroblasts of an acrogeria patient produce normal amounts of type I and III collagen. *Dermatology* 1987; 174: 157–65.
8 Meurer A, Lohmoller G, Keller C. Gottron's acrogeria and sarcoidosis. *Clin Invest* 1993; 71: 387–91.
9 Ho A, White SJ, Rasmussen JE. Skeletal abnormalities of acrogeria, a progeroid syndrome. *Skel Radiol* 1987; 16: 463–8.

Mandibuloacral dysplasia

Definition

This condition is characterized by the combination of short stature, progressive skeletal changes and skin abnormalities.

History

Cavallazzi *et al.* [1] first described this condition as an atypical form of cleidocranial dysostosis. Young *et al.* [2] termed this condition mandibuloacral dysplasia (MAD). Danks *et al.* [3] recognized that Cavallazzi *et al.*'s patient had MAD.

Aetiology and pathogenesis

The condition is inherited as an autosomal recessive trait, which seems to be most commonly reported in Italy [4–6]. The basic defect is unknown, but Friedenberg *et al.* [7] suggested that MAD is a form of lipoatrophic insulin-resistant diabetes mellitus. It has also been suggested that MAD may be heterogeneous [8], so multiple genetic defects may be responsible.

Pathology

Skin biopsy results described by Welsh [9] included moderate homogenization of the dermis and mild elastosis. Zina *et al.* [6] noted loss of rete pegs, but normal dermis and well-developed elastic fibres.

Clinical features

In the more typical cases, age of onset is between 3 and 14 years, with facial and digital changes occurring first. The phenotype consists of short stature; thin, hyperpigmented skin; partial alopecia; prominent eyes; beaked nose; tooth loss; micrognathia; short fingers; and on X-ray, evidence of bone resorption of the clavicles and distal phalanges. In areas of alopecia, prominent scalp veins are present. The skin is described as sclerodermoid in areas, and fingernails and toenails can be dystrophic or absent. Individuals with earlier onset of symptoms and more severe manifestations may be indicative of heterogeneity, or simply variability. These severely affected individuals tend to have most of the manifestations by 5 years of age, including total resorption of clavicles. Two have developed hard subcutaneous lumps which ultimately extrude through the skin [3,10]. The older of the two also had areas of subcutaneous tissue necrosis, and at the age of 27 years, had a tracheostomy for airway management and renal transplant for failure secondary to focal sclerosis. Finally, there exists a group of patients who have some manifestations of MAD, but are missing cardinal findings and have the presence of atypical manifestations. For example, some of the patients described by Friedenberg *et al.* [7] had normal stature, hearing loss and hepatomegaly.

Prognosis

Lifespan appears to be normal for individuals with a more typical presentation of MAD. It is unknown for those with a more severe phenotype. Intellect is unimpaired in any form.

Differential diagnosis

The most important condition to distinguish is cleidocranial dysostosis. In that condition, no skin changes occur, and the bony manifestations are present at birth. Pycnodysostosis should also be considered in the differential diagnosis, but as in cleidocranial dysostosis, no skin changes occur. There have also been descriptions of individuals with the diagnosis of progeria, but in whom MAD is suspected to be the correct diagnosis [11].

Treatment

There is none known.

REFERENCES

1 Cavallazzi C, Cremoncini R, Quadri A. Si du caso di disostosi cledio-cranica. *Rev Clin Pediatr* 1960; 65: 313–26.
2 Young LW, Radebaugh JF, Rubin P, Sensenbrenner JA, Fiorelli G. New syndrome manifested by mandibular hypoplasia, acroosteolysis, stiff joints and cutaneous atrophy (mandibulo-acral dysplasia) in two unrelated boys. *BDOAS* 1971; 7: 291–7.
3 Danks DM, Mayne V, Wettenhall HNB, Hall RK. Craniomandibular dermatodysostosis. *BDOAS* 1974; X: 99–105.
4 Tenconi R, Miotti F, Miotti A, Audino G, Ferro R, Clemente M. Another Italian family with mandibuloacral dysplasia: why does it seem more frequent in Italy? *Am J Med Genet* 1986; 24: 357–64.
5 Pallotta R, Morgese G. Mandibuloacral dysplasia: a rare progeroid syndrome. *Clin Genet* 1984; 26: 133–8.
6 Zina AM, Cravario A, Bundino S. Familial mandibuloacral dysplasia. *Br J Dermatol* 1981; 105: 719–23.
7 Friedenberg GR, Cutler DL, Jones MC *et al.* Severe insulin resistance and diabetes mellitus in mandibuloacral dysplasia. *Am J Dis Child* 1992; 146: 93–9.
8 Toriello HV. Mandibulo-acral dysplasia: heterogeneity versus variability. *Clin Dysmorph* 1995; 4: 12–24.
9 Welsh O. Study of a family with a new progeroid syndrome. *BDOAS* 1975; XI: 25–38.
10 Schrander-Stumpel C, Spaepen A, Fryns J-C, Dumon J. A severe case of mandibuloacral dysplasia in a girl. *Am J Med Genet* 1992; 43: 877–81.
11 Ramesh V, Jain RK. Progeria in two brothers. *Aust J Derm* 1987; 28: 33–5.

Lenz–Majewski syndrome

Definition

The Lenz–Majewski syndrome is a rare disorder of

progeroid appearance, facial and limb defects and skeletal anomalies.

History

Lenz and Majewski [1] first recognized that this condition, which had previously been described by Braham [2] and MacPherson [3] in patients diagnosed with craniodiaphyseal or diaphyseal dysplasia was a distinct entity. Robinow *et al.* [4] suggested the eponym. Gorlin and Whitley [5] and Chrzanowska *et al.* [6] also reported patients.

Aetiology and pathogenesis

Inheritance is unknown, but all previously reported patients had negative family histories for similarly affected individuals. This is probably an autosomal dominant trait, with all patients representing fresh mutations.

Pathology

Hood *et al.* [7] described the absence of elastin fibres in a child reported as a new syndrome who was later recognized as having Lenz–Majewski syndrome.

Clinical features

Affected individuals have pre- and postnatal growth retardation; a characteristic face with relative macrocephaly, frontal bossing, midface hypoplasia, short nose, long philtrum, thin upper lip and large posteriorly rotated ears; short hands and feet with marked cutaneous syndactyly; and loose, atrophic skin with prominent venous patterns. Mental retardation is present, and sensorineural deafness can also occur. Skeletal manifestations include sclerosis of the skull base, bone remodelling in tubular bones, various synostoses, and rib and vertebral anomalies.

Prognosis

The lifespan is unknown. Mental retardation can range from mild to severe. The bone changes are progressive.

Differential diagnosis

The conditions which need to be considered in the differential diagnosis, radiographically, include craniometaphyseal dysplasia, diaphyseal dysplasia and craniodiaphyseal dysplasia. However, other phenotypic manifestations should distinguish among these.

REFERENCES

1 Lenz WD, Majewski F. A generalized disorder of the connective tissues with progeria, choanal atresia, symphalangism, hypoplasia of the dentine, and craniodiaphyseal hypostosis. *BDOAS* 1974; X: 133–6.
2 Braham RL. Multiple congenital abnormalities with diaphyseal dysplasia (Camurati–Engelmann's syndrome). *Oral Surg* 1969; 27: 20–6.
3 MacPherson RI. Craniodiaphyseal dysplasia, a disease or group of diseases. *J Canad Assoc Radiol* 1974; 25: 22–3.
4 Robinow M, Johanson AJ, Smith T. The Lenz–Majewski hyperostotic dwarfism. *J Pediatr* 1977; 91: 417–21.
5 Gorlin RJ, Whitley CB. Lenz–Majewski syndrome. *Radiology* 1983; 149: 129–31.
6 Chrzanowska KH, Fryns J-P, Krajewska-Walasek M, Van den Berghe H, Wisniewski L. Skeletal dysplasia syndrome with progeriod appearance, characteristic facial and limb anomalies, multiple synostoses, and distinct skeletal changes: a variant example of the Lenz–Majewski syndrome. *Am J Med Genet* 1989; 32: 470–4.
7 Hood OJ, Lockhart LH, Hughes TE. Cutis laxa with craniofacial, limb, genital, and brain defects. *J Clin Dysmorph* 1984; 2: 23–6.

Mulvihill–Smith syndrome

Definition

A rare syndrome in which short stature, minor craniofacial anomalies, postnatal onset naevi and immunodeficiency occur.

History

The Mulvihill–Smith syndrome was described in 1975 [1] by the two authors after whom this condition is named, although Shepard [2] is now recognized as having published the first description of this rare syndrome. Elliott reported on the same patient in 1975 [3]. Since then, descriptions of three other definite [4–6] and one possible [7] patients have been published.

Aetiology and pathogenesis

The cause of this condition is unknown; all reported individuals have been the only such affected family member.

Pathology

Studies on skin have not been done.

Clinical features

Mulvihill–Smith syndrome is characterized by low birth weight in all but two patients, with subsequent short stature in all but the patient described by Ohashi *et al.* [7]. Microcephaly affected five out of six. The face is distinctive, with relative lack of subcutaneous fat, broad forehead, malar flattening, small and pointed chin and prominent ears. The voice is often highly pitched; hypodontia and irregular teeth are common. Most have sensorineural hearing loss.

The most characteristic finding is the pigmented naevi, which occur on all parts of the body. However, age at the appearance of the naevi is variable, with the naevi noted in the patient of Bartsch *et al.* [6] at the age of 1 year, in the patient of Baraitser *et al.* [5] at the age of 5–6 years and in the patient of Ohashi *et al.* [7] at the age of 25 years. Additional skin manifestations include normal subcutaneous fat distribution on the trunk and limbs, dryness and increased hirsutism. Immunodeficiency has been reported occasionally, with decreased levels of immunoglobulin A (IgA) and IgG. Advanced bone age was reported in one patient [5]. Mental retardation is an inconstant finding, ranging from severe to mild in those with this manifestation.

Prognosis

Lifespan is unknown, although several patients were adults at the time of the reports.

Differential diagnosis

Other progeroid syndromes need to be ruled out, although definitive diagnosis is difficult prior to the appearance of the naevi. The LEOPARD syndrome includes lentigines and short stature in the phenotype (plus electrocardiogram abnormalities, ocular hypertelorism, pulmonary stenosis, abnormalities of the genitalia and deafness), but can be distinguished by the characteristic facial appearance in Mulvihill–Smith syndrome.

Treatment

None is known, other than for infections when they occur.

REFERENCES

1 Mulvihill JJ, Smith DW. Another disorder with prenatal shortness of stature and premature ageing. *BDOAS* 1975; XI: 368–71.
2 Shepard MK. An unidentified syndrome with abnormality of skin and hair. *BDOAS* 1971; VII: 353–4.
3 Elliott DE. Undiagnosed syndrome of psychomotor retardation, low birthweight dwarfism, skeletal, dental, dermal and genital anomalies. *BDOAS* 1975; XI: 364–7.
4 Wong W, Cohen MM, Miller M, Pruzansky S, Rosenthal IM, Solomon LM. Case report for syndrome identification. *Cleft Palate J* 1979; 16: 286–90.
5 Baraitser M, Insley J, Winter RM. A recognisable short stature syndrome with premature ageing and pigmented naevi. *J Med Genet* 1986; 25: 53–6.
6 Bartsch O, Tympner K-D, Schwinger E, Gorlin RJ. Mulvihill–Smith syndrome: case report and review. *J Med Genet* 1994; 31: 707–11.
7 Ohashi H, Tsukahara M, Murano I *et al.* Premature ageing and immunodeficiency: Mulvihill–Smith syndrome? *Am J Med Genet* 1993; 45: 597–600.

Lenaert syndrome

Definition

This is a rare hereditary syndrome which includes premature ageing, joint dislocations and minor craniofacial anomalies among the phenotypic manifestations.

History

Only one family has been described, by Lenaerts *et al.* in 1994 [1].

Aetiology and pathogenesis

This condition is likely inherited as an autosomal dominant trait, although X-linked dominant inheritance cannot be excluded. The basic genetic defect is unknown.

Pathology

None is known.

Clinical features

Full expression of this condition is characterized by short stature; sparse hair and blue sclerae; thin nose; thin lips; joint anomalies, including large joint hyperlaxity; subluxation of the interphalangeal joints of the hands and feet, and talipes equinovarus; carpal synostosis; and thin skin with lower extremity livedo reticularis. Documented panhypogammaglobulinaemia developed during adulthood in the proposita, but may have affected others in the family as well.

Prognosis

This is apparently normal for lifespan and intellectual functioning.

Differential diagnosis

This condition most closely resembles Larsen's syndrome with regards to joint dislocations, but can be distinguished by the additional skin and immune system findings.

Treatment

Antibiotics for infections or intravenous provision of γ-globulin may be indicated.

REFERENCE

1 Lenaerts J, Fryns JP, Westhovens R, Dequeker J. A familial syndrome of dwarfism, bilateral club feet, premature ageing and progressive panhypogammaglobulinemia. *J Rheumatol* 1994; 21: 961–3.

Conditions with skin laxity

Cutis laxa (see Chapter 19.18)

Cutis laxa refers to loose skin which tends to hang in folds and may be inherited or acquired. Autosomal dominant and recessive forms have been described. Alibert [1] is attributed with the first description of autosomal recessive cutis laxa, which was published in 1833. Rossbach [2] described the first instance of autosomal dominant cutis laxa in 1884.

REFERENCES

1 Alibert JL. Histoire d'un berger des invirons de Gisore (dermatose hypermorphe). *Monogr Dermatol* 1833; 2: 719.
2 Rossbach MJ. Ein merkwurdiger Fall von greisenhafter Veranderung der allgemeinen Korperdecke bei einem achtzehnjahrigen Jungling. *Dtsch Arch Klin Med* 1884; 36: 197–203.

Cutis laxa–mental retardation syndrome

Definition

This is a form of cutis laxa which accompanies growth retardation, ligamentous laxity, joint dislocation and developmental delay.

History

This entity was first delineated as a distinct condition in 1971 [1], although other patients had been previously reported under different diagnoses [2–4]. Since then over 25 patients have been described [5–13].

Aetiology and pathogenesis

The cause is thought to be either an X-linked dominant gene mutation or homozygosity for an autosomal recessive condition. The former suggestion is based on a significant preponderance of affected females among reported females. The presence of several sibling pairs indicates an autosomal recessive inheritance.

Skin biopsies have generally shown decreased or absent elastin. A detailed description of skin biopsy findings included loose and dispersed papillary and upper reticular dermis. Elastic fibres were absent in this part of the dermis and upper corium. In the lower dermis, elastic fibres were malformed. Electron microscopy demonstrated sparse microfibrillar bundles. The reticular dermis contained only primitive elastic tissue with loose granular fibrillar material replacing the normal peripheral elastic microfibrils [12].

Clinical features

Affected individuals usually have prenatal and postnatal growth retardation, with weight more severely affected than height. Congenital hip dislocation is common. Cutis laxa and ligamentous laxity affects all reported individuals to some degree; prominent vasculature and/or telangiectasias on the abdomen have also been described in some. Craniofacial anomalies are common, and include large fontanelles which show delayed closure, blue sclerae, broad nasal bridge, downslanting palpebral fissures, prominent nose, long philtrum, highly arched palate and apparently low-set ears. Inguinal and/or umbilical hernias are common; hydronephrosis also occurs.

Prognosis

The lifespan is unknown. Mental retardation is variable, with severe to mild degrees of retardation reported.

Differential diagnosis

This includes other forms of cutis laxa and DeBarsy's syndrome, but can be distinguished by the presence and pattern of other phenotypic manifestations.

Treatment

None is known.

REFERENCES

1 Reisner SH, Seelenfreund M, Ben-Bassat M. Cutis laxa associated with severe intrauterine growth retardation and congenital dislocation of the hip. *Acta Paediatr Scand* 1971; 60: 357–60.
2 Debre R, Marie J, Seringe P. Cutis laxa avec dystrophies osseuses. *Bull Soc Med Hop Paris* 1937; 53: 1038.
3 Fittke H. Uber eine ungewohnliche form 'multipler Erbartung' (Chalodermie und Dysostose). *Z Kinderheilk* 1943; 63: 510.
4 Bittel-Dobrzynska N, Sinieki B. 'Cutis Laxa' (Zespol Ehlers–Danlos) Z Wrobzonym Zwichnieciem Stawow Biodrowych. *Endokrynol Pol* 1964; 15: 469–79.
5 Allanson J, Austin W, Hecht F. Congenital cutis laxa with retardation of growth and motor development: a recessively inherited disorder of connective tissue with male lethality. *Clin Genet* 1986; 29: 133–6.
6 Fitzsimmons JS, Fitzsimmons EM, Guibert PR, Zaldua V, Dodd KL. Variable clinical presentation of cutis laxa. *Clin Genet* 1985; 28: 284–95.
7 Karrar ZA. Letter to the editor: cutis laxa, ligamentous laxity and delayed development. *Pediatrics* 1984; 74: 903–4.
8 Lambert D, Beer F, Jeannin-Magnificat C *et al*. Cutis laxa generalisee congenitale. *Ann Dermatol Vénéréol* 1983; 110: 129–38.
9 Patton MA, Tolmie J, Ruthnum P, Bamforth S, Baraitser M, Pembrey M. Congenital cutis laxa with retardation of growth and development. *J Med Genet* 1987; 24: 556–61.
10 Philip AGS. Cutis laxa with intrauterine growth retardation in a male. *J Pediatr* 1978; 93: 150–1.
11 Sakati NO, Nyhan WL, Shear CS *et al*. Syndrome of cutis laxa, ligamentous laxity, and delayed development. *Pediatrics* 1983; 72: 850–6.
12 Ogur G, Yuksel-Apak M, Demiryont M. Syndrome of congenital cutis laxa with ligamentous laxity and delayed development: report of a brother and sister from Turkey. *Am J Med Genet* 1990; 37: 6–9.

13 Goldblatt J, Wallis C, Viljoen D, Beighton P. Cutis laxa, retarded development and joint hypermobility syndrome. *Dysmorph Clin Genet* 1988; 1: 142–4.

Wrinkly skin syndrome

Definition

This is a relatively rare condition characterized by wrinkled skin on the hands, feet and abdomen, multiple skeletal anomalies, microcephaly and mental retardation.

History

Gazit *et al.* [1] first described three siblings with this entity and recognized it as a unique syndrome. Since then, at least six other patients have been described [2–5], almost exclusively in individuals of Middle Eastern ethnic origin.

Aetiology and pathogenesis

The condition is inherited as an autosomal recessive trait, although the exact gene defect is unknown.

Pathology

Skin biopsy findings were described by Casamassima *et al.* [4]. The only abnormality seen was decreased number of shorter than average dermal elastic fibres. Fragmentation of the fibres was not present. Electron microscopy did not show any unusual findings.

Clinical features

Children may have microcephaly, facial asymmetry and relatively expressionless face. Skeletal findings include hip dislocation, kyphosis and/or scoliosis. Hypotonia is common, but not always associated with mental retardation which can also occur. Skin findings are striking, and include a prominent venous pattern on the chest, hands and feet; wrinkled skin on the dorsum of the hands, feet and abdomen; increased palmar creases; and poor elasticity, as evidenced by decreased recoil. Joint hypermobility has also been described.

Prognosis

This is unknown, since all patients were children at the time of the report. One child developed an atrial septal aneurysm by 5.5 years [4], so cardiac complications could potentially shorten the lifespan. Mental retardation, when present, was in the moderate to mild range. It did not correlate with the presence of microcephaly.

Differential diagnosis

Other syndromes with wrinkly skin, such as DeBarsy's syndrome, gerodermia osteodysplastica, cutis laxa and cutis laxa with mental retardation can all resemble the wrinkly skin syndrome, but can be distinguished by other phenotypic manifestations and/or skin biopsy findings. Kreuz and Wittwer [5] described a mother and two sons with chromosome 2q deletions (del(2)(q32)). These individuals had wrinkly skin, but also had more craniofacial anomalies, ataxic gait and an unusual grimace. However, this suggests that a child with wrinkly skin merits a karyotype test.

Treatment

None is known.

REFERENCES

1 Gazit E, Goodman RM, Bat-Miriam Katznelson M, Rotem Y. The wrinkly skin syndrome: a new heritable connective tissue disorder. *Clin Genet* 1973; 4: 186–92.
2 Karrar ZA, Elidrissy ATH, Al Arabi K, Adam A. The wrinkly skin syndrome: a report of two siblings from Saudi Arabia. *Clin Genet* 1983; 23: 308–10.
3 Hurvitz SA, Baumgarten A, Goodman RM. The wrinkly skin syndrome: a report of a case and review of the literature. *Clin Genet* 1990; 38: 307–13.
4 Casamassima AC, Wesson SK, Conlon CJ, Weiss FH. Wrinkly skin syndrome: phenotype and additional manifestations. *Am J Med Genet* 1987; 27: 885–93.
5 Kreuz FR, Wittwer BH. Del(2q)—cause of the wrinkly skin syndrome? *Clin Genet* 1993; 43: 132–8.

Gerodermia osteodysplastica

Definition

The phenotype of this condition includes characteristic face, growth retardation and skin and joint hyperlaxity [1].

Pathology

Skin biopsy findings reported by Hunter [8] included non-specific fragmentation of osteodysplastica.

History

Bamatter *et al.* [2] described an affected family first in 1949, and subsequently over the next 20 years [3–5].

Aetiology and pathogenesis

The inheritance was considered to be X-linked originally [5], but is now known to be autosomal recessive [6,7]. The basic gene defect is unknown.

Clinical features

Facial manifestations include what has been described as a sad appearance, probably attributable to the sagging skin. More specifically, eyelids and cheeks droop, and the lower lip is downturned. There is also a prominent forehead, flat midface, prominent fleshy nose and relative prognathism. Malocclusion and highly arched palate are common. The skin on the rest of the body is thin and wrinkled without recoil. Musculoskeletal manifestations include hypotonia, inguinal herniae, joint laxity and osteoporosis. Fractures are common. Approximately one-third of patients have stature below the third centile; in the remaining patients, upper segment/lower segment or span/height ratios are outside the normal range, with upper segment/lower segment <1 and span/height >1.

Prognosis

Lifespan is unknown. Although gross motor delays are common, cognitive function is probably normal [8].

Differential diagnosis

Other cutis laxa syndromes should be considered in the differential diagnosis. Cutis laxa with mental retardation is especially similar, to the point that Hunter [8] suggests that two of the patients diagnosed with cutis laxa–mental retardation reported by Patton *et al*. [9] actually had gerodermia osteodysplastica.

REFERENCES

1 Gorlin RJ, Cohen MM Jr. Craniofacial manifestations of Ehlers–Danlos syndromes, cutis laxa syndromes, and cutis laxa-like syndromes. *BDOAS* 1989; XXV: 39–71.
2 Bamatter F, Franschetti A, Klein D *et al*. Gerodermie osteodysplastique hereditaire. Un noveau biotype de la progeria. *Confin Neurol* 1949; 9: 397.
3 Bamatter F, Franschetti A, Klein D *et al*. Gerodermie osteodysplastique hereditaire. *Ann Paediatr* 1950; 174: 126–7.
4 Boreux G. La gerodermie osteodysplastique a heredite liee au sexe nouvelle entite clinique et genetique. *J Genet Hum* 1969; 17: 137–8.
5 Klein D, Bamatter F, Franschetti A *et al*. Une affection liee au sexe: la gerodermie osteodysplastique hereditaire (20 ans d'observation). *Rev Otoneuro-ophthalmol* 1968; 40: 415–21.
6 Hunter AGW, Martsolf JT, Baker CG. Gerodermal osteodysplastica—report of two affected families. *Hum Genet* 1978; 40: 311–24.
7 Hall BD. Geroderma osteodysplastica: a rare autosomal recessive connective tissue disorder with either variability or heterogeneity or both. *Proc Greenwood Genet Cent* 1983; 2: 101–2.
8 Hunter AGW. Is geroderma osteodysplastica underdiagnosed? *J Med Genet* 1988; 25: 854–6.
9 Patton MA, Tolmie J, Ruthnum P *et al*. Congenital cutis laxa with retardation of growth and development. *J Med Genet* 1987; 24: 556–61.

Costello syndrome

Definition

Costello syndrome is a multiple congenital anomaly syndrome characterized by the combination of postnatal onset poor growth, typical facial appearance, developmental delay and nasal papillomas. The skin exhibits cutis laxa.

History

Two children were first described in 1971 and again in 1977 by Costello [1,2]. Subsequently, other examples have been reported in the literature [3–7] with debate regarding whether children described by Borochowitz *et al*. [8–13] had Costello syndrome or a distinct entity. Resolution of this issue is important, because the two conditions probably have different modes of inheritance.

Aetiology and pathogenesis

Inheritance of this condition appears to be autosomal recessive, if the cases described by Borochowitz *et al*. [8] and Berberich *et al*. [14] are accepted as having Costello syndrome. If the conditions are deemed to be distinct, then Costello syndrome could be caused by fresh mutations for an autosomal dominant gene or submicroscopic chromosome deletion. The basic genetic defect is unknown.

Pathology

Skin biopsy has demonstrated normal elastic tissue.

Clinical features

Because of postnatal failure to thrive, the head looks too large for the body, leading to the appearance of relative macrocephaly. Ectodermal defects include slow-growing brittle hair which tends to become curly; soft, slow-growing nails; lax skin particularly on the hands and feet, with deep palmar and plantar creases; and papillomas which occur not only in the perinasal region, but also in other areas (e.g. perianal, perioral, etc.); and development of pigmented naevi and acanthosis nigricans. The voice is often hoarse.

Prognosis

Developmental delay is significant, with IQ scores in a 10-year-old child of 40–49. Lifespan is unknown, but cardiac defects or cardiomyopathy, when present, may affect this. There have also been reports of tumours in children with this condition.

Differential diagnosis

There are several similarities to the Noonan and cardiofaciocutaneous syndromes, but phenotypic differences should distinguish among them. As noted above, it is unresolved whether the children reported by Borochowitz *et al.* [8] have the same condition.

Treatment

Nutritional support does not alleviate growth failure. Orthopaedic intervention may be necessary for valgus deformities or hip dislocation.

REFERENCES

1 Costello JM. A new syndrome. *NZ Med J* 1971; 74: 397.
2 Costello JM. A new syndrome: mental subnormality and nasal papillomata. *Aust Paediatr J* 1977; 13: 114–18.
3 Der Kaloustian VM, Noroz B, McIntosh N, Watters AK, Blaichman S. Costello syndrome. *Am J Med Genet* 1991; 41: 69–73.
4 Martin RA, Jones KL. Delineation of Costello syndrome. *Am J Med Genet* 1991; 41: 346–9.
5 Say B, Gucsavas M, Morgan H, York C. The Costello syndrome. *Am J Med Genet* 1993; 47: 163–5.
6 Teebi AS, Shabaani IS. Further delineation of Costello syndrome. *Am J Med Genet* 1993; 47: 166–8.
7 Zampino G, Mastroiacovo P, Ricci R *et al.* Costello syndrome: further clinical delineation, natural history, genetic definition, and nosology. *Am J Med Genet* 1993; 47: 176–83.
8 Borochowitz Z, Pavone L, Mazor G, Rizzo R, Dar H. New multiple congenital anomalies: mental retardation syndrome (MCA/MR) with facio-cutaneous-skeletal involvement. *Am J Med Genet* 1992; 42: 678–85.
9 Philip N, Mancini J. Costello syndrome and facio-cutaneous-skeletal syndrome. *Am J Med Genet* 1993; 47: 176–83.
10 Martin RA, Jones KL. Facio-cutaneous-skeletal syndrome is the Costello syndrome. *Am J Med Genet* 1993; 47: 169.
11 Der Kaloustian VM. Not a new MCA/MR syndrome but probably Costello syndrome? *Am J Med Genet* 1993; 47: 170–1.
12 Teebi AS. Costello or facio-cutaneous-skeletal syndrome? *Am J Med Genet* 1993; 47: 172.
13 Borochowitz Z, Pavone L, Mazor G, Rizzo R, Dar H. Facio-cutaneous-skeletal syndrome. *Am J Med Genet* 193; 47: 173.
14 Berberich MS, Carey JC, Hall BD. Resolution of the perinatal and infantile failure to thrive in a new autosomal recessive syndrome with the phenotype of a storage disorder and furrowing of the palmar creases. *Proc Greenwood Genet Cent* 1991; 10: 98.

Hernandez (Ehlers–Danlos-like) syndrome

Definition

This rare condition includes Ehlers–Danlos-like skin changes, mild mental retardation, multiple naevi and progeroid face in the phenotype.

History

This condition was first described by Hernandez *et al.* in 1979 [1], and further delineated in 1981 and 1986 [2,3].

Aetiology and pathogenesis

The inheritance is unknown, but presumed to be autosomal dominant with all reported cases representing fresh mutations. A connective tissue defect is thought to be the cause of this condition.

Pathology

A skin biopsy was done on one patient, and did not demonstrate epidermal or dermal defects at the light microscopic level. Using electron microscopy, there was slight distension of intracellular spaces in the epidermal spinous layer, and fragmentation of elastic fibres.

Clinical features

Birth weight was normal, but subsequent growth was slow, with short stature present in all but one affected patient. Hair was curly and fine, with partial alopecia of the eyebrows and eyelashes. The face was characterized by telecanthus, wrinkling of the skin and periodontitis/multiple caries. Ears were low set and prominent. Other manifestations included pectus excavatum, winged scapulae, cryptorchidism, inguinal herniae, hypospadias, pes planus, joint hypermobility and varicose veins. One patient each had aortic stenosis and brachydactyly E. Dermatological findings included skin hyperextensibility, dermatorrhexis, easy bruising, papyraceous scars and multiple naevi.

Prognosis

The lifespan is unknown; the oldest patient was 15 years at the time of the report. The IQ was 55–70 (mild mental retardation).

Differential diagnosis

Other forms of Ehlers–Danlos syndrome most clearly resemble this condition, but mental retardation, naevi and minor facial anomalies do not occur with the former.

Treatment

None is known.

REFERENCES

1 Hernandez A, Aguirre-Negrete MG, Ramirez-Soltero S *et al.* A distinct variant of the Ehlers–Danlos syndrome. *Clin Genet* 1979; 16: 335–9.
2 Hernandez A, Aguirre-Negrete MG, Liparoli JC, Cantu JM. Third case of a distinct variant of the Ehlers–Danlos syndrome. *Clin Genet* 1981; 20: 222–4.
3 Hernandez A, Aguirre-Negrete MG, Gonzalez-Flores S *et al.* Ehlers–Danlos features with progeroid facies and mild mental retardation. *Clin Genet* 1986; 30: 456–61.

Kresse syndrome

Definition

This is a provisionally unique syndrome consisting of

growth and developmental delay, hypotonia and multiple connective tissue disorders.

History

Kresse *et al.* [1] described a male patient with a progeroid appearance, mental retardation, and multiple other anomalies. Quentin *et al.* [2] later studied the biochemical defect in this patient.

Aetiology and pathogenesis

The condition is inherited as an autosomal recessive trait. Quentin *et al.* [2] demonstrated that cultured fibroblasts from the child were severely deficient in galactosyltransferase I, and partially deficient in galactosyltransferase II. The authors suggested the gene coded for a subunit common to both galactosyltransferases.

Pathology

None is described.

Clinical features

At birth, the proband had normal birth weight, length and head circumference, although some minor dysmorphic features were noted. Failure to thrive was present, and by the end of the first year, development was delayed. Craniofacial manifestations included triangular face, prominent eyes, small mouth, highly arched palate, hypoplastic uvula and small earlobes. The skin was loose and elastic. Wound healing was abnormal, with formation of atrophic scars. Skin on the palms and soles was thick; sweating was normal. Hair was scanty, and teeth were brown and carious. Minor skeletal anomalies included short clavicles with broad ends, splaying of ribs and postnatal onset osteopenia. Bone age was advanced.

Prognosis

Moderate mental retardation and hypotonia occurred. No health concerns were present, so lifespan is likely to be within normal limits.

Differential diagnosis

The skin manifestations resemble Ehlers–Danlos syndrome, whereas facial appearance may resemble Russell–Silver syndrome. Other progeroid syndromes such as DeBarsy's or Cockayne's syndrome, or progeria, can also be distinguished.

Treatment

None is known, other than symptomatic, such as orthopaedic intervention if indicated.

REFERENCES

1 Kresse H, Rosthoj S, Quentin E *et al.* Glycosaminoglycan-free small proteoglycan core protein is secreted by fibroblasts from a patient with a syndrome resembling progeroid. *Am J Hum Genet* 1987; 41: 436–53.
2 Quentin E, Gladen A, Roden L, Kresse H. A genetic defect in the biosynthesis of dermatan sulfate proteoglycan: galactosyltransferase I deficiency in fibroblasts from a patient with a progeroid syndrome. *Proc Natl Acad Sci* 1990; 87: 1342–6.

Conditions in which individuals appear aged

Marfanoid ageing syndrome

Definition

This is a provisionally unique condition present in a single patient, which is characterized by a marfanoid appearance, premature ageing and primary hypogonadism.

History

This was described in a single patient by Gershoni-Baruch *et al.* [1], although the authors cite a previous report of a similarly affected patient [2].

Aetiology and pathogenesis

The cause of this condition is unknown; both affected individuals had negative family histories.

Pathology

None is described.

Clinical features

The reported individual had a so-called marfanoid habitus, with altered upper segment/lower segment and span/height ratios consistent with those found in individuals with Marfan's syndrome; however, it is noteworthy that the patient's height was only at the 5th centile for Marfan individuals. Other marfanoid manifestations included pectus excavatum, kyphoscoliosis, per planus, camptodactyly and arachnodactyly. The face was characterized by elongation, deviation of the nasal septum, highly arched palate, prognathism and prominent ears. Premature ageing was characterized merely as the man looking 'older than his age'. Additional manifestations included fatty nodules on the back, recurrent inguinal hernias and small testes. Bilateral anterior subluxation of cataractous lenses were diagnosed at the age of 26 years. Aortic stenosis and insufficiency were also noted at this time. During aortic valve replacement surgery, an ascending aortic enlargement and a bicuspid aortic valve were found. Infertility evaluation documented primary hypogonadism. Pertinent dermatological findings included non-hyperextensible skin and no history of easy bruising.

Prognosis

Lifespan is unknown. The described patient died at the age of 44 years of a suspected pulmonary embolus.

Differential diagnosis

Marfan's syndrome is the primary condition to consider in the differential diagnosis, but can be distinguished by the presence of hypogonadism and premature ageing. Homocystinuria, Ehlers–Danlos syndrome and cutis laxa also need to be considered in the differential diagnosis.

Treatment

Treatment is dependent on the symptoms.

REFERENCES

1 Gershoni-Baruch R, Moor EV, Enat R. Marfan syndrome associated with bicuspid aortic valve, premature ageing, and primary hypogonadism. *Am J Med Genet* 1990; 37: 169–72.
2 Nagant de Deuxchaisnes C, Huaux JP, Vandooren-Deflorenne R, LaChapelle JM. Pachydermoperiostose, cryptorchidie, et aspect marfanoiide. *Arch Belg Dermatol Syph* 1967; 23: 121–5.

Lee syndrome

Definition

This is a unique genetic condition characterized by branchial cleft sinuses, pre- and postaxial growth retardation and premature ageing.

History

This combination has only been reported in a mother and son [1].

Aetiology and pathogenesis

Autosomal dominant inheritance is suggested by the presence of the condition in mother and son.

Pathology

Skin biopsies done on both individuals were histologically normal, although actinic changes were present in the mother's specimen.

Clinical features

Pre- and postnatal growth deficiency occur, with adult height in the mother being 146.7 cm. Bilateral branchial cleft sinuses and nasolacrimal duct obstruction were present in both. Craniofacial anomalies include upslanting, short palpebral fissures, broad nose, protruding upper lip, downturned corners of the mouth and prominent ears. The mother had premature greying of the hair at age 18 years of age and aged appearance, as manifested by multiple fine facial wrinkles by the age of 38 years. Cataracts and bilateral deafness had already developed by this age. Intelligence was normal.

Prognosis

This is apparently normal for lifespan and intellectual development.

Differential diagnosis

Other branchial arch syndromes such as branchio-otodysplasia and branchio-otorenal dysplasia need to be considered, but can be distinguished by lack of short stature in those syndromes. There are also superficial similarities to WS and Rothmund–Thomson syndromes.

Treatment

Surgical excision of branchial cleft sinuses and relief of nasolacrimal duct obstruction may be indicated.

REFERENCE

1 Lee WK, Root AW, Fenske N. Bilateral branchial cleft sinuses associated with intrauterine and postnatal growth retardation, premature ageing, and unusual facial appearance: a new syndrome with dominant transmission. *Am J Med Genet* 1982; 11: 345–52.

Berlin syndrome

Definition

The combination of ectodermal defects, growth and mental retardation, and minor facial and genital anomalies characterize this rare syndrome.

History

The condition was first described in four siblings by Berlin in 1961 [1]. It is considered by the London Dysmorphology Database to be provisionally unique.

Aetiology and pathogenesis

A skin biopsy demonstrated normal stratum corneum but reduced thickness of the Malpighian layer. The papillary border was flattened; it and the cutis contained chromatophores. Abnormal pigment distribution was noted in the basal layer and upper epidermis.

Clinical features

The affected individuals are short, with a thin habitus. Scalp hair is dry with a tendency to premature greyness. Eyebrows are sparse, the nose is flat and there are deep furrows around the eyes and mouth. Telangiectasias are present on the lips. The number of teeth is reduced, with the first and second dentition delayed. Females have normal sexual development, whereas males have hypospadias and small external genitalia. The skin is pale, dry and thin, with generalized hyper- and hypopigmentation. Poikiloderma-like lesions occur on the elbows, knees and proximal interphalangeal joints. The palms and soles have hyperkeratosis with mild hyperhidrosis. Sweating is normal elsewhere.

Prognosis

Mild mental retardation affected all patients. The oldest was 29 years at the time of the report, and had no significant health problems.

Differential diagnosis

WS and Rothmund–Thomson syndrome resemble this condition most closely, but can be distinguished from them by the lack of leg ulcers and cataracts.

Treatment

None is known.

REFERENCE

1 Berlin C. Congenital generalized melanoleucoderma associated with hypodontia, hypotrichosis, stunted growth and mental retardation occurring in two brothers and two sisters. *Dermatologica* 1961; 123: 227.

19.22   Xeroderma Pigmentosum, Cockayne's Syndrome and Trichothiodystrophy

ANNETTE WAGNER

Xeroderma pigmentosum
De Sanctis–Cacchione syndrome
Complementation group A
Complementation group B
Complementation group C
Complementation group D
Complementation group E, F and G
Variant complementation group

Cockayne's syndrome

Trichothiodystrophy (Tay's syndrome, BIDS, IBIDS, PIBIDS)

Xeroderma pigmentosum

Definition

Xeroderma pigmentosum (XP) is a rare, autosomal recessive disease characterized by photosensitivity, photodamage, cutaneous malignancies, severe ophthalmological abnormalities and, often, early death from malignancy. Neurological complications are present in 20% of patients [1]. The cells of patients with XP are defective in DNA repair resulting in clinical and cellular hypersensitivity to ultraviolet (UV) radiation.

History

XP was first described by Hebra and Kaposi in 1874 in a series of six young patients with photodistributed pigmentation and skin atrophy [2]. In 1882, Kaposi introduced the term 'XP', emphasizing the pigmented dry skin seen in these patients [3]. Although he recognized the inherited nature of the disease and the localization of the multiple skin tumours to sun-exposed areas of the body, he could not speculate on the underlying cause of the disease.

It was not until 1968 that the pathogenic defect was identified. Cleaver found that cells from individuals with this syndrome were defective in DNA excision repair [4]. Irradiation of fibroblasts from patients with XP with UV light forms covalently linked ring structures called dimers. These dimers modify the structure of the DNA and interfere with vital cell function such as DNA replica-

tion and transcription. Normal cells repair such altered DNA by excising these dimers and replacing them with single-stranded segments of newly synthesized DNA in a complex series of enzymatic reactions. DNA replication is normally restricted to the S phase of the cell cycle, just prior to cell division. Excision repair, however, can occur at any time during the cycle, and is called 'unscheduled'. Compared with normal cells, Cleaver found that XP cells exhibited decreased rates and extents of unscheduled DNA synthesis. Setlow *et al.* went on to produce evidence that XP cells were defective in the first step in repair of UV damage to DNA, the removal of pyrimidine dimers [5–7].

The excision repair defect was demonstated *in vivo* by Epstein *et al.* in 1970 [8]. All cell types were shown to be affected including epidermal cells, fibroblasts, conjunctival cells, corneal cells and lymphocytes.

In 1972, de Weerd-Kastelein *et al.* fused together fibroblasts from different patients with XP to form heteropolykaryons (multinucleated cells containing nuclei from the two different strains) [9]. They were able to demonstrate correction of the excision repair defect in these heteropolykaryons suggesting that different genetic defects could produce similar phenotypic disease [9]. Groups of patients whose cells failed to complement each other in culture were placed within a single complementation group. In this manner, seven complementation groups of XP have now been identified and are designated A–G [10]. Two additional groups, H and I, were originally described [11,12], but have subsequently been found to overlap with previous groups and have been reassigned to groups D and C, respectively [13–15]. A variant complementation group has also been identified with similar clinical disease but normal unscheduled DNA synthesis [16,17]. It is possible that the defect in these patients is in postreplication repair or in a totally different pathway [18].

Although patients with XP within different complementation groups clearly have different genetic defects, the converse is not true. Identical repair defects are not necessarily present in all members of one complementation group. Clinical variability within complementation groups suggests differences exist that are not detectable with complementation assays.

Much has been learned about the details of excision repair in mammalian cells since Bootsma first described the complementation groups of XP. More than 20 polypeptides are now known to participate in the complete process [19]. The genes or proteins for most of the complementation groups have been identified within the past 7 years. XPA is a 31-kDa polypeptide that preferentially binds damaged DNA [20,21]. XPB and XPD are adenosine triphosphate (ATP)-dependent DNA helicases that may be involved in recognition of DNA damage and unwinding of the double helix [22–24]. XPC is a heterodimeric complex of two proteins that is essential only in the repair of sections of the genome that are not undergoing active transcription [25–28]. The gene for XPE has been recently cloned encoding a protein that binds damaged DNA preferentially at the sites of UV photoproducts [29–32]. XPF forms part of a protein complex with endonuclease activity that can nick negatively supercoiled double-stranded DNA and single-stranded DNA [33,34]. XPG is another DNA endonuclease [35,36,37].

Our current understanding of the role that these proteins play in the complex process of DNA repair is discussed below (Table 19.22.1). As we continue to unravel the intricacies of this complex process, we may begin to understand the complexities of the clinical syndromes characterized by defects in DNA repair.

Aetiology

XP affects all races with equal sex incidence. It occurs with a frequency of 1 in 250 000 in the USA and Europe. Higher frequencies (1 in 40 000) have been reported in Japan and Egypt [38].

All patients with XP have an autosomal recessively inherited defect in DNA repair. Parents of affected individuals have a higher incidence of skin cancer, but no other manifestation of the disease [39]. There is variability both in the clinical manifestations of affected individuals and the underlying genetic defects that produce the disease. An understanding of the specific biochemical defects that characterize the various subtypes of XP requires basic knowledge of UV light-induced DNA damage and the mechanisms used in the repair of this damage.

Table 19.22.1 Clinical and genetic characteristics of XP complementation groups. Modified from Lambert *et al.* [10] p. 91 and Wood [19] p. 70

Complementation group	Frequency	Country of origin of patients*	No. of patients reported	Clinical features Skin findings	Neurological findings	Gene cloned	Chromosome	Function of gene product
XPA	Common	Japan Europe USA Middle East	159	Yes	Most severe Some mild	Yes	9q34	Initiation step of DNA repair; binds damaged DNA
XPB	V. rare	Europe Japan	3	Yes	Moderate/severe XPCS	Yes	2q21	DNA helicase; part of initiation complex
XPC	Common largest group	Europe USA Middle East Japan	191	Yes	No (subclinical in adulthood reported)	Yes	5	Early repair binds to ssDNA allowing stable incisions in damaged DNA
XPD	Less common	Europe USA Japan	52	Yes	Moderate/severe	Yes	9q13	DNA helicase; part of RNA polymerase transcription initiation complex
		France	1	Yes	XPCS			
		USA, Europe	6	No	Trichothiodystrophy			
XPE	Rare	Europe Japan	13	Yes	No	Yes	—	Enzyme that cleves pyrimidine dimers; part of endonuclease
XPF	Rare	Japan Europe	16	Yes	No	Possibly	(?)16	Unknown
XPG	V. rare	USA Europe	5	Yes	No except XPCS	Yes	—	Endonuclease; makes DNA incisions
XPV	Common	Japan Europe USA Middle East	130	Yes	No	No	No	Postreplication repair defect

*Listed in decreasing order of frequency.
XP–CS, complex of XP and CS.

Repair of ultraviolet light damage to DNA

When UV light is absorbed by skin many effects are noted. Pigmentation is stimulated and immunosuppression occurs. More importantly, light energy is absorbed by cellular DNA-producing photoproducts or DNA adducts that interfere with the normal processes of DNA replication and transcription [10]. The type of adducts formed depends on the wavelengths of photons that are absorbed. Longer wavelengths produce free radicals that alter bases and produce protein–DNA cross-links [40]. Shorter wavelengths are more energetic and destructive, producing adducts by direct action as well as by the generation of free radicals. Two types of paired pyrimidine base adducts, the cyclobutane-ring-pyrimidine-dimer and the pyrimidine-(6-4)-pyrimidone photoproduct are the most important [41]. Both have carcinogenic potential and the latter produces marked distortion in the architecture of the affected strand of DNA [42].

Several mechanisms are present in injured cells to repair the effects of UV light damage. Altered bases are cleaved by an endonuclease called the FAPY protein (formamidopyrimidine–DNA endonuclease) [40]. Abnormalities in this system have recently been described in a subset of XP patients, but most XP cells repair damaged bases normally [43].

Nucleotide excision repair is the most critical system for repairing the adducts created by UV radiation. The first step in removal of abnormal adducts is cleavage of the DNA molecule at or near the site of damage [42,44]. A DNA endonuclease performs this function. Many of the complementation groups in XP involve a defect in this initiation step. Endonuclease specific for UV-irradiated DNA and for specific adducts have been identified [45].

Once the affected DNA strand is cut, the adduct is removed. Two possible mechanisms are used to remove the abnormal DNA. Firstly, a DNA exonuclease degrades the DNA digesting that portion containing the adduct in one direction, one nucleotide at a time. This results in a gap in one strand of the DNA which is filled in by a DNA polymerase using the opposite strand as a template. A DNA ligase then seals the nick, following the completion of repair synthesis [42]. Secondly, an enzyme complex incises the DNA on both sides of the adduct, removing an intact oligonucleotide structure, followed by filling of the gap with the DNA polymerase and ligase [46] (Fig. 19.22.1).

If an adduct is not repaired before replication, postreplication repair can occur [47]. This is a very complex and error-prone process that may be deficient in the variant complementation group of XP.

Studies of DNA repair in XP have looked at four different repair processes: (a) repair of pyrimidine dimers in active and in (b) inactive genes, and (c) repair of (6-4) photoproducts in active and (d) inactive genes [41,42,48].

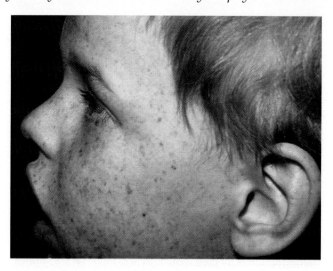

Fig. 19.22.1 XP: typical pigmentary skin changes.

Repair of these two adducts differs in different complementation groups and even within complementation groups and may help to explain some of the clinical variation seen in this disease.

Repair defects in specific complementation groups

Within complementation groups, patients with XP show a number of similar characteristics. The degree of depression of unscheduled DNA synthesis and the hypersensitivity to exposure to UV light *in vitro* are consistent. In addition, different groups preferentially repair active or inactive genes [10]. Our current knowledge of the defect responsible for each complementation group is discussed below.

Complementation group A. The gene for the defective protein responsible for this variant of XP has been identified on chromosome 9q34 [49]. It contains 273 amino acids and binds specifically to damaged DNA [50,51]. Excision repair of (6-4) photoproducts is more efficient than cyclobutane ring pyrimidine dimer in cells from patients with this defect, as the former are better substrates for this protein [21]. Point mutations producing the gene defect have been identified in 63 Japanese patients [52]. Fourteen separate mutations have been identified. Attempts to correlate different mutations in the gene with clinical characteristics have produced mixed results [53]. The XPA protein is felt to be critical in the initiation step of DNA repair with recognition of the damaged DNA adduct [54].

A different human gene, on chromosome 8, has been identified, which also partially corrects the deficient response of group A cells [55]. Different genes may play important roles in expression of the disease.

Complementation group B. Only three patients have been identified in this complementation group [10]. The gene for this protein has been localized to chromosome 2q21 [56]. It encodes a protein of 782 amino acids that has similarities in sequence to a DNA helicase found in yeast [57]. ATPase activity of this protein has also been demonstrated [57]. Helicases function to unwind double-stranded DNA. XPB may be involved in the recognition of damaged DNA and/or in the displacement of the damaged oligonucleotides after incision and before repair synthesis [58].

XPB also forms part of the RNA polymerase II basal transcription initiation complex. Functional protein XPB (and XPD, see below) is needed for repair of non-transcribed as well as transcribed DNA [24,33,58]. This dual function may help to explain the more severe clinical presentation of XPB patients.

Complementation group C. XP patients in this complementation group represent the largest group worldwide [59]. A gene was cloned by Legerski and Peterson encoding a 92-kDa polypeptide that corrects the DNA repair defect and UV hypersensitivity of cells from patients in this group [60]. Located on chromosome 5, this polypeptide is part of a heterodimeric complex that is thought to be involved in an early stage of repair, before initiation of gap filling by the DNA polymerase [19,28]. In addition, cells from patients in complementation group C are deficient in a DNA-dependent ATPase [61].

Complementation group D. Approximately 20% of cases of XP fall into this complementation group [10]. Like XPB, this protein is a DNA helicase involved in the recognition of damaged DNA, unwinding of DNA and removal of the abnormal adduct oligonucleotide prior to repair synthesis [22–24].

The XPD gene was simultaneously cloned by two groups, mapping to chromosome 9q13 [62,63]. This protein has homology with both a rodent and a yeast protein that functions dually in DNA repair and as part of an initiation complex that is specific for RNA polymerase II [64,65]. RNA polymerase II synthesizes most of the mitochondrial RNA (mRNA) within cells. It is activated by phosphorylation by protein kinases or initiation factors such as the XPD protein. The dual role of XPD (and XPB) in transcription initiation, as well as DNA repair, may explain the broader spectrum of clinical symptoms in this subset of patients, which includes developmental delay and neurological impairment as well as evidence of the repair deficiency [19].

Cells from patients in this complementation group have deficiency in repair of damaged bases as well as nucleotide excision repair. This combination of defects, along with marked hypersensitivity to UV light are seen in cells from some patients with Cockayne's syndrome (CS) and trichothiodystrophy with photosensitivity [66].

Complementation group E. In this relatively rare group of patients with XP, the cells lack an enzyme that binds selectively to UV light-damaged DNA [67]. This protein is thought to be homologous with a yeast photolyase that is activated by visible light to cleave the cyclobutane ring of pyrimidine dimers formed by UV damage, yielding normal DNA without incision and repair [67,68]. Not all patients within this complementation group lack this factor, however, and the exact role that this protein plays in repair has yet to be defined [67,69].

The gene encoding this 125-kDa protein was recently cloned [29]. A second 41-kDa protein co-purifies with the XPE protein and this two protein complex is needed to restore full repair synthesis in affected cells [31,32].

Complementation group F. This group of XP patients is rare and comprises mostly Japanese patients. The gene product that is responsible for the defect in these patients has not been conclusively found. A group of proteins has been identified in humans, encoded by the excision repair cross-complementing (ERCC) genes, that can restore repair defects in rodents in the laboratory [19]. A complex containing the gene products from ERCC1, ERCC4 and a factor that can correct the defect in XPF cells has been isolated [34,70]. It is currently postulated that ERCC4, located on chromosome 16, may be analogous to the XPF gene [71]. Another proposed candidate is ERCC11 [70].

Complementation group G. Five patients have been identified in this rare group of XP. The gene encoding a small protein that complements the defect in XPG cells was cloned in 1993 [72]. This gene product has 39% homology to a yeast gene, RAD2, and DNA sequencing of the gene demonstrated homology to the previously described gene ERCC5 [37,72]. The protein product from this gene is an endonuclease that functions to make repair incisions in the DNA flanking a UV-damaged DNA adduct.

Variant complementation group. About one-third of all patients with XP fall into this complementation group. Cells from patients with this variant show normal levels of unscheduled DNA synthesis following UV light exposure. There is no defect in repair of (6-4) photoadducts in these cells [73]. However, a slower rate of recovery following UV light injury is observed. Cells are less viable and show more marked mutagenesis than normal cells after UV injury [74]. UV-irradiated cells produce newly synthesized DNA of a reduced molecular weight and demonstrate a delay in the production of intact high molecular weight DNA strands following UV injury. These differences are more pronounced when cells are treated with

UV light and caffeine [75]. Caffeine may act by inhibiting the activity of a topoisomerase [76]. The defect in repair in patients with this variant is thought to represent a postreplication event or defective daughter-strand repair that has not been further defined, leading to the same clinical phenotype as patients with excision repair defects [77].

Despite the enormous increase in our understanding of the basic genetic defects that are present in patients with XP, we are still far from comprehending how these defects relate to the clinical diversity seen in patients with this condition. There remains marked heterogeneity within members of each group that cannot be easily explained by the biochemical differences as we know them. Clinical expression of sun sensitivity does not always correlate with biological cell culture assays of light sensitivity. Neoplasms occur predominantly, but not exclusively, in sun-exposed areas and are presumed to be the result of UV-induced mutations. Evidence in cell culture of increased UV-induced mutagenesis is present in all groups, but variation in the degree of susceptibility to UV-induced damage is also present. The relationship between abnormal UV excision repair and increased malignancy on non-UV-exposed areas is not clear. Nor can the neurological complications or the complexity of the De Sanctis–Cacchione syndrome be easily explained. New evidence that some of the defective proteins in XP may have dual roles as transcription initiators as well as in excision repair may shed some light on the diverse and complex clinical features of these variants. Perhaps DNA repair mechanisms are essential to maintain the integrity and function of neurones. We remain far from a complete understanding of the pathogenesis of this complex genetic disease.

Pathology

The histological features of severely affected patients with XP are those of severe sun damage. There is hyperkeratosis, atrophy of the epidermis and irregular elongation or atrophy of the rete ridges [78]. There is irregular and marked hyperpigmentation of the basal cell layer and the rete ridges, either with or without an increase in the number of melanocytes [38]. Electron microscopic studies have confirmed the presence of abnormal, polymorphic melanosomes with giant pigment granules in melanocytes and keratinocytes. Melanophages are laden with pigment and dermal fibroblasts appear to behave like macrophages engulfing melanosomes to form pigment vacuoles within their cytoplasm [79].

Epidermal nuclei may show a disordered arrangement with maturation disarray. Atypical downward growth histologically indistinguishable from solar keratoses are prominent. A non-specific chronic inflammatory infiltrate

may be present in the upper dermis. Basophilic degeneration of collagen is present but there is a conspicuous absence of solar elastosis of the upper dermis relative to that seen in older patients with chronic sun exposure producing these changes [10].

Hypopigmented macules show decreased numbers of melanocytes with an increase in Langerhans' cells [80].

Although non-specific, the presence of this combination of histological features in the skin of a young person suggests the diagnosis of XP [78].

Histological evidence of various malignant tumours including basal cell carcinoma, squamous cell carcinoma, keratoacanthoma and, rarely, fibrosarcoma can be seen beginning in the first decade of life. Malignant melanoma is seen in over 20%.

Neuropathological examination, at autopsy, in patients affected with the neurological complications of XP, reveals loss or absence of neurones, particularly of the cerebrum and cerebellum. There is a primary degeneration of axons present in these patients [81,82].

Clinical features (Figs 19.22.1–19.22.3)

The skin of patients with this disorder is normal at birth. The changes that occur are the direct result of UV light injury and therefore are seen almost exclusively in chronically sun-exposed areas of the body. The first manifestations of the disease are usually noted by the third year of life, but may occur very early in infancy or later in childhood. The median age of onset of tumours is 8 years. The timing and degree of changes noted varies between complementation groups (see below). Even within complementation groups, however, there is great individual variation in the time of onset and severity of disease. Changes are progressive and relentless, but the rate of

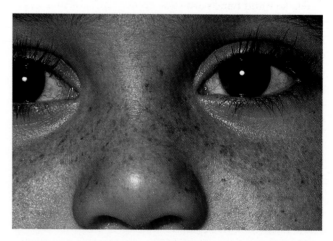

Fig. 19.22.2 XP: early presentation with photosensitivity and freckling across the bridge of the nose and cheeks. Courtesy of Dr J. Harper.

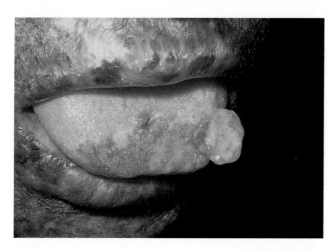

Fig. 19.22.3 XP: carcinoma of the tip of the tongue. Courtesy of Dr J. Harper.

progression is not predictable, even within families. There is no method to predict severity based on age of symptom onset. Fair-skinned patients may be more severely affected than their more darkly pigmented siblings, but the degree of damage and progression to malignancy is more closely related to sun exposure than skin type. XP has been reported in black people [83].

The earliest lesions noted are usually irregular freckling and marked dryness of the sun-exposed areas of skin. Freckling can be associated with sunburn and persistent erythema can be noted. Freckles are small at first, varying in pigmentation with evidence of fading in the winter months, but they soon become permanent and more widespread. There is a tendency towards merging of freckles to form irregular mottled hyperpigmented patches with telangiectasias and small spider angiomas interspersed among them. Atrophic hypopigmented guttate macules also appear within the mottled pigmentation.

The face and hands are affected first, but the neck, lips, conjunctiva and lower extremities become involved over time. In severe cases, even the trunk is affected. Mottled hyperpigmentation, telangiectasias, atrophy and scarring also develop.

By the age of 8 years, over 50% of patients with XP will develop one or more basal cell or squamous cell carcinomas [84]. Recent results reported by the Xeroderma Pigmentosum Registry on 132 patients with XP clearly demonstrated that sunlight exposure is the most important aetiological factor in the development of cutaneous malignancies [84]. Basal cell carcinomas and squamous cell carcinomas of the face, head and neck account for 80% of all cutaneous malignancies in the USA. In patients with XP, 97% arise on these sun-exposed skin sites [84]. Onset of these tumours occurs 50 years before onset in the general population. The risk of developing a cutaneous malignancy, including melanoma, as well as anterior eye

and tongue cancer under 20 years of age is increased 1000-fold in patients with XP [84,85].

Patients with XP are at great risk of developing cutaneous melanoma. In some studies 50% of patients have developed melanoma [86]. The relationship between sun exposure and melanoma is not well understood. Intermittent, but severe sun injury, in the form of repeated blistering sunburns, seems to be a more important factor than chronic sun exposure in the pathogenesis of melanoma in the general population [87]. The most common type of melanoma, the superficial spreading type, is seen on the upper body of men and on the legs of women [88]. This type of melanoma may be most closely related to that seen in XP. The combined carcinogenic effects of DNA damage and stimulation of melanocyte proliferation from acute sunlight injury are felt to play important roles in the pathogenesis of this disease [10].

Distinct clinical and histopathological subsets of melanoma exist in the general population that may differ in pathogenesis. Melanoma in XP patients shares some features with other, less common, subtypes of melanoma. In the report of the Xeroderma Pigmentosum Registry, a higher proportion of melanomas occurred on the face, head and neck, with fewer on the trunk and legs than in the general population [84]. Otherwise, the distribution of melanomas resembled that seen in the general population. Facial melanomas are more commonly of the lentigo maligna melanoma type, occurring exclusively on chronically sun-exposed skin in normal individuals. The pathogenesis of these melanomas is felt to more closely resemble that of non-melanoma sun cancer [89]. Like lentigo maligna melanoma, the majority of melanomas in XP are of the spindle cell variety. However, the histological changes of a solar lentigo have been found contiguous to 88% of melanomas in XP patients [90]. This change is not thought to be a precursor of cutaneous melanoma in the general population. The mechanism of melanoma formation may be completely different in patients with XP than that seen in any subset of the general population.

Ocular abnormalities are an important feature of XP and are almost as common as the cutaneous findings. Since changes are induced by sunlight, they are limited to the anterior portion of the eye including the lids, cornea and conjunctiva [85]. The earliest ocular symptom is photophobia which has been reported in up to 50% of patients [91]. Photophobia is seen more commonly in younger children than in adults [81]. Lid freckles and atrophic skin changes are almost constant features. Loss of lashes and ectropion are common findings. Complete loss of lids can be seen. Benign papillomas as well as squamous and basal cell carcinomas occur more commonly on the lower lids.

Conjunctival involvement including telangiectasis, xerosis, chronic congestion and pigmentation are most prominent in the palpebral fissure and seen in 20–40% of patients [85,91]. The cornea may show xerosis, haziness, exposure keratitis, scarring, ulceration and even perforation leading to corneal opacities and vascularization. Pterygium formation is common (40%) [85]. Direct DNA damage from UV radiation is believed to be responsible for inducing these changes [92]. Corneal transplants have limited success due to corneal vascularization, xerosis and, in some patients, inadequate lid coverage. Iris involvement is rare and usually limited to pigment alteration or iritis of the lower half.

Visual impairment usually results from severe corneal damage or pterygium formation and is seen in approximately 12% of patients [85]. Squamous cell carcinoma (most frequent), basal cell carcinoma and melanoma all occur on the ocular surface with a predilection for the limbal area.

In addition to cutaneous and ocular malignancies, patients with XP are at increased risk for internal malignancies. It has been estimated that the overall risk of non-cutaneous malignancy is approximately 10- to 20-fold [85]. Oral cavity neoplasms, particularly squamous cell carcinoma of the tip of the tongue, are the most common. Sarcoma and medulloblastoma of the brain, astrocytoma of the spinal cord, lung, uterine, breast, pancreatic, gastric, renal and testicular tumours and leukaemias have all been reported [85,93–96].

XP patients can also manifest a progressive neurological deficiency, usually presenting in the first two decades of life [95]. Abnormalities have been reported in approximately 30% of patients [81,85]. Not all complementation groups are at risk for these changes (see below). Patients in complementation group A, a few in complementation group D and rarely other groups are most affected [1,82].

Neurological deficiency in XP was first reported by DeSanctis and Cacchione in 1932 [97]. The patients described were three severely affected Italian brothers with intellectual impairment, microcephaly, delayed motor development, sensorineural deafness, peripheral neuropathy and finally dementia, beginning at 2 years of age.

Few patients with XP have the full-blown De Sanctis–Cacchione syndrome. More commonly, the neurological impairment is much milder, and may consist only of partial sensorineural hearing loss. Severe forms start in early childhood, but mild forms may manifest only as absence of deep tendon reflexes near the end of the first decade of life [1].

Robbins classified neurological XP according to the age of symptomatic onset of the disease with the early onset juvenile form appearing before the age of 7 years, intermediate onset juvenile form appearing between 7 and 12 years of age and the late onset juvenile form appearing after 12 years of age [98]. A late (adult onset) patient with only slight impairment has been identified in complementation group C with symptoms appearing in the fourth decade [82].

Neurological impairment in XP occurs irrespective of exposure to UV light [10]. Although the mechanism of neuronal injury is not known, it has been proposed that transcribed genes in neuronal cells are continuously damaged by endogenous DNA-damaging agents and metabolic stress. Accumulation of unrepaired, damaged DNA occurs due to the biochemical defect in XP [1]. This impairs the transcription, and consequently, the synthesis of proteins necessary to neuronal survival. Cells degenerate and die prematurely. Since different neuronal groups probably possess various degrees of DNA damage (and of DNA repair machinery), selective loss occurs in certain neuronal systems [98]. DNA damage is manifested as clinical disease in neural tissue because, unlike other tissues, neither the function of the damaged cells nor the cell itself can easily be replaced by other cells in the same tissue [82].

De Sanctis–Cacchione syndrome

Patients with De Sanctis–Cacchione syndrome have XP and severe neurological deficiencies. These patients represent a subgroup of complementation group A [10]. Like the three brothers originally described by De Sanctis and Cacchione in 1932, patients have early onset severe and progressive neurological disease. Onset of disease symptoms occurs earlier in this group with the mean onset at 6 months (versus 2 years for other patients with XP). Most report a history of acute sun sensitivity that is born out in laboratory studies that show marked killing of cell cultures by UV irradiation. Moderate to severe mental retardation with a median IQ of 45 has been reported in 80% of these patients. Spasticity and ataxia are present in 30%, sensorineural deafness in 7% and impaired hearing in 18%. Microcephaly is present in 24% with abnormal reflexes and electroencephalogram (EEGs) in 20% [85].

Patients with De Sanctis–Cacchione syndrome are often growth retarded with heights and weights beneath the third percentile in 25%. Secondary sexual characteristics are delayed or absent and no patients with this severe disease have had children [85].

Skin findings, the frequency and distribution of malignancies and ocular complications in these patients are comparable to those seen in other patients with XP. All ethnic groups are represented in this subset, although one-third of reported patients are Japanese [85].

The manifestations of XP and the severity of clinical disease varies between complementation groups. A brief summary of the major differences is presented below.

Complementation group A

XP patients in this group represent the second largest

group worldwide. Patients are reported from Japan, the USA, Europe and the Middle East. Typically, severe skin disease is seen in this group with an early age of onset [52]. Cutaneous malignancy in childhood is the rule unless patients are strictly photoprotected. Neurological disease is common, although a subset of patients within this group have been reported to develop little or no neurological sequelae [10]. Onset of the neurological symptoms is early in life and the most severely affected patients, those with the De Sanctis–Cacchione syndrome, are represented in this group [85]. The defective gene, XPA, is located on chromosome 9q34 [19].

Complementation group B

Only three patients have been reported with this complementation group, worldwide. The one American patient was very severely affected, whereas the two European cases had much milder disease [10]. Stigmata of CS were noted in all cases with typical ocular and neurological findings of this syndrome. The defective gene, XPB, also known as ERCC3, maps to chromosome 2q21 [55].

Complementation group C

This group of patients represents the largest group worldwide and is particularly common in the USA, Europe and the Middle East. It has rarely been seen in Japan. Patients are less severely affected than in complementation group A. Skin and ocular findings are moderately severe, but neurological disease is not seen. Robbins *et al.* reported a single patient in this group with very mild, late onset neurological deficiencies [99].

Repair of actively transcribed genes in patients of this group is usually normal. This may account for the decreased severity of clinical findings reported. The XPC gene is a DNA-dependent ATPase on chromosome 5 [19].

Complementation group D

Patients in this group comprise approximately 20% of all patients with XP worldwide. Compared to patients in group A, their disease is relatively mild. Photosensitivity is present and manifests early in life. Moderately severe skin problems are seen.

Neurological complications are characteristic of this complementation group. Although these can be quite severe, the onset is later in life than that seen in patients in group A. No patients with De Sanctis–Cacchione syndrome have been identified in this group. In general, neurological symptoms are less severe than those reported in group A patients and many patients have mild complications only [100]. A patient with the stigmata of CS and XP as well as several patients with the photosensitive form of trichothiodystrophy without XP have been demonstrated

to share this complementation group defect [101–103]. The gene for this complementation group is found on chromosome 9q13 and is homologous to the rodent gene ERCC2 [104].

Complementation group E, F and G

Few patients have been reported in these complementation groups. Those in group E have mild cutaneous findings and no neurological deficiency [105]. A total of 20 patients from Europe and Japan have been identified. Heterogeneity among patients has been noted both clinically and in laboratory studies [69]. The gene or genes for this group have not been identified.

Cells from patients in group F are more photosensitive than those from group E patients but only a few skin tumours have been noted clinically [106]. No neurological deficits are reported in most patients, although one patient from Japan was recently reported with severe neurological disease [107]. Most patients in this group are Japanese, with a few patients reported from Europe. The XPF gene may be homologous to the ERCC4 gene in rodents. This gene is located on the short arm of chromosome 16 [71].

Only five patients in complementation group G have been reported from Europe, Japan and the USA [108]. One American and one European patient had stigmata of CS. Neurological disease is present in those patients with the stigmata of CS only. No gene for this defect has yet been identified.

Variant complementation group

One-third of all patients with XP fall into this group. It is the most common group in Japan. Patients have also been identified from the USA and Europe. Variant patients have skin disease ranging from very mild to severe [109]. There have been no reports of neurological disease [10]. Unlike all other groups with XP, cells from patients in this group have normal levels of unscheduled DNA synthesis after UV exposure [110] (see above). The genetic defect in this group has not yet been identified.

Prognosis

Our current understanding of the pathogenesis of XP suggests that a favourable prognosis for these patients must rely on strict avoidance of environmental agents that produce DNA damage, particularly UV radiation. Most patients with this disease have shown relentless worsening of the cutaneous, ocular and neurological symptoms with increasing age. Rigorous protection from sunlight beginning in early infancy has been shown to slow the progression of serious cutaneous and ocular abnormalities [111]. The degree of sun protection necessary is extreme and families are forced to make difficult choices in order to provide such protection. The consequences of such choices affect the parents and other non-affected siblings often leading to serious lifestyle changes and neglect of non-affected family members. Some parents choose to provide limited protection only, for these reasons, especially if the affected individual has neurological involvement and a generally poor prognosis.

For those patients with neurological manifestations of the disease, UV exposure impacts little on the dismal prognosis. Progressive deterioration of severely affected patients leads to loss of functions ranging from ambulation to communication skills. The lack of regenerative powers of neurones, affected by exogenous and endogenous agents that cause irreparable DNA damage, leads to cell death and neuronal degeneration.

Differential diagnosis

Although the diagnosis of fully developed XP is evident, early manifestations of the disease in infancy can be less diagnostic. Except for third or fourth affected siblings, it is rare to make the diagnosis early enough to allow prevention of the devastating complications of sunlight exposure. Photosensitivity, often expressed as crying on exposure to sunlight in an infant, and sunburn, are manifestations of erythropoietic protoporphyria, erythropoietic porphyria, polymorphous light eruption, CS, Rothmund–Thomson syndrome and Hartnup's or Bloom's syndrome. Drug-induced photosensitivity or severe sunburn may also produce this symptom. Biopsies and examination of the urine, stool and blood for porphyrins should be performed to aid in clarifying these diagnoses.

As pigmentation is noted other disease possibilities enter the differential diagnosis. Generalized lentigines or a variation of PIBIDS (photosensitivity, ichthyosis, brittle hair, impaired intelligence, decreased fertility and short stature syndrome) may be considered. Urticaria pigmentosa can produce hyperpigmented macules in the early years of life. Poikilodermatous changes may mimic poikiloderma atrophicans, dyskeratosis congenita or radiodermatitis.

Photodamage can produce a clinical picture indistinguishable from the premature ageing syndromes including progeria and acrogeria. Neurological manifestations can further confuse the clinical picture.

Finally, the onset of cutaneous malignancies in childhood can be seen in the basal cell naevus syndrome, epidermodysplasia verruciformis and in the large atypical mole syndrome. Other features of these diseases and biopsies should allow distinction.

Confirmation of XP requires demonstration of the DNA repair defect in cultured fibroblasts from skin biopsy. The unscheduled DNA synthesis test and exposure of cell from patients suspected of having the disease to UV light

and other agents remains the most definitive diagnostic test [44,112]. Other diagnostic tests are currently being developed [113,114]. Molecular probes have been used to look for the XPA gene in the Japanese population. Prenatal diagnosis by amniocentesis in future pregnancies is available by culturing cells from amniotic fluid and measuring the rate of UV-induced, unscheduled DNA synthesis [115,116].

Treatment

The mainstay of therapy for this disease is prevention of the damaging effects of UV irradiation. Children should be kept indoors during midday and rigorously protected from sunlight whenever possible. Multiple layers of sun-protective clothing, hats and sunscreens that combine chemical blockers with physical barriers (such as titanium dioxide or zinc oxide) with skin protection factor (SPF) of over 30 are optimal [117]. Sunscreens should be reapplied frequently. Long hair is preferred to help protect the posterior neck. UV-absorbing sunglasses with side shields are essential to prevent the severe ocular changes. A lifestyle that minimizes outdoor activities should be encouraged [10].

Patients, and in the early years, parents, should be encouraged to examine the sun-exposed skin carefully and frequently to facilitate early detection of cutaneous malignancies. Doctors should instruct family members in the recognition of cutaneous neoplasms. Colour photographs of the entire skin surface with close-ups of lesions can be helpful to parents and doctors. Frequent examinations by a dermatologist once evidence of premalignant skin changes becomes apparent are essential. Routine deep tendon reflexes along with screening audiometry can alert the practitioner to the early onset of neurological disease in otherwise asymptomatic patients.

Special attention should be paid to eye care and an ophthalmologist should be involved early in caring for these patients. In addition to protective sunglasses, artificial tears, steroid drops and bland ointment at night can be helpful [91]. Photophobia and ocular irritation in patients exposed to UV light can be relieved with eye-drops containing quinoline derivatives [118]. UV-absorbing contact lenses have been shown to protect against UV-induced retinopathy and may be helpful in preventing corneal and iris damage in XP patients [119].

Patients should be protected from cigarette smoke and discouraged from smoking since cell cultures show increased sensitivity to benzo[a]pyrene found in cigarette smoke. At least one patient has been reported who smoked for more than 10 years and died of bronchogenic carcinoma of the lungs at the age of 35 years [85].

Premalignant lesions such as actinic keratosis should be treated with cryotherapy, topical 5-fluorouracil or dermabrasion.

Early and complete treatment of all tumours by curettage and electrodesiccation or surgical excision should be performed with avoidance of radiotherapy due to the atrophic and degenerate nature of the sun-damaged skin. Patients with XP are not abnormally sensitive to therapeutic X-rays but cell cultures from a few patients have demonstrated abnormal sensitivity to X-irradiation. Mohs micrographic surgery can be used to spare normal tissue and skin grafts from non-sun-exposed sites can be utilized in filling defects if skin damage becomes extensive and severe [120].

Ocular surgery may be necessary for removal of neoplasms involving the eye, as well as release of symblepharon, and keratoplasty for corneal opacification [121,122].

High-dose isotretinoin has been successfully used in the prevention of cutaneous neoplasms in patients with XP [94,123–126]. Cutaneous neoplasms are reduced by four- to five-fold while on this drug [94,124]. Toxicity in the form of increased serum triglycerides, cutaneous xanthomas, xerosis and skeletal abnormalities limits the use of retinoids to patients with multiple skin cancers. Retinoids are extremely teratogenic and effective birth control is mandatory. Doses of 0.5 mg/kg/day increasing to 1.5 mg/kg/day, depending on tolerance and efficacy are recommended [10,125]. Cessation of these drugs has been associated with an eight-fold increase in the rate of appearance of these tumours to a rate twice that of untreated patients.

A patient with XP and melanoma *in situ* was successfully treated with intralesional interferon-α [127].

REFERENCES

1 Mazzarello P, Poloni M, Spadari S et al. DNA repair mechanisms in neurological diseases: facts and hypotheses. *J Neurol Sci* 1992; 112: 4–14.

2 Hebra F, Kaposi M. *On Diseases of the Skin Including the Exanthemata*, vol. 3 (Tay W, trans). London: New Sydenham Society, 1874: 252–8.

3 Kaposi M. Xeoderma pigmentosum. *Med Jahrb Wien* 1882; 11: 619–33.

4 Cleaver JE. Defective repair replication of DNA in xeroderma pigmentosum. *Nature* 1968; 218: 652–6.

5 Cleaver JE. DNA damage and repair in light-sensitive human skin disease. *J Invest Dermatol* 1970; 54: 181–955.

6 Cleaver JE, Carter DM. Xeroderma pigmentosum variants: influence of temperature on DNA repair. *J Invest Dermatol* 1973; 60: 29–32.

7 Cleaver JE. Xeroderma pigmentosum—progress and regress. *J Invest Dermatol* 1973; 60: 374–80.

8 Epstein JH, Fukuyame K, Reed WWB et al. Defect in DNA synthesis in skin of patients with xeroderma pigmentosum demonstrated *in vivo*. *Science* 1970; 168: 1477–8.

9 deWeerd-Kastelein EA, Keijzer W, Bootsma D. Genetic heterogeneity of xeroderma pigmentosum demonstrated by somatic cell hibridization. *Nature* 1972; 238: 893.

10 Lambert WC, Kuo H-R, Lambert MW. Xeroderma pigmentosum. *Dermatol Clin* 1995; 13: 169–209.

11 Moshell AN, Ganges MB, Lutzner MA et al. A new patient with both xeroderma pigmentosum and Cockayne syndrome establishes the new xeroderma pigmentosum complementation group H. In: Friedberg E, Bridges B, eds. *Cellular Responses to DNA Damage*. New York: Alan R. Liss, 1983: 209–13.

12 Fischer E, Keijzer W, Theilmann HW et al. A ninth complementation group in xeroderma pigmentosum, XPI. *Mutat Res* 1985; 145: 217–25.

13 Bootsma D, Keijzer W, Jung EG et al. Xeroderma pigmentosum complementation group XP-I withdrawn. *Mutat Res* 1989; 218: 149–51.

14 Johnson RT, Elliott GC, Squires S et al. Lack of complementation between xeroderma pigmentosum complementation groups D and H. *Hum Genet* 1989; 81: 203–10.

15 Robbins JH. Xeroderma pigmentosum group H is withdrawn and reassigned to group D. *Hum Genet* 1991; 88: 242.

16 Burk PG, Lutzner M, Clark PD et al. Ultraviolet-stimulated thymidine incorporation in xeroderma pigmentosum lymphocytes. *J Lab Clin Med* 1971; 77: 759.

17 Ichihashi M, Fujiwara Y. Clinical and photobiological characteristics of Japanese xeroderma pigmentosum variant. *Br J Dermatol* 1981; 105: 1–12.

18 Boyer JC, Kaufmann WK, Brylawski BP, Condeiro-Stone M. Defective postreplication repair in xeroderma pigmentosum variant fibroblasts. *Cancer Res* 1990; 50: 2593.

19 Wood RD. Proteins that participate in nucleotide excision repair of DNA in mammalian cells. *Phil Trans Roy Soc Lond B* 1995; 347: 69–74.

20 Miyamoto I, Miura N, Niwa H et al. Mutational analysis of the structure and function of the xeroderma-pigmentosum group-A complementing protein—identification of essential domains for nuclear-localization and DNA excision repair. *J Biol Chem* 1992; 267: 12182–7.

21 Jones CJ, Wood RD. Preferential binding of the xeroderma pigmentosum group A complementing protein to damaged DNA. *Biochemistry* 1993; 32: 12096–104.

22 Schaeffer L, Roy R, Humbert S et al. DNA repair helicase: a component of BTF2 (TFIIH) basic transcription factor. *Science* 1993; 260: 58–63.

23 Sung P, Bailly V, Weber C et al. Human xeroderma pigmentosum group D gene encodes in DNA helicase. *Nature, Lond* 1993; 365: 852–5.

24 Schaeffer L, Moncollin V, Roy R et al. The ERCC2/DNA repair protein is associated with the class-II BTF2/TFIIH transcription factor. *EMBO J* 1994; 13: 2388–92.

25 Venema J, vanHoffen A, Karcagi V et al. Xeroderma pigmentosum complementation group-C cells remove pyrimidine dimers selectively from the transcribed strand of active genes. *Molec Cell Biol* 1991; 11: 4128–34.

26 Shiuji MKK, Eker APM, Wood RD. The DNA repair defect in xeroderma pigmentosum group C and a complementing factor from HeLa cells. *J Biol Chem* 1994; 269: 22749–57.

27 Legerski R, Peterson C. Expression cloning of a human DNA-repair gene involved in xeroderma pigmentosum group C. *Nature, Lond* 1992; 359: 70–3.

28 Masutani C, Sugasawa K, Yanagisawa J et al. Purification and cloning of a nucleotide excision repair complex involving the xeroderma pigmentosum group C protein and a human homologue of yeast RAD23. *EMBO J* 1994; 13: 1831–43.

29 Takao M, Abramic M, Moos M et al. A 127-kDa component of a UV-damaged DNA-binding complex, which is defective in some xeroderma pigmentosum group E patients, is homologous to a slime-mold protein. *Nucl Acids Res* 1993; 21: 4111–18.

30 Treiber DK, Chen ZH, Essigmann JM. An ultraviolet light-damaged DNA recognition protein absent in xeroderma pigmentosum group E cell binds selectively to pyrimidine (6-4) pyrimidone photoproducts. *Nucl Acids Res* 1992; 20: 5805–10.

31 Keeney S, Chang GJ, Linn S. Characterization of a human DNA-damage binding protein implicated in xeroderma pigmentosum E. *J Biol Chem* 1993; 268: 21293–300.

32 Keeney S, Eker APM, Brody T et al. Correction of the DNA-repair defect in xeroderma-pigmentosum group-E by injection of a DNA damage-binding protein. *Proc Natl Acad Sci, USA* 1994; 91: 4053–6.

33 vanVuuren AJ, Vermeulen W, Weeda G et al. Correction of xeroderma pigmentosum repair defect by basal transcription factor BTF2 (TFIIH). *EMBO J* 1994; 13: 1645–53.

34 Biggerstaff M, Szymkowski DE, Wood RD. Co-correction of the ERCC1, ERCC4 and xeroderma pigmentosum group F DNA repair defects in vitro. *EMBO J* 1993; 12: 3685–92.

35 O'Donovan A, Wood RD. Identical defects in DNA repair in xeroderma pigmentosum group G and rodent ERCC group 5. *Nature, Lond* 1993; 363: 185–8.

36 O'Donovan A, Scherly D, Clarkson SG et al. Isolation of active recombinant XPG protein, a human DNA repair endonuclease. *J Biol Chem* 1994; 269: 15961–4.

37 Shiomi T, Harada Y, Saito T *et al*. An ERCC5 gene with homology to yeast RAD2 is involved in group G xeroderma pigmentosum. *Mutat Res* 1994; 314: 167–75.

38 Harper J. Genetics and genodermatoses. In: Champion RH, Burton JL, Burns DA, eds. *Rook Textbook of Dermatology*, vol. 1. Oxford: Blackwell Science, 1998: 357–436.

39 Swift M, Chase C. Cancer in families with xeroderma pigmentosum. *J Natl Cancer Inst* 1979; 62: 1415–21.

40 Pflaum M, Boiteux S, Epe B. Visible light generates oxidative DNA base modifications in high excess of strand breaks in mammalian cells. *Carcinogenesis* 1994; 15: 297–300.

41 Mitchell DL. The relative cytotoxicity of (6-4) photoproducts and cyclobutane dimers in mammalian cells. *Photochem Photobiol* 1988; 48: 51–7.

42 Mitchell DL, Nairn RS. The biology of the (6-4) photoproduct. *Photochem Photobiol* 1989; 49: 805–19.

43 Le Doux SP, Patton NJ, Avery LJ *et al*. Repair of *N*-methylpurines in the mitochondrial DNA of xeroderma pigmentosum complementation group D cells. *Carcinogenesis* 1993; 14: 913–17.

44 Lambert WC, Lambert MW. Diseases associated with DNA and chromosomal instability. In: Alper JC, ed. *Genetic Diseases of the Skin*. St Louis: Mosby Year Book, 1991: 320–58.

45 Tomura T, Van Lancker JL. Purification of human and monkey endonucleases acting on ultraviolet irradiated DNA. *Arch Biochem Biophys* 1980; 201: 636–9.

46 Huang JC, Svoboda DL, Rardon JT *et al*. Human nucleotide excision nuclease removes thymine dimers from DNA by incising the twenty-second phosphodiester bond 5' and the sixth phosphodiester bond 3' to the photodimer. *Proc Natl Acad Sci USA* 1992; 89: 3664–8.

47 Lambert WC, Hanawalt PC. DNA repair mechanisms and their biological implications in mammalian cells. *J Am Acad Dermatol* 1990; 22: 299–308.

48 Galloway AM, Liuzzi M, Paterson MC. Metabolic processing of cyclobutyl pyrimidine dimers and (6-4) photoproducts in UV-treated human cells; Evidence for distinct excision-repair pathways. *J Biol Chem* 1994; 269: 974–80.

49 Henning KA, Schultz RA, Sekhon GS *et al*. Gene complementing xeroderma pigmentosum group A cells maps to distal human chromosome 9q. *Somat Cell Mol Genet* 1990; 16: 395–400.

50 Miura M, Miyamoto I, Asahina H *et al*. Identification and characterization of xpac protein, the gene product of the human XPAC (xeroderma pigmentosum complementation group A complementing) gene. *J Biol Chem* 1991; 266: 19786–9.

51 Tanaka K, Miura N, Satokata I *et al*. Analysis of a human DNA excision repair gene involved in group A xeroderma pigmentosum and containing a zinc-finger domain. *Nature* 1990; 348: 73–6.

52 Satokata I, Tanaka K, Miura N *et al*. Three nonsense mutations responsible for group A xeroderma. *Mutat Res* 1992; 273: 193–202.

53 Mimaki T, Tanaka K, Okada Y *et al*. Allelic heterogeneity in group A xeroderma pigmentosum. *Acta Neurol Scand* 1992; 85: 327–30.

54 Miura M, Domon M, Sasaki T *et al*. Restoration of proliferating cell nuclear antigen (PCNA) complex-formation in xeroderma-pigmentosum group-A cells following *cis*-diammine-dichloroplatinum (II)-treatment by cell-fusion with normal-cells. *J Cell Physiol* 1992; 152: 639–45.

55 Kaur G, Rinaldy A, Lloyd R *et al*. A gene that partially complements xeroderma pigmentosum group A cells maps to human chromosome 8. *Somat Cell Mol Genet* 1992; 18: 371–9.

56 Weeda G, Wiegant J, van der Ploeg M *et al*. Localization of the xeroderma pigmentosum group B-correcting gene ERCC-3 to human chromosome 2q21. *Genomics* 1991; 10: 1035–40.

57 Weeda G, Ma L, van Ham RCA *et al*. Characterization of the mouse homolog of the XPBC/ERCC-3 gene implicated in xeroderma pigmentosum and Cockayne's syndrome. *Carcinogenesis* 1991; 12: 2361–8.

58 Biggerstaff M, Wood RD. Requirement for ERCC1 and ERCC3 gene products in DNA excision repair *in vitro*: complementation using rodent and human cell extracts. *J Biol Chem* 1992; 267: 6879–85.

59 Kraemer KH, Lee MM, Scotto J. Xeroderma pigmentosum: cutaneous, ocular, and neurologic abnormalities in 830 published cases. *Arch Dermatol* 1987; 123: 241.

60 Legerski R, Peterson C. Expression cloning of a human DNA repair gene involved in xeroderma pigmentosum group C. *Nature* 1992; 359: 70–3.

61 Yanagisawa J, Seki M, Ui M *et al*. Alteration of a DNA-dependent ATPase activity in xeroderma pigmentosum complementation group C cells. *J Biol Chem* 1992; 267: 3585–8.

62 Arrand JE, Bone NM, Johnson RT. Molecular cloning and characterization of a mammalian excision repair gene that partially restores UV resistance to xeroderma pigmentosum complementation group D cells. *Proc Natl Acad Sci USA* 1989; 86: 6997–7001.

63 Flejter WL, McDaniel LD, Askari M *et al*. Characterization of a complex chromosomal rearrangement maps the locus for *in vitro* complementation of xeroderma pigmentosum group D to human chromosome band 19q13. *Genes Chrom Cancer* 1992; 5: 335–42.

64 Bootsma D, Hoeijmakers JHJ. Engagement with transcription. *Nature* 1993; 363: 114–15.

65 Guzder SN, Qiu H, Sommers CH *et al*. DNA repair gene *RAD 3* of *S. cerevisiae* is essential for transcription by RNA polymerase II. *Nature* 1994; 367: 91–4.

66 Johnson RT, Squires S. The XPD complementation group: insights into xeroderma pigmentosum, Cockayne's syndrome and trichothiodystrophy. *Mutat Res* 1992; 273: 97–118.

67 Treiber DK, Chen Z, Essigmann JM. An ultraviolet light-damaged DNA recognition protein absent in xeroderma pigmentosum group E cells binds selectively to pyrimidine (604) pyrimidone photoproducts. *Nucleic Acids Res* 1992; 20: 5805–10.

68 Patterson M, Chu G. Evidence that xeroderma pigmentosum cells from complementation group E are deficient in a homology of yeast photolyase. *Mol Cell Biol* 1989; 9: 5105–12.

69 Keeney S, Wein H, Linn S. Biochemical heterogeneity in xeroderma pigmentosum complementation group E. *Mutat Res* 1992; 273: 49–56.

70 van Vuuren AJ, Appeldoorn E, Odijk H *et al*. Evidence for a repair enzyme complex involving ERCC1, ERCC4, ERCC11 and the xeroderma pigmentosum group F proteins. *EMBO J* 1993; 12: 3693–701.

71 Liu P, Callen DF, Reeders ST *et al*. Human DNA excision repair gene ERCC4 is located on chromosome 16 short arm 16p13.13–p13.3. *Cytogenet Cell Genet* 1989; 51: 1035.

72 Scherly D, Nouspikel T, Corlet J *et al*. Complementation of the DNA repair defect in xeroderma pigmentosum group G cells by a human cDNA related to yeast *RAD 2*. *Nature* 1993; 363: 182–5.

73 Mitchell DL, Haipek CA, Clarkson JM. Xeroderma pigmentosum variant cells are not defective in the repair of (604) photoproducts. *Int J Radiat Biol* 1987; 52: 201–5.

74 Waters HL, Seetharam S, Seidman MM *et al*. Ultraviolet hypermutability of a shuttle vector propagated in xeroderma pigmentosum variant cells. *J Invest Dermatol* 1993; 101: 744–8.

75 Fujiwara Y, Ichihashi M, Matsumoto A *et al*. A mechanism for relief of replication blocks by activation of unused origin and age-dependent change in the caffeine susceptibility in xeroderma pigmentosum variant. *Mutat Res* 1991; 254: 79–87.

76 Tohda H, Zhao JH, Oikawa A. A possible involvement of DNA topoisomerase I in 'caffeine effect' after ultraviolet irradiation. *Tokyo J Exp Med* 1992; 168: 129–32.

77 Griffiths TD, Ling SY. Effect of UV light on DNA chain growth and replicon initiation in xeroderma pigmentosum variant cells. *Mutagenesis* 1991; 6: 247–51.

78 Lever WF, Schaumberg-Lever G. *Histopathology of the Skin*, 7th edn. Philadelphia: JB Lippincott, 1990: 72–3.

79 Plotnick H, Lupalescu A. Ultrastructural studies of xeroderma pigmentosum. *J Am Acad Dermatol* 1983; 9: 876–82.

80 Cesarini JP, Bioulac G, Moreno G *et al*. Hypopigmented macules of sun-exposed skin in xeroderma pigmentosum. An electron microscopic study. *J Cutan Pathol* 1975; 2: 128–39.

81 Robbins JH, Kraemer KH, Lutzner MA, Festoof BW, Coon HG. Xeroderma pigmentosum: an inherited disease with sun sensitivity, multiple cutaneous neoplasms and abnormal DNA repair. *Ann Intern Med* 1974; 80: 221.

82 Robbins JH, Brumback RA, Mediones M *et al*. Neurologic disease in xeroderma pigmentosum—Documentation of a late onset type of the juvenile onset form. *Brain* 1991; 114: 1335–61.

83 Loewenthal LJA, Trowell HC. Xeroderma pigmentosum in African Negroes. *Br J Dermatol* 1938; 50: 66–71.

84 Kraemer KH, Lee M-M, Andrews AD *et al*. The role of sunlight and DNA repair in melanoma and skin cancer: the xeroderma pigmentosum paradigm. *Arch Dermatol* 1994; 130: 1018–21.

85 Kraemer KH, Lee MM, Scotto J. Xeroderma pigmentosum: cutaneous ocular and neurologic abnormalities in 830 published cases. *Arch Dermatol* 1987; 123: 241–50.

86 Ariel IM. Theories regarding the cause of malignant melanoma. *Surg Gynecol Obstet* 1980; 150: 907.

87 Holman CDJ, Armstrong BK, Heenan PJ. Relationship of cutaneous malig-

nant melanoma to individual sunlight-exposed habits. *J Natl Cancer Inst* 1986; 76: 403.

88 NIH Consensus Development Conference Statement. *Sunlight, Ultraviolet Radiation and the Skin*. Bethesda: National Institutes of Health, 1989.

89 Elwood JM, Gallagher RP, Roth AJ *et al*. Etiological differences between subtypes of cutaneous malignant melanoma: western Canada melanoma study. *J Natl Cancer Inst* 1987; 78: 37–44.

90 Stern JB, Peck GL, Haupt HM *et al*. Malignant melanoma in xeroderma pigmentosum: search for a precursor lesion. *J Am Acad Dermatol* 1993; 28: 591–4.

91 Goyal JL, Rao VA, Srinivasan R *et al*. Oculocutaneous manifestations in xeroderma pigmentosum. *Br J Ophthal* 1994; 78: 295–7.

92 Applegate LA, Ley RD. DNA damage is involved in the induction of opacification and neovascularization of the cornea by ultraviolet light. *Exp Eye Res* 1991; 52: 493–7.

93 Keukens F, van Voorst Vader PC, Panders AK *et al*. Xeroderma pigmento-sum: squamous cell carcinoma of the tongue. *Acta Derm Venereol (Stockl)* 1989; 69: 530.

94 Kraemer KH, DiGiovanna JJ, Mashell AN *et al*. Prevention of skin cancer with oral 13-*ris* retinoic acid in xeroderma pigmentosum. *N Engl J Med* 1988; 318: 1633.

95 Tomas M, Salinas AS, Moreno J, Server G. Renal leiomyosarcoma associated with xeroderma pigmentosum. *Arch Esp Urol* 1989; 42: 484.

96 Mamada A, Miuva K, Tsunoda K *et al*. Xeroderma pigmentosum variant associated with multiple skin cancers and a lung cancer. *Dermatologica* 1992; 184: 177–81.

97 De Sanctis C, Cacchione A. L'idiozia xerodermica. *Riv Sper Freniatr* 1932; 56: 269–92.

98 Robbins JH. A childhood neurodegeneration due to defective DNA repair: a novel concept of disease based on studies of xeroderma pigmentosum. *J Child Neurol* 1989; 4: 143–6.

99 Robbins JH, Brumbach RA, Moschell AN. Clinically asymptomatic xeroderma pigmentosum neurologic disease in an adult: evidence for a neurodegeneration in later life caused by defective DNA repair. *Eur Neurol* 1993; 33: 188–90.

100 Fukuro S, Yamaguchi J, Mamada A *et al*. Xeroderma pigmentosum group D patient bearing lentigo maligna without neurological symptoms. *Dermatologica* 1990; 181: 129–33.

101 Stefanini M *et al*. Xeroderma pigmentosum (complementation group D) mutation is present in patients affected by trichothiodystrophy with photosensitivity. *Hum Genet* 1986; 74: 107.

102 Lehmann AR *et al*. Trichothiodystrophy, a human DNA repair disorder with heterogeneity in the cellular response to ultraviolet light. *Cancer Res* 1988; 48: 6090.

103 Rebora A, Crovato F. PIBI(D)S syndrome: trichothiodystrophy with xeroderma pigmentosum (group D) mutation. *J Am Acad Dermatol* 1987; 16: 940.

104 Weber CA, Solazar EP, Stewart SA *et al*. Molecular cloning and biological characterization of a human gene, ERCC2, that corrects the nucleotide excision repair defect in CHO UV5 cells. *Mol Cell Biol* 1990; 8: 1137–46.

105 Kondo S, Fukuro S, Nishioka K. Age-related changes in photosensitivity and cellular sensitivity to ultraviolet B in a xeroderma pigmentosum group E patient. *Photodermatol Photoimmunol Photomed* 1991; 8: 79–83.

106 Kondo S, Mamada A, Miyamoto C *et al*. Late onset of skin cancers in two xeroderma pigmentosum group F siblings and a review of 30 Japanese xeroderma pigmentosum patients in groups D, E and F. *Photodermatology* 1989; 6: 89.

107 Moriwaki S, Nishigori C, Imamura S *et al*. A case of xeroderma pigmentosum complementation group F with neurologic abnormalities. *Br J Dermatol* 1993; 128: 91–4.

108 Norris PG, Hawk JL, Avery JA *et al*. Xeroderma pigmentosum complementation group G: report of two cases. *Br J Dermatol* 1987; 116: 861–6.

109 Jung EG, Bohnert E, Fischer E *et al*. Heterogeneity of xeroderma pigmentosum (XP) variability and stability within and between the complementation groups C, D, E, I and variants. *Photodermatology* 1986; 3: 125.

110 Lehmann AR, Kirk-Bell S, Arlett CF *et al*. Xeroderma pigmentosum cells with normal levels of excision repair have a defect in DNA synthesis after UV irradiation. *Proc Natl Acad Sci USA* 1975; 72: 219–23.

111 Lynch HT, Frichot III BC, Lynch JF. Cancer control in xeroderma pigmentosum. *Arch Dermatol* 1977; 113: 193.

112 Cleaver JE, Cortes F, Lutze LH *et al*. Unique DNA repair properties of a xeroderma pigmentosum revertant cell line. *Mol Cell Biol* 1987; 7: 3353–7.

113 Greene MHL, Lowe JE, Harcourt SA *et al*. UV-C sensitivity of unstimulated

114 Parshad R, Tarone RE, Price FM *et al*. Cytogenetic evidence for differences in DNA incision activity in xeroderma pigmentosum group A, C and D cells after X-irradiation during G_1 phase. *Mutat Res* 1993; 294: 149–55.

115 Regan JD, Setlow RB, Kaback MM *et al*. Xeroderma pigmentosum: a rapid sensitive method for prenatal diagnosis. *Science* 1971; 174: 147–50.

116 Ramsay CA, Coltart TM, Blunt S *et al*. Prenatal diagnosis of xeroderma pigmentosum: report of the first successful case. *Lancet* 1974; ii: 1109.

117 Bech-Thomsen N, Wulf HC, Ullman S *et al*. Xeroderma pigmentosum lesions related to ultraviolet transmittance by clothes. *J Am Acad Dermatol* 1991; 24: 364.

118 Florani M, Malaguti C, Boero A, Germogli R. The treatment of photophobia and ocular irritations caused by intense light. *Ann Ophthalmol Clin Oculist* 1990; 116: 85–9.

119 Lao GU, Chuanico RU. Ophthalmic instruments; their ultraviolet hazards. *Philipp J Ophthalmol* 1990; 19: 142–7.

120 Atabay K, Celebi C, Cenetoglu S *et al*. Facial resurfacing in xeroderma pigmentosum with monoblock full-thickness skin graft. *Plast Reconstr Surg* 1991; 6: 1121–5.

121 Jung EG. Xeroderma pigmentosum. *Int J Dermatol* 1986; 25: 629–33.

122 Hertle RW, Durso F, Metzler JP *et al*. Epibulbar squamous cell carcinomas in brothers with xeroderma pigmentosa. *J Pediatr Ophthalmol Strabismus* 1991; 28: 350–3.

123 Berth-Jones J, Graham-Brown RAC. Xeroderma pigmentosum variant: response to etretinate. *Br J Dermatol* 1990; 122: 559–61.

124 Berth-Jones J, Cole J, Lehmann AR *et al*. Xeroderma pigmentosum variant: 5 years of tumor suppression by etretinate. *J Roy Soc Med* 1993; 86: 355–6.

125 Kraemer KH, Di Giovanna JJ, Peck GL. Chemoprevention of skin cancer in xeroderma pigmentosum. *J Dermatol* 1992; 19: 715–18.

126 Kraemer KH, DiGiovanna JJ, Peck GL. Isotretinoin does prevent skin cancer. *Arch Dermatol* 1993; 129: 43 (letter; comment).

127 Turner ML, Moshell AN, Corbett DW *et al*. Clearing of melanoma in situ with intralesional interferon alfa in a patient with xeroderma pigmentosum. *Arch Dermatol* 1994; 130: 1491–4.

Cockayne's syndrome

Definition

CS is a rare autosomal dominant genetic disorder characterized by growth failure, progressive neurological dysfunction, cutaneous photosensitivity and early death. Other common manifestations include cataracts, sensorineural hearing loss, pigmentary retinopathy, skeletal abnormalities and dental caries [1]. The pathogenesis of this disorder is not known, but cells from patients with CS show increased sensitivity to UV light. Unlike patients with XP, they have defective DNA repair only of active genes following UV light injury [2]. In addition, patients with CS have no predisposition to cutaneous cancer [3].

History

In 1936, Cockayne reported two siblings with cachectic dwarfism, progressive mental retardation, an erythematous dermatitis, and an odd facial appearance where loss of subcutaneous fat resulted in a 'wizened' appearance with typical 'bird-headed' facies and prominent 'Mickey Mouse' ears [4]. He reported further details on these patients in 1946, describing loss of vision associated with an unusual pigmentary degeneration of the retina, and progressive hearing loss, emphasizing the progressive nature of the disease [5]. Neil and Dingwall described two siblings with similar clinical features in 1950 [6]. Subsequently, CS has been reported in over 170 patients [1]. A wide spectrum of symptoms and severity of the disease suggests that biochemical and genetic heterogeneity exists in this syndrome.

Because of the dermatological similarities recognized in some patients with CS and XP, the discovery of defective DNA repair in XP resulted in a search for an underlying defect in DNA repair in CS. Although the usual assays of DNA excision repair were found to be normal, it was soon discovered that CS cells were delayed in recovery of DNA and RNA synthesis following UV irradiation [7,8]. Three complementation groups were subsequently identified, including one group of patients with an overlap syndrome consisting of clinical and laboratory features of XP group B and clinical features of CS [9]. Other patients with overlap features have been identified in XP complementation groups D and G [10–13].

In addition to subclassification into complementation groups, a recent attempt has been made to subclassify patients with CS into clinical subtypes [1,14]. These classifications are valuable in providing diagnostic and prognostic assessments of affected patients. Unfortunately, insufficient complementation studies and biochemical assays have been performed, to date, to allow a correlation between the various clinical and complementation subgroups. Results of some studies suggest that there is genetic heterogeneity within the subset of severely affected patients with CS. Cells from some patients in this group show defective excision repair while others do not [15–17].

Aetiology

CS affects males and females with almost equal frequency [1]. Most reported patients have been Caucasian or Japanese [1,18,19]. Two black patients have been reported as well as patients from Argentina, India, Saudi Arabia and Iraq [20–22]. Parental consanguinity has been reported in many cases. The suggested pattern of inheritance is autosomal recessive and over half of reported individuals have at least one other affected family member.

The pathogenesis of CS is unknown. Chromosome karyotype and sister chromatid exchange frequency is normal in untreated cells. Two patients with chromosome abnormalities have been reported; one patient had an extra F group chromosome [23] and another had a deletion of a portion of chromosome 10 [24].

Cultured fibroblasts and lymphocytes from patients with CS are hypersensitive to UV irradiation [7,8]. Recovery of DNA and RNA synthesis is delayed following UV injury. Using this assay, three complementation groups of CS have been described [9]. The defect in group A has

not yet been defined. The defect in group B is a protein encoded by the gene ERCC6 found on chromosome 10 [25–27]. This gene product corrects the defect in hamster complementation group 6, and appears to assist in transcription of damaged genes [28]. Complementation group C comprises patients with CS and XP in group XPB.

CS cells do not have the same DNA repair defects as XP cells. Repair of total genomic DNA is normal in CS, but there is defective repair of actively transcribing genes [2,8]. Transcriptionally active genes are normally repaired at a faster rate than are inactive genes. In addition, CS cells, like XP cells, are not able to repair cyclobutane dimers in DNA [29]. Non-dimer photoproducts are repaired normally in CS [30]. The UV cancer resistance in CS may relate, in part, to the ability of cells from these patients to repair non-dimer photoproducts in active genes normally, a function that is absent in patients with XP.

It is hypothesized that the inability to repair cyclobutane dimers in damaged DNA may result in repeated injury to myelin-producing cells that is not fully repaired [31]. Such cells eventually die from this damage. Mature neurones lack the ability to divide, resulting in progressive loss of myelinated neurones and neurological function. The nature of the damage that occurs in these cells and the reason that damage occurs in such a specific anatomical location is not understood.

Pathology

Few reports of histological findings in CS have appeared in the literature. Biopsies of the facial photosensitivity eruption have been reported as normal or as non-specific dermatitis [32,33]. There is one report of biopsies of four patients with CS who had abnormally small eccrine glands for age [34]. The authors suggested that this histological feature might be a helpful diagnostic aid in some patients. Another study examined the synthesis of collagen in CS patients but could find no detectable abnormality [22].

Neuropathologically, patients show cerebral and cerebellar atrophy, patchy or diffuse demyelination in the central and peripheral nervous system, and pericapillary calcification in the basal ganglia and in the cortex of the cerebrum and cerebellum [3,35].

Clinical features (Fig. 19.22.4)

CS is a multisystem disorder with marked variation in the extent and severity of clinical symptoms. Parents of affected children are asymptomatic [3]. During the first year of life, appearance and development are often normal. Onset of symptoms in the second year of life is heralded by a scaly, erythematous eruption in the sun-exposed areas that may resolve, leaving hyperpigmentation or scarring [36,37]. This is seen in 75% of patients with

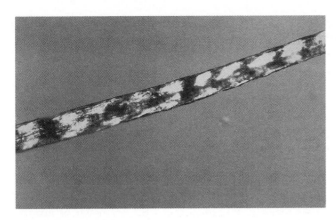

Fig. 19.22.4 Trichothiodystrophy: abnormal striped pattern under polarized light. Courtesy of Dr John Harper.

CS [1]. Growth failure may be noted before the first birthday and involves height, weight and head circumference. Weight is more affected than length, hence the use of the term 'cachectic dwarfism'. All affected patients have height and weight measurements below the fifth percentile by 2 years of age. Few patients with this syndrome exceed heights or weights beyond the 50th percentile for a normal 6-year-old child [1].

All patients with CS develop neurological manifestations. The earliest neurological symptom is delayed psychomotor development with delayed milestones for speech and ambulation [1]. Infants may be noted to feed poorly or have weak cries but this is infrequently attributed to this syndrome until a diagnosis is made later in life. All patients are mentally retarded with reported IQ scores ranging from the borderline to the profoundly retarded range [14–19,21–23,33,36,38,39]. Rarely, a patient with normal intelligence has been reported [40]. For those patients who are higher functioning, deterioration in the teenage years is expected [41].

Microcephaly is radiologically apparent during the second and third years of life [42,43]. The earlier the onset of this finding, the more severe the disease course [1]. Cerebellar signs are usually the first noted on neurological examination. The gait disorder in ambulatory patients is striking and progressive resulting from leg spasticity, ataxia and contractures of the hips, knees and ankles. Tremor, incoordination and dysarthric speech are other common findings. Seizures occur in 5–10% of patients but are usually later complications [1].

Computed tomography (CT) scans and even plain films have demonstrated calcification, usually of the basal ganglia [42,43]. Newer studies of patients using magnetic resonance imaging (MRI) have demonstrated mild ventricular enlargement and delay in myelination of the cerebrum and cerebellum. Other brain structures appear normally myelinated [44].

Most patients with CS have progressive ophthalmological deterioration [19,21,45]. Pigmentary degeneration of the retina has been considered one of the hallmarks of the disease. This 'salt and pepper' retinal change is the most frequently seen ophthalmological complication [45]. Cataracts, optic atrophy and optic disc pallor are also common. Unusual findings such as iris hypoplasia and microphthalmos have been reported but are most common in severe, early onset disease (see below). Cataracts are also a severe prognostic indicator [1].

Sensorineural hearing loss is seen in the majority of CS patients. This may not manifest until the teenage years, but, like the ophthalmological complications, it is usually progressive [41]. Pathological descriptions have confirmed loss of auditory neurones with retrograde atrophy of the auditory pathways in the brainstem as the source of this hearing loss [46,47].

Dental problems are common in CS, consisting of severe caries and malocclusion. The oral cavity and mandible are frequently small resulting in the appearance of large permanent teeth [48].

Renal disease has been reported in 10% of CS patients. Most patients have decreased creatinine clearance and require no medical intervention. Hypertension has also occurred, at times with a documented renal basis. Rarely, renal failure has been reported [16,49].

One-third of males with CS have undescended testes [1]. With the exception of a single female patient with normal intelligence, no retinal changes, mild dwarfism and other mild features, no patient with this disease has had offspring [40]. Females are typically 'underdeveloped' with irregular menses. Other organ systems such as the gastrointestinal (GI) tract and liver have occasionally been involved.

Patients with CS are not at risk for infection. Immune function is normal in this disease [50]. However, severely debilitated patients with neurological deterioration and inadequate nutrition have developed infections.

Patients with CS develop a photosensitivity eruption early in life [3]. Acute sensitivity leads to erythema that desquamates leaving postinflammatory hyperpigmentation and even scarring. This becomes more prominent with time. The freckles and dyspigmentation seen in XP are not features of this disease. With the exception of patients who fall into the CS–XP overlap syndrome, cutaneous malignancies are not reported in this syndrome [3,51].

Other skin manifestations include thin, dry hair and dry, scaly skin. These findings, coupled with the diminution of subcutaneous fat contribute to the 'aged' or progeric appearance of these patients. Characteristic features include a thin prominent nose, prognathism, sunken eyes and large appearing teeth in a small mouth. Hands and limbs are disproportionately large when contrasted with the small trunk. Kyphosis combined with progressive hip, knee and ankle contractures gives a distinctive body habitus [1].

Premature death is a feature of CS. The mean age of death in 140 recently reported patients was 12 years [1]. Causes of death included infections, status epilepticus, cachexia, hypertensive crisis and renal failure. Early death and poor prognosis is associated with low birth weight, microcephaly, structural anomalies of the eye at birth or neurological impairment before the age of 1 year [1].

The variability of severity of this syndrome has led to classification of patients into clinical subgroups to provide guidelines for clinical management and prognosis. The characteristics of these four subgroups are described below.

Classical Cockayne's syndrome

Classical CS or CS I is diagnosed after the first year of life with severe growth failure and neurodevelopmental dysfunction. These two features, accompanied by one other of the following features is sufficient for diagnosis, although most patients have more than one feature: progressive retinitis pigmentosa or cataracts, sensorineural hearing loss or dental caries [1]. Cutaneous photosensitivity is a prominent feature and patients develop the typical physical appearance of 'cachectic dwarfism'. CT or MRI to document white matter abnormalities, or auditory or visual evoked potentials are tests which can corroborate a tentative diagnosis [42–44].

Severe Cockayne's syndrome

Severe CS or CS II has been reported in over 20 patients [1,15–17,43,49,52]. These patients have earlier onset of symptoms and are more severely affected than typical patients. Most die by 6 or 7 years of age. Low birth weight is common with little growth noted postnatally. Final weight does not exceed 8 kg. Neurological development is absent in these patients. Typical progeric, dwarf-like features are noted before the age of 2 years. Structural abnormalities of the eye and early or congenital cataracts are present in 30%. Dental, auditory and cutaneous complications are less commonly noted.

Several other syndromes that share features with this severe form of CS have been described. These include cerebro-oculofacial-skeletal syndrome (COFS), Pena–Shokeir II and CAMFAK syndromes (Congenital cataracts, microcephaly, failure to thrive and kyphoscoliosis) [1,53–56]. All three of these disorders are characterized by prenatal growth failure, microcephaly, cataracts, joint deformities, abnormal myelinization of the brain and early death. Additional anomalies, not typical of severe CS, are also seen. Some patients within these groups demonstrate abnormalities of nucleic acid metabolism and cellular hypersensitivity to UV light and may represent allelic variations of CS.

Mild Cockayne's syndrome

Another group of patients has been described who have some of the clinical features of CS, but lack one of the cardinal features of abnormal growth and intelligence [40,57,58]. Symptoms are typically mild and late in onset. These patients may have normal intelligence, growth and reproductive capacity. One such patient was clearly demonstrated to have the DNA and RNA metabolic abnormalities seen in Cockayne's syndrome [40]. It should be cautioned, however, that patients with features of growth retardation, ophthalmological complications or other major characteristics of CS I are never of normal intelligence or reproductive capacity and parents should be counselled appropriately.

Cockayne syndrome–xeroderma pigmentosum overlap syndrome

A few patients have recently been described with CS accompanied by clinical features of XP [3,9,51,59,60]. Skin manifestations including freckling, hyperpigmentation and cutaneous neoplasms on sun-exposed skin have been reported. These patients are distinguishable, clinically, from XP patients with the De Sanctis–Cacchione syndrome because they lack the typical neurological features of primary neuronal degeneration. The neurological symptoms seen are those of demyelination and cerebellar dysfunction as is typical of CS. In addition, affected patients have other features of CS including pigmentary retinal degeneration, calcification of the basal ganglia, normal pressure hydrocephalus and hyperreflexia [3].

Cells from these patients have reduced DNA excision repair and fall into three different XP complementation groups (B, D and G). The gene that corrects the defect in patients with CS who have overlap with XPB has been identified as ERCC3 on chromosome 2 [61].

Prognosis

The prognosis for patients with CS is poor. In classical CS progressive deterioration of neurological, ophthalmological and auditory function occurs. Early closure of growth plates results in severe dwarfism with progressive contractures and kyphoscoliosis limiting ambulation in the teens, even in those who learn to walk. Death occurs in the early teens in most patients (see above) [1].

Those patients who fall into the severe category of CS II have an even worse prognosis. Here minimal growth from birth is noted with a maximum final weight of 8 kg. There is no neurological development evident and cataracts and eye anomalies limit vision. Death commonly occurs by the age of 6–7 years [1,15–17,43,49,52–56].

Patients who have been reported with mild or atypical CS have a better prognosis. These patients are diagnosed later in life, lacking the severe growth retardation and intellectual impairment. Only a handful of patients have been reported with these findings [40,57,58].

Several features have been identified that predict an unfavourable prognosis for patients with CS. The presence of growth retardation at birth, the presence of neonatal cataracts or early onset cataract formation, eye anomalies, absence of neurological progression in the first year of life and onset of the typical facies and body habitus before the first 2 years of life are all poor prognostic indicators [1].

Differential diagnosis

The differential diagnosis of CS depends on the presenting features and the age of the patient at the time of diagnosis. In the older typical patient, there are few diagnostic considerations. In younger infants and children, the typical presentation is short stature and/or failure to thrive with developmental delay. It is essential that a complete examination be performed to document abnormalities of the skin, eyes, ears, teeth, skeletal system and neurological function. Limb and trunk contractures and the 'cachectic' facial appearance that is diagnostic are not typically identifiable in the first several years of life.

Profound growth failure usually suggests a chromosomal abnormality, or a genetic syndrome such as Hallermann–Streiff, Russell–Silver, Brachmann–deLange, Dubowitz or others. Endocrine, metabolic and gastrointestinal disorders leading to malabsorption must all be considered. The onset of growth failure after birth without physical anomalies makes chromosomal abnormalities less likely. Skeletal dysplasias can be ruled out with routine X-rays. Endocrine and metabolic testing is indicated and feeding history is helpful to exclude GI problems.

The presence of photosensitivity, a facial rash and dry or atrophic hair suggests XP, Bloom's syndrome, dyskeratosis congenita or the premature ageing syndromes such as progeria, Werner's syndrome, Rothmund–Thompson syndrome or tyrosinaemia. Appropriate diagnostic tests can look for chromosome breakage. DNA repair in fibroblasts or other diagnostic features.

If the presentation is seizures or neurological deterioration, an MRI will show primary involvement of the white matter. None of the leucodystrophies cause severe growth failure. Intracranial calcifications might suggest congenital infections or disorders of calcium or phosphate metabolism, but these should be easily eliminated by examination of other organ systems.

Finally, the presence of retinitis pigmentosum with neurological abnormalities might be seen in peroxisomal disorders and mitochondrial encephalomyopathy with ragged-red fibres. These conditions lack the growth, cutaneous and dental finding of CS [1].

The diagnosis of CS relies primarily on the presence of a typical clinical picture that includes the two most diagnostic features, growth retardation and neurological impairment, in combination with one of the other clinical features (see above). Corroborative tests in cases where the diagnosis is uncertain would include a CT or MRI of the brain, auditory or visual evoked potentials, electromyogram (EMG) or nerve conduction velocity (NCV), audiometry and the analysis of the sensitivity of fibroblasts to UV light in combination with other assays of DNA metabolism.

Treatment

There is no medical or surgical treatment for patients with CS. Management is purely symptomatic and supportive. All patients should practice photoprotection to avoid exacerbation of the cutaneous photosensitivity. Sunscreens, especially physical blockers that contain titanium dioxide, may be helpful. Growth failure warrants gastrostomy placement only in those individuals with poor oral intake due to neurological compromise. Longitudinal growth will not improve with this intervention.

Routine paediatric follow-up including periodic formal assessment of neurological impairment, social, auditory and visual function to facilitate providing appropriate placement and services is recommended. Optimizing the potential of patients with deteriorating neurological function is important since this syndrome is characterized by life expectancy into the teens or even 20s. Treatable complications such as hypertension, tooth decay, hearing impairment and contractures should be addressed. Early intervention with physical therapy can help prevent the development and progression of contractures.

Prenatal diagnosis of CS by assay of fetal amniocytes has been performed [62,63]. Carrier testing is not yet possible. Genetic counselling is advised since the risk of a subsequent child being affected is 25%. Reports in the literature of families with multiple affected offspring suggest autosomal recessive inheritance in this disease [64].

REFERENCES

1 Nance MA, Berry SA. Cockayne syndrome: review of 140 cases. *Am J Med Genet* 1992; 42: 68–84.
2 Kraemer KH, Levy DD, Parris CN *et al.* Xeroderma pigmentosum and related disorders: examining the linkage between defective DNA repair and cancer. *J Invest Dermatol* 1994; 103: 96–101.
3 Otsuka F, Robbins JH. The Cockayne syndrome—an inherited multisystem disorder with cutaneous photosensitivity and defective repair of DNA. *Am J Dermatopathol* 1985; 7: 387–92.
4 Cockayne EA. Dwarfism with retinal atrophy and deafness. *Arch Dis Child* 1936; 11: 1–8.
5 Cockayne EA. Dwarfism with retinal atrophy and deafness. *Arch Dis Child* 1946; 21: 52–4.
6 Neil CS, Dingwall MM. A syndrome resembling progeria. A review of two cases. *Arch Dis Child* 1950; 25: 213–21.
7 Tanaka K, Kawai K, Kumahara Y *et al.* Genetic complementation groups in Cockayne syndrome. *Somatic Cell Genet* 1981; 7: 445–55.
8 Venema J, Mullenders LH, Natarajan AT *et al.* The genetic defect in Cockayne syndrome is associated with a defect in repair of UV-induced

DNA damage in transcriptionally active DNA. *Proc Natl Acad Sci USA* 1990; 87: 4707–11.

9 Lehmann AR. Three complementation groups in Cockayne syndrome. *Mutat Res* 1982; 106: 347–56.

10 Cooper PK, Leadon SA. Defective repair of ionizing radiation damage in Cockayne's syndrome and xeroderma pigmentosum group G. *Ann NY Acad Sci* 1994; 726: 330–2.

11 Cleaver JE, Kraemer KH. Xeroderma pigmentosum. In: Scriver CR, Beaudet AL, Sly WS, Valle D, eds. *The Metabolic Basis of Inherited Disease*, 6th edn. New York: McGraw Hill, 1989; 2949–71.

12 Scott RJ, Itin P, Kleijer WJ *et al*. Xeroderma pigmentosum–Cockayne syndrome complex in two patients; absence of skin tumors despite severe deficiency of DNA excision repair. *J Am Acad Dermatol* 1993; 29 (suppl): 883–9.

13 Vermeulen W, Jaeken J, Jaspers NG *et al*. Xeroderma pigmentosum complementation group G associated with Cockayne syndrome. *Am J Hum Genet* 1993; 53: 185–92.

14 Lowry RB. Invited editorial comment: early onset of Cockayne syndrome. *Am J Med Genet* 1982; 13: 209–10.

15 Jaeken J, Klocker H, Schwaiger H *et al*. Clinical and biochemical studies in three patients with severe early infantile Cockayne syndrome. *Hum Genet* 1989; 83: 339–46.

16 Leech RW, Brumback RA, Miller RH *et al*. Cockayne syndrome: clinicopathologic and tissue culture studies of affected siblings. *J Neuropathol Exp Neurol* 1985; 44: 507–19.

17 Patton MA, Giannelli F, Francis AJ *et al*. Early onset Cockayne's syndrome: case reports with neuropathological and fibroblast studies. *J Med Genet* 1989; 26: 154–9.

18 Hashimoto T, Hiura K, Kobayashi Y *et al*. Cockayne's syndrome: report of two sisters and review of the literature in Japan. *Brain Dev* 1978; 10: 465–72.

19 Jin K, Handa T, Ishihara T *et al*. Cockayne syndrome: report of two cases and review of the literature in Japan. *Brain Dev* 1979; 1: 305–12.

20 Cotton RB, Keats TE, McCoy EE. Abnormal blood glucose regulation in Cockayne's syndrome. *Pediatrics* 1970; 46: 54–60.

21 Levin PS, Green WR, Victor DI *et al*. Histopathology of the eye in Cockayne's syndrome. *Arch Ophthalmol* 1983; 101: 1093–7.

22 Keren G, Duksin D, Cohen BE *et al*. Collagen synthesis by fibroblasts in a patient with the Cockayne syndrome. *Eur J Pediatr* 1981; 137: 339–42.

23 Civantos F. Human chromosomal abnormalities. *Bull Tulane Med Fac* 1961; 20: 241–53.

24 Fryns JP, Bulcke J, Verdu P *et al*. Apparent late-onset Cockayne syndrome and interstitial deletion of the long arm of chromosome 10 (del(10)(q11.23q21.2)). *Am J Med Genet* 1991; 40: 343.

25 Troelstra C, Lansvater RM, Wiegant J *et al*. Localization of the nucleotide excision repair gene ERCC6 to human chromosome 10q11–q21. *Genomics* 1992; 12: 745–9.

26 Troelstra C, Van Gool A, De Wit J *et al*. ERCC6, a member of a subfamily of putative helicases, is involved in Cockayne's syndrome and preferential repair of active genes. *Cell* 1992; 71: 939–53.

27 Troelstra C, Hesen W, Bootsma D *et al*. Structure and expression of the excision repair gene ERCC6, involved in the human disorder Cockayne's syndrome group B. *Nucl Acids Res* 1993; 21: 419–26.

28 Sancar A, Tang M. Nucleotide excision repair. *Photochem Photobiol* 1993; 57: 905–21.

29 Barrett SF, Robbins JH, Tarone RE *et al*. Evidence for defective repair of cyclobutane pyrimidine dimers with normal repair of other DNA photoproducts in a transcriptionally active gene transfected into Cockayne syndrome cells. *Mutat Res* 1991; 255: 281–91.

30 Parris CN, Kraemer KH, Ultraviolet-induced mutations in Cockayne syndrome cells are primarily caused by cyclobutane dimer photoproducts while repair of other photoproducts is normal. *Proc Natl Acad Sci USA* 1993; 90: 7260–4.

31 Brumback RA, Yoder FW, Andrews AD *et al*. Normal pressure hydrocephalus: recognition and relationship to neurological abnormalities in Cockayne's syndrome. *Arch Neurol* 1978; 35: 337.

32 MacDonald WB, Fitch KD, Lewis IC. Cockayne's syndrome. An heredofamilial disorder of growth and development. *Pediatrics* 1960; 25: 997–1007.

33 Srivastava RN, Gupta PC, Mayekar G at al. Case report. Cockayne's syndrome in two sisters. *Acta Paediatr Scand* 1974; 63: 461–4.

34 Landing BH, Sugarman G, Dixon LG. Eccrine sweat gland anatomy in Cockayne syndrome: a possible diagnostic aid. *Pediatr Pathol* 1983; 1: 349–53.

35 Pinckers AJL, Hombergen GCJ, Notermans SLH *et al*. Peripheral and central myelinopathy in Cockayne's syndrome. *Neuropediatrics* 1982; 13: 161–7.

36 Lasser AE. Cockayne's syndrome. *Cutis* 1972; 10: 143–8.

37 Proops R, Taylor AMR, Insley J. A clinical study of a family with Cockayne's syndrome. *J Med Genet* 1981; 18: 288–93.

38 Mayne LV, Broughton BL, Lehmann AR. The ultraviolet sensitivity of Cockayne syndrome cells is not a consequence of reduced cellular NAD⁺ content. *Am J Hum Genet* 1984; 36: 311–19.

39 Harbord MG, Finn JP, Hall-Craggs MA *et al*. Early onset leukodystrophy with distinct facial features in two siblings. *Neuropediatrics* 1989; 20: 154–7.

40 Kennedy RM, Rowe VD, Kepes JJ. Cockayne syndrome: an atypical case. *Neurology* 1980; 30: 1268–72.

41 Windmiller J, Whalley PJ, Fink CW. Cockayne's syndrome with chromosomal analysis. *Am J Dis Child* 1963; 105: 204–8.

42 Bensman A, Faure C, Kaufman HJ. The spectrum of X-ray manifestations in Cockayne syndrome. *Skelet Radiol* 1981; 7: 173–7.

43 Riggs W, Seibert J. Cockayne's syndrome. Roentgen findings. *Am J Roentgenol* 1972; 116: 623–33.

44 Dabbagh O, Swaiman KF. Cockayne syndrome: MRI correlates of hypomyelination. *Pediatr Neurol* 1988; 4: 113–16.

45 Coles WH. Ocular manifestations of Cockayne's syndrome. *Am J Ophthalmol* 1969; 67: 762–4.

46 Gandolfi A, Horoupian D, Rapin I *et al*. Deafness in Cockayne's syndrome: morphological, morphometric, and quantitative study of the auditory pathway. *Ann Neurol* 1984; 15: 135–43.

47 Shemen LJ, Mitchell DP, Farkashidy J. Cockayne syndrome—an audiologic and temporal bone analysis. *Am J Otol* 1984; 5: 300–7.

48 Schneider PE. Dental findings in a child with Cockayne's syndrome. *J Dent Child* 1983; 30: 58–64.

49 Higginbottom MC, Griswold WR, Jones KL *et al*. The Cockayne syndrome: an evaluation of hypertension and studies of renal pathology. *Pediatrics* 1979; 64: 929–34.

50 Norris PG, Limb GA, Hamblin AS *et al*. Immune function, mutant frequency, and cancer risk in the DNA repair defective genodermatoses xeroderma pigmentosum, Cockayne's syndrome, and trichothiodystrophy. *J Invest Dermatol* 1990; 94: 94–100.

51 Wood RD. Seven genes for three diseases. *Nature* 1991; 350: 190.

52 Nishio H, Kodama S, Matsuo T *et al*. Cockayne syndrome: magnetic resonance images of the brain in a severe form with early onset. *J Inher Metab Dis* 1988; 11: 88–102.

53 Gorlin RJ, Cohen MM, Levin LS. *Syndromes of the Head and Neck*, 3rd edn. New York: Oxford University Press, 1990; 295–321, 623–4.

54 Lowry RB, McLean R, Maclean DM *et al*. Cataracts, microcephaly, kyphosis, and limited joint movement in two siblings: a new syndrome. *J Pediatr* 1971; 79: 282–4.

55 Scott-Emuankpor AB, Heffelfinger J, Higgins JV. A syndrome of microcephaly and cataracts in four siblings: a new genetic syndrome? *Am J Dis Child* 1977; 131: 167–9.

56 Talwar D, Smith SA. CAMFAX syndrome: a demyelinating inherited disease similar to Cockayne syndrome. *Am J Med Genet* 1989; 34: 194–8.

57 Fujiwara Y, Ichihashi M, Kano Y *et al*. A new human photosensitive subject with a defect in the recovery of DNA synthesis after ultraviolet-light irradiation. *J Invest Dermatol* 1981; 77: 256–63.

58 Lanning M, Simila S. Cockayne's syndrome: report of a case with normal intelligence. *Z Kinderheilk* 1970; 109: 70–5.

59 Robbins JH, Kraemer KH, Lutzner MA *et al*. Xeroderma pigmentosum. An inherited disease with sun sensitivity, multiple cutaneous neoplasms, and abnormal DNA repair. *Ann Intern Med* 1974; 80: 221–48.

60 Venema J, Mullenders LHF, Natarajan AT *et al*. The genetic defect in Cockayne syndrome is associated with a defect in repair of UV-induced DNA damage in transcriptionally active DNA. *Proc Natl Acad Sci USA* 1990; 87: 4707–11.

61 Moshell AN, Ganges MB, Lutzner MA *et al*. A new patient with both xeroderma pigmentosum and Cockayne syndrome establishes the new xeroderma pigmentosum complementation group H. In: Friedberg EC, Bridges BR, eds. *Cellular Response to DNA Damage*. New York: Alan R. Liss, 1983: 209–13.

62 Weeda G, Vantham RC, Vermeulen W *et al*. A presumed DNA helicase encoded by ERCC-3 is involved in the human repair disorders xeroderma pigmentosum and Cockayne's syndrome. *Cell* 1990; 62: 777.

63 Sugita T, Ikenaga M, Suehara N *et al*. Prenatal diagnosis of Cockayne syn-

drome using assay of colony-forming ability in ultraviolet light irradiated cells. *Clin Genet* 1982; 22: 137–42.

64 Lehmann AR, Francis AJ, Giannelli F. Prenatal diagnosis of Cockayne's syndrome. *Lancet* 1985; 1: 486–8.

Trichothiodystrophy (Tay's syndrome, BIDS, IBIDS, PIBIDS)

Definition

Trichothiodystrophy is a rare, autosomal recessive disease characterized by sulphur-deficient brittle hair and a constellation of neuroectodermal symptoms [1]. Many acronyms have been suggested to describe the associated ectodermal and neuroectodermal findings in these patients including BIDS (brittle hair, intellectual impairment, decreased fertility, and short stature), IBIDS (BIDS with ichthyosis) and PIBIDS (IBIDS with photosensitivity) [2–4]. A recent review of the literature identified 95 cases of trichothiodystrophy [5]. In this review, the authors emphasize that sulphur-deficient hair is essential but insufficient to make a diagnosis of trichothiodystrophy. The findings of one of trichoschisis, alternating light and dark bands by polarizing microscope or an absent or severely damaged hair cuticle by scanning electron microscope, are necessary to make the diagnosis. The other clinical manifestations vary widely with no constant features [6]. Other frequent findings include nail dystrophy, growth and mental retardation, ichthyosis, photosensitivity, collodion baby, erythroderma, eczema, cataracts, recurrent infections, sparse axillary hair, defective DNA repair and microcephaly [5]. A typical facies is present in many patients.

History

The term trichothiodystrophy was proposed by Price *et al.* in 1979 and 1980 [1,7]. They suggested that sulphur-deficient brittle hair was a marker for the association of ectodermal and neuroectodermal defects. The first reported cases of trichothiodystrophy appeared a decade before when Pollitt *et al.* described patients with trichorrhexis nodosa, low sulphur content of hair, and associated mental and physical retardation [8]. Two years later, Brown *et al.* reported a case of tricoschisis with the typical pattern of sulphur-deficient hair seen on polarized light microscopy [9]. Tay reported three patients with ichthyosiform erythroderma, hair shaft abnormalities and mental and growth retardation [10]. Other authors have since reported cases of Tay's syndrome with trichothiodystrophy [5,11–13].

Photosensitivity as a prominent feature in trichothiodystrophy was first suggested by Price *et al.* in 1980 [1]. Crovato *et al.* suggested the acronym PIBIDS in 1983 [4]. Further studies on patients with photosensitivity demonstrated a defect in DNA repair [14–16]. Subsequently,

Lehmann *et al.* demonstrated abnormal responses to UV light in three patients with trichothiodystrophy without photosensitivity [17,18].

Cells cultured from patients with trichothiodystrophy, both with and without photosensitivity, have demonstrated responses similar to the impaired DNA excision defect seen in XP complementation group D [16,18–23]. Patients with this overlap syndrome have no increased frequency of skin cancer and are clinically different than patients with XP group D.

Others have reported patients with trichothiodystrophy without photosensitivity but with impaired DNA repair [24], and with different DNA repair defects than those seen in XP group D [18].

Aetiology

All patients with trichothiodystrophy have a single, common hair defect [1]. Samples of hair are abnormally low in sulphur content [25,26]. Biochemical studies have shown that the abnormal hair has less than half of the normal content of cystine. Normal hair and nails contain 40–45% of constituent high-sulphur matrix proteins that lend strength to hair shafts. In trichothiodystrophy, there is a reduction in the amount of these constituent proteins to less than 10% and altered amino acid composition demonstrated on two-dimensional gel electrophoresis [27]. There is also an abnormal distribution of the sulphur-rich, intermicrofibrillar, globular proteins of the cortex and the sulphur-rich proteins of the hair shaft [28,29]. Hairs are abnormally brittle with an absent or greatly reduced cuticle that results in fragile, uneven and easily broken hairs. The low-sulphur proteins are increased in amount and normal in composition [27]. Nails also show a decrease in cystine and sulphur content [1,2,25].

The relationship between the metabolically abnormal hair shafts in trichothiodystrophy and the other ectodermal and neuroectodermal defects remains unclear. Expression of abnormal genes that specifically affect sulphur-rich proteins of keratinization may be pathogenic [26]. It has been speculated that the changed pattern of synthesis of high-sulphur matrix proteins may affect not only hair and nail synthesis, but synthesis of similar matrix proteins in other tissues as well [30]. This may account for the marked biochemical and clinical heterogeneity seen in this disease.

The relationship between trichothiodystrophy patients whose cells demonstrate the excison repair defect seen in group D XP and other patients with XP is also unknown. One explanation is that trichothiodystrophy is part of the spectrum of excision repair disorders which includes XP and CS, and that trichothiodystrophy reflects allelic heterogeneity at the XPD locus [31]. With allelic heterogeneity, a spectrum of clinical phenotypes derives from varying degrees of inactivation of the functional attributes of a single-gene product. Alternately, the excision repair defect may be a marker for one or two subsets of trichothiodystrophy patients with mutations in a gene that maps close to an XP locus [32]. Finally, it is possible that there is a genetic mutation present in an isolated gene in trichothiodystropy at a locus that is unlinked to the XPD locus, which exerts an effect on both the XPD and the trichothiodystrophy gene products [32].

Pathology

On light microscope examination, hair shafts from patients with trichothiodystrophy have a wavy, irregular outline with ribbon-like flattening. Trichoschisis (clean breaks) and trichorrhexis nodosa-like fractures are seen, but there is an absence of the typical release of spindle cells that is seen in true trichorrhexis nodosa [1,33].

The pattern on polarizing microscope is even more distinctive. Using crossed polarizers in the position of extinction, hair shafts show striking alternating bright and dark bands [1,33].

Scanning electron microscopy has demonstrated severe cuticular and secondary cortical degeneration along the entire length of the flattened hair shaft [34,35]. Flattened hairs are seen folding ribbon-like onto themselves [36]. Longitudinal ridging, cuticle loss, trichorrhexis nodosa formation and trichoschisis are also demonstrated [34].

Transmission electron microscopy has demonstrated a quantitative decrease in high-sulphur protein in the hair shaft and a failure of this protein to migrate to the exocuticular part of the cuticle cells [2,29,37]. This results in cuticular weathering and weakness of the hair shaft. Microfibrils are arranged abnormally [2].

Clinical features

All patients with trichothiodystrophy have clinically abnormal hair on the scalp, eyelashes and eyebrows. Hairs are brittle, unruly, of variable lengths, easily broken, sparse and dry. Hypotrichosis, patchy scalp alopecia, scarce eyebrows and eyelashes and sparse axillary and pubic hairs are typical. Other body hair may be scant or absent [5,30]. Hair colour does not seem to be affected [5].

Patients with trichothiodystrophy often resemble one another. They have receding chins, protruding ears, a raspy voice, microcephaly and a sociable, outgoing personality [30].

The range and spectrum of other clinical features in this disease is very broad. Van Neste *et al.* [6,38,39] proposed a system of classification for patients according to the severity of clinical findings in organs derived from ectoderm and neural crest elements as follows: (a) isolated hair defect; (b) onychodystrophy; (c) mental retardation (Sabinas' syndrome); (d) growth retardation (Amish brittle hair syndrome, BIDS); (e) icthyosis (IBIDS, Tay's syndrome); and (f) photosensitivity (PIBIDS). Itin *et al.* added another category (g) to include patients with chronic neutropenia [40]. An extensive review of the literature and clinical manifestations can be found in Itin and Pittelkow [5].

The most common cutaneous features are collodion baby, ichthyosis, erythroderma and eczema [1,3–5,8, 10–13,17,24,28]. Photosensitivity is also seen commonly, especially in association with DNA repair defects and XP group D overlap [5,14,15,24,41]. No increase in malignancies has been demonstrated in this group.

Nail dystrophy is frequent and longitudinal ridging and splitting along with koilonychia are the most common findings [1,5,8,12,40,42]. Dental anomalies such as enamel hypoplasia, caries and a high-arched palate are seen [1,4,5,8,12]. Cataracts are the most frequent eye finding followed by conjunctivitis, epicanthal folds and photophobia [1,3–5,12,15,17,35,40–42].

Mental and growth retardation are typical features of patients with this syndrome [1,3–5,8,10–15,17,24, 35,40–42]. Nystagmus, intention tremor, spasticity and ataxia are the most commonly reported neurological findings [1,4,5,11,12,17,28,41,43]. Growth retarded individuals often have an alteration in body proportions giving the distinctive phenotype [43].

Finally, recurrent infections are another common manifestation of this disease [5,40,42–45]. Chronic neutropenia with monocytosis and disturbed intracellular killing during phagocytosis has been reported [5,40].

Prognosis

Prognosis in trichothiodystrophy is a function of the extent and severity of the neurological and ectodermal components of the disease. Patients that are severely affected die prematurely of causes ranging from infection to complications of surgery. There is no increased incidence of malignancy in trichothiodystrophy. Patients have been described with normal intelligence who are mildly affected and have lived a normal lifespan [6,39].

Differential diagnosis

Not all patients with abnormal sulphur content of hair have trichothiodystrophy. Patients with ichthyosis have been demonstrated to have decreased cystine and other amino acids in hair [46]. Three patients with Clouston's ectodermal dysplasia have been reported with cystine content of hydrolysed hair in the 25% range [47]. Nutrition can influence the sulphur content of hair, with normalization after treatment of the nutritional deficiency [48]. Many products used in the hair industry such as cold-waving lotions, hair bleaching solutions and synthetic organic hair dyes can change the cystine content of hair [49].

The pattern of trichoschisis and alternating bands of light and dark on polarizing microscopy have also been described in patients with other genetic hair abnormalities that do not have low sulphur content [50–52].

Since patients with trichothiodystrophy often have abnormalities of other ectodermal structures, the differential diagnosis includes the other ectodermal dysplasias. By definition, ectodermal dysplasias are disorders characterized by genetic defects in two ectodermally derived structures: hair, nails, teeth and sweat glands [53]. Nail findings and dental abnormalities are frequent in the trichothiodystrophies so overlap with the ectodermal dysplasias exists. Evaluation of the sulphur content of hair in patients with features of ectodermal dysplasia will help to define these overlapping syndromes. Clinical presentations in these syndromes may represent different closely related or linked genetic alterations that regulate keratinization in hair and other ectodermal structures [5].

All patients with congenitally brittle hair should undergo sulphur analysis of hair to look for trichothiodystrophy. Evaluation of clipped hairs under light, polarized, scanning electron and transmission electron microscopy can all aid in establishing the diagnosis.

Treatment

There is no treatment for the underlying deficiency in sulphur that is present in the hair of patients with trichothiodystrophy. It is not associated with any abnormality of serum or urine levels of sulphur-containing amino acids [5]. Since hair is brittle and less strong than normal hair, trauma should be minimized.

The associated neuroectodermal abnormalities should prompt medical examination and pertinent evaluations to diagnose problems that may be treatable. Investigation for photosensitivity and possible DNA repair defects may be helpful in better defining the manifestations of the syndrome that are expressed in a patient. Trichothiodystrophy appears to be inherited as an autosomal recessive syndrome. Prenatal diagnosis can be made in some cases [24].

REFERENCES

1 Price VH, Odom RB, Ward WH *et al.* Trichothiodystrophy. Sulfur-deficient brittle hair as a marker for a neuroectodermal symptom complex. *Arch Dermatol* 1980; 116: 1375–84.
2 Baden HP, Jackson CE, Weiss L *et al.* The physicochemical properties of hair in the BIDS syndrome. *Am J Hum Genet* 1976; 28: 514–21.
3 Jorizzo JL, Atherton DJ, Crounse RG *et al.* Ichthyosis, brittle hair, impaired intelligence, decreased fertility and short stature (IBIDS syndrome). *Br J Dermatol* 1982; 106: 705–10.
4 Crovato F, Borrone C, Rebora A. Trichothiodystrophy–BIDS, IBIDS and PIBIDS? *Br J Dermatol* 1983; 108: 247 (letter).
5 Itin PH, Pittelkow MR. Trichothiodystrophy: review of sulfur-deficient

brittle hair syndromes and association with the ectodermal dysplasias. *J Am Acad Dermatol* 1990; 22: 705–17.
6 Van Neste D, Miller X, Bohnert E. Clinical symptoms associated with trichothiodystrophy: a review of the literature with special emphasis on light sensitivity and the association with xeroderma pigmentosum (complementation group D). In: Van Neste D, Lachapelle JM, Antoine JL, eds. *Trends in Human Hair Growth and Alopecia Research.* Dordrecht: Kluwer Academic Publishers, 1989: 183–93.
7 Price VH. Brüchiges Schwefelmangelhaar: trichothiodystrophie. In: Orfanos CE, ed. *Haar und Haarkrankheiten.* Stuttgart: Gustav Fischer Verlag, 1979: 413–21.
8 Pollitt RJ, Jennfer FA, Davies M. Sibs with mental and physical retardation and trichorrhexis nodosa with abnormal amino acid composition of the hair. *Arch Dis Child* 1968; 43: 211–16.
9 Brown AC, Belser RB, Crounse RG *et al.* A congenital hair defect: trichoschisis with alternating birefringence and low sulfur content. *J Invest Dermatol* 1970; 54: 496–509.
10 Tay CH. Ichthyosiform erythroderma, hair shaft abnormalities, and mental and growth retardation. A new recessive disorder. *Arch Dermatol* 1971; 104: 4–13.
11 Motley RJ, Finlay AY. A patient with Tay's syndrome. *Pediatr Dermatol* 1989; 6: 202–5.
12 Kousseff BG, Esterly NB. Trichothiodystrophy: IBIDS syndrome of Tay syndrome? *Birth Defects* 1988; 24: 169–81.
13 Happle R, Traupe H, Gröbe H *et al.* The Tay syndrome (congenital ichthyosis with trichothiodystrophy). *Eur J Pediatr* 1984; 141: 147–52.
14 Crovato F, Rebora A. PIBI(D)S syndrome: a new entity with defect of the deoxyribonucleic acid excision repair system. *J Am Acad Dermatol* 1985; 13: 683–5.
15 Van Neste D, Caulier B, Thomas P, Vasseur F. Tay's syndrome and xeroderma pigmentosum. *J Am Acad Dermatol* 1985; 12: 372–3.
16 Stefanini M, Giliani S, Nardo T *et al.* DNA repair investigations in nine Italian patients affected by trichothiodystrophy. *Mutat Res, DNA Repair* 1992; 273: 119–25.
17 Lehmann AR. Cockayne's syndrome and trichothiodystrophy: defective repair without cancer. *Cancer Rev* 1987; 7: 82–103.
18 Lehmann AR, Arlett CF, Broughton BC *et al.* Trichothiodystrophy, a human DNA repair disorder with heterogeneity in the cellular response to ultraviolet light. *Cancer Res* 1988; 48: 6090–6.
19 Stefanini M, Lagomarsini P, Fois A *et al.* Sensitivity to sunlight in patients affected by trichothiodystrophy is related to the capacity to repair the UV-induced DNA damage. *Br J Cancer* 1986; 54: 355 (abstract).
20 Stefanini M, Collins AR, Riboni R *et al.* Novel Chinese hamster ultraviolet-sensitive mutants for excision repair form complementation groups 9 and 10. *Cancer Res* 1991; 51: 3965–71.
21 Nuzzo F, Stefanini M. The association of xeroderma pigmentosum with trichothiodystrophy: a clue to a better understanding of XP-D? In: Castellani A, ed. *DNA Damage and Repair.* New York: Plenum Press, 1989: 61–72.
22 Nuzzo F, Stefanini M, Rocchi M *et al.* Chromosome and blood marker studies in families of patients affected by xeroderma pigmentosum and trichothiodystrophy. *Mutat Res* 1988; 208: 159–61.
23 Van Neste D, Caulier B, Thomas P. PIBI(D)S syndrome: a new entity with defect of the deoxyribonucleic acid excision repair system. *J Am Acad Dermatol* 1985; 13 (letter): 685.
24 Blanchet-Bardon C, Sarrasin A, Renault G *et al.* Prenatal diagnosis of BIDS and IBIDS syndromes: trichothiodystrophies with DNA repair defect. *Br J Dermatol* 1989; 123 (suppl 34): 18 (abstract).
25 Pollitt RJ, Stonier PD. Proteins of normal hair and of cystine-deficient hair from mentally retarded siblings. *Biochem J* 1971; 122: 433–4.
26 Gillespie JM, Marshall RC. A comparison of the proteins of normal and trichothiodystrophic human hair. *J Invest Dermatol* 1983; 80: 195–202.
27 Gillespie JM, Marshall RC, Rogers M. Trichothiodystrophy-biochemical and clinical studies. *Aust J Dermatol* 1988; 29: 85–93.
28 Gummer CL, Dawber RPR. Trichothiodystrophy: an ultrastructural study of the hair follicle. *Br J Dermatol* 1985; 113: 273–80.
29 Gummer CL, Dawber RPR, Price VH. Trichothiodystrophy: an electron-histochemical study of the hair shaft. *Br J Dermatol* 1984; 110: 439–49.
30 Price VH. Trichothiodystrophy: update. *Pediatr Dermatol* 1992; 9: 369–70.
31 Friedberg EC, Henning KA. The conundrum of xeroderma pigmentosum—a rare disease with frequent complexities. *Mutat Res* 1993; 289: 47–53.
32 Wood RD. Human diseases associated with defective DNA excision repair. *J Roy Coll Phys Lond* 1991; 24: 300.

33 Price VH. Structural anomalies of the hair shaft. In: Orfanos CE, Happle R, eds. *Hair and Hair Diseases*. Berlin: Springer-Verlag, 1990: 363–422.

34 Meyvisch K, Song M, Dourov N. Review and new case reports on scanning electron microscopy of pili annulati, monilethrix and trichothiodystrophy. *Scann Microsc* 1992; 6: 537–41.

35 Van Neste D, Bore P. Trichothiodystrophy: a morphological and biochemical study. *Ann Dermatol Vénéréol* 1983; 110: 409–17.

36 Van Neste D, Degreef H, van Haute N *et al*. High sulfur protein deficient hair. *J Am Acad Dermatol* 1989; 20: 195–202.

37 Vanning VA, Dawber RPR, Ferguson DJP, Kanan MW. Weathering of hair in trichodystrophy. *Br J Dermatol* 1986; 114: 591–5.

38 Van Neste DJ, Antoine JL, Vasseur F *et al*. Tay's syndrome and xeroderma pigmentosum. *Seventeenth World Congress of Dermatology*, Part 1, 1987: WS-18 (abstract).

39 Alfandari S, Delaporte E, Van Neste D, Lucidarme-Delespierre E, Piette F, Bergoend H. A new case of isolated trichothiodystrophy. *Dermatologica* 1993; 186: 197–200.

40 Itin PH, Pittelkow MR. Trichothiodystrophy with chronic neutropenia and mild mental retardation. *J Am Acad Dermatol* 1991; 24: 356–8.

41 Stefanini M, Lagomarsini P, Arlett CF *et al*. Xeroderma pigmentosum (complementation group D) mutation is present in patients affected by trichothiodystrophy with photosensitivity. *Hum Genet* 1986; 74: 107–12.

42 Cantu JM, Arisas J, Foncerrada M *et al*. Syndrome of onychotrichodysplasia with chronic neutropenia in an infant from consanguineous parents. *Birth Defects* 1975; 11: 63–5.

43 Meynadier J, Guillot B, Barneon G *et al*. Trichothiodystrophie. *Ann Dermatol Vénéréol* 1987; 114: 1529–36.

44 Baden HP, Katz A. Trichothiodystrophy without retardation: one patient exhibiting transient combined immunodeficiency syndrome. *Pediatr Dermatol* 1988; 5: 257–9.

45 Hernandez A, Olivares F, Cantu JM. Autosomal recessive onychotrichodysplasia, chronic neutropenia and mild mental retardation. Delineation of the syndrome. *Clin Genet* 1979; 15: 147–52.

46 Morganti P, Muscardin L, Avido U *et al*. Abnormal amino acid changes in human hair associated with rare congenital syndromes. In: Orfanos CE, Montagna W, Stüttgen G, eds. *Hair Research: Status and Future Aspects*. Berlin: Springer-Verlag, 1981: 442–5.

47 Gold RJM, Scriver CR. The characterization of hereditary abnormalities of keratin: Clouston's ectodermal dysplasia. *Birth Defects* 1971; 7: 91–5.

48 Gillespie JM. The dietary regulation of the synthesis of hair keratin. In: Crewther WG, ed. *Symposium on Fibrous Proteins*. London: Butterworths, 1968: 362–3.

49 Miyazawa F, Tamura T, Nozaki F. Alteration of amino acid composition and keratinolysis of hair due to chemical damage. In: Kobori T, Montagna W, eds. *Biology and Disease of the Hair*. Baltimore: University Park Press, 1976: 659–67.

50 Brown AC. Congenital hair defects. *Birth Defects* 1971; 7: 52–68.

51 Whiting DA. Structural abnormalities of the hair shaft. *J Am Acad Dermatol* 1987; 16: 1–25.

52 Van Neste D. Congenital hair dysplasia: management and value of various diagnostic methods. *Ann Dermatol Vénéréol* 1989; 116: 251–63 (in French).

53 Freire-Maia N, Pinheiro M. Ectodermal dysplasias—some recollections and a classification. *Birth Defects* 1988; 24: 3–14.

Rothmund–Thomson Syndrome, Bloom's Syndrome, Dyskeratosis Congenita and Fanconi's Syndrome

CELIA MOSS

Rothmund–Thomson syndrome

Bloom's syndrome

Dyskeratosis congenita

Fanconi's syndrome

Rothmund–Thomson syndrome

Definition

Rothmund–Thomson syndrome is a rare genetic disorder characterized by poikiloderma affecting particularly the cheeks and backs of the hands. Variable features include short stature, sparse hair, cataract, hypogonadism and mid-face hypoplasia. There is an increased incidence of squamous carcinoma of the skin, and of osteogenic sarcoma.

History

In 1868, Rothmund, a German ophthalmologist, reported several related individuals from an isolated Bavarian village, with poikiloderma often associated with juvenile cataract [1]. In 1923, Thomson, a British dermatologist, reported three similar patients with a 'hitherto undescribed familial disease' [2], which he subsequently named 'poikiloderma congenitale' [3]. It is now widely believed that all of these patients had the same disorder, and by 1992 over 200 cases had been reported in the world literature [4].

Inheritance

This is an autosomal recessive condition. Early reports suggested a 4:1 female predominance, but more recent figures show equal sex incidence, excluding X-linked inheritance [4]. The gene locus is unknown.

Pathogenesis

The increased incidence of dysplasia and malignancy in Rothmund–Thomson syndrome has provoked studies of chromosomal stability and DNA repair. Several patients have been reported with various karyotypic abnormalities including trisomy 15 and 22 [5], and mosaic trisomy 8 [6], and this may reflect a tendency to chromosome breakage [7]. Reduced repair of hypoxic γ-irradiation damage to DNA in cultured fibroblasts [8], and sensitivity to ultraviolet C (UVC) irradiation with impaired DNA repair [9] have been reported in individual patients, but DNA repair has been normal in others [10].

Joint laxity and blue sclerae in some patients have suggested a collagen defect, but none has so far been identified [11].

Kitao *et al.* [12] have reported compound heterozygous mutations in the human helicase gene RECQL4 at chromosome locus 8q24.3 in three patients with Rothmund–Thomson syndrome.

Pathology

Early on, the affected skin is oedematous with a perivascular lymphocytic infiltrate. Later, the poikilodermatous skin shows hyperkeratosis, epidermal atrophy, vasodilatation, pigmentary incontinence, fragmentation of elastic tissue and loss of appendages. The keratoses show dysplastic and bowenoid changes [13].

Clinical features [4,11]

The characteristic poikiloderma is never congenital, but develops at a few months of age. It appears first on the cheeks, and by the end of the first year usually affects also the backs of the hands and extensor forearms, the buttocks and the tops of the feet. Lesions may appear later on the ear margins. Initially, the affected areas appear inflamed (Fig. 19.23.1) and even blistered, but after a few weeks or months the inflammation settles, leaving the characteristic atrophic, pigmented telangiectasia (poikiloderma). Clear areas of normal skin within the affected areas produce a reticulate pattern (Fig. 19.23.2).

Transient photosensitivity has been reported in early childhood, but the typical distribution of inflammatory lesions on the face and backs of the hands may have been

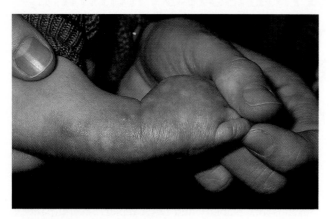

Fig. 19.23.1 Rothmund–Thomson syndrome: early reticulate erythematous areas.

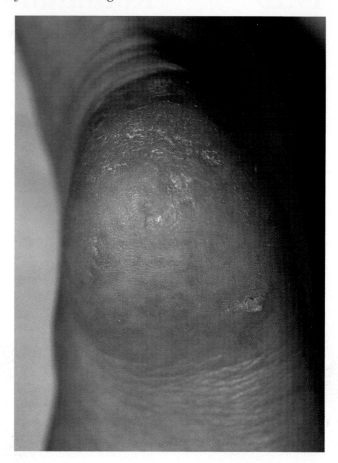

Fig. 19.23.3 Rothmund–Thomson syndrome: hyperkeratosis on the heel.

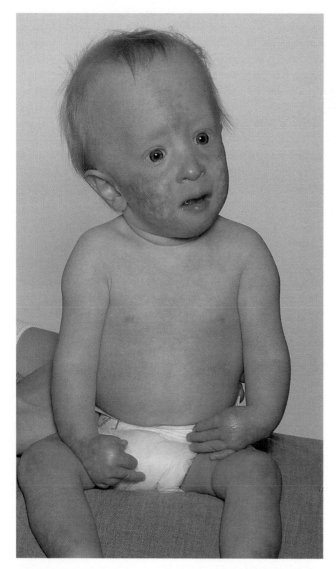

Fig. 19.23.2 Rothmund–Thomson syndrome: typical appearance of poikilodermatous changes mainly on the face, hands and legs.

misinterpreted as photosensitivity. The occurrence of poikiloderma on the buttocks makes it unlikely that photosensitivity plays any part in the pathogenesis of this disorder.

Keratoses are commonly found on the extremities of older children and adults (Fig. 19.23.3), and are considered premalignant [13].

Sparse hair affecting particularly the scalp, eyebrows and eyelashes is commonly reported (see Fig. 19.23.2). Body hair may also be reduced. The nails are usually slow growing and hypotrophic (Fig. 19.23.4). A variety of dental anomalies has been reported [14], none of them characteristic.

Juvenile cataracts develop in about half of patients with Rothmund–Thomson syndrome, and usually occur in all affected members of a sibship. They are generally of rapid onset, bilateral and of the subcapsular type; 73% develop before the age of 6 years [4]. A variety of other ocular abnormalities has been reported occasionally, particularly corneal atrophy and blue sclerae.

Skeletal dysplasia is an important feature of Rothmund–Thomson syndrome. Proportional short stature is common and may be severe. Radial ray defect is the commonest specific skeletal abnormality and presents as thumb hypoplasia or aplasia, with reduction or even

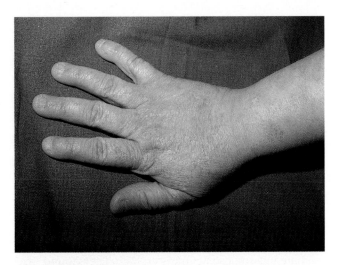

Fig. 19.23.4 Rothmund–Thomson syndrome: hypoplastic nails.

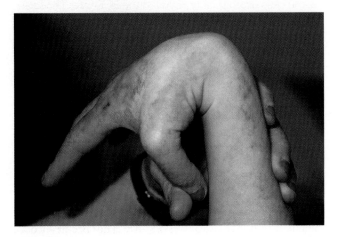

Fig. 19.23.5 Rothmund–Thomson syndrome: acral hypermobile joints.

complete absence of the radius. Some patients simply have an abnormal radial head, limiting joint movement. The knees commonly show genu valgum and occasionally subluxation. Radiologically, metaphyseal chondrodysplasia, sclerosis and undertubulation of long bones are common, sometimes with a striking linear sclerosis affecting the femoral and tibial metaphyses, which may be a precursor to the development of osteosarcoma (see below). Mid-face hypoplasia with 'saddle-nose' may be a marker for pituitary hypogonadism, having been reported in 10 out of 25 hypogonadal patients, but none out of 34 endocrinologically normal patients with Rothmund–Thomson syndrome [11].

Acral hypermobility has been reported in several patients (Fig. 19.23.5). Multiple fractures, again mostly acral, and occasional blue sclerae also suggest a collagen defect but none has been identified [11].

About 40% of adult patients show delayed puberty or hypogonadism. Investigations have usually shown low or normal gonadotrophins suggestive of a primary pituitary defect. This may be structurally related to the mid-face hypoplasia [11].

An association between osteosarcoma and Rothmund–Thomson syndrome was first noted in 1990 [11], and has now been reported in 12 patients [15]. Ages at presentation ranged from 5 to 19 years, and in 75% of patients the tumour was below the knee, usually in the tibia. One patient had two primary tumours, in the tibia and humerus. Four out of five patients showed abnormal sensitivity to chemotherapy, with prolonged myelosuppression and severe mucosal ulceration. Many patients had previously abnormal bone with metaphyseal dysplasia and prominent longitudinal trabeculae. The other malignancy associated with Rothmund–Thomson syndrome is squamous carcinoma of the skin, which again tends to appear in previously dysplastic (keratotic) tissue. Several other malignancies have been reported, but none more than once.

Patients with Rothmund–Thomson syndrome are generally of normal intelligence, with no particular neurological problems.

Prognosis

Unless osteosarcoma develops, life expectancy is normal.

Differential diagnosis

Radial hypoplasia in a child too young to have developed the characteristic skin changes may be misdiagnosed as Fanconi's syndrome or Holt–Oram syndrome [16]. The initial inflammation on light-exposed areas may be mistaken for photosensitivity. Blistering at the onset of poikiloderma may suggest Weary–Kindler syndrome. Later, the atrophic poikilodermatous skin and telangiectasia can mimic the premature ageing syndromes and Bloom's syndrome, respectively.

Treatment

Treatment is largely symptomatic. Retinoids may improve the keratotic lesions [17].

REFERENCES

1 Rothmund A. Uber Kataract in Verbindung mit einer eigentumliche Haut Degenerationen. *Arch Ophthal* 1988; 14: 159–82.
2 Thomson MS. A hitherto undescribed familial disease. *Br J Dermatol* 1923; 35: 455.
3 Thomson MS. Poikiloderma congenitale. *Br J Dermatol* 1936; 48: 221.
4 Vennos EM, Collins M, James WD. Rothmund–Thomson syndrome: review of the world literature. *J Am Acad Dermatol* 1992; 27: 750–62.
5 Koch F, Santamouris C, Ulbrich F. D + G Trisomie bei einem Patienten mit Rothmund-Syndrome. *Zeitschr Kinderheilk* 1967; 99: 1–13.
6 Ying KL, Olzumi J, Curry CJ. Rothmund–Thomson syndrome associated with trisomy 8 mosaicism. *J Med Genet* 1990; 27: 258–60.
7 Orstavik KH, McFadden N, Hagelsteen J et al. Instability of lymphocyte chromosomes in a girl with Rothmund–Thomson syndrome. *J Med Genet* 1994; 31: 570–2.

8 Smith PJ, Paterson MC. Enhanced radiosensitivity and defective DNA repair in cultured fibroblasts derived from Rothmund–Thomson patients. *Mutat Res* 1982; 94: 213–28.

9 Shinya A, Nishigori C, Moriwaki S et al. A case of Rothmund–Thomson syndrome with reduced DNA repair capacity. *Arch Dermatol* 1993; 129: 332–6.

10 Judge MR, Kilby A, Harper JI. Rothmund–Thomson syndrome and osteosarcoma. *Br J Dermatol* 1993; 129: 723–5.

11 Moss C. Rothmund–Thomson syndrome: a report of two patients and a review of the literature. *Br J Dermatol* 1990; 122: 821–9.

12 Kitao S, Shimamoto A, Goto M et al. Mutations in RECQL4 cause a subset of cases of Rothmund–Thomson Syndrome. *Nature Genet* 1999; 22: 82–4.

13 Shuttleworth D, Marks R. Epidermal dysplasia and skeletal deformity in congenital poikiloderma (Rothmund–Thomson syndrome). *Br J Dermatol* 1987; 117: 377–84.

14 Bottomley WK, Box JM. Dental anomalies in the Rothmund–Thomson syndrome. *Oral Surg Oral Med Oral Pathol* 1976; 41: 321–6.

15 Leonard A, Craft AW, Moss C, Malcolm AJ. Osteogenic sarcoma in the Rothmund–Thomson syndrome. *Med Pediatr Oncol* 1996; 26: 249–53.

16 Moss C, Bacon CJ, Mueller RF. 'Isolated' radial ray defect may be due to Rothmund–Thomson syndrome. *Clin Genet* 1990; 38: 318–19.

17 Shuttleworth D, Marks R. Congenital poikiloderma: treatment with etretinate. *Br J Dermatol* 1988; 118: 729–30.

Bloom's syndrome

Definition

Bloom's syndrome is a rare inherited disorder characterized by growth retardation, immunodeficiency, photosensitivity, telangiectasia and pigmentary abnormalities.

History

Bloom, a New York City dermatologist, first described this syndrome in 1966 [1], and contributed to a Bloom Syndrome Registry subsequently set up by Dr James German. The registry closed to new accessions in 1991, and the 165 catalogued patients, mostly Ashkenazi Jews, have provided an invaluable source of data: German observed the first case of leukaemia in a Bloom's syndrome patient in 1963, and correctly deduced, from the fact that this patient was already known to have excessive chromosome breakage, that this was a significant association [2].

Pathogenesis and genetics

The first cellular abnormalities identified in Bloom's syndrome were increased sensitivity to UV light [3] and increased sister chromatid exchange (SCE) [4]. SCE refers to exchange of material between pairs of chromosomes newly replicated from the same parent chromosome in mitosis: there is no loss of genetic material so it may be of little pathogenetic importance, but it is useful as a diagnostic test, and may reflect increased mutagenicity. Other relevant findings include increased chromosomal breakage, susceptibility of Bloom's syndrome cells to oxidative stress, the SCE rate being reduced by antioxidants, and expression of an activated *c-myc* oncogene in Bloom's syndrome lymphoblastoid cells [5]. There is increased expres-

sion of a common fragile site at 5q31 [6]. The normal accumulation of the p53 tumour suppressor protein following DNA damage is reduced [7], but this is not specific for Bloom's syndrome [8]. There is reduced activity of DNA ligase 1, but no mutation has been found in the DNA ligase 1 gene [9]. The primary genetic defect in Bloom's syndrome has not yet been identified.

Bloom's syndrome is inherited as an autosomal recessive trait. Most patients are of Ashkenazi Jewish extraction, the gene frequency in this population being about 1 in 110 [10]. Quantitative SCE facilitated the mapping of Bloom's syndrome to the long arm of chromosome 15 by McDaniel and Schuftz, who carried out complementation studies using a Bloom's syndrome cell line with a stable SCE rate 10-fold higher than normal, and microcell-mediated chromosome transfer [11]. They found that insertion of a normal chromosome 15 into Bloom's syndrome cells dramatically reduced the SCE rate. The localization of Bloom's syndrome to chromosome 15 has been confirmed by two different techniques. Homozygosity mapping in patients with Bloom's syndrome and consanguineous parents showed a common homozygous section at 15q26.1 in 25 out of 26 cases, strongly suggesting the presence of the recessive Bloom's syndrome gene at that locus [12]. Disomy analysis in a single patient with Prader–Willi syndrome and Bloom's syndrome showed that the distal part of the long arm of both chromosome 15s were derived from the mother (maternal isodisomy for distal 15q) so that the patient was homozygous for all genes in this region which presumably includes the recessive Bloom's syndrome gene [13]. The Bloom's syndrome gene is tightly linked to (but distinct from) the FES oncogene, and linkage disequilibrium between these two loci in Ashkenazi Jews is strongly suggestive of a founder effect, i.e. all affected individuals inherited the mutation from a common ancestor [10].

Although there is no reliable method of detecting heterozygous carriers, two fathers of patients with Bloom's syndrome showed an increase in chromosomal structural abnormalities in sperm [14]. SCE rate is increased in cultured chorionic villus cells from Bloom's syndrome fetuses and this test can be used for antenatal diagnosis in a pregnancy at risk [15].

In 1995, Ellis et al. [16] identified the Bloom syndrome gene as RecQL which maps to 15q26.1. The product of this gene probably stabilises other enzymes that participate in DNA replication and repair.

Pathology

This histology of telangiectatic skin is non-specific, with epidermal atrophy, telangiectasia and a mild perivascular inflammatory infiltrate. Immunologically there is reduced immunoglobulin M (IgM), due possibly to a failure of maturation of IgM-bearing B lymphocytes [17].

Clinical features [2]

Affected individuals show growth retardation both pre- and postnatally. The body proportions are normal apart from a characteristic facies with an elongated face and rather beaked nose.

During the first or second summer a slowly fading erythema appears on the cheeks and nose. Later this becomes fixed and telangiectatic, affecting not only the central face but spreading to the ears, neck, dorsa of hands and forearms and sometimes the shoulders and chest. Facial photosensitivity reduces with age. Well-demarcated areas of hyper- and hypopigmentation develop on the trunk and extremities during childhood, and are more obvious in darker skinned people.

The cancer predisposition of Bloom's syndrome was first reported in 1964. Eighty-six malignant tumours have been recorded in 150 patients with Bloom's syndrome, the mean age at diagnosis being 24.4 years; 21 were leukaemias, 20 were lymphomas or Hodgkin's disease. The 41 carcinomas arose in a variety of common sites, nine being in the skin. Seventeen patients had more than one primary tumour [2].

Immunodeficiency, particularly of IgA and IgM leads to recurrent bacterial infections from early childhood. Delayed-type hypersensitivity is impaired. Other abnormalities include reduced sperm count in affected males. Menarche occurs at the normal age but periods are sparse and the menopause is early. Affected women have borne normal children. Twenty patients with Bloom's syndrome and diabetes have been reported. Neurological development and intelligence are normal but there is usually some degree of learning disability.

Prognosis

Life expectancy is reduced by the increased risk of malignancy.

Differential diagnosis

The short stature and facial telangiectasia may be confused with Rothmund–Thomson syndrome. Café-au-lait macules with immunodeficiency are also seen in Fanconi's syndrome. The dwarfism and facial phenotype may resemble progeria. However, the SCE rate provides a specific diagnostic test for Bloom's syndrome.

Treatment

There is no effective treatment for this disorder. Affected individuals should be protected from UV light and ionizing radiation. They should undergo regular haematological and physical examination to detect leukaemia and other malignancies, and infections should be treated promptly.

REFERENCES

1 Bloom D. The syndrome of congenital telangiectatic erythema and stunted growth. *J Pediatr* 1966; 68: 103–13.
2 German J. Bloom syndrome: a mendelian prototype of somatic mutational disease. *Medicine* 1993; 72: 393–405.
3 Gianelli F, Benson PF, Pawsey SA *et al*. Ultraviolet light sensitivity and delayed DNA chain maturation in Bloom's syndrome fibroblasts. *Nature* 1977; 265: 466–9.
4 Dicken CH, Dewald G, Gordon H. Sister chromatid exchanges in Bloom's syndrome. *Arch Dermatol* 1978; 114: 755–60.
5 Nicotera TM. Molecular and biochemical aspects of Bloom syndrome. *Cancer Genet Cytogenet* 1991; 53: 1–13.
6 Fundia AF, Gorla NB, Bonduel MM *et al*. Increased expression of 5q31 fragile site in a Bloom syndrome family. *Hum Genet* 1992; 89: 569–72.
7 Lu X, Lane DP. Differential induction of transcriptionally active p53 following UV or ionizing radiation: defects in chromosome instability syndromes? *Cell* 1993; 75: 765–8.
8 van Laar T, Steegenga WT, Jochemsen AG *et al*. Bloom's syndrome cells GM1492 lack detectable p53 protein but exhibit normal G1 cycle arrest after UV irradiation. *Oncogene* 1994; 9: 981–3.
9 Petrini JHJ, Huwiler KJ, Weaver DT. A wild-type DNA ligase 1 gene is expressed in Bloom's syndrome cells. *Proc Natl Acad Sci USA* 1991; 88: 7615–19.
10 Ellis NA, Roe AM, Kozloski J *et al*. Linkage disequilibrium between the FES, D15S127, and BLM loci in Ashkenazi Jews with Bloom syndrome. *Am J Hum Genet* 1994; 55: 453–60.
11 McDaniel LD, Schultz RA. Elevated sister chromatid exchange phenotype of Bloom syndrome cells is complemented by human chromosome 15. *Proc Natl Acad Sci* 1992; 89: 7968–72.
12 German J, Roe AM, Leppert MF, Ellis NA. Bloom syndrome: an analysis of consanguineous families assigns the locus mutated to chromosome band 15q26.1 *Proc Natl Acad Sci* 1994; 91; 6669–73.
13 Woodage T, Prasad M, Dixon JW *et al*. Bloom syndrome and maternal uniparental disomy for chromosome 15. *Am J Hum Genet* 1994; 55: 74–80.
14 Martin RH, Rademaker A, German J. Chromosomal breakage in human spermatozoa, a heterozygous effect of the Bloom syndrome mutation. *Am J Hum Genet* 1994; 55: 1242–6.
15 Howell RT, Davies T. Diagnosis of Bloom's syndrome by sister chromatid exchange evaluation in chorionic villus cultures. *Prenatal Diagn* 1994; 14: 1071–3.
16 Ellis NA, Groden J, Ye TZ *et al*. The Bloom's syndrome gene product is homologous to RecQ helicases. *Cell* 1995; 83: 655–66.
17 Kondo N, Ozawa T, Kato Y *et al*. Reduced secreted mu mRNA synthesis in selective IgM deficiency of Bloom syndrome. *Clin Exp Immunol* 1992; 88: 35–40.

Dyskeratosis congenita

Definition

Dyskeratosis congenita is a degenerative disorder, characterized by reticulate skin pigmentation, atrophic nails, leucoplakia and bone marrow failure.

History

The eponym Zinsser–Engman–Cole syndrome has been applied to dyskeratosis congenita, following the first description of a patient in 1910 by Zinsser [1], and further delineation of the disorder by Engman [2] and Cole *et al*. [3] in the 1920s. About 200 cases have now been reported in the literature [4].

Inheritance

Dyskeratosis congenita appears to be genetically heterogeneous: three different patterns of inheritance have been reported. Of the 215 patients reviewed by Drachtman and Alter [4], 175 (81%) were male; 155 males were thought to have the X-linked form (MIM no. 305000), eight males and 25 females the autosomal recessive form (MIM no. 224 230) and 12 males and 15 females the autosomal dominant form [5] (MIM no. 127550). The onset of skin and nail changes is later, and life expectancy greater, in patients with the autosomal dominant form [4].

Gutman *et al.* [6] showed cosegregation of X-linked dyskeratosis congenita with glucose-6-phosphate dehydrogenase (G-6-PD), which maps to Xq28. Linkage analysis in a large X-linked pedigree using multiple DNA polymorphisms also assigned the locus to Xq28 [7], and this was subsequently confirmed in other families [8], bringing the LOD score to 5.33 at zero recombination. One boy with dyskeratosis congenita also had X-linked ocular albinism [9]: this is difficult to explain as a contiguous gene syndrome because X-linked ocular albinism maps to the short arm of the X chromosome (Xp).

The autosomal forms of dyskeratosis congenita have not been mapped.

Pathogenesis

Dyskeratosis congenita is a progressive degenerative disorder: the cutaneous and mucosal abnormalities develop during childhood, with marrow failure and malignant changes supervening during the second and third decades.

Because of the haematological similarities with the chromosomal instability disorder Fanconi's anaemia, cytogenetic studies have been carried out in several patients. Aguilar-Martinez *et al.* [10], using lymphocytes, showed increased levels of chromosomal breaks in five affected men aged 24–39 years, and referred to three other patients with increased chromosome breaks, and two with increased SCE. Dokal and Luzzatto [11] showed chromosomal rearrangements in skin fibroblasts and bone marrow cells, but not in blood lymphocytes, with a higher rate of abnormalities in older patients. Kehrer *et al.* [12] also found increased chromosomal aberrations in cultured fibroblasts. However, cytogenetic studies in most patients are normal.

Haematopoiesis has been studied in dyskeratosis congenita patients using a long-term bone marrow culture system [13]. The defect in cell production is maintained in culture. Bone marrow stroma from dyskeratosis congenita patients can support growth of haematopoietic progenitors from normal marrows, but dyskeratosis congenita stem cells seeded on to normal stroma fail to grow, showing that the defect is in the stem cells.

The increased incidence of malignancy in dyskeratosis congenita has prompted studies of p53 gene expression, which was found to increase in hyperkeratotic tongue epithelium biopsied serially over a 5-year period, its appearance preceding that of histological dysplasia [14].

In 1998 Heiss *et al.* [15] identified the dyskeratosis congenita gene at Xq82 and demonstrated missense mutations in five unrelated patients. The gene product, dyskerin, is probably a nucleolar protein with a role in the biogenesis of ribosomes.

Pathology

Histology of pigmented skin shows non-specific changes including epidermal atrophy, a mild chronic inflammatory infiltrate, dilated capillaries and pigment-laden macrophages in the upper dermis [16,17]. Serial biopsies of leucoplakia of the tongue in one boy with X-linked inheritance showed epithelial dysplasia at age 11 and 13 years, and carcinoma *in situ* at 15 years [14]. The haematological abnormality is a pancytopenia due to marrow failure. In one patient immunodeficiency due to severely depressed CD4:CD8 ratio (0.38) was demonstrated [18].

Clinical features [4,15]

The characteristic skin abnormality is reticulate hyperpigmentation affecting the flexures, particularly the neck (see Fig. 19.23.6), axillae and the inner upper thighs. Patients usually present in childhood with a 'dirty neck' appearance. The affected skin varies from grey to red in colour, with spared areas producing a reticulate or mottled pattern (Fig. 19.23.7). The affected skin may show the features of poikiloderma (pigmentation, telangiectasia and atrophy).

The palms and soles sometimes show hyperhidrosis, loss of dermatoglyphics or keratoderma.

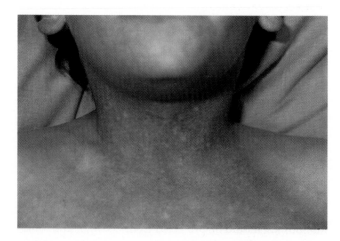

Fig. 19.23.6 Dyskeratosis congenita: reticulate hyperpigmentation on the neck.

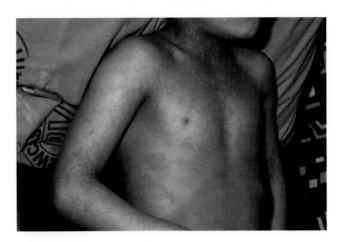

Fig. 19.23.7 Dyskeratosis congenita: more extensive mottled pigmentation.

Nail dystrophy may be congenital but usually appears in childhood, with longitudinal ridging and progressive atrophic changes including koilonychia. Teeth may also appear poorly formed with thin enamel, early decay and periodontitis [19]. Hair may be sparse and show early greying and loss. One female patient had unusual tufts of hair on the limbs [17].

Leucoplakia can affect any of the peripheral mucosal surfaces, but most commonly presents in the mouth. The raised white patches appear later in childhood than the pigmentation and nail dystrophy. Development of squamous carcinoma is not uncommon. The same mucosal abnormality may be responsible for lacrimal duct obstruction, and oesophageal [20] and urethral stenosis.

Fifty per cent of patients develop bone marrow failure which presents, in late childhood or adolescence, as bleeding, anaemia or opportunistic infection. Chronic respiratory disease probably results from immunodeficiency [21,22].

There is an increased risk of malignancy, usually squamous carcinoma arising on mucous membranes at sites of leucoplakia. Hodgkin's disease, acute myeloid leukaemia and pancreatic and bronchial carcinoma have each been reported once in dyskeratosis congenita.

Short stature and delayed development are occasionally found. One woman had colitis and portal hypertension [23].

Prognosis

Projected median survival in X-linked and autosomal recessive dyskeratosis congenita is 33 years, most deaths being due to haematological complications or malignancy [4]. The autosomal dominant form is milder, median survival being greater than 50 years with no reported deaths due directly to the dyskeratosis congenita [4].

Differential diagnosis

Other causes of poikiloderma must be considered, such as Weary–Kindler syndrome, and Rothmund–Thomson syndrome in which the affected skin may also show a reticulate pattern with spared areas. The latter can usually be distinguished by the earlier onset of poikiloderma, and its distribution on the cheeks and extensor surfaces of the hands and forearms. Abnormal pigmentation also occurs in Fanconi's anaemia (which may be haematologically indistinguishable from dyskeratosis congenita) but usually takes the form of café-au-lait macules. Bloom's syndrome also shows patchy dyspigmentation, telangiectasia and chromosomal instability, but more specifically increased SCE. The skin changes of chronic graft-versus-host disease in one boy previously transplanted for aplastic anaemia were difficult to differentiate from dyskeratosis congenita [24].

Treatment

Leucoplakia should be documented, biopsied and closely monitored, and areas showing clinical or histological dysplasia should be excised. Etretinate has been reported to cause regression in leucoplakia of the mouth [25], and retinoids might theoretically defer malignant degeneration. Marrow aplasia is treated initially by transfusion of blood products, and occasionally with androgenic steroids. Granulocyte colony-stimulating factor has produced moderate increases in neutrophil count [26]. Allogeneic bone marrow transplantation has been used [27] but six out of 10 patients died from graft-versus-host disease, veno-occlusive disease, liver failure or pulmonary fibrosis [4].

Given that 50% of patients with dyskeratosis congenita die from marrow failure, it might be worth storing the patient's own marrow cells extracted while the child is still 'well', for subsequent autologous transplantation when required: theoretically this could double survival time from presentation, although the transplanted cells would eventually succumb to the same pathology. Another reason for storing 'pre-aplastic' marrow cells is the possible future development of gene therapy for this disorder.

REFERENCES

1 Zinsser F. Atrophia cutis reticularis cum pigmentatione, dystrophia et leukoplakia oris. *Ikonogr Dermat* 1910; 5: 219–23.
2 Engman FM. A unique case of reticular pigmentation of the skin with atrophy. *Arch Dermatol* 1926; 13: 685–7.
3 Cole HN, Rauschkolb JE, Toomey J. Dyskeratosis congenita with pigmentation, dystrophia unguis, and leukokeratosis oris. *Arch Dermatol* 1929; 21: 71–95.
4 Drachtman RA, Alter BP. Dyskeratosis congenita. *Dermatol Clin* 1995; 13: 33–9.
5 Tchou PK, Kohn T. Dyskeratosis congenita: an autosomal dominant disorder. *J Am Acad Dermatol* 1982; 6: 1034–9.

6 Gutman A, Frumkin A, Adam A *et al*. X-linked dyskeratosis congenita with pancytopenia. *Arch Dermatol* 1978; 114: 1667–71.

7 Connor JM, Gathere D, Gray FC *et al*. Assignment of the gene for dyskeratosis congenita to Xq28. *Hum Genet* 1986; 72: 348–51.

8 Arngrimsson R, Dokal I, Luzzatto L, Connor JM. Dyskeratosis congenita: three additional families show linkage to a locus in Xq28. *J Med Genet* 1993; 30: 618–19.

9 Reichel M, Grix AC, Isseroff RR. Dyskeratosis congenita associated with elevated fetal hemoglobin, X-linked ocular albinism, and juvenile diabetes mellitus. *Paediatr Dermatol* 1992; 9: 103–6.

10 Aguilar-Martinez A, Lautre-Ecenarro MJ, Urbina-Gonzalez F *et al*. Cytogenetic abnormalities in dyskeratosis congenita—report of five cases. *Clin Exp Dermatol* 1988; 13: 100–4.

11 Dokal I, Luzzatto L. Dyskeratosis congenita is a chromosomal instability disorder. *Leuk Lymph* 1994; 15: 1–7.

12 Kehrer H, Krone W, Schindler D *et al*. Cytogenetic studies of skin fibroblast cultures from a karyotypically normal female with dyskeratosis congenita. *Clin Genet* 1992; 41: 129–34.

13 Marsh JC, Will AJ, Hows JM *et al*. 'Stem cell' origin of the haematopoietic defect in dyskeratosis congenita. *Blood* 1992; 79: 3138–44.

14 Ogden GR, Lane DP, Chisholm DM. p53 expression in dyskeratosis congenita: a marker for oral premalignancy? *J Clin Pathol* 1993; 46: 169–70.

15 Heiss NS, Knight SW, Vulliamy TJ *et al*. X-linked dyskeratosis is caused by mutations in a highly conserved gene with putative nucleolar functions. *Nat Genet* 1998; 19: 32–8.

16 Davidson HR, Connor JM. Syndrome of the month: dyskeratosis congenita. *J Med Genet* 1988; 25: 843–6.

17 Joshi RK, Atukorala DN, Abanmi A, Kudwah A. Dyskeratosis congenita in a female. *Br J Dermatol* 1994; 130: 520–2.

18 Lee BW, Yap HK, Quah TC *et al*. T cell immunodeficiency in dyskeratosis congenita. *Arch Dis Child* 1992; 67: 524–6.

19 Yavuzyilmaz E, Yamalik N, Yetgin S, Kansu O. Oral-dental findings in dyskeratosis congenita. *J Oral Pathol Med* 1992; 21: 280–4.

20 Sawant P, Chpda NM, Desai DC *et al*. Dyskeratosis congenita with oesophageal stricture and dermatological manifestations. *Endoscopy* 1994; 26: 711–12.

21 Verra F, Kouzan S, Saiag P *et al*. Bronchoalveolar disease in dyskeratosis congenita. *Eur Resp J* 1992; 5: 497–9.

22 Imokawa S, Sato A, Toyoshima M *et al*. Dyskeratosis congenita showing usual interstitial pneumonia. *Int Med* 1994; 33: 226–30.

23 Brown KE, Kelly TE, Myers BM. Gastrointestinal involvement in a woman with dyskeratosis congenita. *Digest Dis Sci* 1993; 38: 181–4.

24 Ivker RA, Woosley J, Resnick SD. Dyskeratosis congenita or graft versus host disease? A diagnostic dilemma in a child 8 years after bone marrow transplantation for aplastic anaemia. *Paediatr Dermatol* 1993; 10: 362–5.

25 Koch HF. In: Orfanos O *et al*. eds. *Retinoids. Advances in Basic Research and Therapy*. Berlin: Springer-Verlag, 1981: 307–12.

26 Oehler L, Reiter E, Friedl J *et al*. Effective stimulation of neutropoiesis with rh G-CSF in dyskeratosis congenita: a case report. *Ann Hematol* 1994; 69: 325–7.

27 Phillips RJ, Judge M, Webb D, Harper JI. Dyskeratosis congenita: delay in diagnosis and successful treatment of pancytopenia by bone marrow transplantation. *Br J Dermatol* 1992; 127: 278–80.

Fanconi's syndrome

Definition

Fanconi's syndrome is a rare inherited degenerative disorder characterized by pancytopenia, radial ray hypoplasia, pigmentation, susceptibility to malignancy and sometimes renal, cardiac and central nervous system (CNS) anomalies.

History

Fanconi first reported this syndrome in 1927 in three brothers [1]. There are now just under 400 patients enrolled with the International Fanconi Anaemia Registry set up in 1982 [2].

Pathogenesis and genetics

Fanconi's syndrome is inherited in an autosomal recessive manner. Patients' lymphocytes are characterized by increased chromosomal breakage, and sensitivity to cross-linking agents such as nitrogen mustard, mitomycin C and di-epoxybutane [3]. There is evidence for at least eight complementation groups [4], one of which (group C) has been mapped to chromosome 9q22.3 [5], and another to chromosome 16q24.3 [6]. The complementary DNA (cDNA) defective in group C has been cloned and shown to complement the defect in other group C cells [7]. Disease-associated mutations in this gene were identified in 25 of 174 Fanconi's syndrome families screened by Verlander *et al*. [8]. However, the precise function of the gene product is unknown. Levran [9] suggested that the group A gene is a 'caretaker' gene, inactivation of which results in a higher mutation ratio in all genes. Interestingly 9q22.3 is also the locus for three other tumour-prone disorders: xeroderma pigmentosum group A, multiple self-healing epithelioma and naevoid basal cell carcinoma syndrome [3].

The skeletal anomalies characteristic of Fanconi's syndrome have been reported in one family with normal chromosome studies [10].

Clinical features [2,11]

The phenotype is extremely variable, even within families. Skeletal anomalies present at birth include defects of the radius and thumb, but 25% of affected children have no bony abnormalities [11]. Some patients have supernumerary thumbs. Most patients with Fanconi's syndrome show growth retardation both pre- and postnatally. Microcephaly and congenital hip dislocation may be associated with Fanconi's syndrome. Urogenital anomalies found in 33.8% include hypoplastic kidneys, horseshoe kidney, double ureters and small genitalia. Heart defects (patent ductus, aortic stenosis and atrial septal defect) occurred in 13.2%, deafness in 11.3% and gastrointestinal anomalies (usually anorectal defects, duodenal atresia or tracheo-oesophageal fistula) in 14.3%. CNS abnormalities, particularly hydrocephalus, were found in 25.9%.

About 64% of patients show pigmentary anomalies, which become more apparent with time. Usually there is dusky pigmentation distributed proximally and in the flexures. Macules of lighter and darker pigmentation may be superimposed on this background. The dyspigmentation is similar to that seen in dyskeratosis congenita. Café-au-lait macules also occur and may be the sole cutaneous feature.

Analysis of International Fanconi Anemia Registry data showed haematological abnormalities in 332 of 388 patients, developing at a median age of 7 years (range birth to 31 years) [12]. Common abnormalities included pancytopenia and thrombocytopenia, associated with decreased bone marrow cellularity. Fifty-nine patients developed myelodysplastic syndrome or acute myelogenous leukaemia, and 120 patients died of haematological causes.

Patients with Fanconi's anaemia also have a higher incidence of non-haematological malignancy, particularly hepatocellular tumours and squamous carcinomas, notably of the head and neck [13]. One lymphopenic patient had multiple lesions of vulvoanal Bowen's disease and undetectable natural killer (NK) cytotoxicity [14].

Prognosis

There is a 98% risk of developing haematological abnormalities, and 81% risk of dying from them, by 40 years of age [12].

Differential diagnosis

The progressive marrow aplasia and flexural pigmentation can lead to confusion with dyskeratosis congenita. Rothmund–Thomson syndrome presenting in a neonate as radial ray aplasia, before the characteristic poikiloderma has developed, may be misdiagnosed as Fanconi's syndrome [15].

Treatment

Standard treatment includes blood transfusion and supportive therapy for neutropenia and thrombocytopenia. Recombinant human granulocyte–macrophage colony-stimulating factor (GM-CSF) is helpful in severely neutropenic patients [16]. Bone marrow transplantation from an HLA-identical sibling donor carries a 66% probability of 2-year survival [17], and survival is better with lower doses of cyclophosphamide in the conditioning regimen as Fanconi's anaemia patients are unusually susceptible to this drug [18]. In families with Fanconi's anaemia, the deliberate conception of a fetus for the possibility of providing a transplant donor is often undertaken [19]: if antenatal tests have shown that the fetus is unaffected by Fanconi's syndrome and HLA identical to an affected sibling, umbilical cord blood can be used for stem/progenitor cell transplantation [19]. The possibility of effective gene therapy is raised by the successful *in vitro* phenotypic correction of lymphoblastoid cell lines from Fanconi's anaemia group C patients, using a recombinant adeno-associated virus containing the Fanconi's anaemia group C gene [20].

REFERENCES

1 Fanconi G. Familiare infantile pernizosaaritige anamie. *Z Kinderheild* 1927; 117: 257.
2 Giampetro PF, Adler-Brecher B, Verlander PC *et al.* The need for more accurate and timely diagnosis in Fanconi anaemia: a report from the International Fanconi Anaemia Registry. *Pediatrics* 1993; 91: 1116–20.
3 Taylor AMR, McConville CM, Byrd PJ. Cancer and DNA processing disorders. *Br Med Bull* 1994; 50: 708–17.
4 Joenje H, Oostra AB, Wijker M *et al.* Evidence for at least eight Fanconi anemia genes. *Am J Hum Genet* 1997; 61: 940–4.
5 Strathdee CA, Duncan AMV, Buchwald M. Evidence for at least four Fanconi anaemia genes, including FACC on chromosome 9. *Nature Genet* 1992; 1: 196–8.
6 Gschwend M, Levran O, Kruglyak L *et al.* A locus for Fanconi anemia on 16q determined by homozygosity mapping. *Am J Hum Genet* 1996; 59: 377–84.
7 Strathdee CA, Gavish H, Shannon WR, Buchwald M. Cloning of cDNAs for Fanconi's anaemia by functional complementation. *Nature* 1992; 356: 763–7.
8 Verlander PC, Lin JD, Udono MU *et al.* Mutation analysis of the Fanconi anaemia gene FACC. *Am J Hum Genet* 1994; 54: 595–601.
9 Levran O, Erlich T, Magdalena N *et al.* Sequence variation in the Fanconi anemia gene FAA. *Proc Natl Acad Sci* 1997; 94: 13051–6.
10 Milner RD, Khallouf KA, Gibson R *et al.* A new autosomal recessive anomaly mimicking Fanconi's anaemia phenotype. *Arch Dis Child* 1993; 68: 101–3.
11 Glanz A, Fraser FC. Spectrum of anomalies in Fanconi anaemia. *J Med Genet* 1982; 19: 412–16.
12 Butturini A, Gale RP, Verlander PC *et al.* Haematologic abnormalities in Fanconi anemia: an International Fanconi Anemia Registry study. *Blood* 1994; 84: 1650–5.
13 Lustig JP, Lugassy G, Neder A, Sigler E. Head and neck carcinoma in Fanconi's anaemia—report of a case and review of the literature. *Eur J Cancer* 1995; 31B: 68–72.
14 Lebbe C, Pinquier L, Rybojad M *et al.* Fanconi's anaemia associated with multicentric Bowen's disease and decreased NK cytotoxicity. *Br J Dermatol* 1993; 129: 615–18.
15 Moss C, Bacon CJ, Mueller RF. 'Isolated' radial ray defect may be due to Rothmund–Thomson syndrome. *Clin Genet* 1990; 38: 318–19.
16 Kemahli S, Canatan D, Uysal Z *et al.* GM-CSF in the treatment of Fanconi's anaemia. *Br J Haematol* 1994; 87: 871–2.
17 Gluckman E, Auerbach AD, Horowitz MM *et al.* Bone marrow transplantation for Fanconi anaemia. *Blood* 1995; 86: 2856–62.
18 Zanis-Neto J, Ribeiro RC, Madeiros C *et al.* Bone marrow transplantation for patients with Fanconi anaemia: a study of 24 cases from a single institution. *Bone Marrow Trans* 1995; 15: 293–8.
19 Auerbach AD. Umbilical cord blood transplants for genetic disease: diagnostic and ethical issues in fetal studies. *Blood Cells* 1994; 20: 303–9.
20 Walsh CE, Nienhuis AW, Samulski RJ *et al.* Phenotypic correction of Fanconi anaemia in human haemopoietic cells with a recombinant adeno-associated virus vector. *J Clin Invest* 1994; 94: 1440–8.

Genetic Diseases which Predispose to Malignancy

JOHN HARPER

Bazex–Dupré–Christol syndrome

Beckwith–Wiedemann syndrome

Cowden's syndrome

Epidermodysplasia verruciformis

Gardner's syndrome

Peutz–Jeghers syndrome

Genetic diseases which predispose to malignancy fall into several groups: (a) those disorders with a predisposition to specific skin cancers, in which there are premalignant skin lesions; (b) those disorders with a predisposition to skin and systemic malignancies; and (c) those disorders with a predisposition to systemic malignancies but with cutaneous stigmata. Table 19.24.1 details those genetic diseases relevant to dermatology which predispose to malignancy. Selected genetic diseases are discussed in this chapter, others are discussed in more detail elsewhere in this book.

Bazex–Dupré–Christol syndrome [1–11]

Definition

The Bazex–Dupré-Christol syndrome is characterized by follicular atrophoderma, congenital hypotrichosis and the early onset of multiple basal cell carcinomas.

Aetiology

First described in 1964 [1], this rare syndrome is inherited by a presumed X-linked dominant trait. The gene for Bazex–Dupré–Christol syndrome maps to chromosome Xq24–q27 [10]. From a clinical and morphological point of view, it seems to be a disorder of the hair follicle.

Clinical features (Fig. 19.24.1)

The essential features are follicular atrophoderma, present from birth or in early infancy, and the development of multiple basal cell carcinomas on the face from adolescence onwards. The follicular atrophoderma typically affects the dorsa of the hands and feet, and sometimes the extensor limbs, lower back and face. The exaggerated follicular funnels ('ice-pick' marks) are caused by deep and lax follicular ostia rather than a true atrophy. The basal cell carcinomas present as lightly pigmented papules which resemble melanocytic naevi. Inconstant features include facial hypohidrosis with or without generalized hypohidrosis. Hypotrichosis is another feature; in males the hair loss is diffuse, whereas in females, who may not exhibit any clinical evidence of hypotrichosis, normal hairs are intermingled with abnormal hairs. The hair shafts are defective and may show pili torti or trichorrhexis nodosa. In infancy and childhood multiple milia are present.

Differential diagnosis

The condition should be distinguished from the basal cell naevus syndrome (Gorlin's syndrome). It must not be confused with a completely different disorder, acrokeratosis paraneoplastica, a cutaneous marker of malignancy, often referred to as Bazex's syndrome [12]. The Bazex–Dupré–Christol syndrome is more difficult to differentiate from Rombo's syndrome, which includes multiple facial milia, vermiculate atrophoderma, hypotrichosis, multiple basal cell carcinoma, trichoepitheliomas and peripheral vasodilatation with cyanosis. Although clinically very close, the Bazex–Dupré–Christol syndrome and Rombo's syndrome seem to represent distinct disorders. In the latter, follicular atrophoderma is absent, the various abnormalities appear only in late childhood, and the inheritance is autosomal dominant [13].

Treatment

Early diagnosis, which necessitates examining carefully all the family members, is important with regular follow-up. The basal cell carcinomas which usually develop from the second decade, require treatment, preferably by surgical excision.

Table 19.24.1 Genetic diseases which predispose to malignancy

Genetic skin diseases	Tumour susceptibility	Inheritance	Gene localization
Albinism, several forms	Squamous cell carcinoma; basal cell carcinoma, malignant melanoma	Mainly AR	11q14–q21
Ataxia telangiectasia	Lymphoma; leukaemia; epithelial carcinomas	AR	11q22–23
Bazex–Dupré–Christol syndrome*	Basal cell carcinoma	AD	Xq24–q27
Beckwith–Wiedemann syndrome*	Wilms' tumour; adrenal carcinoma; hepatoblastomas	AD	11p15
Bloom's syndrome	Leukaemia; lymphoma; carcinoma of the gastrointestinal tract, cervix and larynx; Wilms' tumour	AR	15q26.1
Cowden's syndrome*	Carcinoma of the breast, uterus and thyroid	AD	10q23.3
Dyskeratosis congenita	Leucoplakia; squamous cell carcinoma	XLR	Xq28
Epidermolysis bullosa dystrophica	Squamous cell carcinoma	AR	3p21.3
Familial atypical mole–malignant melanoma (FAMMM) (dysplastic naevus syndrome)	Cutaneous malignant melanoma	AD	1p36
Epidermodysplasia verruciformis*	Squamous cell carcinoma	?AR	?
Fanconi's anaemia	Leukaemia; hepatic carcinoma	AR	20q12–13.3
Ferguson–Smith type self-healing epithelioma	Self-healing 'squamous cell carcinomas'	AD	9q31
Gardner's syndrome*	Adenocarcinoma of the colon	AD	5q21–22
Gorlin syndrome (naevoid basal cell carcinoma syndrome)	Basal cell carcinomas; other internal malignancies	AD	9q22.3
KID syndrome (keratitis, ichthyosis and deafness)	Squamous cell carcinoma	AD	?
Maffucci's syndrome	Chondrosarcoma; ovarian tumours; gliomas	?AD	?
Muir–Torre syndrome	Sebaceous tumours; keratoacanthomas; adenocarcinoma of the colon; other internal malignancies	AD	2p22–p21
Neurofibromatosis types 1 and 2	CNS tumours; neurofibrosarcoma	AD	type I: 17q11.2 type II: 22q
Peutz–Jeghers syndrome*	Adenocarcinoma of the bowel; tumours at other sites include breast, ovary and testis	AD	19p13.3
Porokeratosis of Mibelli	Squamous cell carcinoma; basal cell carcinoma	AD	?
Rothmund–Thomson syndrome	Squamous cell carcinoma; osteosarcoma	AR	chr 8
Sclerotylosis	Squamous cell carcinoma of the skin, tongue and tonsil; bowel carcinoma	AD	4q28
Tuberous sclerosis complex	CNS, renal and cardiac tumours	AD	TSC1: 9q34 TSC2: 16p13.3
Turcot's syndrome	Adenocarcinoma of the colon; CNS tumours	AR	5q21–q22
Tylosis	Oesophageal carcinoma	AD	17q24
Von Hippel–Lindau disease	Renal cell carcinoma	AD	3p26–p25
Werner's syndrome	Tumours of connective tissue or mesenchymal origin	AR	8p12–p11.2
Wiskott–Aldrich syndrome	Lymphoma; leukaemia	XLR	Xp11.23–p11.22
Xeroderma pigmentosum, several forms (types A–G)	Squamous cell carcinoma; basal cell carcinoma; malignant melanoma; other internal malignancies	AR	A: 9q22.3–q31 B: 2q21 C: 3p25 D: 19q13.2–q13.3 E: 11p12–p11 F: 16p13.3–p13.13 G: 13q33

*Genetic disorders discussed more fully in this chapter.
AD, autosomal dominant; AR, autosomal recessive; XLR, X-linked recessive.

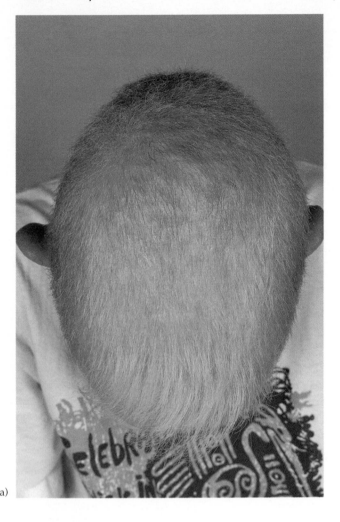

(a)

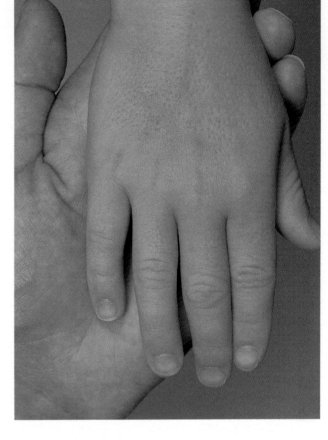

(b)

Fig. 19.24.1 Bazex–Dupré–Christol syndrome: (a) hypotrichosis, and (b) follicular atrophoderma. Courtesy of Dr A.P. Oranje.

REFERENCES

1 Bazex A, Dupré A, Christol B. Genodermatose complexe de type indetermine associant une hypotrichose, un etat atrophodermique generalise et des degenerescences cutanees multiples (epitheliomas-basocellulaires). *Bull Soc Fr Dermat Syph* 1964; 71: 206.

2 Viksnins P, Berlin A. Follicular atrophoderma and basal cell carcinomas. The Bazex syndrome. *Arch Dermatol* 1977; 113: 948–51.

3 Gould DJ, Barker DJ. Follicular atrophoderma with multiple basal cell carcinomas (Bazex). *Br J Dermatol* 1978; 99: 431–5.

4 Plosila M, Kiistala R, Niemi KM. The Bazex syndrome: follicular atrophoderma with multiple basal cell carcinomas, hypotrichosis and hypohidrosis. *Clin Exp Dermatol* 1981; 6: 31–41.

5 Meynadier J, Guilhou J-J, Barneon G, Malbros S, Guillot B. Atrophodermie folliculaire, hypotrichose, grains de milium multiples associés a des dystrophies ostéo-cartilagineuses minimes. Etude familiale de 3 cas. *Ann Dermatol Syph Vénéréol* 1979; 106: 497–501.

6 Mehta VR, Potdar R. Bazex syndrome: follicular atrophoderma and basal cell epitheliomas. *Int J Dermatol* 1985; 24: 444–6.

7 Herges A, Stieler W, Stadler R. Bazex–Dupré–Christol syndrome. Follicular atrophoderma, multiple basal cell carcinomas and hypotrichosis. *Hautarzt* 1993; 44: 385–91.

8 Goeteyn M, Geerts ML, Kint A *et al*. The Bazex–Dupré–Christol syndrome. *Arch Dermatol* 1994; 130: 337–42.

9 Moreau-Cabarrot A, Bonafe JL, Hachich N *et al*. Follicular atrophoderma, multiple basal cell carcinomas and hypotrichosis (Bazex–Dupré–Christol syndrome). A study in two families. *Ann Dermatol Vénéréol* 1994; 121: 297–301.

10 Vabres P, Lacombe D, Rabinowitz LG *et al*. The gene for Bazex–Dupré–Christol syndrome maps to chromosome Xq. *J Invest Dermatol* 1995; 105: 87–91.

11 Kidd A, Carson L, Gregory DW *et al*. A Scottish family with Bazex–Dupré–Christol syndrome: follicular atrophoderma, hypotrichosis and basal cell carcinoma. *J Med Genet* 1996; 33: 493–7.

12 Pecora AL, Landsman L, Imgrund SP, Lambert WC. Acrokeratosis paraneoplastica (Bazex syndrome). *Arch Dermatol* 1983; 119: 820–6.

13 Rabinovitz L, Williams L, Kline T *et al*. Rombo syndrome vs. Bazex syndrome. *Pediatr Dermatol* 1992; 9: 223.

Beckwith–Wiedemann syndrome [1–3]

(SYN: EXOMPHALOS–MACROGLOSSIA–GIGANTISM SYNDROME)

Definition

Beckwith–Wiedemann syndrome is a complex birth defect characterized by visceral and somatic overgrowth and exomphalmos.

Aetiology

Wiedemann's original report concerned three affected siblings [1]; however, most cases are sporadic. A review of the literature in 1970 concluded that autosomal recessive inheritance was usual [4]. Other pedigrees have favoured dominant inheritance, or even a delayed mutation requiring two mutational steps to allow expression of the abnormal gene. The finding of discordancy for the syndrome in a pair of monozygotic twins suggests that multifactorial control is more likely [5]. Genetic linkage studies have mapped Beckwith–Wiedemann syndrome to chromosome 11p15 [6]. It has been suggested that a placental endocrine defect may produce visceromegaly, which leads to various other complications.

Pathology

There is hyperplasia of the adrenals, kidneys, pancreas and Leydig cells [2]. Thickening of subcutaneous tissue and enlarged muscle bulk are also prominent. The macroglossia, which is an essential feature of the syndrome, is often histologically normal.

Clinical features

The characteristic cutaneous changes are ear lobe grooves and circular depressions on the rim of the helices, but the full syndrome includes macroglossia, exomphalmos, visceromegaly (liver, spleen, pancreas, kidney, etc.), anomalies of intestinal rotation. Neonatal hypoglycaemia, somatic gigantism, microcephaly and facial naevus flammeus. Many other metabolic and anatomical abnormalities have also been recorded, including immunodeficiency and a zosteriform rash at birth.

The hypoglycaemia, which is severe and resists simple therapy, is due to excessive insulin production by the enlarged pancreas. In some cases pancreatectomy may be necessary to save the baby.

Children with this syndrome have an increased risk of developing hepatoblastoma, rhabdomyosarcoma and Wilms' tumour.

Treatment

There is no specific treatment apart from the management of problems as and when they arise. Counselling should be given appropriately. Ultrasound prenatal diagnosis is possible.

REFERENCES

1 Wiedemann HR. Complexe malformatif familial avec hernie ombilicale et macroglossie—un 'syndrome nouveau'? *J Genet Hum* 1964; 13: 223–32.
2 Beckwith JB. Macroglossia, omphalocele, adrenal cytomegaly, gigantism, and hyperplastic visceromegaly. *Birth Defects* 1969; V: 188–96.
3 Cohen MM, Gorlin RJ, Feingold M, Ten Bensel RW. The Beckwith–Wiedemann syndrome. Seven new cases. *Am J Dis Child* 1971; 122: 515–19.
4 Filippe G, McKusick VA. The Beckwith–Wiedemann syndrome: report of two cases and review of the literature. *Medicine* 1970; 49: 279–98.
5 Best LG, Hoekstra RE. Wiedemann–Beckwith syndrome: autosomal dominant inheritance in a family. *Am J Med Genet* 1981; 9: 291–9.
6 Konfos A, Grundy P, Morgan K *et al.* Familial Wiedemann–Beckwith syndrome and a second Wilms' tumor locus both map to 11p15.5. *Am J Hum Genet* 1989; 44: 711–19.

Cowden's syndrome
(SYN: MULTIPLE HAMARTOMA SYNDROME)

Definition

In this rare disorder, multiple hamartomatous lesions of the skin, mucous membranes, breast and thyroid are associated with a predisposition to malignant tumours, in particular of the breast. Cowden was the name of the family in whom the disease was first described [1].

Aetiology

Inheritance of the disease appears to be determined by an autosomal dominant gene of variable expressivity. A series of germ-line mutations in a gene known as PTEN/MMAC1/TEP1 have been identified in families with Cowden's syndrome, and mapped to chromosome 10q23.3 [2]. It is a tumour suppressor gene which is likely to have a role in the pathogenesis of human malignancies.

Pathology [3,4]

The skin lesions around the mouth, eyes and chin are trichilemmomas [5]. The breast lesions are fibroadenomas which are liable to undergo malignant degeneration. A unique fibroma on the face and other sites has been described [4,6], composed of broad acellular collagen bundles in a lamellar or whorl-like pattern with occasional giant cells. This has been referred to as 'Cowden's fibroma' [7]. There is a report of amyloid in association with multiple hamartoma syndrome [7].

Clinical features [8–13]

Skin-coloured papules up to 4 mm in diameter, tending to coalesce to give a cobblestone appearance, are distributed on and around the eyes and mouth. On the dorsa of hands and wrists are lesions like those of acrokeratosis verruciformis. On the palms and soles, fingers and toes there are small translucent keratoses. Multiple angiomas and lipomas have been found in several cases. Malignant melanoma has occurred [14].

Verrucous and papillomatous lesions are seen in some patients on the labial and buccal mucosa, fauces and oropharynx, and may extend to the larynx.

In a series of patients [13], craniomegaly was noted to be the most frequent extracutaneous finding, affecting 70% of patients.

Of the many other abnormalities which have been reported in this syndrome, the most frequent involve the thyroid and breasts. Approximately 30% of reported female cases developed breast cancer [13]. Fibrocystic disease of the breast sometimes leads to massive hyperplasia. Goitre or thyroid adenoma are present in many cases and thyroid carcinoma has been reported [6,8]. Adenocarcinoma of the uterus has been reported in 6% of women with multiple hamartoma syndrome [13]. Less frequent associations include adenoid facies, high arched palate, vitiligo, café-au-lait spots, skeletal abnormalities, retinal glioma, pseudotumour cerebri, gastrointestinal polyposis and various gynaecological disorders (menstrual irregularity, uterine fibroids).

Ruschak *et al.* [15] described a patient with this syndrome, who had a deficiency of T-lymphocyte function with recurrent cellulitis and abscess formation and the eventual development of acute myeloid leukaemia.

Differential diagnosis

The skin lesions may be confused with Darier's disease or tuberous sclerosis.

Treatment

Cosmetic surgery may be helpful. The possibility of carcinoma of the breast or thyroid must be borne in mind. Female patients with this syndrome should avoid oestrogen therapy and should have frequent breast checks, including mammography, or even prophylactic mastectomy [16]. DNA testing is theoretically possible [17].

REFERENCES

1 Lloyd KM, Dennis M. Cowden's disease: a possible new symptom complex with multiple system involvement. *Ann Intern Med* 1963; 58: 136–42.
2 Tsou HC, Ping XL, Xie XX et al. The genetic basis of Cowden's syndrome: three novel mutations in PTEN/MMAC1/TEP1. *Hum Genet* 1998; 102: 467–73.
3 Brownstein MH, Mehregan AM, Bikowski B, Lupulescu A, Patterson J. The dermatopathology of Cowden's syndrome. *Br J Dermatol* 1979; 100: 667–73.
4 Starink TM, Meijer CJLM, Brownstein MH. The cutaneous pathology of Cowden's disease: new findings. *J Cutan Pathol* 1985; 12: 83–93.
5 Salem OS, Steck WD. Cowden's disease (multiple hamartoma and neoplasia syndrome). *J Am Acad Dermatol* 1983; 8: 686–96.
6 Weary PE, Gorlin RJ, Gentry WC, Comer JE, Greer KE. Multiple hamartoma syndrome (Cowden's disease). *Arch Dermatol* 1972; 106: 682–90.
7 Barax CN, Lebwohl M, Phelps RG. Multiple hamartoma syndrome. *J Am Acad Dermatol* 1987; 17: 342–6.
8 Burnett JW, Goldner R, Calton GJ. Cowden disease. Report of two additional cases. *Br J Dermatol* 1975; 93: 329–36.
9 Gentry WC, Eskitt NR, Gorlin RJ. Multiple hamartoma syndrome (Cowden disease). *Arch Dermatol* 1974; 109: 521–5.
10 Nuss DD, Aeling JL, Clemons DE, Weber WN. Multiple hamartoma syndrome (Cowden's disease). *Arch Dermatol* 1978; 114: 743–6.
11 Ocana Sierra J. Cowden's syndrome. *Acta Dermosifil* 1974; 65: 117–28.
12 Starink TM. Cowden's disease: analysis of 14 new cases. *J Am Acad Dermatol* 1984; 11: 1127–41.
13 Starink TM, Van der Veen JPW, Arwert F et al. The Cowden syndrome: a clinical and genetic study in 21 patients. *Clin Genet* 1986; 29: 222–33.
14 Siegel JM. Cowden's disease: report of a case with malignant melanoma. *Cutis* 1975; 16: 255–8.
15 Ruschak PJ, Kauh TC, Luscombe HA. Cowden's disease associated with immunodeficiency. *Arch Dermatol* 1981; 117: 573–5.
16 Walton BJ, Morain WD, Baughman RD, Jordan A, Crichlow RW. Cowden's disease: a further indication for prophylactic mastectomy. *Surgery* 1986; 99: 82–6.
17 Eng C. Genetics of Cowden syndrome: through the looking glass of oncology. *Int J Oncol* 1998; 12: 701–10.

Epidermodysplasia verruciformis [1,2]

Definition

Epidermodysplasia verruciformis (EV) is due to a genetic susceptibility to human papilloma virus (HPV), with a risk of malignant transformation.

Aetiology and pathogenesis

The condition is autosomal recessive and seems to represent a specific susceptibility to infection with certain HPVs. The cutaneous neoplasms are associated with HPV-5, HPV-8 or HPV-14, as well as some others, with the implication that these viruses are potentially oncogenic.

Pathology

The histology is that of a viral wart, intraepidermal or squamous cell carcinoma depending on the lesion biopsied.

Clinical features

Lesions on the face and neck are indistinguishable from plane warts. Those on the trunk and extremeties are larger and may coalesce to form plaques. They usually develop in childhood though they may develop at any age. Intraepidermal carcinoma and squamous cell carcinoma frequently develop, usually in light-exposed areas, often during the third decade but it has been recorded before the age of 20 years. There is a report of two siblings, aged 14 and 18 years, both with classical skin lesions of EV together with neurological manifestations and deafness [3].

Differential diagnosis

Immunosuppressed patients, particularly those with renal transplants, commonly have extensive viral warts and other keratotic skin lesions. Acrokeratosis verruciformis may be similar but is normally confined to the hands, feet, knees and elbows. The lesions can look like tinea versicolor.

Treatment

Treatment with retinoids and interferon may be considered. Any lesion suggestive of squamous cell carcinoma should be excised.

REFERENCES

1 Lutzner MA, Blanchet-Bardon C, Orth G. Clinical observations, virologic studies and treatment trials in patients with epidermodysplasia verruciformis, a disease induced by specific human papilloma-viruses. *J Invest Dermatol* 1984; 83: 18–25.
2 de Villiers. Human papillomavirus infections in skin cancers. *Biomed Pharmacother* 1998; 52: 26–33.
3 Al Rubaie S, Breuer J, Inshasi J *et al*. Epidermodysplasia verruciformis with neurological manifestations. *Int J Dermatol* 1998; 37: 766–71.

Gardner's syndrome

Definition

The syndrome comprises multiple epidermoid cysts, fibrous tissue tumours, osteomas and polyposis of the colon. This syndrome was described in 1953 by Gardner and Richards [1].

Aetiology

Inheritance is determined by an autosomal dominant gene of variable expressivity. Gardner's syndrome is located on chromosome 5q, near bands 5q 21–22 [2,3]. It is now thought that Gardner's syndrome and familial polyposis coli are allelic disorders.

Pathology

The pathology and natural history of the polyposes are essentially similar to familial polyposis coli. Several groups have reported the association of hepatoblastoma with polyposis coli [4,5].

Clinical features [1,6–11] (Fig. 19.24.2)

Polyposis of the colon or rectum usually arises during the second decade, but may occur in early childhood. It is present in about 50% of cases by the age of 20 years. There are few symptoms and intussusception is not a feature. Malignant change develops some 15–20 years later in over 40% of reported cases. Sebaceous or epidermoid cysts, which may be numerous, are usually irregularly distributed on the face, scalp and extremities, and are less frequent on the trunk. They may first appear between the ages of 4 and 10 years, but often considerably later, and are ultimately present in almost all cases. Osteomas develop mainly in the maxilla, mandible and sphenoid bones, but also in other bones of the skull, and less frequently in the long bones. They are usually small, multiple and are

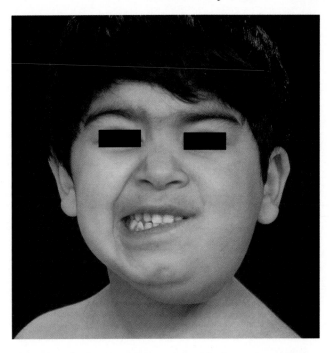

Fig. 19.24.2 Gardner's syndrome: a boy with a large submandibular tumour.

present in some 50% of cases. The age of onset is often not accurately known, but they may be present at puberty. Fibromas or desmoid tumours are less frequently present. They are usually poorly localized tumours in incisional scars of the abdomen, but may occur at other sites. Fibrosarcomas have also been associated with the syndrome. Fibromatous growths of the mesentery may be discovered at operation, and severe peritoneal scarring may follow surgery. Lipomas in the subcutaneous tissues, and in other organs, have frequently been noted. Leiomyomas of the stomach or ileum, or retroperitoneal, are sometimes present. The variable expressivity of the gene must be remembered when a family is investigated [8]. Cutaneous and skeletal changes may be present without polyposis and polyposis may be present when one or more of the other features of the syndrome is lacking [9]. Congenital hypertrophy of the retinal pigment epithelium is a frequent finding in Gardner's syndrome and is a valuable clue to the presence of the gene in people who have not yet developed other manifestations [12,13].

Differential diagnosis

Multiple epidermoid or sebaceous cysts may be inherited as an isolated abnormality and may thus have no sinister significance. Their discovery is an indication for a detailed family history and a careful examination for osteomas, including radiological examination of the skull, and for other dermal tumours. The cutaneous lesions are an important indicator of possible asymptomatic polyposis.

Treatment

Early detection of disease may allow earlier prophylactic colectomy before malignant transformation of polyps. Genetic counselling is crucial. All members of the family should be carefully examined and those at risk should be monitored carefully at regular intervals by both a dermatologist and a gastroenterologist. DNA testing is possible and requires liaison with a genetics laboratory with an interest in this condition.

REFERENCES

1 Gardner EJ, Richards RC. Multiple cutaneous and subcutaneous lesions occurring simultaneously with hereditary polyposis and osteomatosis. *Am J Hum Genet* 1953; 5: 139–47.
2 Bodmer WF, Bailey CJ, Bodmer J et al. Localisation of the gene for familial adenomatous polyposis on chromosome 5. *Nature* 1987; 328: 614–16.
3 Leppert M, Dobbs M, Scambler P et al. The gene for familial polyposis coli maps to the long arm of chromosome 5. *Science* 1987; 238: 1411–13.
4 Kingston JE, Draper GJ, Mann JR. Hepatoblastoma and polyposis coli. *Lancet* 1982; i: 475.
5 Li FP, Thurber WA, Seddon J, Holmes GE. Hepatoblastoma in families with polyposis coli. *J Am Med Assoc* 1987; 257: 2475–7.
6 Danes BS. The Gardner syndrome. *Cancer* 1975; 36: 2327–33.
7 Hornstein OP, Knickenberg M. Perifollicular fibromatosis cutis with polyps of the colon—a cutaneo-intestinal syndrome sui generis. *Arch Dermatol Res* 1975; 253: 161–75.
8 McKusick VA. Genetic factors in intestinal polyposis. *J Am Med Assoc* 1962; 182: 271–7.
9 Weary PE, Linthicum A, Cawley EP, Coleman CC, Graham GF. Gardner's syndrome: a family group study and review. *Arch Dermatol* 1964; 90: 20–30.
10 Danes BS. The Gardner's syndrome: increased tetraploidy in cultured skin fibroblasts. *J Med Genet* 1976; 13: 52–6.
11 Thomas KE, Watne AL, Johnson JG, Roth E, Zimmermann B. Natural history of Gardner's syndrome. *Am J Surg* 1968; 115: 218–26.
12 Blair NP, Trempe CL. Hypertrophy of the retinal pigment epithelium associated with Gardner's syndrome. *Am J Ophthal* 1980; 90: 661–7.
13 Traboulsi EI, Krush AJ, Gardner EJ et al. Prevalence and importance of pigmented ocular fundus lesions in Gardner's syndrome. *N Engl J Med* 1987; 316: 661–7.

Peutz–Jeghers syndrome

(SYN. PERIORIFACIAL LENTIGINOSIS)

Definition

Peutz–Jeghers syndrome is characterized by pigmented macules on the skin and oral mucosa and by gastrointestinal hamartomatous polyps. There is an increased incidence of gastrointestinal malignancy as well as malignancies elsewhere.

Aetiology

The first reported case of Peutz–Jeghers syndrome is believed to be that described by Hutchinson in 1896 [1] in which twin sisters presented with pigmented spots on the lips. In 1921, Peutz [2] described a case of familial intestinal polyposis and hyperpigmentation of the skin and mucous membranes. In 1949, Jeghers et al. [3] confirmed the association and described its familial characteristics. The syndrome is inherited as an autosomal dominant condition with a high degree of penetrance. All races are affected. In about 40% of cases there is no family history and these represent new mutations. It is now known to be due to mutations in the serine/threonine kinase STK11 gene on chromosome 19p13.3 [4,5].

Pathology

The histopathology of the cutaneous macules shows an increase in the amount of melanin in the basal layer of the epidermis, particularly at the tips of the rete pegs and in the melanophores in the adjacent connective tissue. Giant melanin granules have not been observed. A histical hallmark of the gastrointestinal polyps is the pattern of benign glands being surrounded by smooth muscle extending into the submucosa or muscularis propria [4].

Clinical features

The pigmented macules may be present at birth but can develop later in life. They are particularly arranged around the mouth (Fig. 19.24.3), but can involve the palms, soles and mucosae [3]. The condition is associated with hamartomas of the entire bowel and these polyps can be the cause of intestinal obstruction and bleeding. Haemangiomas of the small intestine have been described with mucocutaneous pigmentation [5].

There is an increased risk of malignancy, estimated at 2–3% [6]. Malignant change has been found through the gastrointestinal tract, but mainly in the stomach and duodenum. Other associated tumours include ovarian, breast, testis, pancreas and gallbladder.

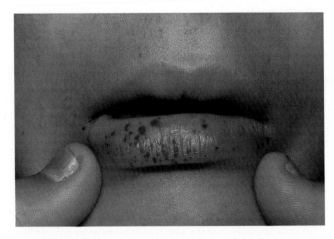

Fig. 19.24.3 Peutz–Jeghers syndrome: pigmented macules on the lip.

Treatment

Regular screening is essential for the early detection and treatment of malignancies.

REFERENCES

1 Hutchinson J. Pigmented spots on the lips in twin sisters. *Arch Surg* 1896; 7: 290.
2 Peutz JLA. Very remarkable case of familial polyposis of mucous membrane of intestinal tract and nasopharynx accompanied by peculiar pigmentations of skin and mucous membrane. *Ned Maandschr Geneeskd* 1921; 10: 134.
3 Jeghers H, McKusick BA, Katz KH. Generalised intestinal polyposis and melanin spots of the oral mucosa, lips and digits. *N Engl J Med* 1949; 241: 1031.
4 Hemminki A, Tomlinson I, Markie D *et al.* Localization of a susceptibility locus for Peutz–Jeghers syndrome to 19p using comparative genomic hybridization and tkage analysis. *Nature Genet* 1997; 15: 87–90.
5 Hemminki A, Markie D, Tomlinson I *et al.* A serine/threonine kinase gene defective in Peutz–Jeghers syndrome. *Nature* 1998; 391: 184–7.
6 Burt RW. Polyposis syndromes. In: Yamada T, ed. *Textbook of Gastroenterology*. Philadelphia: JB Lippincott, 1991: 1684.
7 Bandler M. Haemangiomas of the small intestine associated with mucocutaneous pigmentation. *Gastroenterology* 1960; 38: 641–5.
8 Giardello FM, Welsh SB, Hamilton SR *et al.* Increased risk of cancer in Peutz–Jeghers syndrome. *N Engl J Med* 1987; 316: 1511–14.

19.25 Prenatal Diagnosis of Inherited Skin Disorders

INGRUN ANTON-LAMPRECHT

Prerequisites for prenatal diagnosis

Indications and timing for prenatal diagnosis

Methodology of prenatal diagnosis from fetal skin biopsy
Fetal skin biopsy
Handling of fetal skin samples and preparation for light and electron microscopy
Time requirement

Normal fetal skin development in the second trimester

Prenatal diagnosis of epidermolysis bullosa
Epidermolysis bullosa simplex group
Junctional epidermolysis bullosa or epidermolysis bullosa atrophicans group
Scarring or dystrophic epidermolysis bullosa, epidermolysis bullosa dystrophica group
Transient bullous dermolysis of the newborn
Alpha-fetoprotein and acetylcholinesterase values in amniotic fluid of epidermolysis bullosa fetuses

Prenatal diagnosis of keratinization disorders
Dominantly inherited congenital ichthyoses
Recessively inherited congenital ichthyoses

Prenatal diagnosis of ectodermal dysplasias

Prenatal diagnosis of oculocutaneous albinism and related pigmentary disorders
Menkes' kinky hair syndrome

Prenatal diagnosis of storage disorders or inborn errors of metabolism
Mucopolysaccharidoses
Angiokeratoma corporis diffusum (Fabry's disease)
Neuronal ceroid lipofuscinosis

Disorders that cannot be diagnosed at present from fetal tissues
Chondrodysplasia punctata of the rhizomelic type
Netherton's syndrome
Restrictive dermopathy
Hereditary connective tissue disorders (HCTD)

Conclusion

Genetic skin disorders or genodermatoses are mostly rare diseases, the more severe ones ranging from about 1 in 100 000 to 1 in 500 000. Genodermatoses contribute significantly to the daily practice of the paediatric dermatologist. Most genetic skin diseases are severe chronic disorders for which a specific treatment is not yet available. Several of the severest have a grave, often lethal prognosis, such as the Herlitz type of epidermolysis bullosa (EB), ichthyosis congenita gravis (or harlequin ichthyosis), restrictive dermopathy or some of the most severe connective tissue disorders (neonatal Marfan's syndrome, osteogenesis imperfecta type I, Ehlers–Danlos syndrome type IV in the most severe expression or cutis laxa type II). Others result in severely disabling conditions, such as the mutilating subtype of recessive dystrophic EB (Hallopeau–Siemens or HS). Gene therapy may become available for some of these genodermatoses [1–3]. Prenatal diagnosis (PD) of at-risk pregnancies may be an option for such families with the possibility of terminating a pregnancy if shown to carry an affected fetus. In the past, many healthy fetuses have been aborted solely because of statistical risks of recurrence [4].

All the disorders discussed in this chapter are monogenic disorders following mendelian inheritance, in which karyotype analysis and cytogenetics are uninformative. For many of the genodermatoses, biochemical abnormalities are unknown or cannot be assessed from amniotic fluid or from chorionic villus samples. Exceptions are X-linked ichthyosis with steroid sulphatase deficiency, or Fabry's disease (angiokeratoma corporis diffusum) with lack of α-galactosidase, and some other related inborn errors of metabolism, that can be diagnosed from the amniotic fluid.

Conversely, the pathomorphogenetic patterns and basic structural abnormalities are well known for most of the important types of genodermatoses from systematic ultrastructural studies of large series of patients, such as EB or inherited ichthyoses [5–10]. These ultrastructural criteria have become important markers not only in their early postnatal distinction, diagnosis and classification; many of these markers can be similarly applied to PD on fetal skin samples obtained intrauterinely via fetoscopy under real-time sonography [6–8,11–13]. PD by morphological means is performed in those genodermatoses that cannot be identified by biochemical or cytogenetic means from amniotic fluid or chorionic villus samples. Since the first reports in 1980 and 1981 [11,14–16], experience has accumulated demonstrating that several of the most important genodermatoses can be safely diagnosed prenatally from fetal skin samples, while others cannot, as their specific markers are not expressed early enough during fetal skin development [13,17–19].

The period available for this approach to PD is mid pregnancy, as most of the markers required are not yet expressed in chorionic villus samples or early fetal skin but develop sequentially during the second trimester. This late time bares considerable ethical and psychological problems that have to be taken into account when counselling at-risk families.

Recently considerable progress has been achieved in the understanding of genodermatoses on the molecular genetic level, especially in the three large groups of EB, and increasing numbers of mutations are currently being identified. In such disorders PD may be performed in early pregnancy by molecular genetic means [20], provided that the molecular basis of the genodermatosis at risk has been resolved, and provided that the individual mutation (or at least specific haplotypes) are known for the respective risk family to permit an unequivocal decision on whether or not the fetus is affected. Therefore, PD based on the DNA or molecular level is still restricted to those families in whom the underlying basic abnormalities have been fully resolved. At present, it has to be checked carefully in each individual case whether PD can be performed by molecular genetic means—and in this case in the early pregnancy—or whether fetal skin samples have to be evaluated by morphological means—and in that case in the mid pregnancy.

REFERENCES

1 Taichman LB. Epithelial gene therapy. In: Leigh IM, Lane EB, Watt FM, eds. *The Keratinocyte Handbook*. Cambridge: Cambridge University Press, 1994: 543–51.
2 Fenjves ES. Approaches to gene transfer in keratinocytes. *J Invest Dermatol* 1994; 103: 70S–5S.
3 Greenhalgh DA, Rothnagel JA, Roop DR. Epidermis. An attractive target tissue for gene therapy. *J Invest Dermatol* 1994; 103: 63S–9S.
4 Bandmann HJ, von Ingersleben M, eds. Die Dermatologische Indikation zur Interruptio. 105. Tagung der Vereinigung Südwestdeutscher Dermatologen, München 1978. *Hautarzt* 1980; 31 (suppl. IV).
5 Anton-Lamprecht I. Electron microscopy in the early diagnosis of genetic disorders of the skin. *Dermatologica* 1978; 157: 65–85.
6 Anton-Lamprecht I. Genetically induced abnormalities of epidermal differentiation and ultrastructure in ichthyoses and epidermolyses: pathogenesis, heterogeneity, fetal manifestation, and prenatal diagnosis. *J Invest Dermatol* 1983; 81: 149S–56S.
7 Anton-Lamprecht I. Heterogeneity and prenatal diagnosis of congenital ichthyosis. In: Fabrizi G, Serri F, Cerimele D, eds. *Dermatologia Pediatrica. 4th International Symposium on Pediatric Dermatology, Selinunte (Trapani) 25–28 September 1991*. Naples: Casa Editrice l'Antologia, 1991.
8 Anton-Lamprecht I. The Skin. In: Papadimitriou JM, Henderson DW, Spag-
nolo DV, eds. *Diagnostic Ultrastructure of Non-neoplastic Diseases*. Edinburgh: Churchill Livingstone, 1992: 459–550.
9 Anton-Lamprecht I. Ultrastructural identification of basic abnormalities as clues to genetic disorders of the epidermis. *J Invest Dermatol* 1994; 103: 6S–12S.
10 Gedde-Dahl T Jr, Anton-Lamprecht I. Epidermolysis bullosa. In: Rimoin DL, Connor JM, Pyeritz RE, Emery AEH, eds. *Emery and Rimoin's Principles and Practice of Medical Genetics*, 3rd edn. Edinburgh: Churchill Livingstone, 1996: 1225–78.
11 Anton-Lamprecht I. Prenatal diagnosis of genetic disorders of the skin by means of electron microscopy. *Hum Genet* 1981; 59: 392–405.
12 Anton-Lamprecht I. Prenatal diagnosis of epidermolysis bullosa hereditaria: a review. *Semin Dermatol* 1984; 3: 229–40.
13 Anton-Lamprecht I. Prenatal diagnosis of genodermatoses. In: Dagna Bricarelli F, Casini Lemmi M, Storti G, eds. *La diagnosi fetale*. Suppl *Analysis*, 1992; 7: 131–54.
14 Elias S, Mazur M, Sabaggha R, Esterly NB, Simpson JL. Prenatal diagnosis of harlequin ichthyosis. *Clin Genet* 1980; 17: 275–80.
15 Golbus MS, Sagebiel RW, Filly RA, Gindhart TD, Hall JG. Prenatal diagnosis of bullous congenital ichthyosiform erythroderma (epidermolytic hyperkeratosis) by fetal skin biopsy. *N Engl J Med* 1980; 302: 93–5.
16 Rodeck CH, Eady RAJ, Gosden CM. Prenatal diagnosis of epidermolysis bullosa letalis. *Lancet* 1980; i: 949–52.
17 Anton-Lamprecht I. Prenatal diagnosis of genodermatoses. In: Harahap M, Wallach RC, eds. *Skin Changes and Diseases in Pregnancy*. New York: Marcel Dekker, 1996: 333–84.
18 Holbrook KA, Smith LT, Elias S. Prenatal diagnosis of genetic skin disease using fetal skin biopsy samples. *Arch Dermatol* 1993; 129: 1437–54.
19 Brusasco A, Nicolini U, Cavalli R *et al.* Diagnosi prenatale mediante biopsia cutanea fetale. Esperienza di 12 casi. *G Ital Dermatol Venereol* 1994; 129: 135–42.
20 Christiano AM, Uitto J. DNA-based prenatal diagnosis of heritable skin diseases. *Arch Dermatol* 1993; 129: 1455–9.

Prerequisites for prenatal diagnosis

PD of genodermatoses is no screening method. A clearly defined genetic risk and the exact diagnosis and classification of the disorder are required, based on careful investigation of index cases or affected family members.

Fetal skin sampling, and similarly chorionic villus biopsy, are invasive techniques. Therefore, PD should only be performed if the severity of the disorder at risk justifies termination of the pregnancy in case of an affected fetus. Mild disorders with good postnatal treatment response are no indication for PD, even with a high risk of recurrence (e.g. autosomal dominant ichthyosis vulgaris: 50%; X-linked ichthyosis: 50% in male pregnancies).

The underlying genetic defect must be detectable by morphological, biochemical or molecular genetic means that permit a clear decision on whether or not the fetus is affected. In those families in which the causative mutations are known, DNA-based PD can be performed in early pregnancy.

The developmental state of the organ, cellular or subcellular target structure that later manifests the genetic disorder should have a sufficient degree of maturity to permit a clear decision upon normality or abnormality of fetal skin (e.g. hemidesmosomes, keratinization, skin appendages).

The mutant gene should manifest early enough before the time limit of legal abortion (mostly corresponding to week 22 of fetal life, generally week 24 of the pregnancy). Some of the keratinization disorders, for example, may be expressed only after this time limit and therefore cannot be safely diagnosed from fetal skin samples in due time.

Significant personal experience of the investigator with the normal fetal skin development and ultrastructure as well as with the diagnostic criteria and specific markers of the genodermatosis at risk is required.

The fetal skin samples need to be of excellent quality to permit evaluation of the specific markers at the ultrastructural level and at high resolution. Therefore, the sampling procedure has to be restricted to experienced fetoscopy specialists. Chorionic villus samples need to be free of maternal tissue for DNA extraction and mutational analysis.

Extensive counselling of the at-risk family and detailed information is necessary on the severity and prognosis of the condition, and the risks and reliability of PD in their specific case, to enable them to decide early enough about whether they can accept termination of the pregnancy if their baby is found to be affected. At present, prenatal intrauterine therapy is not available for any of the disorders discussed in this chapter.

Indications and timing for prenatal diagnosis

The main indications among genodermatoses are the severe forms of EB, several but not all types of congenital ichthyoses and ectodermal dysplasias (ED). Other severe genodermatoses for which PD would be desirable, cannot be safely excluded as their mutant genes do not manifest early enough to be detectable on fetal skin samples. Examples are restrictive dermopathy, chondrodysplasia punctata of the rhizomelic type, Netherton's syndrome and most connective tissue disorders (Ehlers–Danlos syndrome, Marfan's syndrome, cutis laxa, pseudoxanthoma elasticum), that all have to await molecular analysis for DNA-based PD.

Therefore, the timing for PD of genodermatoses depends on the time of the first manifestation of the respective disorder and varies between weeks 17 and 19 (EB) and weeks 20 to 22 (congenital ichthyoses, ED syndromes); it should be selected according to the earliest and the optimal time of expression of the diagnostic marker in all those cases where PD is performed by morphological means from fetal skin samples. In at-risk pregnancies for which the underlying mutations have been identified, PD can be performed in the early stages of pregnancy by molecular genetic means, mostly from chorionic villus samples, but also from amniotic fluid cells, if necessary; in the future even earlier times for PD on the DNA level may perhaps become available (e.g. pre-implantation PD) [1–4].

REFERENCES

1 Christiano AM, Uitto U. DNA-based prenatal diagnosis of heritable skin diseases. *Arch Dermatol* 1993; 129: 1455–9.

2 Yerlinsky Y, Kuliev AM. *Preimplantation Diagnosis of Genetic Diseases. A New Technique in Assisted Reproduction*. New York: Wiley-Liss, 1993: 1–144.

3 Delhanty JD. Preimplantation diagnosis. *Prenat Diagn* 1994; 14: 1217–27.

4 McGrath JA, Handyside AH. Preimplantation genetic diagnosis of severe inherited skin diseases. *Exp Dermatol* 1998; 7: 65–72.

Methodology of prenatal diagnosis from fetal skin biopsy

Fetal skin biopsy

Fetoscopy and fetal skin sampling have been well established for about 20 years [1–4], as are intrauterine sampling techniques (amniotic fluid, fetal blood, fetal skin, muscle or liver biopsy). These techniques must be performed by an experienced, specialized gynaecologist. For fetal skin sampling, a trocar is introduced transabdominally into the amniotic cavity under real-time ultrasound guidance after local anaesthesia of the abdominal skin, passing the abdominal and uterine walls and the fetal membranes, chorion and amnion. The trocar is then exchanged either against an endoscope, the fetoscope, or directly against the forceps (or needle) for tissue sampling. With the fetoscope, direct visual inspection of parts of the fetal body or skin is possible. The diameter of the forceps determines the sizes of the fetal skin samples. Forceps of too small a diameter are unstable and thus of too high risk; diameters of 1.7 mm have been found to be optimal [4] yielding skin samples of about 1 mm in diameter. The whole sampling procedure is performed under real-time ultrasound control; the modern ultrasound scanner with its high resolution may allow the omission of the fetoscope entirely, except in cases where malformations (clefting, syndactyly) or facial abnormalitites [4] may be expected in conjunction with the specific genodermatosis (e.g. harlequin ichthyosis [5]). In conjunction with fetal skin sampling, amniotic fluid is collected for chromosome analysis (karyotyping, exclusion of trisomies and other chromosomal aberrations), screening tests such as α-fetoprotein (AFP), acetylcholinesterase (ACHE) and others, and controls for microbial infection.

Biopsy sites for fetal skin sampling depend on the position of the fetus and placenta [4]. Ideally, skin from the fetal back, close to the spine, at the height of the shoulders, heart or kidney, or from the buttocks, should be sampled. Scar formation is less on the buttocks. The lateral thorax can be biopsied when the fetus is in a less optimal position, but will result in more pronounced scarring. The extremities should be avoided, and biopsy on the abdominal skin, palms and soles is contraindicated.

Handling of fetal skin samples and preparation for light and electron microscopy

Fetal skin samples, even those obtained in the late second trimester, are extremely sensitive to desiccation and any kind of mechanical stress and damage. They must be removed from the forceps immediately and without squeezing. To maintain sterility of the instrument, the samples should be cleaned from the tip of the forceps by floating them off into sterile physiological sodium chloride solution, from where they must be transferred immediately to the fixation solution.

Fixation and embedding procedures are principally the same as for postnatal skin samples [6,7]. Fetal skin samples normally are round or ovoid; the samples are subdivided into about three or four blocks before final embedding to ensure their optimal utilization. Well-oriented consecutive tissue blocks may be obtained by embedding in flat silicon moulds.

Extensive experience is required for the evaluation and interpretation of fetal skin sections, so as to avoid pitfalls that may occur and artefactual changes due to the sampling procedure (e.g. suprabasal split formation) [6].

Time requirement

Preparation of fetal skin samples, embedding and curing of the final blocks and sectioning for light and electron microscopy (EM) requires 2 days after receipt of the samples. Light microscopy is sufficient for PD of EDs but EM is indispensable in cases of EB and the congenital ichthyoses; much more time is required in these cases. Samples of a fetus at risk of a keratinization disorder may have to be checked for normality or abnormality in the follicular duct orifices of many or all blocks to prove or exclude the disorder at risk, and subtle abnormalities must be demonstrated to identify an affected fetus. Such investigations are very time-consuming and may need more than 1 day at the EM. However, most PDs may be completed within 3 days.

REFERENCES

1 Valenti C. Endoamnioscopy and fetal biopsy: a new technique. *Am J Obstet Gynecol* 1972; 114: 561–4.
2 Rauskolb R. Fetoscopy. *J Perinat Med* 1983; 11: 223–31.
3 Perry TB. Clinical procedures for prenatal diagnosis of inherited skin disease: amniocentesis, ultrasound, fetoscopy and fetal skin biopsy and blood sampling, chorionic villus sampling. *Semin Dermatol* 1984; 3: 155–66.
4 Rauskolb R, Anton-Lamprecht I. Pränatale Diagnostik von erblichen Hautkrankheiten durch Fetoskopie und Elektronenmikroskopie. In: Holzgreve W, ed. *Pränatale Medizin*. Berlin: Springer, 1987: 80–104.
5 Blanchet-Bardon C, Dumez Y. Prenatal diagnosis of a harlequin fetus. *Semin Dermatol* 1984; 3: 225–8.
6 Anton-Lamprecht I, Arnold M-L, Holbrook KA. Methodology in sampling of fetal skin and pitfalls in the interpretation of fetal skin biopsy specimens. *Semin Dermatol* 1984; 3: 203–15.
7 Anton-Lamprecht I. The skin. In: Papadimitriou JM, Henderson DW, Spagnolo DV, eds. *Diagnostic Ultrastructure of Non-neoplastic Diseases*. Edinburgh: Churchill Livingstone, 1992: 459–550.

Normal fetal skin development in the second trimester (see also Chapter 1.1)

The first stages of human skin development are identifiable already in embryos of 30 days estimated gestational age. At this age, epidermis, dermoepidermal junction (DEJ), dermis and subcutaneous connective tissue have been organized and may be distinguished morphologically [1].

The embryonal epidermis consists of two layers, basal cells and periderm cells. The periderm covers the entire body surface of the developing embryo and fetus as a continuous unicellular layer and persists until the end of the second trimester, when keratinization of the fetal epithelium becomes complete. In the third trimester, the fetal epidermis is principally organized as in postnatal skin [1–4].

In the second trimester between weeks 12 and 24, all of the important structures, proteins and markers (with very few exceptions) are organized in the fetal skin. During the third trimester, these structures increase in number and gradually mature to reach the perinatal stage [4].

In addition to this general developmental progress and maturation of fetal skin, several developmental gradients exist on the fetal body surface that must be considered for diagnostic evaluation of fetal skin samples. Fetal skin development follows a craniocaudal gradient, with the earliest onset of a given developmental sequence on the fetal scalp and a delay of over 1 week down to the buttocks and upper thighs. This craniocaudal gradient is most clearly expressed by the appearance and maturation of the epidermal appendages, hair follicles and sweat glands, but also by the onset and progress of keratinization. Another gradient exists in a more or less horizontal extension from the spine over the back skin and lateral thorax to the chest and abdominal skin. Keratinization does not only follow these two gradients, but may additionally show an irregular patchy onset demonstrable on the lateral thorax and upper back skin from about week 21 or 22 [5,6]; it may not be mistaken as indicating a keratinization disorder. On the face, the earliest onset of keratinization (and the most pronounced hyperkeratosis in ichthyosis fetuses) occurs in the area of the eyebrows and around the vermilion border. A significantly earlier timing concerns ridged skin of palms and soles; formation of the epidermal ridges, development of sweat glands and onset of keratinization begin and become complete about 6 weeks earlier than in the (nonridged) remainder of the fetal skin [2] (for details see [1], [2] and [4]).

Sections of well-oriented fetal skin samples obtained intrauterinely via fetoscope forceps look like little mushrooms (Fig. 19.25.1); they are more or less round with a small 'rootlet' where the sample has been pinched off from the surrounding skin by the forceps [5,7,8]. Cell damage is normally restricted to the area adjacent to this rootlet but may also be seen at the apex of the sample due to the tearing forces when the sample rounds up during biopsy. The best preservation is generally found in the lateral parts of the fetal skin samples [8].

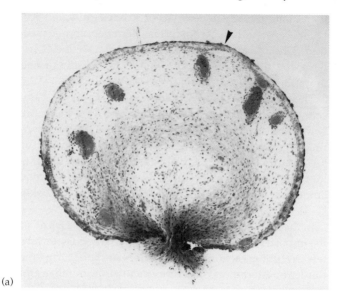

(a)

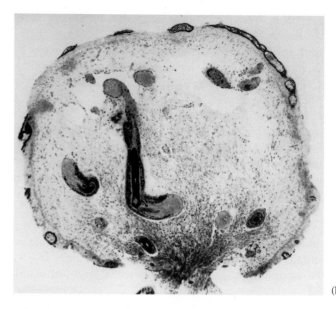

(b)

Fig. 19.25.1 Fetal skin samples look like little mushrooms in well-oriented sections. (a) Normal-appearing nearly unsplit skin sample of a fetus affected with Herlitz type JEB at week 16+6; note the slender profiles of the hair follicles, loose connective tissue and unkeratinized epithelium with small junctional split (arrowhead). (b) Fetus at week 20+6, born healthy; note prominent hair follicle in the centre and keratinized portions of the distal hair canals especially on upper right (see Fig. 19.25.5c). (×60.)

The fetal epithelium, increasing from two to about five cell layers until week 20 or 21, covers a loose connective tissue with scattered fibroblasts, few indeterminate cells (lymphocytes, macrophage and mast cell precursors), ingrowing small blood vessels and accompanying unmyelinated nerve fibre bundles (Fig. 19.25.2). Small fat droplets appear at the subcutaneous borderline. Collagen fibrils are of a uniformly small diameter and form tiny collagen bundles. No differences between the superficial and deep dermal collagen are present as is later typical of postnatal skin. Large empty spaces, probably rich in water and proteoglycans, still predominate in the fetal connective tissue. Elastic fibres are not formed before the end of the second trimester, although elastic stains become positive in this part of fetal life [1]. These histological stains react with the elastic microfibrils, the major protein of which is fibrillin. Tiny bundles of elastic microfibrils appear at about week 20 in the fetal dermis, but no elastin deposition occurs before the end of the second trimester, when some small deposits are first demonstrable in the deep dermis together with the appearance of the first subcutaneous fat droplets. The fetal connective tissue elements are still immature and clearly different from the postnatal stage. This immaturity largely limits the possibility of PD of heritable connective tissue disorders by morphological means, even those present at birth (cutis laxa, EDS type IV, osteogenesis imperfecta). Others that do not manifest before later childhood or even in adult age such as pseudoxanthoma elasticum cannot be diagnosed prenatally on fetal skin samples by light microscopy and EM.

About week 20, the major time of PD of genoder-

matoses, the fetal epithelium is still unkeratinized and covered with periderm (Fig. 19.25.3). It consists of a basal cell layer, two to three intermediate cell layers rich in glycogen, and the periderm facing the amniotic cavity, to which periderm cells form multiple microvilli covered with the surface coat or glycocalyx (Fig. 19.25.4). Basal cells are more or less cuboidal cells with central large nuclei, the normal composition of cell organelles including centrioles and frequent non-motile, sensory single cilia, desmosomes and hemidesmosomes, some lipid droplets, but only low amounts of glycogen. The amount of keratin filaments is still low in basal and suprabasal intermediate cells; here the keratin filaments are mainly located on the cell periphery because of the accumulation of glycogen, which is similarly preserved in the periderm layer.

At this time, keratinization—the most important 'invention' in the evolution of vertebrates including humans, permitting the passage from aquatic to terrestrial life and survival in a dry, arid environment—is not yet necessary for the 20-week fetus in its aquatic intrauterine environment. At the end of the second trimester, keratinization gradually begins to develop with the first stages of keratinized cells becoming demonstrable around the orifices of the pilosebaceous follicles (Fig. 19.25.5a) and in the developing hair roots.

Between week 20 and 22, the number of keratinized cells lining the follicular orifices increases gradually, together with the synthesis of keratohyalin and the formation of barrier lipids in keratinosomes (Odland bodies or lamellar granules) in the cells surrounding these horn

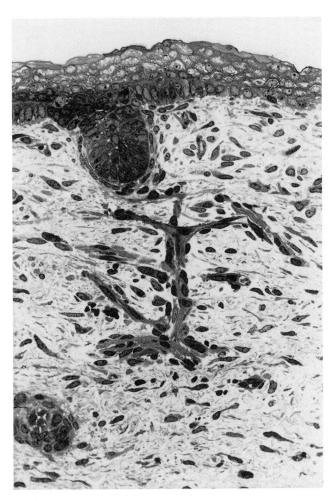

Fig. 19.25.2 Fetal skin sample at week 20; the fetus was born healthy; note the well-developed unkeratinized epithelium with basal layer, 3–4 intermediate cell layers and periderm; downgrowing hair bud and sweat gland primordia on either side; a well-demarcated DEJ and small blood vessels and nerve bundles growing upwards together in a straight branching fashion in the centre of the connective tissue rich in fibroblasts. (×324.)

cells (Fig. 19.25.5b), while the interfollicular epidermis remains unkeratinized until the end of the second trimester, when a continuous cornified layer replaces the periderm. Thus, this important step in fetal development from the second to the third trimester is characterized by the same transition between the unkeratinized fetal epithelium and a keratinized epidermis that marks the aquatic to terrestrial transition in the evolution of vertebrates. Prematurely born neonates of the early third trimester are principally viable due to the protection of the keratinized skin surface.

The late appearance of keratinization-specific markers is a considerable problem in PD of inborn errors of keratinization, such as the severe types of congenital ichthyoses [9]. It must be emphasized that only a few of the severe keratinization disorders may be identified early enough by specific markers. Other types of ichthyoses do

not manifest early enough—only after keratinization is complete or late in the third trimester. These disorders bare the risk of a false-negative PD as the fetal skin appears normal at the end of the second trimester; they have to await molecular genetic identification of the underlying mutations to permit safe prenatal exclusion or identification of the disease.

The patchy onset of keratinization [5,6] discussed above, and the fact that the keratinized portions of the follicular ducts run in parallel with the skin surface over long areas in penetrating the periderm (Fig. 19.25.5c) (visible on the surface of fetal skin samples as regular small ridges), may lead to false-positive diagnoses, when they are mistaken for hyperkeratinization. Therefore, specific reliable markers at high magnification EM are required for safe PD (see below).

In contrast, the boundary between the fetal epithelium and the superficial dermal connective tissue, the DEJ, develops by the beginning of the second trimester. It is complete by about the 20th week (Fig. 19.25.6), differing only quantitatively from the neonatal stage [5,7,10]. Hemidesmosomes are present at the dermal surface of the basal cells, many of them still immature among fully mature, complete hemidesmosomes with attachment plates and sub-basal dense plates identical to the postnatal stage. Their distribution is still irregular: hemidesmosomes are predominantly formed below the nucleus and close to the lateral cell membrane. The basal lamina is thicker underneath the hemidesmosomes, and anchoring fibrils (AF) are found here in their highest frequency. They have the same length and specific banding pattern as found in postnatal skin. It is in this area of the DEJ where blister formation occurs in the various types of EB. Therefore, the severe types of EB are safely identifiable from fetal skin samples with absolute reliability by about week 20 or earlier [10]. Analogous junctions are already present in chorionic villi; however, the specific markers of EB, hemidesmosomes and AFs, are not yet expressed and therefore PD cannot be performed morphologically in the first trimester [11].

In addition to keratinocytes, melanocytes, Langerhans' cells and Merkel cells may be identified in the epithelium of fetal skin samples of the second trimester. Many epidermal melanocytes are still found in a slightly suprabasal position (Fig. 19.25.7). Melanin synthesis and transfer to basal keratinocytes belongs to the late onset developmental processes [2]. Depending on the ethnic background and the family-specific degree of pigmentation of the skin, hair and eyes, the first stages of melanin synthesis may be demonstrable in epidermal melanocytes by about week 20–22, while fully pigmented melanosomes and melanin transfer generally do not appear before the end of the second trimester [6]. Hair bulb melanocytes precede epidermal melanocytes for about 2 weeks with their pigment-synthesizing capacity. Therefore PD of

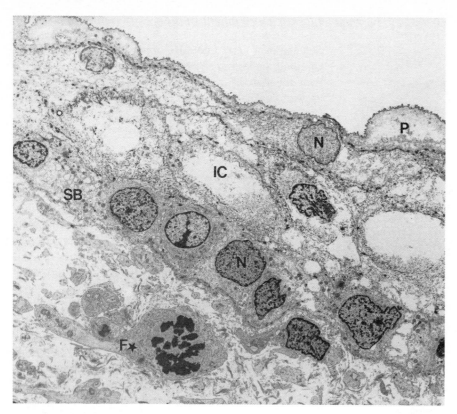

Fig. 19.25.3 Normal fetal epithelium at week 19+0, with basal cell layer (SB), 2–3 layers of intermediate cells (IC) and periderm (P); mitotic stage of a fibroblast (F*) subjacent to the DEJ; loose connective tissue. N, nuclei. (×2600.)

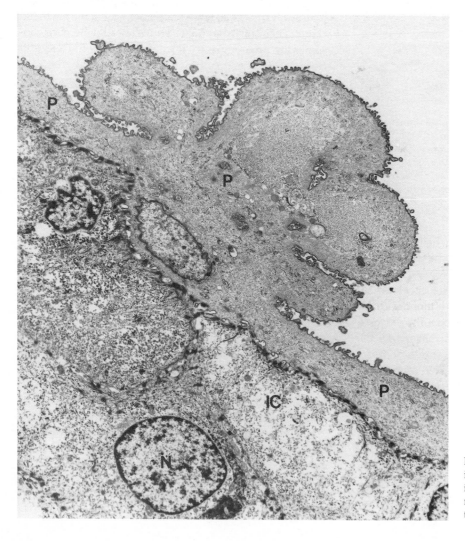

Fig. 19.25.4 Periderm cell (P) 'blebbing' off into the amniotic fluid and superficial intermediate cells (IC) filled with glycogen; note the microvilli with surface coat lining the periderm cell surface. (×5100.)

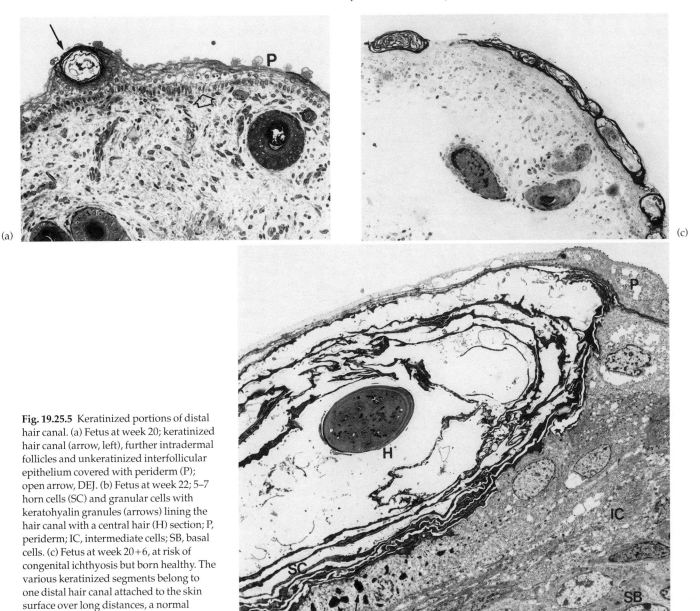

(a)

(c)

Fig. 19.25.5 Keratinized portions of distal hair canal. (a) Fetus at week 20; keratinized hair canal (arrow, left), further intradermal follicles and unkeratinized interfollicular epithelium covered with periderm (P); open arrow, DEJ. (b) Fetus at week 22; 5–7 horn cells (SC) and granular cells with keratohyalin granules (arrows) lining the hair canal with a central hair (H) section; P, periderm; IC, intermediate cells; SB, basal cells. (c) Fetus at week 20 + 6, at risk of congenital ichthyosis but born healthy. The various keratinized segments belong to one distal hair canal attached to the skin surface over long distances, a normal finding at this fetal age. (a, ×165; b, ×2100; c, ×151.)

(b)

oculocutaneous albinism (OCA) [12] is possible at an earlier fetal age in at-risk fetuses from dark-tanning ethnic groups and populations (African black, Japanese, Turks or other Mediterranean groups) than in fetuses from fair northern European populations or families.

Skin appendages (hair follicles, sebaceous glands, eccrine sweat glands and apocrine glands) develop gradually and at different times over a long period of fetal life, following most clearly the various developmental gradients described above [1,2]. Hair follicles with hair shaft, bulb and sheath, with the bulge and associated sebaceous gland, are regularly demonstrable in the fifth month. Their density varies largely with the location on the body surface, being high on the scalp, neck, shoulders and along the spine, and lower on the lateral thorax. Their developmental degree increases together with their growth downward from week to week. At week 16–17, the developing follicles are no more than short, slender tubes (see Fig. 19.25.1a). At week 18 and 19, differentiation of the follicular structures is obvious, but keratinization is still low. At week 20, the intraepidermal portions of the hair canal, the hair shaft and parts of the growing hair bulbs are keratinized (see Fig. 19.25.1b). Sebaceous glands are active in sebum synthesis (Fig. 19.25.8) with their central portions filled with large droplets of sebum lipid. At the same time, the first primordia of eccrine sweat glands begin to organize (see Fig. 19.25.2), while apocrine glands are not formed before the sixth month. The much earlier

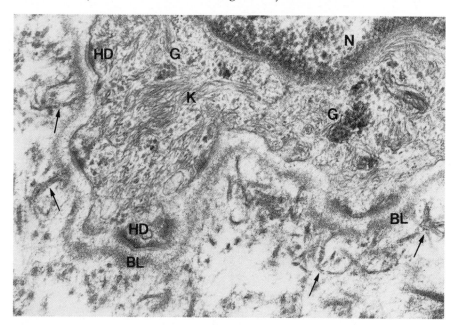

Fig. 19.25.6 DEJ in a fetus at 20 weeks—at risk of EB but born healthy. Basal lamina (BL) with focal thickenings below hemidesmosomes (HD) with clear sub-basal dense plates, anchoring fibrils (AF) (arrows) with band-like structure and cross-banding attached to the basal lamina. G, glycogen; K, keratin filaments; N, nucleus of basal cell. (×72 000.)

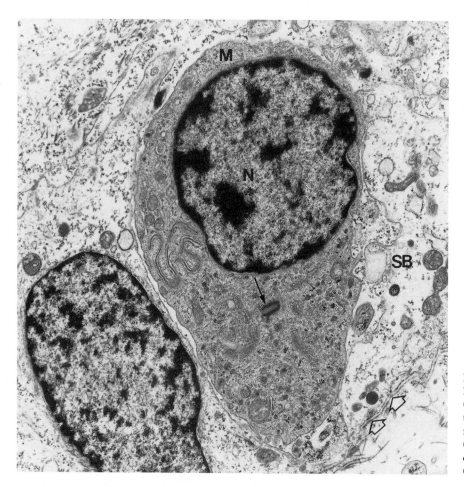

Fig. 19.25.7 Melanocyte (M) in the basal layer (SB) of a fetus at 19+0 weeks; centriol (arrow) in the centre of the Golgi area below the nucleus (N) with many Golgi bodies and numerous yet unmelanized melanosomes (stages I and II, lower right) and paired cisternae at the left; open arrows, DEJ. (×11 400.)

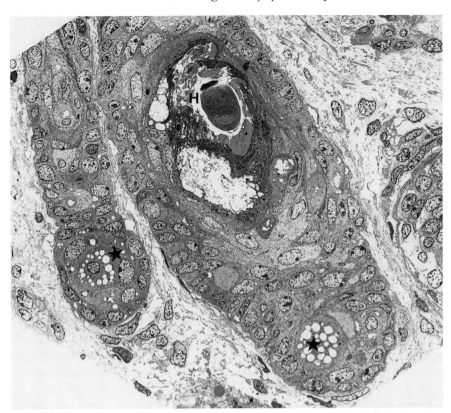

Fig. 19.25.8 Pilosebaceous follicle in a fetus at week 21/22; central duct with cross-sectioned hair (H), sebaceous glands with sebum synthesis (★). (×800.)

timing of the palms and soles has already been mentioned. This gradual and consecutive development of the various skin appendages has to be kept in mind in cases of PD in fetuses at risk for EDs [13]. Lack of sweat glands in a fetal skin sample of 18 weeks is a normal finding and may not be mistaken for indicating an ED.

REFERENCES

1 Holbrook KA, Sybert VP. Basic science. In: Schachner LA, Hansen RC, eds. *Paediatric Dermatology*. Edinburgh: Churchill Livingstone, 1996: 1–70.
2 Holbrook KA, Hoff MS. Structure of the developing human embryonic and fetal skin. *Semin Dermatol* 1984; 3: 185–202.
3 Holbrook KA, Dale BA, Smith LT *et al*. Markers of adult skin expressed in the skin of the first trimester fetus. *Curr Prob Derm* 1987; 16: 94–108.
4 Holbrook KA, Smith LT. Ultrastructural aspects of human skin during the embryonic, fetal, premature, neonatal, and adult periods of life. In: Blandau RJ, ed. *Morphogenesis and Malformation of the Skin. Birth Defects: Original Article Series*. New York: March of Dimes Birth Defects Foundation, Alan R. Liss, 1981; 17 (2): 9–13.
5 Anton-Lamprecht I. Prenatal diagnosis of genodermatoses. In: Harahap M, Wallach RC, eds. *Skin Changes and Diseases in Pregnancy*. New York: Marcel Dekker, 1996: 333–84.
6 Anton-Lamprecht I, Arnold M-L. Prenatal diagnosis of severe genetic disorders of the skin. In: Happle R, Grosshans E, eds. *Pediatric Dermatology. Advances in Diagnosis and Treatment*. Berlin: Springer, 1987: 3–22.
7 Anton-Lamprecht I. Prenatal diagnosis of genodermatoses. In: Dagna Bricarelli F, Casini Lemmi M, Storti G, eds. *La Diagnosi Fetale*. Suppl Analysis 1992; 7: 131–54.
8 Anton-Lamprecht I, Arnold M-L, Holbrook KA. Methodology in sampling of fetal skin and pitfalls in the interpretation of fetal skin biopsy specimens. *Semin Dermatol* 1984; 3: 203–15.
9 Arnold M-L, Anton-Lamprecht I. Problems in the prenatal diagnosis of the ichthyosis congenita group. *Human Genet* 1985; 71: 301–11.
10 Anton-Lamprecht I. Prenatal diagnosis of epidermolysis bullosa hereditaria: a review. *Semin Dermatol* 1984; 3: 229–40.
11 Hausser I, Anton-Lamprecht I. Ultrastructure of first trimester chorionic villi with regard to the prenatal diagnosis of genodermatoses. *Prenat Diagn* 1988; 8: 511–24.
12 Eady RAJ. Prenatal diagnosis of oculocutaneous albinism: implications for other hereditary disorders of pigmentation. *Semin Dermatol* 1984; 3: 241–6.
13 Arnold M-L, Rauskolb R, Anton-Lamprecht I, Schinzel A, Schmid W. Prenatal diagnosis of anhidrotic ectodermal dysplasia. *Prenat Diagn* 1984; 4: 85–98.

Prenatal diagnosis of epidermolysis bullosa

The severe forms of EB have contributed the majority of cases since the development of PD because of their peculiar problems: early death in the lethal Herlitz type and progressive handicap and other complications in the non-lethal mutilating Hallopeau–Siemans (HS) type of EB dystrophica (EBD).

According to clinical features and to the specific plane of blister formation, three major groups of EB have been distinguished: (a) the EB simplex (EBS) group with intraepidermal cleavage; (b) the EB atrophicans group with junctional separation (JEB); and (c) the EBD group with dermolytic cleavage [1]. Ultrastructural analysis of large patient series demonstrated that the various subtypes of these three groups share common target structures that express the type-specific basic defects; recent progress in molecular genetics and mutational analysis have confirmed these ultrastructural data: EBS subtypes are caused by mutations in the genes of basal keratins K5 and K14, JEB subtypes by hemidesmosome hypoplasia and mutations in one of a series of genes of intra- and extracellular constituents of hemidesmosomes, and EBD subtypes by defects of AFs and mutations in the COL7A1 gene encoding collagen VII, the major AF protein. Thus, molecular genetics has confirmed that the classification of EB, based on ultrastructural criteria, is a natural, biological classification. The distinctive ultrastructural markers applied to postnatal diagnosis of EB are similarly used on fetal skin samples for PD. In cases in which the individual causative mutations are known, PD can be performed by mutational screening in early pregnancy.

Epidermolysis bullosa simplex group

Abnormalities of the cytoskeleton of basal cells, the keratin filaments, underlie the process of cytolysis and intraepidermal blister formation. These disturbances are due to mutations in the basal cell-specific keratin genes K5 and K14 on chromosomes 12 and 17, respectively. The site of the mutation within the keratin gene decides the resulting protein abnormality. Point mutations in the highly conserved *N*- and *C*-terminal segments of the rod domain lead to clumping of basal keratins and collapse of the cytoskeleton [2], a unique diagnostic feature of the Dowling–Meara type (EB herpetiformis) [3,4]. Mutations in other positions of the rod domain or in the head or tail domain mainly cause instability of the keratin cytoskeleton typical of milder EBS types such as the Koebner type. In addition to the position, the kind of mutation (amino acid exchange) influences the severity and EBS subtype [5].

The classical EBS types are dominant traits. No experience exists with PD of the Koebner type and the (mostly much milder) Weber–Cockayne type. As generally no constant and specific ultrastructural changes are present before blister formation, safe PD or exclusion of these EBS types from fetal skin seems problematic. In severe cases that would justify termination of a pregnancy, the identification of the individual mutation and PD at the DNA level should be attempted.

The Dowling–Meara type is generally much more severe than the Koebner type and may be an indication for PD. Clumping of basal keratins was clearly demonstrable in fetal skin samples of one fetus at risk of the Dowling–Meara type [6]. In postnatal cases basal keratin clumping is most pronounced in the perilesional inflammatory margin, but may be lacking in normal-appearing skin, indicating additional realization factors required for gene expression. Safe exclusion of the Dowling–Meara type by morphological means may therefore be a problem in at-risk pregnancies. DNA-based PD at the molecular genetic level should be attempted in the future in severely affected Dowling–Meara cases including mutational analysis of the index case. As most cases are dominant new mutations, PD is only required if one of the parents is affected, while healthy parents with an affected child do not have a measurable risk for recurrence. Gonadal mosaicism has not been reported so far for the Dowling–Meara type.

Rare, exceptional cases of recessively inherited EBS (Koebner type) have been identified recently, in whom basal cells are devoid of their keratin cytoskeleton; in the author's Heidelberg series, three out of 45 Koebner cases belong to this subtype [1,3]. In two such cases including one of ours, the underlying mutations have been identified; in our case, born to consanguineous parents, a homozygous point mutation (T to A transition) in helix 1B of the K14 gene leads to a premature termination codon and to lack of measurable K14 protein [7]. K14 was also missing in two other cases identified so far [8,9]. In normal basal cells, K5 and K14 form heterodimers that align to form the keratin filaments of the cytoskeleton. Although K5 is normal in these patients, lack of its natural partner explains instability of K5 and lack of a regular keratin network and cytoskeleton in basal cells (for details see [7]). This recessive subtype of EBS might be another indication for PD, which can be safely performed at the ultrastructural and DNA/mutational level.

Junctional epidermolysis bullosa or epidermolysis bullosa atrophicans group

The Herlitz type, EB atrophicans generalisata gravis, is the major subtype of JEB and the most severe genetic type of EB. It carries a grave prognosis and generalized involvement of the skin and mucous membranes, rapid progression and mostly a rapid lethal outcome. Because of the severity and the early death of affected babies, the Herlitz type is the most frequent at-risk diagnosis for which PD is requested. This lethal Herlitz type is much more frequent than assumed in previous years: among newborns with EB, it may account for up to 40–50% of all cases [10]. In the author's large Heidelberg series of EB cases analysed ultrastructurally for diagnosis and classification, 121 cases out of a total of 627 were identified as Herlitz cases (December 1995; see [1]).

Various defects of hemidesmosomes and their constituents at the DEJ have been identified in the different subtypes of JEB that cause junctional blister formation, i.e. cleavage in the plane of the lamina rara [1]. Hemidesmosomes are important contact structures of basal cells facing the basal lamina and the superficial connective tissue [1,4,11,12]. They have a complex composition, consisting ultrastructurally of an attachment plate on the cytoplasmic face of the plasma membrane, and filamentous extracellular structures in the space of the lamina rara. The attachment plates are related to but not identical with the corresponding plaque structures of desmosomes, into which keratin filaments insert. The extracellular anchoring filaments (AFs) traverse the lamina rara between the plasma membrane and the basal lamina. A specific interdigitation zone, the sub-basal dense plate, runs strictly parallel to the attachment plate in the upper third of the lamina rara (see Fig. 19.25.6). In maturing fetal hemidesmosomes, it is formed by the fusion of small knob-like globular endings of short filaments projecting from the plasma membrane down into the lamina rara [10,13].

Various intracellular, transmembraneous and extracellular proteins are currently being identified as constituting the complex structure of hemidesmosomes that act as targets for mutations in JEB and for binding of antibodies in cases of autoimmune bullous diseases. These are the attachment plate proteins HD1, identical with plectin, the intermediate filament-associated protein IFAP and the bullous pemphigoid antigen BPAG1; the transmembraneous proteins BPAG2 (collagen 17) and the α6β4-integrin which both have extracellular (collagenous) domains projecting into the lamina rara; and the extracellular proteins laminin-5, laminin-6 and ladinin, the autoantigen of linear immunoglobulin A (IgA) bullous dermatosis. Laminin-5 and laminin-6 both consist of three subunit chains that are coded for by three different genes, respectively. Thus, at present at least 13 different genes are known to contribute to the organization of hemidesmosomes and may be candidate genes for JEB [1,11,14]. The NU-T2 antigen is another recently identified novel antigen of the DEJ that may be relevant for JEB [15].

Defective hemidesmosomes are responsible for junctional separation in all JEB subtypes. Distinctive differences in the kind and degree of hemidesmosome hypoplasia serve as a basis for their classification and prognosis on the ultrastructural level [1,4]. In the Herlitz type, hemidesmosomes are generally drastically reduced in number and severely hypoplastic with faint attachment plates, lack of anchoring filaments and lack of sub-basal dense plates. Herlitz children with longer times of survival may develop more prominent attachment plates, but sub-basal dense plates are constantly lacking in all cases. Skin samples fail binding of anti-laminin-5 antibodies (GB3 and others) [16], and mutations in each of the genes for the three chains α3, β3 and γ2 of laminin-5 have been identified in Herlitz children [1,14].

In contrast, in JEB with pyloric obstruction, hemidesmosomes have severely hypoplastic attachment plates and lack sub-basal dense plates, but anchoring filaments are normally expressed [1,4]. These cases show normal binding of anti-laminin-5 antibodies [16] but are negative for the α6β4-integrin, and mutations both in the β4-integrin subunit gene and the α6 subunit gene have been identified [17,18]. Children with this potentially lethal type of JEB are usually born prematurely, mostly with large congenital epithelial defects (often mistaken as aplasia cutis), and may reveal duodenal, urethral or oesophageal obstructions in addition to or instead of pyloric obstruction [1].

Milder, non-lethal JEB types such as JEB inversa and the JEB mitis type reveal different patterns of hemidesmosome hypoplasia (for details see Figs 57–10 and 57–11 in [1]). The expression may be reminiscent of the Herlitz type, but in the mitis type some hemidesmosomes may develop well-formed attachment plates and clear though immature sub-basal dense plates. The (Norwegian) JEB inversa cases have been assigned by haplotyping to LAMC2 encoding the laminin-5 γ2-chain [19]. In the mitis type, mutations have not only been identified for the β3-chain of laminin-5, but also for BPAG2 (and its collagenous domain) [1,20,21]. Recent immunofluorescence studies indicate ladinin and the NU-T2 DEJ Ag antigen as further candidate genes for the mitis type [15,22], stressing the considerable heterogeneity of the JEB group in general and of the mitis type in particular.

All of these criteria—ultrastructural markers, antibody binding and mutational analysis—have now been applied to PD of JEB. Most PDs performed ultrastructurally in Heidelberg and internationally from fetal skin samples [4,10,13,23] concerned the Herlitz type. In addition, the author has been able to exclude both, the inversa and the mitis type, prenatally from fetal skin samples in risk pregnancies. Further cases concerned JEB with pyloric obstruction with two out of eight risk fetuses affected; one of these two affected fetuses was later investigated by Fine *et al.* [24] and shown to lack binding of the 19-DEJ-1 antibody, directed against uncein, another hemidesmosome-related antigen. 19-DEJ-1 is negative in all types of JEB [25]. Twin pregnancies (two at risk of the Herlitz type in the author's series with both fetuses unaffected in each pregnancy) require separate fetal skin sampling of both fetuses. Skin of affected fetuses reacts to the biopsy trauma with fresh dermoepidermal separation (Fig. 19.25.9a). Demonstration of the specific cleavage plane (Fig. 19.25.9b,c) and of hemidesmosome hypoplasia in intact junctions (Fig. 19.25.9d) are the basis of an unequivocal PD of JEB based on the *mutant gene action*; demonstration of normal hemidesmosome ultrastructure with fully mature sub-basal dense plates permits a safe prenatal exclusion of JEB (see Fig. 19.25.6) with absolute reliability [10,13]. Timing of fetal skin sampling for JEB is possible from week 16 or 17 (see Fig. 19.25.1a) onwards; for practical and safety reasons, fetal skin sampling is preferred after week 18, as high fetal mobility and possible unsuited positions of the fetus may interfere with the sampling attempts, and may result in sampling fetal membranes erroneously instead of fetal skin. In exceptional cases, PD by ultrastructural means can also be performed from amnion membrane samples, if no fetal skin is available [26]; however, before week 18 such samples are not reliable enough, as hemidesmosomes formed by amnion

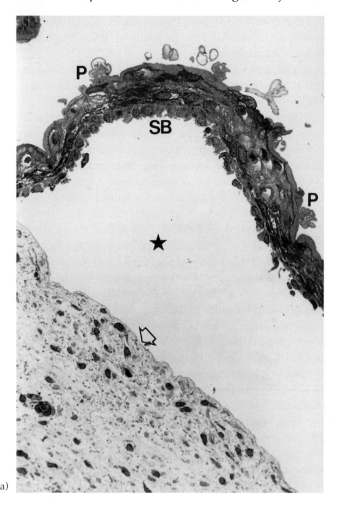

(a)

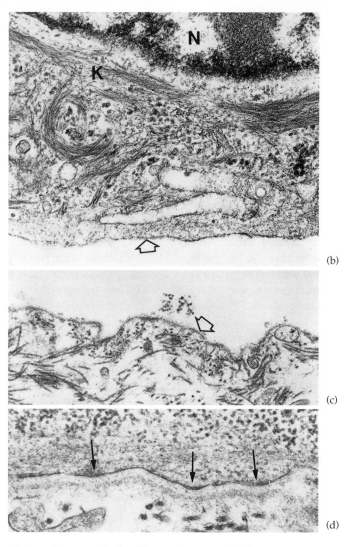

(b)

(c)

(d)

Fig. 19.25.9 Fetal expression of JEB Herlitz. (a) Junctional split in a fetus at week 19; open arrow, basal lamina at blister floor; SB basal cells; P, periderm at blister roof. (b) Undersurface of blister roof (open arrow) in a fetus at 18+0 weeks, lacking hemidesmosomes; N, nucleus of basal cell; K, keratin filaments. (c) Blister floor in a fetus at 19+4 weeks covered by basal lamina (open arrow). (d) Intact junction of affected fetus at 20+6 weeks with pronounced hemidesmosome hypoplasia (arrows); see also Fig. 19.25.1a. (a, ×405; b and d, ×43 000; c, ×19 800.)

epithelium are smaller and less well organized compared to skin. In the previously reported cases of PD from amniotic membranes [26] the failure to obtain fetal skin was mainly due to technical problems; these may be increased at earlier stages of the pregnancy. Epithelial detachment simulating JEB may occur in the amniotic membranes of healthy fetuses; conversely, affected JEB fetuses may not have any clefting in their amniotic membrane samples. Therefore, high-resolution EM is also indispensable in these cases.

Monoclonal and polyclonal antibodies directed against epitopes of the DEJ, especially GB3 (anti-laminin-5) and 19-DEJ-1 (anti-uncein), have been applied to PD of JEB [24,27]. Regarding the large number of possible candidate genes and proteins for JEB it is essential that the validity of

the respective antibody has been proved for the individual risk family. This may often be difficult because of the early death of the index cases, as for mutational analysis as well. In such a case of unclassified EB, a combination of EM with the whole panel of DEJ antibodies by immunofluorescence was applied for safe prenatal exclusion [28].

PD on the molecular genetic level can be safely performed in early pregnancy in all those families for whom the individual underlying mutations have been identified, and experience is presently accumulating [14,29–31]. In view of this progress and the chance of performing PD much earlier in at-risk pregnancies, a reliable and detailed diagnosis at the clinical, ultrastructural, antibody and DNA levels should be attempted as early as possible for each EB baby and the family as a basis for genetic counselling and PD in future pregnancies.

PD by means of ultrastructural analysis of fetal skin biopsies is based on the gene action of the mutant gene, irrespective of the kind and nature of the candidate gene or protein, its antigenicity and individual mutation. It can therefore also be performed in those cases where a previous classification of EB in a deceased index case had not been possible. The fetal skin, if affected, will show the specific ultrastructural markers, at the same time permitting a retrospective classification [10,13].

Scarring or dystrophic epidermolysis bullosa, epidermolysis bullosa dystrophica group

Dominant and recessive types of EBD are known. The recessive Hallopeau–Siemons type (EBD-HS) is the most frequent of this group with a broad range of severity ranging from mild and localized disease to generalized severely mutilating cases. Mutilating EBD-HS in general is non-lethal, and affected individuals survive to adulthood. With its many cutaneous and extracutaneous complications, involving almost all medical disciplines, this is the most severe of all the surviving EB types, affecting skin and mucous membranes. With early development of synechias (bridge-scarring) and mutilations of the phalanges, resulting in 'mitten' hands and feet; oesophageal stenosis; kidney involvement (glomerulonephritis); anaemia; early loss of teeth; possible eye involvement; and risk for amyloidosis and scar carcinoma (skin and oesophagus), affected individuals become increasingly handicapped, and early invalidity is frequent [1]. Survival of patients (in contrast to the lethal Herlitz type) and the need for demanding intensive nursing care of affected children may constitute reasons that parents find it difficult to face a new pregnancy. Although nearly 30% of all EB newborns have EBD-HS [10], PD of EBD-HS ranges far behind the Herlitz type in the author's Heidelberg series and internationally [1,32]. There is no doubt about the justification for PD and termination of affected pregnancies, therefore EBD-HS was among the first cases of PD from fetal skin samples [33].

PD may similarly be justified for the recessive EBD inversa type that lacks synechias and mutilations but otherwise may develop most of the complications of EBD-HS, especially oesophageal stenosis and scar carcinoma [1]. Some severe dominant types, such as the Pasini type, may be further indications for PD. Conversely, the dominant Kuske–Portugal type or pretibial dystrophic EB often ends up with a severe phenotype, developing extensive hyperplastic scarring on the lower legs up to the thighs that may develop carcinoma, with the possible consequence of amputation. Nevertheless, this type of EB shows mild involvement in childhood and adolescence, becoming problematic only in or after the fourth decade

[1]. Therefore the justification for PD and termination of pregnancy has to be discussed very carefully in each individual case. It should be kept in mind that it is the patient and family who have to decide, who must estimate the burden of the disease; it is the counsellor's task to provide all the available information to help the family make their own decision.

Both dominant and recessive types are characterized by dermolytic blister formation immediately underneath the basal lamina, and various degrees of defective AFs [1,11,12]. AFs are important contact devices connecting the basal lamina with the superficial papillary dermis. They have a band-like structure and a specific, non-periodical banding pattern and are formed by the lateral alignment of dimers of triple helices consisting of three identical α1-chains of collagen VII, encoded for by the COL7A1 gene on 3p21.1.

Ultrastructurally, AFs are more or less entirely missing in mutilating EBD-HS while small amounts of hypoplastic AFs are present in the non-mutilating generalized cases [1]. Both fail binding of anti-collagen VII antibodies (e.g. LH7: 2). [1,34]. Affected fetuses react to the sampling procedure with fresh subepidermal blisters in the EBD-specific cleavage plane (Fig. 19.25.10a,b), reveal the same degree of AF hypoplasia as the index cases (Fig. 19.25.10c) and are negative to anti-collagen VII antibodies. EBD inversa shows normal-appearing AFs in uninvolved skin and normal collagen VII immunoreaction, but reduced amounts of AFs and hypoplasia of AFs in atrophic skin, together with destruction of AFs in lesional skin and at the blister roof [1,35]. No experience with PD of the inversa type has been reported, and safe exclusion seems problematic from morphological and immunological criteria. Mild localized EBD-HS cases reveal almost normal AFs and normal immunofluorescence; these cases normally are no indication for terminating a pregnancy, and thus no need for PD.

In the dominant Pasini type, a broad range of AF hypoplasia was found between families, with the most severe cases lacking AFs entirely, and most of the others showing significant hypoplasia [1,36]. Prenatal exclusion has been performed [32]. Affected fetuses are expected to react to the sampling procedure with specific cleavage as in case of EBD-HS. Pretibial EB has well-formed AFs with a typical banding pattern but looser lateral alignment; AFs are retained at the blister roof and may reveal signs of breaking in the distal end of the fibril [1]. No experience with PD has been reported (for ethical problems see above).

Significant progress has been achieved with the molecular analysis of the mutations underlying EBD. All involve the COL7A1 gene, encoding collagen VII, the protein of AFs. In the recessive types, truly homozygous patients have been identified mainly from consanguineous marriages, while the majority of cases are compound het-

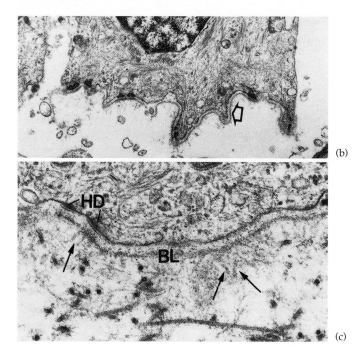

(a)

(b)

(c)

Fig. 19.25.10 Fetal expression of EBD-HS. (a) Subepidermal blister (★) in a fetus at week 21 with the basal lamina at the blister roof (open arrow) below basal cells (SB) but lacking at the blister floor (arrowhead); N, nuclei; IC, intermediate cells; SC, horn cells of follicle ostium. (b) Basal lamina at blister roof (open arrow) in a fetus at week 22 + 5. (c) Intact junction of fetus in (a) with faint hypoplastic AFs (arrows) below basal lamina (BL) and hemidesmosomes (HD). (a, ×3200; b, ×9500; c, ×43 000.)

erozygotes carrying two different (paternal and maternal) COL7A1 gene mutations. In the severest mutilating EBD-HS cases premature termination codons (PTC) explain the lack of any measurable protein and AF, while milder cases may be due to mutations disturbing the association of triple helices into dimers. Finally, dominant mutations were identified as substitutions of glycine to another amino acid leading to various degrees of protein and AF instability [14,37,38]. Increasing numbers of COL7A1 mutations have been identified, and PD of pregnancies at risk of severe EBD types can now safely be performed in the early stages of pregnancy based on the knowledge of the individual mutations [39,40]. If these mutations cannot be fully clarified and intragenic linkage analysis is applied to PD, a positive diagnosis should be controlled by fetal skin biopsy before terminating a pregnancy [13]. In an at-risk family with only one of the two suspected recessive mutations identified, a fetus showed the same intragenic haplotype combination as the affected sibling and due to formal genetics was correctly diagnosed as being affected; however, fetal skin samples taken before the planned termination were completely normal, and a healthy child was born at term (see [1,13]; A.M. Christiano and I. Anton-Lamprecht, unpublished observations, 1994). Cases like this may be due to the combination of a recessive mutation inherited from one side of the family and a spontaneous (?dominant) new mutation. Christiano et al. [41] have identified compound heterozygosity between a recessive paternal PTC in COL7A1 and a very mild dominant maternal glycine substitution that together resulted in a very severe phenotype in monozygotic EBD twins. In the future, PD of pregnancies at risk for EBD will be performed by molecular genetic means in early pregnancy. Only in cases where this is not possible or where doubts may arise because of special problems, will fetal skin biopsy demonstrating or excluding the mutant gene action be performed. The timing should be the same as discussed for the Herlitz type.

Transient bullous dermolysis of the newborn

This is a distinct subtype of EBD [42]. Children may be born with uni- or bilateral epithelial defects of the lower legs but cease to get blisters within weeks or a few months. The pathomorphogenetic abnormality identifying this type as a specific EBD entity is retention of collagen VII in cisternae of the endoplasmic reticulum of basal cells in a very peculiar manner, resulting in impairment of AFs and dermolytic blistering. Normalization within months or after the first year of life [1,43] is the rule. Glycine substitution in the collagenous domain of collagen VII has been identified in one family [44]; this mutation should interfere with post-translational modification of procollagen VII and result in peptide changes that prevent secretion of the triple-helical molecule from basal cells. The ultrastructural changes [42] are highly specific among EB types (see Fig. 57–19 in [1]); the nature of the inclusions in the endoplasmic reticulum as collagen VII has been clarified by immunolabelling with anti-collagen VII antibodies on the light microscopic level [45,46].

Because of the good prognosis, this type of EBD should not be an indication for PD. In two (exceptional) cases affected fetuses have been identified [1,45]. They express retention of collagen VII in basal cell endoplasmic reticulum cisternae even more clearly than affected newborns.

REFERENCES

1 Gedde-Dahl T Jr, Anton-Lamprecht I. Epidermolysis bullosa. In: Rimoin DL, Connor JM, Pyeritz RE, Emery AEH, eds. Emery and Rimoin's *Principles and Practice of Medical Genetics*, 3rd edn. Edinburgh: Churchill Livingstone, 1996: 1225–78.

2 Fuchs E. Intermediate filaments and disease. Mutations that cripple cell strength. Mini-review on the cellular mechanisms of disease. *J Cell Biol* 1994; 125: 511–16.

3 Anton-Lamprecht I. Ultrastructural identification of basic abnormalities as clues to genetic disorders of the epidermis. *J Invest Dermatol* 1994; 103: 6S–12S.

4 Anton-Lamprecht I. The skin. In: Papadimitriou JM, Henderson DW, Spagnolo DV, eds. *Diagnostic Ultrastructure of Non-neoplastic Diseases*. Edinburgh: Churchill Livingstone, 1992: 459–550.

5 Soerensen CB, Ladekkjaer-Mikkelsen A-S, Andresen BS *et al*. Identification of novel and known mutations in the genes for keratin 5 and 14 in Danish patients with epidermolysis bullosa simplex. Correlation between genotype and phenotype. *J Invest Dermatol* 1999; 112: 184–90.

6 Holbrook KA, Wapner R, Jackson L *et al*. Diagnosis and prenatal diagnosis of epidermolysis bullosa herpetiformis (Dowling–Meara) of a mother, two affected children and an affected fetus. *Prenatal Diagn* 1992; 12: 725.

7 Chan Y, Anton-Lamprecht I, Yu QC *et al*. A human keratin 14 'knockout': the absence of K14 leads to severe epidermolysis bullosa simplex and a function for an intermediate filament protein. *Genes Devel* 1994; 8: 2574–87.

8 Rugg EL, McLean WHI, Lane EB *et al*. A functional 'knockout' of human keratin 14. *Genes Devel* 1994; 8: 2563–73.

9 Jonkman MF, De Jong MCJM, Heeres K *et al*. Absence of keratin 14 and of intermediate filaments in basal cells in autosomal recessive epidermolysis bullosa simplex herpetiformis. *J Invest Dermatol* 1994; 103: 262 (abstract) (Presented at the 21st Annual Meeting of the Society of Cutaneous Research, Leiden, 21–24 April.)

10 Anton-Lamprecht I. Prenatal diagnosis of epidermolysis bullosa hereditaria: a review. *Semin Dermatol* 1984; 3: 229–40.

11 Marinkovich MP. The molecular genetics of basement membrane diseases. *Arch Dermatol* 1993; 129: 1557–65.

12 Eady RAJ, McGrath JA, McMillan JR. Ultrastructural clues to genetic disorders of skin: the dermal-epidermal junction. *J Invest Dermatol* 1994; 103: 13S–18S.

13 Anton-Lamprecht I. Prenatal diagnosis of genodermatoses. In: Harahap M, Wallach RC, eds. *Skin Changes and Diseases in Pregnancy*. New York: Marcel Dekker, 1996: 333–84.

14 Christiano AM, Uitto J. Molecular complexity of the cutaneous basement membrane zone. Revelations from the paradigms of epidermolysis bullosa. *Exp Dermatol* 1996; 5: 1–11.

15 Tadini G, Kanitakis J, Cavalli R *et al*. Altered expression of a new antigen of the dermo-epidermal junction (NU-T2 DEJ Ag) in junctional epidermolysis bullosa. *Arch Dermatol Res* 1995; 287: 699–704.

16 Meneguzzi G, Marinkovich MP, Aberdam D *et al*. Kalinin is abnormally expressed in epithelial basement membranes of Herlitz's junctional epidermolysis bullosa patients. *Exp Dermatol* 1992; 1: 221–9.

17 Gil SG, Brown TA, Ryan MC *et al*. Junctional epidermolysis bullosis: defects in expression of epiligrin/nicein/kalinin and integrin β4 that inhibit hemidesmosome formation. *J Invest Dermatol* 1994; 103: 31S–8S.

18 Shimizu H, Suzumori K, Hatta N *et al*. Absence of detectable alpha 6 integrin in pyloric atresia–junctional epidermolysis bullosa syndrome. Application for prenatal diagnosis in a family at risk for recurrence. *Arch Dermatol* 1996; 132: 919–25.

19 Gedde-Dahl T Jr, Dupuy BM, Jonassen R *et al*. Junctional epidermolysis bullosa inversa (locus EBR2A) assigned to 1q31 by linkage and association to LAMC1. *Hum Molec Genet* 1994; 3: 1387–91.

20 McGrath JA, Pulkkinen L, Christiano AM *et al*. Altered laminin 5 expression due to mutations in the gene encoding the β3 chain (LAMB3) in generalized atrophic benign epidermolysis bullosa. *J Invest Dermatol* 1995; 104: 467–74.

21 McGrath JA, Darling T, Gatalica B *et al*. A homozygous deletion mutation in the gene encoding the 180-kD bullous pemphigoid antigen (BPAG2) in a family with generalized atrophic benign epidermolysis bullosa. *J Invest Dermatol* 1996; 106: 771–4.

22 Marinkovich MP, Tran HH, Rao SK *et al*. LAD-1 is absent in a subset of generalized atrophic benign junctional epidermolysis bullosa patients. *J Invest Dermatol* 1996; 106: 852.

23 Rodeck CH, Eady RAJ, Gosden CM. Prenatal diagnosis of epidermolysis bullosa letalis. *Lancet* 1980; i: 949–52.

24 Fine JD, Holbrook KA, Elias S *et al*. Applicability of 19-DEJ-1 monoclonal antibody for the prenatal diagnosis or exclusion of junctional epidermolysis bullosa. *Prenatal Diagn* 1990; 10: 219–29.

25 Fine JD. 19-DEJ-1, a monoclonal antibody to the hemidesmosome anchoring filament complex, is the only reliable immunohistochemical probe for all major forms of junctional epidermolysis bullosa. *Arch Dermatol* 1990; 126: 1187–90.

26 Hausser I, Anton-Lamprecht I. Prenatal diagnosis of genodermatoses by ultrastructural diagnostic markers in extra-embryonic tissues: defective hemidesmosomes in amnion epithelium of fetuses affected with epidermolysis bullosa Herlitz type (an alternative prenatal diagnosis in certain cases). *Hum Genet* 1990; 85: 367–75.

27 Heagerty AH, Eady RAJ, Kennedy AR *et al*. Rapid prenatal diagnosis of epidermolysis bullosa letalis using GB3 monoclonal antibody. *Br J Dermatol* 1987; 117: 271–5.

28 Shimizu H, Horiguchi Y, Suzumori K *et al*. Successful prenatal exclusion of an unspecified subtype of severe epidermolysis bullosa. *Int J Dermatol* 1998; 37: 364–9.

29 Vailly J, Pulkkinen L, Miquel C *et al*. Identification of a homozygous one basepair deletion in exon 14 of the LAMB3 gene in a patient with Herlitz junctional epidermolysis bullosa for recurrence and prenatal diagnosis in a family at risk. *J Invest Dermatol* 1994; 104: 462–6.

30 McGrath JA, Kivirikko S, Ciatti S *et al*. A homozygous nonsense mutation in the α3 chain gene of laminin 5 (LAMA3) in Herlitz junctional epidermolysis bullosa: prenatal exclusion in a fetus at risk. *Genomics* 1995; 29: 282–4.

31 Christiano AM, Pulkkinen L, McGrath JA *et al*. Mutation-based prenatal diagnosis of Herlitz junctional epidermolysis bullosa. *Prenat Diagn* 1997; 17: 343–54.

32 Eady RAJ, Holbrook KA, Blanchet-Bardon C *et al*. Chair's summary. Prenatal diagnosis of skin diseases (Workshop) In: Burgdorf WHC, Katz SI, eds. *Dermatology. Progress and Perspectives. The Proceedings of the 18th*

World Congress of Dermatology. New York: Parthenon Publishing, 1993: 1159–65.

33 Anton-Lamprecht I, Rauskolb R, Jovanovic V *et al*. Prenatal diagnosis of epidermolysis bullosa dystrophica Hallopeau–Siemens with electron microscopy of fetal skin. *Lancet* 1981; 14: 1077–9.

34 Heagerty AHM, Kennedy AR, Leigh IM *et al*. Identification of an epidermal basement membrane defect in recessive dystrophic epidermolysis bullosa by LH7:2 monoclonal antibody: use in diagnosis. *Br J Dermatol* 1986; 115: 125–31.

35 Bruckner-Tuderman L, Winberg JO, Anton-Lamprecht I *et al*. Anchoring fibrils, collagen VII, and neutral metalloproteases in recessive dystrophic epidermolysis bullosa inversa. *J Invest Dermatol* 1992; 99: 550–8.

36 Anton-Lamprecht I, Hashimoto I. Epidermolysis bullosa dystrophica dominans (Pasini)—a primary structural defect of the anchoring fibrils. *Hum Genet* 1976; 32: 69–76.

37 Uitto J, Christiano AM. Molecular basis for the dystrophic forms of epidermolysis bullosa: mutations in the type VII collagen gene. *Arch Dermatol Res* 1994; 287: 16–22.

38 Christiano AM, McGrath JA, Uitto J. Influence of the second COL7A1 mutation in determining the phenotypic severity of recessive dystrophic epidermolysis bullosa. *J Invest Dermatol* 1996; 106: 766–70.

39 Christiano AM, Uitto J. Molecular diagnosis of inherited skin diseases: the paradigm of dystrophic epidermolysis bullosa. *Adv Dermatol* 1996; 11: 199–213.

40 Christiano AM, LaForgia S, Paller AS *et al*. Prenatal diagnosis for recessive dystrophic epidermolysis bullosa in 10 families by mutation and haplotype analysis in the type VII collagen gene (COL7A1). *Mol Med* 1996; 2: 59–76.

41 Christiano AM, Anton-Lamprecht I, Amano S *et al*. Compound heterozygosity for COL7A1 mutations in twins with dystrophic epidermolysis bullosa: a recessive paternal deletion/insertion mutation and a dominant negative maternal glycine substitution result in a severe phenotype. *Am J Hum Genet* 1996; 58: 682–93.

42 Hashimoto K, Matsumoto M, Iacobelli D. Transient bullous dermolysis of the newborn. *Arch Dermatol* 1985; 121: 1429–38.

43 Hatta N, Takata M, Shimizu H. Spontaneous disappearance of intraepidermal type VII collagen in a patient with dystrophic epidermolysis bullosa. *Br J Dermatol* 1995; 133: 619–24.

44 Christiano AM, Fine JD, Uitto J. Genetic basis of dominantly inherited transient bullous dermolysis of the newborn: a splice site mutation in the type VII collagen gene. *J Invest Dermatol* 1997; 109: 811–14.

45 Fine JD, Horiguchi Y, Stein DH *et al*. Intraepidermal type VII collagen. Evidence for abnormal intracytoplasmic processing of a major basement membrane protein in rare patients with dominant and possibly localized recessive forms of dystrophic epidermolysis bullosa. *J Am Acad Dermatol* 1990; 22: 188–95.

46 Phillips RJ, Harper JI, Lake BD. Intraepidermal collagen type VII in dystrophic epidermolysis bullosa: report of five new cases. *Br J Dermatol* 1992; 126: 222–30.

Alpha-fetoprotein and acetylcholinesterase values in amniotic fluid of epidermolysis bullosa fetuses

Maternal serum AFP screening is used routinely for the detection of neural tube defects. Elevated levels of AFP and ACHE have also been observed in amniotic fluid and maternal serum in pregnancies carrying fetuses affected with various types of EB, such as severe EBS [1], JEB with pyloric obstruction [2,3] or recessive EBD [4]. In these cases extensive intrauterine blistering and/or epithelial detachment are to be assumed. Children affected with JEB and pyloric obstruction, and many severe recessive EBD cases, are born with large epithelial defects which probably exist for months prenatally as seen after elective abortion in our first affected EBD fetus at 23 weeks [5]. In contrast, many Herlitz children are born with normal-appearing, intact skin and develop blisters only hours after birth. This explains normal AFP and ACHE values in pregnancies with Herlitz fetuses [6]. Increased amniotic fluid values for AFP and ACHE in pregnancies at risk of EB may indicate an affected fetus but do not replace verification by fetal skin analysis or DNA-based PD, and normal values do not safely exclude EB. In the author's series of affected EB fetuses of whom data are available (consisting of 12 Herlitz, one JEB with pyloric obstruction and five EBD-HS fetuses) only the severe EBD-HS case [5] had slightly elevated amniotic fluid AFP values (3.2 MOM, multiple of median value) while AFP was normal and ACHE negative in all others (I. Anton-Lamprecht, unpublished data, 1996).

REFERENCES

1 Yacoub T, Campbell CA, Gordon YB, Kirby JD, Kitau MJ. Maternal serum and amniotic fluid concentrations of alphafetoprotein in epidermolysis bullosa simplex. *Br Med J* 1979; 3: 307.

2 Dolan CR, Smith LT, Sybert VP. Prenatal detection of epidermolysis bullosa letalis with pyloric atresia in a fetus by abnormal ultrasound and elevated alpha-fetoprotein. *Am J Med Genet* 1993; 47: 395–400.

3 Nesin M, Seymour C, Kim Y. Role of elevated alpha-fetoprotein in prenatal diagnosis of junctional epidermolysis bullosa and pyloric atresia. *Am J Perinatol* 1994; 11: 286–7.

4 Drugan A, Vadas A, Sujov P, Gershoni-Baruch R. Markedly elevated alpha-fetoprotein and positive acetylcholinesterase in amniotic fluid from a pregnancy affected with dystrophic epidermolysis bullosa. *Fetal Diagn Ther* 1995; 10: 37–40.

5 Anton-Lamprecht I, Rauskolb R, Jovanovic V, Kern B, Arnold M-L, Schenck W. Prenatal diagnosis of epidermolysis bullosa dystrophica Hallopeau–Siemens with electron microscopy of fetal skin. *Lancet* 1981; 14: 1077–9.

6 Shulman LP, Elias S, Andersen RN *et al*. Alpha-fetoprotein and acetylcholinesterase are not predictive of fetal junctional epidermolysis bullosa, Herlitz variant. *Prenat Diagn* 1991; 11: 813–18.

Prenatal diagnosis of keratinization disorders

Major indications for PD in this group of genodermatoses are severe, congenital ichthyoses with dominant or recessive inheritance [1]. In the case of dominant disorders, PD is indicated when one of the parents is affected, while healthy parents of a child with a dominant ichthyosis have no increased risk for recurrence, as gonadal mosaicism has not been reported for the ichthyoses in question. Parents of a child with recessive congenital ichthyosis have a 25% risk of another affected child. PD of keratinization disorders has special problems [2], as keratinization has a late onset during fetal skin development and is restricted to the pilosebaceous follicles around week 20, while the interfollicular epithelium retains its periderm until the end of the second trimester. Therefore, only those congenital ichthyoses that express distinctive markers within the second trimester can be diagnosed early enough and be safely excluded [3,4]. Some of the severe recessive types do not have such ultrastructural markers, and no biochemical abnormalities have yet been identified. In the experience of the author and others, skin samples of such at-risk fetuses may appear completely normal during the second trimester although the fetus is affected. Preinvestigation of index cases and exact classification by morphological means [1,5] is therefore of significant importance in counselling families and discussing the possibility of PD (see above).

Dominantly inherited congenital ichthyoses

Bullous congenital ichthyosiform erythroderma of Brocq or epidermolytic hyperkeratosis

Among the dominantly inherited congenital ichthyoses, bullous congenital ichthyosiform erythroderma (bullous CIE) is the only one for which PD has been applied [1,3,4,6–8]. Patients with bullous CIE have a 50% risk of recurrence for their offspring. Because of the pronounced severity in most cases, PD is justified in at-risk pregnancies. As the genes responsible (see below) have a high mutation rate, many solitary cases exist that represent new dominant mutations.

Bullous CIE is characterized postnatally by suprabasal clumping of keratin filaments of the epidermal cytoskeleton, while basal cells are normal [5]. This type of aggregation and clumping of the keratin network is similar to EB herpetiformis Dowling–Meara, where basal keratins are involved and suprabasal cells develop normally. Round and ovoid clumps predominate in basal cells of the Dowling–Meara type, whereas such clumps are intermingled with all kinds of looser and denser aggregates, tangled masses and perinuclear shells of collapsed keratins in the suprabasal cells of bullous CIE. In both disorders, segregation of the cytoplasm of affected cell layers and loss of the normal cytoskeleton function are the reasons for cytolysis and blister formation after minor mechanical stress and trauma; in the Dowling–Meara type, blisters predominate clinically, while in bullous CIE blistering decreases gradually soon after birth with the compensatory development of ichthyosiform hyperkeratosis. The main differences between both disorders are the keratin types and the cell layers involved: basal keratin clumping leads to EB, suprabasal keratin clumping leads to a hyperkeratotic congenital ichthyosis [9].

Molecular genetics have confirmed this concept demonstrating that mutations in K5 and K14 underlie the Dowling–Meara type of EB, while mutations of K1 and K10, the major suprabasal keratins, are responsible for bullous CIE. In addition, mutations in the late-appearing, high-level K2 underlie ichthyosis bullosa Siemens with keratin clumping restricted to the granular layer, and mutations in K9, specifically expressed in the ridged skin of palms and soles, underlie the Voerner type of palmoplantar keratoderma where suprabasal keratin clumping is restricted to the palms and soles. In all these disorders the mutations themselves are located in so-called hotspots in the highly conserved terminal segments of the rod domain, and point mutations resulting in substitution of an arginine into other amino acids such as histidin, cystein or lysine, have been found for bullous CIE in K10 or K1 [10–14].

PD can be performed on fetal skin samples from the 18th week [4,8], or by molecular genetic means in early pregnancy as soon as the individual mutations have been identified [15].

Skin samples of affected fetuses (three out of five in the author's Heidelberg PD series, all from the same family) reveal the same cytolysis of suprabasal cells as found in newborn skin biopsies (Fig. 19.25.11a), while the typical keratin clumping is not yet expressed before the onset of keratinization; it may therefore be lacking in diagnostic skin samples, e.g. from the fetal back. At the same time, the palms and soles of affected fetuses have already developed massive hyperkeratoses, and suprabasal keratin clumping (Fig. 19.25.11b) and cytolysis are demonstrable in these areas with their much earlier timing [1,3,5].

Amniotic fluid samples of some (but not all) affected fetuses contained the specific keratin clumps already in some of their cells [8,16]. It must be stressed, however, that lack of clumping in amniotic fluid cells does not permit safe exclusion of bullous CIE for the at-risk fetus.

REFERENCES

1 Anton-Lamprecht I. Heterogeneity and prenatal diagnosis of congenital ichthyosis. In: Fabrizi G, Serri F, Cerimele D, eds. *Dermatologia Pediatrica. 4th International Symposium on Pediatric Dermatology, Selinunte (Trapani) 25–28 September 1991*. Naples: Casa Editrice l'Antologia, 1991.

2 Arnold M-L, Anton-Lamprecht I. Problems in the prenatal diagnosis of the ichthyosis congenita group. *Hum Genet* 1985; 71: 301–11.

3 Anton-Lamprecht I. Prenatal diagnosis of genodermatoses. In: Dagna Bricarelli F, Casini Lemmi M, Storti G, eds. *La Diagnosi Fetale*. Suppl *Analysis* 1992; 7: 131–54.

4 Anton-Lamprecht I. Prenatal diagnosis of genodermatoses. In: Harahap M, Wallach RC, eds. *Skin Changes and Diseases in Pregnancy*. New York: Marcel Dekker, 1996: 333–84.

5 Anton-Lamprecht I. The skin. In: Papadimitriou JM, Henderson DW, Spagnolo DV, eds. *Diagnostic Ultrastructure of Non-neoplastic Diseases*. Edinburgh: Churchill Livingstone, 1992: 459–550.

6 Golbus MS, Sagebiel RW, Filly RA, Gindhart TD, Hall JG. Prenatal diagnosis of bullous congenital ichthyosiform erythroderma (epidermolytic hyperkeratosis) by fetal skin biopsy. *N Engl J Med* 1980; 302: 93–5.

7 Anton-Lamprecht I. Prenatal diagnosis of genetic disorders of the skin by means of electron microscopy. *Hum Genet* 1981; 59: 392–405.

8 Holbrook KA. Progress in prenatal diagnosis of bullous congenital ichthyosiform erythroderma (epidermolytic hyperkeratosis). *Semin Dermatol* 1984; 3: 216–20.

9 Anton-Lamprecht I. Ultrastructural identification of basic abnormalities as clues to genetic disorders of the epidermis. *J Invest Dermatol* 1994; 103: 6S–12S.

10 Fuchs E. Intermediate filaments and disease: mutations that cripple cell strength. Mini-review on the cellular mechanisms of disease. *J Cell Biol* 1994; 125: 511–16.

11 Cheng J, Syder AJ, Yu QC, Letai A, Paller AS, Fuchs E. The genetic basis of epidermolytic hyperkeratosis: a disorder of differentiation-specific epidermal keratin genes. *Cell* 1992; 70: 811–19.

12 Rothnagel JA, Fisher MP, Axtell SM *et al*. A mutational hot spot in keratin 10

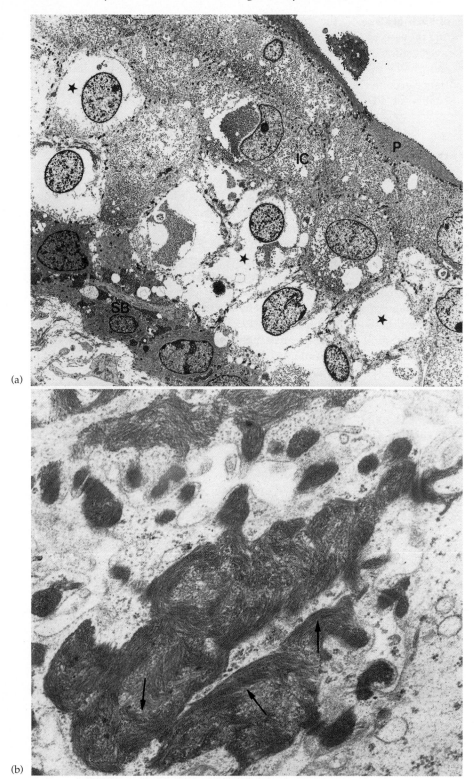

(a)

(b)

Fig. 19.25.11 Fetal expression of bullous CIE. (a) Suprabasal cytolysis (★) of intermediate cells (IC) but normal basal cell layer (SB) and periderm (P) in a fetus at week 20, sibling of (b). (b) Keratin clumps in suprabasal cells of palmar skin after termination in a fetus at week 22, sibling of (a); arrows indicate a periodic banding pattern in the keratin aggregates. (a, ×2100; b, ×28 000.)

(KRT 10) in patients with epidermolytic hyperkeratosis. *Hum Mol Genet* 1993; 2: 2147–50.

13 Rothnagel JA, Traupe H, Wojcik S *et al*. Mutations in the rod domain of keratin 2e in patients with ichthyosis bullosa of Siemens. *Nat Genet* 1994; 7: 485–90.

14 Reis A, Hennies HC, Langbein L *et al*. Keratin 9 mutations in epidermolytic palmoplantar keratoderma (EPPK). *Nat Genet* 1994; 6: 174–9.

15 Rothnagel JA, Longley MA, Holder RA, Küester W, Roop DR. Prenatal diagnosis of epidermolytic hyperkeratosis by direct gene sequencing. *J Invest Dermatol* 1994; 102: 13–16.

16 Eady RAJ, Gunner DB, Carbone LD, Bricarelli FD, Gosden CM, Rodeck CH. Prenatal diagnosis of bullous ichthyosiform erythroderma: detection of tonofilament clumps in fetal epidermal and amniotic cells. *J Med Genet* 1986; 23: 46–51.

Recessively inherited congenital ichthyoses

Harlequin ichthyosis or ichthyosis congenita gravis
(see also Chapter 1.10)

Harlequin ichthyosis is the most severe form of all keratinization disorders, mostly with a lethal course. Affected babies are usually born prematurely around weeks 32–34 with armour-like hyperkeratosis and deep fissures covering the whole skin. Grossly abnormal facial appearance with severe ectropion and eclabion, lack of ear helix development, dermatogenic contractures of large and small joints, and oedema of the hands and feet are consequences of the increasing thickness of hyperkeratoses of the skin. Most of these infants die within a few hours or days, due to respiratory distress or cardiac failure. Surviving cases develop a severely scaling erythrodermic ichthyosis after shedding the perinatal horn masses. In view of the severity of this keratinization disorder, there is no doubt about it being an indication for PD [1–3].

The underlying abnormality is unknown on the biochemical and molecular genetic level. However, ultrastructural expression is unique among the ichthyoses which allows unequivocal postnatal and prenatal identification, whilst emphasizing that harlequin ichthyosis represents an independent nosological entity [2,3].

The target structure of the underlying gene mutations are the keratinosomes (Odland bodies, lamellar granules) which normally accumulate the epidermal barrier lipids, mostly ceramides, during terminal differentiation. Their stacks of polar lipids are discharged into the intercellular spaces at the granular–horny layer interface to be transformed into large non-polar lipid sheets. The 'mortar' of the intercellular barrier lipids and the 'bricks' of cornified cells in the horny layer together act as a very effective barrier preventing transepidermal water loss and penetration of water-soluble substances into the skin.

Keratinosomes are constantly defective in harlequin ichthyosis both in affected fetuses and newborn infants. Although many vesicular keratinosomes are formed, they fail to accumulate barrier lipids; they appear empty or contain small amounts of glycogen-like granules (Fig. 19.25.12a) [2–5]. Glycogen is known to serve as a precursor of lipid synthesis. It is therefore likely that an enzyme deficiency is responsible for an early block of barrier lipid synthesis from glycogen and other precursors in harlequin ichthyosis. The defective keratinosomes are not discharged normally into the intercellular spaces but accumulate in the lowermost cells of the compact horny layer and in the deep follicular plugs (Fig. 19.25.12b–d).

With the ultrastructural demonstration of these defective keratinosomes, a safe and distinctive diagnosis of harlequin ichthyosis is possible [2,4], as all other types of congenital ichthyoses have normal keratinosomes and the capability of barrier lipid synthesis.

Affected fetuses reveal the same peculiar keratinosome abnormality (Fig. 19.25.12a), as soon as keratinization becomes demonstrable with the first appearance of keratohyalin granules and keratinized cells around the distal hair canal; consequently, harlequin ichthyosis can be safely excluded prenatally (Fig. 19.25.12e) by demonstrating the normal lamellated ultrastructure of keratinosomes at about the same time (Fig. 19.25.12a inset), i.e. about week 18–19. Before this time, PD of harlequin ichthyosis is presently not possible. However, in contrast to statements in the literature, it is not necessary to perform PD as late as week 23 [1].

Amniotic fluid cell samples of affected fetuses contain stacks and ring-like aggregates of flat, partly keratinized cells that correspond to the horn cells of follicular plugs and reveal lipid droplets and the remainders of defective keratinosomes (see Figs 9f and 9g in [5]). Follicular plugging is striking in affected fetuses (Fig. 19.25.12b) even before the onset of keratinization in the interfollicular portions of the fetal epithelium. By about week 23, the interfollicular epithelium also reveals pronounced hyperkeratosis [1–5]. The amount of keratohyalin differs between affected fetuses and individuals, but is mostly higher in the plugged follicles.

In the first case of a fetus at risk of harlequin ichthyosis [6] the keratinized portions of normal hair follicles were erroneously interpreted as indicating an affected fetus. With the first true positive PD of harlequin ichthyosis Blanchet-Bardon and Dumez [1] impressively demonstrated the specific facial appearance already expressed in week 23. Another affected fetus identified in Heidelberg (Fig. 19.25.12a–d) was clinically less grossly abnormal at the same age but showed the developing hyperkeratoses on the face (front skin, eyebrows, perioral skin), palms and soles, and the beginning ear malformation [5]. Thus some variation exists in the onset of the clinical expression. Further cases have been identified prenatally by fetal skin biopsy, amniotic fluid cells and ultrasonography [7–10].

The family investigated prenatally by Holbrook *et al.* [11,12] in four subsequent pregnancies (two fetuses judged normal and born healthy at term, two fetuses affected, one of them false negative and born prematurely) is a harlequin ichthyosis family, based on the clinical and ultrastructural features of the affected fetuses, but does not represent congenital ichthyosiform erythroderma as assumed and diagnosed by the authors [11] (for more detailed discussion see [5]). The false-negative evaluation in fetus 3 was explained by the pronounced

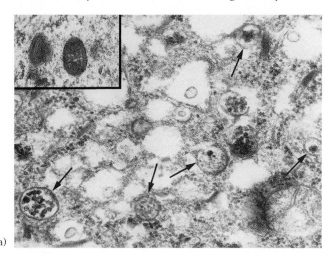

(a)

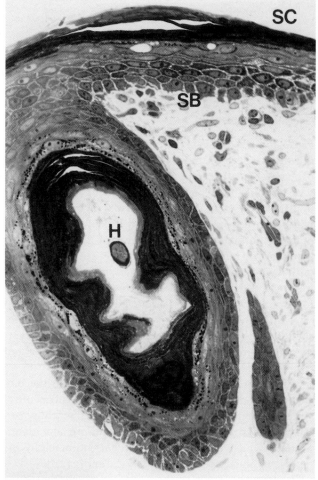

(b)

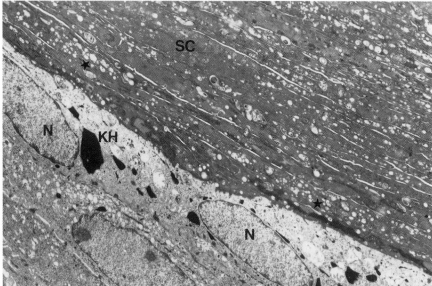

(c)

Fig. 19.25.12 Fetal expression of harlequin ichthyosis at 23 weeks. (a) Defective vesicular keratinosomes (arrows) with few glycogen-like granules but lacking the stacks of barrier lipids present in normal fetal skin (inset, 20 weeks). (b) Follicular plugging and interfollicular hyperkeratosis (SC); note the prominent granular layer lining the follicle. H, hair-shaft section; SB, basal layer. (c, d) Granular and horny layer (SC) lining a follicle, with accumulation of defective keratinosomes (arrows in d) in lowermost horn cells (★). KH, keratohyalin; N, nuclei. (a, ×43 000; b, ×425; c, ×4500; d, ×35 500; e, ×2100.) (e) Exclusion of harlequin ichthyosis at 22 weeks: fetus at risk had normal keratinosomes and large distal hair canals loosely filled with normal horn lamellae (SC); compare with Figs 19.25.12b, 19.25.12c and 19.25.13b. H, hair shaft section; arrow, small keratohyalin granule. *Continued opposite.*

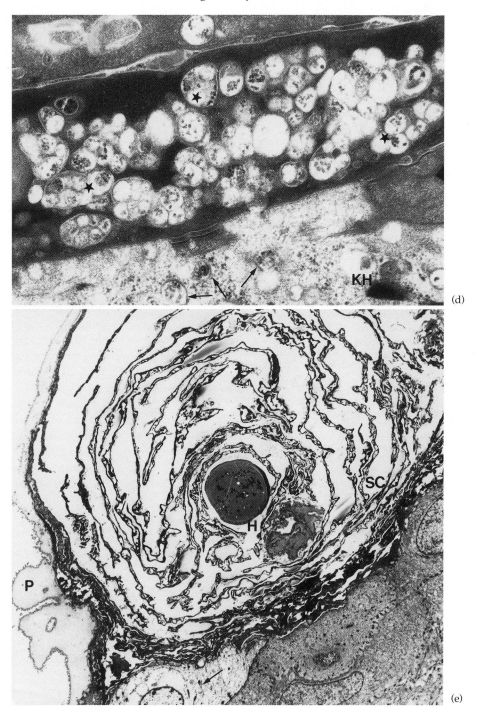

(d)

(e)

Fig. 19.25.12 *Continued*

regional differences because of the patchy onset of keratinization [11,12] (see above). Detailed investigations have been devoted to keratin and keratohyalin expression in this family [11,12], following the previous proposal [13] to classify harlequin ichthyosis according to these parameters, but the basic abnormality is in the keratinosomes. Control of the keratinizing portions of fetal (and postnatal) skin samples at high EM magnifications for the normal

or abnormal ultrastructure of keratinosomes should have helped to avoid a false-negative diagnosis and allowed a correct diagnosis of harlequin ichthyosis in this family [5].

Keratins, filaggrin/profilaggrin and cornified envelope proteins as well as expression of transglutaminase 1 (TGM1) were shown to be normal in harlequin ichthyosis [14,15].

REFERENCES

1 Blanchet-Bardon C, Dumez Y. Prenatal diagnosis of a harlequin fetus. *Semin Dermatol* 1984; 3: 225–8.
2 Anton-Lamprecht I. Heterogeneity and prenatal diagnosis of congenital ichthyosis. In: Fabrizi G, Serri F, Cerimele D, eds. *Dermatologia Pediatrica. 4th International Symposium on Pediatric Dermatology, Selinunte (Trapani) 25–28 September 1991.* Naples: Casa Editrice l'Antologia, 1991.
3 Anton-Lamprecht I. Prenatal diagnosis of genodermatoses. In: Dagna Bricarelli F, Casini Lemmi M, Storti G, eds. *La Diagnosi Fetale.* Suppl *Analysis,* 1992; 7: 131–54.
4 Anton-Lamprecht I. The skin. In: Papadimitriou JM, Henderson DW, Spagnolo DV, eds. *Diagnostic Ultrastructure of Non-neoplastic Diseases.* Edinburgh: Churchill Livingstone, 1992: 459–550.
5 Anton-Lamprecht I. Prenatal diagnosis of genodermatoses. In: Harahap M, Wallach RC, eds. *Skin Changes and Diseases in Pregnancy.* New York: Marcel Dekker, 1996: 333–84.
6 Elias S, Mazur M, Sabaggha R, Esterly NB, Simpson JL. Prenatal diagnosis of harlequin ichthyosis. *Clin Genet* 1980; 17: 275–80.
7 Suzumori K, Kanzaki T. Prenatal diagnosis of harlequin ichthyosis by fetal skin biopsy: report of two cases. *Prenat Diagn* 1991; 11: 451–7.
8 Akiyama M, Kim DK, Main DM, Otto CE, Holbrook KA. Characteristic morphologic abnormality of harlequin ichthyosis detected in amniotic fluid cells. *J Invest Dermatol* 1994; 102: 210–13.
9 Akiyama M, Holbrook KA. Analysis of skin-derived amniotic fluid cells in the second trimester; detection of severe genodermatoses expressed in the fetal period. *J Invest Dermatol* 1994; 103: 674–7.
10 Watson WJ, Mabee LM Jr. Prenatal diagnosis of severe congenital ichthyosis (harlequin fetus) by ultrasonography. *J Ultrasound Med* 1995; 14: 241–3.
11 Holbrook KA, Dale BA, Williams ML *et al.* The expression of congenital ichthyosiform erythroderma in second trimester fetuses of the same family: morphologic and biochemical studies. *J Invest Dermatol* 1988; 91: 521–31.
12 Holbrook KA, Smith LT, Elias S. Prenatal diagnosis of genetic skin disease using fetal skin biopsy samples. *Arch Dermatol* 1993; 129: 1437–54.
13 Dale BA, Holbrook KA, Fleckman P, Kimball JR, Brumbaugh S, Sybert VP. Heterogeneity in harlequin ichthyosis, an inborn error of epidermal keratinization: variable morphology and structural protein expression and a defect in lamellar granules. *J Invest Dermatol* 1990; 94: 6–18.
14 Akiyama M, Yoneda K, Kim S-Y *et al.* Cornified cell envelope proteins and keratins are normally distributed in harlequin ichthyosis. *J Cutan Pathol* 1996; 23: 571–5.
15 Akiyama M, Kim S-Y, Yoneda K *et al.* Expression of transglutaminase 1 (transglutaminase K) in harlequin ichthyosis. *Arch Derm Res* 1997; 289: 116–19.

Autosomal recessive ichthyoses (see also Chapter 19.5)

Congenital ichthyoses with recessive inheritance are far more heterogeneous than previously assumed. In addition to the lethal harlequin ichthyosis type (ichthyosis congenita gravis, see above), this group comprises various non-lethal genetic types that were considered as one entity until about 1985 [1]. Terms such as lamellar ichthyosis and non-bullous CIE are mostly used synonymously and collectively. Distinction into erythrodermic and non-erythrodermic types of lamellar ichthyosis (ELI and NELI) [2] is not reliable as erythroderma may vary considerably even within families and affected individuals [3–5]. Their considerable heterogeneity became apparent during the systematic ultrastructural analysis of large series of ichthyosis patients in Heidelberg [3–5], soon confirmed by EM from Finland [6,7] and later from Italy [8,9], as well as clinically from Norway [10]. Traupe [1] introduced subtypes to ELI and NELI that roughly par-

allel the ultrastructural subtypes. These are based on specific deviations from the normal keratinization process with distinct patterns of lipid deposition in the uppermost living and cornified cells; they have been termed ichthyosis congenita types I–IV [3–5] as follows.

Ichthyosis congenita type I—storage of non-polar lipids in lipid droplets in the horn lamellae. This is the classical type of hyperproliferation hyperkeratosis that may be combined with pronounced erythroderma and fine scaling.

Ichthyosis congenita type II—storage of islands of cholesterol clefts in the horny layer, especially pronounced in the massive follicular plugs (cholesterol type). Pronounced or mild polygonal scaling, with or without erythroderma.

Ichthyosis congenita type III—distended perinuclear membranes, probably consisting of polar lipids, vesicular keratinosome complexes and membrane-bound vacuoles in the granular and horny layer. These patients present with a very characteristic reticular scaling pattern, normally without erythroderma.

Ichthyosis congenita type IV—lentiform paranuclear cell regions of granular cells filled with dense, tangled aggregations of shorter membrane profiles probably also of polar lipids, that are retained in the horn cells. Born premature about week 32–34, these infants are at risk of perinatal death because of considerable shedding of horn cells into the amniotic cavity and risk of asphyxia. Surviving cases develop a mild, mostly follicular keratinization disorder.

A total of 330 patients with autosomal recessive ichthyosis congenita was investigated by EM in Heidelberg up to September 1997. Their relative frequencies were as follows: type I—22.4%; type II—35.2%; type III—15.5%; type IV—4.9%; unclassifiable by EM—21.2% (I. Anton-Lamprecht and coworkers, unpublished data, 1997). This underlines the considerable heterogeneity of these diseases.

Babies of all four types may be born with a collodion skin, which is most pronounced in type II and mild in types III and IV. Severity can vary from very mild to very severe in each of these four types, and erythroderma may or may not be present in all of them.

Deficiency of TGM1, an enzyme cross-linking involucrin and loricrin, precursor proteins of the cornified envelope, was demonstrated in 'severe cases' of lamellar ichthyosis, but normal expression was seen in others, confirming their heterogeneity [11,12]. These patients had not been classified by EM. Meanwhile, correlation of ultrastructural data, linkage analyses and TGM1 expression proved TGM1 deficiency to be linked to ichthyosis congenita type II [10,13,14]. The TGM1 gene has been mapped to 14q11 [15], and mutations have been identified [11,16–18]. Attempts to develop models for gene therapy of TGM1-deficient congenital ichthyosis have been reported [19,20]. DNA-based PD can be performed in early pregnancy in those families in whom the mutations are known; the first case of PD in a pregnancy at risk of congenital ichthyosis type II and TGM1 deficiency by mutational analysis allowed the exclusion of both mutations for the fetus [21]. DNA-based PD and prenatal exclusion of congenital ichthyosis via TGM1 mutational analysis have been published [22,23].

A second gene locus linked to ichthyosis congenita has been mapped to chromosome 2q33–35, but a candidate gene has not yet been identified. Thus, in the majority of cases DNA-based PD is not yet available. However, fetal skin samples can be used for PD by ultrastructural analysis in the middle stages of pregnancy [3,4].

As discussed above, keratinization is one of the late developmental processes in fetal life and is not complete before the end of the second trimester (see above). Therefore, only those congenital ichthyoses that are characterized by disease-specific ultrastructural markers expressed early enough in the keratinizing follicular orifices can be identified prenatally. These are types II and IV (see below). Fetal skin samples of type I fetuses do not show deviations from normal up to about week 22 and thus do not permit distinction of affected fetuses. False-negative PDs resulting in the birth of affected infants have been documented [4,24,25]. PD type I must await the identification of the underlying gene mutations.

No affected type III fetus has been identified so far, and the gene defect is unknown. Therefore it is not known whether type III [5] can be identified prenatally at present.

Type II fetuses develop follicular hyperkeratosis and plugging from about week 20–21; the ultrastructural abnormalities increase from week to week (Fig. 19.25.13). Safe identification is possible at about week 21. Plugging of the distal hair canal increases steadily with a specific pattern of irregular membrane proliferation of the horn cells (Fig. 19.25.13d) lining the follicular orifices. This pattern is most easily demonstrated in tangential sections of plugged follicles (Fig. 19.25.13a,c) and allows the

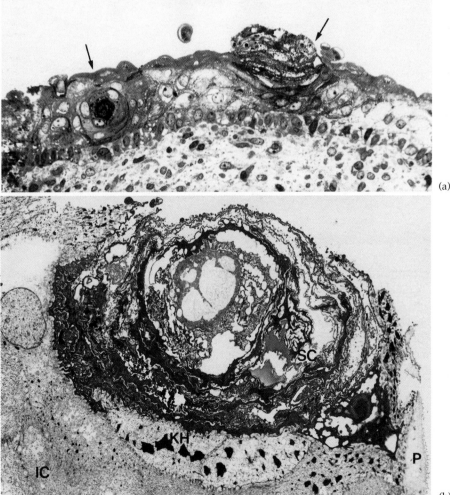

(a)

(b)

Fig. 19.25.13 Fetal expression of ichthyosis congenita type II in two affected fetuses of the same family (fetus 1, 21 + 5 weeks: a, c, d; fetus 2, 21 + 1 weeks: b). Hyperkeratosis and follicular plugging (a–c, arrows in a) of distal hair canal, interfollicular epidermis unkeratinized (a); tangential sections (c, same as in (a) left) most clearly show the irregular pattern of membrane proliferation specific of type II (d). Compare Figs 12.25.5b and 12.25.12e. KH, keratohyalin; L, lipid droplet; N, nuclei; IC, intermediate cells; P, periderm; SC, horn cells. (a, ×404; b, ×2100; c, 4500; d, ×35000.) *Continued on p. 1382.*

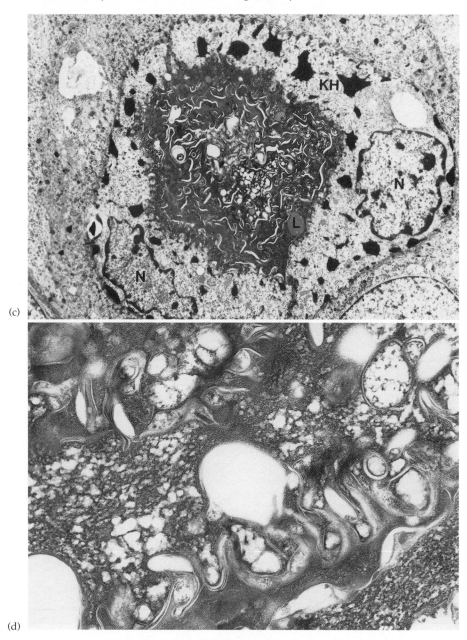

(c)

(d)

Fig. 19.25.13 *Continued*

identification of affected fetuses [3,4,24,26,27]. It is often retained in the collodion membrane of type II neonates and may serve as the first postnatal marker. The islands of cholesterol crystals that characterize type II postnatally are not yet demonstrable in fetal skin at the time of PD and mostly appear only after shedding of the collodion skin. The youngest type II case with cholesterol clefts already demonstrable was a preterm baby at 30 days (I. Anton-Lamprecht, unpublished data, 1997). Occasionally, post-natal diagnosis is possible by EM of desquamated horn lamellae demonstrating the cholesterol islands. The relationship of cholesterol deposition to deficient cor-nified envelope cross-linking due to TGM1 deficiency is unknown.

Type IV can be safely identified in fetal skin as soon as the distal hair canal becomes keratinized (Fig. 19.25.14a):

the specific tangled masses of short (lipid) membranes (Fig. 19.25.14b) appear together with keratohyalin gran-ules and keratinosomes and fill the central lentiform swollen portion of the periluminal horn lamellae (Fig. 19.25.14a). In fetal skin it is much easier to identify these membranes in granular cells than postnatally because of their low amount of keratins (Fig. 19.25.14c). Only one type IV fetus has been diagnosed prenatally [3,26–28]. PD was requested because of asphyxia and perinatal death of the sibling, at a time when the benign course of surviving cases was still unknown. With the ultrastructural identification of further patients [3,7,9,27] it now seems questionable whether termination of a type IV pregnancy is justifiable.

Thus, in families at risk of autosomal recessive congeni-tal ichthyoses, diagnostic classification of index cases with

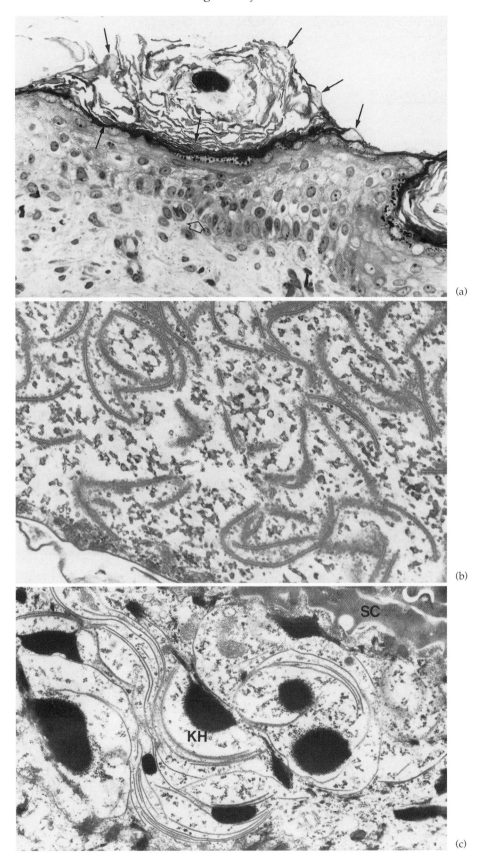

(a)

(b)

(c)

Fig. 19.25.14 Fetal expression of ichthyosis congenita type IV at 22+4 weeks: presence of lentiform swollen parts of loose hyperkeratotic horn cells lining the distal hair canal (a, arrows), filled with tangled masses of lipid membranes (b) that appear during onset of keratinization together with keratohyalin granules (KH) (c); SC, horn cell; open arrow, DEJ. (a, ×400; b, ×26 100; c, ×20 000.)

ultrastructural, enzyme biochemical and molecular genetic means is indispensable to clarify whether or not PD is possible.

REFERENCES

1 Traupe H. *The Ichthyoses. A Guide to Clinical Diagnosis, Genetic Counseling, and Therapy*. Berlin: Springer, 1989.

2 Williams ML, Elias PM. Heterogeneity of autosomal recessive ichthyosis. Clinical and biochemical differentiation of lamellar ichthyosis and nonbullous ichthyosiform erythroderma. *Arch Dermatol* 1985; 121: 477–88.

3 Anton-Lamprecht I. Heterogeneity and prenatal diagnosis of congenital ichthyosis. In: Fabrizi G, Serri F, Cerimele D, eds. *Dermatologia Pediatrica*. 4th *International Symposium on Pediatric Dermatology, Selinunte (Trapani) 25–28 September 1991*. Naples: Casa Editrice l'Antologia, 1991.

4 Arnold M-L, Anton-Lamprecht I. Problems in the prenatal diagnosis of the ichthyosis congenita group. *Hum Genet* 1985; 71: 301–11.

5 Arnold M-L, Anton-Lamprecht I, Melz-Rothfuss B, Hartschuh W. Ichthyosis congenita type III. Clinical and ultrastructural characteristics and distinction within the heterogeneous ichthyosis congenita group. *Arch Dermatol Res* 1988; 280: 268–78.

6 Niemi KM, Kanerva L, Kuokkanen K. Recessive ichthyosis congenita type II. *Arch Dermatol Res* 1991; 283: 211–18.

7 Niemi KM, Kanerva L. Ichthyosis with laminated membrane structures. *Am J Dermatopathol* 1989; 11: 149–56.

8 Patrizi A, Neri I, Di Lernia V, Pasquinelli G, Badiali De Giorgi L. Lamellar ichthyosis with laminated membrane structures. *Br J Dermatol* 1993; 128: 348–51.

9 Brusasco A, Gelmetti C, Tadini G, Caputo R. Ichthyosis congenita type IV: a new case resembling a diffuse cutaneous mastocytosis. *Br J Dermatol* 1997; 136: 377–9.

10 Gedde-Dahl T, Anton-Lamprecht I, Hausser I, Arnold M-L. Nosology of autosomal recessive ichthyosis. (submitted) (letter to the editor).

11 Huber M, Rettler I, Bernasconi K *et al*. Mutations of keratinocyte transglutaminase in lamellar ichthyosis. *Science* 1995; 267: 525–8.

12 Huber M, Rettler I, Bernasconi K, Wyss M, Hohl D. Lamellar ichthyosis is genetically heterogeneous—cases with normal keratinocyte transglutaminase. *J Invest Dermatol* 1995; 105: 653–4.

13 Niemi KM. Electron microscopic and genetic study of ichthyosis congenita types I–IV. SCUR meeting Gardone Riviera, 1996. *J Invest Dermatol* 1996; 107: 659.

14 Hohl D, Huber M, Arnold M-L, Anton-Lamprecht I. In preparation.

15 Russell LJ, DiGiovanna JJ, Hashem N, Compton JG, Bale SJ. Linkage of autosomal recessive lamellar ichthyosis to chromosome 14q. *Am J Hum Genet* 1994; 55: 1146–52.

16 Russell LJ, DiGiovanna JJ, Rogers GR *et al*. Mutations in the gene for transglutaminase 1 in autosomal recessive lamellar ichthyosis. *Nat Genet* 1995; 9: 279–83.

17 Parmentier L, Blanchet-Bardon C, Nguyen S, Prud'homme JF, Dubertret L, Weissenbach J. Autosomal recessive lamellar ichthyosis: identification of a new mutation in trasglutaminase 1 and evidence for genetic heterogeneity. *Hum Mol Genet* 1995; 4: 1391–5.

18 Reis A, Hennies H, Mackova A, Ehrig T, Küster W. Molecular heterogeneity and mutation detection in autosomal recessive lamellar ichthyosis. *Am J Hum Genet* 1995; 57: A46.

19 Huber M, Rettler I, Wagner E, Hohl D. Highly efficient repair of the enzyme defect in lamellar ichthyosis cells. *J Invest Dermatol* 1996; 106: 807.

20 Choate KA, Kinsella TM, Williams ML, Nolan GP, Khavari PA. Corrective gene delivery in lamellar ichthyosis. *J Invest Dermatol* 1996; 106: 807.

21 Hennies HC, Wiebe V, Anton-Lamprecht I *et al*. Prenatal diagnosis of autosomal recessive lamellar ichthyosis (ARLI). *Med Genet* 1997; 2: 286.

22 Schroderet DF, Huber M, Laurini RN *et al*. Prenatal diagnosis of lamellar ichthyosis by direct mutational analysis of the keratinocyte transglutaminase gene. *Prenat Diagn* 1997; 17: 483–6.

23 Bichakjian CK, Nair RP, Wu WW *et al*. Prenatal exclusion of lamellar ichthyosis based on identification of two new mutations in the transglutaminase I gene. *J Invest Dermatol* 1998; 110: 179–82.

24 Arnold M-L, Anton-Lamprecht I. Prenatal diagnosis of epidermal disorders. *Curr Probl Dermatol* 1987; 16: 120–8.

25 Blanchet-Bardon C, Nazzaro V. Use of morphological markers in carriers as an aid in genetic counselling and prenatal diagnosis. *Curr Probl Dermatol* 1987; 16: 109–19.

26 Anton-Lamprecht I. Prenatal diagnosis of genodermatoses. In: Dagna Bricarelli F, Casini Lemmi M, Storti G, eds. *La Diagnosi Fetale*. Suppl *Analysis* 1992; 7: 131–54.

27 Anton-Lamprecht I. The skin. In: Papadimitriou JM, Henderson DW, Spagnolo DV, eds. *Diagnostic Ultrastructure of Non-neoplastic Diseases*. Edinburgh: Churchill Livingstone, 1992: 459–550.

28 Anton-Lamprecht I. Prenatal diagnosis of genodermatoses. In: Harahap M, Wallach RC, eds. *Skin Changes and Diseases in Pregnancy*. New York: Marcel Dekker, 1996: 333–84.

Sjögren–Larsson syndrome

Sjögren–Larsson syndrome (SLS) is a severe, autosomal recessive neurocutaneous disorder characterized by the triad of congenital ichthyosis, spastic diplegia or tetraplegia and mental retardation. The specific 'serrated' epidermal appearance with papillomatosis, acanthosis and prominent hyperkeratosis distinguishes SLS from the various types of ichthyosis congenita (see above). SLS is due to impaired fatty alcohol oxidation based on deficiency of an enzyme of lipid metabolism, fatty aldehyde dehydrogenase (FALDH), a component of fatty alcohol: NAD$^+$ oxidoreductase (FAO) [1]. The FALDH gene maps to chromosome 17p11.2, as does SLS, and mutations including point mutations, deletions and insertions mostly resulting in PTCs, have been identified in homozygous and compound heterozygous SLS patients [2]. The organization of the FALDH gene has also been characterized to facilitate genomic DNA-based mutational analysis [3].

PD of SLS has been performed on fetal skin samples by light microscopy (week 23) [4], by EM [5], by measuring FAO and FALDH values using cultured amniocytes or chorionic villus cells [6] and by polymerase chain reaction (PCR)-based mutational analysis [7]. Fetal skin samples at 19+5 weeks [5] were completely normal, although at the same time FAO values were clearly deficient, indicating SLS in the fetus; SLS was confirmed with repeat biopsy at 23+5 weeks and after termination [5]. DNA-based PD on chorionic villus samples is now possible in pregnancies at risk of SLS. Therefore, mutational analysis should be attempted in all SLS patients to verify the diagnosis and provide the basis for early PD. The first DNA-based PD of SLS has been reported from Sweden [7] with the highest incidence of SLS and predominance of the mutation C943T in the FALDH gene, for which the fetus at risk was homozygous.

REFERENCES

1 Rizzo WB, Craft DA. Sjögren–Larsson syndrome: deficient activity of the fatty aldehyde dehydrogenase component of fatty alcohol: NAD$^+$ oxidoreductase in cultured fibroblasts. *J Clin Invest* 1991; 88: 1643–8.

2 De Laurenzi V, Rogers GR, Hamrock DJ *et al*. Sjögren–Larsson syndrome (SLS) is caused by mutations in the fatty aldehyde dehydrogenase gene. *J Invest Dermatol* 1996; 106: 811.

3 Rogers GR, De Laurenzi V, Bale SJ, Markova N, Rizzo WB, Compton JG.

Genomic organization of the fatty aldehyde dehydrogenase gene for DNA-based mutation analysis in Sjögren–Larsson syndrome. *J Invest Dermatol* 1996; 106: 904.

4 Trepeta R, Stenn KS, Mahoney MJ. Prenatal diagnosis of Sjögren–Larsson syndrome. *Semin Dermatol* 1984; 3: 221–4.

5 Holbrook KA, Smith LT, Elias S. Prenatal diagnosis of genetic skin disease using fetal skin biopsy samples. *Arch Dermatol* 1993; 129: 1437–54.

6 Rizzo WB, Craft DA, Kelson TL *et al.* Prenatal diagnosis of Sjögren–Larsson syndrome using enzymatic methods. *Prenat Diagn* 1994; 14: 577–81.

7 Sillen A, Holmgren G, Wadelius C. First prenatal diagnosis by mutation analysis in a family with Sjögren–Larsson syndrome. *Prenat Diagn* 1997; 17: 1147–9.

Prenatal diagnosis of ectodermal dysplasias

ED represents a very large and highly heterogeneous group of genetic disorders affecting ectodermally derived structures: skin, hairs, nails, teeth, sweat glands and related glandular structures [1]. They have therefore been defined as genetic disorders of the appendages. Most of them are rare and not well understood.

The most important and most frequent is X-linked anhidrotic ED (X-AED), the Christ–Siemens–Touraine syndrome. The gene locus (EDA) has been mapped to Xq12–q13.1; a region of less than 1 million base pairs [2–4] where the closest marker, the DXS732 locus, may contain candidate sequences for the EDA gene [3]. High-resolution mapping permits DNA-based carrier detection, prenatal and postnatal testing [2]. X-autosomal translocations (X;1 [5], X;9, X;12 [6]), molecular deletions (at the DXS732 locus [7]), and *de novo* mutations [8] have been identified in affected males, females and carriers. Isolation and sequencing of the gene by means of positional cloning disclosed the genomic structure to consist of two exons, separated by a single 200-kb intron, encoding a small protein of 135 (or 140) residues predicted to be a novel class II transmembrane protein that may have important functions in epithelial–mesenchymal interaction or signalling [9]. The gene is expressed in fetal and postnatal cells of ectodermal origin. Direct mutational analysis is now possible.

Rare autosomal recessive anhidrotic EDs (R-AED) exist, that are still heterogeneous [10]; the genes and their location in the human genome are unresolved. Clouston's dominant hidrotic ED with pronounced hair and nail abnormalities and prominent hyperkeratosis mainly of the palms and soles, but normal sweating capacity, is similarly unresolved at the molecular level; linkage analyses have excluded the keratin clusters on chromosomes 12 and 17 and various keratin-associated proteins as candidate genes [11].

Experience with PD of EDs has only been reported for the anhidrotic EDs, X-AED and R-AED [10,12–15]. As discussed above, sweat gland primordia appear late in the second trimester, and apocrine glands are not formed before week 26. Lack of these appendages in fetal skin samples at 16–18 weeks may therefore not be taken as a sign of AED (see above). Both, X-AED (in male pregnancies) and R-AED (in both sexes) can be identified or excluded from fetal skin in the late second trimester (about week 21). Affected fetuses lack hair follicles, sebaceous glands and sweat gland primordia (Fig. 19.25.15), although some few hair follicles, often of low developmental degree, may occasionally be present in fetal skin specimens [12,13]. It is therefore essential that multiple skin samples from various locations are investigated. As AED patients are hypotrichotic but not entirely bald, scalp skin biopsy should be avoided because of the risk of false-negative PD.

Interestingly, adult X-AED males may have normal beard hair growth indicating specific gene action in an especially sensitive developmental period (e.g. between weeks 12 and 26), but inactivity in adolescence and adult life.

Skin samples of affected fetuses often react to the squeezing forces of the forceps with suprabasal cleft formation [13]. These clefts are artefactual, but may result from lack of strengthening of the fetal skin from downgrowing hair follicles.

As far as possible, PD of X-AED should now be attempted on the molecular level. Linkage analysis, using closely flanking markers, has been performed in the first trimester from chorionic villus samples [15]. This requires informative marker combinations in the at-risk family. DNA-based prenatal diagnosis and direct mutational

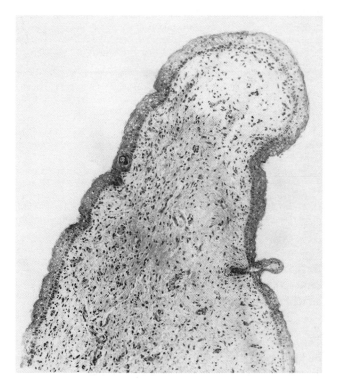

Fig. 19.25.15 Fetal expression of X-AED at week 21. Fetal skin is devoid of appendages. Compare Figs 19.25.1a,b. (×82.)

testing will become increasingly available for X-AED [2]. In cases of remaining uncertainty, fetal skin samples can be checked for gene action as an additional step (at about week 21). PD of R-AED is restricted to fetal skin biopsy analysis. Light microscopic investigation allows the identification or exclusion of both X-AED and R-AED in at-risk fetuses [10,12,13].

REFERENCES

1 Freire-Maia N, Pinheiro M. *Ectodermal Dysplasias: a Clinical and Genetic Study*. New York: Alan R. Liss, 1984.

2 Zonana J. Hypohidrotic (anhidrotic) ectodermal dysplasia: molecular genetic research and its clinical applications. *Semin Dermatol* 1993; 12: 241–6.

3 Zonana J, Jones M, Browne D *et al*. High-resolution mapping of the X-linked hypohidrotic ectodermal dysplasia (EDA) locus. *Am J Hum Genet* 1992; 51: 1036–46.

4 Thomas NS, Chelly J, Zonana J *et al*. Characterisation of molecular DNA rearrangements within the Xq12–q13.1 region, in three patients with X-linked hypohidrotic ectodermal dysplasia (EDA). *Hum Mol Genet* 1993; 2: 1679–85.

5 Limon J, Filipiuk J, Nedoszytko B *et al*. X-linked anhidrotic ectodermal dysplasia and *de novo* t (X;1) in a female. *Hum Genet* 1991; 87: 338–40.

6 Plougastel B, Couillin P, Blanquet V *et al*. Mapping around the Xq13.1 breakpoints of two X/A translocations in hypohidrotic ectodermal dysplasia (EDA) female patients. *Genomics* 1992; 14: 523–5.

7 Zonana J, Gault J, Davies KJ *et al*. Detection of a molecular deletion at the DXS732 locus in a patient with X-linked hypohidrotic ectodermal dysplasia (EDA), with the identification of a unique junctional fragment. *Am J Hum Genet* 1993; 52: 78–84.

8 Zonana J, Jones M, Clarke A, Gault J, Muller B, Thomas NS. Detection of *de novo* mutations and analysis of their origin in families with X-linked hypohidrotic ectodermal dysplasia. *J Med Genet* 1994; 31: 287–92.

9 Kere J, Srivastava AK, Montonen O *et al*. X-linked anhidrotic (hypohidrotic) ectodermal dysplasia is caused by mutation in a novel transmembrane protein. *Nat Genet* 1996; 13: 409–16.

10 Anton-Lamprecht I, Schleiermacher E, Wolf M. Autosomal recessive anhidrotic ectodermal dysplasia: report of a case and discrimination of diagnostic features. In: Salinas CF, Opitz JM, Paul NW, eds. *Recent Advances in Ectodermal Dysplasias. Birth Defects: Original Article Series*, vol. 24, no. 2. New York: Alan R. Liss, 1988: 183–95.

11 Hayflick SJ, Taylor T, McKinnon W, Guttmacher AE, Litt M, Zonana J. Clouston syndrome (hidrotic ectodermal dysplasia) is not linked to keratin gene clusters on chromosomes 12 and 17. *J Invest Dermatol* 1996; 107: 11–14.

12 Arnold M-L, Anton-Lamprecht I, Rauskolb R. Prenatal diagnosis of ectodermal dysplasias. *Semin Dermatol* 1984; 3: 247–52.

13 Arnold M-L, Rauskolb R, Anton-Lamprecht I, Schinzel A, Schmid W. Prenatal diagnosis of anhidrotic ectodermal dysplasia. *Prenat Diagn* 1984; 4: 85–98.

14 Blanchet-Bardon C, Nazzaro V. Use of morphological markers in carriers as an aid in genetic counselling and prenatal diagnosis. *Curr Probl Dermatol* 1987; 16: 109–19.

15 Zonana J, Schinzel A, Upadhyaya M, Thomas NST, Anton-Lamprecht I, Harper PS. Prenatal diagnosis of X-linked hypohidrotic ectodermal dysplasia by linkage analysis. *Am J Med Genet* 1990; 35: 132–5.

Prenatal diagnosis of oculocutaneous albinism and related pigmentary disorders
(see Chapter 14.1)

The various forms of OCA are primary abnormalities of melanin synthesis in the melanocyte, among which tyrosinase-negative and tyrosinase-positive types (OCA I and OCA II) are distinguished [1]. Typing and classification are difficult on the clinical level and demand qualitative tyrosinase tests (DOPA reaction on hair bulb or skin melanocytes) and measurement of enzyme activity [2]. A wide range of residual tyrosinase activities was found in patients with OCA I that helped in the understanding of the clinical variation and the classification of variants of OCA I (yellow pigment, minimal pigment, temperature-sensitive tyrosinase) [2]. The ethnic background and genetic constitution of the individual further contribute to the phenotype and resulting pigmentation. This is especially true for tyrosinase-positive OCA II where some pigment may be formed during the lifetime and hypopigmentation may be less evident.

The gene for tyrosinase-negative OCA I, TYR, has been mapped to chromosome 11q14–q21 [3], possibly close to 11q15.5 [1], isolated and sequenced [4], and large series of mutations have been identified [2,5] that either lead to lack of enzyme protein or to a certain extent abolish tyrosinase activity [2,6]. Clusters of mutations have been found close to the active and substrate binding sites of the enzyme molecule; the complex molecular organization of the active centre with its two copper atoms and functional aspects have been outlined by Oetting and King [2]. Variants of OCA I are all caused by mutations in the TYR locus [2].

OCA type II with normal tyrosinase activity seems to be caused by mutations in the P locus, encoding the P protein, a possible tyrosine transporter in the melanosomes [2,7]. OCA II and the P locus have both been mapped to chromosome 15q11.2–q12 [8], the molecular analysis of which is proceeding [2].

PD of OCA has so far only been performed for the tyrosinase-negative type OCA IA [5,9–11]. As discussed above, melanin synthesis and transfer to keratinocytes (skin and hair bulbs) are late developmental processes in fetal life, modified further by ethnic background and genetic constitution (see above). The first PD of (undetermined, probably tyrosinase-negative) OCA used EM analysis of fetal skin and hair bulb melanocytes [9]. Application of the DOPA technique on the ultrastructural level to demonstrate the presence or absence of tyrosinase activitiy in fetal epidermal melanocytes may facilitate PD of tyrosinase-negative OCA I [10]; in those cases in which the individual mutations have been identified PD may now be performed in early pregnancy on the DNA level by mutational analysis of the tyrosinase gene [5,11,12]. No experience with PD of OCA II has so far been reported.

Chediak–Higashi syndrome with recessive inheritance is characterized by OCA due to pigment dilution, and by functional impairment of leucocyte lysosomes [1]. A membrane abnormality is assumed to cause giant melanosomes and giant lysosomes by the fusion of initially normal-sized organelles. The gene has not yet been mapped. Chediak–Higashi syndrome can be identified or excluded prenatally by the presence or absence of these giant melanosomes and lysosomes [13].

Griscelli's syndrome is characterized by partial albinism and immunodeficiency. It can be differentiated from Chediak–Higashi syndrome by the abundance of normal mature melanosomes in melanocytes and drastically reduced pigmentation of basal keratinocytes as well as by the specific pattern of impaired cellular immunoreactions and recurrent infections [14]. Inheritance is autosomal recessive, but the gene is as yet unknown. Skin biopsy and hair shaft analysis in at-risk fetuses have been used for PD [13].

REFERENCES

1 Witkop CJ. Abnormalities of pigmentation. In: Emery AEH, Rimoin DL, eds. *The Principles and Practice of Medical Genetics*, 2nd edn. Edinburgh: Churchill Livingstone, 1990: 797–833.

2 Oetting WS, King RA. Molecular basis of oculocutaneous albinism. *J Invest Dermatol* 1994; 103: 131S–6S.

3 Barton DE, Kwon BS, Francke U. Human tyrosinase gene, mapped to chromosome 11 (q14–q21), defines second region of homology with mouse chromosome 7. *Genomics* 1988; 3: 17–24.

4 Kwon BS, Haq AK, Pomerantz SH, Halaban R. Isolation and sequence of a putative cDNA clone for human tyrosinase that maps at the mouse *c*-albino locus. *Proc Natl Acad Sci USA* 1987; 84: 7473–7.

5 Falik-Borenstein TC, Holmes SA, Borochowitz Z, Levin A, Rosenmann A, Spritz RA. DNA-based carrier detection and prenatal diagnosis of tyrosinase-negative oculocutaneous albinism (OCA1A). *Prenat Diagn* 1995; 15: 345–9.

6 Oetting WS, King RA. Molecular analysis of type I-A (tyrosinase negative) oculocutaneous albinism. *Hum Genet* 1992; 90: 258–62.

7 Spritz RA. Molecular genetics of oculocutaneous albinism. *Hum Mol Genet* 1994; 3: 1469–75.

8 Ramsay M, Colman MA, Stevens G *et al*. The tyrosinase-positive oculocutaneous albinism locus maps to chromosome 15q11.2–q12. *Am J Hum Genet* 1992; 51: 879–84.

9 Eady RAJ. Prenatal diagnosis of oculocutaneous albinism: implications for other hereditary disorders of pigmentation. *Semin Dermatol* 1984; 3: 241–6.

10 Shimizu H, Ishiko A, Kikuchi A, Akiyama M, Suzumori K, Nishikawa T. Prenatal diagnosis of tyrosinase-negative oculocutaneous albinism. *Lancet* 1992; 340: 739–40.

11 Shimizu H, Niizeki H, Suzumori K *et al*. Prenatal diagnosis of oculocutaneous albinism by analysis of the fetal tyrosinase gene. *J Invest Dermatol* 1994; 103: 104–6.

12 Shimizu H. Technical advances in prenatal diagnosis of tyrosinase-negative oculocutaneous albinism. *Acta Derm Venereol* 1997; 77: 10–13.

13 Durandy A, Breton Gorius J, Guy G and D, Dumez C, Griscelli C. Prenatal diagnosis of syndromes associating albinism and immune deficiences (Chediak–Higashi syndrome and variant). *Prenat Diagn* 1993; 13: 13–20.

14 Klein C, Philippe N, Le Deist F *et al*. Partial albinism with immunodeficiency (Griscelli syndrome). *J Pediatr* 1994; 125: 886–95.

Menkes' kinky hair syndrome

Menkes' syndrome is an X-linked disorder of copper metabolism with progressive multisystem involvement, affecting skin and hair, connective tissue and the central nervous system (CNS). The skin becomes progressively hypopigmented, the hair shafts show kinking (pili torti) and fractures (trichorrhexis nodosa). Cutis laxa-like changes develop in the connective tissue. Myoclonic seizures, spastic paresis, growth retardation and early death are the rule in affected male infants. A copper transport defect has been assumed [1]. Intracellular copper accumulation (in most organs, but depletion in the CNS) has been found and was used for diagnosis [2].

The gene has been isolated and mapped to Xq12–q13. The gene product is assumed to be a copper transporting adenosine triphosphatase (ATPase) [3]. Many of the clinical abnormalities can be ascribed to the functional deficiency of enzymes requiring copper as a cofactor, such as the copper-dependent lysyloxidase responsible for cross-linking of elastin and collagen, copper-dependent formation of disulphide bonds in keratins, and tyrosinase with two copper atoms in its active centre. Copper content measurement on chorionic villi and copper incorporation into cultured cells have been used for PD in Menkes' syndrome [4,5].

By cloning the gene and defining the individual molecular defects, DNA-based carrier detection and PD have become possible. The first PD by direct mutational analysis was performed in a family with a maternal partial deletion [3]. DNA-based PD should be attempted for Menkes' syndrome in the future.

REFERENCES

1 Danks DM. Disorders of copper transport. In: Scriver C, Beaudet A, Sly WS, Valle D, eds. *The metabolic basis of inherited disease*. New York: McGraw-Hill, 1989: 1411–31.

2 Horn N, Heydorn K, Damsgaard E, Tygstrup I, Vestermark S. Is Menkes syndrome a copper storage disease? *Clin Genet* 1978; 14: 186–7.

3 Tumer Z, Tønnesen T, Bohmann J, Marg W, Horn N. First trimester prenatal diagnosis of Menkes disease by DNA analysis. *J Med Genet* 1994; 31: 615–17.

4 Horn N. Menkes' X-linked disease: prenatal diagnosis and carrier detection. *J Inherit Metab Dis* 1983; 6: 59–62.

5 Tønnesen T, Horn N. Prenatal and postnatal diagnosis of Menkes' disease, an inherited disorder of copper metabolism. *J Inherit Metab Dis* 1989; 12 (suppl 1): 207–14.

Prenatal diagnosis of storage disorders or inborn errors of metabolism

Most of these diseases are enzymopathies with well-known enzyme deficiencies. PD has been possible from amniotic fluid by biochemical testing for many years. Some of them are of interest to paediatric dermatology (mucopolysaccharidoses or MPS); in some disorders dermatological features can provide the first hint of the correct diagnosis (Fabry' disease), whilst in others, in which the underlying biochemical and molecular abnormalities are known, a skin biopsy may serve to identify a severe neurodegenerative storage disorder (neuronal ceroid lipofuscinoses (NCL), neuroaxonal dystrophies). Selected examples are discussed below.

Mucopolysaccharidoses

MPS is a large heterogeneous group of inborn errors of glycosaminoglycan metabolism caused by excessive intralysosomal accumulation of different type-specific incomplete degradation products of normal glycosaminoglycans [1]. A series of enzymes is involved in the normal stepwise degradation. Lack of activity of these lysosomal enzymes results in gradual progressive accumulation within lysosomes which increasingly interfere with normal cell function. Most MPSs are autosomal recessive traits except for the X-linked recessive MPS II Hunter type [1]. PD can be done by biochemical testing of amniotic fluid and by S^{35} incorporation studies in cultured amniotic or chorionic villus cells [2,3]. PD by mutational analysis of the iduronate-2-sulphatase (IDS) gene in three fetuses at risk of MPS II Hunter (two affected) has been reported [4].

REFERENCES

1 Spranger J. The mucopolysaccharidoses. In: Emery AEH, Rimoin DL, eds. *The Principles and Practice of Medical Genetics*, 2nd edn. Edinburgh: Churchill Livingstone, 1990: 1797–806.
2 Liebaers I, DiNatale P, Neufeld EF. Iduronate sulphatase in amniotic fluid: an aid in the prenatal diagnosis of the Hunter syndrome. *J Pediatr* 1977; 90: 423–5.
3 Pannone N, Gatti R, Lombardo C, DiNatale P. Prenatal diagnosis of Hunter syndrome using chorionic villi. *Prenat Diagn* 1986; 6: 207–10.
4 Bunge S, Steglich C, Lorenz P, Beck M, Xu S, Hopwood JJ, Gal A. Prenatal diagnosis and carrier detection in mucopolysaccharidosis type II by mutation analysis. A 47, XXY male heterozygous for a missense point mutation. *Prenat Diagn* 1994; 14: 777–80.

Angiokeratoma corporis diffusum (Fabry's disease)

Fabry's disease is a lysosomal storage disorder due to an X-linked inborn error of glycosphingolipid catabolism, i.e. deficiency of α-galactosidase A and accumulation of ceramides in lysosomes of vascular endothelia. The skin, heart, kidneys and CNS are especially involved clinically. Diagnosis is possible by ultrastructural analysis of skin lesions and non-lesional skin of affected males and by enzyme activity measurements. Female carriers normally do not accumulate ceramides and therefore have either no skin lesions or only a few.

The α-galactosidase A gene is located on Xq22.1, and a series of mutations have been identified [1]. PD is already possibe by enzyme activity measurements of amniotic fluid samples or by EM of amniotic fluid cells. The identification of the mutation in a given family now permits carrier detection and DNA-based PD in early pregnancy [1].

REFERENCE

1 Eng CM, Desnick RJ. Molecular basis of Fabry disease: mutations and polymorphisms in the human alpha-galactosidase A gene. *Hum Mutat* 1994; 3: 103–11.

Neuronal ceroid lipofuscinosis

NCLs are heterogeneous autosomal recessive storage diseases with deposition of type-specific lipopigments of unknown enzymatic origin in various cell types of probably all organs, resulting in severe cortical atrophy due to loss of neurones, retinal atrophy, amaurosis and mostly early death [1,2]. Infantile (INCL), late-infantile (LINCL), juvenile (JNCL) and adult onset (ANCL) types have been identified. Their diagnosis is based on the ultrastructural demonstration of their specific granular (INCL), curvilinear (LINCL) or fingerprint profile (JNCL) inclusions in peripheral lymphocytes, skin or other organs; no biochemical criteria are available [2].

INCL has been mapped to chromosome 1p32 [3] with several closely flanking markers available at this site [4], JNCL has been mapped to chromosome 16p12 [5], while LINCL is non-allelic to both [6]. This obvious heterogeneity is underlined by the ultrastructural differences of the specific lipopigment deposits. The genes are termed CLN1, CLN2 and CLN3 [3,5,6].

PD is possible for all three childhood types of NCL by means of EM demonstration of specific lipopigment deposition in vascular cells of chorionic villi, in amniotic fluid cells and fetal skin, combined as far as possible (not for LINCL) with DNA-based haplotype analysis of flanking markers and polymorphisms [2,4,7–11].

REFERENCES

1 Percy AK. Gangliosidoses and related lipid storage diseases. In: Emery AEH, Rimoin DL, eds. *Principles and Practice of Medical Genetics*, 2nd edn. Edinburgh: Churchill Livingstone, 1990: 1827–56.
2 Goebel HH. Prenatal ultrastructural diagnosis in the neuronal ceroid-lipofuscinoses. *Path Res Pract* 1994; 190: 728–33.
3 Järvelä I, Schleutker J, Haataja L *et al*. Infantile form of neuronal ceroid lipofuscinosis (CLN1) maps to the short arm of chromosome 1. *Genomics* 1991; 9: 170–3.
4 Goebel HH, Vesa J, Reitter B, Goecke TO, Schneider-Rätzke B, Merz E. Prenatal diagnosis of infantile neuronal ceroid-lipofuscinosis: a combined electron microscopic and molecular genetic approach. *Brain Devel* 1995; 17: 83–8.
5 Mitchison H, Thompson AD, Mulley JC *et al*. Fine genetic mapping of the Batten disease locus (CLN3) by haplotype analysis and demonstration of allelic association with chromosome 16p microsatellite loci. *Genomics* 1993; 16: 455–60.
6 Williams R, Vesa J, Järvelä I *et al*. Genetic heterogeneity in neuronal ceroid-lipofuscinosis: evidence that the late-infantile subtype (Jansky–Bielschowsky disease, CLN2) is not an allelic form of the juvenile or infantile subtypes. *Am J Hum Genet* 1993; 53: 931–5.
7 MacLeod PM, Nag S, Berry C. Ultrastructural studies as a method of prenatal diagnosis of neuronal ceroid-lipofuscinosis. *Am J Med Genet* 1988; 5: 93–7.
8 Chow CW, Borg J, Billson VR, Lake BD. Fetal tissue involvement in the late infantile type of neuronal ceroid lipofuscinosis. *Prenat Diagn* 1993; 13: 833–41.
9 Lake BD. Morphological approaches to the prenatal diagnosis of late-infantile and juvenile Batten disease. *J Inher Metab Dis* 1993; 16: 345–8.
10 Conradi NG, Uvebrant P, Hökegård KH, Wahlstrom J, Mellqvist L. First-trimester diagnosis of juvenile neuronal ceroid-lipofuscinosis by demonstration of fingerprint inclusions in chorionic villi. *Prenat Diagn* 1989; 9: 283–7.
11 Kohlschütter A, Rauskolb R, Goebel HH, Anton-Lamprecht I, Albrecht R, Klein H. Probable exclusion of juvenile neuronal ceroidlipofuscinosis in a fetus at risk: an interim report. *Prenat Diagn* 1989; 9: 289–92.

Disorders that cannot be diagnosed at present from fetal tissues

In several genodermatoses, it is now clear that their specific abnormalities are not expressed early enough in fetal life to be tested by PD, or they appear later than previously assumed. Examples include ichthyosis congenita type I (see above) and three other genodermatoses with disturbed keratinization, as follows.

Chondrodysplasia punctata of the rhizomelic type

Although presenting with an ichthyosis at birth, this disease entity cannot be diagnosed from fetal skin as the keratinization disturbance is not expressed before week 24 in affected fetuses. PD is possible by control measurements of long bones [1].

Netherton's syndrome

This syndrome which is characterized by the triad of erythrodermic ichthyosiform scaling, trichorrhexis invaginata and atopy cannot be identified prenatally from fetal skin samples or fetal hair, according to the author's Heidelberg experience [2]. Skin and hair abnormalities are only expressed at or after delivery and are probably not present in the middle stages of pregnancy [3].

Restrictive dermopathy

Always a lethal disorder with recessive inheritance, this is another one of those genodermatoses that are not manifest before week 24 [4]. The dramatic pathological process starts only in the third trimester; before week 24, fetal skin development is completely normal and according to fetal age. The previous assumption of a primary arrest in the development of skin and appendages at about week 12–15, thought to be suitable as a criterion for PD [5], does not hold true [2].

Hereditary connective tissue disorders (HCTD)

HCTDs such as Ehlers–Danlos syndrome, cutis laxa, Marfan's syndrome or pseudoxanthoma elasticum [6], also cannot be identified or excluded prenatally from fetal skin samples in the second trimester, as the matrix constituents of the dermal connective tissue are either synthesized only after the 24th week (elastin), or differ specifically from postnatal skin in the fetus (collagen) (for details see [6–9]). As in many other groups of genodermatoses, the underlying mutations are increasingly being identified in HCTDs and may be used for PD in early pregnancy of at-risk fetuses.

REFERENCES

1 Arnold M-L, Anton-Lamprecht I. Problems in the prenatal diagnosis of the ichthyosis congenita group. *Hum Genet* 1985; 71: 301–11.
2 Anton-Lamprecht I. Prenatal diagnosis of genodermatoses. In: Dagna Bricarelli F, Casini Lemmi M, Storti G, eds. *La Diagnosi Fetale*. Suppl *Analysis* No. 7, 1992: 131–54.
3 Hausser I, Anton-Lamprecht I. Severe congenital generalized exfoliative erythroderma in newborns and infants: a possible sign of Netherton syndrome. *Pediatr Dermatol* 1996; 13: 183–99.
4 Happle R, Schuurmans-Stekhoven JH, Hamel BCJ *et al*. Restrictive dermopathy in two brothers. *Arch Dermatol* 1992; 128: 232–5.
5 Holbrook KA, Dale BA, Witt DR, Hayden MR, Toriello HV. Arrested epidermal morphogenesis in three newborn infants with a fatal genetic disorder (restrictive dermopathy). *J Invest Dermatol* 1987; 88: 330–9.
6 Royce PM, Steinmann B, eds. *Connective Tissue and its Heritable Disorders. Molecular, Genetic and Medical Aspects*. New York: Wiley-Liss, 1993.
7 Smith LTL, Holbrook KA, Byers PH. Structure of the dermal matrix during development and in the adult. *J Invest Dermatol* 1982; 79: 93S–104S.
8 Byers PH, Wenstrup RJ. Prenatal diagnosis of inherited connective tissue disorders. *Semin Dermatol* 1984; 3: 257–64.
9 Byers PH, Wenstrup RJ, Bonadio JE, Starman B, Cohn DH. Molecular basis of inherited disorders of collagen biosynthesis: implication for prenatal diagnosis. *Curr Probl Dermatol* 1987; 16: 158–74.

Conclusion

With advancing progress in the understanding and clarification of the basic abnormalities underlying genetic skin disorders at the DNA level, and with the increasing identification of specific mutations in individual patients and families, the focus of PD will be shifted increasingly towards early pregnancy. This will make it easier for the families to accept the considerable ethical problems related to the consequence of terminating a pregnancy. Therefore, detailed diagnosis with exact classification and subtyping by means of ultrastructural and immunohistochemical criteria, and mutational analysis should be attempted as a basis for genetic counselling and PD.

However, as long as DNA-based PD in early pregnancy is still restricted to some families, fetal skin biopsy offers a chance for PD to many families with severe genodermatoses.

19.26 DNA and Gene Analysis in Prenatal Diagnosis

JOHN A. McGRATH

Clinical relevance of molecular gene cloning

The human genome contains approximately 100 000 individual genes of which some 16 000 have already been identified through the Human Genome Project and other molecular cloning studies. Specific functions have been determined for several of these genes including a number involved in the pathogenesis of certain inherited skin disorders [1,2]. Recent identification of abnormalities in single genes in some genodermatoses has led to considerable medical and patient-related benefits. For example, advances in understanding the molecular basis of the inherited blistering skin disorder, dystrophic epidermolysis bullosa, have enhanced approaches to genetic counselling [2,3]. Clinically, it has often previously been difficult to determine whether a child with moderately severe blistering and scarring born to unaffected parents represents sporadic dominant or autosomal recessive disease [4]. However, recent molecular analyses have helped to provide genotype–phenotype information based on mutation detection in the type VII collagen gene (COL7A1 on 3p21.3). Specifically, the identification of pathogenetic glycine substitution mutations in dominant dystrophic epidermolysis bullosa or premature termination codons of translation in recessive disease has helped to clarify most diagnostic dilemmas [5]. Delineation of the molecular pathology in dystrophic epidermolysis bullosa and a number of other inherited skin disorders has also set the stage for the future development of newer forms of treatment, including gene therapy. Although considerable technical and practical obstacles will need to be overcome, genodermatoses characterized by nonsense or premature termination codon mutations on one or both mutant alleles might be suitable diseases for the design of gene replacement therapy, either as *in vivo* or *ex vivo* procedures. Likewise, autosomal dominant disorders, in which there is dominant-negative interference between the wild-type and the mutant protein, may be potential targets for antisense approaches designed to silence the mutant allele.

Development of DNA-based prenatal diagnostic testing

The immediate major benefit of the recent advances in unravelling the molecular basis of the genodermatoses has been in the development of DNA-based prenatal diagnosis in families at risk for recurrence of particular disorders. Established methods of prenatal diagnosis, such as fetoscopy and fetal skin biopsy, are gradually being superseded by gene analysis. A number of inherited skin disorders in which specific gene mutations have been identified and used as a basis for first-trimester DNA-based prenatal diagnosis have been documented and are shown in Table 19.26.1, and an example of DNA analysis for one of these conditions is illustrated in Fig. 19.26.1. To these disorders, several further conditions might be added in the near future based on recent disclosures of pathogenetic molecular events. These include epidermolysis bullosa associated with muscular dystrophy which results from mutations in the plectin gene (PLN on 8q24) [25,26], and junctional epidermolysis bullosa associated with pyloric atresia which is caused by mutations in the genes encoding the α6β4-integrin (ITGA6 and ITGB4, on 2q and 17q11-qter, respectively) [19,20]. Other inherited skin disorders suitable for DNA-based prenatal testing include Sjögren–Larsson syndrome (fatty aldehyde dehydrogenase gene, FALDH, on 17p11) [27], Wiskott–Aldrich syndrome (WASP gene on Xp11.23–p11.22) [28], Chediak–Higashi syndrome (LYST gene on 1q42) [29], pachyonychia congenita (keratins 16 or 17 genes on 17q21–22) [30,31] and Fabry's disease (angiokeratoderma corporis diffusum, α-galactosidase A gene on Xq22.1) [32].

Table 19.26.1 DNA-based prenatal diagnosis by mutation analysis

Genodermatosis	Gene	Gene locus	References
Junctional epidermolysis bullosa* (Herlitz subtype)	Laminin 5 α3 chain (LAMA3)	18q11.2	[6,7]
	Laminin 5 β3 chain (LAMB3)	1q32	[7,8]
	Laminin 5 γ2 chain (LAMC2)	1q25–31	[7]
Dystrophic epidermolysis bullosa (recessive)†	Type VII collagen (COL7A1)	3p21.3	[9–11]
Epidermolysis bullosa simplex (Dowling–Meara)‡	Keratin 14 (KRT14)	17q21–22	[12]
Bullous congenital ichthyosiform erythroderma§	Keratin 10 (KRT10)	17q21–22	[13]
Oculocutaneous albinism (tyrosinase-negative, OCA1A)	Tyrosinase (TYR)	11q14–21	[14,15]
Lamellar ichthyosis**	Transglutaminase 1 (TGM1)	14q11	[16,17]
Mucopolysaccharidosis (Hunter, type II)	Iduronate-2-sulphatase (IDS)	Xq27.3–q28	[18]

*Junctional epidermolysis bullosa is a heterogeneous condition. Other subtypes of this disorder may result from mutations in the genes encoding α6β4 integrin (ITGA6, ITGB4 on 2q and 17q11-qter, respectively) or type XVII collagen (COL17A1/BPAG2 on 10q24.3) [19–21].
† Autosomal dominant forms of dystrophic epidermolysis bullosa also result from mutations in the type VII collagen gene (COL7A1 on 3p21.3) [5,22].
‡ Some cases of epidermolysis bullosa simplex are caused by mutations in the keratin 5 gene on 12q11–q13 [23].
§ Some cases of bullous congenital ichthyosiform erythroderma arise because of mutations in the gene encoding keratin 1 on 12q11–q13 [24].
** Some cases of lamellar ichthyosis show linkage to a different locus on 2q33–35 [17].

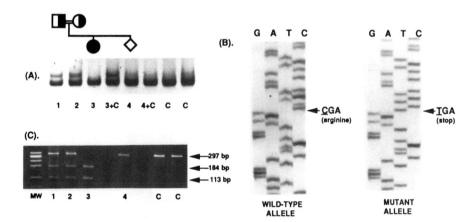

Fig. 19.26.1 Prenatal exclusion of junctional epidermolysis bullosa by *LAMA3* (GenBank no. L34155) mutation analysis. (A) Heteroduplex analysis of polymerase chain reaction (PCR) products spanning part of the *LAMA3* gene reveals heteroduplex and homoduplex bandshifts (two bands) in the paternal and maternal DNA (lanes 1 and 2), but only a homoduplex bandshift (single lower band) in the affected child (lane 3). However, when the affected child's amplified DNA is mixed with control DNA, a separate heteroduplex bandshift is seen (lane 3+C). Only a single homoduplex band is noted in the fetal DNA (lane 4), even with the addition of control DNA (lane 4+C). (B) Nucleotide sequencing of the affected child's DNA reveals a C-to-T transition that converts an arginine residue (CGA) to a stop codon (TGA). (C) Verification of the mutation by *Dde* I restriction endonuclease digestion. The mutation results in a new cut site for *Dde* I. The previously affected child is homozygous for a new restriction site, whilst the parents are heterozygous for the mutation. In contrast, the fetal DNA is not digested and is identical to the control DNA with no evidence for a novel *Dde* I site. This indicates that the fetus is genotypically normal with respect to this *LAMA3* mutation and is predicted to be unaffected with junctional epidermolysis bullosa. Redrawn from [5] with permission.

Prenatal diagnosis in heterogeneous genodermatoses

Further conditions such as lamellar ichthyosis are also suitable for DNA-based prenatal testing [16,17], but this disorder shows molecular heterogeneity and therefore keratinocyte transglutaminase abnormalities should first be identified in the proband before any prenatal test analysing keratinocyte transglutaminase gene (*TGM1* on 14q11) pathology is pursued [33,34]. Similar comments apply to X-linked hypohidrotic ectodermal dysplasia. Although pathogenetic mutations have been identified in the EDA protein gene (on Xq12.2–q13.1) in several affected individuals [35], the disorder is heterogeneous at a molecular level and a number of other candidate genes for disease-associated mutations are likely to exist. Certain other inherited disorders can be tested for prenatally by examination of fetal DNA, although not necessarily involving gene analysis. Prenatal diagnosis has been performed for xeroderma pigmentosum and related disorders which are caused by nucleotide excision repair defects. Approaches to diagnosis have usually been based on analysis of unscheduled DNA synthesis [36], although tests have often taken several weeks to conclude. Recently, more rapid testing for some forms of xeroderma pigmentosum and trichothiodystrophy have been developed using single cell gel electrophoresis assays, enabling prenatal diagnostic testing to be completed within 1–2 days [37].

Preimplantation genetic diagnosis for inherited skin disorders

Knowledge of precise molecular defects in particular inherited skin disorders also enables prenatal testing to be done at a much earlier stage using preimplantation genetic diagnosis. This approach involves *in vitro* fertilization and sampling of a single cell at the eight cell stage of embryonic development [38,39]. Nested polymerase chain reactions on DNA extracted from the single embryonic cell can be designed to test for the presence or absence of the pathogenetic mutation(s) or alternatively for X-linked disorders (for example, incontinentia pigmenti, gene locus Xq28), fluorescent *in situ* hybridization chromosome markers can be used to identify karyotypes [39]. Genotypically selected embryos can then be used for transfer and implantation. Although the first successful application of preimplantation genetic diagnosis was reported for cystic fibrosis in 1992 (cystic fibrosis transmembrane conductance regulator gene on 7q31.2) [40], prenatal testing using this technique has not yet been reported for any of the inherited skin disorders. Nevertheless, unlike chorionic villus sampling at 10–11 weeks gestation, the preimplantation approach obviates the need for possible termination of pregnancy of an affected fetus and may be more acceptable to many couples at risk for further affected children.

Ethical issues in prenatal testing for genetic skin disease

The development of DNA-based prenatal testing for genodermatoses raises several important ethical issues. For example, until recently in epidermolysis bullosa only the severe forms of the disease could be tested for prenatally using fetal skin biopsy and analysis of the skin samples by immunohistochemistry and electron microscopy [41]. Now, not only is it possible to test for the Herlitz (lethal) subtype of junctional epidermolysis bullosa and the mutilating Hallopeau–Siemens form of recessive dystrophic epidermolysis bullosa using DNA analysis [7,10], but several of the milder subtypes such as autosomal dominant or localized recessive dystrophic epidermolysis bullosa (type VII collagen gene, *COL7A1* on 3p21.3) or generalized atrophic benign epidermolysis bullosa (type XVII collagen gene, *COL17A1* on 10q24.3) can now also be assessed by gene analysis. Clearly, given the rapid accumulation of new genetic information the clinical indications for undertaking prenatal diagnosis need to be carefully considered and precisely defined [7,10].

Practical aspects of DNA-based prenatal diagnosis

The feasibility of DNA-based prenatal testing has had substantial benefits for families at risk for recurrence of further affected children with inherited skin disorders in subsequent pregnancies. Compared to fetal skin biopsy sampling, the tests can be done at a much earlier gestation (10–11 weeks) and there is usually no need to travel to specialist centres: many obstetricians are experienced in chorionic villus sampling and the specimens can then be sent to the DNA laboratory. It should be emphasized that careful cleaning of the chorionic villi is necessary to remove maternal decidua and thereby avoid potential contamination of the fetal sample from the mother's DNA. In addition, samples for the laboratory should not be sent in any heparin-containing medium as this will inhibit subsequent polymerase chain reactions used for the mutational analysis. A transport medium such as RPMI (Roswell Park Memorial Institute medium) is suitable, or samples can be shipped directly in a proteinase K buffer after cleaning of the villi. An important prerequisite to undertaking any DNA-based prenatal test procedure is the delineation of informative genetic markers. In most instances it is important to have DNA samples from both parents and the affected individual to determine the pathogenetic mutations [7,10]. Other considerations such as the occurrence of *de novo* mutations, non-paternity, uniparental disomy and germ-line mosaicism can then all be addressed more fully and the suitability of the prenatal diagnosis can be determined. In most inherited skin disorders it is important to base the test on mutational analysis, but for some disorders, such as dystrophic epidermolysis bullosa, indirect linkage analysis using intragenic and flanking type VII collagen gene markers may be appropriate [9,42]. It is also important to stress that in most instances, molecular markers are family-specific and are best determined before pregnancy is contemplated as it may take several weeks or months to complete the DNA screening analysis. Several condition-specific guidelines for prenatal testing in inherited skin disorders have been published [7,10], and will form a useful basis for planning prenatal testing in other genodermatoses as the molecular basis for these disorders is elucidated and DNA-based prenatal diagnosis becomes feasible.

REFERENCES

1 Uitto J, Pulkkinen L, McLean WHI. Epidermolysis bullosa: a spectrum of clinical phenotypes explained by molecular heterogeneity. *Mol Med Today* 1997; 3: 457–65.

2 Korge BP, Krieg T. The molecular basis for inherited bullous diseases. *J Mol Med* 1996; 74: 59–70.

3 Kon A, McGrath JA, Pulkkinen L et al. Glycine substitution mutations in the type VII collagen gene (COL7A1) in dystrophic epidermolysis bullosa: implications for genetic counseling. *J Invest Dermatol* 1997; 108: 224–8.

4 Fine J-D, Bauer E, Briggaman R et al. Revised clinical and laboratory criteria for subtype of epidermolysis bullosa: a consensus report by the subcommittee on diagnosis and classification of the National Epidermolysis Bullosa Registry. *J Am Acad Dermatol* 1991; 24: 119–35.

5 Christiano AM, Uitto J. Molecular diagnosis of inherited skin disease: the paradigm of dystrophic epidermolysis bullosa. *Adv Dermatol* 1996; 11: 199–213.

6 McGrath JA, Kivirikko S, Ciatti S et al. A homozygous nonsense mutation in the α3 chain gene of laminin 5 (LAMA3) in Herlitz junctional epidermolysis bullosa: prenatal exclusion in a fetus at risk. *Genomics* 1995; 29: 282–4.

7 Christiano AM, Pulkkinen L, McGrath JA, Uitto J. Mutation based prenatal diagnosis of Herlitz junctional epidermolysis bullosa. *Prenat Diagn* 1997; 17: 343–54.

8 Vailly J, Pulkkinen L, Miquel C et al. Identification of a homozygous one-base pair deletion in exon 14 of the LAMB3 gene in a patient with Herlitz junctional epidermolysis bullosa and prenatal diagnosis in a family at risk for recurrence. *J Invest Dermatol* 1995; 104: 462–6.

9 Hovnanian A, Hilal L, Blanchet-Bardon C et al. DNA-based prenatal diagnosis of generalized recessive dystrophic epidermolysis bullosa in six pregnancies at risk for recurrence. *J Invest Dermatol* 1995; 104: 456–61.

10 Christiano AM, LaForgia S, Paller AS, McGuire J, Shimizu H, Uitto J. Prenatal diagnosis for recessive dystrophic epidermolysis bullosa in 10 families by mutation and haplotype analysis in the type VII collagen gene (COL7A1). *Molec Med* 1996; 2: 59–76.

11 McGrath JA, Dunnill MG, Christiano AM et al. First trimester DNA-based exclusion of recessive dystrophic epidermolysis bullosa from chorionic villus sampling. *Br J Dermatol* 1996; 134: 734–9.

12 Rugg EL, Shemanko CS, Magee GJ, Batty D, Boxer M, Lane EB. Taking epidermolysis bullosa simplex from mutation analysis to prenatal diagnosis. *J Invest Dermatol* 1997; 108: 597 (abstract).

13 Rothnagel JA, Longley NA, Holder RA, Kuster W, Roop DR. Prenatal diagnosis of epidermolytic hyperkeratosis by direct gene sequencing. *J Invest Dermatol* 1994; 102: 13–16.

14 Shimizu H, Niizeki H, Suzumori K et al. Prenatal diagnosis of oculocutaneous albinism by analysis of the fetal tyrosinase gene. *J Invest Dermatol* 1994; 103: 104–6.

15 Falik-Borenstein TC, Holmes SA, Borochowitz Z, Levin A, Rosenmann A, Spritz RA. DNA-based carrier detection and prenatal diagnosis of tyrosinase-negative oculocutaneous albinism (OCA1A). *Prenat Diagn* 1995; 15: 345–9.

16 Schorderet DF, Huber M, Laurini RN et al. Prenatal diagnosis of lamellar ichthyosis by direct mutational analysis of the keratinocyte transglutaminase gene. *Prenat Diagn* 1997; 17: 483–6.

17 Bichakjian CK, Nair RP, Wu WW, Goldberg S, Elder JT. Prenatal exclusion of lamellar ichthyosis based on identification of two new mutations in the transglutaminase 1 gene. *J Invest Dermatol* 1998; 110: 179–82.

18 Bunge S, Steglich C, Lorenz P et al. Prenatal diagnosis and carrier detection in mucopolysaccharidosis type II by mutation analysis. A 47, XXY male heterozygous for a missense point mutation. *Prenat Diagn* 1994; 14: 777–80.

19 Pulkkinen L, Kimonis VE, Xu Y, Spanou EN, McLean WHI, Uitto J. Homozygous α6 integrin mutation in junctional epidermolysis bullosa with congenital duodenal atresia. *Hum Mol Genet* 1997; 6: 669–74.

20 Vidal F, Aberdam D, Miquel C et al. Integrin β4 mutations associated with junctional epidermolysis bullosa with pyloric atresia. *Nature Genet* 1995; 10: 229–34.

21 Gatalica B, Pulkkinen L, Li K, Christiano AM, McGrath JA, Uitto J. Cloning of the type XVII collagen gene (COL17A1), and detection of novel mutations in generalized atrophic benign epidermolysis bullosa. *Am J Hum Genet* 1997; 60: 352–65.

22 Christiano AM, Ryynanen M, Uitto J. Dominant dystrophic epidermolysis bullosa: identification of a Gly–Ser substitution in the triple-helical domain of type VII collagen. *Proc Natl Acad Sci USA* 1994; 91: 3549–53.

23 Lane EB, Rugg EL, Navsaria H et al. A mutation in the conserved helix termination peptide of keratin 5 in hereditary skin blistering. *Nature* 1992; 356: 244–6.

24 Syder AJ, Yu QC, Paller AS, Giudice G, Pearson R, Fuchs E. Genetic mutations in the K1 and K10 genes of patients with epidermolytic hyperkeratosis. Correlation between location and disease severity. *J Clin Invest* 1994; 93: 1533–42.

25 McLean WHI, Pulkkinen L, Smith FJD et al. Loss of plectin (HD1) causes epidermolysis bullosa with muscular dystrophy: cDNA cloning and genomic organisation. *Genes Dev* 1996; 10: 1724–35.

26 Smith FJD, Eady RAJ, Leigh IM et al. Plectin deficiency results in muscular dystrophy with epidermolysis bullosa. *Nature Genet* 1996; 13: 450–6.

27 De Laurenzi V, Rogers GR, Hamrock DJ et al. Sjögren–Larsson syndrome is caused by mutations in the fatty aldehyde dehydrogenase gene. *Nature Genet* 1996; 12: 52–7.

28 Schwartz M, Bekassy A, Donner M et al. Mutation spectrum in patients with Wiskott–Aldrich syndrome and X-linked thrombocytopenia: identification of 12 different mutations in the WASP gene. *Thromb Haemost* 1996; 75: 546–50.

29 Nagle DL, Karim MA, Woolf EA et al. Identification and mutation analysis of the complete gene for Chediak–Higashi syndrome. *Nature Genet* 1996; 14: 307–11.

30 McLean WHI, Rugg EL, Lunny DP et al. Keratin 16 and keratin 17 mutations cause pachyonychia congenita. *Nature Genet* 1995; 9: 273–8.

31 Smith FJ, Corden LD, Rugg EL et al. Missense mutations in keratin 17 cause either pachyonychia congenita type 2 or a phenotype resembling steatocystoma multiplex. *J Invest Dermatol* 1997; 108: 220–3.

32 Eng CM, Desnick RJ. Molecular basis of Fabry disease: mutations and polymorphisms in the human alpha-galactosidase A gene. *Hum Mutat* 1994; 3: 103–11.

33 Huber M, Rettler I, Bernasconi K et al. Mutations of keratinocyte transglutaminase in lamellar ichthyosis. *Science* 1995; 267: 525–8.

34 Russell LJ, Di Giovanna JJ, Rogers GR et al. Mutations in the gene for transglutaminase I in autosomal recessive lamellar ichthyosis. *Nature Genet* 1995; 9: 279–83.

35 Kere J, Srivastava AK, Montonen O et al. X-linked anhidrotic (hypohidrotic) ectodermal dysplasia is caused by mutations in a novel transmembrane protein. *Nature Genet* 1996; 13: 409–16.

36 Savary JB, Vasseur F, Deminatti MM. Routine autoradiographic analysis of DNA excision-repair. Report of prenatal and postnatal diagnosis in 11 families. *Ann Genet* 1991; 34: 76–81.

37 Alapetite C, Benoit A, Moustacchi E, Sarasin A. The comet assay as a repair test for prenatal diagnosis of xeroderma pigmentosum and trichothiodystrophy. *J Invest Dermatol* 1997; 108: 154–9.

38 Handyside AH. Preimplantation genetic diagnosis today. *Hum Reprod* 1996; 11 (suppl. 1): 139–51.

39 McGrath JA, Handyside AH. Preimplantation genetic diagnosis of severe inherited skin diseases. *Exp Dermatol* 1998; 7: 65–72.

40 Handyside AH, Lesko JG, Tarin JJ, Winston RM, Hughes MR. Birth of a normal girl after *in vitro* fertilization and preimplantation genetic testing for cystic fibrosis. *N Engl J Med* 1992; 327: 905–9.

41 Eady RAJ, Holbrook KA, Blanchet-Bardon C *et al.* Prenatal diagnosis of skin diseases. In: Burgdorf WHC, Katz SI, eds. *Dermatology: Progress and Perspectives. Proceedings of the 18th World Congress of Dermatology.* Carnforth, Lancashire: Pantheon Publishing, 1993: 1159–65.

42 Dunnill MG, Richards AJ, Milana G, Mollica F, Eady RA, Pope FM. Use of type VII collagen gene (COL7A1) markers in prenatal diagnosis of recessive dystrophic epidermolysis bullosa. *J Med Genet* 1995; 32: 749–50.

Section 20
Disorders of Fat Tissue

20.1 Disorders of Fat Tissue

MARC LACOUR

Lipomas and variants
'Solitary' lipoma
Lipoblastoma and lipoblastomatosis
Angiolipomas and others
Hibernoma

Lipomatoses
Encephalocraniocutaneous lipomatosis
Familial multiple lipomatosis
Other syndromes associated with cutaneous lipomatosis

Lipodystrophies
Fat hypertrophy
Fat atrophy

This chapter has been designed to include mainly non-inflammatory disorders of fat tissue. The reader interested in other disorders of fat, such as panniculitis, sclerema neonatorum, fat necrosis, and so on, will be referred to other chapters.

Lipomas and variants

'Solitary' lipoma

Definition

Solitary lipomas are benign tumours of mature adipocytes with a ubiquitous localization. Classically they are well circumscribed and develop slowly.

Aetiology

Lipomas are common connective tissue tumours, representing 25–50% of all soft tissue masses [1] and 80% of all lipomatous tumours [2]. They occur rarely in the first two decades of life and most often appear between 30 and 60 years. There is no ethnic predisposition. The pathogenesis of subcutaneous lipomas remains obscure except in a few situations: post trauma [3,4]; diabetes and obesity; and a genetic predisposition (familial multiple lipomatosis). Similarly the origin of visceral lipomas remains obscure in most cases except for the development of epidural lipomatosis following prolonged corticosteroid treatment [5,6].

Probably the most interesting finding in recent years is the extremely high incidence of chromosomal abnormalities in lipomatous tumours [7]. Of 93 subcutaneous and intramuscular lipomas 80% were shown to harbour specific karyotypic aberrations affecting mainly 12q, 6p and 13q. Other distinct karyotypic abnormalities were found in other types of lipomatous tumours. If such a specificity is confirmed, karyotype analysis of lipoma and related tumours may become a valuable diagnostic and prognostic tool.

Histopathology

Lipomas are usually composed of univacuolated mature adipocytes, the nucleus of which is compressed in the cellular periphery. These features are indistinguishable from adult adipose tissue. Tumours are encapsulated by fibrous tissue and may be uni- or multilobulated. Adipocytes and lobules are thinly divided by a rich vasculature. Degenerative features within the tumour are frequent, and so are foci of fibrous tissue, such as in cervical fibrolipoma [8]. Histological variants are discussed below.

Clinical features

Two main groups of lipoma can be defined according to their localization: superficial or cutaneous lipomas which will be reviewed here, and deeply located lipomas. The latter can arise in any visceral localization such as the anterior mediastin, bones, brain, retroperitoneal area and periarticular regions.

Superficial lipomas appear as a painless subcutaneous mass which develops slowly, reaching a size up to 20 cm. Typically, the tumour is soft and freely mobile and the overlying skin remains perfectly normal. Most lipomas are found (in descending order of frequency) on the neck, scapular regions, back, abdomen, buttocks and upper thighs. More rarely they can occupy the scalp, face or extremities.

Individuals may develop one or multiple lesions. Giant lipoma can occur in children [9] but are more common in adulthood, reaching between 4.5 and as much as 58.5 kg [10].

1397

Congenital lumbosacral lipomas can be a marker of occult spinal dysraphism [11]. In a series of 200 patients with spinal dysraphism, 41 had subcutaneous lipomas in the lumbosacral region, and intracanal extension of the lipoma was seen in all of them [12]. Similarly 75% of 73 patients with intraspinal lipomas were found to have a subcutaneous lipoma [13]. Lipomas can also reveal other types of spinal abnormalities such as filum terminale with tethered conus, and hydrosyringomyelia [14]. Lumbosacral lipomas have specific histological features including lack of capsule, large amounts of fibrous tissue and a variety of ectopic neuroectodermal and mesodermal tissue. This association should be suspected in even minute bulging over the lower spine in a neonate [15]. Rarely, the lipoma may not develop before puberty [16]. Treatment is surgical after a careful neurological assessment and magnetic resonance imaging (MRI) scan [17].

Diagnosis

Clinical findings are usually sufficient to give a diagnosis of subcutaneous lipoma. In difficult cases in children, Doppler-coupled ultrasonography (exclusion of vascular tumour) and MRI scan (presence of fat) will confirm the diagnosis [18]. When presented with a child with an unusual lipoma (localization, number, shape, size) one should be cautious to exclude associated syndromes (see below).

The differential diagnosis of a subcutaneous soft tissue mass appearing in childhood or adolescence, is quite large (see Chapter 13.1).

Treatment

Most lipomas found in children are small, slow growing and of little cosmetic significance. They can be left alone. If necessary, surgical excision with minimal incision on the skin or liposuction are both effective, provided that a skilled hand carefully removes all the tumoral tissue to avoid recurrence [19–24].

REFERENCES

1 Rydholm A, Berg NO. Size, site and clinical incidence of lipoma. *Acta Orthop Scand* 1983; 54: 929–34.
2 Enzinger FM, Weiss SW. *Soft Tissue Tumors.* St Louis: CV Mosby, 1983.
3 Penoff JH. Traumatic lipomas–pseudolipomas. *J Traumatol* 1982; 22: 63–5.
4 Meggit BF. The battered buttock syndrome. A report of a group of traumatic lipoma. *Br J Surg* 1972; 59: 165–9.
5 Crayton HE, Partington CR, Bell CL. Spinal cord compression by epidural lipomatosis in a patient with systemic lupus erythematosus. *Arthritis Rheum* 1992; 35: 482–4.
6 Arroyo IL, Barron KS, Brewer EJ Jr. Spinal cord compression by epidural lipomatosis in juvenile rheumatoid arthritis. *Arthritis Rheum* 1988; 31: 447–51.
7 Fletcher CDM, Akerman M, Dal Cin P *et al.* Correlation between clinico-pathological features and karyotype in lipomatous tumors. *Am J Pathol* 1996; 148: 623–30.
8 Abensour M, Jeandel C, Heid E. Lipomes et lipomatoses cutanés. *Ann Dermatol Vénéréol* 1987; 114: 873–82.
9 N'Diaye B, Guiraud M, Kane A *et al.* Naevus lipomateux tumoral. A propos d'un cas. *Ann Dermatol Vénéréol* 1984; 111: 737–8.
10 Sanchez MR, Golomb FM, Moy JA *et al.* Giant lipoma: case report and review of the literature. *J Am Acad Dermatol* 1993; 28: 266–8.
11 Serna MJ, Vazquez Doval J, Vanaclocha V *et al.* Occult spinal dysraphism: a neurosurgical problem with a dermatologic hallmark. *Pediatr Dermatol* 1993; 10: 149–52.
12 Tavafoghi V, Ghandchi A, Hambrick GW Jr *et al.* Cutaneous signs of spinal dysraphism. *Arch Dermatol* 1978; 114: 573–7.
13 Pierre-Kahn JW, Lacombe J, Pichon J *et al.* Intraspinal lipomas with spina bifida. Prognosis and treatment in 73 cases. *J Neurosurg* 1986; 65: 756–61.
14 Davis DA, Cohen PR, George RE. Cutaneous stigmata of occult spinal dysraphism. *J Am Acad Dermatol* 1994; 31: 892–6.
15 Bodemer C, Durand C, Brunel F *et al.* Lipome sous-cutané révélateur d'un lipome intradural. *Ann Dermatol Vénéréol* 1988; 115: 1130–2.
16 Ryan TJ, Curri SB. Hypertrophy and atrophy of fat. *Clin Dermatol* 1989; 7: 93–106.
17 Hakuba A, Fujitani K, Hoda K *et al.* Lumbosacral lipoma, the timing of the operation and morphological classification. *Neuroorthopedics* 1986; 2: 34–42.
18 Boothroyd AE, Carty H. The painless soft tissue mass in childhood—tumour or not? *Postgrad Med J* 1995; 71: 10–16.
19 Kenawi MM. 'Squeeze delivery' excision of subcutaneous lipoma related to anatomic site. *Br J Surg* 1995; 82: 1649–50.
20 Monfrecola G, Riccio G, Viola L *et al.* A simple cryo-technique for the treatment of cutaneous soft fibromas. *J Dermatol Surg Oncol* 1994; 20: 151–2.
21 Sharma PK, Janniger CK, Schwartz RA *et al.* The treatment of atypical lipoma with liposuction. *J Dermatol Surg Oncol* 1991; 17: 332–4.
22 Apesos J, Chami R. Functional applications of suction-assisted lipectomy: a new treatment for old disorders. *Aesthetic Plast Surg* 1991; 15: 73–9.
23 Pinski KS, Roenigk HH Jr. Liposuction of lipomas. *Dermatol Clin* 1990 8:483–92.
24 Spinowitz AL. The treatment of multiple lipomas by liposuction surgery. *J Dermatol Surg Oncol* 1989; 15: 538–40.

Lipoblastoma and lipoblastomatosis

Definition

Lipoblastomas are rare benign tumours of adipocytes and their mesenchymal precursor cells that occur almost exclusively in early childhood. The term lipoblastoma is reserved for the common type in which the tumour is well encapsulated. Lipoblastomatosis represents the diffuse infiltrating variety which is more difficult to resect completely [1–4].

Aetiology

This is unknown. These lesions probably represent persistence or reactivation of fetal fat proliferation in the postnatal period. Tumoral transformation is likely since in three cases where chromosomal analysis was performed, a rearrangement 8q was found [5].

Histology

A lipoblastoma consists of mature adipocytes, lipoblasts and prelipoblasts arranged in a lobulated pattern and separated by loose fibrous connective tissue, thus recapitulating developing fat. Peripherally, spindle-shaped tumour cells (precursors) can be found in increased numbers.

Clinical features

About 100 cases have been reported with a male to female ratio of 3 : 1. Almost all cases presented before the age of 3 years. Predominantly involved sites are the limbs or back. Typically, lipoblastoma consists of a rapidly enlarging subcutaneous tumour, usually soft and painless. As opposed to common lipomas, which are extremely rare in this age group, the tumour rapidly becomes less mobile and so large that it interferes with local structures. Despite the infiltrating nature of the lipoblastomatosis form, malignant transformation of the disorder has never been reported. Local regrowth can occur after surgery, usually within the first postoperative year. Finally, mediastinal forms can occur [6].

Diagnosis and treatment

A clinical diagnosis of lipoma is insufficient in this age group and all subcutaneous masses must be investigated. MRI has the advantage of confirming a mass of adipose tissue and delineating the extent of the infiltrating forms, thus avoiding other unnecessary 'invasive' investigations [7]. Conservative excision should be carefully planned in order to remove the lesion *in toto*, therefore avoiding recurrence.

REFERENCES

1 Chung EB, Enzinger FM. Benign lipoblastomas: an analysis of 35 cases. *Cancer* 1973; 32: 482–92.
2 Federici S, Cuoghi D, Sciutti R. Benign mediastinal lipoblastoma in a 14-month-old infant. *Pediatr Radiol* 1992; 22: 150–1.
3 Jimenez JF. Lipoblastoma in infancy and childhood. *J Surg Oncol* 1986; 32: 238–44.
4 Stringel G, Shandling B, Mancer K *et al.* Lipoblastoma in infants and children. *J Pediatr Surg* 1982; 17: 277–80.
5 Fletcher CDM, Akerman M, Dal Cin P *et al.* Correlation between clinico-pathological features and karyotype in lipomatous tumors. *Am J Pathol* 1996; 148: 623–30.
6 Whyte AM, Powell N. Case report: mediastinal lipoblastoma in infancy. *Clin Radiol* 1990; 42: 205–6.
7 Norton KI, Glajchen N, Dolgin SE. Magnetic resonance appearance in a case of lipoblastomatosis. *Pediatr Surg Int* 1996; 11: 286–7.

Angiolipomas [1,2], chondroid lipomas [3], adenolipomas [4], spindle cell lipomas [5,6], pleiomorphic lipomas [7,8] and liposarcomas [9,10]

These can occur in children, but mostly arise in adulthood. Angiomyolipoma is a rare benign vascular tumour almost exclusively found in the kidneys and often in association with tuberous sclerosis. Skin angiomyolipomas have also been described [11,12]. Cytogenetic analysis shows that most of these tumours harbour specific karyotypic abnormalities [13].

REFERENCES

1 Belcher RW, Czarnetzki BM, Carnery JF *et al.* Multiple (subcutaneous) angiolipomas. *Arch Dermatol* 1974; 110: 583–5.
2 Shea CR, Prieto VG. Mast cells in angiolipomas and hemangiomas of human skin: are they important for angiogenesis? *J Cutan Pathol* 1994; 21: 247–51.
3 Nielsen GP, O'Connell JX, Dickersin GR *et al.* Chondroid lipoma, a tumor of white fat cells. *Am J Surg Pathol* 1995; 19: 1272–6.
4 Hitchcock MG, Hurt MA, Santa Cruz DJ. Adenolipoma of the skin: a report of nine cases. *J Am Acad Dermatol* 1993; 29: 82–5.
5 Eckert F, Landthaler M, Braun Falco O. Spindle cell lipoma. *Hautarzt* 1989; 40: 161–3.
6 Mehregan DR, Mehregan DA, Mehregan AH *et al.* Spindle cell lipomas. *Dermatol Surg* 1995; 21: 796–8.
7 Nigro MA, Chieregato GC, Querci della Rovere G. Pleomorphic lipoma of the dermis. *Br J Dermatol* 1987; 116: 713–17.
8 Shitabata PK, Ritter JH, Fitzgibbon JF *et al.* Pleomorphic hamartoma of the subcutis: a lesion with possible myogenous and neural lineages. *J Cutan Pathol* 1995; 22: 269–75.
9 Enzinger FM, Winslow DJ. Liposarcoma. A study of 103 cases. *Virchows Arch Pathol Anat* 1962; 335: 367–88.
10 Mrozek K, Karakousis CP, Bloomfield CD. Chromosome 12 breakpoints are cytogenetically different in benign and malignant lipogenic tumors: localization of breakpoints in lipoma to 12q15 and in myxoid liposarcoma to 12q13. *Cancer Res* 1993;53: 1670–5.
11 Mehregan DA, Mehregan DR, Mehregan AH. Angiomyolipoma. *J Am Acad Dermatol* 1992; 27: 331–3.
12 Rodriguez Fernandez A, Caro Mancilla A. Cutaneous angiomyolipoma with pleomorphic changes. *J Am Acad Dermatol* 1993; 29: 115–16.
13 Fletcher CDM, Akerman M, Dal Cin P *et al.* Correlation between clinico-pathological features and karyotype in lipomatous tumors. *Am J Pathol* 1996; 148: 623–30.

Hibernoma

(SYN: FETAL LIPOMA, EMBRYONARY FAT LIPOMA, GRANULAR CELL LIPOMA)

Definition

The term hibernoma was proposed in 1914 by Gery [1] to describe tumours derived from brown fat or embryonary fat.

Aetiology

Brown fat is a specialized form of adipose tissue which is prominent in hibernating animals. In these animals, brown fat mostly consists of two symmetrical masses on either side of the midline between the scapulae, and is thought to serve as a heat-producing tissue. Pathologically, hibernomas are tumours of brown fat. Karyotypic abnormalities (on 11q) have been reported [2].

Histopathology

The tumour is usually well encapsulated, being yellow–brown to red in colour. This brown–tan is due to increased vascularization which also causes the tumour to be warm. The tumour mass consists of round cells with a multivacuolated or granular cytoplasm and central nuclei.

Clinical features

Hibernomas are well-defined mobile, rather hard, painless and often warm subcutaneous nodules of 5–10 cm in diameter. Their elective localization is between the scapulae, but they can occur in the head and neck [3–5], thigh [6] or, rarely, mediastinal region. In a series of 67 patients, median age at diagnosis was 33 years with a female predominance [7]. Hibernomas reported in children are few. The youngest patient was 6 weeks old [8]. Another child's lesion was unusually superficial [9].

The tumour is unlikely to be clinically diagnosed as it often presents as a benign lipoma. Thus, diagnosis has been histological in most reports. Treatment is surgical. Complications from local compression of the surrounding structures can occur. Malignant transformation has been reported only once.

REFERENCES

1 Gery L. Discussion. *Bull Mem Soc Anat Paris* 1914; 89: 110–11.
2 Fletcher CDM, Akerman M, Dal Cin P *et al*. Correlation between clinicopathological features and karyotype in lipomatous tumors. *Am J Pathol* 1996; 148: 623–30.
3 Wilhelm KP, Eisenbeiss W, Wolff HH. Hibernoma of the forehead. *Hautarzt* 1993; 44: 735–7.
4 Abemayor E, McClean P, Cobb CJ *et al*. Hibernomas of the head and neck. *Head Neck Surg* 1987; 9: 362–7.
5 Muszynski CA, Robertson DP, Goodman JC *et al*. Scalp hibernoma: case report and literature review. *Surg Neurol* 1994; 42: 343–5.
6 Merlino AF, Pike RF. Hibernoma of the thigh. A case report. *J Bone Joint Surg* 1973; 55: 406–8.
7 McLane RC, Meyer LC. Axillary hibernoma: review of the literature with report of a case examined angiographically. *Radiology* 1978; 127: 673–4.
8 Cox RW. 'Hibernoma': the lipoma of immature adipose tissue. *J Pathol Bact* 1954; 68: 511–24.
9 Bonifazi E, Meneghini CL. A case of hibernoma in a child. *Dermatologica* 1982; 165: 647–52.

Lipomatoses

The term lipomatosis has been applied to several disorders to describe either abnormal deposition of fat tissue or multiple lipomas. Lipomatoses presenting in children are rare and include the encephalocraniocutaneous lipomatosis, diagnosed soon after birth, and several congenital syndromes such as Proteus syndrome, Cowden's disease or the Bannayan–Riley–Ruvalcaba syndrome.

Encephalocraniocutaneous lipomatosis

Definition

The encephalocraniocutaneous lipomatosis (ECCL), first described in 1970 [1], is a rare congenital hamartomatous disorder classified in the neurocutaneous syndromes and characterized by unilateral skin lesions, lipomas and ipsilateral ophthalmic and cerebral malformations.

Aetiology

Although the course of ECCL is unknown, several mechanisms have been proposed. A maternal viral infection, described in two cases [2,3] is probably incidental. The most widely accepted theory involves dysgenesis of the cephalic neural crest and anterior neural tube. Somatic mosaicism is the most likely explanation [4,5] as in the Proteus syndrome [6]. Indeed ECCL and Proteus syndrome have many overlapping manifestations and ECCL can be considered as either a localized form of Proteus syndrome [7] or as a distinct entity in the same spectrum of mosaic overgrowth [8].

The finding of a mutation in the neurofibromatosis type 1 (NF1) gene in an affected child, who also has café-au-lait patches, suggests a role for this gene, either alone or in combination with another genetic or non-genetic event [7]. Further investigation is needed to confirm this somewhat surprising result. Finally, among lipomatoses, the pathogenic mechanism leading to the development of ECCL is probably similar to the one involved in the association of a cutaneous lipoma with an underlying intradural lipoma [9,10].

Histopathology

Both the subcutaneous soft masses and the intracranial tumours are typical lipomas. The two most common ocular findings in ECCL are epibulbar choristomas, consisting of dermal elements, fatty tissue and cartilage, and small skin nodules around the eyelids which histologically represent connective tissue naevi [11].

Clinical features

The multiple craniofacial abnormalities of ECCL are present at birth, usually consisting of a lipoma of the scalp or forehead with overlying alopecia, ocular lesions and intracranial malformations associated with a cerebral lipoma. Mental retardation and epilepsy closely correlates to the severity of intracranial lesions (hemispherical atrophy, polygyria, porencephaly, distortion of the ventricular system).

There is no geographic, racial or sex predilection in the less than 20 reported cases [12]. Similarly either side of the head can be involved. Intracranial involvement is usually unilateral, except in three children with bilateral lesions [13–15] and one with midline lesions [9].

Diagnosis

Establishing the diagnosis poses few problems because other neurocutaneous syndromes accompanied by cranial, cerebral and ocular malformations are not associated with the characteristic lipomas and alopecia seen in ECCL. Proteus syndrome with similar lesions in other parts of the body, the sebaceous naevus syndrome, and the Bannayan–Riley–Ruvalcaba syndrome with macrocephaly and intestinal polyposis are distinguishable. On the basis of the ocular abnormalities, one should consider, focal dermal hypoplasia (Goltz's syndrome), oculoauricular vertebral dysplasia (Goldenhar's syndrome) and oculocerebrocutaneous (Delleman's) syndrome, the latter sharing several overlapping features [16].

Treatment

Early surgical removal of the subcutaneous and cerebral (when feasible) lipomas, as well as the epibulbar choristomas is advised, but will not likely alter the ultimate prognosis which mainly depends on the extent of the intracranial malformations.

REFERENCES

1 Haberland C, Perou M. Encephalocraniocutaneous lipomatosis. *Arch Neurol* 1970; 22: 144–55.
2 Fishman MA, Chang CS, Miller JE. Encephalocraniocutaneous lipomatosis. *Pediatrics* 1978; 61: 580–2.
3 Alfonso I, Lopez PF, Cullen RF Jr *et al.* Spinal cord involvement in encephalocraniocutaneous lipomatosis. *Pediatr Neurol* 1986; 2: 380–4.
4 Rizzo R, Pavone L, Micali G *et al.* Encephalocraniocutaneous lipomatosis, Proteus syndrome, and somatic mosaicism. *Am J Med Genet* 1993; 47: 653–5.
5 Happle R, Steijlen PM. Enzephalokraniokutane Lipomatose. Ein nicht erblicher Mosaikphänotyp. *Hautarzt* 1993; 44: 19–22.
6 Cohen MM Jr. Proteus syndrome: clinical evidence for somatic mosaicism and selective review. *Neurofibromatosis* 1988; 1: 260–80.
7 Legius E, Wu R, Eyssen M *et al.* Encephalocraniocutaneous lipomatosis with a mutation in the NF1 gene. *J Med Genet* 1995; 32: 316–19.
8 McCall S, Ramzy MI, Cure JK *et al.* Encephalocraniocutaneous lipomatosis and the Proteus syndrome: distinct entities with overlapping manifestations. *Am J Med Genet* 1992; 43: 662–8.
9 Venencie PY, Husson B, Lacroix C *et al.* Lipomatose encéphalo-craniocutanée: une observation. *Ann Dermatol Vénéréol* 1993; 120: 766–7.
10 Bodemer C, Durand C, Brunel F *et al.* Lipome sous-cutané révélateur d'un lipome intradural. *Ann Dermatol Vénéréol* 1988; 115: 1130–2.
11 Kodsi SR, Bloom KE, Egbert JE *et al.* Ocular and systemic manifestations of encephalocraniocutaneous lipomatosis. *Am J Ophthalmol* 1994; 118: 77–82.
12 Nosti Martinez D, del Castillo V, Duran Mckinster C *et al.* Encephalocraniocutaneous lipomatosis: an uncommon neurocutaneous syndrome. *J Am Acad Dermatol* 1995; 32: 387–9.
13 Sanchez NP, Rhodes AR, Mandell F *et al.* Encephalocraniocutaneous lipomatosis: a new neurocutaneous syndrome. *Br J Dermatol* 1981; 104: 89–96.
14 Grimalt R, Ermacora E, Mistura L *et al.* Encephalocraniocutaneous lipomatosis: case report and review of the literature. *Pediatr Dermatol* 1993; 10: 164–8.
15 Al Mefty O, Fox JL, Sakati N *et al.* The multiple manifestations of the encephalocraniocutaneous lipomatosis syndrome. *Childs Nerv Syst* 1987; 3: 132–4.
16 Hennekam RC. Scalp lipomas and cerebral malformations: overlap between encephalocraniocutaneous lipomatosis and oculocerebrocutaneous syndrome. *Clin Dysmorphol* 1994; 3: 87–9 (letter, comment).

Familial multiple lipomatosis

(SYN. FAMILIAL MULTIPLE LIPOMAS, HEREDITARY MULTIPLE LIPOMAS, MULTIPLE CUTANEOUS LIPOMAS, DISCRETE LIPOMATOSIS, LIPOMATOSE DE ROCH–LERI)

Familial multiple lipomatosis [1,2] is characterized by the hereditary occurrence of multiple encapsulated lipomas.

The disorder was first described by Brodie in 1846 and its familial nature was reported by Blaschko in 1911. With a prevalence of 2 in 100000, there is no geographic predilection. Clinically, numerous encapsulated lipomas develop during adulthood and usually remain asymptomatic, their diameter rarely exceeding 5 cm. They occur on the mid level of the body and are predominantly found on the lower arms, forearms, lower chest, abdomen and lumbar region. After a rapid onset lasting 1–2 years, the course of familial multiple lipomatosis is benign in most cases. Both spontaneous resolution and malignant transformation have, however, been described.

Differential diagnosis includes steatoma multiplex (cystic lesions), familial multiple angiolipomas (histologically different) [3], Dercum's disease (painful lesions) and symmetric multiple lipomatosis. The French literature also reports the segmental lipomatosis of Touraine et Renault (1938) which consists of multiple encapsulated lipomas, but is differentiated by its metameric distribution [2].

Treatment requires surgical removal of functionally or aesthetically troublesome lipomas.

REFERENCES

1 Leffell DJ, Braverman IM. Familial multiple lipomatosis. *J Am Acad Dermatol* 1986; 15: 275–9.
2 Abensour M, Jeandel C, Heid E. Lipomes et lipomatoses cutanés. *Ann Dermatol Vénéréol* 1987; 114: 873–82.
3 Kumar R, Pereira BJ, Sakhuja V *et al.* Autosomal dominant inheritance in familial angiolipomatosis. *Clin Genet* 1989; 35: 202–4.

Other syndromes associated with cutaneous lipomatosis

Proteus syndrome

Lipomas often develop in Proteus syndrome [1] which is determined by the association of asymmetrical overgrowth of body parts, vascular malformations, epidermal and naevocellular naevi. For a full description of the syndrome, see Chapter 17.1. Its relationship with encephalocraniocutaneous lipomatosis is discussed above.

Bannayan–Riley–Ruvalcaba syndrome

Bannayan–Riley–Ruvalcaba syndrome is now recognized

to include three phenotypes described earlier by Ruval-caba (macrocephaly, intestinal polyposis, pigmented spot-ting of the penis), Bannayan and later by Zonana (macrocephaly with multiple subcutaneous and visceral lipomas and haemangiomas) and by Riley and Smith (macrocephaly, pseudopapilloedema and multiple hae-mangiomas) [2–5]. All of the phenotypes show an aut-osomal dominant transmission and share overlapping features, such as macrocephaly. Pigmented macules on the penile shaft occur in most males. Other features include cutaneous lipomas, haemangiomas and more commonly lymphangiomas, and multiple hamartous polyps limited to the distal ileum and colon. Hashimoto's thyroiditis has been added as a relatively frequent compli-cation. The syndrome is due to germ line mutations of the PTEN gene [6], as in Cowden's syndrome, and it has recently been proposed to unify these allelic disorders under the heading of PTEN MATCHS syndrome (Macro-cephaly, Autosomal dominant, Thyroid disease, Cancer, Hamartomata and Skin abnormalities) [7]. Prognosis is generally good except in cases who develop aggressive, infiltrating tumours [4]. Differential diagnosis includes Sotos' syndrome and Peutz–Jeghers sydrome; both are easily distinguishable.

Gardner's syndrome

Gardner's syndrome [8,9] is an autosomal dominant dis-order characterized by familial adenomatous polyposis of the colon, osteomas of the skull, mouth and long bones, desmoid tumours (usually as fibromatosis of the mesen-tery), dental abnormalities, epidermoid cysts, lipomas, fibromas and congenital hypertrophy of the retinal pigment epithelium. Mutations of the adenomatous poly-posis coli (APC) gene on chromosome 5q [10] account for the disorder. Lipomas in this syndrome are a secondary feature that appear in early adulthood. This disorder is discussed in more detail in Chapter 19.24.

Cowden's syndrome

Cowden's syndrome, also known as the multiple hamar-toma syndrome, is a rare autosomal dominant condition whereby multiple tumours of ectodermal, mesodermal and endodermal origin occur [9,11] Expression is variable among members of the same family. Mucocutaneous lesions are prominent, including facial trichilemmomas, acral keratoses and oral papillomas. The danger of the disease lies in the development of malignancies in the thyroid, gastrointestinal tract, breasts and female reproductive system. As opposed to Gardner's syndrome, the gastrointestinal polyps of Cowden's syndrome do not represent premalignant lesions. Lipomas occur in about 25% of affected patients, but it is believed that many go unnoticed. Important signs indicating Cowden's disease

in young children include progressive macrocephaly, scrotal tongue and mild to moderate mental retardation. This disorder, due to PTEN gene mutation [7], is discussed in more detail in Chapter 19.24.

REFERENCES

1 Viljoen DL, Saxe N, Temple Camp C. Cutaneous manifestations of the Proteus syndrome. *Pediatr Dermatol* 1988; 5: 14–21.
2 Gorlin RJ, Cohen MM Jr, Levin LS. *Syndromes of the Head and Neck*. New York: Oxford University Press 1990.
3 Gorlin RJ, Cohen MM, Condon LM *et al*. Bannayan–Riley–Ruvalcaba syn-drome. *Am J Med Genet* 1992; 44: 307–14.
4 Hayashi Y, Ohi R, Tomita Y *et al*. Bannayan–Zonana syndrome associated with lipomas, hemangiomas and lymphangiomas. *J Pediatr Surg* 1992; 27: 722–3.
5 Klein JA, Barr RJ. Bannayan–Zonana syndrome associated with lymphan-giomyomatous lesions. *Pediatr Dermatol* 1990; 7: 48–53.
6 Marsh D, Dahia PLM, Zheng Z *et al*. Germline mutations in PTEN are present in Bannayan–Zonona syndrome. *Nature Genet* 1997; 16: 333–4.
7 Diliberty JH. Inherited macrocephaly-hamatomata syndromes. *Am J Med Genet* 1998; 79: 284–90.
8 Pereyo NG. Extra abdominal desmoid tumor. *J Am Acad Dermatol* 1996; 34: 352–6.
9 Rustgi AK. Hereditary gastrointestinal polyposis and non-polyposis syn-dromes. *N Engl J Med* 1994; 331: 1694–702.
10 Olschwang S, Laurent-Puig P, Melot T *et al*. High resolution genetic map of the adenomatous polyposis coli gene (APC) region. *Am J Med Genet* 1995; 56: 413–19.
11 Hanssen AMN, Fryns JP. Cowden syndrome. *J Med Genet* 1995; 32: 117–19.

Lipodystrophies

The term 'lipodystrophy' has traditionally been used as a synonym for lipoatrophy, to describe idiopathic atrophies of the subcutaneous tissue. However, in this chapter the term lipodystrophy, as an abnormality of fat tissue, encompasses both fat hypertrophy and fat atrophy. As stated above, only primary lipodystrophies are discussed here, with the exception of insulin-induced lipodystro-phies. Inflammatory disorders leading to fat atrophy, i.e. panniculitis, are discussed in Chapter 9.4.

Fat hypertrophy

Localized fat hypertrophy

Insulin therapy in diabetes mellitus may result in local or systemic allergic cutaneous reactions, as well as fat hyper-trophy and fat atrophy at sites of injections [1,2]. The prevalence of these reactions overall did decrease, but did not disappear, with the introduction of highly purified bovine/pork insulins and recombinant human insulins [3,4].

Lipohypertrophy follows repeated insulin injections at the same site and is characterized by painless, soft and boggy masses progressively enlarging over several years. It was found in over 20% of diabetic patients having regular insulin injections and, as opposed to insulin lipoatrophy, its prevalence remained above 20% with the introduction of purified insulins [1,5]. Children can be affected. Most patients with lipohypertrophy admit to restricting their injections to anatomically small regions. This is partly due to the fact that the localized swelling is more convenient to aim at and is less painful for injection. Another reason is that restricting injections to one area may result in better metabolic control, since the absorption of insulin varies between anatomical sites [6]. Histologically, the dermis and epidermis are unaltered and the subcutaneous tissue consists of enlarged adipocytes [7]. This lipohypertrophy is regarded as due to a local anabolic effect of insulin, which promotes fat and protein synthesis. The main factor appears to be the constant injections at the same site, rather than the type of insulin. Indeed, all forms of insulin (soluble, isophane, zinc suspension) can cause lipohypertrophy [1,8].

Marked improvement usually follows a switch to human insulin and careful rotation of injection sites [7]. Liposuction can be effective in refractory cases [9].

REFERENCES

1 McNally PG, Jowett NI, Kurinczuk JJ *et al*. Lipohypertrophy and lipoatrophy complicating treatment with highly purified bovine and porcine insulins. *Postgrad Med J* 1988; 64: 850–3.
2 Plantin P, Sassolas B, Guillet MH *et al*. Accidents cutanes allergiques aux insulines. *Ann Dermatol Vénéréol* 1988; 115: 813–17.
3 Payne R, Williams C, Wilson IV. True delayed pressure urticaria induced by human Monotard insulin. *Br J Dermatol* 1996; 134: 184.
4 Goldman JM, Wheeler MF. Lipodystrophy from recombinant DNA human insulin. *Am J Med* 1987; 83: 195–6.
5 Young RJ, Steel JM, Frier BM *et al*. Insulin injection sites in diabetes—a neglected area? *Br Med J* 1981; 283: 349.
6 Koivisto VA, Felig P. Alterations in insulin absorption and in blood glucose control associated with varying insulin injection sites in diabetic patients. *Ann Int Med* 1980; 92: 59–61.
7 Samadaei A, Hashimoto K, Tanay A. Insulin lipodystrophy, lipohypertrophic type. *J Am Acad Dermatol* 1987; 17: 506–7.
8 Meier A, Weerakoon J, Dandona P. Bilateral abdominal lipohypertrophy after continuous subcutaneous infusion of insulin. *Br Med J* 1982; 285: 1539.
9 Field LM. Successful treatment of lipohypertrophic insulin lipodystrophy with liposuction surgery letter. *J Am Acad Dermatol* 1988; 19: 570.

Generalized lipohypertrophy

Obesity is beyond the scope of this chapter and information can be found elsewhere [1–3].

Genetic disorders associated with childhood onset obesity

Prader–Willi syndrome (PWS), with a frequency at about 1 in 25 000 is the most common syndromal cause of human obesity [4] and consists of intrauterine hypotonia, short stature, muscular hypotonia, hypogonadotropic hypogonadism, small hands and feet, fair skin and hair (hypopigmentation), failure to thrive and obesity [5–7]. It is recognized in infancy by a characteristic facies (facial diplegia with flat narrow face and triangular mouth),

hypotonia and feeding problems leading to failure to thrive. During the first year of life, a marked change in activity occurs, the child becomes much more lively and mobile. Hyperphagia/food foraging then develops and results in secondary obesity, with the possible consequence of insulin resistance and glucose intolerance after puberty. Other cutaneous signs include abdominal striae and scars from scratching due to itching after 6 years of age.

There is a male to female predominance of 5:2. The disorder is due to maternal uniparental disomy [8] at the 15q11–113 segment. Of note is that the maternal deletion of the same locus causes Angelman's syndrome (AS), and families with occurrence of both syndromes have been described [9]. Determination of the genes located in the region is under way. Interestingly, one of them is the human homologue for the mouse pink-eyed dilution (p locus). Since mutation in both copies of the P gene were found in a patient with type II oculocutaneous albinism, it has been suggested that deletion of one copy of this gene is the cause of hypopigmentation in PWS and AS [10].

Finally, with abundant fat, muscle hypotonia and small hands and feet, PWS represents the clinical opposite of congenital lipoatrophic diabetes (Seip's syndrome).

Bardet–Biedl syndrome, now considered distinct from Laurence–Moon syndrome [11], is characterized by obesity (predominantly on the trunk and proximal limbs), hypogonadism, mental retardation, blindness due to retinal dystrophy and digital abnormalities (syndactyly, polydactyly). Other cutaneous features are hypertrichosis and web neck [12].

Alström's syndrome is manifested by childhood blindness related to retinal degeneration, infantile obesity, nerve deafness, hypogonadism in males and diabetes mellitus with insulin resistance, acanthosis nigricans and nephropathy [13,14].

Other disorders in which obesity is listed as an associated feature include: X-linked mental retardation with gynecomastia and obesity, also known as the Wilson–Turner syndrome and originally described by Vasquez-Hurst and Sotos [15]; Cohen's syndrome with microcephaly, mental retardation, short stature, facial abnormalities and rather long, fine hands [16]; acrocephalopolysyndactyly type II (Carpenter's syndrome), with mental retardation, acrocephaly, polydactyly, syndactyly and obesity in older patients [17]; and Blount's disease with genua vara, tibial torsion and occasionally obesity.

Non-mendelian disorders should not be forgotten and in clinical practice one should remember that in children, acquired obesity coupled with headaches, growth disorders or endocrine dysfunction merits a lateral X-ray of the head and computed tomography (CT)/MRI scan to search for a craniopharyngioma.

REFERENCES

1 Silva JM, Serra-e-Silva P. Triumph of obesity or of human insanity. *Lancet* 1995; 346: 636–7.

2 Rohner-Jeanrenaud F, Jeanrenaud B. Obesity, leptin, and the brain. *N Engl J Med* 1996; 334: 324–5.

3 Foster DW. Eating disorders: obesity, anorexia nervosa, and bulimia nervosa. In: Wilson JD, Foster DW, eds. *Williams Textbook of Endocrinology*. Philadelphia: WB Saunders, 1992; 1335–65.

4 Butler M. Prader–Willi syndrome: current understanding of cause and diagnosis. *Am J Med Genet* 1990; 35: 319–22.

5 Wiesner GL, Bendel CM, Olds DP *et al.* Hypopigmentation in the Prader–Willi syndrome. *Am J Hum Genet* 1987; 40: 431–42.

6 Prader A, Labhart A, Willi H. Ein Syndrom von Adipositas, Kleinwuchs, Kryptorchismus unf Oligophrenie nach Myatonieartigem Zustand im Neugeborrenealter. *Schweiz Med Wschr* 1956; 86: 1260–1.

7 Holm VA, Cassidy SB, Butler MG *et al.* Prader–Willi syndrome: consensus diagnostic criteria. *Pediatrics* 1993; 91: 398–402.

8 Nichols RD, Knoll JHM, Butler MG *et al.* Genetic imprinting suggested by maternal heterodisomy in non-deletion Prader–Willi syndrome. *Nature* 1989; 342: 281–5.

9 Smeets DFCM, Hamel BCJ, Nelen MR *et al.* Prader–Willi syndrome and Angelman syndrome in cousins from a family with a translocation between chromosomes 6 and 15. *New Engl J Med* 1992; 326: 807–11.

10 Rinchik EM, Bultman SJ, Horsthemke B *et al.* A gene for the mouse pink-eyed dilution locus and for human type II oculocutaneous albinism. *Nature* 1993; 361: 72–6.

11 Schachat AP, Maumenee IH. The Bardet–Biedl syndrome and related disorders. *Arch Ophthal* 1982; 100: 285–8.

12 Green JS, Parfrey PS, Harnett JD *et al.* The cardinal manifestations of Bradet–Biedl syndrome, a form of Laurence–Moon–Biedl syndrome. *N Engl J Med* 1989; 321: 1002–9.

13 Charles SJ, Moore AT, Yates JRW *et al.* Alström's syndrome: further evidence of autosomal recessive inheritance and endocrinological dysfunction. *J Med Genet* 1990; 27: 590–2.

14 Alström CH, Hallgren B, Nilsson LB *et al.* Retinal degeneration combined with obesity, diabetes mellitus and neurogenous deafness: a specific syndrome (not hitherto described) distinct from the Laurence–Moon–Biedl syndrome. *Acta Psychiatr Neurol Scand* 1959; 34 (suppl. 129): 1–35.

15 Wilson M, Mulley J, Gedeon A *et al.* New X-linked syndrome of mental retardation, gynecomastia, and obesity is linked to DXS255. *Am J Med Genet* 1991; 40: 406–13.

16 Cohen MM, Hall BD, Smith DW *et al.* A new syndrome with hypotonia, obesity mental deficiency and facial, oral, ocular and limb anomalies. *J Pediatr* 1973; 83: 280–4.

17 Cohen DM, Green JG, Miller J *et al.* Acrocephalopolysyndactily type II—Caprpenter syndrome: clinical spectrum and an attempt at unification with Goodman and Sumitt syndromes. *Am J Med Genet* 1987; 28: 311–24.

Fat atrophy

Many disorders presenting with fat atrophy (lipoatrophy) have been reported as lipodystrophy. As stated above, the latter denomination will be avoided here in the interest of semantic clarification. Fat atrophy, as the loss of subcutaneous adipose tissue, can result from many congenital or acquired conditions, which can be classified as localized, partial or total lipoatrophies. The most common forms of lipoatrophy in children are localized (Fig. 20.1.1), and follow an inflammatory or scarring process of various origins (Table 20.1.1). In such cases, lipoatrophy may be the only finding; alternatively, other cutaneous modifications may be involved, such as sclerosis in morphoea. These inflammatory disorders are discussed elsewhere (see Chapter 9.4 and 20.1). In this chapter, mainly non-inflammatory, primary or 'idiopathic' lipoatrophies will

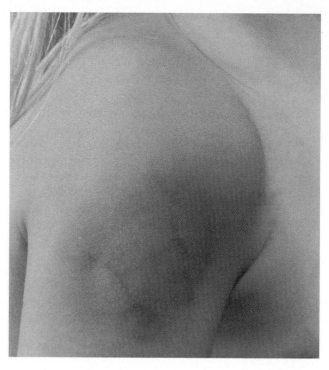

Fig. 20.1.1 Typical appearance of localized lipoatrophy with sharply delineated border and prominent subcutaneous veins.

Table 20.1.1 Acquired localized lipoatrophy

Injections: insulin; corticosteroids
Neonatal subcutaneous necrosis
Postvaccination
Subcutaneous calcification/ossification
Lipoatrophic panniculitis
Infection (bacterial, fungal or parasitic)
Connective tissue diseases
lupus erythematosus
dermatomyositis
morphoea/scleroderma
Thrombophlebitis/liposclerosis
Granuloma necrobiosis
granuloma annulare
necrobiosis lipoidica
rheumatic nodules
Lymphoma, leukaemia, neoplasia

be reviewed, the exception being for lipoatrophy following insulin injection.

Localized lipoatrophies

Localized lipoatrophies correspond to a heterogenic group of disorders whose denomination mainly depicts their clinical appearance. Insulin and centrifugal lipoatrophy can present in childhood. Annular lipoatrophy, semicircular lipoatrophy and lipoatrophy of the ankles are clinically distinct entities mainly seen in adult women and, therefore, will only be briefly mentioned.

Insulin lipoatrophy

Aetiology. Lipoatrophy following subcutaneous insulin injections was probably one of the most common causes of localized fat atrophy, when diabetic patients used conventional bovine—porcine insulin preparations. Since lipoatrophy was more commonly seen with longer-acting insulins rather than soluble ones, and since its occurrence was greatly reduced with the availability in the early 1980s of highly purified porcine insulins [1,2], it is considered to be an immunological reaction to impurities in the insulin preparations and/or to the xenogenic insulin [3,4].

These immunological reactions should be differentiated from allergic reactions to the content of long-acting insulins, which result in generalized urticaria and not lipoatrophy [5,6].

Histopathology. Skin biopsies show a loss of fat tissue. An increase in insulin-binding capacity is found on the edge of lipoatrophic lesions. Inflammatory changes are characteristically scant but immunofluorescence may show deposition of immunoglobulin M (IgM), C3 in the dermis and C3 in dermal blood vessels [4].

Clinical features. Insulin atrophy was previously seen more frequently than insulin hypertrophy, but not now. In a series of 281 patients treated with purified insulins the prevalence of lipohypertrophy was 27% and of lipoatrophy 2.5% [1]. It is a cosmetically distressing complication which presents as a non-inflammatory, painless, small to large dimple at insulin injection sites. It usually develops within 3 years of starting insulin and is more common in children and women. Most cases are associated with higher levels of insulin requirements, since insulin absorption can be delayed or variable due to the formation of avascular, fibrous scar tissue. Lipoatrophic lesions distant to the sites of injection may occur, as well as the coexistence of both fat atrophy and hypertrophy [7].

Treatment. The use of highly purified porcine insulins with a reinforcement of careful rotational routine of injection sites resulted in a marked decrease, but not disappearance, of insulin lipoatrophy. The use of human insulin preparations, injected directly into the lipoatrophic area, is usually curative [7,8]. This often results in both a regression of the localized lipoatrophy and a reduction in insulin requirements. However, cautious optimism should prevail as lipoatrophy may occasionally complicate human insulin injections [9].

REFERENCES

1 McNally PG, Jowett NI, Kurinczuk JJ *et al.* Lipohypertrophy and lipoatrophy complicating treatment with highly purified bovine and porcine insulins. *Postgrad Med J* 1988; 64: 850–3.

2 Young RJ, Steel JM, Frier BM *et al.* Insulin injection sites in diabetes—a neglected area? *Br Med J* 1981; 283: 349.

3 Kahn CR, Rosenthal AS. Immunologic reaction to insulin: insulin allergy, insulin resistance, and the autoimmune insulin syndrome. *Diabetes Care* 1979; 2: 283–95.

4 Reeves WG, Allen BR, Tattersall RB. Insulin-induced lipoatrophy: evidence for an immune pathogenesis. *Br Med J* 1980; 280: 1500–3.

5 Plantin P, Sassolas B, Guillet MH *et al.* Accidents cutanes allergiques aux insulines. *Ann Dermatol Vénéréol* 1988; 115: 813–17.

6 Rowland Payne CME, Williams C, Wilson IV. True delayed pressure urticaria induced by human Monotard insulin. *Br J Dermatol* 1996; 134: 178–92.

7 Valenta LJ, Elias AN. Insulin-induced lipodystrophy in diabetic patients resolved by treatment with human insulin. *Ann Intern Med* 1985; 102: 790–1.

8 Samadaei A, Hashimoto K, Tanay A. Insulin lipodystrophy, lipohypertrophic type. *J Am Acad Dermatol* 1987; 17: 506–7.

9 Chantelau E, Reuter M, Schotes S *et al.* A case of lipoatrophy with human insulin-therapy. *Exp Clin Endocrinol* 1993; 101: 194–6.

Centrifugal lipoatrophy
(SYN: LIPODYSTROPHIA CENTRIFUGALIS ABDOMINALIS INFANTILIS, CENTRIFUGAL LIPODYSTROPHY)

Definition. Described in 1971 by Inamura *et al.* [1] under the name 'lipodystrophia centrifugalis abdominalis infantilis', this form of lipoatrophy is characterized by (a) a localized loss of subcutaneous fat involving the greater part of the abdomen; (b) an onset before 3 years of age; (c) a centrifugal enlargement of the depressed area; (d) slightly reddish and scaly changes in the surrounding area; and (e) no other significant abnormalities. More than 100 cases have been reported to date, mainly in Japanese and rarely in oriental children [2]. Occurrence in Caucasian children appears exceptional [3].

Aetiology. The origin of centrifugal lipoatrophy is uncertain. Although small inflammatory findings, such as lymph node enlargement and peripheral inflammatory cellular infiltrate, are initially present in about two-thirds of cases, systemic signs of inflammation are usually absent [2]. These findings and the fact that corticosteroids do not stop the progressive enlargement of centrifugal lipoatrophy, argue against a primary inflammatory process as in other types of panniculitis. Speculation has covered several possible mechanisms: (a) a primary loss of subcutaneous fat with reactive inflammatory infiltrate and lymphadenopathy; (b) localized trauma such as friction, contusion, inguinal hernia or congenital dislocation of the hip, which have all been reported as possible triggers in some patients; and (c) intercurrent infections. The higher expression of the disorder in Japanese children, together with the description of affected dizygotic twins and siblings [4], may suggest a genetic predisposition.

Histology. Lesions are characterized by a decrease or loss of subcutaneous fat with the presence of inflammatory cells that are more prominent in the surrounding area. The inflammatory cell infiltrate may involve the dermis as well as the subcutaneous tissue and consists of lymphocytes, histiocytes and few plasma cells in most cases

[2,3,5]. Multinucleated giant cells and foamy cells have been reported [5]. Mild vascular changes (endothelial swelling) can occur, but not apparent vasculitis.

Clinical features. With a 2:1 female to male ratio, 90% of cases are characterized by an onset before 8 years of age and an abdominal location, most often the groin or surrounding area. The initial presentation includes erythematous, bluish macules or ecchymoses with regional lymph node enlargement in about half of the cases. In the other half, the parents first notice the lesion only by a well-defined depression or atrophy of the skin. The lesion then spreads centrifugally to leave a central part of lipoatrophy, where subcutaneous veins become easily visible. A few patients have developed two or three lesions. In a follow-up review of cases, it was found that cessation of enlargement occurs within 3 years in 50% of patients and within 8 years in 90%, followed by spontaneous resolution or marked improvement in a majority of cases [2,5–7].

The clinical course appears rather uniform in most cases. However, a few variations were recently reported. These include extra-abdominal locations, such as the head [5], neck [7] and lumbar region [3,6]; and non-regressing cases [8]. Adult cases are extremely rare [9,10], and whether these should be classified as large unusual semicircular lipoatrophies is disputable.

Treatment and prognosis. Topical and oral corticosteroids have been used with little benefit. They are usually effective at decreasing the peripheral inflammation/erythema but do not halt the progressive centrifugal extension [2]. Although most cases spontaneously stop progressing before the age of 13 years and then regress, persistence into adulthood of a lesion further complicated by angioblastoma has been reported [8].

REFERENCES

1 Imamura S, Yamada M, Ikeda T. Lipodystrophia centrifugalis abdominalis infantilis. *Arch Dermatol* 1971; 104: 291–8.
2 Imamura S, Yamada M, Yamamoto K. Lipodystrophia centrifugalis abdominalis infantilis. *J Am Acad Dermatol* 1984; 11: 203–9.
3 Zachary CB, Wells RS. Centrifugal lipodystrophy. *Br J Dermatol* 1984; 110: 107–10.
4 Mizoguchi M, Nanko S. Lipodystrophia centrifugalis abdominalis infantilis in dizygotic twins. *J Dermatol* 1982; 9: 139–43.
5 Hagari Y, Sasaoka R, Nishiura S *et al.* Centrifugal lipodystrophy of the face mimicking progressive lipodystrophy. *Br J Dermatol* 1992; 127: 407–10.
6 Caputo R. Lipodystrophia centrifugalis sacralis infantilis. *Acta Derm Venereol* 1989; 69: 442–3.
7 Higuchi T, Yamakage A, Tamura T *et al.* Lipodystrophia centrifugalis abdominalis infantilis occurring in the neck. *Dermatology* 1994; 188: 142–4.
8 Hiraiwa A, Takai K, Fukui Y *et al.* Nonregressing lipodystrophia centrifugalis abdominalis with angioblastoma (Nakagawa). *Arch Dermatol* 1990; 126: 206–9.
9 Rowland Payne CME, Harper JI, Farthing CE *et al.* Lypodystrophia centrifugalis. *Br J Dermatol* 1985; 113 (suppl): 100–1.
10 Franks A, Verbov JL. Unilateral localized idiopathic lipoatrophy. *Clin Exp Dermatol* 1993; 18: 468–9.

Annular lipoatrophy [1–3]

This entity is characterized by a circular depressed band, 1 cm wide and 0.5–2 cm deep, that encircles an upper limb, usually in women aged 40–70 years. The atrophic lesion is preceded by tenderness and swelling of the entire limb. Unexplained neuralgia and arthralgic pain with muscle weakness or myopathy are frequent. Annular lipoatrophy does not spontaneously regress and may last up to 20 years. Histological findings may be minimal or show polyarteritis and strands of connective tissue replacing the subcutaneous fat. The prevalence of 'rheumatic' pain and associated findings suggests an underlying connective tissue disease.

Atrophy of the ankles [4–6]

This is an extremely rare disorder, mainly characterized by its peculiar location. Less than 10 cases have been described with bilateral circumferential, asymptomatic, lipoatrophic bands, 9–11 cm wide, on the ankles. Local symptomatology and muscle involvement are absent. The disorder should be differentiated from acral lipoatrophy which may develop as an autoimmune process (Fig. 20.1.2).

Semicircular lipoatrophy [2,7–15]

Semicircular lipoatrophy occurs more frequently than annular lipoatrophy and atrophy of the ankles, and it occurs mainly in adults. Patients present with semiannular cutaneous depressions symmetrically distributed on the anterolateral aspects of both thighs. The aetiology remains unclear, probably because the disorder may be heterogeneous; some authors reported trauma or tight jeans. The lesions are asymptomatic and flesh coloured. Spontaneous resolution usually occurs within 3 years of onset. Histological changes include fat atrophy replaced by collagen and mild perivascular cellular infiltrate in the dermis.

In a review of 11 patients with different types of localized lipoatrophies, Peters and Winkelmann [16] found a greater prevalence of inflammatory changes. They suggested that lipoatrophies could be histologically classified as involutional or inflammatory. Lack of correlation between the histological picture and the clinical course, however, limits the value of their findings.

REFERENCES

1 Bruinsma W. Lipoatrophia annularis, an abnormal vulnerability of the fatty tissue. *Dermatologica* 1967; 134: 107–12.
2 Rongioletti F, Rebora A. Annular and semicircular lipoatrophies. *J Am Acad Dermatol* 1989; 20: 433–6.
3 Ferreira-Marques J. Lipoatrophia annularis. Ein Fall einer bisher nicht beschriebenen Krankheit der Haut. *Arch Dermatol Syph (Berlin)* 1953; 195: 479–91.

naevoid disorders such as Becker's naevus [1] or naevoid hypertrichosis [2].

REFERENCES

1 Van Gerwen HJ, Koopman RJ, Steijlen PM *et al.* Becker's naevus with localized lipoatrophy and ipsilateral breast hypoplasia. *Br J Dermatol* 1993; 129: 213.
2 Cox NH, McClure JP, Hardie RA. Naevoid hypertrichosis—report of a patient with multiple lesions. *Clin Exp Dermatol* 1989; 14: 62–4.

Partial lipoatrophy

Familial partial lipodystrophy
(SYN: KÖBBERLING-DUNNIGAN SYNDROME, REVERSE PARTIAL LIPODYSTROPHY, LIPOATROPHIC DIABETES)

Definition and history. Familial partial lipodystrophy (FPL) is an X-linked dominant syndrome comprising at least two clinical phenotypes with progressive loss of subcutaneous fat confined to the limbs (type 1) or also involving the trunk (type 2), starting in childhood. In 1974, Dunnigan *et al.* [1] described three female members of a Scottish family and one female member of another family who showed the complete absence of fat from the limbs and trunk with normal or excessive adipose tissue of the face and neck. All four patients had hyperlipaemia and three had diabetes mellitus. In 1975, Köbberling *et al.* [2] described three female members of a German family who showed complete absence of cutaneous fat from the limbs with normal fat on the face and trunk. Other familial cases were then reported [3,4]. In 1986, Köbberling and Dunnigan reviewed all cases, delineated the two clinical phenotypes and reinterpreted the inheritance as an X-linked dominant syndrome, lethal in the hemizygous state [5].

Aetiology. The disorder remains of an uncertain origin. Post-heparin lipoprotein lipase activity was reduced in some patients with type 1 FPL. Diabetes and hyperlipaemia are frequently present in patients, but do not occur in all cases, and only a few patients exhibit the typical characteristics of acquired lipoatrophic diabetes. This syndrome, however, further suggests a link between the development/maintenance of subcutaneous adipose tissue and insulin resistance as in the recessively inherited congenital total lipodystrophy (Seip–Berardinelli) and the two non-mendelian disorders of progressive partial lipodystrophy (Barraquer–Simmons) and acquired lipoatrophic diabetes (Lawrence).

The X-linked dominance, lethal in the hemizygous state, fits with large pedigrees. However, cases difficult to assign to type 1 or 2 [3], as well as the description of affected males [6,7], indicates a likely heterogeneity

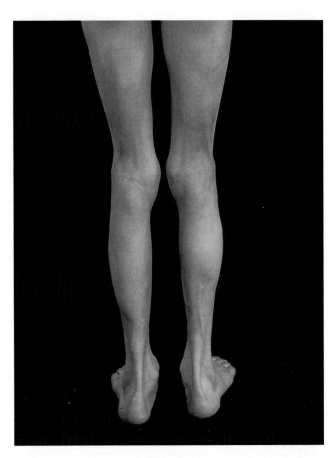

Fig. 20.1.2 Diffuse, predominantly acral lipoatrophy in a girl with autoimmune hepatitis, alopecia and positive antiliver and kidney microsomes antibodies.

4 Jablonska S, Szczepanski A, Gorkiewicz A. Lipoatrophy of the ankles and its relation to other lipoatrophies. *Acta Derm Venereol* 1975; 55: 135–40.
5 Roth DE, Schikler KN, Callen JP. Annular atrophic connective tissue panniculitis of the ankles. *J Am Acad Dermatol* 1989; 21: 1152–6.
6 Shelley WB, Izumi AK. Annular atrophy of the ankles. *Arch Dermatol* 1970; 102: 326–9.
7 Baurle G, Hanke E. Lipodystrophia semicircularis: ein rein kosmetisces Problem? *Artzl Kosmetol* 1983; 13: 135–41.
8 Bloch PH, Runne U. Lipotrophia semicircularis beim Mann. *Hautarzt* 1978; 29: 270–2.
9 Karkavitsas C, Miller JA, Kirby JD. Semicircular lipoatrophy. *Br J Dermatol* 1981; 105: 591–3.
10 Hodak E, David M, Sandbank M. Semicircular lipoatrophy—a pressure-induced lipoatrophy? *Clin Exp Dermatol* 1990; 15: 464–5.
11 Ayala F, Lembo G, Ruggiero F *et al.* Lipoatrophia semicircularis. *Dermatologica* 1985; 170: 101–3.
12 Thiele B, Ippen H. Multilokulare progrediente Lipatrophia semicircularis. *Hautarzt* 1983; 34: 292–2.
13 Mascaro JM, Ferrando J. Lipoatrophia semicircularis: the perils of wearing jeans? *Int J Dermatol* 1982; 21: 138–9.
14 Leonforte JF. Lipoatrophia semicircularis associated with an osseous cyst. *Cutis* 1983; 31: 428,430,435.
15 Gshwandtner WR, Munzberger H. Lipoatrophia semicircularis. *Wien Klin Wochenschr* 1975; 87: 164–8.
16 Peters MS, Winkelmann RK. The histopathology of localized lipoatrophy. *Br J Dermatol* 1986; 114: 27–36.

Naevoid disorders

Localized lipoatrophy can occasionally be associated with

of the disorder and/or occurrence of other familial phenotypes.

Clinical features. Patients with type 1 FPL, (limb dystrophy) show the complete absence of visible or palpable subcutaneous fat on the arms and legs. The subcutaneous veins appear prominent and the muscles hypertrophied. Acanthosis nigricans occurs only in patients with diabetes and hyperlipoproteinaemia. Diabetes can present as the mild maturity onset form or be more severe, complicated by nephropathy and early death [2,4,5]. In type 2 FPL, (limb and trunk lipodystrophy) all three members of the first described family showed the absence of subcutaneous fat from the trunk and limbs, broad facies with short thick-set necks and slight prognathism. Excess fat on the face, neck and supraclavicular fossae can occur. Hands and feet are always normal in size and shape. Associated metabolic abnormalities are mild to severe hyperlipoproteinaemia and insulin-resistant diabetes [1,5].

X-linked familial lipodystrophy can be differentiated from acquired progressive partial lipodystrophy (Barraquer) by the absence of complement system abnormalities or absence of glomerulonephritis; and from the two following forms of total lipoatrophies: acquired lipoatrophic diabetes (Lawrence) by the absence of hepatic impairment and the familial inheritance, and from congenital lipodystrophy (Seip–Berardinelli) by the absence of renal tract and central nervous system (CNS) abnormalities.

REFERENCES

1 Dunnigan MG, Cochrane MA, Kelly A *et al.* Familial lipoatrophic diabetes with dominant transmission. *Q J Med* 1974; 43: 33–48.
2 Köbberling J, Wilms B, Kattermann R *et al.* Lipodystrophy of the extremities. *Humangenetik* 1975; 29: 111–20.
3 Ozer FL, Lichtenstein JR, Kwiterovitch PO *et al.* A 'new' variety of lipodystrophy. *Clin Res* 1973; 21: 533A.
4 Davidson MB, Young RT. Metabolic studies in familial partial lipodystrophy of the lower trunk and extremities. *Diabetologia* 1975; 11: 561–8.
5 Köbberling J, Dunnigan MG. Familial partial lipodystrophy: two types of an X-linked dominant syndrome, lethal in the hemizygous state. *J Med Genet* 1986; 23: 120–7.
6 Reardon W, Temple IK, Mackinnon H *et al.* Partial lipodystrophy syndromes—a further male case. *Clin Genet* 1990; 38: 391–5.
7 Burn J, Baraitser M. Partial lipoatrophy with insulin resistant diabetes and hyperlipidaemia (Dunnigan syndrome). *J Med Genet* 1986; 23: 128–30.

Progressive partial lipodystrophy
(SYN: BARRAQUER–SIMONS DISEASE)

Definition. Progressive partial lipodystrophy (PPL) is a non-mendelian disorder that occurs predominantly in females who exhibit a loss of subcutaneous adipose tissue, starting on the face and progressing downwards to the trunk, and accompanied by normal or excessive fat deposition in the pelvic girdle and lower limbs [1]. Of cases 90% have low C3 levels due to the presence of C3 nephritic factor (C3NeF) and about half of the patients develop

an associated membranoproliferative glomerulonephritis [2].

Aetiology. The disorder may follow an acute specific fever such as measles [2] or dermatomyositis [3,4]. Although the exact cause of PPL remains obscure in most cases, the frequent relationship with C3NeF (an acquired autoantibody that binds to the C3 convertase enzyme) often associated with an immunologically related glomerulonephritis, or other autoimmune diseases [4–8] supports an immunological basis for PPL. The role of C3 deficiency as a primary event in PPL is further supported by the description of PPL in a family with C3 deficiency [9].

Although the link between C3 deficiency (with C3NeF) and glomerulonephritis and/or later onset of systemic lupus erythematosus (SLE) can be explained [2,8], its link with lipoatrophy is unknown.

As opposed to total lipodystrophies, diabetes mellitus is rare in PPL [10]. However, basal hyperinsulinaemia following an oral glucose tolerance test is frequent [11–13] implying a similarity with forms of lipoatrophic diabetes, where insulin and insulin receptor abnormalities have been described.

Clinical features. With a female to male predominance of 5:1, patients usually present in the second decade of life. Onset of PPL earlier in childhood has been well described [8]. PPL is acquired in most cases and has a fairly sudden onset, characterized by the symmetrical disappearance of facial fat, producing a cadaveric-like facies, followed by the progressive loss of subcutaneous fat in the upper half of the body. Some patients may somewhat paradoxically develop fat overgrowth on the lower part of the body. Glomerulonephritis, diabetes mellitus and SLE are the most frequent complications/associations and should be sought. Occasional findings include cutaneous vasculitis and purpura, cirrhosis, myopathy and coeliac disease [14–17].

Treatment. No preventive or therapeutic measures appear effective on the lipoatrophy, and facial reconstruction may be necessary to improve the dramatic facial appearance [18]. Management of the complications (diabetes, nephritis) should follow the usual course. Closely monitored pregnancy can be successful [19].

REFERENCES

1 Barraquer-Ferré L. Lipodystrophie progressive, syndrome de Barraquer et Simons. *Presse Med* 1935; 86: 1672–4.
2 Sissons JG, West RJ, Fallows J *et al.* The complement abnormalities of lipodystrophy. *N Engl J Med* 1976; 294: 461–5.
3 Kavanagh GM, Colaco CB, Kennedy CT. Juvenile dermatomyositis associated with partial lipoatrophy. *J Am Acad Dermatol* 1993; 28: 348–51.
4 Torrelo A, Espana A, Boixeda P *et al.* Partial lipodystrophy and dermatomyositis. *Arch Dermatol* 1991; 127: 1846–7.

5 Alarcon Segovia D, Ramos Niembro F. Association of partial lipodystrophy and Sjögren's syndrome letter. *Ann Intern Med* 1976; 85: 474–5.

6 Font J, Herrero C, Bosch X *et al.* Systemic lupus erythematosus in a patient with partial lipodystrophy. *J Am Acad Dermatol* 1990; 22: 337–40.

7 Hall SW, Gillespie JJ, Tenczynski TF. Generalized lipodystrophy, scleroderma, and Hodgkin's disease letter. *Arch Intern Med* 1978; 138: 1303–4.

8 Walport MJ, Davies KA, Botto M *et al.* C3 nephritic factor and SLE: report of four cases and review of the literature *Q J Med* 1994; 87: 609–15.

9 McLean RH, Hoefnagel D. Partial lipodystrophy and familial C3 deficiency. *Hum Hered* 1980; 30: 149–54.

10 Rifkind BM, Boyle JA, Gale M. Blood lipid levels, thyroid status, and glucose tolerance in progressive partial lipodystrophy. *J Clin Pathol* 1967; 20: 52–5.

11 Boucher BJ, Cohen RD, Frankel RJ *et al.* Partial and total lipodystrophy: changes in circulating sugar, free fatty acids, insulin and growth hormone following the administration of glucose and of insulin. *Clin Endocrinol Oxf* 1973; 2: 111–26.

12 Sissons JG, Liebowitch J, Amos N *et al.* Metabolism of the fifth component of complement, and its relation to metabolism of the third component, in patients with complement activation. *J Clin Invest* 1977; 59: 704–15.

13 West RJ, Fosbrooke AS, Lloyd JK, Metabolic studies and autonomic function in children with partial lipodystrophy. *Arch Dis Child* 1974; 49: 627–32.

14 Robertson DA, Wright R. Cirrhosis in partial lipodystrophy. *Postgrad Med J* 1989; 65: 318–20.

15 O'Mahony D, O'Mahony S, Whelton MJ *et al.* Partial lipodystrophy in coeliac disease. *Gut* 1990; 31: 717–18.

16 Orrell RW, Peatfield RC, Collins CE *et al.* Myopathy in acquired partial lipodystrophy. *Clin Neurol Neurosurg* 1995; 97: 181–6.

17 Perrot H, Delaup JP, Chouvet B. Lipodystrophie de Barraquer et Simons. *Ann Dermatol Vénéréol* 1987; 114: 1083–91.

18 Coessens BC, Van Geertruyden JP. Simultaneous bilateral facial reconstruction of a Barraquer–Simons lipodystrophy with free TRAM flaps. *Plast Reconstr Surg* 1995; 95: 911–15.

19 Akhter J, Qureshi R. Partial lipodystrophy and successful pregnancy outcome. *J Pak Med Assoc* 1995; 45: 24.

Total lipoatrophy

Leprechaunism, congenital lipoatrophic diabetes (Seip–Berardinelli syndrome) and acquired lipoatrophic diabetes (Lawrence's syndrome) are three clinically distinct forms of total lipoatrophies, which belong to a group of disorders associated with severe insulin resistance. These are therefore characterized by diabetes mellitus, acanthosis nigricans and, in female patients, hirsutism and virilization. The term 'lipoatrophic diabetes' is rather confusing in that it is used for disorders that present with either partial (X-linked lipodystrophy) or total lipoatrophy. It will, however, be retained here as it unifies disorders with a common clinical expression. An attempt has been made to mention synonyms of syndromes that are still used in the recent literature.

Leprechaunism
(SYN: DONOHUE'S SYNDROME)

Definition. Leprechaunism is an autosomal recessive disorder due to a mutation of the insulin receptor gene and characterized by intrauterine growth retardation, small elfin-like face with protuberant ears, distended abdomen, large hands, feet and genitalia, abnormal skin with hypertrichosis, acanthosis nigricans and decreased subcutaneous fat [1–3]. Fifty-two cases were recorded in 1993 [4].

Aetiology. The molecular defect in leprechaunism is a mutation in the insulin receptor gene (INSR). More than 10 different mutations have been described [5]. These included both homozygous and combined heterozygous mutations which result in either a decrease in the number of receptors or in a defective function of the receptor. Secondary defective formation of insulin-like growth factor 1 (IGF-1) and epidermal growth factor (EGF) receptors have been described [6,7]. Since IGF-1 receptors are present on the ovary, heart and kidneys, but not fat cells, this could explain ovarian enlargement, myocardial hypertrophy and kidney enlargement reported in some patients. Finally, Psiachou *et al.* [8] suggested that growth hormone (GH) resistance was a secondary effect caused by down-regulation of GH receptor activity in the presence of a high concentration of insulin proximal to the cell membrane, with consequent limitation of IGF-1 formation and cellular growth. Thus, although the primary defect in leprechaunism is in the INSR gene, a secondary defect is probably responsible for an impaired response to endogenous GH and growth failure.

Histopathology. Skin biopsies show the complete absence of fat. Autopsy findings often show pancreatic β-cell hyperplasia in 60% of patients, increased iron deposition in liver, kidney calcifications as well as other rarer features [1].

Clinical features. Leprechaunism is characterized by cessation of intrauterine growth at about 7 months of gestation. The two sisters first described by Donohue [2] also had a peculiar facies, creating a gnome-like appearance leading to the designation. Severe endocrine disturbance was indicated by emaciation and enlargement of the breasts and clitoris. The children died at 46 and 66 days of age, respectively. Unequivocal cases are all characterized in addition by hypertrichosis, acanthosis nigricans and symptomatic hypoglycaemia due to insulin resistance. Most patients die before 1 year of age [1,9].

Variant syndromes with leprechaun features include patients with clinical Cushing's disease, enlarged adrenals and severe bone changes [10,11]; three infants with associated generalized elastic fibre deficiency [12]; and five siblings with less severe leprechaun features, survival beyond 10 years of age, normal subcutaneous fat, kidney enlargement, myocardial hypertrophy and ovarian enlargement in the female case [4].

Diagnosis and treatment. Intrauterine growth retardation, abnormal facies, hirsutism and decreased subcutaneous fat lead to the diagnosis in most cases. Insulin resistance and a rapidly lethal course then follow. In milder cases, differentiation with congenital lipoatrophic diabetes may be difficult. However, in the latter, no mutation on the insulin receptor gene can be found [13].

Rabson–Mendenhall syndrome is another condition presenting with lipoatrophic diabetes and associated insulin receptor gene mutation, which can be differentiated by additional dysmorphic features (short stature, teeth and nail abnormalities) [14].

Treatment in leprechaunism is aimed at avoiding hypoglycaemic attacks that are potentially fatal. However, this may not prevent sudden death at an early age.

REFERENCES

1 Rosenberg AM, Haworth JC, William Degroot G et al. A case of leprechaunism with severe hyperinsulinemia. Am J Dis Child 1980; 134: 170–5.
2 Donohue WL. Leprechaunism. J Pediatr 1954; 45: 505–19.
3 Elsas LJ, Endo F, Strumlauf F et al. Leprechaunism: an inherited defect in a high affinity insulin receptor. Am J Hum Genet 1985; 37: 73–88.
4 al Gazali LI, Khalil M, Devadas K. A syndrome of insulin resistance resembling leprechaunism in five sibs of consanguineous parents. J Med Genet 1993; 30: 470–5.
5 Taylor SI. Diabetes mellitus. In: Scriver CR, Beaudet AL, Sly WS, Valle D, eds. The Metabolic and Molecular Bases of Inherited Disease. New York: McGraw Hill, 1995: 843–96.
6 Van Oberghen-Schilling E, Rechler M, Romanus J et al. Receptors for insulin like growth factor I are defective in fibroblast cultures from a patient with leprechaunism. J Clin Invest 1981; 68; 1358–65.
7 Reddy SS-K, Kahn CR. Epidermal growth factor receptor defects in leprechaunism: a multiple growth factor-resistant syndrome. J Clin Invest 1989; 84: 1569–76.
8 Psiachou H, Mitton S, Alaghband-Zadeh J et al. Leprechaunism and homozygous nonsense mutation in the insulin receptor gene. Lancet 1993; 342: 924.
9 Cantani A, Ziruolo MG, Tacconi ML. A rare polydysmorphic syndrome: leprechaunism — review of 49 cases reported in the literature. Ann Genet 1987; 30: 221–7.
10 David R, Goodman RM. The Patterson syndrome, leprechaunism and pseudo-leprechaunism. J Med Genet 1981; 18: 294–8.
11 Patterson JH, Watkin WL. Leprechaunism in a male infant. J Pediatr 1962; 60: 733–9.
12 Dallaire L, Cantin M, Melancon SB et al. A syndrome of generalized elastic fiber deficiency with leprechaunoid features: a distinct genetic disease with an autosomal recessive mode of inheritance. Clin Genet 1976; 10: 1–11.
13 Desbois Mouthon C, Magre J, Amselem S et al. Lipoatrophic diabetes: genetic exclusion of the insulin receptor gene. J Clin Endocrinol Metab 1995; 80: 314–19.
14 Rabson SM, Mendenhall EN. Familial hypertrophy of pineal body, hyperplasia of adrenal cortex and diabetes mellitus. Am J Clin Pathol 1956; 26: 283.

Congenital lipoatrophic diabetes

(SYN. SEIP–BERARDINELLI SYNDROME, TOTAL LIPODYSTROPHY WITH ACROMEGALOID GIGANTISM)

Definition. Congenital lipoatrophic diabetes (CLD) is a rare autosomal recessive syndrome characterized by extreme paucity of fat in adipose tissue from birth, severe insulin resistance, hyperlipaemia and increased bone growth [1,2].

Aetiology. The syndrome is autosomal recessive; heterozygous subjects may manifest hyperlipaemia. Although the underlying molecular abnormality remains unclear, CLD patients have provided a unique opportunity to study the metabolism of insulin resistance. Marked

insulin resistance was confirmed *in vivo* concerning glucose disposal and hepatic glucose output [3,4]. *In vitro* studies have revealed abnormalities in glucose metabolism [4,5] and in insulin-receptor tyrosine kinase [6]. Mutation of the INSR gene has, however, been excluded [7,8]. Recent observations showed a profound metabolic resistance to the carbohydrate and lipid actions of insulin, with preservation of protein anabolism, thus indicating that the biological effects of insulin on carbohydrate, lipids and proteins are independently distributed [9]. Furthermore, the finding that in affected patients, adipose tissue remained present in particular anatomical sites (i.e. the orbits, palms, soles and periarticular regions) indicate a difference in growth/maintenance between metabolically active adipose tissue (totally absent) and 'mechanical' adipose tissue (preserved) [10].

Clinical features. Complete loss of subcutaneous fat appears at birth or within the first 2 years of life. Nonketotic insulin-resistant diabetes mellitus usually develops during the first or second decade. Other findings include acanthosis nigricans, acromegaloid features, marked hypertriglyceridaemia (± eruptive xanthoma), visceromegaly, hirsutism, virilization in female patients and possible muscular hypertrophy.

A syndrome in every way identical to CLD, but associated with systemic angiomatosis, was reported by Brunzell et al. [11]. Polycystic ovaries and cystic angiomatosis of bones were present. A 13-year-old girl with similar presentation was also reported by Van Maldergem et al. [12], who favoured the distinction of the term Brunzell's syndrome, which they suggested should include polycystic disease.

Treatment. With good control of the diabetes, hyperlipaemia and prevention of their complications, patients reach adult life. Management of pregnancy is difficult, as in acquired lipoatrophic diabetes [13].

REFERENCES

1 Berardinelli W. An undiagnosed endocrinometabolic syndrome: report of two cases. J Clin Endocrinol Metab 1954; 14: 193–204.
2 Seip M. Generalized lipodystrophy. Ergeb Inn Med Kinderheilkd 1971; 31: 59–95.
3 Robert JJ, Rakotoambinina B, Cochet I et al. The development of hyperglycaemia in patients with insulin-resistant generalized lipoatrophic syndromes. Diabetologia 1993; 36: 1288–92.
4 Tsukahara H, Kikuchi K, Kuzuya H et al. Insulin resistance in a boy with congenital generalized lipodystrophy. Pediatr Res 1988; 24: 688–72.
5 Moller DE, Flier JS. Insulin resistance — mechanisms, syndromes and implications. N Engl J Med 1991; 325: 938–48.
6 Kriaciunas KM, Kahn CR, Muller Wieland D et al. Altered expression and function of the insulin receptor in a family with lipoatrophic diabetes. J Clin Endocrinol Metab 1988; 67: 1284–93.
7 van der Vorm ER, Kuipers A, Bonenkamp JW et al. Patients with lipodystrophic diabetes mellitus of the Seip–Berardinelli type, express normal insulin receptors. Diabetologia 1993; 36: 172–4.

8 Desbois Mouthon C, Magre J, Amselem S *et al.* Lipoatrophic diabetes: genetic exclusion of the insulin receptor gene. *J Clin Endocrinol Metab* 1995; 80: 314–19.

9 Copeland KC, Nair KS, Kaplowitz PB *et al.* Discordant metabolic actions of insulin in extreme lipodystrophy of childhood. *J Clin Endocrinol Metab* 1993; 77: 1240–5.

10 Garg A, Fleckenstein JL, Peshock RM *et al.* Peculiar distribution of adipose tissue in patients with congenital generalized lipodystrophy. *J Clin Endocrinol Metab* 1992; 75: 358–61.

11 Brunzell JD, Shankle SW, Bethune JE. Congenital generalized lipodystrophy accompanied by cystic angiomatosis. *Ann Intern Med* 1968; 69: 501–16.

12 Van Maldergem L, Bacq C, Mommen N *et al.* Total lipodystrophy, polycystic ovaries and cystic angiomatosis of bones (Brunzell syndrome): confirmation of a separate entity. *Am J Hum Genet* 1992; 51 (suppl): A109 (abstract).

13 Sturley RH, Stirling C, Reckless JP. Generalised lipodystrophy and pregnancy. *Br J Obstet Gynaecol* 1994; 101: 719–20.

Acquired lipoatrophic diabetes
(SYN. LAWRENCE'S SYNDROME, TOTAL LIPODYSTROPHY)

Acquired lipoatrophic diabetes comprises the same clinical features as congenital lipoatrophic diabetes (Seip–Berardinelli syndrome), with the difference that symptoms develop later in life [1,2]. Lipoatrophy is delayed until adolescence or early adulthood. Lawrence's syndrome was believed to be acquired and restricted to women; however, consanguinity or family antecedents have recently been reported [3,4]. Mutations of the insulin receptor gene have also been excluded [3].

REFERENCES

1 Lawrence RD. Lipodystrophy and hepatomegaly. *Lancet* 1946; i: 724.

2 Sasaki T, Ono H, Nakajima H *et al.* Lipoatrophic diabetes. *J Dermatol* 1992; 19: 246–9.

3 Desbois Mouthon C, Magre J, Amselem S *et al.* Lipoatrophic diabetes: genetic exclusion of the insulin receptor gene. *J Clin Endocrinol Metab* 1995; 80: 314–19.

4 Robert JJ, Rakotoambinina B, Cochet I *et al.* The development of hyperglycaemia in patients with insulin-resistant generalized lipoatrophic syndromes. *Diabetologia* 1993; 36: 1288–92.

Section 21
The Histiocytoses

21.1 Langerhans' Cell and Non-Langerhans' Cell Histiocytosis

FREDERIC CAMBAZARD AND JEAN-LOUIS STEPHAN

Langerhans' cell histiocytosis (class I histiocytosis)

Non-malignant non-Langerhans' cell histiocytosis (class II histiocytosis)
Systemic class II histiocytosis
Cutaneous class II histiocytosis

Class III histiocytosis

Definition

Histiocytes are classified into two major subsets: the mononuclear phagocyte system (circulating monocytes and tissular macrophages) and the dendritic cell system or antigen-presenting cells (APC) [1].

The cells of the histiocytic system (previously named the reticuloendothelial system) originate from a common granulocyte bone marrow precursor: the granulocyte–macrophage colony-forming unit [2].

The term histiocytosis includes all of the proliferative disorders of the bone marrow derived histiocytes and immune-related dendritic cells [3–6].

Three histiocytosis classes were defined in 1987 by the Histiocyte Society [7].

Class I: Langerhans' cell (LC) histiocytosis (LCH), probably due to an uncontrolled antigenic stimulation. Proliferating cells have specific cytoplasmic organelles (Birbeck granules) and specific surface antigens (CD1a).

Class II: histiocytosis of the mononuclear phagocyte system: (infection-associated and familial haemophagocytic syndromes), sinus histiocytosis with massive lymphadenopathy (Dorfman's disease) and benign skin histiocytosis, such as juvenile xanthogranuloma (JXG).

Class III: malignant clonal proliferation, such as acute monocytic leukaemia.

Langerhans' cell histiocytosis (class I histiocytosis)

History

LCH was probably first described by Smith in 1865 [8]. In 1853, Hand reported a syndrome with polyuria, believed at the time to be a form of tuberculosis. In 1915, Schüller described a disease that was characterized by lytic bone lesions in children. In 1920, Christian reported a syndrome with lytic bone lesions, exophthalmos and diabetes insipidus. Letterer in 1924 and Siwe in 1933 described a childhood disorder characterized by reticuloendothelial proliferation. In 1940, Lichtenstein described eosinophilic granuloma of the bone and in 1953 [9] suggested that eosinophilic granuloma, Letterer–Siwe disease and Hand–Schüller–Christian syndrome were manifestations of the same disease process. He named this disease 'histiocytosis X', because the specific nature of the involved histiocytes was not known. In 1965, Basset and Turiaf, and in 1966 Basset and Nezelof [10,11], described specific ultrastructural structures, which they believed were viral inclusions. However, these were in fact identical to the granules described by Birbeck et al. in 1961 [12]. In 1973, Nezelof et al. [13] reported that the lesions of histiocytosis X were due to a proliferation of histiocytic cells of the LC system; the name of this disease was then changed to LCH [14].

Pathogenesis and epidemiology

LCH is a rare disease, estimated to occur in 2–5 children per million per year [15–17]. The incidence is similar in the USA, Denmark and France. No racial predilection has been observed, and there is no evidence for a familial predisposition. In France, fewer than 50 new cases are seen each year [18]. Because spontaneous regression occurs, both skin and bone disease may go unnoticed or misdiagnosed [19].

Boys are affected more often than girls. LCH occurs most frequently in young children (aged 1–4 years), but it can be seen at any age. Children with LCH seem to have a higher incidence of congenital malformations [20]. LCH in twins or siblings is rare [21,22].

Physiology of Langerhans' cells

LCs are skin histiocytes with a specific antigen-presenting function [23,24]. Like all APCs, they have Fc receptors for immunoglobulins and lysosomes with specific enzymes. They express major histocompatibility class (MHC) II molecules. Immunohistochemistry reveals that the histiocytes in LCH are CD1a-antigen positive [25]. Electronmicroscopic (EM) evaluation shows specific bodies in the cytoplasm—Birbeck granules [11].

LCs originate from CD34 haematopoietic precursors that migrate in the suprabasal regions of the malpighian epithelium of the skin and mucous membranes. They are also found in T-cell areas of lymph nodes and the thymus. Like other histiocytes, they are large mononucleated cells with indented nuclei. Their dendritic cytoplasm expands between epithelial cells. On the ultrastructural level, specific cytoplasmic organelles, Birbeck granules, probably represent an invagination of the cell membrane. These organelles have a double membrane, and have been compared in shape to a tennis racket.

LC activation is part of the antigen-specific immune response [26]. Activated LCs take up and process antigens and migrate via lymphatics to the paracortical areas of the draining lymph nodes, where the antigen is presented to T lymphocytes. LCs are potent stimulators of antigen-specific and MHC-restricted T-cell response.

Certain adhesion molecules, such as LFA1, CD4 and B7-1, are normally seen in the T-cell area of the lymph node. These molecules are noted with greater frequency in LCH [27]. A loss of regulation of the cytokine cascade is thought to be responsible of LC proliferation.

Role of cytokines in Langerhans' cell histiocytosis

Proliferation, differentiation and activation of haematopoietic cells is regulated by cytokines [28]. *In vitro*, granulocyte–macrophage colony-stimulating factor (GM-CSF), tumour necrosis factor α (TNF-α), interleukin 4 (IL-4) and stem cell factor stimulate LC formation [29,30]. Normal LCs and LCs of LCH [31] have numerous GM-CSF receptors. GM-CSF induces differentiation and proliferation of human LC from haematopoietic progenitors [32], and can induce the local accumulation of LCs [33]. Children with disseminated and active LCH have elevated serum levels of GM-CSF [34], suggesting that GM-CSF is a growth factor for LCH cells. Other cytokines, including IL-2, may be involved in this process [35]. Most likely, the pathogenesis of LCH is multifactorial, with an underlying antigenic stimulation and an excessive host immune response [36]. LCH may be due to an alteration of adhesion molecule expression [37,38]. Initial LC proliferation may be caused by airborne antigen, such as tobacco smoke in adult pulmonary LCH [39], scabies infection [40] or a virus.

Role of viruses in Langerhans' cell histiocytosis

Several authors have suggested a viral aetiology for LCH. Leahy *et al.* noted the presence of human herpesvirus 6 in the lesional tissue of patients with LCH [41]. However,

this result was not confirmed by McClain *et al.* [42,43]. In addition, ultrastructural studies [44] reveal no evidence of viral infection.

Langerhans' cell histiocytosis as clonal proliferation?

Clonal proliferation was recently detected in LCH by molecular analysis of patterns of chromosome X-inactivation. This monoclonal LCH proliferation was found in both acute disseminated forms and unifocal diseases [45,46].

The presence of clonality does not prove LCH to be a malignant disorder. Clonal cells have been detected in such proliferative lesions as dermopathic lymphadenopathy [47]. The rarity of mitotic figures [14,48] and the highly differentiated appearance of the LC in LCH suggest that LCH is in fact a reactive proliferative disorder [49–52].

Although some patients with LCH have abnormal immunoglobulin levels [53], there is no constant and well-defined immune defect [54,55] in LCH.

Pathology

Light microscopy

The cells [56–69]. LCH is characterized by the presence of many LCs in lesional tissues [48]. The cytoplasm is large, homogeneous, pink with haematoxylin eosin staining and has numerous vacuoles. The nucleus is kidney-shaped, indented and eccentric, with an irregular granular chromatin pattern. Mitotic figures are rare. Histiocytic cells may form granulomas with central necrosis. Polymorphonuclear lymphocytes and mast cells are also found, together with lymphocytes and eosinophils. Eventually macrophages and multinucleated giant cells may predominate, especially in the bone and lymph node lesions.

Involved tissues. The most frequently affected organs are the skin, bone, bone marrow, lymph node, spleen, liver and lungs. In the skin, the infiltrate of abnormal cells is lichenoid, and is confined to the upper dermis. Epidermotropism may be present. The histological diagnosis of LCH must be confirmed by immunohistochemistry or EM [7].

Immunocytochemical studies

LCH cells express antigens present on normal LC (HLA-DR, Dq, CD1a, CD1b, CD1c, CD4, CD11a–LFA1, CD11b, CD24, CD32, CD68, ICAM3–CD50, CD58–LFA3, CD80–B7.1, C3b receptor, protein S100) and determinants of the monocyte macrophage lineage (CD11c, KP1, Mac 387 and others), lymphocytes (T3), natural killer cells (HNK1) and thymic prelymphocytes (OKT10). Other antigens, such as CD14, IL2 receptors and LN2–LN3, are also found [16,60,61].

CD1a antigen is consistently expressed in LCH. This antigen is identified by the use of monoclonal antibodies (obtained either by immunization of mice with human cortical thymocytes (OKT16) [62–65] or with proliferating cells of LCH [66]). In paraffin tissue CD1a may now be identified by monoclonal antibody [67,68]. CD1a antigen is found only on LCs, cortical thymocytes and some leukaemia cells.

Protein S100 (surface antigen) [69] is also positive in paraffin-embedded LCH tissue. Immunohistochemical expression of neurospecific enolase was found in 80% of histiocytic cells in LCH and was absent in non-LCH [70]. HLA-DR antigen is more often expressed in LCH LCs than in normal LCs [27]. LCH tissue produces a plasminogen activator which may facilitate cellular migration and tissue destruction [71]. Gamma interferon is expressed on the LCH cell surface and not on normal LCs [72]. LCH cells are proliferating cells and stain with antibody against antiproliferating cell nuclear antigen Ki 67 and the proliferation markers Ki S1 and PC10 [73].

Ultrastructure [74,75]

Birbeck granules are cytoplasmic lamellar plates with a central striation (rod-shaped bodies), sometimes with a terminal vesicular dilatation (tennis racket appearance). Birbeck granules occur in 20–80% of infiltrating cells in skin lesions and are less common in areas of visceral involvement. Birbeck granules may be localized by specific antibodies, such as anti-Lag [76]. Immunocytochemical stains for CD1a antigen may now be used to diagnose LCH without EM.

Proliferating histiocytic cells differ only slightly from normal LCs. They may be larger and more rounded, and contain fewer dendrites and more vacuoles. They have a more convoluted and clearer nucleus and contain more LC granules in a peripherical location. Cytoplasmic organelles are more numerous and cells are more often in mitosis than normal LCs. These ultrastructural findings are not specific for LCH and identical features are observed in LCs in other inflammatory disorders. Birbeck granules are absolutely specific for LC.

Clinical features

LCH has a wide spectrum of clinical manifestations, acute or chronic, disseminated or localized. Some lesions regress spontaneously and others herald the development of a life-threatening disorder [15,18,19,77–82].

Historical classification [9]

Clinical manifestations are historically separated into four clinical types: eosinophilic granuloma (chronic form), Hand–Schüller–Christian syndrome (subacute form), Letterer–Siwe disease (acute form) and Hashimoto–Pritzker self-healing LCH (benign neonatal form). These syndromes may overlap.

Solitary eosinophilic granuloma of bone is the most frequent and occurs mainly in adolescent boys and young adults. Flat bones (skull, pelvis, scapula, ribs, sternum) are more often involved than long bones (humerus, femur). The patient may have one or several lesions, which are either asymptomatic or cause localized pain. Fractures are rare.

Hand–Schüller–Christian syndrome occurs in children between 2 and 6 years of age. Lytic bone lesions are associated with diabetes insipidus (hypothalamic or pituitary localization) and exophthalmos (due to retro-ocular bone involvement). Skin lesions and other endocrinological manifestations may occur.

Letterer–Siwe disease is an acute and disseminated form of LCH, occurring in young children. Organ involvement may include the skin, bone, bone marrow, spleen, lymph nodes, liver and lung. Fever may be present. Cutaneous lesions are always present and are commonly the initial presentation.

Congenital self-healing histiocytosis (Hashimoto–Pritzker syndrome) (Figs 21.1.1–21.1.3) [83,84] usually features only cutaneous involvement. Skin lesions are nodular and less numerous than in Letterer–Siwe disease. Papulonodules have central necrosis and a characteristic peripheral rolled edge (elevated border) [85–89]. Multiple and superficial necrotic or vesicular lesions or small ulcerations may resemble those of chicken pox or other viral infections [90–92]. Visceral involvement is rare. The lesions may occur in crops, but complete spontaneous regression generally occurs in a few weeks or months [93]. Close follow-up is required over a period of many months, because some patients with the Hashimoto–Pritzker phenotype go on to develop visceral involvement and even the life-threatening Letterer–Siwe disease [91,94–98]. There is no specific histopathological feature of Hashimoto–Pritzker disease. However, LC granules appear to be less numerous (5–20% of histiocytic cells) and histiocytic organelles (e.g. dense or lamellar bodies, pleiomorphic inclusions, comma bodies) are more frequent in Hashimoto–Pritzker syndrome than in other forms of histiocytosis. Birbeck granules may be absent [99].

The clinician must remember that the different forms of LCH have no specific histological, immunological or ultrastructural findings. The clinical presentations may overlap and the disease may occasionally progress from one form to another [100].

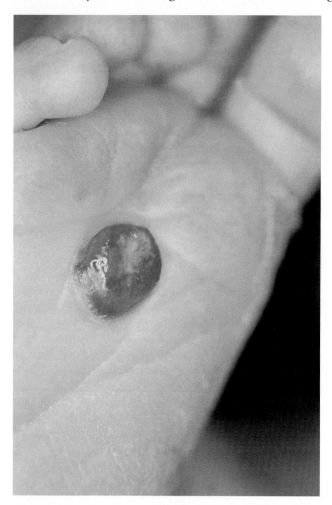

Fig. 21.1.1 Single neonatal lesion of Hashimoto–Pritzker.

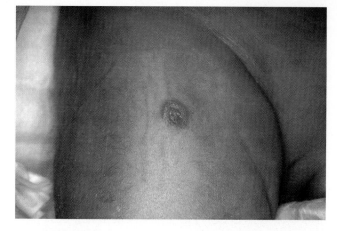

Fig. 21.1.3 Typical lesion of Hashimoto–Pritzker (central necrosis, elevated borders).

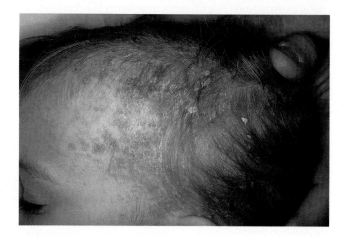

Fig. 21.1.4 LCH: scalp involvement.

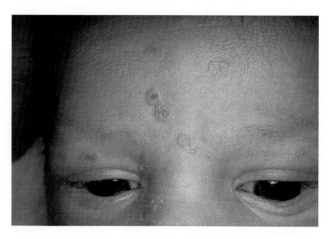

Fig. 21.1.2 Hashimoto–Pritzker: neonatal umbilicated lesion.

Clinical manifestations of LCH (by organ system)

Cutaneous lesions. Skin lesions are common (40% of LCH [18]) and are often the presenting manifestation of LCH [101,102] (Figs 21.1.4–21.1.9). These preferentially involve the trunk, scalp, napkin area and intertriginal folds. On the trunk, lesions may favour the mid-back, sparing the shoulders.

At first presentation, the erythematous pink or brown papules may be subtle and go unnoticed. Over time, these papules may become scaly, crusted or purpuric, and may become confluent. Petechiae and xanthomatous lesions may evolve.

Lesions may be pruritic and are often misdiagnosed as atopic dermatitis or infantile seborrhoeic dermatitis.

On the scalp, the scaly eruption may become exudative and encrusted. Lesions may coalesce and result in alopecia. The removal of the scale or crust may result in bleeding, a helpful diagnostic sign.

In intertriginal areas, papules and vesicles may coalesce to form superficial ulcerations and weeping lesions.

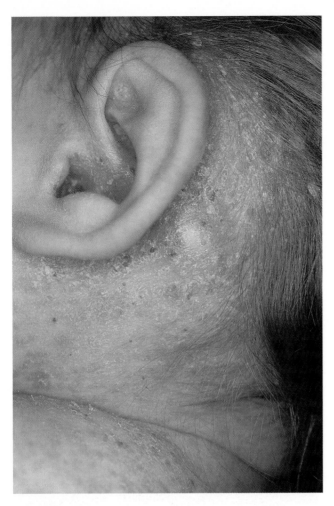

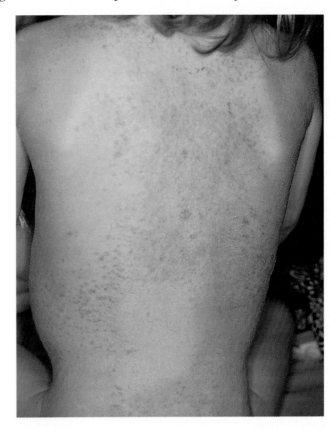

Fig. 21.1.6 LCH: distribution on the back.

Fig. 21.1.5 LCH: periauricular lesions.

graphic evaluation is necessary, and must be repeated at intervals.

Bone lesions [108–111]. Bone lesions are the most frequent manifestation of LCH (80%) [18,82] (Fig. 21.1.10). Bone involvement alone occurs in 50–60% of cases [18] and is seen most commonly in older children and young adults. Bone lesions are often asymptomatic. However, painful swelling, bone deformation, fracture or medullar compression may occur. Only one or two lesions may develop, (30% of LCH) [18] and spontaneous resolution may occur within a few months to a year. Diagnosis may be confirmed by surgical curettage or simple needle aspiration [112].

The skull is the most frequently affected bone. Most characteristically, radiographic examination reveals single or multiple punched-out lesions in the cranial vault. Chronic otitis media with mastoid necrosis, otorrhoea, vestibular syndrome and external otitis may occur [113]. Mastoid involvement resembles infectious mastoiditis and extension to the middle ear causes deafness by destruction of the ossicles. In the jaw bone destruction occurs and is accompanied by gingival swelling, floating teeth and pain. Orbital wall involvement may lead to proptosis.

Fissures are seen behind the ears, in the ear canal and in axillary and inguinal folds. There is often involvement of the perianal area and around the vaginal orifice. Superinfection may occur and older lesions may become verrucous and haemorrhagic.

Nodular lesions may develop in the periorificial areas or on the gums. Necrotic and ulcerative lesions in the mouth may lead to loosening of the teeth [103]. Premature eruption of teeth may be the first manifestation of LCH. Involvement of the female genital tract may occur (vulva, vagina, cervix, endometrium or ovary) [104,105].

Nail involvement is recognized [106,107]. Friable nails, longitudinal grooving, pigmented and purpuric striae, hyperkeratosis, subungual pustules, paronychia, onychorrhexis and onycholysis have all been noted. Permanent nail dystrophy may occur.

Pure cutaneous LCH may spontaneously regress. However, this form may evolve, even after many years, to systemic involvement. Even in the presence of a normal clinical examination, laboratory and radio-

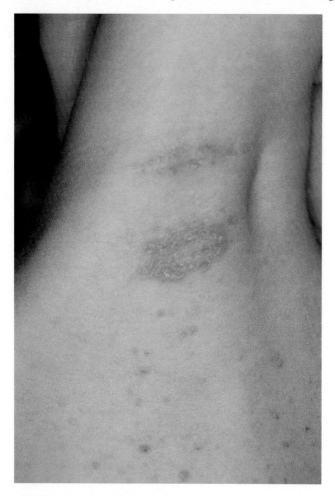

Fig. 21.1.7 LCH: flexural involvement.

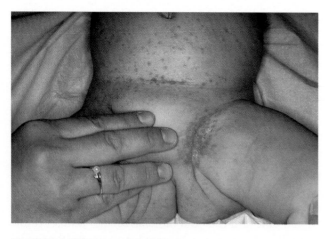

Fig. 21.1.8 LCH: groin and napkin area.

In the spine [114], compression fractures of the vertebral bodies are seen (vertebra plana). The long bone (femur, humerus) may also be involved and lytic lesions with irregular borders are noted.

For the evaluation of bone involvement, magnetic reso-

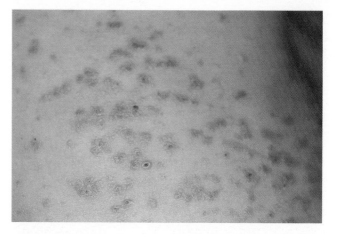

Fig. 21.1.9 LCH: close-up of typical lesions—encrusted papules.

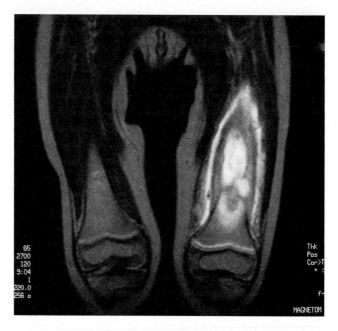

Fig. 21.1.10 LCH: MRI showing bone and muscle involvement.

nance imaging (MRI) has no advantage over conventional X-ray. However, isotopic bone scan is useful in looking for multiple lesions.

Bone marrow involvement is rare and occurs late in the course of the disease [115]. Anaemia, thrombocytopenia, leucopenia or pancytopenia may result from bone marrow dysfunction.

Pulmonary lesions. Pulmonary lesions [116–118] are frequent (12–23% of LCH) [18,80], especially in older patients. Clinical manifestations include cough, thoracic pain, tachypnoea with rib retraction, associated with fever and weight loss. Mediastinal compression may occur [119]. In later disease, bulla formation may lead to

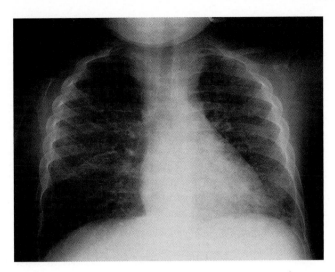

Fig. 21.1.11 LCH: honeycomb lung involvement.

pneumothorax. Emphysematous changes with diffuse interstitial fibrosis may also occur.

Chest X-ray shows diffuse micronodules and later a miliary interstitial or reticulonodular pattern [120–122] (Fig. 21.1.11). Computed tomography (CT) scan is helpful in defining the degree of lung involvement.

To diagnose LCH by bronchoalveolar lavage, more than 5% of LCs must be detected by EM or immunostaining: 1% of LCs may be found in normal lungs and are not indicative of disease [123,124].

Liver/spleen lesions. The liver and spleen are involved in 15–50% of LCH [18,80]. Hepatosplenomegaly may be due to portal infiltration with LCs, Kupffer cell hyperplasia with activation of the cellular immune system or a compression of portal nodes with obstructive hepatopathy. Initial mild cholestasis may progress to sclerosing cholangitis [125,126], severe fibrosis, biliary cirrhosis [127] and liver failure. Hypoalbuminaemia with ascites, jaundice and prolonged prothrombin time may be found. Splenomegaly may increase the severity of thrombocytopenia. Successful liver transplant has been accomplished [128–130].

Gastrointestinal lesions. The frequency of gastrointestinal tract involvement is often underestimated. This may present with non-specific manifestations, such as abdominal pain, vomiting, diarrhoea, duodenal ulcer or protein-losing enteropathy. Failure to thrive may result from malabsorption [131–134]. Symptoms are due to massive mucosal infiltration and this clinical development indicates a poor prognosis.

Radiographic studies may show dilated and stenotic segments in the small and large bowel. Endoscopic biopsy is used to confirm the diagnosis.

Lymph nodes. Cervical lymph nodes are the most often affected. Lymph node involvement may be seen in LCH which is otherwise restricted to bone or skin.

Endocrine glands and growth retardation [135]. Diabetes insipidus [136] is the most common endocrine manifestation and mainly seen in patients with skull involvement and extensive disease. CT examination and gadolinium-enhanced MRI show thickening of the hypothalamopituitary region and bone alterations. Diabetes insipidus must be evaluated by a water deprivation test and measurement of urinary arginine vasopressin.

The pancreas, thyroid and gonads may also be affected by infiltration of LCs. The thymus is often involved and thymic enlargement may be visible on routine chest X-ray [137,138].

Growth hormone deficiency caused by anterior pituitary involvement is rare [139]. However, growth retardation is common in children with LCH and is most often due to steroid therapy and chemotherapy, malabsorption and general illness.

Central nervous system [140,141]. Cerebral LCH is not common. Clinical manifestations are progressive and most frequent in patients with skull involvement and diabetes insipidus. Most commonly the hypothalamo-pituitary region is involved, resulting in various endocrinopathies. Hypothalamic involvement may cause anterior panhypopituitarism without diabetes insipidus [142]. In this case, MRI is used to localize the tumour [143].

Progressive intellectual deficit, encephalopathy, spastic paraplegia and tetraplegia, ataxia, pyramidal tract signs, tremor, dysarthria, blurred vision or cranial nerve deficit can occur [18]. Acute manifestations, such as seizures or intracranial hypertension are unusual. Lesions are found with MRI first in the cerebellum and then in the paraventricular cerebral white matter [144]. Disseminated cerebral LCH may respond to chemotherapy [145].

Prognosis

Prognosis of Langerhans' cell histiocytosis

The evolution of LCH is unpredictable. The prognosis is related to the age of onset, the rate of disease progression and the number of organ systems involved. Organ dysfunction (liver, bone marrow and lung), occurring in about 15% of LCH, is the most important predictor of poor outcome [146–150].

In a large retrospective study [18], the overall survival rate was 90% at 4 years, with a median age at diagnosis of 8.5 months. The median time between diagnosis and death was 1 year. In children under 2 years of age with organ dysfunction, the mortality rate may be as high as 50–65%. In all cases, the histopathological features are not predictive and the prognosis is based on clinical features.

Involutive neonatal LCH generally regresses spontaneously in a few weeks or months. However, no single clinical, histological, immunological or ultrastructural feature rules out the rare evolution to Letterer–Siwe disease.

Solitary eosinophilic granuloma of bone, treated with curettage or radiotherapy, has a favourable prognosis [151]. However, rarely, patients with bone involvement may progress to Letterer–Siwe disease.

In cases of Letterer–Siwe disease which are clinically restricted to the skin, careful initial and follow-up evaluation is required in order to detect the true extent of disease. Forms of organ dysfunction which are associated with a poor prognosis are: (a) lung dysfunction (i.e. cough, dyspnoea or tachypnaea, cyanosis, radiological interstitial syndrome, pneumothorax or pleural effusion); (b) haematopoietic dysfunction (i.e. anaemia not due to infection or iron deficiency, leucopenia, neutropenia or thrombocytopenia); (c) liver dysfunction (i.e. hypoproteinaemia not due to protein-losing enteropathy, ascites, oedema, hyperbilirubinaemia and prolonged prothrombin time); and (d) hypercalcaemia (sometimes due to bone resorption or excess prostaglandin production). For this reason, indomethacin, an inhibitor of prostaglandin production, is sometimes a good treatment for hypercalcaemia and bone pain [152].

Immunolocalization, using an [111]I-labelled murine monoclonal antibody against CD1a antigen, may be used to detect the extent of disease [153,154]. Likewise, serum GM-CSF is elevated in some patients with disseminated disease, but not in those with localized bone disease or disease in remission [34].

The rapidity and the intensity of the clinical response to initial treatment is an indicator of prognosis [18,155]. In one study, only three of 299 patients who responded rapidly to therapy died of their disease. By contrast, LCH was fatal in 12 of 36 patients who had a partial response to treatment and in all 13 patients who had an unfavourable response [18].

After completion of the proliferating and destructive phase, the scarring fibrotic process may lead to severe sequelae. These are often more frequent than originally thought, from 20 to 50%, and do not always correlate with the apparent severity of the disease [18,156].

Hepatic sequelae include sclerosis, cholangitis, cirrhosis and hepatocellular failure. The presence of cholestasis requires the use of echography and transhepatic cholangiography to determine the presence of sclerosing cholangitis. In some cases, ursodesoxycholic acid has prevented the evolution to cirrhosis [157].

Endocrinological sequelae include diabetes insipidus. This complication has a 36% incidence in patients treated conservatively and a 15% incidence following multiple-drug chemotherapy. Diabetes insipidus can be treated with desmopressin (1-desamino-8-D-arginine vasopressin).

Other sequelae are growth hormone deficiency, decreased intelligence, neurological symptoms, pulmonary insufficiency and orthopaedic disabilities.

Careful staging is performed to ensure the absence of disseminated LHC. The extent of evaluation depends on the clinical severity [158]. The older child with bone lesions may require only chest and skeletal radiographs, a complete blood count and assays of liver function. Children with Letterer–Siwe syndrome, and those under the are of 2 years, require a chest CT scan to look for early lung lesions and a bone marrow analysis for the presence of CD1a cells.

Systematic investigation should be repeated at least every 6 months until 2 years after the completion of treatment. This evaluation should include weight, height, sedimentation rate, serum glucose, C-reactive protein, haemoglobin, leucocyte and platelet count, liver function tests, coagulation studies, iron, ferritin, chest radiograph and abdominal ultrasonography. Other investigations that are required under specific circumstances are bone marrow aspiration or biopsy, skeletal survey, urine osmolality after water deprivation, growth hormone, thyroid-stimulating hormone, ear, nose and throat examination, audiogram, brain MRI, bronchoalveolar lavage, lung biopsy, small bowel biopsy and liver biopsy (Table 21.1.1).

Prognosis of intercurrent diseases

A large number of other diseases have been described in association with LCH, although some of these may be coincidental. These include benign mediastinal teratoma, neonatal encephalopathy, Hirschsprung's disease, von Willebrand's disease, myasthenia gravis, multicystic renal dysplasia and intestinal fistula [18].

The association of LCH with malignant neoplasms is not unusual. In 1991, 10 cases of solid tumours were reported [159]. Egeler *et al.* [160] described 30 solid tumours associated with LCH, including 12 lung tumours. Half of the tumours occurred after resolution of LCH and 70% in radiation fields. Other tumours reported include coeliomesenteric neuroblastoma [18] or apudoma [161]. Malignant lymphomas and acute leukaemias are also associated with LCH [162]. In 1991, four malignant lymphomas and 13 acute leukaemias were noted by the Histiocyte Society [159]. Acute lymphoblastic leukaemias may precede LCH (four out of five). In these cases, LCH may be a reactive process. Acute myeloid leukaemias, probably a result of therapy, usually follow LCH and may occur more than 2 years after the resolution of histiocytosis. The French LCH study group [18] reported a case of acute T-lymphoblastic leukaemia 3 years after a single

Table 21.1.1 Investigations in LCH

Systematic investigations		Specific investigations	Indication
Every 6 months	Every month if involved		
		Small bowel series and biopsy	Malabsorption
Hb, leucocyte, platelet count	Hb, leucocyte, platelet count	Bone marrow biopsy	
Liver function tests	Liver function tests	Liver biopsy	To determine LCH cirrhosis
Coagulation studies	Coagulation studies		
Chest radiograph	Chest radiograph	Pulmonary function tests Bronchoalveolar lavage	Tachypnoea; before chemotherapy
		Lung biopsy	To exclude opportunistic infection
Skeletal radiograph survey			
Urine osmolality after water deprivation		Brain MRI	Hormonal abnormalities; visual abnormalities; neurological abnormalities
		Endocrine evaluation; growth hormone; thyroid-stimulating hormone	Short stature; hypothalamic syndrome; galactorrhoea, precocious puberty
		Otorhinolaryngology, audiogram	Aural discharge, deafness

untreated episode of bone involvement. Similarly, Arico *et al.* [163] reported a case of acute lymphoblastic leukaemia after untreated LCH. In 1993, Egeler *et al.* [160] found 39 malignant lymphomas (25 Hodgkin's lymphomas); 11 lymphomas were followed by LCH (1–33 years after); 24 lymphomas occurred concurrently with LCH; and four lymphomas occurred 0.5–2 years after LCH. Leukaemias were found in 22 cases: LCH was followed by leukaemia in 14 cases (1–17 years after); leukaemia preceded LCH in two cases and both occurred concurrently in six cases.

In conclusion, LCH may in some cases be considered as a reactive process associated with malignancy. Neoplasms may also be related to chemotherapy [164] or radiotherapy [165] for LCH.

Differential diagnosis

The clinical appearance of LCH is distinctive. However, it is a rare disease and is often misdiagnosed early in its course.

LCH is most often confused with seborrhoeic dermatitis. This disorder is characterized by superficial crusts in the scalp and intertriginal areas. However, it lacks the discrete clusters of purpuric and encrusted lesions seen in LCH.

Atopic dermatitis is generally more pruritic than LCH. In addition, it tends to resolve dramatically in response to topical corticosteroids. The lesions are more superficial, less infiltrated and rarely purpuric.

Candidiasis and tinea capitis both may cause scaling and erythema in areas typically affected by LCH. Both

may superinfect lesions of histiocytosis [166]. In the newborn, vesicular lesions of LCH may be confused with varicella or herpes simplex infection. In more unusual cases, LCH has been noted to resemble lichen aureus [167], cherry angioma [168], flat warts [169], hidradenitis suppurativa [170] or other skin tumours [171]. In these cases careful skin examination and skin or bone biopsy allow for the correct diagnosis.

Treatment

Treatment of LCH is determined by the extent of visceral organ involvement. As LCH is a rare disease, with variable clinical manifestations and prognosis, treatments are diverse. A standardized staging classification has facilitated the evaluation of treatments in multicentre studies.

Isolated skin involvement may regress spontaneously especially in infants. When treatment is elected, topical steroids may be effective. Topical therapy with nitrogen mustard is often effective and may succeed even after failure of systemic therapy [172–176]. Generally, improvement occurs within 10 days and resolution between 2 or 3 weeks. Erythema or irritation may occur, but hypersensitivity reactions, such as urticaria or contact dermatitis, are rare. Nitrogen mustard may cause skin pigmentation. Psoralens and ultraviolet A (PUVA) therapy [177] and irradiation [178,179] are also effective, but may be unwise in the treatment of children.

Isolated bone involvement may resolve spontaneously and resolution of lesions may follow bone biopsy (with or without curettage). In the presence of one or two lesions, therapy may be deferred. Other possible approaches include intratumoural steroid or interferon injection [179–184]. Active therapy is especially indicated if the lesions are painful. Bernstrand *et al.* [182] treated six children from 6 months to 7 years of age with intralesional steroids. The time to relief of symptoms was from 1 day to 1 month and the radiographic resolution from 1 to 8 months. Injection into jaw lesions was somewhat less successful. No complications were observed.

Surgical treatment may be used in cases of deformity or fracture. Radiation therapy [178,179] is used less frequently, and carries significant danger of a delayed secondary tumour within the radiation field (malignant meningioma, thyroid cancer) [18] and growth impairment.

In cases where there is neurological risk (e.g. compressive vertebral lesion or ocular compression), possibilities include surgical decompression [185], or if the lesion is inoperable, radiation therapy or systemic steroid and chemotherapy. Additional treatment is also required in cases of bone growth impairment, loss of permanent teeth and hearing loss.

If LCH is present in more than three sites, systemic therapy is required. Children with severe bone or multivisceral involvement have been treated with either monotherapy or combination therapy [149,150]. Agents include vinblastine (VBL) [145,186–189], vincristine [189, 190], steroids [188], methotrexate [190], chlorambucil [191], cyclophosphamide [189], cytarabine [161], daunorubicine, chlormetine, procarbazine, 6-mercaptopurine (6-MP) [186,188], VP16 (etoposide) [81,187] and more recently cyclosporin and interferon.

Because of the heterogeneity of LCH, objective response to various regimens of chemotherapy is difficult to evaluate and compare. In all cases after chemotherapy, GM-CSF should be avoided as it may cause LC proliferation [20].

The combination of VBL and steroids is often used [18]. Lahey's non-randomized study [188] (83 patients) showed no appreciable difference between treatment with VBL alone, VBL plus steroids and 6-MP plus steroids.

In 1990, McLelland [192] attempted a more conservative treatment protocol. Among 58 LCH patients, 44 had multisystem disease (22 with vital organ dysfunction). Seventeen patients were treated with prednisone alone, and 19 with short-term chemotherapy. Eight patients died, 24 had sequelae and 12 no long-term sequelae. These results were felt to be equivalent to those achieved by more aggressive treatment with longer term combination chemotherapy.

In 1993, Egeler *et al.* [161] observed complete remission in 63% of eight patients with multiorgan dysfunction. The treatment regimen consisted of cytosine arabinoside, vincristine and prednisolone. The Italian Cooperative Study [81] of 1993 (91 patients) noted 45% survival at 48 months among 11 patients with organ dysfunction. All were treated with vincristine, doxorubicine and prednisone. There was 100% survival among 79 patients with good prognosis; 59 of them were treated with VBL and then, if necessary, doxorubicine and VP16.

The multicentre prospective German study (DAL HX-83 study group) of 106 patients [186] showed that early treatment with long-term maintenance therapy improves the outcome of LCH. Patients were divided into three groups: A (multifocal bone disease, $n = 28$), B (soft tissue involvement with or without bone involvement, $n = 56$); and C (organ dysfunction, $n = 21$). Induction therapy for all groups consisted of VP16, followd by VP16, VBL and prednisone for 6 weeks. Subsequently, all groups received 6-MP and VBL for 1 year. Group B also received VP16, and group C also received VP16 and methotrexate. The initial response rate was high (85%) and the recurrence rate was low (23% versus 65% in other studies). In the high-risk group, survival was 62% (versus 30–50% in other studies), late complications were 15% (versus 50% in other studies) and iatrogenic complications were rare (no leukaemia after 7 years).

The iatrogenic complications of chemotherapy may be signficant. Inhibitors of topoisomerase II (epipodophyllotoxins—etoposide, teniposide—and anthracyclines) which are very effective in the treatment of malignancies of the monocyte–macrophage lineage have been successful in the treatment of LCH [193–197]. However, the combination of etoposide and prednisolone may induce hypofibrinogenaemia [198], most likely be reducing the production of fibrinogen in the liver. Most importantly, this drug especially if cumulative doses exceed 4000 mg/m^2, carries a significant risk of causing acute myeloid leukaemia [159,164,199,200]. Therefore, this drug should be reserved for the treatment of LCH which is severe and resistant to other therapies [201,202].

Cyclosporin may act by its action on transcription and synthesis of lymphokines, inhibition of IL2 and interferon-γ secretion and its consequent effect on dendritic cells. Since its first use in 1991 [203,204], it has been used effectively in some patients. Chlorodeoxyadenosine has a specific cytotoxic effect on monocytes and control of immune-mediated cytokine release. It may be effective for refractory LH [205–207]. Interferon has been used [22,208–210], alone or in combination with etretinate [211]. Administrations of thymic extract [55,212,213] did not result in reproducible positive outcomes. Thalidomide has been shown to be effective in the treatment of skin lesions in adults [214,215]. The use of monoclonal antibody against the CD1a antigen [216] requires further investigation.

Bone marrow transplantation from identical HLA donors, or autotransplantation with CD1$^+$ depleted bone marrow, was effective in six of eight cases of severe LCH [18,217–219]. Liver transplantation has been performed to treat major hepatic sclerotic sequelae [128–130].

Non-malignant non-Langerhans' cell histiocytosis (class II histiocytosis)

Class II histiocytoses are separated into the systemic and cutaneous histiocytoses.

Systemic class II histiocytosis

These histiocytoses are generally treated by paediatric oncologists. A brief classification follows [5,6].

Acquired haemophagocytic syndromes (HS). HSs are forms of histiocytic hyperplasia with medullary haemophagocytosis, with or without immunodeficiency. They may be due to a viral infection—mainly Epstein–Barr virus (EBV) and other herpes virus, including cytomegalovirus (CMV)—other serious infections (such as brucellosis, tuberculosis and kala-azar), inflammatory diseases (juvenile chronic arthritis, systemic lupus erythematosus) or to primary immunodeficiency (severe combined immunodeficiency, Chediak–Higashi disease with accelerated lymphoma phase, X-linked lymphoproliferative syndrome and others) to pre-existing malignancies (acute lymphoblastic leukaemia, Hodgkin's disease, acute non-lymphoblastic leukaemia) or only to long-term use of lipid emulsion.

Inappropriate activation of the macrophage lineage and a primary or acquired T-cell disorder leads to a hypercytokinetic state. Hypofibrinogenaemia results from increased plasminogen activator, hypertriglyceridaemia from TNF-β and cytopenia from inflammatory cytokines.

The severe clinical features consist of high spiking fever, failure to thrive, hepatomegaly, generalized lymphadenopathy, haemorrhage and jaundice. Therapy depends on aetiological factors. Treatment of a documented infection, high-dose steroids, etoposide, plasmapheresis and intravenous immunoglobulins may be beneficial. Lipid macrophage activation is reversible by steroids. Chediak–Higashi syndrome should be treated by bone marrow transplantation.

Familial haemophagocytic lymphohistiocytosis is a rapidly fatal autosomal recessive inherited condition. It is apparently due to an intrinsic T-cell defect and an uncontrolled secretion of cytokines, with resultant proliferation of the macrophage–phagocyte system. Clinical features are identical to infection-associated HS: fever, haemorrhagic diathesis, pancytopenia and neurological deterioration. Histiocytic infiltration of multiple organs is noted. Therapy consists of steroids, etoposide, intrathecal infiltration of methotrexate or antithymocyte globulins and cyclosporin. Bone marrow transplantation offers the only possibility of cure.

Rosai–Dorfman disease (RDD) (or sinusal histiocytosis with massive lymphadenopathy) is a benign disorder which most often resolves after several months without treatment [220]. Rarely, it can evolve to malignant lymphoma. RDD seems to be due to a viral agent, perhaps EBV. Clinical signs include a massive indolent cervical lymphadenopathy with low-grade fever and night sweats, weight loss and malaise. Eyelid, orbital and mediastinal sites of involvement have been reported.

Skin lesions consist of well-circumscribed red–brown or red–yellow papules, nodules or plaques, sometimes with a lumpy appearance [221].

An associated inflammatory syndrome consists of elevated white blood count, polyclonal hypergammaglobulinaemia, haemolytic anaemia and glomerulopathy.

Lymph node biopsy is characterized by a histiocytic sinusal infiltration of benign cells with lymphocytophagocytosis and plasmocyte infiltration.

Progressive forms are treated with chemotherapy or radiation therapy. Aciclovir is sometimes effective [222].

Multicentric reticulohistiocytosis is rare in children [223]. Skin lesions consist of papules or nodules, which occasionally evolve to form mutilating sclerosing lesions. Pathology shows a histiocytic granuloma associated with giant cells, activated T lymphocytes and macrophages. This reactive histiocytic proliferation may regress spontaneously.

Arthritis, occurring a few years before or a few months after the skin lesions, affects the interphalangeal joints of the hands, knees, shoulders and wrists. Joint destruction may occur. Other abnormalities include elevated erythrocyte sedimentation rate [50%], anaemia and hypercholesterolaemia [30%].

Therapy with non-steroidal anti-inflammatory drugs, cyclosporin and immunosuppressive agents are disappointing. Steroids and alkylating agents may be effective. Methotrexate is sometimes effective in adult patients [224].

Cutaneous class II histiocytosis

The cutaneous class II histiocytoses are biologically benign and often regress spontaneously [3,4,225–227]. The pathophysiology of these lesions is unknown and their classification is based on clinical and pathological description.

Juvenile xanthogranuloma

Definition

JXG is a benign self-healing non-LCH characterized by an accumulation of lipid-laden macrophages. JXG is not associated with disorders of lipid metabolism.

History

Helwig and Hackney (1954) introduced the term JXG as an alternative to the term naevoxanthoendothelioma.

Pathogenesis

JXG occurs in young children with an equal sex ratio. The involved cells are dermal macrophages.

Pathology

In early lesions, histiocytes predominate. Other inflammatory cells (lymphocytes, eosinophils, plasma cells and neutrophils) may be present [228–230]. CD1a staining is negative and Birbeck granules are not found on EM.

In well-developed lesions, histiocytes have foamy cytoplasm and multinucleated Touton giant cells are present. These cells express Ki M1P, KP1 and anticathepsin B. Eosinophils and neutrophils are scattered throughout the infiltrate. In long-standing lesions, fibroblasts are conspicuous with areas of fibrosis.

Clinical features

The lesions typically appear before the age of 1 year and they may be present at birth (Figs 21.1.12). The number and size tends to increase during the first 18 months of life.

Lesions are smooth, firm, dome-shaped papules or nodules. Initially red (Fig. 21.1.13), they eventually develop the typical yellow–orange coloration (Fig. 21.1.14) [229,230]. Lesions may be single or multiple, congenital [20%] or acquired. Size varies from a few millimetres to several centimetres. Lesions are often localized to the head and neck and occur less often on the trunk and the extensor surface of the extremities. Two main clinical forms have been described. A small nodular form (60%)

and a large nodular form (40%). Mixed forms and JXG 'en plaque' have been described [231].

The solitary giant congenital form is initially shiny and purple–red in colour [232–234]. There is often central ulceration, crusting and peripheral telangiectasia.

Prognosis

JXG most often regresses spontaneously over a period of 3–6 years. Lesions become more yellow and brown, less elevated and result in a small area of scarring. Systemic involvement of the lung [235,236], spleen or liver [237]

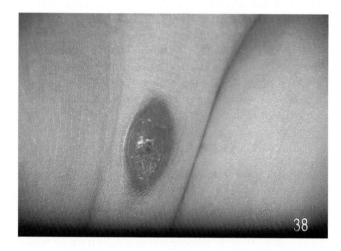

Fig. 21.1.13 Red colour of an early JXG.

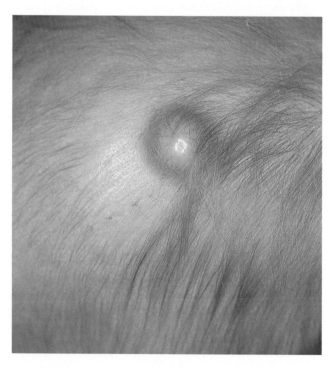

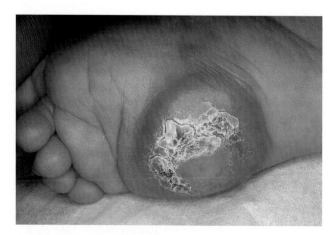

Fig. 21.1.12 Giant congenital JXG.

Fig. 21.1.14 Typical yellow appearance of a mature JXG.

(spontaneous regression of hepatic nodules) or central nervous system [238] is rare. A lethal form, with aggressive nervous system lesions, hypertension and hydrocephalus, has been described.

Eye involvement results in ocular hypertonia and hyphema; these may regress with systemic steroid therapy [239].

The combined occurrence of JXG and café-au-lait spots (neurofibromatosis type 1) suggests an increased risk for myelomonocytic leukaemia [240,241].

Benign cephalic histiocytosis

Benign cephalic histiocytosis (BCH) [242–244] was described by Gianotti and Caputo in 1971. Skin lesions occur between 2 and 34 months of age, with a male to female ratio of 2:1.

Lesions occur initially on the head (forehead and cheeks) (Fig. 21.1.15) and sometimes spread to the neck and shoulders. There are no mucosal or visceral lesions. Maculopapules are yellow–brown, and range from 2 to 4 mm in diameter. They flatten with time, and over years resolve into atrophic pigmented macules.

Histological studies show a histiocytic infiltrate in the

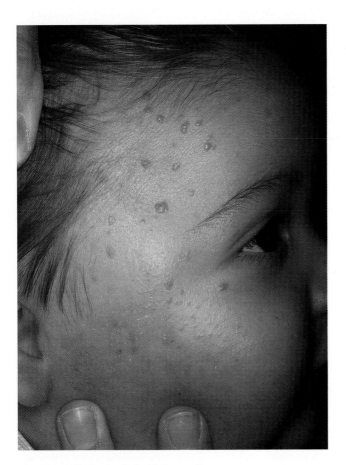

Fig. 21.1.15 Benign cephalic histiocytosis.

upper and middle dermis that is S100 and CD1a negative, and OKM and Leu 3 positive. Lymphocytes and a few eosinophils are also present. EM shows histiocytic organelles, comma-shaped or S-shaped worm-like bodies and desmosome-like junctions. Birbeck granules and lipid droplets are absent.

The main differential diagnoses are the micronodular form of xanthogranuloma (where foamy cells and Touton giant multinucleated cells are present) and generalized eruptive histiocytoma. BCH may be confused with facial flat warts.

This asymptomatic and self-healing disorder does not require treatment.

Generalized eruptive histiocytoma

Generalized eruptive histiocytoma (GEH) [245,246] is a self-healing histiocytosis that is uncommon in children. Skin lesions consist of numerous (50 to 1000) small, smooth, yellow or pink–brown papules that appear in successive crops, mainly on the trunk, face and proximal limbs. There is no pruritus or visceral involvement. The disorder resolves spontaneously over a period of several years.

GEH has the same histology as benign cephalic histiocytosis, but lesions are more extensive and mucosal membranes can be involved. On EM, no desmosome-like intercellular junctions are present. However, dense lamina and worm-like bodies and pleiomorphic inclusions are seen.

Papular xanthoma

Skin lesions [3] are yellowish papulonodular lesions from 2 to 15 mm in diameter. These non-coalescent lesions occur on skin or mucous membranes. Histological features are those of mature JXG. Involution occurs in several years.

Xanthema disseminatum

Xanthema disseminatum (XD) [3] is a rare benign form of histiocytoxanthomatosis. Skin involvement consists of hundreds of red–brown and then yellowish papules on the trunk, face and flexures. These lesions may merge into plaques. The eyelids, conjunctivae, lips, pharynx and larynx are typically infiltrated with red or yellow plaques. Diabetes insipidus is present in half of the cases. Lipid metabolism is often normal. Foamy cells and histiocytes are seen on histopathological studies. In the self-healing form, skin lesions and endocrine abnormalities resolve in several years. However, persistent and disfiguring forms do exist.

Unclassified histiocytosis

Various distinctive nodular histiocytoses have been described. These may be self-healing or require steroid therapy [247,248]. The progressive nodular form [249] may result in leonine facial features, and peculiar cytoplasmic inclusions have been reported [250]. The term multiple reticulohistiocytoma [251] has been replaced by progressive nodular histiocytosis [3].

Class III histiocytosis

True histiocytic lymphomas [252,253], that are clonal proliferations of malignant histiocytosis, are very rare in childhood. They have to be differentiated from monocytic leukaemias.

Acute monocytic leukaemia (M5) and acute myelomonocytic leukaemia (M4) show specific cutaneous lesions in 20% of cases. This is the highest incidence of specific cutaneous infiltrations among all leukaemias. Clinical manifestations are light-red or brown macules to red–violet macules with rapid development and spontaneous involution. Gingival infiltration is frequent (50%). Cutaneous and mucosal infiltrations are not related to the number of leucocytes in the peripheral blood and local factors seem to interfere.

Malignant histiocytosis [254–257] was previously considered to be a malignant proliferation of monocyte–macrophage origin. In fact, this proliferation is of lymphoid origin as proved by immunocytochemical and molecular investigation: they are Ki+ (CD30+ anaplastic large cell lymphoma, most of them of T-cell lineage [258,259].

Although rare, histiocytic malignancies do exist, but this diagnosis should be made only after careful correlation of atypical tumour cells in sections stained immunohistochemically: CD45 (leucocyte common antigen), CD20 (L26) for B cells, CD3 and CD45 Ro (UCHL-1) for T cells, CD68 (KP-1) and lysozyme for histiocyte, CD30 (Ber H2) for Ki-1 positive cells.

REFERENCES

1 Cline MJ. Histiocytes and histiocytosis. *Blood* 1994; 84: 2840–53.
2 Foucar K, Foucar E. The mononuclear phagocyte and immunoregulatory effector (M-PIRE) system: evolving concepts. *Semin Diagn Pathol* 1990; 7: 4–18.
3 Gianotti F, Caputo R. Histiocytic syndromes: a review. *J Am Acad Dermatol* 1985; 13: 383–404.
4 Roper SS, Spraker MK. Cutaneous histiocytosis syndromes. *Pediatr Dermatol* 1985; 3: 19–30.
5 Stephan JL. Histiocytoses. *Eur J Pediatr* 1995; 154: 600–9.
6 Snow JL, Su WP. Histiocytic diseases. *J Am Acad Dermatol* 1995; 33: 111–16.
7 Writing Group of the Histiocyte Society (Chu T, D'Angio GJ, Favara B, Ladisch S, Nesbit M, Pritchard J). Histiocytosis syndromes in children. *Lancet* 1987; i: 208–9.
8 Komp DK. Historical perspectives of Langerhans' cell histiocytosis. *Hematol Oncol Clin N Am* 1987; 1: 9–21.
9 Lichtenstein L. Histiocytosis X: integration of eosinophilic granuloma of bone, 'Letterer–Siwe disease' and 'Schüller–Christian disease' as related manifestations of a single nosologic entity. *Am Med Assoc Arch Pathol* 1953; 56: 84–102.
10 Basset F, Turiaf J. Identification par la microscopie électronique de particules probablement virales dans les lésions granulomateuses d'une histiocytose X pulmonaire. *CR Acad Sci (Paris)* 1965; 261: 3701–3.
11 Basset F, Nezelof C. Présence au microscope électronique de structures filamenteuses originales dans les lesions pulmonaires et osseuses de l'histiocytosis X. *Bull soc Med Hop (Paris)* 1966; 117: 413–26.
12 Birbeck MS, Breathnach AS, Everall JD. An electron microscope study of basal melanocytes and high-level clear cells (Langerhans' cells) in vitiligo. *J Invest Dermatol* 1961; 37: 51–63.
13 Nezelof C, Basset F, Rousseau MF. Histiocytosis X: histogenetic arguments for a Langerhans' cell origin. *Biomedicine* 1973; 18: 365–71.
14 Risdall RJ, Dehner LP, Duray P, Kobinsky N, Robinson L, Nesbit ME. Histiocytosis X (Langerhans' cell histiocytosis). *Arch Pathol Lab Med* 1983; 107: 59–63.
15 Raney RB, d'Angio GJ. Langerhans' cell histiocytosis (histiocytosis X): experience at the Children's Hospital of Philadelphia, 1970–1984. *Med Pediatr Oncol* 1989; 17: 20–8.
16 Favara BE, McCarthy RC, Mierau GW. Histiocytosis X. *Hum Pathol* 1983; 14: 663–76.
17 Cartensen H, Ornvold K. The epidemiology of Langerhans' cell histiocytosis in children in Denmark 1975–1989. *Med Pediatr Oncol* 1993; 21: 387–8.
18 The French Langerhans' Cell Histiocytosis Study Group. A multicentre retrospective survey of Langerhans' cell histiocytosis: 348 cases observed between 1983 and 1993. *Arch Dis Child* 1996; 75: 17–24.
19 Broadbent V, Egeler RM, Nesbit ME. Langerhans' cell histiocytosis: clinical and epidemiological aspects. *Br J Cancer* 1994; 70vc(SXXIII): S11–16.
20 Sheils C, Dover GJ. Frequency of congenital anomalies in patients with histiocytosis X. *Am J Hematol* 1989; 31: 91–5.
21 Katz AM, Rosenthal D, Jakubovic HR, Pai M, Quinonez GE, Sauder DN. Langerhans' cell histiocytosis in monozygotic twins. *J Am Acad Dermatol* 1991; 24: 32–7.
22 Halton J, Whitton A, Wiernikowski J, Barr RD. Disseminated Langerhans' cell histiocytosis in identical twins unresponsive to recombinant human alpha-interferon and total body irradiation. *Am J Pediatr Hematol Oncol* 1992; 14: 269–72.
23 Schmitt D, Dezutter-Dambuyant C, Staquet MJ, Thivolet J. La cellule de Langerhans. *Med Sci* 1989; 5: 103–11.
24 Emile JF, Donadieu J, Thomas C, Brousse N. L'histiocytose langerhansienne. Données récentes sur le diagnostic et la physiopathologie. *Ann Pathol* 1995; 15: 252–9.
25 Harrist TJ, Bhan AK, Murphy G, Sato S, Mihm MC. Histiocytosis X: *in situ* characterization of cutaneous lesions. *J Invest Dermatol* 1982; 78: 354–5.
26 Bos JD, Kapsenberg ML. The skin immune system: progress in cutaneous biology. *Immunol Today* 1993; 14: 75–8.
27 Emile JF, Fraitag S, Leborgne M, De Prost Y, Brousse N. Langerhans' cell histiocytosis cells are activated Langerhans' cells. *J Pathol* 1994; 174: 71–6.
28 Kannourakis G, Abbas A. The role of cytokines in the pathogenesis of Langerhans' cell histiocytosis. *Br J Cancer* 1994; 70(SXXIII): S37–40.
29 Emile JF, Peuchmaur M, Brousse N. Controle des cellules de Langerhans par le GM-CSF. *Med Sci* 1994; 10: 171–5.
30 Caux C, Dezutter-Dambuyant C, Schmitt D, Banchereau J. GM-CSF and TNF-α cooperate in the generation of dendritic Langerhans' cells. *Nature* 1992; 360: 258–61.
31 Emile JF, Fraitag S, Andry P, Leborgne M, Lellouch-Tubiana A, Brousse N. Expression of Gm-CSF receptor by Langerhans' cell histiocytosis cells. *Virchows Arch* 1995; 427: 125–9.
32 Romani N, Gruner S, Brang D et al. Proliferating dendritic cell progenitors in human blood. *J Exp Med* 1994; 180: 83–93.
33 Kaplan G, Walsh G, Guido LS et al. Novel responses of human skin to intradermal recombinant granulocyte/macrophage colony stimulating factor: Langerhans' cell recruitment, keratinocyte growth, and enhanced wound healing. *J Exp Med* 1992; 175: 1717–28.
34 Emile JF, Tartour E, Brugieres L et al. Detection of GM-CSF in the sera of children with disseminated Langerhans' cell histiocytosis. *Pediatr Allerg Immunol* 1994; 5: 162–3.
35 Barbey S, Gane P, Le Pelletier O, Nezelof C. Histiocytosis X Langerhans' cells react with anti-interleukin-2 receptor monoclonal antibody. *Pediatr Pathol* 1987; 7: 569–74.
36 Favara BE. Langerhans' cell histiocytosis pathobiology and pathogenesis. *Semin Oncol* 1991; 18: 3–7.

37 Ruco LP, Stoppacciaro A, Vitolo D, Uccini S, Baroni CD. Expression of adhesion molecules in Langerhans' cell histiocytosis. *Histopathology* 1993; 23: 29–37.

38 De Graaf JH, Tamminga RYJ, Kamps WA, Timens W. Langerhans' cell histiocytosis: expression of leucocyte cellular adhesion molecules suggests abnormal homing and differentiation. *Am J Pathol* 1994; 144: 466–72.

39 Casolaro MA, Bernaudin JF, Saltini C, Ferrans VJ, Crystal RG. Accumulation of Langerhans' cells on the epithelial surface of the lower respiratory tract in normal subjects in association with cigarette smoking. *Am Rev Respir Dis* 1988; 137: 406–11.

40 Talanin NY, Smith SS, Shelley ED, Moores WB. Cutaneous histiocytosis with Langerhans' cell features induced by scabies: a case report. *Pediatr Dermatol* 1994; 11: 327–30.

41 Leahy MA, Krejci SM, Friednash M et al. Human herpes virus 6 is present in the lesions of Langerhans' cell histiocytosis. *J Invest Dermatol* 1993; 101: 642–5.

42 McClain K, Jin H, Gresik V, Favara B. Langerhans' cell histiocytosis: lack of viral etiology. *Am J Hematol* 1994; 47: 16–20.

43 McClain K, Weiss RA. Viruses and Langerhans' cell histiocytosis: is there a link? *Br J Cancer* 1994; 70: 34–6.

44 Mierau GW, Wills EJ, Steele PO. Ultrastructural studies in Langerhans' cell histiocytosis: a search for evidence of viral etiology. *Pediatr Pathol* 1994; 14: 895–904.

45 Yu RC, Chu C, Buluwela L, Chu AC. Clonal proliferation of Langerhans' cells in Langerhans' cell histiocytosis. *Lancet* 1994; 343: 767–8.

46 Willman CL, Busque L, Griffith BB et al. Langerhans' cell histiocytosis (histiocytosis X): a clonal proliferative disease. *N Engl J Med* 1994; 331: 154–60.

47 Weiss LM, Wood GS, Trela M. Clonal T cell populations in lymphomatoid papulosis: evidence of a lymphoproliferative origin for a clinically benign disease. *N Engl J Med* 1986; 315: 475–9.

48 Van Heerde P, Egeler RM. Cytology of Langerhans' cell histiocytosis (histiocytosis X). *Cytopathology* 1991; 2: 149–58.

49 Rabkin MS, Wittwer CT, Kjeldsberg CR, Piepkorn MW. Flow-cytometric DNA content of histiocytosis X (Langerhans' cell histiocytosis). *Am J Pathol* 1988; 131: 283–9.

50 Ornvold K, Carstensen H, Larsen JK, Christensen IJ, Ralfkiaer E. Flow cytometric DNA analysis of lesions from 18 children with Langerhans' cell histiocytosis (histiocytosis X). *Am J Pathol* 1990; 136: 1301–7.

51 Goldberg NS, Bauer K, Rosen ST et al. Histiocytosis X: flow cytometric DNA-content and immunohistochemical and ultra-structural analysis. *Arch Dermatol* 1986; 122: 446–50.

52 MacLelland J, Newton JA, Malone M, Camplejohn RS, Chu AC. A flow cytometric study of LC histiocytosis. *Br J Dermatol* 1989; 120: 485–91.

53 Lahey ME, Heyn R, Ladisch S et al. Hypergammaglobulinemia in histiocytosis X. *J Pediatr* 1985; 107: 572–4.

54 Nesbit M, O'Leary M, Dehner LP, Ramsay NKC. Histiocytosis continued: the immune system and the histiocytosis syndromes. *Am J Pediatr Hematol Oncol* 1981; 3: 141–9.

55 Osband ME, Lipton JM, Lavin P et al. Histiocytosis X: demonstration of abnormal immunity, T-cell histamine H2-receptor deficiency, and successful treatment with thymic extract. *N Engl J Med* 1981; 304: 146–53.

56 Nezelof C, Barbey S. Histiocytosis nosology and pathobiology. *Pediatr Pathol* 1985; 3: 1–41.

57 Peters MS. Histiocytic and Langerhans' cell reactions. In: Farmer ER, Hood AF, eds. *Pathology of the skin*. Norwalk: Appleton & Lange, 1990: 249–72.

58 Malone M. The histiocytoses of childhood. *Histopathology* 1991; 19: 105–19.

59 Favara BE, Jaffe R. The histopathology of Langerhans' cell histiocytosis. *Br J Cancer* 1994; 70(SXXIII): S17–23.

60 Romani N, Lenz A, Glassel H et al. Cultured human Langerhans' cells resemble lymphoid dendritic cells in phenotype and function. *J Invest Dermatol* 1989; 93: 600–9.

61 Misery L, Lyonnet S, Cambazard F, Faure M. *Histiocytose langerhansienne.* Encycl Med Chin (Paris, France). Dermatologie 12798 A10, 1993; 12: 798.

62 Chollet S, Dournovo P, Richards MS. Reactivity of histiocytosis X cells with monoclonal anti-T6 antibody. *N Engl J Med* 1982; 307: 685 (letter).

63 Cambazard F, Fernandez-Bussy R, Schmitt D, Thivolet J. Identification immunohistologique des cellules de l'histiocytosis X. *Ann Dermatol Vénéréol* 1983; 110: 33–40.

64 Harrist TJ, Bhan AK, Murphy GS et al. Histiocytosis X: *in situ* characterization of cutaneous infiltrates with monoclonal antibodies. *Am J Clin Pathol* 1983; 79: 294–300.

65 Fumio I, Taikoshi I, Ichiso S, Umemura S, Nakajima T. Immunohistochemical and ultrastructural analysis of the proliferating cells in histiocytosis X. *Cancer* 1984; 53: 917–21.

66 Cambazard F, Dezutter-Dambuyant C, Staquet MJ, Schmitt D, Thivolet J. Eosinophilic granuloma of bone and biochemical demonstration of 49 kDa molecule expression by Langerhans' cell histiocytosis. *Clin Exp Dermatol* 1991; 16: 377–82.

67 Krenacs L, Tiszalvicz L, Krenacs T, Boumsell L. Immunohistochemical detection of CD1a antigen in formalin-fixed and paraffin-embedded tissue sections with monoclonal antibody 010. *J Pathol* 1993; 171: 99–104.

68 Emile JF, Wechsler J, Brousse N et al. Langerhans' cell histiocytosis: definitive diagnosis with the use of monoclonal antibody 010 on routinely paraffin-embedded samples. *Am J Surg Pathol* 1995; 19: 636–41.

69 Rowden G, Connelly EM, Winkelman RK. Cutaneous histiocytosis X: the presence of S-100 protein and its use in diagnosis. *Arch Dermatol* 1983; 119: 553–9.

70 Kanitakis J, Fantini F, Pincelli C, Hermier C, Schmitt D, Thivolet J. Neuron-specific enolase is a marker of cutaneous Langerhans' cell histiocytosis ('X')—A comparative study with S100 protein. *Anticancer Res* 1991; 11: 635–9.

71 Burg G, Stunkel KG, Bieber T, Opitz U, Kaudewitz P. Cutaneous infiltrates of HX contain plasminogen activator-bearing epidermotropic dendritic cells different from Langerhans' cells. *Arch Dermatol Res* 1987; 279: 588–91.

72 Neumann C, Schaumberg-Lever G, Dopfer R, Kolde G. Interferon gamma is marker for histiocytosis X cells in the skin. *J Invest Dermatol* 1988; 91: 280–2.

73 Hage C, Willman CL, Favara BE, Isaacson PG. Langerhans' cell histiocytosis (histiocytosis X), immunophenotype and growth fraction. *Hum Pathol* 1993; 24: 840–5.

74 Mierau GW, Favara BE, Brenman JM. Electron microscopy in histiocytosis X. *Ultrastruct Pathol* 1986; 3: 137–42.

75 Shamoto M. Langerhans cell granule in Letterer–Siwe disease. An electron microscopy study. *Cancer* 1990; 26: 1102–8.

76 Kashimara-Sawami M, Horiguchi Y, Ikai K et al. Letterer–Siwe disease: immunopathologic study with a new monoclonal antibody. *J Am Acad Dermatol* 1988; 18: 646–54.

77 Leahy MA, Brice SL, Weston WL. Langerhans' cell histiocytosis. *Curr Probl Dermatol* 1994; 6: 1–25.

78 Egeler RM, D'Angio GJ. Langerhans' cell histiocytosis. *J Pediatr* 1995; 127: 1–11.

79 Berry DH, Gresik MV, Humphrey GB. Natural history of histiocytosis X: a pediatric oncology group study. *Med Pediatr Oncol* 1986; 14: 1–5.

80 Rivera-Luna R, Martinez-Guerra G, Altamirano-Alvarez E et al. Langerhans' cell histiocytosis: clinical experience with 124 patients. *Pediatr Dermatol* 1988; 5: 145–50.

81 Ceci A, De Terlizzi M, Colella R et al. Langerhans' cell histiocytosis in childhood: results from the Italian Cooperative AIEOP—CNR-H.X 83 study. *Med Pediatr Oncol* 1993; 21: 259–64.

82 Estery NB, Maurer HS, Gonzalez-Crussi F. Histiocytosis X: a 7-year experience at a children's hospital. *J Am Acad Dermatol* 1985; 13: 481–96.

83 Hashimoto K, Pritzker MS. Electron microscopy study of reticulohistiocytoma: an unusual case of self-healing reticulohistiocytosis. *Arch Dermatol* 1973; 170: 263–70.

84 Hashimoto K, Takahashi S, Lee RG, Krull EA. Congenital self-healing reticulohistiocytosis: report of the seventh case with histochemical and ultrastructural studies. *J Am Acad Dermatol* 1984; 11: 447–54.

85 Kanitakis J, Zambruno G, Schmitt D, Cambazard F, Jacquemier D, Thivolet J. Congenital self-healing histiocytosis (Hashimoto–Pritzker): an ultrastructural and immunohistochemical study. *Cancer* 1988; 61: 508–16.

86 Bunse T, Kuhn A, Mahrle G, Krieg T, Oeding-Erdel C, Weltersbach W. Congenital self-healing reticulohistiocytosis: a clinical, histochemical and electron microscope study. *Eur J Dermatol* 1993; 3: 531–5.

87 Bernstein EF, Resnik KS, Loose JH, Halcin C, Kauh YC. Solitary congenital self healing reticulohistiocytosis. *Br J Dermatol* 1993; 129: 449–54.

88 Paquet P, Hermanns-Le T, Pierard GE. Reticulohistiocytose auto-involutive de Hashimoto–Pritzker et les histiocytoses congénitales. *Arch Pediatr* 1994; 1: 578–81.

89 Cambazard F, Kanatikis J, Michel JL, Boucheron S, Thivolet J. Les différentes manifestations cliniques des histiocytoses congènitales involutives. *Ann Dermatol Vénéréol* 1995; 122: S75–6.

90 Herman LE, Rothman KF, Harawi S, Gonzalez-Serva A. Congenital self healing reticulohistiocytosis. A new entity in the differential diagnosis of neonatal papulovesicular eruptions. *Arch Dermatol* 1990; 126: 210–12.

91 Johno M, Oishi M, Kohmaru M, Yoshimura K, Ono T. Langerhans' cell histiocytosis presenting as a varicelliform eruption over the entire skin. *J Dermatol* 1994; 21: 197–204.

92 Cambazard F, Blanc JF, Perrot JL, Boucheron S. Eruption vésiculeuse congénitale révélatrice d'une histiocytose langerhansienne d'évolution spontanément favorable. *Ann Dermatol Vénéréol* 1996; 123: S90–1.

93 Whitehead B, Michaels M, Sahni R, Stroebel S, Harper JI. Congenital self-healing Langerhans' cell histiocytosis with persistent cellular immunological abnormalities. *Br J Dermatol* 1990; 122: 563–8.

94 Garcia Muret MP, Fernandez-Figueras MT, Gonzalez MJ, De Moragas JM. Histiocytose langerhansienne congénitale cutanée auto-involutive avec atteinte osseuse. *Ann Dermatol Vénéréol* 1995; 122: 612–14.

95 Longaker MA, Frieden IJ, Leboit PE, Sheretz EF. Congenital 'self-healing' Langerhans' cell histiocytosis: the need for long-term follow-up. *J Am Acad Dermatol* 1994; 31: 910–16.

96 Kodet R, Elleder M, De Wolf-Peeters C, Mottl H. Congenital histiocytosis. A heterogeneous group of diseases, one presenting as so-called congenital self-healing histiocytosis. *Pathol Res Pract* 1991; 187: 458–66.

97 Enjolras O, Leibowitch M, Bonacini F, Vacher-Lavenu MC, Escande JP. Histiocytoses langerhansiennes congénitales cutanées. A propos de 7 cas. *Ann Dermatol* 1992; 119: 111–17.

98 Tamura T, Umetsu M, Motoya H, Yokoyama S. Congenital Letterer–Siwe disease associated with protein losing enteropathy. *Eur J Pediatr* 1980; 135: 77–80.

99 Levisohn D, Seidel D, Phelps A, Burgdorf W. Solitary congenital indeterminate cell histiocytoma. *Arch Dermatol* 1993; 129: 81–5.

100 Komp DM. Concepts in staging and clinical studies for treatment of Langerhans' cell histiocytosis. *Semin Oncol* 1991; 18: 18–23.

101 Wolfson S, Botero F, Hurwitz S, Pearson H. 'Pure' cutaneous histiocytosis X. *Cancer* 1981; 48: 2236–8.

102 Magana-Garcia M. Pure cutaneous histiocytosis X. *Int J Dermatol* 1986; 25: 106–8.

103 Hartman KS. Histiocytosis. Review of 114 cases with oral involvement of LCH. *Oral Surg* 1980; 49: 38–54.

104 Otis CN, Fisher RA, Johnson N, Kelleher JF, Powell JL. Histiocytosis X of the vulva: a case report and review of the literature. *Obstet Gynecol* 1990; 75: 555–8.

105 Axiotis CA, Merino MJ, Duray PH. Langerhans' cell histiocytosis of the female genital tract. *Cancer* 1991; 67: 1650–60.

106 Alsina MM, Zamora E, Ferramso J, Mascaro J, Conget JL. Nail changes in histiocytosis X. *Arch Dermatol* 1991; 127: 1741.

107 De Berker D, Lever LR, Windebank K. Nail features in Langerhans' cell histiocytosis. *Br J Dermatol* 1994; 130: 523–7.

108 Slater JM. Eosinophilic granuloma of bone. *Med Pediatr Oncol* 1980; 8: 151–5.

109 Sessa S, Sommelet D, Gabet F, Cavare S, Lascombes P, Prevot J. Les localisations osseuses de l'histiocytose X. *Rev Chir Orthop Repar Appar Mot* 1992; 78: 112–23.

110 Fiorillo A, Sadile F, De Chiara C et al. Bone lesions in Langerhans' cell histiocytosis. *Clin Pediatr Phila* 1993; 32: 118–20.

111 Kilpatrick SE, Wenger DE, Gilchrist GS, Shives TC, Wollan PC. Langerhans' cell histiocytosis (histiocytosis X) of bone. *Cancer* 1995; 76: 2471–84.

112 Elsheikh T, Silverman JF, Wakely PE Jr, Holbrook CT, Joshi VV. Fine-needle aspiration cytology of LCH (eosinophilic granuloma) of bone in children. *Diagn Cytopathol* 1991; 7: 261–6.

113 Cunnigham MJ, Curtin HD, Jaffe R, Stool SE. Otologic manifestations of LCH. *Arch Otolaryngol Head Neck Surg* 1989; 115: 807–13.

114 Jouve JL, Bollini G, Jacquemier M, Bouyala JM. Quinze cas de localisation vertebrale de l'histiocytose X chez l'enfant. *Ann Pediatr* 1991; 38: 167–74.

115 McClain K, Ramsay NKC, Robinson L, Sundberg RD, Nesbit ME. Bone marrow involvement in histiocytosis X. *Med Pediatr Oncol* 1983; 11: 167–71.

116 Nondahl SR, Finlay JL, Farrell PM, Warner TF, Hong R. A case report and literature review of 'primary' pulmonary histiocytosis X of childhood. *Med Pediatr Oncol* 1986; 14: 57–62.

117 Ha SY, Helms P, Fletcher M et al. Lung involvement in Langerhans 'cell histiocytosis: prevalence, clinical features and outcome. *Pediatrics* 1992; 89: 466–9.

118 Travis WD, Borok Z, Roum JH et al. Pulmonary Langerhans' cell granulomatoses: a clinicopathologic study of 48 cases. *Am J Surg Pathol* 1993; 17: 971–86.

119 Mogul M, Hartman G, Donaldson S et al. Langerhans' cell histiocytosis presenting with the superior vena cava syndrome: a case report. *Med Pediatr Oncol* 1993; 21: 456–9.

120 Brauner MW, Grenier P, Mouelhi MM, Mompoint D, Lenoir S. Pulmonary histiocytosis X: evalutation with high resolution CT. *Radiology* 1989; 172: 255–8.

121 Moore AD, Godwin JD, Muller NL et al. Pulmonary histiocytosis X: comparison of radiographic and CT findings. *Radiology* 1989; 172: 249–54.

122 Kulwiec EL, Lynch DA, Aguayo SM, Schwarz MI, King TE. Imaging of pulmonary histiocytosis X. *Radiographics* 1992; 12: 515–26.

123 Bonnet D, Kermaree J, Marotel C et al. Données du lavage bronchoéalvéolaire et histiocytose X pulmonaire. *Rev Pneumol Clin* 1987; 43: 121–30.

124 Auerswald U, Barth J, Magnussen H. Value of CD1 positive cells in bronchoalveolar lavage fluid for the diagnosis of pulmonary histiocytosis X. *Lungs* 1991; 169: 305–9.

125 Neveu I, Labrune P, Huguet P, Musset D, Chaussain JL, Odievre M. Cholangite sclérosante revelatrice d'une histiocytose X. *Arch Fr Pediatr* 1990; 47: 197–9.

126 Soua H, Poousse H, Ladeb F et al. Histiocytose X et cholangite sclérosante. *Ann Pediatr Paris* 1993; 40: 316–19.

127 Pirovino M, Jeanneret C, Lang H, Luisier J, Bianchi L, Spichtin H. Liver cirrhosis in histiocytosis X. *Liver* 1988; 8: 293–8.

128 Mahmoud H, Gaber O, Wang W, Whintington G, Vera S, Murphy SB. Successful orthotopic liver transplantation in a child with Langerhans' cell histiocytosis. *Transplantation* 1991; 51: 278–80.

129 Concepcion W, Esquivel CO, Terry A et al. Liver transplantation in Langerhans' cell histiocytosis. *Semin Oncol* 1991; 18: 24–8.

130 Sommeraver JF, Atkinson P, Andrews W, Moor P, Wall W. Liver transplantation for Langerhans' cell histiocytosis and immunomodulation of disease pre and post transplant. *Transplant Proc* 1994; 26: 178–9.

131 Egeler RM, Schipper ME, Heymans HS. Gastrointestinal involvement in Langerhans' cell histiocytosis (histiocytosis X): a clinical report of three cases. *Eur J Pediatr* 1990; 149: 325–9.

132 Boccon Gibod LA, Krichen HA, Carlier-Mercier LM, Salaun JF, Fontaine JL, Leverger GR. Digestive tract involvement with exudative enteropathy in Langerhans' cell histiocytosis. *Pediatr Pathol* 1992; 12: 515–24.

133 Stuphen JL, Fechner RE. Case report: chronic gastroenteritis in a patient with histiocytosis X. *J Pediatr Gastroenterol Nutr* 1986; 5: 324–8.

134 Hyams JS, Haswell JE, Gerber MA, Berman MM. Case report: colonic ulceration in histiocytosis X. *J Pediatr Gastroenterol Nutr* 1985; 4: 286–90.

135 Braunstein GD, Kohler PO. Endocrine manifestations of histiocytosis. *Am J Pediatr Hematol Oncol* 1981; 3: 67–75.

136 Dunger DB, Broadbent V, Yeoman E et al. The frequency and natural history of diabetes insipidus in children with Langerhans' cell histiocytosis. *N Engl J Med* 1989; 321: 1157–62.

137 Newton WA, Hamoudi AB, Shannon BT. Role of the thymus in histiocytosis X. *Hematol Oncol Clin N Am* 1987; 1: 63–74.

138 Hamoudi AB, Newton WA, Mancer K, Penn GM. Thymic changes in histiocytosis. *Am J Clin Pathol* 1982; 77: 169–73.

139 Dean HJ, Bishop A, Winter JSD. Growth hormone deficiency in patients with histiocytosis X. *J Pediatr* 1986; 109: 615–18.

140 Grois N, Barkovich AJ, Rosenau W, Ablin AR. Central nervous system disease associated with Langerhans' cell histiocytosis. *Am J Pediatr Hematol Oncol* 1993; 15: 245–54.

141 Grois N, Tsunematsu Y, Barkovich AJ, Favara BE. Central nervous system disease in Langerhans' cell histiocytosis. *Br J Cancer* 1994; 70 (suppl XXIII): S24–8.

142 Tabarin A, Corcuff JB, Dautheribes M et al. Histiocytosis X of the hypothalamus. *J Endocrinol Invest* 1991; 14: 139–45.

143 Rosenfield NS, Abrahams J, Komp D. Brain MR in patients with Langerhans' cell histiocytosis: findings and enhancement with Gd-DTPA. *Pediatr Radiol* 1990; 20: 433–6.

144 Braunstein GD, Whitaker NJ, Kohler PO. Cerebellar dysfunction in Hand–Schuller–Christian disease. *Arch Intern Med* 1973; 132: 387–90.

145 Carpentier MA, Maheut J, Grangeponte MC, Billard C, Santini JJ. Disseminated cerebral histiocytosis X responding to vinblastine therapy: a case report. *Brain Dev* 1991; 13: 193–5.

146 Nezelof C, Frileux-Herbert F, Cronier-Sachot J. Disseminated histiocytosis X. Analysis of prognostic factors based on a retrospective study of 50 cases. *Cancer* 1979; 44: 1824–38.

147 Lahey ME. Prognostic factors in histiocytosis X. *Am J Pediatr Hematol Oncol* 1981; 3: 57–60.

148 Benz-Lemoine E. Facteurs de pronostic dans l'histiocytose X. *Ann Pediatr* 1989; 36: 499–503.

149 Ladisch S, Gadner H. Treatment of Langerhans' cell histiocytosis. Evolution and current approaches. *Br J Cancer* 1994; 70: 41–6.

150 Greenberger J, Crocker A, Vawter G, Jaffe N, Cassady JR. Results of treatment of 127 patients with systemic histiocytosis (Letterer–Siwe syndrome, Schüller–Christian syndrome and multifocal eosinophilic granuloma). *Medicine* 1981; 60: 311–38.

151 Broadbent V. Favorable prognostic features in histiocytosis X bone involvement and absence of skin disease. *Arch Dis Child* 1986; 61: 1219–21.

152 McLean T, Pritchard J. Langerhans' cell histiocytosis and hypercalcemia: clinical response to indomethacin. *J Pediatr Hematol Oncol* 1996; 18: 318–20.

153 Pritchard J, Gordon I, Beverley PC, Chu AC. CD1 antibody immunolocalization in Langerhans' cell histiocytosis. *Lancet* 1993; 342: 367–8 (letter).

154 Kelly KM, Beverley PCL, Chu AC et al. Successful *in vivo* immunolocalization of Langerhans' cell histiocytosis with use of a monoclonal antibody. NA1/34 *J Pediatr* 1994; 125: 717–22.

155 Lavin PT, Osband ME. Evaluating the role of therapy in histiocytosis X: clinical, studies, staging and scoring. *Hematol Oncol Clin N Am* 1987; 1: 46–51.

156 Komp DM, El-Madhi A, Starling KA et al. Long-term sequelae of histiocytosis X. *Am J Pediatr Hematol Oncol* 1981; 3: 165–8.

157 Poupon RE et al. Ursodiol for long-term treatment of primary biliary cirrhosis. *N Engl J Med* 1994; 330: 1342–7.

158 Clinical Writing Group of the Histiocyte Society (Broadbent V, Gadner H, Komp DM, Ladisch S). Histiocytosis syndrome in children. II. Approach to the clinical and laboratory evaluation of children with Langerhans' cell histiocytosis. *Med Pediatr Oncol* 1989; 17: 492–5.

159 Egeler RM, Neglia JP, Arico M, Favara BE, Heitger A, Nesbit ME. Acute leukemia in association with Langerhans' cell histiocytosis. *Med Pediatr Oncol* 1994; 23: 81–5.

160 Egeler RM, Neglia JP, Pucetti DM, Brennan C, Nesbit ME. The association of Langerhans' cell histiocytosis with malignant neoplasms. *Cancer* 1993; 71: 865–73.

161 Egeler RM, De Kraker J, Voute PA. Cytosine-arabinoside, vincristine, and prednisolone in the treatment of children with disseminated Langerhans' cell histiocytosis with organ dysfunction: experience at a single institution. *Med Pediatr Oncol* 1993; 21: 265–70.

162 Ben Ezra JM, Koo CH. Langerhans' cell histiocytosis and malignancies of the M-PIRE system. *Am J Clin Pathol* 1993; 99: 464–71.

163 Arico M, Comelli A, Bossi G, Raiteri E, Piombo M, Egeler RM. Langerhans' cell histiocytosis and acute leukemia: unusual association in two cases. *Med Pediatr Oncol* 1993; 21: 271–3.

164 Horibe K, Matsushita T, Numata SI et al. Acute promyelocytic leukemia with t(15;17) abnormality after chemotherapy containing etoposide for Langerhans' cell histiocytosis. *Cancer* 1993; 72: 3723–6.

165 Chap L, Nimer SD. Chronic myelogenous leukemia following repeated radiation therapy for histiocytosis X. *Leuk Lymphoma* 1994; 12: 315–16.

166 Pakula AS, Paller AS. Langerhans' cell histiocytosis and dermatophytosis. *J Am Acad Dermatol* 1993; 29: 340–3.

167 Megahed M, Sschuppe HC, Holzle E, Jurgens H, Plewig G. Langerhans' cell histiocytosis masquerading as lichen aureus. *Pediatr Dermatol* 1991; 8: 213–16.

168 Messenger GG, Kamei R, Honig PJ. Histiocytosis X resembling cherry angiomas. *Pediatr Dermatol* 1985; 3: 75–8.

169 Nagy-Vezekenyi K, Makai A, Ambro I, Nagy E. Histiocytosis with unusual skin symptoms. *Acta Derm Venereol* 1981; 61: 447–51.

170 Dufresne AG, Malcomb AW, Salhany KE, King LE. Histiocytosis X mimicking the follicular occlusion syndrome: response to local therapy. *J Am Acad Dermatol* 1987; 16: 385–6.

171 Santhosh-Kumar CR, Almomen A, Ajarim DSS, Shipkey FH, Kyriacou KC. Unusual skin tumors in Langerhans' cell histiocytosis. *Arch Dermatol* 1990; 126: 1617–20.

172 Zachariae H. Histiocytosis X in two infants treated with topical nitrogen mustard. *Br J Dermatol* 1979; 100: 433–8.

173 Lemarchand-Venencie F, Saurat JH. Traitement local des lésions cutanées d'histiocytosis X par la moutarde a l'azote. *Ann Pediatr* 1982; 29: 70–3.

174 Thivolet J, Cambazard F, Euvrard S, Hermier M, Kanitakis J. Histiocytose langerhansienne cutanée isolée. Amélioration clinique et immunologique apres applications locales de moutarde a l'azote. *Ann Dermatol Vénéréol* 1984; 11: 765–6.

175 Wong E, Holden CA, Broadbent V, Atherton DJ. Histiocytosis X presenting as intertrigo and responding to topical nitrogen mustard. *Clin Exp Dermatol* 1986; 11: 183–7.

176 Sheehan MP, Atherton DJ, Broadbent V, Pritchard J. Topical nitrogen mustard: an effective treatment for cutaneous Langerhans' cell histiocytosis. *J Pediatr* 1991; 119: 317–21.

177 Kaudewitz P, Przybilla B, Chmoeckel C, Gollhausen R. Cutaneous lesions in histiocytosis X: successful treatment with PUVA. *J Invest Dermatol* 1986; 86: 324–5.

178 Selch MT, Parker RG. Radiation therapy in the management of Langerhans' cell histiocytosis. *Med Pediatr Oncol* 1990; 18: 97–102.

179 Minehan KJ, Chen MG, Zimmerman D, Su JQ, Colby TV, Shaw EG. Radiation therapy for diabetes insipidus caused by Langerhans' cell histiocytosis. *Int J Radiat Oncol Biol Phys* 1992; 23: 519–24.

180 Cohen M, Zornoza J, Cangir A, Murray JA, Wallace S. Direct injection of methylsodium succinate in the treatment of solitary eosinophilic granuloma of bone. *Radiology* 1980; 136: 289–93.

181 Wirtschafter JD, Nesbit M, Anderson P, McClain K. Intralesional methylprednisolone for Langerhans' cell histiocytosis of the orbit and cranium. *J Pediatr Ophthalmol Strabismus* 1987; 24: 194–7.

182 Bernstrand C, Bjork O, Ahstrom L, Henter JI. Intralesional steroids in Langerhans' cell histiocytosis of bone. *Acta Paediatr* 1996; 85: 502–4.

183 Egeler RM, Thompson RC Jr, Voute PA, Nesbit ME Jr. Intralesional infiltration of corticosteroids in localized Langerhans' cell histiocytosis. *J Pediatr Orthop* 1992; 12: 811–14.

184 Goihman-Yahr M. Resolution of cutaneous lesions of histiocytosis X by intralesional injections of interferon beta. *Int J Dermatol* 1991; 30: 373–4.

185 Martinez-Lage JF, Poza M, Cartagena J, Vicente JP, Biec F, De Las Heras M. Solitary eosinophilic granuloma of the pediatric skull and spine. The role of surgery. *Child Nerv Syst* 1991; 7: 448–51.

186 Gadner H, Heitger A, Grois N, Gatterer-Menz I, Ladisch S. (for the DAL HX-83 Study Group). Treatment strategy for disseminated Langerhans' cell histiocytosis. *Med Pediatr Oncol* 1994; 23: 72–80.

187 Ladisch S, Gadner H, Arico M et al. (for the Histiocyte Society). LCH-I. A randomized trial of etoposide vs. vinblastine in disseminated Langerhans' cell histiocytosis. *Med Pediatr Oncol* 1994; 23: 107–10.

188 Lahey ME. Histiocytosis X. Comparison of three treatment regimens. *J Pediatr* 1975; 87: 170–83.

189 Starling JS. Therapy of histiocytosis X with vincristine, vinblastine and cyclophosphamide. *Am J Dis Child* 1972; 123: 105–10.

190 Jones B. Chemotherapy of reticuloendotheliosis. Comparison of methotrexate plus prednisolone vs vincristine plus prednisolone. *Cancer* 1974; 34: 1011–16.

191 Lahey ME. Histiocytosis X: clinical trial of chlorambucil a report from children study group. *Med Pediatr Oncol* 1979; 7: 197–203.

192 McLelland J, Broadbent V, Yeomans E, Malone M, Pritchard J. Langerhans' cell histiocytosis: the case for conservative treatment. *Arch Dis child* 1990; 65: 301–3.

193 Ceci A. Etoposide in recurrent childhood Langerhans' cell histiocytosis: an Italian Cooperative Study. *Cancer* 1988; 62: 2528–31.

194 Sheehan MP, Chu AC. Oral, skin and bone multisystem Langerhans' cell histiocytosis and its response to etoposide. A case report. *Clin Exp Dermatol* 1991; 16: 463–6.

195 Viana MB, Oliveira BM, Silva CM, Rios Leite VH. Etoposide in the treatment of six children with Langerhans' cell histiocytosis (histiocytosis X). *Med Pediatr Oncol* 1991; 19: 289–94.

196 Ishii E, Matsuzaki A, Okamura J et al. Treatment of Langerhans' cell histiocytosis in children with etoposide. *Am J Clin Oncol* 1992; 15: 515–17.

197 Yu LC, Shenoy S, Ward K, Warrier RP. Successful treatment of multisystem Langerhans' cell histiocytosis with etoposide. *Am J Pediatr Hematol Oncol* 1993; 16: 275–7.

198 Miura T, Nakamura M, Tsunematsu Y, Fujimoto J, Meguro T, Yamada K. Hypofibrinogenemia in a girl with Langerhans' cell histiocytosis during etoposide and prednisolone therapy. *Acta Paediatr Jpn* 1993; 35: 148–50.

199 Pui CH, Ribeiro RC, Hancock M et al. Acute myeloid leukemia in children treated with epipodophyllotoxins for acute lymphoblastic leukemia. *N Engl J Med* 1991; 325: 1682–7.

200 Haupt R, Comelli A, Rosanda C, Sessarego M, De Bernardi B. Acute myeloid leukemia after single-agent treatment with etoposide for Langerhans' cell histiocytosis of bone. *Am J Pediatr Hematol Oncol* 1993; 15: 255–7.

201 Smith MA, Rubinstein L, Ungerleider RS. Therapy-related acute myeloid leukemia following treatment with epipodophyllotoxins: estimating the risk. *Med Pediatr Oncol* 1994; 23: 86–98.

202 D'Angio GJ. Langerhans' cell histiocytosis and etoposide: risks vs benefits. *Med Pediatr Oncol* 1994; 23: 69–71.

203 Mahmoud HH, Wang WC, Murphy SB. Cyclosporine therapy for advanced Langerhans' cells histiocytosis. *Blood* 1991; 77: 721–5.

204 Sawamura M, Yamaguchi S, Marayama K *et al*. Cyclosporine therapy for Langerhans' cell histiocytosis. *Br J Haematol* 1993; 83: 178–9 (letter).

205 Seto S, Carrera CJ, Kubota M, Wasson DB, Carson DA *et al*. Mechanism of deoxyadenosine and 2-chloro-deoxyadenosine toxicity to non-dividing human lymphocytes. *J Clin Invest* 1985; 75: 377–83.

206 Carrera CJ, Terai C, Lotz M *et al*. Potent toxicity of 2-chlorodeoxyadenosine towards human monocytes *in vitro* and *in vivo*: a novel approach to immunosuppressive therapy. *J Clin Invest* 1990; 86: 1480–8.

207 Saven A, Figueroa ML, Piro LD, Rosenblatt JD. 2-chlorodeoxyadenosine to treat refractory histiocytosis X. *N Engl J Med* 1993; 329: 734–5 (letter).

208 Jakobson AM, Kreuger A, Hagberg H, Sundstrom C. Treatment of Langerhans' cell histiocytosis with alpha interferon. *Lancet* 1987; 8574: 1520–1.

209 Sato Y, Ikeda Y, Ito E *et al*. Histiocytosis X: successful treatment with recombinant interferon alpha. *Acta Paediatr J* 1990; 32: 151–4.

210 Bellmunt J, Albanell J, Salud A, Espanol T, Morales S, Sole-Calvo LA. Interferon and disseminated Langerhans' cell histiocytosis. *Med Pediatr Oncol* 1992; 20: 336–7.

211 Tiedemann KH, Bandmann J, Stuttgen G. Successful therapy of histiocytosis X with etretinate and alpha 2B interferon. *J Invest Dermatol* 1989; 93: 582.

212 Davies EG, Levinski RJ, Butler M, Broadbent V, Pritchard J, Chessels J. Thymic hormone therapy for histiocytosis X. *N Engl J Med* 1983; 309: 493–4.

213 Nicolas JF, Thivolet J. Les hormones thymiques en Dermatologie. *Ann Dermatol Vénéréol* 1989; 116: 681–4.

214 Gnassia AN, Gnassia RT, Bonvalet D, Puissant A, Goudal H. Histiocytose X avec 'granulome eosinophile vulvaire': effet spectaculaire de la thalidomide. *Ann Dermatol Vénéréol* 1987; 114: 1387–9.

215 Thomas L, Ducros B, Secchi T, Balme B, Moulin G. Successful treatment of adult's Langerhans' cell histiocytosis with thalidomide. *Arch Dermatol* 1993; 129: 1261–4.

216 Kelly KM, Pritchard J. Monoclonal antibody therapy in Langerhans' cell histiocytosis—feasible and reasonable? *Br J Cancer* 1994; 70 (SXXIII): S54–5.

217 Ringden O, Ahstrom L, Lonnquist B, Baryd I, Svedmyr E, Gahrton G. Allogeneic bone marrow transplantation in a patient with chemotherapy-resistant progressive histiocytosis X. *N Engl J Med* 1987; 316: 733–5.

218 Stoll M, Freund M, Schmid H *et al*. Allogeneic bone marrow transplantation for Langerhans' cell histiocytois. *Cancer* 1990; 66: 284–8.

219 Greinix HT, Storb R, Sanders JE, Petersen FB. Marrow transplantation for treatment of multisystem progressive Langerhans' cell histiocytosis. *Bone Marrow Transplant* 1992; 10: 39–44.

220 Foucar E, Rosai J, Dorfman R. Sinus histiocytosis with massive lymphadenopathy (Rosai–Dorfman disease): review of the entity. *Semin Diagn Pathol* 1990; 7: 19–73.

221 Lazar AP, Esterly NB, Gonzales-Crussi F. Sinus histiocytosis clinically limited to the skin. *Pediatr Dermatol* 1987; 4: 247–53.

222 Baildam EM, Ewing CI, D'Souza SW, Stevens RF. Sinus histiocytosis with massive lymphadenopathy (Rosai–Dorfman disease): response to acyclovir. *J Roy Soc Med* 1992; 85: 179–80.

223 Kuramoto Y, Iizawa O, Aiba S, Makino Y, Tagami H. Multicentric reticulohistiocytosis in a child with sclerosing lesion of the leg. *J Am Acad Dermatol* 1989; 20: 329–35.

224 Frank N, Amor B, Ayral X *et al*. Multicentric reticulohistiocytosis and methotrexate. *J Am Acad Dermatol* 1995; 33: 524–5.

225 Mullans EA, Helm TN, Taylor JS, Helm KF, Olin JW, Bergfeld WF. Generalized non-Langerhans' cell histiocytosis: four cases illustrate a spectrum of disease. *Int J Dermatol* 1995; 34: 106–12.

226 Winkelman RK. Cutaneous syndromes of non-X histiocytoses. *Arch Dermatol* 1981; 117: 667–72.

227 Ringel E, Moshella S. Primary histiocytic dermatoses. *Arch Dermatol* 1985; 121: 1531–9.

228 Seo IS, Min KW, Mirkin OL. Juvenile xanthogranuloma. *Arch Pathol Lab Med* 1986; 110: 911–15.

229 Cohen BA, Hood A. Xanthogranuloma: report on clinical and histologic findings in 64 patients. *Pediatr Dermatol* 1989; 6: 262–6.

230 Sonoda T, Hashimoto K, Enjoli M. Juvenile xanthogranuloma. Clinicopathologic analysis and immunohistochemical study of 57 patients. *Cancer* 1985; 56: 2280–6.

231 Caputo R, Grimalt R, Gelmetti C, Cottoni F. Unusual aspects of juvenile xanthogranuloma. *J Am Acad Dermatol* 1993; 28: 868–70.

232 Resnick SD, Woosley J, Azizkhan RF. Giant juvenile xanthogranuloma: exophytic and endophytic variants. *Pediatr Dermatol* 1990; 7: 185–8.

233 Magana M, Vazquez R, Fernandez-Diez J, Flores-Villa R, Cazarin J. Giant congenital juvenile xanthogranuloma. *Pediatr Dermatol* 1994; 11: 227–30.

234 Labbe L, Bioulac-Sage P, Taïeb A. Xanthogranulome juvénile: une forme géante congénitale. *Ann Dermatol Vénéréol* 1995; 122: 678–81.

235 Diard F, Cadier L, Billaud C, Trojani M. Xanthogranulome juvenile a expression neonatale avec atteinte pulmonaire, extrapleurale et hepatique. *Ann Radiol* 1982; 25: 113–18.

236 Lottsfeldt FE, Good RA. Juvenile xanthogranuloma with pulmonary lesions. *Pediatrics* 1964; 33: 233–8.

237 Di Blasi A, De Seta L, Marsilia GM, Coletta S, Siani P, De Rosa I. Xantogranuloma giovanile. Descrizione di un caso con interessamento epatico. *Pathologica* 1993; 85: 85–90.

238 Flach DB, Winkelman RK. Juvenile xanthogranuloma with central nervous system lesions. *J Am Acad Dermatol* 1986; 14: 405–11.

239 Amoric JC, Stalder JF, Schmuck C, Bureau B, Litoux P. Complication oculaire révélatrice d'un xanthogranulome juvénile. *Ann Dermatol Vénéréol* 1991; 118: 629–32.

240 Morier P, Merot Y, Paccaud D, Beck D, Frenk E. Juvenile chronic granulocytic leukemia and juvenile xanthogranuloma and neurofibromatosis. *J Am Acad Dermatol* 1990; 22: 962–5.

241 Rotte JJ, De Vaan GAM, Koopman RJJ. Juvenile xanthogranuloma and acute leukemia: a case report. *Med Pediatr Oncol* 1994; 23: 57–9.

242 Gianotti F, Caputo R, Ermacora E, Gianni E. Benign cephalic histiocytosis. *Arch Dermatol* 1986; 122: 1038–43.

243 Godfrey KM, James MP. Benign cephalic histiocytosis. *Br J Dermatol* 1990; 123: 245–8.

244 Pena Penabad C, Unamuno P, Garcia Silva J, Ludena D, Armijo M. Benign cephalic histiocytosis: case report and literature review. *Pediatr Dermatol* 1994; 11: 164–7.

245 Caputo R, Ermacora E, Gelmetti C, Berti E, Gianni E, Nigro A. Generalized eruptive histiocytoma in children. *J Am Acad Dermatol* 1987; 17: 449–54.

246 Umbert IJ, Winkelman RK. Eruptive histiocytoma. *J Am Acad Dermatol* 1988; 20: 958–64.

247 Van Haselen CW, Toonstra J, Den Hengst CW, Van Vloten WA. An unusual form of localized papulonodular cutaneous histiocytosis in a 6-month-old boy. *Br J Dermatol* 1995; 133: 444–8.

248 Caputo R, Grimalt R, Ermacora E, Cavicchini S, Portaleone D. Unusual case of non-Langerhans' cell histiocytosis. *J Am Acad Dermatol* 1994; 30: 367–70.

249 Torres L, Sanchez J, Rivera A, Gonzalez A. Progressive nodular histiocytosis. *J Am Acad Dermatol* 1993; 29: 278–80.

250 Caputo R, Crosti C, Cainelli T. A unique cytoplasmic structure in papular histiocytoma. *J Invest Dermatol* 1997; 68: 98–104.

251 Toporcer MB, Kantor GR, Benedetto AV. Multiple cutaneous reticulohistiocytomas (reticulohistiocytic granulomas). *J Am Acad Dermatol* 1991; 25: 948–51.

252 Levine EG, Hanson CA, Jaszez W, Peterson BA. True histiocytic lymphoma. *Semin Oncol* 1991; 18: 39–49.

253 Hsu SM, Ho YS, Hsu PL. Lymphomas of true histiocytic origin: expression of different phenotypes in so called histiocytic lymphoma and malignant histiocytosis. *Am J Pathol* 1991; 138: 1389–404.

254 Laroche L, Leverger G, Cazin B *et al*. Forme bulleuse d'histiocytose maligne. *Ann Dermatol Vénéréol* 1985; 112: 729–30.

255 Wilson MS, Weiss LM, Gatter KC, Mason DY, Dorfman RF, Warnke RA. Malignant histiocytosis: a reassessment of cases previously reported in 1975 based on paraffin section immunophenotyping studies. *Cancer* 1990; 66: 530–6.

256 Arai E, Su WP, Roche PC, Li CY. Cutaneous histiocytic malignancy. Immunohistochemical re-examination of cases previously diagnosed as cutaneous 'histiocytic lymphoma' and 'malignant histiocytosis'. *J Cutan Pathol* 1993; 20: 115–20.

257 Jaffe ES, Costa J, Fauci AS, Cossman J, Tsokos M. Malignant lymphoma and erythrophagocytosis simulating malignant histiocytosis. *Am J Med* 1983; 75: 741–9.

258 Bucksy P, Favara B, Feller AC *et al*. Malignant histiocytosis and large cell anaplastic (Ki-1) lymphoma in childhood: guidelines for differential diagnosis. Report of the Histiocyte Society. *Med Pediatr Oncol* 1994; 22: 200–3.

259 Ferster A, Corazza F, Heimann P *et al*. Anaplastic large cell lymphoma of true histiocytosis origin in an infant: unusual clinical, haematological and cytogenetic features. *Med Pediatr Oncol* 1994; 22: 147–52.

Section 22
The Oral Cavity

22.1 Diseases of the Oral Mucosa and Tongue

JANE LUKER

Mouth ulcers/sore mouth
Recurrent aphthous stomatitis (RAS)
Minor aphthous stomatitis
Major aphthous stomatitis
Herpetiform ulceration
Behçet's syndrome
MAGIC syndrome
Traumatic ulceration
Infections
Oral ulceration in association with neoplasia
Oral ulceration associated with systemic disease

White patches
Normal anatomy
Congenital causes of white patches
Acquired transient white lesions
Acquired persistent white lesions

Red and pigmented lesions
Localized lesions
Generalized lesions
Pigmentation of the teeth

Swellings/lumps in and around the mouth
Developmental soft tissue swellings
Acquired soft tissue swellings
Bony swellings
Generalized gingival swelling
Salivary gland swelling

Lesions of the tongue
Congenital/developmental lesions
Acquired lesions

Lesions of the oral mucosa may occur in isolation, as a specific disease entity, or as a manifestation of a systemic disease process. Oral lesions may on occasion be the presenting feature of a systemic disease. This chapter describes oral conditions occurring in childhood that may present to the dermatologist, or may be noted on examination by the dermatologist. It is beyond the scope of this chapter to discuss all of the conditions mentioned in great detail, this may be found in specialist textbooks on the oral mucosa; for this reason there is no mention of disease affecting the teeth. The chapter is divided into sections depending upon the most likely presenting symptoms and signs and not aetiology.

Mouth ulcers/sore mouth

Stomatitis is a term used for diseases of the oral mucosa of an inflammatory nature be it either acute or chronic. The symptom of sore mouth is usually caused by some form of stomatitis, the most common of which is oral ulceration, defined as a local discontinuity of the oral epithelium. This section deals with the various causes of oral ulceration including those related to systemic disease.

Recurrent aphthous stomatitis (RAS)

Definition

After caries and periodontal disease RAS is the most common disease affecting the mouth with up to 20% of the population being affected. The condition is characterized by painful shallow ulcers which heal and recur at fairly regular intervals.

Aetiology

The aetiology of RAS is not known [1]. There does appear to be a genetic predisposition with a third of patients having a positive family history, and an increased frequency of HLA-A2, HLA-A11, HLA-B12 and HLA-DR2. Reports of immunological phenomena are either unconfirmed or disputed. There is no evidence to suggest that RAS is an autoimmune disease. In some patients there appears to be a relationship with stress and some females exhibit ulceration in the luteal phase of their menstrual cycle, suggesting a hormonal association. Some patients relate their RAS to the ingestion of particular foodstuffs such as cheese and chocolate.

About 10–20% of patients investigated with RAS have an underlying haematinic deficiency usually a low serum ferritin, vitamin B_{12} or red cell folate [2]. Some 3% of patients with RAS have been found to have coeliac disease. Other gastrointestinal diseases which cause malabsorption may also present with RAS, such as Crohn's disease and pernicious anaemia. RAS-like ulceration has also been described in association with human immunodeficiency virus (HIV) infection, Behçet's syndrome and Sweet's syndrome.

Table 22.1.1 Clinical features of RAS

	Minor	Major	Herpetiform
Incidence	80%	10%	10%
Age (years)	10–19	10–19	20–29
Sex (F : M)	1.3 : 1	0.8 : 1	2.6 : 1
Site	Non-keratinized mucous	Anywhere	Anywhere
Number	1–5	1–10	1–100
Size	< 10 mm	> 10 mm	1–2 mm
Duration (days)	7–10	> 20	7–10
Scarring	8%	64%	32%
Recurrence	1–4 months	< 1 month	> 1 month
Duration of disease (years)	< 5	> 15	> 5

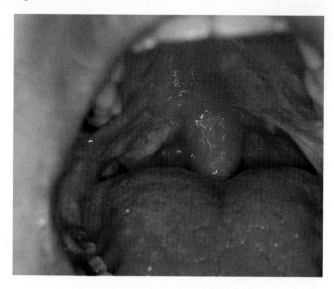

Fig. 22.1.1 Major aphthous ulceration of the palate.

Pathology

Ulceration is thought to be preceded by lymphocytic infiltration of the basal cell layer, and perivascular accumulation of monocytes in the connective tissue, although this is seldom seen. Once the epithelium has ulcerated the surface of the ulcer is covered by a fibrinous exudate (slough) and there is a superficial infiltrate of neutrophils. Monocytes predominate more deeply.

Histopathology is not diagnostic and the diagnosis is primarily dependent upon the clinical history.

Clinical features

RAS can be divided into three clinical types which are summarized in Table 22.1.1.

Minor aphthous stomatitis
(SYN. MIKULICZ ULCERS)

Minor aphthae are the most common accounting for 80% of RAS. Ulceration usually begins in childhood or adolescence, there is a slight female sex predilection of 1:3. The lesions are usually less than 10 mm, an average size being 3–4 mm in diameter and occur in crops of between one and five ulcers on non-keratinized mobile mucosa, i.e. floor of mouth, buccal or labial mucosa. The ulcers are round or ovoid, are shallow and have a white slough with an erythematous inflammatory halo. They heal within 7–10 days and rarely cause scarring (8%). They recur at intervals of between 1 and 4 months. However, crops of ulceration may be so frequent that the patient may never be ulcer free. With increasing age of the patient minor RAS tends to occur less frequently and may cease to be a problem.

Major aphthous stomatitis
(SYN. SUTTON'S ULCERS, PERIADENITIS MUCOSA NECROTICA RECURRENS)

Major aphthae account for about 10% of all RAS. They initially occur in childhood or adolescence, with a slight male predilection of 1:0.8. They are much larger than minor apthae being greater than 10 mm in diameter, typically 1.5–3.0 cm in diameter. They can occur anywhere in the mouth in crops of one to six ulcers and are much more painful than minor apthae. They may have a firm raised margin but otherwise apart from their size have a similar clinical appearance to minor apthae (Fig. 22.1.1). They take a month or more to heal. Healing often occurs with fibrosis resulting in scarring (64%). The rate of recurrence is usually of a shorter interval (within 4 weeks) than that of minor apthae.

Herpetiform ulceration

Herpetiform ulceration affects a slightly older age group (20–29 years). The clinical features are shown in Table 22.1.1.

Differential diagnosis

The diagnosis is made on the clinical appearance of the lesions and the clinical history. It is important to eliminate any underlying predisposing factors such as haematinic deficiencies, and to ask if genital ulceration is present in order to exclude Behçet's syndrome. Biopsy is rarely indicated but may be carried out on major apthae that have failed to heal to eliminate neoplasia.

Treatment

Treatment is symptomatic and often unsuccessful, unless an underlying predisposing factor is identified and corrected. In the majority of patients RAS resolves spontaneously with age. If symptomatic treatment is required it is best to approach therapy systematically, working through a variety of agents beginning with those that have little or no side-effects until one is found that provides symptomatic relief.

Chlorhexidine gluconate (0.2%) or bezydhamine hydrochloride mouthwashes or sprays are a good starting point and often give good symptomatic relief. The spray forms of these agents are particularly useful in children.

Topical tetracycline mouthwash, made up from a 250 mg capsule of tetracycline in 5 ml of water, may be useful particularly in herpetiform ulceration. However, it is unsuitable for young children as they may ingest some of the mouthwash.

Topical steroids such as hydrocortisone hemisuccinate pellets (Corlan) 2.5 mg or triamcinolone acetonide in carboxymethyl cellulose (Adcortyl A in Orabase) applied to the ulcers four times daily.

Becotide 50 or 100 inhaler may be used as a topical mouthspray four to six times a day. Soluble betamethasone tablets (0.5 mg) made up as a mouthwash with 15–20 ml of water and held in the mouth for 3 min four times a day is not suitable for young children but may be of benefit to adolescents. Very occasionally systemic steroids or other immunosuppressive agents such as azathioprine and thalidomide have been necessary to control ulceration; their use in children must be carefully monitored and they should only be used as a last resort.

REFERENCES

1 Scully C, Porter SR. Recurrent aphthous stomatitis current concepts of etiology pathogenesis and management. *J Oral Pathol Med* 1989; 18: 21–7.
2 Field AE, Brookes V, Tyldesley W. Recurrent aphthous ulceration in children—a review. *Int J Paediatr Dent* 1992; 2: 1–10.

Behçet's syndrome

Definition

Behçet's disease is a multisystem disease in which nearly 100% of cases affects the mouth. Mouth lesions manifest as RAS. Other sites that may be affected include the genitals, eyes, skin and joints. There may be a number of other systemic or cutaneous manifestations. Clinical diagnosis of Behçet's syndrome is dependent on the presence of at least three or more possible clinical manifestations, e.g. orogenital ulceration and uveitis (see Chapter 25.8).

Aetiology

The aetiology of Behçet's syndrome is unknown. There is increasing evidence to suggest an immunological aetiology; however, immunological findings appear to vary considerably and therefore cannot be used for the diagnosis or management of the disease. HLA-B5, HLA-BW51 and HLA-DR7 appear to be associated with Behçet's syndrome.

The condition predominantly affects young males, there is often a positive family history. There is also a higher prevalence of the disease in certain geographical areas, which include Japan, China, the Mediterranean and Middle East [1].

Clinical features

Behçet's syndrome can occur in any age group but most commonly affects adult males in their third decade, although it may occur in childhood. The most common clinical feature is that of oral ulceration (90–100%) which may involve the posterior pharynx, and is indistinguishable clinically and histopathologically from recurrent aphthous stomatitis (Figs 22.1.1, 22.1.2). Ulcers may occur at other sites including the anus and genitals. Skin lesions such as erythema nodusum, pustules and pathergy are also common findings. The disease process is transient and subject to spontaneous remissions.

Differential diagnosis

Recurrent oral ulceration may be the first and only initial clinical feature of Behçet's syndrome, but only a very few patients with RAS develop Behçet's syndrome; however, Behçet's syndrome must always be excluded when considering a diagnosis of RAS as unlike RAS it is not self-limiting.

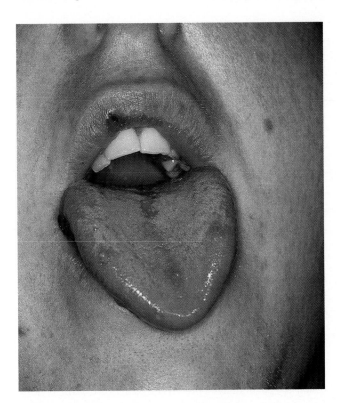

Fig. 22.1.2 Ulceration of the tongue and labial mucosa due to primary herpes virus infection.

Oral and genital ulceration may result from folate deficiency, and together with ocular lesions may occur in erythema multiforme and ulcerative colitis.

Treatment

Oral ulceration can be managed symptomatically as in RAS. Immunosuppressive treatment is required for those with other lesions. Results using cyclosporin and dapsone have been inconclusive, colchicine appears to be of value and thalidomide may be required in cases of recalcitrant orogenital ulceration, but requires extreme caution as it is teratogenic.

MAGIC syndrome

A condition which overlaps with Behçet's syndrome and causes large joint arthropathies, consists of mouth and genital ulcers with inflamed cartilage (MAGIC) [2].

REFERENCES

1 Abesfeld SJ, Kurban AK. Behçet's disease. New perspectives on an enigmatic syndrome. *Am J Dermatol* 1988; 19: 767–79.
2 Firestein GS, Gruber HE, Weisman MH, Zvaifler NJ, Barber J, O'Duffy JD. Mouth and genital ulcers with inflamed cartilage: MAGIC syndrome. *Am J Med* 1985; 79: 65–71.

Traumatic ulceration

Trauma to the oral mucosa is common and may cause localized ulceration, which resolves as long as the causative agent is removed. The trauma may be physical, thermal or chemical, it may be self-inflicted particularly with disorders such as congenital insensitivity to pain, Lesch–Nyhan syndrome, epilepsy, athetosis and mental handicap. Oral ulceration may also be caused by non-accidental injury.

Clinical features

The clinical appearance of a traumatic ulcer is dependent upon the causative agent. Physical trauma gives rise to a localized ulcer which may resemble a minor or major apthous ulcer. Tongue or cheek biting gives rise to more irregularly shaped ulcer. Thermal and chemical trauma caused by the ingestion of hot food or drinking caustic/acidic agents gives rise to more generalized ulceration which tends to affect the tongue and palate. Ulcers may heal with scarring especially if loss of connective tissue has occurred.

Oral ulceration due to non-accidental injury often occurs around the mouth and may involve the labial mucosa, particularly the labial fraenum which may become torn and ulcerated by attempts to silence a child with a hand across the mouth.

Differential diagnosis

The possibility of other causes of oral ulceration should always be considered as described in this section.

Treatment

Usually no treatment is required other than reassurance. If soreness is a problem benzydamine hydrochloride may be useful as either a mouthwash or spray. If the ulcer has been caused by a sharp tooth or orthodontic appliance appropriate modification should be carried out. If self-mutilation is a problem the provision of polyvinyl occlusal splints may be useful. If an ulcer fails to heal within 2–3 weeks, after the causative agent has been removed, a biopsy should be considered to exclude neoplasia.

If child abuse is suspected appropriate action should be taken which is usually dependent upon local guidelines.

Infections

A variety of infections may give rise to oral ulceration/stomatitis; this will be considered under three main groups, viral, fungal and bacterial.

Viral infections

The acute viral infections of childhood may give rise to oral symptoms and ulceration. Due to vaccination programmes measles and rubella are rarely seen in the Western world. The symptoms of acute viral infections affecting the mouth are all very similar but the distribution of lesions may vary. Generally, if a viral infection is suspected the diagnosis is made on clinical and epidemiological information, it is only where virus identification is of importance, such as in immunocompromised patients, that culture and antibody titres to identify the virus are undertaken.

Herpetic gingivostomatitis (see Chapter 5.2)

Aetiology. Herpes simplex virus type 1 and increasingly type 2 causes primary herpetic gingivostomatitis and reactivation of latent virus causes recurrent herpes labialis. Primary herpes most commonly occurs in young children (2–4 years) and is often subclinical; however, many children now reach maturity without acquiring immunity to the virus, giving rise to an increased incidence of primary herpes infections in young adults. Primary herpes infection is twice as common in lower socioeconomic groups. Herpes simplex virus is found in the saliva in both primary and secondary infections, and may be spread in this way. The incubation period is 3–7 days.

Pathology. Well-defined fluid-filled vesicles form in the upper epithelium. The vesicles rupture infecting the epithelium throughout its entire thickness. Ulceration is caused by shedding of the viral damaged epithelial cells.

Clinical features. The lesions consist of well-defined vesicles about 2 mm in diameter, which may coalesce to form larger irregular lesions that may be distributed over the entire oral mucosa and gingivae, but are commonly seen on the dorsum of the tongue and the hard palate. The vesicles rapidly rupture to form circular, sharply defined shallow ulcers with a yellowish-grey floor and erythematous margin (Fig. 22.1.2). The ulcers are very painful. The gingival margins are usually enlarged and inflamed. There is often associated cervical lymphadenopathy, pyrexia and general malaise. Diagnosis is usually made on the clinical features but may be confirmed by either a direct smear or a rise in titre of antibody in an acute and convalescent serum sample.

Differential diagnosis. Acute ulcerative gingivitis and erythema multiforme may occasionally give a similar clinical appearance, as may hand–foot and mouth disease and herpangina (see below). Gingival enlargement similar to that caused by primary herpes may be seen in acute childhood leukaemia particularly the myeloid type.

Treatment. In most cases the infection resolves spontaneously with 7–10 days. For the majority of patients the management is supportive, with antipyretic analgesics (e.g. paracetamol), bed rest and adequate fluid intake. Chlorhexidine gluconate 0.2% mouthwash or spray may help to prevent secondary infection of the ulcers.

Systemic aciclovir hastens recovery but is only really useful if used in the vesicular stage of infection. As most cases present in the ulcerative phase it is of little benefit. Aciclovir does have a role to play if patients are immunocompromised, and in rare complications such as encephalitis and neuropathy.

Recurrent herpes simplex

Following primary infection the herpes virus remains latent in the trigeminal ganglion. About one-third of patients experience recurrent herpes infections, the most common form of which is herpes labialis (cold sore). Typical triggering events include exposure to sunlight, infections such as the common cold, stress and trauma.

Intraoral recurrence often manifests as a dendritic ulcer on the tongue or palate. Chronic ulceration of this type or nodular lesions can occur in immunosuppressed individuals and may require treatment with systemic aciclovir.

Chickenpox

Chickenpox is caused by the varicella-zoster virus and is one of the few remaining common, childhood infections without a vaccine. Lesions occur mainly over the trunk but may also occur intraorally. The oral lesions appear as vesicles that break down to form discrete well-defined ulcers; they are usually fewer in number than in primary herpes and there is no associated gingival enlargement.

Herpes zoster (shingles)

Herpes zoster may give rise to oral lesions if the maxillary or mandibular branch of the trigeminal nerve is involved. Ulcers appear in the distribution of the affected nerve, the lesions do not cross the midline and are preceded by a toothache-like pain. It is rare to see herpes zoster in childhood unless the child is immunocompromised.

Herpangina

Herpangina is caused by a coxsackie A virus. The infection is usually confined to children and presents as an acute pharyngitis with lymphadenopathy and pyrexia. Oral lesions are localized to the soft palate; they resemble those of primary herpes. There is no gingival involvement. The infection resolves spontaneously in 10–14 days. Treatment is supportive as described for primary herpes.

Hand–foot and mouth disease

Hand–foot and mouth disease often causes minor epidemics among schoolchildren. It is caused by a coxsackie A virus usually A10 or A16 or occasionally a coxsackie B or enterovirus.

Clinically, the oral lesions resemble those of primary herpes although they occur in much smaller numbers and cause few symptoms. As in herpangina the gingivae are not involved. Cutaneous lesions affect the hands and feet and consist of small deep-seated vesicles with surrounding erythema situated on the digits or base of the phalanges. Management is as for herpangina.

Infectious mononucleosis (Epstein–Barr viral infection)

Infectious mononucleosis is caused by the Epstein–Barr virus (EBV). In the Western world it is more common in teenagers and young adults, but it may occur in children. Oral symptoms include sore throat, and palatal petechiae is often evident. Occasionally there may be severe ulceration of the fauces, less severe non-specific oral ulceration and pericornitis may also occur.

Cytomegalovirus infection

Cytomegalovirus (CMV) may cause a glandular fever type illness but rarely causes oral ulceration. Persistent CMV-induced ulcers have been described in immunosuppressed patients [1]. Persistent oral ulcers in immunosuppressed patients should be biopsied and sent for histopathology and microbiological culture.

REFERENCE

1 Epstein J, Scully C. Cytomegalovirus: a virus of increasing relevance to oral medicine. *J Oral Pathol Med* 1993; 22: 348–53.

Human immunodeficiency virus

Oral ulceration may occur in children who are HIV positive. Clinically they are often aphthous-like [1] and may be treated as such; however the possibility of an infective cause should always be considered, e.g. CMV.

REFERENCE

1 Scully C, Laskaris G, Porter SR. Oral manifestations of HIV infection and their management. II. Less common lesions. *Oral Surg Oral Med Oral Pathol* 1991; 71: 167–71.

Fungal infections

Oral fungal infections rarely cause ulceration of the oral mucosa in the Western world except in immunocompromised or debilitated patients. In the tropics otherwise healthy individuals may occasionally present with oral fungal lesions.

Deep mycoses

Deep mycoses infections are uncommon in the UK but they are seen in South America and some parts of the southern USA where the climate is warmer and more moist. Oral lesions are most common in histoplasmosis and paracoccidioidomycosis, but have been described in all of them. The oral lesions are not distinctive and diagnosis is usually made on biopsy.

The following deep mycoses may give rise to oral ulceration in the immunocompromised child, particularly those undergoing cytotoxic chemotherapy or bone marrow transplantation, or in patients with acquired immune deficiency syndrome (AIDS). They should always be considered as part of the differential diagnosis in the immunocompromised, and if necessary biopsied to exclude them as causative agents.

Aspergillosis may causes black necrotic ulceration of the palate (Fig. 22.1.3). The infection usually originates from infection in the maxillary sinuses and is caused by direct invasion of the palate. Diagnosis is made from

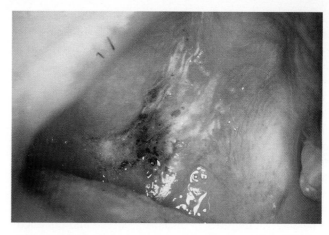

Fig. 22.1.3 Necrotic ulceration of the hard palate due to antral aspergillosis in a child following bone marrow transplantation.

biopsy and radiographic examination of the paranasal air sinuses. Treatment is usually with intravenous ictraconazole or amphotericin.

Mucormycosis (zygomycosis, phycomycosis), a fungus associated with mouldy bread, may give rise to a similar clinical picture as aspergillosis. It is a condition which has been associated with uncontrolled diabetes mellitus.

Histoplasmosis oral lesions are uncommon and present as a non-specific ulcer or lump. They are usually seen in chronic disseminated histoplasmosis.

Bacterial infections

Acute ulcerative gingivitis

Acute ulcerative gingivitis (AUG) is an uncommon disease in childhood and may be associated with immune deficiency such as AIDS and cytotoxic chemotherapy. In countries where nutrition is poor it can manifest as cancrum oris (noma) causing massive soft tissue destruction.

Aetiology. It is thought to be caused by a proliferation of two normal oral commensals, the Gram-negative anaerobes *Borrelia vincentii* and *Fusobacterium nucleatum*.

Clinical and pathological features. Classically, AUG begins on the tips of the interdental papillae causing intense pain and halitosis. Spontaneous bleeding of the gingivae may occur. The ulceration spreads along the gingival margin but is well localized. In the immunocompromised child the ulceration may be far more destructive and spread onto the palate and buccal sulci may occur. Histologically, there is intense inflammation and destruction of the epithelium and connective tissue.

Differential diagnosis. When occurring in a young child primary herpetic gingivostomatitis may give a similar gingival appearance, but it is unusual for ulceration to be localized to the gingivae. Systemic upset is usually more severe in primary herpes.

Treatment. AUG responds rapidly to metronidazole therapy three times daily for 3 days, the dose depending upon age. If the child is immunocompromised a longer course and higher dose may be indicated. Local measures such as improving oral hygiene and the use of an antibacterial mouthwash (e.g. chlorhexidine gluconate 0.2%) should also be considered.

Oral ulceration in association with neoplasia

Oral carcinoma is extremely rare in children. Very occasionally oral ulceration may be the presenting feature of a malignant lesion, particularly lymphoma or histiocytosis. Any chronic oral ulcer in a child with no obvious causative factors should therefore be biopsied.

Oral ulceration associated with systemic disease

Oral ulceration may occasionally be the presenting feature of a systemic disease. The relationship of oral ulceration to systemic diseases will be discussed in this section with reference only to the systemic disease and oral features.

Haematological disorders

Haematinic deficiencies are discussed above. Immunodeficiencies, whether congenital or acquired, may also give rise to oral ulceration. These ulcers usually resemble recurrent aphthae but if a neutropenia is present they lack the erythematous inflammatory halo, as in hereditary benign neutropenia (Fig. 22.1.4).

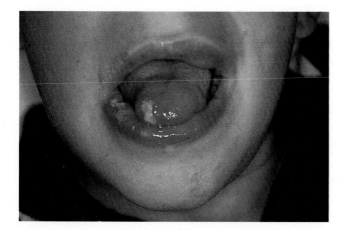

Fig. 22.1.4 Neutropenic ulcers in a child with familial chronic neutropenia. Note the lack of inflammation surrounding the ulcers.

Gastrointestinal disease

As discussed with RAS haematinic deficiencies may give rise to oral ulceration, therefore any gastrointestinal disease causing malabsorption predisposes the child to oral ulceration.

Coeliac disease (gluten sensitivity enteropathy)

Coeliac disease after cystic fibrosis is the commonest gastrointestinal cause of failure to thrive. The greatest prevalency occurring in Irish, British, German and Italian families; it is rare in black and oriental people. Of affected individuals 50% present before 18 months of age. Older children and adolescents with undiagnosed coeliac disease may occasionally present with sore mouths.

Oral manifestations of coeliac disease include recurrent aphthous ulcers, glossitis, angular stomatitis and dental hypoplasia, related to underlying haematinic and vitamin deficiencies.

Crohn's disease

Crohn's disease is a chronic inflammatory disease of the gastrointestinal tract, the aetiology of which is unknown. It is characterized by granulomatous inflammation which may affect any part of the gastrointestinal tract (often the terminal ileum), causing ulceration, fissuring and fibrosis of the mucosa. Crohn's disease may occur in any age group but most commonly affects young adults. When a child is affected by an inflammatory bowel disease there is a 20–30% likelihood that there is a family history of the disease.

Oral lesions related to Crohn's disease include facial or labial swelling (orofacial granulomatosis), oral ulcers which may be large and ragged or linear in appearance, mucosal tagging or proliferation of the oral mucosa to give a 'cobblestone' appearance, other lesions such as RAS and glossitis may be due to an associated nutritional deficiency caused by malabsorption or may be coincidental.

Oral lesions may occur prior to any gastrointestinal symptoms. Biopsy of the oral lesions will confirm the diagnosis, histology showing non-caseating granulomas in the corium with an overlying normal or ulcerated epithelium. Differential diagnosis includes sarcoidosis and tuberculosis.

Treatment of the oral lesions is dependent upon whether there is active gastrointestinal disease, if systemic corticosteroid or aminosalicylate therapy for active gastrointestinal disease is used the oral lesions may also improve. If oral lesions remain symptomatic or occur in isolation local measures to control the symptoms such as those used in RAS may be adequate.

Orofacial granulomatosis is a term given to labial or gingival swelling due to a granulomatous reaction but without any detectable systemic cause, e.g. Crohn's disease, sarcoidosis.

Some patients with this diagnosis will go on to develop a systemic disease some time later. In some cases the granulomatous reaction is thought to be due to a food allergy, particularly cinnamon-containing foodstuffs. Exclusion of cinnamon from the diet of these individuals causes resolution of the lesions. A short course of high-dose or intralesional steroids may reduce swelling [1].

REFERENCES

1 Williams PM, Greenberg S. Management of cheilitis granulomatosa. *Oral Surg Oral Med Oral Pathol* 1991; 72: 436–9.

Ulcerative colitis

Ulcerative colitis is a chronic inflammatory disease of the gastrointestinal tract of unknown aetiology which affects the mucosa of the large bowel, causing diffuse inflammation and ulceration. The prevalence of the condition has a large geographic variance occurring most frequently in Western societies. The disease may occur at any age but the majority of cases occur in late adolescence.

Oral lesions associated with ulcerative colitis include aphthous-type ulceration and glossitis, which may be associated with anaemia. Other oral lesions are rare and include, haemorrhagic ulceration of the mucosa, chronic oral ulceration resembling pyostomatitis gangrenosum of the skin and pyostomatitis vegetans, which clinically gives rise to hyperplastic folds of the oral mucosa between which microabscesses or fissures form; multiple yellowish pustules may also form on the mucosa.

Behçet's syndrome should be considered in the differential diagnosis of oral lesions. Treatment is the same as in Crohn's disease, oral lesions being more apparent with exacerbations of bowel inflammation.

Dermatological disorders

Dermatological disorders rarely cause mouth ulcers in children, if they do occur skin lesions can aid diagnosis.

Lichen planus, lichenoid reactions and chronic graft-versus-host disease

Lichen planus is rare in childhood. Drug-induced lichenoid lesions may occur — they are particularly associated with the use of anti-inflammatory agents, antihypertensives and antimalarial drugs. Graft-versus-host disease (GVHD) following organ or bone marrow transplantation may also give rise to lichenoid lesions.

Clinically, several forms of lichen planus may be observed. Reticular lichen planus is usually asymptomatic and is usually symmetrically distributed on the buccal mucosa and lateral borders of the tongue. It may resemble oral thrush, particularly if plaque-like in appearance. This form of lichen planus requires no treatment.

Atrophic or erosive lichen planus is symptomatic and may be seen in GVHD. It presents as erosive often linear ulcers which affect any site but commonly the tongue and buccal mucosa (Fig. 22.1.5). It is unlikely to be the only clinical manifestation of GVHD. Skin and liver GVHD are often concurrent requiring the use of immunosuppressive therapy. The immunosuppressive therapy does not always resolve the oral GVHD and topical steroid therapy using Becotide 50 or 100 inhaler as a topical mouth spray four to six times a day together with soluble betamethasone 0.5 mg (Betnesol), used as a mouthwash (dissolved in 25 mls of water) and held in the mouth for 2–3 min four times a day, may aid healing and improve symptoms. Benzydamine hydrochloride mouthwash or spray may also be of symptomatic use. It is also important to keep the mouth as clean as possible, to prevent secondary infection. As toothbrushing may be painful, the use of chlorhexidine gluconate mouthwash 0.2% or spray twice daily may be helpful. As the GVHD responds to the immunosuppressive therapy oral lesions usually resolve.

Vesiculobullous disorders

The more common dermatological conditions that cause vesiculobullous lesions in the mouth, such as pemphigus vulgaris and benign mucous membrane pemphigoid, are rare in childhood and will not be discussed. Oral vesicles or bullae may occur in childhood in benign familial chronic pemphigoid which break down to form well-demarcated ulcers.

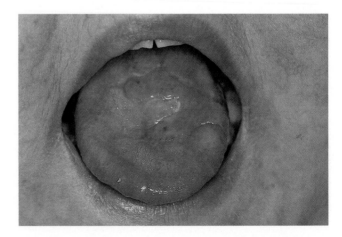

Fig. 22.1.5 Erosive lichen planus-like lesions of the tongue due to GVHD. Note also the depapillation of the tongue.

Epidermolysis bullosa. Epidermolysis bullosa (EB) is discussed in Chapter 19.4. In most forms of the disease bullae will form on the oral mucosa. They usually appear in infancy and may be precipitated by suckling. The bullae break down to form ulcers which heal slowly usually with scarring, The tongue becomes depapillated. Because of the sensitivity of the mucosa to trauma oral hygiene is usually poor and the incidence of caries and periodontal disease is high.

Dermatitis herpetiformis and linear immunoglobulin A disease. Dermatitis herpetiformis may occur in childhood and is often associated with gluten enteropathy (see Chapter 12.4). Oral lesions may occur and include erythematous papules and macules, petechia, vesicles, bullae and erosions. Similar oral lesions may occur in linear immunoglobulin A (IgA) disease. Oral lesions rarely occur in isolation and will respond to therapy for cutaneous lesions, dapsone or sulphapyridine. Diagnosis is made on biopsy.

Erythema multiforme. Erythema multiforme is discussed in Chapter 9.5. Oral features characteristically include swollen, bleeding, crusted lips and widespread oral ulceration. Oral ulcers are preceded by erythematous macules which become vesicles. Intact vesicles are rarely seen as they rapidly break down to form ill-defined ulcers. The tongue is often furred and there may be regional lymphadenitis. Oral lesions may occur in isolation or with a skin rash, which characteristically consists of 'target' lesions and ocular involvement.

The combination of oral lesions, skin lesions and conjunctivitis is referred to as Stevens–Johnson syndrome.

Biopsy may be necessary in less characteristic cases and will exclude other vesiculobullous disorders and Behçet's syndrome.

Aciclovir may be beneficial prophylactically in herpes precipitated erythema multiforme.

Connective tissue disorders

Connective tissue disorders that give rise to oral ulceration rarely occur in children, e.g. systemic and discoid lupus erythematoses. Juvenile rheumatoid arthritis may be associated with anaemia that may predispose to RAS. Behçet's syndrome may occur in childhood and is discussed above.

Iatrogenic oral ulceration

Oral ulceration may be caused by certain drugs, e.g. cytotoxic agents, Septrin. The ulceration is usually aphthous-like in appearance but may lack an inflammatory halo if associated with neutropenia. It is self-limiting and heals within 7–10 days. It is now less commonly seen in association with methotrexate as folinic acid rescue (calcium leucovorin) is usually always given with high-dose methotrexate therapy. Aphthous-type ulceration can occur in long-term use of some antibiotics, such as Septrin, which inter-fere with folate metabolism giving rise to a macrocytic anaemia and predisposing to RAS. Aplastic anaemia may also be drug induced and give rise to oral ulceration and purpura.

Radiation to the head and neck, and total body irradiation for bone marrow transplantation, gives rise to mucositis. Mucositis occurs 7–10 days after beginning radiotherapy to the head and neck, and lasts for up to 4 weeks of completion of treatment. Those undergoing total body irradiation experience mucositis within 5–10 days and the mucositis heals within 2–3 weeks of treatment.

Various agents have been used to decrease the amount of mucositis and improve healing; however, none have been particularly successful. Treatment therefore remains symptomatic, benzhydamine hydrochloride and Corsodyl may help alleviate symptoms. The use of antibiotics to decrease the numbers of oral Gram-negative bacteria in mucositis may be of benefit [1].

REFERENCE

1 Spijkervet FKL, van Saene HKF, van Saene JJM *et al*. Mucositis prevention by selective elimination of oral flora in irradiated head and neck cancer patients. *J Oral Pathol Med* 1990; 19: 486–9.

White patches

Definition of leucoplakia

The term leucoplakia is often used clinically to describe a chronic white lesion of the oral mucosa. It should really be restricted to those white lesions for which there is no identifiable cause or underlying disease process.

Normal anatomy

Fordyce's spots or granules

Fordyce's spots are sebaceous glands that are present beneath the oral mucosa. Although they are present at birth they do not usually become clinically apparent until puberty.

They appear as asymptomatic slightly raised yellowish nodules usually on the buccal mucosa just inside the commissure, or the labial and retromolar mucosa. They may be discrete or coalesce.

Diagnosis is made on the clinical appearance. Treatment involves reassurance that they are a normal feature of the oral mucosa.

Gingival cysts of infancy (Epstein's pearls and Bohn's nodules)

These cysts are commonly seen in the newborn. They either rupture spontaneously or involute and are rarely apparent after 3 months or age. They arise from remnants of the dental laminae on the alveolus (Epstein's pearls) or epithelial inclusion at a site of fusion, e.g. midline of the palate (Bohn's nodules).

Clinically, they appear as 2–3 mm diameter white nodules on the crests of the alveolar ridge or the midline of the palate. As they resolve spontaneously no treatment is required.

Congenital causes of white patches

White sponge naevus (familial white folded gingivostomatitis)

Aetiology

This is a rare condition inherited as an autosomal dominant trait which results in the formation of widespread white plaques of the oral mucosa caused by abnormal tonofilament organization. Other mucosae may be affected.

Pathology

The epithelium appears hyperplastic and has a thick irregular parakeratotic layer which, due to epithelial odema, has a so-called 'basket-weave appearance'.

Clinical features

The clinical appearance is very distinctive and is often first noticed in childhood. The oral mucosa is irregularly thickened, folded and appears white. Unlike other white lesions there is no clear margin to the lesion and it merges imperceptibly with normal mucosa. The buccal mucosa is usually affected but the entire oral mucosa may be involved, the attached gingivae are usually spared.

Differential diagnosis

The clinical appearance is usually sufficient to diagnose the condition, and a positive family history is helpful. Biopsy may be necessary to eliminate other causes of white patches in less classical cases.

Treatment

As the condition is asymptomatic and benign, no treatment is required other than reassurance.

Darier–White disease (dyskeratosis follicularis)

Inherited as an autosomal dominant disorder of keratinization, this condition manifests in early adolescence (see Chapter 19.9). Oral lesions occur in about 50% of affected individuals and their appearance bears no significance to the intensity of the skin involvement.

Clinically, the lesions consist of flattish initially erythematous papules which coalesce to give a cobblestone appearance. The lesions become progressively paler until they are white. The lesions tend to occur on the tongue, palate and gingivae [1]. Palatal lesions can resemble nicotinic stomatitis.

REFERENCE

1 Macleod RI, Munro CS. The incidence and distribution of oral lesions in patients with Darier's disease. *Br Dent J* 1991; 177: 133–6.

Tylosis (palmoplantar keratoderma) and Clouston's syndrome

Tylosis is inherited as an autosomal dominant trait and is discussed in Chapter 19.6. Orally preleucoplakia lesions have been reported in most affected children [1]. These lesions are diffuse and greyish in colour; they go on to form non-specific leucoplakia with increasing age. These lesions do not appear to be premalignant.

Clouston's syndrome (hidrotic ectodermal dysplasia) which also causes palmoplantar hyperkeratosis may also give rise to oral leucoplakia [2].

REFERENCES

1 Tyldesley WR. Oral leukoplakia associated with tylosis and oesophageal carcinoma. *J Oral Pathol* 1974; 3: 62–70.
2 George DI, Escobar VH. Oral findings of Clouston's syndrome. *Oral Surg Oral Med Oral Pathol* 1984; 57: 258–62.

Pachyonychia congenita

Pachyonychia congenita is discussed in Chapter 23.2. Oral lesions occur in 60% of affected individuals and present as focal or generalized greyish white thickening of the oral mucosa. They do not have an increased malignant potential [1]. Vesicular and ulcerative oral lesions have also been described. Of affected individuals 10% have angular cheilitis, and there is an increased risk of chronic candidiasis in this group. Natal or neonatal teeth, may also be present in 16% of individuals.

REFERENCE

1 Feinstein A, Friedman J, Schewach-Millet M. Pachyonychia congenita. *J Am Acad Dermatol* 1988; 19: 705–11.

Dyskeratosis congenita

This is a rare disorder with both a sex-linked and a recessive form. The main features include dysplastic lesions of the oral mucosa, dermal pigmentation, nail dystrophy and aplastic anaemia (see Chapter 19.23).

Oral lesions usually occur between the ages of 5 and 10 years and consist of white patches, usually affecting the palate or tongue, which may be preceded by vesicles or erosions [1]. Oral lesions may also manifest as small erythematous areas. Biopsy of the lesion shows dysplasia and there is a high risk of malignant change. Regular review and rebiopsy of lesions is essential.

REFERENCE

1 Cannell H. Dyskeratosis congenita. *Br J Oral Surg* 1971; 9: 8–20.

Hereditary benign intraepithelial dyskeratosis

This is a very rare autosomal dominant condition in which oral lesions occur in childhood and become more obvious by adolescence. They consist of milky white smooth translucent plaques which predominantly affect the buccal mucosa, lips and ventrum of the tongue. Biopsy may be necessary to differentiate from white sponge naevus and other white lesions. No treatment is required.

Acquired transient white lesions

Traumatic/frictional keratosis

Frictional keratosis is caused by chronic irritation of the oral epithelium which causes hyperkeratosis. It is often caused by a sharp tooth or restoration, or by a habit such as cheek biting. Clinically, the relationship of the keratosis to a causative factor should be established. On removal of the causative agent or cessation of the habit resolution of the keratosis should occur.

Chemical trauma to the oral mucosa may also lead to a transient white lesion. Children may occasionally ingest caustic or acidic agents, e.g. household cleaning agents, which cause epithelial cell death that clinically appears as a soft white patch. Aspirin burns result from an aspirin being placed next to a painful tooth. In this case the white plaque is localized.

Furred/hairy tongue

See lesions of the tongue (below).

Koplik's spots

Koplik's spots are an oral manifestation of measles. They appear as small white lesions resembling grains of salt on the buccal mucosa. Their appearance may precede the cutaneous skin rash by 1–2 days. Measles is an uncommon childhood infectious illness in areas where there is a measles immunization programme.

Candidiasis

Definition

This is an acute or chronic infection of the oral mucosa caused by invasion of the epithelium by candidal hyphae, which usually induces a proliferative response and causes a plaque to form.

Aetiology

Candida species are isolated in about 50% of the population as a normal oral commensal organism, the commonest species being *Candida albicans*. *C. krusei*, *C. guilliermondii*, *C. tropicalis* and *C. parapsilosis* may also be implicated especially in the immunocompromised patient. Should the balance of the oral environment be disturbed (e.g. systemic infection, use of an orthodontic appliance, suppression of cell-mediated immunity, iron deficiency) candidal organisms may proliferate and give rise to infection. Candidiasis is the commonest oral manifestation of HIV disease.

Chronic mucocutaneous candidiasis is characterized by persistent candidiasis which usually begins in early childhood, involving the skin, mucous membranes and nails. About 50% of patients have an associated endocrinopathy, which is usually preceded by candidiasis. Of patients 20% have a family history.

Clinical features, pathology, diagnosis and treatment

The clinical features of oral candidiasis are dependent upon whether the infection is acute or chronic. The various clinical entities are discussed below.

Acute pseudomembranous candidiasis (thrush). Thrush is typically seen in the neonatal period when immune mechanisms have not fully developed. It may also be seen in children who are compromised in some way. The lesions are usually asymptomatic and manifest as thick creamy plaques which are easily wiped off the oral mucosa leaving an erythematous area of mucosa. The lesions may occur in any area of the mouth, but are commonly seen on the soft palate and fauces (Fig. 22.1.6).

On direct smear with a Gram stain masses of candidal hyphae may be seen with a few yeast cells.

The plaques are formed by proliferation of the epithelium in response to invasion by candidal hyphae. The plaque consists of epithelial cells which are separated by inflammatory infiltrate making the plaque friable.

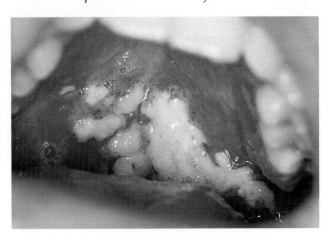

Fig. 22.1.6 Acute pseudomembranous candidiasis in a child undergoing chemotherapy for acute leukaemia.

The deeper epithelium is hyperplastic and there is an acute inflammatory reaction in the connective tissue. Sections stained with periodic acid–Schiff (PAS) show candidal hyphae growing downwards through the epithelium.

If no predisposing factor is evident investigation should be undertaken to establish why candidiasis has occurred, e.g. anaemia, diabetes mellitus or immunodeficency. If the child is known to be immunocompromised it is important to culture the lesions for species other than *C. albicans*, such as *C. kruseii* which is inherently resistant to some antifungal agents [1].

In the majority of cases topical antifungal therapy is usually adequate to treat the infection. Nystatin suspension or pastilles can be used or amphotericin B lozenges or miconazole oral gel used four times a day for 10–14 days. If the lesions fail to respond to topical antifungals, systemic use of fluconazole or itraconazole should be considered.

Erythematous candidiasis. Candidal infection may cause erythematous lesions such as in chronic denture stomatitis, and candidiasis associated with xerostomia and the use of topical steroid inhalers. However, the term erythematous candidiasis is now frequently used to describe the patchy erythematous lesions associated with HIV infection. Treatment is as for thrush.

Chronic atrophic candidiasis (chronic denture stomatitis). This condition is often seen under the fitting surface of upper dentures, hence the term denture stomatitis. It may also occur under a removable orthodontic appliance. It is bright red in appearance and is clearly defined to the area under the appliance. Candidal hyphae can be isolated from the mucosa and the porous acrylic surface of the appliance. The infection is caused by the continual wearing of the appliance which prevents debridement of the covered mucosa and forms a warm moist environment which favours the proliferation of candidal organisms.

Histologically, the epithelium exhibits acanthosis with an oedematous superficial layer. The underlying connective tissue contains a chronic inflammatory cell infiltrate.

Chronic atrophic candidiasis usually resolves if the appliance is removed from the mouth for a few hours each day cleaned thoroughly and soaked in a mild hypochlorite solution, e.g. Milton. If this is not possible miconazole gel can be applied to the mucosal surface of the appliance four times a day. Once the appliance is no longer needed the candidiasis will resolve spontaneously.

Angular stomatitis. Angular stomatitis describes an inflammatory lesion at the angle of the mouth, it is often bilateral and may be asymptomatic or painful. It can occur with any concurrent intraoral candidiasis but is not always due to candidal infection. *Staphylococcus aureus* may also cause angular stomatitis, the organisms often originating from the nares. Angular stomatitis may also be non-infective and may be due to persistent dribbling causing maceration of the tissues.

Diagnosis of the causative organism will require a microbiological swab which should be cultured for *S. aureus* and *Candida* species.

Treatment is dependent on the causative factor. Both candidal and staphylococcal infections will respond to miconazole gel. If *Staphylococcus* is isolated a more rapid resolution may occur with Fucidin cream and the nose may also need to be treated. If no organisms are cultured, and maceration is the cause, a barrier ointment may be of use.

REFERENCE

1 Johnson EM, Warnock DW, Luker J, Porter SR, Scully C. Emergence of azole resistance in *Candida* species from HIV-infected patients receiving prolonged fluconazole therapy for oral candidosis. *J Antimicrob Chemother* 1995; 35: 103–14.

Acquired persistent white lesions

Chronic hyperplastic candidiasis (candidal leucoplakia)

Chronic hyperplastic candidiasis in childhood is unusual and most often seen in mucocutaneous candidiasis, congenital immunodeficiencies and AIDS. Clinically, the oral lesions all have similar features: they are white, tough and firmly adherent to the underlying mucosa. They are often of irregular thickness and outline. Common sites include the buccal mucosa and dorsum of the tongue.

There are four main clinical variants of chronic mucocutaneous candidiasis.
1 Candidal leucoplakia (idiopathic limited type).
2 Familial chronic mucocutaneous candidiasis.
3 Diffuse-type chronic mucocutaneous candidiasis.
4 Endocrine candidiasis syndrome.

All give rise to persistent candidiasis in which the mouth is the sole or main site of infection. The lesions do not respond to topical antifungal therapy.

Histologically, the features are similar to those seen in thrush. The plaques consist of thick layers of parakeratotic epithelium invaded by candidal hyphae. There is an inflammatory infiltrate within the plaque which is concentrated at its base. The underlying epithelium is hyperplastic and there are chronic inflammatory changes in the dermis.

Diagnosis of chronic hyperplastic candidiasis is confirmed by biopsy.

Treatment is difficult and topical antifungal agents are rarely of use. Systemic agents such as fluconazole and itraconazole are beneficial but may require continued prophylactic administration if mucocutaneous candidiasis syndrome is diagnosed. If recurrence occurs with use of long-term azole antifungals is used recurrence of the lesions should be cultured to check for azole resistance.

Lichen planus, lichenoid lesions and chronic graft-versus-host disease

See Mouth ulcers/sore mouths, p. 1435.

Psoriasis

Oral lesions are extremely rare in psoriasis and are usually only associated with pustular psoriasis. The lesions may resemble erythema migrans (see p. 1448) or take the form of translucent plaques. Macules, diffuse erythema and pustules have also been reported.

Lupus erythematosus

This is a connective tissue disorder which is very rare in childhood but may give rise to oral lesions that resemble lichen planus, particularly the atrophic type. The lesions are not symmetrical in distribution and the white striae tend to radiate centrifugally.

Hairy leucoplakia

Hairy leucoplakia may be seen in children with severe immune defects particularly HIV infection. EBV has been shown to be present in the epithelium, and the lesions have been reported to regress with aciclovir therapy. Histological features include severe parakeratosis, hyperplasia, koilocyte-like cells and an absence of inflammatory infiltrate.

Clinically, the lesion appears more corrugated in appearance than hairy, and is most often seen on the lateral borders of the tongue [1]. It is symptomless and no treatment is required.

Biopsy may be necessary to confirm the diagnosis.

REFERENCE

1 Scully C, Laskaris G, Porter SR. Oral manifestations of HIV infection and their management. I. More common lesions. *Oral Surg Oral Med Oral Pathol* 1991; 71: 158–66.

Chronic renal failure

Stomatitis is commonly seen in uraemic patients. Leucoplakias have also been reported [1]. Clinically, the lesions resemble congenital white sponge naevus, although the lesions have well-defined margins. The ventral surface of the tongue is often the main site affected.

REFERENCE

1 Kellet M. Oral white patches in uraemic patients. *Br Dent J* 1983; 154: 366–8.

Leucoplakia of unknown cause

Leucoplakia is uncommon in childhood. The clinical appearance is highly variable as is the size of the lesion (Fig. 22.1.7). Histologically, they range from simple hyperkeratosis to atrophic parakeratotic epithelium with severe dysplasia. Although the clinical appearance is no indication of the underlying histology speckled lesions are more likely to show dysplastic changes.

Any leucoplakia of unknown cause should be biopsied and kept under regular 3-monthly review. If the lesion changes in character it should be rebiopsied because of the risk of malignant change.

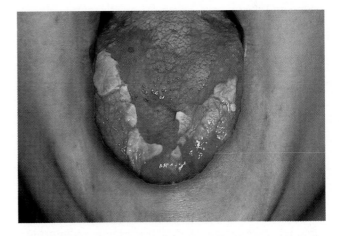

Fig. 22.1.7 Leucoplakia of the tongue. Clinically, this lesion resembles lichen planus, but histologically showed only hyperkeratosis. The 17-year-old patient had undergone bone marrow transplantation some 8 years previously, suggesting that the lesion may have been initially due to GVHD.

Red and pigmented lesions

Localized lesions

Amalgam tattoo

Amalgam tattoos are the most common cause of localized oral pigmentation. They can occur at any age, and result from minor trauma to the oral mucosa during the placement of an amalgam restoration or during the extraction of a tooth containing an amalgam restoration, which allows amalgam particles to penetrate into the epithelium. The amalgam particles are deposited in the corium. A foreign body giant cell reaction or macrophage accumulation occurs in about 55% of cases.

Clinically, they are most commonly seen on the gingivae, alveolar mucosa, floor of the mouth and buccal mucosa. They appear as symptomless blue–black macules the margins of which may be well defined or diffuse. They may vary in size from 1 to 20 mm.

Radiography may aid the diagnosis as many lesions are radio-opaque. If any doubt exists as to the diagnosis biopsy should be performed.

Oral pigmented naevi

Melanocytic naevi are rare in the mouth when compared to the occurrence on the skin (see Chapter 16.1). They are twice as common in females and tend to occur in the 30–50-year-old age group, although they may be seen in childhood. They range in size from 1 to 30 mm the majority being less than 6 mm. They may be grey, brown, black or blue in colour; about 20% are non-pigmented. The hard palate and buccal mucosa are the most common sites of occurrence.

Histologically, several types of naevi can be identified: junctional, compound, intramucosal, blue oral melanotic macule and melanoacanthoma. They are all benign. Malignant melanoma is rare in childhood. Diagnosis may be confirmed by biopsy.

Melanotic neuroectodermal tumour of infancy

This is a rare tumour occurring in the first year of life. It is thought to arise from neural crest tissue. Clinically, lesions occur in the anterior maxilla as painless, non-tender enlarging dark masses. Growth may be rapid. Radiographic examination shows underlying radiolucency and displacement of developing teeth. The lesion is benign and conservative surgical excision is curative.

Peutz–Jeghers syndrome

This autosomal dominant syndrome comprises of intestinal polyposis and melanotic pigmentation of the face and mouth (see Chapter 19.24). Oral pigmentation is usually confined to the lower lip and buccal mucosa.

Haemangiomas

Haemangiomas are localized congenital vascular hamatomas (described more fully in Chapter 18.2.) Clinically, oral haemangiomas appear as superficial purple/bluish nodules or macules that blanch on pressure, the common sites of occurrence being the lips (Fig. 22.1.8), tongue, palate and buccal mucosa. Intraoral haemangiomas are also associated with certain syndromes including Sturge–Weber syndrome, Klippel–Trenaunay–Weber syndrome and Maffucci's syndrome.

Excision or biopsy of the lesion may be necessary if the diagnosis is unclear or the lesion is enlarging to eliminate neoplasia. Surgery or cryotherapy may be required if repeated haemorrhage is a problem. Very large haemangiomas are difficult to treat surgically and sclerosing agents may be of benefit.

Hereditary mucoepithelial dysplasia

This is a rare autosomal dominant trait which results in abnormal desmosome and gap junctions. Clinically, oral lesions appear in infancy as red macules or papules on the palate and gingivae. They are painless and may persist throughout life.

Erythema migrans

See lesions of the tongue (below).

Kaposi's sarcoma

Rarely Kaposi's sarcoma may occur intraorally in children with AIDS, particularly in Africa [1]. Lesions are most

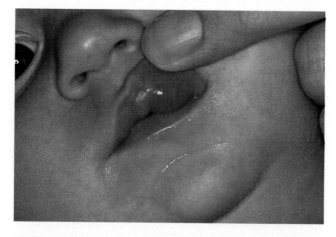

Fig. 22.1.8 Haemangioma of the upper lip in a 6-month-old baby. The lesion was surgically excised as it was enlarging and causing lip distortion.

common on the palate and present as purple/red nodules or macules. They rarely require treatment.

REFERENCE

1 Ficarra G, Berson AM, Silverman S *et al.* Kaposi's sarcoma of the oral cavity: a study of 134 patients with a review of the pathogenesis, epidemiology, clinical aspects and treatment. *Oral Surg Oral Med Oral Pathol* 1988; 66: 543–50.

Chronic atrophic candidiasis

See acquired transient white lesions (candidiasis) above.

Gingivitis

Gingivitis is uncommon in preschool children (with the exception of acute viral infections) and an underlying systemic disease should always be considered in a differential diagnosis, particularly immunological deficiencies such as neutropenia (Fig. 22.1.9).

In older children gingivitis is usually concurrent with poor oral hygiene; however, if associated with destruction of the periodontium (the supportive tissues of the teeth) underlying disease should be eliminated particularly diabetes mellitus and immunodeficiency.

Gingivitis presents clinically as redness of the gingivae surrounding the tooth, it is usually painless but the child may report bleeding of the gingivae on toothbrushing. There is usually a heavy accumulation of plaque around the necks of the teeth.

Treatment involves removal of plaque, instigation of good oral hygiene and the use of chlorhexidine gluconate mouthwash 0.2% twice daily until gingivitis resolves.

Allergic gingivostomatitis

Occasionally gingivitis may be caused by an allergic reaction. The gingivitis tends to be diffuse and oral hygiene is

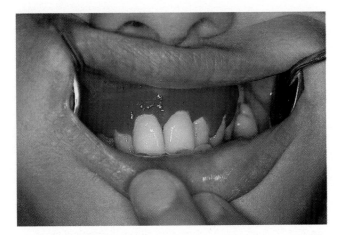

Fig. 22.1.9 Acute gingivitis and periodontitis in a child with familial chronic neutropenia.

often very good. Common causative agents include cinnamon-containing toothpastes, certain chewing gums and mints. The gingivitis resolves when the causal agent is removed and recurs when rechallenged.

Generalized lesions

Racial pigmentation is the most common cause of generalized pigmentation of the oral mucosa in both children and adults; however, other causes such as those discussed below should be eliminated from the differential diagnosis. Other rare causes of generalized oral pigmentation include haemochromatosis, neurofibromatosis and incontinentia pigmenti.

Racial pigmentation

Racial pigmentation mainly occurs in individuals of black, Asian or Mediterranean descent and 5% of Caucasians. It varies in colour from light brown to black and may occur anywhere in the mouth particularly the gingivae and tongue.

Drug-induced hyperpigmentation

Drugs such as anticonvulsants, cytotoxic agents (especially busulphan), adrenocorticotropic hormone (ACTH) therapy and oral contraceptives may cause brown oral pigmentation. Antimalarial drugs produce a range of mucosal pigmentation from yellow to blue/black depending on the drug used.

Minocycline has also been reported to cause a blue/grey staining of the gingival margins [1].

REFERENCE

1 Berger RS, Mandel EB, Hayes TJ *et al.* Minocycline staining of the oral cavity. *J Am Acad Dermatol* 1989; 21: 432–42.

Addison's disease

Oral hyperpigmentation ranging from light brown to almost black may be seen in Addison's disease or in ectopic ACTH production. The pigmentation is variable in its distribution but often affects the soft palate, buccal mucosa, lateral borders of the tongue, gingivae and lips. Addison's disease may be associated with chronic mucocutaneous candidiasis (see above).

Albright's syndrome

Pigmentation of the oral mucosa has been reported in Albright's syndrome, which consists of polyostotic fibrous dysplasia (facial bones affected in 25% of cases), pigmentation of the skin and precocious puberty in females.

Hereditary haemorrhagic telangiectasia (Osler–Weber–Rendu disease)

This is an autosomal dominant trait characterized by multiple telangiectasia of the skin and mucous membranes. Lesions do not normally become apparent until the second or third decade. Any area of the mouth may be affected, the lesions appear as red spots or spider-like lesions which empty on applying pressure, they are caused by the superficial dilation of small blood vessels. If traumatized they may cause bleeding which may be difficult to control. Laser therapy to the lesions may be required.

Oral telangiectasia may also be seen following radiotherapy to the head and neck region.

Thrombocytopenic purpura

Thrombocytopenia whatever its aetiology (idiopathic, drug induced, etc.) may cause oral purpura or petechiae at a platelet count of below $50 \times 10/l$. Lesions commonly occur on mucosa that is easily traumatized such as the tongue, palate and buccal mucosa. They are reddish/purple in colour and vary in size (Fig. 22.1.10). They do not blanch on pressure. Oral purpura may be the first clinical manifestation of leukaemia, aplastic anaemia or HIV disease.

Pigmentation of the teeth

Pigmentation or discoloration of the teeth may be due to intrinsic or extrinsic staining (Table 22.1.2; Fig. 22.1.11).

Swellings/lumps in and around the mouth

Lumps in the mouth may have a variety of causes ranging from normal anatomy to neoplasia. In this section they are considered in three main groups: soft tissue swellings, bony swellings and gingival swelling.

Developmental soft tissue swellings

Cogenital granular cell epulis of the newborn

The congenital epulis is a rare tumour occurring on the alveolar ridge which as its name implies is present at birth. It may form a soft rounded pedunculated swelling of a few millimetres in diameter or be so large as to protrude from the mouth. The aetiology is unclear but they are thought to be mesenchymal in origin and may be a hamartoma. Eighty per cent of lesions occur in females and are more common on the maxillary alveolar ridge than the mandibular. Treatment is by excision and recurrence is very uncommon.

Lingual thyroid

See lesions of the tongue (below).

Table 22.1.2 Causes of pigmentation of the teeth

Extrinsic
Chromogenic bacteria
Chlorhexidine gluconate
Iron preparations
Intrinsic
Amelogenesis imperfecta
Dentinogenesis imperfecta
Tetracycline staining
Fluorosis
Porphyria
Erythroblastosis fetalis
Chronological hypoplasia
Trauma

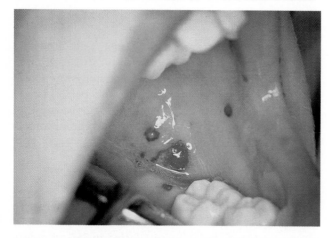

Fig. 22.1.10 Oral purpura in a child with thrombocytopenia caused by Wiskott–Aldrich syndrome.

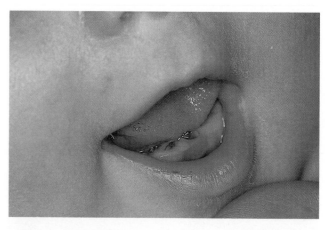

Fig. 22.1.11 Porphyria. A baby with the lower first deciduous incisors erupting. Note the red colour due to porphyrin deposition in the dentine.

Dermoid cyst

See lesions of the tongue (below).

Lingual tonsil

See lesions of the tongue (below).

Eruption cyst

Eruption cysts are soft tissue follicular cysts that form over the crowns of erupting teeth of children particularly deciduous teeth or permanent molar teeth. They appear as rounded smooth bluish swellings on the alveolar ridge. They are usually asymptomatic and resolve spontaneously as the tooth erupts. If they cause symptoms or become infected marsupialization may be necessary.

Lymphangioma

Lymphangiomas are hamartomas that bear a close structural resemblance to cavernous haemangiomas, but contain lymph instead of blood. They are often present at birth and usually manifest before 10 years of age. Intraoral lymphangiomas are uncommon but are most likely to occur on the tongue. Clinically, they appear as a sessile swelling with a pale translucent appearance with a finely nodular surface. They may appear to turn black if bleeding occurs into the lesion, and simulate a haemangioma. Treatment if the lesion is symptomatic and involves surgical excision, although cryosurgery may be useful for small lesions.

Haemangioma

See pigmented and red lesions (above).

Von Recklinghausen's neurofibromatosis
(see Chapter 19.13)

This is syndrome comprising of multiple neurofibromas, cutaneous pigmentation in the form of café-au-lait spots and skeletal abnormalities. Oral neurofibromas occur in about 10% of cases and may involve any oral soft tissues.

Tuberous sclerosis (epiloia) (see Chapter 19.14)

This is an autosomal dominant condition of mental handicap, epilepsy and cutaneous angiofibromas. Oral lesions consisting of fibrous outgrowths of the oral mucosa, particularly affecting the anterior gingivae have been described in this condition [1].

REFERENCE

1 Murti PR, Bhonsle RB, Mehta FS, Daftary DK. Oro-facial lesions of tuberous sclerosis. *Int J Oral Surg* 1980; 9: 292–7.

Multiple hamartoma and neoplasia syndrome (Cowden's syndrome) (see Chapter 19.24)

Papillomatous outgrowths from the buccal mucosa and papular lesions of the palate, lips and gingivae have been described in this syndrome. Other oral lesions may include fissured tongue and hypoplasia of the maxillae, mandible and uvula.

Acquired soft tissue swellings

Abscesses

Intraoral abscesses are almost always dental in origin. They usually present as painful fluctuant soft tissue swellings of the gingivae, palatal mucosa or buccal sulci (Fig. 21.1.12). An associated cellulitis may also occur giving rise to facial swelling. The abscess is often preceded by toothache and the offending tooth is usually carious and tender to pressure.

The diagnosis is made on clinical findings and treatment involves draining the abscess via the tooth itself or the soft tissue. Antibiotics may be required if there is an associated regional lymphadenopathy or if treatment is delayed, as a general anaesthetic may be required to treat very young children.

Fibroepithelial polyp/nodule

Fibroepithelial polyps or nodules are the most common type of tumour-like swelling found in the mouth. They are usually considered to be caused by chronic low-grade trauma. Often a source of trauma cannot be found.

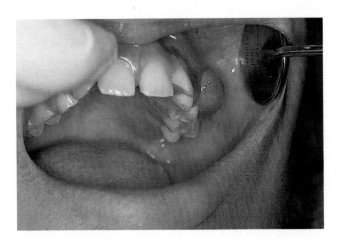

Fig. 22.1.12 Dental abscess causing soft tissue swelling in the upper left quadrant of a 12-year-old child.

Histologically, these lesions consist of stratified squamous keratinized epithelium with underlying dense bundles of collagenous connective tissue in continuity with the corium. They are not encapsulated. There may be an inflammatory exudate and occasionally dystrophic calcification occurs.

Clinically, they appear as either sessile or pedunculated soft pink swellings. They may occur on the gingivae, where they are referred to as epulides, palate and buccal mucosa or tongue. They are usually painless.

Treatment involves surgical excision with curettage of the underlying periostium to prevent recurrence.

Pyogenic granuloma

Pyogenic granulomas are soft tissue swellings which are highly vascular and have a tendency to haemorrhage. They are caused by a tissue reaction to non-specific infection as a result of minor trauma to the oral mucosa. Histologically, they contain numerous thin-walled blood vessels in a loose, moderately cellular fibrous stroma.

Clinically, they usually present as a painless swelling on the gingival margin, but may occur at other sites, e.g. buccal mucosa, palate. The swelling may be sessile or pedunculated with either a smooth, lobulated or warty surface. They are red in colour and soft to palpation. They are variable in size from a few millimetres to a few centimetres. Differential diagnosis includes a fibroepithelial polyp and giant cell epulis. Treatment is by surgical excision.

Giant cell epulis/granuloma

A giant cell granuloma is a non-neoplastic swelling of proliferating fibroblasts in a vascular stroma containing multinucleate giant cells. Its aetiology is unknown. It is more commonly seen in children than adults and presents as a deep red/purple soft swelling which often arises interdentally adjacent to permanent incisor or premolar teeth. Hyperparathyroidism (brown tumours) should always be considered when a lesion containing giant cells is diagnosed.

Treatment is by surgical excision and curettage of the underlying bone.

Squamous papilloma

Squamous cell papillomas are common benign oral lesions caused by human papilloma virus (HPV types 11a or 11b). They may occur at any age. Clinically, they present as a well-defined exophytic mass with a warty surface. If the surface epithelium is keratinized they appear white. Although they may occur anywhere in the mouth they are most commonly seen at the junction of the hard and soft palate. Oral papillomas should be excised and examined histologically to confirm the diagnosis, as they may resemble a fibroepithelial polyp. Treatment is by total excision to prevent recurrence.

HPV types 2a–e may also cause common warts and oral papillomas, particularly on the lips, and often seen in association with verruca vulgaris of the skin. HPV 12 or 32 are also implicated in focal epithelial hyperplasia (Heck's disease) which presents as multiple sessile soft papules, usually on the lower labial and buccal mucosa.

Molluscum contagiosum

Molluscum contagiosum may occasionally affect the mouth, particularly the lips, as a result of autoinoculation from cutaneous lesions. Facial and perioral molluscum contagiosum is frequently seen in patients with AIDS.

Orofacial granulomatosis and Crohn's disease

See gastrointestinal diseases (above).

Melkersson–Rosenthal syndrome

See lesions of the tongue (below).

Lymphoma

Lymphomas are the third most common malignant disease of childhood, although it is unusual for them to occur in the mouth and jaw (with the exception of Burkitt's lymphoma). They may present as a soft tissue enlargement, non-healing ulcer and occasionally loosening of the teeth. Radiographically, there may be evidence of bone resorption. Most lymphomas presenting in children under 10 years of age are of the non-Hodgkin's type.

Any swelling of the oral tissues without obvious cause should be biopsied.

Burkitt's lymphoma

African Burkitt's lymphoma typically affects preteenage children and is strongly associated with EBV. The jaw, particularly the mandible, is a common site of presentation. Clinically, there is massive swelling which may ulcerate into the mouth.

Langerhans' cell histiocytosis (histiocytosis X, eosinophilic granuloma) (see Chapter 21.1)

This condition refers to a neoplastic-like proliferation of Langerhans' cells. The spectrum of Langerhans' cell histiocytosis ranges from isolated lesions which spontaneously regress to widespread fatal disease. Multifocal eosinophilic granuloma presents in young children and often gives rise to lytic lesions in the skull and mandible which may involve oral soft tissue resulting in swelling. Treatment is dependent upon the extent of dissemination of the disease and may involve surgery, chemotherapy and radiotherapy.

Sarcomas and related conditions

Oral facial sarcomas are rare tumours of childhood, the most common being rhabdomyosarcoma. Locally invasive tumours such as infantile fibromatosis may also give rise to intraoral swelling, which presents as a progressively enlarging mass. Biopsy of lesions of doubtful diagnosis should always be performed to eliminate neoplasia. Salivary gland tumours are also uncommon in childhood, but should be considered in the differential diagnosis particularly in swellings involving the upper lip where mucoceles are uncommon.

Bony swellings

The majority of intraoral bony swellings in children are caused by unerupted teeth, supernumerary teeth, cysts and odontomes.

Tori

Tori are slow-growing exostoses that are thought to be inherited as a dominant trait. The torus palatinus occurs in the midline of the hard palate and the torus mandibularis lingually in the premolar area of the mandible; 80% of cases are bilateral. Although they may be seen in childhood the peak incidence is around 30 years of age.

Fibrous dysplasia

Fibrous dysplasias which include familial fibrous dysplasia (cherubism), monostotic polyostotic and Albright's syndrome may all give rise to expansile lesions of the jaws. On skeletal maturation the lesions tend to cease growth (see also pigmented and red lesions above).

Odontogenic cysts

Odontogenic cysts refer to a group of jaw cysts which are derived from the epithelium of the dental laminae. Follicular cysts are the most common odontogenic cysts seen in childhood (see eruption cyst above). Gorlin–Goltz syndrome, an autosomal dominant trait with variable expression, comprises of multiple basal cell carcinomas, odontogenic keratocysts that may become apparent in childhood, bifid ribs and calcification of the falx cerebri (see Chapter 19.16).

Gardner's syndrome

Gardner's syndrome is an autosomal dominant trait consisting of colonic polyps, which often undergo malignant change, epidermoid or sebaceous cysts, dermoid tumours, multiple supernumerary and impacted teeth and osteomas that may cause swellings of the jaw or cranium.

Bone cysts

Bone cysts, such as the aneurysmal bone cyst and solitary bone cyst, are seen almost exclusively in children and adolescents. They may occasionally present as a bony swelling of the mandible, but most are found as an incidental finding on routine radiography of the jaws.

Osteomyelitis

Osteomyelitis affecting the jaw is rare in the UK but is occasionally seen following radiotherapy to the head and neck as a result of endarteritis obliterans. Osteosarcoma may occur in the jaw of children who have undergone irradiation of the jaw for sarcomas.

Juvenile active ossifying fibroma

Juvenile active ossifying fibroma is occasionally seen in children under 15 years of age. Unlike the ossifying fibromas of adults it is very cellular and locally aggressive.

Generalized gingival swelling

Gingivitis is the most common cause of generalized gingival enlargement. Gingival enlargement may be aggravated by local factors such as mouth breathing. Enlarged gingivae without evidence of poor oral hygiene or in preschool children may be indicative of a systemic disorder, e.g. aplastic anaemia (Fig. 22.1.13) or sarcoidosis.

Hereditary gingival fibromatosis

Hereditary gingival fibromatosis is an autosomal dominant trait in which there is fibrous gingival enlargement, hypertrichosis and coarseness of facial features. It is occasionally associated with epilepsy and mental retardation. Clinically, the gingivae begin to enlarge around the time of tooth eruption. The gingivae are usual firm, pink and stippled, although if oral hygiene is poor inflammation may be concurrent. The teeth may eventually be buried by the gingivae. Treatment is by maintenance of good oral hygiene and when aesthetically necessary gingivectomy. Growth of the gingivae slows after puberty.

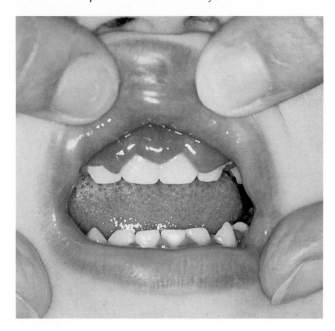

Fig. 22.1.13 Gingival enlargement due to acute inflammation in a 3-year-old child with aplastic anaemia.

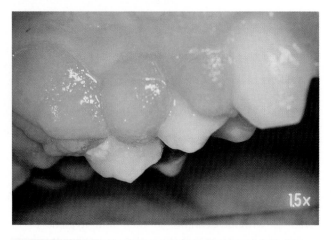

Fig. 22.1.14 Drug-induced (phenytoin) gingival hyperplasia. Note the enlargement is particularly apparent at the interdental papillae.

Drug-induced gingival hyperplasia

Drug-induced gingival hyperplasia is associated with several drugs including phenytoin, cyclosporin and the calcium channel blockers nifedipine and diltiazem. Clinically, the hyperplasia resembles that of hereditary gingival fibromatosis although hyperplasia is particularly apparent at the interdental papillae and gingival stippling is exaggerated (Fig. 22.1.14). Poor oral hygiene aggravates the hyperplasia. The history and clinical features should help to distinguish it from the hereditary form.

Acute leukaemia

Generalized gingival swelling may occur with acute

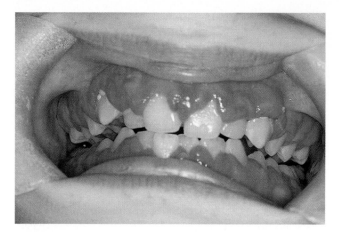

Fig. 22.1.15 Generalized gingival swelling in a child with acute myeloid leukaemia.

leukaemia. It is more frequently reported in association with acute myeloid leukaemia but may also be apparent in other forms, e.g. acute lymphoblastic leukaemia. The swelling is produced by leukaemic cell infiltrate in response to bacteria in dental plaque. The gingivae appear swollen, soft and may have a bluish/purple colour (Fig. 22.1.15). The surrounding mucosa may be pale (anaemia) and there may be petechiae or purpura present (thrombocytopenia).

Salivary gland swelling

The most common cause of salivary gland swelling in children was mumps. However, with the introduction of measles/mumps/rubella (MMR) vaccine, mumps is uncommon in young children in the Western world. Mumps usually gives rise to bilateral parotid swelling causing eversion of the ear lobe. Occasionally the swelling begins unilaterally. Parotitis may be caused by other viruses including coxsackie A, echo virus, parainfluenza, EBV and CMV. Treatment is symptomatic. Other causes of salivary gland swelling are discussed below and listed in Table 22.1.3 [1]. Salivary gland malignancy in childhood is rare [2].

Chronic recurrent sialadenitis

Chronic recurrent sialadenitis presents with recurrent painful swelling of one or more major salivary glands, usually the parotid. The attacks vary in frequency and the gland may remain enlarged between attacks. The aetiology is unclear but EBV may be involved. The condition usually resolves spontaneously at puberty.

Mucocele/ranula

Mucoceles are mucous extravasation cysts often resulting from trauma to the minor salivary glands. They most com-

Table 22.1.3 Causes of salivary gland swelling in childhood

Mumps
Chronic recurrent sialadenitis
Ascending parotitis
Calculi
HIV disease
Cystic fibrosis
Sjögren's syndrome
Sarcoidosis plus other granulomatosis
Mikulicz's disease
Sialosis
Drugs, e.g. chlorhexidine, sulphonamides, iodine
Salivary gland neoplasia, e.g. juvenile haemangioma
Lymphoma

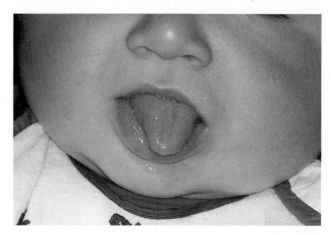

Fig. 22.1.17 Macroglossia in a baby with Beckwith–Wiedemann syndrome.

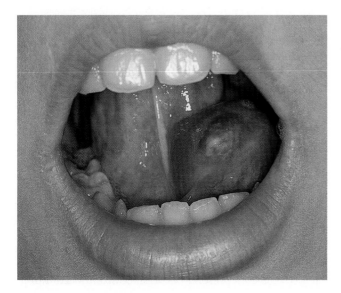

Fig. 22.1.16 A ranula, sublingual mucous retention cyst.

monly occur on the lower lip but may occur on the palate, upper lip and buccal mucosa. They usually present as a tense localized fluid-filled swelling. The lesion may burst due to trauma from the teeth. Recurrence is common and may lead to fibrosis.

The diagnosis is usually made on the history and clinical appearance. Treatment is either by cryosurgery or surgical removal of the cyst together with the offending minor salivary gland.

A ranula is a form of mucous retention cyst arising in the floor of the mouth often involving the sublingual salivary gland. It may cause both intra- and extraoral swelling (Fig. 22.1.16). It is usually treated by marsupialization.

Human immunodeficiency virus infection

Cystic enlargement of the major salivary glands has been reported in HIV disease together with lymphocytic infiltration, giving a Sjögren's syndrome appearance histologically, which may give rise to xerostomia. Swellings

of this nature should be regularly observed because of the increased risk of lymphoma development.

Cystic fibrosis

Enlargement of the salivary glands, particularly the submandibular gland may occasionally be seen in patients with cystic fibrosis.

Sarcoidosis

Sarcoidosis is a chronic granulomatous disease of unknown aetiology described more fully in Chapter 25.1. Sarcoidosis causes asymptomatic enlargement of the major salivary glands in 6% of cases and involvement of the facial nerve may lead to facial palsy. Gingival enlargement may also occur. Biopsy of affected gingivae or minor salivary glands show typical granulomas.

REFERENCES

1 Lamey PJ, Lewis MAO. Oral medicine in practice: salivary gland disease. *Br Dent J* 1990; 168: 237–43.
2 Baker SR, Malone B. Salivary gland malignancies in children. *Cancer* 1985; 55: 1730–6.

Lesions of the tongue

Congenital/developmental lesions

Macroglossia

The majority of cases of macroglossia, enlargement of the tongue, are congenital and most commonly associated with syndromes, e.g. Down's syndrome, Beckwith–Wiedemann syndrome (Fig. 22.1.17), Hurler's syndrome, cretinism and Rubenstein–Taybi syndrome. Congenital macroglossia is due to muscle hypertrophy. Secondary macroglossia may occur and is caused by tumours or hamartomas, the most common of which in childhood is a lymphangioma. Congenital macroglossia is not usually treated, the only option being surgical.

Microglossia

Microglossia, small tongue, is a rare congenital anomaly which occasionally causes difficulty in talking and eating. Only a few cases of aglossia have ever been reported.

Ankyloglossia

Ankyloglossia or tongue tie affects up to 1.7% of children and is usually caused by a short lingual fraenum. Surgical intervention is rarely necessary as it is usually of little consequence and does not interfere with speech. However, the scavenging action of the tongue may be impaired.

Fissured/scrotal tongue

Definition

This is a tongue with multiple small fissures or grooves on the dorsal surface which may have a scrotal appearance (Fig. 22.1.18).

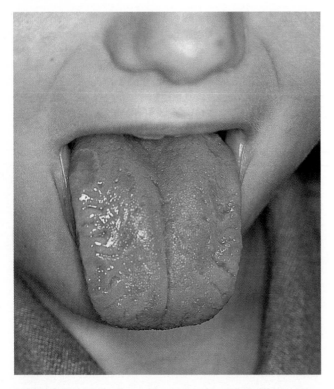

Fig. 22.1.18 A child with a mildly fissured tongue with concurrent erythema migrans which is most apparent on the right lateral border of the tongue just anterior to the commissure.

Aetiology

This is thought to be a developmental anomaly affecting about 1% of children although it is rarely seen before the age of 4 years. In surveys of the adult population the reported frequency is between 3 and 5% suggesting that it may not be developmental. It has an increased frequency of occurrence in children who suffer from mental retardation particularly Down's syndrome.

Fissured tongue is one of the features of Melkerson–Rosenthal syndrome; the other features include facial swelling and facial palsy. This syndrome may possibly be an incomplete manifestation of oral Crohn's disease.

Pathology and clinical features

The histopathology of fissured tongue is essentially normal. Clinically, fissured tongue is usually asymptomatic except on occasions when food and debris collect in the fissures giving rise to irritation.

Treatment

If irritation occurs food and debris should be removed by stretching and flattening the fissures and using a toothbrush, gauze or sponge to cleanse the surface.

Lingual thyroid

Ectopic thyroid tissue may occasionally be found at the base of the tongue at the site of the foramen caecum. Clinically, the lesion presents as a smooth surfaced lump. Symptoms of dysphagia may occur but the lesion is often asymptomatic. If surgery is indicated it is important to establish that there is normal thyroid tissue in the neck.

Lingual tonsil

The lingual tonsil is a mass of lymphoid tissue, divided into two parts by a midline ligament, situated between the epiglottis and circumvallate papillae. If the lingual tonsil is enlarged as in tonsillitis or in atopic individuals symptoms such as a lump in the throat, dyspnoea and dysphonia may occur. The condition may be distinguished from other lesions of the tongue by its site, symmetry and midline ligament.

The foliate papillae on the lateral border also contains lymphoid tissue which may undergo reactive hyperplasia during upper respiratory tract infections, causing the papillae to enlarge and rub against the teeth causing inflammation (foliate papillitis).

Sublingual dermoid cyst

This is a developmental cyst derived from embryonic

germinal epithelium. They usually occur in the midline above the mylohyoid muscles. Although they do not occur in the tongue they cause elevation of the tongue and may be associated with symptoms of dysphagia and dysphonia. Unlike other dermoid cysts, those arising in the floor of the mouth are seldom present at birth, becoming clinically obvious in the second decade.

The histological appearance of a dermoid cyst is very variable. It is usually lined by stratified squamous epithelium and is surrounded by lymphoid tissue. The cyst wall may contain sweat and sebaceous glands and hair follicles. Its contents may include keratin, sebum and matted hair.

Clinically, the lesions are variable in size. They may be fluctulant to palpation or have a 'dough like' feel, depending on the contents of the cyst.

Several lesions may resemble a sublingual dermoid cyst including a ranula, obstruction of the submandibular duct, thyroglossal tract cyst, cystic hygroma, branchial cleft cyst and cellulitis of the floor of the mouth.

Acquired lesions

Glossitis

Glossitis describes an acute inflammatory reaction of the tongue. It may be localized to a particular area of the tongue or generalized. There may or may not be associated symptoms.

Median rhomboid glossitis

Definition

A central rhomboid shaped area of depapillation anterior to the sulcus terminalis. Seldom seen in children.

History and aetiology

Debate exists over the aetiology of median rhomboid glossitis which affects 0.2% of the population. It was originally considered to be developmental in origin resulting from the persistence of the tuberculum impar. However, as it is less commonly seen in children than adults this aetiology is unlikely. It is now thought to be infective in nature and caused by *Candida* (40% of lesions exhibit candidal colonization). The consistent positioning of this condition does, however, support a developmental aetiology and it has been hypothesized that there may be a vascular anomaly in this area.

Pathology

Histologically, the epithelium shows loss of papillae and parakeratosis of the epithelium, with acanthosis and downward growth of the rete ridges. Polymorphonuclear lymphocytes may be seen in the superficial epithelium and candidal hyphae may be present. The underlying connective tissue is vascular and infiltrated with chronic inflammatory cells.

Clinical features

It is usually asymptomatic but soreness may be reported particularly after consumption of salty or spicy foods. The lesion presents as a rhomboid-shaped area of depapillation immediately anterior to the sulcus terminalis. The lesion may vary in colour from pale pink to bright red. The surrounding lingual epithelium appears normal (Fig. 22.1.19).

Treatment

A swab should be taken for candidal culture. If *Candida* is identified a topical antifungal agent should be prescribed, e.g. miconazole gel, nystatin suspension or pastilles or amphotericin B lozenges. If *Candida* is isolated underlying systemic conditions predisposing to candidal infections should be eliminated.

Deficiency states

Nutritional deficiency in the Western world is rare in childhood and usually the result of malabsorption. Haematinic deficiencies (vitamin B_{12}, ferritin, folate) may give rise to a sore tongue and atrophic glossitis. The symptoms may precede the clinical features. Classically, vitamin B_{12} deficiency causes a raw beefy tongue. Clinically, other oral signs of deficiency may be apparent (see oral ulceration and candidal infection above). If a nutritional deficiency is suspected it is important to establish that the child is obtaining adequate dietary intake (is not

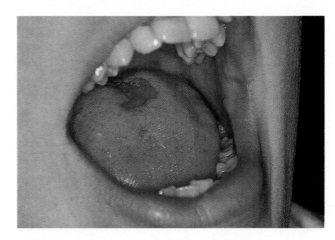

Fig. 22.1.19 Median rhomboid glossitis in a child using a steroid inhaler for asthma. In this case the lesion is due to candidal infection of the lingual mucosa.

vegetarian or anorexic) and to eliminate causes of malabsorption, e.g. Crohn's disease, coeliac disease. If a deficiency is suspected it may be prudent to carry out a full blood count, haemoglobin, serum ferritin, serum vitamin B_{12} and red cell folate as a deficiency in a haematinic that has not yet given rise to anaemia may cause oral symptoms and give rise to glossitis.

Infections

Scarlet fever, a *Streptococcus pyogenes* infection, and Kawasaki's disease (mucocutaneous lymph node syndrome [1]), of uncertain but possibly infectious aetiology may both cause furring of the tongue and prominence of the fungiform papillae, a so-called 'strawberry tongue' appearance. In scarlet fever the coating on the tongue is rapidly lost, and the tongue becomes smooth and deep red in colour (raspberry tongue).

REFERENCE

1 Ogden GR, Kerr M. Kawasaki syndrome. *Br Dent J* 1988; 165: 327–8.

Erythema migrans (geographical tongue, benign migratory glossitis)

Defintion

This is a benign condition which gives rise to well-defined areas of depapillation of the tongue which heal and recur at a different site, hence the term migratory.

Aetiology

Erythema migrans is a common condition affecting 1–2% of the population. The aetiology is unclear. There is often a positive family history and it is often associated with fissured tongue and possibly with psoriasis [1].

Pathology

Histologically, erythema migrans bears a striking resemblance to oral psoriasis. The lesions exhibit thinning of the epithelium, elongation of the rete ridges and a polymorphonuclear infiltrate of the superficial epithelium.

Clinical features

The lesions may occur at any age and are often symptomless. Soreness may be a presenting symptom which is usually aggravated by eating salty or spicy foods. Typically erythema migrans presents on the dorsum of the tongue as well-defined erythematous areas of depapillation, surrounded by a slightly raised white margin (see Fig. 22.1.18). The lesions are usually serpiginous in shape

giving rise to a map-like appearance; they may, however, be rounded or scalloped. The appearance of the lesions may change from day to day, hence the term migratory. Rarely erythema migrans has been described in other sites such as the labial mucosa and the palate [2]. Usually the diagnosis can be made from the history and clinical appearance of the lesions.

Treatment

If the lesions are causing symptoms benzydamine hydrochloride mouthrinse or spray may be of use.

REFERENCES

1 Morris LF, Phillips CM, Binnie WH, Sander HM, Silverman HK, Menter MA. Oral lesions in patients with psoriasis: a controlled study. *Cutis* 1992; 49: 339–44.
2 Luker J, Scully C. Erythema migrans affecting the palate. *Br Dent J* 1983; 155: 385.

Localized enlargement of the tongue

The commonest cause of localized enlargement of the tongue in children is acute inflammation caused by tongue biting. Persistent localized swellings are uncommon and are most likely to be due to a lymphangioma (see soft tissue swellings above) or a haemangioma (see red and pigmented lesions above).

Hairy and furred tongue

Hairy tongue is not commonly seen in childhood; it results from excessive elongation of the filiform papillae of the posterior dorsum of the tongue, caused by chronic irritation, but may be idiopathic particularly when seen in young children (Fig. 21.1.20). It is asymptomatic but if it is causing aesthetic problems brushing the dorsum of the tongue with a toothbrush, sucking a peach stone or the use

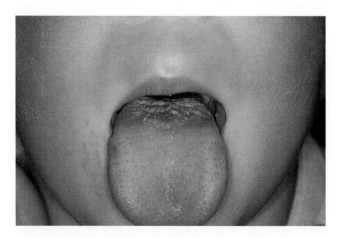

Fig. 22.1.20 Hairy tongue in a young preschool child.

of an effervescent vitamin C tablet on the tongue may be beneficial.

Furring of the tongue resulting from an accumulation of squames rarely occurs in healthy children, but is often seen in association with acute systemic illness particularly scarlet fever. It results from a lack of mechanical debridement and changes in the oral flora. It may be precipitated by the use of broad-spectrum antimicrobial agents.

Brown or black discoloration of the tongue may occur with either a furred or coated tongue. The staining may be caused by chromogenic bacteria within the oral cavity or by extrinsic agents such as iron supplements or chlorhexidine gluconate.

Section 23
Hair and Nails

23.1 Hair Disorders

ELISE A. OLSEN

Hair loss in childhood is usually fraught with overwhelming concern by parents that the condition will be permanent and/or leave psychological scars in the affected child. Conversely, physicians are more likely to focus on the potential relatedness of the hair loss to an underlying medical problem. The concerns of both are valid. There is great value in diagnosing a given case of childhood alopecia since herein may be the necessary clue to an otherwise unfathomable multisystem illness or an explanation for an unexplained developmental delay. The treatment of hair loss presenting in childhood does include disorders for which no good therapy yet exists but there are many conditions in which specific treatment can either reverse the hair loss or make the hair more manageable and, hence, more cosmetically acceptable.

Hypertrichosis specifically refers to hair density or length beyond the accepted limits of normal for a particular age, race and sex and does not imply, as does the term hirsutism, a particular distribution of hair or a hormonal aetiology. Hypertrichosis may be generalized or localized, and may consist of lanugo, vellus or terminal hair. The presence of hypertrichosis in a child may signify an underlying physical abnormality, an associated metabolic disorder, a genetic multifocal syndrome or merely a cosmetic problem.

This chapter presents an effective approach to the diagnosis of the various types of alopecia and hypertrichosis presenting in childhood. Aetiologies of hair loss or hypertrichosis presented in detail in other chapters (e.g. alopecia areata, trichotillomania, ectodermal dysplasia, tinea capitis, Cornelia–de Lange syndrome, porphyria, etc.) will be mentioned only briefly and the reader is referred to these other sources of information.

Normal hair loss/growth in childhood

To fully understand hair loss or excess growth in childhood, a basic working knowledge of normal hair growth is necessary including the embryology and cycling of hair. Hair development begins *in utero* at 9–12 weeks with the follicular units composed of epidermally derived follicles and mesodermally derived papillae [1] (Fig. 23.1.1). By 18–20 weeks of gestation, fine lanugo (unpigmented, unmedullated fine hair that may grow several centimetres in length [2,3]) hairs in anagen (active growth) cover the scalp and proceed to appear elsewhere in a cephalocaudal direction, eventually covering the entire fetus. This hair is normally shed at the seventh or eighth month [2,4] and is rapidly replaced by vellus hair on the body and vellus or terminal hair on the scalp. The transition wave from anagen to telogen in the occipital area is delayed, however, and the expected telogen shedding in the occiput occurs at 2–4 months postpartum [2,4], accounting for the occipital alopecia normally seen in infants of this age (Fig. 23.1.2). Lanugo hair may also be seen on the limbs and shoulders of full-term, normally developed newborns but this should be shed by 1–2 months of age.

For the remainder of the first year of life, scalp hair growth is synchronous, only taking on the adult mosaic pattern towards the end of the first year [2]. The number of follicles does not change after birth but rather the follicular density decreases as the skin expands to cover an increasing surface area. The follicular density of the scalp at birth is $1135/cm^2$ decreasing to $615/cm^2$ by young adulthood [4,5]. There is a gradual transition from vellus (unmedullated, lightly pigmented hair, final length less than 2cm [5]) to terminal (usually pigmented, usually medullated, generally thicker shafts with longer anagen phase and thus longer ultimate length) hair over the scalp during the first year or two. Hair colour tends to darken with age [6].

All human scalp hairs regularly cycle through various stages of growth. In anagen, or the active growth phase, the follicular bulb embraces the dermal papillae in the

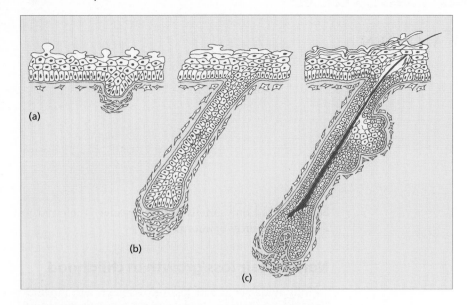

Fig. 23.1.1 Embryology of the hair follicle. (a) Follicular germ illustrating the condensing mesenchyme proximal to the epidermally derived follicle cells. (b) Follicle peg stage illustrating the organization of keratinocytes in the follicle and the mesenchyme of the follicle sheath and presumptive dermal papillae. (c) Bulbous hair peg stage illustrating the regions of the differentiated follicle. The upper bulge on the right represents the sebaceous gland and duct. The 'Bulge' area where the arrector pili muscle will insert is below this.

periods of time based on the area of the body the hair resides in: the normal anagen time for scalp hair is 3+ years [9].

When a particular hair has completed its sojourn in anagen, it begins to assume the physical characteristics and location of a resting (telogen) hair. The follicular bulb moves up in the dermis with the dermal papillae no longer intimately associated but lagging behind (Fig. 23.1.3). The attachment of the root sheaths to the hair shaft loosens and the telogen hair is now subject to being dislodged with simple pressure or traction. Once telogen is completed, and the time in telogen varies with body site, being 3–4 months for the scalp, the process is reversed. Specialized cells in the *Bulge* region of the sebaceous gland may carry the stem cell capacity for follicular regeneration, providing the cell population necessary to lengthen and deepen the follicle so it can once again assume the physical properties of anagen [9,10]. The spontaneous loss of a telogen hair generally signals the presence in the follicular canal of a new growing anagen hair.

Hair loss

Evaluation of the child with hair loss

History

The evaluation of a child with scalp hair loss should always include a history, physical examination and microscopic examination of the hair bulb and/or shaft. The history should differentiate between hair never coming in fully from hair that once covered the scalp but was later lost or shed. However, it is entirely within the range of normal for either the so-called second pelage, the second wave of anagen scalp hair, or the transition from vellus to terminal hair to be delayed up to 1 year of age, making

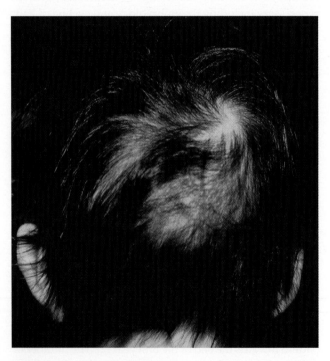

Fig. 23.1.2 Occipital alopecia in 4-month-old infant.

dermis or subcutaneous tissue (Fig. 23.1.3). The division and maturation of the matrix (those cells in the centre of the hair bulb contiguous to the dermal papillae) produce columns of cells which stream superficially into the central portion of the bulb and then enter the straight linear portion of the follicle [7]. The cellular keratin filaments (protein) organize into larger aggregates that become progressively more compact as the shaft moves upwards and away from the bulb [8]. For much of the length of the follicle, the hair shaft is attached to layers of root sheaths which serve both to anchor and mould the newly formed hair. Anagen lasts for predetermined

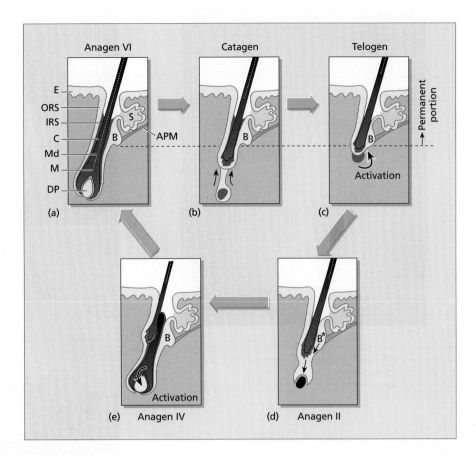

Fig. 23.1.3 Normal cycling of hair. Follicular structures above the dashed line form the permanent part of the follicle. Keratinocytes below the bulge (B) degenerate during catagen and telogen. Note that during catagen, the dermal papillae (DP) lags behind the ascending terminal bulb and that cells in the bulge region are poised for downward proliferation in early anagen (anagen II). When the germinative epithelium is once again in close approximation to the dermal papillae, the anagen growth cycle begins again. The preceding hair is lost as the new hair begins its growth phase. APM, arrector pili muscle; C, cortex; E, epidermis; IRS, inner root sheath; M, matrix; Md, medulla; ORS, outer root sheath; S, sebaceous gland.

it falsely appear that the affected child has congenital alopecia. Hair that never comes in is generally genetic in origin.

Diffuse scalp hair loss that has a hereditary basis usually manifests itself by the first or second year of life but in some genetically based disorders, the associated hair loss only becomes obvious later (e.g. dyskeratosis congenita [11], Jorgensen's syndrome [12], Beare's pili torti [13], androgenetic alopecia). Obviously, family history is key in determining the exact mode of inheritance of a suspected genetic disorder but family members may only have some but not all of the features associated with a particular syndrome, and alopecia may not be one of them. Therefore, when suspecting a familial syndrome, or probing for one that has alopecia as one feature, multi-organ signs and symptoms should be enquired about. Since the group of disorders collectively called ectodermal dysplasia commonly involve hair loss (and effects on the teeth, nails and sweating), this should particularly be looked for. Dental X-rays may be necessary to exclude tooth involvement in the very young and formal sweat testing may be necessary to document decreased sweating. Currently, there is no standardized test protocol for the evaluation of sweating in ectodermal dysplasia syndromes but recommended techniques are those that assess both sweat gland number and function postsweat induction [14].

Physical examination

A physical examination should be performed in all children with hair loss of uncertain aetiology. The possibility of a syndrome must be entertained and multisystem abnormalities sought for and catalogued: those of ectodermally derived organs (epidermis derived, teeth, ears, eyes, central nervous system, mammary glands), bone, cleft lip and/or cleft palate are frequently associated with scalp hair loss. Particular attention should be paid to the child's facial features and whether a distinctive facies is present.

The scalp examination should first conclude whether the hair loss is diffuse (or global) or focal (Fig. 23.1.4). A diffuse loss could be secondary to an inherited problem of abnormal follicular or hair shaft development or an acquired problem (e.g. alopecia areata, anagen effluvium, telogen effluvium). Focal alopecia is less likely to be inherited and much more likely to be acquired (Fig. 23.1.5a).

The scalp in the areas of alopecia should be evaluated for the preservation of follicular openings (implying a non-scarring potentially reversible process; Fig. 23.1.5a) versus smooth, poreless skin indicating attrition of follicular units and a potentially irreversible or scarring process (Fig. 23.1.5b). Scarring alopecia is rare in children outside of congenital focal scalp abnormalities, tumours or trauma.

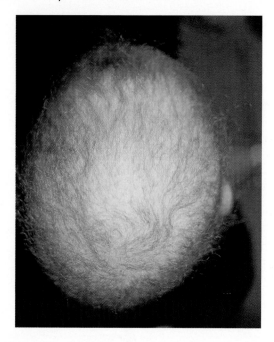

Fig. 23.1.4 Diffuse (global) hair loss in child with Rosselli–Gulienetti syndrome (palate–popliteal pterygia syndrome) type of subgroup 1, 2, 3, and 4 ectodermal dysplasia.

Further differentiation can be made between hair growth abnormalities secondary to (a) failure to initiate production; (b) intrinsic breakage; (c) unruly hair; and (d) abnormalities of cycling (increased shedding). To determine if hair is currently growing at the normal rate of 1 cm per month, a simple hair window can be performed. In this procedure, hair is clipped flush with the scalp in an arbitrarily determined target area (generally at the back of the scalp to prevent manipulation by the patient and in a shape unlikely to occur naturally such as a square or rectangle) and the hair length in this area observed a few weeks later. Even if there is an underlying hair shaft fragility problem that precludes the hair growing long, the hair should be able to attain a length of 0.5 cm in 2–3 weeks.

To determine whether abnormal shedding is occurring, a simple hair pull is performed. Approximately 50 to 100 hairs are grasped at the base between the thumb and forefinger and gently pulled proximally to distally. This procedure is repeated in various sections of the scalp, six to eight times total. The number and type of shed hairs are counted: greater than six to eight telogen hairs total is abnormal. A few anagen hairs on a gentle hair pull in a young child is common and most of these hairs assume the microscopic appearance of 'loose anagen' (LA) hairs. Anagen hairs on a hair pull are unusual in normal post-pubescent children.

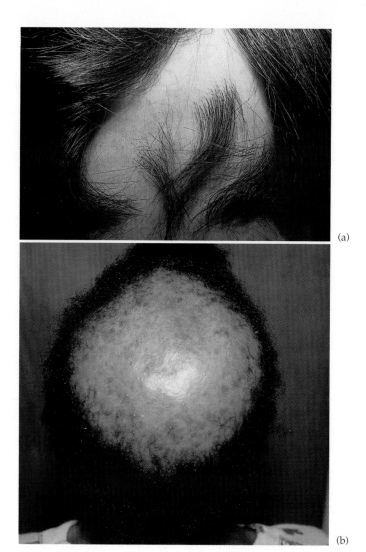

(a)

(b)

Fig. 23.1.5 (a) Focal, non-scarring hair loss of alopecia areata. (b) Scarring (permanent) hair loss in a 10-year-old child with dyspigmentation and follicular papules.

Microscopic examination

If abnormal shedding is occurring, the shed hairs should be examined under the light microscope. One to two drops of cyanoacrylic glue (e.g. Acrytol, Surgipath Medical Industries, Illinois) are placed on a slide and the proximal hair bulbs are lined up in the glue and a cover-slip placed over them: this facilitates orientation, decreases distortion and provides a permanent record of the hairs in question. The bulbs are then examined to determine if the loss is telogen or anagen. Telogen bulbs are unpigmented, rounded up and devoid of attached root sheath (Fig. 23.1.6a). Conversely, anagen bulbs are pigmented, somewhat distorted in appearance and normally surrounded by attached inner root sheath (Fig. 23.1.6b). Loose anagen (LA) hairs are generally devoid of inner root sheath and the attached cuticle assumes a ruffled or 'floppy sock' appearance (Fig. 23.1.6c). Each type of shed-

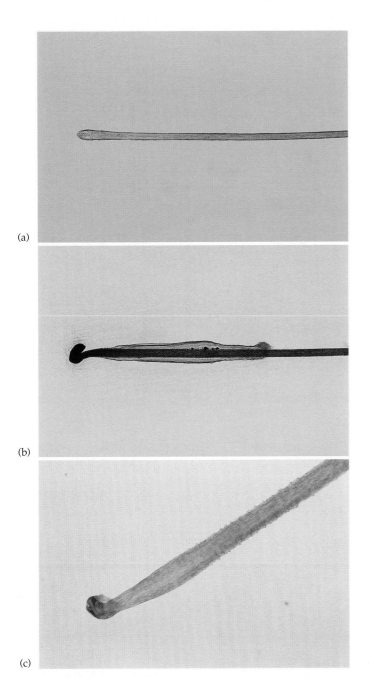

(a)

(b)

(c)

Fig. 23.1.6 (a) Telogen bulb (light micrograph, ×40). (b) Anagen bulb (light micrograph, ×40). (c) Loose anagen syndrome (light micrograph, ×100).

ding should trigger a very different type of work-up and the differential diagnosis is almost mutually exclusive.

If no abnormal shedding is occurring but instead the hair is fracturing with simple trauma (rubbing the hair between the fingers is one way of precipitating this in susceptible patients) or has an abnormal texture or dullness resulting in unruliness, a sample of affected hairs should be clipped and the distal portion examined under the microscope. Most hair shaft abnormalities can be diag-

nosed in this manner although some will require further examination by scanning electron microscopy to confirm findings only hinted at under light microscopy (e.g. longitudinal grooving). Polariscopic examination is necessary in cases where the particular light microscopic findings of trichoschisis with or without trichorrhexis nodosa are seen, making the diagnosis of trichothiodystrophy a possibility. The aetiology of brittle hair can be further pursued by chemical analysis of the hair for sulphur content and/or quantitation of individual amino acids.

Together these simple tools—history, physical examination and microscopic examination of the hair—will help narrow the differential diagnosis. The various aetiologies of childhood alopecia are discussed below in further detail.

Types of hair loss

Abnormality in initiation of hair growth

Diffuse loss

Near or complete universal atrichia as an isolated event generally develops within the first 1–2 years of life or may be present at birth. This is usually autosomal dominant in inheritance but X-linked and autosomal recessive inheritance patterns have also been reported [15]. Universal alopecia may also occur with mental retardation and either talipes [16] or seizures [17–19]. Patients with the X-linked recessive condition Mendes da Costa–van der Valk genodermatosis present with universal alopecia at birth or within the first few months of life accompanied by reticular brown–red pigmentation on the face and extremities [20]. During the first few years of life, these patients develop recurrent non-traumatic intraepidermal blisters and may have associated acrocyanosis, microcephaly with mental retardation, dwarfism, short conic fingers and nail dystrophy [21]. Patients with atrichia with papular lesions have early onset universal alopecia but do not generally develop the characteristic keratin-filled epithelial cysts until at least age 5 years [22–24]. A list of conditions presenting with alopecia and associated with follicular hyperkeratosis are presented in Table 23.1.1.

A few of the ectodermal dysplasias present with universal or near total alopecia in infancy: those with hair, nail and sweating abnormalities include odonto-onychodysplasia with alopecia [12,46], Hayden's syndrome [12], alopecia–onychodysplasia–hypohidrosis syndrome [12,47], ectodermal alopecia with severe mental retardation [12] and dermotrichic syndrome [12]; those with hair and teeth abnormalities include: alopecia, unusual facies and preaxial polydactyly (Wilson's syndrome) [48]; those with hair and nail abnormalities: tricho-onychodysplasia with xeroderma [13,49], skeletal anomalies–ectodermal dysplasia–growth and mental

Table 23.1.1 Follicular hyperkeratosis with scalp alopecia. Modified from Olsen EA. Hair loss in Childhood. In: Olsen EA, ed. *Disorders of Hair Growth: Diagnosis and Treatment.* New York: McGraw-Hill, 1994: 150–67.

	Inheritance	Hair	Teeth	Nails	Sweating	Skin	Other	References
Atrichia with papular lesions	?AR, ?AD	Born with normal, partial or absent scalp coverage but shed by 2 years; lashes ± sparse; usually absent brows; absent body hair	Normal	Normal	±↓	Keratin-filled epithelial cysts from age 2 years	Psychomotor retardation; ataxia; hypogonadism; all symptoms may be delayed a few years	[22–26]
Ichthyosis follicularis	AD or X-linked recessive	Sparse, short or absent scalp hair; sparse or absent lashes, brows, body hair	Normal	± Dystrophy in childhood (?secondary to infections)	Normal	Extensive follicular hyperkeratosis; chronic skin infections; hyperkeratotic plaques extensor extremities, hands, groin	Marked photophobia ± conjunctivitis, blepharitis, corneal abnormalities; ± hearing loss	[26–28]
Keratosis follicularis spinulosa decalvans	X-linked recessive or dominant; ?AD	Progressive scarring; loss of scalp hair, lashes, brows, body hair during childhood and adolescence	Normal	Normal	Normal	Generalized follicular hyperkeratosis with marked plugging, especially head and dorsum hands, fingers; these may become atrophic at puberty; palmoplantar hyperkeratosis; may develop telangiectatic pigmentation cheeks and brows late	Atopy; conjunctivitis; photophobia; corneal defects	[26, 28]
Alopecia, keratosis pilaris, cataracts and psoriasis	AD	Childhood onset hair loss without preceding inflammation or lesions → scarring alopecia; sparse lashes, brows, body hair	Caries	Small and pitted	Normal	Childhood psoriasis; diffuse follicular hyperkeratosis sparing face and scalp	Keratoconjunctivitis; cataracts	[29]
Marie–Unna hypotrichosis	AD	Scalp hair sparse or absent at birth, coarse hair grows in early childhood, diffuse loss (especially over vertex) at puberty; hair shaft; cuticle abnormal, longitudinal ridging and irregular twisting; sparse or absent brows, lashes, body hair	No	Normal	Normal	Diffuse follicular hyperkeratosis with milia-like facial lesions	± Atopy	[30–33]
Perniola's syndrome	AR	Near universal alopecia with sparse brittle lanugo hairs	Normal	Normal	Normal	Hyperkeratotic follicular papules	Seizures; ± sensorineural deafness	[19]
Dwarfism, cerebral atrophy and keratosis pilaris	X-linked	Almost complete absence of hair	Delayed eruption	Normal	Normal	Generalized keratosis follicularis	Physical and psychomotor retardation, dwarfism	[34]
Keratitis-Ichthyosiform Erythroderma–Deafness Syndrome (KID syndrome)	AR? AD?	Diffuse, fine, sparse or absent scalp hair; +/− patchy, scarring alopecia; sparse lashes, brows; hair shaft: trichorrhexis nodosa	+/− caries; brittle, malformed, delayed	Leukonychia, +/− thickened, hypoplastic	+/−↓	Diffuse follicular hyperkeratosis; leathery erythroderma (not scaly) from birth including keratoderma; plaques on face in infancy; verrucous hyperkeratosis over knees	Neurosensory deafness; keratitis	[35–38]

Condition	Inheritance	Hair	Teeth	Nails		Skin	Other	References
Onychotrichodysplasia with neutropenia (Cantu's syndrome)	AR	Brittle, lusterless, sparse, short, curly scalp hair; scanty eyebrows, lashes, body hair; microscopic exam hair: trichorrhexis nodosa; sparse to absent pubic, axillary hair at puberty	Normal	Dystrophic; koilonychia and onychorrhexis	Normal	Follicular hyperkeratosis	Chronic neutropenia and recurrent infections; mild hypotonia	[13,39,40]
Pachyonychia congenita	AD	Generalized hypotrichosis, dry hair	Natal teeth; +/- caries; malformation	Yellowish-brown discoloration; thickened nails (distal 2/3) with pinched margins and upward tilt of distal tips (all cases); paronychial infections	↑	Palmer-plantar hyperkeratosis; follicular keratosis, esp. knees and elbows; asteatosis; painful bullae or ulceration palms and soles; verrucous lesions extremities; +/- epidermal cysts	Cataracts; hoarseness; +/- oral leukokeratosis; corneal dyskeratosis	[41–44]
Cystic eyelids, palmoplantar keratosis, hypodontia and hypotrichosis (Schöpf–Schulz–Passarge's syndrome)	AR	Marked hypotrichosis, especially scalp; eyebrows and lashes coarse, sparse	Hypodontia; central incisors	Onychodystrophy; longitudinal ridging; splitting; onycholysis	Normal	Follicular hyperkeratosis; palmoplantar hyperkeratosis; late development eyelid aprocrine hidrocystomas		[45]

retardation [12,50], cataracts–alopecia–sclerodactyly [51].

Alopecia areata is the only potentially completely reversible universal alopecia that may present in infancy. This is rare in the first year of life.

There is a very long list of conditions that present with 'hypotrichosis', but not complete alopecia, in infancy. The hypotrichosis may be secondary to follicular hypoplasia or to faulty hair shaft production and breakage. Many of the ectodermal dysplasias have associated 'hypotrichosis', but unfortunately most of the hair shaft abnormalities have not been well characterized: the abnormal hair is generally only described clinically as 'brittle', 'sparse' or 'lustreless'. (The ectodermal dysplasias are discussed in further detail in Chapter 19.11.) There are other non-ectodermal dysplasia syndromes that present in infancy with sparse, lustreless hair as one part of multiorgan abnormalities (e.g. cartilage–hair hypoplasia [52]; hypomilia–hypotrichosis–facial haemangioma [53], regional choroidal atrophy and alopecia [54]). The diagnosis of the primary condition in these cases is rarely suggested by the hair abnormality, probably secondary to the dearth of available information on the hair.

There are, however, a number of conditions that *can* be diagnosed by microscopic evaluation of the hair shaft. Depending on the type of hair shaft abnormality, they generally present as fragile or unruly hair. These will be presented here according to their microscopic description.

Hair shaft abnormalities presenting with hair breakage

Trichorrhexis nodosa

The most common defect of the hair shaft leading to hair breakage is trichorrhexis nodosa [55]. The primary abnormality is a focal loss of the cuticle that leads to exposed and eventually frayed cortical fibres [56,57]. This appears initially microscopically as a nodal swelling and is followed by fracturing and splaying of the exposed fibres in a fan-like array (Fig. 23.1.7). Trichorrhexis nodosa can occur in normal hair that has been abused by excessive repetitive chemicals or physical trauma but more commonly occurs in inherently weak hairs after trivial trauma (e.g. brushing, combing).

Although trichorrhexis nodosa can present at birth as an isolated problem [58] or with teeth with or without nail abnormalities [59], its presence in an infant or young child should trigger a search for an underlying metabolic problem. One association is with argininosuccinic aciduria in which the absence of the enzyme argininosuccinase, which normally splits argininosuccinic acid into arginine and fumaric acids, leads to acidosis, hyperammonaemia, low serum arginine, increased serum and urine citrulline and argininosuccinic acid [60]. In these children, symptoms of psychomotor retardation, ataxia and dull brittle hair (with microscopic trichorrhexis

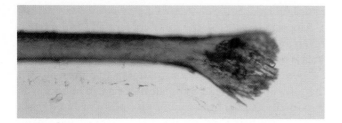

Fig. 23.1.7 Trichorrhexis nodosa (light micrograph, ×100).

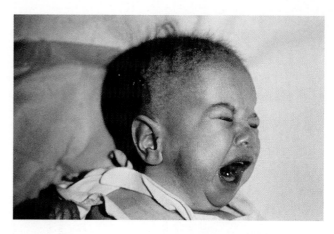

Fig. 23.1.8 Menke's syndrome. Courtesy of Dr Janet L. Roberts.

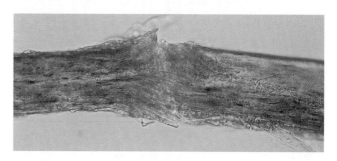

Fig. 23.1.9 Trichoschisis (light micrograph, ×400). Reprinted from Whiting [55].

nodosa) begin to develop after age 2 years [61,62].

Citrullinaemia, in which there is a deficiency of the enzyme argininosuccinic acid synthetase [63], may also present with increased serum citrulline and low arginine. Children with citrullinaemia may present with a scaly skin eruption and hair fragility with trichorrhexis nodosa and pili torti on microscopic examination of the hair [63–66].

Patients with Menke's syndrome, or trichopoliodystrophy, an X-linked disorder of copper transport, also have trichorrhexis nodosa and pili torti on microscopic examination of the hair [67,68]. The defective gene, MKN or ATP7A, encodes a copper translocating membrane protein adenosine triphosphatase (ATPase) that disturbs intracellular copper homoeostasis and the function of copper-requiring enzymes [69,70]. Systemic copper deficiency occurs from trapping of copper in some tissues, particularly the intestine, kidney, fibroblasts and red blood cells, leading to failure of copper delivery to other tissues [71–74]. In affected children, the hair is normal at birth but is replaced in early infancy by sparse, brittle, depigmented hair which feels like steel wool, hence the colloquial term of 'steely hair syndrome' [74–76] (Fig. 23.1.8). The skin is characteristically pale and lax, the face expressionless and the child drowsy and/or listless. There may be associated hypothermia, mental retardation and degeneration of cerebral, cerebellar, bone and connective tissue. A low serum ceruloplasmin is diagnostic of Menke's syndrome. Treatment with copper is usually ineffective and most affected children die by the age of 3 years [77]. However, recent reports of immediate postpartum treatment with copper–histidine show a prevention or diminution in the severe neurodegeneration typical of the disease [69].

Trichoschisis

Trichoschisis is a clear transverse fracture through the entire hair shaft (Fig. 23.1.9). Under the light microscope, the affected hairs often appear flat and may be folded over as well [78]. Trichorrhexis nodosa may also be present. Under scanning electron microscopy, the areas of fracture are associated with localized absence of the cuticle [79].

Trichoschisis, although not absolutely pathognomonic, is nonetheless seen only with regularity in the condition termed trichothiodystrophy.

Trichothiodystrophy is an autosomal recessive disorder characterized by sulphur-deficient brittle hair that may occur alone or in conjunction with other neuroectodermal abnormalities [78]. The hair abnormality identifies a group of genetic disorders in which acronyms or eponyms identify particular constellations of extratrichological findings (Table 23.1.2). Clinically, the patients with trichothiodystrophy have, since early infancy, short brittle hair on the scalp, eyelashes or eyebrows (Fig. 23.1.10). The cystine content of the hair is about half of normal primarily from a major reduction and altered composition of the high sulphur matrix proteins [98–101]. Polariscopic examination of affected hairs characteristically show alternating dark and light bands (Fig. 23.1.11), presumably secondary to alternating sulphur content [97]. Sulphur and/or amino acid analysis of the hair is diagnostic.

Other abnormalities should be sought in those patients with trichothiodystrophy (Table 23.1.2) particularly the presence of photosensitivity. Patients with trichothiodystrophy, particularly the 50% with photosensitivity, may have a defect in excision repair of ultraviolet damage but

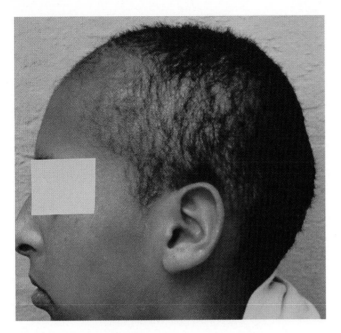

Fig. 23.1.10 Trichothiodystrophy. Reprinted from Whiting [55], courtesy of Dr Vera H. Price.

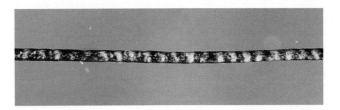

Fig. 23.1.11 Trichothiodystrophy polariscopic micrograph (×40). Note alternating light and dark bands. Courtesy of Dr David A. Whiting.

without an increased risk of skin cancer [102]. It has recently been determined that the various clinical presentations and DNA repair characteristics of both trichothiodystrophy and xeroderma pigmentosa can be correlated with mutations found in the ERCC2 locus—trichothiodystrophy due primarily to mutations that affect the transcriptional role of ERCC2 and xeroderma pigmentosa due to mutations that primarily alter the repair role of ERCC2 [102].

Table 23.1.2 Syndromes associated with trichothiodystrophy. Modified from Whiting [55]

Group	Brittle hair	Brittle nails	Intellectual impairment	Decreased fertility	Short stature	Ichthyosis	Photo-sensitivity	Neutropenia	Other findings	Acronym/eponym
(a) Isolated hair defect	+									Trichoschisis [80]
(b) Hair and nail dystrophy	+	+								Trichoschisis/Onychodystrophy [78,81]
(c) Above and mental retardation, infertility	+	+	+	+					Astigmatism, pale optic discs, retinopathy	Sabinas syndrome [82,83]
(d) Above and growth retardation	+	+	+	+	+				Quadriplegia, seizures, microcephaly	BIDS, Amish brittle hair syndrome [84,85]
(e) Above and ichthyosis	+	+	+	+	+	+			Abnormal teeth, tongue plaques, cataract, VSD	IBIDS [86,87] Tay's syndrome [88,89] Pollitt syndrome [90]
(f) Above and photosensitivity	+	+	+	+	+	+	+		Abnormal repair UV-induced DNA damage	PIBI(D)S [91–94]
(g) Most of above and chronic neutropenia	+	+	+		+	+		+	Recurrent infections, folliculitis, conjunctivitis	ONMR, [95] onychotrichodysplasia neutropenia, mental retardation [84]
(h) Marinesco–Sjögren syndrome	+	+	+		+				Ataxia, dysarthria, cataracts, abnormal teeth (primarily non-ectodermal)	Marinesco–Sjögren syndrome [64,84,96,97]

VSD, ventricular septal defect.

Trichorrhexis invaginata

Trichorrhexis invaginata (bamboo hair) clinically presents in infancy with short, brittle often sparse hair [103] (Fig. 23.1.12). The primary defect appears to be abnormal keratinization of the hair shaft in the keratogenous zone allowing intussusception of the fully keratinized and hard distal shaft into the incompletely keratinized and soft proximal portion of the shaft [104,105]. This leads to a proximal 'cup-like' or 'socket-like' expansion embracing a 'ball', the typical 'ball and socket' deformity (Fig. 23.1.13). Fracture of the shaft through this area is common but there may also be disarticulation of the distal 'ball' leaving a golf-tee or tulip-shaped end to the abnormal hair [106] (Fig. 23.1.14). Pili torti and trichorrhexis nodosa may also be seen with the trichorrhexis invaginata. Sulphur content is normal in trichorrhexis invaginata and no scanning electron microscopic studies are necessary to make this diagnosis. However, the abnormal hairs may be present only in certain sections of the scalp so many areas of the scalp may need to be evaluated to make a definitive diagnosis.

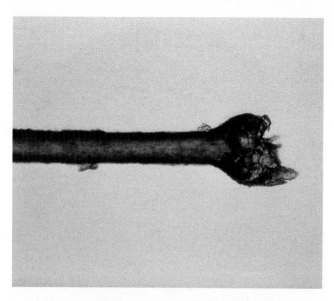

Fig. 23.1.14 Trichorrhexis invaginata, golf-tee fracture (light micrograph, ×200). Reprinted from Whiting [55].

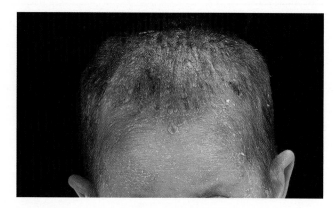

Fig. 23.1.12 Netherton's syndrome. Courtesy of Dr John Harper.

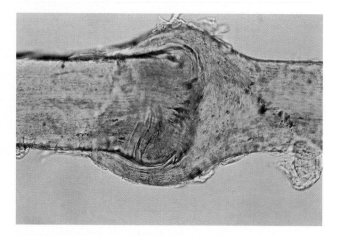

Fig. 23.1.13 Trichorrhexis invaginata (light micrograph, ×400). Reprinted from Whiting [55].

Trichorrhexis invaginata can rarely occur in traumatized, otherwise normal hair or with other congenital hair shaft abnormalities. Usually, however, the hair abnormality is associated with Netherton's syndrome, an autosomal recessive inherited disorder which consists of the triad of ichthyosis, atopic diathesis and trichorrhexis invaginata [107–109]. The ichthyosis is most commonly ichthyosis linearis circumflexa, a polycyclic, ever-transforming scaly eruption with a double-edged scale on the leading edge [105,110,111] (Fig. 23.1.15). However, some cases of trichorrhexis invaginata have instead been associated with lamellar ichthyosis, or less commonly, ichthyosis vulgaris or X-linked ichthyosis [109,112]. The atopic diathesis usually includes persistent xerosis and may include erythroderma [108,113]. The diagnosis of Netherton's syndrome should always be entertained in 'red scaly babies' who have sparse hair. Recurrent infections, short stature and mental retardation have been reported rarely in Netherton's syndrome [114].

There is no specific treatment for trichorrhexis invaginata. Retinoids and photochemotherapy have been reported to be of some value and the condition may spontaneously improve with age [115–117].

Pili torti

Patients with pili torti typically present with short, brittle hair. Microscopically, the hair is flattened and twisted on its own axis anywhere from 90 to 360° [118]. Twisted hairs on the scalp may normally be seen sporadically in Caucasians and are the norm in black people and in the pubic/axillary hair of both races. For pili torti to be diag-

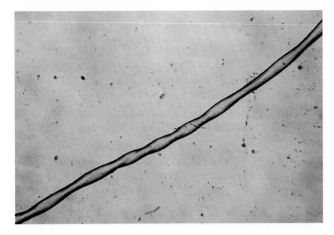

Fig. 23.1.16 Pili torti. Reprinted from Whiting [55].

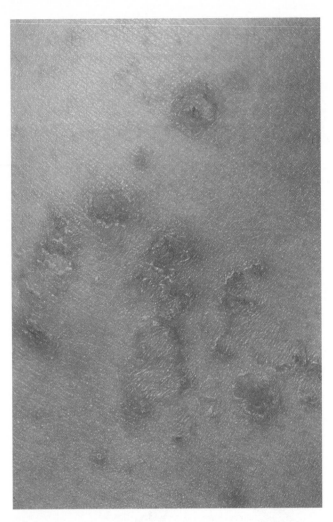

Fig. 23.1.15 Ichthyosis linearis circumflexa. Courtesy of Dr Neil S. Prose.

been described in a number of cases and early auditory testing should be done in all children with pili torti [127,128]. Pili torti may also be present in many other syndromes which are summarized in Table 23.1.3. The hair abnormality in these conditions may persist indefinitely or improve at puberty.

Pili torti may also present as a focal area of abnormal hair. This is usually secondary to trauma or to an underlying scarring condition of the scalp.

Table 23.1.3 Infantile hair loss associated with pili torti. Modified from Olsen [209]

Ectodermal dysplasia
  Rapp–Hodgkins syndrome
  Sălamon's syndrome
  Arthrogryposis and ectodermal dysplasia
  Ectodermal dysplasia with syndactyly
  Tricho-odonto-onychodysplasia with pili torti
  Pili torti and enamel hypoplasia (Ronchese type)
  Pili torti and onychodysplasia (Beare's type)
  Ankyloblepharon–ectodermal defects with cleft lip and palate
    syndrome
Björnstad's dysplasia
Salti and Salem syndrome
Crandall's syndrome
Menke's kinky hair syndrome
Tay's syndrome and other cases of trichothiodystrophy
Chondrodysplasia punctata
Bazex's syndrome
Citrullinaemia

nosed, there must be multiple twists at irregular intervals on a given hair (Fig. 23.1.16). The affected hairs generally fracture through the twists.

Pili torti, like trichorrhexis nodosa, can occur in the presence of other hair shaft abnormalities either as an inherited or acquired finding and is also present in many different syndromes. It has been reported to occur in association with monilethrix [119], pseudomonilethrix [120], wooly hair [121], longitudinal grooving [122], trichorrhexis nodosa [57] and trichorrhexis invaginata [123]. In the classic Ronchese type of pili torti, the inheritance is usually autosomal dominant, but autosomal recessive and sporadic inheritance have been also reported [118,124–126]. The hair abnormality usually presents in infancy [124]; however, as with many inherited hair abnormalities, the first and second pelages may be normal with the pili torti not developing until the second year. Pili torti may be an isolated finding or part of an ectodermal dysplasia complex of findings. Sensorineural deafness has

Monilethrix

The hairs of monilethrix macroscopically appear beaded which is explained microscopically by the presence of elliptical nodes occurring with regular periodicity every 0.7–1 mm [55] (Fig. 23.1.17). In between the nodes, the hair shaft is constricted and it is at these points that the hairs usually fracture. Pili torti is often mistaken for monilethrix by the uninitiated due to the microscopic illusion of variation in diameter of the shaft due to twisting. On scanning electron microscopy of monilethrix hairs, there are both structural abnormalities of the cortex and cuticle in the zone of keratinization [129].

Recessively inherited cases are reported but most pedigrees show autosomal dominant inheritance with high penetrance [119,130]. The disorder has been found to be closely linked to the type II keratin gene cluster on chromosome 12q13 implicating a mutation in the structure or regulation of a trichocyte keratin gene in the pathogenesis of this disorder [131]. The condition may have a delayed onset of hair loss with presentation anywhere from infancy to the teens. Expression is variable with a spectrum of localized to total alopecia [131]. The clinical picture of monilethrix, however, is very distinctive secondary to the usual appearance of extremely short brittle hairs emerging through keratotic follicular papules (Fig. 23.1.18). The occiput and nape of the neck are especially affected.

The hair defect may occur alone or in association with keratosis pilaris, physical retardation, syndactyly, cataracts and nail/teeth abnormalities [132]. Improvement in the hair brittleness may occur during summer and with age [44]. Etretinate and topical minoxidil may potentially be useful therapies [133–135].

Pseudomonilethrix

Pseudomonilethrix is microscopic irregular beading along the hair shaft as opposed to the regular beading seen in monilethrix (Fig. 23.1.19) [120]. Although it has been

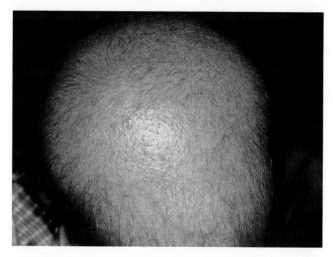

Fig. 23.1.18 Monilethrix. Reprinted from Whiting [55].

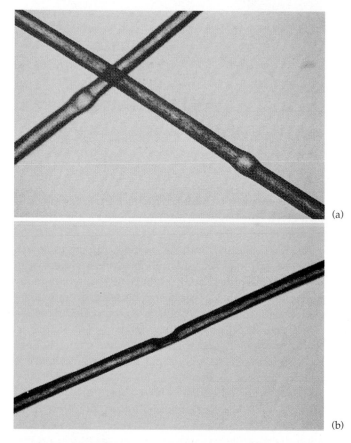

(a)

(b)

Fig. 23.1.19 Pseudomonilethrix (light micrographs, ×200). Reprinted from Zitelli [137]. (a) Shows pseudomonilethrix induced by pressure on overlapped normal hairs. (b) Rotated 90° to demonstrate indentation.

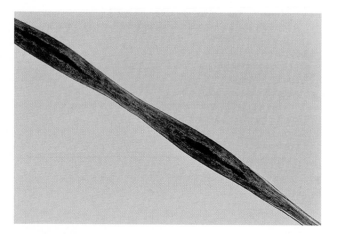

Fig. 23.1.17 Monilethrix (light micrograph, ×100). Courtesy of Dr David A. Whiting.

reported in patients with fragile hair [120,136], the appearance of pseudomonilethrix can be produced in normal hairs by compressing two hairs together between two glass slides [137,138]. It is likely that the nodes in pseudomonilethrix are artefactual [55].

Hair shaft abnormalities associated with unruly hair

Uncombable hair syndrome

Children with uncombable hair syndrome present in infancy up to puberty with slow-growing, silvery-blonde 'spun-glass' hair that is disorderly and unmanageable [139–142] (Fig. 23.1.20). Under light microscopy, the hairs may appear normal or may have some midline darkening suggestive of the typical longitudinal grooves so clearly seen on scanning electron microscopy [143–145]. Longitudinal grooving in itself is a relatively common hair shaft abnormality being seen in normal hair and in many cases of ectodermal dysplasia along with other hair shaft abnormalities [55]. On scanning electron microscopy of hairs in unmanageable hair syndrome, the longitudinal grooving is generally seen in conjunction with a cross-sectional triangular shape, the basis for the term pili trianguli et canaliculi [142] (Figs 23.1.21, 23.1.22). One potential explanation for the hair shaft abnormality is premature keratinization of the inner root sheath: normally, the inner root sheath forms a rigid casing that influences the resultant shape of the hair shaft (normally round or oval) [140]. By itself, pili trianguli et canaliculi does not lead to hair fragility.

The condition may be sporadic or autosomal dominant inheritance [143,146] and is generally without other associations or abnormalities. The condition of uncombable hair syndrome may improve with age. Supplemental biotin has been reported to be of use in one case [147] but

generally does not affect the process. Conditioners are helpful.

Woolly hair

Woolly hair is the presence of Negroid hair on the scalp of non-Negroid persons. Microscopically, the hair is tightly coiled without generally going to the extremes of pili torti. However, pili torti and pili annulati (blonde hair with both the clinical and microscopic findings of alternating bands of light and dark on the hair shaft) may be seen with this condition [121].

The hair in woolly hair is unruly only in the sense that it is difficult to manage but probably not more so than the hair normally occurring in black people of African extraction. The aberrant hair growth begins at birth or infancy with excessively tight curls making the hair appear bushy or frizzy. Hair length may be decreased secondary to brit-

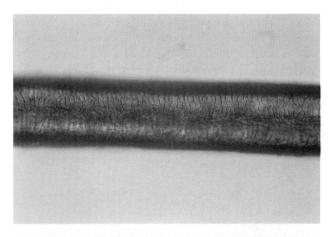
Fig. 23.1.21 Longitudinal grooving (light micrograph, ×400). Courtesy of Dr David A. Whiting.

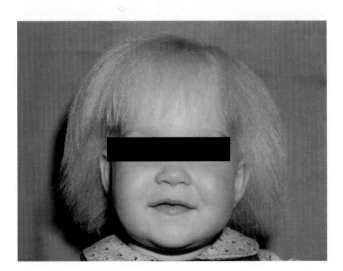
Fig. 23.1.20 Uncombable Hair Syndrome.

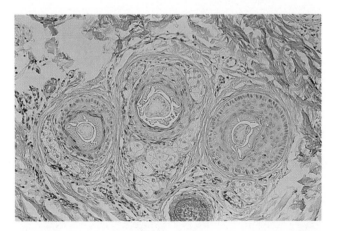
Fig. 23.1.22 Cross-section of hairs on scalp biopsy of child with Uncombable Hair Syndrome. Note triangular cross-section of affected hair (horizontal section, H & E). Courtesy of Dr David A. Whiting.

tleness, a common problem with Negroid hair in general. Woolly hair may go from curly to wavy as the child ages.

Woolly hair usually appears as a solitary problem inherited in an autosomal dominant fashion [121] but has been reported in conjunction with enamel hypoplasia [148], ocular defects [149,150], deafness and ichthyosis vulgaris [151], keratosis pilaris atrophicans [152] and Noonan's syndrome [153]. It has been reported to occur in a sporadic recessive form and in these cases, the scalp hair is usually fine and white–blonde [121]. With excessively curly hair in a non-Negroid infant, one must also consider the following syndromes: trichodento-osseous syndrome (small widely spaced teeth, frontal bossing and dolichocephaly [154],) and CHAND (curly hair, ankyloblepheron and nail dysplasia) syndrome [155].

Marie–Unna type of hereditary hypotrichosis

This autosomal dominantly inherited condition has a distinctive type of hair loss which varies with the child's age [30–33]. The hair is sparse or absent at birth with variable abnormal coarse hair regrowth in childhood and potential loss again at puberty (Fig. 23.1.23). The coarse, wiry, twisted hair is very distinctive. Hair shaft examination shows irregular twisting and by scanning electron microscopy, longitudinal ridging and peeling of the cuticle. Diffuse follicular hyperkeratosis with milia-like

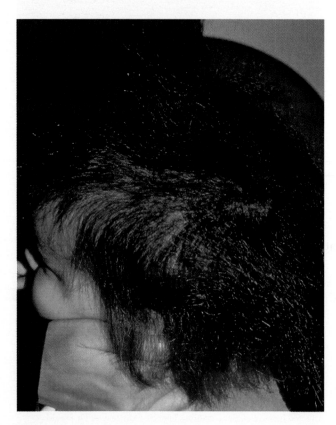

Fig. 23.1.23 Marie–Unna hypotrichosis.

facial lesions may be present.

Acquired localized unruly hair

Four non-inherited conditions may present as patches of scalp hair that differ from the normal for that individual. The most common is X-ray therapy-related with the hair that regrows after treatment (and epilation) being different in quality from that seen pretreatment. Localized woolly hair naevus, occurring only in non-Negroid persons, usually develops within the first 2 years of life (although this has been first reported in adolescence) with the affected hair being finer, lighter and more tightly curled than that of the rest of the scalp hair [156,157] (Fig. 23.1.24). Microscopically, the hairs may show trichorrhexis nodosa, longitudinal grooving, flattening and twisting [158–160]. Almost 50% of patients with woolly hair naevus have an underlying linear epidermal naevus or pigmented naevus [161,162].

Straight hair naevus, in which a localized portion of the normally curled or kinky hair is straight, has been noted only in Negroid persons. This may also have an association with an underlying epidermal naevus [163,164]. Acquired progressive kinking occurs after puberty, generally in males with androgenetic alopecia, and presents as gradual curling and darkening of the frontal, temporal, auricular and vertex hairs [165–168]. Microscopically, the hairs of acquired progressive kinking are short with kinks and twists and may show longitudinal grooving.

Localized tufts of hair

In pili multigemini, hairs from two to eight follicular bulbs, each with their own inner root sheath but surrounded by a

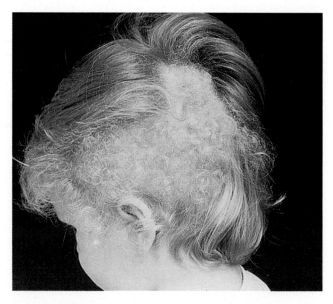

Fig. 23.1.24 Woolly hair naevus. Courtesy of Dr Vera H. Price.

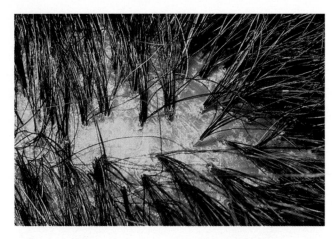

Fig. 23.1.25 Tufted folliculitis. Reprinted from Baden [172].

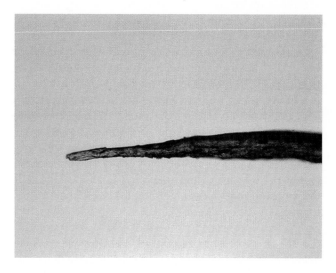

Fig. 23.1.26 Tapered proximal portion and point of breakage in hairs involved in an anagen effluvium (light micrograph, ×100). Courtesy of Dr David A. Whiting.

common outer root sheath, emerge from one follicular canal [169]. In children, this condition may appear as an isolated scalp problem or may occur with classic pili torti [124] or in cleidocranial dysostosis [170]. Although compound follicles may appear similar to pili multigemini, in this condition two to three different hair shafts, each with their own inner root sheath and outer root sheath, eventually emerge from the same follicular opening. These two non-scarring entities must be differentiated from tufted folliculitis in which scalp inflammation is prominent and leads to focal scarring with units of 10–15 hairs, each from their own follicle, emerging as tufts of hair from a single follicular canal [171,172] (Fig. 23.1.25).

Abnormal cycling

For the purposes of facilitating diagnosis, there are two main types of abnormal hair cycling and, hence there are two types of hair loss, i.e. anagen loss or telogen loss. Both are suspected by the clinical presentation of abnormal shedding and confirmed by histological evaluation of the proximal hair shaft/bulb. The differential diagnosis and consequent evaluation and treatment varies greatly, however, between these two conditions.

Anagen loss

Anagen effluvium. Anagen loss is *always* abnormal and with the exception of loose anagen syndrome, scalp anagen hair loss generally implies a toxic exposure. The most common and easily recognizable cause of anagen loss (or effluvium) is that related to oncological treatment, either X-ray therapy or chemotherapy. In both cases, there is generally immediate cessation of mitosis, and hence hair shaft production, that can either produce a hair shaft with a focal weakened point, if the duration of treatment is brief, or discontinuation of growth if the treatment persists for any length of time. In either case, the

damaged hair shaft will break off within the first few millimetres of protruding from the scalp (Fig. 23.1.26). Hair loss is profound since over 80% of scalp hair is normally in anagen at any given time. Telogen hairs may remain in place.

The hair loss from chemotherapy is reversible when treatment stops. The potential for regrowth after X-ray therapy will depend on the type, depth and dose–fractionation of the X-rays. Regrowth after loss from either chemotherapy or X-ray therapy may produce hair that is different in colour, curl or texture than that seen pretreatment.

In the absence of the above history, anagen effluvium in children should lead one to consider toxic exposure to boric acid or heavy metals. Boric acid is the main ingredient in some common household pesticides and is also used as a preservative in some household products [173,174]. Boric acid poisoning is suggested by gastrointestinal, central nervous system and renal symptoms, skin findings of exfoliation, erythroderma and bullae, and a haemorrhagic diathesis [173,175,176]. Confirmation is by measuring blood boric acid levels [175].

Mercury intoxication is primarily through chronic industrial exposure, consumption of industrially polluted water or affected seafood or inadvertent exposure to mercury used as a fungicide or antiseptic [177]. Hair loss may occur with or without the other common symptoms (particularly neurological) of mercury intoxication [178–180]. Acrodynia is a particular constellation of findings (pain in the abdomen, extremities and joints, pink scaly palms and soles, headache, photophobia, irritability, hyperhidrosis and hair loss) that can occur with chronic exposure to inorganic mercury [181]. Diagnosis of mercury intoxication is made by measuring urine, blood or hair levels of mercury [180,182].

Acute toxicity to arsenic may occur with suicidal or homicidal attempts or with accidental ingestion or exposure [177]. Inorganic arsenic compounds are found in insecticides, rodenticides, fungicides, herbicides and wood preservatives [182]. Acute arsenic toxication presents with gastrointestinal symptoms, hypotension, shortness of breath, central nervous system changes, haemolysis and acute tubular necrosis [183]. Approximately 6 weeks later, white transverse lines on all the nails (Mees' lines) may appear. The importance of hair in this diagnosis is not alopecia (which is rare) but rather that arsenic is concentrated in the hair and is detectable for months after exposure (as opposed to being detectable in urine for 7–10 days after exposure), facilitating a diagnosis even while symptoms improve or after the patient's demise [183,184].

The symptoms of acute thallium poisoning are insomnia, irritability, pain in the hands and feet and abdominal colic [185]. Two to three weeks later, there is a precipitous loss of all scalp hair together with peripheral and autonomic nervous system symptoms. Mees' lines develop later. Blood and urine levels are diagnostic but must be done as soon as possible as thallium levels tend to decrease rapidly.

Very severe protein malnutrition may also give an anagen effluvium as can the exposure to colchicine. Ingestion of certain plants, *Lecythis ollaria* and *Leucaena glauca*, can also lead to anagen hair loss [177].

Loose anagen syndromem (LAS). LAS was originally coined to describe a condition in children who had sparse hair that did not grow long, often with patches of dull matted hair, in whom unusual anagen hairs were easily extracted (Figure 23.1.27a). These anagen hairs had misshapen bulbs, absent root sheaths and ruffled cuticles (Figure 23.1.6c) [186–188]. The term loose anagen syndrome has also come to incorporate the easy extractability of these abnormal hairs in children with patchy unruly hair (Figure 23.1.27b) and otherwise clinically normal hair with increased shedding in subjects of any age [189]. It is now clear that normal prepubescent children commonly have a few loose anagen hairs found on a gentle hair pull and that the criteria for diagnosis of loose anagen syndrome must include a designated number of loose anagen hairs, ≥ 3 and perhaps ≥ 10, per hair pull [189,190]. Whether the presence of loose anagen hairs on hair pull is a marker for one or several distinct or overlapping hair disorders is currently unclear.

A report of two siblings with ocular colobomas, anagen hair shedding and decreased hair growth rate has been described [191]. However, the hairs in these cases did not attain the length normally seen in the loose anagen syndrome.

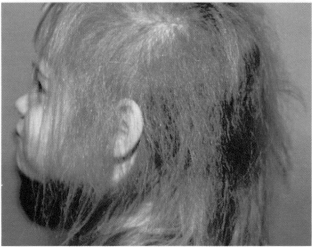

(a)

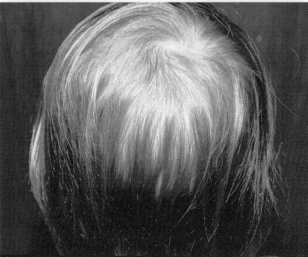

(b)

Fig. 23.1.27 (a) Loose anagen syndrome in child with easily extractable hair. (b) Loose anagen syndrome in child with unruly hair. (With permission from *J Invest Dermatol*. Olsen EA, Bettencourt MS, Cote NL. The presence of loose anagen hairs obtained by hair pull in the normal population, 1999).

Telogen loss

Telogen effluvium. The stress on the anagen hair follicle necessary to cause a telogen effluvium is milder than that with an anagen effluvium and precipitates an abrupt end to anagen and transformation to telogen versus the inherent damage or weakening of the shaft seen in an anagen effluvium. In a telogen effluvium, about 10–40%, rarely more, of the scalp anagen hairs suddenly move in concert through the physical transformation to telogen and are shed together after the usual obligatory time in telogen. Thus, a patient with a telogen effluvium generally experiences a sudden increase in hair shedding diffusely over the scalp 3–4 months after an inciting event. In the situation where the aetiological factor has been removed (e.g. recovery from a severe infection), the telogen loss would be followed by a recapitulation of anagen in the affected follicles and regrowth of hair over the ensuing 6 months.

In cases where the aetiological factor remains (e.g. untreated thyroid disease), the continued effect on the anagen follicles would cause persistence of the increased percentage of telogen hairs even while those telogen hairs that are shed are being replaced in the normal cycle with anagen hairs. Once the inciting factor(s) is removed, a telogen effluvium generally will resolve over the next 6–12 months.

The diagnosis of telogen effluvium is confirmed by finding a positive hair pull and confirmation that the shed hair bulbs are telogen by microscopic examination. Fifty to 100 telogen hairs are normally shed per day, reflecting the 10–15% of scalp hairs in telogen at any one time [192]. In a telogen effluvium, 100–300 hairs per day are usually shed and 20–50% of the scalp hairs may be in telogen at a given time. Telogen effluvium is less common in children than adults, and in children is more likely to be related to a sudden and transient illness than the drugs and hormonal fluctuations that commonly trigger this in adults (Table 23.1.4). It must be emphasized that any drug can trigger a telogen effluvium just as any drug can cause a cutaneous allergic reaction. However, there are certain drugs that cause this more commonly than others and these are listed in Table 23.1.4. Only those causes of telogen effluvium related to nutrition will be discussed here.

Protein malnutrition (kwashiorkor) and caloric malnutrition (marasmus) usually occur concurrently and are common in children living in developing nations [193,194]. The hair in affected individuals is slow growing, sparse and dyspigmented (Fig. 23.1.28). The increased telogen percentage is accompanied by relative anagen bulb atrophy and a concomitant diminution in hair shaft diameter and stability [194,198].

Zinc deficiency in childhood can lead to sparse and slow hair growth. The low plasma zinc levels are caused by either an autosomal recessive inherited disorder of intestinal absorption of zinc (acrodermatitis enteropathica) or may be acquired in the situation of general intestinal malabsorption with inadequate zinc replacement [199]. The hair loss may be accompanied by acral and periorificial vesiculobullous or eczematoid plaques, glossitis, stomatitis, nail dystrophy and diarrhoea [200]. Oral zinc supplementation will reverse all findings.

Essential fatty acid deficiency in children usually occurs with prolonged parenteral alimentation with inadequate inclusion of supplemental essential fatty acids. The hair becomes sparse and less pigmented, and a generalized and periorifical dermatitis and thrombocytopenia may develop [201–203]. The skin returns to normal within weeks and the hair within months of either intravenous essential fatty acid replacement or treatment with topical linoleic acid [202].

Biotin deficiency may be secondary to either dietary deficiency or hereditary multiple carboxylase deficiency. In the autosomal recessive infantile form of multiple carboxylase deficiency (the neonatal form is usually rapidly fatal), infants develop the first symptoms at 2–3 months of age [204–207]. The genetic abnormality is a deficiency (<5% normal) of biotinidase leading to impaired biotin absorption and reutilization [204,207,208]. Hair may be sparse and fine, and a distinctive sharply marginated dermatitis of the face, groin and periorifical areas reminiscent of acrodermatitis entropathica may develop (Fig. 23.1.29) together with central nervous system dysfunction and recurrent infections. A partial deficiency (15–40% of normal) of biotinidase may exist and appears

Table 23.1.4 Causes of telogen effluvium in children and adolescents

Medical illness
  Severe infections, usually associated with high fever
  Other systemic illnesses, acute or chronic
  Hypo- or hyperthyroidism
Postpartum
Surgery
Medications (including but not limited to)
  Anticoagulants
  β-blockers
  Lithium
  Oral contraceptive pills—during or after discontinuation
  Retinoids and excess vitamin A
  Valproic acid
Nutritional
  Precipitous diminution calories or protein
  Iron deficiency
  Zinc deficiency
  Essential fatty acid deficiency
  Biotin deficiency
Psychological stress

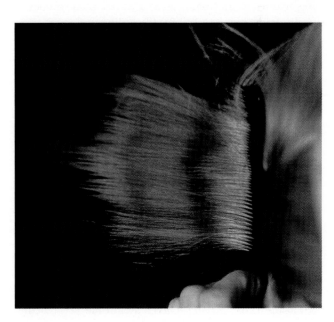

Fig. 23.1.28 Protein malnutrition: flag sign. Courtesy of Dr Nancy B. Esterly.

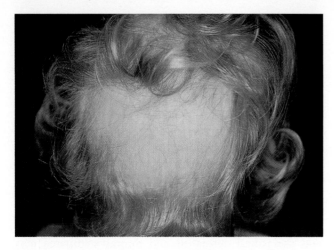

Fig. 23.1.29 Biotin deficiency. Courtesy of Dr Nancy B. Esterly.

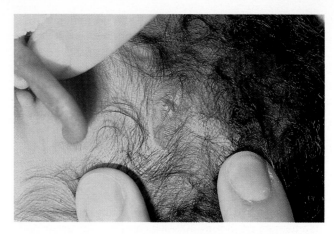

Fig. 23.1.30 Aplasia cutis congenita. Courtesy of Dr Neil S. Prose.

Table 23.1.5 Conditions associated with focal scarring hair loss in children. Modified from Olsen [209]

Ankyloblepharon–ectodermal defects–cleft lip/palate syndrome
Aplasia cutis congenita
Single anomaly
Associated with other anomalies
Associated with limb abnormalities
46XY genotype/gonadal dysgenesis
'Lumpy' scalp syndrome
Trisomy 13
4p – syndrome
Ectodermal dysplasia of Carey
Ectodermal dysplasia of Tuffli
Hallermann–Streiff syndrome
ANOTHER syndrome
Focal dermal hypoplasia
Johanson–Blizzard syndrome
Birth trauma
Congenital ectodermal dysplasia of the face
Conradi–Hünermann chondrodysplasia punctata
Epidermal or organoid naevus
CHILD syndrome (congenital hemidysplasia with ichthyosiform erythroderma and limb defects)
Epidermolysis bullosa
Hallermann–Streiff syndrome
Incontinentia pigmenti
Keratosis follicularis spinulosa decalvans
Kerion
KID syndrome (keratitis, ichthyosis, deafness)
Neoplasia
Prolonged pressure
Primary cutaneous disease
Tufted folliculitis

to be associated with lesser symptoms, i.e. mild hair loss and eczema [208]. The diagnosis is made by finding hyperammonuria, ketoacidosis and lactic acidosis, organic acidosis and/or low serum biotin (however, biotin level may be normal) [205,206]. The biotinidase deficiency can be overcome with biotin replacements and all changes are potentially reversible if the biotin deficiency is treated early [206].

Focal alopecia

Focal scarring alopecia

Focal alopecia can either be of a potentially transient non-scarring nature or of a potentially permanent or scarring nature. In an infant, there are four main causes of focal scarring hair loss: trauma (including prolonged pressure), aplasia cutis congenita, underlying naevus (or neoplasia) or as part of a syndrome. Those conditions associated with focal scarring alopecia are shown in Table 23.1.5.

Aplasia cutis congenita is the focal absence of epidermis plus or minus other layers of the skin: the hair follicles are variably affected [210]. Eighty-five per cent of aplasia cutis congenita presents on the scalp and 70% of patients have only a single lesion [210,211]. Usually aplasia cutis congenita lesions are small and round unless they are in one of the cranial suture lines in which case they may be quite large and can extend to the dura or meninges [210,211]. At birth, aplasia cutis congenita may present as ulcerations or with a crust, scar or parchment-like membrane secondary to *in utero* healing [210] (Fig. 23.1.30). Aplasia cutis congenita may present alone or with various other abnormalities [211–216], including trisomy 13 syndrome [216], 4p–syndrome [216], Adams–Oliver syndrome [217] oculocerebrocutaneous syndrome [218] or various ectodermal dysplasias [12,216–222]. No specific therapy is necessary except in cases of large or deep lesions which may require surgical correction.

Hair generally does not grow in an area affected by an epidermal naevus, regardless of whether the clinical subtype is inflammatory linear epidermal, comedonal or sebaceous naevus. Other causes of scarring alopecia which are primary aetiological factors in adults, i.e. lupus erythematosus, lichen planus, folliculitis decalvans and pseudopelade of Brocq, are rare in children. A kerion can

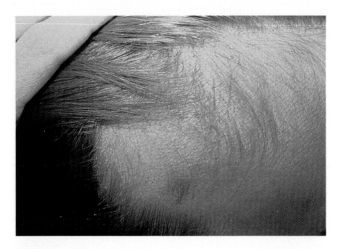

Fig. 23.1.31 Triangular alopecia. Courtesy of Dr Jerry Shapiro.

leave the permanent sequelae of hair loss in the affected area but this is a rare occurrence in developed nations. Areas of tufted folliculitis display both aberrant hairs and scarring alopecia.

Focal non-scarring hair loss

These conditions are common and include alopecia areata, tinea capitis, traction alopecia, trichotillomania and pityriasis amiantacea. Triangular alopecia is also a potentially reversible type of acquired focal hair loss, usually presenting in early childhood but potentially occurring at any age [223,224]. The temporal areas is the most common location and the lesions may be unilateral or bilateral. The area of alopecia may be roughly triangular in shape with the base of the triangle at the junction of the frontal and temporal hairline (Fig. 23.1.31) or may be oval or lancet shaped. The area may be hairless or vellus hair may be present. Histologically, there is a transition of hairs from terminal to vellus. The alopecia is usually persistent [225].

Familial focal alopecia is the name proposed for the recently described patchy non-scarring areas of decreased hair density in the scalp in a mother and daughter [226]. On biopsy, there was telogen arrest, absence of inflammation and preservation of sebaceous epithelium.

Hypertrichosis

Generalized hypertrichosis

Hereditary hypertrichosis

Congenital hypertrichosis lanuginosa implies a rare generalized and confluent overgrowth (or persistence) of lanugo hair in all hair-bearing areas [227,228]. The condition is thought to be inherited as an autosomal dominant with variable expressivity [227,230]. The excess hair is

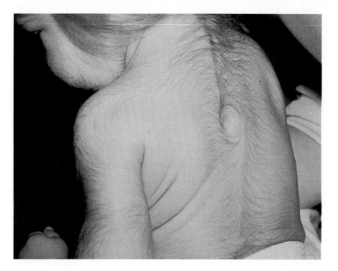

Fig. 23.1.32 Congenital hypertrichosis lanuginosa. Reprinted Olsen [229].

usually silvery grey to blond in colour and is either apparent at birth or within the first few months of life (Fig. 23.1.32). Children are generally otherwise normal except for possible anomalous dental development [227]. The hypertrichosis may persist, decrease or increase with age [227].

The other types of generalized hereditary hypertrichosis seen in childhood do not generally have the even confluent hair growth as seen in congenital hypertrichosis lanuginosa. Infants with Ambras syndrome may have a generalized hypertrichosis at birth but the hair is generally much longer and thicker on the face, ears and shoulders, and converges in the midline on the back [231]. Facial dysmorphism and dental abnormalities are common. Inheritance is presumed to be autosomal dominant. Whether the affected children in a large five-generation Mexican family with congenital generalized hypertrichosis, described by Macias-Flores, have a different condition is unclear [232]. These children were born with excessive terminal hair on their face and upper body but the hair growth was generally more excessive in males than females and the inheritance was ascribed to X-linked dominant [233].

Gingival fibromatosis—autosomal dominant, autosomal recessive or sporadic in inheritance—is characterized by marked gingival hypertrophy, which is usually apparent at birth or within the first year of life, although it can be delayed until puberty [234–237]. Associated hypertrichosis is inconstant but when it occurs, presents as dark hair mainly confined to the eyebrows, face, limbs and mid-back. These patients may also have oligophrenia and epilepsy, or a particular constellation of findings including hypoplastic phalanges, hepatosplenomegaly and facial dysmorphism (the latter termed Laband's syndrome). A related condition, congenital macrogingiva and giant fibrodenomas, may also have associated generalized, but not confluent, hypertrichosis [236,237]. There is obvious overlap of features in many of these conditions.

The hypertrichosis in Cornelia de Lange's syndrome is nowhere as confluent as that seen in congenital hypertrichosis lanuginosa but consists of persistent excess lanugo hair over the forehead, nape of neck, back, shoulders and extremities [238,239]. The eyebrows are bushy and confluent and the lashes are very long. The syndrome commonly is sporadic in inheritance but the exact genetic nature remains to be determined [229,240]. The children with Cornelia de Lange's syndrome have distinctive facies, mental and growth retardation, limb abnormalities and a low pitched cry [238,241,242]. Typical laboratory findings are hyperglutamic acidaemia, hypoamino-aciduria and elevated serum and ketoglutarate [243].

Children with the autosomal recessive Hurler's syndrome also have distinctive ('gargoyle') faces, and may have the trunk and extremities covered with dense lanugo hair [244].

Patients with one of four different types of porphyria can develop generalized hypertrichosis. Children with the autosomal recessive erythropoetic protoporphyria usually develop widespread hypertrichosis by the age of 5–6 years [245]. The excess hair is usually mainly on the limbs and trunk, may be downy or coarse, and is generally pigmented. Other cutaneous findings include photosensitivity and vesiculobullous lesions. Hypertrichosis is also common in porphyria cutanea tarda but presents on the temples, cheeks, eyebrows and hairline—more so than on the trunk and extremities [246]. Although the manifestations of this hereditary enzymatic disorder usually first appear in adulthood, an acquired form of porphyria cutanea tarda secondary to the inadvertant ingestion of hexachlorobenzene or chlorinated phenols can be seen in all ages [246,247]. Variegate porphyria may cause similar cutaneous findings to those seen with porphyria cutanea tarda but is distinguished by intermittent gastrointestinal and neurological symptoms after exposure to certain provoking medications. Variegate porphyria has a different urine and stool porphyrin profile from porphyria cutanea tarda. Porphyrias are discussed in further detail in Chapter 15.2.

Acquired hypertrichosis

Drug related

Generalized hypertrichosis, typically of vellus versus lanugo hair, may be an acquired problem caused by several drugs. Minoxidil, a piperidinopyrimidine derivative used to treat hypertension, causes hypertrichosis in about 70% of users [248,249]. The excess hair is especially prominent over the face, shoulders and extremities and

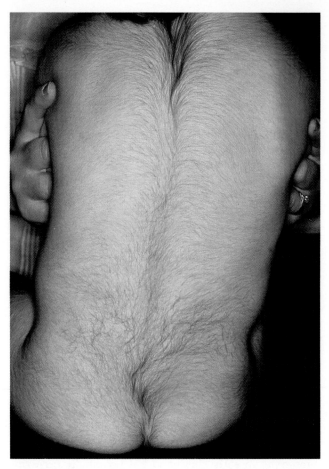

Fig. 23.1.33 Minoxidil-induced hypertrichosis. Courtesy of Dr Nancy B. Esterly.

develops weeks to months after starting treatment (Fig. 23.1.33). The hypertrichosis regresses within months of discontinuing the drug.

Hypertrichosis is seen in up to 60% of patients given cyclosporine to prevent organ rejection [250]. Hypertrichosis is even more common in patients given cyclosporine to treat graft-versus-host disease or insulin-dependent diabetes mellitus [251,252]. The hair growth is diffuse and begins within 2–4 weeks of starting the drug [245]. Children and adolescents are at the greatest risk of developing moderate to severe hypertrichosis [247]. Usually the hypertrichosis resolves 1–2 months after discontinuing the drug [250,252].

Diazoxide is a benzothiadiazine used to treat idiopathic hypoglycaemia of childhood. Lanugo hair growth is commonly seen in children usually beginning 6 weeks after the start of treatment and demonstrated most prominently on the forehead, nape of the neck, eyebrows, eyelashes and dorsum of the trunk and limbs [253–256]. The excess hair growth usually regresses 2–5 months after discontinuation of the drug but may take longer. Infants born to women given diazoxide for hypertension during pregnancy have a high incidence of hair abnormalities including hypertrichosis lanuginosa and focal alopecia [257].

Hypertrichosis occurs in 5–12% of patients on phenytoin, usually most prominently on the extremities versus the face and trunk [258,259]. The hair growth usually regresses within 1 year after treatment stops but can persist [260,261].

Although uncommonly used in children, psoralens and ultraviolet A (PUVA) [262,263] and acetozolamide have both been reported to cause hypertrichosis [264]. Streptomycin used to treat tuberculosis also has been associated with hypertrichosis [265].

Other illnesses/conditions associated with hypertrichosis

Certain acquired medical conditions have been associated with diffuse hypertrichosis. *POEMS* is an acronym for peripheral neuropathy, organomegaly, endocrine dysfunction, monoclonal gammopathy and skin changes, the latter including hypertrichosis primarily on the extensor surfaces, malar region and forehead [266–268]. Patients with hypothyroidism, acrodynia (mercury poisoning), tuberculosis or head trauma may also have a generalized increase in hair growth [229]. There have been several reports of hypertrichosis in children with a variety of gastrointestinal problems including coeliac disease, infantile steatorrhoea and failure to thrive: the primary mechanism is unknown [229]. Children with juvenile dermatomyositis, may have a concomitant hypertrichosis which may diminish with treatment of the dermatomyositis [269,270].

Localized hypertrichosis

There are several causes of localized hypertrichosis in childhood, some of which are isolated anomalies and others which are indicative of either underlying anatomical abnormalities or other anomalies.

Congenital localized hypertrichosis

Congenital hair on the elbows, usually lanugo at birth, may become terminal and more dense in early childhood and then regress with age [271,272]. Short stature has been associated in some cases [273,274]. Congenital hair on the external ears in children can be seen as an isolated anomaly in some Pacific Islanders or in patients with XYY syndrome or offspring of diabetic mothers [275–277]. Congenital trichomegaly of the eyelashes can occur as an isolated event or as part of one of several syndromes including Cornelia de Lange's syndrome, Rubenstein–Taybi syndrome, congenital hypertrichosis lanuginosa and a syndrome described by Oliver and McFarlane that

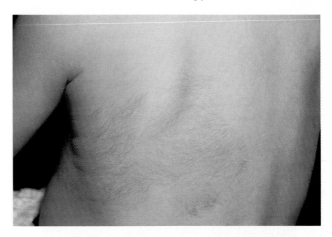

Fig. 23.1.34 Congenital smooth muscle hamartoma. Courtesy of Dr Nancy B. Esterly.

includes dwarfism, mental retardation and pigmentary degeneration of the retina [229,278].

Naevoid hypertrichosis is an uncommon congenital disorder consisting of terminal hair growth in usually a solitary area but rarely in multiple patches of normal underlying skin [279]. However, localized hypertrichosis can be associated with underlying abnormalities and should be further evaluated by biopsy. Localized areas of either hypertrichosis or alopecia at birth can overlie primary cutaneous meningiomas [280]. These may occur on the scalp, midline or paravertebral area of the back or face. Histologically, these show polygonal to fusiform cells with syncytial appearance, eosinophilic cytoplasm and regular nuclei plus/minus psammoma bodies. Clinically, these are benign neoplasms.

Localized hypertrichosis and hyperpigmentation may be seen in both congenital smooth muscle hamartomas and congenital pigmented hairy naevi. These two conditions are easily distinguished both clinically and by biopsy [281]. Congenital smooth muscle hamartomas histologically show smooth muscle bundles varying in size, shape and orientation. The lesions clinically may be single or multiple (Fig. 23.1.34), are usually indurated and show transient raising upon rubbing (pseudo-Darier's sign) [281,282]. The lesions tend to decrease with time [282,283]. Generalized congenital smooth muscle hamartomas with extensive hypertrichosis and an increase in skin folds may be seen in the Michelin Tire syndrome [282].

In contradistinction, congenital hairy naevi histologically demonstrate a naevocellular naevus. They are usually solitary, are not indurated and have a negative pseudo-Darier's sign [229] (Fig. 23.1.35). Congenital hairy naevi tend to persist and have a potential for malignant degeneration.

The Winchester syndrome may also present with irregular patches of thickened skin, hyperpigmentation and hypertrichosis but biopsy here shows fibroblastic proliferation with homogenized bundles of collagen [284].

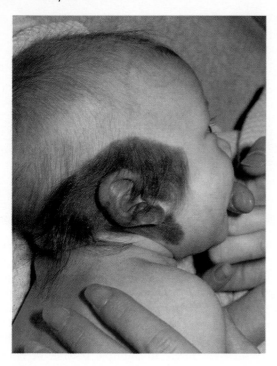

Fig. 23.1.35 Congenital hairy naevus. Courtesy of Dr Nancy B. Esterly.

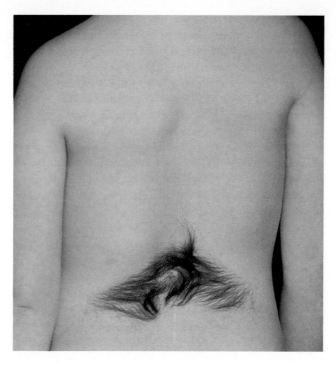

Fig. 23.1.36 Faun-tail. Courtesy of Dr Janet L. Roberts.

Affected children will develop short stature secondary to osteoporosis, osteolysis and periarticular and intra-articular joint erosions.

The presence of localized hypertrichosis over the spinal column, most common in the lumbar or sacral area, is a cause for concern. Infants born with a so-called 'faun-tail' (Fig. 23.1.36) may have an underlying spina bifida occulta, spina bifida, traction band or diastematomyelia [229,285]. A traction band can tether the cord or its appendages or the cauda equina to bone or skin through attachment to the meninges or through a tight filium terminale [229]. Diastematomyelia is duplication or splitting of a portion of the spinal cord through which a bony spur or fibrous band passes and attaches to the vertebral body anteriorly or neural arch posteriorly [286]. In the latter two conditions, neurological symptoms may not appear until the child is a toddler or older when dissimilar growth of the cord and its bony housing causes the spinal cord to ascend in the vertebral column [286,287]. The localized hypertrichosis may not, therefore, be at the level of a neural defect if one occurs [288].

Midback hypertrichosis may accompany other cutaneous abnormalities that may signal either a primary or secondary (from pressure) underlying neurological abnormality. Dermal sinuses, often associated with protrusion of hair from the sinus and pigmentation or port-wine discoloration, can extend into the spinal canal or may expand into an epidermoid or dermal cyst. Midline lipomas are frequently attached to the cord, cauda equina, filium terminalis or conus medullaris.

Inadvertant manipulation of these lesions could lead to a portal of entry for infection in the central nervous system or neurological deficit. No excision or manipulation of an area of hypertrichosis over the spinal cord should be carried out without first evaluating the underlying cord or spinal column, preferably by non-invasive techniques.

Acquired localized hypertrichosis

Any repeated irritation, inflammation or trauma may cause localized hypertrichosis by transformation of vellus to terminal hair [229]. The classic example is the localized hypertrichosis that develops under a casted appendage. The increased length of the hair that occurs in this situation is quickly lost when the cast is removed. Although localized hypertrichosis may be seen with morphoea [229], in general chronic dermatoses do *not* stimulate hair growth.

Terminal hair growth on the scrotum has been described in otherwise normal male infants at 2–4 months of age which generally goes away by 15 months [289,290]. This probably represents hypersensitivity to transiently elevated androgen levels.

Interferon and cyclosporine have each been associated with localized hypertrichosis of the eyelashes, although the latter is not surprising given that cyclosporine is frequently associated with a diffuse hypertrichosis [291–293]. A localized increase in the length of hairs on the ear, eyebrows and/or eyelashes has also been reported in

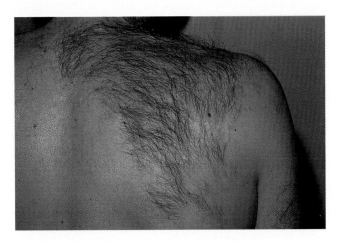

Fig. 23.1.37 Becker's naevus. Reprinted from Olsen [229].

patients with AIDS but the aetiology remains unclear [294–296].

Becker's naevus usually first appears in adolescence but has been reported from infancy to middle age (Fig. 23.1.37) [297]. These lesions may rarely have a familial incidence. The term 'naevus' is a misnomer as there are no naevus cells histologically but rather variable hyperkeratosis and marked hyperpigmentation in the basal layers of the epidermis with varying amounts of melanophages in the papillary dermis [297,298]. Hair follicles are normal or enlarged [297,299]. Some cases may also show an increase in smooth muscle bundles and in these cases clinically one may see perifollicular papules [298,300]. The question of why these lesions appear in adolescence may be related to the presence of androgen cytosol receptors in involved areas similar to genital skin [301].

The hyperpigmentation of Becker's naevus usually appears first and may fade with time [299,302]. The associated localized hypertrichosis may take years to develop [298,302]. Males are preferentially affected. Usually the lesions are single around the shoulders and at least palm sized but occasionally an unusual size or location can cause confusion with a naevus. In most cases, there are no other associated problems or abnormalities although there have been rare reports of hypoplasia of an ipsilateral limb or breast, pectus carinatum, spina bifida and accessory scrotum [229,303].

Treatment of hypertrichosis

In acquired hypertrichosis secondary to a drug or underlying disease, removal of the inciting cause will generally lead to loss of the increased hair growth and resumption of the normal type of hair growth, length of hair and cycle. In the case of hereditary or developmental hypertrichosis, treatment must be directed at either psychological acceptance or cosmetic removal of the increased hair growth. Shaving and chemical depilatories

serve to temporarily remove the offending hairs from sight without physically affecting the growth of the hairs. Plucking and wax epilation only temporarily remove the hair and can be quite painful. Each of these techniques run the risk of pseudofolliculitis barbae in those with very curly or kinky hair and chemical depilatories can be very irritating.

Electrolysis refers to electrochemical destruction of the hair follicle, either through thermolysis (AC current with destruction of the hair by local heat production) or 'the blend', a combination of thermolysis and galvanic DC current (which produces destruction of the hair by local production of caustic lye and H_2 gas) [218]. The current used is generally low intensity and high frequency to minimize tissue destruction and pain. Electrolysis varies greatly in terms of technique, machines and probes used, and results (permanent hair removal) may vary widely. Potential but controllable side effects are pain, scarring, infection and folliculitis. Some new information suggests laser destruction of hairs can be targeted and permanent [304] but little published data is available.

Summary

The diagnosis of alopecia in children is important both in order to direct treatment and to rule out extracutaneous disease. Many cases of alopecia in infancy and even childhood are part of a larger constellation of symptoms and signs indicative of an inherited syndrome and the associated hair abnormality may be the necessary clue to the diagnosis. The evaluation of a child with hair loss can be straightforward and the differential diagnosis can be significantly narrowed using the simple tools of history, physical examination and microscopic examination of the hair. Effective treatment is not available for all causes of hair loss but many conditions can be corrected and if not fully reversed, information about prognosis and management given to parents.

Hypertrichosis in childhood is generally a hereditary or developmental problem with a risk of other organ anomalies. Correct diagnosis can facilitate early interventional therapy for the underlying disease. As with alopecia, reversal of the hair abnormality may not be possible but discussion of psychological and physical management issues for the child with the parents is paramount and can only be done with assurance when a correct diagnosis is in place.

REFERENCES

1 Pinkus H. Embryology of hair. In: Montagna W, Ellis RA, eds. *The Biology of Hair Growth*. New York: Academic Press, 1958: 1–32.
2 Barth JH. Normal hair growth in children. *Pediatr Dermatol* 1987; 4: 173–84.
3 Danforth CH. Studies on hair. *Arch Dermatol Syph* 1925; 11: 804–21.
4 Barman JM, Pecoraro V, Astore I, Ferrer J. The first stage in the natural history of the human scalp hair cycle. *J Invest Dermatol* 1967; 48: 138–42.

5 Giacometti L. The anatomy of the human scalp. In: *Advances in Biology of Skin*, vol. 6. Oxford: Pergamon Press, 1965: 97–120.

6 Price ML, Griffiths WAD. Normal body hair: a review. *Clin Exp Dermatol* 1985; 10: 87–97.

7 Abel E. Embryology and anatomy of the hair follicle. In: Olsen EA, ed. *Disorders of Hair Growth: Diagnosis and Treatment*. New York: McGraw-Hill, 1994: 1–19.

8 Bertolino A, O'Guin WM. Differentiation of the hair shaft. In: Olsen EA, ed. *Disorders of Hair Growth: Diagnosis and Treatment*. New York: McGraw-Hill, 1994: 22–5.

9 Montagna W, Parakkal PF. *The Structure and Function of the Skin*, 3rd edn. New York: Academic Press, 1974: 172–258.

10 Cotsarelis G, Sun T-T, Lavker RM. Label retaining cells reside in the Bulge area of pilosebaceous unit: implication for follicular stem cells, hair cycle, and skin carcinogenesis. *Cell* 1990; 61: 1329–37.

11 Sirinavin C, Trowbridge AA. Dyskeratosis congenita: clinical features and genetic aspects: report of a family and review of the literature. *J Med Genet* 1975; 12: 339–54.

12 Freire-Maia N, Pinheiro M. *Ectodermal Dysplasias: a Clinical and Genetic Study*. New York: Alan R. Liss, 1984.

13 Beare JM. Congenital pilar defect showing features of pili torti. *Br J Dermatol* 1952; 64: 366–72.

14 Berg D, Weingold DH, Abson KG, Olsen EA. Sweating in ectodermal dysplasia syndromes. *Arch Dermatol* 1990; 6: 1075–9.

15 Lundbäck H. Total congenital hereditary alopecia. *Acta Derm Venereol* 1945; 25: 189–206.

16 Baraitser M, Carter CO, Brett EM. A new alopecia/mental retardation syndrome. *J Med Genet* 1983; 20: 64–75.

17 Shokeir MHK. Universal permanent alopecia, psychomotor epilepsy, pyorrhea and mental subnormality. *Clin Genet* 1977; 11: 13–17.

18 Moynahan EJ. Familial congenital alopecia, epilepsy, mental retardation with unusual electroencephalograms. *Proc Roy Soc Med* 1962; 55: 411–12.

19 Perniola T, Krajewska G, Carnevali F, Lospalluti M. Congenital alopecia, psychomotor retardation, convulsions in two sibs of a consanguineous marriage. *J Inher Metab Dis* 1980; 3: 49–53.

20 Hassing JH, Doeglas HMG. Dystrophia bullosa hereditaria, typus maculatus (Mendes da Costa–van der Valk): a rare genodermatosis. *Br J Dermatol* 1980; 102: 474–6.

21 Carol WLL, Rooij R. Typus Maculatus der Bullosen Hereditaren Dystrophie. *Acta Derm Venereol* 1937; 18: 265–83.

22 Loewenthal LJA, Prakken JR. Atrichia with papular lesions. *Dermatologica* 1961; 122: 85–9.

23 del Castillo V, Ruiz-Maldonado R, Carnevale A. Atrichia with papular lesions and mental retardation in two sisters. *Int J Dermatol* 1974; 13: 261–5.

24 Kanzler MH, Rasmussen JE. Atrichia with papular lesions. *Arch Dermatol* 1986; 122: 565–7.

25 Damsté TJ, Prakken JR. Atrichia with papular lesions, a variant of congenital ectodermal dysplasia. *Dermatologica* 1954; 108: 114–21.

26 Eramo LR, Esterly NB, Zieserl EJ, Stock EL, Herrmann J. Ichthyosis follicularis with alopecia and photophobia. *Arch Dermatol* 1985; 121: 1167–74.

27 Rothe MJ *et al.* Ichthyosis follicularis in two girls: an autosomal dominant disorder. *Pediatr Dermatol* 1990; 7: 287–92.

28 Rand R, Baden HP. Keratosis follicularis spinulosa decalvans: report of two cases and literature review. *Arch Dermatol* 1983; 119: 22–6.

29 Appell ML, Sherertz EF. A kindred with alopecia, keratosis pilaris, cataracts, and psoriasis. *J Am Acad Dermatol* 1987; 16: 89–95.

30 Stevanovic DV. Hereditary hypotrichosis congenita: Marie Unna type. *Br J Dermatol* 1970; 83: 331–7.

31 Wirth G, Bindewald I, Küster W, Goerz G. Hypotrichosis congenital hereditaria Marie Unna. *Hautarzt* 1985; 36: 577–80.

32 Mende B, Kreysel HW. Hypotrichosis Congenita Hereditaria Marie Unna mit Ehlers–Danlos-Syndrom und Atopie. *Hautarzt* 1987; 38: 532–5.

33 Solomon LM, Esterly NB, Medenica M. Hereditary trichodysplasia: Marie Unna's hypertrichosis. *J Invest Dermatol* 1971; 57: 389–400.

34 Cantu JM, Hernandez A, Larracilla J *et al.* A new X-linked recessive disorder with dwarfism, cerebral atrophy, and generalized keratosis follicularis. *J Pediatr* 1974; 84: 564–7.

35 McGrae JD Jr. Keratitis, ichthyosis, and deafness (KID) syndrome. *Int J Dermatol* 1990; 29: 89–92.

36 Cram DL, Resneck JS, Jackson WB. A congenital ichthyosiform syndrome with deafness and keratitis. *Arch Dermatol* 1979; 115: 467–71.

37 Senter TP, Jones KL, Sakati N, Nyhan WL. Atypical ichthyosiform erythroderma and congenital neurosensory deafness—A distinct syndrome. *J Pediatr* 1978; 92: 68–72.

38 Rycroft RJG, Moynahan EJ, Wells RS. Atypical ichthyosiform erythroderma, deafness and keratitis. *Br J Dermatol* 1976; 94: 211–17.

39 Hernandez A, Olivares F, Cantu J-M. Autosomal recessive onychotrichodysplasia, chronic neutropenia and mild mental retardation. *Clin Genet* 1979; 15: 147–52.

40 Verhage J *et al.* A patient with onychotrichodysplasia, neutropenia and normal intelligence. *Clin Genet* 1987; 31: 374–80.

41 Soderquist NA, Reed WB. Pachyonychia congenita with epidermal cysts and other congenital dyskeratoses. *Arch Dermatol* 1968; 97: 31–3.

42 Su WPD, Chun SI, Hammond DE, Gordon H. Pachyonychia congenita: a clinical study of 12 cases and review of the literature. *Pediatr Dermatol* 1990; 7: 33–8.

43 Tidman MJ, Wells RS, MacDonald DM. Pachyonychia congenita with cutaneous amyloidosis and hyperpigmentation—A distinct variant. *J Am Acad Dermatol* 1987; 16: 935–40.

44 Feinstein A, Friedman J, Schewach-Millet M. Pachyonychia congenita. *J Am Acad Dermatol* 1988; 19: 705–11.

45 Burket JM, Burket BJ, Burket DA. Eyelid cysts, hypodontia, and hypotrichosis. *J Am Acad Dermatol* 1984; 10: 922–5.

46 Pinheiro M, Freire-Maia N, Gollop TR. Odonto-onychodysplasia with alopecia: a new pure ectodermal dysplasia with probable autosomal recessive inheritance. *Am J Med Genet* 1985; 20: 197–202.

47 Freire-Maia N, Cat I, Rapone-Gaidzinski R. An ectodermal dysplasia syndrome of alopecia, onychodysplasia, hypohidrosis, hyperkeratosis, deafness and other manifestations. *Hum Hered* 1977; 27: 127–33.

48 Wilson WG *et al.* 'New' ectodermal dysplasia syndrome with distinctive facial appearance and preaxial polydactyly of feet. *Am J Med Genet* 1989; 34: 227–9.

49 Freire-Maia N, Pinheiro M, Fernandes-dos-Santos A. Xerodermia como sinal mais grave num quandro de displasia ectodérmica pura com etiologia genética. *Cienc Cult Suppl* 1982; 34: 764.

50 Schinzel A. A case of multiple skeletal anomalies, ectodermal dysplasia, and severe growth and mental retardation. *Helv Paediatr Acta* 1980; 35: 243–51.

51 Wallis C, Ip FS, Beighton P. Cataracts, alopecia, and sclerodactyly: a previously apparently undescribed ectodermal dysplasia syndrome on the island of Rodrigues. *Am J Med Genet* 1989; 32: 500–3.

52 Blackston RD, Brown AC. Cartilage–hair hypoplasia. In: Brown AC, Crounse RG, eds. *Hair, Trace Elements and Human Illness*. New York: Praeger, 1980: 257–72.

53 Hall BD, Greenberg MH. Hypomelia–hypotrichosis–facial hemangioma syndrome. *Am J Dis Child* 1972; 123: 602–4.

54 Moloney J. Regional choroidal atrophy and alopecia: a new syndrome. *Bull Soc Belge Ophthalmol* 1987; 224: 39–41.

55 Whiting DA. Hair shaft defects. In: Olsen EA, ed. *Disorders of Hair Growth: Diagnosis and Treatment*. New York: McGraw-Hill, 1994: 91–137.

56 Dawber RPR, Comaish S. Scanning electron microscopy of normal and abnormal hair shafts. *Arch Dermatol* 1970; 101: 316–22.

57 Chernosky ME, Owens DW. Trichorrhexis nodosa: clinical and investigative studies. *Arch Dermatol* 1966; 94: 577–85.

58 Wolff HH, Vigl E, Braun-Falco O. Trichorrhexis congenita. *Hautarzt* 1975; 26: 576–80.

59 Rousset MJ. Genodermatose difficilement classable (trichorrhexis nodosa) predominant chez les males dans quatre generations. *Bull Soc Fr Dermatol Syph* 1952; 59: 298–300.

60 Batshaw ML, Thomas GH, Brusilow SW. New approaches to the diagnosis and treatment of inborn errors of urea synthesis. *Pediatrics* 1981; 68: 290–7.

61 Shih VE. Early dietary management in an infant with argininosuccinase deficiency: preliminary report. *J Pediatr* 1972; 80: 645–8.

62 Rauschkolb EW, Chernosky ME, Knox JM, Owens DW. Trichorrhexis nodosa—an error of amino acid metabolism? *J Invest Dermatol* 1967; 48: 260–3.

63 Goldblum OM, Brusilow SW, Maldonado YA, Farmer ER. Neonatal citrullinemia associated with cutaneous manifestations and arginine deficiency. *J Am Acad Dermatol* 1986; 14: 321–6.

64 Porter PS. The genetics of human hair growth. In: Bergsma D, ed. *Birth Defects, Original Article Series*. Baltimore: Williams & Wilkins, 1972: 69–85.

65 Danks DM, Tippett P, Zentner G. Severe neonatal citrullinemia. *Arch Dis Child* 1974; 49: 579–81.

66 Patel HP, Unis ME. Pili torti in association with citrullinemia. *J Am Acad Dermatol* 1985; 12: 203–6.

67 Menkes JH *et al.* A sex-linked recessive disorder with retardation of growth, peculiar hair and focal cerebral and cerebellar degeneration. *Peditrics* 1962; 29: 764–79.

68 Menkes JH. Kinky hair disease. *Pediatrics* 1972; 50: 181–3.

69 Tümer Z, Horn N, Tonnesen T *et al.* Early copper–histidine treatment for Menkes disease. *Nature Genetics* 1996; 12: 11–13.

70 Davies K. Cloning the Menkes disease gene. *Nature* 1993; 361: 98.

71 Danks DM *et al.* Menkes' kinky hair syndrome. *Lancet* 1972; i: 1100–3.

72 Horn N. Copper incorporation studies on cultured cells for prenatal diagnosis of Menkes' disease. *Lancet* 1976; i: 1156–8.

73 Kodama H. Recent developments in Menkes disease. *J Inher Metab Dis* 1993; 16: 791–9.

74 Danks DM *et al.* Menkes' kinky hair syndrome. An inherited defect in copper absorption with widespread effects. *Pediatrics* 1972; 50: 188–201.

75 French JH *et al.* Trichopoliodystrophy. *Arch Neurol* 1972; 26: 229–44.

76 Goka TJ, Stevenson RE, Hefferan PM, Howell RR. Menkes' disease: a biochemical abnormality in cultured human fibroblasts. *Proc Natl Acad Sci USA* 1976; 73: 604–6.

77 Wheeler EM, Roberts PF. Menkes's steely hair syndrome. *Arch Dis Child* 1976; 51: 269–74.

78 Price VH, Odom RB, Ward WH, Jones FT. Trichothiodystrophy: sulfur-deficient brittle hair as a marker for a neuroectodermal symptom complex. *Arch Dermatol* 1980; 116: 1375–84.

79 Venning VA, Dawber RPR, Ferguson DJP, Kanan MW. Weathering of hair in trichothiodystrophy (abstract). *Br J Dermatol* 1986; 114: 591–5.

80 Brown AC, Belser RB, Crouses RG, Wehr RF. A congenital hair defect: trichoschisis and alternating birefringence and low sulfur content. *J Invest Dermatol* 1970; 54: 496–509.

81 Van Neste D, Miller X, Bohnert E. Clinical symptoms associated with trichothiodystrophy: A review of the literature with special emphasis on light sensitivity and the association with xeroderma pigmentosum (complementation group D). In: Van Neste D, Lachapelle JM, Antoine JL, eds. *Trends in Human Hair Growth and Alopecia Research.* Dordrecht: Kluwer Academic, 1989: 183–93.

82 Arbisser AI *et al.* A syndrome manifested by brittle hair with morphologic and biochemical abnormalities, developmental delay and normal stature. *Birth Defects* 1976; 12: 219–28.

83 Howell RR *et al.* The Sabinas brittle hair syndrome. In: Brown AC, Crounse RG, eds. *Hair, Trace Elements and Human Illness.* New York: Praeger, 1980: 210–19.

84 Baden HP *et al.* The physicochemical properties of hair in the BIDS syndrome. *Am J Hum Genet* 1976; 28: 514–21.

85 Jackson CE, Weiss L, Watson JHL. 'Brittle' hair with short stature, intellectual impairment and decreased fertility: an autosomal recessive syndrome in an Amish kindred. *Pediatrics* 1974; 54: 201–7.

86 Jorizzo JL, Crounse RG, Wheeler CE Jr. Lamellar ichthyosis, dwarfism, mental retardation and hair shaft abnormalities; a link between the ichthyosis-associated and BIDS syndromes. *J Am Acad Dermatol* 1980; 2: 309–17.

87 Jorizzo JL, Atherton DJ, Crounse RG, Wells RS. Ichthyosis, brittle hair, impaired intelligence, decreased fertility and short stature (IBIDS syndrome). *Br J Dermatol* 1982; 106: 705–10.

88 Tay CH. Ichthyosiform erythroderma, hair shaft abnormalities, and mental and growth retardation: a new recessive disorder. *Arch Dermatol* 1971; 104: 4–13.

89 Happle R, Traupe H, Grobe H, Bonsmann G. The Tay syndrome (congenital ichthyosis with trichothiodystrophy). *Eur J Pediatr* 1984; 141: 147–52.

90 Pollitt RJ, Jenner FA, Davies M. Sibs with mental and physical retardation and trichorrhexis nodosa with abnormal amino acid composition of the hair. *Arch Dis Child* 1968; 43: 211–16.

91 Crovato F, Borrone C, Rebora A. Trichothiodystrophy—BIDS, IBIDS and PIBIDS? *Br J Dermatol* 1983; 108: 247–51.

92 Crovato F, Rebora A. PIBI(D)S syndrome: a new entity with defect of the deoxyribonucleic acid excision repair system. *J Am Acad Dermatol* 1985; 13: 683–5.

93 Lucky PA, Kirsch N, Lucky AW, Carter DM. Low-sulfur hair syndrome associated with UVB photosensitivity and testicular failure. *J Am Acad Dermatol* 1984; 11: 340–6.

94 Rebora A, Guarrera M, Crovato F. Amino-acid analysis in hair from PIBI(D)S syndrome. *J Am Acad Dermatol* 1986; 15: 109–11.

95 Itin PH, Pittelkow MR. Trichothiodystrophy with chronic neutropenia and mild mental retardation. *J Am Acad Dermatol* 1991; 24: 356–8.

96 Norwood WF. The Marinesco–Sjögren syndrome. *J Pediatr* 1964; 65: 431–7.

97 Itin PH, Pittelkow MR. Trichothiodystrophy: review of sulfur-deficient brittle hair syndromes and association with ectodermal dysplasias. *J Am Acad Dermatol* 1990; 22: 705–17.

98 Gillespie JM, Marshall RC A comparison of the proteins of normal and trichothiodystrophic human hair. *J Invest Dermatol* 1983; 80: 195–202.

99 Gummer CL, Dawber RPR, Price VH. Trichothiodystrophy: an electron-histochemical study of the hair shaft. *Br J Dermatol* 1984; 110: 439–49.

100 Chen E, Cleaver JE, Weber CA *et al.* Trichothiodystrophy: clinical spectrum, central nervous system imaging, and biochemical characterization of two siblings. *J Invest Dermatol* 1994; 103: 154S–8S.

101 Gillespie JM, Marshall RC. Effect of mutations on the proteins of wool and hair. In: Rogers GE *et al.*, eds. *The Biology of Wool and Hair.* London: Chapman & Hall, 1989: 257–73.

102 Takayama K, Salazar EP, Broughton BC *et al.* Defects in the DNA repair and transcription Gene ERCC2(XPD) in trichothiodystrophy. *Am J Hum Genet* 1996; 58: 263–70.

103 Netherton EW. A unique case of trichorrhexis nodosa—'bamboo hairs'. *Arch Dermatol* 1958; 78: 483–7.

104 Ito M, Ito K, Hashimoto K. Pathogenesis in trichorrhexis invaginata (bamboo hair). *J Invest Dermatol* 1984; 83: 1–6.

105 Mevorah B, Frenk E. Ichthyosis linearis circumflexa comel with trichorrhexis invaginata (Netherton's syndrome): a light microscopical study of the skin changes. *Dermatologica* 1974; 149: 193–200.

106 De Berker D, Paige D, Harper J, Dawber RPR. Golf tee hairs: a new sign in Netherton's syndrome. *Br J Dermatol* 1992; 127 (suppl 40): 30.

107 Netherton EW. A unique case of trichorrhexis nodosa 'bamboo hairs'. *Arch Dermatol* 1958; 78: 483–7.

108 Wilkinson RD, Curtis GH, Hawk WA. Netherton's disease. *Arch Dermatol* 1964; 89: 106–13.

109 Greene SL, Muller SA. Netherton's syndrome. *J Am Acad Dermatol* 1985; 13: 329–37.

110 Orfanos CE, Mahrle G, Salamon T. Netherton-Syndrome. Ichthyosiforme Hautveranderungen un Trichorrhexis invaginata, Nachweis eines krankhaft veranderten Cortexkeratins im Harr. *Hautarzt* 1971; 22: 397–409.

111 Comel M. Ichthyosis linearis circumflexa. *Dermatologica* 1949; 98: 133–6.

112 Hurwitz S, Kirsch N, McGuire J. Re-evaluation of ichthyosis and hair shaft abnormalities. *Arch Dermatol* 1971; 103: 266–71.

113 Krafchik BR. Netherton syndrome. *Pediatr Dermatol* 1992; 9: 158–60.

114 Greig D, Wishart J. Growth abnormality in Netherton's syndrome. *Aust J Dermatol* 1982; 23: 27–30.

115 Hausser I, Anton-Lamprecht I, Hartschuh W, Petzoldt D. Netherton's syndrome: Ultrastructure of the active lesion under retinoid therapy. *Arch Dermatol Res* 1989; 281: 165–72.

116 Happle R, Traupe H. Etretinat bei Genodermatosen und verschiedenen entzundlichen Hautkrankheiten. In: Bauer RH, Gollnick H, eds. *Retinoide in der Praxis.* Berlin: Grosse, 1984: 35–49.

117 Nagata T. Netherton's syndrome which responded to photochemotherapy. *Dermatologica* 1980; 161: 51–6.

118 Hellier RR, Astbury WT, Bell FO. A case of pili torti. *Br J Dermatol Syph* 1940; 52: 173–82.

119 Summerly R, Donaldson EM. Monilethrix: a family study. *Br J Dermatol* 1962; 74: 387–91.

120 Bentley-Phillips B, Bayles MAH. A previously undescribed hereditary hair anomaly (pseudo-monilethrix). *Br J Dermatol* 1973; 89: 159–67.

121 Hutchinson PE, Cairns RJ, Wells RS. Woolly hair: clinical and genetic aspects. *Trans St John's Hosp Dermatol Soc* 1974; 60: 160–77.

122 Peachey RDG, Wells RS. Hereditary hypotrichosis (Marie–Unna type). *Trans St John's Hosp Dermatol Soc* 1971; 57: 157–66.

123 Stevanovic DV. Multiple defects of the hair shaft in Netherton's disease; association with ichthyosis linearis circumflexa. *Br J Dermatol* 1969; 81: 851–7.

124 Ronchese F. Twisted hairs (pili torti). *Arch Dermatol Syph* 1932; 26: 98–109.

125 Kurwa AR, Abdel-Aziz AM. Pili torti—congenital and acquired. *Acta Derm Venereol (Stockh)* 1973; 53: 385–92.

126 Lyon JB, Dawber RPR. A sporadic case of dystrophic pili torti. *Br J Dermatol* 1977; 96: 197–8.

127 Björnstad R. *Pili Torti and Sensory-Neural Loss of Hearing.* Copenhagen: Proceedings of the 17th Meeting of the Fennoscandinavian Association of Dermatologists, 1965: 3.

128 Robinson GC, Johnston MM. Pili torti and sensory neural hearing loss. *J Pediatr* 1967; 70: 621–3.

129 Gummer CL, Dawber RPR, Swift JA. Monilethrix: An electron microscopic and electron histochemical study. *Br J Dermatol* 1981; 105: 529–41.

130 Healy E, Holmes SC, Belgaid CE *et al*. A gene for monilethrix is closely linked to the type II keratin gene cluster at 12q13. *Hum Molec Genet* 1995; 4: 2399–402.

131 Stevens HP, Kelsell DP, Bryant SP *et al*. Linkage of monilethrix to the trichocyte and epithelial keratin gene cluster on 12q11–q13. *J Invest Dermatol* 1996; 106: 795–7.

132 Salamon T, Schnyder UW. Uber die Monilethrix. *Arch Klin Exp Dermatol* 1962; 215: 105.

133 Tamayo L. Monilethrix treated with the oral retinoid RO 10-9359 (Tegison). *Clin Exp Dermatol* 1983; 8: 393–6.

134 de Berker D, Dawber RPR. Monilethrix treated with oral retinoids. *Clin Exp Dermatol* 1990; 16: 226–8.

135 Saxena U, Ramesh V, Misra RS. Topical minoxidil in monilethrix. *Dermatologica* 1991; 182: 252–3 (letter).

136 Bentley-Phillips B, Bayles MAH. Pseudo-monilethrix. *Br J Dermatol* 1975; 92: 113–15.

137 Zitelli JA. Pseudomonilethrix: an artifact. *Arch Dermatol* 1986; 122: 688–90.

138 Whiting DA. Structural abnormalities of hair shaft. *J Am Acad Dermatol* 1987; 16: 1–25.

139 Dupre A, Rochiccidi P, Bonafe JL. 'Cheveux incoiffable': anomalie congenitale des cheveux. *Bull Soc Fr Dermatol Syph* 1973; 80: 111–12.

140 Stroud JD, Mehregan AH. 'Spun glass' hair: a clinicopathologic study of an unusual hair defect. In: Brown AC, ed. *The First Human Hair Symposium*. New York: Medcom, 1974: 103–7.

141 Dupre A, Bonafe JL, Litoux F, Victor M. Le syndrome des cheveux incoiffables; pili tranguli et canaliculi. *Ann Dermatol Vénéréol (Paris)* 1978; 105: 627–30.

142 Ferrando J, Fontarnau R, Gratacos MR, Mascaro JM. Pili canaliculi ('cheveuxincoiffables' ou 'cheveux en fibre de verre'): dix nouveaux cas avec etude au microscope electronique a balayage. *Ann Dermatol Vénéréol (Paris)* 1980; 107: 243–8.

143 Garty B, Metzker A, Mimouni M, Varsano L. Uncombable hair: a condition with autosomal dominant inheritance. *Arch Dis Child* 1982; 57: 710–12.

144 Hebert AA, Charrow J, Esterly NB, Fretzin DF. Uncombable hair (pili triangui et canaliculi): evidence for dominant inheritance with complete penetrance based on scanning electron microscopy. *Am J Med Genet* 1987; 28: 185–93.

145 Matis WL *et al*. Uncombable-hair syndrome. *Pediatr Dermatol* 1987; 4: 215–19.

146 Rest EB, Fretzin DF. Quantitative assessment of scanning electron microscope defects in uncombable-hair syndrome. *Pediatr Dermatol* 1990; 7: 93–6.

147 Shelley WB, Shelley ED. Uncombable hair syndrome: observation on response to biotin and occurrence in siblings with ectodermal dysplasia. *J Am Acad Dermatol* 1985; 13: 97–102.

148 Robinson GC, Miller JR. Hereditary enamel hypoplasia: its association with characteristic hair structure. *Pediatrics* 1966; 37: 498–502.

149 Jacobsen KU, Lowes M. Woolly hair nevus with ocular involvement: Report of a case. *Dermatologica* 1975; 151: 249–52.

150 Taylor AEM. Hereditary woolly hair with ocular involvement. *Br J Dermatol* 1990; 123: 523–5.

151 Verbov J. Woolly hair—study of a family. *Dermatologica* 1978; 157: 42–7.

152 McHenry PM, Nevin NC, Bingham EA. The association of keratosis pilaris atrophicans with hereditary woolly hair. *Pediatr Dermatol* 1990; 7: 202–4.

153 Neild VS, Pegum JS, Wells RS. The association of keratosis pilaris atrophicans and woolly hair, with and without Noonan's syndrome. *Br J Dermatol* 1984; 110: 357–62.

154 Lichtenstein J *et al*. The tricho-dento-osseous (TDO) syndrome. *Am J Hum Genet* 1972; 24: 569–82.

155 Baughman FA. CHANDS: the curly hair–ankyloblepharon–nail dysplasia syndrome. *Birth Defects* 1971; 7: 100–2.

156 Wise F. Woolly hair nevus. A peculiar form of birthmark of hair of the scalp, hitherto undescribed, with report of two cases. *Med J Rec* 1927; 125: 545–7.

157 Reda AM, Rogers RS, Peters MS. Woolly hair nevus. *J Am Acad Dermatol* 1990; 22: 337–80.

158 Crosti C, Menni S. Woolly hair nevus: osservazion sutre casi clinici. *Minerva Dermatol* 1979; 114: 45–9.

159 Harper MF, Klokke AH. Woolly hair nevus with triangular hairs (abstract). *Br J Dermatol* 1983; 111–13.

160 Goldin HM, Branson DM, Fretzin DF. Woolly-hair nevus: a case report and study by scanning electron microscopy. *Pediatr Dermatol* 1984; 2: 41–4.

161 Wright S, Lemoine NR, Leigh IM. Woolly hair naevi with systematized linear epidermal naevus. *Clin Exp Dermatol* 1986; 11: 179–82.

162 Peteiro C, Oliva NP, Zulaica A, Toribio J. Woolly-hair nevus: report of a case associated with a verrucous epidermal nevus in the same area. *Pediatr Dermatol* 1989; 6: 188–90.

163 Day TI. Straight-hair nevus, ichthyosis hystrix, leukokeratosis of the tongue. *Arch Dermatol* 1967; 96: 606.

164 Gibbs RC, Berger RA. The straight hair nevus. *Int J Dermatol* 1970; 9: 47.

165 Coupe RL, Johnston MM. Acquired progressive kinking of the hair: structural changes and growth dynamics of affected hairs. *Arch Dermatol* 1969; 100: 191–5.

166 Mortimer PS, Gummer C, English J, Dawber RPR. Acquired progresive kinking of hair: report of six cases and review of literature. *Arch Dermatol* 1985; 121; 1031–3.

167 Balsa RE, Ingratta SM, Alvarez AG. Acquired kinking of the hair: a methodologic approach. *J Am Acad Dermatol* 1986; 15: 1133–6.

168 Esterly NB, Lavin MP, Garancis JC. Acquired progressive kinking of the hair. *Arch Dermatol* 1989; 125: 813–15.

169 Pinkus H. Multiple hairs (Flemming–Giovannini): report of two cases of pili multigemini and discussion of some other anomalies of the pilary complex. *J Invest Dermatol* 1951; 17: 291–301.

170 Mehregan AH, Thompson WS. Pili multigemini: report of a case in association with cleidocranial dysostosis. *Br J Dermatol* 1979; 100: 315–22.

171 Dalziel KL, Telfer NR, Wilson CL, Dawber RPR. Tufted folliculitis: a specific bacterial disease? *Am J Dermatopathol* 1990; 12: 37–41.

172 Tong AKF, Baden HP. Tufted hair folliculitis. *J Am Dermatol* 1989; 21: 1096–9.

173 Tan TG. Occupational toxic alopecia due to borax. *Acta Derm Venereol* 1970; 50: 55–8.

174 Schillinger BM, Berstein M, Goldberg LA, Shalita AR. Boric acid poisoning. *J Am Acad Dermatol* 1982; 7: 667–73.

175 Stein KM *et al*. Toxic alopecia from ingestion of boric acid. *Arch Dermatol* 1973; 108: 95–7.

176 Rubenstein AD, Musher DM. Epidemic boric acid poisoning simulating staphylococcal toxic epidermal necrolysis of the newborn infant: Ritters disease. *J Pediatr* 1970; 77: 884–7.

177 Grossman KL, Kvedar JC. Anagen hair loss. In: Olsen EA, ed. *Disorders of Hair Growth: Diagnosis and Treatment*. New York: McGraw-Hill, 1994: 223–39.

178 Pierard GE. Toxic effects of metals from the environment on hair growth and structure. *J Cutan Pathol* 1979; 6: 237–42.

179 Elhassani SB. The many faces of methylmercury poisoning. *J Toxicol* 1982; 19: 875–906.

180 *An Assessment of Mercury in the Environment. A Report Prepared by the Panel on Mercury of the Coordinating Committee for Scientific and Technical Assessments of Environmental Pollutants, National Research Council*. Washington: National Academy of Sciences, 1978.

181 Hirschman SZ, Feingold M, Boylen G. Mercury in house paint as a cause of acrodynia: Effect of therapy with N-acetyl-D, L-penicillamine. *N Engl J Med* 1963; 65: 889–93.

182 Graef JW, Lovejoy FJ Jr. Heavy metal poisoning. In: Braunwald E *et al*. eds. *Harrison's Principles of Internal Medicine*, 11th edn. New York: McGraw-Hill, 1987: 850–5.

183 Heyman A, Pfeiffer JB Jr, Willett RW, Taylor HM. Peripheral neuropathy caused by arsenical intoxication. *N Engl J Med* 1956; 254: 401–9.

184 Peters HA *et al*. Hematological, dermal and neuropsychological disease from burning and power sawing chromium–copper–arsenic (CCA)-treated wood. *Acta Pharmacol Toxicol* 1986; 59: 39–43.

185 Herrero F, Fernandez E, Gomez J *et al*. Thallium poisoning presenting with abdominal colic, paresthesia, and irritability. *Clin Toxicol* 1995; 33: 261–4.

186 Nodl F, Zaun H, Zinn HK. Gesteigerte Epilierbarkeit von Anagenhaaren bei Kindernals Folge eines Reifungsdefekts der Follikel mit Gestorter Verhaftung von Haarschaft und Wurzelscheiden: Das Phanomen der Leicht Ausziehbaren Haare. *Aktüel Dermatol* 1986; 12: 55–7.

187 Hamm H, Traupe H. Loose anagen hair of childhood: the phenomenon of easily pluckable hair. *J Am Acad Dermatol* 1989; 20: 242–8.

188 Price VH, Gummer CL. Loose anagen syndrome. *J Am Acad Dermatol* 1989; 20: 249–56.

189 Olsen EA, Bettencourt MS, Coté N. The presence of loose anagen hairs obtained by hair pull in the normal population. *J Invest Dermatol* 1999; 4.

190 Tosti A, Peluso AM, Miscali C, Venturo N, Patrizi A, Fanti PA. Loose Anagen Hair. *Arch Dermatol* 1997; 133: 1089–93.

191 Murphy MF, McGinnity FG, Allen GE. New familial association between ocular coloboma and loose anagen syndrome. *Clin Genet* 1995; 47: 214–16.

192 Olsen EA. Clinical tools for assessing hair loss. In: Olsen EA, ed. *Disorders of Hair Growth: Diagnosis and Treatment*. New York: McGraw-Hill, 1994: 59–69.

193 Sims RT. Hair growth in kwashiorkor. *Arch Dis Child* 1967; 42: 397–400.

194 Bradfield RB, Jelliffe EFP. Early assessment of malnutrition. *Nature* 1970; 225: 283–4.

195 Bradfield RB, Baily MA, Cordano A. Hair-root changes in Andean Indian children during marasmic kwashiorkor. *Lancet* 1968; ii: 1169–70.

196 Bradfield RB, Cordano A, Graham GG. Hair-root adaptation to marasmus in Andean Indian children. *Lancet* 1969; ii: 1395–7.

197 Bradfield RB, Bailey MA, Margen S. Morphological changes in human scalp hair roots during deprivation of protein. *Science* 1967; 157: 438–9.

198 Johnson AA, Latham MC, Roe DA. An evaluation of the use of changes in hair root morphology in the assessment of protein-calorie malnutrition. *Am J Clin Nutr* 1976; 29: 502–11.

199 Neldner KH, Hambidge KM, Walravens PA. Acrodermatitis enteropathica. *Int J Dermatol* 1978; 17: 380–7.

200 Tucker SB, Schroeter AL, Brown PW, McCall JT. Acquired zinc deficiency: cutaneous manifestations typical of acrodermatitis enteropathica. *J Am Med Assoc* 1976; 235: 2399–402.

201 Caldwell MD, Jonsson HT, Othersen HB Jr. Essential fatty acid deficiency in an infant receiving prolonged parenteral alimentation. *J Pediatr* 1972; 81: 894–8.

202 Skolnik P, Eaglstein WH, Ziboh VA. Human essential fatty acid deficiency: treatment by topical application of linoleic acid. *Arch Dermatol* 1977; 113: 939–41.

203 Hansen AE *et al.* Role of linoleic acid in infant nutrition. *Pediatrics* 1963; 31: 171–92.

204 Burlina AB *et al.* Neonatal screening for biotinidase deficiency in north eastern Italy. *Eur J Pediatr* 1988; 147: 317–18.

205 Williams ML, Packman S, Cowan MJ. Alopecia and periorificial dermatitis in biotin-responsive multiple carboxylase deficiency. *J Am Acad Dermatol* 1983; 9: 97–103.

206 Wolf B *et al.* Neonatal screening for biotinidase deficiency: an update. *J Inher Metab Dis* 1986; 9(suppl 2): 303–6.

207 Thoene J, Baker H, Yoshino M, Sweetman L. Biotin-responsive carboxylase deficiency associated with subnormal plasma and urinary biotin. *N Engl J Med* 1981; 304: 817–20.

208 Burlina AB, Sherwood WG, Zacchello LF. Partial biotinidase deficiency associated with Coffin–Siris syndrome. *Eur J Pediatr* 1990; 149: 628–9.

209 Olsen EA. Hair loss in childhood. In: Olsen EA, ed. *Disorders of Hair Growth. Diagnosis and Treatment*. New York: McGraw-Hill, 1994; 141: 173.

210 Frienden IJ. Aplasia cutis congenita: a clinical review and proposal for classification. *J Am Acad Dermatol* 1986; 14: 646–60.

211 Peer La, van Duyn J. Congenital defect of the scalp: report of a case with fatal termination. *Plast Reconstr Surg* 1948; 3: 722–6.

212 Ruiz-Maldonado R, Tamayo L. Aplasia cutis congenita, spastic paralysis, and mental retardation. *Am J Dis Child* 1974; 128: 699–701.

213 Sybert VP. Congenital scalp defects with distal limb anomalies (Adams–Oliver syndrome—McKusick 100300): further suggestion of autosomal recessive inheritance. *Am J Med Genet* 1989; 32: 266–7 (letter).

214 Brosnan PG *et al.* A new familial syndrome of 45,XY gonadal dysgenesis with anomalies of ectodermal and mesodermal structures. *J Pediatr* 1980; 97: 586–90.

215 Finlay AY, Marks R. An hereditary syndrome of lumpy scalp, odd ears and rudimentary nipples. *Br J Dermatol* 1978; 99: 423–30.

216 Mardini MK, Ghandour M, Sakati NA, Nyhan WL. Johanson–Blizzard syndrome in a large inbred kindred with three involved members. *Clin Genet* 1978; 14: 247–50.

217 Zapata HH, Sletten LJ, Pierpont MEM. Congenital cardiac malformations in Adams–Oliver syndrome. *Clin Genet* 1995; 47: 80–4.

218 Baruchin AM, Nahieli O, Golan Y. Oculo-cerebro-cutaneous syndrome: first description in an adult. *J Cranio-Maxillo-Facial Surg* 1992; 20: 70–2.

219 Tuffli GA, Laxova R. Brief clinical report: new, autosomal dominant form of ectodermal dysplasia. *Am J Med Genet* 1983; 14: 381–4.

220 Pinheiro M, Penna FJ, Freire-Maia N. Two other cases of ANOTHER syndrome: family report and update. *Clin Genet* 1989; 35: 237–42.

221 Goltz RW, Henderson RR, Hitch JM, Ott JE. Focal dermal hypoplasia syndrome: a review of the literature and report of two cases. *Arch Dermatol* 1970; 101: 1–11.

222 Gershoni-Baruch R *et al.* Johanson–Blizzard syndrome: clinical spectrum and further delineation of the syndrome. *Am J Med Genet* 1990; 35: 546–51.

223 Kubba R, Rook A. Congenital triangular alopecia. *Br J Dermatol* 1976; 95: 657–9.

224 Trakimas C, Sperling LC, Skelton HG *et al.* Clinical and histologic findings in temporal triangular alopecia. *J Am Acad Dermatol* 1994; 31: 205–9.

225 Minars N. Congenital temporal alopecia. *Arch Dermatol* 1974; 109: 395–6.

226 Headington JT, Astle N. Familial focal alopecia. A new disorder of hair growth clinically resembling pseudopelade. *Arch Dermatol* 1989; 123: 234–7.

227 Partridge JW. Congenital hypertrichosis lanuginosa: neonatal shaving. *Arch Dis Child* 1987; 62: 623–5.

228 Ravin JG, Hodge GP. Hypertrichosis portrayed in art. *J Am Med Assoc* 1969; 207: 533–5.

229 Olsen EA. Hypertrichosis. In: Olsen EA, ed. *Disorders of Hair Growth: Diagnosis and Treatment*. New York: McGraw-Hill, 1994: 315–36.

230 Beighton P. Congenital hypertrichosis lanuginosa. *Arch Dermatol* 1970; 101: 669–72.

231 Baumeister FAM, Egger J, Schildhauer MT *et al.* Ambras syndrome: delineation of a unique hypertrichosis universalis congenita and association with a balanced pericentric inversion (8) (P11.2;q22). *Clin Genet* 1993; 44: 121–8.

232 Figuera LE, Pandolfo M, Dunne PW *et al.* Mapping of the congenital generalized hypertrichosis locus to chromosome Xq24–q27.1. *Nature Genet* 1995; 10: 202–7.

233 Macias-Flores MA *et al.* A new form of hypertrichosis inherited as an X-linked dominant trait. *Hum Genet* 1984; 66: 66–70.

234 Laband PF, Habib G, Humphreys BS. Hereditary gingival fibromatosis: report of an affected family with associated splenomegaly and skeletal and soft-tissue abnormalities. *Oral Pathol* 1964; 17: 339–51.

235 Winter GB, Simpkiss MJ. Hypertrichosis with hereditary gingival hyperplasia. *Arch Dis Child* 1974; 49: 394–9.

236 Witkop CJ Jr. Heterogeneity in gingival fibromatosis. *Birth Defects: Original Article Series* 1971; 7: 210–21.

237 LaCombe D, Bioulac-Sage P, Sibout M *et al.* Congenital marked hypertrichosis and Laband syndrome in a child: overlap between the gingival fibromatosis-hypertrichosis and Laband syndromes. *Genet Counsel* 1994; 5: 251–6.

238 De Lange C. Memoires Originaux: Sur un Type Nouveau de dégénération (Typus Amstelodamensis). *Arch Méd* 1933; 36: 713–19.

239 Ptacek LJ *et al.* The Cornelia–de Lange syndrome. *J Pediatr* 1963; 635: 1000–20.

240 Beck B. Familial occurrence of Cornelia–de Lange's syndrome. *Acta Paediatr Scand* 1974; 63: 225–31.

241 Pashayan H, Whelan D, Guttman S, Fraser FC. Variability of the de Lange syndrome: Report of three cases and genetic analysis of 54 families. *J Pediatr* 1969; 75: 853–8.

242 Soderquist NA, Reed WB. Cornelia–de Lange syndrome. *Cutis* 1968; 4: 1333–5.

243 Daniel WL, Higgins JV. Biochemical and genetic investigation of the de Lange syndrome. *Am J Dis Child* 1971; 121: 401–5.

244 Hambrick GW Jr, Scheie HG. Studies of the skin in Hurler's syndrome. *Arch Dermatol* 1962; 85: 455–70.

245 Magnus IA. The cutaneous porphyrias. *Semin Hematol* 1968; 5: 380–408.

246 Grossman ME *et al.* Porphyria cutanea tarda: clinical features and laboratory findings in 40 patients. *Am J Med* 1979; 67: 277–85.

247 Bleiberg J, Wallen M, Brodkin R, Applebaum IL. Industrially acquired prophyria. *Arch Dermatol* 1964; 89: 793–7.

248 Earhart RN, Ball J, Nuss DD, Aeling JL. Minoxidil-induced hypertrichosis: treatment with calcium thioglycolate depilatory. *South Med J* 1977; 70: 442–3.

249 Olsen EA *et al.* Topical minoxidil in early male pattern baldness. *J Am Acad Dermatol* 1985; 13: 185–92.

250 Cohen DJ *et al.* Cyclosporine: a new immunosuppressive agent for organ transplantation. *Ann Intern Med* 1984; 101: 667–82.

251 Harper JI *et al.* Dermatological aspects of the use of cyclosporin A for prophylaxis of graft-versus-host disease. *Br J Dermatol* 1984; 110: 469–74.

252 Wysocki GP, Daley TD. Hypertrichosis in patients receiving cyclosporine therapy. *Clin Exp Dermatol* 1987; 12: 191–6.

253 Burton JL, Scutt WH, Caldwell IW. Hypertrichosis due to diazoxide. *Br J Dermatol* 1975; 93: 707–11.

254 Okun R, Russell RP, Wilson WR. Use of diazoxide with trichlormethiazide for hypertension. *Arch Intern Med* 1963; 112: 882–8.

255 Baker L, Kaye R, Root AW, Prasad ALN. Diazoxide treatment of idiopathic hypoglycemia of infancy. *J Pediatr* 1967; 71: 494–505.

256 Menter MA (for Wells RS). Hypertrichosis lanuginosa and a lichenoid eruption due to diazoxide therapy. *Proc Roy Soc Med* 1973; 66: 16–17.

257 Milner RDG, Chouksey SK. Effects of fetal exposure to diazoxide in man. *Arch Dis Child* 1972; 47: 537–43.

258 Herberg K-P. Effects of diphenylhydantoin in 41 epileptics institutionalized since childhood. *South Med J* 1977; 70: 19–24.

259 Livingston S, Pauli LL, Pruce I, Kramer II. Phenobarbital vs. phenytoin for grand mal epilepsy. *Am Fam Phys* 1980; 22: 123–7.

260 Livingston S, Petersen D, Boks LL. Hypertrichosis occurring in association with dilantin therapy. *J Pediatr* 1955; 47: 351–2.

261 Bartuska DG. Hypertrichosis in a brain damaged child. *J Am Med Wom Assoc* 1963; 18: 711–13.

262 Elliott JA Jr. Clinical experiences with methoxsalen in the treatment of vitiligo. *J Invest Dermatol* 1959; 32: 311–13.

263 Rampen FHJ. Hypertrichosis in PUVA-treated patients. *Br J Dermatol* 1983; 109: 657–60.

264 Weiss IS. Hirsutism after chronic administration of acetazolamide. *Am J Ophthalmol* 1974; 78: 327–8.

265 Fono R. Appearance of hypertrichosis during streptomycin treatment. *Ann Paediatr* 1950; 174: 389–92.

266 Bosco J, Pathmanathan R. POEMS syndrome presenting as systemic sclerosis. *Am J Med* 1988; 84: 524–8.

267 Feddersen RM *et al.* Plasma cell dyscrasia: a case of POEMS syndrome with a unique dermatologic presentation. *J Am Acad Dermatol* 1989; 21: 1061–8.

268 Viard J-P *et al.* POEMS syndrome presenting as systemic sclerosis. *Am J Med* 1988; 84: 524–8.

269 Pope DN, Strimling RB, Mallory SB. Hypertrichosis in juvenile dermatomyositis. *J Am Acad Dermatol* 1994; 31: 383–7.

270 Fontenla MAF. Severe hypertrichosis as an uncommon feature of juvenile dermatomyositis. *J Am Acad Dermatol* 1995; 33: 691.

271 Andreev VC, Stransky L. Hairy elbows. *Arch Dermatol* 1979; 115: 761.

272 Beighton P. Familial hypertrichosis cubiti: hairy elbows syndrome. *J Med Genet* 1970; 7: 158–60.

273 Miller ML, Yeager JK. Hairy elbows. *Arch Dermatol* 1995; 131: 858–9.

274 Di Lernia V, Neri I, Trevisi P *et al.* Hypertrichosis cubiti. *Arch Dermatol* 1996; 132: 589.

275 Rafaat M. Hypertrichosis pinnae in babies of diabetic mothers (letter). *Pediatrics* 1981; 65: 745–6 (letter).

276 Singh M, Kumar A, Paul VK. Hairy pinna: a pathognomonic sign in infants of diabetic mothers. *Indian Pediatr* 1987; 24: 87–9.

277 Woods DL, Malan AF, Coetzee EJ. Intra-uterine growth in infants of diabetic mothers. *S Afr Med J* 1980; 58: 441–3.

278 Oliver GL, McFarlane DC. Congenital trichomegaly with associated pigmentary degeneration of the retina, dwarfism, and mental retardation. *Arch Ophthalmol* 1965; 74: 169–74.

279 Rupert LS, Bechtel M, Pellegrini A. Nevoid hypertrichosis: multiple patches associated with premature graying of lesional hair. *Pediatr Dermatol* 1994; 11: 49–51.

280 Peñas PA, Jones-Caballero M, Amigo A *et al.* Cutaneous meningiomas underlying congenital localized hypertrichosis. *J Am Acad Dermatol* 1994; 30: 363–6.

281 Slifman NR, Harrist TJ, Rhodes AR. Congenital arrector pili hamartoma. *Arch Dermatol* 1985; 121: 1034–7.

282 Glover MT, Malone M, Atherton DJ. Michelin tire baby syndrome resulting from diffuse smooth muscle hamartoma. *Pediatr Dermatol* 1989; 6: 329–31.

283 Metzer A, Amir J, Rotem A, Merlob P. Congenital smooth muscle hamartoma of the skin. *Pediatr Dermatol* 1994; 2: 45–8.

284 Cohen AH, Hollister DW, Reed WB. The skin in the Winchester syndrome. *Arch Dermatol* 1975; 111: 230–6.

285 Haris HW, Miller OF. Midline cutaneous and spinal defects *Arch Dermatol* 1976; 112: 1724–8.

286 Thursfield WRR, Ross AA. Faun tail (sacral hirsuties) and diastematomyelia. *Br J Dermatol* 1961; 73: 328–36.

287 James CCM, Lassman LP. Spinal dysraphism: an orthopaedic syndrome in children accompanying occult forms. *Arch Dis Child* 1960; 35: 315–27.

288 Perret G. Diagnosis and treatment of diastematomyelia. *Surg Gynecol Obstet* 1957; 105: 69–83.

289 Slyper AH, Easterly NB. Non-progressive scrotal hair growth in two infants. *Pediatr Dermatol* 1993; 10: 34–5.

290 Francis JS, Ruvalcaba RH. Scrotal hair growth in infancy. *Pediatr Dermatol* 1993; 10: 389–90.

291 Berglund EF, Burton GV, Mills GM, Nichols GM. Hypertrichosis of the eyelashes associated with interferon-α therapy for chronic granulocytic leukemia. *South Med J* 1990; 83: 363.

292 Foon KA. Increased growth of eyelashes in a patient given leukocyte A interferon. *N Engl J Med* 1984; 311: 1259.

293 Weaver DT, Bartley GB. Cyclosporine-induced trichomegaly. *Am J Ophthalmol* 1990; 109: 239.

294 Casanova JM, Puig T, Rubio M. Hypertrichosis of the eyelashes in acquired immunodeficiency syndrome. *Arch Dermatol* 1987; 123: 1599–601.

295 Tosti A, Gaddoni G, Peluso AM *et al.* Acquired hairy pinnae in a patient infected with the human immunodeficiency virus. *J Am Acad Dermatol* 1993; 28: 513.

296 Vélez A, Kindelán JM, García-Herola A *et al.* Acquired trichomegaly and hypertrichosis in metastatic adenocarcinoma. *Clin Exp Dermatol* 1995; 20: 237–9.

297 Glinick SE, Alper JC, Bogaars H, Brown JA. Becker's melanosis: associated abnormalities. *J Am Acad Dermatol* 1983; 9: 509–14.

298 Haneke E. The dermal component in melanosis naeviformis Becker. *J Cutan Pathol* 1979; 5: 53–8.

299 Poomeechaiwong S, Golitz LE. Hamartomas. *Adv Dermatol* 1990; 5: 257–88.

300 Urbanek RD, Johnson WC. Smooth muscle hamartoma associated with Becker's nevus. *Arch Dermatol* 1978; 114: 104–6.

301 Person JR, Longcope C. Becker's nevus: an androgen-mediated hyperplasia with increased androgen receptors. *J Am Acad Dermatol* 1984; 10: 235–8.

302 Bhawan J, Chang WH. Becker's melanosis: an ultrastructural study. *Dermatologica* 1979; 159: 221–30.

303 Lambert JR, Willems P, Abs R *et al.* Becker's nevus associated with chromosomal mosaicism and congenital adrenal hyperplasia. *J Am Acad Dermatol* 1994; 30: 655–7.

304 Grossman MC, Dierickx C, Ferinelli W *et al.* Damage to hair follicles by normal-mode ruby laser pulses. *J Am Acad Dermatol* 1996; 35: 889–94.

Nail Disorders

ANTONELLA TOSTI AND
BIANCA MARIA PIRACCINI

Common nail disorders
Acute paronychia
Atopic dermatitis
Congenital malalignment of the big toenail
Ingrown nails
Nail biting and onychotillomania
Parakeratosis pustulosa
Psoriasis
Transitory koilonychia
Punctate leuconychia
Twenty-nail dystrophy (trachyonychia)
Warts

Uncommon nail disorders
Lichen planus
Lichen striatus
Periungual fibromas
Subungual exostosis
Nail matrix naevi
Anonychia/micronychia
Iso–Kikuchi syndrome
Nail–patella syndrome
Polydactyly
Epidermolysis bullosa
Ectodermal dysplasias
Pachyonychia congenita
Chronic mucocutaneous candidiasis

Anatomy

The nail unit consists of four specialized epithelia: the nail matrix, the nail bed, the proximal nail fold and the hyponychium. The nail matrix is a germinative epithelial structure that gives rise to a fully keratinized multilayered sheet of cornified cells: the nail plate. In longitudinal sections the nail matrix consists of a proximal and a distal region. Because the vertical axes of the nail matrix cells are oriented diagonally and distally, proximal nail matrix keratinocytes produce the upper portion of the nail plate while distal nail matrix keratinocytes produce the lower portion of the nail plate [1]. The peculiar kinetics of nail matrix keratinization explain why diseases of the proximal nail matrix result in nail plate surface abnormalities whereas diseases of the distal matrix result in abnormalities of the ventral nail plate or the nail free edge or both. Nail plate corneocytes are tightly connected by desmosomes and complex digitations.

The nail plate is a rectangular, translucent and transparent structure that appears pink because of the vessels of the underlying nail bed. The proximal part of the nail plate of the fingernails, especially those of the thumbs, shows a whitish, opaque, half-moon shaped area, the lunula, that corresponds to the visible portion of the distal nail matrix. The shape of the lunula determines the shape of the free edge of the plate. The nail plate is firmly attached to the nail bed, which partially contributes to nail formation along its length. The longitudinal orientation of the capillary vessels in the nail bed explains the linear pattern of the nail bed haemorrhages. Proximally and laterally the nail plate is surrounded by the nail folds. The horny layer of the proximal nail fold forms the cuticle, which intimately adheres to the underlying nail plate and prevents its separation from the proximal nail fold. Distally the nail bed continues with the hyponychium, which marks the separation of the nail plate from the digit. The nail plate grows continuously and uniformly throughout life. Average nail growth is faster in fingernails (3 mm/month) than in toenails (1–1.5 mm/month) [2].

The nails of newborns are thin and soft, and frequently present a certain degree of koilonychia that is especially evident in toenails. Since the nail plate of the great toenail may be relatively short a mild distal embedding is frequently observed as soon as the nail grows. This is transitory unless the presence of congenital malalignment. Nail growth rate in children is comparable to the values observed in young adults, the fastest values of nail growth (150 mm/day) being reached between the age of 10–14 years. The thickness and breadth of the nail plate increase rapidly in the first two decades of life [3].

The brief arrest of growth that characterizes the first days of life may involve the nail unit and result in a transitory arrest of the nail growth with development of Beau's lines that become visible at the base of the nails after the age of about 4 weeks. These physiological lines, however, are an inconstant phenomenon that occurs only in about 20–25% of healthy newborns [4].

Common nail disorders

Nail diseases are a rather uncommon cause of dermatological consultation in children. They may be present at birth or be acquired. Nail signs of congenital and hereditary nail diseases usually develop during childhood and their presence may be a clue for the diagnosis of a syndrome or a systemic disorder.

Although the acquired nail conditions observed in childhood are similar to those of adults, the prevalence of several diseases may vary in the different age groups. For instance there are some conditions that are exclusively or typically seen in children such as parakeratosis pustulosa and twenty-nail dystrophy (TND), whereas other disorders such as onychomycosis are only exceptionally encountered in the first 10 years of life. The common disorders and traumatic nail abnormalities account for 90–95% of all nail abnormalities in children.

This chapter reviews the nail disorders which are most commonly observed in childhood, then discusses some nail diseases that although uncommon are of diagnostic significance. The nail disorders that are most frequently diagnosed in children are listed in Table 23.2.1.

Acute paronychia

Acute paronychia is usually caused by *Staphylococcus aureus* although other bacteria and herpes simplex virus may be responsible. A minor trauma commonly precedes the development of the infection.

The affected digit shows acute inflammatory changes of the nail folds, with erythema, swelling, pus formation and pain (Fig. 23.2.1). Whenever possible cultures should be taken to identify the responsible organism. Treatment includes prompt incision and drainage of the abscess, local medications with antiseptics and administration of systemic antibiotics or aciclovir depending on the causative agent.

Table 23.2.1 Common nail disorders in childhood

Acute paronychia
Congenital malalignment of the big toenail
Eczema
Ingrown nail
Nail biting
Parakeratosis pustulosa
Psoriasis
Transitory koilonychia
Traumatic fingernail abnormalities
TND
Warts

Atopic dermatitis

The nails in children with atopic dermatitis may present nail plate surface abnormalities due to eczematous involvement of the nail matrix. These include irregular pitting and Beau's lines. Onycholysis may occasionally occur as a consequence of eczematous involvement of the fingertips.

Congenital malalignment of the big toenail

In congenital malalignment the nail plate of the big toenail deviates laterally from the longitudinal axis of the distal phalanx. This congenital abnormality deserves attention because it is almost always complicated by the development of lateral or distal nail embedding.

The affected nail has a triangular shape and frequently shows dystrophic changes due to repetitive traumatic injuries. The nail plate may be thickened, yellow–brown in colour and present transverse ridging due to intermittent nail matrix damage. Onycholysis is frequent. This diagnosis should always be considered in children with dystrophic or ingrowing toenails. The condition is probably inherited with an autosomal dominant pattern.

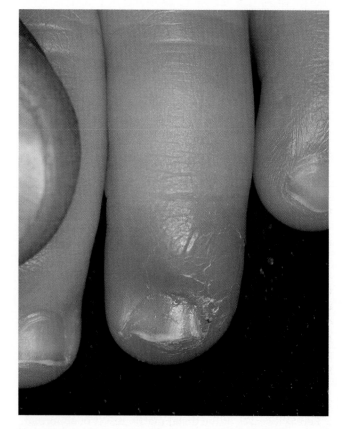

Fig. 23.2.1 Acute paronychia due to primary herpes simplex infection.

Spontaneous improvement with complete resolution can occur. Surgical treatment produces the best results when performed before the age of 2 years [5].

Ingrown nails

Ingrown nails are a common complaint and usually affect the great toe of teenagers and young adults. The presence of a congenital malalignment of the great toenails is an important predisposing factor. The development of nail ingrowing may be favoured by improper nail trimming, traumatic injuries and occlusive footwear.

The clinical manifestations of ingrown toenails can be divided into three stages.

Stage 1. Embedding of the nail spicula within the lateral nail fold produces painful erythema and swelling of the nail fold. Treatment is conservative with extraction of the embedded spicula and introduction of a package of non-absorbent cotton under the lateral corner of the nail. This medication should be replaced every few days.

Stage 2. Characterized by the formation of granulation tissue that covers the nail plate. The affected nail is very painful and the nail fold presents a pseudopyogenic granuloma with seropurulent exudation. In this stage the topical application of high-potency steroids under occlusion for a few days can reduce the overgrowth of granulation tissue. Conservative treatment as for stage 1 can then be utilized.

Stage 3. The granulation tissue is covered by the epidermis of the lateral nail fold. This stage requires surgical treatment with selective destruction of the lateral horn of the nail matrix.

Nail biting and onychotillomania

Nail biting is common in childhood affecting up to 60% of children. Conversely, onychotillomania is rather uncommon and usually associated with underlying psychological disorders. Nail biting produces short and irregular nails that show depressions and scratches.

Secondary bacterial infections of the periungual tissues are common, as are periungual warts. Apical root resorption may occasionally occur. The habit of picking, breaking or chewing the skin over the proximal nail fold is occasionally associated with nail biting. This may produce nail matrix injury with nail plate surface abnormalities and longitudinal melanonychia due to matrix melanocyte stimulation [6].

Most children discontinue nail biting when they grow up. Frequent application of distasteful topical preparations on the nail and periungual skin can discourage patients from biting and chewing their fingernails.

Parakeratosis pustulosa

Parakeratosis pustulosa is a chronic condition that exclusively affects children and usually involves a single finger, most commonly a thumb or an index [7]. In the early phases the affected digit shows eczematous changes associated with mild distal subungual hyperkeratosis and onycholysis. Nail abnormalities are usually more marked on a corner of the nail. Pitting of the nail plate may be present (Fig. 23.2.2).

Whether parakeratosis pustulosa is a limited form of nail psoriasis or a clinical manifestation of other conditions such as contact and atopic dermatitis is still being discussed. In the author's experience most of the children with parakeratosis pustulosa develop a mild nail psoriasis when they grow up [8]. Since parakeratosis pustulosa and nail psoriasis produce similar nail changes the diagnosis of parakeratosis pustulosa is based on the localization of the disease to a single digit rather than on the morphology of the nail lesions. This diagnosis should always be considered in a child with psoriasiform nail changes limited to a single finger. Patch tests can be useful to rule out contact dermatitis. The nail lesions usually resolve spontaneously. Topical treatment with steroids and/or retinoic acid may induce partial remission of the nail changes.

Psoriasis

The prevalence of nail involvement in children with psoriasis ranges from 7 to 39% according to the different studies. The clinical manifestations of nail psoriasis in children are quite similar to those of adults except for the fact that nail bed involvement is usually absent or mild. Fingernails are much more commonly affected than toenails [9–11].

Nail pitting is the most common sign of psoriasis in

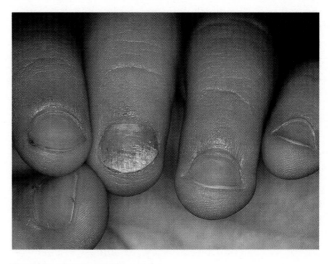

Fig. 23.2.2 Parakeratosis pustulosa.

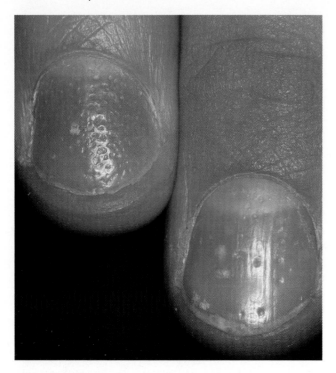

Fig. 23.2.3 Nail pitting due to psoriasis.

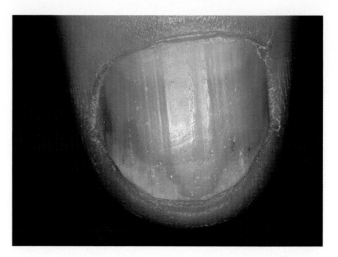

Fig. 23.2.4 Nail psoriasis: the onycholytic area is surrounded by an erythematous border.

children (Fig. 23.2.3). Pitting is the consequence of a focal psoriatic inflammatory involvement of the proximal nail matrix that results in the persistence of clusters of parakeratotic cells within the upper layers of the nail plate. Pits usually look shiny because they reflect light. Psoriatic pits are usually large, deep and randomly scattered within the nail plate. They are rarely found in toenails. Pits may be the sole manifestation of nail psoriasis or they may be associated with distal onycholysis and sometimes salmon patches of the nail bed.

Onycholysis is the detachment of the nail plate from the nail bed. The onycholytic area looks whitish because of the presence of air under the detached nail plate. In psoriasis the onycholytic area is typically separated from the normal nail plate by an erythematous border (Fig. 23.2.4). Oily patches appear as yellowish or pink salmon areas easily visible through the transparent nail plate. They result from a focal psoriatic involvement of the nail bed.

Subungual hyperkeratosis and splinter haemorrhages, which are commonly observed in adults with nail psoriasis, are rarely seen in children.

Subungual hyperkeratosis describes the accumulation of parakeratotic cells under the distal portion of the nail plate.

Splinter haemorrhages appear as longitudinal linear red–brown haemorrhages. They are almost exclusively seen in fingernails and are usually located in the distal portion of the nail plate. Splinter haemorrhages are a con-

sequence of psoriatic involvement of the nail bed capillary loops that run in a longitudinal direction along the nail bed dermal ridges.

The following nail findings strongly suggest the diagnosis of nail psoriasis.
1 Onycholysis surrounded by an erythematous border.
2 Salmon patches of the nail bed.
3 Irregular pitting associated with onycholysis and/or subungual hyperkeratosis and/or splinter haemorrhages. The differential diagnosis of nail psoriasis in children mainly includes eczema and parakeratosis pustulosa. Although onychomycosis may produce nail changes very similar to nail bed psoriasis, this condition is exceedingly rare in children.

Nail psoriasis has an unpredictable course but in most cases the disease is chronic and complete remissions are uncommon.

The favourable effects of environmental factors such as sunlight and hot weather are less evident than in skin psoriasis. Stressful events may precipitate relapses.

Transitory koilonychia

Transitory koilonychia is a physiological phenomenon in children most commonly affecting the toenails. The nail plate, which is flat, thin and soft, presents everted edges resulting in a spoon-shaped appearance (Fig. 23.2.5). Lateral embedding may occur and produce mild nail ingrowing. Distal embedding can also be observed.

The condition spontaneously regresses when the nail plate thickens with age.

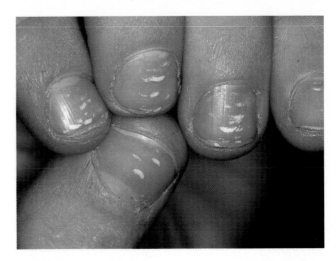

Fig. 23.2.6 Punctate leuconychia.

Twenty-nail dystrophy (trachyonychia)

The term TND or trachyonychia describes a spectrum of nail plate surface abnormalities that produce nail roughness. This nail symptom may be the clinical manifestation of numerous inflammatory nail diseases including alopecia areata, lichen planus and psoriasis. The nail pathology permits the definitive diagnosis by showing the typical features of lichen planus or psoriasis in trachyonychia due to these conditions, or spongiotic changes in trachyonychia due to alopecia areata [12].

Patients affected by TND may be divided into two major groups.

1 Patients with personal history or clinical evidence of alopecia areata.

2 Patients with isolated nail involvement (idiopathic trachyonychia).

Up to 12% of children with alopecia areata present with this nail disorder which may precede or follow the onset of hair loss even by years.

The frequency of idiopathic trachyonychia is unknown but it is almost exclusively seen in children. In most cases idiopathic trachyonychia is a clinical manifestation of alopecia areata limited to the nails. Two varieties of trachyonychia, opaque trachyonychia and shiny trachyonychia were originally described by Baran *et al.* in 1978. Both varieties may occur in association with alopecia areata or be idiopathic. In opaque trachyonychia the affected nails show excessive longitudinal striations with loss of nail lustre (vertical striated sandpapered nails) (Fig. 23.2.7). The nail plate surface is brittle, friable and covered with small scales of keratin. Koilonychia may be present. In shiny trachyonychia nail roughness is less severe and caused by numerous small superficial pits. The disorder is symptomless and patients only complain of brittleness and cosmetic discomfort.

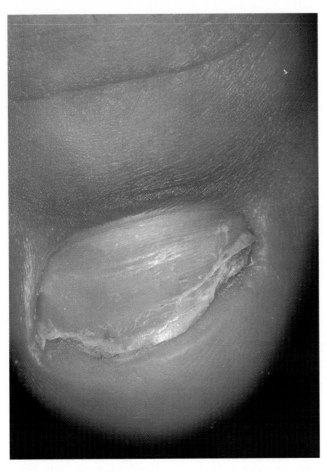

Fig. 23.2.5 Transitory koilonychia.

Punctate leuconychia

Punctate leuconychia is a traumatic fingernail abnormality which is almost exclusively seen in children. Punctate leuconychia is usually caused by repetitive minor traumatic injuries to the nail matrix producing a disturbance in the nail matrix keratinization.

The incomplete keratinization of the distal matrix determines the presence of parakeratotic cells in the ventral nail plate. These modify the transparency of the nail plate and appear as white spots. The affected nails show single or multiple opaque small white spots which move distally with nail growth (Fig. 23.2.6).

The condition may involve a few or all the fingernails with a variable number of white opaque spots that may disappear before reaching the distal nail margin. Although punctate leuconychia is commonly believed to be caused by calcium deficiency there are no relationships between this condition and the calcium content of the nail.

Punctate leuconychia spontaneously regresses by avoiding traumas.

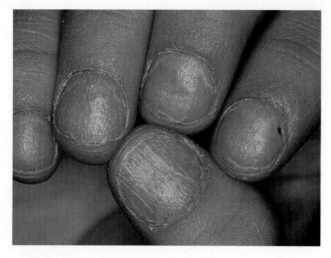

Fig. 23.2.7 Trachyonychia: sandpapered nails.

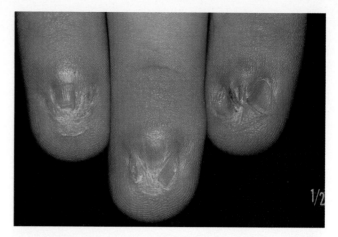

Fig. 23.2.8 Lichen planus: severe nail pterygium.

Despite the term TND, the nail changes do not necessarily involve all 20 nails. TND is a benign condition that usually regresses spontaneously over the years. Even in patients with TND due to lichen planus, the prognosis is favourable and nail scarring is never observed. Treatment is not necessary. Nail fragility may be improved by the application of topical emollients and systemic administration of biotin.

Warts

Periungual and subungual warts are very common in children, usually affecting more than one digit and frequently recurring. Large subungual warts may uplift the nail plate and be painful. In young children surgical procedures should be avoided and treatment should be as conservative as possible.

Since cryotherapy in the periungual area may be associated with considerable morbidity this technique should be not be used for treating multiple periungual warts in children. Topical antiwart solutions containing salicylic and lactic acids can be prescribed even though their efficacy is usually limited. Topical immunotherapy with strong sensitizers (squaric acid dibutylester (SADBE) or diphencyprone) is an effective and painless modality of treatment for multiple warts [13]. SADBE or diphencyprone 2% in acetone are used for sensitization. After 21 days weekly applications are carried out with dilutions selected according to the patient's response. Complete cure usually requires 3–4 months.

Uncommon nail disorders

Lichen planus

Nail lichen planus is very rare in children where it produces clinical signs identical to those seen in adults [14].

Most frequently the nails are thinned and show longitudinal ridging and splitting of the nail plate. Dorsal pterygium due to nail matrix destruction is a common occurrence. Pterygium appears as a V-shaped extension of the skin of the proximal nail fold. The nail plate is split into two portions that progressively decrease in size as the pterygium widens. In some cases, when the nail matrix has been completely destroyed, the pterygium substitutes the whole nail (Fig. 23.2.8).

In some children nail lichen planus produces a rapid and complete atrophy of the nail apparatus with permanent destruction of the nail plate of several digits (idiopathic atrophy of the nail). The diagnosis of nail lichen planus should be considered when nail thinning is associated with longitudinal ridging and splitting. The presence of nail pterygium is quite diagnostic. If lichen planus is correctly diagnosed and treated, permanent damage to the nail unit is rare even in patients with diffuse involvement of the nail matrix [15].

Systemic steroids are effective in treating nail lichen planus and prevent destruction of the nail matrix. Oral prednisone 0.5 mg/kg every other day for 2–6 weeks usually produces recovery of the nail abnormalities.

Lichen striatus

Nail lichen striatus is rare and almost exclusively seen in children. It is usually associated with typical skin lesions on the affected extremity but may occur in isolation [16]. It is almost always limited to a single nail. The nail abnormalities closely resemble those of nail matrix lichen planus with nail thinning associated with longitudinal ridging and splitting [17]. However, they do not involve the whole nail plate but are frequently restricted to its medial or lateral portion.

Onycholysis, leuconychia, longitudinal melanonychia and nail loss can occasionally occur. The presence of linearly arranged papules which may present verrucous scaling along the affected extremity suggests the diagnosis. The nail lesions regress spontaneously in a few years and require no treatment. The nail pathology reveals changes similar to those of lichen planus in the nail matrix.

Periungual fibromas

Periungual fibromas in children are usually a sign of tuberous sclerosis (Koenen's tumour). Periungual fibromas appear as a firm, flesh-coloured, smooth growth that originates in the periungual groove and usually extends outwards over the nail plate. Compression of the nail matrix may produce a groove in the nail plate.

In tuberous sclerosis periungual fibromas are commonly associated with other skin signs including facial angiofibromas, hypomelanotic macules, shagreen patches and forehead plaques. Periungual fibromas are asymptomatic and usually require no treatment. Large lesions can be surgically excised.

Subungual exostosis

Subungual exostoses are not uncommon in teenagers where they are frequently precipitated by a trauma. They almost exclusively involve the toenails, most commonly the great toe where they are usually localized on the dorsomedial aspect of the distal phalanx. Subungual exostosis appears as a firm tender subungual nodule that elevates the nail plate producing distal or lateral onycholysis. Because of the gradual enlargement of the excess bone, the nail plate may be deformed or destroyed.

X-ray is diagnostic showing an exophytic lesion on the distal phalangeal bone. The lesion should be surgically excised [18].

Nail matrix naevi

Nail matrix naevi in Caucasians are uncommon but not exceptional and are usually seen in childhood [19]. Nail matrix naevi may be congenital or acquired and usually produce a pigmented longitudinal band in the nail plate (longitudinal melanonychia) (Fig. 23.2.9).

Nail matrix naevi occur more frequently in fingernails than in toenails, the thumb being affected in about half of the cases. Nail pigmentation due to nail matrix naevi may be associated with a naevus of the periungual skin. From a clinical point of view it may be difficult to distinguish longitudinal melanonychia due to a naevus from longitudinal melanonychia due to other conditions including nail melanoma. Nail matrix naevi have variable features. The size as well as the degree of pigmentation of the band of longitudinal melanonychia varies considerably between patients. In most cases the naevus produces a heavily pigmented band, but it can also cause a scarcely pigmented

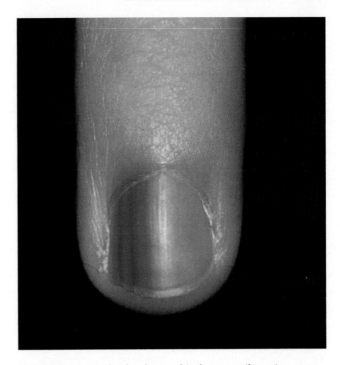

Fig. 23.2.9 Longitudinal melanonychia due to a nail matrix naevus.

light or brown band that may even undergo spontaneous fading.

A possible diagnosis of nail matrix naevus should always be considered in the case of a single pigmented band. A nail biopsy is necessary for a definitive diagnosis. Nail pigmentation due to congenital nail matrix naevi may spontaneously regress. This phenomenon, which has been exclusively reported in children, may be erroneously interpreted as a benign clinical sign [20]. However, this is not the case, since fading of the pigmentation only indicates a decreased activity of the naevus cells and not a regression of the naevus itself [21]. The frequency of progression from nail matrix naevi to nail matrix melanoma is not known but some cases have been documented. The author advises the excision of nail matrix naevi as a preventive measure after puberty.

Anonychia/micronychia

Total or partial absence of the nail at birth is rare. It may be a consequence of fetal exposure to systemic medications in early pregnancy or be a sign of numerous syndromes.

Hypoplasia of the nails and terminal phalanges can occur in children whose mothers have been exposed to anticonvulsant drugs, alcohol or warfarin. Congenital syndromes associated with anonychia include DOOR syndrome (deafness, onycho-osteodystrophy, mental retardation), Iso–Kikuchy syndrome and some ectodermal dysplasias.

Iso–Kikuchi syndrome

This congenital nail deformity affects one or both index fingers and occasionally other fingers [22]. The affected nails most commonly show micronychia or hemionychogryphosis. Anonychia may also be present. X-ray shows a Y-shaped bifurcation of the distal phalanx on lateral pictures.

Nail–patella syndrome

In this condition, which is inherited with an autosomal dominant pattern, nail hypoplasia is associated with bone and kidney abnormalities. The nail abnormalities may be limited to the thumbs or affect all fingernails, the thumb, however, being more severely affected. The affected digits show absence or hypoplasia of the nail plate. This is usually more marked on the medial portion of the nail. The bone abnormalities characteristic of nail–patella syndrome include absent or hypoplastic patella, radial head abnormalities and iliac crest exostosis. In 40% of all cases of nail–patella syndrome a nephropathy develops. In 5.5–8% of cases, the disease leads to the necessity of haemodialysis because of renal insufficiency.

Polydactyly

The frequency of polydactyly of the hands has been estimated to be 0.37% and it is more common than polydactyly of the feet. Duplication of the thumb is a manifestation of congenital polydactyly, one of the most common anomalies of the hand. Patients with type 1 and 2 thumb polydactyly may have two distinct nails separated by a longitudinal incision or a single nail with a central indentation of the distal margin when the bone duplication is limited to the distal phalanx [23].

Thumb polydactyly may be sporadic or transmitted as an autosomal dominant trait with variable expressivity. X-ray shows bone bifurcation. Early surgical treatment is important to maximize functional restoration and aesthetic results.

Epidermolysis bullosa

In epidermolysis bullosa nail changes are common even though not specific to the epidermolysis bullosa subtypes. Extensive and repetitive blistering may produce permanent nail loss. In epidermolysis bullosa junctionalis progressiva, a rare form of junctional epidermolysis inherited as an autosomal recessive trait, nail lesions, which normally develop during childhood, usually precede the other clinical manifestations of the disease. The nails appear thick and short, and develop recurrent periungual and subungual haemorrhagic blisters.

Other clinical features include non-scarring blisters on the hands, feet, elbows, knees and mouth, the loss of finger patterns, hypodontia and dental caries [24].

Ectodermal dysplasias

Patients with ectodermal dysplasia present dystrophic nails, the presence of nail abnormalities being a major criterion for the classification of these conditions (subclass 3). The nails show variable features depending on the different syndromes. Nail hypoplasia is frequently associated with thickening of the nail plate.

Pachyonychia congenita

Pachyonychia congenita is an autosomal dominant disorder characterized by severe nail thickening due to nail bed hyperkeratosis. Three different types of pachyonychia congenita have been recognized depending on the clinical features and biochemical defect. Nail abnormalities are a constant feature and usually develop during childhood [25]. All the nails are thickened, difficult to trim and show an increase in the lateral curvature of the nail plate. The condition can be treated surgically or using a carbon dioxide laser with excision of the hyperkeratotic nail bed.

Chronic mucocutaneous candidiasis

This condition is characterized by recurrent *Candida* infection of the skin, mucous membranes and nails. In patients with this condition, *Candida* invades the nails producing a total onychomycosis. The affected nails are markedly thickened, crumbly and yellow–brown in colour. The digit usually presents a bulbous appearance due to severe oedema of the periungual tissues. Although the nail abnormalities can be cured with systemic antifungals, recurrences are frequent due to underlying immunological defects.

REFERENCES

1 Zaias N. *The Nail in Health and Disease*, 2nd edn. Norwalk: Appleton & Lange, 1990.
2 Runne U, Orfanos CE. The human nail. *Curr Prob Dermatol* 1981; 9: 102–49.
3 Hamilton JB, Terada H, Mestler GE. Studies of growth throughout the lifespan in Japanese: growth and size of nails and their relationship to age, sex, heredity and other factors. *J Gerontol* 1995; 10: 401–15.
4 Sibinga MS. Observations on growth of fingernails in health and disease. *Pediatrics* 1959; 24: 225–33.
5 Baran R. Significance and management of congenital malalignment of the big toenails. *Cutis* 1996; 58: 181–4.
6 Tosti A, Baran R, Dawber RPR. The nail in systemic diseases and drug-induced changes. In: Baran R, Dawber RPR, eds. *Diseases of the Nails and their Management*, 2nd edn. Oxford: Blackwell Scientific Publications, 1994: 175–261.
7 Hjorth N, Thomsen K. Parakeratosis pustolosa. *Br J Dermatol* 1967; 79: 527.
8 Tosti A, Peluso AM, Zucchelli V. Clinical feature and long term follow-up of 20 cases of parakeratosis pustolosa. *Pediatr Dermatol* 1998; 15: 259–63.
9 Farber EJ, Jacobs AH. Nail infantile psoriasis. *Am J Dis Child* 1977; 131: 1266.

10 Baran R, Dawber RPR. The nail in dermatological diseases. In: Baran R, Dawber RPR, eds. *Diseases of the Nails and their Management*, 2nd edn. Oxford: Blackwell Scientific Publications, 1994: 135–73.

11 Nanda A, Kaur S, Kaur I *et al.* Childhood psoriasis: an epidemiologic survey of 112 patients. *Pediatr Dermatol* 1990; 7: 19–21.

12 Tosti A, Piraccini BM. Trachyonychia or twenty-nail dystrophy. *Curr Opin Dermatol* 1996; 3: 83–6.

13 Iijima S, Otsuka F. Contact immunotherapy with squaric acid dibutylester for warts. *Dermatology* 1993; 187: 115–18.

14 Peluso AM, Piraccini BM, Cameli N *et al.* Lichen planus limited to the nails in childhood: report of a case and review of the literature. *Pedriatr Dermatol* 1992; 10: 36–9.

15 Tosti A, Peluso AM, Fanti PA *et al.* Nail lichen planus: clinical study of 24 patients. *J Am Acad Dermatol* 1993; 28: 724–30.

16 Tosti A, Peluso AM, Misciali C *et al.* Nail lichen striatus: clinical features and long-term follow-up of five cases. *J Am Acad Dermatol* 1997; 36: 908–13.

17 Baran R, Dupré A, Lauret P *et al.* Le lichen striatus onychodystrophique. *Ann Dermatol Vénéréol* 1979; 106: 885–91.

18 Lemont H, Christman RA. Subungual exostosis and nail disease and radio-logical aspects. In: Scher RK, Daniel III CR. *Nails: Therapy Diagnosis Surgery*. Philadelphia: WB Saunders, 1990: 250–7.

19 Tosti A, Baran R, Piraccini BM *et al.* Nail matrix nevi: a clinical and pathological study of 22 patients. *J Am Acad Dermatol* 1996; 34: 765–71.

20 Kikuchi I, Inoue S, Sakaguchi E *et al.* Nevoid area melanosis in childhood (cases which showed spontaneous regression). *Dermatology* 1993; 186: 88–93.

21 Tosti A, Baran R, Morelli R *et al.* Progressive fading of longitudinal melanonychia due to a nail matrix melanocytic naevus in a child. *Arch Dermatol* 1994; 130: 1076–7.

22 Baran R. Syndrome d'Iso et Kikuchi. *Ann Dermatol Vénéréol* 1980; 107: 431.

23 Tosti A, Paoluzzi P, Baran R. Doubled nail of the thumb: a rare form of polydactyly. *Dermatology* 1992; 184: 216–18.

24 Bruckner-Tuderman L, Schnyder UW, Baran R. Nail changes in epidermolysis bullosa: clinical and pathogenetic considerations. *Br J Dermatol* 1995; 132: 339–44.

25 Samman PD. Developmental anomalies. In: Samman PD, Fenton DA, eds. *Samman's The Nails in Disease*, 5th edn. Oxford: Butterworth-Heinemann, 1995: 183–208.

Section 24
Genitourinary Problems

24.1 Vulvovaginitis and Lichen Sclerosus

SALLIE M. NEILL

Vulvovaginitis

Lichen sclerosus

Vulvovaginitis

Definition

Vulvovaginitis is defined as inflammation involving both the vulval and vaginal epithelia. However, in clinical practice this term is often incorrectly applied to cases where there is vulval inflammation alone, vulvitis. Inflammation of the vagina (vaginitis) does not always occur in isolation as the associated discharge that accompanies it usually results in contamination of the perineum with consequent irritation and inflammation of the vulva.

It is important in assessing the patient to ascertain whether there is both vulval and vaginal involvement in order to narrow down the possible diagnoses.

Anatomy and physiology

The vulva in the pubescent girl is comprised of various anatomical sites which include the mons pubis, paired labia majora, the labia minora, the glans clitoris and the inner vulval vestibule. The epithelium throughout is cornified and stratified with the exception of the vestibule which is still stratified but non-cornified, i.e. mucosal. The entire length of the vagina is lined with stratified non-cornified epithelium.

In the premenarchal girl the labia minora are only partly developed as the hood over the glans clitoris, the labia majora, have only sparse fine hair and are less rounded as the subcutaneous fat pads are undeveloped. The unoestrogenized vestibule is covered with a thinned epithelium and the underlying vasculature is clearly visible giving it a bright red appearance which is often misdiagnosed as pathological inflammation by the inexperienced examiner.

This thinned epithelium is more sensitive to irritants. The vaginal pH is neutral to alkaline and lactobacilli are absent, the common commensal organisms being *Staphylococcus epidermidis* and diphtheroids [1]. The higher pH, while offering some protection against can-

didal infection, leaves the epithelium more susceptible to bacterial infection. Moreover, the vestibule and vaginal opening are more exposed in the child, not being afforded the protection of the rounded contours of the fully developed, hairy labia majora. In addition the anus lies in close proximity to the vestibule and very often perineal hygiene is inadequate with habits such as back to front wiping after opening the bowels leading to bacterial contamination or irritation from faecal material. Following the thelarche oestrogen stimulates the endocervical glands to produce mucus, the labia enlarge, sebaceous gland activity is promoted, hair develops on the mons pubis and the labia majora and labia minora develop around the vestibule. The vagina becomes thickened and rugose and the vaginal and vestibular epithelial cells become glycogenated. The neutral pH of the vagina becomes acidic due to the fermentation of glycogen in the oestrogenized epithelium lowering the pH to 4.0–4.5 which then supports the normal flora of lactobacilli, haemolytic streptococci and diphtheroids.

Aetiology and pathogenesis

In considering the pathogenesis of vulvovaginitis it is helpful to categorize it into that associated with a vaginal discharge and that without.

Vulvovaginitis associated with a discharge

This is most likely to be due to an infection or a retained foreign body. In prepubertal girls the recognized pathogenic organisms include *Haemophilus influenzae* [2], *Shigella* and groups A and B β-haemolytic streptococci. Until recently, group A haemolytic *Streptococcus* was not considered important in the cause of symptomatic vulvovaginitis but recent studies have shown an increasing incidence of this organism associated with symptomatic disease [3,4]. The commonest enteric pathogen is *Shigella* which frequently occurs in the absence of diarrhoea [5].

Candidal infection is the commonest cause of vulvovaginitis in postpubertal children presumably due to the effects of oestrogen on the vaginal epithelium increasing the glycogen content of the epithelial cells of both the vestibule and vagina. The rare occurrence of candidal infection in early infancy may be explained by the fact that maternal oestrogens still exert an effect on the infants mucosae from birth to 2 months [6]. An overgrowth of *Candida* may, however, be a complication in all children with vulval skin affected with a pre-existent dermatoses. Candidiasis in this situation is a secondary phenomenon and once the underlying dermatosis is treated the *Candida* is no longer a problem. A foreign body in the vagina can give rise to a vaginal discharge and secondary vulval irritation. In premenarchal girls one of the commonest items found was toilet paper [7].

Sexually transmitted infections are confined to sexually active teenagers or to younger children who are being abused (see Chapter 24.3). The commonest bacterial pathogens in this situation are *Neisseria gonorrhoeae*, *Chlamydia trachomatis* and *Trichomonas*. The two commonest viral infections are herpes simplex and human papilloma virus; however, it should be appreciated that neither of these infections are always sexually transmitted.

Vulvovaginitis without a discharge

This usually occurs when there is inflammation of the vulva alone and it would be more accurate to refer to the problem as vulvitis. Vulvitis may be caused by any dermatosis occurring at this site in isolation or as part of a generalized eruption. Diagnostic difficulties arise most frequently when vulvitis occurs in isolation because the typical morphological signs that aid in diagnosis are often lost due to the occlusive effect at this natural flexural site. The most common dermatological disorders seen in the vulva are eczema and psoriasis and there is normally evidence of these disorders at extragenital sites.

Lichen sclerosus is the commonest skin disorder to affect this site exclusively as extragenital lesions are uncommon in children. Cutaneous lichen planus is very rare in childhood. Most of the cases reported occur after the age of 10 years and there are no descriptions of genital involvement. Blistering disorders may also present as vulval inflammation in the prebullous phase, and include the immunobullous diseases, chronic bullous disease of childhood and bullous pemphigoid (see Chapters 12.3 and 12.5). Erythema and bullous lesions may also involve the vulval skin either as part of the prodrome or simultaneously when the rest of the skin is affected by erythema multiforme, Stevens–Johnson syndrome and Kawasaki's disease. A fixed drug eruption may affect the vulval skin alone. Rarer dermatoses presenting as vulvitis include acrodermatitis enteropathica, Crohn's disease, Langerhans' cell histiocytosis (Letterer–Siwe disease) and Darier's disease.

Irritant eczema and inflammation of the vulval skin associated with play are recognized after playing in sand ('sand pit vulvitis'), swimming in chlorinated pools and

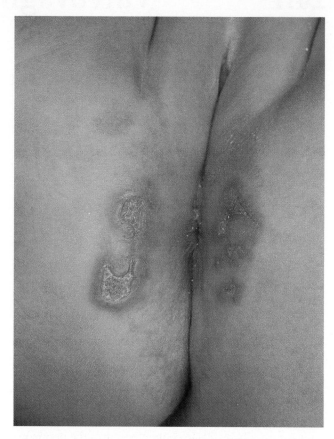

Fig. 24.1.1 Jacquet's dermatitis showing healing lesions which had been ulcerated nodules.

bathing in bubble baths [8]. True allergic contact dermatitis of the vulva is rarely seen in childhood.

Jacquet's irritant erosive dermatitis describes a condition with ulcerated papules and pustules on the labia of the vulval skin of infants and is believed to be due to prolonged contact with soiled napkins (Fig. 24.1.1). This is seen less frequently with the use of disposable nappies and the recently improved absorbancy of the materials used in their manufacture. A similar but quite separate entity, granuloma gluteale infantum, was first described in 1971 [9]. This condition is seen almost exclusively in infants treated with a topical corticosteroid and consists of larger non-ulcerating nodules usually on the convexities of the nappy area.

Congenital cavernous haemangiomas may occur on the vulval skin where they are more likely to become ulcerated due to the chafing effect of napkins. A further complication with a large haemangioma in this area is obstruction of the free flow of the urine leading to pooling and bacterial contamination. The other causes of urinary pooling are labial adhesions and a microperforate hymen. In the latter the normal escape of urine that enters the vagina on micturition is obstructed [10]. Thread worm infestations are a common cause of vulvovaginitis and reported in nearly a third of the cases of vulvovaginitis in one series and in half of these there was also a positive vaginal swab culture for bacteria [11].

Finally, the trauma of sexual abuse may result in inflammation with or without an associated sexually transmitted infection.

Clinical features

The skin signs seen in vulvovaginitis usually include erythema, oedema and fissuring. If the underlying condition is itchy there will also be lichenification and excoriations. In severe inflammation, blisters and erosions develop. In the absence of a vaginal discharge a vaginal infection is extremely unlikely.

The main symptoms that the child complains of include itch, vulval soreness, dysuria and discharge. These symptoms may be severe enough to interfere with sleep and the parents may notice blood or evidence of a discharge on the child's underwear. Confirmation of the discharge is important as it is often reported but found infrequently on examination. In one study only half of those reportedly having a discharge were found to have one when examined [12]. The discharge due to a foreign body often has an unpleasant odour.

Diagnosis

A careful history and thorough examination are essential to establish an accurate diagnosis. Any discharge must be fully investigated with samples for wet preparations to examine for trichomonads and candidiasis, and further samples for Gram staining and bacterial culture. If herpes simplex is suspected then viral culture and smear preparations for electron microscopy should be performed. Any vaginal samples can be obtained atraumatically using a catheter within a catheter technique [13]. In this technique the hub of a butterfly infusion set with only the first 11.25 cm of the tubing still attached to it, the needle end having been cut off, is threaded into the distal end of a FG No. 12 bladder catheter which has been shortened to 10 cm. The butterfly hub is then attached to a 1-ml syringe filled with sterile saline. The uncut proximal end of the catheter is inserted into the vagina and the saline is then gently flushed through and reaspirated. This aspirate is then examined and cultured. If intestinal worms are suspected a sticky tape test should be done in the morning to try and detect parasitic ova (Fig. 24.1.2).

In cases where candidiasis recurs without a background dermatosis, diabetes or immune deficiency must be excluded.

Treatment

Treatment is dependent upon the diagnosis. If it is due to a dermatosis, appropriate treatment will be neces-

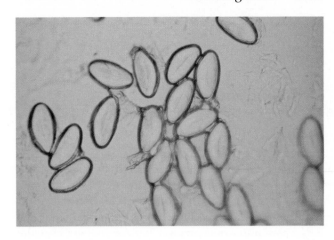

Fig. 24.1.2 Ova of *Enterobius vermicularis*.

sary. General measures to prevent irritation include washing with a soap substitute such as aqueous cream or emulsifying ointment, avoiding bubble baths and using Vaseline petroleum jelly as a barrier when swimming in chlorinated pools. If there is a proven infection or infestation, the appropriate antibiotic or antihelminthic agent should be prescribed. However, a change in perineal hygiene alone may be extremely effective in treating the immediate problem and preventing further episodes.

Foreign bodies may be removed with gentle vaginal lavage after first anaesthetizing the vulva with topical lignocaine but in those cases where the object is firmly imbedded in the vaginal wall an examination under general anaesthesia will usually be required to remove it atraumatically [14].

REFERENCES

1 Hammersclagg MR, Alpert S, Rosner I *et al*. Microbiology of the vagina in children. Normal and potential pathogenic organisms. *Pediatrics* 1978; 62: 57–62.
2 Macfarlane DE, Sharma DP. *Haemophilus influenzae* and genital tract infections in children. *Acta Paediatr Scand* 1987; 76: 363–4.
3 Murphy TV, Nelson JD. *Shigella* vaginitis: report of a case and review of the literature. *Pediatrics* 1979; 63: 511–16.
4 Donald FE, Slack DB, Colman G. *Streptococcus pyogenes* vulvovaginitis in children in Nottingham. *Epidemiol Infect* 1991; 106: 459–65.
5 Dhar V, Roker K, Adhami Z, McKenzie S. Streptococcal vulvovaginitis in girls. *Pediatr Dermatol* 1993; 10: 366–7.
6 Bennett D, Kearney. Vulvovaginitis and vaginal pH. *Arch Dis Child* 1992; 67: 1520.
7 Pokorny SF. Long-term intravaginal presence of foreign bodies in children. A preliminary study. *J Reprod Med* 1994; 39: 931–5.
8 Heller RH, Joseph JM, Davis HJ. Vulvovaginitis in the premenarchal child. *J Pediatr* 1969; 74: 370–77.
9 Tappeiner J, Pfleger L. Granuloma gluteale infantum. *Hautartz* 1971; 22: 383–8.
10 Caparro VJ, Dillon WP, Gallego MB. Microperforate hymen. A distinct clinical entitiy. *Obstet Gynecol* 1974; 44: 903–5.
11 Pierce AM, Hart CA. Vulvovaginitis: causes and management. *Arch Dis Child* 1992; 67: 509–12.
12 Paradise JE, Campos JM, Friedman HM, Frishmuth G. Vulvovaginitis in premenarchal girls: clinical features and diagnostic evaluation. *Paediatrics* 1982; 70: 193–8.

13 Pokorny SF, Stormer J. Atraumatic removal of secretion from the prepubertal vagina. *Am J Obstet Gynecol* 1987; 156: 581–2.

14 Pokorny S. Prepubertal vulvovaginopathies. *Obstet Gynecol Clin N Am* 1992; 19: 39–58.

Lichen sclerosus

Definition

Lichen sclerosus is a chronic, lymphocyte-mediated inflammatory dermatosis characterized by shiny, white, atrophic patches with a predilection for the genital and perianal skin (Fig. 24.1.3). It occurs in children and adults with two peaks of age of presentation, prepubertal and either peri- or postmenopausal. It is commoner in females than males and was originally described in 1887 by Hallopeau as a variant of lichen planus [1].

Aetiology and pathogenesis

The aetiology is unknown but familial cases are now recognized [2]. The evidence is increasing that it is an autoimmune-related disorder [3–5] with many patients having lichen sclerosus and at least one other autoimmune disorder, the most frequently reported being vitiligo, morphoea and thyroid disease. There have been conflicting results of an association with particular HLA types [6,7]. Some evidence suggests that there is an association of positive *Borrelia burgdorferi* serology with both morphoea and lichen sclerosus [8] but this proposed aetiology is still unclear and controversial.

The incidence of lichen sclerosus is unknown but it has been estimated that the prevalence may be between 1 in 300 and 1 in 1000 of the population [9].

Pathology

The histopathological features were first described by Darier [10] and later by Hewitt [11]. The typical histological findings include a thinned, effaced epidermis with or without an overlying hyperkeratosis. In the reticular dermis, immediately beneath the epidermis, there is a broad band of homogenized collagen. A lymphocytic infiltrate may be present just below the abnormal dermis (Fig. 24.1.4). In some areas this infiltrate can be seen along the dermoepidermal junction with areas of liquefactive degeneration very similar to those changes seen in lichen planus.

Clinical features

The main symptom in girls is itch, but dysuria and difficulty with defaecation are not uncommon if there is vulval or perianal fissuring. The condition is reportedly rarer in boys occurring most frequently on the prepuce. However, the condition may be underrecognized as a study demonstrated that 14% of prepubertal boys requiring a circumcision for medical reasons had evidence of

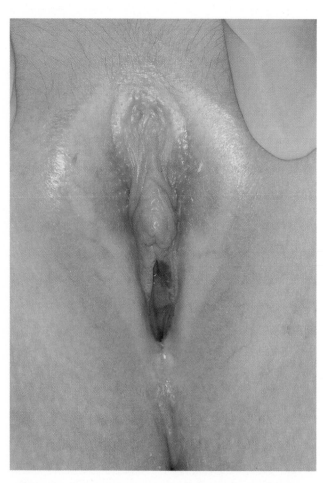

Fig. 24.1.3 Lichen sclerosus showing characteristic white atrophic skin with some purpura around the introitus.

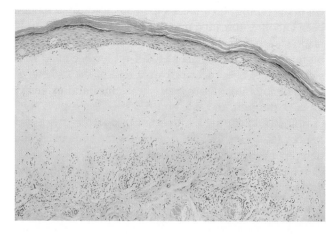

Fig. 24.1.4 Histology of lichen sclerosus. The epidermis is thinned and effaced. The superficial dermis is hyalinized and there is a lymphocytic infiltrate immediately beneath this zone.

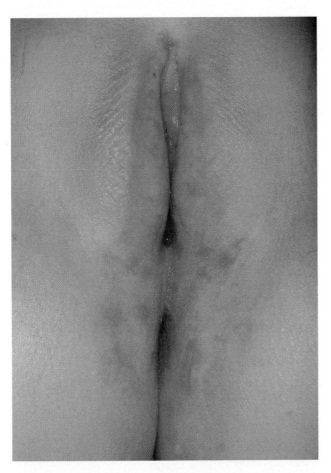

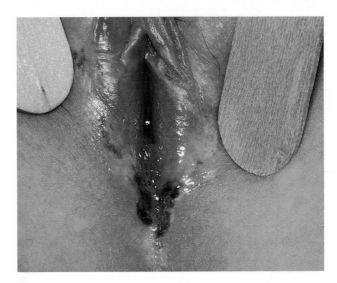

Fig. 24.1.6 Ecchymoses of introital skin. Courtesy of Dr C.M. Ridley.

Fig. 24.1.5 Early, erythematous phase of lichen sclerosus involving the vulval and perianal skin in a figure of eight configuration.

lichen sclerosus [12]. The usual presentation in young boys is a history of recurrent balanitis with erythema, fissuring and tightening of the foreskin which can eventually lead to phimosis. Difficulty micturating may occur because of the phimosis or more rarely from meatal narrowing if the glans and urethral meatus are involved.

In girls the initial cutaneous signs are erythema, excoriations and lichenification which settle with loss of pigmentation and an acquired atrophic appearance often described in appearance as 'cigarette paper' wrinkling (Fig. 24.1.5). There may be purpura and extensive ecchymoses which can be mistaken for child abuse [13] (Fig. 24.1.6). This is not usually the case but it must be appreciated that lichen sclerosus can koebnerize and if a child was the subject of abuse it could possibly exacerbate the symptoms and signs. Blistering may be seen but it is very unusual. In postpubertal girls there may be architectural distortion with resorption of the labia minora and burying of the clitoris leading to a loss of the usual anatomical features of the vulva. Introital narrowing is an unusual complication as lichen sclerosus rarely affects the vestibule and never affects the vagina as it appears to

be confined to cornified stratified squamous epithelium, sparing non-cornified (mucosal) squamous epithelium. The lesions often extend in a figure of eight configuration to involve the perianal skin in girls but not in boys [14] (Fig. 24.1.5). If involvement is severe, perianal fissuring results in painful defaecation which can subsequently lead to constipation and faecal retention. Extragenital involvement is rare in children occurring in less than 10%.

Prognosis

It was believed that lichen sclerosus remitted spontaneously at puberty but this has now been disputed and many children still continue to have the disease beyond menarche [14]. Interestingly these children are often asymptomatic which may be one explanation for the mistaken belief that resolution occurred at puberty. Longitudinal studies will hopefully settle this.

Architectural destruction is irreversible and those children that have the disease before the minora develop fully and are untreated will have underdeveloped labia minora. The disease often continues unremittingly without treatment for many years.

Differential diagnosis

In the early stages the disease can be mistaken for psoriasis or eczema but once the characteristic whitening occurs these diseases can easily be excluded (Fig. 24.1.7). Vitiligo enters into the differential diagnosis but this does not involve a textural change in the skin as it is only a loss of pigmentation (Fig. 24.1.8).

At the stage where there is no evidence of activity and the signs include atrophy and scarring the differen-

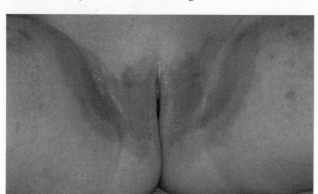

Fig. 24.1.7 Differential diagnosis: psoriasis extending into the genitocrural folds.

tial diagnosis for the previous inflammatory disorder would have to include the blistering disorders such as chronic bullous disease of childhood or cicatricial pemphigoid. Finally, as already mentioned, if there is extensive ecchymoses a mistaken diagnosis of child abuse may be made.

Treatment

Medical

The treatment of choice is a potent topical corticosteroid such as clobetasol propionate 0.05% [15]. This is applied to the affected skin once daily usually at night taking care to avoid smearing onto the inner upper thighs where striae are likely to develop with the injudicious use of a very potent steroid. Nightly application is carried out for 4 weeks and then reduced to alternate nights for a further 4 weeks. The final 4 weeks requires application twice a week. The majority of children respond to this and then use the steroid cream as and when required which is usually infrequently. A 30-g tube of clobetasol will usually last a year and the child should not have any side-effects with this regimen. Topical testosterone and progesterone are no longer recognized treatments and have no place in the management of lichen sclerosus in children.

Oral steroids are not required and failure to respond to a topical steroid ointment should raise the possibility of another diagnosis. A soap substitute such as aqueous cream is also a useful adjunct to treatment.

Surgical

There are only rare instances where surgery is indicated in the treatment of girls with lichen sclerosus as surgical excision may result in koebnerization and exacerbation of the disease postoperatively. In a very small number of cases, surgical division of persistent fusion of the labia minora

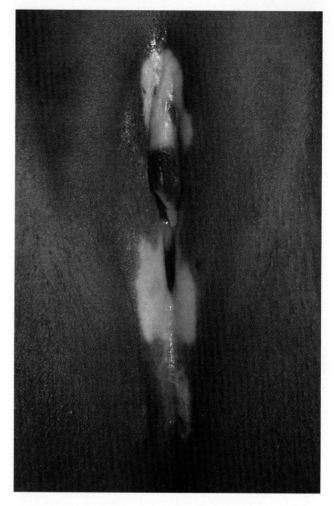

Fig. 24.1.8 Differential diagnosis: vitiligo results in loss of pigmentation only with no textural change in the skin.

may be necessary if there is interference with micturition or menstruation. Surgery is obviously required in the extremely rare event of a squamous cell carcinoma occurring. In boys who develop phimosis of the prepuce, circumcision is the treatment of choice and it is extremely unusual for the disease to affect the glans postoperatively if there was no involvement before.

REFERENCES

1 Hallopeau H. Lichen plan sclereux. *Ann Dermatol Syph* 1887; 10: 447–9.
2 Sahn ES, Bluestein EL, Oliva S. Familial lichen sclerosus et atrophicus in childhood. *Paediatr Dermatol* 1994; 11: 160–3.
3 Goolamali SK, Barnes EW, Irvine WJ *et al*. Organ-specific antibodies in patients with lichen sclerosus. *Br Med J* 1974; iv: 78–9.
4 Harrington CI, Dunsmore IR. An investigation into the incidence of autoimmune disorders in patients with lichen sclerosus et atrophicus. *Br J Dermatol* 1981; 104: 563–6.
5 Meyrick-Thomas RH, Ridley CM, McGibbon DH, Black MM. Lichen sclerosus et atrophicus and autoimmunity—a study of 350 women. *Br J Dermatol* 1988; 118: 41–6.
6 Sideri M, Rognoni M, Rizzolo L *et al*. Antigens of the HLA system in women with vulvar lichen sclerosus. Association with HLA-B21. *J Reprod Med* 1994; 88: 551–4.

7 Marren P, Yell J, Bunce M *et al*. The association between lichen sclerosus and antigens of the HLA system. *Br J Dermatol* 1995; 132: 197–203.

8 Schempp C, Bocklage H, Lange R, Komel HW, Orfanos CE, Gollnick H. Further evidence for *Borrelia burgdorferi* infection in morphoea and lichen sclerosus et atrophicus confirmed by DNA amplification. *J Invest Dermatol* 1993; 100: 717–20.

9 Wallace HJ. Lichen sclerosus et atrophicus. *Trans St John's Dermatol Soc* 1971; 57: 9–30.

10 Darier J. Lichen plan sclereux. *Ann Dermatol Syph* 1892; 3: 833–7.

11 Hewitt J. Histologic criteria for lichen sclerosus of the vulva. *J Reprod Med* 1986; 31: 781–7.

12 Chalmers RJG, Burton PA, Goring C *et al*. Lichen sclerosus et atrophicus — a common and distinctive cause of phimosis in boys. *Arch Dermatol* 1984; 120: 1025–7.

13 Handfield-Jones SE, Hinde FRJ, Kennedy CTC. Lichen sclerosus et atrophicus in children misdiagnosed as sexual abuse. *Br Med J* 1987; 294: 1404–5.

14 Ridley CM. Genital lichen sclerosus (lichen sclerosus et atrophicus) in childhood and adolescence. *J Roy Soc Med* 1993; 86: 69–75.

15 Dalziel K, Millard PR, Wojnarowska F. The treatment of vulval lichen sclerosus with a very potent topical corticosteroid (clobetasol propionate 0.05%) cream. *Br J Dermatol* 1991; 124: 461–4.

24.2 Sexually Transmitted Diseases in Children and Adolescents

KENNETH BROMBERG, MARGARET
HAMMERSCHLAG, SARAH A. RAWSTRON,
ROBERT A.C. BILO AND ARNOLD P. ORANJE

Syphilis

Gonorrhoea

Chlamydia trachomatis infections

Condyloma acuminata

Hepatitis B in children

Genital herpes simplex virus infection

Human immunodeficiency virus

Trichomonas vaginalis infection

Bacterial vaginitis

Sexually transmitted diseases (STDs) in childhood occur as a result of intrauterine infections, vertical transmission and postnatal infection [1]. STDs have a special implication in pregnancy [2]. They may influence the course of pregnancy and, for example, cause premature birth due to chorioamnionitis or polyhydramnios. STDs may also pose a threat to the unborn and the newborn. A number of STDs such as syphilis may transplacentally infect and damage the fetus. The newborn may become infected during passage through the birth canal. These include *Chlamydia trachomatis* (CT) infections, gonorrhoea, human immuno-deficiency virus (HIV) infection and primary genital herpes simplex virus (HSV) infections. The newborn may also be infected with HIV via breast-feeding or from bystanders as in herpes labialis. Establishing a diagnosis of STD in a newborn forces investigation into the contacts and sexual partner(s) of the mother. It is evident that such an investigation may pose extra problems.

Concerning acquired infections, various modes of transmission of infection must be considered. The child may become infected via everyday contact with an infected adult, for example, through intimate non-sexual physical contact. Infections may also occur as a result of medical interventions. The child may acquire the infection via voluntary or involuntary sexual contact. Theoretically, STDs can also be transmitted during normal sexual exploratory behaviour between an infected and a non-infected child. An adolescent may also acquire STDs by voluntary sexual contact with another individual from their peer group. However, if STD is established in a young child sexual abuse must always be suspected.

The occurrence of STDs in abused children has been reported to vary from 3 to 13% in the available literature [3,4]. Infection may sometimes be the presenting feature, although it is more often encountered during routine physical examination in suspected cases of abuse. Dealing with these problems requires particular care and expertise.

A number of factors influence the risk that a child runs of acquiring STD infection during abuse. The chance that a child acquires STD infection from sexual abuse outside the family is higher than that from abuse within the family. The final factor that is important in evaluating the manner in which the child could have acquired STD is the occurrence of the intercultural differences in the mode of transmission. Whittle *et al.* [5], for example, have described that at present, horizontal transmission of hepatitis B from child to child is most common in certain developing countries, whereas vertical transmission from mother to child is more common in other countries.

Policy on sexually transmitted diseases in childhood

STDs in children have two important implications: first, it is essential that the correct diagnosis be made speedily and that adequate treatment is provided; second, STDs provide a signal for imperative further investigation into the mode of transmission whereby sexual abuse must be excluded. Therefore, a multidisciplinary approach is important in dealing with STDs in children (Table 24.2.1).

Tracing of (sexual) contacts should be undertaken for epidemiological reasons. The primary aim is the diagnosis and treatment of STD and to prevent further spread [5].

REFERENCES

1 Bilo RAC, Oranje AP. STD in childhood: the clinical and social context. *SOA Vademecum* 1997; D7: 1–17 (in Dutch).
2 Hartwig NG, Oranje AP, Groot de R, Dekker JH. STD and the newborn. *SOA Vademecum* 1997; D5: 1–12 (in Dutch).

Table 24.2.1 Policy on STDs in childhood

Phase 1

Referral to a (paediatric) dermatologist and/or a paediatrician and eventually a (paediatric) gynaecologist

Contact with a child abuse doctor in suspected sexual abuse

Phase 2

Investigation and treatment of STD by a (paediatric) dermatologist and/or a paediatrician and eventually a (paediatric) gynaecologist; to ascertain the source of infection, mode of transmission, elimination of other STDs, examination of the parents and other members of the family

Supplementary examination and diagnosis by a paediatrician in connection with other physical abnormalities and psychosocial problems, in cooperation with a (medical) social worker

On indication

(a) hospitalization for observation, supplemented if appropriate by a paediatric psychological examination; and

(b) gynaecological examination and investigation by a (paediatric) gynaecologist in older girls; to note any congenital abnormalities and abnormalities considered to be the result of sexual contacts/sexual abuse

Involvement of a child abuse doctor in suspected sexual abuse

3 Hobbs CJ, Wynne JM. Child sexual abuse: an increasing rate of diagnosis. *Lancet* 1987; ii: 837–41.
4 White ST, Leda FA, Ingram DL, Pearson A. Sexually transmitted diseases in sexually abused children. *Pediatrics* 1983; 72: 16–21.
5 Whittle HC, Inskip H, Hall AJ *et al.* Vaccination against hepatitis B and protection against viral carriage in the Gambia. *Lancet* 1991; 337: 747–50.

Syphilis

Definition

Infection with *Treponema pallidum* causes syphilis. Infection can be transmitted transplacentally (congenital syphilis) or postnatally (acquired syphilis). Congenital syphilis is always caused by maternal syphilis. Almost all acquired syphilis in children is associated with sexual contact which by definition involves abuse.

History

Caspar Torella in 1498 suggested that syphilis in nursing infants was acquired from syphilitic wet nurses [1]. Paracelsus in the early part of the 16th century felt that syphilis could be acquired *in utero*, describing the condition as hereditary syphilis. Even as late as 1901, Carpenter [2] made reference to hereditary syphilis. The pathogenesis of congenital syphilis and a clear distinction between acquired and congenital syphilis was not possible until the identification of *T. pallidum* by Schaudinn and Hofman in 1905, and the development of a serological test for syphilis by von Wassermann in 1906.

Published reports from 1906 until 1940 mostly described childhood syphilis in the first few years of life or after the initiation of sexual activity. Cases of syphilis in the first few years of life were either congenital or acquired. Most cases seen after the initiation of sexual activity were probably acquired and unlikely to be congenital.

However, if the presentation of syphilis was that of a neurological illness, the distinction between the sequelae of congenital syphilis and acquired syphilis was and still is not always possible to make. In the 1920s and 1930s, some but not all of the cases of syphilis described in children between the first year of life and the onset of sexual activity were reported to be associated with sexual abuse. A changing view of abuse requires a reinterpretation of these reports. It is likely that almost all cases of acquired syphilis in children were associated with abuse.

REFERENCES

1 Dennie CC. *A History of Syphilis*. Springfield, Illinois: C.C. Thomas, 1962.
2 Carpenter G. *The Syphilis of Children in Every-Day Practice*. New York: William Wood, 1901.

Pathology

Vasculitis and plasma cell infiltration are the hallmark of infection with *T. pallidum*. However, atypical findings may be seen in early fetal death [1] or with secondary syphilis. Identification of *T. pallidum* in suspicious cases may clarify the issue [2].

REFERENCES

1 Harter CA, Benirschke K. Fetal syphilis in the first trimester. *Obstet Gynecol* 1976; 124: 705–11.
2 Jeerapaet P, Ackerman AB. Histologic patterns of secondary syphilis. *Arch Dermatol* 1973; 107: 373–7.

Clinical features of acquired syphilis

Acquired syphilis is unique in children in that transmission as now reported is almost always associated with abuse. Exceptions include transmission from breastfeeding, and the rare instance where a primary chancre is identified at a non-genital site together with a plausible explanation such as a neck chancre from an innocent kiss. The following clinical descriptions of primary and secondary syphilis are based on data from adults with specific examples from children cited when available.

Primary syphilis

The initial hallmark of acquired syphilis is the chancre. Chancres are seen at the site of contact. Since transmission is usually sexual, chancres are seen on the penis, vagina and anus. Lesions can also be seen on the lips and breasts. After an incubation period of between 10 and 90 days (average 3 weeks), this usually single but occasionally multiple lesion develops at the site of initial infection. The chancre begins as an erythematous macule which becomes papular and then ulcerates. The resultant painless chancre has well-defined borders and a rubbery base. Associated with the chancre is regional non-tender adenopathy. Without treatment, the chancre heals within 6–12 weeks [1,2]. In children, chancres are said to be smaller than in adults and less likely to be recognized. However, in adults as in children the presentation may be very atypical. Frequently in adults, chancres are not recognized either because they are atypical, or because they are hidden (e.g. cervical or anal).

Secondary syphilis

Six weeks after the development of a chancre (2 weeks to 6 months), the rash of secondary syphilis develops as a consequence of generalized *T. pallidum* dissemination. The initial chancre may still be present when the secondary eruption occurs. The rash of secondary syphilis is macular, progressing to a papular eruption with a scaly component. The rash can be seen on both flexor and extensor surfaces. Associated with the rash are flat wart-like eruptions (condyloma lata) in intertriginous areas, especially the perineum. Alopecia is also associated with the secondary stage. Constitutional symptoms such as fever and malaise are common [3,4]. The descriptions of acquired syphilis in children include both papular and papulosquamous eruptions with a typical adult distribution including palms and soles as well as a description of moist verrucous plaques in the perianal area and mucous patches in the mouth [5,6]. Rash is a common initial complaint for paediatric patients with acquired syphilis.

Latent syphilis

By definition, syphilis becomes latent after the fading of the secondary rash. The stages are divided into early latent (<1 year) and late latent (>1 year), based on the lower level of transmissability in late latent syphilis. Latent syphilis in children has not been well described.

Acquired syphilis in children is infrequently reported [7–16]. Most cases of acquired syphilis are consistent with abuse. A few cases had a plausible non-abuse related explanation for transmission. Since a modern interpretation of the older literature strongly suggests that most syphilis in children was associated with abuse, most evaluations of sexual abuse now involve an evaluation for syphilis [7–16]. Given the lag between infection and the presence of detectable non-treponemal antibodies, it is suggested that a syphilis serology be performed 6 weeks after an acute episode of sexual abuse to detect a serological response. However, since much sexual abuse is chronic, even a single serological test for syphilis would detect some cases of syphilis if the infection were commonly seen in abused children. Rimsza and Niggemann [16] performed a medical evaluation on 311 sexually abused children who were seen in an emergency room over a 3-year period of time. A Venereal Disease Research Laboratory (VDRL) test was obtained on any patient who was a victim of vaginal intercourse or sodomy. None of the 104 patients who had this test performed had a reactive test. No follow-up serological tests for syphilis were performed. It should be noted that antibiotics which could have had an effect on *T. pallidum* were given to 83 of the 311 patients.

De Jong [17] evaluated 532 victims of sexual abuse over a 3-year period. Patients were evaluated for syphilis on the initial visit and at follow-up. Only one patient had syphilis.

White *et al.* [18] evaluated 409 cases of sexual abuse. In Wake County, North Carolina, 62 of 99 patients were evaluated for syphilis and in other counties, 46 of 310 were evaluated. Five patients had a diagnosis of syphilis in Wake County and one in the other counties. Tests were performed because of the presence of other sexually transmitted diseases in four of the children and because of a chancre in the other. Follow-up testing was not performed [18].

Congenital syphilis

Congenital syphilis is transplacentally acquired and presents either early (<2 years of age) or late (≥2 years of age). The presentation of congenital syphilis can be either a syphilitic stillbirth, an infant with signs and symptoms presenting at birth or an infant with delayed presentation who gradually develops signs and symptoms over the first few months of life. Late congenital syphilis presents with some characteristic finding such as interstitial keratitis. According to the older literature, it is possible to develop late congenital syphilis without any of the signs or symptoms of early congenital syphilis [1,2].

Congenital syphilis is an infection caused by maternal syphilis. At birth, if a mother lacks serological evidence of syphilis, then the signs and symptoms in her infant are not from congenital syphilis. While the presence of non-treponemal antibodies in an infant at birth suggests the diagnosis of passive transfer of maternal antibodies, the rate of false positive and false negative results in infant cord blood and serum would suggest that only a negative maternal test for syphilis at delivery should be used to eliminate congenital syphilis as a diagnostic possibility in the infant [19]. However, there are two flaws in this approach. If the maternal titre is extremely high a false negative result can be obtained (prozone effect). Thus, if an infant has signs and symptoms of congenital syphilis and the mother's serology is reported as negative, that test should be repeated after serial dilution. It is also possible that a mother incubating syphilis will have a negative serology but an infant infected with *T. pallidum*. However, that infant will not have symptoms at birth and by the time the infant presents with symptoms, the mother's serological test should be reactive [20].

In the penicillin era, almost all deaths from congenital syphilis are seen in either stillbirths or those infants who present at birth. While the diagnosis of delayed onset congenital syphilis may not immediately be made, most often therapy is successful since the diagnosis is usually made before the infant becomes seriously ill. In the prepenicillin era, because therapy was not as effective as with penicillin, some infant deaths beyond the first few months of life were associated with early congenital syphilis. In the early 1900s, the death rate for congenital syphilis approached 80% [21].

The diagnosis of congenital syphilis in stillbirths can be made presumptively by performing a syphilis serology on all mothers who have had stillbirths. Serological titres that indicate recent syphilis (rapid plasmin reagin test >1 : 64) probably implicate syphilis as a cause of the fetal death [22]. However, syphilitic stillbirths can be associated with lower titres. Identification of *T. pallidum* in fetal tissue can be used to make a definitive diagnosis.

Syphilis is a multisystem disease. Congenital syphilis presents with similar features to secondary syphilis. Patients can have a rash, hepatosplenomegaly and central nervous system involvement. Although uncommon in secondary syphilis, bone findings are common in congenital syphilis and have been used to make a diagnosis before the other signs of congenital syphilis have developed [23,24].

The rash of congenital syphilis can resemble the papulosquamous eruption of secondary syphilis (Fig. 24.2.1) and features include condyloma lata. Palm and sole involvement (Fig. 24.2.2) may be prominent. In addition, unlike in secondary syphilis, the rash can be vesicular or bullous [1,2]. The presence of snuffles, a muccid sometimes bloody nasal discharge was frequently reported in the prepenicillin era but has not been common in recent congenital syphilis outbreaks [25]. The skin lesions and nasal discharge will reveal the presence of *T. pallidum* and may be a source of infection. Hepatosplenomegaly and findings of abnormal levels of liver enzymes or evidence of cholestasis are seen in congenital syphilis [25]. Many now believe that the hepatic abnormalities are initially made worse by therapy [26]. The liver findings are not specific enough to distinguish congenital syphilis from a number of other congenital infections.

A positive cerebrospinal fluid (CSF) VDRL test in a newborn establishes a diagnosis of congenital syphilis but the overlap between CSF cell counts and protein determinations in infants with and without syphilis is so broad as to make the cell count and protein determination of no

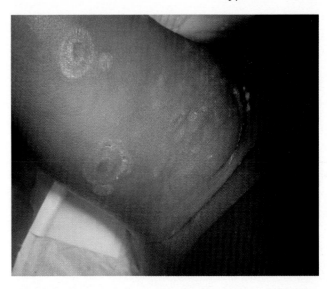

Fig. 24.2.1 Congenital syphilis: papulosquamous rash similar to secondary syphilis.

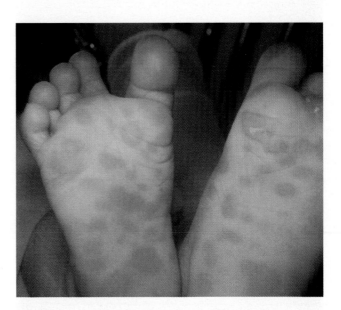

Fig. 24.2.2 Congenital syphilis: involvement of the soles.

value [29]. Detection of *T. pallidum* may also be diagnostic [27,28] (Fig. 24.2.3). The bone lesions of congenital syphilis are those of a metaphysitis with either lucency or increased density seen in the long bones. The development of further involvement with erosion is a later finding. Erosion of the tibia is known as the cat bite or Wimberger's sign. Periosteal involvement is also seen with congenital syphilis [28] (Fig. 24.2.4). Inflammation of bone associated with congenital syphilis can cause pain and impairment of movement. This is known as the pseudoparalysis of Parrot. Occasionally, fractures are seen. Similar findings can be seen in child abuse. Diffuse bone involvement suggests congenital syphilis whilst an asymmetrical finding favours trauma [29]. A serological

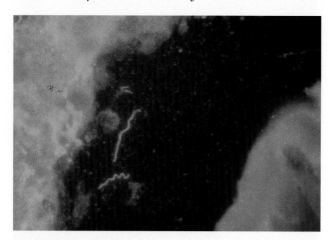

Fig. 24.2.3 Diagnosis by detection of *Treponema pallidum*.

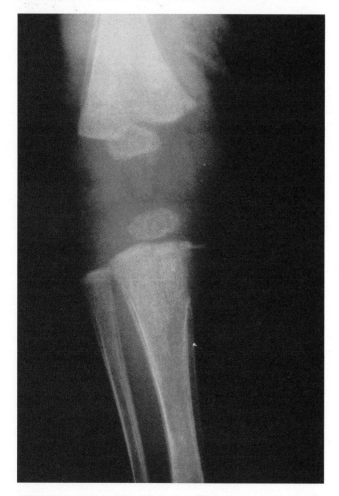

Fig. 24.2.4 Syphilitic periosteal involvement.

test for syphilis performed on the infant's serum will be reactive in cases of congenital syphilis associated with significant bone pathology.

Late onset congenital syphilis is manifest by evidence of continuing infection or evidence of stigmata. Most stigmata of congenital syphilis should be avoidable by adequate treatment but since an infant with late onset congenital syphilis may never exhibit the early signs of congenital syphilis, and since 60% of cases of late onset congenital syphilis were initially detected by serology alone, stigmata could theoretically develop because of treatment failure or lack of therapy. The findings of late onset congenital syphilis as summarized by the American public health service include the following.

1 Interstitial keratitis, a condition which leads to bilateral blindness and tends to develop around the time of puberty.

2 Hutchinson's teeth, a developmental abnormality of the upper and sometimes lower central incisors in which the teeth are notched and small, resulting in a gap between them.

3 Mulberry molars in which the first molars show maldevelopment of the cusps and look like a mulberry.

4 Eighth nerve deafness, which is infrequent and tends to develop around puberty.

5 Neurosyphilis which has all of the manifestations of neurosyphilis in acquired syphilis including meningovascular, parenchymatous and gummatous neurosyphilis.

6 Bone involvement which can be sclerotic (sabre shins, frontal bossing), or lytic (gummas resulting in destruction of the nasal bridge or the palate).

7 Cutaneous involvement from healed syphilitic rhinitis (rhagades or cracks and fissures around the mouth).

8 Cardiovascular lesions as seen in acquired lesions are reported but rare.

9 Clutton's joints, the painless hydrarthrosis of the knees. Hutchinson's triad consists of keratitis, dental abnormalities and deafness. Clutton's joints, interstitital keratitis and deafness are not infectious and do not respond to penicillin.

Diagnosis

Testing of women during pregnancy and at delivery will identify women with syphilis and those infants at risk for congenital syphilis [30–32]. It is more difficult to eliminate the possible diagnosis of congenital syphilis in an infant born to a mother with a reactive test for syphilis, especially if previous test information is not available. Results of serological tests based on endemic treponematoses are not distinguishable from syphilis, and may lead to misinterpretation (see Chapter 5.13). Endemic treponematoses never lead to congenital infections. Those antibodies are always passively acquired. Without a careful history, neither reactive maternal serological findings nor the height of the maternal titre can determine infectivity [32,33]. Following the American Centers for Disease Control (CDC) criteria for STDs one will overtreat some children, but will almost never miss one possible case [20]. These criteria were developed to overcome the missing of a definitive test to identify the still symptom-free infected infant [33].

A diagnosis of infection with *T. pallidum* is made by either the detection of non-specific antibodies (non-treponemal antibodies) with confirmation by the detection of specific antibodies (treponemal antibodies) or the detection of *T. pallidum*. Non-treponemal antibodies are detected using the rapid plasma reagin card or the VDRL test. The tests are reactive, a quantitative titre obtained and the results are confirmed with a specific treponemal test. The specific treponemal tests are considered as confirmatory tests. Current tests include the fluorescent treponemal antibody absorbed (FTA-ABS) test or the microhaemagglutination assay for antibody to *T. pallidum* (MHA-TP). In Europe, immunoglobulin G (IgG) and IgM enzyme immunoassays (EIAs) are also used for the diagnosis of syphilis. Non-standardized immunoblot assays are also used by some investigators [27,28]. The IgM assays have the potential to detect cases of congenital syphilis as well as cases of acquired syphilis. The IgM test may not detect cases of congenital syphilis in which the patient has yet to develop symptoms [28]. *T. pallidum* is detected by either dark-field examination, immunofluorescent antigen detection, the polymerase chain reaction (PCR) or the rabbit infectivity test. These tests approach 100% specificity but have variable sensitivity. They are of most value in the diagnosis of the early stages of congenital and acquired syphilis. The rabbit infectivity test is a useful standard against which to measure these other tests but it is only available in a research setting [27].

Prognosis

Both untreated congenital and acquired syphilis share some sequelae. Early and appropriate therapy results in a good outcome [31]. Whilst there is not a large enough experience with late congenital syphilis to evaluate the effectiveness of penicillin therapy, case reports have not shown penicillin to be helpful [34]. Failures from appropriate therapy of congenital syphilis are not reported but there have been short-term failures of benzathine penicillin therapy. All of the patients have been retreated appropriately [35]. Careful follow-up of all infants at risk of congenital syphilis is essential to ensure that the given treatment was effective [33].

REFERENCES

1 US Public Health Service. *Syphilis: a synopsis*. Washington, DC, US Public Health Service, 1968.
2 Schulz KP *et al.* In: Holmes *et al.*, ed. *Sexually Transmitted Diseases*. New York: McGraw-Hill, 1990.
3 Chapel TA. The signs and symptoms of secondary syphilis. *Sex Transm Dis* 1980; 7: 161–4.
4 Fiumara N. Treatment of secondary syphilis: an evaluation of 204 patients. *Sex Transm Dis* 1977; 4: 96–9.
5 Echols SK, Shupp DL, Schroeter AL. Acquired secondary syphilis in a child. *J Am Acad Dermatol* 1990; 22(2 Pt 1): 313–14.
6 Horowitz S, Chadwick DL. Syphilis as a sole indicator of sexual abuse: two cases with no intervention. *Child Abuse Negl* 1990; 14: 129–32.
7 Waugh JR. Acquired syphilis of infancy and childhood. *Am J Syph Gon Ven Dis* 1938; 22: 607–22.
8 Schoch AG, Long WE. Acquired syphilis in children. *Am J Syph Gon Ven Dis* 1939; 23: 186–7.
9 Smith FR. Acquired syphilis in children. *Am J Gon Ven Dis* 1938; 23: 165–85.
10 Ackerman AB, Goldfaden G, Cosrnides JC. Acquired syphilis in early childhood. *Arch Dermatol* 1972; 106: 92–3.
11 Ginsburg CM. Acquired syphilis in prepubertal children. *Pediatr Infect Dis* 1983; 2: 232–4.
12 Aloi F. Lip syphilitic chancre in a child. *Pediatr Dermatol* 1987; 4: 63 (letter).
13 Goldenring JM. Secondary syphilis in a prepubertal child. Differentiating condylomata lata from condylomata acuminata. *NY State J Med* 1989; 89: 180–1.
14 Tomeh MO, Wilfert CM. Venereal diseases of infants and children at Duke University Medical Center. *N C Med J* 1973; 34: 109–13.
15 Schwarcz SK, Whittington WL. Sexual assault and sexually transmitted diseases: detection and management in adults and children. *Rev Infect Dis* 1990; 12(Suppl. 6): S682–90.
16 Rimsza ME, Niggemann EH. Medical evaluation of sexually abused children: a review of 311 cases. *Pediatrics* 1982; 69: 9–14.
17 De Jong AR. Sexually transmitted diseases in sexually abused children. *Sex Transm Dis* 1986; 13: 123–6.
18 White ST, Loda FA, Ingram DL *et al.* Sexually transmitted diseases in sexually abused children. *Pediatrics* 1983; 72: 16–21.
19 Rawstron SA, Bromberg K. Comparison of maternal and newborn serologic tests for syphilis. *Am J Dis Child* 1991; 145: 1383–8.
20 Dorfman DR, Claser JH. Congenital syphilis presenting in infants after the newborn period. *N Engl J Med* 1990; 323: 1299–302.
21 Carpenter G. *The Syphilis of Children in Every-Day Practice*. New York: William Wood, 1901.
22 Centers for Disease Control and Prevention (1998) Sexually Transmitted diseases treatment guidelines. *MMWR* 1998; 47: 1–111.
23 Ingraham NR. The diagnosis of infantile congenital syphilis during the period of doubt. *Am J Syph Neurol* 1935; 19: 547–80.
24 Cremin BJ, Fisher RM. The lesions of congenital syphilis. *Br J Radiol* 1970; 43: 333–41.
25 Rawstron SA, Jenkins S, Blanchard S, Li PW, Bromberg K. Maternal and congenital syphilis in Brooklyn, NY. Epidemiology, transmission, and diagnosis. *Am J Dis Child* 1983; 147: 727–31.
26 Shah MC, Barton LL. Congenital syphilitic hepatitis. *Pediatr Infect Dis J* 1989; 8: 891–2.
27 Sanchez PJ, Wendel GD Jr, Grimprel E *et al.* Evaluation of molecular methodologies and rabbit infectivity testing for the diagnosis of congenital syphilis and neonatal central nervous system invasion by *Treponema pallidum*. *J Infect Dis* 1993; 167: 148–57.
28 Bromberg K, Rawstron S, Tannis G. Diagnosis of congenital syphilis by combining *Treponema pallidum*-specific IgM detection with immunofluorescent antigen detection for *T. pallidum*. *J Infect Dis* 1993; 168: 238–42.
29 Fiser RH, Kaplan J, Holder JC. Congenital syphilis mimicking the battered child syndrome. How does one tell them apart? *Clin Pediatr (Phila)* 1972; 11: 305–7.
30 Boot JM, Oranje AP, de Groot R *et al.* Congenital syphilis. *Int J STD AIDS* 1992; 3: 161–7.
31 Boot JM, Menke HE, Eijk van RVW *et al.* Congenital syphilis in The Netherlands: cause and parental characteristics. *Genito Urin Med* 1988; 64: 298–302.
32 Boot JM, Oranje AP, Menke HE *et al.* Congenital syphilis in The Netherlands: diagnosis and clinical features. *Genito Urin Med* 1989; 65: 300–3.
33 Glaser JH. Centers for Disease Control and prevention guidelines for congenital syphilis. *J Pediatr* 1996; 129: 488–90.
34 Wiggelinkhuizen J, Mason R. Congenital neurosyphilis and juvenile paresis: a forgotten entity? *Clin Pediatr* 1980; 19: 142.
35 Beck-Sague C, Alexander ER. Failure of benzathine penicillin G treatment in early congenital syphilis. *Pediatr Infect Dis* 1987; 6: 1061–4.

Differential diagnosis

Syphilis is the great imitator. When acquired syphilis in children presents with a primary chancre, the differential diagnosis would include a bacterial skin infection which does not respond to treatment, HSV and chancroid. The rash of secondary syphilis can be confused with any of the papulosquamous disorders with the greatest likelihood of confusion with pityriasis rosea. The systemic manifestations of acquired syphilis are non-specific except for such findings as epitrochlear adenopathy.

Either congenital or acquired syphilis can present with a cerebrospinal pleocytosis. There are very few findings in the CSF that would specifically indicate syphilis other than tabes dorsalis.

The bullous skin findings of congenital syphilis can be seen with epidermolysis bullosa, dermatitis herpetiformis or staphylococcal infection [1]. Hepatosplenomegaly can be seen in any of the congenital infections such as toxoplasmosis, rubella or cytomegalovirus. The anaemia of congenital syphilis can be seen in any other cause of hydrops fetalis, especially parvovirus infection. The bone lesions of congenital syphilis can be confused with either infection or child abuse.

REFERENCE

1 Schulz KF *et al.* In: Holmes *et al.*, ed. Sexually Transmitted Diseases. New York: McGraw-Hill, 1990.

Treatment

Treatment of congenital syphilis either involves:

1 adequate treatment of the mother before pregnancy;

2 adequate treatment of the mother during pregnancy, preferably in the first half of pregnancy but definitely before the last month of pregnancy; or

3 adequate treatment of the infant either at delivery or postnatally when symptoms develop. Any strategy involving maternal therapy must involve therapy of all sexual partners or the treated mother will become reinfected.

Adequate maternal therapy is defined as either one injection of benzathine penicillin (2.4 million units) for early syphilis (primary and secondary syphilis), or 3 weekly injections of benzathine penicillin to a total dose of 7.2 million units. As a result of this therapy, patients with early syphilis should show a fourfold decrease in nontreponemal titre or return to become negative. Patients with late syphilis should have stable or declining titres of less than or equal to 1:4 [1].

Most pregnant women with reactive syphilis serologies do not fit into any of these categories, frequently because an appropriate fall in titre is not documentable before delivery. Thus, many infants at risk for congenital syphilis are treated for congenital syphilis because adequate therapy in their mother cannot be established with certainty.

The therapy of congenital syphilis is 10–14 days of penicillin G (50 000/kg/dose every 12 h for the first week of life and every 8 h thereafter). Although therapy with intravenous penicillin G is one option, the authors' experience with procaine penicillin 50 000 units/kg given intramuscularly daily for 10 days has been good. There have been no reported treatment failures with either penicillin G or procaine penicillin while therapy with benzathine penicillin as a single injection has resulted in some treatment failures [2,3]. The cost–benefit analysis of treatment with benzathine penicillin with discharge thereafter versus 10 days of parenteral therapy has yet to be determined [4]. As in acquired syphilis, an appropriate fall in the nontreponemal serology is expected. Infants who are treated late in the course of their disease may never become seronegative [5]. Non-penicillin therapies of congenital syphilis have not been evaluated and should not be used. Appropriate doses of ampicillin can be considered as equivalent to penicillin [1].

REFERENCES

1 Centers for Disease Control. 1993 sexually transmitted diseases treatment guidelines. Centers for Disease Control and Prevention. *MMWR* 1993; 42(RR-14): 1–102.

2 Beck-Sague C, Alexander ER. Failure of benzathine penicillin G treatment in early congenital syphilis. *Pediatr Infect Dis J* 1987; 6: 1061–4.

3 Hardy JB, Hardy PH. Oppenheimer EH, Ryan SJ Jr, Sheff RN. Failure of penicillin in a newborn with congenital syphilis. *J Am Med Assoc* 1970; 212: 1345–9.

4 de Lissovoy G, Zenilman J, Nelson KE, Ahmed F, Celentano DD. The cost of a preventable disease: estimated US national medical expenditures for congenital syphilis, 1990. *Publ Health Rep* 1995; 110: 403–9.

5 Smith FRJ. Congenital syphilis children, results of treatment, 521 patients. Part I. *Am J Syph Neurol* 1935; 532–46.

Gonorrhoea

Definition

Neisseria gonorrhoeae (gonococci) are non-motile, non-spore-forming Gram-negative diplococci (they grow in pairs). Gonococcal infection in children is acquired either perinatally, from an infected mother to a newborn, or by intimate contact (almost always sexual) in older children.

History

Gonorrhoea is one of the oldest known human illnesses. While references to urethral discharge are made in the Old Testament, and in the fourth and fifth centuries BC Hippocrates wrote of gonorrhoea, the term gonorrhoea ('flow of seed/semen') was not introduced until the second century by Galen. The causal organism of gonorrhoea was finally identified in 1879 by Neisser, who also discovered that the agent could be found in cases of ophthalmia neonatorum. Leistikow and Loeffler in 1882 were the first to culture the organism, and around the same time in 1881 Credé, who had been working on neonatal ophthalmia, started to use silver nitrate instillation into the eyes of newborns to prevent gonococcal ophthalmia, a common cause of blindness. The use of silver nitrate prophylaxis reduced the incidence of neonatal gonococcal ophthalmia from more than 10% to 0.5% [1]. Epidemic vulvovaginitis in girls was a common disease in the early 20th century before the advent of penicillin therapy, and was believed to be extremely contagious, requiring only superficial contact for transmission [2]. However, careful study of infected girls in controlled circumstances showed that gonococcal vulvovaginitis was not contagious (no transmission was seen from infected to non-infected girls on a ward, although there was no effective treatment at that time) [2]. The conclusion that 'transmission of the disease requires intimate contact between an infected adult or child and non-infected child', remains today.

Aetiology and pathogenesis

Gonorrhoea is an STD which can only be acquired by intimate contact, almost always sexual [3]. Humans are the only natural host and direct mucous membrane contact is necessary to spread disease [4]. Studies of STDs in various populations of children being evaluated for sexual abuse have shown rates varying from 2.8% [5], 4.7% [6], 7.4% [7] to 18.2% and 36.8% [8] the range being a function of the prevalence of *N. gonorrhoeae* in the community. In addition a heightened suspicion for sexual abuse in recent times has resulted in an apparent decreased prevalence due to more evaluations in asymptomatic children.

In the neonatal period infection is acquired perinatally from the mother by passage through an infected birth canal. In older prepubertal children, the infection is almost always sexually acquired, usually by sexual abuse from an adult, occasionally by sexual play between children [9], although even in these cases there is often abuse or exploitation of younger children by older ones who introduce the infection [10]. In older postpubertal children, consensual sexual activity is the usual source of infection, although the sexual activity can still be associated with abuse [11]. The role of fomites in the spread of disease is not clear, but is probably extremely uncommon. The only well-documented spread of gonococcal infection in a non-sexual manner was a hospital outbreak of neonatal gonococcal infection probably spread by contaminated rectal thermometers [12].

Careful interviewing enabled a history of sexual contact to be elicited in 44 of 45 1–9 year olds with gonorrhoea [13]. Similarly, a history of sexual contact was obtained in 90–100% [5,14] of children 5–12 years of age with gonorrhoea, and 35–75% [5,14] of children 1–5 years of age. If gonorrhoea is highly associated with sexual contact in verbal children, it follows that this is the most likely mode of transmission in non-verbal children. Repeated interviews by sympathetic and skilled workers may be necessary to elicit a history of abuse [15]. Sometimes the history of abuse may not be revealed until years later [16].

Pathology

Gonococcal infections start with the organism adhering to the mucosal cells which is mediated by pili and other surface proteins. Stratified squamous cells can resist invasion, but columnar epithelium is susceptible. This explains the distribution of infection: urethra, Skene's and Bartholin's glands, cervix and fallopian tubes in females; urethra, prostate, seminal vesicles and epididymis in males; and rectum, pharynx and conjunctivae in both sexes. Prepubertal girls are susceptible to vaginal infections with *N. gonorrhoeae* because of the alkaline pH and lack of oestrogenization, whereas postpubertal girls develop cervical not vaginal infections. The organism is engulfed by endocytosis of the cell into vacuoles, where they may replicate and eventually exit from the basal surface of the epithelial cell to the subepithelial tissues [17]. There is a marked inflammatory response at the site of inoculation with a polymorphonuclear leucocyte response, purulent material being exuded from the surface and submucosal microabscess formation.

The pathology of the skin lesions in disseminated gonococcal infection (DGI) consists of haemorrhage, vasculitis and a moderately heavy inflammatory cell presence, mostly polymorphonuclear leucocytes but a variable presence of mononuclear cells [18]. Thrombosis of the small venules and arterioles of the dermis is common. Epidermal changes range from minimal oedema with few polymorphonuclear cells and red blood cells to intradermal vesicles or pustules. The organisms are only detected in the skin lesions by Gram stain or culture in about 10% of cases [19]. However, the presence of organisms can be detected in about 57% of skin lesions with the use of immunofluorescent stains [19].

Clinical features

Infection in infants

In newborns, the disease is acquired perinatally from an infected mother during delivery through an infected birth canal with direct mucosal contact from infected cervical secretions of the mother to mucous membranes (conjunctiva, pharynx) of the baby. Without prophylaxis, neonatal gonococcal conjunctivitis occurred in 42% of babies born to mothers with gonorrhoea, with 7% also having orogastric contamination with *N. gonorrhoeae* [20]. The prevalence of maternal disease varies depending on the prevalence of gonorrhoea in the community at any particular time. The rate of maternal gonorrhoea in most American populations is less than 5%, though rates in Africa are higher (5–10% or more). Prenatal care with screening and treatment is effective at preventing neonatal infections in high-risk populations. In addition, neonatal ocular prophylaxis can reduce the incidence of gonococcal ophthalmia in newborns with infected mothers by 83–93% [21]. However, universal screening of all pregnant women and neonatal ocular prophylaxis are not cost-effective when maternal gonococcal infections are infrequent (<1%) as is found in many industrialized countries. In the USA both universal maternal screening and neonatal ocular prophylaxis are used to decrease the likelihood of neonatal infection, with neonatal ocular prophylaxis required by law in most states.

Conjunctivitis is the most common manifestation in newborns [22]. The conjunctivitis usually presents at 2–5 days of life (range 0–28 days), initially as a watery conjunctival exudate which rapidly becomes purulent, thick and may be blood-tinged. The conjunctiva and eyelid are oedematous, and if the infection goes untreated keratitis, iridocyclitis, corneal ulceration and perforation can ensue with blindness as a consequence. Other manifestations seen at this age are other local infections such as scalp abscesses (associated with scalp electrodes), or systemic infections caused by gonococcaemia and subsequent seeding of organisms to other areas, for example sepsis, arthritis, meningitis and pneumonia. Gonococcal infections may also be asymptomatic, with cultures positive from the oropharynx, vagina and rectum. The most common manifestation of systemic infections in neonates is arthritis. This presents between 1 and 4 weeks after delivery. In the largest series [12], the neonates were often irritable and febrile, but neonates may also present with joint swelling alone, with no systemic findings [23]. Some had skin lesions (not described) and superficial abscesses before they developed arthritis. The arthritis was usually polyarticular, with wrists, knee and shoulder joints most commonly affected.

Older children

Gonococcal infections in older children are usually local infections (vaginitis, urethritis, conjunctivitis). Disseminated infections are uncommon but do occur in preadolescent children, with arthritis and DGI being the most common manifestations. However, many gonococcal infections are asymptomatic, with 15–44% of genital infections in children being asymptomatic [5,6].

The most common manifestation is vulvovaginitis. This usually presents as a profuse purulent vaginal discharge ranging from white, cream, yellow or green in colour which stains the underwear. However, the vaginal

discharge may be minimal and confused with a benign discharge [24]. Associated pruritus, vulval erythema and dysuria may also by present [25]. Rarely prepubertal girls may have lower abdominal pain and fever in association with gonococcal vaginitis suggesting ascending pelvic infection [26]. Symptoms are usually present for less than a week (median 3 days), but some children have symptoms for more than 2 weeks or even months before they are brought for evaluation. Gonococcal infections are less frequent in boys and the usual presentation is a urethral discharge associated with urethritis. The discharge may be copious or scant, and rarely may be associated with penile oedema [27] or the testicular swelling of epididymitis [25]. Dysuria may also be present. Gonococcal conjunctivitis can also present outside the neonatal period, usually in association with autoinoculation from a genital infection in the same patient. Conjunctivitis is often severe with profuse purulent discharge, chemosis, eyelid oedema and ulcerative keratitis, and presentations may mimic orbital cellulitis. On rare occasions, the conjunctivitis is the only gonococcal infection present, and the source of the infection is obviously from another person, often in the family [28]. The method of transmission in these cases is not clear, but non-sexual transmission is unlikely.

Pharyngeal and rectal infections are fairly common, but prevalence varies in different populations [25], probably reflecting sexual practices. Pharyngeal infections are seen in 15–54% of children with gonococcal infections [25,29]. Almost all pharyngeal and rectal infections are asymptomatic, and are detected by routinely screening these sites in children who are suspected to have been sexually abused, or who have genital discharges [30]. Rarely, pharyngeal infections are symptomatic [31]. Rectal infections are common in girls, probably due to the proximity of the vagina and anus with the possibility of contamination of the anus with vaginal discharge. Rectal cultures may be positive in up to 50% of girls with positive vaginal gonococcal cultures [25]. Most rectal infections in girls are asymptomatic, but occasionally there are symptoms [32]. The symptoms seen are of a purulent rectal discharge with rectal pain, blood or mucus in the stools and perianal itching or burning. Symptomatic rectal infections are associated with penile-rectal penetration. Rectal infections are rarely seen in boys, and are associated with anal intercourse.

Infection in adolescents is very similar to that seen in adults. In girls, the presentation is with cervicitis, DGI, perihepatitis (Fitz–Hugh–Curtis syndrome), salpingitis and occasionally proctitis. In boys, urethritis, epididymitis and occasionally proctitis are the usual presentations. The most serious potential complication of gonococcal infection in adolescent girls is salpingitis and pelvic inflammatory disease (PID), which is seen in about 15% of adolescent girls with gonococcal infections.

DGI can be seen in the adolescent population, although it is more common in adults, with ages 15–35 years having the highest risk for DGI. DGI is more common in women than men, and more common during the first few days of menstruation and during pregnancy. DGI can result from a primary infection at any site including the cervix, urethra, anal canal, pharynx and conjunctiva. The presentation of DGI is usually with dermatitis, arthropathy or both. Skin involvement is seen in about 50–70% of patients with DGI [33]. The skin lesions are usually multiple, erythematous, maculopapular, vesicular, haemorrhagic, pustular or necrotic lesions. They often progress from papules to pustular, haemorrhagic or necrotic lesions, and the presence of lesions in different stages of evolution is typical of DGI [33]. The lesions are usually on the extremities and number from between one and 40, and range in size from 1 to 20 mm [34].

Joint symptoms are seen at the initial presentation of DGI in more than 90% of patients [33]. The most commonly involved joints are the knees, ankles, wrists, elbows and the small joints of the hands and feet. Polyarthralgia is common and may be migratory. The symptoms range from mild to severe and include arthralgias with no inflammation to arthritis with synovial effusion and even joint destruction. Tenosynovitis is frequent [35]. It has been hypothesized that DGI consists of an early bacteraemic stage which if left untreated leads to a septic joint stage [33,35], though not all patients fit this picture. Some bacteriological findings are consistent with this hypothesis, for example blood cultures are often positive in the early phase and joint fluid may be culture positive in the later stage. Positive blood and synovial fluid cultures are almost always mututally exclusive [35].

Diagnosis

Since the diagnosis of gonococcal infections in children has serious medicolegal implications, it is essential to use only standard culture systems for diagnostic purposes in children [36]. Non-culture gonococcal tests such as Gram-stained smears, EIA tests and DNA probes should not be used for diagnostic purposes in children. Although Gram-stained smears of specimens can be useful in clinical practice, and are recommended for screening, they are inadequate for definitive diagnostic purposes. Gonococci have complex growth requirements, but grow well on enriched chocolate agar. However, isolating gonococci from sites with many saprophytic bacteria is easier with selective media containing antimicrobial agents that inhibit the growth of saprophytic bacteria, but permit the growth of most gonococci. Therefore, specimens from the vagina, urethra, pharynx, rectum or conjunctiva should be streaked onto selective media for isolation of *N. Gonorrhoeae*, such as Thayer–Martin media or modified Thayer–Martin media. Specimens from normally sterile sites such as synovial fluid, blood or CSF should only be inoculated onto non-selective media (enriched chocolate agar). Whenever possible, the culture plate should be inoculated immediately with the specimen at room temperature, and placed in a carbon dioxide enriched environment (a candle extinction jar or carbon dioxide incubator) for incubation. Confirmation of isolates as *N. gonorrhoeae* should include at least two tests that include different principles, for example, biochemical, enzyme substrate or serological. Misidentification of organisms as *N. gonorrhoeae* has occurred and confirmation of isolates is essential before action is taken regarding accusations of sexual abuse [37]. In addition, all isolates should be preserved to allow for repeated testing or additional testing in the future. This can be useful in individual cases or outbreak situations to determine the likely perpetrator [38]. All gonococcal isolates should be tested for β-lactamase production as well as screened for additional resistance to penicillin and tetracycline.

Prognosis

The prognosis for most children with gonococcal disease is excellent, but complications can occur, especially when the child is not brought to medical attention promptly. In neonates with conjunctivitis, the prognosis for normal eyesight is excellent providing therapy is given in a timely fashion. Previously, neonatal gonococcal conjunctivitis was a significant cause of blindness, but this is no longer seen. The prognosis for preadolescent children with gonococcal infections from sexual abuse is again excellent. Young girls with gonococcal vaginitis rarely have any complications, although ascending pelvic infections have been described which responded well to parenteral antibiotics. Unfortunately, the psychological sequelae of sexual abuse, and the turmoil in the family produced by suspicions and allegations are largely unknown, but are probably lifelong. The prognosis for gonococcal infections in adolescent girls is not as good. Many gonococcal infections are associated with salpingitis, and sequelae of this can include ectopic pregnancies and infertility. DGI sequelae are uncommon even with significant joint involvement.

Differential diagnosis

In the newborn period, gonococcal conjunctivitis may be confused with conjunctivitis caused by other bacteria or viruses or even chemical conjunctivitis secondary to prophylactic medication instilled in the eye at birth. The most common organism responsible for neonatal conjunctivitis is CT. Other bacteria responsible for neonatal conjunctivitis are *Staphylococcus aureus*, *Haemophilus* species, *S. pneumoniae*, *Streptococcus* group A, *Pseudomonas* and enteric Gram-negative organisms. Viral conjunctivitis can be caused by HSV type 1 and 2. It is more likely to be associated with keratitis.

The differential diagnosis of vulvovaginitis in prepubescent girls includes infection with group A *Streptococcus*, *N. meningitidis*, *H. influenzae*, pathogenic enteric organisms such as *Shigella* species and *Yersinia*, and non-specific vaginitis caused by poor hygiene and growth of usually non-pathogenic bowel flora in the vagina. Foreign bodies in the vagina can also give a similar picture as can threadworm (*Enterobius vermicularis*) infestation.

The differential diagnosis for urethritis and epididymitis in boys includes other STDs, such as CT and *Ureaplasma urealyticum*, as well as enteric Gram-negative infections.

Cervicitis, salpingitis and PID in adolescent girls can also be seen with infection with CT, and anaerobic infections.

Treatment

Penicillin was the treatment of choice until the spread of β-lactamase producing gonorrhoea worldwide precluded this as an initial treatment option. However, third-generation cephalosporins are now first-line therapy in children and experience with these drugs has been very favourable. In adults, quinolones are also first-line therapy, but these are not approved for use in children less than 18 years of age due to effects on growth cartilage seen in animal experiments.

In infants with gonococcal ophthalmia neonatorum, the recommended regimen is ceftriaxone 25–50 mg/kg given intravenously or intramuscularly in a single dose not to exceed 125 mg [36]. Although one dose of ceftriaxone is sufficient for gonococcal conjunctivitis, some paediatricians prefer to continue the antibiotics until cultures are negative at 48–72 h. Frequent irrigation of the eye with topical saline is also recommended. Topical antibiotics are not necessary [36].

Disseminated gonococcal infection in infants is also treated with ceftriaxone 25–50 mg/kg/day given intravenously or intramuscularly in a single daily dose, but here treatment is continued for 7 days, or 10–14 days if meningitis is documented. Alternative treatment is cefotaxime 25 mg/kg given intravenously every 12 h for 7 days, with duration of 10–14 days if meningitis is documented [36].

Infants born to mothers with untreated gonococcal infections are at high risk for infection and it is therefore recommended that they received prophylactic therapy with a single dose of ceftriaxone 25–50 mg/kg not exceeding 125 mg [36].

Prophylaxis for gonococcal ophthalmia neonatorum is recommended for all newborns in the USA, and is required by law in most American states. Recommended ocular prophylaxis includes silver nitrate (1%) aqueous solution or erythromycin (0.5%) ophthalmic ointment or tetracycline (1%) ointment each in a single application instilled into the eyes of every neonate as soon as possible after delivery, regardless of the type of delivery [36]. In some countries (e.g. The Netherlands), this approach is not recommended, because too often toxic side-effects (etching), of the (concentrated) aqueous solution are observed.

Gonococcal infections in older prepubertal children with uncomplicated vulvovaginitis, cervicitis, urethritis, pharyngitis or proctitis is with a single dose of ceftriaxone. The dose of ceftriaxone is 125 mg in those weighing less than 45 kg, and 250 mg in those weighing more than 45 kg. An alternative regimen for patients allergic to ceftriaxone is spectinomycin 40 mg/kg (maximum 2 g) given intramuscularly in a single dose. Spectinomycin is not as effective for pharyngeal gonococcal infections [37].

In children who have disseminated gonococcal infections with bacteraemia, arthritis or meningitis, the recommended regimen for children weighing less than 45 kg is ceftriaxone 50 mg/kg/day (maximum 1 g) given intramuscularly or intravenously in a single dose daily for 7 days. For children with meningitis the maximum dose is 2 g and the duration is extended to 10–14 days [36].

Follow-up cultures from infected sites should be repeated to document adequate therapy. This is important since reinfection is not uncommon. Parenteral third-generation cephalosporins and spectinomycin are the only recommended therapies in children. Oral cephalosporins have been successfully used in adults, but have not been adequately evaluated to recommend their use in children. In addition to treatment for their gonococcal infection, children should be evaluted for coinfection with other STDs, particularly CT and syphilis.

REFERENCES

1 Forbes GB, Forbes GM. Silver nitrate and the eyes of the newborn. *Am J Dis Child* 1971; 121: 1–4.
2 Rice JL, Cohn A, Steer A, Adler EL. Recent investigations on gonococcal vaginitis. *J Am Med Assoc* 1941; 117: 1766–9.
3 Neinstein LS, Goldenring J, Carpenter S. Nonsexual transmission of sexually transmitted diseases: an infrequent occurrence. *Pediatrics* 1984; 74: 67–76.
4 Nazarian LF. The current prevalence of gonococcal infections in children. *Pediatrics* 1967; 39: 372–7.
5 Ingram DL, Everett VD, Lyna PR *et al.* Epidemiology of adult sexually transmitted disease agents in children being evaluated for sexual abuse. *Pediatr Infect Dis J* 1992; 11: 945–50.
6 DeJong AR. Sexually transmitted diseases in sexually abused children. *Sex Trans Dis* 1986; 13: 123–6.
7 Rimsza ME, Niggemann EH. Medical evaluation of sexually abused children: a review of 311 cases. *Pediatrics* 1982; 69: 8–14.
8 White ST, Loda FA, Ingram DL, Pearson A. Sexually transmitted diseases in sexually abused children. *Pediatrics* 1983; 72: 16–21.
9 Potterat JJ, Markewich GS, King RD, Merecicky LR. Child-to-child transmission of gonorrhea: report of asymptomatic genital infection in a boy. *Pediatrics* 1986; 78: 711–12.
10 Gunby P. Childhood gonorrhea—but no sexual abuse. *J Am Med Assoc* 1980; 244: 1652.
11 Vermund SH, Alexander-Rodriguez T, Macleod S. History of sexual abuse in incarcerated adolescents with gonorrhea or syphilis. *J Adolesc Health Care* 1990; 11: 449–52.

12 Cooperman MB. Gonococcus arthritis in infancy. *Am J Dis Child* 1927; 33: 932–48.

13 Branch G, Paxton R. A study of gonococcal infections among infants and children. *Publ Health Rep* 1965; 80: 347–52.

14 Ingram DL, White ST, Durfee MF, Pearson AW. Sexual contact in children with gonorrhea. *Am J Dis Child* 1982; 136: 994–6.

15 Farrell MK, Billmire E, Shamroy JA, Hammond JG. Prepubertal gonorrhea: a multidisciplinary approach. *Pediatrics* 1981; 67: 151–3.

16 Ingram DL. The gonococcus and the toilet seat revisited. *Pediatr Infect Dis J* 1989; 8: 191.

17 Dallabetta G, Hook EW. Gonococcal infections. *Infect Dis Clin NA* 1987; 1: 25–54.

18 Shapiro L, Teisch JA, Brownstein MH. Dermatopathology of chronic gonococcal sepsis. *Arch Dermatol* 1973; 107: 403–6.

19 Tronca E, Handsfield HH, Wiesner PJ *et al.* Demonstration of *N. gonorrhoeae* with fluorescent antibody in patients with disseminated gonococcal infection. *J Infect Dis* 1974; 129: 583–6.

20 Laga M, Nzanze H, Brunham R *et al.* Epidemiology of ophthalmia neonatorum in Kenya. *Lancet* 1986; ii: 1145–9.

21 Laga M, Plummer FA, Piot P *et al.* Prophylaxis of gonococcal and chlamydial ophthalmia neonatorum. A comparison of silver nitrate and tetracycline. *N Engl J Med* 1988; 318: 653–7.

22 Desenclos J-C, Garrity D, Scaggs M *et al.* Gonococcal infection of the newborn in Florida, 1984–89. *Sex Transm Dis J* 1992; 19: 105–10.

23 Kleiman MB, Lamb GA. Gonococcal arthritis in a newborn infant. *Pediatrics* 1973; 52: 265–86.

24 Michalowski B. Difficulties of diagnosis and treatment of gonorrhoea in young girls. *Br J Vener Dis* 1961; 37: 142–4.

25 Nelson JD, Mohs E, Dajani A, Plotkin S. Gonorrhea in preschool and school-aged children. Report of the Prepubertal Gonorrhea Cooperative Study Group. *J Am Med Assoc* 976; 236: 1359–64.

26 Burry VF. Gonococcal vulvovaginitis and possible peritonitis in prepubertal girls. *Am J Dis Child* 1971; 121: 536–7.

27 Fleisher G, Hodge D, Cromie W. Penile edema in childhood gonorrhea. *Ann Emerg Med* 1908; 9: 314–15.

28 Lewis LS, Glauser TA, Joffe MD. Gonococcal conjunctivitis in prepubertal children. *Am J Dis Child* 1990; 144: 546–8.

29 Groothuis JR, Bischoff MC, Jauregui LE. Pharyngeal gonorrhea in young children. *Pediatr Infect Dis J* 1983; 2: 99–101.

30 Rawstron SA, Hammerschlag MR, Gullans C, Cuffnings M, Sierra M. Ceftriaxone treatment of penicillinase-producing *Neisseria gonorrhoeae* infections in children. *Pediatr Infect Dis J* 1989; 8: 445–8.

31 Abbott SL. Gonococcal tonsillitis—pharyngitis in a 5-year-old girl. *Pediatrics* 1973; 52: 287–9.

32 Speck WT, Lawsky AR. Symptomatic anorectal gonorrhea in an adolescent female. *Am J Dis Child* 1971; 122: 438–9.

33 Ahmed H, Ilardi I, Antognoli A, Leone F, Sebastiani A, Amiconi G. An epidemic of 33. Disseminated gonococcal infection. *Clin Obstet Gynecol* 1975; 18: 131–43.

34 Barr J, Danielson D. Septic gonococcal dermatitis. *Br Med J* 1971; 1: 482–5.

35 O'Brien JP, Goldenberg DL, Rice PA. Disseminated gonococcal infection: a prospective analysis of 49 patients and a review of pathophysiology and immune mechanisms. *Medicine* 1983; 62: 395–406.

36 Centers for Disease Control and Prevention. 1993 Sexually Transmitted Diseases Treatment Guidelines. *MMWR* 1993; 42 (no. RR14)56–67: 99–102.

37 Whittington WL, Rice RJ, Biddle JW, Knapp JS. Incorrect identification of *Neisseria gonorroeae* from infants and children. *Pediatr Infect Dis J* 1988; 7: 3–10.

38 Ahmed Hi, Ilardi I, Antognoli A, Leone F, Sebastiani A, Amiconi G. An epidemic of *Neisseria gonorroeae* in a Somali orphanage. *Int J STD AIDS* 1992; 3: 52–3.

39 Judson FN, Ehret JM, Handsfield HH. Comparative study of ceftriaxone and spectinomycin for treatment of pharyngeal and anorectal gonorrhea. *J Am Med Assoc* 1985; 253: 1417–19.

Chlamydia trachomatis infections

Definition and microbiology

CT causes urethritis in males and urethritis and cervicitis in females. Complications include ascending infections.

The genus *Chlamydia* is a group of obligate intracellular parasites with a unique developmental cycle with morphologically distinct infectious and reproductive forms. All members of the genus have a Gram-negative envelope without peptidoglycan, share a genus-specific lipopolysaccharide antigen and utilize host adenosine triphosphate (ATP) for the synthesis of chlamydial protein [1]. The genus now contains three species: *C. psittaci, C. pneumoniae* and *C. pecorum.* There are 15 known serotypes of CT. A chlamydial developmental cycle involves an infectious, metabolically inactive extracellular form (elementary body) and a non-infectious, metabolically active intracellular form (reticulate body). Elementary bodies, which are 200–400 mm in diameter, attach to the host cell by a process of electrostatic binding and are taken into the cell by endocytosis that is not dependent on the microtubule system. Within the host cell, the elementary body remains within a membrane-lined phagosome. Fusion of the phagosome with the host cell lysosome does not occur. The elementary bodies then differentiate into reticulate bodies that undergo binary fusion. After approximately 36 h the reticulate bodies differentiate into elementary bodies. At about 48 h, release may occur by cytolysis, or by a process of exocytosis or extrusion of the whole inclusion, leaving the host cell intact [1].

REFERENCE

1 Schachter J. The intracellular life of *Chlamydia. Curr Top Microbiol Immunol* 1988; 138: 109–39.

History

At the turn of the 20th century, there was no screening of expectant mothers for STDs, no instillation of prophylactic eyedrops and no antibiotic treatment for established infections. In this period, the term ophthalmia neonatorum was for all practical purposes synonymous with gonococcal conjunctivitis. As neonatal conjunctivitis came under control with silver nitrate prophylaxis, the importance of another form of ophthalmia neonatorum termed 'inclusion blennorrhoea' was noted. The relationship between maternal genital infection and conjunctivitis of the newborn associated with inclusion bodies within epithelial cells was established by Lindner, Halberstader, Von Prowazek and others [1]. It was not until the 1950s that CT was isolated from an infant with inclusion blennorrhoea [2]. In 1967, Schachter *et al.* further emphasized the relationship of sexual transmission of the infection in the parents of infants of inclusion conjunctivitis [3].

Respiratory infection in infants due to CT was probably first reported by Botsztejn in 1941 who described an entity he called pertussoid eosinophilic pneumonia [4]. However, it was not until 1975 that Schachter *et al.* [5]

isolated CT from the respiratory tract of an infant with pneumonia. The syndrome of infantile chlamydial pneumonia was further characterized by Beem and Saxon in 1977 [6]. CT pneumonia is probably the most prevalent sexually transmitted infection in the USA today [7]. The American CDC estimates that the number of new CT infections exceeds 4 million, annually [6]. The prevalence of chlamydial infection is more weakly associated with socioeconomic status, urban/rural residence and race/ethnicity than gonorrhoea and syphilis. Prevalences of CT infection are consistently greater than 5% among sexually active, adolescent and young adult women attending outpatient clinics, regardless of the region of the country, location of the clinic (urban/rural) and the race or ethnicity of the population. Among sexually active adolescents, prevalences commonly exceed 10% and may exceed 20% [8]. Decreasing age at first intercourse and increasing age of marriage have contributed importantly to the higher prevalence of CT infection. Infection with CT tends to be asymptomatic and of long duration. If a pregnant woman has an active infection during delivery, the infant may acquire the infection, developing either conjunctivitis or pneumoniae. Rarely, children may also acquire chlamydial infection as a result of sexual abuse.

REFERENCES

1 Thygeson P, Stone W. Epidemiology of inclusion conjunctivitis. *Arch Ophthalmol* 1942; 27: 91–122.
2 Jones BR, Collier LH, Smith CH *et al*. Isolation of virus from inclusion blennorrhoea. *Lancet* 1959; i: 902–5.
3 Schachter J, Rose L, Dawson CR *et al*. Comparison of procedures for laboratory diagnosis of oculogenital infections with inclusion conjunctivitis agents. *Am J Epidemiol* 1967; 85: 443–8.
4 Botsztejn A. Die pertussoide, eosinophile pneumonie des Sauglings. Benigne subakute afebrile hilifugale pneumonie des untergewichtigen Sauglings im ersten trimeron mit starker eosinophilie und pertussisahnlichem husten. *Ann Paediatr* 1941; 157: 28–46.
5 Schachter J, Lum L, Gooding CA *et al*. *J Pediatr* 1975; 87: 779–80.
6 Beem MO, Saxon EM. Respiratory tract colonization and a distinctive pneumonia syndrome in infants infected with *Chlamydia trachomatis*. *N Engl J Med* 1977; 296: 306–10.
7 Centers for Disease Control and Prevention. Recommendations for the prevention and management of *Chlamydia trachomatis* infections. *MMWR* 1993; 42(RR-12): 1–39.
8 Hammerschlag MR, Golden NH, Oh MK *et al*. Single dose azithromycin for the treatment of genital chlamydial infections in adolescents. *J Pediatr* 1993; 122: 961–5.

Clinical features

Infections in infants

Pregnant women who have cervical infection with CT can transmit the infection to their infants who may subsequently develop neonatal conjunctivitis and pneumonia. Epidemiological evidence strongly suggests that the infant acquires chlamydial infection from the mother during vaginal delivery [1]. Infection after caesarean section is rare and usually occurs after early rupture of the amniotic membrane. There is no evidence supporting postnatal acquisition from the mother or other family members. Approximately 50–75% of infants born to infected women will become infected at one or more anatomical sites, including the conjunctiva, nasopharynx, rectum and vagina.

Inclusion conjunctivitis

CT is the most frequent identifiable infectious cause of neonatal conjunctivitis and the major clinical manifestation of neonatal chlamydial infection. Approximately 30–50% of infants born to *Chlamydia*-positive mothers will develop conjunctivitis. CT is identified in 30–40% of infants less than 1 month of age presenting with conjunctivitis [2]. The incubation period is 5–14 days after delivery, or earlier if there has been premature rupture of membranes. Infection is rare following caesarean section with intact membranes but can happen. At least 50% of infants with chlamydial conjunctivitis will also have nasopharyngeal infection. The presentation is extremely variable ranging from mild conjunctival infection with scant mucoid discharge to severe conjunctivitis with copious purulent discharge, chemosis and pseudomembrane formation. The conjunctiva can be very friable and may bleed when stroked with a swab. Chlamydial conjunctivitis needs to be differentiated from gonococcal ophthalmia in some infants, especially those born to mothers who did not receive any prenatal care, had gonorrhoea during pregnancy or abused drugs. There can be an overlap in both incubation periods and presentation.

Pneumonia

The nasopharynx is the most frequent site of perinatally acquired chlamydial infection. Approximately 70% of infected infants will have positive cultures at this site. The majority of these nasopharyngeal infections are asymptomatic and may persist for 3 years or more [1,3,4]. Chlamydial pneumonia develops in only about 30% of infants with nasopharyngeal infection. In those who develop pneumonia, the presentation and clinical findings are very characteristic. The children usually present between 4 and 12 weeks of age. A few cases have been reported presenting as early as 2 weeks of age, but no cases have been seen beyond 4 months. The infants frequently have a history of cough and congestion with an absence of fever. On physical examination the infant is tachypnoeic and rales are heard on auscultation of the chest; wheezing is distinctly uncommon. There are no specific radiographic findings except hyperinflation [5,6]. Significant laboratory findings include peripheral eosinophilia (>300 cells/cm^3) and elevated serum immunoglobulins [6].

Infections at other sites

Infants born to *Chlamydia*-positive mothers may also become infected in the rectum and vagina [7]. Although infection at these sites appears to be totally asymptomatic, the infection may cause confusion if detected at a later date. Schachter *et al.* [7] reported finding subclinical rectal and vaginal infection in 14% of infants born to *Chlamydia*-positive women; some of these infants were still culture positive at 18 months of age. Bell *et al.* [6] were able to follow 22 infants born to women with culture-proven chlamydial infections and found that positive cultures were detected in these children as late as 28.5 months after birth: this was the longest duration of perinatally acquired infection and it occurred in the nasopharynx or oropharynx. Nine infants had rectal or vaginal infections which persisted for slightly over 12 months. There are other anecdotal reports of perinatally acquired rectal, vaginal and nasopharyngeal infections persisting for at least 3 years [3]. This needs to be kept in mind when evaluating children for suspected sexual abuse [3].

REFERENCES

1 Alexander ER, Harrison HR. Role of *Chlamydia trachomatis* in perinatal infection. *Rev Infect Dis* 1983; 5: 713–19.
2 Hammerschlag MR. Neonatal conjunctivitis. *Pediatr Ann* 1993; 22: 346–51.
3 Bell TA, Stamm WE, Wang SP *et al. J Am Med Assoc* 1992; 267: 400–2.
4 Hammerschlag MR. Chlamydial infections. *J Pediatr* 1989; 114: 727–34.
5 Beem MO, Saxon EM. Respiratory tract colonization and a distinctive pneumonia syndrome in infants infected with *Chlamydia trachomatis*. *N Engl J Med* 1977; 296: 306–10.
6 Harrison HR, English MG, Lee CK *et al. N Engl J Med* 1978; 298: 702–8.
7 Schachter J, Grossman M, Sweet RL *et al.* Prospective study of perinatal transmission of *Chlamydia trachomatis*. *J Am Med Assoc* 1986; 255: 3374–7.

Infections in older children

CT has not been associated with any specific clinical syndrome in older infants and children. Most attention to CT infection in these children has concentrated on the relationship to child sexual abuse. It has been suggested that the isolation of CT from a rectal or genital site in children without prior sexual activity may be a marker of sexual abuse. Although evidence for other modes of spread, such as through fomites, is lacking for this organism, as previously mentioned, perinatal maternal–infant transmission resulting in vaginal and/or rectal infection has been documented with prolonged infection for periods of up to 3 years. This is an important confounding variable.

Chlamydia trachomatis infection and sexual abuse

Vaginal infection with CT was uncommonly reported in prepubertal children before 1980. The possibility of sexual contact was frequently not even discussed. In 1981, Rettig

et al. reported concurrent or subsequent chlamydial infection in nine of 33 (27%) episodes of gonorrhoea in a group of prepubertal children [1]. This compares with rates of concurrent infection in men and women of 11–62%, depending on the study. However, CT was not found in any of 31 children presenting with urethritis or vaginitis that was not gonococcal. No information was given about possible sexual activity. Studies have identified rectogenital chlamydial infection in 2–13% of sexually abused children, when these children were routinely cultured for the organism. The majority of those with chlamydial infection were asymptomatic. In two early studies that had control groups, similar percentages of control patients were also infected [2,3]. The control group in one study consisted of children who were also referred for evaluation of possible sexual abuse but were found to have no history of sexual contact, and siblings of abused children. The mean age of this group was 4.5 years as compared to 7.5 years for the group with a history of sexual contact, thus suggesting a bias related to the inability to elicit a history of sexual contact from young children. In the second study the control group was selected from a well-child clinic. Three girls in this group were found to have positive chlamydial cultures; two who had positive vaginal cultures were sisters who had been sexually abused 3 years previously and had not received interim treatment with antibiotics. The implication of this observation was that these children were infected for at least 3 years and were totally asymptomatic. The remaining control child had CT isolated from her throat and rectum; no history of sexual contact could be elicited. A subsequent larger study by Ingram *et al.* [4,5] found a stronger association between vaginal chlamydial infection and a history of sexual abuse, but not with pharyngeal infection, which was found in a similar number of controls. Rectal infection was detected in only one of 124 abused children. The possibility of prolonged perinatally acquired vaginal or rectal carriage in the sexually abused group was minimized in the study of Hammerschlag *et al.* [3] since the chlamydial cultures obtained at the initial examination were negative and the infection was only detected at follow-up examination 2–4 weeks later. However, the two abused girls who developed chlamydial infection were victims of a single assault by a stranger. In the setting of repeated abuse by a family member, over long periods of time, development of infection would be difficult to demonstrate. Even among adolescents and adults who are victims of sexual assault, acquisition of CT is uncommon, less than 2% over the rate found at baseline [2,6]. The 1993 STD treatment guidelines have dropped the recommendation that cultures for CT be obtained routinely from the pharynx and urethra in children who are suspected as victims of sexual abuse [7]. The major reasons were the low yield from the urethra, the tendency for longer persistence of perinatally acquired pharyngeal infection and the potential confusion with *C. pneumoniae*.

REFERENCES

1 Rettig PJ, Nelson JD. Genital tract infection with *Chlamydia trachomatis* in prepubertal children. *J Pediatr* 1981; 99: 206–10.
2 Glaser JD, Schachter J, Benes S *et al*. Sexually transmitted diseases in postpubertal female rape victims. *J Infect Dis* 1991; 167: 726–30.
3 Hammerschlag MR, Doraiswamy B, Alexander ER *et al*. Are rectogenital chlamydial infections a marker of sexual abuse in children? *Pediatr Infect Dis* 1984; 3: 100–4.
4 Ingram DL, Runyan DK, Collins AD *et al*. Vaginal *Chlamydia trachomatis* infection in children with sexual contact. *Pediatr Infect Dis* 1984; 3: 97–9.
5 Ingram DL, White ST, Occhiuti AR *et al*. *Pediatr Infect Dis* 1986; 5: 226–9.
6 Jenny C, Hooton TM, Bowers A *et al*. Sexually transmitted diseases in victims of rape. *N Engl J Med* 1990; 322: 713–16.
7 Centers for Disease Control. 1993 Sexually transmitted diseases treatment guidelines. Centers for Disease Control and Prevention. *MMWR* 1993; 42(RR-14): 1–102.

Diagnosis

The 'gold standard' remains isolation by culture of CT from the conjunctiva, nasopharynx, vagina or rectum. *Chlamydia* culture has been further defined by the CDC as isolation of the organism in tissue culture and confirmation by microscopic identification of the characteristic inclusions by fluorescent antibody staining [1]. Several non-culture methods have the American Food and Drink Administration (FDA) approval for diagnosis of chlamydial conjunctivitis. They include EIA, specifically Chlamydiazyme (Abbott Diagnostics, Illinois), Pathfinder (Sanofi-Pasteur, Minnesota) and SureCell (Kodak, New York) and direct fluorescent antibody tests (DFA) including Syva Micro Trak (Genetic Systems, Washington) and Pathfinder (Sanofi-Pasteur). These tests appear to perform very well with conjunctival specimens with sensitivities over 90% and specificities over 95% compared to culture [2]. Unfortunately, the performance with nasopharyngeal specimens has not been as good with sensitivities in infants with pneumonia at 79%, but only 30–60% in nasopharyngeal specimens from infants with conjunctivitis. The recently approved PCR assay, Amplicor (Roche, New Jersey) has approval only for genital sites in adults. Preliminary studies suggest PCR is equivalent to culture for conjunctival specimens and possibly superior for respiratory specimens [3]. Non-culture tests should never be used for rectal or vaginal sites in children, or for any forensic purposes in adolescents and adults. This is stated clearly in the CDC 1993 *Chlamydia* guidelines and the CDC 1993 STD treatment guidelines [1,4]. Use of these tests for vaginal and rectal specimens has been associated with a large number of false positive tests [5–7]. Faecal material can give false-positive reactions with any EIA; none are approved for this site in adults. Common bowel organisms, including *Escherichia coli*, *Proteus* species, vaginal organisms such as group B *Streptococcus* and *Gardnerella vaginalis* and even some respiratory flora such as group A *Streptococcus* can also give positive reactions with EIAs [7]. These types of test are best for screening infection in adolescents and adults in high prevalence populations (prevalence of infection >7%) [1]. There are very few reports on the performance of the DNA probe, but it appears to be equivalent to most available EIAs, in terms of sensitivity and specificity compared to culture for genital specimens. Another potential problem can occur with use of an EIA for respiratory specimens. As all of the available EIAs use genus-specific antibodies, if used for respiratory specimens, these tests will also detect *C. pneumoniae*. Even though culture is considered the gold standard, culture of CT is not regulated and sensitivity may vary between laboratories [8].

PCR techniques are currently more reliable [9]. PCR is the gold standard for diagnosis in adults. To date, this is unclear in children. The CDC advises the isolation of CT from tissue culture as a standard determination in cases of suspected sexual abuse [9]. Cultures may be positive after 2–7 days. Serological investigation in suspected cases is not meaningful because of the limited reliability [10]. Culturing samples from the pharynx for CT in children is also not meaningful considering the possibility of a persistent perinatal infection and confusion with *C. pneumoniae* [9].

REFERENCES

1 Centers for Disease Control and Prevention. Recommendations for the prevention and management of *Chlamydia trachomatis* infections. *MMWR* 1993; 42(RR-12): 1–39.
2 Hammerschlag MR. *Pediatr Ann* 1993; 22: 346.
3 Roblin PM, Sokolovskaya N, Gelling M. Comparison of Amplicor *Chlamydia trachomatis* test and culture for detection of *Chlamydia trachomatis* in ocular and nasopharyn of specimens from infants with conjunctivitis. *Pediatr Res* 1996; 39: 301A.
4 Centers for Disease Control. 1993 Sexually transmitted diseases treatment guidelines. Centers for Disease Control and Prevention. *MMWR* 1993; 42(RR-14): 1–102.
5 Hammerschlag MR, Rettig PJ, Shields ME. False positive results with the use of chlamydial antigen detection tests in the evaluation of suspected sexual abuse in children. *Pediatr Infect Dis J* 1988; 7: 11–14.
6 Hauger SB, Brown J, Agre F *et al*. Failure of direct fluorescent antibody staining to detect *Chlamydia trachomatis* from genital tract sites of prepubertal children at risk for sexual abuse. *Pediatr Infect Dis J* 1988; 7: 660–2.
7 Porder K, Sanchez N, Roblin PM *et al*. Lack of specificity of Chlamydiazyme for detection of vaginal chlamydia infection in prepubertal girls. *Pediatr Infect Dis J* 1989; 8: 358–60.
8 Pate MS, Hook EW III. Laboratory to laboratory variation in *Chlamydia trachomatis* culture practices. *Sex Transm Dis* 1995; 22: 322–6.
9 Centres for Disease Control/MMWR Sexually transmitted diseases treatment guidelines. *Atlanta: US Publ Health* 1993; 38: 98–102.
10 Lacey CJN. Sexually transmitted diseases in the prepubertal child. *Clin Pediatr* 1993; 1: 165–83.

Treatment

Because of its long growth cycle, treatment of chlamydial infections requires multiple dose regimens. None of the currently recommended single-dose regimens for gonor-rhoea are effective against CT.

Treatment of Chlamydia *conjunctivitis and pneumonia in infants*

Oral erythromycin suspension (ethylsuccinate or sterate) 50 mg/kg/day for 10–14 days is the therapy of choice. It provides better and faster resolution of the conjunctivitis as well as treating any concurrent nasopharyngeal infection, which will prevent the development of pneumonia.

Additional topical therapy is not needed [1]. The efficacy of this regimen has been reported to range from 80 to 90%, thus as many as 20% of infants may require another course of therapy [1]. Erythromycin at the same dose for 2–3 weeks is the treatment of choice for pneumonia and does result in clinical improvement as well as elimination of the organism from the respiratory tract.

Treatment of older children

Chlamydial infections may be treated with oral ery-thromycin 50 mg/kg/day four times a day orally to a maximum of 2 g/day for 7–14 days. Children over 12 years of age may be treated with tetracycline 50 mg/kg/day four times a day orally for 7 days. The new macrolide antibiotic, azithromycin is very effective as single-dose treatment for uncomplicated chlamydial urethral and cervical infection in men and non-pregnant women [2]. Single-dose azithromycin has also been shown to be effective in adolescents [3]. However, there are no data on its use for this indication in children.

REFERENCES

1 Hammerschlag MR. Chlamydial infections. *J Pediatr* 1989; 114: 727–34.
2 Centers for Disease Control and Prevention. Recommendations for the prevention and management of *Chlamydia trachomatis* infections. *MMWR* 1993; 42(RR-12): 1–39
3 Hammerschlag MR. Neonatal conjunctivitis. *Pediatr Ann* 1993; 22: 346–51.

Condyloma acuminata (see also Chapter 5.1)

Definition

Condyloma acuminata (CA) are anogenital warts (Fig. 24.2.5) caused by human papillomavirus (HPV) infection. Most commonly these warts are caused by HPV types 6, 11, 16 and 18, though type 2 is also found. In the last instance these infections are caused by manual transmission [1–3].

Aetiology

The majority of the CA in children younger than 3 years is due to vertical transmission during birth. However,

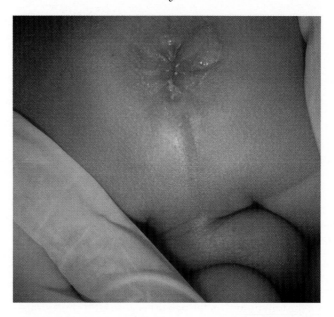

Fig. 24.2.5 Condyloma acuminatum.

within this age group, there is suspected sexual abuse in a number of cases which is difficult to estimate. Sexual transmission has been reported to be up to one in two or three children older than 3 years of age [1]. Non-sexual infection via child–child contact (e.g. via exploratory sexual games) or non-sexual intimate contacts between adults and children is possible [1,4]. A careful derma-tological and paediatric examination is imperative in all children with CA. Modes of non-sexual transmission include:

1 hand–genital contact via an infected carer of the child;
2 non-sexual intimate behaviour; or
3 inadequate hygiene, for example via contaminated objects such as a towel.

All HPV types can infect the epithelium of the anogeni-tal region, the mucous membranes in the mouth and the adjoining skin. Typing of HPV from the warts located in the anogenital region is therefore also indicated. This typing should be done with formalin-fixed or preferably with cryobiopsies supplemented with PCR. If HPV types 6, 11, 16, 18 or (very rarely) 31 are found, then one may speak of a sexually transmissible form of the HPV types [1–3]. However, this is no proof for sexual abuse. In prepubertal children with anogenital warts, besides these HPV types, type 2 is also regularly encountered. Usually, this type is also found in the warts on the hands [1,3].

Clinical features

The incubation period of HPV infections varies from 1.5 to 8 months with a peak at 3 months. However, incubation periods of up to 20 months have been reported [2]. Such a long incubation period poses difficulty in establishing the exact aetiology [3]. The average incubation period from birth is about 3 months, with a maximum of about 2 years.

Usually, CAs cause no complaints and are generally noticed by chance by the parents or by a doctor during physical examination [5]. CAs are usually encountered in the mucocutaneous or intertriginous areas such as the anogenital region, the perineum, on the labia, around the vaginal entrance, around the anus and in the rectum. CAs are rarely found intravaginally in young girls. Moreover, CA may occur in and around the mouth, and in the throat cavity and between the toes. CAs are predominantly encountered in the perianal region (57% of the CA in boys, 37% in girls). CAs are seen on the labia in 23% of the girls and on the penis and scrotum in 17% of the boys [5]. CAs occur more frequently in girls than in boys (2.5:1). The majority are children younger than 3 years of age [6]. CA may also be encountered on the lips, on the tongue and on the palate because HPV can be transmitted via orogenital contact between the victim and the perpetrator [7].

The warts usually have the shape of a cauliflower or are stemmed, although flat forms may be encountered. They are red, pink or skin-coloured. Subclinical infections may occur in teenagers and adults. Probably, such infections also occur in children. Extremely large CAs may occur in children with HIV infection [8].

CAs as a result of a perinatal infection occur in the larynx and in the anogenital region. Juvenile papillomas of the respiratory tract (oral cavity, vocal chords, epiglottis, trachea and lungs) are a rare manifestation of such HPV infections. These are caused by HPV types 6 and 11 [9,10]. The majority of the children with juvenile papillomas are diagnosed between the age of 1 and 3 years, although the disorder has been observed regularly in other children [1]. The infection presents as hoarseness or respiratory problems.

In any case, the virus may remain latent in an apparently normal skin. Therefore, new lesions may develop several months after treatment [6].

Treatment

The treatment of CA is difficult because of moderate response to topical medication. The treatment of choice for large CAs is surgery and cauterization or treatment with a CO_2 laser [1].

Prognosis

CAs may disappear spontaneously after 3–5 years so that a 'wait and see policy' is possible [1]. Malignant transformation in young children has not been described.

REFERENCES

1 Oranje AP, Waard-van der Spek FB de, Bilo RAC. Condylomata acuminata in children. *Int STD AIDS* 1990; 1: 250–5 (editorial review).
2 Stewart D. Sexually transmitted diseases. In: Heger A, Emans SJ. *Evaluation of the Sexually Abused Child—a Medical Textbook and Photographic Atlas.* Oxford: Oxford University Press, 1992: 155–6.
3 Armstrong DKB. Anogenital warts in prepubertal children: pathogenesis, HPV typing and management. *Int J STD AIDS* 1997; 8: 78–81.
4 Herman-Giddens ME, Gutman LT, Berson NL. Association of coexisting vaginal infections and multiple abusers in female children with genital warts. *Sex Transm Dis* 1988; 15: 63–7.
5 Finkel MA, DeJong AR. Medical findings in child sexual abuse. In: Reece RM. *Child Abuse—Medical Diagnosis and Management.* Lea & Febiger, 1994: 229–30.
6 Lacey CJN. Sexually transmitted diseases in the prepubertal child. *Clin Pediatr* 1993; 1: 165–83.
7 Blackwell AL. Paediatric gonorrhoea: non venereal epidemic in a household. *Genitourin Med* 1986; 62: 228–9.
8 Shelton TB, Jerkins GR, Noe HN. Condylomata acuminata in the pediatric patient. *J Urol* 1986; 135: 548–9.
9 Lindeberg H, Elbrond O. Laryngeal papillomas: the epidemiology in a Danish subpopulation 1965–1984. *Clin Otolaryngol* 1990; 15: 125–31.
10 Terry RM, Lewis FA, Robertson S *et al.* Juvenile and adult laryngeal papillomata: classification by *in-situ* hybridization for human papilloma virus. *Clin Otolaryngol* 1989; 14: 135–9.

Hepatitis B in children

Hepatitis B virus (HBV) infection can be due to transplacental transmission, a non-sexual transmission and transmission via sexual contact. The incubation period is 3–6 months. Criteria for testing children for HBV in suspected sexual abuse are:

1 a homosexual or heterosexual perpetrator with multiple sexual contacts with various partners; or
2 a perpetrator who is an intravenous drug abuser or has a partner who is an intravenous drug abuser [1].

Most children acquire HBV infection via non-sexual contacts with infected individuals from their peer group or infected adults [1].

An HBV infection has been proven if antigens (HBsAg and HBeAg) and antibodies (anti-HBs, anti-HBc (IgM or IgG), anti-HBe) have been demonstrated. The direct (non-sexual) contacts of the child should also be tested if a child is HBsAg- and HBeAg-positive. Antiviral therapy for hepatitis B is still experimental. Vaccination may be considered [2]. Immunization and vaccination are standard in children born to HBV-positive mothers.

REFERENCES

1 Finkel MA, DeJong AR. Medical findings in child sexual abuse. In: Reece RM. *Child Abuse—Medical Diagnosis and Management.* Lea & Febiger, 1994: 229–30.
2 Whittle HC, Inskip H, Hall AJ *et al.* Vaccination against hepatitis B and protection against viral carriage in the Gambia. *Lancet* 1991; 337: 747–50.

Genital herpes simplex virus infection
(see also Chapter 5.2)

Definition

Genital HSV infections are caused by HSV type 2 and less commonly type 1.

Aetiology

The transmission of HSV may occur in various manners such as intrauterine (transplacental or via an ascending infection), during delivery, after delivery via a sexual contact and via non-sexual contacts.

Sexual contact should be definitely considered in acquired HSV-2 and HSV-1 genital infections in children. Transmission occurs via close contact with an infected individual from an active lesion, mucosa or secretion. It is not necessary to have a clinically recognizable lesion to be infectious [1]. Autoinoculation via the fingers from the mouth to the genitalia is also possible. Autoinoculation is less probable if there has been recovery from the primary infection or in a recurrent infection [1]. In autoinoculation, the genital infection will occur simultaneously or soon after the oral infection. It should be noted that the simultaneous occurrence of an oral and a genital infection may also be the result of orogenital and genitogenital contact.

HSV can survive for some time, for example, on a speculum or glass slide, or on plastic and rubber objects for a maximum of 4h [2–4]. However, transmission in this manner is unlikely because for an infection, direct contact between live virus and the mucosa or damaged skin is essential [2]. HSV is rapidly inactivated at room temperature and through drying.

Clinical presentation

The incubation period of acquired infection is 4–20 days. HSV causes painful vesicular or ulcerating lesions on the skin or mucosae, often with fever. Sometimes, there is itch. An acquired infection in children is usually located around the mouth or on the fingers. Genital HSV infections are rare in children. An acute napkin rash and vulval ulceration have been reported.

Neonatal herpes

In a neonatal HSV infection, several days or weeks after delivery, the infant develops one or more of the following illnesses whereby fever is not prominent:
1 local skin infection (blisters), eyes (keratoconjunctivitis) and/or mouth;
2 disseminated infection with the appearance of neonatal sepsis;

3 meningoencephalitis with reduced consciousness, convulsions and/or general sickness; or
4 pneumonia with (serious) respiratory problems (cough, tachypnoea) [5].

The last three disorders have a high mortality rate because the diagnosis of 'HSV infection' may be delayed and only considered after an unsuccessful clinical response to empirically chosen antibiotic treatment. The consequence is a delay in initiating adequate therapy [6]. In particular, residual abnormalities may be observed after meningoencephalitis or disseminated infection [7]. Moreover, it appeared that neurological damage had still occurred in about 10% of the cases also after local infections without neurological abnormalities and with a normal CSF [7]. The residual complaints after an infection with HSV-2 are generally more severe than those after infection with HSV-1.

Diagnosis

In principle, the same diagnostics are used in children with an acquired HSV infection as that used in a neonatal infection (see Chapter 5.2).

Treatment

An uncomplicated HSV infection is usually not treated. A primary infection with severe symptoms is treated orally with 500mg valaciclovir twice a day for 5 days. For very severe symptoms, including neonatal infection, intravenous treatment with aciclovir is mandatory (10 mg/kg/dose three times daily for 5–10 days).

REFERENCES

1 Finkel MA, DeJong AR. Medical findings in child sexual abuse. In: Reece RM. *Child Abuse—Medical Diagnosis and Management*. Lea & Febiger, 1994: 229–30.
2 Gardner M, Jones JG. Genital herpes acquired by sexual abuse of children. *J Pediatr* 1984; 104: 243–4.
3 Larson T, Bryson YJ. Fomites and herpes simplex virus. *J Infect Dis* 1985; 151: 746–7 (letter).
4 Neinstein LS, Goldenring J, Carpenter S. Nonsexual transmission of sexually transmitted diseases: an infrequent occurrence. *Pediatrics* 1984; 74: 67–9.
5 Sullivan Bolyai JZ, Hull HF, Wilson C, Smith AL, Corey L. Presentation of neonatal herpes simplex virus infections: implications for a change in therapeutic strategy. *Pediatr Infect Dis J* 1986; 5: 309–14.
6 Hubell C, Dominguez R, Kohl S. Neonatal herpes simplex pneumonitis. *Rev Infect Dis* 1988; 10: 431–8.
7 Whitley R, Arvin A, Prober C *et al*. Predictors of morbidity and mortality in neonates with herpes simplex virus infections. *N Engl J Med* 1991; 324: 450–4.

Human immunodeficiency virus
(see also Chapter 5.6)

HIV infections in children are the result of medical intervention such as administration of infected blood products in haemophilia patients, via mother–child transmission, through intravenous drug abuse and through sexual contact. Since 1989, several reports have been published in which attention has been drawn to the dangers of HIV infection through sexual abuse of children [1–3]. In most countries, the risk that a child runs of HIV infection as a result of sexual violence, considering the epidemiological state of affairs, is still small [4]. Therefore, at present there are no reasons for routinely testing for HIV in cases of suspected sexual abuse. The diagnosis of HIV may be essential on indication. The criteria for HIV testing in children [4] are as follows:

1 a request from the victim, parents or guardians;

2 serious concern for the possibility of infection;

3 the child has symptoms which may be due to HIV infection;

4 the suspicion or assurance of seropositiveness of the perpetrator or risky sexual contacts of the perpetrator;

5 intravenous drug abuse by the perpetrator;

6 frequently occurring abuse with vaginal/anal contact;

7 additional 'unknown' perpetrators (e.g. in child prostitution); or

8 the suspicion or assurance that the perpetrator has been to high-risk areas such as Thailand and the Philippines and has had sexual contact there.

An ethical problem may arise when it is decided to test a child for HIV for whatever reason. An objection may be raised against such a test because a child is being tested for a lethal illness for which there is no treatment available. Therefore, children should not be tested without extensive prior consultation with others and only when appropriate guidance is available if the results are positive. Testing may only be undertaken after either the parents or guardians (*loco parentis*) have given permission. The incubation period of HIV in children may vary considerably. Generally, seroconversion occurs within 3 months. This does not mean that the first signs of acquired immune deficiency syndrome (AIDS) also appear. The period between seroconversion and the manifestation of signs and symptoms may be between 8 and 9 years. This makes it extremely difficult to obtain a reliable history concerning transmission at the time the symptoms develop.

The treatment of HIV infection in childhood must be left to a paediatrician with specialized expertise in infectious diseases. Cutaneous abnormalities should be referred to and treated by a dermatologist familiar with paediatric skin diseases.

REFERENCES

1 Gellert GA, Mascola L. Rape and AIDS. *Pediatrics* 1989; 83: 644.

2 Gutman LT, St Claire KK, Weedy C *et al*. Human immunodeficiency virus transmission by child sexual abuse. *Am J Dis Child* 1991; 145: 137–41.

3 Murtagh C, Hammill H. Sexual abuse of children: a new risk factor for HIV transmission. *Adolesc Pediatr Gynecol* 1993; 6: 33–5.

4 National Committee on the Prevention of AIDS. Children, HIV infection and AIDS. *NCAB* 1989.

Trichomonas vaginalis infection
(see also Chapter 24.1)

There is a difference of opinion on the occurrence of *Trichomonas vaginalis* (TV) in women after puberty. Pokorny [1] reported that the frequency of TV infections in adults had decreased to such an extent that one would be rarely confronted with such a problem in children. However, in a recent publication from the Royal College of Physicians, it was reported that TV infection occurs very regularly in women after puberty [2]. An infection with TV in adults is only possible through sexual contact. There are several possible explanations for infections in children [3]. Contamination of the nose/throat cavity and also of the vagina may occur during delivery. Acquired TV infections are rare before puberty because the environment in the prepubertal vagina (hypertrophic epithelium, non-glycogen-containing and alkaline environment) is a poor source of nutrition whereby growth and colonization are not possible. A sexual contact between a child and an adult is suspected if a TV infection is encountered in a child older than 1 year. Moreover, it indicates that the contact has occurred recently because the organism of TV does not survive for long in the prepubertal vagina. Non-sexual transmission in prepubertal children is probably very rare because the organism is highly location specific [2]. Nevertheless, in principle, non-sexual transmission because of inadequate hygiene should be excluded if abuse is suspected: the organism of TV can survive for several hours on wet towels and clothing which have been used by infected women [2]. The organism also appeared to be able to survive in samples of urine and sperm even after they had been exposed to air for several hours [2].

The period of incubation is 1–4 weeks. In adolescents there may be vulvovaginitis with purulent discharge, urethritis and cystitis. The infection may be asymptomatic. Transient vulvovaginitis is the most probable complaint in prepubertal children.

TV is demonstrated by means of a direct preparation of the exudate to which physiological saline has been added (sampling with a moist cotton-wool swab). The preparation must be evaluated directly. The sensitivity of a direct preparation is moderate, but the specificity is very high; a TV culture has a sensitivity of 95% [3].

The first choice in the treatment of TV infection is metronidazole 30 mg/kg/day in three doses given orally for 7 days. Tinidazole 50–75 mg/kg in a single dose is an alternative choice; this may be repeated once.

REFERENCES

1 Pokorny SF. Child abuse and infections. *Obstet Gynecol Clin N Am* 1989; 16: 401–15.

2 Royal College of Physicians. *Physical Signs of Sexual Abuse in Children*. Royal College of Physicians of London, 1991.

3 Stewart D. Sexually transmitted diseases. In: Heger A, Emans SJ. *Evaluation of the Sexually Abused Child—a Medical Textbook and Photographic Atlas.* Oxford: Oxford University Press, 1992: 155–6.

Bacterial vaginitis (see also Chapter 24.1)

Bacterial vaginitis (BV) is encountered regularly in adult women and has also been reported in prepubertal girls. It is a polymicrobial disorder, whereby various bacteria such as *G. vaginalis*, anaerobes (among others, *Bacteroides* and *Peptococcus* varieties), *Mobiluncus* species and *Mycoplasma hominis* are present in excess, whereas the number of lactobacilli is highly reduced. The incidence in prepubertal girls is low. Although, BV is encountered more often in abused than in non-abused girls, it cannot be regarded as strong evidence for abuse [1,2]. The pathogenesis, both in adults and children is only partially known. It is unclear whether BV can be transmitted during delivery. The length of time that BV can remain asymptomatic is also unclear. Complaints of vulvovaginitis, a thin, homogenous grey–white to yellow discharge or a typical odour, may be the result of BV.

BV is thought to be present if there is a homogenous discharge, a pH of higher than 4.5, a positive amine test and 'clue cells' in the physiological saline preparation. Measuring the vaginal pH is only meaningful in postpubertal girls. In younger girls, measuring the pH as a diagnostic criterium for BV is unreliable because the pH in these girls is always higher than 4.5. Demonstration of *G. vaginalis* in culture is unnecessary for the diagnosis. Spontaneous recovery is possible. If treatment is opted for then the first choice is 30 mg/kg/day metronidazole in three doses given orally for 7 days. Amoxicillin 50 mg/kg/day in four doses for 7 days is an alternative choice.

REFERENCES

1 Bartley DL, Morgan L, Rimsza M. *Gardnerella vaginalis* in prepubertal girls. *Am J Dis Child* 1987; 141: 1014–17.
2 Hammerschlag M, Cummings M, Doraiswamy B *et al.* Nonspecific vaginitis following sexual abuse in children. *Pediatrics* 1985; 75: 1028–31.

Physical and Sexual Abuse

VIC LARCHER

> Child abuse is the difference between a hand on the bottom and a fist in the face. (Henry Kempe)

Abuse, neglect and exploitation remain important causes of mortality and morbidity for the world's children irrespective of ethnicity, social status or religious belief. Identification and prevention of abuse continue to be impeded by difficulties in recognition and ownership, professional accountability and responsibility, and by lack of resources.

Dermatologists may find themselves involved in child abuse cases because:
1 a child discloses abuse to them;
2 a child's skin condition is likely to have been the result of abuse or neglect; or
3 an expert opinion is sought as to the nature of a child's skin lesions.
For a more detailed general account of child abuse, specific texts should be consulted [1–3]. It is important to be familiar with local guidelines, policies and procedures for interagency cooperation in the diagnosis and management of child abuse. Cases should be discussed with, or referred to, colleagues with particular expertise in child abuse; appropriate agencies (e.g. social work, child protection) should be involved at an early stage.

This chapter considers physical and sexual abuse separately, except for the principles of management and legal considerations which are common to both.

Physical abuse

Definition

Physical abuse is an injury caused to a child by a carer for any reason. Tissue damage so produced includes bruises, burns, punctures, fractures, ruptures of organs and disruption of function. The use of an instrument on any part of the body is abuse [4,5].

History

Forensic accounts of cruelty to children were first published by Tardieu in Paris in 1860. Subsequent public concern in the English-speaking world led to the establishment of societies for the prevention of cruelty to children and widespread, specific, regularly reviewed legislation to make child cruelty and neglect a criminal offence.

By the early 20th century it was established that in many cases the perpetrators were parents or caregivers.

Current awareness of the prevalence of physical abuse stems from Caffe's description of radiological features [6] and Kempe et al.'s demonstration that a large number of supposedly accidental injuries to children in hospital had been deliberately inflicted [7]. In the USA legislation was passed creating an obligation on professionals to report suspicions of abuse to authorities. In the UK a series of incidents involving abuse and death of children led to reforms in the management of such cases, emphasizing the need for multidisciplinary working between agencies, i.e. health, social services, police and education. Internationally the 1980s saw increased acknowledgement of children's rights and autonomy culminating in the United Nations (UN) Convention of Children's Rights and the recognition of other forms of abuse, e.g. Munchausen syndrome by proxy (MSBP) or factitious illness [8].

Incidence and prevalence

True incidence and prevalence of physical abuse depends upon its definition and the extent to which minor degrees of abuse are reported. Slapping, sufficient to leave a bruise, may be regarded as inappropriate by doctors but not reported as abuse [9]. Under-reporting and under-recognition are therefore likely [4,5].

Statistics may be obtained from (a) criminal prosecution records; (b) records of protection agencies or social services; and (c) national survey. In the UK 4% of under 18

Table 24.3.1 Risk factors for physical abuse

Teenage pregnancy
Unwanted pregnancy
Prematurity
Developmental disorders and/or chronic illness
Twin pregnancy
Substance abuse
Poverty
Lack of knowledge of parenting, child health and development

year olds are reported annually to child protection agencies; 1–2% of UK children are abused [10]. In the USA a similar percentage are maltreated (16.2 in 1000) of whom 9.2 of 1000 were physically, emotionally or sexually abused [5]. Surveys from both the USA and UK indicate that 1 in 1000 children are seriously injured and 1 in 10 000 die [4,5,10].

Demographical characteristics

Both boys and girls are abused. Within a family the first-born child is more often affected and only one child of the family may be abused. The mean age of abused children is approximately 6 years, but children under 2 years of age are most at risk from serious injury with death being uncommon after 1 year [4]. The preponderance in lower socioeconomic groups may reflect higher detection rates in such groups.

Known risk factors are shown in Table 24.3.1. Most abuse is inflicted by parents; men constitute over half of the abusers and are more likely to injure children fatally [11].

Partners or cohabitees who are not related to the child are also likely perpetrators [4]. Abusers may have personality traits which predispose them to violent behaviour but defined mental illness is rare. Poor parenting skills in young parents and a history of abuse on behalf of one of the parents are also associated factors.

Clinical indicators

A number of features may lead to suspicion that a child's injuries are non-accidental:
1 Delay or failure in seeking medical help.
2 A history which is vague and temporally and factually inconsistent.
3 A history incompatible with the child's injuries and/or their known and verified state of development (or that of the alleged perpetrator).
4 Abnormal parental affect—more concerned with their own problems than those of the child.
5 Parental hostility and non-cooperation with the investigating process.
6 Abnormal appearance of the child (sad, withdrawn, frightened, frozen watchfulness), abnormal interreaction with parents.
7 Presence of injuries of different ages.

Children may disclose abuse; all such disclosures must be investigated.

Patterns of injury

Two types of physical injury may be seen by dermatologists; (a) bruises and skin marks; and (b) burns and scalds. A detailed consideration of fractures is beyond the scope of this chapter, though some conditions which predispose to fractures, e.g. osteogenesis imperfecta, may have skin stigmata [12,13].

Bruises and skin marks

Aetiology

These may be caused by direct blows from an assailant or by an object. Finger tip bruising (induced by gripping), punch marks (leaving knuckle prints) and slap marks are characteristics of abuse. Slap marks produce linear patterns in which petechial bruising occurs between points of impact of the finger pulps (Figs 24.3.1–24.3.4).

Objects leave characteristic 'brand' marks, e.g. linear marks from sticks, buckle marks from belts and looped scars from electrical cords [14,15].

Bites are rarer but a study of imprints may yield useful information about the perpetrator and be of forensic value. Direct trauma may only produce marks over bony prominences, e.g. spinous processes because of compression of soft tissues between the source of trauma and underlying bone. The degree of force necessary to produce any given injury depends on a number of complex variables involving the child, the abuser and the implement used. In assessing causation developmental capabilities of the child must be considered.

Sites

Some sites of injury have high specificity for physical abuse, e.g. torn frenulum. Although buttocks or hips are the most common site of injury, over 60% of deliberate injuries occur on the upper body and head [5,14]. Blows to ears may produce subperichondrial haematomas which may be associated with retinal haemorrhages and cerebral oedema [16].

Age of bruises

Bruises of different ages are highly suspicious of child abuse in the absence of adequate explanation. Bruises change colour and fade over time, a property used in esti-

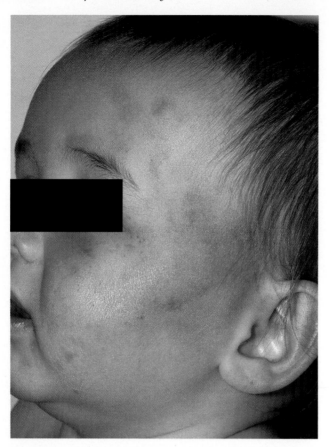

Fig. 24.3.1 Face of toddler showing purple–red bruising of recent onset. Linear pattern of bruising over outer canthus of eye suggests that injury was produced by a slap.

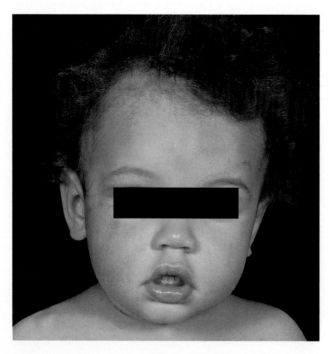

Fig. 24.3.2 Face of infant showing multiple bruises of differing ages. Note yellowish appearance to those on the forehead.

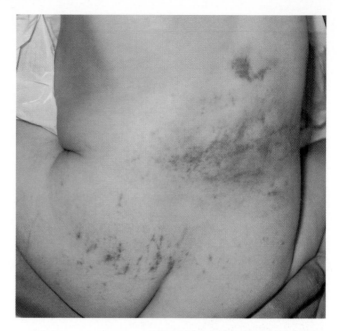

Fig. 24.3.3 Back of toddler showing linear slap marks with distinct impression of pulps of the fingers being left as paler areas. Linear petechial marks delineate interdigit species and interphalangeal areas.

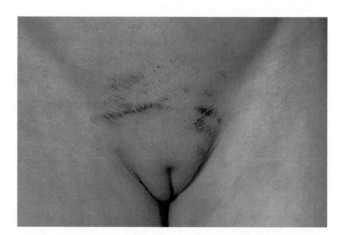

Fig. 24.3.4 Pubic area of a 7-year-old girl, showing transverse healing scratches and some bruising. This girl had been the subject of penile penetration of the anus and digital vaginal interference.

mating their age (Table 24.3.2) [17,18]. Cutaneous bruising depends on the amount and density of connective tissue; with loose tissues, e.g. periorbital and genitalia, being subject to ready and extensive bruising. Cutaneous signs of bleeding into deep tissues may take some time to emerge, making estimating the age of bruises difficult [19].

Non-visible bruises and those in pigmented skin may be demonstrated by ultraviolet (UV) light [20].

Differential diagnosis

A history of easy bruising and bleeding may indicate bleeding disorder [21,22]. Children with haemophilia may

Table 24.3.2 Age of bruising by colour change

Day	1–2	3–5	6–7	8–10	13–28
Colour	Red/blue	Blue/purple	Green	Yellow/brown	Resolved

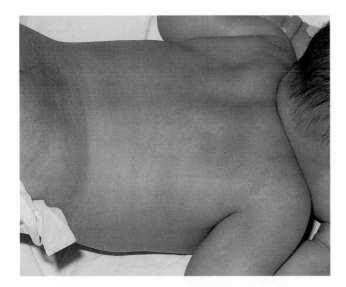

Fig. 24.3.5 Mongolian blue spots on back of Asian child; confusion with finger bruising.

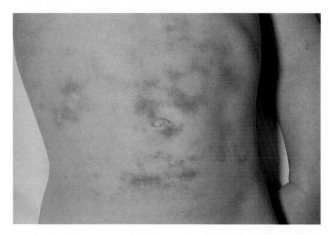

Fig. 24.3.6 Vasculitic skin lesions on the abdomen of a 19-month-girl, resembling bruising.

present with deep bruising or haemarthroses. Bleeding due to quantitative or qualitative disorders of platelets should be excluded. Investigations should include full blood count, platelet count, bleeding time, prothrombin time, partial thromboplastin time and thrombin time. Abnormalities of screening tests should trigger a more detailed evaluation. Viral infection can produce transient clotting dysfunction; drugs, e.g. penicillin, can induce platelet dysfunction [22]. However, non-accidental injury may occur in children with bleeding disorders because of the latter's stress-provoking nature [23].

Easy bruising may be due to vitamin K deficiency, e.g. haemorrhagic disease of the newborn or liver disease; it may also occur with collagen disorders, e.g. osteogenesis imperfecta, Ehlers–Danlos syndrome [24,25].

Other conditions which may be confused with bruising due to abuse are as follows.
1 Mongolian blue sports: pigmented cell naevi found usually over the sacrum and back in children with skin pigment and rarely in Caucasians (Fig. 24.3.5). They do not show the temporal colour changes associated with bruising.
2 Pigment cell or blue naevi which occur on the face following the branches of the fifth cranial nerve. They do not show the temporal colour changes associated with bruising.
3 Angioedema, characterized by sudden swelling around the face or limb, which may be secondary to type 1 hypersensitivity reactions. There may be no urticaria but absence of skin markings suggests diagnosis.

4 Vasculitic lesions associated with viral or streptococcal infection or drug therapy, e.g. Henoch–Shönlein purpura [26], erythema multiforme [27], meningococcal sepsis or disseminated intravascular coagulation (DIC) (Fig. 24.3.6).
5 Infection—staphylococcal scalded skin syndrome, parvovirus (slapped cheek syndrome) [28], haemorrhagic chicken pox.
6 Self-inflicted injuries associated with depression or mental retardation, e.g. Cornelia de Lange, Lesch–Nyhan and Riley–Day syndromes, and temper tantrums.
7 Cultural practices, e.g. *cia gao* [29] (the Vietnamese practice of rubbing a spoon heated in oil on the spine, ribs and neck of children producing burns and abrasions) or cupping [30].

Burns and scalds

Thermal injury may follow lapses in normal protection given to children, or be due to negligent or inadequate parenting. Burns may be deliberately inflicted by hot liquids or objects [5,14,31,32]. Significant mortality and morbidity result from children burned in house fires resulting from neglect [33].

Prevalence

Thermal injuries comprise about 10% of injuries of physically abused children [14,32] and 5% of those who are sexually abused. Deliberate burns may comprise 1–16% of all children with burns or scalds but because of difficulty in diagnosis this form of abuse is probably under-reported and under-recognized.

Demography

Accidental burns occur when a child is exploring their environment, giving a peak age in their second year; the peak age for deliberate burns is in the third [32].

Table 24.3.3 Thermal injury in children

Type	How produced	Characteristics
Scald	Hot liquid	'Wet', burn with blistering and splash marks (if accidental)
Contact	Contact with hot object	Brand-like dry burn of uniform depth (Fig. 24.3.7)
Cigarette	Contact with cigarette	Circular burn, often deep, may have a tail (Fig. 24.3.8)
Flame	Exposure to flame	Dry burn, variable depth, skin charring (Fig. 24.3.9)
Friction	Abrasion of skin	Over bony prominences, broken blisters
Chemical	Exposure to chemicals	Staining, scarring, blistering
Radiant	Exposure to radiation	Extensive injury, protected by clothing

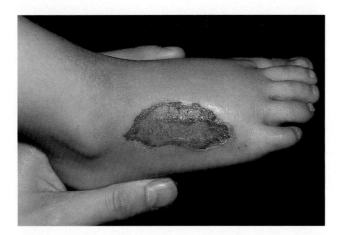

Fig. 24.3.7 Contact burn on the dorsum of the foot of a 28-month-old child. No history available. Likely to be due to non-accidental injury.

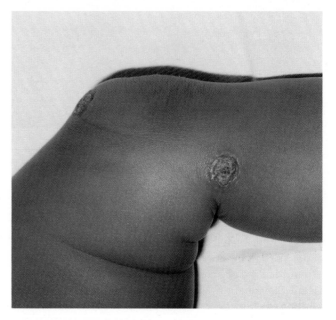

Fig. 24.3.8 Cigarette burns on the knee and leg of 10-month-old infant showing scarred burns with scabs. Such burns are typical of non-accidental injury.

Clinical indicators

Delay in presentation with accidental burns may be due to the care-giver being unaware of the seriousness of first-degree burns or a minor second-degree burn.

Types of burns

Causation and characteristics are shown in Table 24.3.3 (Figs 24.3.7–24.3.9); all have been implicated in non-accidental injury in children. Deliberate microwave burns are rare but produce deep burns which involve greater damage to tissues with a high water content whilst sparing others [34].

Both temperature and time of exposure affect the depth of the burn produced. First- and second-degree burns can be produced by a three second exposure to water at 60°C (the temperature of domestic hot water supplies) and full thickness burns in approximately five times this [35]. However, these figures were derived from experiments with adults or animals and the time taken to damage a child's skin is likely to be less.

Distinction between accidental and non-accidental thermal injury

Accidental scalds may occur when a child pulls a container of hot liquid from a higher surface over their face, shoulders and chest. Splashing is a feature and, dependent on the type of clothing worn, a glove and stocking distribution can occur. Similarly, accidental scalds in baths produce an irregular injury with splash marks. Accidental contact burns are superficial except when a hot object is gripped.

In contrast non-accidental thermal injuries tend to involve the face, head, perineum, buttocks, genitalia, feet and legs. Scalds due to forcible immersion injury may involve lower limbs, with flexural sparing. With further immersion the centre of the buttocks may be pressed against a cold bath producing a central sparing ('hole in

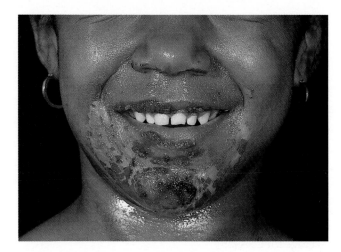

Fig. 24.3.9 Flame burns to chin and upper chest in an 8-year-old girl. Her older brothers were playing 'flame throwing' with an aerosol and matches. Note charring of skin and sparing of area covered when chin was flexed. Injuries thought consistent with history.

Table 24.3.4 Differential diagnosis of thermal injury

Dermatological conditions
Impetigo
Epidermolysis bullosa
Papular urticaria
Contact dermatitis
Severe nappy rash

Medical conditions which may predispose to thermal injury
Anaesthesia
Movement disorders, e.g. cerebral palsy
Neurological defects, e.g. syringomyelia, Riley–Day syndrome

doughnut effect'). Glove and stocking injuries without splashing may occur. Cigarette burns may be inflicted on the face, dorsum of the hands and soles of feet, as may contact burns. Burns to the perineum and genitalia are associated with sexual abuse.

Differential diagnosis

Dermatological conditions which may be confused with thermal injury and medical conditions which predispose to thermal injury are shown in Table 24.3.4.

Impetigo is the commonest cause of mistaken diagnosis of cigarette burn injury and is more likely to occur in children from poor social circumstances [22]. Crops of irregular, superficial, crusted erosions occur on the face, arms and legs; they heal promptly without scarring when treated with antibiotics. However, if cigarette burns are secondarily infected distinction may be difficult.

Other forms of abuse which may be associated with skin lesions

Factitious illness or Munchausen's syndrome by proxy

In MSBP or factitious illness there is:
1 fabrication of symptoms and signs by parent/carer;
2 repeated presentation with symptoms for which treatment is ineffective;
3 denial; and
4 resolution following separation from the perpetrator.
The perpetrator is motivated by the need to assume the sick person's role by proxy or other attention-seeking behaviour [8].

Skin rashes form 9% of reported cases [36] and may be produced by drug poisoning, scratching, application of caustics or painting the skin. There may be demands that a child be placed on a restricted diet because of claimed allergy which may be alleged to produce other symptoms, e.g. diarrhoea, which cannot be verified.

Detection depends on clinical suspicion and liaison with colleagues having necessary expertise. A careful, multidisciplinary approach is essential. Appropriate assays of blood, urine and skin washings may detect administered drugs or locally applied chemicals. Other skin conditions should be actively excluded as should claimed allergies. Evidence of other forms of abuse should be sought because of their increased prevalence in MSBP or factitious illness [37].

Emotional abuse and neglect

Failure to meet a child's emotional needs, e.g. by subjecting children to verbal abuse, disparagement, criticism, threat and ridicule, results in impaired development [38]. Neglect involves lack of physical care taking and supervision, and failing to provide the developmental needs of a child, but is often only identified when there is an adverse outcome [39,40]. Both emotional abuse and neglect may precede or accompany other forms of abuse and may be present in children referred to dermatology departments.

Severe napkin dermatitis may, for example, be the result of deliberate neglect or poor parenting; other features, e.g. poor cognitive development or failure to thrive, may be present. Parents may fail to follow treatment regimes through ignorance or malintent. In circumstances where neglect is suspected a full medical, developmental and psychosocial assessment are required.

Dermatological symptoms, e.g. trichotillomania, may rarely accompany emotional abuse [40]. Such children present with hair loss which is often frontoparietal, and they and their parents may be unaware that it is self-inflicted. In children referred to dermatological departments, hair pulling is usually a sign of chronic social and emotional deprivation, especially involving the maternal relationship. Twisted and broken hairs are usually visible. Differential diagnosis includes ring worm and alopecia areata. Management depends on causation for which psychosocial assessment is necessary.

Child sexual abuse

Definition

Child sexual abuse (CSA) is the involvement of dependent developmentally immature children and adolescents in sexual activities that they do not fully comprehend, to which they are unable to give informed consent and which violate the social taboos of family roles [41]. CSA may be categorized as exposure, molestation, sexual intercourse or rape [42].

History

The first forensic descriptions of CSA were published in France. Tardieu (1857), Bernard and Lacassagne argued that (a) sexual acts against children were frequent and often accompanied by no physical signs; (b) children's reports were largely truthful; (c) fathers and brothers were often the perpetrators; and (d) higher education was no protection. Counter views held that children lied and made false allegations based on hysteria, hallucinations and as part of attention-seeking behaviour. Freud initially believed that much mental illness in adult life resulted from psychological effects of CSA, but subsequently reversed his view, proposing that children fantasized about their sexual relationships with adults [43].

Since the 1980s increased awareness of CSA has resulted from Kempe's work with physical abuse and the obligation to report all abuse. Retrospective prevalence studies in the USA [44–46] and the UK [47,48] have shown that a significant proportion of adults have been the subject of abuse. Both short-term [49] and long-term adverse psychiatric effects of CSA, e.g. depression, personality disorder and alcoholism, are now well recognized [50,51].

In contrast it has been suggested that CSA is over-reported and over-recognized, the result of false allegation or false memory syndrome, and that certain types of minor sexual abuse are the norm for society.

Incidence and prevalence

Self-reporting surveys indicate that 1 in 10 of UK adults have been subject to some form of sexual abuse at the hands of an adult before the age of 16 years [48]. Half had been subject to non-contact exposure but 1 in 200 had experienced full sexual intercourse and 1 in 400 incest. Approximately 1% of American children will experience some form of sexual abuse each year. Prevalence estimates in community surveys range from 6 to 62% for females and 3 to 16% for males [52].

Demographic characteristics

More reported cases involve girls, the female to male ratio being 2.5:1. The risk of sexual abuse rises in preadolescence (>10 years) [53] but children under 6 years of age comprise 10% of all victims [52]. Reported cases show a disproportionate representation in children from lower socioeconomic groups but retrospective community surveys show neither class nor ethnic differences [53]. In some ethnic groups CSA may be under-reported [54] and 98% may be unreported.

Approximately 1 in 6 of physically abused and 1 in 7 of sexually abused children have suffered both kinds of abuse; the children involved are often younger than average for CSA [55].

Although a variety of long-term psychological disorders of CSA been reported [56], a minority of victims have somatic symptoms such as abdominal pain which persist into adulthood [57,58].

Risk factors

Most perpetrators are male and likely to be trusted by the victim. Some features of family structure are associated with a *small* increased risk of CSA [52] as follows:
1 presence of a step-father;
2 children living without one or both natural parents;
3 maternal disablement or absence; or
4 poor or punitive parenting.

A child is more vulnerable to abuse if their activities and contacts are inadequately monitored and supervised; an emotionally neglected or otherwise abused child is also at greater risk of extrafamilial abuse [52]. A prior history of CSA by parents may also be associated [59].

Clinical and historical indicators

Allegations of CSA must be investigated. The diagnosis is based on history, physical examination and appropriate laboratory tests [60,61]. Even in the absence of disclosure there may be other indicators of CSA which may be specific or diagnostic and/or carry a high moderate or low index of suspicion [60,61].

Findings specific or diagnostic of child sexual abuse even in the absence of history

1 Presence of semen/sperm/acid phosphatase in the vagina, anus or external genitalia.
2 Pregnancy.
3 Fresh genital or anal injury (lacerations, abrasions, contusion, trans-section, avulsions, bruises, etc.) in the absence of any other credible explanation.
4 Positive evidence of gonorrhoea or syphilis in the absence of perinatal transmission.

5 Human immunodeficiency syndrome (HIV) infection not acquired through perinatal or intravenous routes.
6 Either or both of the following:
  (a) a markedly enlarged hymenal opening with features of disruption; or
  (b) scarring of the anal mucosa extending beyond the anal margin.

Findings which are highly suspicious but require clarification by history

1 Evidence of sexually transmitted disease (STD) in the absence of perinatal acquisition.
2 Disruption of hymen tissue (trans-section, attenuation, scars).
3 Reflex anal dilatation (RAD) >1.5–2 cm without evidence of stool in the ampulla and if accompanied by irregularity of the orifice.
4 Anal scars or skin tags outside the mid-line.
5 Marked and persistent dilatation of hymenal opening.
6 Repeated and frequent exhibition of sexualized behaviour.

Findings which are moderately suspicious and require multidisciplinary evaluation

1 Repeated perineal symptoms, especially if accompanied by signs compatible with trauma. Repeated RAD of <1.5 cm in the absence of constipation, perianal oedema, fissures and infection.
2 Psychiatric disturbances especially mutism, anorexia and attempted suicide.
3 Child hints repeatedly at undisclosed and awful secrets.
4 Inappropriate behavioural patterns with other children or adults.

Features which arouse a low suspicion of child sexual abuse—monitoring advisable

1 Recurrent urinary tract infections, persistent constipation.
2 Recurrent psychosomatic illness, e.g. abdominal pain, headaches.
3 Isolated observation of sexualized behaviour.
4 Isolated but eccentric family patterns of sexual interaction.

Specific clinical features

Normal physical findings occur in 26–73% of girls and 17–82% of boys [60]. Diagnostic findings, namely semen, genital trauma or STD, occur in 3–10%. The reasons for this include delay in seeking medical examination; rapid healing [62–64]; failure of sperm to be identified if 72 h have elapsed or if the child is washed; occurrence of rape without hymenal damage; 'conditioning' of children by perpetrators; and ability of the anus to pass large stools without obvious injury. Use of the colposcope may enable more subtle changes to be identified [65,66]. Hymenal appearances vary naturally with age and the effects of oestrogen. The hymenal aperture depends on the child's age and the examination technique used. Congenital absence of the hymen is rare and a hymenal aperture which exceeds by two standard deviations of the mean for age is highly suspicious of CSA [60].

Signs of anal abuse may be more difficult to interpret. RAD is dilation of the external anal sphincter followed by the internal sphincter on gentle buttock traction for up to 30 s [61,67]. The test is positive in 42% of British sexually abused children [68] but is also found in up to 18% of controls and 15–18% of those with constipation [61,69]. In the USA the incidence of anal findings in children with gastrointestinal symptoms is less than 5% [70].

Differential diagnosis of child sexual abuse and congenital variations

Congenital variations of normal which lead to misdiagnosis include periurethral bands, intravaginal ridges, midline perianal skinfolds, perineal grooves, diastasis ani, smooth wedge-shaped areas in the midline of the anal verge, abnormalities of the bulbocavernosus muscle and a white linea vestibularis [60,65].

Accidental trauma

The genitalia, perineum or anus may be injured accidentally by blunt trauma, e.g. straddle injury. In girls the pubic bone and labia usually protect the hymen and other internal structures from injury. Superficial bruising involves the mons pubis and labia, or male genitalia or buttocks. Penetrating injuries are rare and more likely to involve the lateral walls of the introitus than the hymen [71].

Lichen sclerosis et atrophicus (see Chapter 24.1)

Lichen sclerosis et atrophicus (LSA) is a degenerative condition of unknown cause which primarily involves the anogenital region. Both sexes may be involved; boys may develop phimosis. The condition produces epidermal thinning beginning as pink to ivory flat-topped papules which coalesce into pearly atrophic plaques with wrinkling and increased fragility. Affected areas are susceptible to trauma; minor injuries produce haemorrhage, vesicular and bullous lesions. Fissures and secondary infections, including vulvovaginitis, are common. The area involved is restricted to the labia majora and perianal tissues; bruising outside of this area requires an explanation.

Diagnosis is confirmed by tissue biopsy; therapy is by local glucocorticoids, but response rate may be variable.

Although the pitfalls of confusing LSA with CSA are well recognized [72], the two conditions are not mutually exclusive [73]. Physical trauma of CSA may arguably induce LSA; other clinical features of CSA, e.g. hymenal damage, should be actively excluded [74].

Threadworms

Threadworm infestation may produce severe itching and vulvovaginitis leading to concerns about CSA; hymenal damage is rare.

Diagnosis is established by clinical suspicion and identification of threadworms or their ova in stools or on the anal margin. Treatment is Mebendazole (two doses 2 weeks apart) or piperazine (single dose); other family members should be treated.

Group A streptococci

Group A streptococcal infection produces mainly perianal symptoms, which may be protracted and include discomfort, pruritis, discharge, localized bleeding and an erythematous rash. Systemic symptoms, e.g. headaches, fever or abdominal pain, may occur [61,74].

Examination reveals marked perianal inflammation, with areas of bleeding, a purulent discharge and radial fissuring. Other evidence of abuse is lacking.

Diagnosis is confirmed by culture. Treatment is by appropriate antibiotics and results in rapid and complete resolution.

Vulvovaginitis

Vulvovaginitis produces symptoms of vaginal discharge, localized discomfort and dysuria which may be associated with poor hygiene and the wearing of tight, occlusive clothing. Specific irritants, e.g. bubble baths or shampoos, may cause symptoms. Vaginal discharge may be physiological, or associated with *Candida albicans*, or orovaginal transmission of organisms, e.g. *Haemophilus influenzae* or *Streptococcus pneumoniae*. Diagnosis is confirmed by finding a non-sexually transmitted organism in the absence of features of CSA.

Foreign bodies and masturbation

Insertion of foreign bodies, e.g. tissue paper or cotton wool, into the vagina produces an offensive bloody discharge [75]. Injury to the hymen is uncommon and if present should alert the clinician to the possibility of CSA, as should repeated episodes or concommitant STD. Examination under anaesthesia to confirm diagnosis and remove all foreign material, together with appropriate antibiotic therapy, is required.

Although persistent masturbation may be associated with CSA, prepubertal tampon usage [76], clitoral masturbation [71] and persistent masturbation and insertion of foreign bodies by children with learning difficulties [77] seldom produce evidence of anogenital injury. Similarly boys who self-inject water per urethram seldom have genital injuries [78].

Labial adhesions

Variable degrees of posterior labial fusion may occur, especially in nappy wearers, in response to inflammation produced by poor hygiene, but must be distinguished from posterior fourchette scars produced by sexual abuse [60,61]. Adhesions occurring in girls out of nappies for several years who have no features of poor hygiene should be regarded as suspicious. Labial adhesions respond to endogenous or exogenous oestrogen.

Other abnormalities

Urethral caruncle and prolapse, Crohn's disease, haemolytic uraemic syndrome and neurogenic anus have all produced anogenital appearances which have been confused with CSA [60,74,79].

Sexually transmitted diseases and child abuse (see also Chapter 24.2)

General considerations

Identification of organisms responsible for STDs in children outside the perinatal period raises the suspicion of CSA [60,61]. The possibility of congenital or perinatal infection or infection by direct contact, self-inoculation or formites (issues seldom arising when adults are infected) requires knowledge of the characteristics of infecting organisms, the epidemiology of the illness caused, and the specificity and sensitivity of detection methods [60,61,80–82].

Perinatal transmission of *Neisseria gonorrhoeae*, *Chlamydia*, *Trichomonas*, syphilis, human papillomavirus (HPV), herpes simplex virus (HSV), HIV and hepatitis B are well recognized. Persistence of organisms for months or years may occur [83], e.g. *Chlamydia* or untreated *Trichomonas*, as may delayed presentation, e.g. HIV or HPV [60,82]. Fomite transmission and autoinoculation with HPV are recorded.

Obtaining a history of abuse from a child with STD may be difficult [82] but this neither excludes CSA nor makes fomite or perinatal transmission more likely. Particular caution is required in children under 18 months in whom the possibility of persistent neonatal infection is strongest but who will be unable to give a detailed history. Furthermore, a child may have been the subject of CSA but also acquired a perinatal STD.

False positive tests may occur in a population with a low prevalence of STD resulting in avoidable errors in the identification of *Neisseria* and *Chlamydia* infection [84,85]. Since the implications of positive results are serious it is important that positive identification is made by appropriate culture techniques.

Despite these caveats the presence of STD in a child under 3 years of age is an indication for full exploration of the possibility of sexual abuse, including behavioural assessment, structured interview, medical examination and appropriate microbiology. The presence of one STD is an indication to look for others. Conversely, suspected CSA is an indication to screen for STD even in an asymptomatic child.

Gonorrhoea

Presumptive identification of *N. gonorrhoeae* in a Gram-stained smear must be confirmed by specific microbiological techniques [84]. Transmission occurs by intimate contact with epithelial or mucus-secreting cells and may involve multiple sites, e.g. the rectum, vagina, urethra or orpharynx, from which swabs should be taken. Oropharyngeal infection may be asymptomatic. Over 50% of infected children have symptoms, e.g. vaginal/rectal discharge [86], but frequency of infection in children presenting to sexual assault centres varies from 2.3 to 11.2% and is most likely in multiple episodes of abuse [86,87].

Gonococci may survive for 24h on toilet seats and 72h on other materials, e.g. cardboard or swabs, but in adults non-sexual transmission is unlikely. Although not all cases in children can positively be attributed to CSA [88] the identification of gonococci in children outside the perinatal period is highly suggestive of abuse [61,81].

Syphilis

Some abused children have positive serology for syphilis, though few will present with primary or secondary disease [86]. The predominant mode of spread is by sexual contact. If there is suspicion of CSA and syphilis is a risk, serological tests should be taken immediately and repeated at 3 months. Dark-ground microscopy of suspect material may demonstrate the organisms. Prepubertal children with early syphilis are presumed victims of CSA [61,81].

Chlamydia trachomatis

Prolonged periods of subclinical infection characterize human chlamydial disease. Manifestations of the disease may be ocular or genital and are associated with different serotypes of *Chlamydia trachomatis* (CT).

Reliable diagnosis of chlamydial infection depends on special handling of specimens and culture techniques, since enzyme immunoassays and direct immunofluorescence antibody tests may lack sensitivity and specificity. False positives from rectal swabs have been reported in children [61].

Over 50% of infants born to infected mothers will acquire symptomatic infection, commonly ophthalmia, during vaginal delivery but asymptomatic rectal or vaginal infection may occur in up to 15%. Rectovaginal infection may persist for months or years, so that neonatally acquired infection may be a differential diagnosis of CT acquired from CSA. Supportive evidence of CSA includes absence of asymptomatic maternal CT infection and the presence of culture confirmed urethral infection in an alleged perpetrator.

Rectogenital CT infections were found in 4–17% of sexually abused children [89,90]. Vaginal CT infection in prepubertal children is largely asymptomatic.

Trichomonas vaginalis

Non-sexual transmission of *Trichomonas vaginalis* (TV) is rare because of its specificity for the genitourinary tract; TV can survive on damp towels and clothing. Neonatal transmission can occur in 5% of infants born to infected women and may persist for 3–6 weeks because of the residual effect of maternal oestrogen. However, because TV does not survive in the prepubertal vagina, the presence of culture-proven vaginal infection after the perinatal period strongly suggests sexual abuse [60,61].

Herpes simplex virus

Both HSV types 1 and 2 may be associated with genital disease [61]. Transmission may occur by mouth to mouth, genital to genital or orogenital and anogenital contact with an incubation period of 2–20 days. Seemingly asymptomatic patients may shed the virus. Transmission via inanimate objects has been postulated but requires such an unlikely sequence of events as to be implausible.

Primary genital herpes produces vesicular or ulcerated lesions with tender inguinal lymphadenopathy; there may be systemic features, e.g. fever, malaise or myalgia.

HSV is detected by viral culture from swabs of specimens of vesicular fluid transported in Hank's balanced salt solution. Restriction enzyme technology may demonstrate uniqueness of HSV isolates; discovery of identical strains in an abused child and an alleged perpetrator would provide presumptive evidence of CSA. In contrast serological testing is of little value because of extensive cross-reactivity and the high prevalence of HSV antibodies in the population.

Genital warts (human papillomavirus)

In adults anogenital warts, are mainly transmitted by sexual intercourse [91]. Typing by DNA hybridization suggests site specificity in adults which may apply only partly in children [92]. HPV types 6 and 11 (and to a lesser extent 16 and 18) are associated with adult genital warts, but may produce laryngeal lesions in children [61].

Perinatal transmission of HPV can produce warts up to 2 years later [93,94]; transmission by autoinoculation and fomites also occurs [95,96,97].

However, anogenital warts in children can result from CSA and simultaneous presence of another STD would make this diagnosis virtually certain. Presence of anogenital warts in children over 2 years of age should trigger full evaluation for CSA [60,98]. HPV typing may enable identification of an anogenital-specific serotype and be of epidemiological use but may not be of value in identifying the perpetrator.

Bacterial vaginosis

Bacterial vaginosis, a polymicrobial infection by vaginal anaerobes and *Gardnerella vaginalis* (GV), is a common cause of vulvovaginitis in adults [99]. Although the role of sexual transmission is not yet well defined, GV is rare in virgins and can be recovered from sexual partners of women with GV [61].

In children GV prevalence rates of 14.6–25% have been recorded in sexually abused girls compared with 3–4% in controls [99,100]. GV isolates may be more likely in victims of multiple sexual abuse; transhymenal cultures may be helpful [99]. However, concerns exist about the age matching of controls and currently most authorities regard GV infection as suspicious but not diagnostic of CSA.

Screening for sexually transmitted diseases

Screening of sexually abused children for STD is recommended [60,61,82]. As in adults gonorrhoea and *Chlamydia* are the most prevalent STD organisms [82].

The timing, number and nature of specimens obtained depends on the nature and timing of abuse, the age of the child and the need to obtain concomitant forensic specimens. Some young children who have been recently abused may be distressed at the need to obtain multiple specimens which should include, oral, external and internal anal and vaginal swabs, and urethral swabs. Appropriate swabs and culture medium must be used [60,61,82].

Children and adolescents presenting more than 1 week after an episode of abuse should be tested, as a minimum, for gonorrhoea and chlamydial infection. Prompt screening may fail to detect incubating infection in prepubertal children seen immediately after sexual contact and screening should be deferred accordingly. Adolescents should be screened for gonorrhoea and *Chlamydia* at presentation because of the risk of ascending pelvic disease. Adolescents screened immediately and not given prophylaxis should be retested at 7 days to detect incubating infection. Those given prophylaxis should be retested 1 week after completing treatment [82].

Selection of other screening tests is dependent upon the child's estimated risk of acquiring specific infections. Information about the perpetrator's STD status is seldom available. However, it is reasonable to obtain blood for syphilis serology and to arrange for serum to be stored for possible use for HIV and hepatitis B testing [61,82]. Although the abused child's risk of acquiring HIV is small [101], the perpetrator's status is seldom known. Therefore parents should be given the opportunity to make informed decisions about HIV and hepatitis B testing after formal counselling. If the child has been the subject of recent abuse by a person from a population with a high prevalence of hepatitis B it would be prudent to begin active immunization subject to the child's hepatitis B status being determined. Similarly, if there is a high risk of transmission of HIV, appropriate anti-viral therapy, together with serology and techniques to detect viral nucleic acid, should be considered.

Prophylaxis

Prophylactic antibiotic therapy is not recommended [60,82,102] in CSA since the risk of developing infection is low. In adolescents prophylaxis against syphilis, *Chlamydia* and gonorrhoea may be indicated to reduce the risk of pelvic inflammatory disease. Prophylaxis should also be considered if the patient or child requests it, if it is felt that to do so would aid psychological healing, and if there are no facilities to obtain cultures [82].

Pregnancy testing and/or postcoital contraception should be offered if appropriate [82].

Management of suspected or actual child abuse

Many hospital, community units and local authorities have published guidelines or policies for management which may have statutory force, so the management of individual cases will depend on local practice. However, the following general principles apply [1–3].

Medical management

All injuries should be carefully documented by timed, dated, signed and contemporaneous records, supported where necessary by photographs for which consent is required. Differential diagnoses considered should be recorded. Injuries should be treated, using appropriate specialist expertise, e.g. general, plastic, orthopaedic and gynaecological surgery. Urgent medical treatment may have to be given without consent if clinically necessary. The need to obtain forensic specimens should be considered.

Determination of level of medical suspicion

This is a medical rather than legal concern [103,104]. It includes (a) consultation with colleagues having specific expertise; (b) consideration of the explanation given for the child's injuries and condition in the light of their known physical and developmental characteristics; and (c) consideration of differential diagnoses and any specific investigations needed to clarify these [5,10,60].

The multidisciplinary child abuse investigation

In all child abuse investigations the welfare of the child is paramount [105,106]. If there are immediate concerns about the child's safety such statutory action as is necessary to protect him or her and other family members should be taken. If the level of concern is less a number of agencies including health, social services, law enforcement and education will share information about the child and family prior to planning an investigation. Issues of gender, race, culture, religion, language and disability should be taken into account [105].

Attempts are made to carry out investigations in partnership with parents or carers, who should be consulted and informed at all stages unless it is against the best interests and the welfare of the child. Interviews and/or examination of the child should be the minimum required to clarify the child's situation.

An initial assessment interview with the child may be held in the absence of parents or carers to (a) obtain an account of what has happened; and (b) ascertain the child's wishes and feelings. Where criminal proceedings are contemplated such interviews should comply with local rules of evidence and may be videotaped. Information is also gathered from others personally and professionally involved with the child to identify the source and level of risk to the child and others in the family.

Professionals' meetings

The functions of professionals' meetings are as follows:
1 to share and evaluate information gathered during the investigation;
2 to make decisions about the level of risk to the child and others in the family;
3 to make plans for the child's future management; and
4 to make recommendations about the nature of any legal action [1–3,107].

Treatment and prevention

A detailed discussion of treatment strategies for victims and abusers is beyond the scope of this chapter. Removal of children from the non-abusing members of the family may reinforce feelings of victimization and guilt but may be necessary if the child's welfare cannot be safeguarded by other means. Treatment strategies include group psychotherapy and counselling for victims, self-help and anger management programmes, education in parenting skills and family therapy for perpetrators [108–110].

Prevention strategies are hampered by lack of funds, difficulties in recognition and lack of case–controlled studies [111,112]. Regular visiting of families by professionals may prevent accidents, but has a less clear role in prevention of abuse [113]; epidemiological studies do not specifically identify at risk individuals [52].

Child abuse—legal considerations

Cases of abuse in which the perpetrator cooperates fully with child protection agencies may not require legal intervention. However, some general legal issues need consideration.

Consent

All medical examinations or treatment require valid consent. For consent to be valid the consent giver must be competent to understand what is intended, have adequate information on which to base a rational choice and be free from coercion [114]. Children may not be competent and in normal circumstances consent is obtained from a proxy who possesses parental power/rights or has been granted or acquired parental responsibility. Whilst a child's view is important, it is not determinative in most legal systems [105,115].

Examination and treatment may proceed without consent if clinically necessary, e.g. in life-threatening situations.

For general medical assessment (which may give rise to suspicions of abuse), the child's presentation to doctors by a person with parental responsibility may imply consent. For more detailed assessment, e.g. of sexual abuse, specific consent is required and this may be unobtainable in the presence of a possible perpetrator. It may therefore be necessary to obtain some kind of statutory order to enable the examination or assessment to proceed.

If consent is withdrawn at any stage examination should cease immediately and legal advice be obtained.

Confidentiality

A doctor has a duty to 'respect the secrets which are confided in me, even after the patient has died' (Declaration of Helsinki as modified in Sydney in 1968) [116]. However, an absolute duty of confidentiality may place children at risk of further serious injury or death.

In some countries, e.g. the USA, there is a legal obligation for doctors to report suspicions of child abuse [5]; in others professional regulations permit breach of confidentiality in specific circumstances (including child abuse) when non-disclosure would place the patient at risk. Courts may have powers to compel disclosure of information.

Doctors have a defence against breach of confidentiality and defamation in abuse cases if they (a) reasonably believed their suspicions were true; and (b) communicated with a person with a legitimate interest in the information.

Specific legal considerations

Contemporary management of child abuse follows principles embodied in the UN Convention of Rights of the Child [106] including the following.

1 The need to take any decisions affecting children with their best interests as the paramount consideration (A3).

2 The right of a child not to be separated from parents or carers unless it is in their best interests (A9).

3 The right of families to support, advice and services to enable them to fulfil their obligations (A5, 18).

4 The right of children to protection and support, care and rehabilitation if they suffer from abuse or neglect (A19).

5 'A child who is capable of forming his or her own views has the right to express those views freely . . . the views of the child being given due weight in accordance with the age and maturity of the child' (A12).

The Convention has no legal force but many governments having ratified it are committed to its implementation, usually by statute.

Contemporary management of child abuse usually requires partnership between parents and professionals.

Where the risk to children is great, or their best interests are not protected, or society feels it important to punish perpetrators, the law will be involved.

Civil and criminal law and child abuse

The primary function of the law is child protection [105,107]. The mechanism whereby it achieves this will depend on whether civil or criminal law is involved. Criminal law is concerned with the punishment of perpetrators. Significant differences in criminal law practice exist between the inquisitorial system (used in much of Europe) and the adversarial system (used in much of the English-speaking world). The major differences between criminal and civil proceedings are shown in Table 24.3.5. A crucial difference is that in civil proceedings the welfare of the child is paramount; no such conditions apply in criminal proceedings where the function of the court is to decide the guilt or innocence of the accused.

The adversarial and inquisitorial system [117]

In the adversarial system each side presents a case to the court by means of witnesses who give evidence on which they are cross-examined in the presence of each other and the accused. The function of the judge is to see that rules are kept and to sum up the points each side has made. He or she takes no part in preliminary enquiries or establishing the truth.

In the inquisitorial system the court is a public agency whose function is to ascertain the truth. It gathers information, questions those who have useful information (including the accused in criminal cases) and then applies reasoning powers to elucidate the truth.

Increasingly civil courts in English-speaking areas use the inquisitorial approach to child abuse cases; criminal courts do not.

Table 24.3.5 Comparison between civil and criminal proceedings

	Types of proceedings	
	Civil	Criminal
Who needs to establish proof	Plaintiff	Prosecution
Standard of proof	Balance of probabilities	Beyond reasonable doubt
Grounds for making orders/bringing verdict	The child's actual or likely risk of harm	The accused committed the offence
Competence of child witness	The child understands the need to speak the truth	Assumed
Attendance in court	Dependent on child's wishes and welfare	Required for cross-examination, perhaps by video link
Rules of evidence	May be relaxed	Apply, with few exceptions
Video recording of evidence	Often admissible	May replace child's evidence

NB: These comments apply to the adversarial (English/US) system.

The child as a witness

For children (who may be the only witnesses to abuse) the adversarial proceedings are stressful because of (a) delay in organizing the trial; (b) cross-examination; (c) the presence of perpetrator; and (d) embarrassment at public recounting of events. These factors reduce the number of prosecutions and affect the quality of children's evidence [118]. A number of reforms have been made in most jurisdictions [119], and are listed below.

Children's competency

A child is usually allowed to give 'unsworn' (no oath) evidence providing that they can give a coherent account of events. The onus is now to prove a child's incompetence rather than assume it [117].

Corroboration

The need for a child's evidence to be corroborated in sexual abuse (where there may be no witnesses and no physical signs) has largely disappeared though courts may warn jurors of the dangers of convicting on uncorroborated evidence [117].

Alternatives to live evidence

In the adversarial system, videotaping of children's evidence is often accepted provided that rules of evidence are kept; a child will still face cross-examination in open court or by video link. In countries following the inquisitorial system the judge may question all parties in the case separately but can arrange for a confrontation between the child and the accused. Alternatively, special tribunals may avoid the need for cross-examination, and exclude both public and defendant if their presence is likely to harm the child. Such manoeuvres are more in keeping with the best interests approach of civil law but are not used worldwide [119,120].

Expert witnesses

Expert witnesses who may include dermatologists are used in both criminal and civil proceedings to provide informed opinion on technical matters relating to issues which courts have to decide. Their opinion may be sought by either party in a dispute, the child's legal representative or the court, or at their own initiation [1,121].

An expert witness should have sufficient knowledge skill, experience, training or education. In child abuse this includes knowledge of normal and abnormal findings, and of normal mechanisms of accidental injury to children. In sexual abuse cases expertise of other professionals may be involved but some kind of medical substantiation is required if a child is to be protected by law [103,104].

Experts may interview and examine a child but may need the courts' consent (as well as that of the parents or carers). Alternatively, case notes and pathological and radiological data may be supplied for review. Experts can favour an inquisitorial process by insisting their reports be disclosed to all parties concerned. They may also give opinions on facts and can use information which would not be available independently as evidence.

Broad guidelines for expert witnesses have been suggested [121] as follows.

1 Experts should present a straightforward and non-misleading opinion giving arguments objectively and impartially. Hypotheses which are untested or not accepted by medical peers should not be presented to courts.

2 Experts should not suppress material which does not support their opinion. The courts will wish to know how this opinion was reached.

3 Experts should be properly researched, i.e. in possession of all the relevant facts required to reach an opinion.

Doctors should not be asked to express certainty of opinion according to degree of proof, which is a legal rather than a clinical construct.

REFERENCES

1 Meadow R, ed. *ABC of Child Abuse*, 2nd edn. London: British Medical Association Publications, 1993.
2 Reece RM, ed. *The Pediatric Clinics of North America: Child Abuse*, vol. 37, no. 4. Philadelphia: WB Saunders, 1990.
3 Hobbs CJ, Hanks HGI, Wynne JM, eds. *Child Abuse and Neglect*. Edinburgh: Churchill Livingstone, 1993.
4 Meadow R. Epidemiology in ABC of Child Abuse. *Br Med J* 1989; 298: 727–9.
5 Johnston CF. Inflicted injury versus accidental injury. *Pediatr Clin N Am* 1990; 37: 791–814.
6 Caffe J. Multiple fractures of the long bones in infants suffering from chronic subdural haematomas. *Am J Roentgenol* 1946; 56: 143–50.
7 Kempe CH, Silverman FN, Steele BF, Droegmueller W, Silver HK. The battered child syndrome. *J Am Med Assoc* 1962; 181: 17–24.
8 Meadow R. What is and what is not Munchaussen syndrome by proxy? *Arch Dis Child* 1995; 72: 534–8.
9 Morris JL, Johnson CF, Clasen M. To report or not to report; physicians attitudes towards discipline and child abuse. *Am J Dis Child* 1985; 139: 194–7.
10 Hobbs CJ. Physical abuse. In: Hobbs CJ, Hankes HGI, Wynne JM, eds. *Child Abuse and Neglect*. Edinburgh: Churchill Livingstone, 1993: 47–75.
11 Rivara FP, Di Guiseppi C, Thompson RS *et al.* Risk of injury to children less than 5 years of age in day care versus home care settings. *Pediatrics* 1989; 84: 1011–16.
12 Taitz LS. Child abuse and osteogenesis imperfecta. *Br Med J* 1987; 295: 1082–3.
13 Smith R. Osteogenesis imperfecta non-accidental injury and temporary brittle bones disease. *Arch Dis Child* 1995; 72: 169–76 (plus commentaries).
14 Johnson CF, Showers J. Injury variables in child abuse. *Child Abuse Negl* 1985; 9: 207–15.
15 Showers J, Bandman RL. Scarring for life: abuse with electric cords. *Child Abuse Negl* 1986; 10: 25–31.
16 Hanigan WC, Peterson RA, Njus G. Tin ear syndrome. Rotational acceleration paediatric head injuries. *Pediatrics* 1987; 80: 618–20.
17 Wilson EF. Estimation of the age of cutaneous contusions in child abuse. *Pediatrics* 1977; 60: 750–2.

18 Langlois NEI, Greshan GA. The ageing of bruises: a review and study of colour changes with time. *Forensic Sci Int* 1991; 50: 227–38.

19 Stephenson T, Bialas Y. Estimation of age of bruising. *Arch Dis Child* 1996; 74: 53–5.

20 Hempling SM. The application of ultra violet photography in clinical forensic medicine. *Med Sci Law* 1981; 21: 215–22.

21 O'Hare AE, Eden OB. Bleeding disorders and non-accidental injury. *Arch Dis Child* 1984; 59: 860–4.

22 Wheeler DM, Hobbs CJ. Mistakes in diagnosing non-accidental injury: 10 years experience. *Br Med J* 1988; 296: 1233–6.

23 Johnson CF, Goury DL. Bruising and haemophillia: accident or child abuse? *Child Abuse Negl* 1988; 12: 409–15.

24 Ellerstein NS. The cutaneous manifestations of child abuse and neglect. *Am J Dis Child* 1979; 133: 906–9.

25 Roberts DLL, Pope FM, Nicholls AC, Narcisi P. Ehlers–Danlos syndrome type IV mimicking non-accidental injury in a child. *Br J Dermatol* 1984; 111: 341–5.

26 Brown J, Melinkovich P. Schonlein–Henoch purpura misdiagnosed as suspected child abuse. A case report and literature review. *J Am Med Assoc* 1986; 256: 617–18.

27 Adler R, Kane-Nussen B. Erythema multiforme: confusion with child battering syndrome. *Pediatrics* 1983; 72: 718–20.

28 Cohen B. Parvovirus B19: an expanding spectrum of disease. *Br Med J* 1995; 311: 1549–52.

29 Yeatman GW, Shaw C, Barlow MJ *et al*. Pseudo-battering in Vietnamese children. *Pediatrics* 1976; 58: 616–18.

30 Asnes RS, Wisotsky DH. Cupping lesions simulating child abuse. *J Pediatr* 1981; 99: 267–8.

31 Showers J, Garrison KM. Burn abuse: a 4 year study. *J Trauma* 1988; 28: 1581–3.

32 Hobbs CJ. ABC of child abuse: burns and scalds. *Br Med J* 1989; 298: 1302–5.

33 Roberts I. Deaths of children in house fires. *Br Med J* 1995; 311: 1381.

34 Alexander RC, Surrell JA, Cohle SD. Microwave oven burns to children: an unusual manifestation of child abuse. *Pediatrics* 1987; 79: 255–60.

35 Moritz AR, Henrigues FC. Studies of thermal injury. Pathology and pathogenesis of cutaneous burns: an experimental study. *Am J Pathol* 1947; 23: 915–41.

36 Rosenberg DA. Web of deceit; a literature review of Munchausen syndrome by proxy. *Child Abuse Negl* 1987; 11: 547–63.

37 Bools C, Neale BA, Meadow SR. Follow-up of victims of fabricated illness (Munchausen syndrome by proxy). *Arch Dis Child* 1993; 69: 625–30.

38 Helfer RE. The neglect of our children. *Pediatr Clin N Am* 1990; 37: 923–42.

39 Skuse D. Emotional abuse and neglect. *Br Med J* 1989; 298: 1692–3.

40 Verbov J. Hair loss in children. *Arch Dis Child* 1993; 68: 702–6.

41 Schechter MD, Roberge L. Sexual exploitation. In: Helfer RE, Kempe CH, eds. *Child Abuse and Neglect: the Family and the Community*. Cambridge: Ballinger, 1976: 127–42.

42 Mrazeck D, Mrazeck P. Child maltreatment. In: Rutter M, Hersov L, eds. *Child and Adolescent Psychiatry—Modern Approaches*. Oxford: Blackwell Scientific Publications, 1985.

43 Olafson E, Corwin DL, Summit RC. Modern history of child sexual abuse awareness: cycles of discovery and suppression. *Child Abuse Negl* 1993; 17: 7–24.

44 Finkelhor D. *Sexually Victimised Children*. New York: Free Press, 1979.

45 Finkelhor D. *Child Sexual Abuse: New Therapy and Research*. New York: Free Press Macmillan, 1984.

46 Russell D. The incidence and prevalence of intrafamilial sexual abuse of female children. *Child Abuse Negl* 1983; 7: 133–46.

47 *Child Sexual Abuse Within the Family*. London: CIBA Foundation, 1984.

48 Baker AW, Duncan SP. The incidence and prevalence of intrafamilial sexual abuses of female children in Great Britian. *Child Abuse Negl* 1985; 9: 457–67.

49 Beitchman JH, Zucker KJ, Hood JE, Da Costa GA, Akman D. A review of the short term effects of child sexual abuse. *Child Abuse Negl* 1991; 15: 537–56.

50 Miller BA, Downs WR, Gondoli DM, Keil A. The role of childhood sexual abuse in the development of alcoholism in women. *Violence Victims* 1987; 2: 157–72.

51 Glaser D, Frosh S. *Child Sexual Abuse*. London: Macmillan, 1988.

52 Finkelhor D. Epidemiological factors in the clinical identification of child sexual abuse. *Child Abuse Negl* 1993; 17: 67–70.

53 Finkelhor D, Baron L. High risk children. In: Finkelhor D *et al.*, eds. *Source Book of Child Sexual Abuse*. Beverley Hills: Sage, 1986: 60–88.

54 Moghal NE, Notal K, Hobbs CJ. A study of sexual abuse in an Asian community. *Arch Dis Child* 1995; 72: 346–7.

55 Hobbs CJ, Wynne JM. The sexually abused battered child. *Arch Dis Child* 1990; 65: 423–7.

56 West DJ. Incest in childhood and adolescence: long term effects and therapy. *Br J Hosp Med* 1988; 40: 352–60.

57 Arnold RP, Rogers D, Cook DAG. Medical problems in adults who were sexually abused in childhood. *Br Med J* 1990; 300: 705–8.

58 Briere J, Runtz M. Symptomatology associated with childhood sexual experience in a non-clinical female population. *Child Abuse Negl* 1988; 12: 51–9.

59 Bentovim A. Why do adults sexually abuse children? *Br Med J* 1993; 307: 144–5.

60 Bays J, Chadwick D. Medical diagnosis of the sexually abused child. *Child Abuse Negl* 1993; 17: 91–110.

61 Royal College of Physicians. *Physical Signs of Sexual Abuse in Children*. London: Royal College of Physicians, 1991.

62 Adams JA, Harper K, Krudson S, Revilla J. Examination findings in legally confirmed sexual abuse; it's normal to be normal. *Pediatrics* 1994; 94: 310–17.

63 Finkel MA. Anogenital trauma in sexually abused children. *Pediatrics* 1989; 84: 317–22.

64 McCann J, Voris J, Simon M. Genital lesions resulting from sexual abuse; a longitudinal study. *Pediatrics* 1992; 89: 307–17.

65 McCann J. Use of the colposcope in childhood sexual abuse examination. *Pediatr Clin N Am* 1990; 378: 63–80.

66 Hobbs CJ, Wynne JM, Thomas AJ. Colposcopic genital findings in prepubertal girls assessed for sexual abuse. *Arch Dis Child* 1995; 73: 465–71.

67 Hobbs CJ, Wynne JM. Buggery in childhood a common syndrome of child abuse. *Lancet* 1986; 11: 792–6.

68 Hobbs CJ, Wynne JM. Sexual abuse of English boys and girls: the importance of anal examination. *Child Abuse Negl* 1989; 13: 195–210.

69 Agnarrson U, Warde C, McCarthy G, Evans N. Perianal appearances associated with constipation. *Arch Dis Child* 1990; 65: 1231–4.

70 Lazar LF, Muram D. The prevalence of perianal and anal abnormalities in a paediatric population referred for gastrointestinal complaints. *Adolesc Paediatr Gynaecol* 1989; 2: 37–9.

71 Hobbs CJ, Wynne JM. Child sexual abuse—an increasing rate of diagnosis. *Lancet* 1987; 11: 837–41.

72 Handfield-Jones SE, Hinde FRJ, Kennedy CTC. Lichen sclerosis et atrophicus in children misdiagnosed as sexual abuse. *Br Med J* 1987; 294: 1404–5.

73 Priestly B, Bleehen S. Lichen sclerosis and sexual abuse. *Arch Dis Child* 1990; 65: 335.

74 Bays J, Jenny C. Genital and anal conditions confused with child sexual abuse trauma. *Am J Dis Child* 1990; 144: 1319–22.

75 Paradise JE, Willis E. Probability of vaginal foreign body in girls with genital complaints. *Am J Dis Child* 1985; 139: 472–6.

76 Woodling BA, Kissons PD. Sexual misuse, rape, molestation and incest. *Pediatr Clin N Am* 1981; 28: 481–99.

77 Hyman SL, Fisher W, Mercugliano A, Cataldo MF. Children with self-injurious behaviour. *Pediatrics* 1990; 85: 437–41.

78 Labbe J. Self-induced urinary tract infections in school aged boys. *Pediatrics* 1990; 86: 703–6.

79 Johnson CF. Prolapse of the urethra: confusion of clinical and anatomic characteristics with sexual abuse. *Pediatrics* 1991; 87: 722–5.

80 DeJong AR, Finkel M. Sexual abuse of children. *Curr Probl Pediatr* 1990; XX: 490–567.

81 Neinstein LS, Golden-Ring J, Carpenter S. Non-sexual transmission of sexually transmitted diseases; an infrequent occurrence. *Pediatrics* 1984; 74: 67–76.

82 Paradise JE. The medical evaluation of the sexually abused child. *Pediatr Clin N Am* 1990; 37: 839–62.

83 Schachter J, Pattel BJ. Sexually transmitted diseases in victims of sexual assault. *N Eng J Med* 1987; 316: 1023–7.

84 Whittington WL, Rice RJ, Biddle JW *et al*. Correct identification of *Neisseria gonorrhoea* from infants and children. *Pediatr Infect Dis* 1988; 7: 3–10.

85 Hammerschlag MR, Rettig PJ, Shields ME. False positive results with the use of chlamydial antigen detection tests in the evaluation of suspected sexual abuse in children. *Pediatr Dis J* 1988; 7: 11.

86 DeJong A. Sexually transmitted diseases in sexually abused children. *Sexually Trans Dis* 1986; 13: 123–6.

87 Tilelli JA, Thurek D, Jaffe AC. Sexual abuse in children; clinical findings and implications for management. *N Engl J Med* 1980; 302: 319–23.

88 Fairell MK, Billmen E, Shamroy JA, Hammond RN. Prepubertal gonorrhoea; a multidisciplinary approach. *Pediatrics* 1981; 37: 151–3.

89 Fuster CD, Neinstein LS. Vaginal chlamydial trachomatis infection; prevalence in sexually abused prepubertal girls. *Pediatrics* 1987; 79: 235–8.

90 Hammerschlag MR, Doraiswany B, Alexander ER, Cox P, Price W, Gleyzer BG. Are retrogenital chlamydial infections a marker of sexual abuse in children. *Pediatr Infect Dis* 1984; 3: 100–4.

91 Giardino AP, Fuikel MA, Giardino ER, Seidi T, Ludwig S, eds. Sexually transmitted disease. In: *A Practrical Guide to the Evaluation of Sexual Abuse in Prepubertal Women.* London: Sage, 1992: 100–12.

92 Stewart D. Sexually transmitted diseases. In: Heger A, Emon SJ, eds. *Evaluation of the Sexually Abused Child.* Oxford: Oxford University Press, 1992: 145–69.

93 DeJong AR, Weiss JC, Brent RL. Condyloma acuminata in children. *Am J Dis Child* 1982; 136: 704–6.

94 Gutman LT, Herman-Giddens ME, Phelps WC. Transmission of human genital papilloma virus disease. Comparison of data from adults and children. *Pediatrics* 1993; 91: 31–8.

95 Bergeron C, Fernizy A, Richart R. Underwear: contamination by human papilloma viruses. *Am J Obstet Gynaecol* 1990; 162: 25–9.

96 Fleming KA, Vening V, Evans M. DNA typing of genital warts and diagnosis of sexual abuse of children. *Lancet* 1987; 11: 454.

97 Pacheco BP, DiPaola G, Ribas JM, Viglu S, Rueda NG. Vulval infections caused by human papilloma virus in children and adolescents without sexual contact. *Adoles Pediatr Gynaecol* 1991; 4: 136–42.

98 Herman-Giddens ME, Gutman LT, Berson NL, and the Duke Child Protection Team. Association of coexisting vaginal infections and multiple abusers in female children with genital warts. *Sexually Transm Dis* 1988; 15: 63–7.

99 Steele AM, De San Lazaro C. Transhymenal cultures for sexually transmitted organisms. *Arch Dis Child* 1994; 71: 423–7.

100 Ingram DL, White ST, Lyna PR *et al. Gardnerella vaginalis* infection and sexual contact in female children. *Child Abuse Negl* 1992; 16: 847–52.

101 Gutman LT, St Claire KK, Weedy C *et al.* Human immunodeficiency virus transmission by child sexual abuse. *Am J Dis Child* 1991; 145: 137–41.

102 Glaser JB, Hammerschlag MR, McCormack WM. Sexually transmitted diseases in victims of sexual assault. *N Engl J Med* 1986; 315: 625–7.

103 Chadwick DL. Preparation for court testimony in child abuse cases. *Pediatr Clin N Am* 1990; 37: 955–70.

104 Myers JE. Expert testimony regarding child sexual abuse. *Child Abuse Negl* 1993; 17: 175–85.

105 Stainton-Rogers W, Roche J. Child welfare law; how the legal system operates. In: *Children's Welfare and Children's Rights.* London: Hodder & Stoughton, 1994: 21–41.

106 *United Nations Convention on the Rights of the Child,* Article 3. London: HMSO, 1991.

107 Stainton Rogers W, Roche J. Child protection. In: *Children's Welfare and Children's Rights.* London: Hodder and Stoughton, 1994: 93–117.

108 Corby B. Research into child protection practice. In: *Child Abuse Towards a Knowledge Base.* Buckingham: Open University Press, 1993: 127–43.

109 Jones DPH. Professional and clinical challenges to protection of children. *Child Abuse Negl* 1991; 15: 57–66.

110 Doek JE. Management of child abuse and neglect at the international level; trends and perspectives. *Child Abuse Negl* 1991; 15: 51–6.

111 Altemeier WA, O'Connor S, Vietze PM *et al.* Behavioural paediatrics. antecedents of child abuse. *Pediatrics* 1982; 100: 823–9.

112 Dubowitz H. Prevention of child maltreatment. What is known. *Pediatrics* 1989; 83: 570–7.

113 Roberts I, Kramer MS, Suissa S. Does home visiting prevent childhood injury? A systematic review of randomised controlled trials. *Br Med J* 1996; 312: 29–33.

114 Kennedy I, Grubb A. Consent. In: *Medical Law Text and Materials.* London: Butterworth, 1994.

115 Devereux JA, Jones DPH, Dickenson DL. Can children withold consent to treatment. *Br Med J* 1993; 306: 1459–61.

116 British Medical Association. *The Handbook of Medical Ethics.* London: BMA Publications, 1984: 69–81.

117 Spencer JR, Flin R. The accusatorial system. In: *The Evidence of Children. The Law and the Psychology.* London: Blackstone Press, 1990: 65–99.

118 Saywitz KJ, Nathanson R. Children's testimony and their perception of stress in and out of the court room. *Child Abuse Negl* 1993; 17: 613–22.

119 Spencer JR, Flin R. The evidence of children in other legal systems. In: *The Evidence of Children. The Law and the Psychology.* London: Blackstone Press, 1990: 306–16.

120 Stainton Rogers W, Roche J. Is the law good for children. In: *Children's Welfare and Children's Rights.* London: Hodder & Stoughton. 1994: 210–25.

121 Williams C. Expert evidence in the case of child abuse. *Arch Dis Child* 1993; 68: 712–14.

Section 25
Systemic Diseases

25.1

Sarcoidosis, Pyoderma Gangrenosum, Crohn's Disease and Granulomatous Cheilitis

KAREN WISS

Sarcoidosis

Pyoderma gangrenosum

Crohn's disease

Granulomatous cheilitis

Sarcoidosis

Definition

Sarcoidosis is a systemic disease of unknown aetiology that is characterized by the presence of non-caseating granulomas primarily in the lungs, eyes, skin and lymph nodes. It is rare in children and more typically affects young adults.

History

Hutchinson, a London surgeon and dermatologist, described the first cases of sarcoidosis in the 1870s with emphasis on the impressive cutaneous manifestations. In 1892, he described a young girl with a 'relapsing iritis of inherited gout' [1] which most historians view as a child with sarcoidosis. Besnier in 1889 [2], described a case of what he called 'lupus pernio', a violaceous chilblain-like swelling of the nose and fingers. In 1899, Boeck [3], a Norwegian dermatologist, recorded a patient with multiple skin nodules and striking lymphadenopathy. Histologically, the lesions resembled a sarcoma. Hence the name 'multiple benign sarkoid'. The first international conference on sarcoidosis was held in 1934 [4] and at that time the disease was recognized as a distinct entity.

Aetiology and pathogenesis

The aetiology of sarcoidosis is not known. The disease is thought to represent a reaction pattern to one or several infectious agents or allergens that have not yet been identified [5]. The histopathological features are similar to those seen with mycobacterial infections, some fungi and with inhaled exposure to zirconium and beryllium.

However, none of these agents has been identified in patients with sarcoidosis.

A family tendency towards sarcoidosis exists [6] although no mode of inheritance has been determined. Human leucocyte antigen (HLA) typing has revealed an association between HLA-A1B8 and acute episodes of sarcoidosis with uveitis and arthritis [7]. Individuals with HLA-B8 seem to have an increased risk of developing the disease [8]. HLA-B13 is associated with a particularly chronic form of the disease [9]. It is possible that a genetically predisposed host responds to some incompletely degraded antigen (that has not been identified) by forming a specific reaction pattern of granulomas in various organs [5].

An assortment of immunological abnormalities has been found in various tissues. The most characteristic findings are elevated serum immunoglobulins, circulating immune complexes and depressed cell-mediated immunity with cutaneous anergy [10]. The granulomas contain CD4 positive T-helper lymphocytes and macrophages in the centre and CD8 T-suppressor lymphocytes at the periphery [11,12]. Because there is an excess of T-helper cells at sites of disease activity [12], circulating T-helper cells are decreased. This leads to an imbalance in T-cell subpopulations that seems responsible for some of the abnormalities noted [11]. T-helper cells typically stimulate B lymphocytes to produce immunoglobulins so their excess in tissue may be responsible for the polyclonal hyperglobulinaemia seen [9]. The movement of T-helper lymphocytes to tissue leaving behind T-suppressor cells in the blood may be responsible for the anergy to skin test antigens that is frequently observed [9].

Pathology

The classic histopathological features include non-caseating granulomas comprised of tightly packed epithelioid cells and Langhans' giant cells. Lymphocytes, macrophages and fibroblasts surround these granulomas [13]. The granulomas can be found in almost any organ. Common sites for biopsy include the bronchus, lymph nodes, conjunctiva, minor salivary glands and the skin. Three types of inclusion bodies have been described in the skin: Schaumann bodies (calcium carbonate, phosphate and iron), asteroid bodies (lipoprotein) and residual bodies (lipomucoprotein granules) [14]. Special stains for fungi and mycobacteria plus polarization for foreign bodies will be negative and are important tests in excluding other causes of granulomatous inflammation.

Clinical features

Sarcoidosis is rare in children [15] and reported more frequently in young adults. It has been reported primarily in the USA, England, Japan and Scandinavia. In the USA, it is most prevalent in the south-eastern portion, the so-called 'sarcoid belt'.

Sarcoidosis is a multisystem disease with numerous presentations and as a result has been nicknamed 'the great pretender' [15]. While any organ can be involved, the joints, skin and eyes are typically affected in young children [16]. Older children usually have disease that is similar to that in adults with involvement of the lungs, lymph nodes and eyes [16]. Other areas affected include calcium metabolism, serum protein, salivary glands, heart, liver, spleen, musculoskeletal, haematological system, kidneys and central nervous system [17]. In one series, 75% of children had five or more areas of involvement [17]. Young children frequently present with non-specific symptoms of fatigue, anorexia, weight loss and fever. Older children, like adults, often describe fatigue, lethargy, malaise, cough and dyspnoea [18].

Sarcoidosis in young children

'Preschool sarcoidosis', seen in children under 6 years of age, characteristically involves the skin, joints and eyes [19]. The lungs and other organs are infrequently involved [17]. An asymptomatic eczematous dermatitis or infiltrative plaques are often the initial complaints [18]. An eruption of slightly scaly erythematous macules and papules that starts peripherally is common in this population [16]. These young children have a polyarthritis consisting of non-deforming and painless swelling of the fingers and wrists [20]. Granulomatous uveitis and keratitis are the ocular manifestations seen in this age group and can result in serious and progressive eye disease [19].

Cutaneous features

An extensive spectrum of cutaneous lesions of sarcoidosis has been reported. These lesions can be specific for sarcoidosis with histological features of non-caseating granulomas or non-specific as a reaction to sarcoidosis elsewhere. The most typical lesions with specific histology are firm flesh-coloured red or yellow–brown papules that appear on the face, especially the nares, nasolabial folds and eyelids [21]. However, any region of the body can be involved. The papules are frequently in an annular or serpiginous pattern. Diascopy reveals an apple jelly colour that is seen with a variety of cutaneous granulomatous infiltrates. Indurated plaques are common and have been referred to as Hutchinson's plaques [21]. When prominent telangiectatic vessels are seen within the papules or plaques, the lesions are termed 'angiolupoid'. Cutaneous sarcoidosis regularly appears in old scars and resembles a keloid [21]. Other cutaneous lesions reported that demonstrate granulomas histologically include generalized erythematous macules and papules [16,22], an acquired ichthyosis [23], erythroderma [24], hypopigmented macules, papules, plaques or nodules [25], ulcers [26], scarring alopecia [27], a psoriasiform dermatitis [21] and granulomatous cheilitis [28]. Erythema nodosum is a common non-specific presentation seen in patients with acute sarcoidosis [29]. Patients present with fever, malaise and polyarthralgias. The prognosis with erythema nodosum is favourable with a high rate of spontaneous resolution. Erythema nodosum is unusual in children with sarcoidosis.

There are several unique forms of cutaneous sarcoidosis. Lupus pernio, the most distinctive sarcoidal skin lesion, manifests as violaceous papules, nodules or plaques on the nose, cheeks and ears [30]. This presentation is usually seen in women, is associated with involvement of the upper respiratory tract [30], and often results in nasal deformity. Darier–Roussy sarcoidosis refers to sarcoidal granulomas in the subcutaneous fat [31]. Patients present with firm nodules on the trunk and extremities. Lofgren's syndrome includes the sudden onset of erythema nodosum, fever, uveitis, polyarthralgia and bilateral hilar adenopathy [32].

Intrathoracic features

The lung is the most frequently involved organ in older children as well as in adults [33]. Patients may present with mild cough and exertional dyspnoea. Bilateral hilar adenopathy is the most common intrathoracic finding [33]. The lung parenchyma may be involved with interstitial fibrosis resulting in restrictive pulmonary disease [33].

Ocular features

Approximately one-third of patients with systemic disease have ocular involvement [34]. Uveitis, especially chronic anterior granulomatous uveitis, is the most typical finding [34]. Also seen are iritis, involvement of the lacrimal gland, chorioretinitis, periphlebitis and glaucoma [34]. Conjunctival granulomas can be found in many patients. Biopsy of the conjunctivae even when there is no obvious ocular disease can aid in diagnosis [35].

Rheumatological features

In older children, the joint findings are similar to juvenile rheumatoid arthritis with morning stiffness, pain and restricted movement [20]. Preschool sarcoidosis can also be confused with juvenile rheumatoid arthritis because uveitis and arthritis are features common to both diseases [36].

Other organs

Lymphatic involvement is quite common with generalized enlargement of lymph nodes [33]. Parotitis, especially as part of uveoparotid fever or Heerfordt's syndrome, is seen in combination with uveitis, facial nerve palsy and fever [37]. Cardiac involvement results from granulomatous infiltration leading primarily to arrhythmias [38]. Neurosarcoidosis may present as meningitis, cranial nerve palsies, peripheral neuropathy, myopathy [39], diabetes insipidus or a seizure disorder [15]. Renal disease, which is not common in children, occurs secondary to hypercalcaemia, granulomatous infiltration or glomerulonephritis [15].

Laboratory findings

There is no laboratory test that will diagnose sarcoidosis, rather there are tests that will lend support to the diagnosis. Biopsy of the skin, peripheral lymph nodes, liver, conjunctiva, salivary glands and lacrimal glands can all be of benefit. Chest radiographs are frequently useful [17], especially in older children. Hypercalcaemia and hypercalciuria are common findings [17]. Angiotensin-converting enzyme (ACE) can be of benefit in patients with sarcoidosis. The test is not specific for sarcoidosis but is frequently elevated in the disease [40]. When ACE levels are elevated, the test can be used to follow disease activity and assist in decisions about systemic treatment [40]. There is also evidence that maximum serum ACE levels may aid in assessing prognosis [41]. Other common abnormalities include an elevated erythrocyte sedimentation rate, elevated immunoglobulins, leucopenia, eosinophilia, haematuria, proteinuria, pyuria and abnormal liver function test [17].

The Kveim test is of historical interest and not currently recommended [42]. Sarcoidal tissue is injected intracutaneously. If a cutaneous reaction occurs, a biopsy is performed to look for sarcoidal granulomas. The Kveim test is not standardized and it is perhaps ill-advised to inject a tissue homogenate of uncertain aetiological nature into a subject's skin [42].

Prognosis

There is insufficient data regarding the long-term conse-quences of sarcoidosis on children [43]. It appears that most children with sarcoidosis improve with time [17]. Some have complications of persistent restrictive lung disease and blindness [17].

Differential diagnosis

Sarcoidosis has numerous presentations and can mimic multiple disorders. The differential diagnosis of papules would include xanthelasmas, syringomas, trichoepitheliomas and angiofibromas [21]. When multiple annular collections of papules are evident, granuloma annulare is considered [21]. With arthritis and uveitis, juvenile rheumatoid arthritis may be entertained as a diagnosis. The granulomatous form of perioral dermatitis can mimic sarcoidosis. Deep fungal and mycobacterial infections are included in the histological differential diagnosis.

Treatment

Therapy is aimed at reducing symptoms and preventing disease progression. Systemic corticosteroids are the mainstay of therapy, usually with prednisone at a starting dose of 1 mg/kg/day [17]. Treatment with systemic corticosteroids is indicated if progressive lung disease, disfiguring cutaneous lesions, renal insufficiency, myocardial involvement, neurological disease, eye disease or abnormal calcium metabolism are present [17]. Other treatment modalities that may be of benefit include non-steroidal anti-inflammatory drugs for arthritis and erythema nodosum, methotrexate, azathioprine and cyclosporine [44]. Topical or intralesional corticosteroids may be useful when treating cutaneous lesions. Antimalarials [45] and isotretinoin [46] may eliminate skin lesions.

Children need evaluation of the eyes with slit-lamp examination and determination of calcium metabolism by measuring serum calcium and 24-h urinary calcium excretion. Pulmonary activity should be evaluated by pulmonary function tests and chest radiographs.

REFERENCES

1 Hutchinson J. Recurring ophthalmitis with opacities in the vitreous: Mabey's malady. *Arch Surg* 1892; 4: 361.

2 Besnier E. Lupus pernio de la face: synovites fongueuses symetriques des extremites superieures. *Ann Dermatol Syph* 1889; 10: 333–6.

3 Boeck C. Multiple benign sarkoid of the skin. *J Cutan Genitourin Dis* 1899; 17: 543–50.

4 Reunion Dermatologique de Strasbourg. Seance special du 13 mai 1934 consacree a l'etude des sarcoides. *Bull Soc Fr Dermatol Syph* 1934; 41: 995–1392.

5 Hanno R, Callen JP. Sarcoidosis. A disorder with prominent cutaneous features and their interrelationship with systemic disease. *Med Clin N Am* 1980; 64: 847–66.

6 Sharma OP, Neville E, Walker AN *et al.* Familial sarcoidosis: a possible genetic influence. *Ann NY Acad Sci* 1976; 278: 386–400.

7 Brewerton DA, Cockburn C, James DCO *et al.* HLA antigens in sarcoidosis. *Clin Exp Immunol* 1977; 27: 227–9.

8 Olenchock SA, Heise ER, Marx JJ Jr *et al.* HLA-B8 in sarcoidosis. *Ann Allergy* 1981; 47: 151–3.

9 James DG, Williams WJ. Immunology of sarcoidosis. *Am J Med* 1982; 72: 5–8.

10 Daniele RR, Dauber JH, Rossman MD. Immunologic abnormalities in sarcoidosis. *Ann Intern Med* 1980; 92: 406–16.

11 Semenzato G, Pezzutto A, Agostini C *et al.* Immunoregulation in sarcoidosis. *Clin Immunol Immunopathol* 1981; 19: 416–27.

12 Hunninghake GW, Gadek JE, Young RC *et al.* Maintenance of granuloma formation in pulmonary sarcoidosis by T lymphocytes within the lung. *N Engl J Med* 1980; 302: 594–8.

13 Crystal RG, Roberts WC, Hunninghake GW *et al.* NIH conference. Pulmonary sarcoidosis: a disease characterized and perpetuated by activated lung T-lymphocytes. *Ann Intern Med* 1981; 94: 73–94.

14 Kerdel FA, Moschella SL. Sarcoidosis. An updated review. *J Am Acad Dermatol* 1984; 11: 1–19.

15 Hetherington S. Sarcoidosis in children. *Comp Ther* 1982; 8: 63–8.

16 Hetherington S. Sarcoidosis in young children. *Am J Dis Child* 1982; 136: 13–45.

17 Pattishell EN, Strope GL, Spinola SM *et al.* Childhood sarcoidosis. *Pediatrics* 1986; 108: 169–7.

18 Clark SK. Sarcoidosis in children. *Pediatr Dermatol* 1987; 4: 291–9.

19 Rasmussen JE. Sarcoidosis in young children. *J Am Acad Dermatol* 1981; 5: 566–70.

20 Lindsley CB, Godfrey WA. Childhood sarcoidosis manifesting as juvenile rheumatoid arthritis. *Pediatrics* 1985; 76: 765–8.

21 Elgart ML. Cutaneous sarcoidosis. Definitions and types of lesions. *Clin Dermatol* 1986; 4: 35–45.

22 Sharma OP. Cutaneous sarcoidosis: clinical features and management. *Chest* 1972; 61: 320–5.

23 Kauh YC, Goody HE, Luscombe HA. Ichthyosiform sarcoidosis. *Arch Dermatol* 1978; 114: 100–1.

24 Wigly JEM, Musso LA. A case of sarcoidosis with erythrodermic lesions. Treatment with calciferol. *Br J Dermatol* 1951; 63: 398–407.

25 Cornelius CE, Stein KM, Hanshaw WJ *et al.* Hypopigmentation and sarcoidosis. *Arch Dermatol* 1973; 108: 249–51.

26 Schiffner J, Sharma OP. Ulcerative sarcoidosis: report of an unusual case. *Arch Dermatol* 1977; 113: 676–7.

27 Greer KE, Harman LE Jr, Kayne AL. Unusual cutaneous manifestations of sarcoidosis. *South Med J* 1977; 70: 666–8.

28 Borugeois-Droin C, Havard S, Granier F *et al.* Granulomatous cheilitis in two children with sarcoidosis. *J Am Acad Dermatol* 1993; 29: 822–4.

29 James DG. Erythema nodosum. *Br Med J* 1961; 1: 853–7.

30 Jorizzo JL, Koufman JA, Thompson JN *et al.* Sarcoidosis of the upper respiratory tract in patients with nasal rim lesions: a pilot study. *J Am Acad Dermatol* 1990; 22: 439–43.

31 Vainsencher D, Winkelmann RK. Subcutaneous sarcoidosis. *Arch Dermatol* 1984; 120: 1028–31.

32 Lofgren S. Primary pulmonary sarcoidosis: early signs and symptoms. *Acta Med Scand* 1953; 145: 424–31.

33 Mayock RL, Bertrand P, Morrison CE *et al.* Manifestations of sarcoidosis. Analysis of 145 patients with a review of nine series selected from the literature. *Am J Med* 1963; 35: 67–89.

34 Obenauf CD, Shaw HE, Sydnor CF *et al.* Sarcoidosis and its ophthalmic manifestations. *Am J Ophthal* 1978; 86: 648–55.

35 Khan F, Wessely Z, Chazin SR *et al.* Conjunctival biopsy in sarcoidosis: a simple, safe, and specific diagnostic procedure. *Ann Ophthalmol* 1977; 9: 671–6.

36 Sahn EE, Hampton MT, Garen PD *et al.* Preschool sarcoidosis masquerading as juvenile rheumatoid arthritis: two case reports and a review of the literature. *Pediatr Dermatol* 1990; 7: 208–13.

37 Heerfordt CF. Ueber ein febris uveo-parotidea sub chronica an der glandula patotis unter der uvea des auges lokalisiert und haufig mit paresencerebrospinaler nerven compliziert. *Albrecht V Graefes Arch Ophthal* 1909; 70: 254.

38 Roberts WC, McAllister HA, Ferrans VJ. Sarcoidosis of the heart. A clinicopathologic study of 35 necropsy patients (group I) and review of 78 previously described necropsy patients (group II). *Am J Med* 1977; 63: 86–108.

39 Chapelon C, Ziza JM, Piette JC *et al.* Neurosarcoidosis: signs, course and treatment in 35 confirmed cases. *Medicine* 1990; 69: 261–76.

40 Rodriguez GE, Shin BC, Abernathy RS *et al.* Serum angiotensin-converting enzyme activity in normal children and in those with sarcoidosis. *J Pediatr* 1981; 99: 68–72.

41 Takada K, Ina Y, Noda M *et al.* The clinical course and prognosis of patients with severe, moderate or mild sarcoidosis. *J Clin Epidemiol* 1993; 46: 359–66.

42 Siltzbach LE. An international Kveim test study. *Acta Med Scand* 1964; 176 (suppl 425): 178.

43 Marcille R, McCarthy M, Barton JW *et al.* Long-term outcome of pediatric sarcoidosis with emphasis on pulmonary status. *Chest* 1992; 102: 1444–9.

44 Mathur A, Kremer JM. Immunopathology, rheumatic features, and therapy of sarcoidosis. *Curr Opin Rheumatol* 1992; 4: 76–80.

45 Zic JA, Horowitz DH, Arzubiaga C *et al.* Treatment of cutaneous sarcoidosis with chloroquine. Review of the literature. *Arch Dermatol* 1991; 127: 1034–40.

46 Waldinger TP, Ellis CN, Quint K *et al.* Treatment of cutaneous sarcoidosis with isotretinoin. *Arch Dermatol* 1983; 119: 1003–5.

Pyoderma gangrenosum

Definition

Pyoderma gangrenosum is an uncommon, ulcerative cutaneous disorder of unknown aetiology. The classic ulcer consists of a violaceous undermined border and a necrotic exudative base. Pyoderma gangrenosum is frequently seen in association with an underlying systemic illness, such as inflammatory bowel disease, arthritis or leukaemia.

History

Although it was probably described earlier, Brunsting *et al.* gave the first clear description of what they termed 'pyoderma gangrenosum' in 1930 [1]. The authors reported five cases with extensive cutaneous ulcers thought to be caused by *Staphylococcus* or *Streptococcus*. Four of the patients had ulcerative colitis [1]. Though it is no longer believed that pyoderma gangrenosum represents a true pyoderma, Brunsting's detailed morphological description of the ulcers fits with current understanding of the disease.

Aetiology and pathogenesis

The aetiology of pyoderma gangrenosum is unknown and very little is understood about the pathogenesis. Numerous investigators have searched for a bacterial cause to no avail. Multiple immunological abnormalities have been found in patients with pyoderma gangrenosum but no consistent aberration. The most common defect has been a monoclonal or polyclonal gammapathy [2]. However, this is not seen uniformly in all patients. In fact, congenital hypogammaglobulinaemia has been observed in some children [3]. There have also been reports of impaired neutrophil and monocyte chemotaxis and phagocytosis [2]. Histological studies have supported an immune-mediated vasculitis [4]. It is possible that the ulcers appear because of a cutaneous reaction in a host who is immunologically impaired because of an underlying systemic disease [5].

Pathology

Skin biopsy is often performed in order to exclude other aetiologies, primarily infectious. The histopathological features of pyoderma gangrenosum are non-diagnostic and vary depending on the age of the lesion and the site of the biopsy [4]. Specimens taken from the erythematous region peripheral to the ulcer show a lymphocytic vasculitis with endothelial swelling, vessel thrombosis, haemorrhage, fibrinoid necrosis and lymphocyte predominance [4]. Biopsy from the necrotic undermined edge is likely to demonstrate mixed cellularity, vasculitis and early abscess formation [4]. Samples obtained from the ulcer base reveal a dense dermal neutrophilic infiltrate, abscess formation and necrosis [4]. Direct immunofluorescence is frequently positive with immunoglobulinM (IgM), C3 and fibrin in dermal vessels [4].

Clinical features

The diagnosis of pyoderma gangrenosum is suggested in a patient with the characteristic ulcer appearance, distribution and course. Typically, a collection of painful, erythematous papules, macules, nodules or sterile pustules appears first. Children are more likely to have pustules upon presentation [6]. The collection of pustules rapidly breaks down into an irregular ulcer with a dusky red or violaceous, raised, undermined border. The edge of the ulcer often has perforations that release pus. The ulcer base contains alternating areas of abscesses and granulation tissue and has a purulent, necrotic, haemorrhagic exudate (Fig. 25.1.1). The ulcer expands with haemorrhagic pustules along the undermined border that break down or form a burrowing underneath the border. The ulcers frequently extend into the deep dermis but may extend into fat and fascia. Ulcers are usually solitary and very painful. They often heal with cribriform [2] or parchment-like scarring. Some patients with pyoderma gangrenosum have associated fever and systemic toxicity.

Ulcers may appear anywhere on the body. As in adults, the lower extremities are the region most often affected in children (in 80% in one series) [6]. Otherwise, the distribution differs between children and adults. The head and buttocks are frequently involved in children [6] and infants tend to have lesions in the perianal and genital regions [6] (Fig. 25.1.2). Mucous membranes are rarely affected.

The lesions of pyoderma gangrenosum tend to occur or worsen at sites of minimal cutaneous trauma, a phenomenon termed pathergy. Pathergy occurs in about 25% of adults with pyoderma gangrenosum [31]. It has also been noted in children [6]. This phenomenon can occur after insect bites, needle-stick injury and at biopsy sites. Although rarely reported in children [7], parastomal ulcers can appear as a result of pathergy related to the surgical procedure [8]. Ulcers can also develop secondary to an irritant contact dermatitis that so frequently occurs on peristomal skin.

Pyoderma gangrenosum is usually seen in association with an underlying systemic disease. The most common relationship in children is with inflammatory bowel disease, in particular ulcerative colitis [6]. Leukaemia, usually acute myeloid, is the most common malignancy noted in conjunction with pyoderma gangrenosum [6].

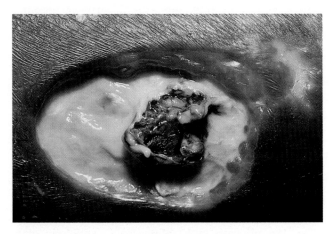

Fig. 25.1.1 A typical ulcer of pyoderma gangrenosum in a 16-year-old boy with systemic lupus erythematosus. This lesion demonstrates the violaceous, raised, undermined border and the necrotic exudative base.

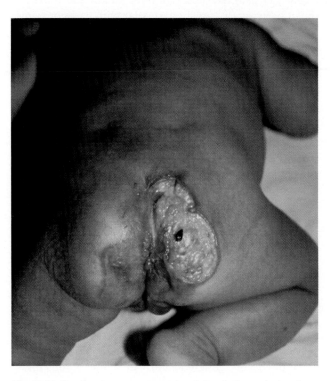

Fig. 25.1.2 Pyoderma gangrenosum involving the buttocks in a 4-month-old infant.

Arthritis (seronegative, rheumatoid and ankylosing spondylitis) is frequently seen with pyoderma gangrenosum in adults and children [6,9,10]. Other associated disorders described in children include human immunodeficiency verus (HIV) infection [11], selective IgA deficiency, [12] impaired leucocyte function [13], hypogammaglobulinaemia [12] and a neutrophil and T-cell deficiency [14]. In a review by Graham *et al.* [6], 27% of children had no underlying disease. This is similar to the percentage of 'idiopathic' cases in adults [15].

Some entities exist that are thought to represent variants of pyoderma gangrenosum. These include malignant pyoderma, an ulcerative and pustular disorder of the head and neck [2,16]; bullous pyoderma gangrenosum [17,2] with haemorrhagic bullae and eventually ulcers; and granulomatous pyoderma gangrenosum with superficial vegetative ulcers [18].

Laboratory evaluation should be targeted at identifying and managing an underlying disease. Most patients will have an elevated erythrocyte sedimentation rate and a neutrophilia.

Prognosis

The course of the ulcers is quite variable. They may expand rapidly or slowly, and may heal in one region while expanding in another. They can heal spontaneously or with treatment. They sometimes recur months or years later with or without cutaneous trauma. The course of pyoderma gangrenosum will often follow the course of the underlying disease, in particular with flares or remissions of inflammatory bowel disease. The ulcers heal with significant scarring.

Differential diagnosis

The diagnosis is made based on the clinical appearance and the exclusion of other causes of cutaneous ulcers, especially infectious aetiologies. Skin biopsy is usually performed from the ulcer border. While not diagnostic, skin biopsy demonstrating a neutrophilic infiltrate can lend support to the diagnosis. The biopsy should be viewed histopathologically with special stains and sent for microbiological culture to look for bacteria, viruses, fungi and mycobacteria.

The lesions of pyoderma gangrenosum can predate the recognition of the underlying systemic disorder. Children without an obvious explanation should be evaluated for inflammatory bowel disease, arthritis and underlying haematological malignancy [6]. Immune evaluation should also be considered.

The pustules or inflammatory papulonodules seen in early pyoderma gangrenosum can mimic a folliculitis, furunculosis, bites or a vasculitis [19]. Entities that could

be considered in the ulcerative stage include deep fungal infections like cryptococcosis, North American blastomycosis, histoplasmosis or sporotrichosis; and atypical mycobacterial infections, Meleney's ulcers, syphilitic gummas, herpes simplex, ulcerating necrobiosis lipoidica diabeticorum, amoebiasis, brown recluse spider bites, bromodermas, pyoderma vegetans, Wegener's granulomatosis and factitial ulcers.

Other neutrophilic dermatoses such as Sweet's syndrome (acute febrile neutrophilic dermatosis) and subcorneal pustular dermatosis often are considered in the differential diagnosis [2].

Treatment

Because of the rarity of pyoderma gangrenosum, there have been very few large series evaluating treatment. Therefore, most published reports are anecdotal, describing response to therapy in one or a small number of patients. It seems clear that in addition to managing the pyoderma gangrenosum, an attempt should be made at diagnosing and controlling the underlying systemic illness. Systemic corticosteroids are thought to be the first line of therapy [6,15]. Usually high doses of oral prednisone are needed to halt disease progression. Large doses of intravenous methylprednisolone have also been used successfully in 5-day pulses [20]. Pulsed corticosteroids may prove to reduce side-effects such as growth impairment seen with chronic oral corticosteroid use. Intralesional corticosteroids have been used successfully in some adults [21].

Sulpha drugs such as dapsone [1], sulphapyridine [22] and sulphasalazine [23] are frequently of benefit. They may be advantageous alone or in combination with systemic corticosteroids. Other treatments that have been successful in some adults and children include cytotoxic agents like cyclophosphamide [24] and chlorambucil [25]. A variety of antibiotics [5,6,26] such as rifampin [27], minocycline, clofazimine [12], vancomycin and mezlocillin have been used successfully. Hyperbaric oxygen [28] may also be useful. Oral cyclosporine has recently emerged as a very effective treatment for pyoderma gangrenosum in adults [29]. However, there have been few published reports of its use in children and adolescents [30].

While local therapy is rarely effective when used alone [31], it can be beneficial in combination with systemic treatment. Some topical treatments that have been useful include topical corticosteroids [6,31] and topical cromolyn sodium [32]. Whirlpool therapy is often beneficial in cleaning and gently debriding the ulcer. Wound care with saline soaks, antibiotic ointments and occlusive dressings may help maintain a clean wound. Aggressive surgical debridement should never be performed because of the likelihood that the ulcer will expand due to pathergy. Similarly, any surgical manipulation such as excision and grafting will tend to worsen the problem [31].

REFERENCES

1 Brunsting LA, Goeckerman WH, O'Leary PA. Pyoderma (ecthyma) gangrenosum. Clinical and experimental observations in five cases occurring in adults. *Arch Dermatol* 1930; 22: 655–80.
2 Malkinson FD. Pyoderma gangrenosum vs malignant pyoderma. *Arch Dermatol* 1987; 123: 333–7.
3 Barriere H, Litoux P, Stalder JF *et al.* Pyoderma gangrenosum au cours d'une hypogammaglobulinemie congenitale. *Ann Dermatol Vénéréol* 1979; 106: 695–6.
4 Su WPD, Schroeter AL, Perry HO *et al.* Histopathologic and immunopathologic study of pyoderma gangrenosum. *J Cutan Pathol* 1986; 13: 323–30.
5 Duguid CM, Powell FC. Pyoderma gangrenosum. *Clin Dermatol* 1993; 11: 129–33.
6 Graham JA, Hansen KK, Rabinowitz LG *et al.* Pyoderma gangrenosum in infants and children. *Pediatr Dermatol* 1994; 11: 10–17.
7 Klein JD, Biller JA, Leape LL *et al.* Pyoderma gangrenosum occurring at multiple surgical incision sites. *Gastroenterology* 1987; 92: 810–13.
8 Cairns BA, Herbst CA, Sartor BR *et al.* Peristomal pyoderma gangrenosum and inflammatory bowel disease. *Arch Surg* 1994; 129: 769–72.
9 Jacobs JC, Goetzl EJ. 'Streaking leukocyte factor', arthritis, and pyoderma gangrenosum. *Pediatrics* 1975; 56: 570–8.
10 Hambidge KM, Norris DA, Githens JH *et al.* Hyperzincemia in a patient with pyoderma gangrenosum. *J Pediatr* 1985; 106: 450–1.
11 Paller AS, Sahn EE, Garen PD *et al.* Pyoderma gangrenosum in pediatric acquired immunodeficiency syndrome. *J Pediatr* 1990; 117: 63–6.
12 Bundino S, Zina AM. Pyoderma gangrenosum associated with selective hereditary IgA deficiency. *Dermatologica* 1984; 168: 230–2.
13 Anderson DC, Springer TA. Leukocyte adhesion deficiency: an inherited defect in the Mac-1, LFA-1, and p 150, 95 glycoproteins. *Ann Rev Med* 1987; 38: 175–94.
14 Robinson MF, McGregor R, Collins R *et al.* Combined neutrophil and T-cell deficiency. Initial report of a kindred with features of the hyper-IgE syndrome and chronic granulomatous disease. *Am J Med* 1982; 73: 63–70.
15 Schwaegerle SM, Bergfeld WF, Senitzer D *et al.* Pyoderma gangrenosum: a review. *J Am Acad Dermatol* 1988; 18: 559–68.
16 Wernikoff S, Merritt C, Briggaman RA *et al.* Malignant pyoderma or pyoderma gangrenosum of the head and neck? *Arch Dermatol* 1987; 123: 371–5.
17 Perry HO, Winkelmann RK. Bullous pyoderma gangrenosum and leukemia. *Arch Dermatol* 1972; 106: 901–5.
18 Wilson-Jones E, Winkelmann RK. Superficial granulomatous pyoderma: a localized vegetative form of pyoderma gangrenosum. *J Am Acad Dermatol* 1988; 18: 511–21.
19 Keltz M, Lebwohl M, Bishop S. Peristomal pyoderma gangrenosum. *J Am Acad Dermatol* 1992; 27: 360–4.
20 Johnson RB, Lazarus GS. Pulse therapy. Therapeutic efficacy in the treatment of pyoderma gangrenosum. *Arch Dermatol* 1982; 118: 76–84.
21 Moschella SL. Pyoderma gangrenosum. A patient successfully treated with intralesional injections of steroid. *Arch Dermatol* 1967; 95: 121–3.
22 Perry HO, Brunsting LA. Pyoderma gangrenosum. A clinical study of 19 cases. *Arch Dermatol* 1957; 75: 380–6.
23 Powell FC, Perry HO. Pyoderma gangrenosum in childhood. *Arch Dermatol* 1984; 120: 757–61.
24 Crawford SE, Sherman R, Favara B. Pyoderma gangrenosum with response to cyclophosphamide therapy. *J Pediatr* 1967; 71: 255–8.
25 Callen JP, Case JD, Sager D. Chlorambucil—an effective corticosteroid-sparing therapy for pyoderma gangrenosum. *J Am Acad Dermatol* 1989; 21: 515–19.
26 Obasi OE. Pyoderma gangrenosum and malignant pyoderma in Nigeria. *Clin Exp Dermatol* 1991; 16: 34–7.
27 Tay CH. Pyoderma gangrenosum and leukemia. *Arch Dermatol* 1973; 108: 580–1.
28 Davis JC, Landeen JM, Levine RA. Pyoderma gangrenosum: skin grafting after preparation with hyperbaric oxygen. *Plast Reconstr Surg* 1987; 79: 200–7.
29 Matis WL, Ellis CN, Griffiths CE *et al.* Treatment of pyoderma gangrenosum with cyclosporine. *Arch Dermatol* 1992; 128: 1060–4.
30 Schmitt EC, Pigatto PD, Boneschi V *et al.* Pyoderma gangrenosum treated with low-dose cyclosporin. *Br J Dermatol* 1993; 128: 230–1 (letter).
31 Powell FC, Schroeter AL, Su WPD *et al.* Pyoderma gangrenosum: a review of 86 patients. *Q J Med* 1985; 55: 173–86.
32 De Cock KM, Thorne MG. The treatment of pyoderma gangrenosum with sodium cromoglycate. *Br J Dermatol* 1980; 102: 231–3.

Crohn's disease

Definition

Crohn's disease is a chronic inflammatory disease of the intestinal tract characterized histologically by non-caseating granulomas. It may affect any region of the gastrointestinal tract from the oropharynx to the perianal region but typically involves the terminal ileum and colon. Crohn's disease may also occur outside the intestinal tract. The disease shares many clinical and pathophysiological features with ulcerative colitis. Crohn's disease and ulcerative colitis comprise the main entities of idiopathic inflammatory bowel disease.

History

The first detailed description of Crohn's disease was in 1913 by Dalziel [1]. This Glasgow surgeon reported nine patients with a chronic granulomatous syndrome of the intestine. In their landmark article in 1932, Crohn *et al.* defined the clinical features of this illness and searched unsuccessfully for a causative agent [2]. Crohn's disease is now recognized as an important chronic disease of childhood and adolescence.

Aetiology and pathogenesis

The cause of Crohn's disease is unknown. An infectious agent is thought to play a role but no single organism has been identified. It has been speculated [3] that several different organisms may be involved in a host who has had some immunological or genetic alteration that makes him predisposed to the disease.

Pathology

Biopsy specimens taken from the bowel in Crohn's disease will show non-caseating granulomas through all layers of the bowel wall [4]. There are often intramural sinuses and fibrosis. Samples taken from the lesions of cutaneous (contiguous to or distant from the gastrointestinal tract) and mucosal Crohn's will demonstrate non-caseating granulomas comprised of epithelioid and giant cells, surrounded by a mononuclear cell infiltrate [5].

Clinical features

The classic presentation for Crohn's disease includes abdominal pain, diarrhoea, anorexia and weight loss [6]. However, children and adolescents often present with extraintestinal manifestations and delayed growth [6]. Hence, symptoms point away from bowel disease and diagnosis is often delayed. The disease more commonly affects adolescents than children [7].

A wide spectrum of extraintestinal manifestations have been reported with Crohn's disease. Large studies have shown that 24–36% of patients with inflammatory bowel disease have at least one associated extraintestinal manifestation [8,9]. Other organs commonly involved include the skin, eyes, joints, blood vessels and liver. Malnutrition is routine in patients with inflammatory bowel disease and in children can result in the growth failure that is so typically seen [6].

Cutaneous manifestations

The skin lesions of Crohn's disease may be non-specific and reactive, or specific with non-caseating granulomas histologically. Three of the most recognized non-specific cutaneous disorders seen with Crohn's disease include erythema nodosum, pyoderma gangrenosum and apthous stomatitis. Erythema nodosum occurs in approximately 7% of patients with Crohn's disease [9]. It is thought to represent a hypersensitivity reaction and may correlate with the presence of arthritis [10]. Pyoderma gangrenosum, also a non-specific finding, occurs in 1.4% of patients with Crohn's disease [9]. Aphthous stomatitis has been reported in up to 20% of patients with inflammatory bowel disease [9]. Tiny superficial linear ulcerations appear on the gingivae, upper and lower lips, palate and uvula [9]. The oral ulcers seem to be somewhat less common in children with inflammatory bowel disease than in adults [10,11]. Oral ulcers frequently precede but may coincide with or follow any gastrointestinal symptoms [9].

Other non-specific skin findings that have been described in association with inflammatory bowel disease include epidermolysis bullosa acquisita [12], vesiculopustular lesions (that may represent a variant of pyoderma gangrenosum) [13], psoriasis [9], vitiligo [14], erythema multiforme [15] and clubbing of the fingers [10].

Specific manifestations of Crohn's disease include perianal disease, perioral disease and metastatic Crohn's disease. Perianal involvement is quite common in Crohn's disease, occurring in 62% of 325 patients reviewed by Palder *et al.* [16]. Perianal skin tags (Fig. 25.1.3), anal fissures, abscesses and fistulas are the typical findings [16]. In this series [16], 49% of patients had perianal lesions as one of the first signs of the disease [16]. As with other cutaneous and oral manifestations, the

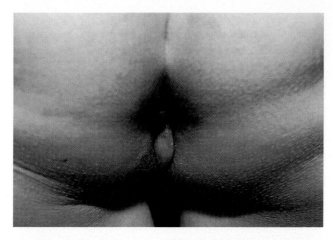

Fig. 25.1.3 Perianal tag in a 13-year-old boy with Crohn's disease.

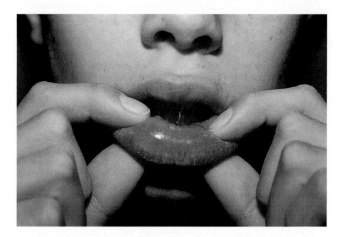

Fig. 25.1.4 Diffuse swelling of the lower lip in a 13-year-old child with Crohn's colitis.

perianal disease can predate the onset of gastrointestinal symptoms.

Besides the non-specific aphthous ulcers, granulomatous infiltration can occur on the oral mucosa. Some oral manifestations can be very suggestive for Crohn's disease. Oedema, ulcers and polypoid papular hyperplasia of the mucosa are the most common types of lesions [17]. Angular cheilitis, epithelial tags and folds, erythema and enlargement of the gingivae, and persistent diffuse swelling of the lips (Fig. 25.1.4) and cheeks have all been described [18]. A pebbly or 'cobblestone' appearance of the mucosae is a characteristic feature [15]. Pyostomatitis vegetans, referring to a vegetative, pustular eruption of the oral mucosa is another manifestation [19]. Frequent sites for oral lesions include the lips, gingiva, vestibular sulci and buccal mucosa [17].

Metastatic Crohn's disease refers to granulomatous infiltration of the skin in sites remote from the gastrointestinal tract [20]. This manifestation of Crohn's disease is rare [20]. Cutaneous lesions may be in the form of nodules, plaques and ulcers (Fig. 25.1.5).

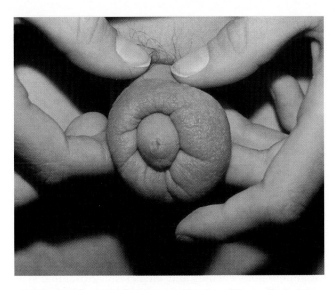

Fig. 25.1.5 Diffuse granulomatous infiltration of the penile shaft in a teenage boy with Crohn's disease.

Extracutaneous manifestations

Arthritis is the most common extraintestinal manifestation in children [11]. The joint findings belong to the seronegative spondyloarthropathies including peripheral arthropathy and ankylosing spondylitis [11]. The most common ocular findings seen in inflammatory bowel disease include conjunctivitis, anterior uveitis and episcleritis [21]. These findings occur in 4% [8] to 11% [21] of patients with inflammatory bowel disease. Patients often present with a red eye.

Prognosis

Crohn's disease is characterized by a chronic [7] and recurrent course with unpredictable periods of remission and exacerbation [22]. Life expectancy is reduced and quality of life affected. The disease in most patients can be controlled [22].

Differential diagnosis

The diagnosis of Crohn's disease is often delayed because the gastrointestinal symptoms may not be obvious initially. Early disease may mimic juvenile rheumatoid arthritis, anorexia nervosa or idiopathic growth failure [6]. The anogenital lesions can masquerade as child sexual abuse [23]. The perianal tags may be confused with haemorrhoids. When oral aphthae are present, Behçet's disease, systemic lupus erythematosus, herpes simplex and complex aphthosis may be included in the differential diagnosis. Crohn's disease should be considered when evaluating a patient for cheilitis granulomatosa (Melkersson–Rosenthal syndrome) since both disorders can present with swelling of the lips and granulomas histolog-ically. Sarcoidosis may be included in the differential diagnosis clinically and histologically.

Treatment

The first-line treatments for the intestinal manifestations of Crohn's disease include aminosalicylic acid derivatives and systemic corticosteroids [24]. Immunosuppressive steroid-sparing agents such as azathioprine, 6-mercaptopurine, cyclosporine plus metronidazole are important second-line treatments [6].

The cutaneous and mucosal manifestations are often difficult to treat [15]. They will often respond to systemic treatment used for Crohn's disease. Orofacial lesions may improve with topical corticosteroids [17]. Systemic steroids and azathioprine have been used successfully for cutaneous disease when topical therapy fails [17]. Perianal disease is treated with conservative perineal care and metronidazole [16]. Nutritional intervention is a crucial part of management, especially in children [16]. While not curative, surgery is often indicated for the acute and chronic complications of Crohn's disease [6].

REFERENCES

1 Dalziel TK. Chronic interstitial enteritis. *Br Med J* 1913; 2: 1068–70.
2 Crohn BB, Ginzburg L, Oppenheimer GD. Regional ileitis. A pathologic and clinical entity. *J Am Med Assoc* 1932; 99: 1323–9.
3 Thayer WR, Chitnavis V. The case for an infectious etiology. *Med Clin N Am* 1994; 78: 1233–47.
4 Lockhart-Mummery HE, Morson BC. Crohn's disease (regional enteritis) of the large intestine and its distinction from ulcerative colitis. *Gut* 1960; 1: 87–105.
5 Witkowski JA, Parish LC, Lewis JE. Crohn's disease—noncaseating granulomas on the legs. *Acta Derm Venereol (Stockh)* 1977; 57: 181–3.
6 Hofley PM, Piccoli DA. Inflammatory bowel disease in children. *Med Clin N Am* 1994; 78: 1281–302.
7 Farmer RG, Michener WM. Prognosis of Crohn's disease with onset in childhood or adolescence. *Dig Dis Sci* 1979; 24: 752–7.
8 Rankin GB, Watts HD, Melnyk CS *et al.* National Cooperative Crohn's Disease Study: extraintestinal manifestations and perianal complications. *Gastroenterology* 1979; 77: 914–20.
9 Greenstein AJ, Janowitz HD, Sachar DB. The extra-intestinal complications of Crohn's disease and ulcerative colitis. A study of 700 patients. *Medicine* 1976; 55: 401–12.
10 Ament ME. Inflammatory disease of the colon: ulcerative colitis and Crohn's colitis. *J Pediatr* 1975; 86: 322–34.
11 Lindsley CB, Schaller JG. Arthritis associated with inflammatory bowel disease in children. *J Pediatr* 1974; 84: 16–20.
12 Ray TL, Levine JB, Weiss W *et al.* Epidermolysis bullosa acquisita and inflammatory bowel disease. *J Am Acad Dermatol* 1982; 6: 242–52.
13 O'Loughlin S, Perry HO. A diffuse pustular eruption associated with ulcerative colitis. *Arch Dermatol* 1978; 114: 1061–4.
14 McPoland PR, Moss RL. Cutaneous Crohn's disease and progressive vitiligo. *J Am Acad Dermatol* 1988; 19: 421–5.
15 Burgdorf W. Cutaneous manifestations of Crohn's dieseace. *J Am Acad Dermatol* 1981; 5: 689–95.
16 Palder SB, Shandling B, Bilik R *et al.* Perianal complications of pediatric Crohn's disease. *J Pediatr Surg* 1991; 26: 513–15.
17 Plauth M, Jenss H, Meyle J. Oral manifestations of Crohn's disease. An analysis of 79 cases. *J Clin Gastroenterol* 1991; 13: 29–37.
18 Ghandour K, Issa M. Oral Crohn's disease with late intestinal manifestations. *Oral Surg Oral Med Oral Pathol* 1991; 72: 565–7.
19 VanHale HM, Rogers RS, Zone JJ *et al.* Pyostomatitis vegetans. A reactive

mucosal marker for inflammatory disease of the gut. *Arch Dermatol* 1985; 121: 94–8.

20 Shum D, Guenther L. Metastatic Crohn's disease. Case report and review of the literature. *Arch Dermatol* 1990; 126: 645–8.

21 Wright R, Lumsden J, Luntz MH *et al.* Abnormalities of the sacroiliac joints and uveitis. *Q J Med* 1965; 34: 229–36.

22 Katz J. The course of inflammatory bowel disease. *Med Clin N Am* 1994; 78: 1275–80.

23 Sellman SPB, Hupertz VF, Reece RM. Crohn's disease presenting as suspected abuse. *Pediatrics* 1996; 97: 272–4.

24 Podolsky DK. Medical progress: inflammatory bowel disease. Part 2. *N Engl J Med* 1991; 325: 1008–16.

Granulomatous cheilitis

Definition

Granulomatous cheilitis or Meischer's granulomatous cheilitis is a condition of recurrent lip swelling and non-caseating granulomatous inflammation. It is frequently seen as part of the Melkersson–Rosenthal syndrome, which includes a triad of relapsing facial paralysis, fissured tongue and recurrent orofacial oedema. However, it can occur as a disease isolated to the lips. The concept of 'orofacial granulomatosis' has been proposed as a unifying term to include all patients with non-caseating granulomas in the orofacial region. This diagnosis encompasses patients with orofacial Crohn's disease, sarcoidosis, Melkersson–Rosenthal syndrome including its monosymptomatic form of granulomatous cheilitis, food or contact allergy, and tooth-associated infections.

History

In 1928, Melkersson [1] described a woman with recurrent perioral oedema and facial nerve paralysis. Subsequently, Rosenthal in 1931 [2] described a patient with the additional finding of lingua plicata (fissured tongue). In 1949, the triad became known as Melkersson–Rosenthal syndrome [3]. In 1945, Miescher described localized, episodic non-inflammatory oedema of the lip as granulomatous cheilitis [4]. It is now believed that granulomatous cheilitis is a limited or monosymptomatic variant of the Melkersson–Rosenthal syndrome. Apparently, the first descriptions in the paediatric literature were in 1962, when the Melkersson–Rosenthal syndrome was described in two children, aged 22 months and 8 years [5].

Aetiology and pathogenesis

The aetiology of granulomatous cheilitis is unknown. Infectious and allergic theories have been proposed but have not been substantiated. There have been numerous reports of familial cases [6], in particular autosomal dominant inheritance [7]. It has recently been suggested that the gene for Melkersson–Rosenthal syndrome is located at 9p11 [8].

Pathology

Biopsy of the lip typically shows non-caseating sarcoidal granulomas. Early in the course of the disease, the granulomas are not always evident. Rather, non-specific dermal oedema with dilated lymphatics, perivascular collections of histiocytes, lymphocytes and plasma cells are seen [9]. With repeated bouts of swelling, the small non-caseating granulomas with Langhans' giant cells are found in the dermis or lamina propria [9]. Fibrosis may also be seen. At times, it can be difficult to find the typical granulomas. Serial sections and repeat biopsies are often necessary.

Clinical features

Granulomatous cheilitis and Melkersson–Rosenthal syndrome often begin in adolescence or young adulthood [9,10]. Of 58 cases of Melkersson–Rosenthal syndrome reported in 1972 by Alexander and James [6], 45% had disease onset before the age of 20 years. In the first two decades of life, the disease is more common in females [10,11].

The clinical features in children are identical to those in adults [12]. The lip swelling is painless, non-pruritic, firm and often asymmetric or unilateral [13]. Either or both lips can be involved (Fig. 25.1.6). The lips may swell to three times their normal size. The lips are often purple, scaly, chapped and fissured. The oedema occurs at irregular intervals and lasts for a few days. After repeated bouts, the swelling becomes persistent, leaving firm, indurated lips. When part of the Melkersson–Rosenthal syndrome, there may also be swelling of the chin, cheeks and periorbital

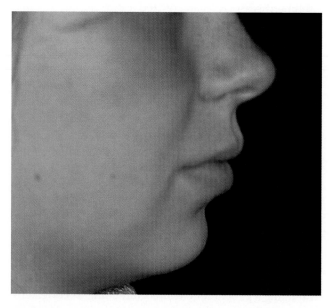

Fig. 25.1.6 Granulomatous cheilitis in a boy. Courtesy of Dr Jane Luker.

regions [13]. Usually, the facial paralysis starts after the orofacial oedema, is abrupt in onset and indistinguishable from a Bell's palsy [11].

Prognosis

The course of granulomatous cheilitis is typically episodic. Eventually, the lip swelling becomes constant. Spontaneous remission is unusual. Patients are typically otherwise healthy.

Differential diagnosis

The diagnosis of granulomatous cheilitis is based on clinical and histopathogical findings. The oral manifestations of sarcoidosis and Crohn's disease can mimic granulomatous cheilitis. Crohn's disease is very important to exclude because of the frequency of oral manifestations and the fact that patients with Crohn's disease can have asymptomatic bowel disease for many years before the diagnosis is made. When the lips are involved with Crohn's disease, they are firm, oedematous and may have a 'cobblestone' pattern. The presence of buccal and/or gingival hyperplasia or aphthous ulcers might suggest a diagnosis of Crohn's disease. The presence of granulomatous inflammation in the bowel would confirm a diagnosis of Crohn's disease. Some authors [14] propose that all patients with granulomatous cheilitis should be evaluated for Crohn's disease before being labelled as having monosymptomatic Melkersson–Rosenthal syndrome. Sarcoidosis, which can mimic granulomatous cheilitis histologically is an extremely rare cause of lip swelling [15]. Discrete sarcoidal papules or nodules are more commonly seen. A search for sarcoidal lesions elsewhere especially in the lung and lymph nodes would aid in the diagnosis. Other conditions that may present in a similar manner to granulomatous cheilitis but could normally be distinguished histologically would include angio-oedema (usually pruritic), trauma, contact dermatitis, insect bite reaction, erysipelas and submucosal neoplasms [13].

Treatment

Short courses of systemic corticosteroids or intralesional steroids can be but are not uniformly of benefit [16]. There have been reports of successful treatment with clofazamine [15,17], broad-spectrum antibiotics [13], dapsone and sulphapyridine [10] and hydroxychloroquine [18]. Cold compresses and lip emollients may be used for symptomatic relief. Disfiguring swelling can be treated successfully with reduction cheiloplasty when swelling is persistent; conservative measures are not effective [16,19]. However, the improvement with surgical resection is often temporary [16].

REFERENCES

1 Melkersson E. Ett fall av recidiverande facialispares i samband med angioneurotisk odem. *Hygiea* 1928; 90: 737–41.
2 Rosenthal C. Klinisch-errbiologischer Beitrag zur Konstitutions-pathologie. Gemeinsames Auftreten von (rezidivierender familiarer) Facialislahmung, angioneurotischem Gesichtsodem und Lingua plicata in Arthritismus-Familien. *Z Ges Neurol Psychiatr* 1931; 131: 475–501.
3 Luscher E. Syndrom von Melkersson–Rosenthal. *Schweiz Med Wochenschr* 1949; 79: 1–3.
4 Miescher G. Uber essentielle granulomatose Makrocheilie (cheilitis granu-lomatosa). *Dermatologica* 1945; 91: 57–85.
5 Ehmann B, Stickl H. Recurring facial paralysis and facial swelling: a pe-diatric contribution to the Melkersson–Rosenthal syndrome. *Z Kinderheilk* 1962; 110: 541–3.
6 Alexander RW, James RB. Melkersson–Rosenthal syndrome: review of the literature and report of a case. *J Oral Surg* 1972; 30: 599–604.
7 Carr RD. Is the Melkersson–Rosenthal syndrome hereditary? *Arch Dermatol* 1966; 93: 426–7.
8 Smeets E, Fryns JR, Van der Berghe H. Melkersson–Rosenthal syndrome and *de novo* autosomal t(9;21) (p11;p11) translocation. *Clin Genet* 1994; 45: 323–4.
9 Worsaae N, Christensen KC, Schiodt M, Reibel J. Melkersson–Rosenthal syndrome and cheilitis granulomatosa. A clinicopathological study of 33 patients with special reference to their oral lesions. *Oral Surg Oral Med Oral Pathol* 1982; 54: 404–13.
10 Greene RM, Rogers III RS. Melkersson–Rosenthal syndrome: a review of 36 patients. *J Am Acad Dermatol* 1989; 21: 1263–70.
11 Zimmer WM, Rogers RS III, Reeve CM, Sheridan PJ. Orofacial manifesta-tions of Melkersson–Rosenthal syndrome. *Oral Surg Oral Med Oral Pathol* 1992; 74: 610–19.
12 Wadlington WB, Riley HD Jr, Lowbeer L. The Melkersson–Rosenthal syn-drome. *Pediatrics* 1984; 73: 502–6.
13 Rogers RS. Melkersson–Rosenthal syndrome and orofacial granulomatosis. *Dermatol Clin* 1996; 14: 371–9.
14 Misra S, Ament ME. Orofacial lesions in Crohn's disease. *Am J Gastro* 1996; 91: 1651–3.
15 Bourgeois-Droin C, Havard S, Granier F *et al.* Granulomatous cheilitis in two children with sarcoidosis. *J Am Acad Dermatol* 1993; 29: 822–4.
16 Glickman LT, Gruss JS, Birt BD, Kohli-Dang N. The surgical management of Melkersson–Rosenthal syndrome. *Plast Reconstr Surg* 1992; 89: 815–21.
17 Sussman GL, Yang WH, Steinberg S. Melkersson–Rosenthal syndrome: clinical, pathologic, and therapeutic considerations. *Ann Allergy* 1992; 69: 187–94.
18 Allen CM, Camisa C, Hamzeh S, Stephens L. Cheilitis granulomatosa: report of six cases and review of the literature. *J Am Acad Dermatol* 1990; 23: 444–50.
19 Ellitsgaard N, Andersson AP, Worsaae N, Medgyesi S. Long-term results after surgical reduction cheiloplasty in patients with Melkersson–Rosenthal syndrome and cheilitis granulomatosa. *Ann Plast Surg* 1993; 31: 413–20.

25.2 Cystic Fibrosis

ROD PHILLIPS

Definition

Cystic fibrosis (mucoviscidosis, fibrocystic disease) is an autosomal recessive disease characterized by increased salt loss from sweat glands and by dysfunction of exocrine glands, especially the lungs and pancreas [1].

History

First recognized in 1936 as 'cystic fibrosis of the pancreas', cystic fibrosis was soon discovered to involve all exocrine glands. The basic pathology was subsequently shown to be obstruction of the exocrine ducts rather than fibrosis but the name cystic fibrosis is now virtually universal. For many years, most children with cystic fibrosis died in early childhood. However, changes in management since the 1970s have led to greatly increased survival and quality of life.

Aetiology and pathogenesis

One of the striking medical achievements of the 1980s was a major international collaboration that led to the isolation and cloning of the cystic fibrosis gene in 1989 [2]. The abnormal gene in cystic fibrosis is located on the long arm of chromosome 7. One mutation, ΔF_{508}, accounts for about 85% of defective genes worldwide. Over 800 other mutations have been identified. In populations of white Caucasians, cystic fibrosis is the most common serious inherited disease with a gene frequency of 1 in 25 (i.e. 1 in 2500 births). It is less common in black Americans (gene frequency 1 in 65) and rare in Asian populations.

The cystic fibrosis gene codes for a protein, cystic fibrosis transmembrane regulator, that plays a key role in regulating chloride ion transport across epithelial cell membranes [3]. In sweat glands, chloride is normally reabsorbed as the sweat passes along the duct to the skin surface. In cystic fibrosis, this absorption is impaired, leading to increased salt loss in sweat. In other glands, impaired transport of chloride into the ducts can lead to abnormally viscous secretions, duct obstruction and progressive organ dysfunction.

Pathology

The pancreas is often the most severely affected of the exocrine glands, possibly because of the proteolytic nature of the blocked secretions. Histological changes progress from eosinophilic material in the duct lumina to formation of dilated cysts in the ducts, surrounding fibrosis and finally replacement of normal pancreatic tissue by fat. Lung involvement is characterized initially by occlusion of bronchioles by mucous and then by air trapping, recurrent and persistent bacterial infection and bronchiectasis. In the liver, mucous plugs in bile ducts can lead to focal biliary cirrhosis and uncommonly to widespread cirrhosis, portal vein obstruction and oesophageal varices. In the gastrointestinal tract, abnormal secretions *in utero* can lead to tenacious meconium. Salivary glands can show inspissation of secretions in ducts but progressive fibrosis does not occur. Despite the abnormal sweat gland function, pathology of skin is generally normal [1].

Clinical features

In countries where there is no neonatal screening programme, diagnosis usually follows the development of pulmonary or pancreatic symptoms or both. Onset of such symptoms with associated failure to thrive often occurs in infancy but may not occur until many years after birth.

Lungs

Pulmonary problems in cystic fibrosis usually begin with repeated episodes of cough and wheeze. With time, the cough becomes increasingly persistent and purulent as bacterial colonization and infection develop, especially with *Pseudomonas aeruginosa*. In later disease, bronchiectasis, gross hyperinflation and chronic hypoxaemia can lead to pulmonary hypertension, right heart failure and death.

Pancreas

Malabsorption secondary to pancreatic disease is the second major manifestation of cystic fibrosis. Steatorrhoea and failure to thrive may commence in the neonatal period or at any time during childhood. In about 10% of cases where diagnosis is delayed, malabsorption is sufficiently severe in infancy to cause secondary anaemia and oedema [4]. Insulin-producing cells in the islets of Langerhans can be affected, leading to secondary diabetes in 5–10% of adolescents with cystic fibrosis.

Gastrointestinal tract

Neonatal bowel obstruction secondary to thick meconium occurs in about 10% of cases. Partial or complete obstruction in older children can be due either to intussusception or to accumulation of faecal material in the lower bowel. Rectal prolapse can occur and cystic fibrosis is the most common cause of this condition in childhood. Biliary cirrhosis occurs in about 2% of cases.

Joints

With increasing life expectancy, more children with cystic fibrosis are developing joint complications. These occur in about 5–10% of children over 10 years old, usually as an episodic, non-erosive arthritis involving the large joints of the limbs [5–8].

Skin

Increased saltiness of the skin can be noted from shortly after birth. In hot, humid weather, increased salt loss can lead to collapse with hyponatraemia, hypochloraemia and alkalosis. This sweat gland dysfunction is the only abnormality that is present in virtually all children with cystic fibrosis from infancy and it forms the basis of a sensitive and specific diagnostic test for the disease. Skin of the hands and feet of children with cystic fibrosis has been shown to wrinkle more rapidly than skin from control children when immersed in water [9]. Digital clubbing is present in most older children with cystic fibrosis.

Several reports have described infants who presented with generalized erythematous rashes and who were subsequently found to have cystic fibrosis [10–15]. In this subgroup of infants, the rash typically began as erythematous papules in the napkin area unresponsive to topical treatments. Over a period of weeks, this became generalized and confluent with well-demarcated, erythematous, scaly plaques covering most of the body (Fig. 25.2.1). Papules and desquamation occurred on palms and soles. Associated findings at presentation included normal mucosal surfaces, sparse hair, oedema, lethargy, anaemia, severe hypoproteinaemia, raised liver enzymes and low levels of trace metals. This constellation of findings has been attributed to kwashiorkor secondary to unrecognized malabsorption [15]. The rash may be caused by free radical

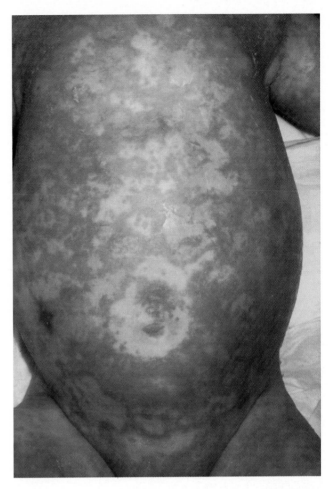

Fig. 25.2.1 Confluent, desquamating, erythematous rash on the abdomen of a 3-month-old boy with cystic fibrosis.

damage to mitochondrial and lipid membranes in the skin, in part due to multiple nutritional deficiencies including zinc and essential fatty acids.

The most common skin problems in treated cystic fibrosis are erythematous, vasculitic or purpuric drug reactions secondary to the multiple antibiotics and other medications used in treatment regimes [16,17]. About 40% of those children who develop arthritis also have an associated rash. This is usually erythematous and maculopapular but purpura, vasculitic nodules and erythema nodosum have also been observed [5–8,18]. Cutaneous reactivity to *Aspergillosis* species is common, particularly in children with more severe lung disease, but the prevalence of cutaneous reactivity to other allergens used to test for atopy is the same as in the normal population [19–23]. A group of 100 children and adults with cystic fibrosis was shown to have a prevalence (not defined in the report) of acute urticaria of 9% and chronic urticaria of 7%. No control group was studied [24]. Isolated associations between cystic fibrosis and Rothmund–Thomson syndrome [25], solar urticaria [26] and albinism [27] have been described. Two children with cystic fibrosis and

Kawasaki's disease have been reported [28,29] but in both cases the diagnosis of Kawasaki's disease is uncertain. Three teenage boys and a girl developed purpura on the lower limbs in conjunction with hypergammaglobulinaemia: all four died within 2 years of onset of purpura [30,31]. Three siblings of consanguineous parents were reported to have generalized follicular hamartoma, alopecia and cystic fibrosis [32].

Other

Nasal polyps are common in cystic fibrosis and if found in a child should always raise the suspicion of this condition. Pansinusitis is seen in most older children. Virtually all males with cystic fibrosis have non-patent vas deferens and hence are infertile.

Prognosis

Untreated, cystic fibrosis usually leads to death during infancy or childhood from malabsorption and/or pulmonary disease. With aggressive treatment, the quality and length of life are greatly improved. Many children live essentially normal childhoods and, in leading centres, median survival of patients now exceeds 30 years. Two young adults with cystic fibrosis and basal cell carcinomas have been reported [33] but the prognostic significance of this observation remains unclear.

Differential diagnosis

Depending on the presentation, the differential diagnosis includes other causes of pulmonary disease, malabsorption or failure to thrive. Thus, recurrent pulmonary infection, asthma, recurrent aspiration, inhaled foreign body, tracheo-oesophageal fistula, immunodeficiency, immotile cilia syndrome, gastrointestinal infection, enteropathy, renal disease, hepatic disease and malnutrition may be considered.

Laboratory diagnosis is by pilocarpine iontophoresis (sweat test) done in an experienced centre. In conjunction with appropriate clinical findings, this test is highly sensitive and specific. However, infants with cystic fibrosis who present with a desquamating rash and/or oedema commonly give false negative results [4,12,15] and need to be retested after treatment of their malabsorption. Alternatively, DNA analysis for common mutations can be used to confirm the diagnosis but this will detect only 80–90% of patients. Prenatal DNA or enzyme analysis can be done in subsequent pregnancies for families with a cystic fibrosis child. Many countries now routinely screen for cystic fibrosis by looking for elevated trypsin levels in neonatal heel prick blood.

Treatment

Treatment requires effective management of malabsorption, pulmonary and other problems by a multidisciplinary team. Malabsorption is controlled by pancreatic enzyme replacement, a high-fat and high-protein diet and supplementation of vitamins and minerals. Pulmonary disease is treated with chest physiotherapy and antibiotics. Exacerbations of chest disease may require intravenous antibiotics for 10–14 days. Lung transplantation can be considered for end-stage pulmonary disease in older children and adults. Gene replacement therapy is being investigated and appears likely to become an effective therapy. With survival into adulthood now the rule, issues such as reproductive health, male infertility, delayed puberty, pregnancy and marriage also need to be addressed during childhood.

REFERENCES

1 Boat TF. Cystic fibrosis. In: Behrman RE, Kliegman RM, Nelson WE, Vaughan VC, eds. *Nelson Textbook of Pediatrics*, 14th edn. Sydney: WB Saunders, 1992: 1106–16.
2 Riordan JR, Rommens JM, Kerem B *et al*. Identification of the cystic fibrosis gene: cloning and characterization of complementary DNA. *Science* 1989; 245: 1066–73.
3 Anderson MP, Gregory RJ, Thompson S *et al*. Demonstration that CFTR is a chloride channel by alteration of its anion selectivity. *Science* 1991; 253: 202–5.
4 Nielsen OH, Larsen BF. The incidence of anaemia, hypoalbuminaemia and oedema in infants as presenting symptoms of cystic fibrosis: a retrospective survey of the frequency of this symptom complex in 130 patients with cystic fibrosis. *J Paediatr Gastroenterol Nutr* 1982; 1: 355–9.
5 Newman AJ, Ansell BM. Episodic arthritis in children with cystic fibrosis. *J Pediatr* 1979; 94: 594–6.
6 Schidlow DV, Goldsmith DP, Palmer J, Huang NN. Arthritis in cystic fibrosis. *Arch Dis Child* 1984; 59: 377–9.
7 Phillips BM, David TJ. Pathogenesis and management of arthropathy in cystic fibrosis. *J Roy Soc Med* 1986; 79(suppl 12): 44–50.
8 Pertuiset BE, Menkes CJ, Lenior G, Jehanne M, Douchain F, Guillot M. Cystic fibrosis arthritis—a report of five cases. *Br J Rheumatol* 1992; 31: 535–8.
9 Johns MK. Skin wrinkling in cystic fibrosis. *Med Biol Illustr* 1975; 25: 205–10.
10 Hansen RC, Lemen R, Revsin B. Cystic fibrosis manifesting with acrodermatitis enteropathica-like eruption. *Arch Dermatol* 1983; 119: 51–5.
11 Rosenblum JL, Schweitzer J, Kissane JM, Cooper TW. Failure to thrive presenting with an unusual skin rash. *J Pediatr* 1985; 107: 149–53.
12 Abman SH, Accurso FJ, Bowman CM. Persistent morbidity and mortality of protein calorie malnutrition in young infants with cystic fibrosis. *J Paediatr Gastroenterol Nutr* 1986; 5: 393–6.
13 Schmidt CP, Tunnessen W. Cystic fibrosis presenting with periorificial dermatitis. *J Am Acad Dermatol* 1991; 25: 896–7.
14 Darmstadt GL, Schmidt CP, Wechsler DS, Tunnessen WW, Rosenstein BJ. Dermatitis as a presenting sign of cystic fibrosis. *Arch Dermatol* 1992; 128: 1358–64.
15 Phillips RJ, Crock CM, Dillon MJ, Clayton PT, Curran A, Harper JI. Cystic fibrosis presenting as kwashiorkor with florid skin rash. *Arch Dis Child* 1993; 69: 446–8.
16 Finnegan MJ, Hinchcliffe J, Russell-Jones D *et al*. Vasculitis complicating cystic fibrosis. *Q J Med New Series* 72, 1989; 267: 609–21.
17 Reed MD, Stern RC, Myers CM, Klinger JD, Yamashita TS, Blumer JL. Therapeutic evaluation of piperacillin in acute pulmonary exacerbations of cystic fibrosis. *Pediatr Pulmonol* 1987; 3: 101–9.
18 Vaze D. Episodic arthritis in cystic fibrosis. *J Pediatr* 1980; 96: 346.
19 Warner JO, Taylor BW, Norman AP, Soothill JF. Association of cystic fibrosis with allergy. *Arch Dis Child* 1976; 51: 507–11.

20 Silverman M, Hobbs FDR, Gordon IRS, Carswell F. Cystic fibrosis, atopy and airways lability. *Arch Dis Child* 1978; 53: 873–7.

21 Allan JD, Moss AD, Wallwork JC, McFarlane H. Immediate hypersensitivity in patients with cystic fibrosis. *Clin Allergy* 1975; 5: 255–61.

22 Laufer P, Fink JN, Bruns WT *et al.* Allergic bronchopulmonary aspergillosis in cystic fibrosis. *J Allerg Clin Immunol* 1984; 73: 44–8.

23 Greally P, Cook AJ, Sampson AP *et al.* Atopic children with cystic fibrosis have increased urinary leukotriene E4 concentrations and more severe pulmonary disease. *J Allergy Clin Immunol* 1994; 93: 100–7.

24 Laufer P. Urticaria in cystic fibrosis. *Cutis* 1985; 36: 245–6.

25 Lewis MB. Rothmund–Thompson syndrome and fibrocystic disease. *Aust J Dermatol* 1972; 13: 105.

26 Laufer P, Laufer R. Solar urticaria in cystic fibrosis. *Cutis* 1983; 31: 665–6.

27 Pruszewicz A, Sokolowski Z, Goncarzewicz A. Mucoviscidosis coexisting with generalised albinism. *Otolaryngol Polska* 1978; 32: 93–5.

28 Rivilla F, Lopez J. Meconium ileus equivalent and Kawasaki syndrome. *Eur J Surg* 1991; 157: 151–2.

29 Ciofu C, Laky D, Geormaneanu M. Kawasaki disease in an infant with cystic fibrosis. *Rom J Morphol Embryol* 1992; 38: 63–6.

30 Nielsen HE, Lundh S, Jacobsen SV, Hoiby N. Hypergammaglobulinemic purpura in cystic fibrosis. *Acta Paediatr Scand* 1978; 67: 443–7.

31 Soter NA, Mihm MC, Colten HR. Cutaneous necrotizing venulitis in patients with cystic fibrosis. *J Pediatr* 1979; 95: 197–201.

32 Mascao JM, Ferrando J, Bombi JA, Lambruschini N, Mascaro JM. Congenital generalised follicular hamartoma associated with alopecia and cystic fibrosis in three siblings. *Arch Dermatol* 1995; 131: 454–8.

33 Healy E, Meenan FOC, Fitzgerald MX, Rogers S. Basal cell carcinoma and cystic fibrosis: a report of two cases. *Br J Dermatol* 1993; 128: 701–9.

25.3 Henoch–Schönlein Purpura

LINDA G. RABINOWITZ

Definition

Henoch–Schönlein purpura (HSP) is an immunologically mediated vasculitis of small blood vessels of the skin, accompanied by involvement of the joints, kidneys, gastrointestinal tract and other organ systems. Clinical manifestations include a purpuric rash, arthritis, abdominal pain and glomerulonephritis. HSP is the most common vasculitis syndrome of childhood. Previously, it has been referred to as anaphylactoid purpura, allergic vasculitis and allergic purpura. These terms are no longer considered appropriate, because there is no evidence that there is an allergic aetiology. HSP is generally a benign, self-limited condition.

History

HSP is named after two 19th century European doctors, although the first case of HSP was described by Heberden in 1801 [1]. This initial patient was a 5-year-old boy who was unable to walk and had severe abdominal pain and bloody stools. He also had a skin rash that featured 'bloody points'. In 1837, Schönlein described a syndrome characterized by acute purpura and arthritis (purpura rheumatica). Subsequently, Henoch, a student of Schönlein, reported a similar syndrome that included nephritis and colicky abdominal pain [2]. This disorder has since become known as HSP. Because Henoch's description followed that of his teacher, some prefer the name Schönlein–Henoch purpura which respects the order of reporters. A subcommittee of the American College of Rheumatology has developed criteria for classification of several major forms of vasculitis. The criteria for diagnosis of HSP were set forth in 1990 [3]. Several review articles and numerous case reports illustrate the expanding clinical spectrum of the disorder.

Aetiology

The precise aetiology of HSP remains unknown. Although the disorder has been shown to be an immunoglobulin A (IgA)- and complement-mediated process affecting small blood vessels, no single stimulus has been identified. The condition occurs all year round, but peak incidences have been described in spring and winter [1]. Clustering of cases in at least one report suggests an infectious aetiology [4]. Schönlein noted that a respiratory tract infection may precede the onset. Multiple organisms have been implicated as causative agents of HSP. Among these are group A β-haemolytic streptococci (GABHS) which are most frequently identified as triggers of the condition. *Mycoplasma pneumoniae*, *Yersinia*, *Legionella*, Epstein–Barr virus, hepatitis B virus, adenovirus, cytomegalovirus, parvovirus B19 and varicella are other suspected infectious trigger factors. There are reports that cite various vaccinations, such as typhoid, measles and cholera, as causes of subsequent HSP. Drugs, especially penicillin, erythromycin, quinine, sulphonamides and anticonvulsants have also been implicated. Occasionally, foods, cold exposure, insect bites and chemical toxins may trigger the disorder.

Pathology

The two major histological features of HSP are vascular changes and a neutrophilic infiltrate, both of which are typical of leucocytoclastic vasculitis. The vascular changes are limited to small blood vessels in the dermis. The capillaries have endothelial cell swelling and deposition of eosinophilic fibrinoid material within and around their walls. If the vascular changes are severe, endothelial cell swelling may cause occlusion of the lumina. There is a predominantly neutrophilic perivascular infiltrate. Fragmentation of nuclei (karyorrhexis) is a characteristic finding. In older, well-developed lesions, the number of neutrophils may be diminished and mononuclear cells may be noted. When the kidneys are involved, there may be a focal or diffuse glomerulitis with occlusion of lobules of glomeruli by fibrin [5].

Results of direct immunofluorescence staining reveal granular deposits of IgA and C3 within the blood vessels of the papillary dermis of both affected and uninvolved skin [6]. This is especially the case when the lesions are of recent onset. These findings are also noted in renal glomeruli. Although it has been traditionally accepted

1564

that the presence of IgA deposition in blood vessel walls is a sensitive and specific marker for HSP, this theory has been challenged. Researchers have found that vascular IgA deposits may be present in patients, particularly adults, who do not have HSP. In addition, some patients who unequivocally have HSP have had immunoreactants other than IgA detected within vessel walls. Thus, some believe that this laboratory finding is sensitive but not specific, and it should not be used as the sole criterion for confirming the diagnosis of HSP [7].

Clinical features

HSP occurs in individuals of all ages, but it is most common in the school-aged child. The mean peak age range is 4–7 years [1]. HSP has been seen in infants less than 1 year of age, but it is rare in this age group. The clinical features of HSP vary with age, and older children and adolescents tend to be more severely affected than infants and young children. HSP is slightly more common in males than females. The incidence in childhood has been estimated to be 14 cases per 100 000 per year [4]. HSP is rare in dark-skinned individuals.

The classic triad of clinical symptoms and signs includes acute onset of a purpuric rash, abdominal cramping and haematuria. However, the clinical expression of HSP may range from a minimal petechial eruption to severe multisystem involvement. Malaise and low-grade fever are seen in approximately one-half of affected patients. HSP often follows an upper respiratory tract infection which precedes the syndrome by 1–3 weeks.

The diagnostic criteria developed by a subcommittee of the American College of Rheumatology for establishing the diagnosis of HSP include the following: (a) palpable purpura; (b) abdominal pain with or without haematochezia; (c) leucocytoclastic vasculitis seen in skin biopsy specimens; (d) age 20 years or under at onset; and (e) renal biopsy findings of mesangioproliferative glomerulonephritis with or without IgA deposits. A firm diagnosis can be made if three of these five criteria are fulfilled [3].

Typically, the cutaneous purpuric eruption is the presenting feature of the disorder. It is present in 100% of patients and is essential for the diagnosis of HSP. In some cases, joint and/or abdominal symptoms may precede the onset of the rash. Oedema of the ears, scalp, hands and feet is a common early finding. Skin lesions may arise as pink or erythematous macules or papules that become purpuric (non-blanching) within a short time. Lesions are distributed over the buttocks and extensor surfaces of the lower limbs but may occur on the upper extremities and trunk (Figs 25.3.1 and 25.3.2). Urticarial wheals, plaques, blisters and ulceration are seen in some cases. The rash may persist for weeks and may reappear. Although the eruption has been described as gravity dependent, it has been proposed that the rash of HSP is a pressure-dependent phenomenon. It has been noted to develop on

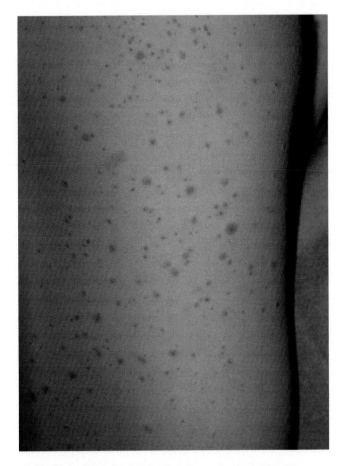

Fig. 25.3.1 A young boy with HSP following a streptococcal infection. Lesions are predominantly petechial and tiny purpuric papules.

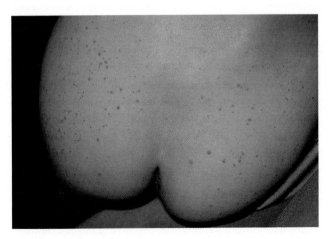

Fig. 25.3.2 Lesions of HSP have a predilection for the buttocks and lower extremities.

the knees of a 10-month-old infant, probably due to pressure effects as a consequence of crawling [8].

A group of Israeli investigators studied the clinical features of HSP in seven infants (aged 5–12 months) and discovered that facial and ear involvement (in addition to limb involvement) was more common in this age group. Oedema associated with the purpuric skin lesions was a prominent feature in all of the infants studied [9]. The syndrome was limited to the skin in all of the infants except one who had joint involvement. In general, infants have a milder course, with only rare involvement of the kidneys and gastrointestinal tract.

Joint manifestations occur in approximately 60–90% of patients with HSP and may develop at any time during the course of illness [2]. Migratory arthralgias or arthritis most often involve the knees and ankles, but joints of the upper extremities may also be affected. Although self-limited, the arthritis can cause difficulty with ambulation. Pelvic and shoulder girdles and small joints of the hands and feet are rarely involved. Joint symptoms may recur but usually resolve completely.

Approximately 50–70% of patients will have gastrointestinal involvement characterized by submucosal vasculitis resulting in oedema and haemorrhage [2]. Very few individuals will have progression to gastrointestinal bleeding or acute pancreatitis. The most common complaint is colicky abdominal pain that is sometimes associated with vomiting. Haematochezia or melena is present in about one-half of patients with abdominal symptomatology. If the skin lesions are not present to aid in determining the diagnosis, the abdominal findings can mimic an acute abdomen. A high index of suspicion and early diagnosis supported by clinical, roentgenographic and laboratory findings may prevent unnecessary surgical procedures in most cases. A small percentage of patients may have life-threatening complications such as haemorrhage, obstruction and intussusception that require early surgical intervention [10]. Endoscopy may be helpful for establishing an early diagnosis of HSP. Characteristic endoscopic findings include haemorrhagic, erosive gastroduodenitis and coin-like lesion [11]. Gastric, jejunal, colonic and rectal erosions have also been reported [12].

The kidneys are affected in up to 60% of patients with HSP [13]. Renal manifestations are more common in older children and may precede or follow other symptoms. The onset of renal involvement may be delayed for weeks to months in many patients but usually occurs within 3 months after the appearance of cutaneous lesions. Haematuria is detected in virtually all patients with nephritis. Proteinuria, hypertension and decreased renal function are less frequently seen. Although most patients present with microscopic haematuria, painless gross haematuria is also common. Haematuria is usually due to glomerulonephritis, and renal biopsy findings are identical to those seen in IgA nephropathy [2]. Non-renal involvement of the urinary tract has been reported to occur but is unusual. Renal colic associated with the passage of tubular-shaped blood clots implies ureteral involvement [13]. Ureteritis, although rare, can be associated with HSP and may be more common than is appreciated.

External genitourinary system involvement in HSP is not rare and is seen in 2–38% of boys with the disease [14]. Scrotal oedema with or without purpura can develop at any time during the illness and may be painless. Testicular pain can be the initial symptom of HSP and represents a diagnostic challenge for the clinician, since it mimics the presentation of testicular torsion, a surgical emergency [15].

Central nervous system manifestations do not occur frequently but, when present, may include headache, mental status changes, seizures, hemiparesis, focal neurological deficits and neuropathy [16]. Seizures may be caused by ischaemia or haemorrhage secondary to the vasculitic process.

Pulmonary involvement is not typical but may occur. Impaired lung diffusion capacity has been demonstrated by a research team in France. This group measured lung transfer of carbon monoxide (TLCO) in 29 patients with HSP. These values were low in 97% of patients during the acute disease process and returned to normal when patients recovered completely. During long-term follow-up, one case of late onset nephritis that was preceded by depressed TLCO levels was detected. It has been speculated that alterations of the alveolocapillary membrane by circulating immune complexes may be responsible for the low TLCO in patients with HSP [17]. Pulmonary haemorrhage has been documented in at least four children with HSP [18]. Periarteriolar infiltrates and fibrinoid necrosis of the lungs have been described on postmortem examination of some patients. Other rare findings associated with HSP include myocarditis, hepatomegaly, parotitis and adrenal necrosis. Gallbladder wall thickening has been reported to occur rarely [19].

The diagnosis of HSP is established by the presence of clinical signs and symptoms. Skin biopsy specimen findings reveal leucocytoclastic vasculitis. Laboratory evaluation is directed towards ruling out other diagnoses and detecting systemic involvement. No laboratory studies are absolutely diagnostic of HSP. Routine laboratory evaluation should include urinalysis, renal function tests, guaiac testing of stool and complete blood cell and platelet counts. The white blood cell count may be elevated. Haemoglobin values are generally normal unless bleeding has resulted in anaemia. Platelet counts and the erythrocyte sedimentation rate may be elevated or normal. Peripheral eosinophilia is rare. Serum IgA levels are inconsistently elevated and are of little diagnostic value. Serum complement levels and prothrombin and partial thromboplastin times are normal. Coagulation factor XIII activity may be decreased in patients with HSP and may be correlated with severity of abdominal symptoms [20]. Although antineutrophil cytoplasmic antibodies (ANCA) have been identified in a wide variety of vasculitic disorders, they have not been demonstrated to be associated with HSP in children [21]. Findings on urinalysis include red blood cells, white blood cells, cellular casts or protein. Abnormal blood urea nitrogen and serum creatinine levels may indicate the presence of glomerulonephritis. Throat cultures are positive for GABHS in up to 75% of patients. Antistreptolysin O and antihyaluronidase titres are increased in up to 60% of patients [1]. Chest radiographs may demonstrate interstitial lung disease. Barium studies can demonstrate the presence of submucosal oedema, haemorrhage and ulceration within the jejunum and ileum, findings known as 'thumbprinting'. According to recent immunological research, it is now possible to correlate clinical disease activity with elevated plasma levels of complement, particularly C3a, C4a and the terminal complement complex [22,23].

Prognosis

Most children have self-limited disease. The average duration of the illness is 4 weeks. Recurrences develop in about 40% of cases and may be multiple over a period of weeks to months before complete remission occurs [24]. Reports of recurrence may be confusing in that there are different definitions of recurrence. Some clinicians believe that symptoms which occur within the first 3 months of onset of disease are part of the original illness [1]. According to this definition, most patients have complete clearing after one to three bouts of purpura. In general, younger children have shorter courses and fewer recurrences.

Once the diagnosis of HSP is established, patients should be evaluated weekly for development of related symptoms and signs. It is important to check urinalyses and blood pressure readings. The need for additional testing is determined by the presence of abnormal findings or symptoms. Long-term follow-up indicates that systemic involvement or serious sequelae do not ordinarily occur. There is no permanent joint disease. Patients with renal involvement may have transient abnormalities or may develop permanent renal insufficiency. HSP-induced nephritis may arise up to 3 years after onset of the illness [1]. Thus, urine dipstick tests must be obtained even after the child appears well. Approximately 5% of individuals with nephritis will develop end-stage kidney disease. Long-term follow-up studies indicate that patients with renal HSP have a higher incidence of hypertension later in life as compared to that for the general population [25].

Mortality is estimated to be 1–2%, strictly due to severe renal involvement and serious gastrointestinal disease.

Differential diagnosis

The differential diagnosis of HSP includes other entities that are characterized by a purpuric skin eruption. Petechial and purpuric lesions may be seen in idiopathic thrombocytopenia, meningococcaemia, bacterial endocarditis, Rocky Mountain spotted fever, leukaemia and disseminated intravascular coagulopathy. Other vasculitic disorders such as lupus erythematosus, polyarteritis nodosa and Wegener's granulomatosis also need to be considered in the differential diagnosis, particularly if the patient is very ill and has widespread organ involvement.

Acute haemorrhagic oedema (AHE) of infancy may or may not represent HSP in infants (see Chapter 25.4). The features of AHE include oedema and ecchymotic targetoid purpuric lesions on the limbs and face. Skin biopsy specimen findings reveal leucocytoclastic vasculitis. It remains unclear whether or not it is an IgA-mediated vasculitis [26].

Hypersensitivity vasculitis is an entity that is distinct from HSP. It can be distinguished from HSP by its more significant organ involvement, relative lack of joint symptomatology and frequent elevations in blood urea nitrogen and serum creatinine levels. The criteria established by the American College of Rheumatology and the recent literature emphasize the distinction between HSP and hypersensitivity vasculitis.

Treatment

Treatment consists of supportive measures such as pain control, hydration, bowel rest, bed rest and attention to nutritional status. Most patients do not require hospitalization. Indications for hospital admission include colicky abdominal pain suggestive of intussusception, gastrointestinal bleeding, severe glomerulonephritis and pulmonary haemorrhage. Salicylates and non-steroidal anti-inflammatory agents should probably not be used for alleviating joint symptoms, as they may increase bleeding from involved organs. Acetaminophen with codeine may be used for pain control. Antibiotic therapy is indicated if a bacterial infection is identified.

The subject of corticosteroid treatment of HSP has been controversial. There is no agreement regarding the role of corticosteroids in the management of this disease. Additionally, the optimal management of HSP nephritis and serious abdominal sequelae is unclear. Prevention of renal complications is one possible benefit of corticosteroids that has been debated in the literature [27]. A retrospective analysis of 50 children revealed that delayed nephritis did develop in patients who had received corticosteroid therapy [28]. This study has been criticized because of the non-random selection of patients, i.e. only the more severely affected patients were treated. In addition, the initiation of steroids was delayed and the treatment course was short and variable [29]. In one prospective controlled study examining the use of systemic corticosteroids, 84 of 168 patients with HSP were treated with systemic corticosteroids. None of these patients developed nephritis, in contrast to 12 of 84 untreated patients who developed nephritis. These researchers believe that early and adequately prolonged treatment with corticosteroids is effective in preventing the development of nephritis in HSP patients [30].

Some uncontrolled studies have supported the use of systemic corticosteroids for treating the abdominal pain. However, the abdominal pain of HSP is believed to be self-limited, and corticosteroids may mask the presence of more ominous abdominal signs. A retrospective analysis of 43 children with HSP and abdominal pain indicates that the only beneficial effect of systemic corticosteroids was a slightly shorter duration of pain in 30% of patients [31]. The decision to treat patients is controversial, but many clinicians believe that abdominal pain resolves more quickly with corticosteroid treatment. Abdominal symptoms have been reported to respond favourably to administration of factor XIII [20], a coagulation factor that is decreased in patients with active HSP.

Despite the controversies surrounding the medical management of HSP, it is common practice to treat patients who have severe abdominal pain or renal involvement with a short course of prednisone (1–2 mg/kg/day).

REFERENCES

1 Robson WL, Leung A. Henoch–Schönlein purpura. *Adv Pediatr* 1994; 41: 163–94.
2 Callen JP. Cutaneous vasculitis: relationship to systemic disease and therapy. *Curr Prob Dermatol* 1993; 5: 45–80.
3 Mills JA, Michel BA, Bloch DA *et al.* The American College of Rheumatology 1990 criteria for the classification of Henoch–Schönlein purpura. *Arthritis Rheum* 1990; 33: 1114–21.
4 Farley TA, Gillespie S, Rasoulpour M *et al.* Epidemiology of a cluster of Henoch–Schönlein purpura. *Am J Dis Child* 1989; 143: 798–803.
5 Lever W, Schaumburg-Lever G. *Histopathology of the Skin*, 7th edn. Philadelphia: JB Lippincott, 1990: 188–91.
6 Van Hale HM, Gibson LE, Schroeter AL. Henoch–Schönlein vasculitis: direct immunofluorescence study of uninvolved skin. *J Am Acad Dermatol* 1986; 15: 665–70.
7 Helander SD, DeCastro FR, Gibson LE. Henoch–Schönlein purpura: clinicopathologic correlation of cutaneous vascular IgA deposits and the relationship to leukocytoclastic vasculitis. *Acta Derm Venereol* 1995; 75: 125–9.

8 Robson WL, Leung AK, Lemay M. The pressure-dependent nature of the rash in Henoch–Schönlein purpura. *J Sing Paediatr Soc* 1992; 34: 230–1.
9 Amitai Y, Gillis D, Wasserman D *et al.* Henoch–Schönlein purpura in infants. *Pediatrics* 1993; 92: 865–7.
10 Katz S, Borst M, Seekri I *et al.* Surgical evaluation of Henoch–Schönlein purpura: experience with 110 children. *Arch Surg* 1991; 126: 849–54.
11 Kato S, Shibuya H, Naganuma H *et al.* Gastrointestinal endoscopy in Henoch–Schönlein purpura. *Eur J Pediatr* 1992; 151: 482–4.
12 Tomomasa T, Hsu JY, Itoh K *et al.* Endoscopic findings in pediatric patients with Henoch–Schönlein purpura and gastrointestinal symptoms. *J Pediatr Gastroenterol Nutr* 1987; 6: 725–9.
13 Robson WL, Leung AK, Mathers MS. Renal colic due to Henoch–Schönlein purpura. *J S Carolina Med Assoc* 1994; 90: 592–5.
14 Singer JI, Kissoon N, Gloor J. Acute testicular pain: Henoch–Schönlein purpura versus testicular torsion. *Pediatr Emerg Care* 1992; 8: 51–3.
15 Chamberlain RS, Greenberg LW. Scrotal involvement in Henoch–Schönlein purpura: a case report and review of the literature. *Pediatr Emerg Care* 1992; 8: 213–15.
16 Belman AL, Leicher CR, Moshe SL *et al.* Neurologic manifestations of Schönlein–Henoch purpura: report of three cases and review of the literature. *Pediatrics* 1985; 75: 687–92.
17 Chaussain M, de Boissieu D, Kalifa G *et al.* Impairment of lung diffusion capacity in Schönlein–Henoch purpura. *J Pediatr* 1992; 121: 12–16.
18 Olson JC, Kelly KJ, Pan CG *et al.* Pulmonary disease with hemorrhage in Henoch–Schönlein purpura. *Pediatrics* 1992; 89: 1177–81.
19 Amemoto K, Nagita A, Aoki S *et al.* Ultrasonographic gallbladder wall thickening in children with Henoch–Schönlein purpura. *J Pediatr Gastroenterol Nutr* 1994; 19: 126–8.
20 Fukui H, Kamitsuji H, Nagao T *et al.* Clinical evaluation of a pasteurized factor XIII concentrate administration in Henoch–Schönlein purpura. *Thromb Res* 1989; 56: 667–75.
21 Robson WL, Leung A, Woodman RC. The absence of anti-neutrophilic cytoplasmic antibodies in patients with Henoch–Schönlein purpura. *Pediatr Nephrol* 1994; 8: 295–8.
22 Kawana S, Nishiyama S. Serum SC5b-9 (terminal complement complex) level, a sensitive indicator of disease activity in patients with Henoch–Schönlein purpura. *Dermatologica* 1992; 184: 171–6.
23 Abou-Ragheb H, Williams A, Brown C *et al.* Plasma levels of the anaphylatoxins C3a and C4a in patients with IgA nephropathy/Henoch–Schönlein nephritis. *Nephron* 1992; 62: 22–6.
24 Allen DM, Diamond LK, Howell DA. Anaphylactoid purpura in children (Schönlein–Henoch syndrome). *Am J Dis Child* 1960; 99: 833–54.
25 Goldstein AR, White RHR, Akuse R *et al.* Long-term follow-up of childhood Henoch–Schönlein nephritis. *Lancet* 1992; 339: 280–2.
26 Legrain V, Lejean S, Taieb A *et al.* Infantile acute hemorrhagic edema of the skin: study of 10 cases. *J Am Acad Dermatol* 1991; 24: 17–22.
27 Raimer SS, Sanchez RL. Vasculitis in children. *Semin Dermatol* 1992; 11: 48–56.
28 Saulsbury FT. Corticosteroid therapy does not prevent nephritis in Henoch–Schönlein purpura. *Pediatr Nephrol* 1993; 7: 69–71.
29 Mollica F, Li Volti S, Garozzo R *et al.* Corticosteroid therapy does not prevent nephritis in Henoch–Schönlein purpura. *Pediatr Nephrol* 1994; 8: 131 (letter).
30 Mollica F, Li Volti S, Garozzo R *et al.* Effectiveness of early prednisone treatment in preventing the development of nephropathy in anaphylactoid purpura. *Eur J Pediatr* 1992; 151: 140–4.
31 Rosenblum HD, Winter HS. Steroid effects on the course of abdominal pain in children with Henoch–Schönlein purpura. *Pediatrics* 1987; 79: 1018–21.

25.4 Acute Haemorrhagic Oedema of the Skin in Infancy

ALAIN TAÏEB AND VALÉRIE LEGRAIN

Definition

Acute haemorrhagic oedema (AHO) in infancy of the skin is a benign cutaneous leucocytoclastic vasculitis of infancy. AHO is a separate entity among leucocytoclastic vasculitides, because of its clinical presentation which is alarming in contrast with its benign course [1]. However, some authors prefer to refer to it as 'infantile Henoch–Schönlein purpura' [2].

REFERENCES

1 Legrain V, Lejean S, Taïeb A et al. Infantile acute hemorrhagic edema of the skin (IAHE): a study of 10 cases. J Am Acad Dermatol 1991; 24: 17–22.
2 Amitai Y, Gillis D, Wasserman D, Kochman RH. Henoch–Schönlein purpura in infants. Pediatrics 1993; 92: 865–7.

History

Although first described by Snow in the USA in 1913 [1], the disease subsequently named infantile acute haemorrhagic (purpuric or ecchymotic would be better, because there is no bleeding) oedema of the skin or postinfectious cockade purpura was not until recently included as a separate entity in the English-language literature. Conversely, AHO is a well-recognized clinical entity in some European countries, most papers on the subject (reviewed in [2]) being written in French or German, even though the name used now first appeared in Spanish [3]. Eponymic designations like Finkelstein's disease [4] or Seidlmayer's disease [5] were used later in the literature as a tribute to these rediscoverers of the disease. Larrègue et al. contributed a comprehensive review of the clinical and histological features of 37 cases [6]. The recent history has been marked by the controversy of this disease versus Henoch–Schönlein purpura (HSP), the bottom line being whether or not the basic immunopathological mechanisms involved in these two vasculitides are the same [2,7,8].

REFERENCES

1 Snow IM. Purpura, urticaria and angioneurotic edema of the hands and feet in a nursing baby. J Am Med Assoc 1913; 61: 18–19.
2 Legrain V, Lejean S, Taïeb A et al. Infantile acute hemorrhagic edema of the skin (IAHE): a study of 10 cases. J Am Acad Dermatol 1991; 24: 17–22.
3 Del Carrel MJ, Diaz Bobillo I, Vidal J. Edema hemoragico agudo en un lactante. Prensa Med Arg 1936; 29: 1719–22.
4 Finkelstein H. Lehrbuch der Säuglingskrankheiten, 4th edn. Amsterdam: 1938: 814–30.
5 Seidlmayer H. Die frühinfantile, postinfectiöse Kokarden-Purpura. Z Kinderheilk 1936; 61: 217–55.
6 Larrègue M, Lesage B, Rossier. Edema agudo hemoragico del lactante (purpura en escarapela con edema postinfeccioso de Seidlmayer) y vascularitis alergica. Med Cutanea 1974; 11: 165–74.
7 Saraclar Y, Tinaztepe K, Adalioglu G, Tuncer A. Acute infantile hemorrhagic edema of infancy (AIHE)—a variant of Henoch–Schönlein purpura or a distinct clinical entity? J Allergy Clin Immunol 1990; 86: 473–83.
8 Amitai Y, Gillis D, Wasserman D, Kochman RH. Henoch–Schönlein purpura in infants. Pediatrics 1993; 92: 865–7.

Aetiology and pathogenesis

AHO is probably an immune complex-mediated vasculitis. However, there is currently no firm evidence that AHO is an immunoglobulin A (IgA) vasculitis in contrast to HSP. Seasonal variation and the frequency of preceding respiratory infection indicates an infective cause, but hypersentitivity to drugs has also been postulated. A history of recent infection mainly respiratory and/or drug intake or immunization is found in three out of four cases [1].

Most classification schemes for vasculitis are based on the calibre of involved vessels and type of inflammation [2]. A major advantage of the term vasculitis is to provide a synthetic entry which avoids the puzzling diversity of (cutaneous) signs of what is thought to be the basic pathological mechanism of lesions. In the skin small dermal vessels that are most commonly involved are the postcapillary venules. Pathological mechanisms are thought to be distinct in the case of neutrophilic (leucocytoclastic vasculitis) and mononuclear cell (lymphocytic vasculitis) infiltrates [3]. Some authors have challenged this view and have reported a continuum of lesions in the skin of the same patient and argue that the type of infiltrate may change over time [4]. In AHO the histological features are mostly those of a leucocytoclastic vasculitis which has been linked pathogenetically to immune complex deposition, complement activation and chemotaxis of neutrophils, with secondary damage to vessel walls due to the release of enzymes by activated neutrophils [5]. However, a lymphocytic vasculitis has already been reported [6]. The location of vasculitis lesions to the extremities and especially the legs in children and adults is thought to be related to increased hydrostatic pressure leading to immune complexes and fibrin deposition. Because of their prone position, lesions are thought to have a reduced gravity-related pattern in infants. Amitai *et al.* [7] have suggested that the proportionally larger head and face in infants corresponds to increased blood supply and susceptibility to facial purpura.

REFERENCES

1 Legrain V, Lejean S, Taïeb A *et al.* Infantile acute hemorrhagic edema of the skin (IAHE): a study of 10 cases. *J Am Acad Dermatol* 1991; 24: 17–22.
2 Mc Cluskey RT, Fineberg R. Vasculitis in primary vasculitides, granulomatoses, and connective-tissue diseases. *Hum Pathol* 1983; 14: 305–15.
3 Smoller BR, McNutt S, Contreras F. The natural history of vasculitis. What the histology tells us about pathogenesis. *Arch Dermatol* 1990; 126: 84–9.
4 Zax RH, Hodge SJ, Callen JP. Cutaneous leukocytoclastic vasculitis. Serial histopathologic evaluation demonstrates the dynamic nature of the infiltrate. *Arch Dermatol* 1990; 126: 69–72.
5 Sams WM Jr. Vasculitis. In: Thiers BH, Dobson RL, eds. *Pathogenesis of Skin Disease.* New York: Churchill Livingstone, 1986: 205–17.
6 Laugier P, Hunziker N, Reiffers J, Rudaz MJ. L'oedème aigu hémorragique du nourrisson (purpura en cocarde avec oedème). *Dermatologica* 1970; 141: 113–18.
7 Amitai Y, Gillis D, Wasserman D, Kochman RH. Henoch–Schönlein purpura in infants. *Pediatrics* 1993; 92: 865–7.

Pathology

Histological examination shows as the most typical finding an intense leucocytoclastic vasculitis with fibrinoid necrosis and erythrocyte extravasation [1–3]. However, lesser specific findings have been reported, i.e. no fibrinoid necrosis or a simple lymphohistiocytic perivascular infiltrate with extravasation of erythrocytes [1]. Perivascular IgA deposits have been found inconsistently in recent reports—around 30% [1–3]. IgM, C1q and fibrinogen are more frequently detected. Occasionally IgG and IgE are also found [2]. When studied, similar deposits have been found in involved and uninvolved skin except for C3 suggesting that the deposition of C3 was necessary to induce clinical lesions [2]. The general impression is that in AHO pathological changes are more intense than in HSP. These changes correlate well with clinical findings.

REFERENCES

1 Legrain V, Lejean S, Taïeb A *et al.* Infantile acute hemorrhagic edema of the skin (IAHE): a study of 10 cases. *J Am Acad Dermatol* 1991; 24: 17–22.
2 Saraclar Y, Tinaztepe K, Adalioglu G *et al.* Acute infantile hemorrhagic edema of infancy (AIHE)—a variant of Henoch–Schönlein purpura or a distinct clinical entity? *J Allergy Clin Immunol* 1990; 86: 473–83.
3 Amitai Y, Gillis D, Wasserman D *et al.* Henoch–Schönlein purpura in infants. *Pediatrics* 1993; 92: 865–7.

Clinical features (Figs 25.4.1–25.4.3)

The low number of reported cases (around 100) and the absence of large series originating from one institution in the literature may reflect a low incidence, but also the fact that AHO was not distinguished from HSP in the English-language literature. Based on a review of 80 cases of the literature [1] AHO affects infants between 4 months and 2 years of age. The most striking feature is the contrast between the acuteness of the cutaneous signs and the good general condition of the child. Fever is mild. The cutaneous features include (a) inflammatory oedema; and (b) ecchymotic purpura of the limbs (mainly the extremities) and face (cheeks, eyelids and ears) which are associated on some sites or separated in others. The trunk is relatively spared. The purpura often appears in a cockade pattern in combined lesions as noted early by Seidlmayer [2]. Oedema resembling nephrotic syndrome may affect the eyelids or more diffusely the face. In half of the patients, swelling of the earlobes also occurs. The oedema can cause weight gain [3]. Other occasional cutaneous signs are petechial or reticulate purpura, necrotic lesions, mainly on the ears, and urticaria. The rarity of visceral involvement is one of the main characteristics of AHO. Although difficult to assess in infants, joint pain has been exceptionally noted. Isolated cases of serosanguinous diarrhoea, of possible infectious origin, and melaena have been reported, but vomiting or abdominal pain are not classical features in contrast with HSP.

Kidney involvement with microscopic haematuria, mild proteinuria or increased blood urea nitrogen levels has always been transient [4].

A limited number of investigations have been reported, including the presence or absence of detectable serum immune complexes and normal serum complement level; no isolated increase in serum IgA has been reported [1].

Some cases are difficult to classify clinically and correspond to an overlap AHO–HSP. Those patients are older than 24 months, and purpura shows a mixed pattern: ecchymotic, reticulated or papular but never with a cockade pattern; localized oedema can occur. Extracutaneous symptoms, such as joint pain and abdominal pain are noted. The duration is longer [1].

REFERENCES

1 Legrain V, Lejean S, Taïeb A *et al.* Infantile acute hemorrhagic edema of the skin (IAHE): a study of 10 cases. *J Am Acad Dermatol* 1991; 24: 17–22.
2 Seidlmayer H. Die frühinfantile, postinfectiöse Kokarden-Purpura. *Z Kinderheilk* 1936; 61: 217–55.
3 Saraclar Y, Tinaztepe K, Adalioglu G *et al.* Acute infantile hemorrhagic edema of infancy (AIHE)—a variant of Henoch–Schönlein purpura or a distinct clinical entity? *J Allergy Clin Immunol* 1990; 86: 473–83.
4 Gelmetti C, Barbagallo C, Cerri D *et al.* Acute haemorrhagic edema of the skin in infants: clinical and pathogenetic observations in seven cases. *Pediatr Dermatol News (Bari)* 1985; 4: 23–34.

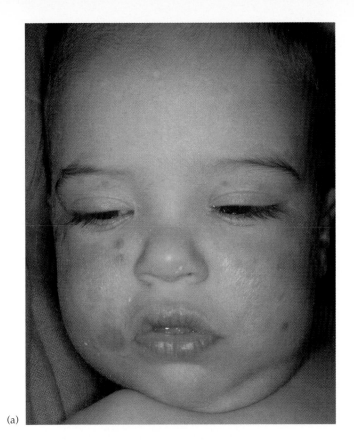

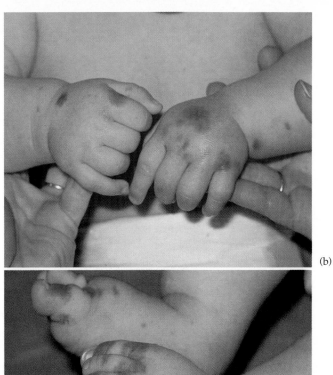

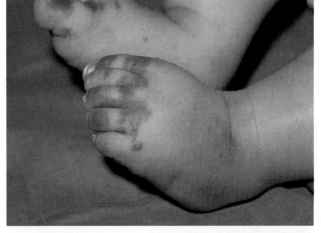

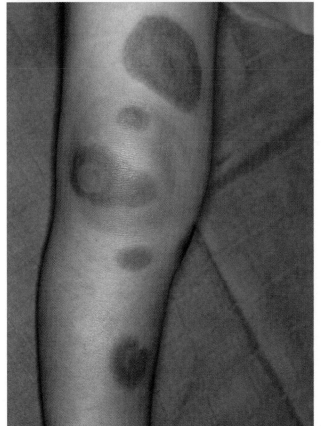

(a)

(b)

(c)

Fig. 25.4.1 AHO in a 7-month-old male; (a) mild facial involvement; and (b,c) oedematous and purpuric involvement of the extremities.

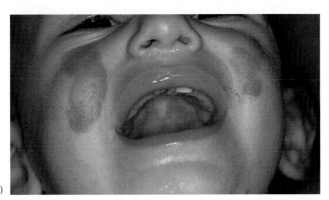

(a)

(b)

Fig. 25.4.2 AHO in a 12-month-old male featuring a typical cockade purpura on (a) the face; and (b) the legs.

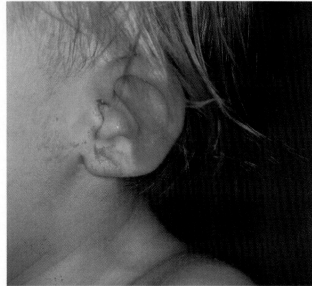

(a)

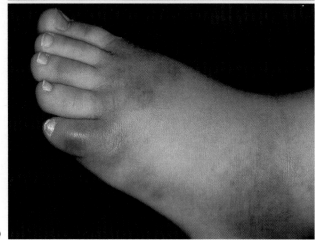

(b)

Fig. 25.4.3 AHO in a 14-month-old male child. Cockades are visible in (a) ear involvement; and (b) foot.

Prognosis

Spontaneous and complete resolution occurs within 1–3 weeks (mean 12 days) after one to three attacks [1]. Long-term follow-up is not available in most cases. However, the absence of reported complications [2] suggest that AHO runs a benign course. However, an intestinal intussusception followed by complications of surgery and death has been described in one case [3]. Torsion of the testis has been reported once [4].

REFERENCES

1 Legrain V, Lejean S, Taïeb A *et al*. Infantile acute hemorrhagic edema of the skin (IAHE): a study of 10 cases. *J Am Acad Dermatol* 1991; 24: 17–22.
2 Ince E, Mumcu Y, Suskan E *et al*. Infantile acute hemorrhagic edema: a variant of leukocytoclastic vasculitis. *Pediatr Dermatol* 1995; 12: 224–7.
3 Larrègue M, Lorette G, Prigent F *et al*. Oedème aigu hémorragique du

nourrisson avec complication léthale digestive. *Ann Dermatol Vénéréol* 1980; 107: 901–5.
4 Gelmetti C, Barbagallo C, Cerri D *et al*. Acute haemorrhagic edema of the skin in infants: clinical and pathogenetic observations in seven cases. *Pediatr Dermatol News (Bari)* 1985; 4: 23–34.

Differential diagnosis

Differential diagnosis includes [1]: necrotic purpuras and especially purpura fulminans, cockade eruptions like erythema multiforme; urticaria [2]; and Kawasaki's disease [3]. It should be stressed that all those disorders may feature a non-pitting oedema of the extremities, which is age specific rather than disease specific. Child abuse should also be considered (personal observations). Can AHO be regarded as a separate clinical entity among leucocytoclastic vasculitides or is it just a clinical variant of HSP? Table 25.4.1 summarizes the differences between the two entities. The immmunopathological studies by Saraclar *et al*. [4] favour a different pathological mechanism for AHO and HSP, since C1q deposits were found constantly in cases of AHO whereas HSP is known for not being associated with such deposits (HSP lesions are thought to be the result of an activation of the complement system via the alternative pathway). In the authors' opinion, there are overlaps between AHO and HSP, but this should not obscure the clinical specificity of these two entities. Both are within the spectrum of leucocytoclastic vasculitides. HSP has been attributed to circulating IgA dimeric complexes but such a mechanism remains to be demonstrated in AHO. Although they do not report AHO as a separate condition, the English literature does state that HSP may take on certain characteristic features when occurring in infants. Subcutaneous oedema is more common and can be extensive; disease course is shorter and visceral involvement uncommon. In Allen *et al*.'s series of 131 patients including 17 patients under 2 years of age [5], a much greater frequency of visceral involvement was noted in infants (renal 23%, gastrointestinal 29%, joint 56%) than mentioned in the AHO literature. The reason for this discrepancy remains unclear. The authors believe that both AHO and HSP in children are distinct clinical entities but that overlap forms exist. The practical benefit of this statement is to allow appropriate prognosis for infants with the full-blown picture of AHO, since the overall course of this disease is benign.

Treatment

There is no specific treatment for AHO. Antibiotics should be given when there is evidence of concurrent (but not necessarily causative) infection. Systemic corticosteroids and antihistamines do not seem to improve the course of the disease. With exceptional complications, close surveillance in hospital is not mandatory when the diagnosis is

Table 25.4.1 Comparison of AHO and HSP

	AHO	HSP
Age	4–24 months	Peak between 3 and 6 years
Purpura	Ecchymotic, cockade pattern limbs and face	Papular, petechial, urticarial, predominantly lower legs
Oedema	Constant, often extensive	Inconsistent
Visceral involvement	Very common	Frequent
Leucocytoclastic vasculitis	+	+
Fibrinoid necrosis	Frequent	Uncommon
Perivascular IgA deposits	Often without (30%+)	+
Perivascular C1q deposits	+	–
Mean duration	12 days	30 days
Relapses	No	Frequent
Sex	Slight male predominance in both entities	
Season	Cold season in both entities	
Prodromes	Respiratory infection, drug intake, immunization in both entities	
Inflammatory syndrome	Frequent in both entities	

made. Follow-up for signs of glomerular disease as in HSP is currently not recommended.

REFERENCES

1 Legrain V, Lejean S, Taïeb A *et al.* Infantile acute hemorrhagic edema of the skin (IAHE): a study of 10 cases. *J Am Acad Dermatol* 1991; 24: 17–22.

2 Legrain V, Taïeb A, Sage T *et al.* Urticaria in infants: a study of 40 patients. *Pediatr Dermatol* 1990; 7: 101–7.

3 Ducos MH, Taïeb A, Sarlangue J *et al.* Signes cutanés de la maladie de Kawasaki. A propos de 30 observations. *Ann Dermatol Vénéréol* 1993; 120: 589–97.

4 Saraclar Y, Tinaztepe K, Adalioglu G *et al.* Acute infantile hemorrhagic edema of infancy (AIHE)—a variant of Henoch–Schönlein purpura or a distinct clinical entity? *J Allergy Clin Immunol* 1990; 86: 473–83.

5 Allen DM, Diamond LK, Howell DA. Anaphylactoid purpura in children (Schönlein–Henoch syndrome). *Am J Dis Child* 1960; 112: 235–40.

Purpura Fulminans

MICHAEL LEVIN AND BRIAN ELEY

Postinfectious purpura fulminans
Congenital purpura fulminans due to defects in the protein C
    or S pathway
Acquired protein C or S deficiency due to drugs or specific diseases
Purpura fulminans associated with the antiphospholipid
    antibody syndrome
Platelet-mediated purpura fulminans occurring during
    heparin therapy
Purpura fulminans following bites or envenomation
Purpura fulminans

Definition

Purpura fulminans is a descriptive term used to describe a heterogeneous group of disorders characterized by rapidly progressive purpuric lesions, which may develop into extensive areas of skin necrosis, and peripheral gangrene (Fig. 25.5.1a). The disorder is associated with laboratory evidence of consumptive coagulopathy. The histopathological features are of widespread thrombosis of the dermal capillaries and venules with haemorrhagic infarction of the surrounding tissues. The condition is often fatal and survivors may suffer loss of digits, limbs or areas of skin [1,2].

History

The term purpura fulminans was first introduced by Henoch in 1887 [3]. Since then an extensive literature on the disorder has been published, containing clear descriptions of the clinical features of the disorder, and its histopathology [1–4]. The term purpura fulminans is now accepted as applying to patients with a devastating illness associated with extensive areas of purpura [2,3]. Despite the large number of cases reported in the literature the cause of the disorder has remained unclear and a confusing and often conflicting array of different theories have been presented on its aetiology and pathogenesis. A large number of different processes have been reported to initiate purpura fulminans, including bacterial and viral infection [4], autoimmune diseases [5], vasculitis and a number of drugs [6]. Several disease mechanisms have been proposed to explain the central features of the disorder: the widespread thrombosis

within dermal blood vessels. These including endothelial injury, primary activation of coagulation pathways, impaired anticoagulation mechanisms or activation of platelets [2,4,6]. Not surprisingly in view of the confusion surrounding the aetiology and the pathogenesis, the literature also contains conflicting recommendations as to treatment. Faced with a progressive and life-threatening illness of unclear aetiology, clinicians have utilized a wide variety of different treatments for the disorder. These include clotting factor replacement [7], anticoagulation [8], antiplatelet agents, glucocorticosteroids and immunosuppression [4], plasma phoresis or whole blood exchange [9], hyperbaric oxygen [10], and fibrinolytic agents [11].

Recognition that congenital deficiencies of protein C or S are associated with purpura fulminans [12], has highlighted the importance of the protein C pathway in the aetiology of the disorder. More recently, reports of purpura fulminans associated with acquired deficiency of protein C or S, either occurring during fulminant sepsis [13,14], or resulting from autoimmune processes [15], have highlighted the importance of primary thrombotic processes in the initiation of the disorder. The reports published in the past few years have not only provided a clearer understanding of the pathogenesis of the disorder, but also increasingly allow purpura fulminans to be understood as a syndrome which can result from several distinct disease processes.

Classification of purpura fulminans based on aetiology and pathogenesis

As with many other clinical disorders which were initially defined simply by description of the major clinical and histopathological features, it is now apparent that purpura fulminans is not a single disease, but a common clinical and histopathological manifestation of a number of distinct disease processes. Thus the major clinical feature (extensive purpura) is the result of a single histopathological process (dermal vascular thrombosis and haemorrhagic infarction of the surrounding tissues). These clinical and histopathological features may be caused by a wide range of different disease processes

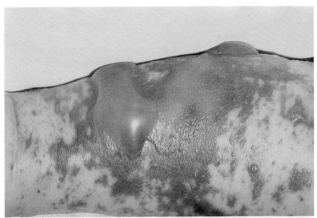

(a)

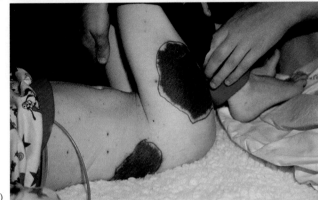

(b)

Fig. 25.5.1 (a) Acute infectious purpura fulminans due to meningococcal sepsis. Sharply demarcated areas of purpura are seen with bullous formation in the overlying skin. (b) Postinfectious purpura fulminans. Large areas of purpura are seen sharply demarcated from the surrounding tissues. Healing varicella vesicles are visible elsewhere on the body.

involving the blood vessel wall, platelets or prothrombotic or antithrombotic pathways.

Effective treatment of individual patients depends on identification of the underlying aetiological and pathophysiological mechanism, and the introduction of specific treatments to correct the disordered physiological process.

In this chapter a classification of purpura fulminans is proposed, which enables patients presenting with purpura fulminans to be classified into one of eight groups, on the basis of clinical and epidemiological criteria, and laboratory findings (Table 25.5.1). Each of these groups has a distinct aetiology and pathogenesis. Treatment recommendations are based on current understanding of the pathophysiological mechanisms.

Acute infectious purpura fulminans

Purpura fulminans occurring in the context of acute bacterial sepsis is the most common form of the disorder. A variety of different bacteria have been associated with

purpura fulminans, including *Staphylococus aureus* [16], groups A and B β-haemolytic streptococci [17,18], *Streptococcus pneumoniae* [19], *Haemophilus influenzae* [20], *H. aegyptius* [21] and *Pseudomonas aeruginosa*. Although purpura fulminans can be seen as an occasional complication of any of these bacterial infections, it occurs so commonly in the context of *Neisseria meningitidis* infection that its presence is considered a cardinal feature of meningococcal septicaemia [11,22,23]. Purpura fulminans associated with acute bacterial sepsis occurs in all age groups, but is most common in children. Patients with purpura fulminans associated with acute bacterial infection such as meningococcaemia invariably present with the features of systemic infection, and the majority will have evidence of shock [11,22]. The presenting features are often high fever, shivering, muscle aches, vomiting and abdominal pain. A particularly common presenting feature of children with severe purpura fulminans in the context of sepsis is intense limb pain which may be an early sign of venous thrombosis. As the disease progresses, confusion, impaired consciousness, laboured breathing and other signs of systemic underperfusion become more apparent. Signs of shock are usually present including tachycardia, delayed capillary refill, a wide gap between central and peripheral temperature, oliguria and elevated respiratory rate. Hypotension ultimately occurs once compensatory vasoconstrictive mechanisms are unable to maintain blood pressure in the face of severe shock. The disorder is frequently associated with multiorgan failure, and a mortality rate of 20–40% has been reported in most cases [11,22,23].

The pathophysiology of sepsis associated with purpura fulminans is complex. Bacteria or their toxins (principally lipo-olygosaccharide in the case of Gram-negative organisms) trigger an intense inflammatory process, with activation of neutrophils, macrophages, compliment and the clotting cascade [11]. Endothelial injury mediated either by bacterial toxins directly, or secondary to host inflammatory factors such as tumour necrosis factor (TNF), interleukin 1 (IL-1), reactive oxygen intermediates or proteolytic enzymes, results in disruption of the endothelium and loss of antithrombotic mechanisms [24]. Endotoxin induces upregulation of adhesion molecules on the endothelial surface which facilitate the attachment of neutrophils to the endothelial surface [24,25]. Upregulation of endothelial procoagulant activities, including tissue factor, occurs [26]. Neutrophils, activated by endotoxin induce loss of the anticoagulant glycosaminoglycans, heparin sulphate and chondroitin sulphate from the endothelial surface [27], downregulation of prostacyclin production [28] and a defect in the activation of antithrombin III by the endothelium [29]. Acquired deficiencies of antithrombin III and proteins C and S are caused by the profound capillary leak, together with consumption of protein C and S by the thrombotic process

Table 25.5.1 Classification of purpura fulminans based on aetiology and pathogenesis

Clinical subgroup	Aetiology	Clinical features	Laboratory features	Pathophysiology	Medical therapy	Outcome
Acute infectious purpura fulminans	*Neisseria meningitidis* *Streptococcus pneumoniae* *Haemophilus influenzae* *Staphylococcus aureus* β-haemolytic streptococci Other bacteria Rickettsiae *Candida albicans*	Any age Acute febrile illness Hypotension Multiorgan failure	Coagulopathy Positive blood culture Other evidence of specific infection	Circulatory insufficiency Endothelial dysfunction Coagulation activation Platelet activation Anticoagulant dysfunction Fibrinolytic dysfunction	*General:* Antimicrobial therapy Treatment of shock Support of multiorgan failure *Specific:* ? Heparin *Experimental:* AT III, protein C concentrates Fibrinolytic agents	Mortality rate 20–40% May require skin grafting, amputation of digits or limbs Long-term orthopaedic problems including disrupted bone growth
Postinfectious purpura fulminans	Varicella Group A β-haemolytic streptococci Other viruses, e.g. rubella	Usually young children Biphasic illness Initial febrile illness Sudden onset of purpura fulminans Haemodynamically stable	Coagulopathy Specific factor deficiency	Acquired protein S or C deficiency Autoantibody-mediated ? Other mechanisms	FFP Heparin ± Fibrinolytics *Speculative:* Factor concentrates Plasmaphoresis Gamma globulin	Self-limiting Mortality rate 15–20% Surgical intervention may be necessary
Congenital protein C or S deficiency	Homozygous or compound heterozygous genetic defects	Usually early neonatal period Spontaneous onset of purpura fulminans Haemodynamically stable Family history of thromboembolism	Coagulopathy Specific factor depletion Specific deficiency in family members	Inherited protein C or S deficiency	*Immediate:* FFP or factor concentrate Heparin *Prophylaxis:* Anticoagulation: warfarin ± Protein C concentrate	Life-long deficiency Fatal if untreated Neurological and ophthalmic sequelae are common Continuous risk of recurrence Surgical intervention may be necessary
Acquired protein C or S deficiency associated with drugs or disease	Coumarin drugs Cholestasis Renal dialysis Nephrotic syndrome Bone marrow transplantation	Any age Predisposing factors: drugs, interventions, hepatic or renal disease	Coagulopathy Specific factor depletion	Acquired protein C or S dysfunction or depletion	FFP or protein C concentrate Heparin Address underlying cause	Usually self-limiting Surgical intervention may be necessary
Antiphospholipid antibody syndrome	Autoimmunity	Usually older children and adults ± Underlying SLE	Prolonged APTT ± Slightly prolonged PT Lupus anticoagulant Antiphospholipid antibodies	Haemostatic dysregulation: multiple autoantibody-mediated mechanisms identified	*Immediate:* Anticoagulation Fibrinolytics Immunosuppression Plasmapheresis *Prophylaxis:* Anticoagulation: warfarin ± Antiplatelet therapy	Fulminant variant is frequently fatal Long-term prophylaxis is required to prevent recurrences Surgical intervention may be necessary
Vasculitic disorders	Polyarteritis Henoch–Schönlein purpura Other systemic vasculitides	Fever Multiorgan involvement Vasculitic rash Arthritis	Acute phase response Leucocytosis Organ dysfunction	Vasculitic damage to blood vessel wall	Immunosuppression steroids Cyclophosphamide ± Anticoagulation Antiplatelet agents	Significant mortality Prognosis depends on response to underlying disease
Platelet-mediated purpura fulminans	Heparin therapy	Usually subcutaneous heparin Purpura fulminans at injection site	± Thrombocytopenia	Antibody-mediated platelet aggregation	Discontinue heparin therapy ± Cyclo-oxengenase inhibitors	Self-limiting Surgical intervention may be necessary
Toxins/poisons	Spider bites Snake bites	History of envenomation Purpura maximum at site of bile	Coagulopathy	Toxic damage to blood vessels Activation of coagulation	Specific antitoxins Supportive treatment	Self limiting Surgical intervention may be required

APTT, activated partial thromboplastin time; ATIII, antithrombin III; PT, plasma thromboplastin.

[13,14,30,31]. Reduced thrombomodulin expression on the endothelium, which has also been reported to be induced by TNF or endotoxin [32], may also play a role in the functional defect in the protein C pathway. Impaired thrombolysis is associated with high levels of plasminogen activator inhibitor, the levels of which increase with increasing severity of the disease [33]. A combination of sluggish vascular circulation due to shock, together with upregulation of procoagulant pathways and downregulation of anticoagulation pathways, contributes to the onset of vascular thrombosis within dermal capillaries and venules [24,34].

Postinfectious purpura fulminans

In contrast to purpura fulminans occurring as a complication of acute bacterial sepsis, 'idiopathic' or 'postinfectious purpura fulminans', characteristically occurs 1–3 weeks after an acute infectious process [4]. The disorder is more common in young children, and varicella and streptococcal infections are the most common antecedents [4], although a variety of other childhood illnesses have been reported to precede the disorder [1,4,15]. The disorder follows a biphasic course. After appearing to recover from an otherwise uncomplicated childhood illness, affected patients suddenly develop extensive areas of purpura, principally affecting the buttocks and lower limbs (Fig. 25.5.1b). Patients are usually afebrile and, except for areas of skin infarction or peripheral gangrene, are well perfused and normotensive. The disease may progress rapidly, to cause extensive areas of skin necrosis, and gangrene of the limbs or digits. Thromboembolic complications of internal organs may subsequently occur. Thrombosis of large vessels may lead to pulmonary emboli, and embolization or thrombosis within the kidneys, brain, heart or other organs [15,35].

Affected patients have laboratory evidence of disseminated intravascular coagulation, with prolongation of prothrombin time, partial thromboplastin time and thrombin time, hypofibrinogenaemia and elevation of fibrin degradation products.

A wide range of different theories on the aetiology of the disorder have been presented. Although it is possible that the purpura fulminans following varicella may be mediated by a different process from that occurring in the context of streptococcal infections or other viral infections [4,6], there is now clear evidence that an acquired deficiency of protein S [35,36], induced by autoantibodies against protein S is a consistent feature of the disorder [15]. In 1993 D'Angelo *et al.* reported a single case of thromboembolic disease occurring in a child who had recently had varicella [37]. The patient had an acquired deficiency of protein S caused by autoantibodies directed against protein S. Although their patient did not have purpura fulminans, or any cutaneous manifestations of

thrombosis, their report led the authors to search for the presence of autoantibodies in similar patients with post-varicella purpura fulminans. In five consecutive children presenting with purpura fulminans following varicella or other viral infections, the authors documented severe acquired protein S deficiency caused by immunoglobulin G (IgG) or IgM autoantibodies directed against protein S, and this now appears to be the common mechanism underlying postinfectious purpura fulminans [15]. Varicella or other bacterial or viral infections, may trigger the production of an autoantibody which cross-reacts with the protein S. As no known varicella proteins exist with similar structure to that of protein S, it is likely that the antibody is directed against a neoantigen exposed during the varicella infection. The antibodies appear to increase the clearance of protein S perhaps by rapid removal of the protein S antibody complex through binding to Fc receptors on the reticuloendothelial system. The enhanced clearance of protein S not only explains the low levels of protein S present at the time of admission, but also explains the difficulties which may be found in restoring protein S levels to normal even following the infusions of large volumes of plasma. Levels of the antiprotein S autoantibodies decline spontaneously within 1–6 weeks after the onset of the disease [15] (Fig. 25.5.2). As IgG responses would normally be expected to be long lasting, the rapid disappearance of the antibody from the circula-

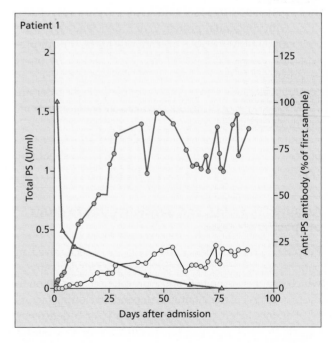

Fig. 25.5.2 Postinfectious purpura fulminans following varicella. The time course of changes in protein S level are shown following admission of a child with purpura fulminans. On admission both free protein S (●) and total protein S (○) levels were undetectable. Levels of antiprotein S antibodies were markedly increased (▲). Over the next 4 weeks antiprotein S antibody levels progressively declined with a concurrent rise in both free and total protein S.

tion may suggest involvement of an anti-idiotype response. Anticardiolipin antibodies are present in some of the patients with postvaricella purpura fulminans, including those with antiprotein S antibodies. Low titres of IgM and IgG anticardiolipin antibodies are detected in some of the patients with antiprotein S antibodies, and may be implicated in the pathogenesis but it is not yet clear whether this represents a cross-reaction or the production of two distinct sorts of cross-reacting antibodies [15,38]. It is also possible that autoantibodies directed against protein C, may cause a similar picture in some cases.

Congenital purpura fulminans due to defects in the protein C or S pathway

Children with congenital protein C and S deficiency, may present in the neonatal period with thrombosis of major organs including the brain with or without the cutaneous manifestations of purpura fulminans [12,39]. Severely affected patients have either homozygous protein C or S deficiency, or are functionally homozygous due to compound heterozygous states. The cutaneous features of purpura fulminans may occur spontaneously either in the neonatal period, or within the first months of life. In some cases cutaneous or internal organ thrombosis occurs spontaneously, but in other cases a precipitating infectious or inflammatory insult appears to trigger the disease. Unlike those patients with acute infectious purpura fulminans, those with congenital protein C or S deficiency are often haemodynamically stable, and afebrile at the time of presentation unless an infection has precipitated the onset of purpura. A family history of thromboembolism is common, as the heterozygous carriers of the disorder are at increased risk of thromboembolism. Any child presenting in the neonatal period or early months of life with purpura fulminans, or thromboembolism, should be suspected as having protein C or S deficiency and should be appropriately investigated [12,39,40–42].

Acquired protein C or S deficiency due to drugs or specific diseases

Purpura fulminans has increasingly been recognized in patients treated with drugs such as coumarin derivatives, which suppress protein C and S production in addition to the production of the vitamin K dependent clotting factors [6]. Patients heterozygous for protein C or S deficiency appear to be at risk [43–45]. Acquired protein C and S deficiency may also occur in patients with cholestatic hepatic disease [46], the nephrotic syndrome, peritoneal dialysis [47] and bone marrow transplantation [48]. The clinical features in this subgroup include the use of drugs which affect protein C or S production, or the presence of underlying predisposing diseases. In the case of coumarin

drug usage, patients developing purpura fulminans appear to have a more rapid decline in protein C and S levels, than the desired depletion of the vitamin K dependent procoagulant factors. Patients heterozygous for protein C or S deficiency are at risk of this complication. Patients with the nephrotic syndrome have increased urinary clearance of protein C and S as part of the generalized proteinuria. Impaired production of protein C and S or increased clearance underlie the association of depletion of these proteins with hepatic disease or dialysis.

Purpura fulminans associated with the antiphospholipid antibody syndrome

Purpura fulminans may occur in patients with systemic autoimmune disease such as systemic lupus erythematosus (SLE) [49], polyarteritis nodosa or Henoch–Schönlein purpura [50]. It may also occur as a component of the antiphospholipid antibody syndrome [51,52] (Fig. 25.5.3). The clinical features of patients presenting with purpura fulminans in the context of these systemic disorders are

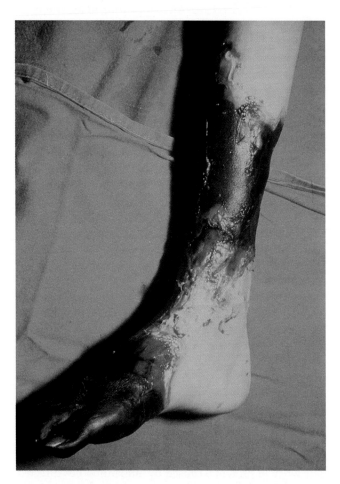

Fig. 25.5.3 Purpura fulminans and peripheral gangrene in a child with SLE and antiphospholipid antibodies.

usually dominated by those of the systemic illness. Patients with SLE or polyarteritis nodosa may have a prolonged febrile illness with evidence of multi-organ involvement including arthritis, nephritis, central nervous system disease or pneumonitis [53,54]. Occasionally patients with antiphospholipid antibodies may have no underlying systemic illness and may present acutely with either purpura fulminans or major organ thrombosis [51,52]. Laboratory features include an acute inflammatory response, with elevation of the erythrocyte sedimentation rate. Neutrophil leucocytosis and elevation of C-reactive protein, is common in the acute vasculitides, whereas in SLE paradoxical depression of C-reactive protein, neutropenia and thrombocytopenia may occur. Antiphospholipid antibodies may occur in association with other markers of SLE including anti-DNA antibodies, antibodies to extractable nuclear antigens and low C3 and C4. A number of antibody-mediated mechanisms initiating thrombosis have been identified in patients with antiphospholipid antibodies, including inhibition of protein C activation by thrombomodulin, inhibition of the anticoagulant action of activated protein C and interference with antithrombin 3 binding to endothelial glycosaminoglycans [51,52]. Platelet activation may also occur. Non-antibody-mediated mechanisms may also be involved including acute vasculitic damage to the vessel wall mediated by neutrophils and the lymphocytes or other inflammatory cells. Patients with systemic vasculitis may have evidence of antineutrophil cytoplasmic antibodies.

Platelet-mediated purpura fulminans occurring during heparin therapy

Heparin-induced skin necrosis, caused by antibody-mediated platelet aggregation, occurs primarily after subcutaneous administration of heparin usually at the injection site [55,56]. Platelet-mediated mechanisms have also been proposed to explain purpura fulminans occurring in the course of thrombotic thrombocytopenic purpura (TTP) [57], or paroxysmal nocturnal haemoglobinuria [58]. Diagnosis of platelet-mediated purpura fulminans is usually suggested by its occurrence in the context of heparin treatment or in patients with TTP. The disease is usually self-limiting once heparin therapy is discontinued, but treatment with alternative anticoagulant agents such as coumarin derivatives, or the use of platelet inhibitors such as non-steroidal anti-inflammatory agents or prostacyclin, may be required in severe cases.

Purpura fulminans following bites or envenomation

Purpura fulminans may occur after a number of toxic insults including snake bites or spider bites (see Chapter 8.3). Activation of coagulation and endothelial injury appears to be the underlying mechanisms. The purpura is usually present locally around the site of the toxin inoculation but in severe cases extensive areas of purpura may be apparent.

Purpura fulminans

Pathology

Although purpura fulminans may be caused by a variety of distinct disease processes, the histopathological findings are common to all patients with the disorder. The hallmark of the disease is thrombotic occlusion of dermal vessels [2,4,6]. In mild cases the process is confined to the dermal capillaries and venules. In more severe cases thrombosis extends into the deeper tissues involving larger vessels and in the most severely affected patients thrombotic occlusion of the major veins draining entire limbs may also occur (Fig. 25.5.4). Veins and small venules are distended and occluded by fibrin thrombi, and large aggregates of red cells. Haemorrhage into the surrounding tissues occurs resulting in oedema, and the appearance of extravascular red blood cells.

The intravascular thrombosis affecting capillaries, veins and venules frequently occurs without any evidence of underlying vasculitis or inflammatory cell-induced disruption of the vessel wall. This is particularly true of postinfectious purpura fulminans which is primarily a thrombotic process. In contrast, patients with purpura fulminans associated with meningococcal sepsis, or in vasculitis-associated purpura fulminans, there may be evidence of vasculitis surrounding areas of venous thrombosis [2]. Even in patients with purpura fulminans associated with meningococcaemia, venous thrombosis

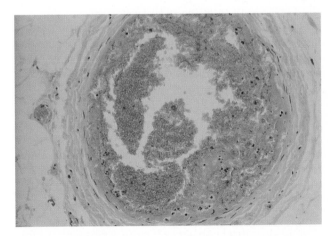

Fig. 25.5.4 Histology of purpura fulminans. Thrombosis within the saphenous vein is visible in a child who required below-knee amputation following meningococcal sepsis. The lumen of the vein is occluded by fibrin/thrombus. No inflammatory infiltrate was visible in the vessel wall.

may occur without any evidence of inflammatory cell infiltrate into the vessel wall [22]. Areas of vasculitis may be interspersed between areas of thrombosis without evidence of underlying vessel wall inflammation. The histopathological findings of widespread vascular thrombosis without evidence of extensive vessel wall inflammation or disruption is one of the most consistent features of the disease.

Clinical features

The major presenting symptoms and clinical signs in purpura fulminans differ amongst clinical subgroups as described in Table 25.5.1, and largely depend on the different aetiological processes. For example, the presenting features of patients with acute infectious purpura fulminans associated with meningococcal sepsis, are dominated by the features of sepsis and septic shock. Similarly patients with purpura fulminans associated with SLE or vasculitic disease will present with features of the underlying disorder. In this section, those clinical features which are common to all patients with purpura fulminans are discussed.

The first cutaneous sign of purpura fulminans is usually the appearance of erythematous or purplish sharply defined skin lesions (Fig. 25.5.5a). These are most common on the periphery but may occur elsewhere on the body and frequently involve the tips of the nose, ears and penis (Fig. 25.5.5b,c). Within a few hours, the initial lesions may progress to sharply defined bruises ranging in size from a few centimetres, to large confluent areas which may affect entire limbs. With time the lesions become black in colour indicating infarction of the affected area of skin (Fig. 25.5.5d). Haemorrhagic bulli or vesicles may be seen in some cases with the accumulation of haemorrhagic oedema fluid round the thrombosed vessels (Fig. 25.5.5e). In patients with progressive disease, lesions at different stages of evolution may be visible at the same time. Early lesions, with erythema and bluish discoloration may coexist with blackened areas of infarcted skin. Well-established lesions frequently have a zone of erythema surrounding the blue–black area of cutaneous infarction (Fig. 25.5.5d,f).

In patients with circumferential lesions of limbs, or those who develop major vein thrombosis, signs of peripheral ischaemia of whole limbs or multiple limbs may become apparent (Fig. 25.5.6). Loss or diminution of pulses in the affected limbs, poor capillary refill, pallor and reduced temperature are signs of impending gangrene. In severely affected cases the disorder may progress to critical ischaemia of entire limbs within a few hours of onset of the disease.

In the days and weeks following the onset of the disease, areas of purpura become sharply demarcated from the surrounding tissues. Whatever the cause of the

purpura fulminans, once the underlying disease process has been treated, and progression of the disease halted (by treatment of sepsis in the case of meningococcaemia, or following the administration of anticoagulants in the case of postinfectious purpura fulminans) the areas of cutaneous purpura persist, surrounded by uninvolved areas of skin which may be warm and well perfused. Where the thrombotic process has extended into the deep tissues, necrosis of the overlying skin will occur. The skin will initially become blackened and mummified. Thrombosed veins are often seen as black lines within the parchment-like dried and thickened skin. With time the thrombosed and blackened dead skin sloughs off, revealing underlying healthy granulation tissue (Fig. 25.5.5f). In superficial lesions blistering or bullous formation may occur but once the surface has been removed or fallen off viable skin may regrow without the need for skin grafting. The underlying depth of the lesions, may be difficult to estimate early in the process, and some patients may show dramatic recoveries without scarring, even when there have been extensive areas of apparent skin necrosis. In contrast patients with deep and extensive lesions will require skin grafting and plastic surgery to cover extensive areas of skin loss, and may be left severely scarred by the disorder (Fig. 25.5.7).

Prognosis

Purpura fulminans remains a devastating condition, which carries a significant mortality, and may cause considerable long-term disability in severe cases. The prognosis of the disorder is largely dependent on the underlying condition (Table 25.5.1). For patients presenting with purpura fulminans as a component of meningococcal septicaemia or other forms of sepsis, the prognosis is largely that of the underlying disorder. With modern aggressive intensive care, a higher proportion of patients with septic shock are now surviving. Mortality rates for patients with meningococcal sepsis range from 10 to 30% depending on the severity of the disease [11,23]. However, with improvements in intensive care, and in the survival rates for patients with severe sepsis, many patients who previously may have died of shock and multiorgan failure, are now surviving, but being left with the consequences of severe purpura fulminans including ischaemia of whole limbs or digits, and loss of extensive areas of skin.

For the other forms of purpura fulminans including postinfectious purpura fulminans, the prognosis has improved as a result of a better understanding of the disease. Reports in the literature of patients with postinfectious purpura fulminans suggested mortality rates of 20–30% [1,4]. With early anticoagulation, and judicious use of fibrinolytic agents, the prognosis has undoubtedly improved, and the majority of patients in whom the

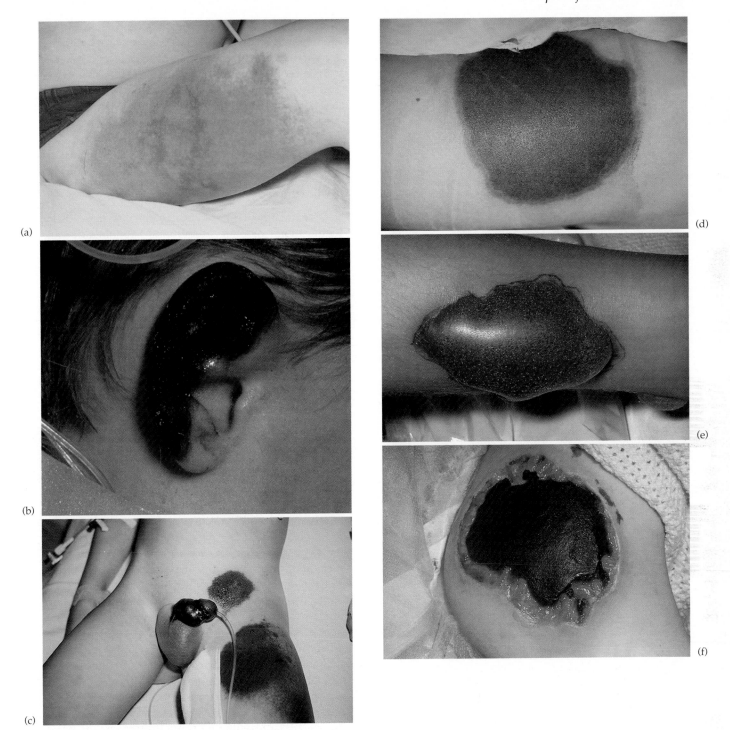

(a)

(b)

(c)

(d)

(e)

(f)

Fig. 25.5.5 (a) Early lesions of purpura fulminans. The child presenting with postinfectious purpura fulminans with early erythematous discoloration is seen with a small area of blue/black bruising in the centre of the lesion. (b,c) Purpura involving the earlobes and penis in a child with postvaricella purpura fulminans (composite). (d) Later lesions in postinfectious purpura fulminans. A sharply demarcated area of purpura is seen separated from surrounding skin by an area of erythema. (e) Haemorrhagic bullous lesions. A large blood-filled bullous area in a child with postinfectious purpura fulminans. (f) Late lesions of postinfectious purpura fulminans. Granulation tissue surrounds a deep area of skin necrosis on the buttock of a child with postvaricella purpura fulminans.

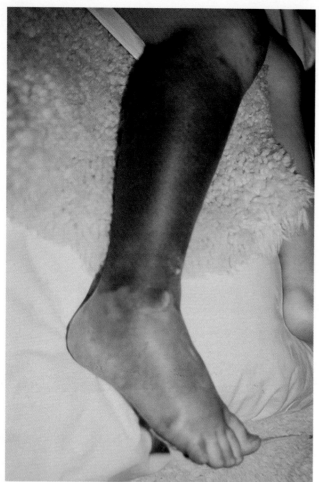

(a)

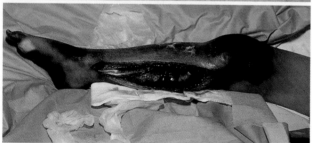

(b)

Fig. 25.5.6 (a) Circumferential areas of purpura in a child with postvaricella purpura fulminans. The foot is pale and pulses were not present. (b) Following fasciotomy, the muscles of the calf can be seen to be black and discolored. Amputation of the leg below the knee was required.

diagnosis is made and appropriate treatment administered should now survive. Clearly those patients in whom the true nature of the illness is not appreciated, and appropriate treatment withheld, continue to have a poor prognosis. Children with congenital protein C and S deficiency continue to have a poor prognosis. Affected children are at life-long risk of major vessel thrombosis, thrombosis of major organs and of recurrence of purpura. The availability of protein C concentrates has dramatically improved

the prognosis for children with this deficiency, but the requirement for life-long replacement therapy, continual vascular access, with the attendant risks of infection and large vessel thrombosis, and the risk of neurological and ophthalmic thrombosis result in these disorders having an uncertain prognosis. Therefore liver transplantation has been considered in some cases.

Treatment

Specific treatment for individual subgroups

Effective treatment of individual patients depends on identification of the underlying aetiological and pathophysiological mechanisms, and the introduction of specific treatments to correct the disordered physiological process. Previously a large number of different therapeutic modalities have been offered to individual patients without a clear understanding of the underlying physiological process. The clinicopathological classification proposed in this chapter now enables patients presenting with purpura fulminans to be assigned at the time of presentation to one of the distinct clinical subgroups based on the history and the presenting features. Treatment can therefore be administered specifically designed to correct the pathophysiological derangement underlying each of the subgroups.

Acute infectious purpura fulminans. The major component of treatment for patients with septic shock and purpura fulminans is directed against treatment of the underlying systemic infection and shock [11]. Patients should be admitted to a paediatric intensive care unit as soon as possible after diagnosis. Patients presenting with shock and purpura fulminans should receive broad-spectrum antibiotics to cover not only *N. meningitidis*, but also the less common organisms associated with purpura fulminans such as *S. pneumoniae*, *P. aeruginosa* and staphylococcal and streptococcal infection. A combination of third-generation cephalosporin and an antipseudomonal agent such as an aminoglycoside, or cefuroxime and an aminoglycoside, would be appropriate.

The main goal of treatment is to improve peripheral and organ perfusion by aggressive treatment of shock. The infusion of large volumes of colloid to correct hypovolaemia, inotropes to improve myocardial output and elective ventilation are indicated. Meticulous attention to fluid and electrolyte balance, and the use of renal replacement therapies are often required. The treatment of shock in meningococcal septicaemia has been described in detail elsewhere [11].

Specific treatments of the purpura fulminans, and the ischaemia of limbs and digits are increasingly used, but there have been few controlled trials to date. Fresh frozen plasma (FFP) infusions are required to correct the severe

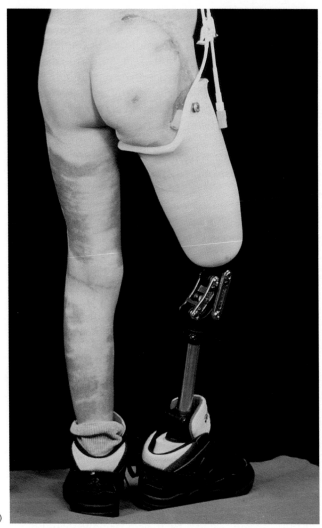

(a)

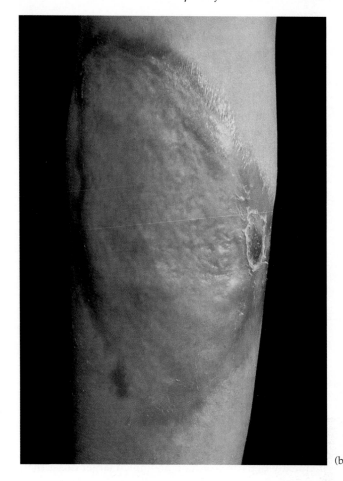

(b)

Fig. 25.5.7 (a,b) Consequences of postinfectious purpura fulminans. The same patient as in Fig. 25.5.6. Amputation of lower leg was required and extensive scarring is seen in other areas.

deficiencies of coagulation factors and to reduce the risk of haemorrhage associated with hypofibrinogenaemia. Despite theoretical concerns that the complement components present in FFP may accentuate the inflammatory process [59,60], FFP is indicated to correct hypofibrinogenaemia and specific clotting factor deficiency, and to reduce the risk of haemorrhage. Improvement of peripheral perfusion by reducing the use of vasoconstrictive agents such as adrenaline, or if this is not possible by the addition of vasodilating agents such as prostacyclin, may help to reduce the risk of peripheral ischaemia [11].

A large number of other modalities of treatment are theoretically attractive based on the growing understanding of the pathophysiology of the disorder, but have not yet been subject to extensive clinical trials. Administration of concentrates of protein C and antithrombin III [61–63] may be beneficial in the face of the depletion of these anticoagulant proteins which have been documented in this disorder [13,14]. There have been a number of case reports of the use of tissue plasminogen activator in patients with

critical limb ischaemia [64]. Such treatment would appear logical in the presence of the high levels of tissue plasminogen activator inhibitor and defective thrombolysis which has been documented in this disorder [64]. Similarly, heparinization may be beneficial in reducing the disseminated intravascular coagulation [65,66]. However, potential beneficial effects of anticoagulant or fibrinolytic agents, must be balanced against the potential risk of haemorrhage around venepuncture sites, or into the gastrointestinal respiratory or central nervous systems. The authors' own policy is to use low-dose heparin (10 units/kg/h) together with a large volume of FFP to replace clotting factors and fibrinogen. In severe cases antithrombin III concentrates and protein C coagulants are given. In patients with impending peripheral gangrene, tissue plasminogen activator is given in a low dose (0.05–0.1 mg/kg/h). Measures aimed at preventing loss of a limb through thrombosis, may not be justified, if the result is a major haemorrhage into the central nervous system. The use of fibrinolytic agents or anticoagulant agents in severe systemic sepsis-associated purpura fulminans should be undertaken only in units familiar with the use of these agents and after careful consideration of the risks and benefits of these treatments. It is likely that in the future with increasing experience of the use of factor replacement with concentrates of antithrombin III or protein C, and experience in fibrinolysis, more patients will be treated with these agents. Controlled trials are needed before the use of these agents is routinely recommended. The role of fasciotomy is discussed below.

Postinfectious purpura fulminans. With the recognition that the pathophysiology of postinfectious purpura fulminans involves acquired deficiency of protein S and that the disorder is primarily a disorder of venous thrombosis, treatment has become much clearer [15,35]. Immediate heparinization should be undertaken in any patient presenting with purpura fulminans following varicella. In patients with severe evidence of disseminated intravascular coagulation, heparinization should be started concurrently with infusions of large volumes of FFP. Correction of hypofibrinogenaemia, and replacement of clotting factors, will usually enable full heparinization to be achieved without major risk of haemorrhage. Heparinization is achieved by immediate administration of 100 units/kg of heparin, followed by a constant infusion of 25 units/kg/h. Patients with purpura fulminans are frequently heparin resistant, and much larger doses may be required to achieve anticoagulation. In most patients heparin alone will be adequate to prevent progression of the disease. However, in patients with critical limb ischaemia or impending infarction of large areas of the body or with evidence of thromboembolism, tissue plasminogen activator (TPA) should be infused in addition to heparin [15,37]. As there is a risk of haemorrhage when combinations of fibrinolytic agents are used together with heparin the dose of TPA should be kept as low as possible (0.05–0.1 mg/kg/h). Our most frequent regime would be to administer FFP on a daily basis (10–20 ml/kg) and to administer heparin continually initially by the intravenous route and once the condition has stabilized by the subcutaneous route. Heparinization is generally indicated until levels of protein S return to normal 2–6 weeks after the onset of the disease [15].

Infection is a common precipitant of purpura fulminans, and may also be a complication occurring in patients with large areas of skin damage. Appropriate antibiotics should be given until the underlying aetiology has been established, and until the sepsis has been excluded.

Although immunosuppression, or plasmapheresis, would theoretically hasten the reduction in plasma levels of antiprotein S antibodies, these treatments are generally not indicated. The antibody levels decline spontaneously within a few weeks and it is dubious whether immuno-

suppression with steroids, or plasmapheresis would result in a decline of the levels much more rapidly. In addition there are significant complications of central venous access which may be required in order to undertake plasmapheresis. In the presence of purpura fulminans and protein S deficiency, major vessel thrombosis including intracardiac thrombosis formation may occur, and central venous cannulation should be avoided if at all possible.

Purpura fulminans associated with the antiphospholipid syndrome or systemic vasculitides. Patients presenting with purpura fulminans in the context of SLE or a systemic vasculitic illness present a complex management problem, as the pathophysiology of the disorder is less clear than in the case of postinfectious purpura fulminans. A combination of platelet-mediated thrombosis, defects in antithrombotic mechanisms including the protein C pathway and damage to the vessel wall by the vasculitic process is common. Immediate therapy for a patient developing critical ischaemia of limbs or large areas of purpura would involve initiating anticoagulation with heparin, and consideration of the use of TPA if critical limb ischaemia is present. In those patients with evidence of arterial occlusion, prostacyclin should be considered in addition. Correction of specific clotting factor deficiencies and hypofibrinogenaemia by infusion of FFP may also be necessary.

Treatment of the underlying disease and the vasculitic process could also be initiated with corticosteroids such as methyl prednisolone, and for those patients with progressive and fulminant disease and evidence of multiorgan involvement, the addition of potent immunosuppressant agents such as cyclophosphamide or azothioprin may also be required. Plasmapheresis may be beneficial for patients with rapidly progressive multiorgan involvement [53].

The long-term treatment of patients with the antiphospholipid syndrome involves maintenance treatment of underlying SLE with steroids and immunosuppressive agents, and the use of oral anticoagulants. Immunosuppressive treatment may not be effective in removing antiphospholipid antibodies, and long-term oral anticoagulation with warfarin has been shown to reduce the risk of venous thrombosis [54].

Surgical, orthopaedic and other aspects of treatment

Patients with extensive purpura fulminans and ischaemia of the limbs or digits require interdisciplinary treatment involving doctors, haematologists and a variety of surgical specialities. Meticulous nursing care, and emotional support to the child and family are required throughout the illness.

Surgical intervention other than fasciotomy is rarely required during the early phases of extensive cutaneous purpura, and debridement and skin grafting to large purpuric areas should be delayed until complete demarcation of the infarcted areas of skin from the surrounding tissues has occurred, and the underlying disease process has been controlled.

For patients developing critical ischaemia of limbs or digits, fasciotomies may be required if there is evidence of compression of the arteries or veins by the oedematous tissues. The venous thrombosis often results in the development of extensive tissue oedema and a compartment syndrome. Fasciotomies, to reduce compression of both veins and arteries may be beneficial in some cases. Although there is a risk of bleeding at the site of the fasciotomy particularly in patients who are treated with anticoagulation, those patients with evidence of vascular compression by the oedematous tissues, may have a rapid improvement in perfusion of the limbs following the fasciotomy. Fasciotomies should therefore be considered early in patients with evidence of increased pressure within the tissues or the muscle compartments (Fig. 25.5.8a). In children with fulminant meningococcal shock, who have a capillary leak syndrome, marked swelling and oedema of the limbs and other tissues may occur extremely rapidly. Compression of the arterial and venous blood supply to the periphery may develop in a period of only a few hours in children who are requiring large volumes of colloid replacement. Careful watch should be kept on the state of perfusion of the periphery in all such patients. Constriction of the blood supply may be further accentuated by plasters and tapes which have been used to secure intravenous cannulae. As the tissues swell, adhesive tapes may produce circumferential constriction of the blood supply and contribute to the peripheral ischaemia. If fasciotomies are required, they should be sufficiently extensive to release any possible constrictions to the major veins or arteries.

Decisions as to the timing and need for skin grafting or amputations should be taken after close interdisciplinary discussion between the paediatric intensive care specialists, orthopaedic and plastic or vascular surgeons. Surgical intervention to remove necrotic skin, or amputate limbs or digits is generally not indicated during the acute phase of the disease for several reasons. First, in patients with shock, multiorgan failure, and severe coagulopathy, major surgical procedures are hazardous, and there will be major risks of bleeding. Second, clear demarcation between viable and dead tissue is extremely difficult in the early days of the illness. The area of skin blackening visible externally, does not give an accurate indication of the condition of the underlying tissue. Because the disease process in all forms of purpura fulminans begins with thrombosis of the dermal vessels, patients may have large areas of blackened and infarcted skin, yet have underlying viable tissues (Fig. 25.5.8a). Even in patients who have evidence of blackening of muscle beds visible at the time of

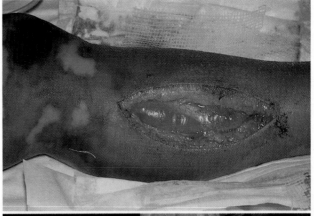

(a)

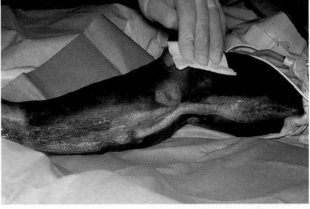

(b)

Fig. 25.5.8 (a) Purpura fulminans in meningococcal infection. A child with extensive purpura of both lower legs following meningococcal sepsis. Despite extensive cutaneous purpura, the muscles exposed by fasciotomy are viable. The oedematous muscle can be seen bulging through the incision site. (b) Meningococcal sepsis. A child with severe purpura fulminans and ischaemia of both lower legs is shown. Despite devitalized appearance of the skin and tissue exposed at fasciotomy, the child survived without loss of limbs, but required extensive skin grafting.

fasciotomy, the muscle infarction may only extend to the superficial visible areas of muscle, with viable tissues being left in deeper layers (Fig. 25.5.8b). For these reasons amputations and skin grafting should be delayed for several days or weeks after the acute onset of the illness. In the case of children with fulminant meningococcal sepsis stabilization of the child's condition, and recovery from multiorgan failure should be allowed to take place before major surgical interventions are undertaken.

Two main considerations have previously favoured early surgery. In patients with large areas of ischaemic tissues, there is a concern that myoglobinuria or the release of other toxic substances from necrotic tissues may result in a deterioration of the child's general condition. Also there is a concern that infection will occur in the devitalized tissues. As purpura fulminans has generally resulted from venous infarction, the ischaemic tissues are seldom in contact with the general circulation, and most patients will not develop evidence of systemic illness as a consequence of the gangrenous tissues. For both patients with acute infectious purpura fulminans, or postinfectious purpura fulminans, a delay of any decision on amputation is generally appropriate for several days or even weeks after the acute illness until complete demarcation has occurred, and signs of shock or multiorgan failure have resolved.

Secondary infection in the devitalized tissues does remain a significant risk. Virtually all patients who have large areas of necrotic skin and ischaemic tissues will have persistent fever, neutrophil leucocytosis and elevation of acute phase proteins. It may be difficult to distinguish fever and an inflammatory response due to the dead tissues from the effects of secondary infection in the devitalized tissues. Antibiotics are generally continued, to cover both aerobic and anaerobic organisms until debridement of the necrotic tissues has been undertaken.

In children who have viable muscles underlying extensive areas of skin necrosis it may be possible to salvage limbs even if the initial appearance of blackening of the entire limbs suggested that amputation may be required. The child shown in Fig. 25.5.8b who appeared to have bilateral ischaemia of both lower limbs, has survived after extensive skin grafting but with lower limbs intact. Although amputation may enable earlier discharge from hospital than is possible with a prolonged period of skin grafting, it may be possible to retain functionally useful limbs and digits even when the initial appearance suggested extensive ischaemia. Close consultation between paediatricians, orthopaedic and plastic surgeons is required in the management of these complex patients.

Differential diagnosis

In children presenting with extensive areas of purpura leading to infarction of areas of the skin or digits, the diagnosis of purpura fulminans is usually obvious, and the major difficulties are therefore in the recognition of the individual disease processes which can lead to purpura fulminans. A number of other conditions may be associated with extensive areas of bruising. These would include subcutaneous bleeding in patients with primary haemostatic defects such as clotting factor deficiencies, anticoagulant overdose or thrombocytopenic disorders. However, in these primary bleeding disorders, although extensive subcutaneous bleeding may occur, infarction of areas of the skin, which is typical of purpura fulminans, does not occur.

The distinction between the different forms of purpura fulminans is made on the basis of the clinical, epidemiological and laboratory features outlined in Table 25.5.1.

REFERENCES

1 Hjort PF, Rapaport SI, Jørgensen L. Purpura fulminans: report of a case successfully treated with heparin and hydrocortisone: review of 50 cases from the literature. *Scand J Haematol* 1964; 1: 169–92.
2 Adcock DM, Hicks MJ. Dermatopathology of skin necrosis associated with purpura fulminans. *Semin Thromb Hemost* 1990; 16: 283–92.
3 Henoch E. Ueber Purpura fulminans. *Berl Klin Wochenschr* 1887; 24: 8–10.
4 Francis RB. Acquired purpura fulminans. *Semin Thromb Hemost* 1990; 16: 310–25.
5 Dodd HJ, Sarkany I, O'Shaughnessy D. Widespread cutaneous necrosis associated with the lupus anticoagulant. *Clin Exp Dermatol* 1985; 10: 581–6.
6 Adcock DM, Bronza J, Marlar RA. Proposed classification and pathologic mechanisms of purpura fulminans and skin necrosis. *Semin Thromb Hemost* 1990; 16: 333–40.
7 Branson HE, Katz J. A structured approach to the management of purpura fulminans. *J Natl Med Assoc* 1983; 75: 821–5.
8 Hatterley PG. Purpura fulminans: complete recovery with intravenously administered heparin. *Am J Dis Child* 1970; 120: 467–71.
9 Daeschner CW, Carpentieri U. Purpura fulminans. *Tex Med* 1981; 77: 62–4.
10 Dudgeon DL, Kellog DR, Gilchrist GS, Woolley MM. Purpura fulminans. *Arch Surg* 1971; 103: 351–8.
11 Nadel S, Levin M, Habibi P. Current management of meningococcal septicaemia and meningitis. In: Cartwright K, ed. *Meningococcal Disease.* Chichester: John Wiley, 1995: 207–43.
12 Marlar RA, Neumann A. Neonatal purpura fulminans due to homozygous protein C and S deficiencies. *Semin Thromb Hemost* 1990; 16: 299–309.
13 Fourrier F, Lestavel P, Chopin C et al. Meningococcaemia and purpura fulminans in adults: acute deficiencies of proteins C and S and early treatment with antithrombin III concentrates. *Intensive Care Med* 1990; 16: 121–4.
14 Powars D, Larsen R, Johnson J et al. Epidemic meningococcaemia and purpura fulminans with induced protein C deficiency. *Clin Infect Dis* 1993; 17: 254–61.
15 Levin M, Eley BS, Louis J, Cohen H, Young L, Heyderman RS. Postinfectious purpura fulminans caused by an antibody directed against protein S. *J Paediatr* 1995; 127: 355–63.
16 Shennan AT. Purpura necrotica as a complication of ventriculoatrial shunts in hydrocephalus. *Arch Dis Child* 1972; 47: 821–3.
17 Isaacman SH, Heroman WM, Lightsey AL. Purpura fulminans following late on-set group B β-hemolytic streptococcal sepsis. *Am J Dis Child* 1984; 138: 915–16.
18 Canale ST, Ikard ST. The orthopaedic implications of purpura fulminans. *J Bone Joint Surg* 1984; 66A: 764–9.
19 Johansen K, Hansen ST. Symmetrical peripheral gangrene (purpura fulminans) complicating pneumococcal sepsis. *Am J Surg* 1993; 165: 612–15.
20 Santamaria JP, Kenney S, Stiles AD. Purpura fulminans associated with *H. influenzae* type b infection. *N C Med J* 1985; 46: 516–17.
21 Brazilian Purpuric Fever Study Group. *Haemophilus aegyptius* bacteremia in Brazilian purpuric fever. *Lancet* 1987; ii: 761–3.
22 Toews WH, Bass JW. Skin manifestations of meningococcal infection: an immediate indicator of prognosis. *Am J Dis Child* 1971; 127: 173–6.
23 Wong VK, Hitchcock W, Mason WH. Meningococcal infections in children: a review of 100 cases. *Pediatr Infect Dis J* 1989; 8: 224–7.
24 Heyderman RS. Sepsis and intravascular thrombosis. *Arch Dis Child* 1993; 68: 621–3.
25 Bone RC. Modulators of coagulation: a critical appraisal of their role in sepsis. *Arch Intern Med* 1992; 152: 1381–9.
26 Heyderman RS, Klein NJ, Daramola O et al. Induction of human endothelial tissue factor expression by *Neisseria meningitidis*: the influence of bacterial killing and adherence to the endothelium. *Microb Pathogen* 1997; 22: 265–74.
27 Klein N, Shennan G, Heyderman R, Levin M. Alteration in glycosaminoglycan metabolism and surface charge on human umbilical vein endothelial cells induced by cytokines, endotoxin and neutrophils. *J Cell Sci* 1992; 102: 821–32.
28 Heyderman RS, Klein NJ, Shennan GI, Levin M. Deficiency of prostacyclin production in meningococcal shock. *Arch Dis Child* 1991; 66: 1296–9.
29 Heyderman RS, Klein NJ, Shennan GI, Levin M. Modulation of the anticoagulant properties of glycosaminoglycans on the surface of the vascular endothelium by endotoxin and neutrophils: evaluation by an amidolytic assay. *Thromb Res* 1992; 67: 677–85.

30 Esmon CT, Taylor FB, Snow RT. Inflammation and coagulation: linked processes potentially regulated through a common pathway mediated by protein C. *Thromb Haemost* 1991; 66: 160–5.

31 Leclerc F, Hazelzet J, Jude B *et al.* Protein C and S deficiency in severe infectious purpura of children: a collaborative study of 40 cases. *Intensive Care Med* 1992; 18: 202–5.

32 Moore K, Esmon CT, Esmon NL. Tumour necrosis factor leads to the internalization and degradation of thrombomodulin from the surface of bovine aortic endothelial cells in culture. *Blood* 1989; 73: 159–65.

33 Brandtzaeg P, Joø G, Brusletto B, Kierulf P. Plasminogen activator inhibitor 1 and 2, alpha-2-antiplasmin, plasminogen and endotoxin levels in systemic meningococcal disease. *Thromb Res* 1990; 57: 271–8.

34 Brandtzaeg P, Sandset PM, Joø GB, Øvstebø R, Abildgaard U, Kierulf P. The quantitative association of plasma endotoxin, antithrombin, protein C, extrinsic pathway inhibitor and fibrinopeptide A in systemic meningococcal disease. *Thromb Res* 1989; 55: 459–70.

35 Nguyên P, Reynaud J, Pouzol P, Munzer M, Richard O, Francois P. Varicella and thrombotic complications associated with transient protein C and protein S deficiencies in children. *Eur J Pediatr* 1994; 153: 646–9.

36 Phillips WG, Marsden JR, Hill FG. Purpura fulminans due to protein S deficiency following chickenpox. *Br J Dermatol* 1992; 127: 30–2.

37 D'Angelo A, Valle PD, Crippa L, Pattarini E, Grimaldi LME, D'Angelo SV. Brief report: autoimmune protein S deficiency in a boy with severe thromboembolic disease. *N Engl J Med* 1993; 328: 1753–7.

38 Manco-Johnson M, Nuss R, Key N *et al.* Lupus anticoagulant and protein S deficiency in children with postvaricella purpura fulminans or thrombosis. *J Pediatr* 1996; 128: 319–23.

39 Marlar RA, Montgomery RR, Bruekmans AW. Diagnosis and treatment of homozygous protein C deficiency. *J Paediatr* 1989; 114: 328–534.

40 Millar DS, Allgrove J, Rodeck C, Kakkar VV, Cooper DN. A homozygous deletion/insertion mutation in the protein C (PROC) gene causing neonatal purpura fulminans: prenatal diagnosis in an at risk pregnancy. *Blood Coag Fibrinol* 1994; 5: 647–9.

41 Dreyfus M, Magny JF, Bridey F *et al.* Treatment of homozygous protein C deficiency and neonatal purpura fulminans with a purified protein C concentrate. *N Engl J Med* 1991; 325: 1565–8.

42 Marlar RA, Sills RH, Groncy PK, Montgomery RR, Madden RM. Protein C survival during replacement therapy in homozygous protein C deficiency. *Am J Hematol* 1992; 41: 24–31.

43 McGehee WG, Klotz TA, Epstein DJ, Rapaport SI. Coumarin necrosis associated with hereditary protein C deficiency. *Ann Intern Med* 1984; 100: 59–60.

44 Teepe RGC, Breikmans AW, Vermeer BJ, Nienhuis AM, Loeglier EA. Recurrent coumarin-induced skin necrosis in a patient with an acquired functional protein C deficiency. *Arch Dermatol* 1986; 122: 1408–12.

45 Friedman KD, Marlar RA, Houston JG, Montgomery RR. Warfarin induced skin necrosis in a patient with protein S deficiency. *Blood* 1986; 68 (Suppl 1): 333a (abstract).

46 Michiels JJ, Bertina RM. Thrombo-haemorrhagic skin necrosis due to rapid development of severe vitamin K deficiency associated with cholestasis. *Thromb Hemost* 1987; 58: 413 (abstract).

47 Kant KS, Glueck HI, Coots MC, Tonne VA, Brubaker R, Penn I. Protein S deficiency and skin necrosis associated with continuous ambulatory peritoneal dialysis. *Am J Kid Dis* 1992; 19: 264–71.

48 Gordon BG, Haire WD, Patton DF, Manno PJ, Reed EC. Thrombotic complications of BMT: association with protein C deficiency. *Bone Marrow Trans* 1993; 11: 61–5.

49 Jindel BK, Martin MFR, Gayner A. Gangrene developing after minor surgery in a patient with undiagnosed systemic lupus erythematosus and lupus anticoagulant. *Ann Rheum Dis* 1983; 42: 347–9.

50 Kisker CT, Glueck H, Kauder E. Anaphylactoid purpura progressing to gangrene and its treatment with heparin. *J Pediatr* 1968; 73: 748–51.

51 Stephens CJM. The antiphospholipid syndrome. Clinical correlations, cutaneous features, mechanism of thrombosis and treatment of patients with the lupus anticoagulant and anticardiolipin antibodies. *Br J Dermatol* 1991; 125: 199–210.

52 Key NS. Toward an understanding of the pathophysiologic mechanism of thrombosis in the antiphospholipid antibody syndrome. *J Lab Clin Med* 1995; 125: 16–17.

53 Asherson RA. The catastrophic antiphospholipid syndrome. *J Rheum* 1992; 19: 508–12.

54 Khamashta MA, Cuadrado MJ, Mujic F, Taub NA, Hunt BJ, Hughes GRV. The management of thrombosis in the antiphospholipid-antibody syndrome. *N Engl J Med* 1995; 332: 993–7.

55 White PW, Sadd JR, Nensel RE. Thrombotic complications of heparin therapy, including six cases of heparin-induced skin necrosis. *Ann Surg* 1979; 190: 595–608.

56 Warkentin TE, Levine MN, Hirsh J *et al.* Heparin-induced thrombocytopenia in patients treated with low-molecular-weight heparin or unfractionated heparin. *N Engl J Med* 1995; 332: 1330–5.

57 Luttengs WF. Skin necrosis in a patient with thrombotic thrombocytopenic purpura. *Ann Intern Med* 1957; 46: 1207–13.

58 Rietschel RL, Lewis CW, Simmons RA, Phyliky RL. Skin lesions in paroxysmal nocturnal hemoglobinuria. *Arch Dermatol* 1978; 114: 560–3.

59 Lehner PJ, Davies KA, Walport MJ *et al.* Meningococcal septicaemia in a C6-deficient patient and effects of plasma transfusion on lipopolysaccharide release. *Lancet* 1992; 340: 1379–81.

60 Busund R, Straume B, Revhaug A. Fatal course in severe meningococcemia: clinical predictors and effect of transfusion therapy. *Crit Care Med* 1993; 21: 1699–705.

61 Lynn WA, Cohen J. Adjunctive therapy for septic shock: a review of experimental approaches. *Clin Infect Dis* 1995; 20: 143–58.

62 Blauhut B, Kramar H, Vinazzer H, Bergman H. Substitution of antithrombin III in shock and DIC: a randomized study. *Thromb Res* 1985; 39: 81–9.

63 Rivard GE, David M, Farrell C, Schwarz HP. Treatment of purpura fulminans in meningococcemia with protein C concentrate. *J Pediatr* 1995; 126: 646–52.

64 Nadel S, De Munter C, Britto J *et al.* Recombinant tissue plasminogen activator restores perfusion in meningococcal purpura fulminans. *Crit Care Med* 1998; 26: 971–2.

65 Kuppermann N, Inkelis SH, Saladino R. The role of heparin in the prevention of extremity and digit necrosis in meningococcal purpura fulminans. *Pediatr Infect Dis J* 1994; 13: 867–73.

66 Feinstein DI. Diagnosis and management of disseminated intravascular coagulation: the role of heparin therapy. *Blood* 1982; 60: 284–7.

25.6 Urticarial Vasculitis

BHAVIK P. SONI AND JOSEPH L. JORIZZO

Definition

Urticarial vasculitis is a small vessel necrotizing vasculitis characterized clinically by urticarial lesions. Urticarial vasculitis may be a manifestation of systemic lupus erythematosus (SLE) as well as other underlying diseases [1]. Urticarial vasculitis, once believed to be an 'SLE-related syndrome', is now recognized as a distinct clinical syndrome [2]. Urticarial vasculitis is actually a disease spectrum ranging from localized cutaneous involvement to severe multisystem disease [2,3]. Although this is primarily a disease of adult women, urticarial vasculitis has been reported in children [4]. Urticarial vasculitis is characterized clinically by generalized erythematous, oedematous wheals which persist longer than 24 h [3]. Associated angio-oedema is often present [3]. Common extracutaneous manifestations include arthralgias and arthritis. More severe multiorgan involvement can occur affecting the ocular, renal, pulmonary, gastrointestinal and central nervous systems. Hypocomplementaemia, particularly affecting Clq and other early complement components C2–C4, is a frequent finding [3].

History

In 1973, McDuffie [5] described four patients with urticarial skin lesions who had skin biopsy specimens which demonstrated leucocytoclastic vasculitis. These four patients were all adult women. Their clinical features included urticarial skin lesions, angio-oedema, arthritis, abdominal pain, mild membranoproliferative glomerulonephritis, hypocomplementaemia and circulating immune complexes. These patients had negative or low titre antinuclear antibodies (ANA) with negative lupus erythematosus (LE) cell preparations and negative anti-DNA [5]. This clinical syndrome was distinct from SLE and termed hypocomplementaemic vasculitis.

Additional patients were described by Agnello et al. [6] and Soter et al. [7]. The literature is now filled with reports of patients with urticarial vasculitis which has previously been termed 'hypocomplementaemic vasculitis', 'an unusual SLE-related syndrome', 'urticaria with vasculitis' and 'hypocomplementaemic vasculitis urticarial syndrome' [8]. Despite these descriptive terms, urticarial vasculitis patients do not have sufficient criteria for a diagnosis of SLE, and not all are hypocomplementaemic [9].

The sera from two of McDuffie's original patients produced bands of precipitation with purified Clq. Agnello et al. [10,11] had reported similar findings. Zeiss et al. [12] observed that the presence of low molecular weight Clq precipitins was a central serological abnormality. Marder et al. [13] demonstrated that these were partially comprised of immunoglobulin G (IgG). Wisnieski and Naff [14] demonstrated that the Clq precipitin is an IgG autoantibody to Clq.

Aetiology and pathogenesis

Currently urticarial vasculitis is believed to be a form of small vessel necrotizing vasculitis mediated by a type 3 circulating immune complex (Arthus-like) reaction [1]. The pathogenesis of small vessel necrotizing vasculitis has been reviewed in detail [15,16]. Circulating immune complexes (antigen–antibody complexes) deposit in postcapillary venules. The trapping of these complexes results in activation of the complement cascade. C5a and other mediators attract neutrophils to the sites of immune complex deposition with subsequent phagocytosis of the complexes by neutrophils. Release of lysosomal enzymes and other products by the neutrophils probably mediates the tissue damage.

Since the vasculitic lesions are urticarial, the possibility of IgE-mediated hypersensitivity involvement has been suggested [3]. Anti-IgE autoantibodies have been reported in patients with urticarial vasculitis [17]. However, other studies have not supported a role for IgE-mediated disease [18].

The IgG anti-Clq antibodies may be pathogenetic, producing antigen–antibody complexes with Clq [14]. Patients with urticarial vasculitis have decreased Clq significantly out of proportion to Clr and Cls (which are relatively normal). This also supports a pathogenetic role for anti-Clq antibodies [14]. Anti-Clq antibodies are not specific for idiopathic urticarial vasculitis. They are also found commonly in patients with SLE and rarely in patients with other autoimmune rheumatic diseases

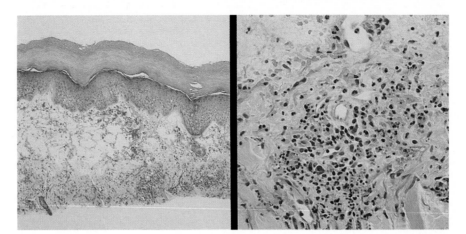

Fig. 25.6.1 Left: urticarial vasculitis with marked papillary oedema. Right: note typical changes of leucocytoclastic vasculitis with neutrophils, extravasated red blood cells and leucocytoclasis. (Haematoxylin and eosin, left × 12, right × 120; Original magnification.) Courtesy of Dr Jeff D. Harvell.

[19,20]. Urticarial vasculitis antibodies to Clq and SLE antibodies to Clq bind to the same collagen-like region of Clq [20]. This may explain the clinical similarity between the two diseases as well as the finding of urticarial vasculitis lesions as a reaction pattern in SLE and other autoimmune diseases. The final role of these anti-Clq autoantibodies in the pathogenesis of urticarial vasculitis remains to be determined [19].

Pathology

Histopathological examination of a skin biopsy specimen can usually distinguish urticarial vasculitis from urticaria [3]. Skin lesions demonstrate leucocytoclastic vasculitis with endothelial cell swelling, neutrophilic infiltration and leucocytoclasis, fibrinoid necrosis and haemorrhage (Fig. 25.6.1) [21]. Papillary dermal oedema is commonly seen [21]. Although the inflammatory infiltrate is usually composed of polymorphonuclear cells, there can be a mixed cellular infiltrate, or even a predominantly lymphocytic infiltrate depending upon the age of the lesion biopsied. Tissue eosinophils can be seen [1,21]. Usually only superficial and mid-dermal vessels are involved, but deep vessels of the dermis can be involved [1]. Some specimens can show hydropic degeneration along the basement membrane zone [1].

Direct immunofluorescence examination of biopsy specimens from patients with urticarial vasculitis usually reveals immunofluorescence staining of blood vessels with either immunoglobulins (IgG and/or IgM) and/or C3 [1,9]. Some biopsy specimens can also show staining along the basement membrane zone with immunoglobulin or C3 in a granular pattern. It is uncommon to have completely negative direct immunofluorescence studies [7]. These findings are not specific [9].

Clinical features

Urticarial vasculitis may occur at any age. There is a

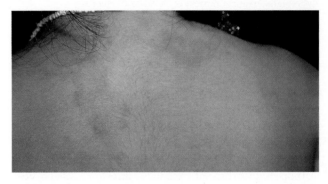

Fig. 25.6.2 Urticarial vasculitis: with lesions persisting for several days or longer.

strong female predominance (female to male ratio 8:1) [22]. A 2-year-old boy is the youngest reported patient [23]. However, there are very few reported children with urticarial vasculitis [23–26]. Urticarial vasculitis is predominantly a disease of adult women with a mean age of onset in the fifth decade, although age at onset has been reported to be as late as 79 years [9]. Duration of disease can range from 1 month to over 20 years [9]. The frequency of attacks of urticarial lesions in urticarial vasculitis is highly variable ranging from daily to monthly [9].

Cutaneous lesions of urticarial vasculitis are erythematous, oedematous papules or wheals (Fig. 25.6.2) [1]. The lesions are usually generalized and may involve the palms and soles [3]. Urticarial vasculitis tends to affect dependent areas such as the legs [27]; however, this is variable [3]. Several clinical features help to distinguish urticarial vasculitis from urticaria. In patients with urticarial vasculitis, individual lesions usually persist for more than 24 h (although usually less than 72h) whereas in true urticaria, individual lesions by definition resolve within 24h [27]. In patients with urticarial vasculitis, resolving lesions may leave purpura [28] or hyperpigmentation (Fig. 25.6.3) [8,9], whereas lesions of urticaria resolve com-

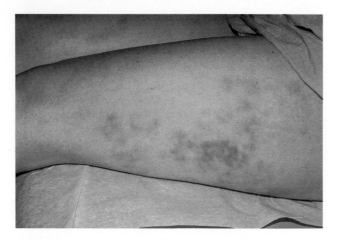

Fig. 25.6.3 Urticarial vasculitis, with areas of residual hyperpigmentation. Courtesy of Dr Adelaide Hebert.

pletely. Lesions of urticarial vasculitis are usually smaller [27]. Patients with urticarial vasculitis have lesions that are slightly more reddish in hue than the pink of true urticaria [27]. Also in urticarial vasculitis close inspection of lesions may reveal foci of non-blanching erythema [3].

In patients with true urticaria, the predominant symptom is itch. In patients with urticarial vasculitis, the lesions are more characteristically painful or burn [9]. Although, in urticarial vasculitis, pruritus is also a very common symptom [1,9]. The lesions may be asymptomatic [3].

Angio-oedema is common and can involve the lips, hands, eyes, tongue or larynx [1,8,9]. The angio-oedema is usually not life threatening [29], but can be [8]. Less common lesions in patients with urticarial vasculitis include purpuric papules, erythema multiforme-like eruptions, vesicles or bullae and livedo reticularis [8]. Raynaud's phenomenon and rheumatoid nodules (without rheumatoid arthritis) have been reported [3,8].

Patients with urticarial vasculitis manifest a spectrum of disease. Some patients have only cutaneous involvement while others can have severe multisystem involvement [9]. Patients with urticarial vasculitis who are hypocomplementaemic are more likely to have systemic involvement than normocomplementaemic patients, and the disease is likely to be more severe [9]. Organs commonly involved include the joints, kidneys and gastrointestinal tract. There is also a high frequency of lung and eye involvement. Less commonly the central nervous system, cardiovascular system and reticuloendothelial system can be affected [3].

Arthralgias and arthritis are the most common extracutaneous manifestations of urticarial vasculitis [1]. The joint symptoms are usually transient and parallel cutaneous disease activity [9]. Commonly affected areas are the hands, elbows, feet, ankles and knees [9]. The joint disease can be persistent. Deforming arthritis has been

reported [3] although there is a question of definition whether this represents an associated disease such as rheumatoid arthritis. Fever and myalgias ('serum-sickness') can occur [9].

Renal involvement is usually benign and tends to remain stable [30]. Evidence of renal involvement is usually manifested by microscopic haematuria and proteinuria [4,9]. Renal biopsies have been performed on many patients and a variety of histological changes have been found with mesangial proliferative glomerulonephritis being the most common [4]. Despite the usually benign course, careful follow-up is required because renal function can deteriorate [4]. Progression to end-stage renal disease requiring dialysis has been reported in adults and children [3,4,25].

Gastrointestinal involvement is usually manifested by abdominal or substernal chest pain [9]. Associated nausea, vomiting and diarrhoea can occur [9]. Abdominal distress is often associated with angio-oedema suggesting intestinal oedema as the aetiology of the gastrointestinal symptoms [3].

Pulmonary involvement can also be present [1]. Chronic obstructive lung disease is a common manifestation [1,9]. Affected patients are often smokers suggesting synergistic damage, but urticarial vasculitis does play a role [30]. Interstitial lung disease such as occurs in connective tissue disorders, and pleural effusions have also been reported [31–33]. Life-threatening pulmonary haemorrhage has been reported in a child [24].

Ocular involvement includes episcleritis, uveitis and conjunctivitis [8,9]. Usually visual acuity is not impaired; however, one patient who developed optic atrophy and blindness has been reported [9]. Pseudotumour cerebri presenting as headaches can occur [9,34]. Aseptic meningitis has been reported [12]. Cardiovascular involvement is unusual, but pericardial effusions have been reported [22]. Other uncommon findings include lymphadenopathy and hepatosplenomegaly [3].

A variety of laboratory abnormalities can occur. The most common are elevated sedimentation rates, hypocomplementaemia and the presence of circulating immune complexes [3]. Increased sedimentation rates are very common but not very specific for urticarial vasculitis [3,9]. However, this test may be used to monitor disease activity.

Hypocomplementaemia is very common, but there are normocomplementaemic patients [3,8,9]. Hypocomplementaemic patients are more likely to have systemic disease and it is more likely to be severe [1,8,9]. Total haemolytic complement (CH50) may be markedly reduced or normal. There is preferential reduction of early complement components, particularly C1q but also C2–C4 [3,8,9]. C1-esterase inhibitor levels are usually normal [8], as are C1r and C1s [29].

The hypocomplementaemia is likely secondary to the

presence of IgG anti-Clq autoantibodies in at least some patients with urticarial vasculitis [29]. This may also explain the presence of circulating immune complexes [3]. These antibodies are not specific to urticarial vasculitis, but are also seen in SLE and other connective tissue diseases [20].

Some patients with idiopathic urticarial vasculitis can have positive ANAs; however, when present they are usually of a low titre. Antibodies to double-stranded DNA are usually negative [8]. Patients can also have false positive non-treponemal tests for syphilis [8].

Prognosis

'Urticarial vasculitis' is a specific disorder as well as a non-specific reaction pattern in the skin caused by multiple aetiological agents [8]. Urticarial lesions which on histological examination reveal leucocytoclastic vasculitis can be a manifestation of SLE, Sjögren's syndrome, complement deficiency, granulomatous vasculitis, IgA multiple myeloma, IgM or IgG gammopathy, viral infections including hepatitis B and C, coxsackie virus, mononucleosis, drug exposure (particularly to cimetidine), cryoglobulinaemia or theoretically any of the causes of necrotizing venulitis [1,15,31,35–37]. Urticarial vasculitis has been reported after sun exposure and in patients with Lyme's disease [38].

The prognosis for patients who have urticarial vasculitis secondary to another disease process is related to the primary process. Drug-induced vasculitis tends to resolve on withdrawal of the drug [39]. True urticarial vasculitis (i.e. 'idiopathic' and a distinct clinical syndrome) tends to have a benign course [1]. However, the disease can be severe, particularly when there is laryngeal oedema or significant internal organ involvement [1,3,9].

Identification of possible causative agents and extent of internal involvement are important parts of the patient evaluation [15]. A complete history and physical examination should be performed. Laboratory screening for extent of disease should include a urinalysis, complete blood cell count and serum chemistry profile [15]. The search for an underlying cause can be viewed as an attempt to discover the antigens present in the immune complexes. An ANA test is a useful screen for collagen vascular diseases. Hepatitis B surface antigen, monospot, antistreptolysin O titre would help exclude common infectious aetiologies. Other tests to consider are cryoglobulins, sedimentation rate and C3 and C4 levels (or CH50) [15].

Differential diagnosis

A patient with an urticarial eruption must be evaluated to distinguish urticarial vasculitis from true urticaria. Individual lesions of true urticaria by definition resolve within 24 h, whereas lesions of urticarial vasculitis persist for more than 24 h [27]. The patient's history is variably reliable. It is often useful to circle individual lesions with a pen and have the patient recheck the site in 24 h. Lesions which last longer than 24 h should be biopsied. Patients with multisystem disease who have urticarial lesions which histologically display leucocytoclastic vasculitis, must be evaluated for SLE. As mentioned, these disease entities may be points along a common disease spectrum [40]. Evidence that patients with urticarial vasculitis have a disease distinct from SLE includes usually negative ANA test, absent antibodies to double-stranded DNA and presence of usually only mild renal disease in patients with systemic involvement [3].

Treatment

The treatment of urticarial vasculitis is challenging. The results of treatment with any agent have been inconsistent and there are no controlled studies [1,3]. Among the drug classes used are systemic corticosteroids [1], antihistamines, (H1- and H2-blockers) [1,3,41], antineutrophilic agents (dapsone [42] sulphapyridine, colchicine [32]), non-steroidal anti-inflammatory agents (indomethacin [21]), antimalarials (hydroxychloroquine [43]) and immunosuppressive agents (azathioprine [41], cyclophosphamide [35], methotrexate [44], gold [45]). Other treatments which have been considered include plasmapheresis [3], danazol [35], pentoxifylline [41], an elimination diet [46], fresh frozen plasma [35], intravenous immunoglobulin [35] and cromoglycate [35]. Aggressiveness of therapy should be tailored to the severity of internal organ involvement [3].

A therapeutic ladder approach is recommended. The urticarial lesions and angio-oedema can be treated with combinations of sedating and non-sedating H1-antihistamines (from different classes). Doxepin can be helpful. Epinephrine (subcutaneous) needs to be employed for life-threatening angio-oedema (laryngeal). Colchicine and dapsone or sulphapyridine can be used as the next step in the therapeutic ladder for patients with only cutaneous vasculitis lesions. Arthralgias can be managed with supportive care and acetaminophen (in general non-steroidal anti-inflammatory agents should be avoided as they can worsen urticarial lesions).

Significant systemic disease should be treated more aggressively. Although no treatment is always beneficial, oral corticosteroids are helpful in the greatest percentage of patients [1]. However, moderately high dosing (up to 1 mg/kg/day) may be needed and prolonged therapy has often been required [3]. Also various immunosuppressive agents can be used as alternatives or as prednisone-sparing agents such as methotrexate, azathioprine or cyclophosphamide. Alternative treatments which have been rarely used include plasmapheresis and immunoglobulin G.

REFERENCES

1 Mehregan DR, Hall MJ, Gibson LE. Urticarial vasculitis: a histopathologic and clinical review of 72 cases. *J Am Acad Dermatol* 1992; 26: 441–8.

2 Wisnieski JJ, Emancipator SN, Korman NJ *et al.* Hypocomplementemic urticarial vasculitis syndrome in identical twins. *Arthr Rheum* 1994; 37: 1105–11.

3 Gammon WR. Urticarial vasculitis. *Dermatol Clin* 1985; 3: 97–105.

4 Kobayashi S, Nagase M, Hidaka S *et al.* Membranous nephropathy associated with hypocomplementemic urticarial vasculitis: report of two cases and a review of the literature. *Nephron* 1994; 66: 1–7.

5 McDuffie FC, Sams WM Jr, Maldonado JE *et al.* Hypocomplementemia with cutaneous vasculitis and arthritis. Possible immune complex syndrome. *Mayo Clin Proc* 1973; 48: 340–8.

6 Agnello V, Ruddy, S, Winchester RJ *et al.* Hereditary C2 deficiency in systemic lupus erythematosus and acquired complement abnormalities in an unusual SLE-related syndrome. *Birth Defects* 1975; 11: 312–17.

7 Soter NA, Austen KF, Gigli I. Urticaria and arthralgias as manifestations of necrotizing angiitis (vasculitis). *J Invest Dermatol* 1974; 63: 485–90.

8 Monroe EW. Urticarial vasculitis: an updated review. *J Am Acad Dermatol* 1981; 5: 88–95.

9 Sanchez NP, Winkelmann RK, Schroeter AL *et al.* The clinical and histopathologic spectrums of urticarial vasculitis: study of 40 cases. *J Am Acad Dermatol* 1982; 7: 599–605.

10 Agnello V, Winchester RJ, Kunkel HG. Precipitin reactions of Clq with various gamma globulins and anionic macromolecules. *J Immunol* 1971; 107: 309.

11 Agnello V, Koffler D, Eisenberg JV *et al.* Clq precipitins in the sera of patients with systemic lupus erythematous and other hypocomplementemic states; characterization of high and low molecular weight types. J Exp Med 1971; 134: 228s–41s.

12 Zeiss CR, Burch FX, Marder RJ *et al.* A hypocomplementemic vasculitic urticarial syndrome. Report of four new cases and definition of the disease. *Am J Med* 1980; 68: 867–75.

13 Marder RJ, Burch FX, Schmid FR *et al.* Low molecular weight Clq precipitins in hypocomplementemic vasculitis–urticaria syndrome: partical purification and characterization as immunoglobulin. *J Immunol* 1978; 121: 613.

14 Wisnieski JJ, Naff GB. Serum IgG antibodies to Clq in hypocomplementemic urticarial vasculitis syndrome. *Arthr Rheum* 1989; 32: 1119–27.

15 Jorizzo JL, Solomon AR, Zanolli MD *et al.* Neutrophilic vascular reactions. *J Am Acad Dermatol* 1988; 19: 983–1005.

16 Sams WM Jr, Thorne EG, Small P *et al.* Leucocytoclastic vasculitis. *Arch Dermatol* 1976; 112: 219–26.

17 Gruber BL, Baeza ML, Marchese MJ *et al.* Prevalence and functional role of anti-IgE autoantibodies in urticarial syndromes. *J Invest Dermatol* 1988; 90: 213–17.

18 Damseaux M, Pierard-Franchimont C, Pierard GE. IgE and immune complexes in the serum of patients with urticaria and urticarial vasculitis. *Dermatologica* 1983; 166: 62–3.

19 Wisnieski JJ, Jones SM. IgG autoantibody to the collagen-like region of Clq in hypocomplementemic urticarial vasculitis syndrome, systemic lupus erythematosus, and six other musculoskeletal or rheumatic diseases. *J Rheumatol* 1992; 19: 884–8.

20 Wisnieski JJ, Jones SM. Comparison of autoantibodies to the collagen-like region of Clq in hypocomplementemic urticarial vasculitis syndrome and systemic lupus erythematosus. *J Immunol* 1992; 148: 1396–403.

21 Millns JL, Randle HW, Solley GO *et al.* The therapeutic response of urticarial vasculitis to indomethacin. *J Am Acad Dermatol* 1980; 3: 349–55.

22 Wisnieski JJ, Baer AN, Christensen J *et al.* Hypocomplementemic urticarial vasculitis syndrome. Clinical and serologic findings in 18 patients. *Medicine* 1995; 74: 24–41.

23 Waldo FB, Leist PA, Strife CF *et al.* Atypical hypocomplementemic vasculitis syndrome in a child. *J Pediatr* 1985; 106: 745–50.

24 Geha R, Akl KF. Shin lesions, angioedema, eosinophilia, and hypocomplementemia. *J Pediatr* 1976; 89: 724–7.

25 Martini A, Ravelli A, Albani S *et al.* Hypocomplementemic urticarial vasculitis syndrome with severe systemic manifestations. *J Pediatr* 1994; 124: 742–4.

26 Stevens HP, Ostlere LS, Rustin MH. Systemic lupus erythematosus in association with ulcerative colitis: related autoimmune diseases. *Br J Dermatol* 1994; 130: 385–9.

27 Dahl MV. Clinical pearl: diascopy helps diagnose urticarial vasculitis. *J Am Acad Dermatol* 1994; 30: 481–2.

28 Callen JP, Kalbfleisch S. Urticarial vasculitis: a report of nine cases and review of the literature. *Br J Dermatol* 1982; 107: 87–93.

29 Bishop PC, Wisnieski JJ, Christensen J. Recurrent angioedema and urticaria. *West J Med* 1993; 159: 605–8.

30 Schwartz HR, McDuffie FC, Black LF *et al.* Hypocomplementemic urticarial vasculitis: association with chronic obstructive pulomonary disease. *Mayo Clin Proc* 1982; 57: 231–8.

31 Lin RY, Caren CB, Menikoff H. Hypocomplementaemic urticarial vasculitis, interstitial lung disease and hepatitis C. *Br J Dermatol* 1995; 132: 821–3.

32 Werni R, Schwarz T, Gschnait F. Colchicine treatment of urticarial vasculitis. *Dermatologica* 1986; 172: 36–40.

33 Paira SO. Bilateral pleural effusion in a patient with urticarial vasculitis. *Clin Rheumatol* 1994; 13: 504–6.

34 Ludivico CL, Myers AR, Maurer K. Hypocomplementemic urticarial vasculitis with glomerulonephritis and pseudotumor cerebri. *Arthr Rheum* 1970; 22: 1024–8.

35 Asherson RA, D'Cruz D, Stephens CJ *et al.* Urticarial vasculitis in a connective tissue disease clinic: patterns, presentations, and treatment. *Semin Arthr Rheum* 1991; 20: 285–96.

36 Knox JP, Welykyj SE, Gradini R *et al.* Procainamide induced urticarial vasculitis. *Cutis* 1988; 42: 469–72.

37 Asherson RA, Sontheimer R. Urticarial vasculitis and syndromes in association with connective tissue disease. *Ann Rheum Dis* 1991; 50: 743–4.

38 Olson JC, Esterly NB. Urticarial vasculitis and Lyme disease. *J Am Acad Dermatol* 1990; 22: 1114–16.

39 Mitchell GG, Magnusson AR, Weiler JM. Cimetidire-induced cutaneous vasculitis. *Am J Med* 1983; 75: 875–6.

40 Bisaccia E, Adamo V, Rozan SW. Urticarial vasculitis progressing to systemic lupus erythematosus. *Arch Dermatol* 1988: 124: 1088–90.

41 Nurnberg W, Grabbe J, Czarnetzki BM. Urticarial vasculitis syndrome effectively treated with dapsone and pentoxifylline. *Acta Derm Venereol* 1995; 75: 54–6.

42 Fortson JS, Zone JJ, Hammon ME *et al.* Hypocomplementemic urticarial vasculitis syndrome responsive to dapsone. *J Am Acad Dermatol* 1986; 15: 1137–42.

43 Lopez LR, Davis KC, Kohler PF *et al.* The hypocomplementemic urticarial–vasculitis syndrome: therapeutic response to hydroxychloroquine. *J Allerg Clin Immunol* 1984; 73: 600–3.

44 Stack PS. Methotrexate for urticarial vasculitis. *Ann Allergy* 1994; 72: 36–8.

45 Handfield-Jones SE, Greaves MW. Urticarial vasculitis—response to gold therapy. *J Roy Soc Med* 1991; 84: 169.

46 Epstein MM, Watsky KL, Lanzi RA. The role of diet in the treatment of a patient with urticaria and urticarial vasculitis. *J Allerg Clin Immunol* 1992; 90: 414–15.

25.7 Erythema Elevatum Diutinum

BHAVIK P. SONI AND JOSEPH L. JORIZZO

Definition

Erythema elevatum diutinum (EED) is a rare disease generally considered to be a chronic localized fibrosing variant of small vessel necrotizing vasculitis [1]. Although EED is predominantly a disease of middle age, it may occur at any age [2]. The disease is characterized by persistent, symmetrical brown–red/purple papules and plaques commonly affecting extensor surfaces with a predilection for skin overlying joints [2]. The backs of the hands, feet, elbows, knees, buttocks and skin overlying the Achilles tendon are common sites. Older lesions become more nodular with a pink/yellow hue [2]. Vesiculation and ulceration can also occur [2].

History

The term EED was first coined by Radcliff-Crocker and Williams [3] in 1894. The term was purely descriptive indicating that the disease was characterized by red (erythema), raised (elevatum), persistent (diutinum) lesions [4]. The condition was originally described by Hutchinson [5] in 1878. Hutchinson [6] described three additional patients in 1888. All of Hutchinson's patients were older males (aged 40–70 years) who had a 'gouty' predisposition. Hutchinson himself was reluctant to give the condition a name [4]. Bury [7] in 1889 described the first child with the disease. He reported a 12-year-old girl with a nodular erythematous eruption of the hands. The patient described by Radcliff-Crocker and Williams [3] was a 6-year-old girl who developed nodules on the knees and then others on the buttocks, elbows and hands.

EED was originally subdivided into a Hutchinson type and a Bury type [4]. The Bury type occurred in young females with a personal or family history of 'gout or rheumatism' [4]. The Hutchinson type occurred entirely in elderly gouty males [4]. This subclassification is no longer valid as evidence indicates that they are the same underlying disease process [8].

Confusion arose in the late 1800s as descriptions of what is now known as granuloma annulare started to appear in the literature. The relationship between granuloma annulare and EED was uncertain, and several doctors considered them to be variants of the same clinical entity [4]. In 1910, Dalla-Favera [9] was the first to set up a clear distinction between EED and granuloma annulare based upon histological criteria. These results were verified by Piccardi [10].

Extracellular cholesterosis was a term coined by Urbach et al. [11] in 1932 to describe the condition of a 68-year-old woman with long-standing orange–red nodules of the face, buttocks and extremities. The term refers to the presence of lipid deposits in the dermis. It is now believed that extracellular cholesterosis represents older lesions of EED [12].

Aetiology and pathogenesis

Currently EED is believed to be a chronic form of small vessel necrotizing vasculitis mediated by a type 3 circulating immune complex (Arthus-like) reaction [2]. Katz et al. [1] first reported the presence of increased C1q-binding activity in some patients with EED. The pathogenesis of small vessel necrotizing vasculitis has been reviewed in detail [13,14]. Circulating immune complexes (antigen–antibody complexes) deposit in postcapillary venules. The trapping of these complexes results in activation of the complement cascade. C5a and other mediators attract neutrophils to the sites of immune complex deposition with subsequent phagocytosis of the complexes by neutrophils. Release of lysosomal enzymes and other products by the neutrophils probably mediates the tissue damage.

Since the initial report of Weidman and Besancon [15], in which they isolated streptococci from an EED lesion, streptococcal infections have been associated with EED [2]. An immune complex reaction to streptococcal antigens has been implicated. Experimentally, lesions may be induced in non-lesional skin of some EED patients by intradermal injection of streptococcal antigens from Lancefield group C strains of streptococci (streptokinase and streptodornase) [16,17]. Additional supportive evidence is the frequency of infections (some streptococcal) in EED patients [1], as well as the association of EED with rheumatic fever [18]. *Escherichia coli* has also been implicated [16]. Not all patients have streptococcal infection, so the exact pathogenesis of EED is still not clearly known.

Histopathology

EED is believed to be part of the spectrum of small vessel necrotizing vasculitis [19,20]. The histopathological features of EED show, at different stages, leucocytoclastic vasculitis, a nodular neutrophilic infiltrate and dermal fibrosis [21]. Some biopsies may show all of these stages in the same lesion [21]. However, the histopathological findings usually correlate to the age of the lesion [19]. The histological changes while characteristic are not diagnostic for EED [4].

Early lesions of EED (Fig. 25.7.1) show a leucocytoclastic vasculitis in which the predominant inflammatory cells are neutrophils [19]. The dermal infiltrate of neutrophils is dense with leucocytoclasis (nuclear dust) [19,21,22]. There is also fibrin deposition in and around vessel walls, endothelial cell swelling and luminal obliteration [19,21,22]. Occasional lymphocytes and histiocytes/macrophages can be found, but eosinophils are rare [21,22]. Increased eosinophils were reported in a patient with EED and hypereosinophilic syndrome [23]. Fully developed nodules show a nodular infiltrate of neutrophils with variable leucocytoclasis and papillary dermal oedema [21]. Epidermal necrosis secondary to the underlying vasculitis and the papillary dermal oedema can lead to vesiculation and ulceration [21].

Late lesions of EED (Fig. 25.7.2) show a predominance of granulation tissue and fibrosis in a nodular arrangement [19,21]. Often the fibrotic nodules are so dominant that serial sections may be needed to demonstrate small foci of persistent vasculitis [21]. Older lesions show an increased number of histiocytes/macrophages [22]. Secondary changes in some older lesions include the deposition of lipid which are believed to be cholesterol esters [19]. This is the origin of the old term extracellular cholesterosis, although recent ultrastructural evidence indicates that the lipid may actually be intracellular [12].

Direct immunofluorescence studies are generally nondiagnostic [19]. However, direct immunofluorescence studies can reveal perivascular deposits of immunoglobulins, fibrin and complement [24]. In a few cases, granular and linear immunoglobulin A (IgA) at the dermoepidermal junction have been noted [25–27].

Clinical features

EED may occur at any age [2]. Age of onset has been reported to be as early as 6 months [28] to as late as 75 years [8]. EED is predominantly a disease of middle age with a peak incidence in the sixth decade; however, there is a smaller peak in childhood with a female preponderance [2,19]. In adults there is an equal sex ratio [2]. There is

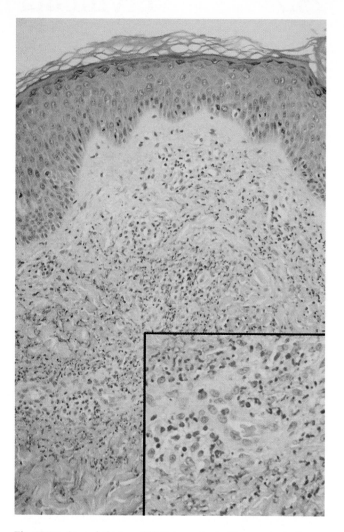

Fig. 25.7.1 An early lesion of EED shows typical leucocytoclastic vasculitis. Inset: note small vessel with plump endothelial cells surrounded by neutrophils and extensive leucocytoclasis. (Haematoxylin and eosin, ×30, inset ×120; original magnification.) Courtesy of Dr Jeff D. Harvell.

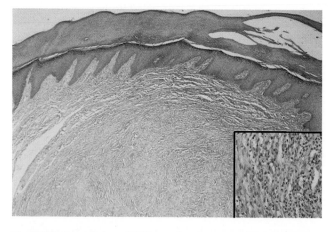

Fig. 25.7.2 A late lesion of EED on volar skin shows a fibrous nodule within the dermis. Inset: residual leucocytoclastic vasculitis is still identifiable in late lesions. (Haematoxylin and eosin, ×12, inset ×120; original magnification.) Courtesy of Dr Jeff D. Harvell.

no familial tendency, but one instance of EED in a mother and daughter has been reported [28,29]. Most reported patients have been Caucasian, although EED has been reported in other ethnic groups [29].

Early lesions of EED typically start as reddish-brown to purple (purpuric) papules or plaques occurring symmetrically over acral and extensor surfaces with a predilection for skin overlying joints [2]. Commonly involved sites include the hands, feet, elbows, knees, buttocks and the Achilles tendons [2] (Fig. 25.7.3). Other sites can be involved but the trunk is nearly universally spared [29]. Earlier lesions are soft to firm in consistency [20]. The lesions can be small or up to several centimetres in diameter, and coalescence of individual lesions may produce irregular, arcuate or gyrate forms [29]. Lesions can be solitary [30]. Vesicular or bullous lesions can occur [19,29]. The lesions can also ulcerate [19].

Later, the lesions become quite hard as fibrosis supervenes [29]. Older lesions become nodular and more pink or yellowish in colour resembling xanthomas [2].

In EED, the lesions are variably symptomatic but are usually asymptomatic [29], though pain (especially of a burning character) and to a lesser extent pruritus have been described [2,4]. The lesions show diurnal and temperature variation [27,31]. In the evening, the lesions become brighter red, more raised and firmer [27]. Lesions and symptoms worsen after cold exposure and improve upon rewarming [27]. Seasonal variation in relapses has been reported [31]. Relapse after pregnancy or menses can occur [29,32].

Constitutional symptoms have been variably reported though they can occur and may be severe, often forming the presenting complaint of the patient. Arthralgias are the most common constitutional symptom [29]. Fever can occur but usually does not [29].

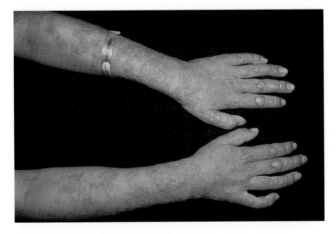

Fig. 25.7.3 EED: reddish-brown papules and plaques located symmetrically over acral and extensor surfaces. Note the predilection for the hands and the skin overlying joints. Courtesy of Dr Stephen I. Katz.

Prognosis

The course of lesions in EED is quite variable. Any individual lesion may arise and persist, arise and permanently resolve or recur after resolution [29]. Lesions that do resolve leave residual hypo- or hyperpigmentation [2,29]. Slight atrophy also occurs [2,29]. Patients who have lesions for longer than 10 years have little chance of permanent resolution and 39 years is the longest recorded duration of illness [2].

EED is considered to be a chronic cutaneous vasculitis usually with no systemic involvement [24]. However, any patient with a small vessel necrotizing vasculitis could have internal organ involvement. A complete history and physical examination should be performed. Screening laboratory studies for extent of disease include a urinalysis, serum chemistry profile and complete blood cell count [14].

Diseases specifically reported in children in association with EED include hyper-IgD syndrome (periodic fever) and coeliac disease (in a patient who also had insulin-dependent diabetes mellitus) [26,33].

Hyper-IgD syndrome is a very rare clinical entity characterized by an elevated serum level of polyclonal IgD and recurrent episodes of high fever [33]. The patient with concomitant hyper-IgD syndrome and EED was a 3-year-old girl who actually had cutaneous lesions since 1.5 years of age. Exacerbations of her cutaneous lesions usually occurred in association with febrile attacks. This patient was controlled with dapsone (25–62.5 mg daily) for over 10 years. Recurrent lesions developed whenever dapsone was discontinued. Although the association may be coincidental, the rarity of both conditions might suggest a pathogenetic relationship [33].

EED associated with coeliac disease has been reported in an 11-year-old girl who also had a history of poorly controlled insulin-dependent diabetes mellitus. This patient also had recurrent haematuria and increased serum IgA values suggesting a diagnosis of IgA nephropathy, but a confirmatory renal biopsy was not done. The cutaneous lesions in this patient preceded the development of recurrent abdominal pain and the diagnosis of coeliac disease. Eight weeks of dapsone therapy at 50 mg/day orally did not improve the cutaneous lesions. After the diagnosis of coeliac disease was confirmed, the dapsone was stopped and a gluten-free diet was instituted. The cutaneous lesions, abdominal pain and haematuria all resolved within 1 month [26].

The literature has many case reports of diseases occurring in association with EED in adult patients. These conditions could represent potential associations in paediatric patients with EED. Haematological abnormalities are the most common, particularly IgA monoclonal gammopathy [19,34]. IgG monoclonal gammopathies, IgA myeloma, multiple myeloma, polycythaemia vera, hairy cell leukaemia, myelodysplastic syndrome, idiopathic hypereosinophilic syndrome, chronic lymphocytic leukaemia and cryoglobulinaemia are other reported haematological diseases [19,34,35]. Chronic and recurrent infections are also very common [1]. Autoimmune diseases such as relapsing polychondritis, rheumatoid arthritis, systemic lupus erythematosus have been reported in association [19,30,36]. Both ulcerative colitis and Crohn's disease have been reported [37,38]. Human immunodeficiency virus (HIV) infection and EED may be a new association [38,39].

Differential diagnosis

The clinical differential diagnosis of EED is extensive. In paediatric patients diagnoses which should be particularly considered include granuloma annulare, xanthomas and multicentric reticulohistiocytosis. The differential diagnosis would also include Sweet's syndrome, hypertrophic lichen planus, cutaneous sarcoidosis and granuloma faciale [1,24,40]. The characteristic colour, symmetric acral location and persistence of lesions are helpful to differentiate EED from these other conditions. EED can develop vesiculobullous lesions [1,31] raising other differential considerations. A case of EED mimicking porphyria cutanea tarda has been reported [41].

EED occurring in a patient with HIV disease raises other diagnostic considerations including bacillary angiomatosis, Kaposi's sarcoma and juxta-articular nodes of syphilis [39,42].

The histological differential diagnosis of EED includes granuloma faciale, other forms of leucocytoclastic vasculitis, Sweet's syndrome, Behçet's syndrome. Older lesions of EED can, particularly at low power, resemble a dermatofibroma or scar tissue [21,24].

Treatment

Dapsone is considered to be the treatment of choice for EED. In some patients, dapsone has been found to produce a dramatic and often immediate response [1,29,31]. Some case reports have not found dapsone to be effective [16,43,44], although Katz *et al.* [1] believes that appropriate dosing is crucial to response. Dapsone treatment is suppressive rather than curative [1,24]. Early withdrawal of dapsone can lead to relapse or more severe exacerbations of EED [1,29]. Important side-effects of dapsone therapy include methaemoglobinaemia and peripheral neuropathy [45]; the glucose-6-phosphate dehydrogenase level should be checked prior to therapy [45].

In patients for whom dapsone is ineffective or in patients who cannot take or tolerate dapsone, there are many other options. Other treatments which have been used include sulphapyridine, colchicine [43], niacinamide and tetracycline [46]—although, tetracycline would be contraindicated in children under the age of 9 years with developing bones and teeth [45]. Chloroquine has been reported to be helpful [47,48], as has clofazimine [27]. One child with EED and coeliac disease did not respond to dapsone, but the cutaneous lesions resolved in response to a gluten-free diet [26].

Corticosteroids are generally believed to be ineffective [1], but there are reports of benefit from topical, intralesional and systemic corticosteroids [2,18]. Despite the association between EED and streptococci, antibiotics have not been shown to be helpful [2].

In older lesions of EED, once fibrosis has supervened, there may be minimal to no response to any standard therapy. Surgical excision has been reported to be of benefit [39].

REFERENCES

1 Katz SI, Gallin JI, Hertz KC *et al.* Erythema elevatum diutinum: skin and systemic manifestations, immunologic studies, and successful treatment with dapsone. *Medicine* 1977; 56: 443–55.
2 Wilkinson SM, English JS, Smith NP *et al.* Erythema elevatum diutinum: a clinicopathological study. *Clin Exp Dermatol* 1992; 17: 87–93.
3 Radcliff-Crocker H, Williams C. Erythema elevatum diutinum. *Br J Dermatol* 1894; 6: 1–9.
4 Haber H. Erythema elevatum diutinum. *Br J Dermatol* 1955; 67: 121–45.
5 Hutchinson J. *Illustrations of Clinical Surgery.* London: J & A Churchill, 1878 (plate VIII, p. 42).
6 Hutchinson J. On two remarkable cases of symmetrical purple congestion of the skin in patches, with induration. *Br J Dermatol* 1888; 1: 10–15.
7 Bury JS. A case of erythema with remarkable nodular thickening and induration of the skin associated with intermittent albuminuria. *Ill Med News* 1889; 3: 145–9.
8 Mraz JP, Newxomer VD. Erythema elevatum diutinum: presentation of a case and evaluation of laboratory and immunological status. *Arch Dermatol* 1967; 96: 235–45.
9 Dalla-Favera GB. Erythema elevatum diutinum und granuloma annulare. *Derm Z* 1910; 17: 541–58.
10 Piccardi G. Erythema elevatum et diutinum. *Derm Wchnschr* 1912; 55: 1115–24.
11 Urbach E, Epstein E, Lorenz K. Beiträger Zq einer Physiologischen und pathologischen Chemie der Haut. IX. Mitteilung. Extracellulärer Cholesterinose. *Arch Dermatol Syph* 1932; 166: 243–72.
12 Kanitakis J, Cozzani E, Lyonnet S *et al.* Ultrastructural study of chronic lesions of erythema elevatum diutinum: 'Extracellular cholesterosis' is a misnomer. *J Am Acad Dermatol* 1993; 29: 363–7.
13 Sams WM Jr, Thorne EG, Small P *et al.* Leukocytoclastic vasculitis. *Arch Dermatol* 1976; 112: 219–26.
14 Jorizzo JL, Solomon AR, Zanolli MD *et al.* Neutrophilic vascular reactions. *J Am Acad Dermatol* 1988; 19: 983–1005.
15 Weidman FD, Besancon JH. Erythema elevatum diutinum: role of streptococci and relationship to other rheumatic dermatoses. *Arch Dermatol* 1929; 20: 593–620.
16 Cream JJ, Levene GM, Calnan CD. Erythema elevatum diutinum: an unusual reaction to streptococcal antigen and response to dapsone. *Br J Dermatol* 1971; 84: 393–9.
17 Wolff HH, Maciejewski W, Scherer R. Erythema elevatum diutinum. Electron microscopy of a case with extracellular cholesterosis. *Arch Dermatol Res* 1978; 261: 7–26.
18 Macotela-Ruiz E, Oliver ON. Eryitema elevatum diutinum: reporte de un caso asociado a fiebre reumatica y co respuesta satis factoria a la cura olusiva con fluocinolona. *Dermatologia* 1971; 15: 42–6.
19 Yiannias JA, el-Azhary RA, Gibson LE. Erythema elevatum diutinumi a clinical and histopathologic study of 13 patients. *J Am Acad Dermatol* 1992; 26: 38–44.

20 Jorizzo JL. Classification of vasculitis. *J Invest Dermatol* 1993; 100: 106S–10S.

21 LeBoit PE, Yen TS, Wintroub B. The evolution of lesions in erythema elevatum diutinum. *Am J Dermatopathol* 1986; 8: 392–402.

22 Lee AY, Nakagawa H, Nogita T *et al.* Erythema elevatum diutinum: an ultrastructural case study. *J Cutan Pathol* 1989; 16: 211–17.

23 Cordier JF, Faure M, Hermier C *et al.* Pleural effusions in an overlap syndrome of idiopathic hyperesoinophilic syndrome and erythema elevatum diutinum. *Eur Resp J* 1990; 3: 115–18.

24 Hansen V, Haerslev T, Knudsen B *et al.* Erythema elevatum diutinum: case report showing an unusual distribution. *Cutis* 1994; 53: 124–6.

25 Morrison JG, Hull PR, Fourie E. Erythema elevatum diutinum, cryoglobulinaemia, and fixed urticaria on cooling. *Br J Dermatol* 1977; 97: 99–104.

26 Rodriguez-Serna M, Fortea JM, Perez A *et al.* Erythema elevatum diutinum associated with celiac disease: response to a gluten-free diet. *Pediatr Dermatol* 1993; 10: 125–8.

27 Farella V, Lotti T, DiFonzo EM *et al.* Erythema elevatum diutinum. *Int J Dermatol* 1994; 33: 638–40.

28 Langhof H, Zabel R. Erythema elevatum et diutinum bet mutter und tochter. *Dermatol Wschr* 1960; 141: 496–503.

29 Fort SL, Rodman OG. Erythema elevatum diutinum. Response to dapsone. *Arch Dermatol* 1977; 113: 819–22.

30 Collier PM, Neill SM, Branfoot AC *et al.* Erythema elevatum diutinum—a solitary lesion in a patient with rheumatoid arthritis. *Clin Exp Dermatol* 1990; 15: 394–5.

31 Vollum DI. Erythema elevatum diutinum—vesicular lesions and sulphone response. *Br J Dermatol* 1968; 80: 178–83.

32 Dowd PM, Munro DD. Erythema elevatum diutinum. *J Roy Soc Med* 1983; 76: 310–13.

33 Miyagawa S, Kitamura W, Morita K *et al.* Association of hyperimmunoglobulinaemia D syndrome with erythema elevatum diutinum. *Br J Dermatol* 1993; 128: 572–4.

34 Aractingi S, Bachmeyer C, Dombret H *et al.* Simultaneous occurrence of two rare cutaneous markers of poor prognosis in myelodysplastic syndrome:

erythema elevatum diutinum and specific lesions. *Br J Dermatol* 1994; 131: 112–17.

35 Delaporte E, Aleandari S, Fenaux P *et al.* Erythema elevatum diutinum and chronic lymphocytic leukemia. *Clin Exp Dermatol* 1994; 19: 188.

36 Bernard P, Bedane C, Delrous JL *et al.* Erythema elevatum diutinum in a patient with relapsing polychondritis. *J Am Acad Dermatol* 1992; 26: 312–15.

37 Buahere K, Hudson M, Mowat A *et al.* Erythema elevatum diutinum—an unusual association with ulcerative colitis. *Clin Exp Dermatol* 1991; 16: 204–6.

38 Walker KD, Badame AJ. Erythema elevatum diutinum in a patient with Crohn's disease. *J Am Acad Dermatol* 1990; 22: 948–52.

39 LeBoit PE, Cockerell CJ. Nodular lesions of erythema elevatum diutinum in patients infected with the human immunodeficiency virus. *J Am Acad Dermatol* 1993; 28: 919–22.

40 Perez IR, Fenske NA. Extensive purpuric and yellowish papules and plaques with an annular configuration. Erythema elevatum diutinum (EED). *Arch Dermatol* 1991; 121: 1399, 1402.

41 Requena L, Barat A, Hasson A *et al.* Erythema elevatum diutinum mimicking porphyria cutanea torda. *Br J Dermatol* 1991; 124: 89–91.

42 Requena L, Sanchez YE, Martin L *et al.* Erythema elevatum diutinum in a patient with acquired immunodeficiency syndrome. Another clinical simulator of Kaposi's sarcoma. *Arch Dermatol* 1991; 127: 1819–22.

43 Henriksson R, Hofer PA, Honqvist R. Erythema elevatum diutinum—a case successfully treated with colchicine. *Clin Exp Dermatol* 1989; 14: 451–3.

44 Lugt LVD. Erythema elevatum et diutinum. *Dermatologica* 1959; 119: 65–74.

45 *Physicians' Desk Reference*, 49th edn. Montvale, New Jersey, USA Medical Economics, 1995.

46 Kohler IK, Lorincz AL. Erythema elevatum diutinum treated with niacinamide and tetracycline. *Arch Dermatol* 1980; 116: 693–5.

47 Kint A, de Cuyper C. Erythema elevatum diutinum. *Hautarzt* 1980; 31: 447–9.

48 Hidano A. Erythema elevatum diutinum: action heurevse de la chloroquine. *Bull Soc Fr Dermatol Syph* 1963; 70: 153–5.

25.8 Wegener's Granulomatosis, Polyarteritis Nodosa, Behçet's Disease and Relapsing Polychondritis

E. JANE TIZARD AND MICHAEL DILLON

Wegener's granulomatosis

Polyarteritis (macroscopic and microscopic)

Behçet's disease

Relapsing polychondritis

Wegener's granulomatosis

Wegener's granulomatosis (WG) is a systemic vasculitis associated with granuloma formation. It is a distinct clinicopathological entity characterized by the classical triad of necrotizing granulomas of the upper and lower respiratory tract, a disseminated small vessel vasculitis involving arteries and veins together with a necrotizing glomerulonephritis. WG was first described by Freidrich Wegener in 1936 based on three similar autopsy cases [1,2]. Nearly 20 years later Godman and Churg named it the 'Wegener triad' [3]. It is a multisystem disease affecting the ears, nose, larynx, eyes, lungs, kidneys, heart, joints, skin and central nervous system (CNS) [4]. It is predominantly a disease of adults, usually 40–50 year olds with a male to female ratio of 1.3–1.6:1. However, the disease does occur in children.

Until recently there were no specific laboratory parameters that significantly contributed to the diagnosis of WG. A mild normochromic normocytic anaemia together with a leucocytosis and thrombocytosis are often found. The erythrocyte sedimentation rate (ESR) and C-reactive protein (CRP) are frequently elevated. Circulating immune complexes and raised immunoglobulins may also support the diagnosis although none are disease specific. The identification of antineutrophil cytoplasmic antibodies (ANCA) has helped not only to identify patients with WG but they may also be useful in monitoring disease activity and may contribute to our understanding of its pathogenesis. Davies et al. in 1982 [5] described antibodies directed against antigenic determinants in the neutrophil cytoplasm of patients with segmental necrotizing glomerulonephritis. Van der Woude et al. [6] demonstrated the presence of these antibodies in adults with WG and correlated their presence with disease activity. It was subsequently found that ANCA

were also commonly found in patients with microscopic polyarteritis (MPA) a systemic vasculitis similar to WG but predominantly affecting the kidney [7]. More detailed research revealed two specific types of ANCA, perinuclear ANCA (pANCA) and cytoplasmic ANCA (cANCA), relating to the pattern of immunofluorescent staining [8] (Fig. 25.8.1). Clinical studies have shown cANCA to be more commonly associated with WG and pANCA to be associated with MPA although there is a degree of overlap. The antigen against which cANCA are directed has been identified as proteinase 3 while that for pANCA is predominantly myeloperoxidase and elastase. The presence of ANCA (especially cANCA) has been found to be highly specific for WG by some authors [9].

Aetiology and pathogenesis

The aetiology of WG is unknown although a hypersensitivity disorder has been suggested. It is clear that infections may precipitate the onset of the disease or relapses. There is evidence that ANCA may be involved in its pathogenesis. WG is often associated with a neutrophilia and ANCA have been shown to activate neutrophils in vitro and produce oxygen radicals that may cause tissue damage [10]. ANCA have also been shown in the presence of low levels of cytokines to stimulate neutrophils to damage endothelial cells giving further evidence that ANCA incite vascular inflammation [11].

Pathology

Wegener's granulomatosis is a necrotizing granulomatous vasculitis, predominantly affecting small arteries and veins, which are infiltrated with polymorphonuclear leucocytes followed by mononuclear cells [12]. Granulomas are particularly seen in the upper and lower airways (Fig. 25.8.2), although there may be an absence of the classical histological changes, with the only abnormality being chronic inflammation. Renal lesions are variable; a focal and segmental glomerulonephritis is most commonly found although a diffuse proliferative glomerulonephritis with crescents is seen in those with a rapidly progressive clinical course and marked renal functional decline.

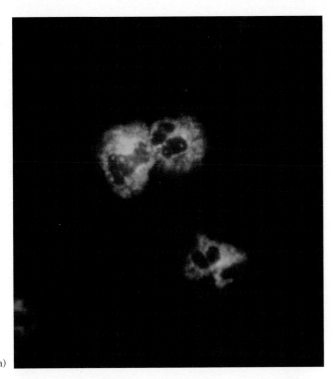

(a)

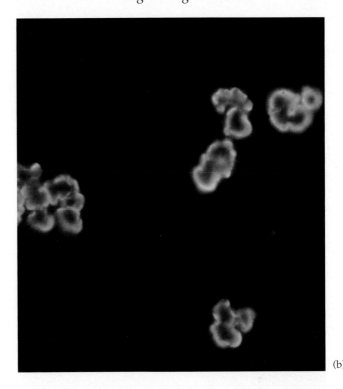

(b)

Fig. 25.8.1 Immunofluorescence pattern of (a) cANCA; and (b) pANCA.

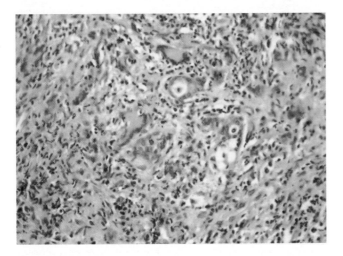

Fig. 25.8.2 Nasal biospy of WG: granulomatous inflammation with giant cells and generalized destructive acute inflammation involving nasal mucous glands.

Granulomas and evidence of vasculitis are often absent in renal biopsies.

Clinical features

The upper respiratory tract and ears are often affected first [13]. Subacute or chronic otitis may cause mastoiditis; hearing loss can be secondary to serous otitis or sensorineural in origin. Nasal congestion and epistaxis are frequent and ulceration and crusting of the mucosa result from the underlying necrotizing inflammatory process that may lead to septum perforation. Chondritis of the nose results in the typical saddle nose deformity (Fig. 25.8.3) [14]. Sinuses are often affected, ranging from mucosal thickening to pansinusitis and bone destruction. Oral features include jaw pain, gingival hyperplasia and palatal ulceration. Subglottic stenosis is the most commonly affected area in the tracheobronchial tree in children (Fig. 25.8.4) [13]. Pulmonary involvement may be asymptomatic. Single or multiple nodular masses with or without cavitation may be seen as can local or diffuse infiltrates [15] (Fig. 25.8.5).

Coronary arteritis, myocardial infarction, granulomatous valvulitis of the aortic or mitral valves, pericarditis or pancarditis are all rare complications. Renal involvement presents as nephritis sometimes with a rapidly progressive clinical picture [16].

Skin disease may present as erythema, urticarial lesions, petechiae, purpura, ulcerative lesions, pyoderma gangrenosum and necrotic lesions [17–24] (Fig. 25.8.6). In both paediatric and adult series skin disease is reported in approximately 50% [4,13]. In one large series of 244 adults 30 (14%) were found to have skin involvement and detailed clinical, histopathological and cANCA findings are reported [17].

Migratory arthralgias may effect several joints and symmetric polyarthritis can occur but destructive arthritis is

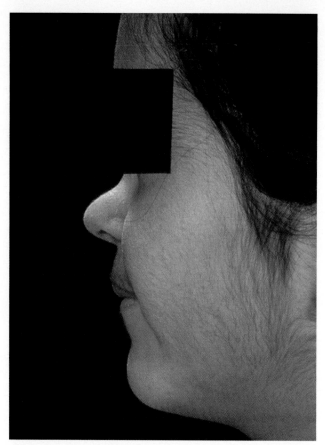

Fig. 25.8.3 Chondritis of the nasal bridge resulting in 'saddle nose' deformity in WG.

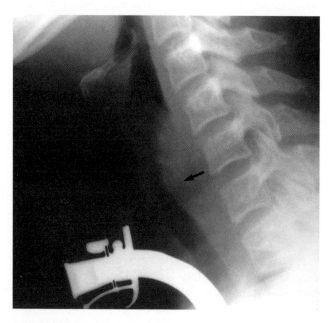

Fig. 25.8.4 X-ray of narrowing of the subglottic region in WG necessitating tracheostomy.

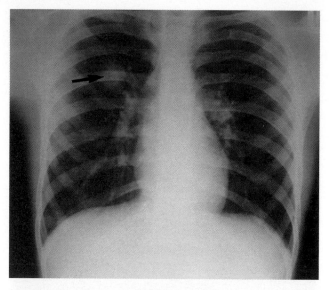

Fig. 25.8.5 Pulmonary nodule in child with WG.

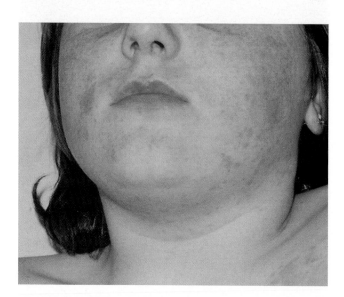

Fig. 25.8.6 Vasculitic rash of the face in WG.

rare. Neurological involvement may result in cranial nerve palsies, mononeuritis multiplex, symmetrical peripheral neuropathy, cerebral infarction and transverse myelitis (Fig. 25.8.7). Ophthalmological disease causing conjunctivitis, episcleritis, corneoscleral ulcers, uveitis, vasculitis of the retina, optic neuritis and central artery occlusion is documented. Unilateral or bilateral proptosis may be caused by granulomatous pseudotumours of the orbit [25,26] (Fig. 25.8.8). Gastrointestinal symptoms are rare although vasculitic ischaemia may result in bowel perforation, and necrotizing vasculitic involvement of the anus and rectum has been seen (Fig. 25.8.9).

It is known that a limited form of WG also exists in which the pathological findings are confined to the

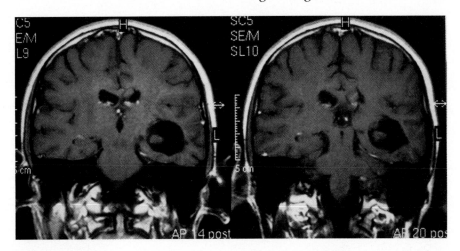

Fig. 25.8.7 MRI of brain cystic dilatation following necrotic haemorrhagic cerebral vasculitis in WG.

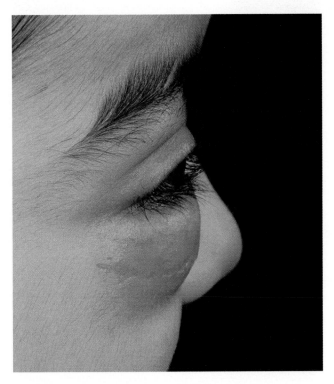

Fig. 25.8.8 Proptosis due to granulomatous pseudotumour of the orbit in WG.

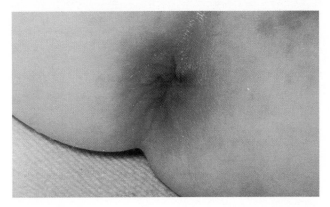

Fig. 25.8.9 Necrotizing vasculitic involvement of the anus and rectum in WG.

respiratory tract [27]. Subglottic stenosis is a feature of WG which has been reported in the absence of other clinical markers but in association with ANCA, demonstrating the benefit of a laboratory marker that allows early diagnosis and intervention with appropriate treatment [28]. A comparison of the clinical findings in children and adults is shown in Table 25.8.1.

In addition to the haematological and immunological investigations discussed above, radiology can be of diagnostic benefit in WG. Chest X-ray may demonstrate pulmonary infiltrates; sinus X-rays may be abnormal and neck views may demonstrate subglottic stenosis [15,29].

Treatment

Prior to the introduction of specific therapy the prognosis of this disease was extremely poor, with a mean survival of 5 months and 90% mortality within 2 years. The introduction of steroids improved the outlook slightly but cytotoxic therapy has had the main impact on the disease [30]. A report of the long-term follow-up over 21 years of patients treated with prednisolone and cyclophosphamide demonstrated complete remission in 79 of 85 (93%) with a mean duration of remission of 48.2 ± 3.6 months [4]. The combination of prednisolone and oral cyclophosphamide therefore remains the standard initial therapy. Other therapy has included intravenous cyclophosphamide, methylprednisolone, plasma exchange, azathioprine, methotrexate and cyclosporin A [13,31–33]. Less aggressive treatment with trimethoprim sulphamethoxasole has been suggested as an alternative for those with limited disease either as monotherapy or in combination with immunosuppressives in those who have failed to respond to routine treatment.

In a series of 23 paediatric onset patients the remission rate was 20 out of 23 (83%). Fifty three per cent of those

Feature	Rottem *et al.* (1993) [13] *n* = 23 children affected % onset	Rottem *et al.* (1993) [13] *n* = 23 children affected % total	Fauci *et al.* 1983 [4] *n* = 85 affected % total
Renal	9	61	85
ENT (total)	87	91	
sinusitis	61	83	91
nasal disease	48	65	64
Lung	22	74	94
Eye disease	13	48	58
Joints	30	78	67
Skin	9	52	45
CNS disease	4	17	22
Heart	9	9	12

Table 25.8.1 Comparison of features of WG in children and adults [4,13]

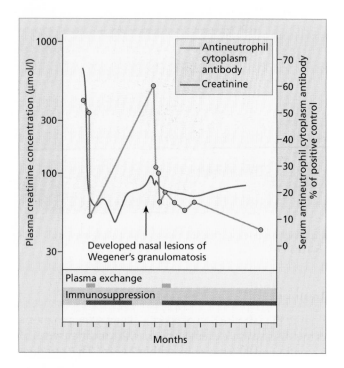

Fig. 25.8.10 ANCA relating to disease activity in a child with WG.

achieving remission had at least one relapse requiring treatment. In some children tracheostomy is necessary to relieve obstruction due to subglottic stenosis [13,33]. In selected patients ANCA titre can be a useful marker of disease activity (Fig. 25.8.10), heralding a relapse for which therapy may be initiated early.

With appropriate treatment, therefore, the outlook for this disease is relatively good although long-term maintenance therapy is often necessary. However, extended follow-up in significant numbers of children is not available at present.

REFERENCES

1 Wegener F. Uber generalisierte, septiche Gerfassekrankungen. *Verhandl Deutsch Path Gesellsch* 1936; 29: 202–8.

2 Wegener F. Uber eine eigenartige rhinogene Granulomatose mit besonderer Beteiligung des Arteriensystems und des Nieren. *Beitr Path Anat Allg Path* 1939; 102: 36–68.

3 Godman GC, Churg J. Wegener's granulomatosis. Pathology and review of the literature. *Am Med Assoc Arch Pathol* 1954; 58: 533–53.

4 Fauci AS, Haynes BF, Katz P, Wolff SM. Wegener's granulomatosis: prospective clinical and therapeutic experience with 85 patients for 21 years. *Ann Intern Med* 1983; 98: 76–85.

5 Davies DJ, Moran JE, Niall JF, Ryan GB. Segmental necrotising glomerulonephritis with antineutrophil antibody: possible arbovirus aetiology. *Br Med J* 1982; 285: 606.

6 Van der Woude FJ, Rasmussen N, Lobatto S et al. Autoantibodies to neutrophils and monocytes: a new tool for diagnosis and marker of disease activity in Wegener's granulomatosis. *Lancet* 1985; i: 425–9.

7 Savage COS, Winearls CG, Jones S, Marshall PD, Lockwood CM. Prospective study of radioimmunoassay for antibodies against neutrophil cytoplasm in diagnosis of systemic vasculitis. *Lancet* 1987; i: 1389–93.

8 Falk RJ, Jennette JC. Anti-neutrophil cytoplasmic antibodies with specificity for myeloperoxidase patients with systemic vasculitis and idiopathic necrotising and crescentic glomerulonephritis. *N Engl J Med* 1988; 318: 1651–7.

9 Venning MC, Quinn A, Broomhead V, Bird AG. Antibodies directed against neutrophils (C-ANCA and P-ANCA) are of distinct diagnostic value in systemic vasculitis. *Q J Med* 1990; 77(284): 1287–96.

10 Falk RJ, Terrell RS, Charles LA, Jeanette JC. Antineutrophil cytoplasmic antibodies induce neutrophils to degranulate and produce oxygen radicals in vitro. *Proc Natl Acad Sci USA* 1990; 87: 4115–19.

11 Ewert BH, Jennette JC, Falk RJ. Anti-myeloperoxidase antibodies stimulate neutrophils to damage human endothelial cells. *Kidney Int* 1992; 41: 375–83.

12 Lieberman K, Churg A. Wegener's granulomatosis. In: Churg A, Churg J, eds. *Systemic Vasculitides*. New York: Igaku-Shoin, 1991: 79–99.

13 Rottem M, Fauci AS, Hallahan CW et al. Wegener's granulomatosis in children and adolescents: clinical presentation and outcome. *J Pediatr* 1993; 122: 26–31.

14 Orlowoski JP, Clough JD, Dyment PG. Wegener's granulomatosis in the pediatric age group. *Pediatrics* 1978; 61: 83–90.

15 Wadsworth DT, Siegel MJ, Day DL. Wegener's granulomatosis in children: chest radiographic manifestations. *Am J Roentgenol* 1994; 163: 901–4.

16 Hall SL, Miller LC, Duggan E, Mauer SM, Beatty EC, Hellerstein S. Wegener granulomatosis in paediatric patients. *J Pediatr* 1985; 106: 739–44.

17 Daoud MS, Gibson LE, DeRemmee RA, Specks U, el-Azhary RA, Su WPD. Cutaneous Wegener's granulomatosis: clinical histopathologic, and immunopathologic features of 30 patients. *J Am Acad Dermatol* 1994; 31: 605–12.

18 Chyu JYH, Hagstrom WJ, Soltani K et al. Wegener's granulomatosis in childhood: cutaneous manifestations as the presenting signs. *J Am Acad Dermatol* 1984; 10: 341–6.

19 Mangold MC, Callen JP. Cutaneous leukocytoclastic vasculitis associated with active Wegener's granulomatosis. *J Am Acad Dermatol* 1992; 52: 535–61.

20 Thomas RHM, Payne CME, Black MM. Wegener's granulomatosis presenting as pyoderma gangrenosum. *Clin Exp Dermatol* 1982; 7: 523–7.

21 Patten SF, Tomecki KJ. Wegener's granulomatosis: cutaneous and oral mucosa disease. *J Am Acad Dermatol* 1993; 28: 710–8.

22 Hisler BM, Saltzman L. Cutaneous involvement in Wegener's granulomatosis. *Cutis* 1991; 48: 460–1.

23 Spigel GT, Krall RA, Hilal A. Limited Wegener's granulomatosis: unusual cutaneous, radiographic, and pathologic manifestations. *Cutis* 1983; 32: 41–51.

24 Camille F, Du LTH, Piette J-C *et al.* Wegener's granulomatosis. Dermatological manifestations in 75 cases with clinicopathologic correlation. *Arch Dermatol* 1994; 130: 861–7.

25 Haynes BF, Fishman ML, Fauci AS, Wolff SM. The ocular manifestations of Wegener's granulomatosis. Fifteen years experience and review of the literature. *Am. J Med* 1977; 63: 131–40.

26 Sacks RD, Stock EL, Crawford SE, Greenwald MJ, O'Grady RB. Scleritis and Wegener's granulomatosis in children. *Am J Ophth* 1991; 111: 430–3.

27 Carrington CB, Liebow AA. Limited forms of angiitis and granulomatosis of Wegener's type. *Am J Med* 1966; 41: 497–527.

28 Hoare TJ, Jayne D, Rhys Evans P, Croft CB, Howard DJ. Wegener's granulomatosis, subglottic stenosis and anti-neutrophil cytoplasm antibodies. *J Laryng Otology* 1989; 103: 1187–91.

29 Neumann G, Benz-Bohm, Rister M. Wegener's granulomatosis in childhood. *Pediatr Radiol* 1984; 14: 267–71.

30 Moorthy AV, Chesney RW, Segar WE, Grosh T. Wegener granulomatosis in childhood: prolonged survival following cytotoxic therapy. *J Pediatr* 1977; 91: 616–18.

31 Harrison HL, Linshaw MA, Lindsley CB, Cuppage FE. Bolus corticosteroids and cyclophosphamide for initial treatment of Wegener's granulomatosis. *J Am Med Assoc* 1980; 244: 1599–980.

32 Tizard EJ, Dillon MJ. Plasmapheresis in childhood. *Care Crit Ill* 1991; 7: 51–5.

33 Tizard EJ, Barratt TM, Dillon MJ. Wegener's granulomatosis in six children. *Am J Kid Dis* 1991; 18: 212.

Polyarteritis (macroscopic and microscopic)

Classic (macroscopic) polyarteritis nodosa (PAN) was first described in 1866 by Kussmaul and Maier in an autopsy of a 27-year-old man who had proteinuria, myalgia, neuritis and abdominal pain [1]. It is a disease of small and medium sized arteries with aneurysmal dilatation especially at arterial branching points. Although it is rare, PAN does occur in childhood [2–4]. There is a debate about the overlap of infantile polyarteritis with Kawasaki disease [5]. Some of the early reports of infantile polyarteritis give classical descriptions of Kawasaki disease [6,7]. PAN may present as multisystem disease but there is also a group of patients in whom the cutaneous manifestations predominate and in whom the prognosis is considerably better [8,9].

Microscopic polyarteritis is a small vessel vasculitis associated with a focal segmental necrotizing glomerulonephritis. Histologically, it is similar to WG without the evidence of granulomas. The renal manifestations predominate and this diagnosis may include what was previously considered to be idiopathic crescentic glomerulonephritis [10,11].

Aetiology and pathogenesis

The cause of PAN is unknown although the association with a previous streptococcal infection is well documented particularly in those with cutaneous involvement [9,12,13]. An immune complex mechanism has been suggested and the finding of immune complexes persisting throughout months of active disease is consistent with this [14]. There is some evidence that autoantibodies to vascular endothelial cells may be involved, again implicating an immunopathogenetic mechanism in the vasculitis [15]. There are reports in the literature of familial PAN suggesting a genetic basis to the disease in some cases but no consistent human leucocyte antigen (HLA) specificity has been identified [16].

Pathology

The classical pathological lesion is of an inflammatory vasculitis of small and medium sized vessels with fibrinoid necrosis of the media and cellular infiltration. There may be evidence of aneurysmal dilatation and arterial thromboses [17].

Clinical features

Classic PAN commonly presents with fever, malaise, weight loss, skin rashes, abdominal pain, myalgia and arthropathy [2–4]. Neurological, particularly peripheral neuropathy rather than CNS involvement is also common. Renal manifestations, which are also frequent findings range from hypertension, haematuria and proteinuria to rapidly progressive nephritis, although this is more likely to be associated with microscopic polyarteritis. Cardiological and thoracic disease are also described, although the latter is far less common than in WG, the main differential diagnosis of PAN. Testicular pain and calf pain are also recognized symptoms of PAN. In a series of 31 children clinical involvement was as shown in Table 25.8.2 [18]. Cutaneous features included livedo reticularis or maculopapular purpuric lesions with or without peripheral gangrene. Nodules were present in two patients and digital infarction was also seen. In a series of 32 patients seen at Great Ormond Street Hospital for Children, London, the clinical features were similar with cardiac and neurological involvement in 28% and renal manifestations in 72% [19].

Others have reported similar cutaneous manifestations including erythematous subcutaneous nodules (Fig. 25.8.11), and livedo reticularis to be common. In addition ulcerated lesions, haemorrhage, bullae, urticaria and petechial lesions have been documented [8,9,20,21] (Figs 25.8.12–25.8.14). Investigations commonly reveal anaemia, polymorph leucocytosis, thrombocythaemia, a raised ESR and CRP [2,3,4,18]. ANCA have been found predominantly in patients with microscopic polyarteritis although they have been identified in some adults and children with 'classic' PAN [22–24]. Microscopic PAN is more commonly associated with pANCA but cANCA may also be detected. In those in whom pANCA is detected the antigen against which the ANCA are directed is most frequently myeloperoxidase [25]. Hepatitis Bs antigen is uncommon in children in contrast to the adult population with PAN [18].

Macroscopic renal disease may be indicated on a technetium-99 dimercaptosuccinic acid (DMSA) scan

Clinical feature	Percentage of patients affected
Fever	65
Skin lesions (including livedo reticularis, maculopapular purpuric lesions, gangrene, nodules, digital infarction)	81
Myalgia, arthralgia	81
Gastrointestinal (abdominal pain/haemorrhage)	61
Neurological (including numbness, paraesthesiae, polyneuropathy, encephalitis, hemiparesis, ptosis, fits)	48
Hypertension	65
Nephrological (including proteinuria/haematuria/rapidly progressive nephritis)	65
Cardiological (including pericarditis, arrhythmias, cardiac failure, myocardial infarction)	16
Pulmonary (including pulmonary infiltrates, pleural effusion, haemoptysis)	10
Anaemia	32
Acute phase reactants (including raised ESR, CRP, leucocytosis)	90
HBsAg	10
Male sex	70

Table 25.8.2 Clinical features of polyarteritis nodosa in 31 patients [18]

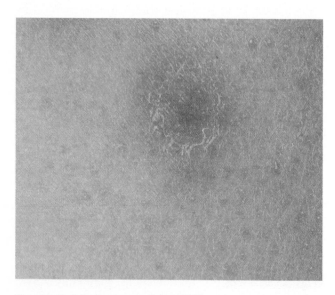

Fig. 25.8.11 Subcutaneous nodule in PAN.

which shows patchy areas of decreased uptake [19]. Renal and hepatic angiography, although invasive, can be an extremely useful investigation in the demonstration of arteritis often showing discrete aneurysms [19,26,27] (Figs 25.8.15, 25.8.16). Biopsies of affected organs, particularly the skin may reveal typical histological appearance. However, the absence of these changes does not exclude the diagnosis of PAN as the patchy nature of the disease may result in the pathological area being missed [2–4].

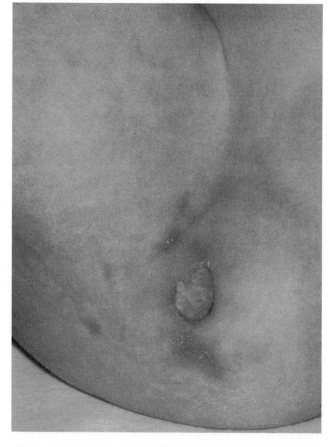

Fig. 25.8.12 Necrotizing lesion of the buttock in PAN.

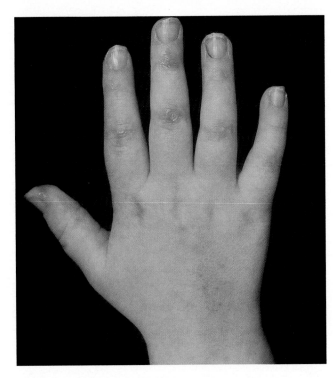

Fig. 25.8.13 Necrotizing vasculitis of the digits in PAN.

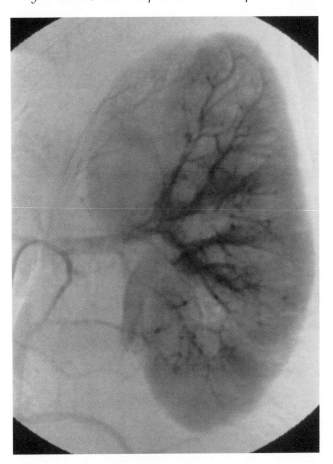

Fig. 25.8.15 Left renal angiogram demonstrating multiple aneurysms in PAN.

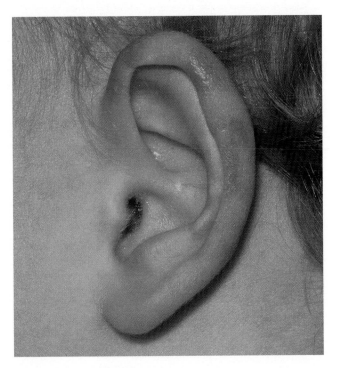

Fig. 25.8.14 Necrotizing vasculitic lesions of the pinna in PAN.

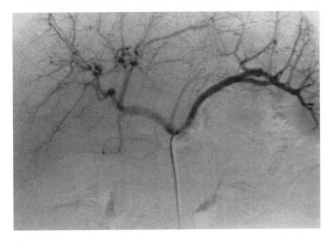

Fig. 25.8.16 Coeliac/hepatic angiogram demonstrating aneurysms in PAN.

Treatment

The treatment of PAN should be tailored to the extent of systemic involvement. In pure cutaneous PAN corticosteroids alone or even anti-inflammatory drugs may suffice [8,9]. In those with systemic involvement corticosteroids and cyclophosphamide are the main therapy of choice, either as oral or pulsed intravenous treatment [2,3,4,18,19,28]. Plasma exchange has been used in severe, life-threatening cases but there are no studies large enough critically to evaluate its use [29]. Azathioprine and cyclosporin A have been used as steroid-sparing agents in the maintenance of remission. Recently high-dose intravenous immunoglobulin has been used with some success [30]. Long-term maintenance therapy may be necessary but it is usually possible to discontinue treatment after 18 months to 2 years.

Prognosis

Prognosis of the systemic form of the disease was extremely poor prior to the introduction of corticosteroid treatment [2]. Royer *et al.* reported 100% mortality in 11 children treated before steroids were available [31]. The outlook remains variable with mortality greater than 20% in some reports despite intensive therapy [32]. It appears that a poor prognosis is related to renal and neurological disease [2,28] and some of the more favourable results may be due to the inclusion of children with cutaneous disease alone which carries a better outlook [8,9]. In some reports a relapsing course of the disease is described, particularly in relation to intercurrent infections [4,12] demonstrating the need for continued surveillance. It remains important to consider investigation in those who present with skin disease alone to allow appropriate intervention with more intensive therapy should other systemic manifestations, especially renal or neurological, be identified.

REFERENCES

1 Kussmaul A, Maier K. Uber eine bischer nicht beschreibene eigenthumliche arterierner Krinkung (Periarteritis nodosa), die mit Morbus Brightii und rapid fortschreitender allgemeiner Muskellahmung einhergeht. *Dtsc Arch Klin Med* 1866; 1: 484–517.

2 Reimold EW, Weinburg AG, Fink CW, Battles ND. Polyarteritis in children. *Am J Dis Child* 1976; 130: 534–41.

3 Blau EB, Morris RF, Yunis EJ. Polyarteritis nodosa in older children. *Pediatrics* 1977; 60: 227–34.

4 Magilavy DB, Petty RE, Cassidy JT, Sullivan DB. A syndrome of childhood polyarteritis. *J Pediatr* 1977; 91: 25–30.

5 Smith AD. Infantile polyarteritis and Kawaski disease. *Acta Paediatr Scand* 1977; 66: 381–4.

6 Roberts EB, Fetterman G. Polyarteritis nodosa in infancy. *J Pediatr* 1963; 63: 519–29.

7 Ahlstrom H, Lundstrom N-R, Mortensson W, Osteberg G, Lantorp K. Infantile periarteritis nodosa or mucocutaneous lymph node syndrome. *Acta Paediatr Scand* 1977; 66: 193–8.

8 Siberry GK, Cohen BA, Johnson B. Cutaneous polyarteritis nodosa. Reports of two cases in children and a review of the literature. *Arch Dermatol* 1994; 130: 884–9.

9 Sheth AP, Olson JC, Esterly NB. Cutaneous polyarteritis nodosa of childhood. *J Am Acad Dermatol* 1994; 31: 561–6.

10 Savage COS, Winearls CG, Evans DJ, Rees AJ, Lockwood CM. Microscopic polyarteritis: presentation, pathology and prognosis. *Q J Med* 1985; 56: 467–83.

11 Jardim HMPF, Leake J, Risdon RA, Barratt TM, Dillon MJ. Crescentic glomerulonephritis in children. *Pediatr Nephrol* 1992; 6: 231–5.

12 David J, Ansell BM, Woo P. Polyarteritis nodosa associated with streptococcus. *Arch Dis Child* 1993; 69: 685–8.

13 Fink CW. The role of the *Streptococcus* in poststreptococcal reactive arthritis and childhood polyarteritis nodosa. *J Rheumatol* 1991; 18(suppl 29): 14–20.

14 Levin M, Holland PC, Nokes TJC *et al.* Platelet immune complex interaction in pathogenesis of Kawasaki disease and childhood polyarteritis. *Br Med J* 1985; 290: 1456–60.

15 Brasile L, Kremer JM, Clarke JL. Identification of and autoantibody to vascular endothelial cell-specific antigens in patients with systemic vasculitis. *Am J Med* 1989; 87: 74–80.

16 Mason JC, Cowie MR, Davies KA *et al.* Familial polyarteritis nodosa. *Arthritis Rheum* 1994; 37: 1249–53.

17 Rosen S, Falk RJ, Jennette JC. Polyarteritis nodosa, including microscopic form and renal vasculitis. In: Churg A, Churg J, eds. *Systemic Vasculitides*. New York: Igaku-Shoin, 1991: 57–77.

18 Ozen S, Besbas N, Saatci U, Bakkaloglu A. Diagnostic criteria for polyarteritis nodosa in childhood. *J Pediatr* 1992; 120: 206–9.

19 Dillon MJ. Vasculitic syndromes. In: Woo P, White PH, Ansell BM, eds. *Paediatric Rheumatology Update*. Oxford: Oxford University Press, 1990: 227–42.

20 Verbov J. Cutaneous polyarteritis nodosa in a young child. *Arch Dis Child* 1980; 55: 569–72.

21 Chen K-R. Cutaneous polyarteritis nodosa: a clinical and histopathological study of 20 cases. *J Dermatol* 1989; 16: 429–42.

22 Dillon MJ, Tizard EJ. Anti-neutrophil cytoplasmic antibodies and anti-endothelial cell antibodies. *Pediatr Nephrol* 1991; 5: 256–9.

23 Gross WL, Schmitt WH, Csernok E. Antineutrophil cytoplasmic autoantibody-associated diseases: a rheumatologist's perspective. *Am J Kid Dis* 1991; 18: 175–9.

24 Wong S-N, Shah V, Dillon MJ. Anti-neutrophil cytoplasmic antibodies (ANCA) in childhood systemic vasculitis. *J Am Soc Nephrol* 1992; 3: 668.

25 Jennette JC, Falk RJ. Antineutrophil cytoplasmic autoantibodies and associated diseases: a review. *Am J Kid Dis* 1990; 15: 517–29.

26 Mc Lain LG, Bookstein JJ, Kelsch RC. Polyarteritis nodosa diagnosed by renal arteriography. *J Pediatr* 1972; 80: 1032–5.

27 Yousefzadeh DK, Chow KC, Benson CA. Polyarteritis nodosa: regression of arterial aneurysms following immunosuppressive and corticosteroid therapy. *Pediatr Radiol* 1981; 10: 139–41.

28 Roberti I, Reisman L, Churg J. Vasculitis in childhood. *Pediatr Nephrol* 1993; 7: 479–89.

29 Tizard EJ, Dillon MJ. Plasmapheresis in childhood. *Care Crit Ill* 1991; 7: 51–5.

30 Jayne DRW, Davies MJ, Fox CJV *et al.* Treatment of systemic vasculitis with pooled intravenous immunoglobulin. *Lancet* 1991; 337: 1137–9.

31 Royer P, Levy M, Gagnodoux MF. Glomerular nephropathies in systemic disease. In: Royer P, Habib R, Mathieu H, Broyer M, eds. *Pediatric Nephrology*. Philadelphia: WB Saunders, 1954: 302–26.

32 Dillon MJ. Classification and pathogenesis of arteritis in children. *Toxicol Pathol* 1989; 17: 214–18.

Behçet's disease

Behçet's disease (BD) was first described in 1937 by Halusi Behçet, a Turkish dermatologist [1]. The classic triad of this disease consists of recurrent aphthous, oral and genital ulceration together with uveitis. However, this is a multisystem disease which may involve the skin, joints, gastrointestinal tract and CNS. Both small and large vessel vasculitis occur and vascular involvement resulting in thromboses is reported [2]. It is rare in children, generally presenting in the twenties or thirties.

Aetiology and pathogenesis

The aetiology of BD is unknown. BD has geographical variability, being more commonly found in the Mediterranean, Middle East and Japan than in the USA and the UK. The predilection for certain ethnic groups and the finding of familial cases supports the contribution of a genetic basis to this disease. HLA-B5 has been found to be more frequent in patients with BD. The split antigens of

HLA-B5 (HLA-B51 and HLA-B52) have been examined in Israeli patients. HLA-B51 was found in 63% of patients compared with 9% of controls and HLA-B52 was found in 21% of patients compared with 9% of controls, giving a relative risk of 18.2 and 2.8 for HLA-B51 and HLA-B52, respectively [3].

It has been suggested that certain factors might trigger the disease in genetically susceptible individuals. Some microbial agents have been implicated but no consistent findings have been documented. Herpes simplex virus (HSV) would appear clinically to be an interesting candidate, which is supported by some immunological and epidemiological studies [4]. The role of *Streptococcus* in the pathogenesis of BD has also has been the subject of considerable debate. In support of an aetiological role is the high incidence of tonsillitis, dental caries and peridontitis, inducement of attacks by tooth extraction, inducement of systemic symptoms by the skin injection of *Streptococcus*, immunological cross-reactivity between streptococcal antigens and human tissue proteins and the production of Behçet-like lesions in animals by streptococci [5].

Immunoregulatory abnormalities have also been reported, including the presence of immune complexes and alterations in T-cell subsets. The pathological findings and response to immunosuppressive therapy is also consistent with an immunological basis to this disease [6].

Pathology

Early or pathergy-induced cutaneous lesions in BD show a neutrophilic vascular reaction. This may be vascular or perivascular with a diffuse dermal neutrophilic infiltrate. Long-standing lesions may show a lymphocytic vasculitis [7,8].

Clinical features

The diagnostic criteria required for the diagnosis of BD are shown in Table 25.8.3 [9]. As BD in children is so rare there are few large series of clinical findings, the majority being case reports. A review of the literature from 1965 to 1990 revealed 37 cases which had similar features to those in adults but a lower incidence of ocular disease [10]. A comparison of the larger documented paediatric series with the analysis of 2176 cases of all ages from Iran is shown in Table 25.8.4 [10–14].

Oral ulcers are the commonest initial major manifestation (Fig. 25.8.17). They are painful and may occur singly or in crops and usually involve the lips, gingivae, buccal mucosa and tongue. They tend to resolve after 1–2 weeks. Genital ulcers in particular should have HSV infection excluded. These lesions mainly affecting the scrotum in males and the vulva in females may result in scarring.

Cutaneous manifestations are variable and may include erythema nodosum like lesions, papulopustular lesions, erythema multiforme-like eruptions (Fig. 25.8.18), folliculitis, thrombophlebitis and abscesses [10,11]. Pyoderma, bullous necrotizing vasculitis [15] and Sweet's syndrome like lesions [16] have also been described.

The skin hyper-reactivity response or pathergy test is not pathognomic of BD but may be an important diagnostic indicator [17]. The skin pathergy test is normally performed with either an intradermal injection of physiological saline or a sterile needle prick. It is normally read at 24–48 h, evaluating the formation of erythema, papules,

Table 25.8.3 International criteria for classification of BD [9]

Recurrence of minor/major aphthous ulceration or herpetiform ulceration at least three times in 1 year plus two of the following

Genital aphthous ulceration

Eye lesions
  anterior/posterior uveitis
  cells in vitreous humour on slit-lamp examination
  retinal vasculitis

Skin lesions
  erythema nodosum
  pseudofolliculitis
  papulopustular
  acneiform nodules

Positive pathergy test results (subcutaneous injection of saline)

Table 25.8.4 Comparison of clinical features in BD (percentage)

Feature	Lang *et al.* (1990) [10] *n* = 37	Kone-Paut and Bernard (1993) [12] *n* = 17	Shafie *et al.* (1993) [13] *n* = 67	Kim *et al.* (1994) [11] *n* = 40	Gharibdoost *et al.* (1993) [14] *n* = 2176
Oral ulcers	100	94	77	100	95
Genital ulcers	75	53	26	83	63
Ocular lesions	30	47	31	28	64
Skin	84	92	61	73	77
Joints	54	69	13	28	47
Gastrointestinal	40	41	—	5	10
Thrombophlebitis	16	—	—	—	10
CNS	32	18	—	3	3
Male to female ratio	19 : 18	11 : 6	33 : 34	16 : 24	1175 : 1000

erythematous papules or pustules. It has been shown that a sharp needle may decrease the sensitivity of the test. Others have used histamine and have found similar results. Positive results have been reported in 84% of adults [18].

Although ocular involvement appears to be less common than in adults the morbidity is significant. Iridocyclitis affecting the anterior segment or chorioretinitis, optic papillitis, retinal thrombophlebitis and arteritis may occur. Long-term sequelae include glaucoma, cataracts and blindness. It has been estimated that in Japan 16% of acquired blindness is due to BD [19].

Arthralgia and arthritis, particularly affecting the knees and ankles are not uncommon in BD. In some cases this may be the presenting complaint. There have been reports of an increase in HLA-B27 in patients with BD-associated arthritis. In the long term the arthritis does not appear to cause significant morbidity. Myositis has also been reported [10,20].

Neurological involvement occurs in a minority of patients but can be life threatening. It can manifest itself as headaches, paralysis, hyperparaesthesia, dementia, behavioural disorders and psychiatric problems. Cerebellar signs and peripheral nerve palsies may also occur. The underlying pathology includes meningoencephalitis, cerebral venous thrombosis and 'benign intracranial hypertension'. It is generally a feature seen late in the disease but may occur in childhood [11,19,21].

Gastrointestinal disease ranges from nausea, vomiting, diarrhoea and weight loss to signs mimicking ulcerative colitis and Crohn's disease. Ulcers may occur throughout the gastrointestinal tract but are more common in the ileum and caecum. Fat malabsorption and lymphangiectasia have also been described [11,22].

Thrombophlebitis is a more common feature in adults than children and is generally confined to boys. Both deep and superficial veins are affected. Arterial involvement may result in aortic aneurysm.

BD is a multisystem disease which affects virtually any organ. Cardiac disease may present as myocarditis and pericarditis. Pulmonary infiltrates may be found and may be associated with pulmonary haemorrhage. Nephrotic syndrome and amyloidosis, haematuria and haematological problems of thrombocytopenia and neutropenia have also been documented in BD.

Prognosis

There are differing views of the prognosis of BD in children. It is in part related to the ophthalmological involvement, which in some reports is less common in children, but when present can lead to severe long-term visual impairment [10,11]. Others have found a more severe course among males and young patients compared with older females [23].

Treatment

The relapsing and remitting nature of this disease has resulted in few controlled trials of therapy and in children the literature is confined to case reports. Treatment has been tailored to the specific organ involvement and the severity of the disease [24]. Oral ulceration is predominantly managed with topical treatment including steroids and antiseptic mouthwash. For more severe disease systemic steroids are effective. Colchicine, sulphasalazine, dapsone and methotrexate have been used in adults with success. Thalidomide has been used successfully particularly for the orogenital ulceration [25]. The risks of teratogenicity and also peripheral nerve conduction

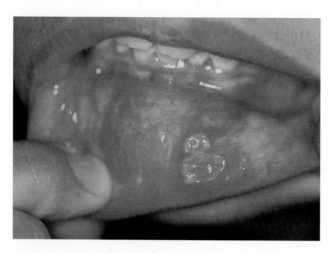

Fig. 25.8.17 Oral ulcers in BD.

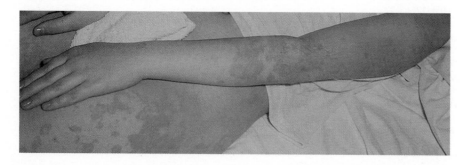

Fig. 25.8.18 Erythema multiforme-like eruptions in BD.

abnormalties must be considered when using this potentially dangerous drug. Skin disease is treated similarly with steroids (topical or systemic) and colchicine is also commonly used.

Ophthalmological BD is normally managed with topical or local intraocular steroids. If this fails systemic steroids, chlorambucil, cyclophosphamide, azathioprine and cyclosporin A have been used [26]. In CNS disease systemic steroids, chlorambucil or cyclophosphamide are recommended.

REFERENCES

1 Behçet H. Uber die rezidivierende ophthose durch ein Virus rerursachte Geschwure am Mund, am Auge und an den Genitalien. *Dermatol Wochenschr* 1937; 105: 1152.

2 Koc Y, Gullu I, Akpek T *et al*. Vascular involvement in Behçet's disease. *J Rheumatol* 1992; 19: 402–10.

3 Arber N, Klein T, Meiner Z, Pras E, Weinberger A. Behçet's syndrome: epidemiology, clinical data, and HLA typing in Israeli patients and their families. In: O'Duffy JD, Kokmen E, eds. *Behçet's Disease*. New York: Marcel Dekker, 1991: 61–6.

4 Denman AM, Pelton BK, Hylton W, Malkowsky M, Dinning WD. Herpes simplex virus infection and Behçet's syndrome. In: O'Duffy JD, Kokmen E, eds. *Behçet's Disease*. New York: Marcel Dekker, 1991: 415–20.

5 Mizushima Y. *Streptococcus* and Behçet's disease. In: O'Duffy JD, Kokmen E, eds. *Behçet's Disease*. New York: Marcel Dekker, 1991: 421–6.

6 O'Duffy JD. Behçet's disease. *Curr Opin Rheumatol* 1994; 6: 39–43.

7 Inoue C, Itoh R, Kawa Y, Mizoguchi M. Pathogenesis of mucocutaneous lesions in Behçet's disease. *J Dermatol* 1994; 21: 474–80.

8 McAlmont TH, Jorizzo JL. Behçet's disease. In: Churg A, Churg J, eds. *Systemic Vasculitides*. New York: Igaku-Shoin, 1991: 219–29.

9 International Study Group for Behçet's disease. Evaluation of diagnostic ('classification') criteria in Behçet's disease: toward internationally agreed criteria. *Lancet* 1990; 335: 1078–80.

10 Lang BA, Laxer RM, Thorner P, Greenberg M, Silverman ED. Paediatric onset of Behçet's syndrome with myositis: case report and literature review illustrating unusual features. *Arthr Rheumatism* 1990; 33: 418–25.

11 Kim D-K, Chang SN, Bang D, Lee ES, Lee S. Clinical analysis of 40 cases of childhood onset Behçet's disease. *Pediatr Dermatol* 1994; 11: 95–101.

12 Kone-Paut I, Bernard JL. Behçet's disease in children: a French nationwide survey. In: Wechsler B, Godeau P, eds. *Behçet's Disease*. Amsterdam: Excerpta Medica, 1993: 385–9.

13 Shafaie N, Shahram, Davatchi F, Akbarian M, Gharibdoost F, Nadji A. Behçet's disease in children. In: Weschler B, Godeau P, eds. *Behçet's Disease*. Amsterdam: Excerpta Medica, 1993: 381–3.

14 Gharibdoost F, Davatchi F, Shahram F *et al*. Clinical manifestations of Behçet's disease in Iran. Analysis of 2176 cases. In: Wechsler B, Godeau P, eds. *Behçet's Disease*. Amsterdam: Excerpta Medica, 1993: 153–8.

15 Lee SH, Chung KY, Lee WS, Lee S. Behçet's syndrome associated with bullous necrotising vasculitis. *J Am Acad Dermatol* 1989; 21: 327–30.

16 Lee ES, Lee SH, Bang D, Lee S. Sweet's syndrome-like skin lesions in Behçet's syndrome: an additional cutaneous manifestation. In: O'Duffy JD, Kokrem E, eds. *Behçet's Disease*. New York: Marcel Dekker, 1991: 223–7.

17 Gilhar A, Winterstein G, Turani H, Landau J, Etzioni A. Skin hyperreactivity response (pathergy) in Behçet's disease. *J Am Acad Dermatol* 1989; 21: 547–52.

18 Tuzun Y, Yazici H, Pozarly H *et al*. The usefulness of non specific skin hyperreactivity (the pathergy test) in Behçet's disease in Turkey. *Acta Derm Venereol (Stockh)* 1978; 59: 77–9.

19 Rakover Y, Adar H, Tal I, Lnag Y, Kedar A. Behçet disease: long-term follow-up of three children and review of the literature. *Pediatrics* 1989; 83: 986–92.

20 Ozdogan H. Behçet's syndrome in children. In: Ansell BM, *et al*. eds. *The Vasculitides*. London: Chapman & Hall, 1996: 417–24.

21 Stern JM, Kesler SM. Raised intracranial pressure in a 16-year-old boy. *S Afr Med J* 1989; 75: 243–4.

22 Chong VFH, Pathmanathan R. Familial Behçet's syndrome with intestinal involvement—case reports and a review of the literature. *Ann Acad Med* 1993; 22: 807–10.

23 Yazici H, Tuzun Y, Pazarli H *et al*. Influence of age of onset and patient's sex on the prevalence and severity of manifestations of Behçet's syndrome. *Ann Rheum Dis* 1984; 43: 783–9.

24 Allen NB. Miscellaneous vasculitic syndromes including Behçet's disease and central nervous system vasculitis. *Curr Opin Rheumatol* 1993; 5: 51–6.

25 Mascaro JM, Lecha M, Torras H. Thalidomide in the treatment of recurrent, necrotic and giant mucocutaneous apthae and apthosis. *Arch Dermatol* 1979; 115: 636–7.

26 Yilmaz O, Sebahattin Y, Hasan Y *et al*. Low dose cyclosporin A versus pulsed cyclophosphamide in Behçet's disease: single masked trial. *Br J Ophthalmol* 1992; 76: 241–3.

Relapsing polychondritis

Relapsing polychondritis (RP) was initially described in 1923 by Jaksch-Wartenhorst [1]. It is characterized by recurrent inflammation and destruction of cartilage. It most commonly affects the ear, nose, trachea and larynx but multiorgan involvement may occur with life-threatening complications. The aetiology of RP remains unknown although an autoimmune phenomena is suspected. There is evidence of antibodies to type II collagen occurring which support this theory [2,3].

Clinical features

This is a disease of adults with about 10% of cases being accounted for by children in whom the literature is confined to case reports [4–7]. There is an equal incidence in both sexes but it is commoner in white people. Diagnos-

Table 25.8.5 Diagnostic criteria for relapsing polychondritis. Diagnosis based on three of these criteria, one clinical criterion plus histological confirmation or chondritis in two or more anatomical sites with response to treatment [8,9]

Recurrent chondritis of both auricles
Non-erosive, inflammatory polyarthritis
Chondritis of nasal cartilages
Inflammation of ocular structures including conjunctivitis, keratitis, scleritis/episcleritis, uveitis
Chondritis of laryngeal or tracheal cartilages
Cochlear or vestibular damage resulting in sensorineural hearing loss, tinnitus and/or vertigo

Table 25.8.6 Clinical manifestations in relapsing polychondritis [8]

Sign/symptom	At presentation (% involvement)	During illness (% involvement)
Auricular chondritis	26	89
Inflammatory arthritis	23	81
Nasal chondritis	13	72
Respiratory involvement	14	56
Audiovestibular abnormalities	6	46
Ocular disease	14	65
Cardiovascular disease	—	24
Dermatological disease	—	17

tic criteria are detailed in Table 25.8.5 and the frequency of clinical manifestations in Table 25.8.6 [8,9]. Inflammation and destruction of the auricular cartilage, inflammatory arthritis and nasal chondritis are the commonest features of RP. Auricular chondritis may manifest itself as pain, erythema and swelling of the cartilaginous portions of both ears (Fig. 25.8.19). The arthritis is variable in its position and number of joints affected [10]. It is thought to start with chondritis of the articular cartilage. Respiratory involvement occurs in about 50% of patients but is a presenting feature in far fewer. Both the upper and lower airways may be affected [11,12]; initial symptoms may include, hoarseness, cough, wheeze and stridor. Tracheal collapse may result in sudden death. Hearing loss, tinnitus and vertigo are also common findings [12].

Ocular disease is usually manifested by episcleritis or conjunctivitis [13]. Valvular heart disease, aortic aneurysms and arrythmias occur, with aortic involvement being the commonest cardiovascular abnormality [12]. Dermatological findings are not particularly common and are variable in their expression, including erythema nodosum and leucocytoclastic vasculitis [14]. Nonspecific symptoms of fever, weight loss and anorexia are also found. The MAGIC (mouth and genital ulcers with inflamed cartilage) syndrome overlaps with Behçet's syndrome [15].

There are no specific diagnostic features of RP. Investigations may demonstrate an elevated ESR, leucocytosis, thrombocytosis, eosinophilia and normocytic, normochromic anaemia. Anti-type II collagen antibodies are found in up to 50% of patients and antinuclear antibodies in about 20% [14]. Urine may demonstrate elevated glycosaminoglycans. Histology of affected cartilage shows loss of the normal basophilic staining of matrix and a cellular infiltrate with polymorphs, lymphocytes, monocytes and plasma cells. Electron microscopy reveals chondrocytes containing large amounts of lysosomes, lipid and glycogen [11].

Treatment

Corticosteroids are the mainstay of treatment of RP. High-dose oral steroids in the initial phase may be converted to low-dose long-term therapy to maintain remission [6,12]. Intravenous methylprednisolone has been used successfully in acute airway obstruction preventing the need for emergency tracheostomy [6]. However, in these severe cases tracheal stenosis may occur in the chronic phase. Immunosuppressive drugs including cyclophosphamide, azathioprine, penicillamine, 6-mercaptopurine and cyclosporin A have been used [4,11–13,16]. In those with mild disease non-steroidal anti-inflammatory drugs or dapsone have been sufficient.

Tracheostomy may be necessary in those with severe tracheal narrowing [4]. Tracheal cartilage may suddenly collapse resulting in acute obstruction and death. However, the diffuse nature of the lesion in RP makes establishing a secure airway difficult and instrumentation and endoscopy may worsen the situation. In the long term tracheal reconstruction may be necessary for chronic strictures. Survival has been reported as 74% at 5 years and 55% at 10 years in adults [17]. Death may be due to tracheal involvement, infections or cardiovascular disease. Appropriate early treatment is necessary to improve outcome.

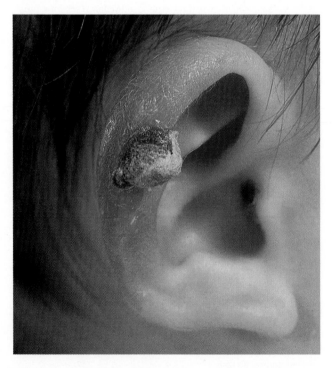

Fig. 25.8.19 Auricular chondritis in RP.

REFERENCES

1 Jaksch-Wartenhorst R. Polychondropathia. *Wiener Arch Inn Med* 1923; 6: 93–100.
2 Foidart JM, Abe S, Martin GR *et al.* Antibodies to type II collagen in relapsing polychondritis. *N Engl J Med* 1978; 299: 1203–7.
3 Meyer O, Cyna J, Dryll A *et al.* Relapsing polychondritis—pathogenic role of anti-native collagen type II antibodies. A case report with immunopathologic studies. *J Rheumatol* 1981; 8: 820–4.
4 Trepel RJ, Lipnick RN, D'Angelo L. Relapsing polychondritis in an adolescent. *J Adolesc Health Care* 1989; 10: 557–60.
5 Oddone M, Toma P, Taccone A, Hanau G, Delogu A, Gemme G. Relapsing polychondritis in childhood: a rare observation studied by CT and MRI. *Pediatr Radiol* 1992; 22: 537–8.
6 Lipnick RN, Fink CW. Acute airway obstruction in relapsing polychondritis: treatment with pulse methylprednisolone. *J Rheumatol* 1991; 18: 98–9.
7 Varanos S, Kostaki M, Tsapra H, Pantelidaki A, Karpathios TH. Polychondritis associated with Schönlein–Henoch purpura: report of a case. *Clin Exp Rheumatol* 1994; 12: 443–5.
8 McAdam LP, O'Hanlan MA, Bluestone R, Pearson CM. Relapsing polychondritis: prospective study of 23 patients and a review of the literature. *Medicine* 1976; 55: 193–215.
9 Damiani JM, Levine HL. Relapsing polychondritis—report of 10 cases. *Laryngoscope* 1979; 89: 929–46.

10 Sartoris DJ, Resnick D. Radiologic vignette: primary disorders of articular cartilage in childhood. *J Rheumatol* 1988; 15: 812–19.

11 Eng J, Sabanthan S. Airway complications in relapsing polychondritis. *Ann Thorac Surg* 1991; 51: 686–92.

12 Clark LJ, Wakeel RA, Ormerod AD. Relapsing polychondritis—two cases with tracheal stenosis and inner ear involvement. *J Laryngol Otol* 1992; 106: 841–4.

13 Trentham DE. Relapsing polychondritis. In: McCarty DJ, Koopman WJ, eds. *Arthritis and Allied Conditions*, vol. 2. Philadelphia: Lea & Febiger, 1993: 1369–75.

14 Maddison PJ. Miscellaneous disorders of bone, cartilage, and synovium. In: Maddison PJ, Isenberg DA, Woo P, Glass DN, eds. *Oxford Textbook of Rheumatology*. Oxford: Oxford University Press, 1993: 1032–42.

15 Orme RL, Nordlund JJ, Barich L, Brown T. The MAGIC syndrome (mouth and genital ulcers with inflamed cartilage). *Arch Dermatol* 1990; 126: 940–4.

16 Gemme G, Hanau G, Mulas R, Delogu A, Moni L. Airway obstruction in relapsing polychondritis: a case in childhood. *Eur J Pediatr* 1992; 151: 388–90.

17 Michet CJ Jr, McKenna CH, Luthra HS, O'Fallen WM. Relapsing polychondritis: survival and predictive roles of early disease manifestations. *Ann Int Med* 1986; 104: 74–8.

25.9 Kawasaki's Disease

TOMISAKU KAWASAKI

Kawasaki disease (KD) is an acute febrile mucocutaneous lymph node syndrome with multisystem vasculitis mainly affecting infants and small children under 5 years of age.

KD is now known to have a worldwide distribution, having been observed on all continents and in all ethnic groups. Although originally believed to be a benign illness, KD is now known to be associated with coronary artery lesions in about 20% of cases. If untreated, patients develop coronary artery changes with a range of severity from asymptomatic coronary artery dilatation or aneurysm to giant coronary artery aneurysms with thrombosis, myocardial infarction and sudden death.

Since the disease was first reported in 1967, significant advances have been made in its clinical, pathological and epidemiological characterization. However, the aetiology, pathogenesis and mechanism of therapeutic effectiveness of intravenous high-dose gammaglobulin (IVGG) in the reduction of coronary artery aneurysm formation, remain unknown. KD appears now to have replaced acute rheumatic fever as the leading cause of acquired heart disease in children in Japan and the USA.

Epidemiology

By the end of December 1994, 13 nationwide surveys [1] had been carried out and there were 128 306 patients registered in Japan. This is the largest number of KD patients internationally. From about 1970 there has been an annual increase in the number of patients (Fig. 25.9.1).

Three nationwide epidemics occurred in 1979, 1982 and 1986. There have been no epidemics from 1987 to 1994. Since 1987 the annual number of KD patients has plateaued at 5000–6000 cases. Of every 100 000 children in the general population under 4 years of age, the number with KD was under 50 until 1980 but after 1981 the number of children with KD rose to between 70 and 90 annually.

The average male to female ratio is 1.4 : 1. The age distribution reaches its peak between 9 and 11 months of age; 50% of children are below 2 years of age and 80% are below 4 years of age (Fig. 25.9.2). Sibling incidence was from 0.7 to 0.9% in the lowest year and between 1.3 and 1.4% in the highest year. The recurrence rate over the past 10 years has been 3–4%. The fatality rate until 1974 was more than 1% but recently the rate has been 0.1–0.2% [2–5].

Research in the USA [6,7] has shown that children of Asian extraction have the highest incidence and children of Caucasian extraction have the lowest incidence. The incidence of KD is low in Europe [8,9] where children of Caucasian extraction are most numerous. Reports of KD are more numerous from the more industrialized countries compared with the developing countries.

REFERENCES

1 Yanagawa H, Nakamura Y, Yashiro M, Ojima T, Koyanagi H, Kawasaki T. Update of the epidemiology of Kawasaki disease in Japan. From the results of 1993–94 nationwide survey. *J Epidemiol* 1996; 6: 148–57.
2 Yanagawa H, Shigematsu I, Kusakawa S, Kawasaki T. Epidemiology of Kawasaki disease in Japan. *Acta Pediatr Jap* 1979; 21: 1–10.
3 Yanagawa H, Nakamura Y, Yashiro M *et al.* A nationwide incidence survey of Kawasaki disease in 1985–1986 in Japan. *J Infect Dis* 1988; 158: 1296–301.
4 Yanagawa H, Kawasaki T, Shigematsu I. Nationwide survey on Kawasaki disease in Japan. *Pediatrics* 1987; 80: 58–62.
5 Yanagawa H, Yashiro M, Nakamura Y *et al.* Results of 12 Nationwide Epidemiological Incidence Surveys of Kawasaki disease in Japan. *Arch Pediatr Adolesc Med* 1995; 149: 779–83.
6 Bell DM, Brink EW, Nitzkin JL *et al.* Kawasaki syndrome: description of two outbreaks in the United States. *N Engl J Med* 1981; 304: 1568–75.
7 Taubert KA, Rowley AH, Shulman ST. Nationwide survey of Kawasaki disease and acute rheumatic fever. *J Pediatr* 1991; 119: 279–82.
8 Salo E, Pelkonen P, Pettay O. Outbreak of Kawasaki syndrome in Finland. *Acta Paediatr Scand* 1986; 75: 75–80.
9 Tizard EJ, Suzuki A, Dillon MJ. Clinical aspects of 100 patients with Kawasaki disease. *Arch Dis Child* 1991; 66: 185–8.

Pathology

The disease course is acute inflammatory process ending in 4–6 weeks. Recurrent angiitis features are rare and fibrinoid necrosis is mild or hardly ever seen. Coronary aneurysms (Fig. 25.9.3) are usually present at autopsy in more than 90% of cases [1–3]. KD could be divided into angiitis and lesions of organs exclusive of vessels in pathological investigations.

The course of angiitis can be classified into four stages according to the duration of illness [3].

Stage 1 is 1–2 weeks from onset. Characteristic features of stage 1 are acute perivasculitis and vasculitis of the

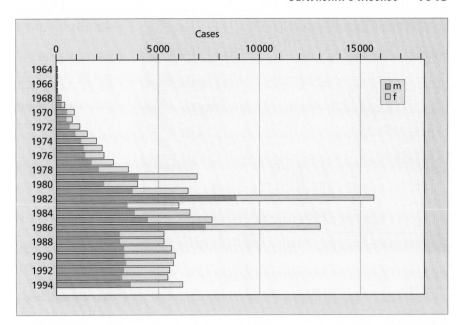

Fig. 25.9.1 Number of patients with KD registered in Japan by year and sex.

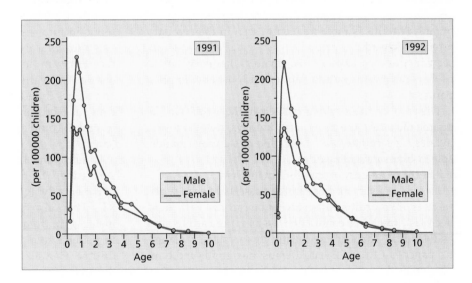

Fig. 25.9.2 Incidence rate of KD in Japan by sex and year.

microvessels, such as arterioles, capillaries and venules, and vasculitis of the veins and small arteries including vasa vasorum of the three main coronary arteries. Another feature is inflammation of intima, externa and perivascular areas in the large and medium sized arteries. There is also oedema and infiltration with leucocytes and lymphocytes. Aneurysm or stenosis is not evident.

Stage 2 is 2–4 weeks from onset. One characteristic feature is less inflammation in the microvessels, small arteries and veins than in stage 1. Another feature is inflammatory changes of intima, media, externa and perivascular areas in the medium sized arteries with focal panvasculitis. Aneurysms with thrombi and stenosis in the medium sized arteries, especially in the coronary arteries, can be seen. Infiltrating cells include neutrophils, eosinophils, lymphocytes, atypical lymphocytes, plasma

cells, monocytes, fibroblasts and fibrocytes. Inflammatory changes of various stages from oedema (exudative stage) and cell infiltration with necrosis (infiltrative stage) to cellular granulation with increase of capillaries can be seen.

Stage 3 is 4–7 weeks from onset. The characteristic feature is subsidence of inflammation in the microvessels, small arteries and veins. There is granulation in the medium sized arteries due to masked intimal thickening.

Stage 4 is more than 7 weeks from onset. There is scar formation and intimal thickening with aneurysms, thrombi and stenosis in the medium sized arteries. In general there is no acute inflammation in the vessels.

These findings persist until adult age, having been seen in some autopsied cases 10 years after onset.

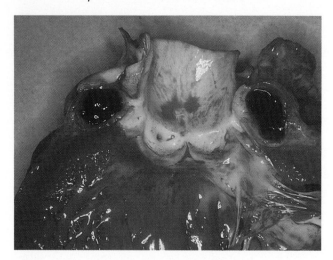

Fig. 25.9.3 Autopsy heart: coronary artery aneurysms with thrombosis.

Angiitis is divided into three categories. First there is angiitis in middle and large sized arteries external to the organs. Arteritis is most frequently seen in the coronary artery (90%) and iliac artery (17–38%). It is less frequently seen in the mesenteric, renal, main pulmonary, aortic, coeliac, intercostal, subclavian, carotid, hepatic, lumbar, pancreatic and splenic arteries.

The second category of angiitis is in the arteries in the organs including the heart, skin, kidneys, tongue, testes, ovaries, gastrointestinal tract, liver, salivary glands, spleen, brain and gallbladder.

The third category of angiitis is in the veins.

Lesions other than those in the vessels are seen when there is myocarditis (interstitial myocarditis with mild necrosis) involving conduction system, pericarditis and endocarditis. There are frequently cholecystitis, cholangitis, pancreatic ductitis, sialoadenitis, meningitis and lymphadenitis. Lesions can be seen in all of them.

Pathological changes can also be seen in the intestines, liver, pancreas, lungs, bronchi, kidneys, ganglion, spleen, thymus, prostate, fatty tissue and muscle. All of these lesions are frequently seen in stages 1 and 2 but rarely in stage 4.

Ischaemic heart disease occurs in stages 1–4. Acute myocardial infarction may not be histologically detectable in some autopsied cases. When sudden death cases are autopsied immediately, arterial obstruction can be seen but myocardial lesions such as necrosis have not yet had time to occur.

Among ischaemic heart disease cases there is fibrosis and/or necrosis of over one-third of the thickness of the left ventricular wall, with marked stenosis or obstruction of the major coronary arteries. These changes are probably due to residual myocardial infarction rather than to myocarditis.

The major causes of death in each stage are as follows.

In stage 1 the major cause is myocarditis, including inflammation of the conduction system. In stages 2 and 3 the major causes are ischaemic heart disease, rupture of an aneurysm and myocarditis. In stage 4 the major cause is ischaemic heart disease.

Arterial lesions were categorized by Amano *et al.* [4], according to the degree of inflammatory change and to the duration of the disease. Six characteristic types of lesions were identified in the arterial system: (a) degeneration of the endothelial cells; (b) oedema and degeneration of the media; (c) necrotizing panarteritis; (d) granulation formation; (e) scar formation; and (f) aneurysm formation.

Amano *et al.* [5] observed the above as a pathological feature of KD. The six types of arteritis changes were not equally distributed throughout the entire arterial system. It was characteristic that these six types of lesions were simultaneously observed not only in various areas of the arterial tree in the same patient but also in different portions of one artery.

In America, Landing and Larson [6,7] suggested that there were 'early' and 'late' stages of arterial lesions found in autopsies of patients dying at various time intervals after clinical onset of their acute KD. It can be thought that Fujiwara and Hamashima's stages [3] can also be divided into early and late. Stages 1 and 2 could be 'early' and stages 3 and 4 could be 'late'. Amano *et al.*'s types could also be thought of in terms of stages. Types (a), (b), (c) and (f) could be 'early' while types (d) and (e) could be 'late'.

Landing and Larson [7] pointed out that there was a surprisingly high incidence of 'late stage' arterial lesions in patients dying within 2 weeks of onset of clinical acute KD. They also pointed out that there was a possible increase in frequency of early stage arterial lesions in patients dying 10–12 weeks from onset of the acute disease. They also added that there was the rare presentation of late stage aneurysms of arteries in patients with no history of an acute phase of disease.

Landing and Larson [7] suggested that more than one of several different patterns or sequences of relation of clinical features to pathological features may occur in KD.

1 A single 'peak' of acute clinical disease and of lesions, with subsequent regression/healing (including scarring) of injured tissues/organs.

2 An acute phase of illness followed by a period of clinical improvement ('convalescence') and then by a second phase of acute illness (the two-peak or the 'camel-back' course).

3 An episode of clinically evident acute disease, followed by a clinically inapparent phase of continued or increased injury of the arteries.

4 A clinically unrecognized or unrecognizable first phase of disease followed by a clinically more overt 'second wave' of disease activity.

5 A single peak of clinically inapparent disease, or two peaks of disease activity, neither clinically appreciated.

Landing and Larson combined pathological findings and considerations of the clinical cause in order to establish their five categories. Their hypothesis can be of use for both clinicians and pathologists.

REFERENCES

1 Tanaka N. Kawasaki disease (acute febrile infantile mucocutaneous lymph node syndrome) in Japan: relationship with infantile periarteritis nodosa. *Pathol Microbiol* 1975; 43: 204–18.
2 Tanaka N, Sekimoto K, Naoe S. Kawasaki disease: relationship with infantile periarteritis nodosa. *Arch Pathol Lab Med* 1976; 100: 81–6.
3 Fujiwara H, Hamashima Y. Pathology of the heart in Kawasaki disease. *Pediatrics* 1978; 61: 100–7.
4 Amano S, Hazama F, Hamashima Y. Pathology of Kawasaki disease. 1. Pathology and morphogenesis of the vascular changes. *Jpn Circ J* 1979; 43: 633–43.
5 Amano S, Hazama F, Hamashima Y. Pathology of Kawasaki disease. 2. Distribution and incidence of the vascular lesions. *Jpn Circ J* 1979; 43: 741–8.
6 Landing BH, Larson EJ. Are infantile periarteritis nodosa with coronary artery involvement and fatal mucocutaneous lymph node syndrome the same? Comparison of 20 patients from North America with patients from Hawaii and Japan. *Pediatrics* 1977; 59: 651–62.
7 Landing BH, Larson EJ. Pathological features of Kawasaki disease (mucocutaneous lymph node syndrome). *Am J Cardiovasc Pathol* 1987; 1: 215–29.

Patterns of relation of clinical features to pathological features

A small but significant fraction of patients with acute KD show exacerbation or recrudescence of sign and symptoms during the subacute or convalescent phase of the disease, within a few to several weeks after initial clinical onset. These patients who show a 'camel-back' clinical course have a poorer prognosis than patients who show only a single peak course [1–3].

REFERENCES

1 Kawasaki T, Kubo N, Sakata G, Kubota S, Iguchi M, Tanaka N. Two autopsy cases of infantile polyarteritis nodosa and their clinical findings: in relation to Kawasaki disease. Part 1. *Chiryo J Ther* 1970; 52: 633–44 (in Japanese).
2 Kawasaki T, Kubo N, Sakata G, Kubota S, Iguchi M, Tanaka N. Two autopsy cases of infantile polyarteritis nodosa and their clinical findings: in relation to Kawasaki disease. Part 2. *Chiryo J Ther* 1970; 52: 811–18 (in Japanese).
3 Landing BH, Larson EJ. Pathological features of Kawasaki disease (mucocutaneous lymph node syndrome). *Am J Cardiovasc Pathol* 1987; 1: 215–29.

Immunopathology of the skin lesion of Kawasaki's disease

In the acute phase of KD, within 5 days after onset, more than 90% of the patients develop polymorphous exanthema on the body trunk or extremities. The most common form of rash is a generalized urticaria-like erythema with large, irregular plaques. The second common form is a maculopapular morbilliform erythema. In rare cases the rash is scarlatiniform erythroderma, erythema marginatum in character or multiform-like with iris lesions.

Histopathologically, the lesion (Fig. 25.9.4) reveals marked oedema of dermal papillae, focal intercellular oedema of the basal cell layer and very slight perivascular infiltration of mononuclear cells in the papillary dermis with the dilatation of small vessels [1,2].

Immunopathologically [3], most of the infiltrates are CD4+ T lymphocytes and CD13+ macrophages. There are few CD8+ T lymphocytes. The expression of the DR locus of human leucocyte antigen is detected not only on the epidermal keratinocyte surface but also on the walls of the small blood vessels and the infiltrating cells around these blood vessels. There are no CD20+ B lymphocytes.

Sato *et al.* [4] used four monoclonal antibodies against cytokines: anti-interferon (IFN)-γ and anti-interleukin 2 (IL-2), anti-IL-1α and anti-TNF-α. As a result, they suggest that (a) IL-1α and TNF-α were strongly positive in all patients with acute KD; and (b) IL-2 and IFN-α were weakly or partially positive. No cytokines were detected in the convalescent phase. They concluded that IL-1α and TNF-α may be involved in the pathogenesis of the inflammation of skin in acute KD.

REFERENCES

1 Hirose S, Hamashima Y. Morphological observations on the vasculitis in the mucocutaneous lymph node syndrome. A skin biopsy study of 27 patients. *Eur J Pediatr* 1978; 129: 17–27.
2 Kawasaki T. Skin lesion of Kawasaki syndrome. In: Urabe H, ed. *Proceedings of the 4th International Pediatric Dermatology*. Tokyo: University of Tokyo Press, 1986: 51–2.
3 Sugawara T, Furukawa S, Yabuta K, Shirai T. Immunopathology of the skin lesions of Kawasaki disease. In: Shulman ST, ed. *Kawasaki Disease*. New York: AR Liss, 1987: 185–92.
4 Sato N, Sagawa K, Sasaguri Y, Inoue O, Kato H. Immunopathology and cytokine detection in the skin lesions of patients with Kawasaki disease. *J Pediatr* 1993; 122: 198–203.

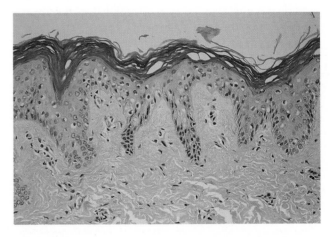

Fig. 25.9.4 Skin histology (of the erythema) showing a sparse mononuclear cell infiltrate in the papillary dermis around small dilated blood vessels.

	Scarlet fever	TSS	KD
Nature of rash	Diffuse, erythema (red punctate or finely papular)	Diffuse, macular erythroderma	Polymorphous erythema
Conjunctival hyperaemia	–	+	+
Erythema of the oral mucosa	–	+	+
Strawberry tongue	+	+	+
Hypotension or shock	–	+	–
Desquamation from finger tips	+	+	+
Aetiological agent	group A *Streptococcus*, SPE-A, SPE-B, SPE-C	*Staphylococcus aureus*, TSST-1	?
Age	>3 years old	All ages	< 5 years old
Recurrence	Rare	30%	3–4%

Table 25.9.1 Comparison of scarlet fever, TSS and KD

Superantigen: aetiological agent of Kawasaki disease?

Table 25.9.1 compares scarlet fever, toxic shock syndrome (TSS) and KD. These three diseases share similar features but there are important differences. The skin rash in scarlet fever is red, punctate, diffuse or finely papular erythema. The TSS rash is diffuse, macular erythroderma. During the state of shock the erythroderma redness becomes faded. In KD the rash is polymorphous as discussed above.

Recently, it has been suggested that superantigens may play an important role in the aetiology of KD. Abe *et al.* and Leung *et al.* [1–3] have suggested that TSS toxin type 1 (TSST-1), SPE-B and SPE-C are the aetiological superantigens of KD. TSST-1 is the aetiological agent of TSS and SPE-A, SPE-B, and SPE-C [4] are the aetiological agents of scarlet fever.

Leung's group base their hypothesis on the expansion of T-cell receptors (TCR) Vβ regions, so Leung's group suggest that a kind of superantigen is the aetiological agent of KD. However, some other researchers [5–8] have recently reported that the TCR Vβ region does not always expand during the acute stage of KD. Thus whether or not superantigens are the aetiological agents of KD remains controversial.

REFERENCES

1 Abe J, Kotzin BL, Jujo K *et al.* Selective expansion of T cells expressing T-cell receptor variable regions Vβ2 and Vβ8 in Kawasaki disease. *Proc Natl Acad Sci* 1992; 89: 4066–70.

2 Abe J, Kotzin BL, Meissner C *et al.* Characterization of T cell repertoire changes in acute Kawasaki disease. *J Exp Med* 1993; 177: 791–6.

3 Leung DYM, Meissner HC, Fulton DR *et al.* Toxic shock syndrome toxin-secreting *Staphylococcus aureus* in Kawasaki disease. *Lancet* 1993; 342: 1385–8.

4 Abe J, Forrester J, Nakahara T *et al.* Selective stimulation of human T cells with streptococcal erythrogenic toxins A and B. *J Immunol* 1991; 146: 3747–50.

5 Melish ME, Parsonett J, Marchette N. Kawasaki syndrome is not caused by toxic shock syndrome toxin-1+staphylococci. *Pediatr Res* 1994; 35: 187A (abstract).

6 Pietra BA, De Inocencio J, Giannini EH *et al.* TCR Vβ family repertoire and T-cell activation markers in Kawasaki disease. *J Immunol* 1994; 153: 1881–8.

7 Terai M, Miwa K, Williams T *et al.* The absence of evidence of staphylococcal toxin involvement in the pathogenesis of Kawasaki disease. *J Infect Dis* 1995; 172: 558–61.

8 Sakaguchi M, Kato H, Nishiyori A *et al.* Characterization of CD4+ T-helper cells in patients with Kawasaki disease: preferential production of tumor necrosis factor-alpha by Vβ2- or Vβ8- CD4+ T-helper cells. *Clin Exp Immunol* 1995; 99: 276–82.

Clinical features and diagnosis [1–7]

In the absence of a diagnostic test for KD, the diagnosis is established by the presence of six principal symptoms [3] (Table 25.9.2).

Table 25.9.2 Diagnostic guidelines for KD. At least five principal symptoms should be satisfied for the diagnosis of KD. However, patients with four of the principal symptoms can be diagnosed as having KD when coronary aneurysm is recognized by two-dimensional echocardiography or coronary angiography

Fever persisting for at least 5 days
Changes in peripheral extremities
   (a) initial stage: reddening of palms and soles, indurative oedema
   (b) convalescent stage: membranous desquamation from finger tips
Polymorphous exanthema
Bilateral conjuctival congestion
Changes of lips and oral cavity: reddening of lips, strawberry tongue, diffuse injection of oral and pharnygeal mucosa
Acute non-purulent cervical lymphadenopathy

1 Fever of unknown aetiology persisting 5 days or more. In general, the patient has remittent or continuous fever ranging from 38 to 40°C but with no prodromal symptoms such as coughing, sneezing or rhinorrhoea. The duration of fever is usually 1–2 weeks in untreated patients. The fever subsides more rapidly when IVGG is administered with aspirin, as compared to therapy with aspirin alone. In KD, the longer the fever continues, the higher the possibility of coronary artery aneurysms. In KD, if fever continues for 10 days or more, severe coronary artery lesions are liable to remain. If fever of unknown origin continues for 1 week to 10 days or longer and if one or two of the principal symptoms are present, then atypical KD can be assumed and IVGG treatment should be considered.

2 Changes in peripheral extremities. The findings on the hands and feet in KD are distinctive. Within 5 days of onset, erythema of the palms and soles (Fig. 25.9.5) and/or indurative oedema of the hands and feet (Fig. 25.9.6) are present. Sometimes the degree of swelling is great and the skin is shining and appears about to burst. After the fever subsides, erythema and swelling disappear in most cases. From 10 to 15 days after the onset, there is fissuring between the nails and the tips of the fingers (Fig. 25.9.7),

after which membranous desquamation spreads over the palm up to the wrist in many cases.

3 Polymorphous erythema. From the first to the fifth day after the onset of fever, polymorphous erythema (Fig. 25.9.8) appears on the body and/or extremities. The

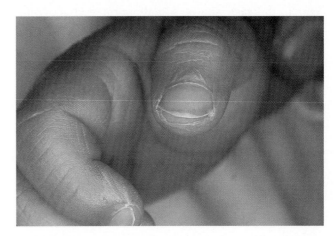

Fig. 25.9.7 Desquamation of the finger tips.

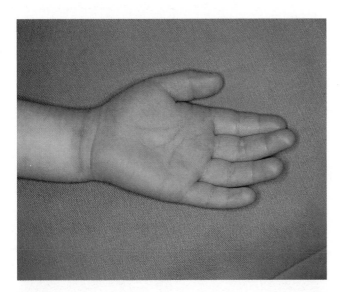

Fig. 25.9.5 Palmar erythema.

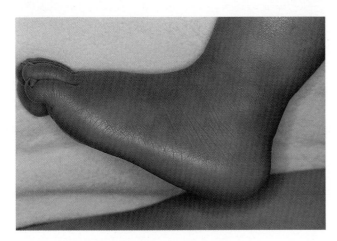

Fig. 25.9.6 Erythema of the sole of the foot.

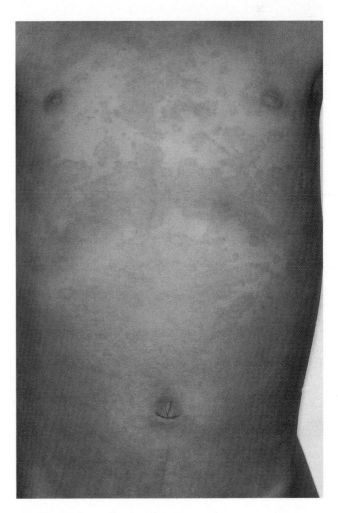

Fig. 25.9.8 Polymorphous erythematous rash.

exanthema can present in many forms: an urticarial exanthema with large erythematous plaques; a morbilliform maculopapular rash; and, in rare cases, erythema multiform-like with central clearing or iris lesions. In each case the exanthema is a different combination of these forms. Each lesion becomes increasingly larger and often coalescent. If the rash shows scarlatiniform erythroderma, careful differentiation is necessary between KD and scarlet fever or TSS [7] (Table 25.9.1). There is no vesicle or bullae formation except at the bacille Calmette–Guérin (BCG) inoculation site. However, about 5% of patients show small aseptic pustules on the knees, buttocks or other sites of the body (Fig. 25.9.9). Desquamation may occur in the perineal region other than on the hands and feet.

4 Bilateral injection of ocular conjunctivae. Within 2–4 days of onset, conjunctival injection develops (Fig. 25.9.10). It is not associated with exudate. Each capillary vessel is clear because of individual capillary dilatation. If there is careful slit-lamp examination early in the course of the disease, anterior uveitis can be discovered in many cases. Conjunctival injection usually subsides within 1–2 weeks but sometimes continues for more than several weeks. With IVGG treatment, conjunctival injection may improve quickly following treatment.

5 Changes in lips and oral cavity. Changes in lips and oral cavity are characterized by redness, dryness, fissuring, peeling and bleeding of the lips, diffuse erythema of the oropharyngeal mucosa, strawberry tongue without pseudomembrane formation, aphtha or ulcerations. Redness of the lips may often continue for 2–3 weeks after the disappearance of other symptoms. Bilateral injection of the eyes together with changes of the lips combine to give the characteristic appearance of KD (Fig. 25.9.11). This appearance can be an important aid to diagnosis.

6 Acute non-purulent cervical adenopathy. Cervical adenopathy is seen in less than 50% of KD patients in the USA and 60–70% in Japan, whereas the other principal symptoms are each observed in 90% or more of all patients. The size of the swelling ranges from 1.5 to 5 cm in diameter and is always a firm, non-fluctuant and painful mass (Fig. 25.9.12). The nodes are unilateral or bilateral and may be misdiagnosed as mumps. There are some patients in whom cervical lymph node adenopathy is the most striking clinical symptom of KD appearing 1 day before the onset of fever or together with fever.

If five or more of the six principal symptoms are present, a diagnosis of KD can be made. However, patients with only four of the principal symptoms can be diagnosed as KD when coronary aneurysm is recognized by two-dimensional echocardiography or coronary angiography (Table 25.9.2).

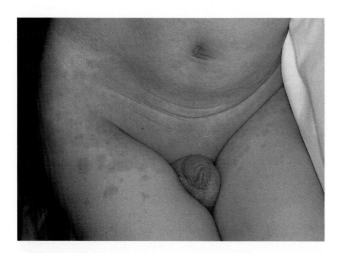

Fig. 25.9.9 Diffuse erythema with small aseptic pustules.

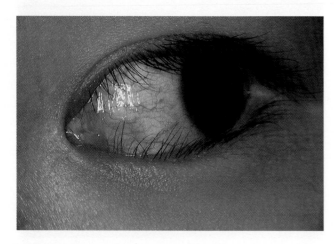

Fig. 25.9.10 Conjunctival injection; no exudate.

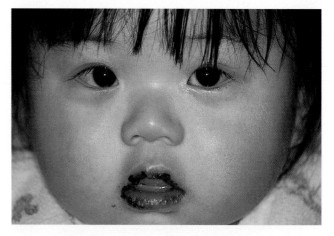

Fig. 25.9.11 Typical appearance of acute KD; redness, dryness, bleeding of the lips with bilateral conjunctival hyperaemia.

REFERENCES

1 Kawasaki T. Febrile oculo-oro-cutaneo-acrodesquamatous syndrome with or without acute non-suppurative cervical lymphadenitis in infancy and

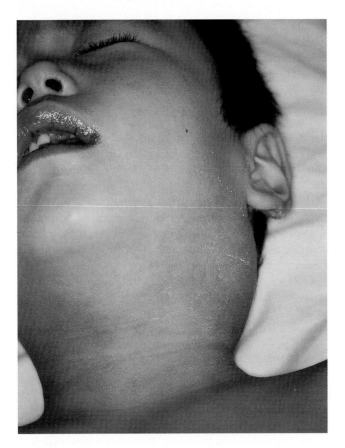

Fig. 25.9.12 Huge cervical lymphadenopathy.

childhood; clinical observations of 50 cases. *Jpn J Allerg* 1967; 16: 178–222 (in Japanese).
2 Kawasaki T, Kosaki F, Okawa S, Shigematsu I, Yanagawa H. A new infantile acute febrile mucocutaneous lymph node syndrome (MCLS) prevailing in Japan. *Pediatrics* 1974; 54: 271–6.
3 Kawasaki T. Clinical features of Kawasaki syndrome. *Acta Paediatr Jpn* 1983; 25: 79–90 (overseas edition).
4 Melish ME, Hicks RV, Larson EJ. Mucocutaneous lymphnode syndrome in the United States. *Am J Dis Child* 1976; 130: 599–607.
5 Melish ME. Kawasaki syndrome (the mucocutaneous lymph node syndrome). *Am Rev Med* 1982; 33: 569–85.
6 Hicks RV, Melish ME. Kawasaki syndrome. *Pediatr Clin N Am* 1986: 1151–75.
7 Behrman RE, Klieqman R, eds. *Essentials of Pediatrics*. Nelson: WB Saunders, 1990: 334–5.

Atypical cases

It is said there are no cases without exceptions and the same can be said about KD. Diagnosis can be made easily for typical cases but atypical cases are sometimes difficult for clinicians.

When KD is taken as a spectrum, the six principal symptoms are at one end while the other end consists of cases with none of the six symptoms. Atypical cases with coronary complications that are either fatal or with remaining aneurysms can be found in KD and these are difficult cases to diagnose [1–3].

Prolonged fever is one symptom that can be seen in atypical cases. Consequently, a case with fever of unknown origin can be considered a possible KD patient. In such cases, if finger tip desquamation is present, even if other principal symptoms are not detected, KD is a strong possibility, especially in infants and small children.

Mild conjunctival injection with prolonged fever can also be KD and possible coronary complications should be checked by two-dimensional echocardiography.

A third example is pale face and red lips with prolonged fever. In this example there is also a strong possibility of KD.

Prolonged fever with one of the principal symptoms can be considered a possible KD case and careful checking is necessary for coronary complications [4].

If the aetiology of KD is made clear, and if it is a micro-organism, early diagnosis will be possible. Until then, we can only depend on diagnosis through symptoms and for atypical cases the guidelines above should be followed (Table 25.9.2).

REFERENCES

1 Fukushige J, Nihill MR, McNamara DG. Spectrum of cardiovascular lesions in mucocutaneous lymph node syndrome: analysis of eight cases. *Am J Cardiol* 1980; 45: 98–107.
2 Rowley AH, Gonzalez-Crussi F, Gidding SS *et al*. Incomplete Kawasaki disease with coronary artery involvement. In: Shulman ST, ed. *Kawasaki Disease*. New York: AR Liss, 1987: 357–65.
3 Sonobe T, Kawasaki T. Atypical Kawasaki disease. In: Shulman ST, ed. *Kawasaki Disease*. New York: AR Liss, 1987: 367–78.
4 Kawasaki T. Comment and discussion: atypical cases. In: Kawasaki T *et al*. *Proceedings of the Third International Kawasaki Disease Symposium*. Tokyo: Japan Heart Foundation, 1988: 224.

Laboratory findings

There are no specific and no diagnostic laboratory findings in KD. A moderate to marked leucocytosis with a shift to the left, elevation of the erythrocyte sedimentation rate and positive C-reactive protein (CRP) are common, CRP is a globulin that forms a precipitate with the C-polysaccharide of the pneumococcus. The thrombocytosis in the acute phase of KD ranges from 50×10^4 to 150×10^4 and begins to rise in the second week, peaking at about 3 weeks, but persisting for several months from onset in some cases. This thrombocytosis is a minor characteristic feature in KD [1].

Aseptic microscopic pyuria is frequently seen in the acute phase in KD and almost always disappears in the convalescent phase.

There are immunoregulatory abnormalities such as imbalance of T-cell population, polyclonal B-cell activation, activated monocytes/macrophages and increased cytokines such as TNF-α, IF-γ, IL-1, IL-2, IL-6, IL-2 receptors and intercellular adhesion molecule type 1 (ICAM-1). However, these cytokines are present in many other disease states that are not associated with the development of arteritis. It therefore appears that 'cytokine activation must act in concert with some other unknown mediator(s) of vascular injury' [2]. The implications of the described immune abnormalities and cytokine activation for the pathogenesis and treatment of KD are unclear [3].

REFERENCES

1 Kawasaki T. Clinical features of Kawasaki syndrome. *Acta Paediatr Jpn* 1983; 25: 79–90 (overseas edition).
2 Rowley AH, Gonzalez-Crussi F, Shulman ST. Kawasaki syndrome. *Curr Prob Pediatr* 1991; 21: 387–415.
3 Terai M, Shulman ST. Immunological features of Kawasaki disease: controversial issues. *Clin Immunol Newsletter* 1995; 15: 93–6.

Cardiovascular complications

The most important clinical problem in KD is cardiovascular lesions, which may cause sudden death or develop into coronary artery diseases [1,2].

In the early phase of the illness pericarditis, myocarditis, endocarditis and coronary arteritis are present and exhibit mild to severe manifestations in most KD patients. The earliest manifestations occur within 10 days of onset and include myocarditis, occasionally with congestive failure manifested by severe tachycardia and gallop rhythm and/or distant heart sounds, severe arrhythmia rarely leading to cardiac arrest, pericarditis with effusion and mitral and/or aortic regurgitation. Electrocardiographic changes show flattening and depression of the ST segment, flattening or inversion of the T wave, decreased voltage and conduction disturbances including heart block.

In Japan, between 1979 and 1982, both two-dimensional echocardiography and coronary angiography were performed just after the acute stage of the illness. Since 1983, patients have had two-dimensional echocardiography which has become the most useful non-invasive method of evaluating coronary aneurysms. Patients found to have medium to large sized aneurysms have had coronary angiography.

From studies employing daily echocardiograms, Hirose *et al.* [3] documented increasing echodensity of the coronary artery wall as early as 7 days after the onset of fever in all cases tested. They also demonstrated that coronary dilatation is first detected at a mean of 10 days of illness and that the peak frequency of coronary dilatation or aneurysm occurs within 3 weeks of onset. The development of echocardiographic coronary artery abnormalities after 4 weeks is rare. Kohata *et al.* [4] reported that myocardial imaging with ^{201}Tl seemed to be more sensitive than stress electrocardiography by treadmill to detect myocardial ischaemia in patients with coronary obstructive lesion after KD. Kondo *et al.* [5] reported that ^{201}Tl myocardial single photon emission computed tomography (SPECT) after dipyridamole infusion is a safe and accurate diagnostic method for identifying coronary stenosis in KD

patients. The fate of coronary aneurysms in KD was well described by Kato *et al.* [6]. One to five months after the onset of KD, 18.7% of all patients in this study had angiographic evidence of coronary aneurysms. Repeated angiography 5–18 months later in those with abnormalities showed that about 57% of the patients had regression of the aneurysms within 2 years of onset. Of those with persistent abnormalities, one-third had disappearance of the aneurysms but developed complete obstruction or marked stenosis of the coronary arteries and the remainder had fine irregularities of the coronary arterial walls without stenosis. If thrombi form in aneurysms, they may increase in size over time and may develop occlusions. It is clear that coronary artery aneurysms, especially giant aneurysms (Fig. 25.9.13), may result in stenosis of the vessels, and that stenosis often leads to significant coronary obstruction and myocardial ischaemia. Kamiya [7] published the diagnostic criteria of cardiovascular lesions in KD in English. This work was the first to standardize coronary artery lesions in KD worldwide.

Based on Kamiya's work, Nakano *et al.* [8] reported that the coronary aneurysms were quantitatively graded as follows.
Grade 0: normal.
Grade 1: less than 4 mm in diameter (mild).
Grade 2: between 4.0 and 8.0 mm in diameter (moderate).
Grade 3: greater than 8.0 mm in diameter (severe; giant).
Nakano *et al.* stated that this grading of the severity of coronary lesions may provide a useful criterion for predicting the prognosis of patients with KD.

Kato *et al.* [9] analysed the clinical data of 195 myocardial infarction cases with KD. They reported that two-thirds of myocardial infarctions in KD patients occurred within the first year of illness. In more than 60% of the patients, myocardial infarction occurred during sleep or at rest. One-third of the myocardial infarctions in KD patients were asymptomatic. In survivors (about 80% of the first attack patients), one-vessel obstruction was frequently recognized, particularly in the right coronary artery.

Suzuki *et al.* [10] reported that they had divided the

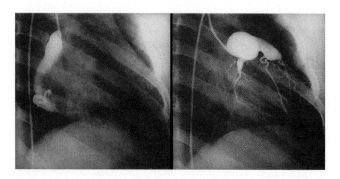

Fig. 25.9.13 Right and left giant coronary aneurysms.

specific coronary artery lesions in KD, known as segmental stenosis, into three groups: braid-like lesions, bridging vessels and pericoronary arterial communications.

Sugimura *et al.* [11] reported that they first applied intravascular ultrasound (IVUS) imaging to evaluate the wall morphology of the regressed coronary artery aneurysms in KD patients and concluded that IVUS was useful and may contribute to the assessment of long-term coronary artery sequelae and the possible development of atherosclerotic changes in KD.

REFERENCES

1 Kato H, Koike S, Yamamoto M, Ito Y, Yano E. Coronary aneurysms in infants and young children with acute febrile mucocutaneous lymph node syndrome. *J Pediatr* 1975; 86: 892–8.

2 Fukushige J, Nihill MR, McNamara DG. Spectrum of cardiovascular lesions in mucocutaneous lymph node syndrome: analysis of eight cases. *Am J Cardiol* 1980; 45: 98–107.

3 Hirose O, Misawa H, Kijima Y *et al.* Two-dimensional echocardiography of coronary artery in Kawasaki disease (MCLS): detection, changes in acute phase, and follow-up observation of the aneurysm. *J Cardiogr* 1981; 11: 89–104 (in Japanese; English abstract).

4 Kohata T, Ono Y, Misawa H *et al.* Myocardial imaging with thallium-201 in the patients with coronary involvement after Kawasaki disease. *J Cardiogr* 1981; 11: 105–14 (in Japanese; English abstract).

5 Kondo C, Hirose M, Nakanishi T, Takao A. Detection of coronary artery stenosis in children with Kawasaki disease: usefulness of pharmacologic stress 201-TI myocardial tomography. *Circulation* 1989; 80: 615–24.

6 Kato H, Ichinose E, Yoshioka F *et al.* Fate of coronary aneurysms in Kawasaki disease: serial coronary angiography and long-term follow-up study. *Am J Cardiol* 1982; 49: 1758–66.

7 Kamiya T. Report of Subcommittee on Standardization of Diagnostic Criteria and Reporting of Coronary Artery Lesions in Kawasaki Disease. *Annual Report of Research Committee on Kawasaki Disease.* Tokyo: Japanese Ministry of Health and Welfare, 1983: 1–13.

8 Nakano H, Ueda K, Saito A, Nojima K. Repeated quantitative angiograms in coronary arterial aneurysms in Kawasaki disease. *Am J Cardiol* 1983; 56: 846–51.

9 Kato H, Ichinose E, Kawasaki T. Myocardial infarction in Kawasaki disease: clinical analyses in 195 cases. *J Pediatr* 1986; 108: 923–7.

10 Suzuki A, Kamiya T, Ono Y, Kinoshita Y, Kawamura S, Kimura K. Clinical significance of morphologic classification of coronary arterial segmental stenosis due to Kawasaki disease. *Am J Cardiol* 1993; 71: 1169–73.

11 Sugimura T, Kato H, Inoue O *et al.* Intravascular ultrasound of coronary arteries in children: assessment of the wall morphology and the lumen after Kawasaki disease. *Circulation* 1994; 89: 258–65.

Treatment and management

At present the most effective treatment in the acute stage is IVGG plus aspirin because clinically it reduces fever and reduces coronary artery aneurysm formation. The IVGG regimen includes the following options.

1 200 mg/kg/day for 5 days.
2 400 mg/kg/day for 4–5 days.
3 1 g/kg/day one infusion.
4 2 g/kg/day (8–12 h) one infusion.
If fever occurs again in all regimens, the dosage should be repeated.

Regimen 1 above [1] is followed in Japan because it has been recognized by the government Japan Health Insurance system and is without fee. Dosage more than the regimen is charged. There have been coronary artery changes in 10–12% of cases under this regimen.

Regimen 2 [2–4] is the original regimen established by Furusho *et al.* [2] and was followed mainly in the USA until 1991. There have been coronary artery changes in approximately 5% of cases. It can be seen that the difference between regimen 1 and 2 is dosage dependent.

Regimen 3 [5,6] was reported by Engle *et al.* Confirmation studies have not yet been made but good results have been reported.

Regimen 4 [7] was established in 1991 by the American Multi-centre Collaborative Controlled Trial and better results than regimen 2 have been reported. At present, this regimen is the main one used in the USA.

The aspirin dosage for Japan [8] is a low dose of 30–50 mg/kg/day for all four regimens. In the USA the aspirin dosage is a high dose of 80–100 mg/kg/day for all four regimens. In both Japan and the USA, if fever subsides, the aspirin dosage is 3–5 mg/kg/day for 2 months.

The choice of regimen will depend on economic circumstances and on the severity of the individual case.

Early diagnosis and early treatment are important. If diagnosis of KD can be given within 1 week from onset and if IVGG treatment can be started, coronary artery changes will be prevented. However, unfortunately, there have been a few cases in which giant aneurysms remained even though IVGG treatment was started within 7 days of onset. If diagnosis is made after 10 days from onset, the risk of coronary artery changes rapidly increases.

In all cases in the acute stage it is important to monitor coronary artery changes through two-dimensional echocardiography. When there are no coronary artery changes such as dilatation or aneurysms 1 month after onset, it can be safely said that coronary artery changes will not occur. The two-dimensional echocardiography data should be technically accurate and should be interpreted by experienced specialists.

When there are coronary artery changes, the prognosis depends on the size of the aneurysms. Small aneurysms (less than 4 mm in diameter) show natural regression within 1 year and prognosis is good in general. Low-dose aspirin treatment (3–5 mg/kg/day) should be continued until regression. Medium sized aneurysms (4–8 mm in diameter) show regression within 2 years in more than half of the cases. In some of the remainder of the cases, there is development of stenosis and development of obstruction despite continued anticoagulant treatment.

Giant aneurysms (more than 8 mm in diameter) almost never show regression. Despite anticoagulant treatment (aspirin, dipyridamole, ticlopidine, warfarin, etc.), within 2 years, there is a strong tendency for development of obstruction or stenosis, especially in the right coronary artery. Obstruction develops sooner in the right coronary artery than in the left coronary artery, usually within 1 year.

It is difficult to interpret obstruction and stenosis through two-dimensional echocardiography for medium and giant sized aneurysms. Thus angiography should be performed and should be repeated in the course of the disease in order to follow the obstruction or stenosis.

If strong anticoagulant treatment is followed for giant aneurysms, and if there is development of obstruction, the process of development is a gradual one. The younger the child the more likely ischaemia will result in collateral circulation. Thus even if there is complete obstruction, the myocardial infarction is asymptomatic. For cases where asymptomatic myocardial infarction is suspected, ^{201}Tl scintigraphy or myocardial imaging should be performed. For older children, exercise electrocardiography (treadmill, etc.) can be performed. However it is important to be aware of the low sensitivity.

For cases of symptomatic myocardial infarction, pericutaneous transluminal coronary recanalization (PTCR) should be done within 6 hours, as in adults.

Some patients with ventricular dysfunction, heart failure, severe arrhythmias or postinfarction angina are managed by surgical treatment. Indications are as follows: (a) three-vessel obstruction; (b) severe occlusion in the left main trunk; and (c) severe occlusion in both the left anterior descending artery and the right coronary artery.

According to Kitamura *et al.* [9], 167 patients with KD in Japan have undergone bypass surgery. The bypass graft using the intrathoracic artery is recommended for left coronary artery bypass because the long-term patency is much more favourable (3 years: 77.1%) than the saphenous vein graft (3 years: 52.8%). The gastroepiploic artery is suitable for right coronary artery bypass graft because it is usually large enough and has sufficient blood flow even in younger children.

Heart transplantation has been performed in a number of cases in the USA and the UK [10]. However, the indications and long-term outcome are not yet certain.

REFERENCES

1 Harada K. Intravenous γ-globulin treatment in Kawasaki disease. *Acta Paediatr Jpn* 1991; 33: 805–10.
2 Furusho K, Kamiya T, Nakano H *et al.* High dose intravenous gamma globulin for Kawasaki disease. *Lancet* 1984; 2: 1055–8.
3 Newburger JW, Takahashi M, Burns JC *et al.* The treatment of Kawasaki syndrome with intravenous gammaglobulin. *N Engl J Med* 1986; 315: 341–7.
4 Morokawa Y, Ohashi Y, Harada K *et al.* A multicenter, randomized, controlled trial of intravenous gamma globulin therapy in children with acute Kawasaki disease. *Acta Paediatr Jpn* 1994; 36: 347–54.
5 Engle MA, Fatica NS, Bussel JB *et al.* Clinical trial of single intravenous gamma globulin in acute Kawasaki disease. *Am J Dis Child* 1989; 143: 1300–4.
6 Barron KS, Daniel JM, Silverman ED *et al.* Treatment of Kawasaki syndrome: a comparison of two dosage regimens of intravenously administered immune globulin. *J Pediatr* 1990; 117: 638–44.
7 Newburger JW, Takahashi M, Beiser AS *et al.* A single infusion of intravenous gamma globulin compared to four daily doses in the treatment of acute Kawasaki syndrome. *N Engl J Med* 1991; 324: 1633–9.
8 Kato H, Koike S, Yokoyama T. Kawasaki disease: effect of treatment on coronary artery involvement. *Pediatrics* 1979; 63: 175–9.
9 Kitamura S, Kameda Y, Seki T *et al.* Long-term outcome of myocardial revascularization in patients with Kawasaki coronary artery disease. A multicenter cooperative study. *J Thorac Cardiovasc Surg* 1994; 107: 663–73.
10 Checchia P, Pahl E, Rosenfeld E, Radley-Smith R, Shulman ST. The worldwide experience with cardiac transplantation for Kawasaki disease. In Kato H, ed. *Kawasaki Disease*. Elsevier Science, 1995: 522–6.

25.10 Cutaneous Manifestations of Endocrine Disease

PETER A. HOGAN

Disorders of thyroid function

Hypothyroidism

Pathogenesis

Congenital hypothyroidism is usually due to hypoplasia or aplasia of the thyroid gland, failure of the thyroid to descend properly during embryogenesis (e.g. lingual thyroid) or an inherited defect in the biosynthesis of thyroid hormone [1–3]. Uncommon causes include endemic iodine deficiency [3], unresponsiveness to thyrotropin [4], hypothalamopituitary dysfunction [5] and infiltration of the thyroid gland with histiocytosis-X [6] and cystinosis [7]. Transient congenital hypothyroidism can occur for no apparent reason [1], can be due to transient hypothalamopituitary dysfunction [8], can follow the use of antithyroid drugs [1] or amiodarone [9] during pregnancy, can follow the cutaneous application of povidone iodine to open wounds in the neonatal period [10] and can be due to transplacental transfer of antithyroid antibodies capable of blocking the thyrotropin receptor [11].

Acquired hypothyroidism is usually due to autoimmune (Hashimoto's) thyroiditis [12], endemic iodine deficiency [3], hypothalamopituitary dysfunction [13] or therapeutic ablation of the thyroid gland (radioactive iodine or surgery). In young infants, hypoplasia of the thyroid gland [12], an ectopic thyroid gland (e.g. lingual) [12], defects in the biosynthesis of thyroid hormone [14] and iodine exposure [15] are additional causes.

The cutaneous findings in hypothyroidism result from alterations in the function and structure of the skin and alterations in the metabolism of bilirubin and β-carotene. In particular, thyroxine deficiency alters cutaneous vascular flow, decreases eccrine and sebaceous gland activity, decreases hair growth, increases production of glycosaminoglycans (GAGs) by dermal fibroblasts, prolongs neonatal jaundice and reduces the conversion of β-carotene to vitamin A.

Pathology

The only distinctive histological finding in the skin of patients with hypothyroidism is the infiltration of the dermis and occasionally the subcutaneous fat with GAGs [16]. The infiltration is most marked around appendageal structures and consists primarily of hyaluronic acid. Identification of the infiltration requires special stains such as toluidine blue or alcian blue.

Clinical features

Congenital hypothyroidism

Newborn screening programmes have found a mean incidence of congenital hypothyroidism of 1 in 3331 births in Australia, 1 in 3801 births in Europe and 1 in 4119 births in the USA [17]. The newborn screening programme in California has found that females are more commonly affected than males in a ratio of 2 : 1 [18]. Most cases of congenital hypothyroidism in the Western world are now diagnosed through newborn screening programmes well before the typical clinical picture develops [2].

Before the introduction of screening programmes, newborn infants with congenital hypothyroidism were typically quiet and initially regarded as good babies. The diagnosis was not considered until other symptoms and signs had developed during infancy and childhood [2,19,20] (Fig. 25.10.1). The characteristic symptoms of congenital hypothyroidism are feeding difficulties, lethargy, constipation, thermal instability with hypothermia and an unusual ('hoarse') cry [2]. Prolonged neonatal jaundice (more than 3 weeks), umbilical hernia, hypotonia, bradycardia and prominent fontanelles are the earliest signs in most cases [3,19]. Linear growth failure, developmental delay and mental retardation are features of well-established cases [20]. Skin involvement is initially characterized by a cool and dry feel on palpation, pronounced cutis marmorata and a translucent pallor resembling alabaster [2]. The pallor results from the combined affect of anaemia, poor peripheral perfusion, prolonged neonatal jaundice, carotenaemia and accumulated GAGs. The accumulation of GAGs in the skin and tongue eventually results in thickening of the skin (myxoedema) and macroglossia. The thickened skin is non-pitting and has a doughy, boggy feel on palpation. The thickening is most prominent around the eyes, lips, supraclavicular fossae, hands and feet. The combination of thickened facial skin, protruding tongue, depressed nasal bridge and mild hypertelorism results in a characteristic facies. Other mucocutaneous findings in established cases include lustreless, slow-growing hair, slow-growing nails and delayed eruption of deciduous teeth.

Although congenital hypothyroidism is an isolated problem in most patients, it has been reported in association with Alström's syndrome [21], the CHARGE association (coloboma, heart disease, atresia choanae, retarded growth and retarded development and/or central nervous system (CNS) anomalies, genital hypoplasia and ear anomalies or deafness) [22], trisomy 4p [23], Wiedemann–Beckwith syndrome [24] and cutis marmorata telangiectatica congenita [25].

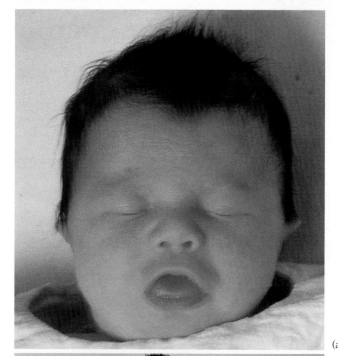

(a)

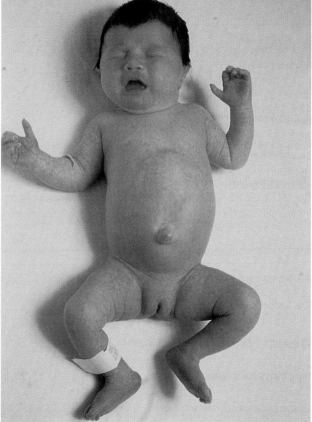

(b)

Fig. 25.10.1 (a, b) A 3-month-old infant with the features of congenital hypothyroidism; myxoedematous facies, macroglossia and umbilical hernia. Courtesy of Dr Geoff Ambler, New Children's Hospital, Sydney, Australia.

Acquired hypothyroidism

Acquired hypothyroidism usually presents with non-specific symptoms such as lethargy, constipation, cold intolerance, arthralgias and myalgias, or with specific problems such as an enlarged thyroid gland, umbilical hernia, poor linear growth, developmental delay, delayed dentition, poor school performance, delayed puberty or a neuropsychiatric illness [26–29]. The mucocutaneous findings will depend on the severity and duration of hypothyroidism at presentation [26,27]. Well-established cases will have cool, dry skin exhibiting a 'yellow tinged' pallor. Myxoedematous changes are evident in the form of macroglossia and thickening of the skin on the face ('expressionless facies'), over the supraclavicular fossae and around the hands and feet. The myxoedematous changes can be associated with purpura and poor wound healing. The lateral third of the eyebrows is characteristically lost and the scalp and body hair is sparse, brittle and lustreless in appearance. Paradoxically, some infants and children develop hypertrichosis on the back and upper arms involving dark, terminal hairs [30]. Nail growth is diminished and is associated with brittleness and ridging of the nail plates.

Acquired hypothyroidism has been reported in association with the Kocher–Debre–Semelgaine syndrome [31], the Wyck–Grumbuch syndrome [32], acanthosis nigricans and insulin resistance [33], acquired von Willebrand's disease [34], precocious puberty [35] and the Schinzel–Giedion syndrome [36]. Patients with hypothyroidism secondary to autoimmune thyroiditis can rarely evolve into hyperthyroidism [37] or develop other autoimmune diseases [38].

Investigations

The clinical diagnosis of hypothyroidism is easily confirmed by measuring serum levels of free thyroxine and/or thyrotropin [1,2]. The thyrotropin level will be high in patients with primary hypothyroidism and low in patients with hypothyroidism secondary to hypothalamo-pituitary dysfunction. Antithyroid antibodies may be found in neonates with transient hypothyroidism secondary to the transplacental transfer of maternal antibodies [11] and in infants and children with autoimmune thyroiditis [27].

Infants with congenital primary hypothyroidism require further evaluation (e.g. radioisotope scan) to determine the presence and location of thyroid tissue [2]. Other investigative findings in patients with congenital hypothyroidism include absence of the long bone epiphyses [2] and pericardial effusions [39].

Prognosis

Newborn screening programmes for congenital hypothyroidism have enabled the early introduction of thyroxine replacement therapy. This has resulted in normal intelligence in infants with mild thyroxine deficiency and a significant reduction in the degree of intellectual impairment in infants with severe thyroxine deficiency [40]. In addition to the resolution of those clinical features directly attributable to thyroxine deficiency (e.g. myxoedema), thyroxine replacement therapy can resolve those clinical features that are not directly attributable to thyroxine deficiency (hypertrichosis [30], acanthosis nigricans (AN) and insulin resistance (IR) [33], precocious puberty [34] and von Willebrand's disease [35]).

Differential diagnosis

The differential diagnosis of congenital hypothyroidism includes trisomy 21, gonadal dysgenesis (Turner's syndrome), mucopolysaccharidoses and Beckwith–Wiedemann syndrome. Trisomy 21 and Turner's syndrome are easily distinguished from congenital hypothyroidism with chromosomal studies. Infants with one of the mucopolysaccharidoses are distinguished by the marked hepatosplenomegaly and normal thyroid function tests. Infants with the Beckwith–Wiedemann syndrome have accelerated growth, an omphalocele rather than an umbilical hernia and normal thyroid function tests.

Management

Congenital and acquired hypothyroidism are treated with L-thyroxine therapy. The dose will vary with the age and weight of the patient and its administration should be supervised by an experienced practitioner (i.e. paediatric endocrinologist). Care must be taken when treating congenital hypothyroidism because of the risk of inducing congestive cardiac disease in the early stages of treatment secondary to the mobilization of fluid from myxoedematous tissues.

REFERENCES

1 Fisher A, Dussault JH, Foley TP *et al.* Screening for congenital hypothyroidism: results of screening 1 million North American infants. *J Pediatr* 1979; 94: 700–5.
2 Grant DB, Smith I, Fuggle PW *et al.* Congenital hypothyroidism detected by neonatal screening: relationship between biochemical severity and early clinical features. *Arch Dis Child* 1992; 67: 87–90.
3 Shanker SM, Menon PSN, Karmarker MG *et al.* Dysgenesis of the thyroid is the common type of childhood hypothyroidism in environmentally iodine deficient areas of North India. *Acta Paediatr* 1994; 83: 1047–51.
4 Takamatsu J, Nishikawa M, Horimoto M *et al.* Familial unresponsiveness to thyrotropin by autosomal recessive inheritance. *J Clin Endocrinol Metab* 1993; 77: 1569–73.
5 Isichei UP, Das SC, Egbuta JO. Central cretinism in four successive siblings. *Postgrad Med J* 1990; 66: 751–6.

6 Braunstein GD, Kohler PD. Endocrine manifestations of histiocytosis-X. *Am J Pediatr Hematol Oncol* 1981; 3: 67–75.

7 Lucky AW, Howley PM, Megyesi K *et al.* Endocrine studies in cystinosis: compensated primary hypothyroidism. *J Pediatr* 1977; 91: 204–10.

8 Jain R, Isaac RM, Gottschalk ME *et al.* Transient central hypothyroidism as a cause of failure to thrive in newborn infants. *J Endocrinol Invest* 1994; 17: 631–4.

9 Magee LA, Downer E, Sermer M *et al.* Pregnancy outcome after gestational exposure to amiodarone in Canada. *Am J Obstet Gynecol* 1995; 172: 1307–11.

10 Barakat M, Carson P, Hetherton AM *et al.* Hypothyroidism secondary to topical iodine treatment in infants with spina bifida. *Acta Paediatr* 1994; 83: 741–3.

11 Matsuura N, Yamada Y, Nohara Y *et al.* Familial neonatal transient hypothyroidism due to maternal TSH binding inhibitor immunoglobulin. *N Engl J Med* 1980; 303: 738–41.

12 Okamura K, Salo K, Ikenoue H *et al.* Primary hypothyroidism manifested in childhood with special reference to various types of reversible hypothyroidism. *Eur J Endocrinol* 1994; 131: 131–7.

13 Samuels MH, Ridgeway EC. Central hypothyroidism. *Endocrinol Metab Clin N Am* 1992; 21: 903–19.

14 De Zegher F, Vanderschueren-Lodeweyckx M, Heinrichs C *et al.* Thyroid dyshormonogenesis: severe hypothyroidism after normal neonatal thyroid stimulating hormone screening. *Acta Paediatr* 1992; 81: 274–6.

15 Vulsma J, Menzel G, Abbad FC *et al.* Iodine induced hypothyroidism in infants treated with continuous cyclic peritoneal dialysis. *Lancet* 1990; 336(8718): 812.

16 Gabrilove JL, Ludwig AW. The histogenesis of myxoedema. *J Clin Endocrinol Metab* 1957; 17: 925–32.

17 Toublanc JE. Comparison of epidemiological data on congenital hypothyroidism in Europe with those of other parts of the world. *Hormone Res* 1992; 38: 230–5.

18 Lorey FW, Cunningham GC. Birth prevalence of primary congenital hypothyroidism by sex and ethnicity. *Hum Biol* 1992; 64: 531–8.

19 Tsai WY, Lee JS, Wang TR *et al.* Clinical characteristics of congenital hypothyroidism detected by neonatal screening. *J Formos Med Assoc* 1993; 92: 20–3.

20 Tarim OF, Yordam N. Congenital hypothyroidism in Turkey: a retrospective evaluation of 1000 cases. *Turk J Pediatr* 1992; 34: 197–202.

21 Charles SJ, Moore AT, Yates JRW *et al.* Alström's syndrome: further evidence of autosomal recessive inheritance and endocrinological dysfunction. *J Med Genet* 1990; 27: 590–2.

22 Marin JF, Garcia B, Quintana A *et al.* The CHARGE association and athyrosis. *J Med Genet* 1991; 28: 207–8.

23 Ioan DM, Ghitan T. Trisomy 4p: a new case of congenital myxedema. *Endocrinologie* 1991; 29: 111–14.

24 Chien CH, Lee JS, Tsai WY *et al.* Wiedemann–Beckwith syndrome with congenital central hypothyroidism in one of monozygotic twins. *J Formos Med Assoc* 1990; 89: 132–6.

25 Pehr K, Moroz B. Cutis marmorata telangiectatica congenita: long-term follow-up, review of the literature and report of a case in conjunction with congenital hypothyroidism. *Pediatr Dermatol* 1993; 10: 6–11.

26 Dallas JS, Foley TP. Hypothyroidism. In: Lifshitz F, ed. *Pediatric Endocrinology: a Clinical Guide*, 2nd edn rev. New York: Dekker, 1990: 478–93.

27 Foley TP, Abbassi V, Copeland KC *et al.* Brief report: hypothyroidism caused by chronic autoimmune thyroiditis in very young infants. *N Engl J Med* 1994; 330: 466–8.

28 Keenan GF, Ostrov BE, Goldsmith DP *et al.* Rheumatic symptoms associated with hypothyroidism in children. *J Pediatr* 1993; 123: 586–8.

29 Chalk JN. Psychosis in a 15-year-old hypothyroid girl: myxoedematous madness. *Aust NZ J Psychiatr* 1991; 25: 561–2.

30 Perloff WH. Hirsutism—a manifestation of juvenile hypothyroidism. *J Am Med Assoc* 1955; 157: 651–2.

31 Najjar SS. Muscular hypertrophy in hypothyroid children: the Kocher–Debre–Semelaigne syndrome. A review of 23 cases. *J Pediatr* 1974; 85: 236–9.

32 Van Wyk JJ, Grumbach MM. Syndrome of precocious menstruation and galactorrhoea in juvenile hypothyroidism: an example of hormonal overlap in pituitary feedback. *J Pediatr* 1960; 57: 416–35.

33 Ober KP. Acanthosis nigricans and insulin resistance associated with hypothyroidism. *Arch Dermatol* 1985; 121: 229–31.

34 Bruggers CS, McElligott K, Rallison ML. Acquired von Willebrand disease in twins with autoimmune hypothyroidism: response to desmopressin and L-thyroxine therapy. *J Pediatr* 1994; 125: 911–13.

35 Bhattacharya M, Mitra A. Regression of precocious puberty in a child with hypothyroidism after thyroxine therapy. *Indian Pediatr* 1992; 29: 96–8.

36 Santos H, Cordeiro I, Medeira A *et al.* Schinzel–Giedion syndrome. A patient with hypothyroidism and diabetes insipidus. *Genet Couns* 1994; 5: 187–9.

37 Maenpaa J. Hypothyroidism preceding hyperthyroid Graves' disease in two children. *Acta Endocrinol* 1983; 251(suppl): 27–31.

38 Wuthrich RP. Pernicious anaemia, autoimmune hypothyroidism and rapidly progressive anti-GBM glomerulonephritis. *Clin Nephrol* 1994; 42: 404.

39 Rondanini GF, De Panizza G, Bollati A *et al.* Congenital hypothyroidism and pericardial effusion. *Horm Res* 1991; 35: 41–4.

40 Tillotson SL, Fuggle PW, Smith I *et al.* Relation between biochemical severity and intelligence in early treated congenital hypothyroidism: a threshold effect. *Br Med J* 1994; 309(6952): 440–5.

Hyperthyroidism

Pathogenesis

Hyperthyroidism in the paediatric population is usually due to autoimmune thyroid disease in the form of Graves' disease (diffuse toxic goitre) [1–3] or Hashimoto's thyroiditis [1]. In both conditions, hypersecretion of thyroxine is due to stimulation of the thyrotropin receptor on the thyroid gland by circulating antibodies. Rarely, hyperthyroidism is due to an overactive thyroid nodule [4], a multinodular goitre in association with the McCune–Albright syndrome [5], increased secretion of thyrotropin from a pituitary adenoma [6], hypersecretion of thyrotropin because of pituitary unresponsiveness to thyroxine [7], iodine exposure [8] or excessive intake of thyroxine. Hyperthyroidism can manifest in newborns secondary to the transplacental transfer of antithyroid antibodies from a thyrotoxic mother [9].

Although most of the cutaneous findings can be directly attributed to the hypermetabolic state induced by the increased levels of thyroxin and triiodothyronine, the development of pretibial myxoedema in Graves' disease does not correlate with elevated thyroxine levels. These patients have a circulating factor which stimulates GAG production by fibroblasts from the pretibial and orbital areas [10]. Fibroblasts from unaffected body parts do not respond to the circulating factor.

Pathology

Pretibial myxoedema is characterized by mucinous deposits that separate collagen in the mid and reticular dermis [11]. The mucinous deposits are acellular and are readily identified with mucin stains such as toluidine blue and alcian blue.

Clinical features

Hyperthyroidism can develop at any age including the newborn period [1–3,8,9]. Females are more commonly affected than males in a ratio of 3–5:1 and there is a family history of thyroid disease in 37–50% of cases [1–3].

The usual presentation of hyperthyroidism is with an obvious goitre or one or more of the following non-specific symptoms: restlessness, nervousness, emotional lability, weight loss despite increased appetite, palpitations, eye prominence and/or stare, hyperactivity with reduced attention span, tremor, heat intolerance and fatigue [1–3]. Many of these symptoms will lead to a deterioration in school performance. Uncommon presenting symptoms include weight gain, amenorrhoea, dyspnoea on exertion and/or at night, hair loss, diarrhoea, polyuria and enuresis [1–3].

Examination reveals a palpable goitre in all patients with an associated bruit in approximately 50% of patients [1,2]. A tremor is usually evident and may be associated with choreoathetoid-like movements of the upper limbs [2]. Cardiovascular examination reveals resting tachycardia, a flow murmur and a pulse pressure of over 50 mmHg in most patients [1–3]. Eye involvement occurs in 60% of cases [1,2] and approximately 66% of prepubertal cases will be above the 75th percentile for height at the time of diagnosis [1]. Eye involvement is usually mild and consists of one or more of the following: conjunctival injection, chemosis, lid fullness, lagophthalmos and increased lacrimation. Cutaneous findings are usually restricted to a flushed appearance of the skin and a warm, clammy feel on palpation. Uncommon skin findings include thinning of the scalp hair, vitiligo, onycholysis (particularly of the fourth finger nail) and hyperpigmentation [1–3].

Paediatric patients with Graves' disease rarely exhibit the characteristic clinical triad of pretibial myxoedema, severe ophthalmopathy and thyroid acropathy [1,2]. Pretibial myxoedema occurs in less than 2% of cases and represents mucinous infiltration of the pretibial skin. Occasionally, other sites can be affected such as the posterior calves, thighs, arms, trunk and the dorsum of the feet. The infiltration is usually bilateral and manifests as non-pitting nodules or plaques that can be skin coloured, yellow, red or brown in colour. The surface characteristically exhibits dilated follicular orifices which convey a peau d'orange appearance. Severe ophthalmopathy usually develops in association with pretibial myxoedema. It is characterized by exophthalmos, diminished eye movements, lid retraction and lid lag. The exophthalmos and diminished eye movements are due to mucinous infiltration within the orbit and extraocular muscles. Thyroid acropathy consists of clubbing and enlargement of the distal extremities. The enlargement is due to a combination of soft tissue hypertrophy and subperiosteal periostosis in the diaphyseal region of the metacarpals, metatarsals, phalanges and distal long bones. It is extremely rare in children.

Investigations

The clinical diagnosis of hyperthyroidism is easily confirmed by measuring free thyroxine and triiodothyronine levels in the serum. The TSH levels are depressed except in those cases due to hypersecretion of thyrotropin [6,7]. Patients with Graves' disease and Hashimoto's thyroiditis will have circulating thyroid-stimulating antibodies. Radioactive iodine test will distinguish Graves' disease (high uptake) from thyroiditis (low uptake). Further investigation is required if an overactive thyroid nodule or pituitary dysfunction is suspected.

Prognosis

The non-specific symptoms and signs of hyperthyroidism will resolve when the thyroxine level returns to normal. Pretibial myxoedema, severe ophthalmopathy and thyroid acropathy usually persist despite reduction in thyroxine levels.

Differential diagnosis

The hyperthyroid child is often labelled as being anxious or suffering from a psychiatric disturbance. The pretibial myxoedema can be confused with scleromyxoedema and lichen amyloidosis. Both conditions can be distinguished on the basis of history, other physical findings and skin biopsy.

Treatment

Patients with Graves' disease can be treated with antithyroid drugs [1–3], subtotal thyroidectomy [12] and/or radioactive iodine [13]. Antithyroid drugs are used initially and approximately 50% of patients will undergo disease remission [1–3,12]. If compliance is poor, side-effects develop to the medication or prolonged therapy fails to induce disease remission, the patient can be treated with subtotal thyroidectomy or radioactive iodine. Patients with Hashimoto's thyroiditis are usually treated with β-blockers because of the self-limited nature of the problem.

Pretibial myxoedema is a difficult problem to treat because of its lack of response to topical steroids, intralesional steroids and oral steroids. A recent report noted clinical and histological improvement with high-dose intravenous gammaglobulin therapy [14].

REFERENCES

1 Vaidya VA, Bongiovanni AM, Parks JS et al. Twenty-two years experience in the medical management of juvenile thyrotoxicosis. *Pediatrics* 1974; 54: 565–70.
2 Barnes HV, Blizzard RM. Antithyroid drug therapy for toxic diffuse goitre (Graves' disease): 30 years experience in children and adolescents. *J Pediatr* 1977; 91: 313–20.
3 Gorton C, Sadeghi-Nejad A, Senior B. Remission in children with hyperthyroidism treated with propylthiouracil. *Am J Dis Child* 1987; 141: 1084–6.
4 Mizukami Y, Michigishi T, Nonomura A et al. Autonomously functioning

(hot) nodule of the thyroid gland. A clinical and histopathological study of 17 cases. *Am J Clin Pathol* 1994; 101: 29–35.

5 Hamilton CR Jr, Maloof F. Unusual types of hypothyroidism. *Medicine (Balt)* 1973; 52: 195–215.

6 Avramides A, Karapiperis A, Triantafyllidou E *et al*. TSH-secreting pituitary macroadenoma in an 11-year-old girl. *Acta Paediatr* 1992; 81: 1058–60.

7 Gershengorn MC, Weintraub BD. Thyrotropin induced hyperthyroidism caused by selective pituitary resistance to thyroid hormone. A new syndrome of inappropriate secretion of TSH. *J Clin Invest* 1975; 56: 633–45.

8 Bryant WP, Zimmerman D. Iodine induced hyperthyroidism in a newborn. *Pediatrics* 1995; 95: 434–6.

9 Smallridge RC, Wartofsky L, Chopra IJ *et al*. Neonatal thyrotoxicosis: alterations in serum concentrations of LATS protector, T4, T3, reverse T3, and 3, 3′T2. *J Pediatr* 1978; 93: 118–20.

10 Cheung HS, Nicoloff JT, Kamiel MB *et al*. Stimulation of fibroblast biosynthetic activity by serum of patients with pretibial myxedema. *J Invest Dermatol* 1978; 71: 12–17.

11 Truhan AP, Roenigk HH Jr. The cutaneous mucinoses. *J Am Acad Dermatol* 1986; 14: 1–18.

12 Desjardins JG. Treatment of hyperthyroidism in children. *Canad J Surg* 1983; 26: 252–3.

13 Clark JD, Gelfand MJ, Elgazzar AH. Iodine-131 therapy of hyperthyroidism in paediatric patients. *J Nucl Med* 1995; 36: 442–5.

14 Antonelli A, Navarrane A, Palla R *et al*. Pretibial myxedema and high dose intravenous immunoglobulin treatment. *Thyroid* 1994; 4: 399–408.

Disorders of the adrenal glands

Cushing's disease and Cushing's syndrome

Pathogenesis

The cushingoid phenotype results from the excessive effect of glucocorticoids on body tissues. Cushing's disease refers to the clinical phenotype resulting from an overproduction of glucocorticoids by the adrenal cortex secondary to hypersecretion of adrenocorticotropic hormone (ACTH) from a pituitary adenoma [1,2]. Cushing's syndrome refers to the clinical phenotype resulting from an overproduction of glucocorticoids by the adrenal cortex because of micronodular adrenal hyperplasia, an adrenal adenoma, an adrenal carcinoma or secondary to stimulation by ectopically prduced ACTH [1,2]. Ectopic ACTH production has been reported in children with thymic carcinoid [1] and bronchial carcinoid [1,2]. Some of the features of Cushing's syndrome can also occur with the overuse of oral steroids, potent topical steroids [3], intralesional steroids [3] and inhaled steroids [4].

Most of the symptoms and signs of Cushing's disease and Cushing's syndrome are due to the direct effect of glucocorticoids on various body tissues. Androgens may contribute to some of the cutaneous findings in patients with Cushing's syndrome due to micronodular adrenal hyperplasia or an adrenal tumour. Hyperpigmentation in patients with Cushing's disease is due to stimulation of melanocytes by ACTH and related peptides.

Clinical features

Cushing's disease can occur at any age with no predilec-

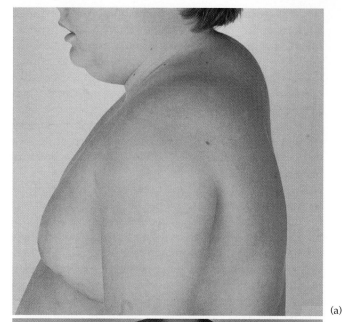

(a)

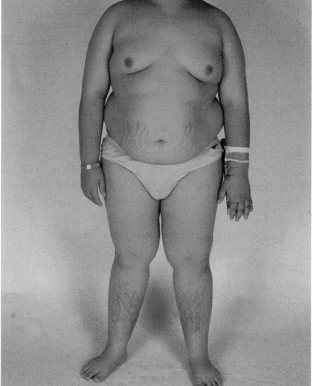

(b)

Fig. 25.10.2 (a) Cushing's disease exhibiting buffalo hump. Courtesy of Dr Geoff Ambler, New Children's Hospital, Sydney, Australia. (b) Cushing's disease exhibiting truncal obesity and abdominal striae. Courtesy of Dr Geoff Ambler, New Children's Hospital, Sydney, Australia.

tion for either sex [1,2] (Fig. 25.10.2). Patients usually present with one or more of the following problems: weight gain, growth retardation in children and young adolescents, delayed sexual maturation in prepubertal patients, menstrual irregularities in postmenarchal females, fatigue, weakness, emotional lability and one or more of the characteristic skin findings [1,2]. The weight gain is associated with redistribution of body fat resulting in a prominent moon face, buffalo hump and truncal obesity with relative thinning of the arms and legs [1,2] (Fig. 25.10.2). The characteristic skin findings are a plethoric facies, broad purple-coloured striae at the sites of skin tension (upper thighs, buttocks, trunk, shoulder girdle, breasts) (Fig. 25.10.2b), skin fragility with poor wound healing, development of purpura with minimal skin trauma, hyperpigmentation, hypertrichosis (vellus-type hair) on the cheeks and forehead of the face, AN and an acneiform eruption on the face and upper trunk [1,2]. The acneiform eruption represents either steroid folliculitis or exacerbation of teenage acne vulgaris. Other clinical findings include hypertension and osteopenia in the majority of patients.

The clinical features of Cushing's syndrome due to ectopic ACTH production are identical to those of Cushing's disease. Cushing's syndrome due to an adrenal tumour or micronodular adrenal hyperplasia is identical to Cushing's disease with the exception of androgen-mediated features such as hirsutism and premature adrenarche and the absence of ACTH-mediated hyperpigmentation. Steroid-induced Cushing's syndrome is characterized by weight gain with redistribution of body fat, striae, skin fragility and an acneiform eruption [3,4].

Nodular adrenal hyperplasia can be associated with myxomatous tumours in the heart, skin and breast, centrofacial lentigines, testicular tumours (Sertoli cell tumour, Leydig cell tumour, adrenocortical rest tumour), pituitary adenomas and peripheral nerve tumours (schwannomas). This constellation of clinical features is referred to as the Carney complex, a multisystem tumour syndrome inherited in an autosomal dominant fashion [5,6].

Investigations

The clinical diagnosis of hypercortisolism is confirmed by measuring free cortisol levels in a 24-h urine specimen and measuring the plasma cortisol levels after the low-dose dexamethasone suppression test [1,2,7]. Patients with hypercortisolism will have elevated free cortisol levels in the urine and no decrease in plasma cortisol levels with low-dose dexamethasone suppression [1,2,7]. ACTH-dependant cases are distinguished from adrenal-mediated cases by measuring ACTH levels. If plasma ACTH levels are elevated, the high-dose dexamethasone suppression test, the corticotropin-releasing hormone (CRH) stimulation test and inferior petrosal sinus sampling will distinguish pituitary and non-pituitary sources of ACTH. If plasma ACTH levels are normal, imaging studies are required of the adrenal glands.

Differential diagnosis

Cushing's disease needs to be excluded from physiological obesity and polycystic ovary disease. The measurement of serum cortisol and the dexamethasone suppression test will distinguish Cushing's disease and Cushing's syndrome from physiological obesity. Polycystic ovary disease is distinguished by ultrasound of the ovaries and the presence of an elevated luteinizing hormone (LH) and depressed follicle-stimulating hormone (FSH) levels.

Prognosis

Provided the cause is identified and removed, the prognosis is good with a gradual reduction in body weight, normal linear growth and the development of normal fertility [1,2].

Treatment

Treatment depends on the underlying aetiology [1,2]. Pituitary tumours are removed surgically through the technique of trans-sphenoidal adenomectomy. Recurrent tumours can be surgically removed or treated with radiotherapy. Nodular adrenal hyperplasia and adrenal tumours are treated surgically. Nelson's syndrome is a potential complication of adrenalectomy [8].

REFERENCES

1 Magiakou MA, Mastorakos G, Oldfield EH *et al.* Cushing's syndrome in children and adolescents. Presentation, diagnosis and therapy. *N Engl J Med* 1994; 331: 629–36.
2 Leinung MC, Zimmerman D. Cushing's disease in children. *Endocrinol Metab Clin N Am* 1994; 23: 629–39.
3 Curtis JA, Cormode E, Laski B *et al.* Endocrine complications of topical and intralesional corticosteroid therapy. *Arch Dis Child* 1982; 57: 204–7.
4 Priftis K, Everard ML, Milner AD. Unexpected side effects of inhaled steroids: a case report. *Eur J Paediatr* 1991; 150: 448–9.
5 Carney JA, Hruska LS, Beauchamp BD *et al.* Dominant inheritance of the complex of myxomas, spotty pigmentation and endocrine over activity. *Mayo Clin Proc* 1986; 61: 165–72.
6 Carney JA, Gordon H, Carpenter PC *et al.* The complex of myxomas, spotty pigmentation and endocrine over activity. *Medicine (Balt)* 1985; 64: 270–83.
7 McLean M, Smith R. Cushing's syndrome: how should we investigate in 1995? *Med J Aust* 1995; 163: 153–4.
8 Thomas CG, Smith AT, Benson M *et al.* Nelson's syndrome after Cushing's disease in childhood: a continuing problem. *Surgery* 1984; 96: 1067–76.

Addison's disease

Pathogenesis

Addison's disease in the paediatric age group can result from reduced secretion of ACTH from the pituitary gland or failure of the adrenal cortex to respond to ACTH. Reduced secretion of ACTH can be due to hypothalamopituitary axis dysfunction (e.g. pituitary tumour) or prolonged steroid therapy [1]. Failure of the adrenal cortex to respond to ACTH can be due to a variety of congenital and acquired conditions. Congenital problems include adrenal hypoplasia [2], congenital unresponsiveness to ACTH [3], adrenal leucodystrophy [4,5] and congenital adrenal hyperplasia [6]. Acquired causes include destruction of the adrenal gland from infection or haemorrhage, surgical removal of the adrenal gland and an idiopathic group. The idiopathic group exhibits a high incidence of circulating autoantibodies, particularly antibodies to the adrenal cortex cells, and most patients have a personal or family history of other autoimmune diseases [7]. The idiopathic group now accounts for most paediatric cases of Addison's disease.

When glucocorticoid deficiency is associated with elevated ACTH levels, hyperpigmentation of the skin is a prominent feature. The pigmentation is due to stimulation of cutaneous melanocytes by ACTH and/or melanocyte-stimulating hormone (MSH) peptides.

Clinical features

The age of the patient at presentation will depend on the cause of the Addison's disease. Patients with adrenal hypoplasia and congenital adrenal hyperplasia usually present shortly after birth. Patients with inadequate ACTH production, adrenal leucodystrophy and the idiopathic form can present at any age.

The usual presentation is with symptoms of lethargy, cyclic vomiting, hypotension and salt craving [6,7]. The onset of symptoms can be precipitated by an intercurrent illness [7]. Patients with gradual onset of the disease will exhibit hyperpigmentation of the skin and mucosal surfaces (gingivae, tongue, hard palate, buccal mucosa, vagina, anus) at the time of presentation [6,7]. The cutaneous pigmentation is diffuse with accentuation on exposed areas (Fig. 25.10.3a), around new scars and over areas of pressure or friction (axillae, elbows, knees and perineum) (Fig. 25.10.3b). The development of mucosal pigmentation and palmoplantar crease pigmentation is restricted to Caucasians because both are normal findings in black patients. The widespread hyperpigmentation is usually accompanied by darkening of the hair, darkening of existing melanocytic naevi and the appearance of longitudinal pigmented bands in the nail plate. Pubic and axillary hair may be lost in postpubertal females and vitiligo can be found in some patients.

Patients with adrenoleucodystrophy will eventually develop the typical neurological features of the disease [4,5] and notably, the diagnosis of Addison's disease can precede the development of the neurological features of the disease by many years [5]. Female patients with congenital adrenal hyperplasia have ambiguous genitalia which alerts the doctor in the newborn period to the possi-

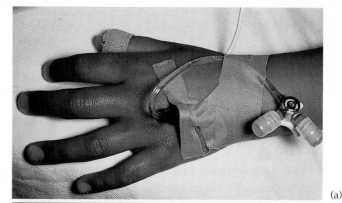

(a)

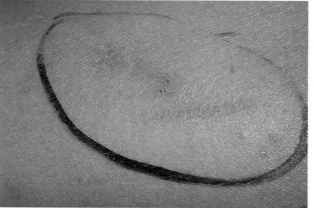

(b)

Fig. 25.10.3 (a) Addison's disease: hyperpigmentation on the dorsal aspect of the hand with accentuation over the knuckles. Courtesy of Dr Geoff Ambler, New Children's Hospital, Sydney, Australia. (b) Hyperpigmented scratch marks in a child with Addison's disease. Courtesy of Dr Geoff Ambler, New Children's Hospital, Sydney, Australia.

bility of adrenal insufficiency. The 3A syndrome refers to an association between glucocorticoid deficiency, alacrima, achalasia of the cardia, fissured palms, cutis anserina, autonomic nerve dysfunction and a variety of neurological abnormalities. Some of these patients also had mineralocorticoid deficiency [8].

Investigations

The clinical diagnosis of Addison's disease is confirmed by measuring the plasma cortisol level and free cortisol levels in a 24-h urine collection [7]. Patients with Addison's disease will have low plasma cortisol and urine free cortisol levels. Measurement of plasma ACTH levels and plasma cortisol levels following ACTH stimulation will distinguish adrenal failure from hypothalamopituitary dysfunction [7]. Most patients with the idiopathic form of Addison's disease will have circulating anti-adrenal antibodies [7]. Patients with adrenoleucodystrophy have raised plasma levels of hexacosanoic acid [5] and characteristic findings with magnetic resonance imaging of the brain [9].

Differential diagnosis

The early non-specific symptoms can be misdiagnosed as a wide variety of conditions. The hyperpigmentation is characteristic and readily distinguishes Addison's disease from other conditions.

Prognosis

All symptoms and signs will clear with appropriate glucocorticoid and mineralocorticoid replacement therapy. Patients with adrenoleucodystrophy will eventually develop neurological impairment.

Treatment

Hydrocortisone and fludrocortisone are administered on a daily basis. The dose will need to be increased during periods of stress and cases associated with circulating autoantibodies will need to be regularly monitored for the development of other autoimmune diseases.

REFERENCES

1 Curtis JA, Cormode E, Laski B *et al*. Endocrine complications of topical and intralesional corticosteroid therapy. *Arch Dis Child* 1982; 57: 204–7.
2 Sperling MA, Wolfsen AR, Fisher DA. Congenital adrenal hypoplasia: an isolated defect of organogenesis. *J Pediatr* 1973; 82: 444–9.
3 Kelch RP, Kaplan SL, Biglieri EG *et al*. Hereditary adrenocortical unresponsiveness to adrenocorticotropic hormone. *J Pediatr* 1972; 81: 726–36.
4 Davis LE, Snyder RD, Orth DN *et al*. Adrenoleukodystrophy and adrenomyeloneuropathy associated with partial adrenal insufficiency in three generations of a kindred. *Am J Med* 1979; 66: 342–7.
5 Sadhegi-Nejad A, Senior B. Adrenomyeloneuropathy presenting as Addison's disease in childhood. *N Engl J Med* 1990; 322: 13–16.
6 Lim YJ, Batch JA, Warne GL. Adrenal 21-hydroxylase deficiency in childhood: 25 years experience. *J Paediatr Child Health* 1995; 31: 222–7.
7 Grant DB, Barnes ND, Moncrieff MW *et al*. Clinical presentation, growth and pubertal development in Addison's disease. *Arch Dis Child* 1985; 60: 925–8.
8 Grant DB, Barnes ND, Dumic M *et al*. Neurological and adrenal dysfunction in the adrenal insufficiency/alacrima/achalasia (3A) syndrome. *Arch Dis Child* 1993; 68: 779–82.
9 Huckman MS, Wong PW, Sullivan T *et al*. Magnetic resonance imaging compared with computed tomography in adrenoleukodystrophy. *Am J Dis Child* 1986; 140: 1001–3.

Disorders of sex hormones

Hypogonadism

Pathogenesis

Hypogonadism in females occurs with deficiency of gonadotrophin secretion, inadequate production of sex hormones by the ovary or secondary to a virilizing disorder, hypothyroidism or hyperprolactinaemia [1].

Hypogonadism in males occurs with deficiency of gonadotrophin secretion, inadequate androgen production by the testis, 5α reductase deficiency or an androgen receptor defect [2].

Clinical features

The clinical features of hypogonadism in both sexes depend on the age of onset of the problem and the severity of the hormone deficiency [1–3]. Hypogonadism in a prepubertal female results in the failure of breast development (thelarche) and the onset of menarche (primary amenorrhoea). Pubic hair, axillary hair, body odour, sebum production and acne will still develop because of the unaltered production and secretion of adrenal androgens (adrenarche). The development of hypogonadism after the onset of puberty limits breast development and results in menstrual irregularities in the form of amenorrhoea, oligomenorrhoea or dysfunctional uterine bleeding. Linear growth is unaffected if growth hormone secretion is unaffected. Additional findings relate to the underlying cause of the hypogonadism (e.g. Turner's syndrome).

In males, hypogonadism *in utero* results in abnormal (e.g. hypospadias) or ambiguous genitalia or infants who are phenotypically female. Prepubertal hypogonadism results in small testes, a small penis, lack of scrotal rugae, feminine fat distribution over the hips, face and chest, arm span 6 cm over height, eunuchoidal skeletal proportions (crown to pubis/pubis to floor ratio <1), decreased muscle mass and delayed bone age. The only notable skin finding is diminished body hair and a smooth, soft skin texture. If androgen deficiency is not corrected by the onset of adolescence, the skin will retain its soft texture and there will be no enlargement of the genitalia (testis, penis) or development of body and facial hair. Pubic and axillary hair may partially develop through the effect of adrenal androgens. Linear growth will continue if growth hormone secretion is normal resulting in eunuchoidal skeletal proportions. If androgen deficiency occurs after the onset of puberty, the clinical signs are more subtle. Established hair on the face, trunk, limbs, axillae and pubic area show very little change although the patient may notice that the interval between shaving gradually increases. The degree of skin oiliness will reduce, acne vulgaris will improve and often clear, and the skin texture becomes smooth with fine wrinkles around the eyes and a decrease in the size of skin pores. Additional clinical findings relate to the underlying cause of the hypogonadism (e.g. Klinefelter's syndrome).

Investigations

Determining the cause of hypogonadism requires a detailed clinical assessment, determination of plasma gonadotropin (LH, FSH) levels, androgen levels, oestrogen levels and response of plasma gonadotropins to gonadotropin-releasing hormone. Imaging studies are needed if a tumour is suspected and chromosomal studies are required if the clinical features suggest Turner's or Klinefelter's syndrome.

Prognosis

The prognosis is determined by the underlying cause.

Treatment

Treatment can involve gonadotropin-releasing hormone, gonadotropins or appropriate sex hormone replacement therapy depending on the cause of the problem.

REFERENCES

1 Rosenfield RL. Puberty and its disorders in girls. *Endocrinol Metab Clin N Am* 1991; 20: 15–42.
2 Styne DM. Puberty and its disorders in boys. *Endocrinol Metab Clinic N Am* 1991; 20: 43–69.
3 Wheeler MD, Styne DM. Diagnosis and management of precocious puberty. *Pediatr Clin N Am* 1990; 37: 1255–71.

Precocious puberty

Definition

Precocious puberty is defined as the appearance of secondary sexual characteristics before the age of 8 years in a female and 9 years in a male [1]. The secondary sexual characteristics are termed isosexual if they are in keeping with the sex of the child. The term contrasexual is used when the secondary sexual characteristics are contrary to the sex of the child (i.e. virilization in a female, feminization in a male). The secondary sexual characteristics are the result of adrenal maturation (adrenarche) and gonadal maturation (gonadarche) [1]. Gonadal maturation is responsible for thelarche (breast development) and menarche (onset of menstruation) in females.

Pathogenesis

Isosexual precocious puberty can develop in response to a wide variety of disease processes. A simple classification divides the causes into gonadotropin-dependent and gonadotropin-independent groups [1]. In the gonadotropin-dependent group, precocious puberty is due to the premature release of gonadotropins from the pituitary gland. This can be constitutional or due to a variety of CNS tumours, CNS infections, head trauma, hydrocephalus, severe hypothyroidism, Addison's disease and following the resolution of a virilizing disorder such as congenital adrenal hyperplasia. In the gonadotropin-independent group precocious puberty is induced through autonomous secretion of gender appropriate sex hormones or the administration of exogenous sex steroids. Autonomous secretion of oestro-

gens in females occurs with follicular cysts, adrenal tumours, ovarian tumours and the McCune–Albright syndrome. Autonomous secretion of androgens in males occurs with congenital adrenal hyperplasia, adrenal tumours, testicular tumours, McCune–Albright syndrome, familial testitoxicosis and in response to secretion of human chorionic gonadotropin by tumours.

Contrasexual precocious puberty in females and males is discussed in the androgen excess and oestrogen excess sections, respectively.

Clinical features

Pubertal development in females is characterized, in order of appearance, by accelerated linear growth, breast development, appearance of pubic and axillary hair and the onset of menstruation [2,3]. Although precocious puberty in females usually involves all of the features of adrenal and gonadal maturation, occasionally it consists of only thelarche, adrenarche or menarche [1]. Premature thelarche usually occurs between 0 and 3 years of age without the other features of oestrogen activity (Fig. 25.10.4a). The timing of the onset of the other features of puberty is unaffected. Premature adrenarche refers to the development of pubic hair, axillary hair, comedones and body odour due to the premature maturation of the adrenal gland and the appearance of dehydroepiandrosterone in the circulation (Fig. 25.10.4b). The skin findings may be accompanied by a slight acceleration of the growth rate and advancement of the bone age. Gonadal maturation in these patients is unaffected. Premature menarche refers to the onset of menstruation between 1 and 9 years of age without any other features of puberty.

Pubertal development in males is characterized, in order of appearance, by testicular enlargement, the appearance of pubic hair, penile enlargement, the appearance of axillary and facial hair, deepening of the voice and acceleration of linear growth with an increase in the muscle mass [4] (Fig. 25.10.4c). Precocious puberty in males usually involves all of the features of adrenal and gonadal maturation. Occasionally, premature adrenarche is the only feature of precocious puberty in males with the clinical findings of pubic hair, axillary hair and body hair.

Accelerated linear growth in children predisposes to premature closure of the epiphyses, resulting in the paradox of a tall child becoming a short adult. Additional clinical findings relate to the underlying cause, e.g. large café-au-lait spots with the McCune–Albright syndrome.

Investigations

Determining the cause of precocious puberty requires a detailed clinical assessment, determination of plasma

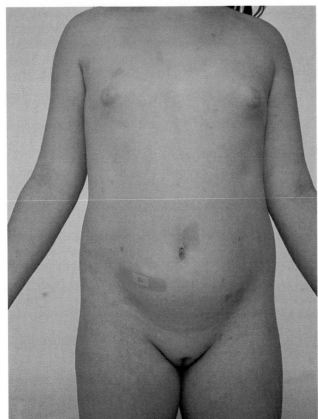

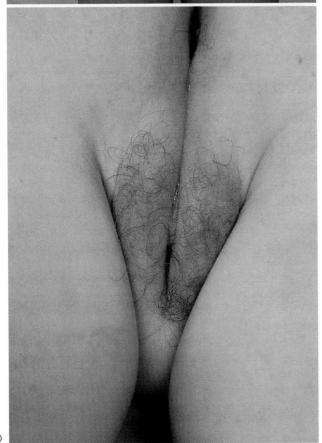

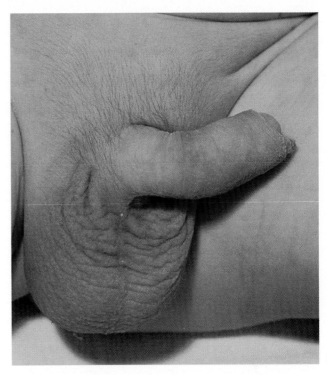

Fig. 25.10.4 (a) Precocious puberty characterized by premature thelarche in a 7-year-old female with neurofibromatosis (note the café-au-lait spots). Courtesy of Dr Geoff Ambler, New Children's Hospital, Sydney, Australia. (b) Premature adrenarche with the development of pubic hair in a 7-year-old female. Courtesy of Dr Christopher Cowell, New Children's Hospital, Sydney, Australia. (c) Precocious puberty in an 8-month-old male with penile enlargement and pubic hair. The precocious puberty was due to a hypothalamic hamartoma. Courtesy of Dr Geoff Ambler, New Children's Hospital, Sydney, Australia.

gonadotropin (LH, FSH) levels, androgen levels, oestrogen levels and response of plasma gonadotropins to gonadotropin-releasing hormone. Imaging studies are required if a tumour is suspected as the underlying cause.

Prognosis

The prognosis is dependent on the underlying cause.

Treatment

Gonadotropin-dependent precocious puberty due to intracranial tumours are treated whenever possible with surgery, radiotherapy and/or chemotherapy. Gonadotropin-dependent precocious puberty not amenable to physical therapy is treated with a gonadotropin-releasing hormone agonist [5]. The regular administration of the agonist has been shown to reduce gonadotropin secretion from the pituitary, reduce sex steroid hormone secretion and slow down advancement of bone age. Gonadotropin secretion returns to normal with cessation of gonadotropin agonist therapy.

Gonadotropin-independent precocious puberty due to a tumour is treated whenever possible with surgery. Congenital adrenal hyperplasia is treated with glucocorticoids. Testolactone, an inhibitor of the enzyme which converts androgens to oestrogens, has been used to treat McCune–Albright syndrome in females [6] and familial testitoxicosis in association with spironolactone [7]. Medroxyprogesterone acetate has been used to treat follicular cysts, McCune–Albright syndrome and familial testitoxicosis [8].

REFERENCES

1 Wheeler MD, Styne DM. Diagnosis and management of precocious puberty. *Pediatr Clin N Am* 1990; 37: 1255–71.
2 Marshall WE, Tanner JM. Variations in the pattern of pubertal changes in girls. *Arch Dis Child* 1969; 44: 291–303.
3 Zacharias L, Rand WM, Wurtman RJ. A prospective study of sexual development and growth in American girls: the statistics of menarche. *Obst Gynecol Surv* 1976; 31: 325–37.
4 Marshall WE, Tanner JM. Variations in the pattern of pubertal changes in boys. *Arch Dis Child* 1970; 45: 13–23.
5 Manasco PK, Pescovitz OH, Hill SC *et al.* Six year results of luteinizing hormone releasing hormone (LHRH) agonist treatment in children with LHRH dependant precocious puberty. *J Pediatr* 1989; 115: 105–8.
6 Feuillan PP, Foster CM, Pescovitz OH *et al.* Treatment of precocious puberty in the McCune–Albright syndrome with the aromatase inhibitor testolactone. *N Engl J Med* 1986; 315: 1115–19.
7 Laue L, Kenigsberg D, Pescovitz OH *et al.* Treatment of familial precocious puberty with spironolactone and testolactone. *N Engl J Med* 1989; 320: 496–502.
8 Grumbach MM, Kaplan SL. Recent advances in the diagnosis and management of sexual precocity. *Acta Paediatr Jpn* 1988; 30(suppl): 155–75 (overseas edition).

Androgen excess

Pathogenesis

Hyperandrogenaemia (HA) can be due to adrenal disease [1], gonadal disease [1], hyperprolactinaemia [1], enhanced peripheral conversion of androstenedione to testosterone in obese females [2] and glucocorticoid receptor defects resulting in hypersecretion of ACTH and increased adrenal androgen production [3]. Adrenal problems capable of producing HA are exaggerated adrenarche [4], congenital adrenal hyperplasia [5–7], Cushing's syndrome [8] and adrenal tumours (adenomas, carcinomas) [9]. Gonad-derived HA is seen in females with hyperinsulinaemia [10–14] and in both sexes with gonadal tumours [15,16].

Congenital adrenal hyperplasia refers to a heterogeneous group of conditions inherited in an autosomal recessive fashion [5–7]. The underlying defect is a deficiency in one of the enzymes involved in the biosynthesis of glucocorticoids and aldosterone. The reduced production of glucocorticoids results in the hypersecretion of ACTH and stimulation of steroid biosynthesis. This results in an accumulation of precursor molecules exhibiting androgenic activity. The clinical picture will depend

on the type and degree of the enzyme deficiency, the degree of glucocorticoid and aldosterone deficiency and the level of androgenic precursors. Severe enzyme deficiency usually presents in early infancy with an addisonian crisis and ambiguous genitalia in females. Mild enzyme deficiency presents later with the clinical features of HA. Most cases of congenital adrenal hyperplasia are due to 21-hydroxylase deficiency [5]. The remaining cases are due to 11β-hydroxylase deficiency [6] or 3β-hydroxysteroid dehydrogenase deficiency [7].

Insulin resistance in females can result in ovarian overproduction of androgens [10–13]. The insulin resistance and HA can be accompanied by menstrual irregularities, obesity, acanthosis nigrican (AN) and a number of ovarian changes (stromal hyperplasia, hyperthecosis, cysts). Patients previously classified with the polycystic ovary syndrome (obesity, menstrual irregularities, hirsutism, polycystic ovaries) [14] are probably a distinct subgroup within the insulin resistance–ovarian hyperandrogenism spectrum of disease.

Clinical features

The symptoms and signs of HA will depend on the age of the patient (prepubertal versus postpubertal), the sex of the patient and the reason for the androgen excess. Furthermore, patients with adrenal tumours may also manifest features of Cushing's syndrome [8] and patients with congenital adrenal hyperplasia may have a past history of an addisonian crisis [5].

Prepubertal patients usually present with accelerated linear growth, significant weight gain, cliteromegaly with varying degrees of posterior labial fusion, penile enlargement without testicular enlargement (Fig. 25.10.5), pubic hair, facial hair, oily skin with facial acne, body odour and a deepening voice [1–16]. Examination usually reveals a muscular habitus with advanced bone age [1–16]. Hypertension is a feature of patients with congenital adrenal hyperplasia due to 11β-hydroxylase deficiency [6]. Premature closure of the epiphyses is a potential problem resulting in decreased adult height. Development of HA around the onset of puberty in females will delay the onset of thelarche and menarche.

Postpubertal females present with hirsutism, difficult to control acne, menstrual irregularities and a deepening voice [1–16]. Examination may reveal a muscular habitus, cliteromegaly with varying degrees of posterior labial fusion, early male pattern alopecia [1–16], hypertension in patients with congenital adrenal hyperplasia due to 11β-hydroxylase deficiency [6] and acanthosis nigricans in patients with insulin resistance and HA [10–12]. Bone age is advanced and premature closure of the epiphyses can occur resulting in decreased adult height. The symptoms and signs of androgen excess in postpubertal males are more subtle and it can be

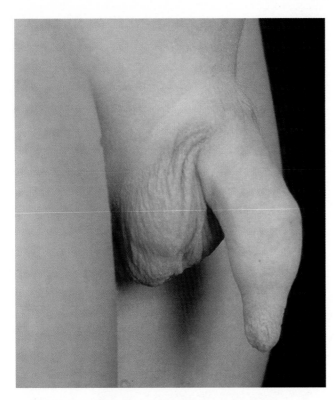

Fig. 25.10.5 Testicular enlargement, penile enlargement and pubic hair in a 2-year-old male with a virilizing adrenal tumour. Courtesy of Dr Geoff Ambler, New Children's Hospital, Sydney, Australia.

difficult to distinguish normal pubertal development from androgen excess.

Investigations

If androgen excess is suspected the most appropriate screening investigation is free plasma testosterone, plasma dehydroepiandrosterone (DHEAS) and plasma androstenedione [17]. Free plasma testosterone is preferred to total testosterone because it takes into consideration the fluctuations in sex hormone binding globulin that can occur for a variety of reasons. Significantly elevated free plasma testosterone levels are indicative of a virilizing gonadal tumour and significantly elevated DHEAS levels are suggestive of an adrenal tumour [17]. Either result requires further investigation with ultrasound, computed tomography and/or magnetic resonance imaging. Individuals with normal levels or mild elevations of plasma androgens should undergo a low-dose dexamethasone suppression test [17]. The response of plasma testosterone, cortisol and DHEAS is usually diagnostic. Suppression of DHEAS and testosterone with insignificant suppression of cortisol indicates Cushing's syndrome [15]. Suppression of DHEAS and cortisol with insignificant suppression of testosterone is seen with the ovarian-mediated HA associated with insulin resistance

or a virilizing tumour [19]. Additional findings with ovarian HA may include an elevated LH level [17], polycystic ovaries on pelvic ultrasound [17] and reduction of plasma testosterone levels with administration of the oral contraceptive. Exclusion of a virilizing tumour requires imaging studies. If plasma DHEAS and testosterone are suppressed with low-dose dexamethasone, ACTH testing is indicated. A marked elevation of 17-hydroxyprogesterone with an intravenous bolus of ACTH is diagnostic of congenital adrenal hyperplasia [15]. A normal ACTH test is seen with abnormal peripheral androgen conversion, hyperprolactinaemia and growth hormone excess.

Prognosis

The prognosis relates to the cause of the HA. The prognosis is good for virilizing adenomas but guarded for virilizing carcinomas because of the risk of metastatic disease. Severe congenital adrenal hyperplasia requires ongoing care to avoid addisonian crises and to minimize the deleterious effects of HA on skeletal development. Mild congenital adrenal hyperplasia and the ovarian HA associated with IR are usually well controlled with medical therapy.

Management

Management depends on the underlying cause [17]. Tumours are surgically excised and postexcision radiotherapy or chemotherapy are undertaken when needed. Congenital adrenal hyperplasia and exaggerated adrenarche requires low-dose glucocorticoid therapy to reduce ACTH stimulation of androgen production. Ovarian HA is treated with an oestrogen-containing oral contraceptive and measures to reduce insulin levels.

REFERENCES

1 Glickman SP, Rosenfield RL, Bergenstal RM *et al*. Multiple androgenic abnormalities including elevated free testosterone in hyperprolactinaemia women. *J Clin Endocrinol Metab* 1982; 55: 251–7.
2 Glass AR. Endocrine function in human obesity. *Metabolism* 1981; 30: 89–104.
3 Moller DE, Flier JS. Insulin resistance-mechanisms, syndromes and implications. *N Engl J Med* 1991; 325: 938–48.
4 Ehrmann DA, Rosenfield RL, Barnes RB *et al*. Detection of functional ovarian hyperandrogenism in women with androgen excess. *N Engl J Med* 1992; 327: 157–62.
5 Lim YJ, Batch JA, Warne GL. Adrenal 21-hydroxylase deficiency in childhood: 25 years experience. *J Paediatr Child Health* 1995; 31: 222–7.
6 Zachmann M, Vollmin JA, New MI *et al*. Congenital adrenal hyperplasia due to deficiency of 11-beta-hydroxylation of 17-alpha-hydroxylated steroids. *J Clin Endocrinol Metab* 1971; 33: 501–8.
7 Pang S, Lerner AJ, Stoner E *et al*. Late onset adrenal steroid 3-beta-hydroxysteroid dehydrogenase deficiency. A cause of hirsutism in pubertal and post pubertal women. *J Clin Endocrinol Metab* 1985; 60: 428–39.
8 Magiakou MA, Mastorakos G, Oldfield EH *et al*. Cushing's syndrome in children and adolescents. Presentation, diagnosis and therapy. *N Engl J Med* 1994; 331: 629–36.
9 Lee PDK, Winter RJ, Green OC. Virilising adrenocortical tumours in

childhood: eight cases and a review of the literature. *Pediatrics* 1985; 76: 437–44.

10 Kahn CR, Flier JS, Bar RS *et al*. The syndromes of insulin resistance and acanthosis nigricans: insulin receptor disorders in man. *N Engl J Med* 1976; 294: 739–45.

11 Taylor SI, Dons RF, Hernandez E *et al*. Insulin resistance associated with androgen excess in women with autoantibodies to the insulin receptor. *Ann Intern Med* 1982; 97: 851–5.

12 Barbieri RL, Makris A, Randall RW *et al*. Insulin stimulates androgen accumulation in incubations of ovarian stroma obtained from women with hyperandrogenism. *J Clin Endocrinol Metab* 1986; 62: 904–10.

13 Nestler JE, Barlascini CO, Matt DW *et al*. Suppression of serum insulin by diazoxide reduces serum testosterone levels in obese women with polycystic ovary syndrome. *J Clin Endocrinol Metab* 1989; 68: 1027–32.

14 Stein IF, Leventhal ML. Amenorrhoea associated with bilateral polycystic ovaries. *Am J Obstet Gynecol* 1935; 29: 181–7.

15 Hatch R, Rosenfield RL, Kim MH *et al*. Hirsutism: implications, etiology, and management. *Am J Obstet Gynecol* 1981; 140: 815–30.

16 Solish SB, Goldsmith MA, Voutilainen R *et al*. Molecular characterization of a Leydig cell tumor presenting as congenital adrenal hyperplasia. *J Clin Endocrinol Metab* 1989; 69: 1148–52.

17 Rosenfield RL, Lucky AW. Acne, hirsutism and alopecia in adolescent girls. *Endocrinol Metab Clin N Am* 1993; 22: 507–32.

Oestrogen excess

Pathogenesis

In males, elevated levels of circulating oestrogen occur with the testicular feminization syndrome [1–3] and oestrogen-producing tumours of the adrenal gland [4–6] or testes [7]. The testicular feminization syndrome involves a failure of testosterone and dihydrotestosterone to bind adequately with the androgen receptor [2]. The absence of androgen effect is compounded by the peripheral conversion of testosterone to oestrogen and the feminizing effect of the oestrogen [3].

In females, elevated levels of oestrogen occur with oral contraceptive use and pregnancy. The appearance of circulating oestrogen in prepubertal females will be discussed with precocious puberty.

Clinical features

In the testicular feminizing syndrome [1–3], babies with an XY karyotype are born phenotypically female with female genitalia that have a normal appearance. The female phenotype continues during puberty with breast development and a female fat distribution. Genital examination at this time will reveal a normal clitoris and external genitalia, a blind vaginal pouch and absent fallopian tubes and ovaries. The testes may be present in the labia or palpable in the groin or abdomen. Testis located in the groin are usually misdiagnosed as inguinal herniae.

Oestrogen-producing tumours in males produce breast enlargement with puffiness and pigmentation of the areolae [4–7] (Fig. 25.10.6). Most oestrogen tumours also produce androgens resulting in the additional findings of axillary hair, pubic hair, mild acne and penile enlargement [1,3].

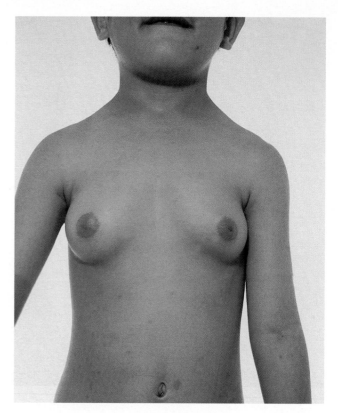

Fig. 25.10.6 Gynaecomastia in a 6-year-old male with an oestrogen-producing adrenal tumour. Courtesy of Dr Geoff Ambler, New Children's Hospital, Sydney, Australia.

Elevated oestrogen levels during pregnancy probably contribute to the development of spider naevi, palmar erythema, chloasma (melasma), darkening of existing melanocytic naevi, hyperpigmentation of the nipples, areolae, genitalia and linea alba and pruritus (± jaundice) secondary to hepatic cholestasis [8]. Oral contraceptive use can be associated with the development of spider naevi, palmar erythema and chloasma. Acne can improve or flare during pregnancy and with oral contraceptive use.

Investigations

The testicular feminization syndrome is characterized by an XY karyotype, normal or slightly elevated plasma levels of testosterone, elevated plasma levels of LH and FSH and elevated plasma levels of oestrogen [1–3]. Pelvic ultrasound will reveal absent ovaries and fallopian tubes. Males with oestrogen-producing tumours will have elevated plasma levels of oestrogen and most will also have elevated plasma androgen levels [4–7].

Prognosis

Patients with the testicular feminization syndrome are usually raised as females and the syndrome is not recognized until they are evaluated for amenorrhoea or a testicle is found. Continuation of the female sex assignment is usually recommended because of their upbringing as females and the absence of any treatment for the infertility. Males with oestrogen-producing tumours do well after removal of the tumour.

Treatment

Patients with the testicular feminizing syndrome should have the testes removed because of the increased risk of testicular malignancy [9]. Oestrogen replacement therapy is required postoperatively because the testis are the principal source of oestrogen through peripheral conversion of testosterone to oestrogen. Oestrogen-producing tumours are surgically excised.

REFERENCES

1 Klinefelter HG Jr, Reifenstein EC Jr, Albright F. Syndrome characterised by gynecomastia, aspermatogenesis without A-leydigism and increased excretion of follicle stimulating hormone. *J Clin Endocrinol Metab* 1942; 2: 615–19.

2 Kovacs WJ, Griffen JE, Weaver DD et al. A mutation that causes lability of the androgen receptor under conditions that normally promote transformation to the DNA-binding state. *J Clin Invest* 1984; 73: 1095–104.

3 MacDonald PC, Madden JD, Brenner OF et al. Origin of oestrogen in normal men and in women with testicular feminization. *J Clin Endocrinol Metab* 1979; 49: 905–16.

4 Mosier HD, Goodwin WE. Feminising adrenal adenoma in a 7-year-old boy. *Pediatrics* 1961; 27: 1016–21.

5 Bhettay E, Bonnici F. Pure oestrogen secreting feminising adrenocortical adenoma. *Arch Dis Child* 1977; 52: 241–3.

6 Itami RM, Amundson GM, Kaplan SA et al. Prepubertal gynecomastia caused by an adrenal tumour: diagnostic value of ultrasonography. *Am J Dis Child* 1982; 136: 584–6.

7 Mostofi FK, Theiss EA, Ashley DJ et al. Tumours of specialised gonadal stroma in human male patients. Andrenoblastoma, sertoli cell tumour, granulosa-theca cell tumour of the testis and gonadal stroma tumour. *Cancer* 1959; 12: 944–57.

8 Wong RC, Ellis CN. Physiologic skin changes in pregnancy. *J Am Acad Dermatol* 1984; 10: 929–40.

9 O'Leary JA. Comparative studies of the gonad in testicular feminization and cryptorchidism. *Fertil Steril* 1965; 16: 813–19.

Insulin resistance

Definition

IR refers to a diminished biological response (glucose clearance) of peripheral tissues to circulating insulin. The diminished peripheral response to circulating insulin results in compensatory hypersecretion of insulin to maintain normal blood glucose levels. The hyperinsulinaemia may or may not be associated with hyperglycaemia. Kahn *et al.* defined two broad categories of IR [1]. Type A is due to an insulin receptor or postreceptor defect [2,3]. Type B is due to blocking of insulin receptors by circulating anti-insulin receptor antibodies [1,4]. These patients may have laboratory (e.g. anti-DNA antibodies) or clinical (e.g. lupus erythematosus) evidence of other autoimmune diseases [5]. The HAIR-AN syndrome refers to type A female patients with HA, IR and AN.

Pathogenesis

IR can result from a primary defect in the insulin receptor [2], a primary defect in the postreceptor pathway [3], blockage of the insulin receptor by circulating anti-insulin receptor antibodies [4] or a reduction in the sensitivity of target tissues due to another process (e.g. obesity, other endocrine diseases) (Table 25.10.1). Patients with IR due to a primary defect in the insulin receptor or postreceptor pathway can be further divided into a number of clinical entities on the basis of clinical findings (Table 25.10.1).

IR and hyperinsulinaemia is usually accompanied by HA and AN in females [1,4,6], and by AN acanthosis nigricans in males [1]. Published data indicates that hyperinsulinaemia is responsible for the development of ovarian-derived HA [7,8] and AN [9]. Stimulation of ovarian androgen production requires the presence of LH and is therefore a feature of postpubertal females [10,11]. The development of AN is probably mediated via a direct or indirect stimulation of receptors for growth factors. Although early reports implicated insulin-like growth factor 1 (IGF-1) receptors [12] in the pathogenesis of IR-associated AN, IR and AN have been reported in patients with decreased IGF-1 receptors [13] suggesting that other receptors are involved.

Clinical features

The characteristic findings of IR are AN in both sexes and the features of HA in postpubertal females [1,4,6]. AN can

Table 25.10.1 Syndromes and diseases associated with IR

Insulin receptor or postreceptor defects
Kahn's type A syndrome
Rabson–Medenhall syndrome
acral enlargement syndrome
leprechaunism
lipodystrophy (complete and partial)
Anti-insulin receptor antibodies
Kahn's type B syndrome
ataxia telangiectasia
Other syndromes (unspecified defect)
polycystic ovary disease
Prader–Willi syndrome
Laurence–Moon–Bardet–Biedel syndrome
Alström's syndrome
streaky gonads
Obesity (unspecified defect)
Endocrine disease (unspecified defect)
gigantism and acromegaly
Cushing's disease
hypothyroidism

manifest before or after the onset of puberty (Fig. 25.10.7). Hyperpigmentation is the earliest feature and parents often mistake the pigmentation for dirty skin. Although the flexures are preferentially involved, the extensor surfaces of the limbs can be involved in severe cases. With the onset of puberty, HA can manifest in females with hirsutism, severe and/or difficult to control acne, oligomenorrhoea or amenorrhoea, cliteromegaly and male pattern alopecia. The degree of virilization will depend on the underlying cause.

Patients with IR related to obesity usually have upper body (shoulders, chest, abdomen) rather than lower body (buttocks, thigh) obesity [14,15]. The degree of IR, AN and HA in females is determined by the degree of obesity. In contrast, patients with the type A IR syndrome typically have severe IR (± hyperglycaemia) with pronounced AN in both sexes and HA in postpubertal females (HAIR-AN syndrome) [1]. Additional findings in established cases may include obesity, serum hyperlipidaemia, non-insulin-dependent diabetes mellitus, essential hypertension and ovarian changes (stromal hyperplasia, hyperthecosis, cysts) [1].

The Rabson–Medenhall syndrome and the acral enlargement syndrome are clinical variants of the type A syndrome. The Rabson–Medenhall syndrome is characterized by type A features combined with pineal hyperplasia, dental hyperplasia and other dysmorphic features [16]. The acral enlargement syndrome (pseudoacromegaly) refers to patients with the features of type A disease and acromegaly (acral enlargement, coarsened facial features, widened spaces between the teeth) despite normal growth hormone levels [17].

A number of syndromes have IR secondary to an insulin receptor or postreceptor defect (Table 25.10.1). Leprechaunism is a rare condition characterized by severe intrauterine and postnatal growth retardation, lipoatrophy, genital enlargement due to HA, AN, a characteristic 'elfin-like' facies, rugation of the perioral skin, cutis verticis gyrata on the scalp, disproportionately large hands and feet, yellow discoloration of the palms and soles and thin dysplastic hyperconvex nails [18–20]. Congenital total lipoatrophy is characterized by the complete absence of subcutaneous fat at birth or the loss of subcutaneous fat by 2 years of age. The lipoatrophy is associated with hirsutism, AN, enlarged genitalia, accelerated somatic growth, advanced bone age, pronounced musculature, enlarged hands and feet, eruptive xanthomas and hepatomegaly secondary to hypertriglyceridaemia [1,21,22]. Partial lipoatrophy is characterized by symmetric loss of fat which can occur in several patterns [1,21,22]. The fat loss may be idiopathic or follow a viral illness. The most common pattern is loss of fat from the head, neck and varying degrees of the trunk and proximal aspects of the limbs. Other patterns include fat loss from the lower half of the body with sparing of the head and neck, fat loss from the limbs with sparing of the

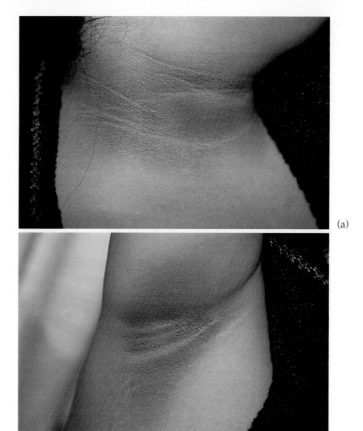

(a)

(b)

Fig. 25.10.7 (a, b) Acanthosis nigricans (AN) of the neck and axillae in a 9-year-old female with severe IR.

trunk, head and neck, and fat loss from the trunk and limbs with sparing of the head and neck. Fat loss from the upper half of the body can be associated with hypertrophy of the soft tissue in the lower half of the body. The presence of hirsutism and AN is variable. Most patients have depressed complement 3 (C3) levels and a circulating immunoglobulin that is capable of activating the alternate complement pathway. This factor is referred to as the C3 nephritic factor [23]. The presence of the C3 nephritic factor is associated with a high incidence of glomerulonephritis [23].

Although the type B IR syndrome usually develops in adult females, it can occur during the adolescent years [4–6]. It is characterized by AN, the features of HA and the laboratory or clinical features of one or more autoimmune diseases, especially lupus erythematosus, Sjögren's syndrome and primary biliary cirrhosis. Type B IR has also been reported in association with ataxia telangiectasia [24].

Prader–Willi [25], Laurence–Moon–Bardet–Biedel [25] and Alström's syndrome [26] are syndromes characterized by IR, obesity, AN and hypogonadism. Other conditions associated with IR include streaky gonads [27], gigantism/acromegaly [28,29], Cushing's disease [30] and hypothyroidism [31].

Laboratory findings

The laboratory findings are diverse and depend on the clinical setting of the IR. A diagnosis of IR is confirmed by elevated serum insulin levels. Patients should have their blood sugar level regularly checked and females need their androgen levels monitored. Specific investigations are required if a co-existent endocrine abnormality (e.g. acromegaly) or autoimmune disease is suspected (e.g. lupus erythematosus).

Treatment

Treatment is determined by the underlying cause. A reduction in the degree of IR will reduce androgen levels and improve AN. The androgen levels can be reduced in patients with the type A form through the use of oral contraceptives and gonadotrophin agonists. Androgen reduction has no effect on IR or AN.

REFERENCES

1 Kahn CR, Flier JS, Bar RS *et al*. The syndromes of insulin resistance and acanthosis nigricans: insulin receptor disorders in man. *N Engl J Med* 1976; 294: 739–45.
2 Shimada M, Taira M, Suzuki Y *et al*. Insulin resistant diabetes associated with partial deletion of insulin receptor gene. *Lancet* 1990; 335: 1179–81.
3 Kusari J, Takata Y, Hatada E *et al*. Insulin resistance and diabetes due to different mutations in the tyrosine kinase domain of both insulin receptor gene alleles. *J Biol Chem* 1991; 266: 5260–7.
4 Flier JS, Kahn CR, Roth J *et al*. Antibodies that impair insulin receptor binding in an unusual diabetic syndrome with severe insulin resistance. *Science* 1975; 190: 63–5.
5 Tsokos GC, Gorden P, Antonovnych T *et al*. Lupus nephritis and other autoimmune features in patients with diabetes mellitus due to auto-antibody to insulin receptors. *Ann Intern Med* 1985; 102: 176–81.
6 Taylor SI, Dons RF, Hernandez E *et al*. Insulin resistance associated with androgen excess in women with autoantibodies to the insulin receptor. *Ann Intern Med* 1982; 97: 851–5.
7 Barbieri RL, Makris A, Randall RW *et al*. Insulin stimulates androgen accumulation in incubations of ovarian stroma obtained from women with hyperandrogenism. *J Clin Endocrinol Metab* 1986; 62: 904–10.
8 Nestler JE, Barlascini CO, Matt DW *et al*. Suppression of serum insulin by diazoxide reduces serum testosterone levels in obese women with polycystic ovary syndrome. *J Clin Endocrinol Metab* 1989; 68: 1027–32.
9 Ober KP. Acanthosis nigricans and insulin resistance associated with hypothyroidism. *Arch Dermatol* 1985; 121: 229–31.
10 Geffner ME, Kaplan SA, Bersch N *et al*. Persistence of insulin resistance in polycystic ovarian disease after inhibition of ovarian steroid secretion. *Fertil Steril* 1986; 45: 327–33.
11 Barbieri RL, Smith S, Ryan KJ. The role of hyperinsulinaemia in the pathogenesis of ovarian hyperandrogenism. *Fertil Steril* 1988; 50: 197–212.
12 Geffner ME, Golde DW. Selective insulin action on skin, ovary, and heart in insulin resistant states. *Diabetes Care* 1988; 11: 500–5.
13 Low L, Chernausek SD, Sperling MA. Acromegaloid patients with type A insulin resistance: parallel defects in insulin and insulin like growth factor-1 receptors and biological responses in cultured fibroblasts. *J Clin Endocrinol Metab* 1989; 69: 329–37.
14 Evans DJ, Hoffman RG, Kalkhoff RK *et al*. Relationship of androgenic activity to body fat topography, fat cell morphology and metabolic alterations in premenopausal women. *J Clin Endocrinol Metab* 1983; 57: 304–10.
15 Kissebah AH, Vydelingum N, Murray R *et al*. Relation of body fat distribution to metabolic complications of obesity. *J Clin Endocrinol Metab* 1982; 54: 254–60.
16 Rabson SM, Medenhall EN. Familial hypertrophy of pineal body, hyperplasia of adrenal cortex and diabetes mellitus: report of three cases. *Am J Clin Pathol* 1956; 26: 283–90.
17 Flier JS, Young JB, Landsberg L. Familial insulin resistance with acanthosis nigricans, acral hypertrophy and muscle cramps. *N Engl J Med* 1980; 303: 970–3.
18 Roth SI, Schedewie HK, Herzberg VK *et al*. Cutaneous manifestations of leprechaunism. *Arch Dermatol* 1981; 117: 531–5.
19 D'Ercole AJ, Underwood LE, Groelke J *et al*. Leprechaunism: studies of the relationship among hyperinsulinism, insulin resistance and growth retardation. *J Clin Endocrinol Metab* 1979; 48: 495–502.
20 Reddy SS, Lauris V, Kahn CR. Insulin receptor function in fibroblasts from patients with leprechaunism: differential alterations in binding, autophosphorylation, kinase activity and receptor mediated internalization. *J Clin Invest* 1988; 82: 1359–65.
21 Senior B, Gellis SS. The syndromes of total lipodystrophy and of partial lipodystrophy. *Paediatrics* 1964; 33: 593–612.
22 Wachslicht-Rodbard H, Muggeo M, Kahn CR *et al*. Heterogeneity of the insulin receptor interaction in lipoatrophic diabetes. *J Clin Endocrinol Metab* 1981; 52: 416–25.
23 Ipp MM, Minta JO, Gelgand EW *et al*. Disorders of the complement system in lipodystrophy. *Immunol Immunopathol* 1976; 7: 281–7.
24 Bar RS, Levis WR, Rechler MM *et al*. Extreme insulin resistance in ataxia telangiectasia: a defect in affinity of insulin receptors. *N Engl J Med* 1978; 298: 1164–71.
25 Reed WD, Ragsdale W Jr, Curtis AC *et al*. Acanthosis nigricans in association with various genodermatoses with emphasis on lipodystrophic diabetes and Prader–Willi syndrome. *Acta Derm Venereol (Stockh)* 1968; 48: 465–73.
26 Goldstein JL, Fialkow PJ. The Alström syndrome: report of three cases with further delineation of the clinical, pathophysiological and genetic aspects of the disorder. *Medicine* 1973; 52: 53–71.
27 Wortsman J, Matsuoka LY, Dietrich J *et al*. Acanthosis nigricans in a patient with streaky gonads. *Arch Intern Med* 1983; 143: 825–7.
28 Brown J, Winkelmann RK. Acanthosis nigricans: a study of 90 cases. *Medicine* 1968; 47: 33–51.
29 Levin SR, Hofeldt FD, Becker N *et al*. Hypersomatotropism and acanthosis nigricans in two brothers. *Arch Intern Med* 1974; 134: 365–7.
30 Curth HO. Pituitary basophilism in the juvenile type of acanthosis nigricans. *J Am Med Assoc* 1955; 157: 266–77.
31 Ober KP. Acanthosis nigricans and insulin resistance associated with hypothyroidism. *Arch Dermatol* 1985; 121: 229–31.

Diabetes mellitus

Pathogenesis

Diabetes mellitus in paediatric patients is usually of the type 1 (insulin-dependent) variety. A minority of patients belong to the type 2 (non-insulin-dependent) variety. Hyperglycaemia, the biochemical hallmark of diabetes mellitus, results from either insulin deficiency or tissue resistance to the effect of circulating insulin. Insulin deficiency is usually due to a failure of the pancreatic islet cells to produce and secrete insulin. This may be an idiopathic problem involving genetic predisposition, viral infection and immunological factors [1–3] or secondary to pancreatic destruction [4]. IR is a feature of a variety of disease processes and is due to an insulin receptor or postreceptor abnormality [5,6] or circulating anti-insulin receptor antibodies [7].

Hyperglycaemia may contribute to some of the cutaneous complications of diabetes mellitus via glycosylation of tissue proteins. Studies have identified glycosylated collagen fibres in the skin of diabetic patients [8]. Glycosylation produces changes in protein solubility, its biological behaviour and its interaction with other proteins and enzymes. In particular, diabetic collagen is less susceptible to collagenase and more susceptible to increased cross-linking than collagen from normal individuals [9]. This structural alteration may contribute to the development of limited joint mobility. The relationship between hyperglycaemia and the other cutaneous findings of diabetes mellitus, including infection, is yet to be determined.

Clinical features

Type 1 diabetes mellitus usually presents in children with a short history of polyuria, polydypsia, polyphagia and weight loss or acutely with frank diabetic ketoacidosis. With the exception of necrobiosis lipoidica diabeticorum (NLD) [10], the cutaneous manifestations of diabetes mellitus usually develop with or after the diagnosis has been made. The cutaneous manifestations of diabetes mellitus in children are listed in Table 25.10.2. Only those findings relevant to the paediatric age group will be discussed. The manifestations can be divided into those that are directly attributable to the metabolic abnormality, skin diseases that are characteristically associated with diabetes mellitus, skin diseases that are commonly associated with diabetes mellitus and skin findings that represent side-effects of diabetes treatment. The clinical features of IR are discussed on pages 1637–9.

Cutaneous manifestations of the metabolic abnormality

Microangiopathy and neuropathy. The cutaneous manifestations of microangiopathy and neuropathy are never seen in prepubertal children and are rarely seen before the onset of adult life [11]. Microangiopathy can manifest in the feet and distal aspects of the lower limbs as coolness and mottling when the legs are in a dependent position. Neuropathy in young patients may involve the autonomic or somatic nervous system. Involvement of the autonomic nervous system can result in anhidrosis with or without compensatory hyperhidrosis [11].

Infection. There is no clear evidence that the incidence of skin infection is greater in diabetic children compared with an age-matched control group. The significance of infection in diabetes mellitus relates to its capacity to interfere with diabetic control and the increased risk of unusual organisms (e.g. mucormycosis) being involved.

Bacterial infection manifests in the usual ways as impetigo, folliculitis, furunculosis, cellulitis and erysipelas [11]. Recurrent folliculitis and furunculosis should raise the possibility of nasal carriage of *Staphylococcus aureus* by

Table 25.10.2 Cutaneous manifestations of diabetes mellitus

Manifestations of the metabolic abnormality
  microangiopathy and neuropathy
  infection
  xanthomas

Manifestations characteristic for the disease
  limited joint mobility and waxy skin thickening
  NLD
  diabetic dermopathy

Adverse reactions to therapy
  local reactions to insulin injection
  generalized reaction to insulin injection

the patient or other family members. Erythrasma may occur, especially in obese patients, and malignant otitis externa due to *Pseudomonas aeruginosa* has been reported in children and teenagers [12,13].

Candida albicans infection is common and can manifest as typical vulvovaginitis, balanitis, angular cheilitis, intra-oral candidiasis, intertrigo and paronychia [11]. All sites of infection respond well to antifungal therapy. Dermatophyte infection in diabetes mellitus is only remarkable for the portal of entry it provides for pathogenic bacteria when the feet are affected.

Poorly controlled diabetic children are predisposed to mucormycosis, a very rare deep fungal infection [14,15]. Primary mucormycosis develops in the skin, as gangrenous ulcers, or in the upper respiratory tract. Upper respiratory tract involvement manifests as black crusting or foul smelling pus on the palatal, buccal or nasal mucosa. Cerebral invasion and/or haematogenous dissemination occurs in two-thirds of cases [16]. Diagnosis requires a biopsy which reveals necrosis, a severe inflammatory reaction involving neutrophilic and granulomatous infiltrates and non-branching septate hyphae with periodic acid–Schiff (PAS) stains.

Eruptive xanthomas. In children with poorly controlled type 1 diabetes mellitus, hypertriglyceridaemia may develop resulting in the appearance of eruptive xanthomas on the buttocks, lumbosacral region of the back and extensor aspects of the limbs [11]. The eruption consists of firm, 1–5 mm wide papules that are initially erythematous before developing the typical yellow/orange colour. The papules may remain discrete, coalesce to form large plaques particularly on the buttocks and may develop along scratch lines as a Koebner phenomenon.

Skin findings characteristic of diabetes mellitus

Limited joint mobility with waxy skin thickening. Limited joint mobility occurs in approximately 30% of type 1 diabetes mellitus patients in the first two decades of life [17–19]. The condition is characterized by flexion contractures of the proximal interphalangeal joints of the fingers, particularly the fourth and fifth fingers [17–19]. This can be easily demonstrated by the inability to flatten the hands on a flat surface or the inability to press the palms together in a praying position (Fig. 25.10.8). In addition to finger involvement there may be similar changes involving the wrists, ankles, elbows, knees, toes and spine [17].

Patients with pronounced limited joint mobility can have waxy thickening of the skin on the dorsum of the hands and fingers [18,19]. The thickening may be diffuse or more discrete, especially on the fingers, conveying a pebbly appearance. Severely affected patients may have short stature and restrictive lung disease [20,21]. Histological examination of affected skin reveals dermal thickening due to increased amounts of collagen [20]. The thickened dermis contains collagen fibres that are heavily glycosylated [20].

Although several reports suggest an association between the onset of limited joint mobility and duration of disease [17,19,22], limited joint mobility has occurred prior to the onset of diabetes or shortly thereafter [18,23]. There does not appear to be any association between the incidence of limited joint mobility and the sex of the patient, the age of onset of the diabetes or the control of the diabetes [18,19]. Notably, one study did find that patients with limited joint mobility were at much higher risk of developing microvascular complications later in life [18].

Necrobiosis lipoidica diabeticorum. NLD usually follows but may precede the diagnosis of diabetes mellitus in children [10]. It is characteristically located over the pretibial areas but may be found elsewhere on the body such as the trunk, limbs, face and scalp. NLD characteristically begins as a well-defined, asymptomatic, erythematous papule or nodule. The lesion slowly enlarges to produce a plaque with a raised rim and slightly depressed centre (Fig. 25.10.9). The edge is usually more erythematous than the centre and may be smooth or scaly in appearance. The slightly depressed centre of the plaque has a waxy, atrophic appearance and can vary from yellowish brown to orange in colour. Atrophy is associated with ulceration that can be slow to heal. NLD can manifest as a solitary lesion or many lesions over the pretibial area.

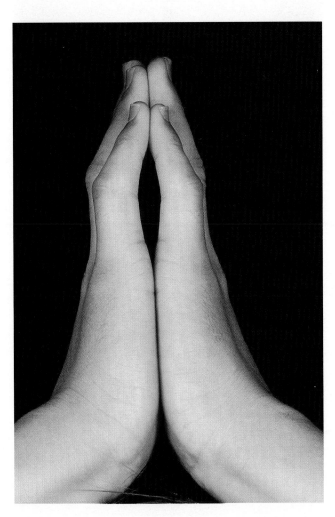

Fig. 25.10.8 Limited joint mobility in a child with insulin-dependent diabetes mellitus. Courtesy of Professor Martin Silink, New Children's Hospital, Sydney, Australia.

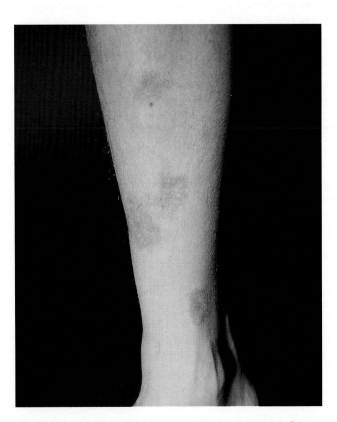

Fig. 25.10.9 Necrobiosis lipoidica on the legs in a teenager with insulin-dependent diabetes mellitus. Courtesy of Professor Martin Silink, New Children's Hospital, Sydney, Australia.

The area of involvement can vary from several centimetres to the entire pretibial region of the leg.

Treatment is required if the lesion has an active, expanding edge or develops surface ulceration. The active edge can be treated with high potency topical steroids under supervision or intralesional steroids. Ulceration is initially treated with regular dressings. Non-healing ulcers may require skin grafting. Although a combination of aspirin and dipyridamole were touted as effective treatments for NLD, a controlled study found no difference between placebo and the combination of aspirin and dipyridamole [24].

Diabetic dermopathy. Although this condition is extremely uncommon in children with diabetes mellitus, it has been reported [25]. The condition is characterized by reddish brown papules measuring less than 1–2 cm in diameter. These papules slowly regress to produce slightly depressed and slightly atrophic reddish brown macules. The macules may persist indefinitely or clear to leave normal skin. The pretibial area is the most commonly affected site but lesions may be found over the arms, thighs and trunk. Histological examination reveals a superficial perivascular infiltrate with overlying epidermal spongiosis and extravasation of red blood cells in some patients. The extravasated red blood cells give rise to haemosiderin pigmentation long term. No treatment is required.

Adverse reactions to therapy

Local side effects of insulin therapy. Local side-effects of insulin therapy manifest at the injection site as an allergic reaction, the development of soft tissue hypertrophy, the development of lipoatrophy or infection.

An allergic reaction at the injection site is characterized by warm, tender, indurated erythema associated with symptoms of burning, stinging and pruritus [26–28]. The reaction can develop immediately (15 min to several hours) after the injection or its onset can be delayed 6–8 h. Immediate reactions last from several hours to several days and delayed reactions usually take several days to settle. A combined reaction involving an immediate and delayed component has been noted in some patients. The diagnosis of insulin allergy can be confirmed by finding serum immunoglobulin E (IgE) antibodies to insulin and positive skin prick tests to the insulin preparation [29].

Soft tissue hypertrophy ('insulin tumours') can develop at sites of insulin injection [11,19,30] (Fig. 25.10.10). The hypertrophy clinically resembles lipomas with firm, non-tender, skin-coloured nodules. Histological examination reveals a mixture of adipose and fibrous tissue. Although the hypertrophy may resolve with rotation of injection sites, it can persist despite this manoeuvre. Diabetic children favour areas of tissue hypertrophy as injection sites because of the hypoaesthetic nature of the area. This should be discouraged because insulin absorption can be erratic from these sites resulting in poor disease control.

Lipoatrophy is more commonly seen in females and in children [11,19,31] (Fig. 25.10.11). Lipoatrophy usually occurs at the site of insulin injection but may develop away from the injection sites on the face, neck and chest. The incidence appears to have decreased with the introduction of highly purified insulin preparations. Some reports suggest that lipoatrophy may resolve with the injection of purified insulin into the periphery of the lipotrophic areas [32].

Poor sterile technique can result in the introduction of

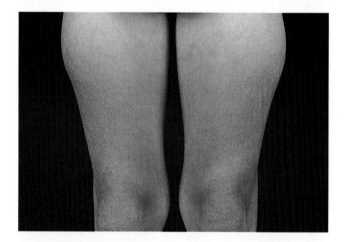

Fig. 25.10.10 Lipohypertrophy at the site of insulin injections. Courtesy of Professor Martin Silink, New Children's Hospital, Sydney, Australia.

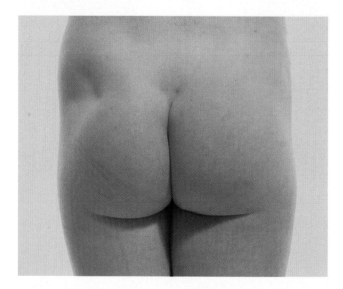

Fig. 25.10.11 Lipoatrophy at the site of insulin injections. Courtesy of Dr Geoff Ambler, New Children's Hospital, Sydney, Australia.

infection at the site of insulin injection. This can manifest as a localized abscess or as erysipelas/cellulitis. *Staphylococcus aureus* and *Streptococcus pyogenes* are the usual organisms. Sterile abscesses can occasionally occur at the site of insulin injection secondary to tissue breakdown.

Generalized reactions to insulin therapy. In contrast to local allergic reactions, generalized allergic reactions to insulin are very uncommon and have been reported with animal and human insulin [33–35]. The reaction usually occurs shortly after starting or restarting treatment and is typically urticarial in appearance. Occasionally, the eruption can be purpuric in appearance, accompanied by the features of a serum sickness-like illness or anaphylactic in type. The widespread reaction can be accompanied by a local reaction at the injection site. If insulin is required for management desensitization can be achieved using increasing doses of the least antigenic regular insulin (determined by prior skin testing) over several hours.

REFERENCES

1 Christy M. Studies of the HLA system and insulin dependent diabetes mellitus. *Diabetes Care* 1979; 2: 209–14.
2 Craighead JE. Viral diabetes mellitus in man and experimental animals. *Am J Med* 1981; 70: 127–35.
3 Lenmark A, Freedman ZR, Hofmann C *et al*. Islet cell surface antibodies in juvenile diabetes mellitus. *N Engl J Med* 1978; 299: 375–80.
4 Cahill GF, McDevitt HO. Insulin dependent diabetes mellitus: the initial lesion. *N Engl J Med* 1981; 304: 1454–65.
5 Shimada M, Taira M, Suzuki Y *et al*. Insulin resistant diabetes associated with partial deletion of insulin receptor gene. *Lancet* 1990; 335: 1179–81.
6 Kusari J, Takata Y, Hatada E *et al*. Insulin resistance and diabetes due to different mutations in the tyrosine kinase domain of both insulin receptor gene alleles. *J Biol Chem* 1991; 266: 5260–7.
7 Flier JS, Kahn CR, Roth J *et al*. Antibodies that impair insulin receptor binding in an unusual diabetic syndrome with severe insulin resistance. *Science* 1975; 190: 63–5.
8 Pusineri S, Alfis M. Presence of glycosylated collagen in the skin of diabetic patients. *Diabetologica* 1982; 23: 303.
9 Chang K, Uitto J, Rowold EA *et al*. Increased collagen cross linkages in experimental diabetes. *Diabetes* 1980; 29: 778–81.
10 Muller SA, Winkelmann RK. Necrobiosis lipoidica diabeticorum: a clinical and pathological investigation of 171 cases. *Arch Dermatol* 1966; 93: 272–81.
11 Edidin DV. Cutaneous manifestations of diabetes mellitus in children. *Pediatr Dermatol* 1985; 2: 161–79.
12 Merritt WT, Bass JW, Bruhn FW. Malignant external otitis in an adolescent with diabetes. *J Pediatr* 1980; 96: 872–3.
13 Joachims HZ. Malignant external otitis in children. *Arch Otolaryngol* 1976; 102: 236–7.
14 Harris JS. Mucormycosis. Report of a case. *Pediatrics* 1955; 16: 857–67.
15 Figueroa-Damian R, Torres-Gonzalez FE. Zygomycosis in childhood. A report of two cases. *Bol Med Hosp Infant Mex* 1993; 50: 813–18.
16 Edwards JE, Tillman DB, Miller ME *et al*. Infection and diabetes mellitus. *West J Med* 1979; 130: 515–21.
17 Grgic A, Rosenblum AL, Weber FT *et al*. Joint contracture—common manifestation of childhood diabetes mellitus. *J Pediatr* 1976; 88: 584–8.
18 Rosenbloom AL, Silverstein JH, Lezotte DC *et al*. Limited joint mobility in childhood diabetes mellitus indicates increased risk for microvascular disease. *N Engl J Med* 1981; 305: 191–4.
19 Kakourou T, Dacou-Voutetakis C, Kavadias G *et al*. Limited joint mobility and lipodystrophy in children and adolescents with insulin dependent diabetes mellitus. *Pediatr Dermatol* 1994; 11: 310–14.
20 Buckingham BA, Uitto J, Sandborg C *et al*. Scleroderma-like syndrome and the non-enzymatic glycosylation of collagen in children with poorly controlled insulin dependent diabetes (IDDM). *Pediatr Res* 1981; 15: 626.
21 Buckingham BA, Uitto J, Sandborg C *et al*. Scleroderma like changes in insulin dependent diabetes mellitus: clinical and biochemical studies. *Diabetes Care* 1984; 7: 163–9.
22 Starkman H, Brink S. Limited joint mobility of the hand in type 1 diabetes mellitus. *Diabetes Care* 1982; 10: 874–8.
23 Sherry DD, Rothstein RRL, Petty RE. Joint contractures preceding insulin dependent diabetes mellitus. *Arthritis Rheum* 1982; 25: 1362–4.
24 Stratham B, Finlay AY, Marks R. A randomised double blind comparison of aspirin and dipyridamole combination versus a placebo in the treatment of necrobiosis lipoidica. *Acta Derm Venereol (Stockh)* 1981; 61: 270–1.
25 Fisher ER, Danowski TS. Histologic, histochemical and electron microscopic features of the shin spots of diabetes mellitus. *Am J Clin Pathol* 1968; 50: 547–54.
26 Palcy RG, Tunbridge RE. Dermal reactions in insulin therapy. *Diabetes* 1952; 1: 22–7.
27 Kahn CR, Rosenthal AS. Immunologic reactions to insulin: insulin allergy, insulin resistance and the autoimmune insulin syndrome. *Diabetes Care* 1979; 2: 283–95.
28 Small P, Lerman S. Human insulin allergy. *Ann Allergy* 1984; 53: 39–41.
29 Patterson R, Mellies CJ, Roberts M. Immunologic reactions against insulin. 2. IgE anti-insulin, insulin allergy and combined IgE and IgG immunologic insulin resistance. *J Immunol* 1973; 110: 1135–45.
30 Johnson DA, Parlette HL. Insulin induced hypertrophic lipodystrophy. *Cutis* 1983; 32: 273–5.
31 Reeves WG, Allen BR, Tattersall RB. Insulin induced lipoatrophy: evidence for an immune pathogenesis. *Br Med J* 1980; 280: 1500–3.
32 Ferland L, Ehrlich RM. Single peak insulin in the treatment of insulin induced fat atrophy. *J Pediatr* 1975; 86: 741–3.
33 Hanauer L, Batson JM. Anaphylactic shock following insulin injection. Case report and review of the literature. *Diabetes* 1961; 10: 105–9.
34 Lieberman P, Patterson R, Metz R *et al*. Allergic reactions to insulin. *J Am Med Assoc* 1971; 215: 1106–12.
35 Galloway JA, Bressler R. Insulin treatment in diabetes. *Med Clin N Am* 1978; 62: 663–80.

Hypopituitarism

Pathogenesis

Hypopituitarism refers to a global decrease in the secretion of pituitary hormones. In children, this is usually due to an adenoma or craniopharyngioma. Uncommon causes include histiocytosis-X, sarcoidosis, a postpartum haemorrhage with hypotension and pituitary infarction and infection (tuberculosis) [1].

Clinical features

The effect of various hormone deficiencies is less pronounced in hypopituitarism compared with individual deficiencies, e.g. thyrotropin deficiency or ACTH deficiency [1]. Prepubertal children usually present with growth failure due to growth hormone deficiency and the features of hypogonadism due to gonadotropin deficiency. Postpubertal individuals usually present with failure of progression of puberty in both sexes and menstrual irregularities in females. The features of hypothyroidism and adrenal insufficiency appear late in the course of the illness.

The mucocutaneous findings relate to specific hormone deficiencies and are only seen with established cases. The skin findings include pallor, soft texture, absence or lack of terminal hair, fine wrinkling, diminished sebaceous gland activity, diminished hair and nail growth, onycholysis and longitudinal ridging of the nail plates. One report noted a solitary, central upper incisor in a boy with growth hormone deficiency [2].

Investigations

The clinical diagnosis is confirmed by measuring the plasma levels of the various anterior pituitary hormones. Imaging studies are usually undertaken to exclude a pituitary tumour.

Prognosis

The prognosis is determined by the underlying cause.

Treatment

Most patients require life-long hormone replacement therapy after treatment for the pituitary lesion.

REFERENCES

1 Thorner MO, Vance ML, Horvall E, Kovacs K. The anterior pituitary. In: Wilson JD, Foster DW, eds. *Williams Textbook of Endocrinology*, 8th edn. Philadelphia: WB Saunders, 1992: 221–310.
2 Rappaport EB, Ulstrom RA, Gorlin RJ *et al*. Solitary maxillary central incisor and short stature. *J Pediatr* 1977; 91: 924–8.

Growth hormone excess

Pathogenesis

Acromegaly and gigantism are terms that are used in relation to the oversecretion of growth hormone from the anterior pituitary gland. Gigantism is used when growth hormone excess occurs in children and adolescence prior to the closure of the epiphyseal plates. Acromegaly refers to the clinical picture that develops with hypersecretion of growth hormone after the closure of the epiphyseal plates.

Hypersecretion of growth hormone is usually due to a benign pituitary adenoma. Approximately 50% of these patients have a mutation in the α-chain of the Gs protein complex within the guanosine triphosphate (GTP) binding domain [1]. This impairs the GTPase activity of Gs-α with a constitutive increase in the production and release of growth hormone. Hypersecretion of growth hormone can also occur with the McCune–Albright syndrome [2], hypothalamic dysfunction [3] and ectopic production of growth hormone-releasing hormone [4].

Clinical features

Gigantism is characterized by excessive linear growth without concomitant advancement of bone age [5–7].

Although acromegalic changes in children are uncommon with growth hormone hypersecretion, they can accompany the gigantism [5–7]. The acromegalic changes consist of enlargement of the hands, feet, ears, nose, lips and tongue, puffiness of the eyelids, mandibular enlargement with separation of the teeth and malocclusion of the bite. The enlargement of facial structures results in a coarsening of facial features. Children with large pituitary tumours may also manifest features of hypogonadism and hypothyroidism [5–7].

Investigations

The diagnosis is easily confirmed by demonstrating elevated plasma growth hormone levels.

Management

The preferred therapy is surgical removal or ablation of the pituitary lesion responsible for the hypersecretion of growth hormone. Postoperative hormone replacement therapy is usually required.

REFERENCES

1 Landis CA, Masters CB, Spada A *et al*. GTPase inhibiting mutations activate the alpha chain of Gs and stimulate adenyl cyclase in human pituitary tumours. *Nature* 1989; 340: 692–6.
2 Cuttler L, Jackson JA, Saeed Us-Zafar *et al*. Hypersecretion of growth hormone and prolactin in McCune–Albright syndrome. *J Clin Endocrinol Metab* 1989; 68: 1148–54.
3 Zimmerman D, Young WF, Ebersold MJ *et al*. *Gigantism due to Growth Hormone-Releasing Hormone (GRH) Excess and Pituitary Hyperplasia with Adenomatous Transformation: Program and Abstracts*. Bethesda, Maryland: Endocrine Society, 1991: 426.
4 Leveston SA, McKeel DW Jr, Buckley PJ *et al*. Acromegaly and Cushing's syndrome associated with a foregut carcinoid tumour. *J Clin Endocrinol Metab* 1981; 52: 682–9.
5 De Majo SF, Onativia A. Acromegaly and gigantism in a boy: comparison with three overgrown non-acromegalic children. *J Pediatr* 1960; 57: 382–90.
6 Spence HJ, Trias EP, Raiti S. Acromegaly in a nine and a half year old boy. Pituitary function studies before and after surgery. *Am J Dis Child* 1972; 123: 504–6.
7 AvRuskin TW, Sau K, Tang S *et al*. Childhood acromegaly: successful therapy with conventional radiation and effects of chlorpromazine on growth hormone and prolactin secretion. *J Clin Endocrinol Metab* 1973; 37: 380–8.

Growth hormone deficiency

See section on hypopituitarism (above).

Disorders of the parathyroid gland

Hypoparathyroidism

Pathogenesis

Hypoparathyroidism may develop as an idiopathic condition, in response to congenital absence of the parathyroid gland and secondary to damage or inadvertent removal of the parathyroids during thyroidectomy. The idiopathic form of hypoparathyroidism is believed to be an autoimmune disease because of the presence of antiparathyroid gland antibodies in the circulation and the well-recognized association between idiopathic hypoparathyroidism and other autoimmune-mediated diseases [1]. This association is referred to as the polyglandular autoimmune syndromes [2]. Hypoparathyroidism due to congenital absence of the parathyroid glands may be associated with hypoplasia of the thymus, immunological defects and cardiovascular defects (Di George's syndrome).

Clinical features

Onset of the symptoms and signs of hypoparathyroidism is determined by the underlying cause. The idiopathic group may appear at any age whilst the group due to congenital absence of the parathyroid gland appear shortly after birth. Hypoparathyroidism usually presents with hypocalcaemia-induced convulsions and/or a history of carpopedal spasm, muscle twitching, paraesthesias and laryngeal stridor [3]. Additional findings may include cataracts, papilloedema, defective dental enamel, dental hypoplasia, failure of adult teeth to erupt, intracranial calcification (especially basal ganglia), mental retardation and a history of constipation, emotional lability and irritability [3]. Cutaneous findings are very uncommon and take the form of dry skin, dry brittle hair, patchy scalp alopecia, thinning of the eyebrows, thin brittle nails with onychorrhexis and transverse leuconychia [4]. Beau's lines may be seen with severe hypocalcaemia following surgical removal of the parathyroid glands.

Paediatric patients with idiopathic hypoparathyroidism should be screened and closely followed for the type 1 polyglandular syndrome [2].

Investigations

The diagnosis is confirmed by measuring the serum calcium, phosphorus and parathyroid hormone levels. The calcium levels will be significantly decreased in association with raised serum phosphorus levels and reduced parathyroid hormone levels.

Management

Treatment is directed at restoring the serum levels of calcium and phosphate to normal. This may require intravenous calcium supplementation in the acute phase and the use of vitamin D preparations and calcium supplements on a long-term basis.

REFERENCES

1 Blizzard RM, Chee D, Davis W. The incidence of parathyroid and other antibodies in the sera of patients with idiopathic hypoparathyroidism. *Clin Exp Immunol* 1966; 1: 119–28.
2 Spinner MW, Blizzard RM, Childs B. Clinical and genetic heterogeneity in idiopathic Addison's disease and hypoparathyroidism. *J Clin Endocrinol* 1968; 28: 795–804.
3 Bronsky D, Kushner DS, Dubin A *et al.* Idiopathic hypoparathyroidism and pseudohypoparathyroidism: case reports and review of the literature. *Medicine* 1958; 37: 317–52.
4 Simpson JA. Dermatological changes in hypocalcaemia. *Br J Dermatol* 1954; 66: 1–15.

Albright's hereditary osteodystrophy, pseudohypoparathyroidism and pseudopseudohypoparathyroidism

Definition

Albright's hereditary osteodystrophy (AHO) is a clinical entity characterized by a particular skeletal phenotype and calcification/ossification of the skin. The skeletal phenotype consists of a round face, short stature, a stocky build and brachydactyly. Pseudohypoparathyroidism (PHP) refers to a clinical setting of hypocalcaemia, hyperphosphataemia and an elevated serum parathyroid level. Most of the patients with PHP exhibit the features of AHO. Pseudopseudohypoparathyroidism (PPHP) refers to patients with the features of AHO and normal serum calcium levels.

Pathogenesis

The metabolic changes of PHP (hypocalcaemia, hyperphosphataemia) are due to a failure of peripheral tissues (kidney, bone) to respond to circulating parathyroid hormone. Parathyroid hormone resistance can result from a variety of defects and patients have been divided into four groups (type 1a, 1b, 1c and 2) on the basis of the underlying defect [1]. The defect can be inherited in an autosomal dominant fashion [2]. Patients in group 1a have a reduction in the activity of a guanine nucleotide binding protein (Gs protein) which links the hormone receptor to the adenylate cyclase system [3]. Deficient Gs protein activity may be non-selective, resulting in tissue resistance to other hormones that operate through the adenylate cyclase system (e.g. thyroid-stimulating hormone, gonadotrophins) [4]. Patients in group 1b have normal Gs protein activity and selective parathyroid hormone resistance. These patients probably have a defect in the parathyroid hormone receptor [5]. Patients in group 1c have a defective adenylate cyclase catalytic subunit resulting in multiple hormone resistance (parathyroid hormone, thyroid-stimulating hormone, gonadotrophins) [6]. Patients in group 2 may have either a defective protein kinase or phosphate transport system distal to the adenylate cyclase system [7].

Although the relationship between PPHP and PHP remains unclear, the former condition is probably an incomplete expression of the latter. Evidence to support this belief is the coexistence of both entities within the same family [8], the presence of reduced Gs protein activity in patients with PPHP [9], the development of resistance to other hormones in patients with PPHP [10] and the report of a female with PPHP giving birth to a male who developed PHP during early infancy [11].

The mechanism involved in calcification and ossification of the skin is unknown. The identification of parathyroid hormone receptors on dermal fibroblasts suggests that parathyroid hormone or related peptides may contribute to the process [12].

Clinical features

Calcification/ossification of the skin can be the presenting feature in patients with PHP and PPHP [10,11,13]. The calcification/ossification can be present at birth or manifest during infancy or childhood as bluish macules, milia-like papules (Fig. 25.10.12), nodules or plaques [10,11,13,14]. Although the calcification/ossification can develop anywhere, there is a predilection for periarticular skin and sites of pressure and trauma [13,14]. The calcification will be accompanied by the other characteristic features of AHO; short stature, stocky build, round face and brachydactyly (particularly of the fourth and fifth fingers) (Fig. 25.10.13) [10,11,13,14]. Additional findings may include cataracts, dental anomalies (enamel defects, hypoplasia, failure of adult teeth to erupt), mental retardation, intracranial calcification (basal ganglia, falx, cerebrum) and the features of hypocalcaemia in patients with PHP (tetany, paraesthesias, muscle twitching, convulsions, laryngospasm) [14].

Patients with PHP can first present with convulsions and/or a history of carpopedal spasm, muscle twitching and paraesthesias induced by hypocalcaemia [14]. Examination will reveal the typical skeletal and cutaneous features of AHO.

Investigation

PHP patients will have hypocalcaemia, hyperphosphataemia, elevated serum parathyroid hormone levels and no increase in plasma and urine cyclic adenosine monophosphate (cAMP) levels with parathyroid injections [1,11,14]. Infants with AHO need close observation because it can take several years for the characteristic laboratory findings of PHP to develop [11,14]. PPHP patients will have normal serum calcium, phosphate and parathyroid hormone levels and an increase in plasma and urine cAMP levels with a parathyroid injection [10,11]. In view of the association between AHO (PHP and PPHP) and multiple hormone resistance [4,10], patients

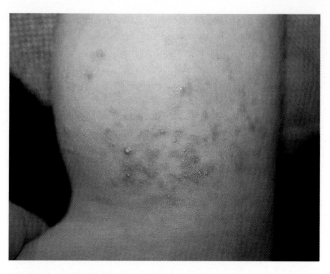

Fig. 25.10.12 Milia-like calcification of the leg in an infant with pseudohypoparathyroidism.

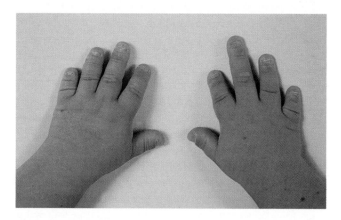

Fig. 25.10.13 Short fourth and fifth metacarpals in an infant with pseudohypoparathyroidism. Courtesy of Dr Geoff Ambler, New Children's Hospital, Sydney, Australia.

should be regularly screened for hypothyroidism and hypogonadism.

Management

Children with PHP require restriction of dietary phosphates and the administration of vitamin D and calcium supplements to increase the serum calcium level.

REFERENCES

1 Breslau NA. Pseudohypoparathyroidism: current concepts. *Am J Med Sci* 1989; 298: 130–40.
2 Van Dop C, Bourne HR, Neer RM. Father to son transmission of decreased N9 activity in pseudohypoparathyroidism type 1a. *J Clin Endocrinol Metab* 1984; 59: 825–8.
3 Spiegel AM, Levine MA, Aurbach GD *et al.* Deficiency of hormone receptor adenylate cyclase coupling protein. Basis for hormone resistance in pseudohypoparathyroidism. *Am J Physiol* 1982; 243: E37–E42.

4 Levine MA, Downs RW Jr, Moses AM *et al*. Resistance to multiple hormones in patients with pseudohypoparathyroidism and deficient guanine nucleotide regulatory protein. *Am J Med* 1983; 74: 545–6.

5 Silve C, Santora A, Breslau N *et al*. Selective resistance to parathyroid hormone in cultured skin fibroblasts in patients with pseudohypoparathyroidism type 1b. *J Clin Endocrinol Metab* 1986; 62: 640–4.

6 Barrett D, Breslau NA, Wax MB *et al*. A new form of pseudohypoparathyroidism with abnormal catalytic adenylate cyclase. *Am J Physiol (Endocrinol Metab)* 1989; 257: E277–E83.

7 Drezner M, Neelon FA. Pseudohypoparathyroidism type 2: a possible defect in the reception of the cyclic AMP signal. *N Engl J Med* 1973; 289: 1056–60.

8 Mann JB, Alterman S, Hills AG. Albright's hereditary osteodystrophy comprising pseudohypoparathyroidism and pseudopseudohypoparathyroidism with a report of two cases representing the complete syndrome occurring in successive generations. *Ann Intern Med* 1962; 56: 315–42.

9 Levine MA, Jap TS, Mauseth RS *et al*. Activity of the stimulatory guanine nucleotide binding protein is reduced in erythrocytes from patients with pseudohypoparathyroidism and pseudopseudohypoparathyroidism: biochemical, endocrine and genetic analysis of Albright hereditary osteodystrophy in six kindreds. *J Clin Endocrinol Metab* 1986; 62: 497–502.

10 Izraeli S, Metzker A, Horev G *et al*. Albright hereditary osteodystrophy with hypothyroidism, normocalcaemia and normal Gs protein activity: a family presenting with congenital osteoma cutis. *Am J Med Genet* 1992; 43: 764–7.

11 Barr DGD, Stirling HF, Darling JAB. Evolution of pseudohypoparathyroidism: an informative family study. *Arch Dis Child* 1994; 70: 337–8.

12 Silve C, Santora A, Spiegel A. A factor produced by cultured rat Leydig tumour (Rice 500) cells associated with humoral hypercalcaemia stimulates adenosine 3'5'-monophosphate production via the parathyroid hormone receptor in human skin fibroblasts. *J Clin Endocrinol Metab* 1985; 60: 1144–7.

13 Prendiville JS, Lucky AW, Mallory SB *et al*. Osteoma cutis as a presenting sign of pseudohypoparathyroidism. *Pediatr Dermatol* 1992; 9: 11–18.

14 Bronsky D, Kushner DS, Dubin A *et al*. Idiopathic hypoparathyroidism and pseudohypoparathyroidism: case reports and review of the literature. *Medicine* 1958; 37: 317–52.

Hyperparathyroidism

Pathogenesis

Primary hyperparathyroidism in the paediatric age group is due to hyperplasia of the parathyroid gland, parathyroid adenoma or rarely, a parathyroid carcinoma [1]. Parathyroid hyperplasia is responsible for most cases of hyperparathyroidism seen during the first 12 months of life [1]. Parathyroid adenoma and rarely carcinoma are responsible for most cases over 12 months of age [1,2]. Hyperparathyroidism due to parathyroid adenoma or hyperplasia may be associated with other endocrine tumours (multiple endocrine neoplasia (MEN) syndromes).

Clinical features

Most paediatric patients with hyperparathyroidism present with non-specific symptoms such as failure to thrive, anorexia, nausea, vomiting, constipation, lethargy, headache, polydipsia, polyuria, irritability and inability to concentrate [1–4]. Occasionally, patients present with bone pain, bone fractures, bone deformities (e.g. genu valgum) or symptoms and signs of nephrolithiasis [1–4]. The skin is rarely affected.

Investigations

The diagnosis of hyperthyroidism is confirmed with elevated serum calcium levels, reduced serum phosphate levels and elevated parathyroid hormone levels. Characteristic radiological findings include demineralization of the bones, destructive changes of the growing ends of long bones and subperiosteal erosions (phalanges, metacarpals and lateral portions of the clavicles). Ultrasound may reveal nephrolithiasis.

Management

The treatment of hyperparathyroidism requires subtotal or complete parathyroidectomy with careful postoperative management of calcium levels.

REFERENCES

1 Norwood S, Andrassy RJ. Primary hyperparathyroidism in children: a review. *Mil Med* 1083; 148: 812–14.

2 Allo M, Thompson NW, Harkness JK *et al*. Primary hyperparathyroidism in children, adolescents and young adults. *World J Surg* 1982; 6: 771–6.

3 Girard RM, Belanger A, Hazel B. Primary hyperparathyroidism in children. *Canad J Surg* 1982; 25: 11–13.

4 Rapaport D, Ziv Y, Rubin M *et al*. Primary hyperparathyroidism in children. *J Pediatr Surg* 1986; 21: 395–7.

Polyglandular autoimmune syndromes

The polyglandular autoimmune syndromes (PGAS) refer to autoimmune-mediated dysfunction of two or more endocrine glands in a particular individual. The endocrine dysfunction involves either an increase or decrease in glandular activity and is associated with circulating autoantibodies specific for the affected gland. The endocrine abnormalities can be accompanied by one or more non-endocrine autoimmune diseases (e.g. pernicious anaemia). The PGAS have been divided into three types on the basis of clinical associations (Table 25.10.3) [1].

Type 1 usually manifests before 15 years of age [2–4]. Hypoparathyroidism (89%) and chronic mucocutaneous candidiasis (CMCC) (75%) are the most common manifestations of the disease and are found together in approximately 70% of patients [4]. The complete triad of hypoparathyroidism, CMCC and Addison's disease (60%) is found in only 30% of patients [4]. Hypoparathyroidism and CMCC usually manifest by 5 years of age and invariably precede the onset of Addison's disease by many years [2–4]. Additional endocrine abnormalities include primary gonadal failure (45%), thyroid disease (usually hypothyroidism: 12%) and rarely, insulin-dependent diabetes mellitus [3,4]. Non-endocrine findings may include malabsorption (25%), alopecia areata (20%), pernicious anaemia (16%), chronic active hepatitis (9%) and vitiligo (4%) [4]. Familial aggregation is found in

Table 25.10.3 Polyglandular autoimmune syndromes

Type 1
  hypopituitarism
  chronic mucocutaneous candidiasis
  Addison's disease
  hypogonadism
  autoimmune thyroid disease
  malabsorption
  pernicious anaemia
  chronic active hepatitis
  alopecia areata
  vitiligo

Type 2
  Addison's disease
  autoimmune disease
  insulin-dependent diabetes mellitus
  hypogonadism
  alopecia areata
  vitiligo
  myasthenia gravis
  Sjögren's syndrome

Table 25.10.4 MEN syndromes

Type 1 (Werner's syndrome)
  parathyroid adenoma or hyperplasia
  pituitary adenoma
  pancreatic islet cell tumours
  carcinoid tumours
  adrenal adenoma
  thyroid adenoma
  facial angiofibromas
  collagenomas

Type 2a (Sipple's syndrome)
  parathyroid hyperplasia
  phaeochromocytoma
  medullary carcinoma of the thyroid
  cutaneous amyloidosis

Type 2b (multiple mucosal neuroma syndrome)
  multiple mucosal neuromas
  phaechromocytoma
  medullary thyroid carcinoma
  marfanoid habitus
  gastrointestinal ganglioneuromatosis
  café-au-lait spots and lentigines

approximately 50% of cases with an autosomal recessive pattern of inheritance [2,4]. Unlike the type 2 form which is associated with HLA antigens B8 and DR3/DR4 [5,6], there are no HLA associations with the type 1 form of PGAS [7]. The prognosis is good provided the endocrine disorders are diagnosed and promptly treated.

The type 2 and type 3 syndromes are principally diseases of the adult population. With the exception of primary gonadal failure (type 2) which can manifest prior to the onset of adult life, all of the other endocrine disorders develop during adult life.

REFERENCES

1 Leshin M. Southwestern internal medicine conference: polyglandular autoimmune syndromes. *Am J Med Sci* 1985; 290: 77–88.
2 Spinner MW, Blizzard RM, Childs B. Clinical and genetic heterogeneity in idiopathic Addison's disease and hypoparathyroidism. *J Clin Endocrinol* 1968; 28: 795–804.
3 Neufeld M, MacLaren NK, Blizzard RM. Two types of autoimmune Addison's disease associated with different polyglandular autoimmune (PGA) syndromes. *Medicine* 1981; 60: 355–62.
4 Brun JM. Juvenile autoimmune polyendocrinopathy. *Hormone Res* 1982; 16: 308–16.
5 Farid NR, Larsen B, Payne R *et al.* Polyglandular autoimmune disease and HLA. *Tissue Antigens* 1980; 16: 23–9.
6 Butler MG, Hodes ME, Conneally PM *et al.* Linkage analysis in a large kindred with autosomal dominant transmission of polyglandular autoimmune disease type 2 (Schmidt syndrome). *Am J Med Genet* 1984; 18: 61–5.
7 Wirfalt A. Genetic heterogeneity in autoimmune polyglandular failure. *Acta Med Scand* 1981; 210: 7–13.

Multiple endocrine neoplasia syndromes

MEN refers to the presence of hyperplastic and/or neoplastic changes in two or more endocrine glands in a particular patient. Three MEN syndromes have been defined on the basis of clinical findings (Table 25.10.4) [1–3]. MEN type 1 is inherited in an autosomal dominant fashion with high penetrance [1]. The genetic defect has been localized to chromosome 11q13[4]. MEN type 2a and 2b are inherited in an autosomal dominant fashion with variable penetrance and expression [2,3]. The genetic defects responsible for type 2a and 2b are located in the pericentromeric region of chromosome 10 [5,6].

Of the three syndromes, type 2b is most relevant to paediatric practice. Type 2b is characterized by mucosal neuromas (100%), medullary thyroid carcinoma (>90%), a marfinoid body habitus (60–75%), phaeochromocytoma (50%) and gastrointestinal ganglioneuromatosis (>30%) [3,7–11]. The mucosal neuromas are evident at birth or appear during infancy or early childhood [3,7–9]. They manifest as a pebbly thickening of the lips and sessile or pedunculated papules on the tongue (Fig. 25.10.14), buccal mucosa, gingivae, palate, pharyngeal mucosa, conjunctiva, eyelid margins and skin. The marfinoid habitus consists of tall stature, long, thin limbs and an elongated face [3,7,10]. Unlike Marfan's syndrome, the patients do not have ectopia lentis or aortic abnormalities. Gastrointestinal ganglioneuromatosis results in chronic constipation or chronic diarrhoea, feeding problems and abdominal pain [3,7,11]. The gastrointestinal symptoms can begin shortly after birth and usually precede the diagnosis of endocrine neoplasia by many years. Additional findings may include circumoral lentiginosis, café-au-lait spots, diffuse pigmentation of the hands and feet, large prominent eyebrows, thickening of the corneal nerves, arched palate and a number of musculoskeletal abnormalities (kyphosis, scoliosis, lordosis, pes cavus,

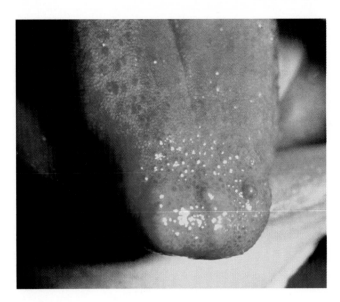

Fig. 25.10.14 Mucosal neuromas on the dorsum of the tongue in a patient with MEN type 2b. Courtesy of Dr Geoff Ambler, New Children's Hospital, Sydney, Australia.

slipped femoral epiphysis, proximal muscle weakness) [3,7,8,11].

A number of reports since 1989 have noted the association between MEN type 2a and cutaneous amyloidosis located unilaterally or bilaterally over the upper back [12–15]. The cutaneous amyloidosis is pruritic and consists of hyperpigmentation, scaling and small papules. Although the clinical appearance fits best with macular amyloidosis, the presence of papules and the histological findings of hyperkeratosis, acanthosis and papillomatosis is more suggestive of lichen amyloidosis. In most patients, the diagnosis of cutaneous amyloidosis preceded the diagnosis of MEN type 2A.

A recent clinical assessment of 30 patients with MEN type 1 found that 87% had multiple facial angiofibromas, 66% had one or more white or skin-coloured collagenomas measuring 3–10 mm in diameter, 40% had café-au-lait spots and 30% had lipomas [16]. The association between facial angiofibromas, collagenomas and MEN type 1 has not been previously reported.

REFERENCES

1 Wermer P. Endocrine adenomatosis and peptic ulcer in a large kindred. Inherited multiple tumours and mosaic pleiotropism in man. *Am J Med* 1963; 35: 205–12.
2 Sipple JH. The association of phaeochromocytoma with carcinoma of the thyroid gland. *Am J Med* 1961; 31: 163–6.
3 Carney JA, Sizemore GW, Hayles AV. C-cell disease of the thyroid gland in multiple endocrine neoplasia type 2B. *Cancer* 1979; 44: 2173–83.
4 Larsson C, Skogseid B, Oberg K *et al*. Multiple endocrine neoplasia type 1 gene maps to chromosome 11 and is lost in insulinoma. *Nature* 1988; 332: 85–7.
5 Simpson NE, Kidd KK, Goodfellow PJ *et al*. Assignment of multiple endocrine neoplasia type 2A to chromosome 10 by linkage. *Nature* 1987; 328: 528–30.
6 Jackson CE, Norum RA. Genetics of the multiple endocrine neoplasia type 2B syndrome. *Henry Ford Hosp Med J* 1992; 40: 232–5.
7 Gorlin RJ, Cohen MM, Levin LS. Hamartoneoplastic syndromes. In: *Syndromes of the Head and Neck*. New York: Oxford University Press, 1990: 385–92.
8 Nasir MA, Yee RW, Piest KL *et al*. Multiple endocrine neoplasia type 3. *Cornea* 1991; 10: 454–9.
9 Schenberg ME, Zajac JD, Lim-Tio S *et al*. Multiple endocrine neoplasia syndrome type 2B. *Int J Oral Maxillofac Surg* 1992; 21: 110–14.
10 Carney JA, Bianco AJJ, Sizemore GW *et al*. Multiple endocrine neoplasia with skeletal manifestations. *J Bone Joint Surg Am* 1981; 3: 405–8.
11 Carney JA, Hayles AB. Alimentary tract manifestations of multiple endocrine neoplasia type 2B. *Mayo Clin Proc* 1977; 52: 543–8.
12 Nunziata V, Di Giovanni G, Lettera AM *et al*. Cutaneous lichen amyloidosis associated with multiple endocrine neoplasia type 2A. *Henry Ford Hosp Med J* 1989; 37: 144–6.
13 Kousseff BG, Espinoza C, Zamore GA. Sipple syndrome with lichen amyloidosis as a paracrinopathy: pleiotropy, heterogeneity or a contiguous gene? *J Am Acad Dermatol* 1991; 25: 651–7.
14 Robinson MF, Furst FJ, Nunziata V *et al*. Characterisation of the clinical features of five families with hereditary primary cutaneous lichen amyloidosis and multiple endocrine neoplasia type 2. *Henry Ford Hosp Med J* 1992; 40: 249–52.
15 Pacini F, Fugazzola L, Bevilacqua G *et al*. Multiple endocrine neoplasia type 2A and cutaneous lichen amyloidosis: description of a new family. *Endocrinol Invest* 1993; 16: 295–6.
16 Turner ML, Darling TN, Skarulis M. Facial angiofibromas and collagenomas in patients with multiple endocrine neoplasia type 1. *J Invest Dermatol* 1996; 106: 889.

The Carney complex

The Carney complex refers to the association of myxomas (cardiac, cutaneous, mammary fibroadenomas), spotty mucocutaneous pigmentation, endocrine abnormalities and psammomatous schwannomas [1–6]. Endocrine abnormalities include Cushing's syndrome secondary to nodular adrenal hyperplasia, androgen excess due to Sertoli cell tumour of the testicle and gigantism/acromegaly due to a pituitary adenoma. Approximately 50% of the patients have a family history of the disease with an autosomal dominant pattern of inheritance [3].

The mucocutaneous features of the disease can be the earliest clinical findings and often manifest during infancy and childhood [1–5]. Lentigines and/or blue naevi are responsible for the spotty mucocutaneous pigmentation [1]. Lesions vary in number and are usually distributed on the face (periocular, nose, perioral), vermilion borders of the lips, eyelids and ears. Some patients will also have lesions on the trunk, limbs, backs of the hands, vulva and conjunctiva. Cutaneous myxoma's manifest as flesh-coloured, sessile or pedunculated papules that are usually less than 1 cm in diameter [1–4]. Although they are usually smooth, they can have a rough, papillomatous surface. Most patients have multiple lesions distributed, in order of frequency, on the eyelid [3], in the external ear canal [4], on the face, neck, trunk, anogenital area, upper limb and lower limb. The hands and feet were notably spared [1,2]. Other cutaneous findings include subcutaneous nodules due to cutaneous psammomatous schwannomas [5,6], the effects of embolization from left ventricular myxomas and the effects of coexistent endocrine disease [1].

REFERENCES

1 Carney JA, Gordon H, Carpenter PC *et al.* The complex of myxomas, spotty pigmentation and endocrine over activity. *Medicine (Balt)* 1985; 64: 270–83.
2 Carney JA, Headington JT, Su DWP. Cutaneous myxomas. A major component of the complex of myxomas, spotty pigmentation and endocrine over activity. *Arch Dermatol* 1986; 122: 790–8.
3 Carney JA, Hruska LS, Beauchamp GD *et al.* Dominant inheritance of the complex of myxomas, spotty pigmentation and endocrine over activity. *Mayo Clin Proc* 1986; 61: 165–72.
4 Kennedy RH, Flanagan JC, Eagles RC Jr *et al.* The Carney complex with ocular signs suggestive of cardiac myxoma. *Am J Ophthalmol* 1991; 111: 699–702.
5 Ferreiro JA, Carney JA. Myxomas of the external ear and their significance. *Am J Surg Pathol* 1994; 18: 274–80.
6 Carney JA. Psammomatous melanotic schwannoma. A distinctive, heritable tumour with special associations, including cardiac myxoma and the Cushing syndrome. *Am J Surg Pathol* 1990; 14: 206–22.

25.11 Morphoea

HELGA ALBRECHT-NEBE
AND JOHN HARPER

Definition

Morphoea or localized scleroderma is a connective tissue disorder of unknown aetiology characterized by sclerosis of the skin and subcutaneous tissue [1–3], often affecting the underlying muscle and bone. It must be distinguished from systemic sclerosis (or scleroderma) which is a multi-system disease; secondary internal organ involvement with morphoea is exceptional [4].

History

In 1854 Addison described areas of induration of the skin, called Addison's keloid. The term 'morphoea' was first introduced by Wilson [5]. However, he interpreted the disorder as leprosy. In 1868 Fagge [6] defined Addison's keloid as morphoea. He differentiated it from Alibert's keloid (true keloid) [5] and described the different forms of localized scleroderma, including the 'en coup de sabre' variant. In 1942 Klemperer *et al.* [7] included scleroderma in the group of collagen diseases. Similarities in the pathogenesis of localized and generalized scleroderma stimulated the discussion on the rare chance of the transfer of morphoea into systemic scleroderma.

REFERENCES

1 Vancheeswaran R, Black CM, David J *et al.* Childhood-onset scleroderma. *Arthritis Rheum* 1996; 39: 1041–9.
2 Jablonska S, Chorzelski T, Blaszczyk M. Pathogenesis of scleroderma. In: Jablonska S, ed. *Scleroderma and Pseudoscleroderma*. Warsaw: Polish Medical Publishers, 1975: 15–138.
3 Falanga V. Localised scleroderma. *Med Clin N Am* 1989; 73: 1143–56.
4 Birdi N, Laxer RM, Thorner P *et al.* Localised scleroderma progressing to systemic disease. Case report and review of the literature. *Arthritis Rheum* 1993; 36: 410–15.
5 Fox TC. Note on the history of scleroderma in England. *Br J Dermatol* 1892; 4: 101–4.
6 Fagge CH. On keloid scleriasis, morphoea. *Guy's Hosp Rep Sev* 1868; 3: 255.
7 Klemperer P, Pollack AD, Baehr G. Diffuse collagen disease. Acute lupus erythematosus and diffuse scleroderma. *J Am Med Assoc* 1942; 119: 331–2.

Pathogenesis

The aetiology of morphoea is still unknown. Correlations between the manifestation of the disease and trauma [1,2], endocrine changes [3], hormonal factors [4] and the coexistence with abnormalities in the vertebral column and the nervous system [5,6] have been documented. Morphoea has also been described after bacille Calmette–Guèrin (BCG) vaccination [7].

Infectious factors have been suspected, because morphoea has been noted to start after viral and bacterial infections, such as *Borrelia burgdorferi* infection and Epstein–Barr virus infection [8]. The detection of spirochaetal organisms in the lesions of morphoea supported the possibility of *B. burgdorferi* infection [9,10]; however, further studies have not substantiated this finding [11,12].

An association with other autoimmune diseases, such as lupus erythematosus [7,13] in relatives of patients, is perhaps indicative of an autoimmune pathogenesis. This hypothesis is also supported by the findings of lympho-histiocytic infiltrates around blood vessels and a high incidence of autoantibodies in this group of patients [14]. However, autoantibodies may be a secondary phenomenon [15].

Another hypothesis is that the collagen synthesis by fibroblasts is stimulated by a soluble factor released by lymphocytes [16]. The findings of elevated serum soluble interleukin-2 receptor (sIL-2R) indicate cell-mediated immune activation. This can cause an overproduction of collagen in the active phase of the disease [17]. Activation of the immune system by an unidentified antigen may result in cytokine release and a cascade of events [17]. This cascade stimulates fibroblast proliferation, excessive collagen production, loss of subcutaneous tissue, fibrosis and secondary deformity. Stimulating factors of fibroblast hyperproliferation, include IL-1 that can modulate fibroblast metabolism [18] and lymphokines and stimulate collagen synthesis [19]. Osteonectin, a potent activator of collagen synthesis, activates fibroblasts [20]. The impairment of collagen metabolism by connective tissue fibroblasts is established [21] by increased accumulation of collagen types I, III and IV and glycosaminoglycan in lesions of morphoea [22]. HLA class II positive fibroblasts in lesions of morphoea synthesize a larger quantity of collagen than HLA class II negative fibroblasts. The expression of HLA class II antigens correlates with activation and proliferation of these cells [23]. Enhanced collagen expression by cytokines elaborated by B cells near the inflammatory cells in skin lesions of localized scleroderma was observed [24]. The transforming growth factor β, elevated in skin lesions in patients with generalized morphoea, and IL-1 may play a role in the pathogenesis of cutaneous scleroderma [21].

Morphoea occurring as part of the spectrum of chronic graft-versus-host disease following bone marrow transplantion is also evidence in favour of an immune-based pathogenesis [25].

Morphoea can be familial, but this is rare. Morphoea was described in siblings [16,26,27] and in three or two generations of families [28,29]. Rees and Bennett have observed the simultaneous appearance of morphoea in a father and his daughter [30].

REFERENCES

1 Varga J, Jimenez SA. Development of severe limited scleroderma in complicated Raynaud's phenomenon after limb immobilization: Report of two cases and study of collagen biosynthesis. *Arthritis Rheum* 1986; 29: 1160–5.
2 Vancheeswaran R, Black CM, David J *et al.* Childhood-onset scleroderma. *Arthritis Rheum* 1996; 39: 1041–9.
3 Curtis AC, Jansen TG. The prognosis of localized scleroderma. *Arch Dermatol* 1958; 78: 749–57.
4 Ghersetich I, Teofoli P, Benci M, Innocenti S, Lotti T. Localized scleroderma. *Clin Dermatol* 1994; 12: 237–42.
5 Cassirer R. *Die vasomotorisch-trophischen Neurosen.* Berlin: Karger, 1912.
6 Littman BH. Linear scleroderma: a response to neurologic injury? Report and literature review. *J Rheumatol* 1989; 16: 1135–40.
7 Mork NJ. Clinical and histopathologic morphoea with immunological evidence of lupus erythematosus. *Acta Derm Vener* 1981; 61: 367–8.
8 Longo F, Saletta S, Lepore L, Pennesi M. Localized scleroderma after infection with Epstein–Barr virus. *Clin Exp Rheumatol* 1993; 11: 681–3.
9 Aberer E, Neumann R, Stanek G. Is localised scleroderma a *Borrelia* infection? *Lancet* 1985; ii: 273 (letter).
10 Aberer E, Stanek G. Histological evidence for spirochetal origin of morphea and lichen sclerosus et atrophicans. *Am J Dermatopathol* 1987; 9: 374–9.
11 Wienecke R, Schlüpen EM, Zöchling N *et al.* No evidence for *Borrelia burgdorferi*-specific DNA in lesions of localized scleroderma. *J Invest Dermatol* 1995; 104: 23–6.
12 Raguin G, Boisnic S, Souteyrand P *et al.* No evidence for a spirochaetal origin of localized scleroderma. *Br J Dermatol* 1992; 127: 218–20.
13 Mackel SE, Kozin F, Ryan LM *et al.* Concurrent linear scleroderma and systemic lupus erythematosus. A report of two cases. *J Invest Dermatol* 1979; 73: 368–72.
14 Krieg H, Meurer M. Systemic scleroderma. *J Am Acad Dermatol* 1988; 18: 457–81.
15 Falanga V, Medsger TA jr, Reichlin M, Rodnan GP. Linear scleroderma—clinical spectrum, prognosis, and laboratory abnormalities. *Ann Intern Med* 1986; 104: 849–57.
16 Panayi GS. *The Immunology of Connective Tissue Disorders.* In: Medicine (series 3, no. 14). London: Medicine Education (International), 1979: 686.
17 Uziel Y, Krafchik BR, Feldman B, Silverman ED, Rubin LA, Laxer RM. Serum levels of soluble interleukin-2 receptor. A marker of disease activity in localized scleroderma. *Arthritis Rheum* 1994; 372: 898–901.
18 Schmidt JA, Mizel SB, Cohen D *et al.* Interleukin 1 a potential regulator of fibroblast proliferation. *J Immunol* 1982; 5: 2177–82.
19 Johnson RL, Ziff M. Lymphokine stimulation of collagen accumulation. *J Clin Invest* 1976; 58: 240–52.
20 Vuorio T, Kahari VM, Black C, Vuorio E. Expression of osteonectin, decorin and transforming growth factor-beta 1 genes in fibroblasts cultured from patients with systemic sclerosis and morphea. *J Rheumatol* 1991; 18: 247–51.
21 Krafchik BR. Localized cutaneous scleroderma. *Semin Dermatol* 1992; 11: 65–72.
22 Perlish JS, Lemlich G, Fleischmajer R. Identification of collagen fibrils in scleroderma skin. *J Invest Dermatol* 1988; 90: 48–54.
23 Branchet MC, Boisnic S, Blétry O, Robert L, Charron D, Frances C. Expression of HLA class II antigens on skin fibroblasts in scleroderma. *Br J Dermatol* 1992; 126: 431–5.
24 Leroy EC, Smith EA, Kahaleh MB, Trojanowska M, Silver RM. A strategy for determining the pathogenesis of systemic sclerosis. Is transforming growth factor beta the answer? *Arthritis Rheum* 1989; 32: 817–25.
25 Harper JI. Graft versus host disease: etiological and clinical aspects in connective tissue diseases. *Semin Dermatol* 1985; 4: 144–51.
26 Burge KM, Perry HO, Stickler GB. 'Familial' scleroderma. *Arch Derm (Chicago)* 1969; 99: 681–7.
27 Kass H, Hanson V, Patrick J. Scleroderma in childhood. *J Pediatr* 1966; 68: 243–56.
28 Kulin P, Sybert VP. Hereditary hypotrichosis and localized morphea: a new clinical entity. *Pediatr Dermatol* 1986; 3: 333–8.
29 Wadud MA, Bose BK, Al Nasir T. Familial localised scleroderma from Bangladesh: two case reports. *Bangladesh Med Res Counc Bull Daeca* 1989; 15: 15–19.
30 Rees RB, Bennett J. Localized scleroderma in father and daughter. *Arch Dermatol* 1953; 68: 360.

Pathology

Morphoea is characterized by an early inflammatory stage with oedema and hyperaemia of the skin followed by fibrosis, sclerosis [1] and finally atrophy [2]. The epidermis may be unchanged or flattened [3]. In the initial stage the dermis shows oedema with swelling and degeneration of collagen fibrils and lymphocytic infiltration around small blood vessels and skin appendages [3,4]. Jablonska [5] described in detail the characteristic histological features in the different variants of the disease. There is a progressive increased thickness of the dermis with condensation of collagen and loss of dermal appendages. Elastic tissue may be fragmented. There is an homogenization of the collagen bundles parallel to the skin. Subcutaneous fat becomes replaced by hyalinized connective tissue. Subcutaneous calcification, myositis or myofibrosis and bone atrophy are possible sequelae. Electron microscopic studies have interpreted the homogenization of collagen as the result of an increased rate of collagen synthesis (neoformation of collagen), with an increased range of variation in the thickness of the collagen fibrils [6]. Immunoglobulin M (IgM) and C3 perivascular and basal membrane located deposits were described in the linear variant of cutaneous scleroderma [7].

REFERENCES

1 Krieg T, Braun-Falco O, Perlish JS, Fleischmajer R. Collagen synthesis in generalized morphea. *Arch Dermatol Res* 1983; 275: 393–6.
2 Black CM. Prognosis and management of scleroderma and scleroderma like disorders in children. *Clin Exp Rheumatol* 1994; 12(suppl 10): 75–81.
3 Ghersetich I, Teofoli P, Benci M *et al.* Localized scleroderma. *Clin Dermatol* 1994; 12: 237–42.
4 Krafchik BR. Localized cutaneous scleroderma. *Semin Dermatol* 1992; 11: 65–72.
5 Jablonska S. Histopathology of scleroderma. In: Jablonska S, ed. *Scleroderma and pseudoscleroderma.* Warsaw: Polish Medical Publishers, 1975: 191–233.

6 Krieg T. Zirhumshripte shlerodermic. In: Braun-Falco O, Plewig G, Wolff HH, eds. *Dermatologie und Venereologie*. Berlin: Springer Verlag, 1996: 724–8.
7 Vincent F, Prokopetz R, Miller RAW. Plasma cell panniculitis: a unique clinical and pathologic presentation of linear scleroderma. *J Am Acad Dermatol* 1989; 21: 357–60.

Clinical features

In childhood, morphoea is more common than systemic sclerosis and shows a greater variety of clinical presentation than in adults. The linear variant is more often found. The different types of morphoea, as discussed in this chapter, are as follows: morphoea 'en plaque'; linear morphoea; 'en coup de sabre' morphoea; generalized morphoea; and the rare disabling pansclerotic morphoea. Other forms which have been described, such as guttate morphoea and subcutaneous morphoea, are to be considered variants of the above subsets and highlight the difficulty in classification and the range of overlap between the different clinical types [1–5].

After an initial erythematous patch, a yellow/white elevated or depressed plaque develops surrounded by a blue/violet erythema (the so-called 'lilac ring'). The process develops into a more solid infiltration of the skin, resulting in atrophy with loss of hair and sebaceous glands and hyper- or hypopigmentation. Morphoea is usually a self-limiting disease. The disease may be associated with joint contractures, extremity deformity and impairment of function. Usually morphoea begins in children at early school age, sometimes even at preschool age, but rarely before then [6,7]. The female to male ratio varies between 1.5 : 1 and 3 : 1 in childhood [8]. The initial stage of the disease may be unnoticed. The progression varies and is dependent on the clinical type; rapidly in the case of the linear variant on the limbs and more gradually with the plaque-type.

Morphoea 'en plaque'

This variant is less common in children than in adults. The skin lesion is most frequently localized on the trunk with preference to the abdominal region, especially over the iliac crests (Fig. 25.11.1). In the initial stage the lesion shows a violaceous border 'the lilac ring' and has a tendency to spread outwards [9]. The patch has a whitish or ivory colour centrally (Fig. 25.11.2). With time the involved skin becomes hairless and anhidrotic, and sclerosis starts to develop [10]. The skin lesion becomes firmer, may show hypo- or hyperpigmentated changes and eventually signs of atrophy.

Dissemination of the lesions is possible and characterized by multiple indurated plaque-like lesions, usually on the upper trunk, abdomen, buttocks and legs, seldom on the face, neck and arms. Associated muscle atrophy may be observed and the joints can be involved depending on the site of the overlying skin.

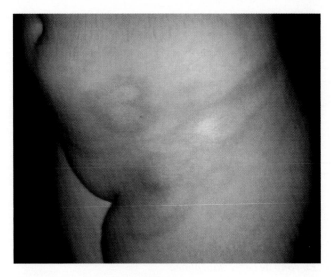

Fig. 25.11.1 Morphoea 'en plaque'.

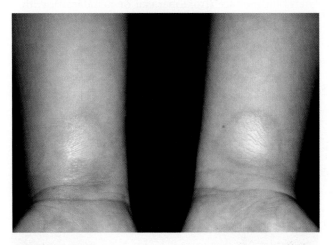

Fig. 25.11.2 Symmetrical lesions on the wrists, illustrating the ivory white sclerotic skin.

Guttate morphoea is a term which has been used to describe multiple small white sclerotic lesions, which may represent disseminated morphoea but need to be differentiated from lichen sclerosus et atrophicus [11]. Coexistence of both diseases has been described [12].

Subcutaneous morphoea, referred to as solitary morphoea profunda, proposed by Whittaker *et al.* [13], is localized on the upper trunk, forearms and lower legs [10,13,14], but can also be unilateral and circular on the thigh and on the buttocks. It involves the deeper layers of the dermis and the subcutaneous fatty tissue [15] giving rise to a peau d'orange effect and sometimes ulceration. The skin is tight and immobile. Arthralgia and joint contractures may result.

Linear morphoea

Linear morphoea is most commonly seen in children,

usually affecting a limb; the legs more than the arms (Fig. 25.11.3). They are usually single and unilateral; occasionally bilateral lesions may occur. Although usually confined to a limb, sometimes the trunk may be affected and rarely, half the body—face, arm, trunk and leg—hemiatrophy.

The linear variant extends along a limb as a sclerotic band in a linear distribution, in a pattern similar to the lines of Blaschko, resulting in deep atrophy involving skin and subcutaneous tissue, muscle and bone. It is more common in girls of early school age. Thinning and shortening of the affected bones may develop, which can result in a shortened wasted limb [16]. If the leg is affected this may have an effect on the spine.

'En coup de sabre' morphoea

The 'en coup de sabre' form in children is most often unilateral on the face (frontoparietal or hemifacial), with a central line of demarcation. After a short phase of erythema and indurated oedema, an atrophic or sclerotic lesion develops with a groove or depression [10] in the form of 'en coup de sabre' (Fig. 25.11.4). The lesions often show hyperpigmentation. After skin and subcutis induration and atrophy, the deeper tissues become affected [17] with the development of facial hemiatrophy.

Apart from the obvious changes in facial appearance, complications depend upon the extent of involvement and can affect the central nervous system with seizures, hemiparesis and headache [18], the eyes [19,20], and the alignment of the jaws with consequent dental problems. Magnetic resonance and/or computed tomography imaging is useful [10,20]; intracranial calcification and white matter abnormality in the ipsilateral frontal lobe and parietal lobe can be detected [21,22].

In Parry–Romberg facial hemiatrophy the subcutaneous tissue, muscles and bones are affected initially. The skin is then lax and movable without pigmentary changes. The nosological position of the disease is not yet clarified; whether it is different or identical with localized scleroderma 'en coup de sabre' is unclear.

Generalized morphoea

Generalized morphoea is defined as a rare condition in which widespread sclerosis of the skin occurs with no systemic involvement. It is mainly seen in adults. It can start insidiously, often on the trunk, with one or more plaques and slowly progress to a much more extensive involvement. Contractures occur in limbs and can give

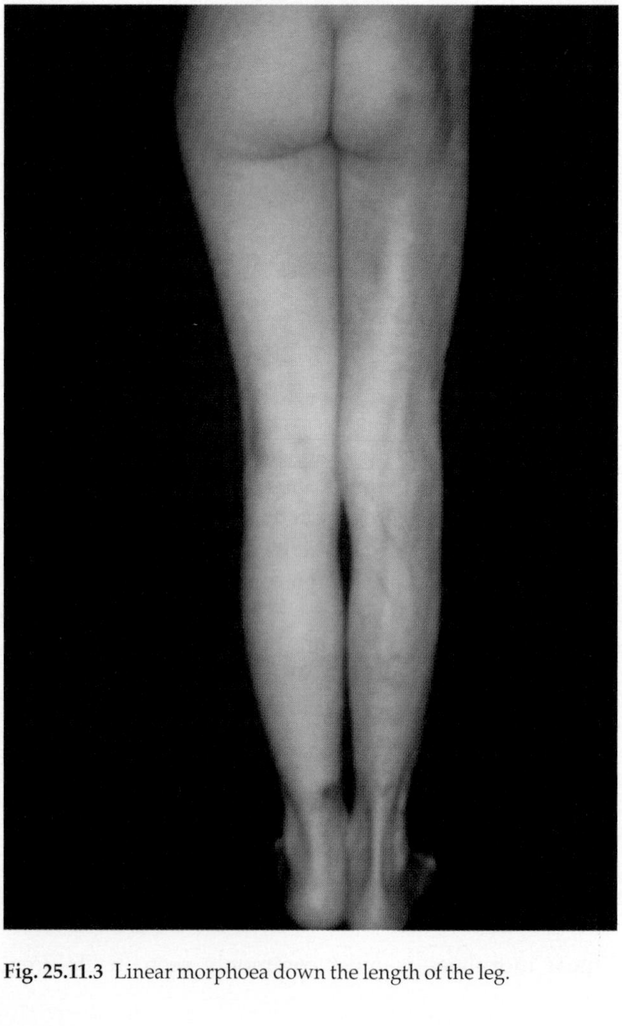

Fig. 25.11.3 Linear morphoea down the length of the leg.

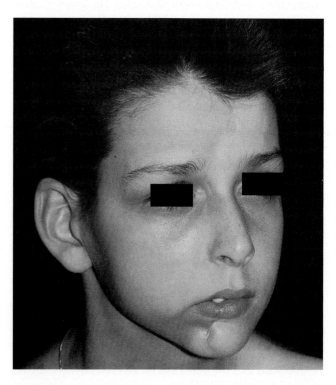

Fig. 25.11.4 'En coup de sabre' morphoea.

rise to joint pains. In contrast to systemic sclerosis, Raynaud's phenomenon, nailfold capillary dilatation and telangiactases are not characteristic features. Chronic graft-versus-host disease may result in generalized morphoea.

Combined forms

Combined forms of plaque and linear morphoea are seen in children. Combinations of plaque-like lesions on the trunk with a linear lesion on the leg or an 'en coup de sabre' lesion are seen. The overlap is indicative of a common pathophysiology and demonstrates the difficulty in classification on solely clinical gounds. The combined types tend to be more aggressive and usually require systemic treatment.

Disabling pansclerotic morphoea

Roudinesco and Vallery-Radot [23] described in 1923 'progressive mutilating scleroderma', characterized by a polymorphous appearance of lesions with involvement of the skin, deep structures, tendons, fascia and muscles. The histological abnormalities include panniculitis and a marked lymphocytic inflammation [24]. The lesions initially occur as a linear variant progressing to generalized lesions [24,25]. Involvement of joints and acral areas leads to arthralgia and joint stiffness. Contractures of the hands and extremities are common features [24]. Systemic involvement in the form of lung fibrosis and oesophageal dysmotility [24] have been described. Raynaud's phenomenon is rare. Eosinophilia, hypergammaglobulinaemia, elevated IgG level, antinuclear antibodies (ANA) have been described [24].

REFERENCES

1 Vancheeswaran R, Black CM, David J *et al.* Childhood-onset scleroderma. *Arthritis Rheum* 1996; 39: 1041–9.
2 Masi AT, Rodnan GP, Medsger TA jr *et al.* Preliminary criteria for the classification of systemic sclerosis (scleroderma). *Bull Rheum Dis* 1981; 31: 1–6.
3 Senff H, Mensing H, Jänner M *et al.* Linear (circumscribed) scleroderma—a case report. Classification and differentiation of circumscribed scleroderma. *Zschr Hautkrankh* 1988; 63: 221–4.
4 Arbeitsgruppe Sclerodermie der Arbeitsgemeinschaft Dermatologische Forschung (ADF). Zur Klassifikation der zirkumskripten Sklerodermie. *Hautarzt* 1990; 41: 16–21.
5 Uziel Y, Krafchik BR, Silverman ED *et al.* Localized scleroderma in childhood: a report of 30 cases. *Semin Arthritis Rheum* 1994; 23: 328–40.
6 Jablonska S. Localized scleroderma. In: Jablonska S, ed. *Scleroderma and Pseudoscleroderma.* Warsaw: Polish Medical Publishers, 1975: 277–303.
7 Albrecht-Nebe H, Laubstein B, Danner R *et al.* Erfahrungen mit der immunsuppressiven Behandlung der zirkumskripten Sklerodermie bei Kindern und Jugendlichen. *Dermatol Monatsschr* 1986; 172: 91–100.
8 Spencer SK. Localized scleroderma: morphea. In: Kelly WN, Harris ED, Ruddy S *et al.*, eds. *Textbook of Rheumatology.* Philadelphia: WB Saunders, 1981: 1231–4.
9 Rosenwasser TA, Eisen AZ. Scleroderma. In: Fitzpatrick B *et al.*, eds. *Dermatology in General Medicine.* New York: McGrawHill, 1993: 2156–67.

10 Krafchik BR. Localized cutaneous scleroderma. *Semin Dermatol* 1992; 11: 65–72.
11 Black CM. Prognosis and management of scleroderma and scleroderma-like disorders in children. *Clin Exp Rheumatol* 1994; 12(suppl 10): 75–81.
12 Uitto J, Santa Cruz DJ, Bauer EA *et al.* Morphea and lichen sclerosus et atrophicus. *J Am Acad Dermatol* 1980; 3: 271–9.
13 Whittaker SJ, Smith NP, Jones RR. Solitary morphoea profunda. *Br J Dermatol* 1989; 120: 431–40.
14 Person JR, Su WPD. Subcutaneous morphoea: a clinical study of sixteen cases. *Br J Dermatol* 1979; 100: 371–80.
15 Stava Z. Zirkumskripte Sklerodermie (klinische Analyse von 50 ausgewählten Fällen). *Dermatol Wschr* 1959; 139: 513–23.
16 Kornreich HK, King KK, Bernstein BH *et al.* Scleroderma in childhood. *Arthritis Rheum* 1977; 20: 343–50.
17 Jablonska S. Facial hemiatrophy and its relation to localized scleroderma. In: Jablonska S, ed. *Scleroderma and Pseudoscleroderma.* Warsaw: Polish Medical Publishers, 1975: 537–48.
18 Moynahan EJ. Morphoea (localized cutaneous scleroderma) treated with low-dosage penicillamine (4 cases including en coup de sabre). *Proc Roy Soc Med* 1973; 66: 49–51.
19 Muchnick RS, Aston SJ, Rees TD. Ocular manifestations and treatment of hemifacial atrophy. *Am J Ophthalmol* 1979; 88: 889–97.
20 Serup J, Aesbirk PH. Localized scleroderma 'en coup de sabre' and iridopalpebral atrophy at the same line. *Acta Derm Venereol (Stockh)* 1983; 63: 75–7.
21 Liu P, Uziel Y, Chuang S *et al.* Localized scleroderma: imaging features. *Pediatr Radiol* 1994; 24: 207–9.
22 David J, Wilson J, Woo P. Scleroderma en coup de sabre. *Ann Rheum Dis* 1991; 50: 260–2.
23 Roudinesco NN, Vallery-Radot P. Sclérodermie mutilante progressive. *Bull Soc Fr Dermatol Syphilol* 1923; 30: 151–4.
24 Diaz-Perez JL, Connolly SM, Winkelmann RK. Disabling pansclerotic morphea of children. *Arch Dermatol* 1980; 116: 169–73.
25 Bourgeois-Drouin C, Touraine R. Sclérodermie en plaques: Perturbations immunologiques et viscérales. *Ann Med Int* 1978; 129: 107–112.

Other findings

Morphoea is usually limited to the skin and subcutaneous tissue [1]. Internal organs are not involved in spite of the very rare progression of a localized form to a diffuse skin involvement [2–4]. The disease in children is only rarely associated with systemic manifestation: arthralgia, Raynaud's like symptoms; migraine; abdominal colic; neurological symptoms including seizures and deafness; a functional defect of the kidneys determined by radioisotope studies, cardiac conduction defects, pericarditis, headaches, transient ischaemic attacks, and non-specific muscle complaints have been described [5–11]. Bone changes in the form of thinning, hypoplasia and shortening are secondary, as are the eye abnormalities in the 'en coup de sabre' variant [12–14].

In children with localized scleroderma, the abnormality is typically localized to the affected skin and subcutis. If complications occur, such as pulmonary disease, pulmonary hypertension, cardiomyopathy and general myopathy, they should be interpreted as a sign of systemic sclerosis [15–21].

Laboratory abnormalities

ANA, anti-Ro/SSA and rheumatoid factor are often found in children with morphoea, the clinical relevance of which is uncertain [7–10,22–28]. The frequency of ANA in children with morphoea differs from study to study and is reported as 25–53%. Eosinophilia may occur [29,30] and reduced complement C2 has been reported [31]. The presence of anti-histone antibodies, in particular antibodies against histone H1 and H3, in morphoea has been reported to correlate with anti-single-stranded-DNA antibodies [32,33]. Anti-topoisomerase I-antibodies, a marker for systemic scleroderma [34], is rarely detected in children with localized scleroderma and then only in the linear and combined variants. Antibodies against extractable nuclear antigens can be detected only in a few children.

The serum concentration of procollagen type I carboxyterminal propeptide (P1cp) has been shown to correlate with the number of sclerotic lesions and the evidence of antisingle-stranded DNA and anti-histone-antibodies in patients with morphoea [35,36]. Therefore the P1cp level in serum may be an important indicator for the severity and progression of localized scleroderma [37]. Another marker of disease activity that has been proposed is serum IL-2R [38], but another study showed no significant difference between the various disease groups and normal controls [22].

There is an increase in C-reactive protein in childhood-onset morphoea, but not paralleled by other acute phase response markers, including erythrocyte sedimentation rate, immunoglobulin and complement [22]. Of interest, this same paper reported abnormal partial thromboplastin time with kaolin (PTTK) values suggesting an abnormal coagulopathy as a result of early endothelial cell damage/activation or tissue factor activation. Other parameters which were normal or negative included: von Willebrand factor, angiotensin-converting enzyme (ACE), E-selectin, endothelin-1 and anti-cardiolipin-antibodies [22].

REFERENCES

1 Masi AT, Rodnan GP, Medsger TA jr *et al*. Preliminary criteria for the classification of systemic sclerosis (scleroderma). *Bull Rheum Dis* 1981; 31: 1–6.
2 Jablonska S. Facial hemiatrophy and its relation to localized scleroderma. In: Jablonska S, ed. *Scleroderma and Pseudoscleroderma*. Warsaw: Polish Medical Publishers, 1975: 537–48.
3 Singsen BH. Scleroderma in childhood. *Pediatr Clin N Am* 1986; 33: 1119–39.
4 Hanson V, Drexler E, Kornreich HK. Rheumatoid factor (antigammaglobulins) in children with focal scleroderma. *Pediatrics* 1974; 53: 945–7.
5 Christianson HB, Dorsey CS, O'Leary PA *et al*. Localized scleroderma. A clinical study of 235 cases. *Am Med Arch Dermatol* 1956; 74: 629–39.
6 Devaux S. Nierenfunktionsdiagnostik in der Kinderheilkunde mit einfachen medizinischen Untersuchungsverfahren. *Kinderärztl Praxis* 1977; 45: 412–20.
7 Albrecht-Nebe H, Stojanow K, Ziegler H *et al*. Zum Aussagewert humoraler Immunphänomäne bei Kindern und Jugendlichen mit zirkumskripter Sklerodermie. *Kinderärztl Praxis* 1989; 57: 315–21.
8 Kornreich HK, King KK, Bernstein BH *et al*. Scleroderma in childhood. *Arthritis Rheum* 1977; 20: 343–50.
9 Goel KM, Shanks RA. Scleroderma in childhood. Report of five cases. *Arch Dis Child* 1974; 49: 861–6.
10 Singsen BH. Scleroderma in childhood. *Pediatr Clin N Am* 1986; 33: 1119–39.
11 Spencer SK. Localized scleroderma: Morphea. In: Kelly WN, Harris ED,

Ruddy S *et al.*, eds. *Textbook of Rheumatology*. Philadelphia: WB Saunders, 1981: 1231–4.
12 Segal P, Jablonska S, Mrzyglod S. Ocular changes in linear scleroderma. *Am J Ophthalmol* 1961; 51: 807–13.
13 Goldenstein-Schainberg C, Pereira RM, Gusukuma MC *et al*. Childhood linear scleroderma 'en coup de sabre' with uveitis. *J Pediatr* 1990; 117: 581–4.
14 Stone RA, Scheie HG. Periorbital scleroderma associated with heterochromia iridis. *Am J Ophthalmol* 1980; 90: 858–61.
15 Birdi N, Laxer RM, Thorner P *et al*. Localized scleroderma progressing to systemic disease. Case report and review of the literature. *Arthritis Rheum* 1993; 36: 410–15.
16 Kass H, Hanson V, Patrick J. Scleroderma in childhood. *J Pediatr* 1966; 68: 243–56.
17 Curtis AC, Jansen TG. The prognosis of localized scleroderma. *Arch Dermatol* 1958; 78: 749–57.
18 Francisco J, Mayorquin TL, McCurley JE *et al*. Progression of childhood linear scleroderma to fatal systemic sclerosis. *J Rheumatol* 1994; 21: 1955–7.
19 Moore EC, Cohen F, Farooki Z, Chang CH. Focal scleroderma and severe cardiomyopathy. Patient report and brief review. *Am J Dis Child* 1991; 145: 229–31.
20 Weidner F, Braun-Falco O. Gleichzeitiges Vorkommen von Symptomen der zirkumskripten und progressiven Sklerodermie. *Hautarzt* 1968; 19: 345–50.
21 Curtis AC, Jansen TG. The prognosis of localized scleroderma. *Arch Dermatol* 1958; 78: 749–55.
22 Vancheeswaran R, Black CM, David J *et al*. Childhood-onset scleroderma. *Arthritis Rheum* 1996; 39: 1041–9.
23 Jablonska S. Histopathology of scleroderma. In: Jablonska S, ed. *Scleroderma and Pseudoscleroderma*. Warsaw: Polish Medical Publishers, 1975: 191–233.
24 Woo TY, Rasmussen JE. Juvenile linear scleroderma associated with serologic abnormalities. *Canad Arch Dermatol* 1985; 121: 1403–5.
25 Black CM. Prognosis and management of scleroderma and scleroderma-like disorders in children. *Clin Exp Rheumatol* 1994; 12(suppl 10): 75–81.
26 Goel KM, Shanks RA. Scleroderma in childhood. Report of 5 cases. *Arch Dis Child* 1974; 49: 861–6.
27 Do Vale E, Gerstmeier H, Meurer M, Krieg T, Braun-Falco O. Spektrum antinuklearer Antikörper bei zirkumskripten Formen der Sklerodermie. *Dtsch Med Wochenschr* 1986; 111: 1922–7.
28 Bernstein RM, Pereira RS, Holden AJ, Black CM, Howard A, Ansell BM. Autoantibodies in childhood scleroderma. *Ann Rheum Dis* 1985; 44: 503–6.
29 Giordano M, Ara M, Valentini G *et al*. Presence of eosinophilia in progressive systemic sclerosis and localized scleroderma. *Arch Dermatol Res* 1981; 271: 411–17.
30 Rodnan GP, Lipinski E, Raben BS *et al*. Eosinophilia serologic abnormalities in localized linear scleroderma. *Arthritis Rheum* 1977; 20: 133.
31 Hulsmans RFHJ, Asghar SS, Siddiqui AH *et al*. Hereditary deficiency of C2 in association with linear scleroderma 'en coup de sabre'. *Arch Dermatol* 1986; 122: 76–9.
32 Sato S, Ihn H, Soma Y *et al*. Antihistone antibodies in patients with localized scleroderma. *Arthritis Rheum* 1993; 36: 1137–41.
33 Ruffatti A, Peserico A, Rondinone R *et al*. Prevalence and characteristics of anti-single-stranded DNA antibodies in localized scleroderma. *Arch Dermatol* 1991; 127: 1180–3.
34 Shero JH, Bordwell B, Rothfield NF *et al*. Antibodies to topoisomerase I in sera from patients with scleroderma. *J Rheumatol* 1987; 14(Suppl 13): 138–40.
35 Keech MK, Reed R, Wood MJ. Further observations on the transformation of collagen fibrils into elastin: an electron microscopic study. *J Path Bact* 1956; 71: 477.
36 Vuorio T, Kahari VM, Black C, Vuorio E. Expression of osteonectin, decorin and transforming growth factor-beta 1 genes in fibroblasts cultured from patients with systemic sclerosis and morphea. *J Rheumatol* 1991; 18: 247–51.
37 Scarola JA, Shulman LE. Serologic abnormalities and their significance in localized scleroderma. *Arthritis Rheum* 1975; 18: 526.
38 Uziel Y, Krafchik BR, Feldman B *et al*. Serum levels of soluble interleukin-2 receptor. A marker of disease activity in localized scleroderma. *Arthritis Rheum* 1994; 37: 898–901.

Prognosis

The course and prognosis of morphoea is unpredictable, depending upon the variant of the disease [1]. Plaque morphoea, isolated, disseminated and guttate types usually show a mild course and are self-limited. The clinical activity generally persists for 3–4 years; new lesions may develop even after a longer time interval, but not usually after puberty [2]. Activity of any ongoing inflammatory changes can be monitored by thermography [3]. The residual inactive lesions often show hyperpigmentation [4]. Progressive generalized morphoea may rarely develop.

The linear variant on the extremity can be responsible for functional impairment, but usually does not progress after 2 or 3 years and ends in residual hyper- or hypopigmentation. The 'en coup de sabre' type can be complicated by bone atrophy, (functional) deformity of the jaws, abnormal position of the teeth and cosmetic impairment by hemiatrophy or deformity of the cranium.

Although the progressive linear variants in children show an extensive spectrum of systemic lupus erythematosus or systemic sclerosis-like humoral immune phenomena, lupus erythematosus or systemic scleroderma rarely develop [5,6].

REFERENCES

1 Black CM. Prognosis and management of scleroderma and scleroderma like disorders in children. *Clin Exp Rheumatol* 1994; 12(Suppl 10): 75–81.
2 Senff H, Mensing H, Jänner M *et al*. Linear (circumscribed) scleroderma—a case report. Classification and differentiation of circumscribed scleroderma. *Zschr Hautkr* 1988; 63: 221–4.
3 Birdi N, Shore A, Rush P *et al*. Childhood linear scleroderma: a possible role of thermography for evaluation. *J Rheumatol* 1992; 19: 968–73.
4 Ghersetich I, Teofoli P, Benci M *et al*. Localized scleroderma. *Clin Dermatol* 1994; 12: 237–42.
5 Súarez-Almazor ME, Catoggio LJ, Maldonadococco JA *et al*. Juvenile progressive systemic sclerosis: Clinical and serologic findings. *Arthritis Rheum* 1985; 28: 699–702.
6 Dubois EL, Chandor S, Friou GJ *et al*. Progressive systemic sclerosis (PSS) and localized scleroderma (morphea) with positive Le cell test and unusual systemic manifestations compatible with SLE. *Medicine* 1971; 50: 199–221.

Differential diagnosis

Morphoea en plaque in its initial stage must be differentiated from annular erythema, erythema migrans and scleroderma [1]. Also morphoea-like sarcoidosis has been described [2]. Isolated atrophic lesions of the plaques-like variant can show a similar clinical picture to the atrophoderma after intramuscular injection of corticosteroids [3] and vitamin K [4]. In the guttate type, lichen sclerosus et atrophicus is clinically similar [4]; however, histological changes are helpful in differentiation.

Hemiatrophy of the face, caused by the 'en coup de sabre' variant, is difficult to differentiate from hemiatrophy without sclerodermatous skin lesions, the so-called Parry–Romberg disease [5]. The nosological position of Parry–Romberg facial hemiatrophy is, however, not well defined.

Linear scleroderma on the extremities in children has to be differentiated from eosinophilic fasciitis (Shulman's syndrome) [6,7]. Eosinophilic fasciitis in children is, however, very rare. The white appearance of linear scleroderma should be easy to differentiate clinically from an achromic naevus [8].

REFERENCES

1 Rower NR, Goodfield MJD. In: Rook AJ, Wilkinson DS, Ebling FJG. *Textbook of Dermatology*, 5th edn. Oxford: Blackwell Scientific Publication, 1992: 2225–35.
2 Hess SP, Agudelo CA, White WL, Jorizzo JL. Ichthyosiform and morpheaform sarcoidosis. *Clin Exp Rheumatol* 1990; 8: 171–5.
3 Holth PJA, Marks R, Waddington E. 'Pseudomorphoea': A side effect of subcutaneous corticosteroid injection. *Br J Dermatol* 1975; 92: 689–91.
4 Texier L, Gendre PH, Gauthier O *et al*. Hypodermites sclérodermiformes lombo-fessieres induites par des injections medicamenteuses intramusculaires associées a la vitamine K. *Ann Dermatol Syph* 1972; 99: 363–7.
5 Fry JA, Alvarellos A, Fink CW *et al*. Intracranial findings in progressive facial hemiatrophy. *J Rheumatol* 1992; 19: 956–8.
6 Miller JJ. The fasciitis morphea complex in children. *Am J Dis Child* 1992; 146: 733–6.
7 Faurrington ML, Haas JE, Nazar-Stewart V *et al*. Eosinophilic fasciitis in children frequently progresses to scleroderma-like cutaneous fibrosis. *J Rheumatol* 1993; 20: 128–32.
8 Gasper S. Naevus depigmentosus. *Dermatol Wochinschr* 1958; 138: 910.

Treatment

Because the aetiology of morphoea is unknown, no specific treatment for the disease is available. Some drugs, topical or systemic, in combination with physiotherapy can be effective in stopping or inhibiting morphoea [1]. Successful treatment leads to softening of the sclerotic areas and prevents functional impairment [2,3]. Thermography can be used for evaluation [4].

Topical treatment

Sometimes encouraging results are obtained in the early stage of the disease, especially in plaque-type morphoea, using a potent corticosteroid ointment [2], until the active inflammatory edge (the lilac ring) has disappeared.

Systemic treatment

Drug treatment is directed towards suppressing inflammation and collagen alteration [5]. The current approach is with steroids, either in the form of intravenous methylprednisolone in the acute phase, and/or oral prednisolone alone or in combination with methotrexate [6,7].

Corticosteroid treatment is indicated for progressive plaque morphoea, which has failed to be controlled by topical therapy [8]; linear morphoea; and the 'en coup de sabre' form [8,9]. Intravenous methylprednisolone is given as an infusion daily for 3 days and then repeated for 3 days the following week. Oral prednisolone alone or in combination with once weekly methotrexate is then started (John Harper, personal communication, 1999).

Penicillamine [10–13] was previously used, but results

are usually disappointing and no controlled trial exists. It also has a high incidence of side-effects in the form of loss of taste [14], leucopenia, thrombocytopenia [15] and an urticaria-like skin rash, as well as renal damage.

Other systemic treatments that have been used include: azathioprine [16], cyclosporin [17], colchicine [18], antimalarials [1], calcitriol [19–21], disodium edetate [22], phenytoin [23], etretinate [24], salazopyrine [25,26], vitamin E, intravenous immunoglobulin and PUVA.

Other treatments

Deep connective tissue massage can be helpful to improve dermal elasticity and joint movement [16]. Regular physiotherapy is essential especially for linear morphoea, to prevent the development of contractures. For established flexion deformities, splinting may be helpful. For those children with leg length shortening, orthopaedic surgical involvement may be necessary [27].

REFERENCES

1 Jablonska S, Szczepanski A. Drugs used in the treatment of systemic a localized scleroderma. In: Jablonska S, ed. *Scleroderma and Pseudoscleroderma*. Warsaw: Polish Medical Publishers, 1979: 610–31.

2 Ghersetich I, Teofoli P, Benci M et al. Localized scleroderma. *Clin Dermatol* 1994; 12: 237–42.

3 Erkrankungen des Bindegewebes. In: Braun-Falco O, Plewig G, Wolff HH, Winkelmann RK, eds. Berlin: Springer Verlag, 1991: 554.

4 Birdi N, Shore A, Rush P et al. Childhood linear scleroderma: a possible role of thermography for evaluation. *J Rheumatol* 1992; 19: 968–73.

5 Black CM. Prognosis and management of scleroderma and scleroderma like disorders in children. *Clin Exp Rheumatol* 1994; 12(suppl 10): 75–81.

6 Van der Hoogen FH, Boerbooms AM, Swaak AJ et al. Comparison of methotrexate with placebo in the treatment of systemic sclerosis: a 24 week randomized double-blind trial, followed by 24 week observational trial. *Br J Rheumatol* 1996; 35: 364–72.

7 Schaller JG. Aggressive treatment in childhood rheumatic diseases. *Clin Exp Rheumatol* 1994; 12(suppl 10): 97–105.

8 Albrecht-Nebe H, Laubstein B, Danner R, Barthelmes H. Erfahrungen mit der immunsuppressiven Behandlung der zirkumscripten Sklerodermie bei Kindern und Jugendlichen. *Dermatol Monatsschr* 1986; 172: 91–100.

9 Rosenwasser TA, Eisen AZ. Scleroderma. In: Fitzpatrick B et al. eds. *Dermatology in General Medicine*. New York: McGraw Hill, 1993: 2156–67.

10 Harris ED, Sjoerdsma A. Effect of penicillamine on human collagen and its possible application to treatment of scleroderma. *Lancet* 1966; ii: 996–9.

11 Fulghum DD, Katz R. Penicillamine for scleroderma. *Arch Derm* 1968; 98: 51–2.

12 Moynahan EJ. D-penicillamine in morphœa (localized scleroderma). *Lancet* 1973; i: 428–9.

13 Falanga V, Medsger TA. D-penicillamine in the treatment of localized scleroderma. *Arch Dermatol* 1990; 126: 609–12.

14 Keiser H. Loss of taste during therapy with penicillamine. *J Am Med Assoc* 1968; 203: 281.

15 Singsen BH. Scleroderma in childhood. *Pediatr Clin N Am* 1986; 33: 1119–39.

16 Black CM. Juvenile scleroderma. In: Woo P, White PH, Ansell BM, eds. *Paediatric Rheumatology Update*. Oxford: Oxford University Press, 1990: 194–208.

17 Follath F, Fontana A, Leumann E et al. Ciclosporin bei Autoimmunkrankheiten. *Schweiz Med Wochenschr* 1994; 124: 1232–9.

18 Alarcon-Segovia D, Ramos-Niembor F, Ibanez de Kasep G et al. Long-term evaluation of colchicine in the treatment of scleroderma. *J Rheumatol* 1979; 6: 705–12.

19 Humbert P, Aubin F, Dupond JL et al. Oral calcitriol as a new therapeutic agent in localized and systemic scleroderma. *Arch Dermatol* 1995; 131: 850.

20 Hulshof MM, Pavel S, Breedveld FC et al. Oral calcitriol as a new therapeutic modality for generalized morphea. *Arch Dermatol* 1994; 130: 1290–3.

21 Bottomley WW, Jutley J, Goodfield MD. The effect of calcipotriol on lesional fibroblasts from patients with active morphoea. *Acta Derm Venereol* 1995; 75: 364–6.

22 Neldner KH, Winkelmann RK, Perry HO. Scleroderma: An evaluation of treatment with disodium edetate. *Arch Dermatol* 1962; 86: 305–9.

23 Neldner KH. Treatment of localized linear scleroderma with phenytoin. *Cutis* 1978; 22: 569–72.

24 Kint A. Behandlung der zirkumskripten Sklerodermie. *Hautarzt* 1980; 31: 284.

25 Leschhorn H. Morphea—Behandlung mit Salazopyrin. *Z Hautkr* 1984; 59: 1108.

26 Czarnecki DB, Taft EH. Generalized morphea successfully treated with salazopyrine. *Acta Derm Venereol* 1982; 62: 81–2.

27 Buckley SL, Skinner S, James P, Ashley RK. Focal scleroderma in children: an orthopaedic perspective. *J Pediatr Orthop* 1993; 13: 784–90.

25.12 Systemic Sclerosis

CAROL M. BLACK AND CHRISTOPHER P. DENTON

'Scleroderma' means hard skin, and is a part of many syndromes including localized, limited and generalized scleroderma. Related to these are undifferentiated connective tissue diseases, overlap syndromes, environmentally induced scleroderma-like diseases and localized fibroses (Table 25.12.1). The disease we call scleroderma or systemic sclerosis (SSc), has been confused with other diseases including sclero-oedema, scleromyxoedema and primary amyloidosis [1]. The pattern of scleroderma occurring in childhood differs from that in the adult [2,3]. Juveniles may develop any form of scleroderma, but fortunately there is a predilection for the localized form, in which the skin, subcutaneous fascia, muscle and bone are the main organs to be attacked [4,5]. Relative to the adult disease and to juvenile chronic arthritis, childhood onset SSc is rare. Less than 3% of all cases are childhood onset [6], and the disease constitutes fewer than 3% of all patients seen in a paediatric rheumatology clinic [7]. In a paediatric rheumatology centre, SSc is seen much less frequently than localized scleroderma, and for every 14 cases of localized disease, there was only one case of systemic disease [8,9]. Ascertainment of SSc in childhood may be biased by referral patterns and subspecialty orientation. Like its adult counterpart, juvenile SSc occurs in all races, with a female predominance. There appears to be no significant familial incidence. HLA studies with sufficient numbers of children in each group are only now being undertaken and so definitive information is awaited. Most of the information relating to pathogenesis of SSc is derived from studies of adult disease, although it is likely that many findings can be extrapolated to childhood onset SSc.

A number of different classification systems for scleroderma have been proposed [10,11]. Central to all of them is the extent of skin involvement. Currently, the most widely used classification defines two subsets based on the extent of skin involvement, together with a number of reliable clinical laboratory and natural history associations. The two subset model divides the disease into diffuse cutaneous SSc (DCSSc) and limited cutaneous SSc (LCSSc) (Table 25.12.2) [11]. In childhood onset SSc the limited cutaneous variant is exeedingly rare, contrasting with its predominance amongst adult SSc cases. The term LCSSc is preferable to CREST, because cutaneous manifestations often extend beyond sclerodactyly, and calcinosis may be present only late or radiologically. DCSSc, the more serious form of the disease is much more rapid in onset, and may lead to organ failure within 5 years of the first symptoms. Within each subset there is often great variability in the speed of the disease, e.g. some patients with LCSSc never develop clinically apparent pulmonary hypertension or mid-gut disease, whereas other individuals develop these complications usually later on, but occasionally as early as 5–7 years after diagnosis. Some patients with DCSSc develop extensive internal organ complications within 2–4 years, whereas others have widespread skin disease but only minimal internal organ complications such as mild interstitial lung disease. Thus, not only is there disease heterogeneity, but differential progression within a subset. Notwithstanding these problems, a useful and practical scheme is to divide the disease into early and late stages (Table 25.12.3). A detailed discussion of the history of this disease is found in the historical review by Rodnan and Benedek [12].

Aetiology and/or pathogenesis

Although the basic aetiology of scleroderma is unknown, it is almost certainly multifactorial with genetic and environmental factors playing a part [13]. The clinical similarities between the systemic forms of scleroderma in adults and children makes it likely that at least some aetiopathogenetic factors are common to both age groups. Many centres, sampling different population groups, have observed abnormal frequencies of the major histocompatibility (MHC) antigens associated with adult scleroderma. The association is complex and the strongest link is between DRw52a and SSc patients with lung fibrosis (relative risk 16.7) [14]. No equivalent information is available on scleroderma in childhood, and although some studies are in progress they are extremely difficult in view of the rarity of childhood onset SSc. There are many reports of chemical agents which may induce adult scleroderma and this may offer some clues towards the underlying disease mechanisms although, as with immunogenetic studies, the rarity of this condition makes formal analysis difficult.

Table 25.12.1 Spectrum of scleroderma and scleroderma-like syndromes

SSc	LCSSc
	DCSSc
	Scleroderma sine scleroderma
Chemically induced SSc	Toxic oil
	Drugs
	L-5-hydroxytryptophan
	pentazocine
	appetite suppressants
	bleomycin
Scleroderma-like diseases	Immunological (chronic graft-versus-host disease)
	Overlap syndromes
	Metabolic
	phenylketonuria
	amyloidosis
	porphyria
Localized scleroderma	Morphoea (plaque, guttate, generalized)
	Linear
	'En coup de sabre'
Raynaud's phenomenon	Primary Raynaud's phenomenon
	Secondary Raynaud's phenomenon (with abnormal nailfold capillaries and autoimmune serology)

Table 25.12.2 Subsets of SSc occurring in childhood

DCSSc
Onset of skin changes (puffy or hidebound) often closely associated with development of Raynaud's phenomenon
Widespread skin involvement including trunk and proximal limbs
Presence of tendon friction rubs
Visceral complications include interstitial lung disease, oliguric renal failure, GI disease and myocardial involvement, usually in first 5 years of disease
Absence of anticentromere antibodies
Nailfold capillary dilatation and capillary destruction*
Antitopoisomerase antibodies (30% of patients)
Anti-RNA polymerase antibodies

LCSSc
Extremely rare in childhood
Long antecedent history of Raynaud's phenomenon
Skin involvement limited to hands, face, feet and forearms (acral) or absent
Subcutaneous calcinosis and visceral fibrosis often occur many years after onset
Dilated nailfold capillary loops, usually without capillary drop-out
Vascular pathology often prominent in established cases, including telangiectasis and pulmonary vascular disease

*Nailfold capillary dilatation and destruction may also be seen in patients with dermatomyositis, overlap syndromes and undifferentiated connective tissue disease. These syndromes may be considered as part of the spectrum of scleroderma-associated disorders.

Some of the agents that can induce a SSc-like disease are listed in Table 25.12.1.

Autoimmune dysfunction

An increasing number of immune abnormalities are being reported in SSc. There is considerable evidence suggesting that abnormalities in both humoral and cell-mediated immunity occur in SSc although the importance of these immunological events in disease pathogenesis is uncertain, particularly in juvenile onset SSc where the hallmark autoantibodies of SSc occur less frequently. Some of this evidence is summarized in Tables 25.12.4 and 25.12.5. The lack of a generalized immune dysfunction in SSc suggests that the derangement of immune cell function may be specific to certain antigens or cell types [15,16]. The relationship of autoantibody production and HLA status is also of increasing interest in scleroderma. It would appear that certain of these antibodies are closely related to particular HLA alleles, for example, it has recently been shown that class II MHC haplotype is an important factor in determining *in vitro* responsiveness to topoisomerase antigen in both SSc patients and healthy control individuals [17]. These antibodies appear also to be mutually exclusive for the different subsets of scleroderma patients, and in addition, mark out within the Raynaud's popula-

tion those patients who are likely to develop SSc. A pathogenic role for the antibodies which target defined epitopes remains unproven. The most obvious targets for the immune response in SSc are endothelial cells and fibroblasts. It is possible that the aberrant properties of connective tissue cells (e.g. excess synthesis of collagen, fibronectin and glycosaminoglycans) and the endothelial cell damage and vasculopathy are in part consequences of immunological events in SSc.

The major pathological processes occurring in SSc are increased deposition of extracellular matrix (ECM) in the skin and internal organs, and vascular damage. It is thought that the processes are closely related. Currently, the most favoured explanation for them implicates widespread intimal vascular damage, with endothelial cell activation, resulting in increased vascular permeability, leucocyte adhesion and subsequent emigration into the interstitium, possibly under the influence of chemotactic stimuli from resident interstitial cells. Following these events, mediators are released from the inflammatory cells and a subset of fibroblasts develop a fibrogenic phenotype [18]. Whether this fibroblast abnormality is wholly acquired or whether it is dependent upon an inherited predisposition is unknown, but the final result is an excess deposition of normal matrix with subsequent organ dysfunction (Fig. 25.12.1).

Skin fibroblasts from scleroderma patients synthesize increased quantities of collagens type I and III and to a

Table 25.12.3 Characteristic findings in the early and late stages of SSc patient subsets. Data from the *Oxford Textbook of Rheumatology*, 2nd edn. Oxford: Oxford University Press, 1996 (with permission).

DCSSc	Early (< 3 years after onset)	Late (> 3 years after onset)
Constitutional	Fatigue and weight loss	Minimal, weight gain typical
Vascular	Raynaud's often relatively mild	Raynaud's more severe, more telangiectasia
Cutaneous	Rapid progression involving arms, trunk, face	Stable or regression
Musculoskeletal	Prominent arthralgia, stiffness, myalgia, muscle weakness, tendon friction rubs	Flexion contractures and deformities, joint/muscle symptoms less prominent
Gastrointestinal	Dysphagia, heartburn	More pronounced symptoms, midgut and anorectal complications more common
Cardiorespiratory	Maximum risk for myocarditis, pericardial effusion, interstitial pulmonary fibrosis	Reduced risk of new involvement but progression of existing established visceral fibrosis
Renal	Maximum risk period for scleroderma renal crisis	Renal crisis less frequent, uncommon after 5 years

LCSSc	Early (< 10 years after onset)	Late (> 10 years after onset)
Constitutional	None	Only secondary to visceral complications
Vascular	Raynaud's typically severe and long-standing telangiectasia	Raynaud's persists, often causing digital ulceration or gangrene
Cutaneous	Mild sclerosis with little progression trunk, face	Stable, calcinosis more prominent
Musculoskeletal	Occasional joint stiffness	Mild flexion contractures
Gastrointestinal	Dysphagia, heartburn	More pronounced symptoms, midgut and anorectal complications more common
Cardiorespiratory	Usually no involvement	Lung fibrosis may develop, but progresses slowly. Maximum risk for developing isolated pulmonary hypertension and secondary right ventricular failure
Renal	No involvement	Rarely involved

Table 25.12.4 Summary of evidence for immune system involvement in SSc

Autoantibody associations (see Table 25.12.5)
Immunogenetic associations
Increased circulating levels of soluble CD4, soluble IL-2 receptor and lymphocyte derived cytokines (IL-2, IL-4, IL-6, IL-8) in *some* patients
Circulating T cells which are reactive to laminin, collagen (type 1) and show increased adhesion to endothelial cells and fibroblasts
Perivascular T-cell infiltrates (DR+, β1, β2 integrin expression) in lesional skin
Increased tissue expression of lymphocyte binding cell surface adhesion molecules in lesional and prelesional skin and lung tissue
Elevated levels of IL-5 and IL-8 in bronchoalveolar lavage fluid
Clinical and pathological similarities with chronic graft-versus-host disease

lesser degree type IV and VI, and also proteoglycan core proteins and fibronectin. Total protein synthesis and growth production are normal. The negative feedback provided by propeptides appears to be normal and these cells are not transformed or immortalized. Scleroderma fibroblasts, however, unlike those from normal skin, display persistent proliferation in serum-free medium, and are without doubt deregulated with respect to ECM synthesis [19,20]. Work in the 1970s by Campbell and LeRoy [21] demonstrated that fibroblasts grown from areas of sclerosis continued to synthesize increased amounts of collagen for several passages *in vitro*. Later, it was demonstrated that the amounts of mRNA for these matrix proteins are increased and localized predominantly to areas surrounding dermal blood vessels. Nucleic acid hybridization techniques have since confirmed that not all fibroblasts are activated, but rather that there is a subset of high collagen producers. The increased collagen RNA levels could arise through increased transcription rate, or by a reduction in mRNA breakdown, and there is evidence that both mechanisms may operate [22]. The transcriptional rate of genes encoding pro-α2(I) collagen (col-IA2) is increased in SSc fibroblasts, suggesting a change in regulatory transcription factors in these cells. Mediators such as transforming growth factor β (TGF-β), platelet-derived growth factor (PDGF), interleukins 1, 4, 6 and 8, insulin-like growth factors (IGFs), fibroblast growth factors (FGFs) and γ-interferons may all be involved in the initiation and/or maintenance of SSc fibroblast activation, possibly through the initiation of autocrine or paracrine loops.

Table 25.12.5 Autoantibodies in scleroderma

Antigen	Molecular identity	Immunofluorescence pattern	Disease subtype and frequency
Scl 70 (topoisomerase)	100 kDa protein degrade 70 kD	Nuclear (diffuse fine speckles)	Up to 40% with diffuse cutaneous SSc 10–15% limited
Kinetochore centromere	17, 80, 140 kDa proteins at inner and outer kinetochore plates	Centromere	70–80% in limited cutaneous SSc 9–29% with primary biliary cirrhosis 10–20% in primary Raynaud's phenomenon
RNA polymerase I, II and III	Complex of 13 proteins 12.5–210 kDa	Nucleolar (punctate)	23% especially diffuse; high prevalence of internal organ involvement
Fibrillarin	34 kDa protein—component of U3RNP†	Nucleolar (clumpy)	6% (immunofluorescence) 60% by fibrillarin fusion protein assay clinical association uncertain ?less articular disease
PM-Scl	Complex of 11 proteins 20–110 kDa	Nucleolar (homogeneous)	3% high prevalence of myositis; more renal involvement
To or Th	40 kDa protein associated with 7–2 & 8–2 kDa RNAs	Nucleolar (homogeneous)	Rare (LCSSC)
Mitochondrial M2	70 kDa protein-dihydrolipoamide acyltransferase	Cytoplasmic (rod like)	25% of CREST* (95% primary biliary cirrhosis)

*CREST, see Table 25.12.4.
†RNP, ribonucleoprotein.

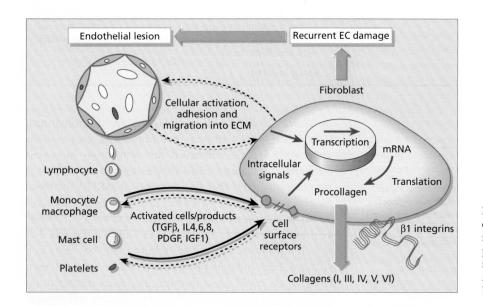

Fig. 25.12.1 Interactions between endothelial cells, leucocytes and fibroblasts in scleroderma and pathogenesis. Modified with permission from (1996) *Oxford Textbook of Rheumatology*, 2nd edn. Oxford: Oxford University Press, 1996.

Vascular lesions

The vascular damage in SSc is widespread and can be recognized as Raynaud's phenomenon, microvascular abnormalities with structural changes characterized by proliferative intimal arterial lesions and obliteration of the vessels leading to chronic ischaemia and intravascular pathology manifest by decreased red cell deformability, increased platelet activation and enhanced thrombus formation. The endothelial cell is thought to have the pivotal role in vascular damage in SSc (Table 25.12.6). The endothelium is now known to produce numerous molecules and to regulate many aspects of vascular stability including control of vascular tone, permeability, thrombotic potential and leucocyte trafficking [23,24].

Vasospasm in SSc is thought to arise due to changes in the levels of a variety of vasoactive mediators including nitric oxide, endothelin-1, prostacyclin, neuropeptides and platelet-released products. The mechanism underlying endothelial cell perturbation is likely to be equally complex. Both immune (cell-mediated and humoral) and non-immune cytotoxicity have been implicated [25,27]. Following injury or activation endothelial cell expression of adhesion molecules, such as E-selectin, vascular cell adhesion molecule type 1 (VCAM-1) and intercellular adhesion molecule type 1 (ICAM-1), is upregulated, usually in response to proinflammatory cytokines. These endothelial adhesion molecules bind to specific ligands on T and B lymphocytes, platelets, neutrophils, monocytes and natural killer cells, facilitating their adhesion to vascular endothelium and subsequent migration through leaky vessels into the ECM, where they may promote fibroblast activation. Therefore, if endothelial changes could be modulated at an early stage in SSc it might influence the clinical expression and progression of the disease.

Clinical features

The recognition of a prescleroderma state is critical, and can be done with some accuracy. The best predictive markers of the subsequent development of scleroderma are abnormal nailfold capillaries (Fig. 25.12.2) and disease-specific antinuclear antibodies, and it has been suggested that the presence of both will detect over 90% of those destined to develop SSc [28,29].

SSc, once established, is a multisystem, multistage disease, and each target organ progresses through stages of inflammation, fibrosis and atrophy, not necessarily at the same time or with the same speed. The eventual effect of these processes is to impede organ function. Cutaneous involvement (Figs 25.12.3, 25.12.4) changes in diffuse disease usually proceeding through three phases: early, classic and late. The early stage is sometimes difficult to diagnose as the puffiness of the hands and feet can be misdiagnosed as early onset inflammatory arthritis. A high level of suspicion is therefore needed. The face may feel slightly taught at this stage, and Raynaud's disease may be present. On examination there is non-pitting oedema, with intact epidermal and dermal appendages. The subsequent, often sudden development of classic scleroderma with firm, taut, hide-bound skin proximal to the metacarpophalangeal joints, permits a definitive diagnosis in over 90% of patients. The skin may be coarse, pigmented and dry at this stage, the epidermis thins, hair growth ceases, sweating is impaired and skin creases disappear.

Changes limited to the fingers alone (sclerodactyly) with minimal facial and foot involvement, defines the limited subset and do not carry the same implications. The classic skin changes in this group of patients once fully developed, can remain static for many years, and the vascular aspects of the disease are usually more troublesome for the patients than the extent of skin involvement. The DCSSc patients have a predominance of visceral involve-

Table 25.12.6 Evidence for endothelial cell dysfunction in SSc

Direct observation of abnormal nailfold capillaries

Increased capillary permeability to tracer molecules with a slowing of flow and increased periods of stasis

Presence of a circulating cytotoxic factor identified as granzyme-1, a serine protease present in granules of activated T cells

Changes in circulating levels of endothelial cell products such as von Willebrand factor, endothelin-1, plasminogen activator, ACE and prostacyclin/thromboxane metabolites

Increased endothelial cell surface expression *in vivo* and elevated circulating levels of the adhesion molecules, ICAM-1, VCAM-1 and E-selectin

The presence of autoantibodies that bind to endothelial cells. These autoantibodies are distinct from other circulating antibodies characteristic of scleroderma

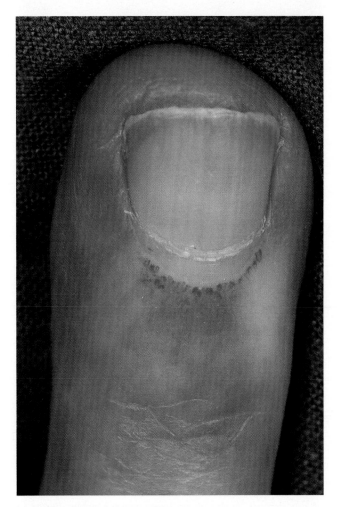

Fig. 25.12.2 Typical macroscopic appearance of dilated abnormal nailfold capillaries in childhood onset scleroderma.

ment in the first 5 years of symptoms. Later, the disease often plateaus and the skin moves into the late or atrophic phase. The taut truncal arm and leg skin may soften and, but for the pigmentation, may return almost to its normal

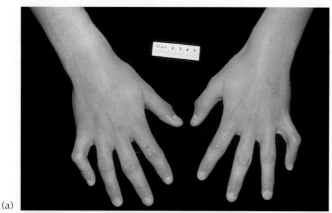

(a)

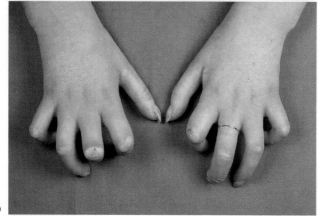

(b)

Fig. 25.12.3 Skin sclerosis and flexion contractures in established childhood onset systemic sclerosis. (a) Mild disease with limited skin sclerosis and mild flexion deformity. (b) More severe flexion contractures in advanced diffuse cutaneous SSc.

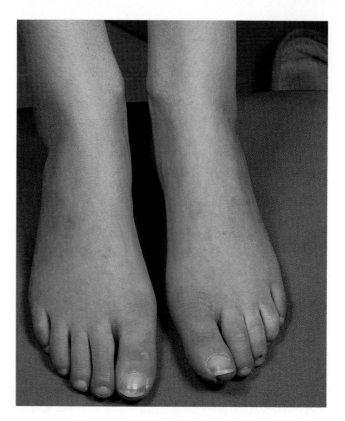

Fig. 25.12.4 Skin changes involving the feet and lower legs in diffuse childhood onset SSc.

texture. Nevertheless, the hands in patients with DCSSc nearly always show the ravages of the early active fibrotic process and contractures usually remain. Other skin manifestations include digital pitting scars, loss of finger pad pulp, ulcers, telangiectasia and calcinosis.

Systemic features of the disease

The patient with SSc has to cope with a complex set of symptoms. Fatigue and lethargy are common throughout the illness, although usually more pronounced in the early phases. Weight loss is almost universal in the diffuse form of the disease and can be quite considerable. Fever is uncommon and anaemia not pronounced. Reactive depression is a frequent accompaniment to this often relentless and disfiguring disorder. In juvenile onset SSc growth impairment is an important consideration. This is probably multifactorial, with anorexia, poor eating habits due to dysphagia, systemic cytokine effects, malabsorption and the effects of therapeutic corticosteroids all being implicated.

Gastrointestinal tract

The gastrointestinal (GI) tract is the most commonly involved internal organ in childhood onset SSc, as in adult disease [30,31]; over 90% of patients have oesophageal hypomotility and serious GI disease has been estimated to occur in up to 50%. It is probable that when the SSc affects an area of the GI tract, it does so in a sequential manner with progressive dysfunction. The earliest event is neural dysfunction, followed by impairment of muscle contractility. These functional changes may remain asymptomatic for a long period and often respond well to prokinetic drugs. Once smooth muscle atrophy is established, symptoms usually appear. The final lesion as with all other organs in SSc is fibrosis, and at this stage restoration of function is not possible.

Pulmonary involvement

Pulmonary disease ranks only second to the gut in frequency of visceral involvement, and with considerable improvements in the management of renal disease, it is now the major cause of death in SSc. Early diagnosis enabling the institution of effective therapy to halt disease progression is therefore a critical aim in the management of the patient with SSc. Fortunately, this is now becoming possible with the aid of modern techniques such as high resolution computed tomography (HRCT) [32] alveolar lavage [33] and DTPA Scanning [34]. There is also evidence that the genetic marker DR3, DR52a [14,35] and specific autoantibodies, antitopoisomerase 1, anti-U3RNP and antihistone antibodies may help separate this group at presentation.

Cardiac disease

Vasospasm, microvascular and larger vessel problems are as in all other organs a feature of cardiac scleroderma [36]. The clinical symptoms are diverse and sometimes difficult to separate from pulmonary or renal disease. They are non-specific including dyspnoea, orthopnoea, paroxysmal nocturnal dyspnoea, oedema, palpitations and atypical chest pain, and as with pulmonary symptoms are often difficult to elicit in a child.

Renal disease

Renal disease, although no longer the major cause of death in SSc, is an important complication, and is amenable to treatment with the outcome critically dependent on early interventional management [37]. The best characterized pattern of renal scleroderma is an acute or subacute renal hypertensive crisis (scleroderma renal crisis) which generally occurs in patients with diffuse SSc within 5 years of onset. Patients usually present with the clinical features of hypertension, headaches, visual disturbances, hypertensive encephalopathy (especially seizures) and pulmonary oedema. Occasionally, a similar pattern of renal dysfunction occurs without hypertension, suggesting that the pathological features are not simply the end-organ consequences of raised arterial pressure. A more benign renal involvement has been reported in which there is a slow reduction in glomerular filtration rate (GFR) accompanied by proteinuria. High-dose steroids have now been formally demonstrated in a case–controlled study to increase the risk of renal crisis in adults with DCSSc [38], and the same risk may exist in juvenile onset disease.

Musculoskeletal system

The skeletal muscle is often involved in scleroderma and many patients have a primary myopathy, which is subtle and distinctive for the disease. Very few patients exhibit an inflammatory myositis. If an inflammatory myopathy is diagnosed, care must be taken when determining treatment, as high-dose steroids might precipitate renal problems. The joints can also be involved in SSc. The arthritis is usually seronegative, non-erosive and in addition to joint disease, the tendons can become inflamed and fibrotic, and ligaments and joint capsules involved with restriction of movement.

Prognosis in scleroderma is dependent on internal organ involvement with the lung, heart and kidney being the major causes of mortality, and the gut the major cause of morbidity.

Differential diagnosis

The differential diagnosis includes the other connective tissue disorders and scleroderma-like diseases (Table 25.12.2).

Treatment

SSc is a chronic disabling disease which needs skilful management in childhood. A team approach is required with input and advice from physiotherapists, occupational therapists, nurse educators, social workers and doctors. The therapy plan must obviously involve the parents and immediate family. Simple measures such as a warm comfortable environment with additional heating aids can make an enormous difference and lubrication of the skin is essential. Early and continuing physical therapy is important in limiting contractures. Both active and passive exercises are necessary with analgesia if required to permit a daily regime. An erratic, irregular regime will not bring about the desired result. Deep connective tissue massage which can be taught to parents is also helpful in improving dermal elasticity and underlying joint movement, where the skin over the joints is involved. Massage can be aided by the use of olive oil or coconut oil, and wax therapy can facilitate hand exercises. The use of corrective splints may also be necessary. Sporting activities at school may also have to be adapted to patient need.

Drug treatment

Although there is currently no cure for SSc, there are therapies available which can offer partial relief, control end-organ damage and improve quality of life. The choice and evaluation of any treatment regime is not easy, and it is additionally difficult in children because of the side-effects of many of the drugs used. The choice is also made more difficult by the heterogeneity of the disease, the variation in its extent, severity and rate of progression, the tendency in some patients towards spontaneous stabilization and the need to consider immune dysfunction, vascular damage and on-going fibrosis. The use of immunosuppression in juvenile scleroderma must be carefully defined. It is essential to consider the potential adverse effects of immunosuppressive therapy and balance these against the likely benefit. As with adult SSc it is likely that immunosuppressive agents will only be effective at stages in the disease in which there is substantial local or systemic immunological activity. Thus early diffuse skin sclerosis, active myositis and lung fibrosis with a predominant inflammatory pathology are the most appropriate targets. The fact that definitive diagnosis is often difficult in early childhood SSc, as with adult disease, has restricted the use of immunosuppressive regimens. Possible agents are methotrexate, cyclophosphamide (oral or parenteral), azathioprine and cyclosporine. Methotrexate has been successfully used in a number of cases of childhood SSc at a dose of 5–10 mg/m^2/week, although there are reports of doses up to 50 mg/week being tolerated by children. There have been no formal trials evaluating any of these immunosuppressive drugs in childhood SSc. Corticosteroids may also be considered, but have a number of specific risks: even at modest doses it has been reported that they may increase the risk of hypertensive renal crisis [42] and there is considerable risk of steroid-induced growth retardation even when an alternate-day regimen is employed. As in adult SSc the benefit of corticosteroid therapy, in the absence of myositis, is unproven.

The choice of antifibrotic agents are very limited. D-penicillamine has been used for many years in the treatment of scleroderma and has been shown to have a promising effect on skin sclerosis in some patients. The dose of the drug in childhood scleroderma is 3 mg/kg/day for the first 2 months, to be increased by 2 mg/kg/day at monthly intervals up to a maximum of 15 mg/kg/day. On retrospective analyses treated groups have had significant reduction in skin thickness relative to non-treated controls. The effect on internal organ involvement is less certain.

The vascular aspects of scleroderma can be extremely troublesome and Raynaud's phenomenon should be treated in the first instance by warm clothing, thermal underwear, heating aids and a steady warm temperature, and if necessary by an oral vasodilator, calcium channel blockers and/or angiotensin-converting enzyme (ACE) inhibitors may be used. If necessary parenteral vasodilatation can be given in the form of iloprost or prostaglandin E1.

REFERENCES

1 Black CM, Stephens CO. Systemic sclerosis (scleroderma) and related disorders. In: Maddison PJ, Isenberg DA, Woo P, Glass DN, eds. *Oxford Textbook of Rheumatology*. Oxford: Oxford Medical Publications, 1993: 771–89.

2 Falanga V. Localised scleroderma. *Med Clin N Am* 1989; 73: 1143–56.

3 Jablonska S. *Scleroderma and Pseudo-scleroderma*. Poland: Warsaw Polish Medical Publishers, 1975.

4 Black CM. Prognosis and management of scleroderma and scleroderma-like disorders in children. *Clin Exp Rheumatol* 1994; 12(suppl 10): S75–81 (review).

5 Ansell BM, Falcini F, Woo P. Scleroderma in childhood. *Clin Dermatol* 1994; 12: 299–307.

6 Dabich L, Sullivan DB, Cassidy JT. Scleroderma in the child. *J Pediatr* 1974; 85: 770–5.

7 Hanson V. Dermatomyositis, scleroderma and polyarteritis nodosa. *Clin Rheum Dis* 1976; 2: 445–67.

8 Dabich L. Scleroderma. In: Cassidy JT, ed. *Textbook of Paediatric Rheumatology*. New York: Wiley, 1982: 433–71.

9 Lehman TJA. The Parry–Romberg syndrome of progressive facial hemiatrophy and linear scleroderma en coup de sabre. Mistaken diagnosis or overlapping conditions? *J Rheumatol* 1992; 19: 844–5 (editorial).

10 Masi AT. Classification of systemic sclerosis (scleroderma): relationship of cutaneous subgroups in early disease to outcome and serologic reactivity. *J Rheumatol* 1988; 15: 894–8.

11 LeRoy EC *et al*. Scleroderma (systemic sclerosis): classification, subsets and pathogenesis. *J Rheumatol* 1988; 15: 202–5.

12 Rodnan GP, Benedek TG. An historical account of the study of progressive systemic sclerosis (diffuse scleroderma). *Ann Intern Med* 1962; 57: 305–19.

13 Silman AJ, Black CM, Welsh KI. Epidemiology, demographics, genetics. In: Philip J, Clements PJ, Furst DE, eds. *Systemic Sclerosis*. Baltimore: William and Wilkins 1995: 23–49.

14 Briggs DC, Vaughan RW, Welsh KI, Myers A, du Bois RM, Black CM. Immunogenetic prediction of pulmonary fibrosis in systemic sclerosis. *Lancet* 1991; 338: 661–2.

15 Padula SJ, Clark RB, Korn JH. Cell mediated immunity in rheumatic diseases. *Human Pathol* 1986; 17: 254–63.

16 Lupoli S, Amlot P, Black CM. Normal immune responses in systemic sclerosis. *J Rheumatol* 1990; 17: 323–37.

17 Kuwana.

18 Black CM. The aetiopathogenesis of systemic sclerosis: thick skin–thin hypotheses. The Parkes Weber Lecture. *J Roy Coll Phys London* 1995; 29: 119–30.

19 Kahari VM. Activation of dermal connective tissue in scleroderma. *Ann Med* 1993; 25: 511–18.

20 de Crombrugghe B, Vuorio T, Karsenty G. Control of type I collagen genes in scleroderma and normal fibroblasts. *Rheum Dis Clin N Am* 1990; 16: 109–23.

21 Campbell PM, LeRoy EC. Pathogenesis of systemic sclerosis a vascular hypothesis. *Semin Arthritis Rheum* 1975; 4: 351–68.

22 Eckes B, Mauch C, Huppe G, Kreig T. Downregulation of collagen synthesis in fibroblasts within three dimensional collagen lattices involves transcriptional and post-transcriptional mechanisms. *FEBS Letts* 1993; 318: 129–33.

23 Pearson JD. The endothelium: its role in systemic sclerosis. *Ann Rheum Dis* 1990; 50: 866–71.

24 Kahaleh B, Matucci-Cerinic M. Raynaud's phenomenon and scleroderma. Disregulation neuroendothelial control of vascular tone. *Arthritis Rheum* 1995; 38: 1–4.

25 Prescot RJ, Freemont AJ, Jones CJ, Hoyland J, Fielding P. Sequential dermal microvascular and perivascular changes in the development of scleroderma. *J Pathol* 1992; 166: 255–63.

26 Harrison NK, Myers AR, Corrin B, Sooray G *et al*. Structural features of interstitial lung disease in systemic sclerosis. *Am Rev Resp Dis* 1991; 144: 706–13.

27 Blann AD, Illingworth K, Jayson MIV. Mechanisms of endothelial cell damage in systemic sclerosis and Raynaud's phenomenon. *J Rheumatol* 1993; 20: 1325–30.

28 Kallenberg CGM, Wouda AA, Hoet MH, van Venrooij OJW. Development of connective tissue disease in patients presenting with Raynaud's phenomenon: a 6-year follow-up with emphasis on the predictive value of antinuclear antibodies as detected by immunoblotting. *Ann Rheum Dis* 1988; 47: 634–41.

29 Zufferey P, Depairon M, Chamot A, Monti M. Prognostic significance of nailfold capillary microscopy in patients with Raynaud's phenomenon and scleroderma-pattern abnormalities: a 6-year follow-up study. *Clin Rheumatol* 1992; 11: 536–41.

30 Jiranek GC, Bredfelt JE. Organ involvement: gut and hepatic manifestations. In: Clements PJ, Furst DE, eds. *Systemic Sclerosis*. Baltimore: Williams and Wilkins 1995: 453–81.

31 Sjogren RW. Gastrointestinal motility disorders in scleroderma. *Arthritis Rheum* 1994; 37: 1265–82.

32 Wells AU, Hansell DM, Rubens MB, Cullinan P, Black CM, du Bois RM. The predictive value of appearances on thin section computed tomography in fibrosing alveolitis. *Am Rev Resp Dis* 1993; 148: 1076–82.

33 Wells AU, Hansell DM, Rubens MR *et al*. Fibrosing alveolitis in systemic sclerosis: bronchoalveolar lavage findings in relation to computed tomographic appearances. *Am J Resp Critical Care Med* 1994; 150: 462–8.

34 Wells AU, Hansell DM, Harrison NK, Lawrence R, Black CM, du Bois RM. Clearance of inhaled 99m-Tc DTPA predicts the clinical course of fibrosing alveolitis. *Eur Respir J* 1993; 6: 797–802.

35 Langevitz P, Buskila D, Gladman DD, Darlington GA, Farewell VT, Lee P. HLA alleles in systemic sclerosis: associations with pulmonary hypertension and outcome. *Br J Rheum* 1992; 31: 609–13.

36 Follansbee WP. Organ involvement: cardiac. In: Clements PJ, Furst DE, eds. *Systemic Sclerosis*. Baltimore: Williams and Wilkins 1995: 333–64.

37 Black CM, Denton CP. In: Davison AM, Cameron JS, Grünfeld J-P, Kerr DNS, Eberhard R, Winearls CG, eds. *Scleroderma—Systemic Sclerosis. Oxford Textbook of Nephrology*. 1998; 961–74.

38 Steen VD, Conte C, Medsger TA Jr. Case–control study of corticosteroid use prior to scleroderma renal crisis. *Arthritis Rheum* 1994; 37(Suppl): S360 (abstract).

25.13 Juvenile Chronic Arthritis, Systemic Lupus Erythematosus and Dermatomyositis

PATRICIA WOO

Juvenile chronic arthritis
Systemic onset juvenile chronic arthritis
Pauciarticular juvenile chronic arthritis
Polyarticular juvenile chronic arthritis

Systemic lupus erythematosus
Neonatal lupus erythematosus

Juvenile dermatomyositis

Juvenile chronic arthritis

The earliest description of arthritis occurring in children was by Phaire in 1545 [1]. Cornil in 1864 described juvenile arthritis for the first time in the French literature [2]. The first comprehensive description of arthritis in children in the UK was first described by Still in 1897 [3]. He described the systemic disease which is now called systemic juvenile chronic arthritis (JCA), as well as other types of arthropathies which were not associated with systemic manifestations. It was not until many years later when Bywaters and Ansell sought to classify children with arthritis seen at the Canadian Red Cross Hospital in the 1950s, and eventually evolved the system of classification which was adopted formally by the European League Against Rheumatism (EULAR) in 1977 [4]. Parallel development in the USA led to a system of classification which was similar to the European one but not exactly the same. Table 25.13.1 shows the similarities and differences between the two classifications. Subsequent research on genetics and immunopathology, as well as clinical observation of disease course, have all shown that these three groups can be further subdivided. Some of the subdivisions do overlap between the groups and therefore there was a need to reclassify the diseases in the light of present knowledge as well as having one internationally agreed classification. A task force convened by the World Health Organization (WHO) and International League Against Rheumatism met in 1994 and proposed a modified classification which has aimed to be flexible and was revised in 1997 [5]. For the purpose of this chapter description of the various arthritides in childhood will be according to the EULAR classification. The diagnosis of JCA is by exclusion (Table 25.13.2). The relative frequency of the different subtypes of JCA as recorded by the National Register of the UK over the past 3 years is shown in Table 25.13.3 [6].

Pathogenesis

In common with idiopathic arthritides of adults, these different types of arthritides in childhood exhibit a chronic immunological inflammatory response in the absence of any known infectious agents, although a history of an infection can often be elicited at the onset of the disease. Therefore, genetic susceptibility for these several groups of diseases have been sought. Analysis of the major histocompatibility complex antigens (HLA antigens) have revealed certain groups which correlate with defined clinical patterns of disease. For example, the early onset (i.e. aged 6 years or under) of the pauciarticular subgroup have been shown in many ethnic groups to be associated with several HLA antigens (Table 25.13.4).

Within the polyarticular group of diseases it is clear that the young onset group have similarities with young onset pauciarticular JCA, with association of HLA-DRB1*0801, a different DP, DPB1*0301. However, when the clinical spectrum of polyarticular disease in the older onset age group is analysed there are many different types which could be subclassified according to the clinical pattern of joint involvement, as well as disease course. Whether these are separate entities from a genetic point of view remains to be seen.

The juvenile onset ankylosing spondylitis (JAS) subgroup can present either as older onset pauciarticular JCA or polyarticular JCA of older onset. The distinguishing feature of this group of diseases is association of the HLA-B27 antigen in the Caucasian population. The clinical pattern is distinct. The role of the HLA-B27 antigen in the pathogenesis of ankylosing spondylitis is still under debate. It has been postulated to be the antigen which causes disease. However, it appears that bacterial antigens may use the B27 as a receptor molecule, which then causes the chronic inflammatory disease.

The search for an association of other candidate genes that might contribute to susceptibility of disease severity, such as cytokine genes, are encouraging; a polymorphism of the interleukin 1α (IL-1α) gene has been associated with the pauciarticular JCA children in a Norwegian population, especially with the group that develop uveitis. Novel polymorphisms of interleukin 6 and 10 which regulate gene expression have been found to be associated with systemic JCA and extended pouciarticular JCA [8,9]. Comprehensive analysis of the genome will ultimately define the number of loci that are associated with JCA, and the contribution of each locus evaluated. The difficulty still remains in the identification of the actual genes in these loci that could cause the diseases. The completion of the sequencing of the human genome in the next few years will make this task much easier.

The type of infectious agents that have been implicated in the aetiology of different JCA subgroups are many. In systemic onset JCA, Epstein–Barr virus, *Mycoplasma*, adenovirus and flu virus have all been implicated in the exacerbation and sometimes onset of the disease. Thus a common pathway rather than a common pathogen is likely to be the trigger to JCA. Bacteria such as *Klebsiella* are historically associated with JAS but the causal link still remains to be established.

Systemic onset juvenile chronic arthritis

This disease typically affects young children, very often below the age of 1 year. Figure 25.13.1 shows the prevalent age of onset of systemic JCA in the UK collected by the National Register over a 3-year period. The male to female ratio is approximately the same. Onset of the disease is typically one of recurrent high fevers up to 40°C and above, often occurring at the same time of day, each day, and in between the temperature is back to normal. Associated with the fever would be seen an evanescent macular rash which often shows target lesions. Sometimes the rash can be urticarial and itchiness is a sensation which is often described by the child (Fig. 25.13.2). The rash occurs usually on the limbs and the cheeks but can be all over the body. There is marked dermographism.

Table 25.13.1 Comparison of classification criteria for chronic arthritis in childhood. Adapted from Prieur and Petty [32]

Characteristic	ACR (JRA)	EULAR (JCA)
Age at onset	< 16 years	< 16 years
Minimum duration of arthritis	6 weeks	3 months
Types	Systemic Pauciarticular Polyarticular	Systemic Pauciarticular Polyarticular
Rheumatoid factor	Does not change classification	Excluded, called JRA
Spondyloarthropathies	Excluded	Not excluded

Table 25.13.2 Differential diagnosis of JCA

Infection
Other inflammatory and non-inflammatory connective tissue diseases
Leukaemia and other malignancies, e.g. neuroblastoma
Haemoglobinopathies
Genetic metabolic diseases, e.g. Hurler's syndrome
Chondrodysplasias

Table 25.13.4 HLA associations with early onset pauciarticular JCA

Present in all ethnic groups studied
DRB1*0801
DPB1*0201
HLA-A2

Other associations with different ethnic groups
DRB1*1201 (Europe)
DRB1*1104 (Texas, Italy, UK)
DRB1*1101 (UK, Greece)
DRB1*1301 (Texas, UK, Norway)
DQA1*0401*0501*0601 (Germany)
DQA1*0501,*0601 (UK)
DQA1*0401,*0501 (Italy, Greece)

Table 25.13.3 Relative frequency of different subtypes of juvenile arthritis (prevalent cases from 18 centres registering 'all' cases). Adapted from Symmons *et al.* [6]

Subtype	No. of cases (%)	No. of females	M : F	Median age at onset	Range
Systemic JCA	201 (11)	111 (54)	1 : 1.2	4.3	1.0–15.0
Pauciarticular JCA	916 (50)	613 (65)	1 : 2.0	5.2	1.0–15.8
Polyarticular JCA	311 (17)	234 (74)	1 : 3.0	6.5	1.1–15.5
Juvenile psoriatic	128 (7)	79 (60)	1 : 1.6	10.1	1.9–14.8
Juvenile spondylarthropathy	146 (8)	35 (24)	1 : 0.3	11.4	4.9–15.0
Juvenile ankylosing spondylitis	37 (2)	9 (21)	1 : 0.3	12.1	6.3–15.1
Reiter's syndrome	19 (1)	10 (43)	1 : 1.1	11.1	2.4–15.7
Arthritis of inflammatory bowel disease	18 (1)	12 (60)	1 : 2.0	10.8	1.4–15.5
Juvenile RA*	55 (3)	51 (93)	1 : 12.8	9.0	1.5–15.9

* Although juvenile RA is not included in the EULAR criteria for JCA, it has been incorporated in this table for completeness and ease of comparison with other studies.

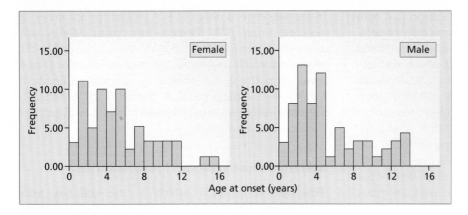

Fig. 25.13.1 Graphs to show the prevalence of systemic JCA in the UK from the National Register of the British Paediatric Rheumatology Group.

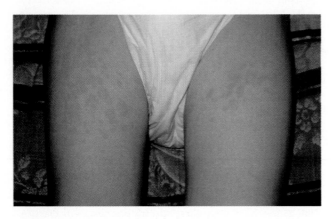

Fig. 25.13.2 A typical rash of systemic JCA.

Although the rash could be mistaken for a drug reaction or viral exanthem, the characteristic of this rash is that it is evanescent.

During the fever phase the child is acutely unwell. There is also associated hepatosplenomegaly, lymphadenopathy, serositis and often pericarditis which can compromise cardiac function. Very often serositis has been mistaken for an acute abdomen. Typically arthritis occurs after the onset of fever and polyarthritis becomes prominent when the fever fades away. The time course of these episodes are highly variable. In one follow-up study at Taplow, Ansell describes remission rates of 50% [10].

The course of disease could be a single episode, relapsing with normal periods in between which can be months or years, and persistent systemic features with arthritis. The latter tend to be of poorer prognosis with destructive changes of the joints. It is often said that if there is aggressive arthritis in conjunction with the onset of fever then the prognosis of these children are usually not so good. This needs to be verified with further prospective multicentre studies.

The mainstay of the management of systemic JCA is still corticosteroid therapy. However, its use has evolved over time. It is imperative to control the disease early and as quickly as possible to prevent complications. Possible complications include macrophage activation syndrome [11]. This consists of rapid deterioration with features of disseminated intravascular coagulation and sometimes frank haemophagocytic syndrome. This is now the most common cause of death. In the 1950s to the 1960s amyloidosis was the major complication and the main cause of death in this disease. Approximately 10% of systemic JCA patients develop this complication [12,13]. The author's system of drug treatment of systemic JCA is illustrated in Fig. 25.13.3.

Pauciarticular juvenile chronic arthritis

This is the commonest form of JCA in children comprising approximately 50–60% of all JCA. A subdivision is commonly made: early onset (up to the age of 6 years) and older onset. The early onset pauciarticular (EOPA) JCA group characteristically affect young girls with a peak age of onset at 3 years. Anterior uveitis has been found associated with this disease in Europe and North America, with a positive antinuclear antibody (ANA) as an associated marker. This may not be the same in all parts of the world. Typically the course of arthritis is mild and 60–70% remit within 2–3 years. The course of uveitis is independent of arthritis and can continue into adulthood. The rest develop polyarthritis, often within 1 or 2 years of onset. The management of pauciarticular JCA is shown in Fig. 25.13.4.

Late onset pauciarticular JCA is a mixed group which have varied disease courses. Many of these have in fact JAS involving lower limb joints asymmetrically, psoriatic arthritis, and rheumatoid factor positive arthritis. They often overlap with some of the polyarticular onset JCA (see below) and often become polyarticular.

Polyarticular juvenile chronic arthritis

The young onset group have similarities with EOPA JCA, associated with uveitis and positive ANA. Later onset groups again are varied and comprise JAS, psoriatics, as

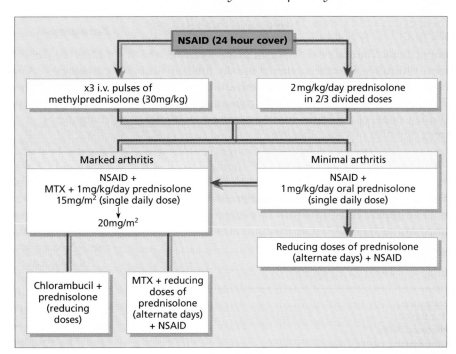

Fig. 25.13.3 Flow diagram of current therapeutic strategy of sytemic JCA employed in the rheumatology unit at Great Ormond Street Hospital for Children, UK. MTX, methotrexate; NSAID.

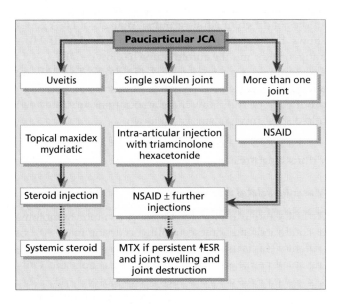

Fig. 25.13.4 Management of pauciarticular JCA. MTX, methotrexate; NSAID. (→ This eventuality is rare.)

well as symmetrical polyarthritis, both rheumatoid factor positive and negative.

Drug management of this group of arthritics is methotrexate, given as a single weekly dose of 15–20 mg/m^2, often as subcutaneous injection due to better absorption profiles.

Treatment

Physiotherapy has a major role in maintaining joint func-

tion and muscle tone during the active disease stage. This includes weight-bearing exercises as it has been shown that if the child is not weight bearing and has hip disease then the acetabulae do not develop normally (reviewed in [14]). However, it is probably important to time the weight-bearing exercises. If the joint is acutely inflamed and under tension it may not be a particularly good time as blood supply to the femoral head could be compromised. Intra-articular steroid therapy has been a major advance in recent years, and early intervention with intra-articular steroids would be highly desirable, especially in joints like the hip joint. If there are radiological changes already in the hip joint affecting the bones intra-articular steroids are contraindicated because it could accelerate avascular necrosis. When physiotherapy and exercise fail to prevent deformity of the joints surgical release of muscle spasm and later joint replacement therapy are all options in further management. Splinting of joints in positions of function are vital during the acute disease phase. Involvement of the chiropodist in correcting hind-foot deformity are important for normal growth of the tibia to prevent tibial torsion as well as maldevelopment of the forefoot.

Systemic lupus erythematosus

Systemic lupus erythematosus (SLE) is a multisystem disease defined by a set of criteria proposed by the American Rheumatism Association (ARA) (now the American College of Rheumatology) (Table 25.13.5). Childhood SLE is rare with an incidence of 10–20 in 100 000 Caucasian children [15] with a male to female ratio of 1:4.5 between the ages of 6 and 18 years. In common with adult disease, the incidence is higher in oriental and Afro-Caribbean populations. The diagnosis of SLE in children can often be more difficult as the criteria are not usually fulfilled all at once. Many patients could present with arthralgia/arthritis which would be mistakenly diagnosed as JCA, until sudden onset of nephritis. Neuropsychiatric manifestations can often precede other symptoms and signs of SLE for years. In particular behavioural changes could be misinterpreted until other signs of SLE appear. The clinical signs and symptoms of SLE are shown in Table 25.13.6. The deterioration of renal function after onset of nephritis is often rapid. Thus urinalysis of patients with JCA is important as this may be the prodrome of SLE.

Table 25.13.5 Revised criteria of the ARA for the classification of SLE

Malar rash
Discoid rash
Photosensitivity
Oral ulcers
Arthritis
Serositis
    (a) pleuritis, or
    (b) pericarditis
Renal disorder
    (a) proteinuria > 0.5 g/24 h or 3+ or,
    (b) cellular casts
Neurological disorders
    (a) seizures
    (b) psychosis
Haematological disorders
    (a) haemolytic anaemia
    (b) leucopenia $< 4 \times 10^9/1$
    (c) lymphopenia $< 1.5 \times 10^9/1$ } on two or more occasions
    (d) thrombocytopenia $< 100 \times 10^9/1$
Immunological disorders
    (a) positive lupus erythematosus cell
    (b) raised anti-DNA
    (c) anti-Sm antibody
    (d) false positive test for syphilis, present for 6 months
ANA in raised titre

Table 25.13.6 Clinical features of SLE. Adapted from Silverman and Eddy [15]

Fever signs	% at diagnosis	% at anytime
Fever	60–90	80–100
Arthritis	60–88	60–90
Skin rash (any)	60–78	60–90
Malar rash	22–60	30–80
Renal	20–80	48–100
Cardiovascular	5–30	25–60
Pulmonary	18–40	18–81
CNS	5–30	26–44
Gastrointestinal	14–30	24–40
Hepatosplenomegaly	16–42	19–43
Lymphadenopathy	13–45	13–45

Pathogenesis

SLE is the clinical manifestation of a number of different pathologies. A small number have complement deficiencies and therefore are unable to handle immune complexes in an efficient manner. Deficiency in early components of the classical complement pathway are characteristically associated, but not always, with this disease. In particular, deficiencies in the C4A and C4B genes and C2 genes, and some deficiency of the late components of complement (C6, C7), also manifest as lupus syndrome, although the latter are usually associated more with susceptibility to *Neisseria* infections. In these complement deficient patients they often do not have high titre ANAs or double-stranded DNA antibodies.

The majority of SLE patients, however, do have the characteristic antibodies as defined by the ARA criteria. Monoclonal anti-DNA antibodies have been found and cloned and shown to produce lupus nephritis in the severe combined immune deficient (SCID) mouse [16]. The tendency to produce autoantibodies suggests immune deregulation. Genetic susceptibility are inferred from animal models and also from epidemiological studies of different ethnic groups. Analysis of HLA genes shows that lupus is associated with the class II HLA antigen DR3, and the autoimmune haplotype DR3, C4QO and tumour necrosis factor α2 (TNF-α2). The TNF-α2 allele has recently been shown to be associated with high production of TNF. How these associations are translated into disease mechanisms is unknown.

Clinical features

Musculoskeletal disease

Arthritis and arthralgia are the most common symptoms in childhood and adolescent SLE, occurring in 60–90% of patients. This is usually a symmetrical polyarthritis affecting small peripheral joints usually, and is episodic. Only 1–2% of patients have destructive changes on X-ray. There have been descriptions of conversion from systemic or polyarticular JCA to SLE.

Mucocutaneous involvement

A classical malar rash in the butterfly distribution (Fig. 25.13.5) is present in 60% of patients at the time of diagnosis. It can be severe with crusting. A true photosensitive rash only occurs in 15–30% of children. This could affect all exposed parts of the body and is maculopapular. Discoid lupus rash is very rare in patients under 18 years of age.

Vasculitis of the skin is seen in SLE, and is reported in 10–20% of patients. It affects the fingers and toes, causing splinter haemophages and digital infarcts (Fig. 25.13.6). Oral or nasal ulcers can also occur.

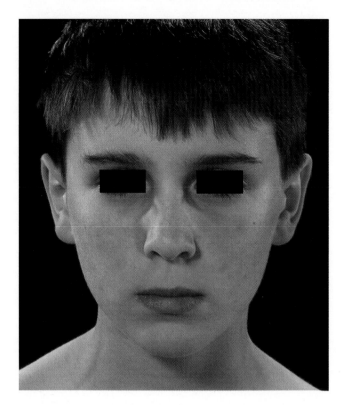

Fig. 25.13.5 Classical malar rash of SLE.

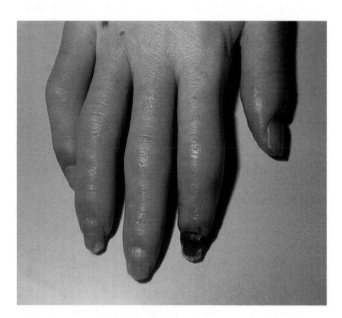

Fig. 25.13.6 Digital infarcts in SLE.

Neuropsychiatric systemic lupus erythematosus

Many patients present with affective or mood disorders which are difficult to differentiate from the effects of steroids or reaction to the illness. This is particularly difficult in the case of the adolescent who will have mood swings irrespective of disease. Cognitive impairment may

Table 25.13.7 International study of kidney disease in children: classification of lupus nephritis. Adapted from Kunkel [33]

I Normal
   IA Nil pathology
   IB Normal by light microscopy but deposits present

II Mesangiopathy only
   IIA Mild
   IIB Moderate

III Segmental and focal proliferative glomerulonephritis
   IIIA Active necrotizing
   IIIB Active and sclerosing
   IIIC Sclerosing

IV Diffuse proliferative glomerulonephritis
   IVA Without segmental necrotizing lesions
   IVB With segmental necrotizing lesions
   IVC With segmental active and sclerotic lesions
   IVD Inactive, sclerotic

V Diffuse membranous glomerulonephritis
   VA Pure membranous
   VB Associated with II (IIA or IIB)
   VC Associated with III (IIIA, IIIB or IIIC)
   VD Associated with IV (IVA, IVB, IVC or IVD)

VI Advanced sclerosing glomerulonephritis

occur in up to 80% of all patients with SLE [17] and is common in children too [18]. Headaches are common. Persistent severe headaches are due to active disease, but migraines can also occur due to vascular instability. It can also be a presenting symptom of pseudotumour cerebri, a presenting symptom of SLE.

Seizures occur in 10–20% and are easily treatable with anticonvulsants. Cranial and peripheral neuropathies can occur. Paresis and transverse myelitis can also occur as a result of vasculitis.

Imaging of the central nervous system (CNS) such as with magnetic resonance imaging (MRI) can show areas of infarct. Abnormalities, however, do not correlate with signs of clinical disease. Antiphospholipid syndrome should be considered in cases of thromboembolism. Lupus anticoagulant and anticardiolipin antibodies are both found in this syndrome.

Renal disease

This is a common manifestation in childhood lupus (Table 25.13.6). Table 25.13.7 shows the classification of renal pathologies. Renal biopsy is necessary to define the renal pathology as well as the degree of active and chronic damage. Semi-quantitative chronicity scores have been developed to predict outcome. The prognosis of the different histological groups are also different, with diffuse proliferative lupus nephritis being the worst. This group can also have associated interstitial inflammation. Patients can present with nephrotic syndrome, haematuria or hypertension.

Treatment

In mild SLE where there is predominantly skin and joint problems, hydroxychloroquine is the drug of choice given at 5 mg/kg in conjunction with non-steroidal anti-inflammatory drugs where appropriate. The arthritis is rarely destructive and does not require any other more potent therapy. Treatment of serositis and other systemic manifestations necessitate corticosteroid treatment with either 2 mg/kg of prednisolone initially or, as is preferred by most doctors, pulse methylprednisolone therapy of 30 mg/kg, given as three doses on consecutive days to achieve an immunosuppressive effect. This is then followed by moderate corticosteroid therapy of 1 mg/kg at slowly reducing doses. Addition of azathioprine up to 3 mg/kg is synergistic in the suppression of lupus manifestations, including lupus nephritis. In fulminating lupus nephritis, however, intravenous cyclophosphamide is preferred, given at approximately 30 mg/kg up to a maximum of 1 g. There is controversy as to how often to repeat cycles of intravenous pulse cyclophosphamide, and also whether continuous oral cyclophosphamide therapy would be preferable. The only study performed was in a small cohort from the American National Institutes of Health where it appeared that intravenous pulse cyclophosphamide was preferable. There are many problems with this study, not least the sequential nature of the study rather than being a concurrent comparative study, as well as the small number of patients involved. Further evaluation using open trial protocol is needed to resolve this issue. Currently the regimen used in the Rheumatology Unit at Great Ormond Street, London, is intravenous pulse cyclophosphamide monthly after initial fortnightly or 3-weekly doses to put the disease into remission. A total of six pulses are then given. Patients then go onto maintenance azathioprine in order to allow further reduction of corticosteroid therapy in the case of remission, or further i.v. cyclophosamide at three-monthly intervals.

Neonatal lupus erythematosus (see Chapter 1.11)

The neonatal lupus erythematosus (NLE) syndrome is a disease of the newborn assumed to be the result of fetal and/or neonatal damage caused by maternal autoantibodies transferred across the placenta. The major clinical manifestations are cardiac and dermatological. The disease is self-limiting.

Clinical features

Cardiac

The characteristic lesion is isolated congenital heart block: Ho *et al.* [19] described the histopathology of eight hearts with complete block and seven were associated with maternal Ro antibodies. In several retrospective and one prospective study the presence of anti-La in association with anti-Ro antibodies is a specific disease marker [20]. The defect is the absence of connection between atrial myocardial tissue and the distal part of the atrioventricular conductive tissue. In some cases, ventricular endomyocardial fibrosis and small inflammatory infiltrates have been described. Immunofluorescence studies have shown deposition of immunoglobulin G (IgG) and complement suggesting an initial inflammatory event.

A long-term follow-up of these children showed six out of 15 required a pacemaker and two neonatal deaths occurred from congestive heart failure [15]. Another series showed three out of 14 neonatal deaths from congestive heart failure and five out of 14 required pacemakers [21].

Skin lesions

The rash is similar to those of subacute cutaneous lupus, in which at least 80% of patients have anti-Ro antibodies [22]. The rash is characteristically photosensitive and ultraviolet (UV) exposure increases the expression of Ro on the surface of keratinocytes.

Liver disease

Enlargement of liver and/or spleen occurred in approximately 30% of babies with NLE [23], with elevation of liver enzymes and cholestasis. Recovery is usual with some residual fibrosis on repeat biopsy.

Treatment

The skin lesions are usually self-limiting without scarring and so topical treatment with steroid is only needed in severe cases.

The prevention of congenital heart block is more controversial. Since only one-third of babies born to mothers at risk will develop heart block, fetal echocardiography could help to screen for heart block/congestive heart failure. Treatment of the mother with dexamethasone and plasmapheresis can reverse the congestive failure but not the heart block. Delivery of such babies should occur in a suitable centre with pacemaker facilities.

Juvenile dermatomyositis

This is an inflammatory vasculitic disease predominantly affecting the skin and muscles. The diagnosis of juvenile dermatomyositis (JDM) is made when three out of four criteria are met in addition to the characteristic rash (Table 25.13.8). It is important to exclude other inflammatory connective tissue diseases which have a myositic component, such as SLE, mixed connective tissue disease, JCA, scleroderma and Sjögren's syndrome.

Table 25.13.8 Criteria for diagnosis of dermatomyositis in childhood. Adapted from Bohan and Peter [34]

Characteristic rash
Symmetrical proximal muscle weakness
Elevated muscle-derived enzymes
Characteristic muscle histopathology
 (inflammatory and atrophy)
EMG changes of inflammatory myopathy
MRI appearance (high signal T2 image)
Exclusion of other rheumatic disease

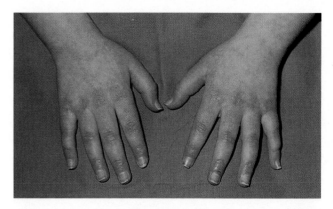

Fig. 25.13.7 Rash of dermatomyositis and Gottron's sign.

Involvement of other organs is evidence of the fulminating type of JDM. In particular vasculitis can lead to infarction of the bowel and can be life threatening.

Pathogenesis

The histopathology of the vascular and muscle lesions are unique. There is usually evidence of damage without prominent inflammatory cellular infiltrates. Small vessel occlusions are uniquely seen in childhood onset dermatomyositis (unlike in adult onset disease). The muscle pathology reflects vascular compromise capillary dropout, perifascicular atrophy of both type 1 and 2 fibres. Histochemical studies reveal HLA class 1 and 2 in the perifascicular area, again suggestive of ischaemia as being a causal factor. Endothelial damage/inflammation is therefore likely to be central to the pathogenesis and serum von Willebrand factor (VWF) reflects disease activity very well.

The link between coxsackie virus and JDM is still controversial. This arose from observations of increased frequency of antibody to coxsackie B and HLA-DR3 in JDM patients in the Chicago area. But attempts to isolate the viral products have so far failed. Other viral illness has been implicated, including hepatitis B [24] and *Toxoplasma* [25]. Of interest is that patients with common variable hypogammaglobulinaemia persistently infected with echo virus also develop dermatomyositis [26].

Clinical features

The skin

The rash can precede or follow muscle weakness. It is characteristically violaceous and typically seen on the eyelid, over the bridge of the nose across the face, over the knuckles of the fingers (Fig. 25.13.7) and the knees. The rash is photosensitive, and skin changes are often seen over the knuckles and knees (Gottron's sign).

Telangiectasia is seen characteristically over the eyelids and nailfolds. The latter has abnormally dilated capillaries. Lipoatrophy of the underlying skin, with panniculitis, is often seen in severe JDM [27].

Calcinosis of soft tissues can occur without obvious muscle weakness. Usually calcinosis is a sequel of tissue damage. It is controversial whether calcinosis is exacerbated by physiotherapy, but chronicity of disease correlates with higher incidence of this complication [28].

Musculoskeletal disease

Muscle weakness occurs initially in the proximal muscle groups, and the neck and abdominal flexors are the first to become weak and the last to recover. Problems with getting up from a chair or the floor, or climbing stairs, are other tell-tale signs of this disease. This weakness is associated with muscular tenderness and the child tends to hold the limb in flexion, thus promoting contractures. Diagnosis is made with the presence of abnormally high muscle enzyme creatine kinase, and muscle histology from a biopsy. MRI is now useful to detect areas of inflammation, shown as high T2 signal, and it is a good test to follow progress as well as being useful in identifying abnormal muscle for biopsy (Fig. 25.13.8).

Arthritis often occurs in severe cases of JDM and osteoporosis occurs in untreated disease, although steroid therapy could also cause osteoporosis.

Gastrointestinal involvement

Decreased oesophageal motility with difficulty in swallowing, reflux with ulceration or aspiration pneumonia and a high-pitched nasal voice are all due to myositis. In addition vasculitis of the mesenteric vessels can cause small bowel angina leading to infarct if untreated. Abdominal pains in JDM patients should therefore be taken seriously, even if there is evidence of reflux and oesophageal ulceration. The areas most commonly affected are the duodenum and upper ileum.

Cardiorespiratory involvement

The electrocardiogram (ECG) is abnormal at the onset in over half of the children [29]. This is usually asymptom-

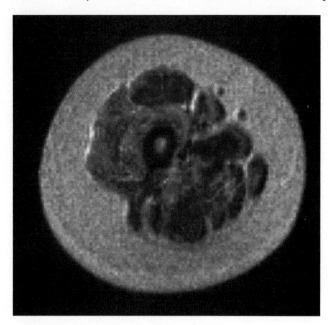

Fig. 25.13.8 MRI of the thigh of a girl with dermatomyositis, showing patchy high signals in many muscle groups.

atic and resolves after remission. The vital capacity is reduced and is usually attributable to myositis of the muscles of the chest wall. Rarely pulmonary fibrosis can occur in the subtypes of patient with RNA synthetase Jo-1 or Mi-2 antibodies. Pulmonary alveolar lipoproteinosis is another rare manifestation of JDM [30].

Genitourinary involvement

Renal ischaemia/vasculopathy can lead to renal failure and necrosis of the ureter has been reported.

Neurological involvement

Vasculitis can lead to vessel thrombosis in the retina and the eyelid. CNS vascular involvement could lead to neuropsychiatric manifestations, as well as epileptic fits.

Treatment and prognosis

Steroid is the drug of choice. With evidence of multi-system involvement, intravenous methylprednisolone is preferable and is given as 3-day pulses of 30 mg/kg. It is worth remembering that intravenous steroid therapy has its own complications such as neurological and gastro-intestinal tract ulceration. This is usually followed by daily oral steroid therapy in divided daily doses. Reduction of steroid therapy should be gradual and monitored by muscle strength. Muscle enzymes are not a good guide after the early phases because of decrease in muscle bulk. Alternate-day steroid does not control the disease well

and so the aim is not to have a differential of more than 5 mg prednisolone on alternate days.

MRI with or without rebiopsy is often needed to assess whether there is continual disease activity.

In the event of life-threatening vasculitis, serum C-reactive protein (CRP) and erythrocyte sedimentation rate (ESR) are also raised. Plasmapheresis and intravenous cyclophosphamide (30 mg/kg) should be instituted. Cyclosporin A is useful as maintenance in steroid 'resistant' subjects but not in the acute phase of vasculitis. Methotrexate is often used too but none of these have undergone comparative open trials or placebo-controlled trials.

Physiotherapy after the acute phase of the disease in the form of passive stretches and graduated muscle strengthening is important in assisting recovery and preventing contractures.

Skin rash is prevented by the use of sunblock and usually recedes with immunosuppressive therapy. Occasionally the rash is the only prominent feature and mepacrine at 5 mg/kg/day is more effective than hydroxychloroquine.

Most cases of JDM have a monocyclic course. But there are relapsing and continuous disease courses as well [31], these are often associated with soft tissue calcinosis. Patients with calcinosis are particularly prone to *Staphylococcus* infection of these sites, and methotrexate can exacerbate this. There is no effective therapy of calcinosis, although etidronate has shown some beneficial effect in a few patients (unpublished data, PW, 1999).

REFERENCES

1 Phaire T. *The Boke of Chyldren*. Edinburgh: E & S Livingston, 1545: 31–2.
2 Cornil PMV. Sur les coincidences pathologiques du rheumatisme articulaire chronique. *Memoire* 1864: 3–25.
3 Still GF. On a form of chronic joint disease in children. *Chirurg Trans* 1897; 80: 47 (reprinted in *Am J Dis Child* 1978; 132: 195–200).
4 Wood PHN. Nomenclature and classification of arthritis in children. In: Munther E, ed. *The Care of Rheumatic Children*. Basel: EULAR, 1978: 47.
5 Petty RE, Southwood TR, Baum J *et al*. Revision of the proposed classification criteria for juvenile idiopathic arthritis: Durban, 1997. *J Rheumatol* 1998; 25(10): 1991–4.
6 Symmons D, Jones MA, Osborne J, Sills J, Southwood T, Woo P. Paediatric rheumatology in the United Kingdom: epidemiological data from the British Paediatric Rheumatology Group National Diagnostic Index. *J Rheumatol* 1996; 23: 1975–80.
7 McDowell TL, Symons JA, Ploski R, Forre O, Duff GW. A genetic association between juvenile rheumatoid arthritis and a novel interleukin-1 alpha polymorphism. *Arthritis Rheum* 1995; 38: 221–8.
8 Fishman D, Faulds G, Jeffery R *et al*. The effect of novel polymorphisms in the interleukin-6 (IL-6) gene on IL-6 transcription and plasma IL-6 levels, and an association with systemic-onset juvenile chronic arthritis. *J Clin Invest* 1998; 102(7): 1369–76.
9 Crawley E, Kay R, Sillibourne J *et al*. Polymorphic haplotypes of the interleukin-10 5′ flanking region determine variable interleukin-10 transcription and are associated with particular phenotypes of juvenile rheumatoid arthritis. *Arthritis Rheum* 1999; 42(6): 1101–8.
10 Ansell BM. Diagnostic criteria, nomenclature, classification. Workshop presentations and discussions. In: Munther E, ed. *The Care of Rheumatic Children*. Basle: EULAR, 1978.
11 Stephan JL, Zeller J, Hubert P, Herbelin C, Dayer JM, Prieur A-M.

Macrophage activation syndrome and rheumatic disease in childhood. *Clin Exp Rheumatol* 1993; 11: 451–6.

12 Schnitzer TJ, Ansell BM. Amyloidosis in juvenile chronic polyarthritis. *Arthritis Rheum* 1977; 20: 245–52.

13 Stoeber E. Progression of juvenile chronic arthritis. *Eur J Pediatr* 1981; 135: 225–8.

14 McCullough CJ. Surgical management of the lipin juvenile chronic arthritis. *Br J Rheumatol* 1994; 33: 178–83.

15 Silverman ED, Eddy A. Systemic lupus erythematosus in childhood and adolescence. In: Maddison P, Isenberg D, Woo P, Glass D, eds. *Oxford Textbook of Rheumatology*. Oxford: Oxford University Press, 1993: 756–71.

16 Mendlovic S, Brooke S, Shoenfeld Y *et al*. Induction of asystemic lupus erythematosus-like disease in mice by a common human anti-DNA idiotype. *Proc Natl Acad Sci (USA)* 1988; 85: 2260–4.

17 Carbotte RM, Denburg SD, Denburg JA. Prevalence of cognitive impairment in systemic lupus erythematosus. *J Nervous Ment Dis* 1986; 174: 357–64.

18 Papero PH, Bluestein HG, White P, Lipnick RN. Neuropsychologic deficits and antineuronal antibodies in pediatric systemic lupus erythematosus. *Clin Exp Rheumatol* 1990; 8: 417–24.

19 Ho YS, Esscher E, Anderson RH, Michaelsson M. Anatomy of clinical complete heartblock and relation to maternal anti-Ro antibodies. *Am J Cardiol* 1986; 58: 291–4.

20 Silverman ED, Mamula M, Hardin JA, Laxer RM. Importance of the immune response to the Ro/La particle in the development of congenital heartblock and neonatal lupus erythematosus. *J Rheumatol* 1991; 18: 120–4.

21 McCune AB, Weston WL, Lee LA. Maternal and fetal outcome in neonatal lupus erythematosus. *Am Int Med* 1987; 106: 518–23.

22 Deng JS, Sontheimer RD, Gilliam JN. Relationships between antinuclear antibodies and anti-Ro/SSA antibodies in subacute cutaneous lupus erythematosus. *J Am Acad Dermatol* 1984; 11: 494–9.

23 Laxer RM, Roberts EA, Gross KR *et al*. Liver disease in neonatal lupus. *J Pediatr* 1990; 116: 238–42.

24 Pittsley PA, Shearer MA, Kaufman MD. Acute hepatitis B stimulating dermatomyositis. *J Am Med Assoc* 1978; 239: 959.

25 Lapetina F. Toxoplasmosis and dermatomyositis. *Pediatr Med Chirurg* 1989; 11: 197–203.

26 Webster ADB. Immunodeficiency. In: Maddison P, Isenberg D, Woo P, Glass D, eds. *Oxford Textbook of Rheumatology*. 1993: 608–13.

27 Commens C, O'Neill P, Walker G. Dermatomyositis associated with multifocal atrophy. *J Am Acad Dermatol* 1990; 22: 966–9.

28 Pachman LM. Polymyositis and dermatomyositis in children. In: Maddison P, Isenberg D, Woo P, Glass D, eds. *Oxford Textbook of Rheumatology*. Oxford: Oxford University Press, 1993: 821–8.

29 Pachman LM, Cooke N. Juvenile dermatomyositis, a clinical and immunological study. *J Pediatr* 1980; 96: 226–34.

30 Samuels MP, Warner JO. Pulmonary alveolar lipoproteinosis complicating juvenile dermatomyositis. *Thorax* 1988; 43: 939–40.

31 Spencer CH, Hanson V, Singsen B, Bernstein BH, Kornreich HD, King KK. Course of treated dermatomyositis. *J Pediatr* 1984; 105: 39–408.

32 Prieur AM, Petty R. *Arthritis in Children and Adolescents*. London: Baillière Tindall, 1993.

33 Kunkel HG. The immunopathology of lupus erythematosus. *Hosp Pract* 1980; 15: 47.

34 Bohan A, Peter JB. Polymyositis and dermatomyositis. *N Engl J Med* 1975; 292: 344–7, 403–7.

25.14 Immunodeficiency Syndromes

AMY S. PALLER

Ataxia telangiectasia

Cartilage–hair hypoplasia syndrome

Chediak–Higashi syndrome

Chronic granulomatous disease

Chronic mucocutaneous candidiasis

Complement deficiency disorders
Hereditary angioneurotic oedema
Other complement deficiencies

DiGeorge's syndrome

Hyperimmunoglobulin E recurrent infection syndrome

Immunoglobulin deficiencies
Immunoglobulin A deficiency
Immunoglobulin M deficiency
X-linked hypogammaglobulinaemia with
    hyperimmunoglobulinaemia M syndrome
Panhypogammaglobulinaemia
X-linked lymphoproliferative disease

Leucocyte adhesion deficiency

Severe combined immunodeficiency

Wiskott–Aldrich syndrome

Several immunodeficiency syndromes are associated with mucocutaneous abnormalities that facilitate early diagnosis or are complications of the immunodeficiency. Since the 1990s tremendous information has accrued to increase the understanding of the pathomechanism of these disorders, diagnosis of patients and carrier mothers, prenatal diagnosis and new means of therapy of selected genetic immunodeficiency diseases (for reviews see [1–3]).

In general, immunodeficiency should be suspected when patients have recurrent infections of increased duration and severity, particularly with unusual organisms. Incomplete clearing of infections or poor response to antibiotics may be associated. The most common non-cutaneous abnormalities are failure to thrive, recurrent infections, diarrhoea, vomiting, hepatosplenomegaly,

arthritis, adenopathy or lack of anticipated nodes and haematological abnormalities. Cutaneous abnormalities may include alopecia, angio-oedema, cutaneous granulomas, cutaneous infections, atopic-like or seborrhoeic-like dermatitis, macular erythemas, lupus-like changes, petechiae, pigmentary dilution, poor wound healing, purpura and telangiectasias. Patients with immunodeficiency disorders have a risk of the development of malignancy (overall 4%) that is 10 000 times higher than that of healthy, age-matched controls. After infection, malignancy is the second leading cause of death in children and adults with congenital immunodeficiency disorders (for review see [4]).

REFERENCES

1 Buckley RH. Breakthroughs in the understanding and therapy of primary immunodeficiency. *Pediatr Clin N Am* 1994; 41: 665–90.
2 Nelson DL, Kurman CC. Molecular genetic analysis of the primary immunodeficiency disorders. *Pediatr Clin N Am* 1994; 41: 657–64.
3 Pacheco SE, Shearer WT. Laboratory aspects of immunology. *Pediatr Clin N Am* 1994; 41: 623–55.
4 Mueller BU, Pizzo PA. Cancer in children with primary or secondary immunodeficiencies. *J Pediatr* 1995; 126: 1–10.

Ataxia telangiectasia

Ataxia telangiectasia (AT) is an autosomal recessive disorder characterized by cerebellar ataxia beginning in early infancy, progressive oculocutaneous telangiectasia, a tendency to sinopulmonary infections, selective immunodeficiencies [1] and chromosomal instability with hypersensitivity to ionizing radiation. The incidence of AT is estimated at about 1 in 40 000 births.

Pathogenesis

Inhibition of semiconservative DNA synthesis and cell cycle progression by ionizing radiation is reduced in AT cells, suggesting defects in the checkpoints at the G1 and G2 phases of the cell cycle. In addition, stability of p53 after irradiation is significantly delayed, further implicating a defective G1 checkpoint that normally allows DNA repair after damage. Using linkage analysis, the gene for AT was localized to 11q22–23 [2]. Recently, the AT gene

(ATM, ataxia telangiectasia, mutated) was identified as a 1708 amino acid protein [3] that resembles phosphatidylinositol (PI)-3 kinases. PI-3 kinases add phosphates to lipid molecules, and thus transmit growth and other regulatory signals. The ATM product is also similar to proteins that control the G1 phase of the cell cycle, and may be essential for DNA repair, meiotic recombination and for the prevention of programmed cell death. Several gene mutations have now been detected in the ATM gene in patients with AT.

Clinical features

The initial manifestation is usually ataxia, which typically becomes apparent when the child begins to walk. The characteristic oculocutaneous features often facilitate the diagnosis, but are usually first noted between 3 and 6 years of age. The telangiectasias first appear at the angles of the eyes and extend medially as bright red, symmetric horizontal streaks on the exposed bulbar conjunctivae (Fig. 25.14.1). During the next few years, patients begin to develop cutaneous telangiectasias, especially on the ears, eyelids, malar prominences, V of the neck and antecubital and popliteal fossae. Less commonly, the dorsum of the hands and feet and the hard and soft palate have telangiectasias. Although the ocular telangiectasias are quite striking, the cutaneous telangiectasias may be subtle and resemble fine petechiae, especially at sites other than the face. Evidence of premature ageing of the skin and hair is noted eventually in almost 90% of children [4]. Subcutaneous fat is lost early and the facial skin tends to become atrophic and sclerotic. Grey hairs may be found in young children and diffuse greying of the hair often occurs by adolescence. Other dermatological changes that appear to be associated specifically with AT are hypertrichosis, especially noticeable on the forearms, chronic seborrhoeic dermatitis with blepharitis, poikilodermatous pigmentary changes, large café-au-lait spots and non-infectious cutaneous granulomas [5]. The granulomatous lesions are tender, erythematous atrophic papules and plaques (Fig. 25.14.2), and are often ulcerated. Biopsy sections of these granulomas show granuloma annulare or granulomatous dermatitis, and cultures and special stains for organisms are negative.

The ataxia is cerebellar, and is characterized by swaying of the head and trunk. Myoclonic jerks, choreoathetosis, oculomotor abnormalities and dysarthric speech become prominent in older children. Ocular apraxia, the inability to follow an object with the eyes, is a reliable neurological finding [1]. Patients are usually confined to a wheelchair by the time they are 11 years old despite good muscular strength. A characteristic facies develops that is dull, sad and hypotonic when relaxed. Later, the face becomes mask-like when progeric changes ensue.

The third feature of AT, sinopulmonary infections,

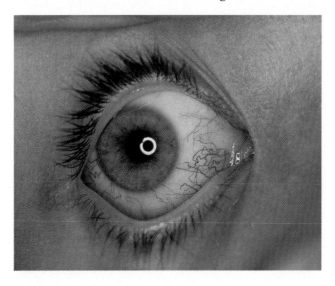

Fig. 25.14.1 Telangiectasias of the bulbar conjuctiva in AT are particularly prominent at the canthi.

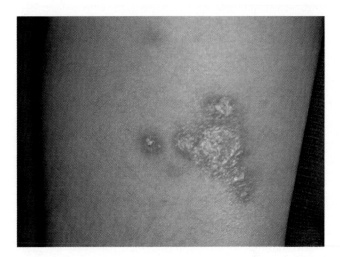

Fig. 25.14.2 Cutaneous granulomas in AT are persistent and may become ulcerated.

occurs in more than 80% of patients in some series. It is the most common cause of death, usually from bronchiectasis and respiratory failure. Other manifestations of AT include retardation of somatic growth (72%), mental retardation (33%) and endocrine abnormalities, especially ovarian agenesis or hypoplasia and insulin-resistant diabetes. Malignancy occurs in up to one-third of patients, and may be the presenting problem, leading to the use of dangerously high doses of radiation therapy. Of malignancies 80% are lymphoreticular, and B-cell lymphomas predominate. However, more than 20% of the malignancies are leukaemias, particularly T-cell leukaemias that involve chromosome 14 translocations or inversions. Spontaneous chromosomal abnormalities (fragments, breaks, gaps and translocations) occur between two and

18 times more frequently in patients with AT than in normal individuals. Rearrangements of chromosomes 7 and 14, and especially 14:14 translocations, seem to predict the development of lymphoreticular malignancy. Fibroblast DNA is extremely sensitive to ionizing radiation and to radiomimetic agents such as bleomycin, probably due to failure to cease DNA synthesis transiently after radiation exposure, and perhaps also due to defective repair. Gastric carcinomas have also been described, always in association with deficient immunoglobulin A (IgA) in AT. Patients with AT also have an increased risk of the development of epithelial malignancy, especially basal cell carcinomas, after 20 years of age.

Heterozygotes for the ATM gene (1% of the US population) are at increased risk for neoplasia, especially breast cancer in female carriers [6]. Heterozygote fibroblasts and lymphocytes demonstrate chromosomal breaks after exposure to ionizing radiation, raising the issue of routine mammography in these patients as a means to screen for breast cancer.

A variety of immunological defects have been described in patients with AT [7]. Approximately 70% of patients have deficient or absent levels of serum IgA, and many patients demonstrate circulating anti-IgA antibodies. Even if the total serum IgA is normal, many patients have demonstrated the specific deficiency of IgA2. Of patients 80% demonstrate deficient to absent levels of IgE. Occasionally, levels of IgM are increased, and 80% of patients show a low molecular weight (8S) serum IgM. IgG is often deficient, especially subgroups IgG2 and IgG4. Not infrequently, patients demonstrate increased levels of T-suppressor cells and decreased T-helper cells. Almost all patients with AT tend to have elevated levels of α-fetoprotein and carcinoembryonic antigen. Defective cell-mediated immunity is noted in 70% of patients. Abnormalities include lymphopenia, delayed allograft rejection, impaired self-response to recall antigens, and a deficient response to specific antigens and mitogens. The majority of patients have an absent or abnormally developed thymus. Other laboratory abnormalities include mildly elevated liver function tests in 40–50% of patients, and evidence of glucose intolerance with hyperinsulinaemia, insulin resistance and hyperglycaemia in over 50% of patients.

Prognosis

Patients with AT have progressive ataxia, often leading to the inability to walk without assistance by the early teenage years. The features of ageing are also progressive and marked by adolescence. Death frequently occurs in late childhood or the early teenage years. The oldest reported patients died at 50 years of age. Of patients 55% die because of chronic sinopulmonary disease and progressive respiratory insufficiency. The second most common cause of death is malignancy, leading to death in 15% of patients. The remaining 30% of patients tend to die because of sinopulmonary infection and respiratory insufficiency, but show evidence of malignancy on autopsy. Some of the patients who survive into their thirties or forties show stabilization of the disorder, with improvement in neurological and immunological status.

Differential diagnosis

The features of AT are similar to those of Nijmegen breakage syndrome (NBS), a rare autosomal recessive disorder in which patients have short stature, a 'bird-like' face, microcephaly from birth and retardation [8]. Immunological, cytogenetic and cell biological findings are almost identical. Patients with NBS do not have the ataxia, telangiectasia or elevated α-fetoprotein levels of AT, but have a greater risk of malignancy and more severe immunodeficiency. Patients with overlap features of both disorders have been described [9].

Treatment

The treatment of patients with AT is supportive. No agent has been demonstrated to control the progressive neurological and cutaneous changes. The infections must be treated appropriately with antibiotics. Avoidance of sun exposure and use of sunscreens may help to prevent the actinic-like changes of ageing. Early physiotherapy should be instituted for patients with pulmonary bronchiectasis and physical therapy appropriate for the neurological dysfunction should be started early to prevent contractures. Radiation and radiomimetic chemotherapeutic agents, especially bleomycin, actinomycin D and cyclophosphamide, may lead to extensive tissue necrosis and should be avoided unless no other alternative is available. If necessary, small doses of chemotherapeutic drugs and radiation doses of less than 20 Gy, in fractions of less than 1 Gy, are the least harmful means of managing these malignancies. AT patients have decreased thresholds for postradiation erythema, tissue necrosis and radiation-induced cutaneous malignancy.

Prenatal diagnosis has been successfully performed to diagnose AT [10–12], including by molecular genetic analysis [13]. In addition, affected fetal cells show increased spontaneous chromosome breakage and lack of control of cell cycling after irradiation damage, particularly during S phase. Bone marrow and fetothymic transplants, transfer factor and levamisole hydrochloride therapy have not resulted in clinical improvement.

REFERENCES

1 Gatti RA. Ataxia-telangiectasia. *Dermatol Clin* 1995; 13: 1–6.

2 Gatti RA, Berkel I, Boder E *et al*. Localization of an ataxia-telangiectasia to chromosome 11q22–23. *Nature* 1988; 336: 577–80.

3 Savitsky K, Bar-Shira A, Gilad S *et al*. A single ataxia-telangiectasia gene with a produce similar to PI-3 kinase. *Science* 1995; 268: 1749–53.

4 Cohen LE, Tanner DJ, Schaefer HG, Levis WR. Common and uncommon cutaneous findings in patients with ataxia telangiectasia. *J Am Acad Dermatol* 1984; 10: 431–7.

5 Paller AS, Massey RB, Curtis MA *et al*. Cutaneous granulomatous lesions in patients with ataxia-telangiectasia. *J Pediatr* 1991; 119: 917–22.

6 Swift M, Morrell D, Massey RB, Chase CL. Incidence of cancer in 161 families affected by ataxia-telangiectasia. *N Engl J Med* 1991; 325: 1831–6.

7 Waldmann TA, Misiti J, Nelson DL, Kraemer KH. Ataxia telangiectasia: a multisystem hereditary disease with immunodeficiency, impaired maturation, X-ray hypersensitivity, and a high incidence of neoplasia. *Ann Intern Med* 1983; 99: 367–79.

8 Weemaes CMR, Smeets DFCM, van der Burgt CJAM. Nijmegen breakage syndrome: a progress report. *Int J Radiat Biol* 1994; 66: S185–8.

9 Jaspers NGJ, Taalman RDFM, Baan C. Patients with an inherited syndrome characterized by immunodeficiency, microcephaly and chromosomal instability: genetic relationship with ataxia-telangiectasia. *Am J Hum Genet* 1988; 42: 66–73.

10 Kleijer WJ, Van der Kraan M, Los FJ, Jaspers NGJ. Prenatal diagnosis of ataxia-telangiectasia and Nijmegen breakage syndrome by the assay of radioresistance DNA analysis. *Int J Radiat Biol* 1994; 66: S167–74.

11 Jaspers NG, van der Kraan M, Linssen PCM, Macek M, Seemanova E, Kleijer WJ. First-trimester prenatal diagnosis of the Nijmegen breakage syndrome and ataxia telangiectasia using an assay radioresistant DNA synthesis. *Prenat Diagn* 1990; 10: 667–74.

12 Llerena J, Murer-Orlando M, McGuire M *et al*. Spontaneous and induced chromosome breakage in chorionic villus samples: a cytogenetic approach to first trimester prenatal diagnosis of ataxia telangiectasia syndrome. *J Med Genet* 1989; 26: 174–8.

13 Gatti RA, Peterson KL, Novak J *et al*. Prenatal genotyping of ataxia-telangiectasia. *Lancet* 1993; 342: 376.

Cartilage–hair hypoplasia syndrome

Cartilage–hair hypoplasia (CHH) syndrome is an autosomal recessive disorder that is most common in Amish individuals and in the Finnish population [1]. Patients have fine, sparse, hypopigmented hair and metaphyseal dysostosis that results in the short-limbed dwarfism. Patients may have soft, doughy skin with degenerated elastic tissue [2]. Growth failure is disproportionate, with a long trunk in relationship to short limbs. Most patients manifest some degree of defective cell-mediated immunity, although 44% of patients show no unusual suscptibility to infections. Varicella infection may be fatal [3]. A minority of affected patients also have defective humoral immunity as well. Malignancy, especially lymphoreticular, occurs in 10% of patients. The CHH gene was recently assigned to chromosome 9, and has allowed prenatal diagnosis in four patients.

REFERENCES

1 Makitie O, Sulisalo T, de la Chapelle A, Kaitila I. Cartilage–hair hypoplasia. *J Med Genet* 1995; 32: 39–43.

2 Brennan T, Pearson R. Abnormal elastic tissue in cartilage–hair hypoplasia. *Arch Dermatol* 1988; 124: 1411–14.

3 Polmar SH, Pierce GF. Cartilage–hair hypoplasia: immunological aspects and their clinical implications. *Clin Immunol Immunopathol* 1986; 40: 87–93.

Chediak–Higashi syndrome

Chediak–Higashi syndrome (CHS) is an autosomal recessive disorder characterized by incomplete oculocutaneous albinism, photophobia and severe recurrent infections [1–3].

Pathogenesis

The giant abnormal granules are the hallmark of CHS, and result from dysregulated fusion of primary lysosomes. They are found in circulating leucocytes, melanocytes, melanosomes of hair, renal tubular epithelial cells, central nervous system (CNS) neurones and other tissues. These giant granules within phagocytic cells of affected children cannot discharge their lysosomal and peroxidative enzymes into phagocytic vacuoles. The dysregulated fusion results from mutations in LYST, a lysosomal transport protein.

Immunological defects of CHS include diminished chemotaxis of polymorphonuclear cells, monocytes and lymphocytes, decreased antibody-dependent cytotoxicity and reduced suppressor cell function. Natural killer cell function is often profoundly decreased, despite a relative increase in the number of γ/Δ T cells [5]. These immune abnormalities have been thought to cause the increased susceptibility to infections and the lymphoma-like phase. Neutrophils show a deficiency of cathepsin G and elastase [6] owing to the presence of excess inhibitors [7]; the inactivation of these enzymes may also contribute to the increased susceptibility to infection.

Clinical features

Patients with CHS usually have a characteristic silvery sheen to the hair and skin, and may demonstrate partial albinism of the hair, skin or eyes when contrasted with other family members. Loss of iris pigmentation results in an increased red reflex and photophobia. Strabismus and nystagmus are common, but visual acuity is usually normal. Inflammation and ulceration of the oral mucosa, especially of the gingivae, have been described.

Many patients with CHS develop progressive neurological deterioration, particularly with clumsiness, abnormal gait, paraesthesias and dysaesthesias. Peripheral and cranial neuropathies and, occasionally, a form of spinocerebellar degeneration may occur [2]. Other findings on physical examination relate to the frequent infections in the accelerated phase of the disease.

Infectious episodes are associated with fever and predominantly involve the skin, lungs and upper respiratory tract. The most common organisms found are *Staphylococcus aureus*, *Streptococcus pyogenes* and *Pneumococcus*. The skin infections are primarily pyodermas, but infections with these organisms that result in deeper ulcerations resembling pyoderma gangrenosum have been reported.

Of patients 85% undergo an accelerated lymphomatous phase, characterized by widespread visceral tissue infiltration with lymphoid and histiocytic cells, which are sometimes atypical in appearance. Hepatosplenomegaly, lymphadenopathy, pancytopenia, jaundice, a leukaemia-like gingivitis and pseudomembranous sloughing of the buccal mucosa are associated features. The thrombocytopenia and depletion of coagulation factors (decreased hepatic synthesis) may lead to petechiae, bruising and gingival bleeding. Granulocytopenia and anaemia are found in 90% of patients during the accelerated phase. Viral infection, particularly due to Epstein–Barr virus (EBV) infection, has been implicated in causing the accelerated lymphomatous phase [8–10].

Prognosis

The mean age of death for patients with CHS is 6 years of age. Fatality usually results from overwhelming infection or haemorrhage during the lymphoma-like accelerated phase.

Differential diagnosis

CHS should be differentiated from other 'silver hair syndromes' [11], particularly Griscelli's syndrome [12,13]. The clinical signs of Griscelli's syndrome include silver–grey hair and a relatively light skin colour, recurrent episodes of fever with or without infection, increasing hepatosplenomegaly due to lymphohistiocytic infiltration and progressive neurological deterioration with hypotonia and motor retardation [13]. Patients have impaired delayed type hypersensitivity, hypogammaglobulinaemia and impaired NK cell function. Blood smears show pancytopenia, but no leucocyte inclusions. Microscopic examination of the hair shows clumping of pigment in the hair shaft, similar to that of CHS, and ultrastructural examination of skin biopsies reveals accumulation of melanosomes in the melanocytes.

Treatment

Bone marrow transplantation is the treatment of choice for patients with an HLA-matched marrow available. Otherwise, management of the disorder is largely supportive. Antibiotics help to control the recurrent infections. Vincristine sulphate and prednisone combination therapy has been beneficial, as have high dosages of aciclovir [14] and gammaglobulin [15] in controlling the accelerated lymphoma-like phase. Splenectomy has been advocated in patients with the accelerated phase unresponsive to other forms of therapy [16]. Ascorbic acid has been administered, and has been found to correct the *in vitro* defect

of microtubular function, perhaps through elevation of cyclic adenosine monophosphate (cAMP). However, when given to patients for weeks to months, it does not appear to decrease the frequency of infections in most cases, nor does it prevent the accelerated phase. Interferon has been demonstrated by some authors to restore partially natural killer cell function.

The profound natural killer defect and immunodeficiency has been reversed by successful bone marrow transplantation, but the partial albinism is not altered [17]. Bone marrow transplantation has also successfully reversed the relentless deterioration of patients with Griscelli's syndrome [12]. Prenatal diagnosis of CHS has been determined by the demonstration of giant melanin granules in the hair of scalp biopsy samples, and confirmation by blood cell analysis [18].

REFERENCES

1 Stegmaier OC, Schneider LA. Chediak–Higashi syndrome: dermatologic manifestations. *Arch Dermatol* 1965; 91: 1–9.
2 Blume RS, Wolff SM. The Chediak–Higashi syndrome: studies in four patients and review of the literature. *Medicine* 1972; 51: 247–80.
3 Anderson LL, Paller AS, Malpass D, Schmidt ML, Berger TG. Chediak–Higashi syndrome in a black child. *Pediatr Dermatol* 1992; 9: 31–6.
4 Barbosa MDFS, Nguyen QA, Tchernev VT *et al.* Identification of the homologous beige and Chediak–Higashi Syndrome genes. *Nature* 1996; 382: 262–4.
5 Holcombe RF, van de Griend R, Ang S-L, Bolhuis RLH, Seidman JG. Gamma-delta T cells in Chediak–Higashi syndrome. *Acta Haematol* 1990; 83: 193–7.
6 Ganz T, Metcalf JA, Gallin JI, Boxer LA, Lehrer RI. Microbicidal/cytotoxic proteins of neutrophils are deficient in two disorders: Chediak–Higashi syndrome and 'specific' granule deficiency. *J Clin Invest* 1988; 82: 552–6.
7 Takeuchi KH, Swank RT. Inhibitors of elastase and cathepsin G in Chediak–Higashi (beige) neutrophils. *J Biol Chem* 1989; 264: 7431–6.
8 Rubin CM, Burke BA, McKenna RW *et al.* The accelerated phase of Chediak–Higashi syndrome: an expression of the virus-associated hemophagocytic syndrome? *Cancer* 1985; 56: 524–30.
9 Merino F, Henle W, Ramirez-Duque P. Chronic active Epstein–Barr virus infection in patients with Chediak–Higashi syndrome. *J Clin Immunol* 1986; 6: 299–305.
10 Kinugawa N. Epstein–Barr virus infection in Chediak–Higashi syndrome mimicking acute lymphocytic leukemia. *Am J Pediatr Hematol/Oncol* 1990; 12: 182–6.
11 Larregue M, Buriot D, Prigent F, Lorette G, Marie M, Degos R. Les cheveux argentes chez l'enfant. Symptome d'appel des maladies leucogranulocytaires et melanocytaires. *Ann Dermatol Vénéréol* 1981; 108: 329–34.
12 Schneider LC, Berman RS, Shea CR, Perez-Atayde AR, Weinstein H, Geha RS. Bone marrow transplantation (BMT) for the syndrome of pigmentary dilution and lymphohistiocytosis (Griscelli's syndrome). *J Clin Immunol* 1990; 10: 146–53.
13 Mancini AJ, Chan LS, Paller AS. Partial albinism with immunodeficiency; Griscelli Syndrome: report of a case and review of the literature. *J Am Acad Dermatol* 1998; 38: 295–300.
14 Conley M, Henle W. Acyclovir in accelerated phase of Chediak–Higashi syndrome. *Lancet* 1987; 1: 212–13.
15 Kinugawa N, Ohtani T. Beneficial effects of high-dose intravenous gammaglobulin on the accelerated phase of Chediak–Higashi syndrome. *Helv Pediatr Acta* 1985; 40: 169–72.
16 Harfi HA, Malik SA. Chediak–Higashi syndrome: clinical, hematologic, and immunologic improvement after splenectomy. *Ann Allergy* 1992; 69: 147–50.
17 Griscelli C, Virelizier J-L. Bone marrow transplantation in a patient with Chediak–Higashi syndrome. *Birth Defects: Orig Article Ser* 1983; 19: 333–4.
18 Durandy A, Breton-Gorius A, Guy-Grand D, Dumez C, Griscelli C. Prenatal diagnosis of syndromes associating albinism and immune deficiencies (Chediak–Higashi syndrome and variant). *Prenat Diagn* 1993; 13: 13–20.

Chronic granulomatous disease

Chronic granulomatous disease (CGD) is a group of disorders characterized by severe recurrent infections due to an inability of phagocytic leucocytes to kill intracellular bacteria by generating oxidative metabolites. The incidence of this rare disease is estimated to be between approximately 1 in 250 000 and 1 in 500 000 people. The disorder is usually inherited by X-linked transmission, and less commonly as an autosomal recessive disorder.

Pathogenesis

For normal bactericidal activity after phagocytosis, cells must respond to phagocytosed organisms with a 'respiratory burst', producing toxic metabolites of oxygen. The defect in CGD involves the nicotinamide adenine dinucleotide (NADPH) oxidase system, which consists of NADPH, an unusual phagocyte cytochrome b and several cytosolic proteins [1]. In most X-linked kindreds (60% of patients), p22-phox or gp91-phox subunits of cytochrome b_{558} are mutated and usually not detectable [2]. Most patients with autosomal recessive CGD (40%) have normal cytochrome b_{558} [3], but are deficient in NADPH oxidase cytosolic factors (47 kDa and, less commonly, 67 kDa) [4]. It is thought that cytochrome b_{558} is the membrane attachment site for the p47 and p67 cytosolic factors that translocate from the cytosol to the plasma membrane and this assembly of oxidase components, including phosphorylation of p47, allows activation.

The laboratory and clinical abnormalities that are seen in CGD may be explained as compensatory reactions after the failure of phagocytic killing. These include the characteristic classes of microbial organisms involved in producing infections, the intensive humoral reaction reflected by hypergammaglobulinaemia and the brisk cellular reaction characterized by cutaneous inflammation. In addition, granulomas are formed around the invading organisms in an attempt to confine them further, but result in visceral impairment. When granulomas involve the skin, a skin biopsy demonstrates histiocytic infiltrates associated with foreign body giant cells, and accumulation of neutrophils with necrosis.

Clinical presentation

The areas of the body that are most often involved in CGD are those that are frequently challenged by bacteria, including the skin, lungs and perianal tissue. The earliest lesions are usually staphylococcal infections of the skin around the ears and nose, and may be present at birth [5,6]. The localized pyodermas may progress in infancy to extensive purulent dermatitis with regional lymphadenopathy. Skin abscesses are common, especially in the perianal region. Inflammatory reactions, often purulent, tend to develop at sites of minor cutaneous trauma or sites of regional lymph node drainage, which heal slowly with scarring. CGD may also present as Sweet's syndrome during infancy [7]. Cutaneous granulomas occur less frequently than cutaneous infections, and are nodular and often necrotic. Seborrhoeic dermatitis, scalp folliculitis, perioral ulcers and intraoral ulcerations, resembling aphthous stomatitis, have been described. Occasionally, patients may have cutaneous features of systemic or discoid lupus erythematosus.

The extracutaneous organs most frequently involved in CGD are the lymph nodes, lungs, liver, spleen and gastrointestinal tract. Suppurative lymphadenitis usually affects the cervical nodes, with abscess and fistula formation. Axillary, inguinal, mesenteric and mediastinal lymph nodes are often involved as well. Bronchopneumonia occurs in almost all children with CGD, and responds slowly and inadequately to appropriate antibacterial therapy. Abscess formation, cavitation and empyema are frequent complications. Hepatosplenomegaly is found in 80–90% of patients. More than one-third of patients develop hepatic abscesses, and granulomas of the liver and spleen are common. These granulomas can occlude vital structures, especially granulomas of the gastrointestinal and genitourinary systems. Gastrointestinal abnormalities in CGD are most commonly characterized by persistent or recurrent diarrhoea and malabsorption. Gastritis, oesophagitis and colitis have been described as well. Osteomyelitis and urinary tract abnormalities are other features of CGD.

The laboratory abnormalities in CGD include leucocytosis, anaemia, elevated erythrocyte sedimentation rate, hypergammaglobulinaemia and an abnormal chest radiograph. Skin testing for delayed hypersensitivity is normal, as is phagocytosis and chemotaxis. The screening test for CGD is the nitroblue tetrazolium (NBT) reduction assay. NBT is yellow in its soluble, oxidized form. When reduced, the dye precipitates and becomes blue–black (formazan). Approximately 80–90% of normal leucocytes are able to reduce NBT during phagocytosis. However, only 50% of leucocytes from carriers of CGD and 5–10% of leucocytes from patients with CGD are able to reduce NBT during phagocytosis. Quantitative NBT tests, chemiluminescence assays, and flow cytometric techniques may also be performed to further verify the diagnosis. Western blotting may distinguish the four subgroups of CGD, using antibodies against p22-phox, gp91-phox, p47-phox and p67-phox.

The organisms associated with CGD are usually *S. aureus* and opportunistic Gram-negative bacteria, including *Klebsiella*, *Pseudomonas*, *Escherichia coli* and *Serratia*. Other organisms involved in the disorder include *Aspergillus*, *Candida*, *Cryptococcus* and *Nocardia*. The generation of oxidative metabolites is necessary for phagocytic leucocytes to kill these microorganisms.

Differential diagnosis

CGD should be suspected in children with recurrent cutaneous, nodal and visceral infections. Laboratory tests allow differentiation of CGD from other disorders with increased susceptibility to bacterial infections, such as hypogammaglobulinaemias and the hyper-IgE (HIE) syndrome.

Treatment

The use of antibiotics has markedly reduced the morbidity and mortality of CGD [8]. Cutaneous or nodal infections may be readily apparent. However, small localized areas of inflammation, with or without fever, may be difficult to detect. Vigorous investigation of the lungs, liver and bones by scans or ultrasound often uncovers an occult focus of inflammation. Cultures should be performed to determine the aetiological agent, and appropriate therapy should be initiated. Invasive surgical procedures may be required for adequate cultures. If culture material cannot be obtained or while awaiting culture results, patients should be treated with parenteral antibiotics, including antibiotics effective for staphylococcal infections, for at least 10–14 days. A course of oral antibiotics should subsequently be continued for weeks. Long-term prophylactic trimethoprim–sulphamethoxazole therapy decreases the incidence of bacterial infection without increasing the incidence of fungal infection [9,10]. Administration of itraconazole diminishes the incidence of *Aspergillus* infection [11]. Surgical intervention can be very important for deeper infections and includes debridement, irrigation and prolonged drainage. Leucocyte transfusions have been used in cases of rapidly progressive, life-threatening infections. Bone marrow transplantation has been employed successfully in CGD [12], but is not appropriate for most patients.

Patients with both X-linked CGD and 'variant' CGD have shown clinical improvement after administration of γ-interferon [13], although the mechanism of action is unclear [14]. One of the compensatory reactions after the failure of phagocytic killing in patients with CGD is the generation of granulomas in viscera and less commonly in the skin. Short courses of systemic corticosteroids have been helpful for patients with obstructive visceral granulomas of the bronchopulmonary, gastrointestinal or genitourinary tracts [15,16]. Preliminary gene therapy studies have shown successful introduction of the normal p47phox gene into cells of deficient patients, but *in vivo* testing has not been performed [17].

The diagnosis of carrier state is important for genetic counselling before pregnancy, including for sisters of the affected male patient. Approximately 50% of women are carriers in families of patients with the X-linked form of CGD. Heterozygous carriers have variable proportions of normal and abnormal cells, and may demonstrate a partial defect in oxidative metabolism and bacterial killing, but generally do not show increased susceptibility to infections. Many carriers have been described with discoid lupus erythematosus, photosensitivity, severe aphthous stomatitis [18,19], Jessner's lymphocytic infiltrate or granulomatous cheilitis [20]. The histopathology of the discoid lupus is not typical, and immunofluorescence examination is negative [19]. The relationship between the development of the lupus-like illness and impaired microbial killing remains unclear. Prenatal diagnosis of CGD has been achieved by the NBT slide test on blood samples obtained by placental vessel puncture from fetuses at risk [21], and may be performed by molecular analysis.

REFERENCES

1 Roos D. The genetic basis of chronic granulomatous disease. *Immunol Rev* 1994; 138: 121–57.
2 Segal AW, Cross AR, Garcia RC *et al.* Absence of cytochrome b245 in chronic granulomatous disease. *N Engl J Med* 1983; 308: 245–51.
3 Weening R, Corbeel L, de Boer M *et al.* Cytochrome b deficiency in an autosomal form of chronic granulomatous disease. *J Clin Invest* 1985; 75: 915–20.
4 Clark RA, Malech HL, Gallin JI *et al.* Genetic variants of chronic granulomatous disease: prevalence of deficiencies of two cytosolic components of the NADPH oxidase system. *N Engl J Med* 1989; 321: 647–52.
5 Windhorst DB, Good RA. Dermatologic manifestations of fatal granulomatous disease of childhood. *Arch Dermatol* 1971; 103: 351–7.
6 Babior BM, Woodman RC. Chronic granulomatous disease. *Semin Hematol* 1990; 27: 247–59.
7 Sedel D, Huguet P, Lebbe C, Donadieu J, Odievre M, Labrune P. Sweet syndrome as the presenting manifestation of chronic granulomatous disease in an infant. *Pediatr Dermatol* 1994; 11: 237–40.
8 Seger RA, Ezekowitz RAB. Treatment of chronic granulomatous disease. *Immunodeficiency* 1994; 5: 113–30.
9 Margolis DM, Melnick DA, Alling DW, Gallin JI. Trimethoprim–sulfamethoxazole prophylaxis in the management of chronic granulomatous disease. *J Infect Dis* 1990; 162: 723–6.
10 Mouy R, Fischer A, Vilmer E, Seger R, Griscelli C. Incidence, severity, and prevention of infections in chronic granulomatous disease. *J Pediatr* 1989; 114: 555–60.
11 Muoy R, Veber F, Blanche S *et al.* Long-term itraconazole prophylaxis against *Aspergillus* infections in 32 patients with chronic granulomatous disease. *J Pediatr* 1994; 125: 998–1003.
12 Kamani N, August CS, Campbell DE, Hassan NF, Douglas SD. Marrow transplantation in chronic granulomatous disease: an update, with 6-year follow-up. *J Pediatr* 1988; 113: 697–700.
13 International Chronic Granulomatous Disease Cooperative Study Group. A controlled trial of interferon gamma to prevent infection in chronic granulomatous disease. *N Engl J Med* 1991; 324: 509–16.
14 Muhlebach TJ, Gabay J, Nathan CF *et al.* Treatment of patients with chronic granulomatous disease with recombinant human interferon-gamma does not improve neutrophil oxidative metabolism, cytochrome b558 content or levels of four anti-microbial proteins. *Clin Exp Immunol* 1992; 88: 203–6.
15 Chin TW, Stiehm ER, Falloon J, Gallin JI. Corticosteroids in treatment of obstructive lesions of chronic granulomatous disease. *J Pediatr* 1989; 111: 349–52.
16 Danziger RN, Goren AT, Becker J, Greene JM, Douglas SD. Outpatient management with oral corticosteroid therapy for obstructive conditions in chronic granulomatous disease. *J Pediatr* 1993; 122: 303–5.
17 Sekhsaria S, Gallin JI, Linton GF, Mallory RM, Mullingan RC, Malech HL. Peripheral blood progenitors as a target for genetic correction of p47phos-deficient CGD. *Proc Natl Acad Sci USA* 1993; 90: 7446–50.
18 Brandrup F, Koch C, Petri M, Schiodt M, Johansen KS. Discoid lupus erythematosus-like lesions and stomatitis in female carriers of X-linked chronic granulomatous disease. *Br J Dermatol* 1981; 104: 495–505.

19 Sillevis Smitt JH, Weening RS, Krieg SR, Bos JD. Discoid lupus erythematosus-like lesions in carriers of X-linked chronic granulomatous disease. *Br J Dermatol* 1990; 122: 643–50.

20 Dusi S, Poli G, Berton G, Catalano P, Fornasa CV, Peserico A. Chronic granulomatous disease in an adult female with granulomatous cheilitis. Evidence for an X-linked pattern of inheritance with extreme lyonization. *Acta Haematol* 1990; 84: 49–56.

21 Newberger PE, Cohen HJ, Rothchild SB, Hobbins JC, Malawista SE, Mahoney MJ. Prenatal diagnosis of chronic granulomatous disease. *N Engl J Med* 1979; 300: 178–81.

Chronic mucocutaneous candidiasis

Patients with chronic mucocutaneous candidiasis (CMC) have recurrent, progressive infections of the skin, nails and mucous membranes most commonly due to *Candida albicans*, and in some cases to dermatophytes as well [1,2]. The clinical features of CMC may be seen as the manifestations of a variety of immunological disorders, all characterized by ineffective defence mechanisms against *Candida*. In general, the patients with an earlier onset and greater severity of cutaneous candidal infections tend to have a more severe immunological alteration.

Pathogenesis

All patients with CMC have a T-cell deficiency that prevents effective handling of candidal organisms. In some patients, the defect is specific to *Candida*, and in others, the immunological response to other organisms is defective as well.

Clinical presentation

The extent of involvement is variable, and ranges from recurrent, recalcitrant thrush to mild erythematous scaling plaques with a few dystrophic nails to severe generalized, crusted granulomatous plaques. The cutaneous plaques tend to occur most commonly in intertriginous and on periorificial sites and the scalp, but may be more generalized (Fig. 25.14.3). Scalp infections may lead to scarring and alopecia. The nails are thickened, brittle and discolored (Fig. 25.14.4), and the paronychial areas are often erythematous, swollen and tender. The oral mucosal is the most frequent site of mucosal alteration (thrush with hyperkeratotic plaques), but the oesophageal, genital and laryngeal mucosae may be affected as well by chronic infection and resultant stricture formation. Patients with CMC do not tend to develop systemic candidiasis [3], but 80% of patients have recurrent or severe infections other than candidal, including bacterial septicaemia [4], particularly if other immune defects are present. Concomitant dermatophyte infections are not uncommon.

Many patients with CMC have candidiasis endocrinopathy syndrome (CES) [5] (see Chapter 25.10). The candidal infections tend to begin by 5 years of age, although the endocrinological dysfunction may not be

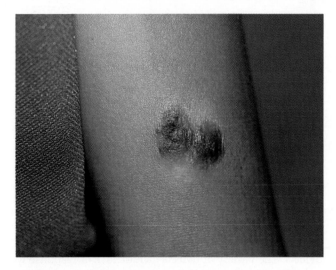

Fig. 25.14.3 Candidal cutaneous granulomas are a feature of patients with more severe CMC.

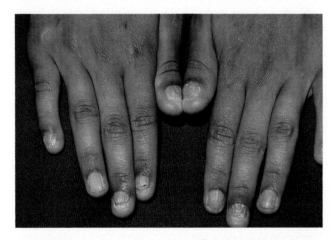

Fig. 25.14.4 Thickening, discoloration and dystrophy of all nails due to candidal infection in a patient with CES. Note the hyperpigmentation of the skin of the hands, particularly overlying the joints in this patient with associated Addison's disease.

apparent until 12–13 years of age. Candidal granulomas, especially of the face and scalp, may be seen. A variety of associated endocrinopathies have been described. Most common are hypoparathyroidism (88%) and hypoadrenocorticism (60%) (Fig. 25.14.4). One-third of patients have candidiasis, hypoparathyroidism and defective adrenal function. Other associated endocrinopathies or autoimmune disorders include gonadal insufficiency (45%), alopecia areata (20%), pernicious anaemia (16%), thyroid abnormalities (12%), chronic active hepatitis or juvenile cirrhosis (9%), vitiligo, diabetes mellitus and hypopituitarism. Chronic diarrhoea and malabsorption have been reported in 25% of patients, and are usually associated with hypoparathyroidism. Some of the affected children also have pulmonary fibrosis, dental enamel hypoplasia and keratoconjunctivitis. Patients with CES often have autoimmune antibodies, including antithyroglobulin, antimicrosomal antibodies, antiadrenal and antimelanocyte antibodies, and rheumatoid factor. Autoantibodies have also been found in patients with CMC who do not have clinical endocrinological disease.

Scrapings and cultures from cutaneous or mucosal lesions demonstrate candidal organisms. Histological examination of skin specimens reveals hyperkeratosis, papillomatosis and infiltration of the dermis with lymphocytes, plasma cells, neutrophils and foreign body giant cells. The candidal organisms are confined to the stratum corneum. The majority of patients with CMC demonstrate defective cell-mediated immunity, although no uniform alteration is found. Between 25 and 35% of patients with CMC have no demonstrable immunological defects. The variety of defects include lack of response to candidal antigens in skin testing, reduced lymphocyte blastogenic transformation response to *Candida*, abnormal lymphokine production in response to *Candida*, serum inhibition factors that alter the response to *Candida*, abnormal monocyte/macrophage chemotaxis, phagocytosis and intracellular killing, and depressed IgA or complement function. Although the frequent candidal infections are generally assumed to result from the immunological deficiency, delayed hypersensitivity to candidal antigens has been restored after antifungal therapy in some patients, suggesting that anergy may result from the candidal infection.

Treatment

The oral imidazole ketoconazole is an effective treatment [6]. With ketoconazole therapy, thrush tends to clear in a week, the skin lesions in 2 months and the nail dystrophy after 5–9 months. The cutaneous granulomas tend to be less responsive, despite clearance of infection. Recurrences are common, and ketoconazole must be used intermittently and with caution in children as in adults. Although side-effects have been less frequent and less severe than with other effective anticandidal agents, hepatitis is a feared side-effect, and has been reported in two children taking ketoconazole for CMC [7,8]. The drug appears to have no effect on the abnormal cell-mediated immunity.

Alternative therapeutic agents are itraconazole [9] and fluconazole [10]. Additional therapy may include supplemental oral and parenteral iron and folate if needed, possible nail avulsion, drainage of cutaneous abscesses, debridement of cutaneous hyperkeratoses and crusts, and endocrinological therapy as indicated.

REFERENCES

1 Dwyer JM. Chronic mucocutaneous candidiasis. *Ann Rev Med* 1981; 32: 491–7.

2 Kirkpatrick CH. Chronic mucocutaneous candidiasis. Antibiotic and immunologic therapy. *Ann NY Acad Sci* 1988; 544: 471–80.

3 Kauffman CA, Shea MJ, Frame PT. Invasive fungal infections in patients with chronic mucocutaneous candidiasis. *Arch Intern Med* 1981; 141: 1076–9.

4 Herrod HG. Chronic mucocutaneous candidiasis in childhood and complications of non-*Candida* infection: a report of the Pediatric Immunodeficiency Collaborative Study Group. *J Pediatr* 1990; 116: 377–82.

5 Ahonen P, Myllärniemi S, Sipilä I, Perheentupa J. Clinical variation of autoimmune polyendocrinopathy–candidiasis–ectodermal dystrophy (APECED) in a series of 68 patients. *N Engl J Med* 1990; 322: 1829–36.

6 Horsburgh CR, Kirkpatrick CH. Long-term therapy of chronic mucocutaneous candidiasis with ketoconazole: experiences with 21 patients. *Am J Med* 1983; 74(suppl): 23–9.

7 Macnair AL, Gascoigne E, Heap J, Schuermans V, Symoens J. Hepatitis and ketoconazole therapy. *Br Med J* 1981; 283: 1058–9.

8 Tkach JR, Rinaldi MG. Severe hepatitis associated with ketoconazole therapy for chronic mucocutaneous candidiasis. *Cutis* 1982; 29: 482–4.

9 Burke WA. Use of itraconazole in a patient with chronic mucocutaneous candidiasis. *J Am Acad Dermatol* 1989; 21: 1309–10.

10 Hay RJ. Overview of studies of fluconazole in oropharyngeal candidiasis. *Rev Infect Dis* 1990; 12(suppl 3): S334–7.

Complement deficiency disorders

Isolated complement component deficiencies often result in autoimmune disorders or unusual susceptibility to recurrent infections [1,2]. Hereditary angioneurotic oedema (HAO) occurs in 1 in 150 000 people [3–5]. Decreased antigenic and functional levels of an inhibitor of C1 esterase are found in 85% of affected individuals. The remaining 15% of patients have normal or elevated antigenic levels of a functionless protein or low levels of a normally functioning C1-esterase inhibitor (C1 INH). In contrast with all other complement disorders, HAO is inherited as an autosomal dominant disorder with incomplete penetrance. C2 deficiency is the most common complement component deficiency. The homozygous form of C2 deficiency occurs in 1 in 10 000 to 1 in 40 000 individuals, and the heterozygous form is found in 1 to 2% of people. Most of the complement defects are inherited as autosomal recessive traits, except for hereditary angioneurotic oedema (C1 INH deficiency or dysfunction).

Hereditary angioneurotic oedema

HAO is a potentially lethal, dominantly inherited form of angio-oedema, characterized by non-pruritic swelling of the face, extremities, gastrointestinal and respiratory tracts without urticaria [3–5].

Pathogenesis

The genetic alterations in HAO affect a structural gene for C1 INH [6] and primarily occur by DNA rearrangements. C1 INH modulates clotting, kinin generation, fibrinolysis and complement pathways. It appears to be produced by hepatocytes, and blocks the generation of C4 and C2 by active C1. The angio-oedema probably results from uncontrolled activation of the complement pathway. In

HAO, C1 becomes activated by proteolytic enzymes, including kallikrein, plasmin and thrombin, which are produced when Hageman factor is activated by trauma. The mechanism of oedema production remains unclear. When purified activated C1 is injected into normal individuals, a wheal develops. In patients with HAO, the injection leads to a typical attack, but patients with homozygous C2 deficiency demonstrate no wheal. This evidence suggests that a polypeptide fragment of C2 with kinin-like activity (C2 kinin) is released, which increases capillary permeability and causes angio-oedema. The reason for normal C3 levels despite classical complement activation remains unclear, but may relate to the site of C1 activation (in blood rather than on cell surfaces).

Clinical presentation

The first episode of angio-oedema tends to occur in early childhood. Since the early episodes most often are manifested as swelling of an extremity following trauma, they are commonly overlooked. The number of attacks usually increases throughout adolescence and young adulthood. The frequency of attacks varies widely among patients; some individuals have only a few attacks over several decades, while others have weekly bouts. No periodicity to the attacks is noted. Although attacks may be spontaneous, approximately 50% of bouts are precipitated by emotional or physical trauma. Dental treatment of patients with HAO can trigger life-threatening pharyngeal oedema [7]. Female patients commonly report more attacks in association with menses or oral contraceptive use. During the last two trimesters of pregnancy, the frequency of attacks appears to wane and the occurrence of angio-oedema at delivery is extremely rare.

Patients should be questioned about the occurrence of swelling in other family members, as well as about prodromal signs including hoarseness, altered taste, difficulty with swallowing and the presence of abdominal pain. Patients may also report a localized tingling or tightening of the skin prior to the onset of swelling. The attack often begins suddenly without a prodrome. The angio-oedema progressively increases for several hours, then stabilizes for 1–2 days before resolution. The total duration of episodes is typically 48–72h, but an attack may last longer. The oedema is non-pitting, non-erythematous and non-pruritic. In about 25% of patients, a transient or erythematous, non-pruritic macular rash resembling erythema marginatum precedes or accompanies the angio-oedema, but typical urticaria is not a feature of HAO. The most common sites of involvement are the extremities, face, oropharyngeal mucosae and gastrointestinal tract. Compromise of the airways due to laryngeal angio-oedema occurs most commonly in adults, and is reported in two-thirds of patients at some time. Often patients are warned of impending obstruction by a voice change or dysphagia. Up to 25% of patients die from airway compromise. Occasionally genitourinary tract oedema occurs and results in urinary retention. Rarely the angio-oedema involves the brain, pleura or joint space, leading to headaches, seizures, paresis, cough, pleuritic chest pain or arthralgias. Manifestations in the gastrointestinal tract depend upon the location and intensity of the visceral swelling. Jejunal swelling leads to bilious vomiting and crampy abdominal pain; colonic involvement results in watery diarrhoea. Rarely the intestinal oedema is so extensive that hypotension results. Contrast studies of the intestines during attacks may show oedematous mucosae. HAO may also be associated with membranoproliferative glomerulonephritis (non-systemic lupus erythematosus (SLE)) [8].

A number of patients with HAO demonstrate features of autoimmune disorders as is seen in deficiencies of early complement components of the classical complement pathway. Most of these patients have systemic or discoid lupus erythematosus (LE) [9]; patients have also been described with scleroderma or focal lipodystrophy in association with HAO.

Laboratory confirmation of the diagnosis depends upon assays of complement pathway proteins. The best screening tests are levels of C4 and C1 INH. Levels of C4 and C2 are low during attacks, since these complement components are the substrates of C1 esterase. The C4 level tends to be depressed when the patient is asymptomatic as well. Total haemolytic complement (CH50) is often normal, and the C3 level is almost always normal as well. Direct measurement of immunoreactive C1 INH can be done by immunodiffusion assay. When the C1 INH level is normal but the C4 level is low in a patient with possible HAO, an immunodiffusion assay of C1 INH function will identify antigenically normal but functionally abnormal protein [10]. Serum C1 levels are normal or minimally depressed in HAO.

Differential diagnosis

The diagnosis of HAO is easily made when a patient complains of angio-oedema with recurrent abdominal pain and reveals a positive family history. However, the clinical diagnosis of HAO in a patient without other affected family members and with a vague history of abdominal discomfort and acral swelling may be difficult. The differential diagnosis includes disorders of painless swelling and recurrent abdominal pain.

The majority of the causes of angio-oedema involve urticaria and are often pruritic. The causes of angio-oedema include allergic factors, immune complex disease, viral infections, drug-induced histamine release and physically induced angio-oedema. In addition, various syndromes may be associated, including urticarial vasculitis, urticaria pigmentosa, capillary leak syndrome, carboxypeptidase B deficiency and C3b activator deficiency.

An acquired deficiency of C1 INH is most commonly associated with lymphomas and cryoglobulinaemia. C1 is consumed and levels of C1 are very low, in contrast to normal levels in HAO. Other disorders with facial swelling are the Melkersson–Rosenthal syndrome with facial palsy and a deeply furrowed tongue, patients with lip infiltration from Crohn's disease and the superior vena cava syndrome associated with cardiovascular manifestations.

Abdominal pain may occur without angio-oedema involving the skin. If intestinal obstruction or appendicitis are suspected, an exploratory laparotomy may be performed and cause the angio-oedema to become exacerbated by the increased trauma. Many patients are called 'hysterical' and the diagnosis of HAO is not made.

Treatment

The mortality of HAO can be reduced significantly by adequate therapy. Patients with mild, infrequent attacks do not require long-term prophylaxis, but patients with frequent life-threatening attacks (one or two per month) should receive prophylactic therapy. Children usually do not need these drugs, but adolescents may have severe attacks. The two groups of drugs used are an analogue of the antifibrinolytic drug ε-aminocaproic acid (EACA), tranexamic acid and androgens. Danazol, a derivative of ethyltestosterone, is the drug of choice and has few masculinizing side-effects [11]. By inducing mRNA synthesis by hepatocytes, danazol stimulates the synthesis of functional C1 INH. Danazol appears to be effective in elevating C1 INH levels and eliminating attacks in both forms of HAO. Irregular menstruation was the only significant side-effect of danazol or stanozolol in a study of 24 patients for more than 5 years. Danazol has also caused hepatic cell necrosis in one patient [12].

Children and adolescents should use short-term prophylaxis before elective traumatic procedures, such as dental treatment or surgery, are performed. Antifibrinolytic components, kallikrein inhibitor, fresh frozen plasma and C1 INH concentrate have been used. Within 15 min of administration of C1 INH concentrate, serum levels of C1 INH increase to 50% above normal values and remain elevated for 1–2 days. If concentrated C1 INH is not available, fresh frozen plasma or high-dose antifibrinolytic agents (EACA) are the drugs of choice. Occasionally, the administration of fresh frozen plasma may aggravate the attack by renewing early complement components. For the patient with laryngeal oedema, antihistamines, corticosteroids and epinephrine may be tried, but are often unsuccessful. Intubation or tracheostomy is life-saving if medical therapy is not effective. Affected individuals should carry a medical alert card describing

the diagnosis and proper therapy. The pain of gastrointestinal oedema may be relieved by aspirin or codeine preparations. Swelling of the extremities does not require intervention.

Other complement deficiencies

Pathogenesis

Defects involving the early components of the classical complement pathway tend to resemble autoimmune disorders, especially SLE. There are a number of possible explanations for the association. Viruses have been implicated in causing SLE. The inability to neutralize and lyse certain viruses because of complement deficiency may increase the risk of SLE. Also, the genes for the production of C2 and C4 are part of the HLA locus, suggesting that the increased frequency of SLE may be due to gene linkage. Finally, complement components participate in the reticuloendothelial system. Both alternate and classical complement pathways are required for the solubilization of immune complexes. Ineffective clearance of immune complexes may result in autoimmune disease manifestations.

The milder course of SLE in patients with complement deficiency may be explained by the lower or absent titres of anti-DNA antibodies and antinuclear antibodies (ANA), and by the inflammatory response that is altered by the complement deficiency. Since skin lesions are common and severe in complement deficiency, other antibodies, such as anti-Ro antibodies, may be more important than complement activation and ANA in the pathogenesis of skin disease.

The variety of recurrent infections associated with complement deficiencies emphasizes the central role of complement components in bacterial clearance. Deficiencies of the early components, especially C2, are associated with infection by encapsulated bacteria, especially *Pneumococcus*. Opsonization of bacteria and fungi may be ineffective in disorders of the classical pathway because of the slow, inadequate formation of C3b. Patients with deficiencies of C5 do not generate chemotactic factors normally and polymorphonuclear leucocyte function may be inadequate. Children with C5–C9 complement deficiencies tend to develop recurrent neisserial infections in their teenage years. Presumably an intact alternate complement pathway is required for destruction of neisserial organisms.

Clinical presentation

Many patients with complement deficiencies are normal. Only patients with clinical disease or family members of patients come to medical attention. Deficiencies of the early components of the classical complement pathway

(C1, C4, C2) tend to be manifested by lupus-like disorders in childhood. Patients demonstrate photosensitivity and skin changes of systemic or subacute LE. Most patients have absent or low ANA titres and mild renal disease. Pyogenic infections occur with increased frequency in some patients with deficiencies of components of the classical complement cascade, but are not as frequent as in complement deficiencies involving the alternate pathway or membrane attack complex.

C2 deficiency is the most prevalent of the homozygous deficiencies of the complement components [13]. Autoimmune disorders occur in almost 50% of people with the homozygous form and in approximately 10% of those with the heterozygous form of C2 deficiency. SLE is more commonly manifested in female patients with homozygous C2 deficiency, 60% of whom show features of SLE. Other disorders have been associated less frequently than lupus with C2 deficiency. They include juvenile rheumatoid arthritis (especially in heterozygous female patients), dermatomyositis, Henoch–Schönlein purpura, glomerulonephritis, vasculitis, atrophoderma, cold urticaria, common variable immunodeficiency (CVI), hypogammaglobulinaemia, Hodgkin's disease and inflammatory bowel disease. The time of onset of lupus-like manifestations varies, even within affected families. Many patients show characteristics in young childhood; others first have symptoms of autoimmune disease as young adults.

The most typical clinical finding in patients with C2 deficiency is a rash that tends to be exacerbated by exposure to sunlight. The skin lesions are frequently papulosquamous plaques, as in subacute LE, but may be more typical of discoid LE or include malar erythema. Skin lesions are often extensive and may be difficult to control. The palmoplantar hyperkeratosis has been noted in C4 deficiency with lupus, but has not been described in C2-deficient patients. Lupus-like alopecia is often reported.

Other features of SLE are often present. Arthritis and arthralgias are found in 80% of patients, as are unexplained fevers. Leucopenia and oral ulcerations are noted in almost 50% of patients. Less frequent manifestations include CNS vasculitis, pleuritis, pericarditis, Raynaud's phenomenon and thrombocytopenia. Renal disease is generally mild or detectable only by biopsy, but occasional patients have severe renal disease.

The most common laboratory abnormality in C2 deficiency is an elevated titre of anti-Ro antibodies, found in 75% of patients with SLE and C2 deficiency [14]. The anti-Ro antibody is also found in 60% of patients with subacute cutaneous LE, a subset of LE with prominent papulosquamous plaques, photosensitivity, milder systemic symptoms and often negative ANA tests. Increased titres of anti-Ro antibodies are not found in homozygous or heterozygous C2 deficiency without LE. Rheumatoid factor is elevated in 40% of patients with C2 deficiency, but ANA and anti-DNA antibodies are usually of low titre or absent. Rarely, elevated levels of Sm and antiribonucleoprotein (RNP) antibodies, circulating immune complexes and a positive RPR have been found in patients with LE and C2 deficiency.

Patients with C2 deficiency are also susceptible to recurrent infections with pyogenic organisms. Most infections are pulmonary, due to *Pneumococcus*, but other encapsulated bacteria have also been implicated.

Patients with complement deficiencies involving the alternate and terminal pathways tend to suffer from disseminated infections of Gram-negative diplococci, especially *Neisseria*, as well as from other pyogenic microorganisms [15,16]. Recurrent respiratory tract infections and peritonitis affect patients with deficiencies of C3 and C3 inactivator. Generalized seborrhoeic erythroderma with failure to thrive, recurrent infections and diarrhoea ('Leiner's phenotype') has been described in patients with C3 or C5 deficiency and in C5 dysfunction. C3 deficiency has also been associated with partial thoracic or cephalothoracic lipodystrophy [17,18], often with mesangioproliferative glomerulonephritis. Patients with deficiencies of components of the membrane attack sequence, C5–C9, have recurrent neisserial infections. These neisserial infections tend to begin approximately around the time of puberty, although other infections, especially pneumococcal, often start earlier in childhood. Patients with deficiencies of the membrane attack complex occasionally have autoimmune disorders as well. Patients with C7 deficiency may have features of the CRST syndrome (Calcinosis, Raynaud's phenomenon, sclerodactyly and telangiectasia).

CH50 is markedly decreased or undetectable in complement deficiencies other than HAO. The single affected complement component may be shown to be decreased by radioimmunodiffusion assay. All other complement components are within the normal range.

Treatment

Conservative therapy is often effective for patients with autoimmune manifestations of complement deficiency. The use of sunscreens and topical corticosteroids and avoidance of sunlight may be sufficient. Antimalarial drugs, systemic corticosteroids and other immunosuppressive medications should be employed in more severe cases. The increased risk of infections in patients with complement deficiencies should be recalled in choosing to use systemic medications. The use of transfusions of plasma to replace the deficient components may activate C3 and C5 and accelerate immune complex deposition in the inflammatory reaction. Vigorous and early use of antibiotics is important in handling the recurrent infections.

REFERENCES

1 Guenther LC. Inherited disorders of complement. *J Am Acad Dermatol* 1983; 9: 815–39.

2 Tappeiner G. Disease states in genetic complement deficiencies. *Int J Dermatol* 1982; 21: 175–91.

3 Agostoni A, Cicardi M. Hereditary and acquired C1-inhibitor deficiency: biological and clinical characteristics in 235 patients. *Medicine* 1992; 71: 206–15.

4 Frank MM, Gelfand JA, Atkinson JP. Hereditary angioedema: the clinical syndrome and its management. *Ann Intern Med* 1976; 84: 580–93.

5 Blok PH, Baarsma EA. Hereditary angio-edema (HAE). *J Laryngol Otol* 1984; 98: 59–63.

6 Stoppa-Lyonnet D, Tosi M, Laurent J, Sobel A, Lagrue G, Meo T. Altered C1 inhibitor genes in type I hereditary angioedema. *N Engl J Med* 1987; 317: 1–6.

7 Atkinson JC, Frank MM. Oral manifestations and dental management of patients with hereditary angioedema. *J Oral Pathol Med* 1991; 20: 139–42.

8 Pan CG, Strife CF, Ward MK, Spitzer RE, McAdams AJ. Long-term follow-up of non-systemic lupus erythematosus glomerulonephritis in patients with hereditary angioedema: report of four cases. *Am J Kidney Dis* 1992; 19: 526–31.

9 Massa MC, Connolly SM. An association between C1 esterase inhibitor deficiency and lupus erythematosus. *J Am Acad Dermatol* 1982; 7: 255–64.

10 Yelvington M, Prograis LJ, Pizzo CJ, Curd JG. Immunodiffusion assay of C1 inhibitor function in serum: prospective analysis in angioedema-urticaria. *Am J Clin Pathol* 1983; 80: 309–13.

11 Rosen FS, Beyler A. Hereditary angioneurotic edema and its correction with androgen therapy. *Birth Defects: Orig Article Ser* 1980; 16: 499–507.

12 Cicardi M, Bergamascini L, Cugno M, Hack E, Agostoni G, Agostoni A. Long-term treatment of hereditary angioedema with attenuated androgens: a survey of a 13-year experience. *J All Clin Immunol* 1991; 87: 768–73.

13 Johnson CA, Densen P, Wetsel RA, Cole FS, Goeken NE, Colten HR. Molecular heterogeneity of C2 deficiency. *N Engl J Med* 1992; 326: 871–4.

14 Provost TT, Arnett FC, Raichlin M. Homozygous C2 deficiency, lupus erythematosus and anti-Ro (SSA) antibodies. *Arthritis Rheum* 1983; 26: 1279–82.

15 Fijen CA, Kuijper EJ, Hannema AJ, Sjoholm AG, van Putten JP. Complement deficiencies in patients over 10 years old with meningococcal disease due to uncommon serogroups. *Lancet* 1989; ii: 585–8.

16 Nagata M, Hara T, Aoki T, Mizuno Y, Akeda H, Inaba S. Inherited deficiency of ninth component of complement: an increased risk of meningococcal meningitis. *J Pediatr* 1989; 114: 260–4.

17 Bier DM, O'Donnell JJ, Kaplan SL. Cephalothoracic lipodystrophy with hypocomplementemic renal disease: discordance in identical twin sisters. *J Clin Endocrinol Metab* 1978; 46: 800–7.

18 Borzy MS, Gewurz A, Wolff L, Houghton D, Lovrien E. Inherited C3 deficiency with recurrent infections and glomerulonephritis. *Am J Dis Child* 1988; 142: 79–83.

DiGeorge's syndrome

DiGeorge's syndrome (congenital thymic aplasia) results from developmental defects of the third and fourth pharyngeal pouches. Although most cases are sporadic, many families with an autosomal dominant form of inheritance have been described [1]. DiGeorge's syndrome is often associated with microdeletions in 22q11 [2]. The immunodeficiency is variable; most patients have T-cell defects, but some have only mild T-cell abnormalities, while others have associated hypogammaglobulinaemia of a severe combined immunodeficiency (SCID) phenotype [3,4], presumably due to the effect of T cells on B-cell function. The thymic shadow is absent or reduced at birth. Infants often have neonatal tetany with hypocalcaemia due to the aplastic parathyroid glands. The cardiac anomalies are most commonly truncus arteriosus, septal defects and abnormal aortic arch vessels. Characteristic facial fea-

tures of DiGeorge's syndrome include a short philtrum, low-set malformed ears and hypertelorism.

Many patients have recurrent mucocutaneous candidal infections as neonates, as well as increased susceptibility to viral infections, *Pneumocystis carinii* and other fungal infections. Graft-versus-host disease (GVHD) may develop in infants who are given non-irradiated blood products. There is considerable clinical overlap between DiGeorge's syndrome and velocardiofacial syndrome [1], an autosomal dominant multiple anomaly disorder characterized by cleft palate, heart defects, cognitive disorder and a typical facial appearance; similar chromosomal abnormalities of 22q11 have been noted in velocardiofacial syndrome [2,5–7]. Bone marrow transplantation has corrected the immune defect in patients with complete DiGeorge's syndrome.

REFERENCES

1 Stevens CA, Carey JC, Shigeoka AO. DiGeorge anomaly and velocardiofacial syndrome. *Pediatrics* 1990; 85: 526–30.

2 Driscoll DA, Salvin J, Sellinger B *et al*. Prevalence of 22q11 microdeletions in DiGeorge and velocardiofacial syndrome: implications for genetic counseling and prenatal diagnosis. *J Med Genet* 1993; 30: 813–17.

3 Muller W, Peter HH, Kallfelz HC, Franz A, Rieger CH. The DiGeorge sequence. II. Immunologic findings in partial and complete forms of the disorder. *Eur J Pediatr* 1989; 149: 96–103.

4 Hong R. The DiGeorge anomaly. *Immunodef Rev* 1991; 3: 1–14.

5 Scambler PJ, Kelly D, Lindsay E *et al*. Velo-cardio-facial syndrome associated with chromosome 22 deletions encompassing the DiGeorge locus. *Lancet* 1992; 339: 1138–9.

6 Fibison WJ. Molecular studies of DiGeorge syndrome. *Am J Hum Genet* 1990; 46: 888–95.

7 Carey AH, Kelly D, Halford S *et al*. Molecular genetic study of the frequency of monosome 22q11 in DiGeorge syndrome. *Am J Hum Genet* 1992; 51: 964–70.

Hyperimmunoglobulin E recurrent infection syndrome

HIE recurrent infection syndrome is characterized by repeated cutaneous and sinopulmonary infections and dermatitis from birth or early childhood, associated with extremely elevated IgE levels (greater than 2000 IU/ml) [1,2]. Job's syndrome is a subgroup of female patients with fair skin, red hair and hyperextensible joints in addition to the general features of HIE [3]. The disorder is rare and usually sporadic. Familial cases have occurred with an inheritance pattern suggestive of an autosomal dominant mode with incomplete penetrance. A family history of atopy is frequently reported.

Pathogenesis

The aetiology for the recurrent infections and dermatitis of HIE remains unclear. The diminished neutrophil chemotaxis found in some patients may explain the recurrent bacterial infections. Chemotaxis may be impaired because of a serum factor produced by patients with HIE that is capable of inhibiting neutrophil chemotaxis of normal individuals [1]. Patients with HIE overproduce IgE antistaphylococcal antibodies, suggesting impaired regulation of humoral function. The frequency of dermatitis may also be related to the elevated levels of IgE, as seen in atopic dermatitis. Stimulation of B cells from patients with HIE syndrome by interleukin 4 (IL-4) fails to increase the production of IgE, in contrast to the stimulatory effect of IL-4 on B cells from normal individuals and patients with atopic dermatitis [4].

Clinical presentation

The dermatitis often begins during the first 6 months of life, and cutaneous candidiasis may also be an early clinical feature. Bacterial infection is a prominent problem after the first 6 months of life. Cutaneous infections may take the form of excoriated crusted plaques, pustules, furuncles, cellulitis, lymphangitis or abscesses. Paronychial infections lead to nail dystrophy. The cutaneous abscesses occur most commonly on the neck, scalp, periorbital areas, axillae and groin, and are often huge (Fig. 25.14.5). The patient is often afebrile, or has a slight temperature elevation. The abscesses are slightly erythematous and tender, but not nearly to the degree expected for a normal individual. Although the abscesses tend to harbour *S. aureus*, many patients have frequent cutaneous infections from *Candida* and *Streptococcus*. Although some patients demonstrate cutaneous manifestations only [5], patients with HIE usually have recurrent bronchitis and pneumonias usually due to *S. aureus* and *H. influenzae*, with resultant empyema, bronchiectasis and pneumatocele formation. The pneumatoceles tend to persist and become the site of further infections with bacterial or fungal organisms. Rarely, massive haemoptysis ensues. Other common sites of infection include the ears, oral mucosae, sinuses and eyes. Visceral infections other than pneumonia are unusual.

The eczematous rash is extremely pruritic and papular with lichenification. Although the rash resembles that of atopic dermatitis, the distribution of the dermatitis may differ in HIE, with accentuation of intertriginous, retroauricular and hairline areas. Superinfection of the dermatitis with *S. aureus* and *S. pyogenes* is common. The eczema is always present in infants and young children, but frequently clears by later childhood. Despite the markedly elevated IgE levels and eczematous rash, patients may not exhibit other signs of atopy, such as a propensity towards hay fever or asthma. Patients with HIE develop an atypical facial appearance, partially due to severe deforming facial abscesses, with progressive facial coarseness, a broad nasal bridge, prominent nose and irregularly proportioned cheeks and jaw. Osteopenia with increased risk of bone fractures has also been described.

Extensive studies of complement levels and activities, polymorphonuclear leucocyte phagocytosis and killing, and lymphocyte subgroup distribution have been normal. All patients, by definition, have markedly elevated levels of polyclonal IgE, but it should be remembered that normal levels of IgE in infants are considerably lower than levels in older children. IgD levels are also increased in the majority of patients, but other immunoglobulin levels are usually normal. Many patients have eosinophilia of the blood and sputum. Abnormal polymorphonuclear leucocyte and monocyte chemotaxis has been noted in a number of patients, but the chemotactic defects have been intermittent and not related to periods of infection. Patients also tend to have positive immediate wheal and flare reactions to a variety of foods and inhalants, as well as to bacteria and fungi, and an impaired anamnestic response to antigens, such as tetanus. Cell-mediated immunity is often abnormal, as manifested by anergy to skin testing, altered responses in mixed leucocyte culture, and impaired blastogenic responses to specific antigens, such as *Candida* and tetanus. In contrast, the blastogenic responses are normal to non-specific mitogens.

Differential diagnosis

HIE syndrome must be differentiated from a number of other disorders in which IgE levels may be elevated. Among these are Wiskott–Aldrich syndrome (WAS), atopic dermatitis, DiGeorge's syndrome, GVHD, Nezelof's syndrome and selected IgA deficiency. Of these, WAS and atopic dermatitis are most easily confused because of the frequent dermatitis with superinfections of *S. aureus*. The coarse facial features and presence of abscesses help to distinguish HIE from atopic dermatitis. Patients with the WAS have thrombocytopenia with cutaneous petechiae and haemorrhagic episodes. Neither disorder demonstrates the cutaneous abscesses that are so

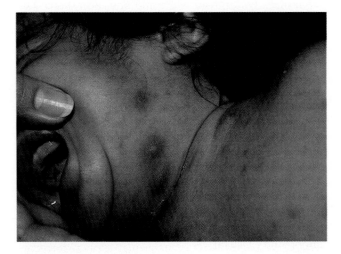

Fig. 25.14.5 Multiple staphylococcal abscesses on the neck region of an infant with HIE syndrome.

prevalent in HIE. Bacterial and candidal abscesses may be features of myeloperoxidase deficiency [6].

Treatment

The mainstay of therapy for HIE is antistaphylococcal antibiotics. When other bacterial or fungal infections develop, the infections must be treated with appropriate antibiotics as well. Recombinant interferon-γ has been shown to increase neutrophil chemotactic responses in patients with HIE and recurrent infections [7]. A number of other agents have been shown to correct the variable chemotactic defects, including ascorbic acid and cimetidine. However, these agents have not altered the clinical course of the disorder. The cutaneous and pulmonary abscesses often require incision and drainage. The pneumatoceles should be removed surgically, especially if present for longer than 6 months, or the patient is at risk for severe superinfection by bacterial or fungal organisms. The long-term prognosis of children with HIE syndrome is unknown, but it is not uncommon for these children to die prematurely due to bacterial or fungal infections of the lungs.

REFERENCES

1 Donabedian H, Gallin JI. Hyperimmunoglobulin-E recurrent infection (Job's) syndrome: review of the NIH experience in the literature. *Medicine* 1983; 62: 195–208.
2 Ring J, Landthaler M. Hyper-IgE syndromes. *Curr Probl Dermatol*, 1989; 18: 79–88.
3 Hill HR, Ochs HD, Quie PG et al. Defect in neutrophil granulocyte chemotaxis in Job's syndrome of recurrent 'cold' staphylococcal abscesses. *Lancet* 1974; ii: 617–19.
4 Claassen JJ, Levine AD, Schiff SE, Buckley RH. Mononuclear cells from patients with the hyper-IgE syndrome produce little IgE when they are stimulated with recombinant human interleukin-4. *J Allergy Clin Immunol* 1991; 88: 713–21.
5 Hochreutener H, Wüthrich B, Huwyler T, Schopfer K, Seger R, Baerlocher K. Variants of Hyper-IgE syndrome: the differentiation from atopic dermatitis is important because of treatment and prognosis. *Dermatologica* 1991; 182: 7–11.
6 Parry MF, Root RK, Metcalf JA, Delaney KK, Kaplow LS, Richard WJ. Myeloperoxidase deficiency: prevalence and significance. *Ann Intern Med* 1991; 95: 293–301.
7 Jeppson JD, Jaffe HS, Hill HR. Use of recombinant human interferon gamma to enhance neutrophil chemotactic responses in Job syndrome of hyperimmunoglobulinemia E and recurrent infections. *J Pediatr* 1991; 118: 383–7.

Immunoglobulin deficiencies

Several primary immunodeficiencies involve low levels of immunoglobulins, and are most commonly diagnosed after 6 months of age, when patients develop recurrent bacterial infections. Immunoglobulin replacement reduces the severity and frequency of infections in these patients. Replacement treatment with intravenous or subcutaneous injections of immunoglobulin [1] can be administered at home.

Immunoglobulin A deficiency

The most common immunoglobulin deficiency is selective IgA deficiency, found in 1 in 500 people. Between 10 and 15% of patients have clinical manifestations. These features usually are sinopulmonary bacterial infections and *Giardia* gastroenteritis. Approximately one-third of patients with clinical disease develop autoimmune disorders, some of which involve the skin. These include SLE, vitiligo, CMC and idiopathic thrombocytopenic purpura. A number of patients have severe atopic-like dermatitis. Patients are at increased risk of developing gastric carcinoma. The treatment of IgA deficiency is vigorous treatment with antibiotics. It is imperative that patients do not receive immune serum globulin or blood products with IgA-bearing lymphocytes. Almost half of patients have serum anti-IgA antibodies, and fatal anaphylactic reactions have occurred from the administration of blood products.

Immunoglobulin M deficiency

An extremely rare selective immunoglobulin deficiency, IgM deficiency is apparently due to an inability of T-helper cell function to stimulate IgM production. In addition to recurrent bacterial infections, severe eczema and extensive large warts have been described. Early and vigorous antibiotic use is the only effective therapy.

X-linked hypogammaglobulinaemia with hyperimmunoglobulinaemia M syndrome

Patients with this X-linked recessive disorder have recurrent infections in association with hepatosplenomegaly, cervical adenitis, autoimmune disorders (especially thyroiditis and haemolytic anaemia) and an increased risk of lymphoma. Cutaneous manifestations include pyodermas, widespread warts and oral ulcerations (Fig. 25.14.6) [2], the latter sometimes due to neutropenia. Patients tend to have deficiencies of IgA and IgG with neutropenia, but increased levels of IgM and isohaemagglutinins. The pathomechanism for this form of hypogammaglobulinaemia is now known and involves a T-cell defect, rather than a primary B-cell defect. Cross-linking of CD40 on B cells induces, in the presence of lymphokines, switching of immunoglobulin classes from IgM to IgG, IgA or IgE. A transmembrane protein—tumour necrosis factor (TNF)-related activation protein (TRAP or gp39)—encoded by a gene at Xq26.3–27.1, is the physiological ligand for CD40. B cells from patients with hyperimmunoglobulinaemia M express functional CD40, but the T cells express defective CD40 ligand (gp39) and cannot bind CD40 [3].

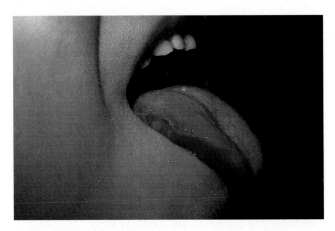

Fig. 25.14.6 Large ulceration on the side of the tongue in a male infant with X-linked hypogammaglobulinaemia with HIE syndrome. These frequent oral ulcerations may result from bouts of neutropenia.

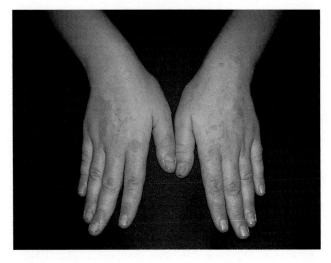

Fig. 25.14.7 Myriads of recalcitrant warts in a teenage girl with CVI.

Panhypogammaglobulinaemia

Hypogammaglobulinaemia is found in 1 in 50 000 people, and is classified into two major subdivisions: Bruton's X-linked hypogammaglobulinaemia and CVI. In Bruton's X-linked hypogammaglobulinaemia, pre-B cells are blocked in their conversion in the bone marrow to B cells, by interference with early B-lineage growth and clonal expansion. X-linked hypogammaglobulinaemia is now known to be caused by a defect in the gene encoding a newly described tyrosine kinase (Btk) involved in B-cell development [4], the activity of which is markedly decreased in the B cells of patients. Patients develop recurrent bacterial infections after the first several months of life. The organisms most commonly involved are *Staphylococcus*, *Streptococcus*, *Haemophilus* and *Pneumococcus*. The skin frequently has multiple furuncles and cellulitis. Echthyma gangrenosum may be the presenting sign [5]. Patients also have an increased risk of developing dermatitis. Non-infectious cutaneous granulomas have been described, as has papular dermatitis due to extensive lymphohistiocytic infiltration of the skin [6]. Patients have increased susceptibility to enterovirus and hepatitis B infections. A small percentage of patients develop a dermatomyositis-like disorder, with slowly progressive neurological involvement usually related to echoviral meningoencephalitis. Up to 6% of patients develop lymphoreticular malignancies.

Female carriers of X-linked hypogammaglobulinaemia may be detected through examination of X-inactivation patterns of maternal B cells using a methylation-sensitive probe [7]. Prenatal diagnosis is possible by detecting restriction fragment length polymorphism in regions surrounding the gene [8]. An autosomal recessive form that resembles X-linked hypogammaglobulinaemia has been described [9].

CVI is a heterogeneous group of disorders [10,11]. The hallmark of the disorder is the deficiency of at least two of the three major serum immunoglobulin isotypes, IgG, IgA and IgM. The average age of onset is 27 years old, but 45% of cases are diagnosed during childhood. The disorder may present as early as 2 years of age, but before that time it is difficult to distinguish from transient hypogammaglobulinaemia (see below). The incidence of the disorder is distributed equally among both sexes. Family members often have evidence of immunodeficiency, including hypogammaglobulinaemia and selective IgA deficiency. Patients are particularly predisposed to pyogenic upper and lower respiratory tract infections. The infectious agents are similar to those of X-linked hypogammaglobulinaemia, but *Giardia* infections are more common in CVI than in the X-linked form. Patients frequently have cutaneous pyodermas and eczema. Abnormalities of cell-mediated immunity occur in many patients in addition to the immunoglobulin deficiency and may manifest in the skin as widespread warts (Fig. 25.14.7) and extensive dermatophyte infections. Patients may develop non-caseating granulomas of the lungs, liver, spleen and/or skin that are not due to microorganisms and may respond to corticosteroids. Patients with CVI have an increased risk of autoimmune diseases [12], including vitiligo and alopecia areata. The incidence of lymphoreticular malignancy is also increased, with an eight to 13 times increased risk of cancer overall and a 438-fold increased risk of lymphoma [13]. Death in patients with CVI usually results from infection, respiratory insufficiency or neoplasia.

Patients with transient hypogammaglobulinaemia of infancy often show early failure to thrive, with recurrent sinopulmonary infections and diarrhoea, particularly beginning at 6–9 months of age when maternal antibody levels wane. Affected infants may have recurrent pyodermas and cutaneous abscesses. Immunoglobulin production is delayed, and begins at 18–30 months of age.

X-linked lymphoproliferative disease

X-linked lymphoproliferative disease (Duncan's disease) is characterized by an inadequate response to EBV infection [14]. Affected boys are healthy until childhood or adolescence when they develop infectious mononucleosis. Clinical features include fever, pharyngitis, maculopapular rash, lymphadenopathy, hepatosplenomegaly, purpura and jaundice. Almost 70% of patients die of the disease due to overwhelming B-cell lymphoma stimulated by the virus, often with superimposed bacterial sepsis. Both humoral and cell-mediated immune responses are diminished. Patients cannot adequately produce EBV-specific antibodies or EBV-specific memory T cells. In addition, the affected boys have increased percentages of suppressor T cells, decreased natural killer function and low antibody-dependent cellular cytotoxicity. Etoposide and/or T-cell immunosuppression, particularly with cyclosporin, have been used successfully to treat the infectious mononucleosis or aplastic exacerbations [15]. Bone marrow transplantation is the only definitive therapy [16]. X-linked lymphoproliferative disease has been mapped to Xq24–27 [17], and prenatal diagnosis has been achieved by chorionic villus sampling and restriction fragment polymorphic markers [18], but carrier females show random X inactivation [19].

REFERENCES

1 Gardulf A, Andersen V, Bjorkander J *et al.* Subcutaneous immunoglobulin replacement in patients with primary antibody deficiencies: safety and costs. *Lancet* 1995; 345: 365–9.

2 Chang MW, Romero R, Scholl PR, Paller AS. Mucocutaneous manifestations of the hyper-IgM immunodeficiency syndrome. *J Am Acad Dermatol* 1998; 38: 191–6.

3 Kroczek RA, Graf D, Brugnoni D *et al.* Defective expression of CD40 ligand on T cells causes 'X-linked immunodeficiency with hyper-IgM (HIGM1)'. *Immunol Rev* 1994; 138: 39–59.

4 Vetrie D, Vorechovsky I, Sideras P *et al.* The gene involved in X-linked agammaglobulinaemia is a member of the src family of protein-tyrosine kinases. *Nature* 1992; 361: 226–33.

5 Nussinovitch M, Frydman M, Cohen HA, Varsano I. Congenital agammaglobulinemia presenting with echthyma gangrenosum. *Acta Paediatr Scand* 1991; 80: 732–4.

6 Bentur L, Shear N, Roifman CM. Cutaneous lymphohistiocytic infiltrates in patients with hypogammaglobulinemia. *J Pediatr* 1990; 116: 68–72.

7 Conley ME, Brown P, Pickard AR *et al.* Expression of the gene defect in X-linked agammaglobulinemia. *N Engl J Med* 1986; 315: 564–7.

8 Journet O, Durandy A, Doussau M *et al.* Carrier detection and prenatal diagnosis of X-linked agammaglobulinemia. *Am J Med Genet* 1992; 43: 885–7.

9 Conley ME, Sweinberg SK. Females with a disorder phenotypically identical to X-linked agammaglobulinemia. *J Clin Immunol* 1992; 12: 139–43.

10 Cunningham-Rungles C. Clinical and immunologic studies of common variable immunodeficiency. *Curr Opin Pediatr* 1994; 6: 676–81.

11 Sneller MC, Strober W, Eisenstein E, Jaffe JS, Cunningham-Rundles C. NIH Conference: new insights into common variable immunodeficiency. *Ann Int Med* 1993; 118: 720–30.

12 Conley ME, Park CL, Douglas SD. Childhood common variable immunodeficiency with autoimmune disease. *J Pediatr* 1986; 108: 915–22.

13 Cunningham-Rundles C, Siegal FP, Cunningham-Rundles S, Lieberman P. Incidence of cancer in 98 patients with common varied immunodeficiency. *J Clin Immunol* 1987; 7: 294–9.

14 Sullivan JL, Woda BA. X-linked lymphoproliferative syndrome. *Immunodef Rev* 1989; 1: 325–47.

15 Seemayer TA, Gross TG, Egeler RM *et al.* X-linked lymphoproliferative disease: 25 years after the discovery. *Pediatr Res* 1995; 38: 471–8.

16 Pracher E, Panzer-Grumayer ER, Zoubek A, Peters C, Gadner H. Successful bone marrow transplantation in a boy with X-linked lymphoproliferative syndrome and acute severe infectious mononucleosis. *Bone Marrow Trans* 1994; 13: 655–8.

17 Skare JC, Milunsky A, Byron KS, Sullivan JL. Mapping the X-linked lymphoproliferative syndrome. *Proc Natl Acad Sci USA* 1987; 84: 2015–18.

18 Skare J, Madan S, Glaser J *et al.* First prenatal diagnosis of X-linked lymphoproliferative disease. *Am J Med Genet* 1992; 44: 79–81.

19 Conley ME, Sullivan JL, Neidich JA, Puck JM. X chromosome inactivation patterns in obligate carriers of X-linked lymphoproliferative syndrome. *Clin Immunol Immunopathol* 1990; 55: 486–91.

Leucocyte adhesion deficiency

Leucocyte adhesion deficiency (LAD) is a rare autosomal recessive disorder that affects the adherence of neutrophils, cytolytic T lymphocytes and monocytes [1–3], resulting in cutaneous and visceral infections. Two subgroups have been described, LAD I and LAD II.

Pathogenesis

The adherence of leucocytes relates in part to a group of cell surface glycoproteins that share a common 95 kDa β-subunit (CD18). LAD I results from mutations in the CD18 gene, located on the distal portion of the long arm of chromosome 21 (21q22.3) [1]. The β-subunit is linked to three distinct α-chains to form three different surface glycoproteins. Because of the deficient or defective β_2-subunit, these glycoproteins, CD11a (lymphocyte function associated antigen 1 or LFA-1), CD11b (iC3b receptor, CR3, Mac-1), and CD11c (CR4, p150,95), are all absent or deficient in affected patients. The principal ligand for these glycoproteins is intracellular adhesion molecule 1 (ICAM-1), which participates actively in the initiation and evolution of localized inflammation in skin and other tissues. As a result, neutrophil and monocyte chemotaxis and phagocytosis are impaired. Infections result from profound impairment of leucocyte mobilization into extravascular inflammatory sites. The degree of glycoprotein deficiency is proportional to the severity of clinical involvement, with 'severe' deficiency patients having undetectable expression and moderate deficiency patients having 2–10% of normal CD18 levels. LAD II is caused by a deficiency of sialyl Lewis X, the neutrophil ligand for selectins [3].

Clinical presentation

Patients with LAD have frequent skin infections, mucositis and otitis. The skin infections often present as necrotic abscesses that resemble pyoderma gangrenosum, but the inflammatory response and production of purulent material are impaired. Gingivitis with periodontitis may result in loss of teeth. Moderately affected patients have been noted to have only recurrent skin infections and mild peri-odontitis or severe gingivitis with only occasional skin infections. Cellulitis of the face and perirectal area is common. Life-threatening severe bacterial or fungal infections may occur. Some patients are susceptible to severe viral infections [4]. Poor wound healing leads to paper-thin or dysplastic cutaneous scars. Patients with LAD I may have delayed separation of the umbilical cord. Patients with LAD II have developmental abnormalities with growth and mental retardation [3].

Affected individuals have marked peripheral blood granulocytosis (five to 20 times normal levels). *In vitro*, leucocytes from patients show defective adhesion-related function, including defective adhesion to endothelial cells, T lymphocyte and natural killer cell-mediated killing, migration and antigen presentation. Cultures of soft tissue infections reveal a variety of causative Gram-positive, Gram-negative or fungal organisms. In LAD I, opsonic activity and T- and B-cell function may be reduced, while in LAD II neutrophil rolling is significantly diminished [3].

Treatment

Therapy of the soft tissue infections includes appropriate antimicrobial agents and, in some cases, debridement of wounds. Scrupulous dental hygiene is important in reducing the severity of the periodontitis. In patients with significant LAD, death usually occurs by 2 years of age unless successful bone marrow transplantation is performed [5,6]. The oldest known living patient, with a moderate deficiency, was 38 years of age. Analysis of cord blood at 18 weeks gestation is possible using monoclonal antibodies against leucocyte adhesion molecules [7]. Somatic gene therapy through introduction into haematopoietic stem cells of the normal CD18 subunit may be sufficient to convert patients with more severe deficiency into patients with a less severe deficiency or even the heterozygote state [8].

REFERENCES

1 Anderson DC, Springer TA. Leukocyte adhesion deficiency: an inherited defect in the Mac-1, LFA-1, and p150,95 glycoproteins. *Ann Rev Med* 1987; 38: 175–94.
2 El Habbal MH, Strobel S. Leukocyte adhesion deficiency. *Arch Dis Child* 1993; 69: 463–6.
3 Etzioni A. Adhesion molecule deficiencies and their clinical significance. *Cell Adhesion Commun* 1994; 2: 257–60.
4 Kohl S, Loo LS, Schmalstieg FS, Anderson DC. The genetic deficiency of leukocyte surface glycoprotein Mac-1, LFA-1, p150,95 in humans is associated with defective antibody-dependent cellular cytotoxicity *in vitro* and defective protection against herpes simplex virus infection *in vivo*. *J Immunol* 1986; 137: 1688–94.
5 Fischer A, Trung PH, Descamps-Latascha B et al. Bone-marrow transplantation for inborn error of phagocytic cells associated with defective adherence, chemotaxis, and oxidative response during opsonized particle phagocytosis. *Lancet* 1983; ii: 473–6.
6 Le Diest F, Blanche S, Keable H *et al*. Successful HLA nonidentical bone marrow transplantation in three patients with the leukocyte adhesion deficiency. *Blood* 1989; 74: 512–16.
7 Weening RS, Bredius RG, Wolf H, van der Schoot CE. Prenatal diagnostic procedure for leukocyte adhesion deficiency. *Prenat Diagn* 1991; 11: 193–7.
8 Hibbs M, Wardlaw A, Stacker S *et al*. Transfection of cells from patients with leukocyte adhesion deficiency with an integrin beta subunit (CD18) restores lymphocyte function-associated antigen-1 expression and function. *J Clin Invest* 1990; 85: 674–81.

Severe combined immunodeficiency

SCID is a group of heterogeneous disorders that have similar clinical manifestations and functional immunological capacity, but differ in biochemical and cellular features. Of patients with SCID 60% have an X-linked recessive form, but inheritance in an autosomal recessive or sporadic mode has also been described. Of affected patients 75% are male. The frequency of SCID is 1 in 500 000 to 1 in 100 000 live births.

Pathogenesis

Patients with SCID have a profound deficiency in both T- and B-lymphocyte function. Most patients also lack antibody-dependent cellular cytotoxicity and natural killer cell function. SCID has been subclassified based upon morphological, biochemical and cellular immunological distinctions. The best defined subgroups are as follows.
1 The most common form, X-linked SCID, caused by mutations in the γ form of the IL-2 receptor [1]. While the lack of functional receptors for IL-2 can easily explain the lack of T-cell response to mitogens, mature T-cell lymphopenia and B-cell defects are not predicted from the known defect. IL-2Rγ is now known to function in receptor complexes of IL-4 (on B-cell lineage) and IL-7 (leading to maturational events) [2].
2 Adenosine deaminase (ADA) deficiency [3], an autosomal recessive disorder, accounts for 20% of patients with SCID. ADA is an enzyme of the purine salvage pathway. In its absence, toxic metabolites such as deoxyadenosine triphosphate (dATP) accumulate, particularly in immature intrathymic lymphocytes, which contain the highest concentration of kinases to convert the adenosine to toxic phosphorylated derivatives. Patients may also have skeletal defects and growth delay. A less severe form results in late onset.
3 Approximately 4% of patients with SCID have purine nucleoside phosphorylase deficiency [4]. Most suffer from neurological changes, particularly of spasticity and retardation. This autosomal recessive disorder results from abnormalities in purine metabolism and predominantly affect lymphocytes.
4 Major histocompatibility complex (MHC) class II deficient SCID [5–7] (bare lymphocyte syndrome) results from a gene defect in transactivating factors that control the expression of HLA class II genes, not in the MHC class II genes themselves. Most patients with class II deficiency

show a characteristic defect in the binding of a nuclear complex, RFX5, to the X box motif of MHC class II promoters. Other patients carry a gene mutation in CIITA, a non-DNA-binding transactivator.

5 T-cell activation defects: in this autosomal recessive form of SCID, cells are deficient in ZAP-70 tyrosine kinase expression [9,10]. CD8+ cells are absent, and CD4+ cells do not respond to mitogenic stimuli mediated through the T-cell receptor.

6 Defects in CD3 expression: mutations in genes encoding CD3γ and ε-chains have been described [11,12].

7 Langerhans' cell histiocytosis X-like (Omenn's syndrome) [13,14].

Clinical presentation

Patients with SCID begin to have recurrent infections, diarrhoea and failure to thrive by 3–6 months of age. Among the common early infections are mucocutaneous candidiasis, viral-induced chronic diarrhoea with malabsorption and pneumonia due to bacteria, *P. carinii* or parainfluenza virus type III [15]. Patients with SCID usually lack tonsillar buds and usually lack palpable lymphoid tissue, despite recurrent infections.

The mucocutaneous manifestations of patients with SCID include cutaneous infections, especially due to *C. albicans*, *S. aureus* and *S. pyogenes*. The most common rashes are morbilliform or similar to seborrhoeic dermatitis [16,17], and the possibility of associated acute GVHD must be considered (see Chapter 25.15). Occasionally, cutaneous lesions that resemble lichen planus, acrodermatitis enteropathica, Langerhans' cell histiocytosis, lamellar ichthyosis and scleroderma may be manifestations of GVHD in infants with SCID. Skin biopsies of lesional skin show the histopathological characteristics of GVHD. Extensive eczematous lesions or severe exfoliative erythroderma, often with alopecia, may occur without GVHD in a subgroup of SCID with reticuloendothelial cell proliferation (Omenn's syndrome) [13,14]. Lymphadenopathy, hepatomegaly, occasionally splenomegaly and eosinophilia are associated.

Prognosis

Patients with SCID usually die by 2 years of age without bone marrow transplantation or other definitive therapy.

Differential diagnosis

SCID must be distinguished from other disorders of immunodeficiency, especially acquired immunodeficiency syndrome (AIDS). Patients with SCID do not have the human immunodeficiency virus (HIV) virus or anti-HIV antibodies, and usually do not have an inverted CD4/CD8 ratio. Patients with SCID do not tend to have

normal or increased levels of immunoglobulins. Patients with Nezelof's syndrome present later in infancy or childhood with infections similar to those of patients with SCID. These patients characteristically have lymphopenia, but other leucocyte counts are normal. T cells are deficient, but immunoglobulin levels are normal or near normal. Despite the presence of immunoglobulin, antibody production in patients with Nezelof's syndrome is suboptimal or absent.

Treatment

Early diagnosis of SCID is imperative, if possible before the administration of live vaccines or unirradiated blood products. Infants with SCID should be kept in protective isolation and watched for the presence of infections, which should be vigorously treated. All blood products should be irradiated to prevent GVHD.

Bone marrow transplantation of infants with SCID is the treatment of choice, since otherwise infants usually die by 2 years of age [18]. In patients without a suitable HLA-identical donor, post-thymic T lymphocytes have been removed with lectins or anti-T-cell antibodies from parental haploidentical marrow and successfully administered. Bone marrow transplantation has been performed as early as 4 days of age in an affected sibling with SCID with rapid reconstitution of immune function and little morbidity. *In utero* transplantation of fetal liver stem cells has also been successful [19].

As little as 5–10% of normal ADA maintains patients, and increases of 30–50 times normal levels of ADA are not toxic. Recently, lymphocyte gene therapy by monthly injection of the patient's ADA gene-corrected T cells has been used to provide helper T-cell function to increase antibody responses [20,21]. ADA enzyme replacement has been successful in many patients, particularly by injection of polyethylene glycol-conjugated ADA [22], but does not usually result in complete restoration of immune function. Administration of recombinant IL-2 has been used in patients who lack IL-2 production and immunoglobulin synthesis to restore T- and B-cell function [23,24].

T and B lymphocytes of female carriers of X-linked SCID exhibit non-random X-chromosome inactivation, a feature that allows proper diagnosis of some boys with 'sporadic' SCID as X-linked disease [25]. Prenatal diagnosis of SCID has been performed in families with a previously affected sibling of known phenotype by analysis levels of ADA or by examination of maternal X-chromosome inactivation and linkage analysis [26].

REFERENCES

1 Noguchi M, Nakamura Y, Russell SM *et al.* Interleukin-2 receptor γ chain: a functional component of the interleukin-4 receptor. *Science* 1993; 262: 1877–90.

2 Kondo M, Takeshita T, Ishii N *et al.* Sharing of the interleukin-2 (IL-2) receptor γ chain between receptors for IL-2 and IL-4. *Science* 1993; 262: 1874–7.

3 Hirschhorn R. Genetic deficiencies of adenosine deaminase and purine nucleoside phosphorylase: overview, genetic heterogeneity and therapy. *Birth Defects: Orig Article Ser* 1983; 19: 73–81.

4 Market L. Purine nucleoside phosphorylase deficiency. *Immunol Rev* 1991; 3: 45–81.

5 Cunningham-Rundles S, Yeger-Arbitman R, Nachman SA, Kaul S, Fotino M. New variant of MHC class II deficiency with interleukin-2 abnormality. *Clin Immunol Immunopathol* 1990; 56: 116–23.

6 Griscelli C. Combined immunodeficiency with defective expression in major histocompatibility complex class II genes. *Clin Immunol Immunopathol* 1991; 61: S106–10.

7 Mach B, Steimle V, Reith W. MHC class II-deficient combined immunodeficiency: a disease of gene regulation. *Immunol Rev* 1994; 138: 207–21.

8 Steimle V, Durand B, Barras E *et al.* A novel DNA-binding regulatory factor is mutated in primary MHC class II deficiency (bare lymphocyte syndrome). *Genes Devel* 1995; 9: 1021–32.

9 Elder ME, Lin D, Clever J *et al.* Human severe combined immunodeficiency due to a defect in ZAP-70, a T cell tyrosine kinase. *Nature* 1994; 264: 1596–9.

10 Chan AC, Kadlecek TA, Elder ME. ZAP-70 deficiency in an autosomal recessive form of severe combined immunodeficiency. *Nature* 1994; 264: 1599–601.

11 Arnaiz-Villena A, Timon M, Corell A, Perez-Aciego P, Martin-Villa JM, Regueiro JR. Primary immunodeficiency caused by mutations in the gene encoding the CD3-γ subunit of the T-lymphocyte receptor. *N Engl J Med* 1992; 327: 529–33.

12 Soudais C, De Villartay JP, Le Diest F, Fischer A, Lisowska-Grospierre B. Independent mutations of the human CD3ε resulting in a T cell receptor/CD3 complex immunodeficiency. *Nature Genet* 1993; 3: 77–81.

13 Cederbaum SD, Niwayama G, Stiehm R, Neerhout RC, Ammann AJ, Berman W. Combined immunodeficiency presenting as the Letterer–Siwe syndrome. *J Pediatr* 1974; 85: 466–71.

14 Omenn GS. Familial reticuloendotheliosis with eosinophilia. *N Engl J Med* 1965; 273: 427–32.

15 Buckley RH. Advances in the diagnosis and treatment of primary immuno-deficiency diseases. *Arch Intern Med* 1986; 146: 377–84.

16 Postigo Llorente C, Ivars Amoros J, Ortiz de Frutos FJ *et al.* Cutaneous lesion in severe combined immunodeficiency: two case reports and a review of the literature. *Pediatr Dermatol* 1991; 8: 314–21.

17 De Raeve L, Song M, Levy J, Mascart-Lemone F. Cutaneous lesions as a clue to severe combined immunodeficiency. *Pediatr Dermatol* 1992; 9: 49–51.

18 Himelstein BP, Puck J, August C, Pierson G, Bunin N. T-cell-depleted maternal bone marrow transplantation for siblings with X-linked severe combined immunodeficiency. *J Pediatr* 1993; 122: 289–91.

19 Touraine JL. New strategies in the treatment of immunological and other inherited diseases: allogeneic stem cell transplantation. *Bone Marrow Trans* 1989; 4(suppl): 139–41.

20 Culver KW, Anderson WF, Blaese RM. Lymphocyte gene therapy. *Hum Gene Ther* 1991; 2: 107–9.

21 Hoogerbrugge PM, Beusechem VW, Kaptein LCM, Einerhand MPW, Valerio D. Gene therapy for adenosine deaminase deficiency. *Br Med Bull* 1995; 51: 72–81.

22 Hershfield MS, Buckley RH, Greenberg ML *et al.* Treatment of adenosine deaminase deficiency with polyethylene glycol-modified adenosine deaminase. *N Engl J Med* 1987; 316: 589–96.

23 Chatila T, Castigli E, Pahwa R *et al.* Recombinant interleukin 2 therapy in severe combined immunodeficiency disease. *Proc Natl Acad Sci USA* 1989; 86: 5069–73.

24 Doi S, Saiki O, Hara T. Administration of recombinant IL-2 augments the level of serum IgM in an IL-2 deficient patient. *Eur J Pediatr* 1989; 148: 630–3.

25 Conley ME, Buckley RH, Hong R *et al.* X-linked severe combined immuno-deficiency: diagnosis in males with sporadic severe combined immuno-deficiency and clarification of clinical findings. *J Clin Invest* 1990; 85: 1548–54.

26 Puck JM, Krauss CM, Puck SM, Buckley RH, Conley ME. Prenatal test for X-linked severe combined immunodeficiency by analysis of maternal X-chromosome inactivation and linkage analysis. *N Engl J Med* 1990; 322: 1063–6.

Wiskott–Aldrich syndrome

WAS is a rare X-linked recessive disorder which in its classic form consists of recurrent pyogenic infections, bleeding due to thrombocytopenia and platelet dysfunction, and recalcitrant dermatitis [1,2]. Only 27% of patients, however, have all three major features at presentation [3], 20% have haematological manifestations only and 5% have only infectious features before diagnosis. The recurrent infections result from immunodeficiency of both humoral and cell-mediated immune responses. The majority of patients are male, but full expression has been reported in a girl [4].

Pathogenesis

The haemorrhagic diathesis is due to both quantitative and qualitative platelet defects. Platelets from most patients are small, abnormal structurally and have a reduced half-life without decreased production. No antiplatelet anti-bodies have been demonstrated. The recurrent infections are secondary to immunodeficiency of both cell-mediated and humoral immune responses.

A lymphocyte and platelet surface sialylated glycoprotein (CD43, sialophorin, leucosialin), a component of the T-lymphocyte activation pathway that binds ICAM-1, is deficient or defective in WAS patients [5–7], and was suspected at first to be the primary defect. Subsequent investigations showed that the gene for CD43 was located on chromosome 16 [8], not at the pericentric region of the X chromosome, the site of the mutations in WAS [9]. The gene that is abnormal in WAS has now been determined. 'WASP' encodes a 501 amino acid proline-rich protein that may serve as a transcription factor important for lymphocyte and platelet function. Several mutations in the WASP gene have now been found in patients with WAS [10,11].

The eczema appears to be related to the T-lymphocyte defect, since it is corrected by T-lymphocyte engraftment (see below). The development of malignancies is poorly understood, but may result from the immunodeficiencies with inadequate immune surveillance, or from the chronic immunostimulation of recurrent infections [12,13].

Clinical manifestation

Since thrombocytopenia and platelet dysfunction are often present from birth, epistaxis and bloody diarrhoea are often the initial manifestations. In addition, mucocutaneous petechiae (Fig. 25.14.8) may appear, consistent with the platelet abnormalities [14]. Spontaneous bleeding from the oral cavity, cutaneous ecchymoses, haematemesis, melaena and haematuria are common but the severity varies. Painful cutaneous vasculitis with significant oedema may also develop, particularly as the disorder progresses.

Dermatitis usually develops during the first few months of life, and fulfils criteria for the definition of atopic dermatitis. The face, scalp and flexural areas are the most severely involved, although patients commonly have widespread involvement with progressive lichenification (Fig. 25.14.9). Excoriated areas frequently have serosanguineous crust and often associated petechiae or purpura. Secondary bacterial infection of eczematous lesions is common, as are eczema herpeticum and molluscum. IgE-mediated allergic problems such as urticaria, food allergies and asthma are also seen with increased frequency.

Recurrent bacterial infections begin in infancy as placentally transmitted maternal antibody levels diminish and include otitis externa and media, pneumonia, pansinusitis, conjunctivitis, furunculosis, meningitis and septicaemia. Infections with encapsulated bacteria such as pneumococcus, *H. influenzae*, and *Neiserria meningitidis* predominate. With advancing age, T-cell function progressively deteriorates and patients become increasingly susceptible to infections due to herpes and other viruses,

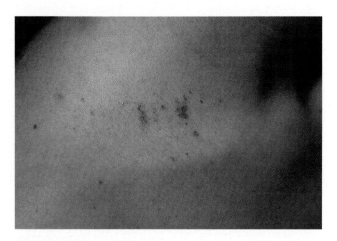

Fig. 25.14.8 Numerous petechiae in a boy with Wiskott–Aldrich syndrome, providing evidence of thrombocytopenia and platelet dysfunction.

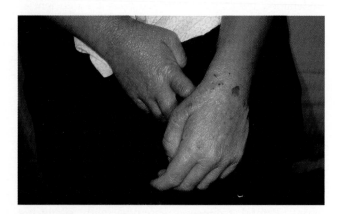

Fig. 25.14.9 Atopic dermatitis with marked lichenification and erosions covered with serosanguineous crust in a boy with Wiskott–Aldrich syndrome.

and to *P. carinii*. Additional clinical features may be hepatosplenomegaly, lymphadenopathy and transient arthritis with joint effusions.

Lymphoreticular malignancies occur overall in 18% of patients [13], with an average age of onset of 9.5 years. Non-Hodgkin's lymphoma [11–13] is the most common malignancy, and extranodal and brain involvement predominate. The risk of developing non-Hodgkin's lymphoma approaches 100% by 30 years of age [11,12]. Malignancy is the most common cause of death in patients with WAS who survive the infections and haemorrhages of early childhood.

Laboratory studies often demonstrate persistent thrombocytopenia, in the range of 1000–80 000 platelets/mm³. Platelets tend to be small and aggregation is sometimes defective [14]. Patients may also have Coomb's positive haemolytic anaemia (14%), leucopenia, lymphopenia and eosinophilia. Total serum gammaglobulin is usually normal, but immunoelectrophoresis shows low levels of IgM and sometimes IgG, and IgM antibodies to blood group antigens (isohaemagglutinins) are absent. Levels of IgA, IgE and IgD tend to be elevated. The number of T lymphocytes and response *in vitro* to mitogens may be normal in early life, but often decreases with advancing age. Delayed hypersensitivity skin test reactions are usually absent, and antibody responses to polysaccharide antigens are markedly diminished. Patients with decreased neutrophil or monocyte chemotaxis have been reported. Proliferative lymphocyte responses to periodate are decreased [15].

Prognosis

The clinical course of WAS is progressive, usually resulting in death by adolescence. Most patients die by 3 years of age. In 55% of patients, infection is the cause of death; 24% die of haemorrhage, usually intracranial, and 10% of malignant neoplasia.

Differential diagnosis

Several conditions may be confused with the WAS. Many of the other immunodeficiencies are characterized by eczema, increased susceptibility to infections and the development of malignancy. Patients with agammaglobulinaemias have no bleeding tendency. In DiGeorge's syndrome, facial anomalies, seizures associated with hypoparathyroidism and hypocalcaemia, and normal humoral immunity help to distinguish the disorder. CHS differs from WAS by the incomplete albinism and giant granules in leucocytes. WAS can also be mistaken for various eczematous processes. The distribution and character of the rash resemble atopic dermatitis. Seborrhoeic dematitis, Leiner's disease and histiocytosis-X may also be confused with WAS. The other clinical findings of haemorrhage, petechiae and recurrent infections in WAS, together with the histopathological examination of skin for histiocytosis-X, help to differentiate the conditions.

Treatment

Bone marrow transplantation with HLA-identical marrow is the treatment of choice for patients with recurrent problems. Full engraftment results in normal platelet numbers and functions, immunological status and, if T lymphocytes engraft, clearance of the dermatitis [15,16]. Splenectomy has been advocated to ameliorate the bleeding abnormality in patients with recurrent severe haemorrhage, although it increases the risk of infection by encapsulated organisms. Splenectomy is probably the treatment of choice in patients with thrombocytopenia who have no HLA-matched bone marrow transplantation donor [17]. Otherwise, therapy for patients has been directed towards the recurrent infections and haemorrhage. Appropriate antibiotics and transfusions of platelets and plasma decrease the risk of fatal infections and haemorrhage. Intravenous infusions of gammaglobulin are also useful in some patients. Transfer factor has also been infused with resultant decreased frequency of infection and improvement of the eczema. Topical corticosteroid preparations and systemic gammaglobulin may improve the dermatitis, and chronic administration of oral acyclovir is appropriate for patients with eczema herpeticum.

Genetic counselling is important in families of patients with WAS, including for sisters of involved patients. Female carriers for WAS may be detected by the selective inactivation of the abnormal X chromosome in T and B cells and in platelets [18,19]. Studies of maternal X chromosome inactivation have also been used to diagnose two boys with atypical WAS [20]. Prenatal diagnosis has been achieved in the first trimester by DNA markers [21].

REFERENCES

1 Perry GS III, Spector BD, Schuman LM *et al*. The Wiskott–Aldrich syndrome in the United States and Canada. *J Pediatr* 1980; 97: 72–8.
2 Peacocke M, Siminovitch KA. Wiskott–Aldrich syndrome: new molecular and biochemical insights. *J Am Acad Dermatol* 1992; 27: 507–29.
3 Sullivan KE, Mullen CA, Blaese RM, Winkelstein JA. A multi-institutional survey of Wiskott–Aldrich syndrome. *J Pediatr* 1994; 125: 876–85.
4 Conley ME, Wang WC, Parolini O, Shapiro DN, Campana D, Siminovitch KA. Atypical Wiskott–Aldrich syndrome in a girl. *Blood* 1992; 80: 1264–9.
5 Mentzer SJ, Remold-O'Donnell, Crimmins AV, Brier BE, Rosen FS, Burakoff SJ. Sialophorin, a surface sialoglycoprotein defective in Wiskott–Aldrich syndrome, is involved in human T lymphocyte proliferation. *J Exp Med* 1987; 165: 1383–92.
6 Park JK, Rosenstein YJ, Remold-O'Donnell E, Bierer BE, Rosen FS, Burakoff SJ. Enhancement of T-cell activation by the CD43 molecule whose expression is defective in Wiskott–Aldrich syndrome. *Nature* 1991; 350: 706–9.
7 Rosenstein Y, Park JK, Hahn WC, Rosen FS, Bierer BE, Burakoff SJ. CD43, a molecule defective in Wiskott–Aldrich syndrome, binds ICAM-1. *Nature* 1991; 354: 233–5.
8 Pallant A, Eskenazi A, Mattei M-G *et al*. Characterization of cDNAs encoding human leukosialin and localization of the leukosialin gene to chromosome 16. *Proc Natl Acad Sci USA* 1989; 86: 1328–32.
9 Peacocke M, Siminovitch KA. Linkage of the Wiskott–Aldrich syndrome with polymorphic DNA sequences from the human X chromosome. *Proc Natl Acad Sci USA* 1987; 84: 3430–3.
10 Derry JM, Ochs HD, Francke U. Isolation of a novel gene mutated in Wiskott–Aldrich syndrome. *Cell* 1994; 78: 635–44.
11 Kwan S-P, Hagemann TL, Radtke BE, Blaese RM, Rosen FS. Identification of mutations in the Wiskott–Aldrich syndrome gene and characterization of a polymorphic dinucleotide repeat at DXS6940, adjacent to the disease gene. *Proc Natl Acad Sci USA* 1995; 92: 4706–10.
12 Filipovich AH, Mathur A, Kamat D, Kersey JH, Shapiro RS. Lymphoproliferative disorders and other tumors complicating immunodeficiencies. *Immunodeficiency* 1994; 5: 91–112.
13 Cotelingam JD, Witebsky FG, Hsu SM, Blaese RM, Jaffe ES. Malignant lymphoma in patients with the Wiskott–Aldrich syndrome. *Cancer Invest* 1985; 3: 515–22.
14 Corash L, Shafer B, Blaese RM. Platelet-associated immunoglobulin, platelet size, and the effect of splenectomy in the Wiskott–Aldrich syndrome. *Blood* 1985; 65: 1439–43.
15 Parkman R, Rappeport J, Geha R *et al*. Complete correction of the Wiskott–Aldrich syndrome by allogeneic bone marrow transplantation. *N Engl J Med* 1978; 298: 921–7.
16 Brochstein JA, Gillio AP, Ruggiero M *et al*. Marrow transplantation from human leukocyte antigen-identical or haploidentical donors for correction of Wiskott–Aldrich syndrome. *J Pediatr* 1991; 119: 907–12.
17 Mullen CA, Anderson KD, Blaese RM. Splenectomy and/or bone marrow transplantation in the management of the Wiskott–Aldrich syndrome: long-term follow-up of 62 cases. *Blood* 1993; 10: 2961–6.
18 Fearon ER, Kohn DB, Winkelstein JA, Vogelstein B, Blaese RM. Carrier detection in the Wiskott–Aldrich syndrome. *Blood* 1988; 72:1735–9.
19 Winkelstein JA, Fearon E. Carrier detection of the X-linked primary immunodeficiency diseases using X-chromosome inactivation analysis. *J Allergy Clin Immunol* 1990; 85: 1090–7.
20 Puck JM, Siminovitch KA, Poncz M, Greenberg CR, Rottem M, Conley ME. Atypical presentation of Wiskott–Aldrich syndrome: diagnosis in two unrelated males based on studies of maternal T cell X chromosome inactivation. *Blood* 1990; 75: 2369–74.
21 Schwartz M, Mibashan RS, Nicolaides KH *et al*. First-trimester diagnosis of Wiskott–Aldrich syndrome by DNA markers. *Lancet* 1989; ii: 1405.

Graft-Versus-Host Disease

JOHN HARPER

Graft-versus-host disease

Definition

Graft-versus-host disease (GVHD) is the term used to describe the clinical manifestations and histopathological features provoked by a graft-versus-host reaction (GVHR). A GVHR occurs when immunocompetent cells of the graft react with the tissues of an immunosuppressed histoincompatible recipient. Although this response has been known for many years and has been studied in several animal species, it has come to the fore as a clinical problem in humans with the development of bone marrow transplantation (BMT).

Billingham [1] described the essential conditions for the occurrence of the reaction as follows.
1 There is a profound depression of cellular immunity of the recipient, otherwise the graft is rejected.
2 The patient must have received an allograft of lymphoid immunocompetent cells in sufficient quantity.
3 There is recognition by the graft of foreign antigens in the tissues of the host.

Histoincompatibility differences may be major, carried on the histocompatibility antigens of the HLA system, the major histocompatibility complex (MHC) in humans, or there may be minor differences which are more difficult to define as in the case of identical twin donors in whom a GVHR may occur despite the graft and recipient having identical HLA mixed lymphocyte reaction (MLR) matching [2,3].

Clinical situations in which graft-versus-host disease may occur

GVHD may occur in a human fetus with a congenital cellular immunodeficiency due to the transplacental passage of maternal lymphocytes [4]. Lymphocytes are known to cross the placental barrier and may react against fetal antigens. GVHD may also be due to an *in utero* transfusion for rhesus incompatibility (erythroblastosis fetalis) [5].

In a neonate or infant with severe immune deficiency, GVHD may be provoked by the therapeutic transfusion of whole blood or by the transfusion of blood products such as packed red cells, platelets and even fresh plasma [6,7]. This risk must be recognized in such neonates and all blood products should be irradiated to prevent a GVHR.

In patients with disseminated malignancy, who have a depressed immune system due to the malignancy itself and to cytotoxic drugs, GVHD may be induced by the administration of non-irradiated blood products [8,9].

GVHD occurs in patients given therapeutic grafts of haemopoietic cells, i.e. bone marrow, placental blood [10], liver and thymus. GVHD is a common and often serious complication of BMT and it is in this clinical context that GVHD is most frequently encountered.

History

Experimental animal models of graft-versus-host disease

In 1916, Murphy [11] was the first to describe the GVHR. He observed that inoculation of the chorioallantoic membranes of young (7 day) chicken embryos with fragments of certain tissues (spleen and bone marrow) from adult chicken donors resulted in enlargement of the host spleen. The effect was misinterpreted as splenic stimulation and the implications of this were not fully realized until the 1950s.

When immunologically competent cells of an adult animal are injected into a newborn of a different strain, immunological immaturity of the recipient allows the graft to take with the development of GVHD, which was originally described by Billingham and Brent [12] as runt disease.

A similar situation is brought about by injecting a first-generation hybrid, resulting from a cross between two pure strains, with lymphoid cells of either parent. The term secondary disease denotes GVHD in a lethally irradiated animal reconstituted by the administration of foreign haematological cells. This experimental model is called a radiation chimera.

The most studied animals are rodents—mice, rats and hamsters. In all these experimental models of GVHD cutaneous lesions have been observed, the severity of which varies with the animal species.

Historical summary of human graft-versus-host disease

The 1960s saw the early attempts at human BMT. Clinical marrow transplant experiments were limited by the frequency and severity of GVHD. The 1970s was an era of clinical trials for GVHD prophylaxis with methotrexate, antithymocyte and antilymphocyte globulin. From the 1980s onwards major advances have occurred in the prophylaxis of GVHD with the introduction of cyclosporin, T-cell depletion of donor marrow and the introduction of specific monoclonal antibodies. A better understanding of GVHD and improved patient care has led to a significant increase in the survival figures of BMT. Also the more recent recognition of the graft-versus-leukaemia (GVL) effect which may be a useful modality of treatment for some patients with leukaemia.

Pathogenesis

Acute disease

The essential hypothesis is that GVHD occurs as a result of an interaction of donor T lymphocytes with recipient histoincompatible antigens. The T lymphocytes become sensitized to recipient antigens, differentiate *in vivo* and then directly, or through secondary mechanisms, attack recipient cells, producing the clinical symptomatology of acute GVHD. In BMT donor lymphocytes are infused into a host that has been profoundly damaged. The effects of the underlying disease, prior infection and the conditioning regime may result in substantial proinflammatory changes in endothelial and epithelial cells. Donor cells rapidly encounter not only a foreign environment, but also one that has been altered to promote the activation and proliferation of inflammatory cells by the increased expression of adhesion molecules [13], cytokines and cell surface recognition molecules [14].

The onset of acute GVHD is determined by the time required for the infused lymphocytes to proliferate and differentiate. Mature donor T cells recognize recipient peptide–HLA complexes (alloantigens) on the surface of antigen-presenting cells (APCs), in which both the HLA molecules and the bound peptides are foreign. The peptides represent minor histocompatibility antigens (mHAs), some of which have been identified [15–17]. In mouse models of GVHD, CD4+ cells induce GVHD to MHC class II (HLA-DR, -DP, -DQ) differences, and CD8+ cells induce GVHD to MHC class I (HLA-A, -B, -C) differ-

ences [18]. In HLA-matched BMTs, GVHD may be induced by either subset or simultaneously by both. Cytokines produced in response to alloantigens are predominantly secreted by the CD4+ (T-helper type 1 or Th1) subset of T cells [19]. Both interleukin 2 (IL-2) and interferon-γ (IFN-γ) play a central role in further T-cell activation, induction of cytotoxic T lymphocytes (CTLs) and natural killer (NK) cell responses, and the priming of additional donor and residual mononuclear phagocytes to produce IL-1 and tumour necrosis factor-α (TNF-α) [20]. The balance in Th1 and Th2 cytokines is critical for the development (or prevention) of acute GVHD.

Keratinocytes have been shown to express DR antigen during early and established GVHD. Keratinocyte DR expression can be induced *in vitro* by γ-interferon [21], suggesting that, during GVHD, sensitized T lymphocytes release cytokines which induce the expression of DR. The induced DR then becomes a target for CTLs directed against class II antigens.

The mechanism leading to tissue damage in GVHD is complex. As well as the cellular damage caused by CTLs and NK cells, inflammatory cytokines play an important role. TNF-α can cause direct tissue damage by inducing necrosis of target cells, or it may induce tissue destruction by apoptosis or programmed cell death. The induction of apoptosis occurs after activation of the TNF-α–Fas antigen pathway [22].

The target organs of GVHD support the close relationship between infection and GVHD. The skin, gastrointestinal tract and liver all share exposure to endotoxin and other bacterial products that can trigger and amplify local inflammation. These tissues have a large proportion of APCs, such as macrophages and dendritic cells that may enhance the GVHR. Similarly viral infections, in particular cytomegalovirus (CMV), herpes viruses and Epstein–Barr virus, are frequent in patients undergoing BMT and may trigger or aggravate GVHD. Cells infected with a viral agent can induce neoantigens on their surface. The immune system may then recognize these cells as foreign and destroy them even when both the infected cells and the immunologically competent donor cells have the same histocompatibility antigens.

Chronic disease

Chronic manifestations of GVHD [23] are thought to be due to the generation of autoreactive T-cell clones [24]. These are derived from the engrafted donor lymphoid stem cells, which differentiate entirely within the recipient. The mechanism of the sclerotic change in the skin most likely relates to the effect of cytokines on collagen synthesis. *In vitro* experiments have shown that collagen synthesis by fibroblasts is increased by the cytokines present in the supernatant of a phytohaemaglutinin (PHA)-stimulated lymphocyte culture [25,26].

Holmes *et al.* [27] reported a patient with disseminated carcinoma who developed cutaneous and systemic features closely resembling those seen in chronic GVHD. The authors suggested the possibility that a GVH-like reaction was induced by alteration of 'self-antigens', consequent upon her malignancy. This case lends support to the suggestion that GVHRs are not simply limited to patients with bone marrow grafts or blood product transfusions but may develop in a situation in which there has been an alteration in self-antigens. Such a change in self-antigens could occur as a result of viral infections, malignant disease or certain drugs. This broader concept of GVHD may help to advance our understanding of the pathogenesis of the so-called 'idiopathic' disorders, lichen planus, toxic epidermal necrolysis (TEN) and scleroderma.

Pathology

Histopathology

Histopathological features of a skin biopsy of GVHD are classified into four grades (Table 25.15.1). The earliest change is perivascular cuffing of lymphocytes often seen around dilated blood vessels and swollen endothelial cells. These changes occur within the first 24 h. The next stage is marked by a mild to moderate lymphocytic infiltrate in the upper dermis and dermoepidermal junction at sites of focal basal cell vacuolation. Established GVHD is characterized by more extensive basal cell vacuolation with disruption of the basement membrane, lymphocytes migrating into the epidermis and intercellular oedema of the epidermis (spongiosis) (Fig. 25.15.1). Degenerate keratinocytes (individual cell necrosis) are seen scattered throughout the epidermis, some with a pyknotic nucleus and eosinophilic, hyalinized cytoplasm. These necrotic keratinocytes were sometimes associated with one or more satellite lymphocytes, an association referred to as satellite cell necrosis [4] (Fig. 25.15.2). In fulminant acute GVHD, there is separation of the epidermis at the dermoepidermal junction with widespread desquamation of skin and necrosis of the overlying epidermis.

Histopathological features of chronic GVHD shows the epidermis to be atrophic with hyperkeratosis, thickening of the basement membrane and condensed/homogeneous connective tissue in the upper dermis. Basal layer vacuolar degeneration, inflammation and eosinophilic body formation are rare or absent. The dermis shows thickened, hyalinized collagen bundles together with destruction of the adnexal structures.

In the setting of BMT, a skin biopsy is the preferred method of establishing a diagnosis of GVHD and in monitoring its course. Although recognized early in its course as an erythematous maculopapular rash, there is no one clinical or pathological feature which is specifically diagnostic of GVHD [28]. Individual keratinocyte cell necrosis may be induced by total body irradiation [29] and various

Table 25.15.1 Histopathological grades of acute cutaneous GVHR

Grade	Definition
1	Focal or diffuse vacuolar alteration of basal epidermal cells
2	Vacuolar alteration of basal epidermal cells; spongiosis and dyskeratosis of epidermal cells
3	Formation of subepidermal cleft in association with spongiosis and dyskeratosis
4	Complete loss of epidermis

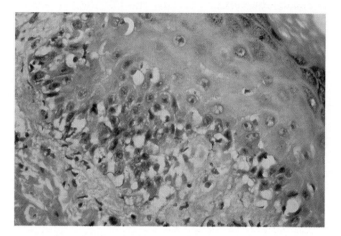

Fig. 25.15.1 Established GVHD: histopathology of the skin showing basal cell vacuolation, lymphocytic infiltrate and individual cell necrosis of keratinocytes (grade 2). (H&E.)

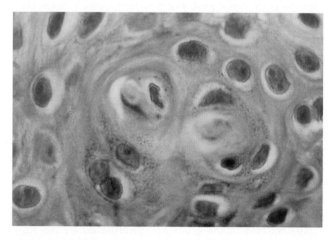

Fig. 25.15.2 Satellite cell necrosis in GVHD. (H&E.)

cytotoxic drugs [30,31]. Evidence that cytotoxic agents can produce mild epidermal damage, including necrosis of occasional keratinocytes in association with a sparse lymphocytic infiltrate and some vacuolar alteration of basal epidermal cells, comes from studies of psoriatic patients treated with methotrexate and hydroxyurea [32,33]. Similar changes have been described with bleomycin, adriamycin and cyclophosphamide [31]. The author's results showed seven of 17 pretransplant skin biopsies to be abnormal [3]. The specificity of the histological features of acute GVHD was questioned by Sale and the Seattle team [31]. Some 49 skin biopsy specimens taken from marrow transplant patients, who received either allogeneic, syngeneic or autologous marrow, were coded and studied 'blindly' by three pathologists. These authors concluded the following.

1 The early cutaneous histological changes do not permit a diagnosis of GVHD except late in its evolution (after the 35–40th day) when the effects of the cytotoxic agents have normally disappeared.

2 The presence of eosinophilic bodies, with or without satellite lymphocytes, is a necessary criterion, but is insufficient to confirm the diagnosis of GVHD since they can be caused by cytotoxic drugs. Their presence is, however, rare after the 19th day in patients who have received only cyclophosphamide and total body irradiation.

3 Certain situations require the repetition of skin biopsies at intervals of a few days. If epidermal lesions persist, the probability that they are due to cytotoxic agents decreases as the probability of GVHD increases. The histological diagnosis of GVHD, therefore, must take into account all other available relevant data. The author's findings stress the importance of taking a pretransplant skin biopsy as a baseline.

Immunopathology

In a study by the author and co-workers 14 skin biopsies of GVHD [34] were examined by an indirect immunoperoxidase technique using a panel of monoclonal antibodies. Controls included pretransplant skin biopsies, skin from normal healthy volunteers and from patients with lichen planus and cutaneous T-cell lymphoma.

The results demonstrated the following immunopathological features of cutaneous GVHD.

1 The lymphoid infiltrate of acute GVHD is composed of mainly T lymphocytes.

2 Helper (CD4+) T lymphocytes, of donor origin, appear early and accumulate around blood vessels.

3 Suppressor/cytotoxic (CD8+) T lymphocytes are found predominantly at the dermoepidermal junction and in the epidermis (Fig. 25.15.3).

4 There is a significant reduction in number of detectable Langerhans' cells in acute GVHD.

5 Acute GVHD is associated with HLA-DR expression of keratinocytes (Fig. 25.15.4).

6 There is a persistence of increased numbers of perivascular helper (CD4+) T lymphocytes in chronic GVHD.

The presence of CD8+ cells in contact with destroyed keratinocytes strongly infers a cytopathic potential of these cells. Anti-Leu-7, which stains human NK cells, as well as a subset of CD8+ cells, were few in number.

HLA-DR (Ia) staining of keratinocytes occurred in acute

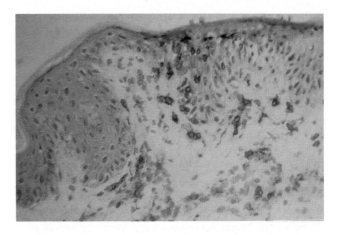

Fig. 25.15.3 CD8+ T lymphocytes at the dermoepidermal junction and in the epidermis demonstrated using an indirect immunoperoxidase technique.

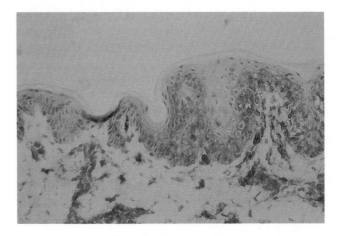

Fig. 25.15.4 HLA-DR expression of basal keratinocytes.

GVHD, lichen planus and in two of the six patients with cutaneous T-cell lymphoma. HLA-DR expression was not observed in normal or pretransplant skin biopsies. Studies in rats have shown that Ia staining can be induced in the skin during contact hypersensitivity reactions but is absent following mechanical or chemical damage to the skin [35]. Scheynius and Tjernlund [36] have demonstrated the induction of HLA-DR on keratinocytes during the tuberculin reaction. These facts suggest that HLA-DR or Ia staining by keratinocytes is a consequence of cellular immunity. Breathnach and Katz [37] have shown, in a murine model of acute cutaneous GVHD, that the keratinocytes themselves synthesize Ia antigen in acute GVHD.

The observation of a reduction in number of Langerhans' cells in acute GVHD was first made by Lampert *et al.* [38] and Mason *et al.* [39] in F1 hybrid rats and subsequently in human GVHD [40]. However, in these studies there were no controls. The author's studies confirmed that there is a significant decrease in the number of CD1-positive dendritic (Langerhans') cells detectable in the skin biopsies of acute GVHD; although there was a slight reduction in the number of Langerhans' cells in pretransplant skin biopsies compared with the normal controls, presumably related to chemotherapy. These results suggest that the Langerhans' cell is a primary target in cutaneous GVHD [3,34].

Clinical features

BMT is now a well-accepted treatment for a variety of severe haematological disorders, such as the acute leukaemias, aplastic anaemia, immunodeficiency diseases and, more recently, it has become recognized that BMT can offer treatment for some of the inborn errors of metabolism [41]. The cutaneous signs are usually the earliest manifestation of GVHD [3,24,42]. Tissues which are primary targets include the epithelium of the skin, gastrointestinal tract and liver. It is traditional to divide the clinical manifestations into acute and chronic phases; this distinction is difficult to define precisely as acute lesions can transform and progress imperceptibly into chronic lesions.

Of the 100 BMT patients studied by the author [3], 76 developed GVHD (Table 25.15.2). Fever and skin rash occurred in all 76 patients (100%); 46 patients (61%) had acute gastrointestinal symptoms and 28 patients (37%) had hepatic involvement. Out of the 76 patients 23 (30%) developed chronic skin changes of GVHD.

Acute disease

The most common presentation is a faint, erythematous maculopapular eruption on the trunk and limbs (Fig. 25.15.5), often starting on the face and affecting the palms (Fig. 25.15.6) and soles. Typically, acute GVHD is seen at the time of haemopoietic reconstitution, 10–14 days post-transplant; in the author's series this ranged from day 5 to day 60 postgraft. The more severe forms of acute GVHD develop an erythroderma and subsequent

epidermal separation, resulting in the appearance of bullae. The occurrence of TEN as a manifestation of fulminant acute GVHD in man was reported by Peck *et al.* [43] and was witnessed in three of the author's 100 patients. This has a high mortality; of the 100 patients, one died as a result of overwhelming acute GVHD and the other two died of septicaemia. In areas of blister formation the sepa-

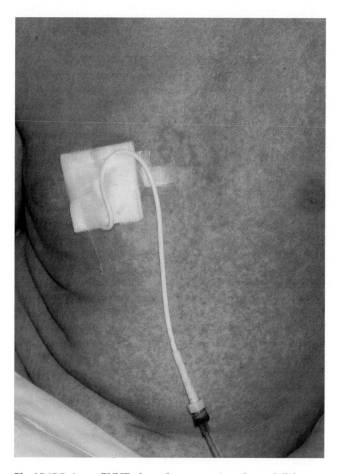

Fig. 25.15.5 Acute GVHD: the early presentation of a morbilliform rash.

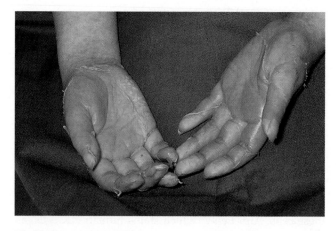

Fig. 25.15.6 Acute GVHD: desquamation of the palms.

Table 25.15.2 Incidence of GVHD in patients after BMT. Adapted from Harper [3]

	No. of patients	GVHD
Aplastic anaemia	16	12
Leukaemias		
ALL	50	42
AML	5	3
Fanconi's anaemia	3	3
Immunodeficiency diseases	11	4
Inborn errors of metabolism	15	12
Total	100	76

ALL, acute lymphocytic leukaemia; AML, acute myelocytic leukaemia.

ration is dermoepidermal, similar to that seen in drug-induced TEN. The severity of acute GVHD is dependent on the degree of histoincompatibility and was inevitably worse when mismatched donors were used.

Other manifestations of acute GVHD include fever, gastrointestinal and liver disturbance. Intestinal involvement is manifested by diarrhoea, nausea and vomiting. Abdominal pains and ileus are indicative of severe disease. Hepatic involvement causes an elevation in aspartate transaminase (AST) and alanine transaminase (ALT), hyperbilirubinaemia of the conjugated type and an elevation of alkaline phosphatase.

Certain factors have been associated with an increased risk of GVHD in humans, including older recipient age [44], female donor [45,46] and HLA-B18 phenotype [47]. The severity of GVHD is related to donor-recipient compatibility, the number of lymphocytes transfused, the bacterial microflora of the gastrointestinal tract, viral infections and pretransplant irradiation.

Chronic disease

When patients survive acute GVHD and other complications, especially infections, the cutaneous lesions either disappear completely or they gradually progress and evolve into the chronic manifestations of GVHD. The incidence of chronic cutaneous GVHD in the author's patients was 30%. All the patients who developed chronic skin changes had had previous acute manifestations. In a series of transplant patients by the Seattle group [47], chronic GVHD proved to be a significant problem in 19 of 92 patients (21%) surviving 150 days or more; in five individuals chronic GVHD apparently occurred without a preceding acute reaction. Chronic skin manifestations of GVHD include lichen planus-like lesions, pigmentary changes and sclerosis.

In the author's series, a variety of lichenoid lesions occurred from day 29 to day 350 postgraft. Involvement of the buccal mucosa is a frequent finding. Saurat and Gluckman [49] stated that oral lesions always preceded the cutaneous lesions of chronic GVHD. However, this was not substantiated by the author's observations. The mucosal lesions are similar to those seen in idiopathic lichen planus, with a white reticulate pattern affecting the buccal mucosa, gingiva, tongue and palate. Lichen planus lesions of the genitalia have also been reported [48,49] and were seen in one patient in the author's series. The appearance of lichen planus papules on the skin shows similarities to that seen in idiopathic lichen planus [50–52] with polygonal, violaceous, shiny papules and Wickham striae. More often, though, the lesions are less typical of lichen planus while remaining lichenoid in nature. Lesions are often seen in a reticulate configuration, especially on the limbs (Fig. 25.15.7), suggesting some relationship to the underlying vascular network. The distribution, when wide-

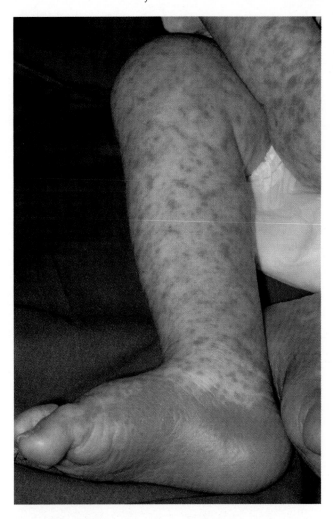

Fig. 25.15.7 Chronic GVHD: lichenoid lesions in a reticulate configuration.

spread, does not tend to affect those areas of predilection seen in idiopathic lichen planus, like the anterior aspects of the wrists. Follicular lesions, resembling lichen planopilaris, are seen as an early manifestation of chronic GVHD. The lichenoid lesions exhibit the Koebner phenomenon, seen in two of the author's patients. There has been the suggestion that the lichenoid lesions occur more often in the zones previously affected by the acute GVHD rash. The author observed no evidence to support this, although one patient in the series did develop tiny lichenoid papules on the palms, which is unusual in idiopathic lichen planus. Nail involvement occurred in two patients. Cicatrical alopecia has been reported by Touraine *et al.* [50] Saurat *et al.* [52] and Shulman *et al.* [48]; but this was not noted in the author's study.

Hyperpigmentation is a frequent finding, which is either diffuse, reticulate or follicular. Lesions may have a poikilodermatous appearance [48,50,53]. Less commonly, areas of hypopigmentation occur. Pigmentary changes precede the development of sclerosis.

Areas of induration and sclerosis of the skin develop as

a late manifestation of GVHD. These sclerotic lesions tend to be localized [4,54,55]; or progress to extensive sclerosis (generalized scleroderma) (Fig. 25.15.8). Ulceration, particularly at pressure points [50,53,56], and flexion contractures with limitation of joint movement [57,58] may result. Four patients in the author's series developed morphoea-like areas of skin and in one boy these were widespread. In these patients the lesions have remained static or have gradually improved; none progressed to the more serious sequelae. This may be related to their long-term treatment with prednisolone and azathioprine. Saurat *et al.* regard [52] these late changes to be more like lichen sclerosus et atrophicus with, in particular, characteristic genital lesions. Shulman *et al.* [48] noted a phimosis in two of their 19 patients, an observation that could possibly reinforce Saurat's hypothesis. However, oesophageal involvement [59] and subcutaneous calcification [60] suggest that this disease process is more like scleroderma.

Other manifestations of chronic disease. Chronic GVHD may manifest as a variety of autoimmune or connnective

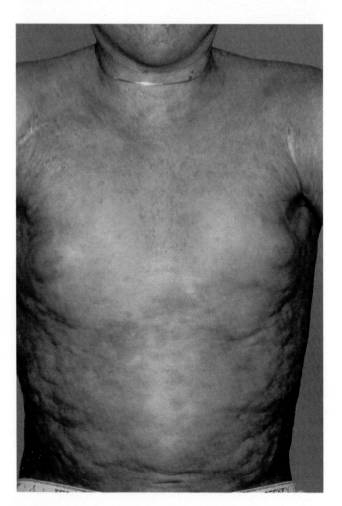

Fig. 25.15.8 Chronic GVHD: generalized scleroderma.

tissue diseases [23], sharing overlapping features with scleroderma, lupus erythematosus, dermatomyositis, polymyositis, primary biliary cirrhosis and chronic active hepatitis. The occurrence of Sjögren's syndrome is well documented [48,60]. Xerophthalmia, conjunctivitis and xerostomia were observed in one patient in the author's study, who also had lichenoid lesions of chronic GVHD. Gratwhol *et al.* [60] reported cutaneous lesions, which, clinically and histologically, resembled discoid lupus erythematosus in one patient, 19 months after transplantation. The author has seen vitiligo and polymyositis associated with chronic GVHD. Visceral manifestations of chronic GVHD are essentially malabsorption and chronic hepatitis. Chronic liver damage with progressive destruction of bile cannaliculi may lead to primary biliary cirrhosis [61] or to a syndrome mimicking chronic active hepatitis. Most patients with chronic GVHD tend to have prolonged humoral and cellular immune defects with an increased susceptibility to bacterial, viral and fungal infections. Laboratory tests in chronic GVHD may show abnormal liver function eosinophilia, hypogammaglobulinaemia with polyclonal elevation of immunoglobulin G (IgG) or IgM, and a variety of circulating autoantibodies, especially antinuclear, antismooth muscle and antimitochondrial antibodies.

Differential diagnosis

The differential diagnosis of acute cutaneous GVHD includes the effects of radiotherapy, drug reactions and infections. Usually, these can be distinguished clinically, but the major practical problems of diagnosis include (a) drug-induced rashes, as a result of immunosuppressive or antibiotic therapy; and (b) a viraemia caused by hepatitis B or CMV, which can exceptionally be responsible for an exanthematous eruption. As detailed in the section on histology, there are no features specifically diagnostic for GVHD; however, a skin biopsy may provide useful information to support the diagnosis.

The diagnosis of chronic GVHD is usually straightforward based on clinical examination of lichenoid or sclerodermatous lesions in a BMT recipient.

Treatment

Prevention

Until 1980, methotrexate was the principal agent used for the prophylaxis of GVHD. Since then cyclosporin has been introduced [62,63]. Cyclosporin has proved to be extremely effective in reducing the severity but not the incidence of GVHD [64]. There has been a better survival rate and decreased severity of GVHD in patients receiving prophylactic cyclosporin compared with methotrexate alone [65]. Cyclosporin can cause renal toxicity, which limits the dose used. Other side effects include hypertension, fits, hypertrichosis, gum hypertrophy and a rare but serious 'capillary leak' syndrome [64]. Often a combination of cyclosporin and methotrexate is used [24].

Another approach to the prophylaxis of GVHD has been the use of a monoclonal antibody to eliminate T lymphocytes from the donor marrow. It has been shown in animal experiments that removal of mature T lymphocytes from the marrow graft will prevent GVHD. The monoclonal antibody developed for this is CAMPATH-1 [66]. CAMPATH-1 is a rat antihuman lymphocyte antibody which lyses cells in the presence of autologous human complement. Results were encouraging with the elimination of lethal GVHD; however, there is now evidence that the use of this monoclonal antibody is associated with an increased risk of failure of engraftment and of leukaemic relapse.

Acute disease

Several agents have been used to treat established acute GVHD, with varying degrees of success. High-dose corticosteroids given as a bolus injection of intravenous methylprednisolone produces a dramatic effect on acute GVHD and is used widely as first-line treatment [67]. While skin GVHD responds rapidly, liver and gut GVHD can be resistant, and some patients become refractory to steroids. Oral corticosteroids used alone in conventional doses are much less effective. Cyclosporin, cyclophosphamide and antithymocyte globulin are given as second-line treatments. In the case of refractory acute GVHD, use of monoclonal antibodies anti-IL-1, anti-IL-2, anti-TNF-α and anti-INF-γ, have each been suggested [68,69]. Other possible treatments include the immunosuppressive agent FK-506 and photophoresis.

Chronic disease

A combination of corticosteroids and cyclosporin is often used or alternatively corticosteroids and azathioprine. Chronic GVHD occurring after stopping cyclosporin will often regress when the drug is reintroduced, but some patients develop chronic GVHD during adequate cyclosporin therapy [62]. Localized morphoea lesions may gradually improve [3]. However, the severe progressive wasting disease with immunodeficiency, liver damage and scleroderma is not always controllable; the sclerodermatous form may produce permanent deformity which persists after the GVHD process has burnt out.

The use of thalidomide has been documented in several case reports and small series showing a favourable response [70,71], but this remains difficult to assess and in the author's experience is more often than not disappointing.

Photochemotherapy (psoralens and vitamin A or PUVA) may be helpful for the treatment of lichenoid GVHD inadequately controlled by systemic therapy [72]. The efficacy of PUVA treatment for sclerodermatous GVHD is more controversial and there is a small but definite risk of developing skin malignancy [73].

Topical treatments that are useful include cyclosporin in solution as a mouthwash [74] or a potent corticosteroid as an inhaler (Becotide) for oral erosive lichen planus; and a potent topical steroid ointment (Dermovate) for phimosis or localized chronic GVHD elsewhere.

Finally, other measures include prevention of infection, physiotherapy, a high-protein diet, the use of artificial tears if necessary and the regular application of a sunscreen.

Graft-versus-leukaemia effect

Evidence supporting the existence of an antileukaemia effect of allogeneic bone marrow has rapidly expanded [75]. Early mice studies demonstrated a 'graft-versus-leukaemia' effect in association with GVHD. One possible explanation is the recognition of altered cell surface antigens by T cells. Progress in this area will provide insights for finding ways to direct the destructive immunological effects against leukaemia cells and not against normal tissues.

In clinical practice this effect is now well established and induction of GVL is a modality of treatment for patients with chronic myeloid leukaemia or juvenile chronic myeloid leukaemia who have relapsed after BMT. This can be achieved by either infusing donor buffy coat cells containing T lymphocytes or by reducing/stopping immunosuppression. Although this may increase the risk of GVHD, it can eliminate residual leukaemia. Immune therapy based on the GVL effect has the potential for being an effective treatment for leukaemia and warrants further study.

Conclusion: why graft-versus-host disease is important to the dermatologist

GVHD is a frequent complication of BMT and is responsible for significant mortality. The rash is usually the first sign of GVHD and early recognition and treatment is imperative. The effect on the skin may be the chief morbid factor, such as TEN. Finally, GVHD is a biological model for other 'idiopathic' skin diseases such as lichen planus, TEN and morphoea/scleroderma. Knowledge of the mechanisms involved in GVHD will hopefully lead to a better understanding of the pathophysiology of these 'idiopathic' diseases.

REFERENCES

1 Billingham RE. The biology of graft versus host reactions. *Harvey Lectures* 1967; 62: 21–78.

2 Rappeport J, Mihm M, Reinherz E *et al*. Acute graft versus host disease in recipients of bone marrow from identical twin donors. *Lancet* 1979; ii: 717–20.

3 Harper JI. *A clinicopathological study of cutaneous graft versus host disease*. MD thesis, University of London, 1985.

4 Grogan TM, Odom RB, Burgess JH. Graft versus host reaction. *Arch Dermatol* 1977; 113: 806–12.

5 Parkman R, Mosier D, Umansky I *et al*. Graft versus host disease after intrauterine and exchange transfusions for haemolytic disease of the newborn. *N Engl J Med* 1974; 290: 359–63.

6 Hathaway WE, Githens JH, Blackburn WR *et al*. Aplastic anaemia, histiocytosis and erythrodermia in immunologically deficient children: probable human runt disease. *N Engl J Med* 1965; 273: 953–8.

7 Park BH, Good RA, Gate J *et al*. Fatal graft versus host reaction following transfusion of allogenic blood and plasma in infants with combined immunodeficiency disease. *Trans Proc* 1974; 6: 385–8.

8 Von Fleidner V, Higby DJ, Kim U. Graft-versus-host reaction following blood product transfusion *Am J Med* 1982; 72: 951–61.

9 Tolbert B, Kaufman CE, Burgdorf WHC *et al*. Graft-versus-host disease from leucocyte transfusions. *J Am Acad Dermatol* 1983; 9: 416–19.

10 Kurtzberg J, Laughlin M, Graham ML *et al*. Placental blood as a source of hematopoietic stem cells for transplantation into unrelated recipients. *N Engl J Med* 1996; 335: 157–66.

11 Murphy JB. The effect of adult chicken grafts on the chick embryo. *J Exp Med* 1916; 24: 1–6.

12 Billingham RE, Brent L. A simple method for inducing tolerance of skin homografts in mice. *Trans Bull* 1957; 4: 67–71.

13 Behar E, Chao NJ, Hiraki DD *et al*. Polymorphism of adhesion molecule CD31 and its role in acute graft versus host disease. *N Engl J Med* 1996; 334: 286–91.

14 Vogelsang GB, Hess AD. Graft versus host disease: new directions for a persistent problem. *J Am Soc Hematol* 1994; 84: 2061–7.

15 Nichols W, Antin J, Lunetta K. Identification of non-HLA loci contributing to graft versus host disease. *Blood* 1995; 86(suppl 1): 630a.

16 Goulmy E, Schipper R, Pool J *et al*. Mismatches of minor histocompatibility antigens between HLA identical donors and recipients and the development of graft versus host disease after bone marrow transplantation. *N Engl J Med* 1996; 334: 281–5.

17 Den Haan JM, Sherman NE, Blokland E *et al*. Identification of a graft versus host disease-associated human minor histocompatibility antigen. *Science* 1995; 268: 1476–80.

18 Korngold R, Sprent J. T cell subsets in graft versus host disease. In: Burakoff SJ, Deeg HJ, Ferrara J, Atkinson K, eds. *Graft versus Host Disease: Immunology, Pathophysiology and Treatment*. New York: Marcel Dekker, 1990: 31–50.

19 Sad S, Marcotte R, Mosmann TR. Cytokine-induced differentiation of precursor mouse CD8+ T cells into cytotoxic CD8+ T cells secreting Th1 or Th2 cytokines. *Immunity* 1995; 2: 271–9.

20 Ferrara JLM. Paradigm shift for graft versus host disease. *Bone Marrow Trans* 1994; 14: 183–4.

21 Morhenn VB, Nickoloff BJ, Merigan TC *et al*. The effect of gamma interferon on cultured human keratinocytes. *J Invest Dermatol* 1984; 82: 410 (abstract).

22 Laster SM, Wood JG, Gooding LR. Tumour necrosis factor can induce both apoptotic and necrotic forms of cell lysis. *J Immunol* 1988; 141: 26–9.

23 Harper JI. Graft versus host disease: etiological and clinical aspects in connective tissue diseases. *Semin Dermatol* 1985; 4: 144–51.

24 Aractingi S, Chosidow O. Cutaneous graft versus host disease. *Arch Dermatol* 1998; 134: 602–12.

25 Johnson RL, Ziff M. Lymphokine stimulation of collagen accumulation. *J Clin Invest* 1976; 58: 240–52.

26 Spielvogel RL, Goltz RW, Kersey JH. Mononuclear cell stimulation of fibroblast collagen synthesis. *Clin Exp Dermatol* 1977; 3: 25–35.

27 Holmes RC, Cooper CB, Jurecka W *et al*. Syndrome resembling graft-versus-host disease in a patient with disseminated carcinoma. *J Roy Soc Med* 1983; 76: 703–5.

28 Darmstadt GL, Donnenberg AD, Vogelsang GB *et al*. Clinical, laboratory, and histopathologic indicators of the development of progressive acute graft versus host disease. *J Invest Dermatol* 1992; 99: 397–402.

29 Woodruff JM, Eltringham JR, Casey HW. Early secondary disease in the rhesus monkey. I. A comparative histologic study. *Lab Invest* 1969; 20: 499–511.

30 Woodruff JM, Hansen JA, Good RA *et al*. The pathology of the graft versus host reaction (GVHR) in adults receiving bone marrow transplants. *Trans Proc* 1976; 8: 675–84.

31 Sale GE, Lerner KG, Barker EA *et al*. The skin biopsy in the diagnosis of acute graft versus host disease in man. *Am J Pathol* 1977; 89: 621–35.

32 Smith C, Gelfant S. Effects of methotrexate and hydroxyurea on psoriatic epidermis. Preferential cytotoxic effects on psoriatic epidermis. *Arch Dermatol* 1974; 110: 70–2.

33 Kennedy BJ, Smith LR, Goltz RW. Skin changes secondary to hydroxyurea therapy. *Arch Dermatol* 1975; 111: 183–7.

34 Harper JI, Zemelman V, Nagvekark NM *et al*. Graft versus host disease: T-lymphocyte subsets, Langerhans' cells and HLADR+ cells in the skin after human bone marrow transplantation. *J Invest Dermatol* 1984; 82: 562–3.

35 Suitters AJ, Lampert IA. Expression of Ia antigen on epidermal keratinocytes is a consequence of cellular immunity. *Br J Exp Pathol* 1982; 63: 207–13.

36 Scheynius A, Tjernlund U. Human keratinocytes express HLA-DR antigens in the tuberculin reaction. *Scand J Immunol* 1984; 19: 141–7.

37 Breathnach SM, Katz SI. Keratinocytes synthesize Ia antigen in acute cutaneous graft versus host disease. *J Immunol* 1983; 131: 2741–5.

38 Lampert IA, Suitters AJ, Chisholm PM. Expression of Ia antigen on epidermal keratinocytes in graft versus host disease. *Nature* 1981; 293: 149–50.

39 Mason DW, Dallman M, Barclay AN. Graft versus host disease induces expression of Ia antigen in rat epidermal cells and gut epithelium. *Nature* 1981; 293: 150–1.

40 Lampert IA, Janossy G, Suitters AJ *et al*. Immunological analysis of the skin in graft versus host disease. *Clin Exp Immunol* 1982; 50: 123–31.

41 Hobbs JR. Bone marrow transplantation for inborn errors. *Lancet* 1981; ii: 735–40.

42 Dinulos JG, Levy M. Graft versus host disease in children. *Semin Dermatol* 1995; 14: 66–9.

43 Peck GL, Herzig GP, Elias PM. Toxic epidermal necrolysis in a patient with graft-vs-host reaction. *Arch Dermatol* 1972; 105: 561–9.

44 Ringden O, Nilsson B. Death by graft versus host disease associated with HLA mismatch, high recipient age, low marrow cell dose and splenectomy. *Transplantation* 1985; 40: 39–44.

45 Storb R, Weiden PL, Graham TC *et al*. Marrow grafts between DLA-identical and homozygous unrelated donors. *Transplantation* 1977; 24: 165.

46 Bortin M, Rimm A. Treatment of 144 patients with severe aplastic anaemia using immunosuppression and allogeneic marrow transplantation. A report from the International Bone Marrow Transplantation Registry. *Trans Proc* 1981; 13: 227–9.

47 Storb R, Hansen JA, Prentice RL *et al*. Association between HLA-B antigens and acute graft versus host disease. *Lancet* 1983; 2: 816–19.

48 Shulman HM, Sale GE, Lerner KG *et al*. Chronic cutaneous graft versus host disease in man. *Am J Pathol* 1978; 91: 545–70.

49 Saurat JH, Gluckman E. Lichen planus-like eruption following bone marrow transplantation: a manifestation of the graft versus host disease. *Clin Exp Dermatol* 1977; 2: 335–44.

50 Touraine R, Revuz J, Dreyfus B *et al*. Graft versus host reaction and lichen planus. *Br J Dermatol* 1975; 92: 589.

51 Saurat JH, Didier-Jean L, Gluckman E *et al*. Graft versus host reaction and lichen planus-like eruption in man. *Br J Dermatol* 1975; 92: 591–2.

52 Saurat JH, Gluckman E, Bussel A *et al*. The lichen planus-like eruption after bone marrow transplantation. *Br J Dermatol* 1975; 93: 675–81.

53 Spielvogel RL, Goltz RW, Keysey JH. Scleroderma-like changes in chronic graft versus host disease. *Arch Dermatol* 1977; 113: 1424–8.

54 Masters R, Hood A, Cosini A. Chronic cutaneous graft-vs-host reaction following bone marrow transplantation. *Arch Dermatol* 1975; 111: 1526.

55 Van Vloten WA, Scheffer E, Dooren LJ. Localised scleroderma-like lesions after bone marrow transplantation in man. *Br J Dermatol* 1977; 96: 337–41.

56 Hood AF, Soter NA, Rappeport J *et al*. Graft versus host reaction. Cutaneous manifestations following bone marrow transplantation. *Arch Dermatol* 1977; 113: 1087–91.

57 Siimes MA, Johansson E, Rapola J. Scleroderma-like graft-versus-host disease as a late consequence of bone marrow grafting. *Lancet* 1977; ii: 831–2.

58 Shulman HM, Sullivan KM, Weiden PL *et al*. Chronic graft-versus-host

syndrome in man. A long-term clinicopathologic study of 20 Seattle patients. *Am J Med* 1980; 69: 204–17.

59 Roujeau JC, Revuz J, Touraine R. Graft versus host reactions. In: Rook A, Savin J, eds. *Recent Advances in Dermatology*, vol. 5. Edinburgh: Churchill Livingstone, 1980: 131–57.

60 Gratwhol AA, Moutsopoulos HM, Chused TM *et al.* Sjögren type syndrome after allogenic bone marrow transplantation. *Ann Intern Med* 1977; 87: 703–70.

61 Epstein O, Thomas HC, Sherlock S. Primary biliary cirrhosis is a dry gland syndrome with features of chronic graft versus host disease. *Lancet* 1980; i: 1166–8.

62 Powles RL, Clink HM, Spence D *et al.* Cyclosporin A to prevent graft versus host disease in man after allogenic bone marrow transplantation. *Lancet* 1980; i: 327–9.

63 Barrett AJ, Kendra JR, Lucas CF *et al.* Cyclosporin A as prophylaxis against graft versus host disease in 36 patients. *Br Med J* 1982; 285: 162–6.

64 Harper JI, Kendra JR, Desai S *et al.* Dermatological aspects of the use of cyclosporin A for prophylaxis of graft versus host disease. *Br J Dermatol* 1984; 110: 469–74.

65 Kendra JR, Barrett AJ, and the Westminster Hospital Bone Marrow Team. Comparison of methotrexate and cyclosporin A in the prevention of graft versus host disease in leukaemia transplants. In: Touraine J-L, Gluckman E, Griscelli C, eds. *Bone Marrow Transplantation in Europe. Proceedings of the Fifth European Symposium on Bone Marrow Transplantation, Courchevel*, vol. 2. Armsterdam: Excerpta Medica, Elsevier, 1981: 165–70.

66 Waldmann H, Hale G, Cividalli G *et al.* Elimination of graft versus host disease by *in-vitro* depletion of alloreactive lymphocytes with a monoclonal rat anti-human lymphocyte antibody (Campath 1). *Lancet* 1984; ii: 483–5.

67 Kendra J, Barrett AJ, Lucas C *et al.* Response of graft versus host disease to high doses of methylprednisolone. *Clin Lab Haematol* 1981; 3: 19–26.

68 Hollar E, Kolb H, Mittermuller J *et al.* Modulation of acute graft versus host disease after allogeneic bone marrow transplantation by TNF release in the course of pretransplant conditioning: role of conditioning regimes and prophylactic application of monoclonal antibody neutralizing human TNF. *Blood* 1995; 85: 890–9.

69 Anasetti C, Hansen J, Waldmann T *et al.* Treatment of acute graft versus host disease with humanized anti-Tac: an antibody that binds to IL-2 receptor. *Blood* 1994; 84: 1320–7.

70 Vogelsang G, Farmer E, Hess A *et al.* Thalidomide for the treatment of chronic graft versus host disease. *N Engl J Med* 1992; 326: 1055–8.

71 Parker P, Chao N, Nademanee A *et al.* Thalidomide as salvage therapy for chronic graft versus host disease. *Blood* 1995; 86: 3604–9.

72 Volc-Platzer A, Hönigsmann H, Hinterberger W *et al.* Photochemotherapy improves chronic cutaneous graft versus host disease. *J Am Acad Dermatol* 1990; 23: 220–8.

73 Altman R, Adler S. Development of multiple cutaneous squamous cell carcinomas during PUVA treatment for cutaneous chronic graft versus host disease. *J Am Acad Dermatol* 1994; 31: 505–7.

74 Eisen D, Ellis C, Duell E *et al.* Effect of topical cyclosporine rinse on oral lichen planus: double-blind analysis. *N Engl J Med* 1990; 323: 290–4.

75 Sosman JA, Sondel PM. The graft-vs-leukemia effect. *Am J Pediatr Hematol Oncol* 1993; 15: 185–95.

Section 26
Psychological Aspects of Skin Disease in Children

26.1 Coping with Chronic Skin Disease

CAROLINE SCOTT KOBLENZER

The patient
Early parent–child interactions, and the developing personality
Age at onset
The nature of the disease

The family

The community

Enhancement of coping skills

When coping fails

When a child is born with, or develops a skin disease that is chronic, a psychosocial impact on patient, family and community is inevitable, though the severity of that impact and the capacity to cope show remarkable variability. This chapter explores the factors that contribute to that variability and describes measures to reduce psychosocial distress and improve coping strategies.

The patient

Early parent–child interactions, and the developing personality [1]

Individual differences in handling adversity depend on complex interactions between the genetic endowment of the person and the early psychological development, tempered by progressive life experience. The capacity to adapt is already determined, in large part, in the very early months of life. That very early experience, in conjunction with genetic endowment, shapes the developing self-esteem, the integrity of the body image, the stability of gender and personal identity and the capacity to modulate emotion effectively [2]. The same elements contribute in major ways to the shaping of personality, and the flexibility of character and coping styles; they help to determine the capacity to capitalize on evolving physical and emotional assets, and to adapt in positive ways to the realities of changing circumstances [3]. The skin, the envelope that contains us, and the boundary that defines us, plays a crucial role in this early experience. In what follows, that role will be

discussed, in relation to self-esteem, body image and the capacity to modulate anxiety.

Self-esteem

Each infant has his or her particular emotional needs; when parental touch and emotional stimulation is in tune with the needs of the infant, in a loving environment, that child will learn to find his or her body and persona as admirable and worthy of respect as do the parents; the child will incorporate and make a part of himself or herself those overt and hidden parental attitudes that are communicated in the early interactions [1,4–6]. The child whose whole body surface is lovingly touched will develop a more favourable view of themselves than will the child for whom skin contact is more restricted [4].

Should skin disease develop, inner strength will then permit toleration of physical discomfort, or cruel and insensitive comments; basic trust will permit an effective doctor–patient relationship to develop, and thus ensure optimal benefit from dermatological treatment; self-worth will permit a realistic appraisal of the circumstances and ensure treatment compliance, while flexibility of personality will allow the channelling of creative energies into alternate pathways for emotional growth and personal gratification, should the illness preclude certain pleasurable activities [7–9]. In the face of illness, the person who is less favoured may feel worthless, as though the diseased skin symbolically represents an inner defectiveness of the whole person [10]; these negative feelings further diminish shaky self-esteem, lead to depressive mood and may set a destructive spiral in motion. The child who does not feel good about themselves may elect not to comply with treatment, and allow the condition to worsen. The patient may then feel angry and helpless, peer and family relationships may suffer and school performance fall off.

Body image

Development of the body image starts within the very early months of life, and is essentially complete by about 4 years of age [11], although final consolidation of personal and gender identity is delayed until the turmoil of adoles-

1713

cence is over [12,13]. The greater the area of skin that is empathically touched during that early developmental phase, the more accurate and stable will be the image [6]; the more clear the physical and emotional boundaries of the self, the more firm the sense of personal and sexual identity [4]. Though body image changes with time, incorporating into itself attitudes and memories associated with those changes [14,15], the capacity to maintain stable boundaries requires the early positive tactile experience, and when this is so, physical change can be integrated without too much stress. A fragile self-image, however, may be associated with heightened anxiety, profound worries about the nature of the disease, even about the very integrity of the self [16]. Dysmorphic obsessions, embarrassment and shame may keep the patient out of school [17,18]; an unshakeable false belief of delusional intensity, that the patient is infested, infected, hideously ugly or seriously deformed may even be triggered [19]. Minor flaws are experienced by these patients as major disasters, and skin disease in general is handled much less adaptively than by those with more stable self-esteem [7–9,16–20].

Modulation of anxiety, and emotional response

Infantile responses are physiological, and total. Through contact with the mother, a capacity to modulate the physiological response gradually evolves; this modulation translates into the baby's internal adaptive regulation first of anxiety, and later of emotion [21,22]. When regulation is not achieved in infancy, emotional discharge will persist through physiological channels, and create a predisposition towards psychophysiological illness [23]. In the genetically predisposed, stress may then precipitate or aggravate skin disease, or may significantly affect its course. A number of associations have been made in the literature, the most prominent being the heightened anxiety, and hyperkinesis frequently found in patients with chronic intractable atopic eczema [1,24–27], and the association of anxiety and depression with psoriasis [1,28–31], chronic urticaria [1,32] and pruritus [32,33].

Age at onset

When present at birth or in very early childhood, abnormal skin is incorporated into the body image as it develops, and is accepted as an integral part of the self. The stable body image and positive self-esteem that come with optimal parenting enable the child to adapt in a positive way to disease or disability [34,35]. The following description of a patient with congenital ichthyosis is an example. In her strongly united family, the patient was never made to feel different, or a bother. Mother patiently and tirelessly scrubbed the scales from the scalp and limbs daily throughout her early childhood, and comforted the patient when she was teased at school. Cheer-leading was encouraged, and gave the patient a sense of mastery, boosting self-esteem and self-confidence, and making her popular, as she became a star. She did not permit her skin to interfere in friendships, or later in sexual relationships. She is currently preparing to enter a 'helping' profession.

Present from birth, the skin condition is an integral part of this patient's body image, while the tactile stimulation from the mother's untiring care helped define her boundaries. Her loving and supportive family ensured the flexibility of character and self-esteem necessary for her to accept herself, and build on her strengths, while her illness has made her sensitive to the pain of others, and perhaps contributed to her choice of a 'helping' profession.

The need to incorporate altered skin into an already developed body image, however, imposes some psychological stress, and disturbing fantasies may result from the altered appearance [16]. This was the case with a 6-year-old girl who presented with severe alopecia areata. For this girl, the bald spots 'showed' that she was a wicked person; deformed and ugly; and magically punished by her mother with whom she was very angry. Both her anger, and her wish to be 'beautiful', and therefore 'good', were expressed in the repeated enactment of traditional fairy tales, as she worked through her conflict in the course of intensive psychotherapy. Whereas supportive psychotherapy is very helpful for children whose appearance is altered by disease, it requires long-term and intensive treatment to help a child to become aware of disturbing fantasies of this type.

Onset in adolescence is particularly stressful because of peer pressures, and the age-related psychological consolidation of personal and gender identity [12,13,16]. This is especially true of lesions that are visible, or affect the face or genitals [4]. If the body image and self-esteem are already fragile, emotional decompensation and mental illness may develop, with depressed mood, dermatitis artefacta, neurotic excoriations, dysmorphic obsessions or delusions, and a further diminution of self-worth. The following history of a 17-year-old girl illustrates these points. The only child of a depressed and anxious mother and distant father, this adolescent girl had received little close parenting in early childhood. Overtly vying for father's attention, she came to believe that only perfection was acceptable; every minor flaw was exaggerated in her mind. At 17, her fragile body image was seriously distorted by minor facial acne. She felt deformed, ugly, ashamed and unlovable. She became depressed and felt socially and sexually unacceptable to such a degree that she would see no one, and refused to leave her room for months. With intensive individual psychotherapy for the patient, and treatment also for her mother, this girl was able to separate from the parents, appraise the severity of her condition more realistically, treat it appropriately and make adaptive behavioural changes. She is now a successful young adult.

The nature of the disease

A visible rash may cause feelings of embarrassment or shame. When compounded by exudates, scales or odour, the negative feelings may be more intense, the child feeling dirty and contaminated, a 'freak', and 'different' at a time when 'sameness' is crucial [10,25,36]. Real or anticipated negative attitudes may arouse a reciprocal negative response in the patient [10,37], which may lead to social withdrawal, school refusal, falling grades and depressive mood. Alternatively, in denial of unhappiness, the child may overcompensate and become loud, pushy and arrogant, behaviour equally unlikely to gain acceptance. Feelings, though more private, are no less intense if the disease is hidden; an embarrassing secret that dare not be shared, while tacit messages that the genitals are shameful or forbidden, may arouse feelings of guilt and sexual unacceptability [4].

The rash itself, its complications or treatment requirements, may disturb sleep, erode school or play-time, preclude pleasurable activities such as athletics, impair performance and cause anger and frustration. Loss of sleep and irritability may generate regressive, demanding, babyish behaviour that is difficult to tolerate, while unaesthetic, time-consuming and rigid treatment schedules preclude full participation in peer-group activities [10,38,39]. All of these increase the sense of being 'freakish' and different, and contribute to social isolation and feelings of diminished self-worth.

Finally, unspoken, irrational thoughts and fears, and unconscious fantasies about causation, may raise questions about infection, contagion, malignancy, whether treatment is indeed possible or even the possibility of death. The guilty may interpret the illness as punishment for forbidden activity, and heightened anxiety may then lead to overtreatment, a reactive non-compliance, unnecessary self-denial or repetitive and ritualistic activities that serve as punishment [10,38].

The story of a 35-year-old man with life-long atopic eczema illustrates some of these points. This man's childhood memories are of shame, embarrassment and guilt, as his weeping limbs were daily bandaged (undoubtedly altering the normal tactile experience for this child) and then unbandaged, for all to see. He describes agonising feelings of abandonment during numerous hospitalizations for exacerbations and infections. An object of ridicule at school, the patient was pitied at home, where the mother tenderly cared for his skin, until he was well into adolescence. In defence against the ever-present fear of abandonment, and the pull to remain dependent on the nurturing mother, the patient became tough, combative and competitive, and despite many absences he did very well in school. Through achievement this patient compensated for the shame and humiliation caused by his skin, and the lurking fear that the rash was punishment for some real or imagined childhood misdeed. Constantly aware of his appearance, the patient carefully monitored the degree of redness, and the response of those around him, angry if the rash was ignored, but shamed if it was observed and pitied. Because of his early experience, the patient could not tolerate passivity, and despite a pervasive anxiety and unhappiness, he coped by succeeding, taking control of his life and of those around him.

The family

A child that is 'imperfect' is a crushing blow to parental self-esteem, a constant reminder that may be viewed by the parents as failure or punishment [3]. These negative interpretations, together with real or inferred judgements by family and friends, impose a stress on the parents, the marital relationship and the siblings. The 'imperfect' child may be subtly or less subtly rejected, and thus deprived of the benefits of an optimal emotional environment as described above. Alternatively, a mistaken sense of guilt may cause parents to be oversolicitous and intrusive, flooding the infant with sensation that may generate chronic anxiety [38]. Or, overwhelmed by her own anxiety in the face of her infant's disability, a mother may fail in helping the child to master the modulation of anxiety, predisposing the child to later somatization and psychophysiological illness [23].

Angry that their child is not normal and healthy, resentful of the cost in time and money, and of the sick child's importunate demands, and irritable from loss of sleep and the stress of coping, the parents feel increasingly guilty, while sensitivity to the parents' ambivalence in turn heightens the child's anxiety, and with it, his or her emotional demands [21,38–42]. In this situation, parents find it difficult to set limits, and may indulge and infantilize the child at the expense of other siblings. Siblings may express their jealousy and resentment of the invalid openly, or covertly, by oversolicitous behaviour or passive–aggressive acts. Subtle and not-so-subtle ways may be found to 'get back' at the affected sibling and the parents, while guilt for the conscious and unconscious anger that motivates the negative behaviour, may lead the siblings to indulge in self-punishing activities.

At 2 and a half years old, one toddler had had recalcitrant atopic eczema since infancy. He was demanding and fractious, and itching prevented sleep at night; for comfort, he shared the mother's bed, the father being relegated to the couch. Mother resented this boy's constant demands, the disruption of her marital relationship and the cost in time and money of his treatments. Sensing her ambivalence, the patient's anxiety increased, and with it, his itching and his demands. Guilty because of her resentment, and fearing that she may in some way be responsible for his illness, the mother could not permit herself to set limits, so that the child was continually pampered and infantilized at the expense of his siblings who, in turn, escalated the situation, feeling resentful and neglected. Only when mother could acknowledge and accept the negative side of her ambivalence, and set appropriate limits for the patient, did his eczema respond to treatment, and his physical and emotional growth move forward normally [38].

The community

Atopic eczema [25,27,38–42], psoriasis [10,31,38–42], and acne vulgaris [55–58] are the conditions most extensively studied, with regard to the relationship between the patient and the community, though the findings can be applied to any chronic skin disorder. A child may be ridiculed by teachers or shunned by peers. In the hair-dressing salon, the barber's shop, the gymnasium, the dance class, the swimming pool or the beach, patients may be subjected to curious stares, insensitive questions or outright rejection. Fears of contagion are not far from the surface. For similar reasons after-school employment in food-handling, or the sale of beauty or fashion items, may be precluded by visible lesions. Patients with acne are less readily employed than those with clear skin [54], and clothing must frequently be restricted as to style and colour, to camouflage the tell-tale signs of dermatitis, the better to avoid anticipated negative comment or rejecting behaviour [10,48].

It is important for doctors to be sensitive to the psychosocial difficulties of patients, who too often feel that adequate time is not allotted for their questions or their feelings, and that their doctors spend a disproportionate amount of the interview in writing prescriptions [43,44].

Enhancement of coping skills

The more that parents know about the cause, expectable course and prognosis of a child's illness, the better they can master their own anxiety, allay the child's fears and avoid the unnecessary disappointment of failed unrealistic goals. Genetic counselling may be needed for optimal planning. Parents need reassurance that the illness is not unique, and that they themselves are in no way to blame. They must be helped to acknowledge and verbalize understandable feelings of guilt and anger in order to avoid the unwitting expression of those feelings in non-adaptive or destructive behaviour. Siblings too must be educated, and permitted to experience occasional resentment and ambivalence towards the sick child. Tension may be reduced, if the abundant energy of the siblings can be used constructively, in helping with some aspect of the care-taking.

Parents must understand the need for unconditional love and acceptance for healthy emotional development. Every aspect of the illness should be handled in a matter of fact way, and the child treated as close to normal as the disease will allow. Creative thinking and flexibility of scheduling may be needed to allow for doctor visits and treatment programmes, while still leaving room for peer-group activities and the separate needs of the siblings. Creative thinking may also be necessary to capitalize on the child's strengths, and to find areas of achievement that are compatible with the child's talents and the nature of the disease.

Support groups offer many benefits [59]. Patients and families feel less uniquely disadvantaged and alienated. The sense of 'family' and 'belonging' enhances self-esteem, while the opportunity to ventilate negative feelings with others similarly placed, relieves stress. Information about scientific advances can be introduced, and individual coping strategies discussed, so that families can learn from each other. Group activities, and summer camps may be organized, and the force of the organization used to educate the community [60–62].

The patients themselves also need information to come to terms realistically with the disease, the limitations that it may impose and what may be expected in the future. Verbal expression of thoughts and feelings should be encouraged, and anxiety allayed, in order to minimize self-destructive or aggressive behaviour, while personal goals and ambitions should also be encouraged and supported realistically. The patient is empowered and in control, when he or she can be given responsibility for carrying out the treatment, which does not then become the focus of a power struggle between patient, parents and doctor.

Information must be given to community leaders to enable them to respond appropriately to the child. Teachers can serve as positive role models in their relationship with the patient. Whereas empathy is helpful, oversolici-tousness or pity are counterproductive. Like the parents, community leaders should foster development of the child's strengths, and strive to promote the child's acceptance in the peer group. Public lectures and newspaper articles are very helpful for dissemination of accurate information.

When coping fails

With the doctor's help, the child and the family can often come to accept realistically the child's condition, and learn optimal modes of coping to improve the quality of life. Unexpected recalcitrance to therapy should alert the doctor to the child at risk; this recalcitrance may result from a psychophysiological response to the stress of coping, from rebellious non-compliance or from dysfunctional interactions within the family. Other warning signs may be unnecessary restrictions in dress or lifestyle that come from shame or embarrassment, overt anxiety, social withdrawal, poor school performance or deteriorating peer and family relationships; depression may sometimes be so severe that suicidal thoughts or even plans, may supervene [10,19,30]. In the face of these, the doctor must be ready to discuss the issues openly, and refer the family to a child psychiatrist or psychoanalyst for evaluation [1].

A thorough evaluation will take into consideration all of the issues that have been discussed above, and treatment recommendations will be made accordingly. Psychoanalysis or intensive psychotherapy may be indicated for the patient, or patient and parents [13,17,38,63]; supportive psychotherapy, group therapy [64], behaviour therapy [65], hypnosis [66,67] and stress management techniques [68,69] all have their place in the treatment of the family at risk.

REFERENCES

1 Koblenzer CS. *Psychocutaneous Disease.* Orlando, FL: Grune & Stratton, 1987.

2 Gottfried AW. Touch as an organiser for learning and development. In: Brown CC, Brazelton TB, eds. *The Many Facets of Touch.* Skillman, New Jersey: Johnson and Johnson Pediatric Round Table Series, 1984; 10: 114–20.

3 Murphy LB, Mintzer D, Lipsitt LP. Psychoanalytic views of infancy. In: Greenspan SI, Pollock GH, eds. *The Course of Life. Vol. 1: Infancy.* Madison, CT: International University Press, 1989: 561–641.

4 Weiss ST. Parental touching: correlates of a child's body concept and body sentiment. In: Barnard KE, Brazelton TB, eds. *Touch. The Foundation of Experience.* Madison, CT: International University Press, 1990: 425–59.

5 Hartman H, Kris E, Lowenstein RM. Comments on the formation of psychic structure. *Psychoanal Stud Child* 1946; 2: 11–38.

6 Hofer W. Development of the Body Ego. *Psychoanal Stud Child* 1950; 5: 18–23.

7 Hill-Beuf A, Porter JDR. Children coping with impaired appearance. Social and psychological influences. *Gen Hosp Psychiatr* 1984; 6: 294–301.

8 Porter J, Beuf AH, Nordlund JJ, Lerner AB. Psychological reaction to chronic skin disorders. A study of patients with vitiligo. *Gen Hosp Psychiatr* 1979; 1: 73–7.

9 Moser DK, Clements PJ, Brecht ML, Weiner SR. Predictors of psychosocial adjustment in systemic sclerosis. *Arthritis Rheum* 1993; 36: 1398–405.

10 Ginsburg IH, Link BG. Feelings of stigmatization in patients with psoriasis. *J Am Acad Dermatol* 1989; 20: 53–63.

11 Greenacre P. Early physical determinants in the development of the sense of identity. *J Am Psychoanal Assoc* 1958; 6: 612–27.

12 Kaplan EH. Adolescents age 15–18: a psychoanalytic developmental view. In: Greenspan SI, Pollock GH, eds. *The Course of Life. Vol. 4: Adolescence.* Madison, CT: International University Press, 1991: 205.

13 Blos P. *The Adolescent Passage. Developmental Issues.* New York: International University Press, 1979: 141–70.

14 Krueger DW. Developmental and psychodynamic perspectives on body-image change. In: Cash TF, Pruzinsky T, eds. *Body Images. Development, Deviance and Change.* New York: Guilford Press, 1990: 255–71.

15 Van der Velde CD. Body image of one's self and of others: developmental and clinical significance. *Am J Psychiatr* 1985; 142: 527–37.

16 Blos P. *On Adolesence. A Psychoanalytic Interpretation.* New York: Free Press, 1962.

17 Koblenzer CS. Psychotherapy in the treatment of intractable inflammatory dermatosis. *J Am Acad Dermatol* 1995; 32: 609–12.

18 Koblenzer CS. The dysmorphic syndrome. *Fitzpatrick's J Clin Dermatol* 1994; March/April: 14–19.

19 Phillips KA. Body dysmorphic disorder: the distress of imagined ugliness. *Am J Psychiatr* 1991; 148: 1138–49.

20 Maffei C, Fossati A, Rinaldi F, Riva E. Personality disorders and pathological symptoms in patients with androgenetic alopecia. *Int J Dermatol* 1994; 130: 868–72.

21 Polan HJ, Ward MJ. Role of the mother's touch in failure to thrive: a preliminary investigation. *J Am Acad Child Adolesc Psychiatr* 1994; 3: 1098–105.

22 Greenspan SI. *The Development of the Ego.* Madison, CT: International University Press, 1989; 2: 27–44.

23 Taylor GT. *Psychosomatic Medicine and Contemporary Psychoanalysis.* Madison, CT: International University Press, 1987: 146.

24 Roth N, Beyreiss J, Schlenka K, Beyer H. Coincidence of attention deficit disorder and atopic disorders in children. *J Abnorm Child Psychol* 1991; 9: 216–19.

25 Cotterill JA. Psychophysiological aspects of eczema. *Semin Dermatol* 1990; 9: 216–19.

26 Panconesi E. Psychosomatic dermatology. In: Panconesi E, ed. *Stress and Skin Disease: Psychosomatic Dermatology. Clinics in Dermatology.* Philadelphia: JB Lippincott, 1984; 2(4): 94–179.

27 Lawson V, Lewis-Jones MS, Reid P *et al.* Family impact of childhood atopic eczema. *Br J Dermatol* 1995; 133 (Suppl. 45): 19.

28 Gupta MA, Gupta AK, Kirkby S *et al.* A psychocutaneous profile of psoriasis patients who are stress reactors. *Gen Hosp Psychiatr* 1989; 11: 166–73.

29 Gupta MA, Gupta AK, Kirkby S *et al.* Pruritus in psoriasis. A prospective study of some psychiatric and dermatologic correlates. *Arch Dermatol* 1988; 124: 1052–7.

30 Gupta MA, Schork NJ, Gupta AK *et al.* Suicidal ideation in psoriasis. *Int J Dermatol* 1993; 32: 188–90.

31 Fried RG, Friedman S, Paradis C *et al.* Trivial or terrible? The psychosocial impact of psoriasis. *Int J Dermatol* 1995; 34: 101–5.

32 Gupta MA, Gupta AK, Schork NJ, Ellis CN. Depression modulates pruritus perception: a study of pruritus in psoriasis, atopic dermatitis and chronic idiopathic urticaria. *Psychosom Med* 1994; 56: 36–40.

33 Koblenzer CS. Psychologic and psychiatric aspects of itching. In: Bernhard JD, ed. *Itch. Mechanisms and Management of Pruritus.* New York: McGraw-Hill, 1994: 347–65.

34 Malm M, Carlberg M. Port-wine stain—a surgical and psychological problem. *Am Plast Surg* 1988; 20: 512–16.

35 Dieterich-Miller CA, Cohen BA, Liggett J. Behavioral adjustment and self-concept of young children with hemangiomas. *Pediatr Dermatol* 1992; 9: 241–5.

36 Gupta MA, Gupta AK, Haberman HF. Psoriasis and psychiatry: an update. *Gen Hosp Psychiatr* 1987; 9: 157–66.

37 Hatfield E. Physical attractiveness in social interaction. In: Graham JA, Kligman AM, eds. *The Psychology of Cosmetic Treatments.* New York: Praeger, 1985: 77–92.

38 Koblenzer CS, Koblenzer PJ. Chronic intractable atopic eczema as a physical sign of impaired parent–child relationships and psychological developmental arrest; improvement through parent insight and education. *Arch Dermatol* 1988; 124: 1673–8.

39 Daud LR, Garralda ME, David TJ. Psychosocial adjustment in pre-school children with atopic eczema. *Arch Dis Child* 1993; 69: 670–6.

40 Spitz RA. *The First Year of Life.* New York: International University Press, 1965: 224–42.

41 Broberg A, Kalimo K, Linblad B *et al.* Parental education in the treatment of childhood atopic eczema. *Acta Dermatol Venereol* 1990; 70: 495–9.

42 Gieler U, Kohnlein B, Schauer U *et al.* Parent counseling for children with atopic dermatitis. *Hautarzt* 1992; 43: 37–42.

43 Jobling RG. Psoriasis—a preliminary questionnaire study of sufferers' subjective experience. *Clin Exp Dermatol* 1976; 1: 233–6.

44 Stankler L. The effect of psoriasis on the sufferer. *Clin Exp Dermatol* 1981; 6: 303–6.

45 Jowett S, Ryan T. Skin disease and handicap: an analysis of the impact of skin conditions. *Soc Sci Med* 1985; 4: 425–9.

46 Finlay AY, Kelly SE. Psoriasis—an index of disability. *Clin Exp Dermatol* 1987; 12: 8–11.

47 Ramsay B, O'Reagan M. A survey of the social and psychological effects of psoriasis. *Br J Dermatol* 1987; 118: 195–201.

48 Ginsburg IH, Link BG. Psychosocial consequences of rejection and stigma feelings in psoriasis patients. *Int J Dermatol* 1993; 32: 587–91.

49 Finlay AY, Coles EC. The effect of severe psoriasis on the quality of life of 369 patients. *Br J Dermatol* 1995; 132: 236–44.

50 Lapidus CS, Schwarz DF, Honig PJ. Atopic dermatitis in children: who cares? Who pays? *J Am Acad Dermatol* 1993; 28: 699–703.

51 Salek MS, Finlay AY, Luscombe DK *et al.* Cyclosporin greatly improves the quality of life in adults with severe atopic dermatitis. *Br J Dermatol* 1993; 129: 422–30.

52 Eun HC, Finlay AY. Measurement of atopic dermatitis disability. *Ann Dermatol* 1990; 15: 301–405.

53 Long CC, Funnell CM, Collard R, Finlay AY. What do members of the Eczema Society really want? *Clin Exp Dermatol* 1993; 18: 516–22.

54 Motley RJ, Finlay AY. Measurement of atopic dermatitis disability. *Ann Dermatol* 1990; 15: 401–5.

55 Motley RJ, Finlay AY. How much disability is caused by acne? *Clin Exp Dermatol* 1989; 14: 194–8.

56 Van der Merren HLM, Van der Schaar WW, Van der Hurk CMAM. The psychological impact of severe acne. *Cutis* 1985; 7: 84–6.

57 Chee-Chong LL, Tah-Chew T. Personality, disability and acne in college students. *Clin Exp Dermatol* 1991; 16: 371–3.

58 Koo J. The psychosocial impact of acne: patients' perceptions. *J Am Acad Dermatol* 1995; 32: 526–30.

59 Lieberman MA, Borman LD, eds. *Self-help Groups for Coping with Crisis.* San Francisco: Jossey-Bass, 1989.

60 Coles RB, Ryan TJ. The psoriasis sufferer in the community. *Br J Dermatol* 1975; 93: 111–13.

61 Ardell L. The National Eczema Society. *Practitioner* 1984; 22: 1059–62.

62 McSkimming J, Gleeson L, Sinclair M. A pilot study of a support group for parents of children with eczema. *Aust J Dermatol* 1984; 25: 8–11.

63 Koblenzer CS. Successful treatment of a chronic and disabling dermatosis by psychotherapy. *J Am Acad Dermatol* 1986; 15: 390–3.

64 Bremer-Schulte M, Cormane RH, van Dijk E, White J. Group therapy for psoriasis. *J Am Acad Dermatol* 1985; 12: 61–6.

65 Waxman D. Behavior therapy of psoriasis—a hypno-analytic and counter-conditioning technique. *Postgrad Med J* 1973; 49: 591–5.

66 Frankel FH, Misch RC. Hypnosis in a case of long-standing psoriasis in a person with character problems. *Int J Clin Exp Hypnosis* 1973; 21: 121–30.

67 Stewart AC, Thomas SE. Hypnotherapy as a treatment for atopic dermatitis in adults and children. *Br J Dermatol* 1995; 132: 778–83.

68 Hughes H, Brown BW, Lawlis GF, Fulton JE. Treatment of acne vulgaris, by biofeedback, relaxation, and cognitive imagery. *J Psychosom Res* 1983; 27: 185–91.

69 Winchell SA, Watts RA. Relaxation therapies in the treatment of psoriasis, and possible pathophysiologic mechanisms. *J Am Acad Dermatol* 1988; 18: 101–4.

26.2 Habit Disorders and Factitious Disease

ARNOLD P. ORANJE AND ROBERT A.C. BILO

Physiological habits
Thumb- and finger-sucking
Other physiological habits

Onychotillomania and onychophagia

Trichotillomania

Dermatitis artefacta

Obsessive–compulsive disorders

Pathomimicry

Definition

The skin, mucous membranes (mouth and genitalia), hair and nails may be direct targets for problems of behaviour. Psychodermatology has emerged as an important subdiscipline of both dermatology and psychiatry. In many clinical situations, cooperation between the psychiatrist or the psychologist and the dermatologist is necessary for treatment.

Three main categories of dermatological disorders with psychological components are recognized [1].
1 Cutaneous disorders which result from underlying primary psychiatric disease.
2 Psychosomatic dermatoses which are mainly caused by stress (such as lichen simplex chronicus).
3 Dermatological disorders in which the course is codetermined by emotional factors (e.g. atopic eczema).

Dermatitis artefacta, habit disorders and obsessive–compulsive disorders belong to the first category. Self-inflicted skin lesions (dermatitis artefacta) may occur in children who inflict the lesions consciously and knowingly, and in children who are satisfying a conscious or unconscious psychological need.

Pathomimicry (simulation of a serious, known disease) is also termed Munchausen's syndrome [2,3]. In children, the 'illness' may be produced by a parent or a parent figure [3] when it is known as Munchausen's syndrome by proxy [2].

In children and adolescents thumb- and finger-sucking, onychotillomania, onychophagia, mutilation of the skin (dermatitis artefacta), trichotillomania, excessive obses-sive hand washing and excoriated acne (acne excoriée de la jeune fille) are most common [4].

In many children, hair pulling (trichotillomania), nail biting and thumb-sucking are habitual activities that are practiced spontaneously and inadvertently [5].

Obsessive–compulsive disorders are characterized by obsessions or compulsions. An obsession is defined as an intrusive thought, urge or impulse that is experienced as repulsive, irrational and ego-distonic. Compulsion is defined by repetitive, often ritualized or stylized behaviour [4,6].

REFERENCES

1 Van Moffaert M. Psychodermatology: an overview. *Psychother Psychosom* 1992; 58: 125–36.
2 Koblenzer C. *Psychocutaneous Disease*. 1987.
3 Reece RM. *Child Abuse—Medical Diagnosis and Management*. Lea & Febiger, 1994: 266–78.
4 Koo JYM, Smith LL. Obsessive–compulsive disorders in the pediatric dermatology practice. *Pediatr Dermatol* 1991; 8: 107–13.
5 Oranje AP, Peereboom-Wynia JDR, De Raeymaecker DMJ. Trichotillomania in childhood. *J Am Acad Dermatol* 1986; 15: 614–19.
6 Stein DJ, Hollander E. Dermatology and conditions related to obsessive–compulsive disorder. *J Am Acad Dermatol* 1992; 26: 237–42.

History

Prior to the 1950s, psychodermatology was confined to the study of the role of psychological factors in dermatological disorders. Diseases like urticaria and lichen simplex were the frequent targets of studies [1,2]. After the 1950s and 1960s, the character of research changed from anecdotes and descriptions to analyses of large patient series evaluated through a standardized protocol [3].

In 1953, the first psychodermatology subunit in The Netherlands was set up at the Department of Dermatology and Venereology in Amsterdam. Professor Musaph, who was a psychologist practising in that clinic, was one of the pioneers in the field. In the last 10 years, the approach to dermatological disorders caused or aggravated by psychological factors has stressed the importance of teamwork (cooperation by the dermatologist, psychiatrist, clinical psychologist, welfare worker and, in children, a child protection specialist) [4].

The term trichotillomania was introduced by Hallopeau in 1889 (the Greek *thrix* means hair, *tillein* means to pull and *mania* means madness). Hallopeau considered trichotillomania as a compulsive trait in otherwise healthy individuals [5].

Little is known about the history of dermatitis artefacta and self-mutilating behaviour. Tuke (1892) stated that self-mutilation was encountered 'not infrequently' [6]. It was concluded that such behaviour was observed mainly in psychotic or mentally retarded subjects. Although a relationship to eating disorders exists, it was described only incidentally [7].

In 1951 Asher used the term Munchausen's syndrome to describe patients exhibiting questionable symptoms and a desire for extensive diagnostic evaluation [8]. Baron Von Munchausen was an 18th-century mercenary who, after his return from the Russian–Turkish war, spent his remaining years concocting embellished tales of his adventures [9,10]. The term pathomimicry, as a synonym of Munchausen's or Munchausen by proxy syndrome, was introduced by Millard in 1984 [9–11].

REFERENCES

1 Wittkower E, Russell B. *Emotional Factors in Skin Diseases.* New York: Hoeber, 1953.
2 Alexander F, French TM. *Studies in Psychosomatic Medicine.* New York: Ronald Press, 1948.
3 Musaph H. *Itching and scratching. Psychodynamics in Dermatology.* Basel: Karger, 1964.
4 Musaph H. Psychodermatology. *Psychother Psychosom* 1974; 24: 79.
5 Tuke DH. *A Dictionary of Psychological Medicine*, Vol. 2, Philadelphia: Blackiston, 1892.
6 Parry-Jones B, Parry-Jones WL. Self-mutilation in four historical cases of bulimia. *Br J Psychiatr* 1993; 163: 394–402.
7 Hallopeau M. Alopecie par grattage (trichomanie ou trichotillomanie). *Ann Dermatol Vénéréol* 1889; 10: 440–1.
8 Asher R. Munchausen syndrome. *Lancet.* 1951; i: 339–41.
9 Millard LG. Dermatologic pathomimicry: a form of patient maladjustment. *Lancet* 1984; ii: 969–71.
10 Rosenberg DA. Munchausen syndrome by proxy. In: Rese R, ed. *Child Abuse.* 1992: 266–78.
11 Meadow R. Munchausen syndrome by proxy: the hinterland of child abuse. *Lancet* 1977; ii: 343–5.

Aetiology and pathogenesis

Various hypotheses have been used to explain the aetiology of self-mutilation disorders, trichotillomania and obsessive–compulsive disorders. These disorders are three times more common in females than in males. Psychoanalytic, developmental, personality and biochemical (serotonin) theories have been postulated [1]. The most serious forms of these disorders may be related to physical, emotional and sexual abuse [2].

The psychoanalytic theory stresses the importance of early emotional traumas such as illness, separation from parents and disturbances in the mother–child relationship [3]. Developmental difficulties (school, coping problems, physical unattractiveness) also play a role.

Developmental disturbances can lead to a poor self-image, or lack of self-esteem. The child lacks positive feelings about his or her own body (even though he or she is not conscious of this problem). The child turns his aggression against self [4]. In children, most cases are related to distortion of the parent–child relationship. Other important factors are marital or domestic strife.

Some of the habit phenomena, such as thumb- or finger(s)-sucking, nail biting and hair-pulling (in toddlers), are of physiological origin. The cause of thumb- or finger(s)-sucking is not fully understood [5]. Anxiety and stress play an important role in the aetiology of nail biting [6].

Trichotillomania in young children is a habit phenomenon that is most often not a sign of serious emotional disturbance. It is comparable with thumb- or finger(s)-sucking and nail biting. Trichotillomania occurring later in life, especially of long duration, tends to be more serious from a psychological perspective. Hair is an important symbol of biological maturity. Therefore, trichotillomania may indicate a unconscious, symbolic effort to deny maturity [4].

Personality characteristics of patients with dermatitis artefacta have been described by many authors without consistent clarity. Most patients suffering from dermatitis artefacta have a borderline personality [1].

A group of patients practice self-mutilation knowingly and consciously for secondary benefits and gain. This phenomenon occurs very rarely in children. Purposeful self-mutilation must be differentiated from self-mutilation that satisfies a psychological need (neurotic excoriation). Contagious self-mutilation behaviour in groups has been described in prisons, schools and psychiatric institutions. These epidemics are more common in females [7] and may occur in young people without clear psychopathology [8].

Lesh–Nyhan syndrome, which is associated with self-mutilation, is an X-linked recessive disorder caused by a deficiency of hypoxanthineguanine phosphoribosyltransferase activity [9].

Prader–Willi syndrome (PWS) is also associated with self-mutilating behaviour. The aetiology of PWS is unknown, but associations with abnormalities of chromosome 15 (of paternal origin) and paternal exposure to hydrocarbons have been reported [10]. In the Gilles de la Tourette's syndrome, also associated with self-mutilation, familial occurrence is found in about 58% of the cases [11].

REFERENCES

1 Koblenzer C. *Psychocutaneous Disease.* 1987.
2 Gupta MA, Gupta AK. Dermatitis artefacta and sexual abuse. *Int J Dermatol* 1993; 32: 825–6.
3 Koo JYM, Smith LL. Obsessive–compulsive disorders in the pediatric dermatology practice. *Pediatr Dermatol* 1991; 8: 107–13.
4 Oranje AP, Peereboom-Wynia JDR, De Raeymaecker DMJ. Trichotillomania in childhood. *J Am Acad Dermatol* 1986; 15: 614–19.

5 Peterson JE, Schneider PE. Oral habits. A behavioral approach. *Pediatr Oral Health* 1991; 38: 1289–307.
6 Leung AKC, Robson WLM. Nail biting. *Clin Pediatr* 1990; 29: 690–2.
7 Ross RR, McKay HB. *Self-Mutilation.* Lexiton, MA: DC Health, 1979.
8 Fennig S, Carlson GA, Fennig S. Contagious self-mutilation. *J Am Acad Child Adoles Psychiatr* 1995; 34: 402–3.
9 Lesh M, Nyhan WL. A familiar disorder or uric acid metabolism and central nervous system function. *Am J Med* 1964; 36: 561–70.
10 Butler MG, Palmer CG. Clinical and cytogenetic survey of 39 individuals with Prader–Labhart–Willi syndrome. *Am J Med Genet* 1986; 23: 793–809.
11 Regeur L, Pakkenberg B, Fog R *et al.* Clinical features and long-term treatment with pimozide in 65 patients with Gilles de La Tourette's syndrome. *J Neurol Neurosurg Psychiatr* 1986; 49: 791–5.

Physiological habits

The physiological habits are listed in Table 26.2.1. Thumb- and finger-sucking is very common in young children and soon becomes a habit, only rarely lasting to adulthood [1,2].

Thumb- and finger-sucking

Thumb- and finger-sucking develops as a habit in 13–45% of children [1]. The habit is physiological in infants from the early months to 4 years (peak age about 20 months). It gives a feeling of warmth, pleasure and certainty. Trichotillomania in toddlers is often associated with thumb- or finger-sucking [3]. In trichotillomania, thumb- and finger-sucking indicate the presence of inner conflicts. Sometimes the reason is simple, for example in order to avoid playing piano [4] or playing an important tennis game.

Clinical features

Sucking of the thumb or the fingers may cause maceration of the finger tips. Among children, thumb-sucking is the most common cause of paronychia. Digit-sucking is also a cause of radial angular deformity, in which a finger or the thumb is abnormally separated from the other fingers [1] (Figs 26.2.1, 26.2.2).

If the habit persists, dental complications can develop [1]. Between the ages of 4 and 14 years, thumb- and finger-sucking may have a deleterious effect on dentofacial development [1,2].

Prognosis

The prognosis is most often excellent. Only rarely will the habit continue into adulthood.

Differential diagnosis

The diagnosis is very easy and simple because the habit is observed. There are no differential diagnostic problems.

Other physiological habits

In neonates, reflex smile, 'sobbing' inspirations and myoclonic twitches are physiological habits. From 0 to 1 year of age sucking of the thumb, finger(s), toe and lips is common. Other common habits are masturbation, rocking and rolling (head banging) and teeth grinding. Head banging is often dramatic and upsetting to the other members of the family. Questions asked by the parents are: (a) 'will it cause brain damage?' (the answer is always no); and (b) 'is it associated with an emotional disorder?' (in most cases the answer is no) [1]. These habits are of pathological significance only when they persist beyond early childhood or occur in combination with other habits.

Table 26.2.1 Dermatitis artefacta and habit phenomenons, obsessive and compulsive disorders

Physiological habit/disorders	Infancy	Childhood	Puberty	Adulthood
Body rocking, head banging, head rolling	++F	+P	—	—
Thumb-sucking	++F	+F	±P	±P
Finger(s)-sucking	++F	+F	±P	±P
Nail biting	±P	+F/P	++F/P	+P
Onychotillomania	—	+F/P	++F/P	+P
Trichotillomania	±P	++F/P	+P	+P
Lip-licking/biting	—	+F/P	+F/P	+P
Cheek biting	—	—	+P	+P
Obsessive hand washing	—	+P	+P	+P
Dermatitis artefacta	—	+P	+P	+P
Excoriated acne	—	—	+P	+P

F, physiological; P, pathological; —, not occurring; ±, infrequent; +, common; ++, frequent.

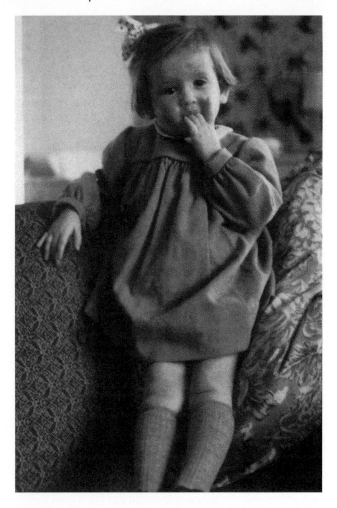

Fig. 26.2.1 Finger-sucking in a girl aged 3 years.

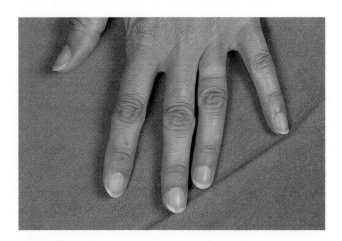

Fig. 26.2.2 Deformity of the fingers of the same girl (as adult woman) as in Fig. 26.2.1 after prolonged sucking.

In children older than 1 year of age, nail biting, nose picking and habit tics may develop. Except for nail biting and nose picking, the symptoms warrant serious attention, because they can be pathological. Males are more

likely to have habit tics. Any stress factor needs to be identified and treated. Habit coughs are typical tics in adolescents. Chronic tic disorders can be the first signs of Gilles de la Tourette's syndrome [5]. In this syndrome, motor and vocal tics of variable intensity develop between the ages of 2 and 15 years.

Prognosis

Many repetitive habits disappear with age and have no pathological importance. However, persistence of these repetitive behaviour problems may be a manifestation of psychological distress, side-effects of drugs or a first sign of physical disease.

Differential diagnosis

The diagnosis is most often simple because the habit is observed. The clinician must distinguish between physiological and pathological behaviour. It may be difficult to diagnose early Gilles de la Tourette's syndrome [5].

REFERENCES

1 Peterson JE, Schneider PE. Oral habits. A behavioral approach. *Pediatr Oral Health* 1991; 38: 1289–307.
2 Lubitz L. Nail biting, thumb sucking, and other irritating behaviours in childhood. *Austr Fam Physician* 1992; 21: 1090–4.
3 Koblenzer C. *Psychocutaneous Disease*. 1987.
4 Spraker MK. Cutaneous artifactual disease: an appeal for help. *Pediatr Clin N Am* 1983; 30: 659–68.
5 Regeur L, Pakkenberg B, Fog R *et al*. Clinical features and long-term treatment with pimozide in 65 patients with Gilles de la Tourette's syndrome. *J Neurol Neurosurg Psychiatr* 1986; 49: 791–5.

Onychotillomania and onychophagia

Nail biting (onychophagia) and nail picking (onychotillomania) are very common, especially among children [1]. The incidence of nail biting has been reported to be 33% in children [2] and 45% in teenagers [2–4]. Before the age of 10 years, the incidence of nail biting in the sexes is relatively equal. Thereafter it is more common in boys [5]. Its incidence in adults is much lower. In most cases, nail biting cannot be categorized as a sign of psychological or psychiatric disease. Trichotillomania can be associated with nail biting, but rarely in children [6].

Clinical features

Damage to the cuticle, bleeding around the nails, distal onycholysis and short irregular nail plates are the clinical clues (Fig. 26.2.3). Nail dystrophy develops in more severe and persistent cases. Secondary periungual bacterial infection may occur as a complication.

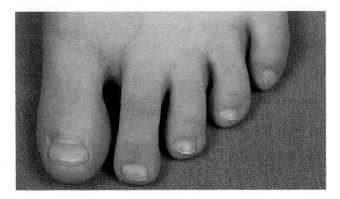

Fig. 26.2.3 Nail biting of the toe nails.

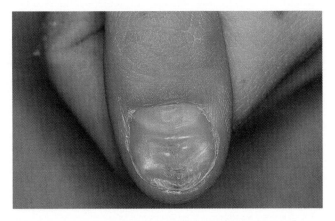

Fig. 26.2.4 Habit phenomenon resulting in median dystrophy.

Other sequelae of persistent nail biting are paronychia, periungual warts, melanonychia and osteomyelitis [1,7,8]. Nail biting may increase nail growth by 20% [2].

Rubbing the thumb nail and proximal nail fold with the index finger of the same hand results in characteristic median dystrophy [9]. A longitudinal depression in the centre of the nail over its entire length is observed (Fig. 26.2.4).

Prognosis

The incidence is highest in children and teenagers. This habit normally disappears in early adult life.

Differential diagnosis

Nail changes because of biting should be distinguished from other physical or chemical trauma, as well as from congenital abnormalities and acquired disorders. Median nail dystrophia should be distinguished from congenital dystrophia mediana canaliformis [9]. In most cases it is not difficult; the history is most helpful.

REFERENCES

1 Oderick L, Brattstrom V. Nail biting: frequency and association with root resorption during orthodontic treatment. *Br J Orthodon* 1985; 12: 78–81.
2 Leung AKC, Robson WLM. Nail biting. *Clin Pediatr* 1990; 29: 690–2.
3 Massler M, Malone AJ. Nail biting — a review. *J Pediatr* 1950; 36: 523–31.
4 Wechsler D. The incidence and significance of finger-nail biting in children. *Psychoanal Rev* 1931; 18: 201–8.
5 Malone AJ, Massler M. Index of nail biting in children. *J Abnorm Soc Psychol* 1952; 47: 193–202.
6 Dimino-Emme L, Carmisa CH. Trichotillomania associated with the 'Friar Tuck sign' and nail biting. *Cutis* 1991; 47: 107–10.
7 Tosti A, Peluso AM, Bardazzi F. Phalangeal osteomyelitis due to nail biting. *Acta Derm Venereol* 1994; 74: 206–7.
8 Baran R. Nail biting and picking as a possible cause of longitudinal melanonychia. *Dermatologica* 1990; 181: 126–8.
9 Baden HP. *Diseases of the Hair and Nails*. Chicago: Year Book Medical Publishers, 1987.

Trichotillomania

Trichotillomania is seven times more common in children than in adults. It is 2.5 times more common in girls than in boys [1–3]. It is the most common form of artefactual disease after thumb- or finger-sucking [4]. The incidence is not really known, but at a child guidance clinic, three cases of trichotillomania were diagnosed among 500 children [5].

Pathology

Microscopic examination of the hair roots (the trichogram), obtained by using a standardized method, shows few telogen or catagen hairs, but there is an increase in dysplastic and/or dystrophic hair shapes [6].

Trichotillomania is characterized by the presence of empty hair follicles among completely normal hairs. Residual fragments of partially extracted hair provides evidence of trauma. Clumped melanin and keratinized material is seen within the disrupted hair follicles (trichomalacia) and this picture is considered pathognomonic [2,7]. Follicular plugging with keratin debris may also be present. Hair shafts within the lower follicular duct appear small and sometimes have a corkscrew appearance. Extravasated erythrocytes are sometimes visible in the epidermis and around the follicles. Usually there is no infiltration of leucocytes, except when secondary infection develops. Completely normal anagen follicles are present in the affected areas.

Clinical features

One or more areas of the scalp are affected. The areas may be quite small, or the process may involve almost the entire scalp [1]. In most cases, the areas of hair loss are not well demarcated. The eyebrows and eyelashes are sometimes affected. Most often, the areas of hair loss are contralateral to the handedness of the patient. Excoriation and crusts are sometimes visible on the scalp. The most typical pattern is an area of patchy alopecia surrounded by a rim of unaffected hair. This is called tonsure pattern alopecia or 'Friar Tuck' sign, for its resemblance to the hair style worn by monks [3,8] (Fig. 26.2.5).

Complications of trichotillomania are a permanent damage to hair, and hair ingestion (trichophagia) leading to a hairball (trichobezoar) in the stomach. Trichobezoar can lead to abdominal pain, nausea, vomiting, foul breath, anorexia, obstipation, flatulence, anaemia, gastric ulcer, bowel obstruction or perforation, intestinal bleeding, obstructive jaundice and pancreatitis [8]. Trichobezoars weighing up to 412 g have been described [9].

Although trichotillomania in children usually presents as an isolated symptom, it may be associated with serious psychopathology such as mental retardation, depression, borderline disorder, schizophrenia, autism, obsessive–compulsive disorder and drug abuse [8]. However, it is commonly an anxiety condition in toddlers and is easily cured [2].

Prognosis

In many cases this symptom disappears with appropriate emotional support and when the child gains insight into the underlying psychological problems. However, one should not assume that trichotillomania will disappear spontaneously, therefore careful follow-up is required to establish resolution [2]. In a selected population, one-third of the patients required psychiatric treatment and guidance [2]. In serious and long-standing cases, psychological or psychiatric treatment is warranted.

Repeated manipulation of the hair in trichotillomania can lead to curly hair, trichorrhexis nodosa, other hair shaft fractures and finally to cicatricial alopecia.

Differential diagnosis

The differential diagnosis includes alopecia areata, psoriasis and tinea capitis. Clinical differential diagnosis between trichotillomania and alopecia areata may be difficult in some cases. History of hair-pulling is often lacking, except in very young children, when the parents report the symptom [2]. The presence of an initial area of almost total hair loss favours alopecia areata. Exclamation hairs, a positive hair plucking test (loss of more than 5 hairs when pulled from the periphery of the bald area), pitting of the nails and depigmentation in regrowing in older children strongly support the diagnosis of alopecia areata. Laboratory examination will exclude tinea capitis.

REFERENCES

1 Stroud JD. Hair loss in children. *Pediatr Clin N Am* 1983; 30: 641–57.
2 Oranje AP, Peereboom-Wynia JDR, De Raeymaecker DMJ. Trichotillomania in childhood. *J Am Acad Dermatol* 1986; 15: 614–19.
3 Muller SA. Trichotillomania. *Dermatol Clin* 1987; 5: 595–601.
4 Spraker MK. Cutaneous artifactual disease: an appeal for help. *Pediatr Clin N Am* 1983; 30: 659–68.
5 Anderson FW, Dean HC. Some aspects of child guidance clinic in policy and practice. *Publ Health Rep* 1956: 71.
6 Peereboom-Wynia JDR. *Hair root characteristics of the human scalp hair in health and disease.* Thesis, Rotterdam 1979.
7 Lachapelle JM, Pierard GE. Traumatic alopecia in trichotillomania. *J Cutan Pathol* 1977; 4: 51–67.
8 Hamdan-Allen G. Trichotillomania in childhood. *Acta Psychiatr Scand* 1991; 83: 241–3.
9 Ewert P, Keim L, Schulte-Markwort M. Der Trichobezoar. *Monatsschr Kinderheilkd* 1992; 140: 811–13.

Dermatitis artefacta

Dermatitis artefacta in childhood can develop under circumstances such as (a) distortion within the parent–child relationship; (b) in homes where there is significant marital and domestic strife; and (c) in children who have been the victims of physical, emotional and sexual abuse. Many patients with dermatitis artefacta have a borderline or hysterical personality disorder [1,2].

Depending on the methods employed by the patient, dermatitis artefacta is characterized by excoriations, ulcerations, purpura or bullae [3,4]. Methods include rubbing, sucking, biting, use of bottles, sucking cups, scratching, picking, cutting, slashing, gouging, punctur-

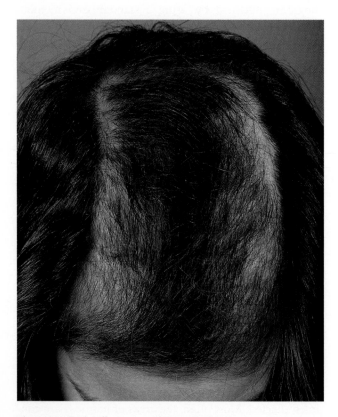

Fig. 26.2.5 Trichotillomania with 'Friar Tuck' sign.

ing, application of caustic or hot agents and injections of various substances [4]. The relationship between self-injury behaviour and child abuse is illustrated by a case report of a mother with dermatitis artefacta on the forearm and lower legs, who produced the same lesions on her child's face [5] (Figs 26.2.6–26.2.9).

Pathology

Dermatitis artefacta shows no characteristic histopathological pattern. The abnormalities are compatible with irritant dermatitis. Severity depends on the techniques used by the patient.

Clinical features

The lesions are single or multiple, and occur in an area accessible to the dominant hand. However, the lesions may be symmetrical and bilateral, especially after the patient has been confronted with the unilateral distribution of lesions. A significant sign is the presence of bizarre and angulated configurations. The incidence is higher in females (adults and children) except for individuals involved in purposeful self-mutilation. The condition can be seen at any age, but is most common in adolescents and young adults [1].

Several subgroups occur [4]. The first group consists of patients with an autoaggressive habitual behaviour and recognized, plausible motives, or those who are neurotic pickers and who readily admit to damaging their skin. The second group consists of patients with hysterical and obsessive impulses. The third group encompasses mentally retarded or psychotic individuals who self-mutilate frequently and in the presence of others. Patients with delusions of parasitosis may also self-mutilate. Self-mutilation, especially of the hands and lips, is characteristic of Lesh–Nyhan syndrome.

Excoriations

Excoriations are probably most common in dermatitis artefacta. Lesions are sometimes deep enough to cause ulceration and scarring. Lesions are often localized (regional), sharply bordered, deep, linear and crusted.

Acne excoriée de la jeune fille (excoriated acne)

Acne patients often pick at their lesions. The majority of such patients are aware of and admit to their behaviour, and can be classified as neurotic excoriators. In extreme cases, the picking is more severe. Often, these patients are pubertal or adolescent girls who have only minimal acne. By manipulating their skin lesions, they transform them into excoriations or ulcers and cause scarring or postinflammatory hyperpigmentation.

Purpura

Purpura can be induced by sucking, cupping, rubbing or biting the skin, or with a bottle or a hard rapidly moving object.

Painting of the skin

A skin disease can be mimicked by painting the skin with a dye. The result of this behaviour may mimic cellulitis or purpura. The diagnosis is established by removing the dye with solvents. In most cases, this behaviour is a form of 'cry for help', but it should not be categorized with Munchausen's syndrome [6].

Burns

Self-induced burns are severe manifestations of a psychiatric disturbance. The skin is usually burned with a hot object, such as a cigarette. Most severe self-induced burns are observed in adolescents, although some occur in children [7]. Burns in children are usually inflicted by another individual and are manifestations of child abuse or Munchausen's syndrome by proxy (see Chapter 24.3).

Other manifestations

Lip-licking is a common and generally insignificant problem. Ligatures applied around a finger, extremity or penis may result in oedema, ulcerations or extreme demarcations and even amputations. Epistaxis and bleeding from other mucous surfaces, such as the gingiva, can be induced [8,9].

Syndromes associated with self-mutilation are Lesh–Nyhan syndrome, PWS, Gilles de la Tourette's syndrome and familial dysautonomia. Self-mutilation is common in mentally retarded children [10–13].

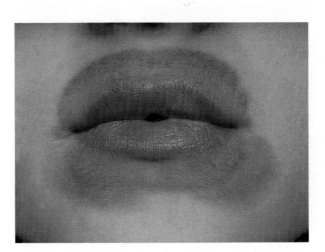

Fig. 26.2.6 Lip-lick dermatitis.

Prognosis

Self-mutilation occurs in all age groups. It is more common in children, and has a significantly better prognosis. In some patients the clinical symptoms and signs are present for years before the diagnosis is made. Careful follow-up is indicated in all cases. Sometimes, severe cases of self-mutilation in adults originate in childhood. However, in most children, the prognosis for complete recovery is excellent.

Diagnosis

The morphology of the lesions and the history will usually indicate the suspected diagnosis. Organic disturbances and systemic diseases should be ruled out. When self-mutilation is denied by the patient, it is possible to establish the diagnosis by careful observation.

Purpuric lesions can also be induced by stress, skin fragility, as side-effects of drugs and by applying a device to the skin (e.g. in Vietnam *cao gio* or coin rubbing). Purpura can be a symptom of thrombocytopenia, 'painful bruising' syndrome or vasculitis. Purpura may also be the result of child abuse.

REFERENCES

1 Koblenzer C. *Psychocutaneous Disease.* 1987.
2 Dulit RA, Fyer MR, Leon AC *et al.* Clinical correlates of self-mutilation in borderline personality disorder. *Am J Psychiatr* 1994; 151: 1305–11.
3 Spraker MK: Cutaneous artifactual disease: an appeal for help. *Pediatr Clin N Am* 1983; 30: 659–68.
4 Hollender MH, Abram HS. Dermatitis factitia. *South Med J* 1973; 66: 1279.
5 Jones DPH. Dermatitis artefacta in a mother and baby as child abuse. *Br J Psychiatr* 1983; 143: 199–200.

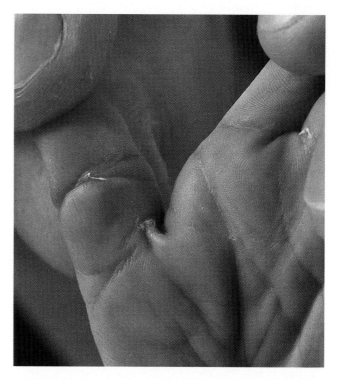

Fig. 26.2.8 Ligature around the thumb resulting in a demarcation.

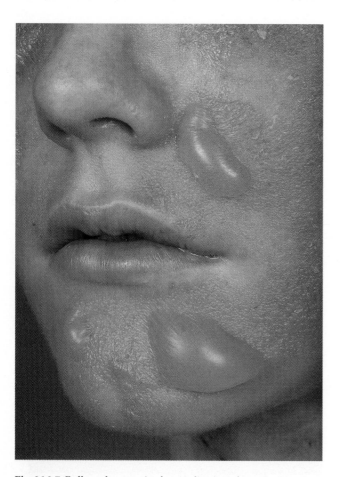

Fig. 26.2.7 Bullous dermatosis after application of caustic substances to the skin.

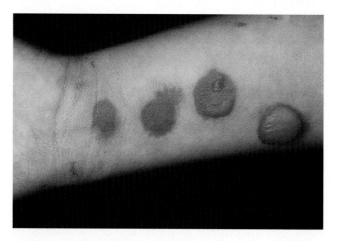

Fig. 26.2.9 Self-inflicted burns on the arms.

6 Schreier HA, Libow JA. Munchausen by proxy syndrome: a modern pediatric challenge. *J Pediatr* 1994; 125: S110–15.
7 Stoddard FJ. A psychiatric perspective on self-inflicted burns. *J Burn Care Rehabil* 1993; 14: 480–2.
8 Tunnessen WW, Chessar IJ. Factitious cutaneous bleeding. *Am J Dis Child* 1984; 138: 354–5.
9 Rodd HD. Self-inflicted gingival injury in a young girl. *Br Dent J* 1995; 178: 28–30.
10 Butler MG, Palmer CG. Clinical and cytogenetic survey of 39 individuals with Prader–Labhart–Willi syndrome. *Am J Med Genet* 1986; 23: 793–809.
11 Prader A, Labhart A, Willi H. Ein Syndrom von Adipositas, Kleinwuchs, Krytorchismus and Oligophrenie nach Myatonieartigem Zustand im Neugeborenalter. *Schweiz Med Wochenschr* 1956; 86: 1260–1.
12 Regeur L, Pakkenberg B, Fog R *et al.* Clinical features and long-term treatment with pimozide in 65 patients with Gilles de La Tourette's syndrome. *J Neurol Neurosurg Psychiatr* 1986; 49: 791–5.
13 Gadoth ME. Oro-dental self-mutilation in familial dysautonomia. *J Oral Pathol Med* 1994; 23: 273–6.

Obsessive–compulsive disorders

Obsessive–compulsive disorders may be difficult to distinguish from other causes of dermatitis artefacta [1]. In a small minority of cases, trichotillomania, onychotillomania, onychophagia and acne excoriée are the result of obsessive and compulsive disorders [2,3]. Repeated hand washing is most often a form of obsessive–compulsive disorder which may lead to irritative hand eczema.

When this hand washing tendency suddenly develops, diabetes mellitus should be ruled out. Differential diagnosis of hand eczema also includes tinea manuum and allergic contact eczema.

One per cent of children and adolescents suffer from obsessive–compulsive disorders [4,5].

Prognosis and treatment

The prognosis of obsessive–compulsive disorder is poor, and the condition often worsens with age. The dermatologist should ask for the help of a paediatric psychiatrist in diagnosis and treatment. Newer drug therapies, such as clomipramine and fluoxetine, have resulted in optimism regarding the treatment of obsessive–compulsive disorders [2].

REFERENCES

1 Koblenzer C. *Psychocutaneous Disease.* 1987.
2 Koo JYM, Smith LL. Obsessive–compulsive disorders in pediatric dermatology practice. *Pediatr Dermatol* 1991; 8: 107–13.
3 Oranje AP, Peereboom-Wynia JDR, De Raeymaecker DMJ. Trichotillomania in childhood. *J Am Acad Dermatol* 1986; 15: 614–19.
4 Leonard HL, Rapoport JL. Pharmacotherapy of obsessive-compulsive disorders. *Psychiatr Clin N Am* 1989; 12: 963–70.
5 Rapoport JL. Annotation: childhood obsessive–compulsive disorder. *J Child Psychol Psychiatr* 1986; 27: 289–95.

Pathomimicry

Pathomimicry (Munchausen's syndrome or Munchausen's syndrome by proxy) simulates a known disease such as asthma, fever, infection, haemorrhagic diathesis and autoimmune disease [1]. Dermatological pathomimicry may also result in apparent recurrences or exacerbations of a pre-existing skin disease [2]. Cases of this type are a form of Munchausen's syndrome [3,4]. Dramatic presentations such as autocastration, penis amputation, kidney extirpation, cardiac failure and death have been described [1,4–6]. This phenomenon is not confined to adults. Children have died after a harmful medication was given by their mother [7,8]. Harmful genital care practices that produce physical and psychoemotional abnormalities have been described in children. These unusual and ritualistic practices may lead to chronic and somatic complaints (e.g. vaginal discharge, enlarged vaginal opening, anal irritation) and unnecessary medical diagnostic procedures. In addition, some of these parents sexually abuse these children [9]. Artefactual cutaneous diseases are uncommon in Munchausen's syndrome by proxy, but this diagnosis should always be considered [10]. The relationship with artefactual disease is illustrated by the authors' observation in a boy with alopecia areata, who pulled out the hair of his younger brother (unpublished observations).

REFERENCES

1 Koblenzer C. *Psychocutaneous Disease.* 1987.
2 Millard LG. Dermatological pathomimicry—a form of patient maladjustment. *Lancet* 1984; ii: 969–71.
3 Rosenberg DA. Munchausen syndrome by proxy. In: Rese R, ed. *Child Abuse.* 1992: 266–78.
4 Meadow R. Munchausen syndrome by proxy: the hinterland of child abuse. *Lancet* 1977; ii: 343–5.
5 Fras I, Coughlin B. The treatment of factitial disease. *Psychosomatics* 1971; 12: 117–22.
6 Hawkins JR, Jones KS, Sim M *et al.* Deliberate disability. *Br Med J* 1956; 1: 361–7.
7 Meadow R. Munchausen syndrome by proxy. *Arch Dis Child* 1982; 57: 92–8.
8 Stankler L. Factitious lesions in a mother and two sons. *Br J Dermatol* 1977; 97: 217–19.
9 Hermans-Giddens ME, Berson NL. Harmful genital care practices in children. A type of child abuse. *J Am Med Assoc* 1989; 261: 577–9.
10 Fays-Bouchon N. Syndrome de Münchausen à révélation dermatologique. *Nouv Dermatol* 1991; 10: 566–71.

Treatment

Treatment approaches for the factitious disorders can be divided into four categories: (a) behavioural modification; (b) treatment devices; (c) pharmacological treatment; and (d) psychotherapy.

Before choosing any treatment modality, it is first necessary to analyse the home and social environments, school and social influences and religious beliefs. Treatment should be directed at the causes of any precipitating stress [1,2]. Simple problems may be handled by the dermatologist [3]. A psychiatrist or psychologist should be consulted if the problem is more serious, or if early therapeutic attempts are not successful.

Behavioural modification

The first step in behavioural modification is focused on building the child's self-confidence and self-esteem [1,2]. The next steps are: (a) dispelling any threats of punishment; (b) improving insight and understanding; (c) maintaining authority; (d) tackling the symptoms; and (e) recognizing positive self-actualizations. The parents are important in these stages of treatment.

Interaction between parent(s) and the child should be monitored, and keeping a diary may be helpful. A schedule of tasks and a change in attitude may have a positive effect on behaviour [1].

Up to 6 years of age the child undergoes psychological development through which children progress. During infancy and early childhood, oral habit phenomena are usually common, physiological and of relatively little importance [1]. In these cases, only limited therapeutic intervention is necessary.

In trichotillomania, behavioural intervention may be successful [4]. In young children, trichotillomania is often accompanied by thumb-sucking. The behavioural intervention may be aimed at the thumb-sucking and include aversive taste treatment and response-dependent alarm [5,6]. Trichotillomania is, however, not always associated with thumb-sucking. Behavioural therapy is still possible in these situations and can include hypnotherapy or intensive parent–child interaction (increased physical contact, frequent praise, avoiding criticism and discussing response prevention) [5]. Nail biting can be treated with bitter-tasting aversive substances and competing response therapies [7].

Use of devices

Use of devices is especially indicated in repetitive habit disorders. In trichotillomania, the child may be taught to pick hairs from a fuzzy toy [3].

Treatment of trichotillomania accompanied by thumb-sucking may also include a response-disrupting thumb-post [6].

Pharmacological treatment

Drugs include clomipramine, desipramine, fluoxetine and pimozide. In a study in 25 serious nail-biting adults, clomipramine was superior to desipramine [8]. The same results were reported in the long-term treatment of serious trichotillomania [9]. Although anecdotal reports indicated that fluoxetine was effective, its efficacy could not be confirmed in a placebo-controlled, double-blind crossover study in 21 adults with trichotillomania [10].

Behavioural treatment can be combined with pharmacological modalities. This approach was reported to be successful, even in an autistic girl [11].

Psychotherapy

Psychotherapy is warranted in cases in which the above approaches are unsuccessful, or after thorough psychological analysis establishes the presence of serious psychopathology. Often, a combined therapy with pharmacological agents and psychotherapy is used. Psychotherapy is more frequently indicated in cases of dermatitis artefacta and in obsessive–compulsive disorders.

REFERENCES

1 Peterson JE, Schneider PE. Oral habits. A behavioral approach. *Pediatr Oral Health* 1991; 38: 1289–307.
2 Leung AKC, Robson WLM. Nail biting. *Clin Pediatr* 1990; 29: 690–2.
3 Oranje AP, Peereboom-Wynia JDR, De Raeymaecker DMJ. Trichotillomania in childhood. *J Am Acad Dermatol* 1986; 15: 614–19.
4 Blum NJ, Barone VJ, Friman PC. A simplified behavioral treatment for trichotillomania: report of two cases. *Pediatrics* 1993; 75: 993–5.
5 Friman PC, Finney JW, Christophersen ER. Behavioral treatment of trichotillomania: an evaluative review. *Behav Ther* 1984; 15: 249–65.
6 Watson TS, Allen KD. Elimination of thumb-sucking as a treatment for severe trichotillomania. *J Am Acad Child Adoles Psychiatr* 1993; 32: 830–4.
7 Silber KP, Haynes CE. Treating nail biting: a comparative analysis of mild aversion and competing response therapies. *Behav Res Ther* 1992; 30: 15–22.
8 Leonard HL, Lenage MC, Swedo SE *et al.* A double-blind comparison of clomipramine and desipramine treatment of severe onychophagia (nail biting). *Arch Gen Psychiatr* 1991; 48: 821–7.
9 Swedo SE, Lenane MC, Leonard HL. Long-term treatment of trichotillomania (hair pulling). *N Engl J Med* 1993; 329: 141–2.
10 Christenson GA, Mackenzie TB, Mitchell JE *et al.* A placebo-controlled double-blind crossover study of fluoxetine in trichotillomania. *Am J Psychiatr* 1991; 148: 1566–71.
11 Holttum JR, Lubetsky MJ, Eastman LE. Comprehensive management of trichotillomania in a young autistic girl. *J Am Acad Child Adoles Psychiatr* 1994; 33: 577–81.

Acknowledgements

The authors are indebted to Dr B. Tank at the Department of Dermato-Venereology, Erasmus University Rotterdam, The Netherlands, for correcting the English.

Section 27
Treatment, Reactions to Drugs and Poisoning

27.1 Principles of Paediatric Dermatological Therapy

DENNIS P. WEST AND GIUSEPPE MICALI

Although general principles for treatment of paediatric skin diseases are similar to that of the adult, several unique aspects regarding dermatological therapeutics in the paediatric patient should be emphasized.

First, the therapeutic approach to a paediatric patient, especially if a newborn or an infant, differs from an older person because of the difficulty in obtaining a detailed medical history, including time of onset of the dermatosis, original morphology of lesions at their onset and primary symptomatology. Although in a majority of cases the parents may be helpful in providing information, important symptoms may be overlooked or misunderstood. In the paediatric population, these issues may pose serious difficulties both at the point of diagnosis and therapeutic decision making.

Second, among a large variety of systemic agents and topical preparations currently available for use in dermatological disorders, only a few pharmaceutical products have been specifically designed or tested for paediatric use.

As a result, specific information for drug formulations and possible side-effects in the paediatric dermatology population is not only desirable but necessary.

In general, treatment of skin disorders in the paediatric patient is aimed at restoring normal appearance and physiological state of the skin. When systemic drugs are used, the skin is just one of several possible target organs even though it may be the only intended target organ. A systemically administered drug typically reaches the skin only after gastrointestinal absorption, biotransformation in the liver and eventual distribution to remote tissues of the body. As would be expected, the pharmacokinetics of a drug following systemic administration differs quite considerably from that following percutaneous administration. In the latter case, a drug is applied directly to the target organ, and the skin is often a preferred route of administration when it is desirable to deliver an optimum concentration of medication.

Barrier properties of skin

To be effective, a topically applied drug must be absorbed through relatively inert stratum corneum and into the metabolically active epidermis and dermis. The outer layer of the skin, the stratum corneum, represents the main barrier to free movement of substances through the skin. It consists of flat, dead keratinocytes arranged in closely packed stacks 10–12 cells deep. The intercellular matrix consists predominantly of lipids while the intracellular space is predominantly proteins. An average composition of stratum corneum is 50% proteins, 20% lipids, 23% water-soluble substances and 7% water.

In general, drugs permeate stratum corneum at rates determined largely by their lipid–water coefficients, water-soluble ions and polar molecules [1]. Permeation through stratum corneum is thought to occur primarily through cell membranes. Studies suggest the existence of a significant intercellular volume which can facilitate diffusion of polar drugs within an aqueous region and non-polar drugs within a lipid region of a bilayered intercellular structure [2].

Whilst the stratum corneum acts as an effective barrier system to the penetration of exogenous substances, it also acts as a barrier to loss of endogenous substances. This is of particular relevance when, due to extensive tissue damage (e.g. severe burns or destruction of the epidermis), the loss of water by evaporation may clinically result in life-threatening problems due to dysregulation of the normal homoeostatic process. Therefore, the rate of transepidermal water loss (TEWL) may provide information on the current status of the skin and, consequently, predictive information on the pharmacokinetics of a transdermal drug [3].

Factors affecting permeation of drugs through skin (Table 27.1.1)

Age

The full-term infant has a well-developed epidermis which, similar to adults, possesses excellent barrier properties. By contrast, the infant who is born prematurely, particularly before 24 weeks of gestation, has a thin epidermis with a poorly developed stratum corneum. Although rapid postnatal maturation of the epidermis occurs over the first 1–3 weeks of age [4] the preterm infant's skin is a poor barrier in this early postnatal period [5,6]. As a consequence, there is an increased TEWL which may lead to fluid imbalance and temperature dysregulation, as well as increased absorption of topically applied agents. The latter may have therapeutic as well as toxicological implications (see Chapter 27.3).

Nachman and Esterly [7] applied a 10% phenylephrine solution on neonatal skin of variable gestational age and compare the degree of skin blanching in an effort to measure relative skin permeability. Infants were divided into three groups: (a) 28–34 weeks; (b) 35–37 weeks; and (c) 38–42 weeks of gestational age. The authors demonstrate that infants in the 28–34 weeks age group had the

most rapid blanching response which lasted from 30 min to several hours. Infants in the 35–37 weeks age group had less response than the first group and infants in the 38–42 weeks age group generally failed to show blanching. After day 21 of postnatal age, most infants showed no blanching response regardless of their gestational age at birth.

Harpin and Rutter [5] modified the study design of Nachman and Esterly by assessing skin blanching response with two different strengths of phenylephrine combined with TEWL determinations. Infants were categorized into four different groups: group A, less than 30 weeks; group B, 30–32 weeks; group C, 33–36 weeks; and group D, 37 weeks or greater gestational age. Their results also showed that full-term infants had no or minimal response to phenylephrine and further demonstrated that TEWL was relatively low. In group C a mild blanching response was observed, which rapidly decreased by 1 week of age. TEWL was slightly greater than in group D, but by 1 week postnatal age it decreased to mature levels. In group B a high blanching response was initially seen, but by 2 weeks postnatal age it had essentially disappeared. TEWL was initially elevated but decreased to normal levels by 10 days postnatal age.

In group A, a very high blanching response, together with a very high TEWL, was seen. However, by 2 weeks postnatal age values were similar to group D. A correlation between response to skin blanching and TEWL was noted in group D.

West *et al.* [8] applied stable, isotope labelled ($^{13}C_6$) benzoic acid to the skin of newborn infants of variable gestational and postnatal ages and measured urinary recovery. Benzoic acid was used since it is found endogenously in mother's milk, is well tolerated by the skin and easily absorbed and rapidly excreted in urine. The results of the study demonstrated that skin absorption in premature infants is most marked in the first postnatal days, and correlates with gestational age, but declines to that expected of a full-term infant over 3 weeks of age [9].

Children may also have an increased risk of systemic toxicity from a topically applied drug because of their greater body surface area to body weight ratio where a given amount of an applied drug represents a proportionately greater dose (in mg/kg) compared to adults [9].

Anatomical region

Drug penetration at different anatomical sites results from variable thickness of stratum corneum. In general, anatomical sites can be ranked in the following order of decreased permeability: postauricular, scrotum, abdomen, scalp, forearm, foot and sole [10].

Skin appendages

Penetration of drugs through skin appendages (shunt

Table 27.1.1 Factors affecting permeation of drugs through skin

Age
Anatomical region
Skin appendages
Skin hydration
Skin damage
Drug type
Vehicle type
Technique of application

routes) is not a major contributory pathway for steady-state diffusion, although it may be important in the very early stages of diffusion and for some ions and larger molecules [1]. Extent of contribution is probably also limited by the fact that appendages cover less than 1% of the skin surface [9]. Extent of appendageal penetrance also depends on the solute. Highly polar non-electrolytes capable of binding to hydrated keratin, thus hindering diffusion across stratum corneum, are more likely to undergo relatively prominent shunt diffusion [12].

In vivo studies have also shown that shunt diffusion could be of significance in penetration of drugs through skin. If appendages are modified by trauma, e.g. burned skin, the short-cut diffusion of drugs through these appendages might be impaired even after wound healing has occurred. There is also the suggestion that targeting of a drug to skin appendages could be important in the treatment of some follicular disorders [13–15].

Skin hydration

Hydration is an important factor in the penetration of drug through skin. Generally, hydration increases the rate of absorption of most substances that permeate the skin, particularly of water-soluble compounds. Immersion of the skin in water results in its uptake by corneocytes and saturation of the intercellular spaces, producing an increased thickness of the stratum corneum. Further exposure to water leads to replacement of lipid covalent bonds between corneocytes by weak hydrogen (water) bonds followed by cell separation. This phenomenon also occurs in occluded body fold areas where evaporation of water is restricted, especially in flexural sites of the axillae and groins where consequently the absorption of drugs is increased [15].

It is also known that elevated ambient temperatures and relative humidity both enhance the toxic effects of chemicals in occupational settings [16].

Skin damage

If the stratum corneum is damaged or removed by stripping, significant increments in drug penetration are observed [17]. Skin diseases which affect stratum corneum may alter barrier function. In ichthyosis, skin permeability is remarkably increased because of changes in stratum corneum which decrease the barrier property of the skin. In the scaly dermatoses, disintegration of the stratum corneum often leads to a dry, scaly skin as a result of contact with solvents and soaps; in this case the damaged barrier is combined with a thick epidermis which is of little importance in the permeation process. In chronic eczema there is frequently a thickened epidermis and stratum corneum, which typically decreases absorption of drugs through skin. The thicker the stratum

corneum, as in orthokeratosis, the lower the rate of diffusion. Psoriasis also involves a thickened stratum corneum and a generally thickened epidermis. However, the presence of parakeratosis enhances permeation, because water content of the still living parakeratotic cells is increased compared to dead corneocytes, so that the skin barrier is less compact [18].

Drug type

Awareness of the pharmacological properties of drugs used in treating dermatological diseases is essential for a rational therapeutic approach. Important determinants for the rate of diffusion of a drug molecule through stratum corneum are size and shape, lipid/water partition coefficient and pH of the drug and surrounding tissue.

Molecular mass and size play a considerable role in stratum corneum penetration. Drug particle size inversely determines rate of cutaneous absorption, such that the smaller the particle the greater the absorption rate. Presence of polar groups in the molecule may significantly impair rate of drug penetration [19]. Many simple polar electrolytes penetrate stratum corneum at the same rate as water with similar diffusion constants, e.g. ethanol and propranolol. A study on a series of corticosteroids showed that the more polar compounds have a much lower diffusion constant, and this seems to be due to increased binding to keratin [20]. For less polar compounds (lipid-soluble non-electrolytes) with similar diffusion constants, permeability must be determined by differences in the partition coefficient (Fick's law) [21].

Vehicle type

The solvent (vehicle) is a substance which forms the medium in which the active medicament is either dissolved or dispersed for application to the skin surface [22]. It is normally intended to be pharmacologically inert but may have some important physical properties. The solvent itself may cause sensitization reactions, but these are relatively uncommon in children. The solvent may have conflicting functions: (a) to increase the penetrance of a substance through the skin; (b) to decrease permeation and hold the substance in upper layers of the skin (i.e. antifungals in the stratum corneum, retinoids in the epidermis); and (c) to target the drug to the skin appendages.

Vehicles that contain oleaginous solids with little or no water are usually called ointments; those with 20–50% water are typically called creams; an even greater amount of water results in a lotion.

Vehicles may be characteristic of the dosage form, as in ointments, emulsions (oil in water, water in oil) and gels. Ointments are usually composed of a fairly lipophilic drug in a base such as petrolatum, mineral oil, waxes or organic alcohols. They spread easily on the skin and are completely water insoluble with maximal water-retaining occlusive properties. These dosage forms usually leave a greasy film on the skin which may cause excessive heat retention, which can be discomforting to the patient.

An emulsion is a two-phase system of otherwise immiscible substances mixed with an oil or an emulsifier. These dosage forms are generally more cosmetically acceptable. They may be water-in-oil (cold creams) or oil-in-water (vanishing creams) systems.

Gels are solubilized solids, usually with no oleaginous phase. They typically consist of fatty alcohols or fatty acids loosely aggregated with water, forming a gelatinous matrix at room temperature. These systems liquefy upon application to the skin and the water phase evaporates, leaving semisolid particles and the active drug on the skin [12]. Other components that may be added to vehicles include emulsifiers, stabilizers, thickening agents and humectants.

It is important to choose an appropriate vehicle on the basis of clinical appearance of skin lesions and their anatomical location. An oozing lesion, e.g. acute weeping eczema, might require a water-based vehicle such as a cream, whereas the dry scaly skin of long-standing eczema might require an oil-based vehicle such as an ointment. Preparations for the scalp and hairy areas are more cosmetically acceptable as creams or gels [15]. Particular care is needed when dealing with body fold areas, where the microenvironment (temperature, humidity, pH) differs from that of other anatomical sites, and percutaneous absorption may be significantly enhanced.

Technique of application

Use of occlusive dressings may increase absorption of some molecules, e.g. corticosteroids, from 10 to 100 times [23]. Occlusion with a plastic film dressing, increases hydration and temperature which leads to enhanced drug permeation. Generally, the increase in drug permeability resulting from the use of occlusive dressings or occlusive formulations is caused by increased hydration of stratum corneum rather than increased temperature [24]. Some compounds, i.e. topically applied corticosteroids, may produce a 'reservoir effect' that can last for several days after application [24].

Systemic delivery of drugs through skin

In humans, plasma levels of drugs are often very low following topical application (often beyond assay detection level) and it may be necessary to use tracer methodology to study skin absorption [25].

Although drug permeability through skin is generally low, some drugs may readily migrate to deeper layers of skin and into the systemic circulation and other tissues or organs. An increase in dermal blood flow and/or skin temperature are important promoting factors [26]. These observations have contributed to recent interest in systemic administration of drugs via the transdermal route [27].

Transdermal delivery of drugs to the systemic circulation can rationally be achieved with transdermal therapeutic delivery systems (TTDS). These devices are designed for delivering drugs through the skin to elicit systemic therapeutic effects. It is the device itself, and not necessarily the stratum corneum, that controls the rate at which the drug is delivered into the skin.

The TTDS usually consists of a microporous polymeric membrane which incorporates the drug. It controls the rate at which the drug is delivered to the skin and thus the rate of absorption. A loading dose is usually contained in the adhesive that affixes the device to the skin [24]. Only certain drugs, however, are suitable for TTDS.

A candidate drug must penetrate skin at adequate rates so that the rate-limiting step is supply of drug from the system and not the ability of the skin to transport drug. This allows drug input to be relatively constant in patients despite individual variations in skin permeability. Usually, agents effective at a parenteral dose of 2 mg/day or less are ideal for TTDS. However, 30 cm^2 systems delivering 15 mg/day nitroglycerin have been successfully accomplished. The less potent a drug, the higher its permeability must be to achieve a therapeutic rate of delivery through a reasonable surface area of skin [12,28]. The therapeutic areas of motion sickness (scopolamine), angina pectoris (nitroglycerin), hypertension (clonidine) and hormone replacement (17β-oestradiol) currently have representative TTDS. To date, there are no commercially available TTDSs for paediatric use, although preliminary studies using theophylline for the treatment of apnoea in premature infants have shown positive data compatible with the development of TTDSs for the paediatric patient [5,9,29].

There are several advantages in using TTDS. Transdermal delivery approaches zero-order drug input, which is similar to the administration of a continuous intravenous infusion, and thereby provides the following advantages.

1 Avoids the need for intravenous therapy, which is both inconvenient and risky.
2 Avoids oral therapy, which is sometimes associated with variable absorption and metabolism.
3 Permits use of drugs with a short half-life.
4 Bypasses hepatic first pass and allows lower daily dosage of drug.
5 Permits reversibility of drug delivery by removal of the system from the skin.
6 Provides a more simplified drug administration routine.
7 Decreases the chance of over- or underdosing.

Metabolism of drugs in skin

Not only may drugs penetrate the skin unchanged, but they may also be metabolized in the skin or interact with receptors present on, or in, epidermal cells. The enzyme system responsible for drug metabolism in skin resembles that of liver. This system is membrane bound and requires reduced nicotinamide adenine dinucleotide phosphate (NADPH) and oxygen for catalytic activity, as well as exhibiting an optimum pH [12]. Oxidative reactions that occur in the skin include alcohol oxidation, hydroxylation of aliphatic and alicyclic carbon atoms, oxidation of aromatic rings, deamination and dealkylation. Reductive reactions also occur in skin [30]. There is little information on conjugation reactions in the skin, but methylation, sulphate conjugation and glucuronide formation have been demonstrated [31]. The skin is also involved in metabolic activation of carcinogens such as benzopyrene by oxidation of aromatic rings [32].

REFERENCES

1 Hadgraft J, Guy RH. *Transdermal Drug Delivery, Developmental Issues and Research Initiatives.* New York: Marcel Dekker, 1989.

2 Sznitowska M, Berner B. Polar pathway for percutaneous absorption. *Curr Prob Dermatol* 1995; 22: 164–70.

3 Aalto-Korte K, Turpeinen M. Transepidermal water loss and absorption of hydrocortisone in widespread dermatitis. *Br J Dermatol* 1993; 128: 633–5.

4 Evans NJ, Rutter N. Development of the epidermis in the newborn. *Biol Neonate* 1986; 49: 74–80.

5 Harpin VA, Rutter N. Barrier properties of the newborn infant's skin. *J Pediatr* 1983; 102: 419–25.

6 Mancini AJ, Sookdeo-Drost S, Madison KC, Smoller BR, Lane AT. Semipermeable dressings improve epidermal barrier function in premature infants. *Pediatr Res* 1994; 36: 306–14.

7 Nachman RL, Esterly NB. Increased skin permeability in preterm infants. *J Pediatr* 1971; 79: 628–32.

8 West DP, Halket JM, Harvey DR, Hadgraft J, Solomon LM, Harper JI. Percutaneous absorption in preterm infants. *Pediatr Dermatol* 1987; 4: 234–7.

9 West DP, Worobec S, Solomon LM. Pharmacology and toxicology of infant skin. *J Invest Dermatol* 1981; 76: 147–50.

10 Rougier A, Dupuis D, Lotte C *et al.* Regional variation in percutaneous absorption in man: measurement by the stripping method. *Arch Dermatol Res* 1986; 278: 465–9.

11 Guy RH, Hadgraft J. Structure activity correlations in percutaneous penetration. In: Bronaugh RL, Maibach HI, eds. *Percutaneous Absorption: Mechanisms, Methodology and Drug Delivery.* New York: Marcel Dekker, 1989.

12 Ghadially R, Shear NH. Topical therapy and percutaneous absorption. In: Yaffe SJ, Aranda JV, eds. *Pediatric Pharmacology. Therapeutic Principles in Practice,* 2nd edn. Philadelphia: WB Saunders, 1992.

13 Schaefer H, Watts F, Brod J, Illel B. Follicular penetration. In: Scott RC, Guy RH, Hadgraft J, eds. *Prediction of Percutaneous Penetration, Methods, Measurements, Modelling.* IBC Technical Services, 1989.

14 Jamoulle JC, Grandjean L, Lamaud E *et al.* Follicular penetration and distribution of topically applied CD-271, a new naphthoic acid derivative intended for topical acne treatment. *J Invest Dermatol* 1990; 94: 731–2.

15 Harper JI. Skin disorders. In: Barltrop D, Brueton MJ, eds. *Paediatric Therapeutics. Principles and Practice.* Oxford: Butterworth-Heinemann, 1990.

16 Bickers DR, Hazen PG, Lynch WS. *Clinical Pharmacology of Skin Disease.* New York: Churchill Livingstone, 1984.

17 Bronaugh RL, Weingarten DP, Lowe NJ. Differential rates of percutaneous absorption through the eczematous and normal skin of a monkey. *J Invest Dermatol* 1986; 87: 451–3.

18 Brandau R, Lippold BH. *Dermal and Transdermal Absorption.* Stuttgart: Wissenschaftliche Verlagsgesellschaft, 1982.

19 Shear NH, Radde IC. Percutaneous drug absorption. In: Radde IC, MacLeod SM, eds. *Pediatric Pharmacology and Therapeutics,* 2nd edn. St Louis: Mosby-Year Book, 1993.

20 Scheuplein RJ, Blank IH, Brauner GJ *et al.* Percutaneous absorption of steroids. *J Invest Dermatol* 1969; 52: 63–70.

21 Scheuplein RJ, Bronaugh RL. Percutaneous absorption. In: Goldsmith LA, ed. *Biochemistry and Physiology of the Skin.* Oxford: Oxford University Press, 1983.

22 Archer CB. The skin as a barrier. In: Champion RH, Burton JL, Burns JL, Breathnach SM. *Textbook of Dermatology,* vol. 1, 6th edn. Oxford: Blackwell Science, 1998: 113–17.

23 Hepburn D, Yohn JJ, Weston WL. Topical steroid treatment in infants, children, and adolescents. In: Callen JP, Dahl MV, Golitz LE, Greenway HT, Schachner LA, eds. *Advances in Dermatology.* St Louis: Mosby-Year Book, 1994.

24 Arndt KA, Mendenhall PV, Sloan KB *et al.* The pharmacology of topical therapy. In: Fitzpatrick TB, Eisen AZ, Wolff K, Freedberg IM, Austen KF, eds. *Dermatology in General Medicine,* 4th edn. New York: McGraw-Hill, 1993.

25 Schaefer H, Lambrey B, Caron D *et al.* Methods in skin pharmacokinetics: introduction. In: Shroot B, Schaefer H, eds. *Skin Pharmacokinetics.* Basel: Karger, 1987.

26 Siddiqui O, Roberts MS, Polack AE. Percutaneous absorption of steroids: relative contributions of epidermal penetration and dermal clearance. *J Pharmacokinet Biopharm* 1989; 17: 405–24.

27 Ridout G, Houk J, Guy RH, Santus GC, Hadgraft J, Hall LL. An evaluation of structure–penetration relationships in percutaneous absorption. *Pharmacokinetics* 1992; 47: 869–92.

28 Chandrasekaran SK, Bayne W, Shaw JE. Pharmacokinetics of drug permeation through human skin. *J Pharm Sci* 1978; 67: 1370–4.

29 Micali G, Bhatt RH, Distefano G *et al.* Evaluation of transdermal theophylline pharmacokinetics in neonates. *Pharmacotherapy* 1993; 13: 386–90.

30 Potts RO, McNeill SC, Desbonnet CR, Wakshull E. Transdermal drug transport and metabolism. II. The role of competing kinetic events. *Pharm Res* 1989; 6: 119–20.

31 Noonan PK, Wester RC. Cutaneous metabolism of xenobiotics. In: Bronaugh RL, Maibach HI, eds. *Percutaneous Absorption.* New York: Marcel Dekker, 1989.

32 Kapitulunik J, Levin W, Conney AH, Yagi H, Jerina DM. Benzo(a)pyrene 7,8-dihydrodiol is more carcinogenic than benzo(a)-pyrene in newborn mice. *Nature* 1977; 266: 378–80.

Topical therapy

Emollients

Emollients are usually bland, fatty or oleaginous substances that hydrate and soften the skin. They are typically occlusive and this results in a decrease of TEWL. Emollients often contain lipids, such as liquid paraffin or soya oil [1]. Those containing fragrances should be used with caution, if at all, since they may cause irritation and/or sensitization.

The use of emollients is indicated in scaly dermatoses and for routine skin care in children with dry skin. Their use in preterm infants may help to prevent the onset of dermatitis [2]. Moreover, emollients are an essential part of the treatment of atopic dermatitis. Petrolatum is quite occlusive and is one of the most widely used emollients. Unfortunately, it is not well accepted by patients because of its greasiness and staining properties.

Emollients can also be used as bath additives, since bathing in water alone may excessively dry the skin. Application of vegetable or mineral oils during or after bathing reduces TEWL, thus having a moisturizing effect

[3]. For this reason, bath oils are particularly useful in children with atopic dermatitis. Bath oils also keep the skin clean and free from debris (crusts and scales). Moreover, in children with atopic dermatitis, the use of over-the-counter soaps should be avoided, as they are alkaline and may contain perfumes or fragrances that irritate the skin [3].

Protectants

These are used to protect the skin against inflammation due to irritating chemicals (i.e. ammonia released by bacteria in infant's urine) or repeated trauma or friction. Zinc oxide (1–25%) in various topical dosage forms is widely used and clinically accepted as a skin protectant. It is also considered to be mildly astringent and antiseptic as well. It is commonly applied as an ingredient in a paste (Lassar's), ointment or lotion (calamine).

Water-repellent protectants may contain substances such as dimethicone or other silicones. These may be irritating to the skin when the concentration of the silicone material is increased, particularly above 20%.

Antiseptics

A 4% solution of chlorhexidine gluconate may be used for the initial bath after a newborn infant's temperature is stable, to decrease colonization by staphylococcal bacteria. The active agent is bactericidal on contact and binds with skin proteins to provide residual, and thus prolonged, duration of antibacterial action. The frequency of bathing may vary according to the presence of outbreaks of staphylococcal infections [4]. This is also useful as an adjunctive measure in managing impetigo. Povidone iodine and hexachlorophene should not be used in routine newborn bathing because of the high risk of percutaneous toxicity (see Chapter 27.3).

Astringents

Astringents produce mild vasoconstriction, reduce cutaneous blood flow and cleanse the skin of exudate, crust and debris. They are often applied as a wet dressing or compress, in an effort to also cool and dry the skin through evaporation. Aluminum subacetate and potassium permanganate solutions are commonly used astringents. Aluminum subacetate solution (5%) is diluted 1 : 10 to 1 : 40 with water before use. It is commercially available as tablets and powders for ready mixing. Potassium permanganate can be administered either as a wet soak or added to the bath in a dilution of 10 ml of 1% concentration diluted to 1 l. The concentrated solutions of these astringent agents are highly irritant, so dilution is essential.

Keratolytics

These substances are used to thin excessively thickened skin. Keratolytics include lactic acid, propylene glycol, sulphur compounds, urea and salicylic acid. These agents are known to dissolve the intercellular matrix and thereby soften hyperkeratotic areas by enhancing the removal of scales [5]. Salicylic acid is available in different formulations including gels, ointments, creams, transdermal patches or plasters, in concentrations ranging from 1 to 40%. Formulations and concentrations vary according to the disorder being treated. Hyperkeratotic conditions such as psoriasis, ichthyosis, warts and acne each require a dosage form and concentration suited to the clinical features of the disease [6]. The use of these agents over extensive areas of the body surface, particularly in children, should involve extreme caution and careful monitoring because of the potential to induce systemic toxicity (see Chapter 27.3).

Corticosteroids

The anti-inflammatory, antipruritic and antiproliferative properties of corticosteroids are well known [7,8]. In treating children with topical corticosteroids, there is as much concern for safety as there is for efficacy. A majority of marketed topical corticosteroid preparations have not been tested in children. Guidelines for their use in paediatric patients (Table 27.1.2) have been largely derived from adult studies [8].

Another important factor to consider is that, although topical corticosteroids are very effective in controlling acute inflammatory dermatoses as well as the aggravating symptoms of chronic dermatoses, they do not necessarily correct the underlying disorder [9]. Therefore, upon discontinuation of topical steroid therapy, the dermatosis

Table 27.1.2 Topical corticosteroids in controlled trials that included paediatric subjects. Adapted from Hepburn *et al.* [8]

Drug name and strength	Clinical potency (United States Pharmacopeia)
Alclometasone dipropionate cream 0.05%	Low
Desonide cream 0.05%	Low
Hydrocortisone ointment 1%	Low
Clobetasone butyrate cream 0.05%	Medium
Diflucortolone valerate cream 0.1%	Medium
Fluocinolone acetonide cream 0.025%	Medium
Fluticasone propionate	Medium
Hydrocortisone butyrate cream, 0.01%	Medium
Mometasone furoate cream 0.1%	Medium
Halcinonide cream 0.1%	High
Betamethasone dipropionate cream 0.05%	Very high
Halobetasol propionate cream 0.05%	Very high
Halobetasol propionate ointment 0.05%	Very high

may recur, sometimes flaring into a state worse than before treatment. Topical corticosteroids are safe and effective when used for brief periods on limited areas without occlusion. Minimizing occlusion in the paediatric population is important, since cutaneous atrophy can be produced within 7 days by superpotent topical corticosteroid under occlusion, and as early as 2 weeks with less potent agents or a superpotent agent without occlusion [10].

Occlusion enhances cutaneous absorption by concentrating topically applied steroid in upper layers of the stratum corneum. When occlusion is removed, the elevated moisture content of the stratum corneum rapidly returns to normal. The stratum corneum also returns to normal but it now contains a relatively high concentration of poorly diffusible, rather insoluble corticosteroid. Upper layers of stratum corneum may be supersaturated with corticosteroid, and some of the drug may precipitate. A fraction of the available molecules may bind to keratin or other tissue components, as the remainder diffuses slowly inward. A dynamic equilibrium is established, for which insoluble and bound steroid serves as a reservoir to replace molecules which are permeating to lower layers of stratum corneum, the viable epidermis and the dermis.

Ideal conditions may exist for some corticosteroids to remain in the stratum corneum for a protracted period of time and to provide a steady low flux of drug to the dermis. As a result, sensitive analytical methods can detect the presence of steroid in the stratum corneum for many days or even a few weeks after application to the skin.

Other complications that may be seen after steroid occlusion include miliaria and microbial overgrowth of yeast and bacteria [11].

Based on these considerations, it is advisable to follow some general guidelines when treating infants and children with topical corticosteroids [8].

1 Choose the corticosteroid potency and dosage form according to the anatomical area being treated. In infants, body fold areas provide a natural occlusive phenomenon such as that found in the napkin area, where the use of low-potency corticosteroids is recommended when steroids are necessary. Treatment of intertriginous areas, such as axillae or groin where the skin is thin, moist and to some degree occluded, also requires particular care. On the trunk and extremities moderate potency corticosteroids can be used, when required, with greater safety.

2 In infants and children, twice a day applications, and therapy durations of 7–14 days is usually sufficient.

3 Do not use superpotent corticosteroids.

4 If the response is inadequate, consider alternative therapies.

In the USA, topical corticosteroids are divided into four groups with respect to clinical potency according to the United States Pharmacopeia (USP). (a) Only those labelled as low potency are acceptable for chronic use in infants and young children. (b) Occasionally, it may be necessary to use a medium potency preparation for acute care of moderate inflammatory dermatoses such as atopic dermatitis. (c) High potency preparations are used in severe inflammatory dermatoses such as psoriasis, and only for short treatment durations. (d) Very high potency products are used primarily as an alternative to systemic corticosteroid therapy when local areas are involved. They may be used for only a short duration of therapy and limited to small surface areas. Protracted use of topical corticosteroids is associated with local as well as systemic side-effects.

Local side-effects, although not life threatening, are more common than systemic side-effects, often insidious in their onset, and frequently troublesome. They include atrophy of the epidermis and dermis, striae, rosacea, tinea incognito, granuloma gluteale infantum, flare of acne, hirsutism and hypopigmentation.

As regards systemic side-effects, infants and toddlers are at high risk as they have a greater surface to body ratio [12] and they may be less able to metabolize potent glucocorticoid quickly. Systemic side-effects from topical corticosteroids include hypothalamopituitary–adrenal axis suppression, failure to thrive, overt Cushing's syndrome, glaucoma and benign cephalic hypertension.

Factors that may influence the risk of systemic side-effects include the amount of drug applied, the extent of skin surface treated, the frequency of application, the length of treatment, the glucocorticoid potency of the individual steroid being used and the use of occlusion.

Intralesional corticosteroids in the paediatric age group should be used with caution by trained doctors only, as the side-effects resulting after incorrect administration may be significant and long lasting.

Coal tar and anthralin

Coal tar is a complex mixture of organic compounds, rich in polycyclic hydrocarbons, that is produced by the distillation of coal. Little is known about its exact mechanism of action. Some studies have shown coal tar to inhibit DNA synthesis thus acting as a cytostatic. Coal tar may be used in different concentrations either alone, in an ointment or paste or included with other substances such as salicylic acid, hydrocortisone or zinc oxide. Scalp preparations and shampoos are also available. Primary uses of coal tar are in the treatment of common skin disorders such as psoriasis and atopic dermatitis where it is considered safe and effective [13]. Its use has been somewhat limited due to cosmetic unacceptability by the patient, since coal tar therapy is malodorous, staining, messy and a burdensome treatment regimen. Improved formulations that are relatively non-staining, with no or minimal tar odour, are now available, thus rendering the use of coal tar, especially among children, more acceptable.

Anthralin (dithranol) is a synthetic anthraquinone that is structurally related to acridine, a component of crude coal tar. The primary indication for anthralin is psoriasis. It is a primary irritant that should be applied to lesional skin only and not to normal skin, the face, genitalia or areas of acute inflammation. Like coal tar, it also stains clothing and skin. Anthralin is used in variable concentrations, particularly in the treatment of psoriasis. Short contact application, such as for 30–60 min daily, is effective and represents a practical approach, especially for children.

Antibacterials

Ideally, bacterial skin infections would be treated with topical antibiotics to minimize systemic exposure. However, their use is limited because of the risks of promoting bacterial resistance and of sensitization reactions. Mupirocin (pseudomonic acid A) is a topical antibacterial that is produced by *Pseudomonas fluorescens*. Few local side-effects result from the use of mupirocin, and there is little systemic absorption. It is effective for the treatment of impetigo caused by *Staphylococcus aureus* and *Streptococcus pyogenes*. Some clinical study data indicate that mupirocin is equivalent in efficacy to systemic erythromycin in the treatment of childhood impetigo and with less frequent adverse reactions. Mupirocin is available as an ointment (2%) that is applied to the affected areas three times a day [6]. Topical fusidic acid is another relatively safe compound that is primarily used for staphylococcal skin infections. Although sensitization by fusidic acid is uncommon, bacterial resistance is documented. Topical antibacterials that are commonly used in the treatment of inflammatory acne in paediatric patients include clindamycin and erythromycin. Tetracycline derivatives should be used with great caution, if at all, in children where dentition and long bone growth are still taking place.

Antifungals

Topical antifungals are used for the treatment of superficial fungal infections of the skin and mucosae. They may be used adjunctively for mycoses of the nail and hair, and adjunctively for the treatment of systemic mycoses, but are not effective as primary agents in these conditions. A plethora of topical antifungal agents are currently available. Preferred formulations for a topical antifungal are usually creams or solutions. Ointments are not as commonly used because they may be too occlusive for macerated or fissured tissue. The use of powders, whether applied by shake containers or aerosols, is largely confined to the feet and moist lesions of the groin and other intertriginous areas. Powders are less effective dosage forms for delivering active ingredients into the stratum corneum and epidermis. A majority of available topical antifungals are imidazole or triazole synthetic agents such as clotrimazole, econazole, miconazole and oxiconazole. Non-imidazole compounds include ciclopirox olamine, haloprogin, tolnaftate, naftifine and terbinafine. In general, topical antifungals are safe for paediatric use although contact sensitization occurs on rare occasions.

Antivirals

Topical antivirals are sometimes used in paediatric patients for the treatment of primary and recurrent herpes simplex virus (HSV) infections. They include aciclovir and idoxuridine. The former is available as 5% cream and may be helpful if frequently applied early in the course. An ophthalmic formulation may be used when appropriate. Idoxuridine (10 or 40% lotion) is used in similar indications as for aciclovir.

Antihistamines

Topical antihistamines are not commonly used by dermatologists because of the high risk of allergic contact sensitization [14].

Vitamin D₃ analogues

Two vitamin D_3 analogues are currently available for topical use, calcitriol and calcipotriol (calcipotriene in the USA).

Calcipotriol is a vitamin D_3 analogue which has a high binding affinity to the cellular receptor for biologically active vitamin D_3 (1,25-dihydroxy-vitamin D_3) (calcitriol). Receptors for calcitriol have been demonstrated in various cells, including keratinocytes and fibroblasts. Calcitriol and calcipotriol produce equivalent dose-dependent inhibition of proliferation, and stimulation of terminal differentiation, in cultured human keratinocytes [15]. Unlike calcitriol, however, calcipotriol presents lower risk of inducing calcium-related side-effects. Favourable results in the treatment of psoriasis in children have been reported with calcitriol [16,17], while calcipotriol has shown to be of some efficacy in the treatment of congenital ichthyoses [15].

Antiparasitic preparations

Antiparasitic preparations may be used for the treatment of scabies and pediculosis. Gamma-benzene hexachloride (lindane) is available in some countries as creams, lotions and shampoos, usually as a 1% concentration. Although it is effective for both scabies and pediculosis, its use is still a matter of debate since central nervous system toxicity has been documented following topical application of lindane [18], particularly in children. Use of lindane during pregnancy and under the age of 6 years is not recommended.

Permethrin as a 5% cream is safe and effective for both scabies and pediculosis. Contraindications for its use include pregnancy and age below 2 months.

Benzoyl benzoate, used widely outside the USA, is available as 28–50% lotion. It may be used in infants, young children, pregnant and nursing women. It may cause irritation and/or contact sensitization in some individuals.

Other antiparasitic preparations include carbaryl, as an acceptable treatment for lice and ticks, and malathion 0.5% in an alcoholic base for use against lice and their ova [19].

Insect repellents

An effective insect repellent should be non-toxic, non-irritant, non-allergenic, harmless to clothing, odourless and easy to apply. It should also be effective against multiple insects and offer protection for several hours in variable weather conditions. One of the more effective repellents is *N,N*-diethyl-*m*-toluamide (DEET). Product forms include aerosols, pump sprays, lotion-creams, liquids, roll-on sticks and impregnated towelettes, in concentrations ranging from 5 to 100% [20]. The maximum suggested concentration for use of DEET in children is 20% [21]. DEET is effective on mosquitoes, biting flies, ticks, gnats, chiggers and fleas. The use of DEET should be used with considerable caution since cases of systemic toxicity have been reported following topical use [22]. Other insect repellents include dimethylphthalate (30–70%) and butopyronoxyl (Indalone), which are particularly effective on mosquitoes and biting flies [21].

Oil of citronella (0.5%) mixed with inert ingredients is aromatically pleasant but it may cause contact sensitization.

EMLA

EMLA cream (eutectic mixture of local anaesthetics) is a topical anesthetic composed of 25 mg lidocaine and 25 mg prilocaine in an oil-in-water emulsion cream. It is mainly used to decrease the pain of venepuncture, myringotomy placement, split-thickness skin grafting, curettage of molluscum contagiosum, cautery of genital warts and laser treatment [23].

Metronidazole

Topical metronidazole gel (0.75%) is a compound for treatment of rosacea that has also shown positive results in the treatment of perioral dermatitis in children [24].

Sunscreens

Chemical sunscreens are characteristically divided into ultraviolet A (UVA) blockers, active in the range 320–360 nm, and UVB blockers, active in the range 290–320 nm [25]. Some products are effective in both ranges and are termed 'broad-spectrum' blockers. The efficiency of each agent is related to the spectrum of wavelengths absorbed and to the resistance to washing off during swimming or sweating [26,27].

REFERENCES

1 Overgaard Olsen L, Jemec GB. The influence of water, glycerin, paraffin oil and ethanol on skin mechanics. *Acta Derm Venereol* 1993; 73: 404–6.

2 Lane AT, Drost SS. Effects of repeated application of emollient cream to premature neonates skin. *Pediatrics* 1993; 92: 415–19.

3 Loden M. The increase in skin hydration after application of emollients with different amounts of lipids. *Acta Derm Venereol* 1992; 72: 327–30.

4 Hodgman JE. Skin disorders of the neonate. In: Burg FO, Ingelfinger JR, Wald ER, Polin RA, eds. *Current Pediatric Therapy*, 15th edn. Philadelphia: WB Saunders, 1996.

5 Loden M, Bostrom P, Kneczke M. Distribution and keratolytic effect of salicylic acid and urea in human skin. *Skin Pharmacol* 1995; 8: 173–8.

6 Guzzo CA, Lazazus GS, Werth VP. Dermatological pharmacology. In: Hardman, Limbird, Molinoff, Ruddon, Gilman, eds. *The Pharmacological Basis of Therapeutics*, 9th edn. New York: McGraw Hill, 1996.

7 Krafchik BR. The use of topical steroids in children. *Semin Dermatol* 1995; 14: 70–4.

8 Hepburn D, Yohn JJ, Weston WL. Topical steroid treatment in infants, children, and adolescents. In: Callen JP, Dahl MV, Golitz LE, Greenway HT, Schachner LA, eds. *Advances in Dermatology*. St Louis: Mosby-Year Book, 1994.

9 Christophers E. Thoughts on the use of topical corticosteroids. In: Christophers E, Schopf E, Kligman AM *et al.*, eds. *Topical Corticosteroid Therapy: a Novel Approach to Safer Drugs*. New York: Raven Press, 1988.

10 Katz HI, Prawer SE, Mooney JJ *et al.* Preatrophy: covert sign of thinned skin. *J Am Acad Dermatol* 1989; 20: 731–5.

11 Sterry W. Therapy with topical corticosteroids. *Arch Dermatol Res* 1992; 284(suppl 1): S27–9.

12 West DP, Worobec S, Solomon LM. Pharmacology and toxicology of infant skin. *J Invest Dermatol* 1981; 76: 147–50.

13 Dodd WA. Tars. Their role in the treatment of psoriasis. *Dermatol Clin* 1993; 11: 131–5.

14 Anonymous. Rash promises for topical antihistamines. *Drug Therap Bull* 1992; 30: 49–50.

15 Lucker GPH, Van de Kerkhof PCM, Van Dijk MR *et al.* Effect of topical calcipotriol on congenital ichthyoses. *Br J Dermatol* 1994; 131: 546–50.

16 Saggese G, Federico G, Battini R. Topical application of 1,25-dihydroxyvitamin D₃ (calcitriol) is an effective and reliable therapy to cure skin lesions in psoriatic children. *Eur J Pediatr* 1993; 152: 389–92.

17 Perez A, Chen TC, Turner A, Holick MF. Pilot study of calcitriol (1,25-dihydroxyvitamin D₃) for treating psoriasis in children. *Arch Dermatol* 1995; 131: 961–2.

18 Solomon LM, Fharner L, West DP. Gamma benzene hexachloride toxicity. *Arch Dermatol* 1977; 113: 353–7.

19 Vander Stichele RH, Dezeure EM, Bogaert MG. Systematic review of clinical efficacy of topical treatments for head lice. *Br Med J* 1995; 311: 604–8.

20 Veltri JC, Osimitz TG, Bradford DC *et al.* Retrospective analysis of calls to poison control centers resulting from exposure to the insect repellent *N,N*-diethyl-*M*-toluamide (DEET) from 1985–1989. *J Toxicol Clin Toxicol* 1994; 32: 1–16.

21 Hebert AA. *Pediatric Dermatology Seminar*. Chicago: American Academy of Dermatology Summer Meeting, 1995.

22 Osimitz TG, Grothaus RH. The present safety assessment of Deet. *J Am Mosquito Control Assoc* 1995; 11: 274–8.

23 Ashinoff R, Geronemus RG. Effect of the topical anesthetic EMLA on the efficacy of pulsed dye laser treatment of port-wine stains. *J Dermatol Surg Oncol* 1990; 16: 1008–11.

24 Miller SR, Shalita AR. Topical metronidazole gel (0.75%) for the treatment of perioral dermatitis in children. *J Am Acad Dermatol* 1994; 31: 847–8.

25 Stern RS. Sunscreens for cancer prevention. *Arch Dermatol* 1995; 131: 220–1.

26 Odio MR, Veres DA, Goodman JJ *et al.* Comparative efficacy of sunscreen reapplication regimens in children exposed to ambient sunlight. *Photodermatol Photoimmunol Photomed* 1994; 10: 118–25.

27 Banks BA, Silverman RA, Schwartz RH, Tunnessen WW Jr. Attitudes of teenagers toward sun exposure and sunscreen use. *Pediatrics* 1992; 89: 40–2.

Systemic therapy

Antihistamines

Antihistamines are not effective for all types of pruritic eruptions even though they may be commonly used without regard to aetiology of the itch. Antihistamines antagonize the peripheral action of histamine and in dermatology are particularly valuable in treating histamine-associated disorders such as urticaria, angio-oedema and insect bites.

They are of limited value in the management of atopic dermatitis. There are numerous H_1-blocking antihistamines commercially available and they differ in duration and side-effects (drowsiness and anticholinergic effects). Those with a significant sedative effect (diphenhydramine, promethazine) may be used to promote sleep especially in those children whose itchy dermatitis may disrupt sleep [1]. Newer generation antihistamines which cause less sedation (astemizole, terfenadine, loratadine, cetirizine) are available, but some of these pose serious drug interaction problems.

H_2-blocking antihistamines are useful to protect vulnerable patients from gastric complications related to systemic corticosteroid or non-steroidal anti-inflammatory drug (NSAID) therapy. Recently, various authors have shown that cimetidine may exhibit an antipruritic effect [2] and has immunomodulating capability as has been demonstrated with cimetidine-augmented cell-mediated immunity [2]. For these reasons, cimetidine has been successfully used for treating common variable immunodeficiency [3], hypergammaglobulin E [4] and to reverse the cutaneous anergy associated with Crohn's disease. Dermatological conditions that may be responsive to cimetidine include mucocutaneous candidiasis [5], herpes zoster, although data are controversial, and a variety of human papillomavirus (HPV) infections ranging from verruca plana to common warts and/or plantar warts to condyloma acuminatum [2,6,7]. In the USA, its use is not specifically approved in children under 12 years of age.

Antibacterials

Systemic antibacterials are used to treat primary and secondary bacterial infections of the skin. Some antibiotics present problems when used in the neonatal period and are best avoided when suitable safer alternatives are available. Among these, tetracyclines are incorporated into developing teeth and bone, resulting in subsequent discoloration of teeth and altered bone growth after exposure during the fetal or neonatal period. Anti-infective sulphonamides may produce kernicterus after fetal or newborn exposure to the drug. Chloramphenicol is known to produce an often fatal 'grey syndrome'.

Examples of systemic antibiotics for paediatric treatment of skin, mucous membranes and soft tissue are penicillin, dicloxacillin, amoxicillin, clavulinic acid, erythromycin, cephalexin and cefadroxil [8]. Azithromycin and clarithromycin are two macrolides that have been shown to be two to four times more active than erythromycin versus staphylococcal and streptococcal infections, but not reliably effective versus erythromycin-resistant organisms or methicillin-resistant *Staphylococcus aureus* [9]. Moreover, they have been not approved for use in children. In Japan, cefditoren has been shown to be effective on streptococci, staphylococci and *Haemophilus influenzae*. A major attribute is its safety in children [9].

Corticosteroids

The use of systemic corticosteroids in children should be limited to appropriate indications in dermatology; some of these are erythema multiforme major, systemic lupus erythematosus, bullous dermatoses, pemphigus disorders and acute allergic reactions such as anaphylactic shock, angioneurotic oedema, multiple bee or wasp stings, poisonous bites and severe allergic contact dermatitis, as from poison ivy. They may also be used for the treatment of large haemangiomas and diffuse neonatal angiomatosis. Their use is not recommended for chronic administration in disorders such as psoriasis and atopic dermatitis.

Retinoids

Retinoids have demonstrated dramatic efficacy in the treatment of severe acne, psoriasis and various disorders of keratinization. Currently available retinoids for systemic administration include isotretinoin, etretinate and its active metabolite acitretin, with others under current investigation. The mode of action of the retinoids has not been completely elucidated, but they have profound effects on differentiation of cell growth and immune response. Recent data suggest a role in cancer prevention as well as cancer therapy.

Isotretinoin (13-*cis*-retinoic acid) is effective in the treatment of severe, recalcitrant, nodular acne. It reversibly decreases the size of sebaceous glands and normalizes keratinization of the glandular acroinfundibulum. It also inhibits the release of arachidonic acid by macrophages, thus contributing to their anti-inflammatory effect [10]. Of great importance is that remissions following therapy are, in a majority of cases, definitive [11]. Isotretinoin may be useful in the prevention of malignant skin tumours in individuals who are predisposed to skin cancers, including individuals previously exposed to arsenic, patients with naevoid basal cell carcinoma syndrome and those patients with xeroderma pigmentosum [11].

Therapy with isotretinoin may be associated with a variety of skin and mucosal side-effects such as xerosis, cheilitis, conjunctival irritation, skin fragility and hair loss. Other side-effects include headache from pseudotumour cerebri, papilloedema, nausea, vomiting, visual disturbances and arthralgia, usually as a result of hyperostosis and tendinous calcifications. Premature epiphyseal closure and pathological fractures have been observed in long-term therapy patients. Hypertriglyceridaemia develops in approximately 25% of patients under treatment and is usually reversible. Depression and suicide ideation is also a recognized side-effect requiring careful monitoring.

Risk of teratogenicity is an extremely important factor to consider when prescribing isotretinoin. Pregnancy is an absolute contraindication to the use of the drug and women should not become pregnant for at least three complete menstrual cycles after the drug has been discontinued. Therefore, the use of contraceptives is advisable. Despite warnings, some women have taken the drug during pregnancy, and several infants with multiple anomalies have been born. A specific syndrome that includes central nervous system, ear and great vessel abnormalities, along with hypoplasia of the thymus and parathyroid gland, has been described. This condition is a phenocopy of the DiGeorge sequence that occurs as a contiguous gene syndrome related to a microdeletion of chromosome 22.

Etretinate, an aromatic retinoid, is effective in the treatment of erythrodermic and generalized pustular psoriasis. It is also indicated for the treatment of palmoplantar pustular forms, especially when associated with marked hyperkeratosis. The efficacy of etretinate in psoriasis is thought to result from its effect on epidermal differentiation and keratinization, although decreased migration of neutrophils and monocytes has also been demonstrated in treated patients [11]. The use of etretinate for psoriasis in children is usually reserved for selected cases where the risks versus benefits have been carefully evaluated.

Beside psoriasis, a wide variety of disorders of keratinization are somewhat responsive to etretinate: epidermolytic hyperkeratosis, keratoderma, X-linked ichthyosis and ichthyosis vulgaris, erythrokeratoderma variabilis, pityriasis rubra pilaris, discoid lupus erythematosus and lichen planus.

Darier's disease, lamellar ichythiosis and non-bullous ichthyosiform erythroderma are responsive to both etretinate and isotretinoin. For these conditions, long-term treatments are required, as remissions following discontinuation of treatment have not been reported.

A successful outcome of cases of harlequin fetus treated with etretinate has been reported by many authors. The toxicity of etretinate is similar to that of isotretinoin with regards to mucocutaneous signs, hyperlipidaemia and abnormal liver function tests. The majority of patients on long-term therapy developed tendinous and ligamentous calcifications and hyperostoses. In children, high-dose and long-term administration has produced a spectrum of skeletal toxicities similar to those seen with hypervitaminosis A in humans and animals [12].

Etretinate is also teratogenic and is highly problematic because of fat storage in the host and slow release over many months and years. Pregnancy should be avoided even after etretinate is discontinued [13]. The active metabolite, acitretin, is more rapidly excreted, but reverse metabolizes to etretinate to some minor degree, creating potential long-term teratogenic hazards.

Acitretin has now superceded etretinate, which is now no longer available in most countries.

Antifungals

The use of systemic antifungals in children should be limited to those fungal infections that are refractory to topical agents or where topical treatment is not feasible to eradicate the disease. Typical conditions that need systemic treatment include tinea capitis, mucocutaneous candidiasis, onychomycoses, systemic infections in severely ill or immunocompromised patients and deep mycoses. There are many systemic agents available, although not all are recommended for paediatric use. Most of them are marketed as oral agents. Among the first-generation compounds are griseofulvin, particularly effective for tinea capitis, and amphotericin B, one of the few drugs available for intravenous administration. Newer systemic antifungals are safer and require shorter treatment schedules. Unfortunately, clinical trials in children are limited. Newer systemic antifungals include fluconazole, itr conazole and terbinafine. The use of ketoconazole is reduced because of its relatively high rate of hepatotoxicity.

Antivirals

Aciclovir is one of the most widely used medications in treating herpes virus infections. It works by inhibition of DNA viral synthesis. Its mode of action involves activation by thymidine kinase and subsequent inhibition of viral polymerase. Aciclovir is available in 200, 400 and 800 mg tablets, and as intravenous infusion. It is very effective on HSV-1 and HSV-2 infections. In children oral aciclovir is particularly indicated for severe herpetic gingivostomatitis and for severe genital HSV infections in adolescents. Intravenous administration is required for eczema herpeticum and for HSV infections in immuno-compromised children. Although aciclovir is more active against HSV infections, it is the preferred drug for varicella and herpes zoster infections. In both conditions, parenteral administration of the drug is recommended in severe cases (immunocompromised children and high-risk infected neonate). In one study, oral aciclovir on varicella in children was beneficial and non-toxic but only when administered within 24h after the onset of the disease. A vaccine for varicella has been recently marketed in the USA [14].

Interferons

The medical literature details the cases of at least 20 paediatric patients with haemangiomas treated with subcutaneous injections of interferon. Patient remissions were noted in at least 90% of these patients. Inclusion criteria for the use of interferon in the treatment of haemangiomas are: corticosteroid therapy proved ineffective, life- or vision-threatening haemangiomas, diffuse neonatal angiomatosis and Kasabach–Merrit syndrome. Interferon may also be effective in severe atopic dermatitis. It should be used in patients unresponsive to corticosteroid therapy and with severe widespread disease. In one study, patients aged 3–20 years showed the highest (67%) rate of improvement with more than 50% skin surface clearing [15]. However, there is now serious concern about spastic diplegia as a complication of interferon therapy [16].

Essential fatty acids

Essential fatty acids (EFA) are those acids which cannot be synthesized by humans and must therefore be a part of the diet. Major essential fatty acids found in humans are linoleic acid and its products, γ-linoleic acid and arachidonic acid.

Deficiency of EFA in the diet leads to a scaly dermatitis and impaired skin-barrier function [17,18]. Oral intake may cause clinical improvement in the skin of patients with atopic dermatitis [19].

The eicopentaenoic acids (EPA) are polyunsaturated fatty acids with a longer chain length than linoleic and more double bonds, and are found in large quantities in fish oils. Long-term administration of fish oil can modify the severity of psoriasis and enhance the efficacy of coadministered conventional psoriatic therapy. EPA have been also proposed as a supplementary treatment for patients receiving cyclosporin for psoriasis and other dermatoses, because of their beneficial effects on renal function [20].

Other drugs

A few drugs are used on a very restricted basis to treat der-matological disorders in paediatric patients. Agents such as dapsone, hydroxychloroquine and cyclosporin are used in children but a narrow margin of safety versus toxicity limits their utility [21–23].

Dapsone has been used, and is recommended, for the treatment of chronic bullous disease of childhood, leprosy and lupus profundus [21]. Hydroxychloroquine is indicated in the treatment of systemic lupus erythematosus in childhood [21]. Cyclosporin has been used with positive results in children with recalcitrant dermatomyositis [22] as well as in severe atopic dermatitis [23].

REFERENCES

1 Adair RH, Bauchner H. Sleep problems in childhood. *Curr Prob Pediatr* 1993; 23: 147–70.
2 Choi YS, Hann SK, Park YK. The effect of cimetidine on verruca plana juvenilis: clinical trials in six patients. *J Dermatol* 1993; 20: 497–500.
3 Wershil DK, Mekery VA, Galli SJ. Cimetidine and common variable hypogammaglobulinemia. *N Engl J Med* 1985; 313: 264–6.
4 Simon GL, Miller HG, Scott SJ. Cimetidine in the treatment of hyper-immunoglobulinemia E with impaired chemotaxis. *J Infect Dis* 1983; 147: 1121–2.
5 Jorizzo JL, Sams WM, Jegasothy BV et al. Cimetidine as an immunomodulator: chronic mucocutaneous candidiasis as a model. *Ann Intern Med* 1980; 92: 192–5.
6 Orlow SJ, Paller A. Cimetidine therapy for multiple viral warts in children. *J Am Acad Dermatol* 1993; 28: 794–6.
7 Rampen FH, van Everdingen JJ. Inefficacy of cimetidine in condylomata acuminata. *Br J Venereol Dis* 1982; 58: 275.
8 Rhodes KH, Henry NK. Antibiotic therapy for severe infections in infants and children. *Mayo Clin Proc* 1992; 67: 59–68.
9 Mirensky Y, Parish LC, Witkowsky JA. Recent advances in antimicrobial therapy of bacterial infections of the skin. In: Dahl MV, Lynch PJ, eds. *Current Opinion in Dermatology.* Philadelphia: Current Science, 1995.
10 Peck GL, Olsen TG, Yoder FW et al. Prolonged remission of cystic acne and conglobate acne with 13-*cis*-retinoic acid. *N Engl J Med* 1979; 300: 329–33.
11 Orfanos CE, Ehlert R, Gollnick H. The retinoids. A review of their clinical pharmacology and therapeutic use. *Drugs* 1987; 34: 459–503.
12 DiGiovanna JJ, Peck GL. Retinoid toxicity. *Progr Dermatol* 1987; 21: 1–8.
13 Guzzo CA, Lazarus GS, Werth VP. Dermatological pharmacology. In: Hardman JG, Limbird LE, Molinoff PB, Ruddon RW, eds. *The Pharmacological Basis of Therapeutics*, 9th edn. New York: McGraw Hill, 1996.
14 DiNicola AF. Varicella vaccine guidelines. *Pediatrics* 1995; 95: 791–6.
15 Landow RK. The use of interferon in dermatology. In: Dahl MV, Lynch PJ, eds. *Current Opinion in Dermatology.* Philadelphia: Current Science, 1995.
16 Barlow CF, Priebe CJ, Mulliken JB et al. Spastic diplegia as a complication of interferon alpha-2a treatment of haemangiomas of infancy. *J Pediatr* 1998; 132: 527–30.
17 Skolnik P, Eaglstein WH, Ziboh VA. Human essential fatty acid deficiency. *Arch Dermatol* 1977; 113: 939–41.
18 Tolesson A, Frithz A, Berg A et al. Essential fatty acid in infantile seborrheic dermatitis. *J Am Acad Dermatol* 1993; 28: 957–61.
19 Fiocchi A, Sala M, Signoroni P, Banderali G, Agostoni C, Riva E. The efficacy and safety of gamma-linolenic acid in the treatment of infantile atopic dermatitis. *Int Med Res* 1994; 22: 24–32.
20 Elzinga L, Kelley VE, Houghton DC et al. Modification of experimental nephrotoxicity with fish oil as the vehicle for cyclosporine. *Transplant* 1987; 43: 271–5.
21 Burg FO, Ingelfinger JR, Wald ER, Polin RA. *Current Pediatric Therapy*, 15th edn. Philadelphia: WB Saunders, 1996.
22 Hechmatt J, Saunders C, Peters AM. Cyclosporin in juvenile dermatomyositis. *Lancet* 1989; i: 1063.
23 Berth-Jones J, Finlay AY, Zaki I et al. Cyclosporin in severe childhood atopic dermatitis. A multicentre study. *J Am Acad Dermatol* 1996; 34: 1016–21.

27.2 Hypersensitivity Reactions to Drugs

NEIL H. SHEAR, MARINA LANDAU AND
LORI E. SHAPIRO

Acneiform drug eruptions

Acute generalized exanthematous pustulosis

Drug-induced lupus

Drug-induced pseudoporphyria

Fixed drug eruption

Hypersensitivity syndrome reaction

Pigmentary disturbances

Serum sickness-like reactions

Definition

Adverse effects from drugs can be broadly categorized into three groups. The most common are simply idiopathic nuisance side-effects such as mild headache or gastrointestinal upset. The next most common group of adverse effects are pharmacologically mediated and are expected as one increases the dose of a drug. There may be a normal variation in good and bad effects in the population. Ultimately a window of safety can be determined at which the serum concentration or effect of the drug is balanced between being helpful and toxicity. The third group of adverse events are idiosyncratic reactions which are unexpected and not predictable based on the pharmacological reaction of the drug. It is this group of drug reactions as a whole that are considered 'hypersensitivity reactions'. Not only are these reactions unexpected, but they may also be the most severe. Many unexpected or idiosyncratic hypersensitivity reactions have manifestations in the skin.

Diagnosis

The proper diagnosis of drug eruptions requires a four-step approach (Table 27.2.1). These are making the best diagnosis of the eruption, determining the differential diagnosis of the event and the causes, finding every drug that the patient was exposed to and estimating the probability that the drug was responsible for the reaction [1].

Making a diagnosis

The first step in managing an adverse drug reaction (ADR) is to make the proper diagnosis. Reactions in the skin can be diagnosed at three different levels. These are based on the determination of a specific morphology, skin disease or syndrome.

Morphology. The morphology of a drug eruption is usually exanthematous, urticarial or blistering. Sometimes it is not possible to be more specific. Synonyms used for exanthematous reactions are morbilliform, scarlatinaform or toxic erythema. These reactions can progress to erythroderma or exfoliative dermatitis.

Urticarial reactions may represent simple urticaria or be in association with other symptoms or pathological changes, or they may represent an urticarial vasculitis or serum sickness-like reaction (SSLR). Until further diagnostic steps are taken, the urticarial morphology is often the only clue to diagnosis.

Skin disease. Specific diseases would include eruptions as diverse as fixed drug eruption (FDE), acute generalized exanthematous pustulosis (AGEP) or urticaria. These are based on cutaneous findings and the specific diagnosis relates to a purely cutaneous manifestation of a drug eruption without internal organ involvement.

Syndrome. There are many syndromes that fall into the hypersensitivity reaction category and these are associated with cutaneous manifestations as well as internal organ involvement. SSLR and hypersensitivity syndrome reaction (HSR) are two examples.

Differential diagnosis

The second step in diagnosing a drug reaction requires an evolution of the differential diagnosis of the rash or syndrome. Aetiologies that may enter into the discussion, include viral exanthems (infectious mononucleosis, human parvovirus infection, etc.), bacterial infections, Kawasaki's disease and collagen vascular diseases. For erythema multiforme, the common alternative causes

Table 27.2.1 Diagnostic approach to hypersensitivity drug reactions

Diagnosis
Determination of the best diagnosis based on
1 Morphology
   (a) exanthematous
   (b) urticarial
   (c) blistering
   (d) photosensitivity
2 Skin disease (examples)
   (a) fixed drug eruption
   (b) hyperpigmentation
   (c) toxic epidermal necrolysis
   (d) acute generalized exanthematous pustulosis
3 Syndrome (examples)
   (a) serum sickness-like reaction
   (b) hypersensitivity syndrome reaction

Differential diagnosis
List of causes of the best diagnosis, for example exanthematous rash:
   infectious exanthem, drug induced and collagen vascular disease

Drug
Complete drug history, including natural/herbal products

---

include herpes virus and *Mycoplasma* infection [2]. The usual dilemma is that the reaction is believed to be due to a drug, but it is not clear which drug caused it.

Drug exposure

The third step in diagnosing a drug reaction is to determine all drug exposures. All new drugs started within the previous 6 weeks are important, but one should also look for drugs that were used intermittently, including over-the-counter, herbal and natural preparations. A careful history from the patient, their doctor and pharmacist is often needed to get the most complete list of drug exposures.

Probability and causation

The final step in the diagnosis of drug reaction is to determine the probability that each possible cause may have caused the reaction seen. This would include an assessment of each potential cause of the reaction. For example, a patient with a HSR may have a combination of fever, rash and hepatitis that could have been caused by a drug, but might also have been caused by a viral infection, such as human parvovirus. It is up to the clinician to decide the likelihood that each possible cause was responsible for the clinical event. There are sophisticated programmes that have been developed to help with this and require an exhaustive evaluation of the existing literature and a careful evaluation of each of the contributing factors. These contributing factors include the result of stopping the drug (dechallenge), the result of restarting the drug (rechallenge) and, most importantly, timing. The distribu-

tion of the time of onset of drug eruptions is often very specific for the drug and the reaction. This information is often critical in defining the likelihood of a drug causing a reaction [3,4].

Epidemiology

Sparse information is available regarding the incidence of the ADRs in children. The results of a voluntary report system in The Netherlands showed that in the 15-year period spanning 1973–88, 4.5% of reported ADRs had occurred in the paediatric population. Of these 40% had cutaneous manifestations [5]. In a study by Kramer *et al.* [6] ADRs were documented in 4.7% of separate drug courses taken by children. Among the most common reactions were antibiotic-associated rashes [6].

REFERENCES

1 Shear NH. Diagnosing cutaneous adverse reactions to drugs. *Arch Dermatol* 1990; 126: 94–7.
2 Lanctôt KL, Ghajar BM, Shear NH, Naranjo CA. Improving the diagnosis of hypersensitivity reactions associated with sulfonamides. *J Clin Pharmacol* 1994; 34: 1228–33.
3 Prussick R, Knowles S, Shear NH. Cutaneous aspects of drug reactions. *Curr Prob Dermatol* 1994; 6: 83–122.
4 Levy M, Shear NH. *Mycoplasma pneumoniae* infections and Stevens–Johnson syndrome: report of eight cases and analysis of the literature with implications to clinical characteristics, pathogenic and diagnositic critieria. *Clin Pediatr* (Phila) 1991; 30: 42–9.
5 Meyboom RH. Adverse drug reaction to drugs in children, experiences with 'spontaneous monitoring' in The Netherlands. *Bratisl Lek Listy* 1991; 92: 554–9.
6 Kramer MS, Hutchinson TA, Flegel KM *et al.* Adverse drug reactions in general pediatric outpatients. *J Pediatr* 1985; 106: 305–10.

Acneiform drug eruptions

Eruptions morphologically mimicking acne vulgaris, may be associated with drug ingestion. Iodides, bromides, adrenocorticotropic hormone (ACTH), corticosteroids, isoniazid, androgens, lithium, actinomycin D and phenytoin are reported to induce acne-like lesions. Drug-induced acne may appear in atypical areas, such as the legs and arms [1], and be monomorphous. Comedones are usually absent. Acneiform eruptions do not affect prepubertal children, indicating that previous hormonal priming is a necessary prerequisite. Topical tretinoin may be useful, if the drug cannot be stopped [2]. Acne fulminans has been induced by testosterone in 1–2% of adolescent boys treated for excessively tall stature [3]. Acne fulminans has to be managed in the usual aggressive way.

REFERENCES

1 Heng MCY. Cutaneous manifestation of lithium toxicity. *Br J Dermatol* 1982; 106: 107–9.
2 Remmer HI, Falk WE. Successful treatment of lithium-induced acne. *J Clin Psychiatr* 1986; 47: 48.

3 Traupe H, von Muhlendahl KE, Bramswig J, Happle R. Acne of the fulminans type following testosterone therapy in three excessively tall boys. *Arch Dermatol* 1988; 124: 414–17.

Acute generalized exanthematous pustulosis

AGEP is a rare drug reaction pattern, occurring mainly in an adult population. Nevertheless, paediatric cases of AGEP are reported [1].

The eruption starts within days of drug ingestion, typically preceded by a high fever. Cutaneous manifestations begin with an erythematous oedema, soon covered by hundreds of non-follicular sterile pustules. In about half of the patients additional cutaneous lesions are found, such as oedema of the face, target lesions, purpura, vasculitis, blisters and mucosal erosions. Two weeks later, generalized desquamation occurs.

Leucocytosis is a common finding, usually subsiding before desquamation begins. Eosinophilia, relative hypocalcaemia and renal failure have been documented.

Skin biopsy demonstrates spongioform superficial pustulosis with papillary oedema and mixed perivascular infiltrates, which is with or without eosinophils.

AGEP is most commonly associated with β-lactam and macrolide antibiotic usage [1–5], although exposure to mercury is considered to be an aetiological factor in some cases [1]. The short interval to onset (about 5 days) may help to differentiate between AGEP and acute pustular psoriasis.

REFERENCES

1 Roujeau JC, Biolac-Sage P, Bourseau C *et al*. Acute generalized exanthematous pustulosis: analysis of 63 cases. *Arch Dermatol* 1991; 127: 1333–8.
2 Kalb RE, Grossman ME. Pustular eruption following administration of cephadrine. *Cutis* 1986; 38: 58–60.
3 Stough D, Guin JD, Baker GF, Haynie L. Pustular eruption following administration of cefazolin: a possible interaction with methyldopa. *J Am Acad Dermatol* 1987; 16: 1051–2.
4 Jackson H, Vion B, Levy PM. Generalized eruptive pustular drug rush due to cephalexin. *Dermatologica* 1988; 177: 292–4.
5 Shelley ED, Shelley WB. The subcorneal pustular drug eruption: an example induced by norfloxacin. *Cutis* 1988; 42: 24–7.

Drug-induced lupus

Drug-induced lupus (DIL) is defined by the absence of idiopathic lupus, development of antinuclear antibodies (ANAs), at least one clinical symptom of lupus and symptom resolution upon drug withdrawal. The literature contains 24 reports of DIL attributable to minocycline with an additional six cases in abstract form. These reactions occur mainly in females on average of 2 years (3 days to 6 years) after initiation of therapy. The clinical findings are commonly arthritis and hepatitis, and a positive ANA in a homogeneous pattern. Cutaneous eruptions occurred in two patients but the details are lacking. Two

of the reported cases occurred in 16-year-old girls [1–3]. No neurological, renal or vasculitic involvement has been reported which are features typically not found in DIL.

To put these reactions into perspective, they occur only rarely. However, when young women present with polyarthritis and a positive ANA, it is likely to be labelled as idiopathic lupus particularly when the patient has been taking a drug for a prolonged interval prior to the onset of symptoms. It may be appropriate to do baseline antinuclear factor and hepatic transaminases in adolescents on long-term minocycline [4].

REFERENCES

1 Gough A, Chapman S, Wagstaff K, Emery P, Elias E. Minocycline induced autoimmune hepatitis and systemic lupus erythematosus-like syndrome. *Br Med J* 1996; 312: 169–72.
2 Byrne P, Williams B, Pritchard M. Minocycline-related lupus. *Br J Rheum* 1994; 33: 674–6.
3 Matsuura T, Shimizu Y, Fujimoto H, Miyazaki T, Kano S. Minocycline-related lupus. *Lancet* 1992; 340: 1553.
4 Knowles S, Shapiro L, Shear N. Serious adverse reactions induced by minocycline: a report of 13 patients and review of the literature. *Arch Dermatol* 1996; 132: 934–9.

Drug-induced pseudoporphyria

Pseudoporphyria is a cutaneous disorder characterized by skin fragility, blister formation and scarring in sun-exposed areas. This occurs in the setting of normal porphyrin metabolism [1]. A recent sudy demonstrates a prevalence of 12% in naproxen-treated children with juvenile rheumatoid arthritis [2]. Other features of porphyria cutanea tarda such as milia, hypertrichosis, hyperpigmentation and scleroderma are not seen [3].

A second clinical pattern of pseudoporphyria mimics erythropoietic protoporphyria manifest as cutaneous burning, erythema, vesiculation, angular scars and waxy thickening of the skin [4].

The propionic group on non-steroidal anti-inflammatory drugs (NSAIDs) is phototoxic and may cause cell membrane damage due to reactive singlet oxygen created after absorption of ultraviolet radiation in the skin. Because of the risk of permanent facial scarring, it is recommended that naproxen therapy be discontinued as soon as this reaction pattern is recognized.

REFERENCES

1 Suarez SM, Cohen PR, Deleo V. Bullous photosensitivity to naproxen: 'pseudoporphyria'. *Arthritis Rheum* 1990; 33: 903–8.
2 Lang B, Finlayson L. Naproxen-induced pseudoporphyria in patients with juvenile rheumatoid arthritis. *J Pediatr* 1994; 124: 639–42.
3 Bigby M, Stern R. Cutaneous reactions to non-steroidal anti-inflammatory drugs. *J Am Acad Dermatol* 1985; 12: 866–76.
4 Kochevar IE. Phototoxicity of non-steroidal anti-inflammatory drugs. *Arch Dermatol* 1989; 125: 824–6.

Fixed drug eruption

This eruption is characterized by lesions which recur at the same sites, whenever the responsible drug is administered. About 10% of FDEs occur in children and adolescents [1], the youngest reported case being in an 8-month-old infant [2].

The lesions of FDE are well-circumscribed, oval oedematous plaques, dusky brown in colour, covered by a large bulla in some cases. The cardinal morphological feature is a persistent pigmentation following the acute stage. This highly typical hyperpigmentation, makes the diagnosis obvious even weeks after the eruption subsides. Nevertheless, non-pigmenting FDEs are reported in children [3]. A generalized bullous variety occurs, causing confusion with Stevens–Johnson syndrome or TEN [4].

The size of the lesions varies, but their number is usually few. The sites of predilection include the lips, trunk, legs, arms and genitals. In male patients the glans penis is often affected. Local symptoms include pruritis and a burning sensation. Systemic symptoms are rare.

Familial cases of FDE have been published [5], and an association with HLA-B22 antigen has been suggested [6].

Once the patient has acquired an FDE to a drug, rechallenge will almost always result in an immediate recurrence of the existing lesions and appearance of new lesions. Cross-reactivity to chemically related drugs is reported [7]. Oral provocative tests have been suggested to be safe and reliable in children [8]. Patch testing on the site is often useful.

Histology reveals hydropic degeneration of the basal layer which results in pigmentary incontinence. Individual dyskeratotic cells may be found in the epidermis, while the dermis demonstrates superficial or deep perivascular lymphohistiocytic infiltrate with scattered eosinophils. Subepidermal bullae may be present [9].

Although the exact pathogenetic mechanism of FDE remains unknown, a few *in vitro* studies implicated a serum factor with T-suppressor cells playing a major role in mediating the reaction [10,11].

The drugs commonly associated with FDE are barbiturates, sulphonamides, phenolphthalein, tetracyclines, paracetomol, salicylates and NSAIDs [12].

REFERENCES

1 Shakla SR. Drugs causing fixed drug eruption. *Dermatologica* 1981; 11: 160–3.
2 Bharija SC, Singh M, Belhaj MS. Fixed drug eruption in an 8-month-old infant. *Dermatologica* 1988; 176: 108.
3 Shelley WB, Shelley ED. Non-pigmenting fixed drug eruption as a distinctive reaction pattern: examples caused by sensitivity to pseudoephedrine and tetrahydrozoline. *J Am Acad Dermatol* 1987; 17: 403–7.
4 Baird BJ, DeVillez RL. Widespread bullous fixed drug eruption mimicking toxic epidermal necrolysis. *Int J Dermatol* 1988; 27: 170–4.
5 Hatzis J, Noutsis K, Hatxidakis E, Bassioukas K, Perissios A. Fixed drug eruption in a mother and her son. *Cutis* 1992; 50: 50–2.
6 Pellicano R, Ciavarella G, Lomuto M, Di Giorgio G. Genetic susceptibility to fixed drug eruption: evidence for a link with HLA-B22. *J Am Acad Dermatol* 1994; 30: 52–4.
7 Pandhi RK, Bedi TR. Fixed drug eruption caused by oxyphenobutazone with cross-reactivity to phenylbutazone. *Arch Dermatol* 1975; 111: 131.
8 Kanwar AJ, Bharija SC, Belhaj MS. Fixed drug eruptions in children: a series of 23 cases with provocative tests. *Dermatologica* 1986; 172: 315–18.
9 Lever WF, Schaumberg-Lever G. Histopathology of the skin, 7th edn. Philadelphia: JB Lippincott, 1990: 284–5.
10 Hindsen M, Christensen OB, Gruic V, Lofberg H. Fixed drug eruption: an immunohistochemical investigation of the acute and healing phase. *Br J Dermatol* 1987; 116: 351–60.
11 Wyatt E, Greaves M, Sondergaard J. Fixed drug eruption (phenolphthalein): evidence for a blood borne mediator. *Arch Dermatol* 1972; 106: 671–3.
12 Sehgal VN, Gangwani OP. Fixed drug eruption. Current concepts. *Int J Dermatol* 1987; 26: 67–74.

Hypersensitivity syndrome reaction [3]

Clinical features

This is a rare but serious syndrome. For most drugs that cause this condition, the estimate is that it occurs in approximately 1 in 10000 exposures. The syndrome is characterized by the initial onset of fever, subsequent development of a skin rash and the possible involvement of internal organs. Skin manifestations are the first dramatic sign, so dermatologists are the specialists most often consulted for HSR.

HSR occurs most often on the first exposure to the drug. Therefore, this can occur at any age. There is a delayed onset of 7–28 days after the initial exposure to the drug and this depends partly on the drug. For sulphonamide antibiotics, the mean time of onset is 14 days, for phenytoin the mean time is 17–21 days and for carbamazepine reactions may be seen as late as 21–28 days.

The first signs are a fever and malaise. This is often followed by oedema and swelling of the face, especially upon rising in the morning. Patients will develop erythema and itching on the face and the erythema will then spread down the body. Pharyngitis and cervical lymphadenopathy are often early manifestations.

Approximately 85% of patients will develop a rash [1]. This is usually an exanthematous eruption which starts on the face and has many of the features of graft-versus-host disease (Fig. 27.2.1). This may also develop first in photo-exposed areas or, in patients who have received X-ray therapy, it may present in the radiation port. The full reaction will evolve but the photo-exposed or photo-recall type of reaction may precede the fever in these patients.

The authors and others have seen patients who have pustular eruptions as part of the HSR. These can be either non-follicular or perifollicular pustules and may be confused with AGEP or pustular psoriasis [2].

A smaller group of patients will develop a severe cutaneous adverse reaction such as erythema multiforme major, Stevens–Johnson syndrome or toxic epidermal necrolysis (TEN) [3] (Figs 27.2.2–27.2.4) as part of the HSR. In children there is an interesting 'bandit' appearance with

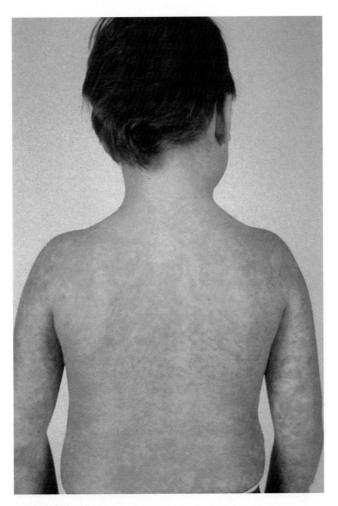

Fig. 27.2.1 A 10-year-old boy who developed fever, an exanthematous eruption and nephritis, 17 days after starting phenobarbital.

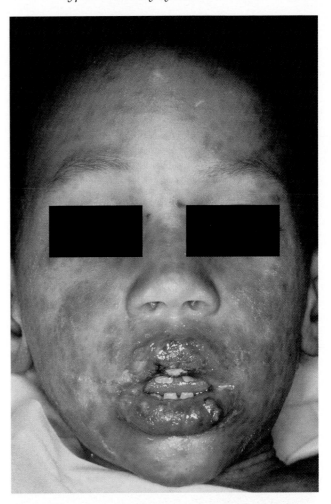

Fig. 27.2.2 A 6-year-old boy who developed Stevens–Johnson syndrome and fever after 10 days of sulphonamide therapy. His rash is characterized by atypical target lesions.

involvement around the eyes and on the hands and feet of severe blistering and epidermal necrosis. This is a form of Stevens–Johnson syndrome that is not usually seen in adults.

There is a reaction with widespread lesions like erythema multiforme minor. These are well-formed, three-ringed, iris lesions that are usually centrifugal, but are more widespread in patients who have the combination of metastatic cancer, cranial X-ray and exposure to phenytoin, and often dexamethasone. This has been reported in adults but could occur in children.

Virtually all patients will have fever and some degree of lymphadenopathy. Fevers can be low grade, but can also be as high as 40°C. The lymphadenopathy is usually cervical, but can be generalized and some patients will have lymph nodes that are then suggestive of the syndrome called pseudolymphoma.

Internal organ involvement may come as late as 1–2 weeks into the reaction, though some patients have had internal organ involvement delayed up to 1 month after

Table 27.2.2 Manifestations of HSR (based on data from anticonvulsant patients) [4]

Reaction	Prevalence (%)
Fever	100
Skin rash	87
Hepatitis	51
Eosinophilia	30
Nephritis	11
Pneumonitis	9
Atypical lymphocytosis	6

the start of the rash. The patterns seen are either inflammatory, reactive or toxic. Patients may have fever, rash and multiple internal organ involvement, or may have a specific organ that is severely affected while others are either mildly affected or spared (Table 27.2.2).

The most common inflammatory reaction is hepatitis. This can range from raised serum transaminases to

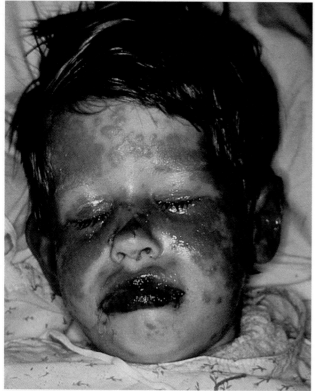

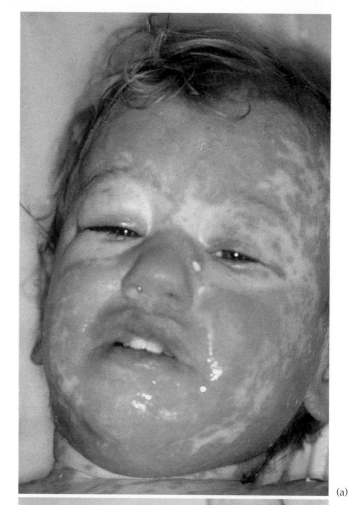

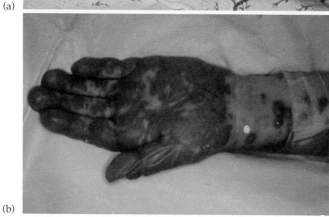

Fig. 27.2.3 (a, b) The face and hand of a 3-year-old boy who developed Stevens–Johnson syndrome, fever and hepatitis after 21 days of phenobarbital therapy. His face shows 'bandit blistering'.

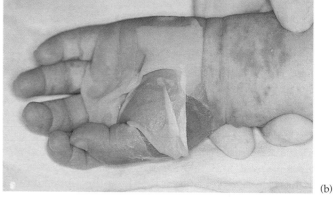

Fig. 27.2.4 (a, b) The face and hand of a 7-year-old boy in whom TEN developed 14 days after starting phenobarbital. He had fever, neutropenia and respiratory distress syndrome.

hepatic necrosis and liver failure. Some patients have had granulomatous hepatitis.

The kidney is the second most common internal organ involved. Patients most often have red cells, white cells or eosinophils in the urine and a renal biopsy compatible with interstitial nephritis. These patients may develop acute renal failure and need transient dialysis. Some patients develop renal vasculitis.

Other less common, but important internal reactions include the central nervous system (encephalitis, aseptic meningitis) and the lungs (mild to severe interstitial pneumonitis, respiratory distress syndrome or vasculitis).

Some patients have had epididymitis and pancreatitis. Patients who complain of limb pain rarely have arthritis, but usually have myositis which can be confirmed by raised serum creatine phosphokinase. Some patients will develop rhabdomyolysis and this can lead to renal failure.

Conjunctivitis can be part of a severe cutaneous reaction, but involvement of the tear ducts leads to a dry-eye syndrome that can ultimately result in corneal scarring and blindness.

Myocarditis is described. Patients have electrocardiographic changes suggestive of pancarditis, but also patients have developed biventricular failure.

Thyroiditis occurs and, early in the reaction, it may be missed because the fever, tachycardia and malaise will appear to be part of the syndrome. At this time, a thyroid-stimulating hormone (TSH) assay will be extremely low and in approximately 2 months, patients will have become hypothyroid as part of an autoimmune-mediated thyroiditis.

Reactive patterns are seen generally in blood tests. While patients have lymphadenopathy, they may also have very raised, atypical lymphocyte counts in the peripheral blood suggesting infectious mononucleosis, but this is part of the drug reaction. Atypical lymphocytosis occurs within the first 2 weeks and a blood or urine eosinophilia generally appears in the second or third week. Some patients have developed ANAs after HSR and it is not clear whether this is an outcome of the disease or an unmasking of an incipient lupus erythematosus.

Toxic changes are seen most commonly in the blood with neutropenia, agranulocytosis or aplastic anaemia. Thrombocytopenia in isolation has also been seen, but may be an autoimmune phenomenon. In patients with aplastic anaemia, an empty bone marrow biopsy will be seen. Patients have also developed Coombs-positive haemolytic anaemia and, because of toxicity to B cells, hypogammaglobulinaemia.

Later findings

In managing patients with this disease, it is not uncommon for the disease to initially improve and then flare 3–4 weeks after the start of the reaction. Patients will redevelop rash, fever, malaise and may have a recurrence of internal organ involvement such as hepatitis. The authors have seen patients who develop a hepatitis that is far worse during recurrence than it was in the original phase.

Between 2 and 3 months after the reaction, some patients will develop hypothyroidism, associated with antimicrosomal antibodies. These are antibodies that are directed against the thyroid peroxidases, oxidative enzymes that were initially involved in the metabolism of the drug [4].

A small group of patients will continue to be troubled with non-specific rashes and malaise for up to 1 year after the reaction. These patients need a lot of reassurance and should be followed closely for the development of longer standing autoimmune diseases such as lupus erythematosus.

In rare instances, where patients have had a second exposure to the drug, the usual reaction is development of fever and erythroderma within hours. This may last for up to a week, but patients generally will recover without sequelae.

Drugs which cause hypersensitivity reaction

Anticonvulsants [1,5]

Phenytoin, phenobarbital and carbamazepine are commonly associated with HSR. There is a risk that if a patient has reacted to one of these three drugs, they will have a 75% chance of also reacting to another. It is not understood how this reaction works, but it does not appear to be an immunological cross-reactivity, but more a shared sensitivity to each compound. Whether there are reactive metabolites that are similar in structure is also not known, but there are clear implications for the management of these patients.

The anticonvulsant lamotrigine is also associated with rashes and most often these are without fever and without incident. However, there are hypersensitivity reactions similar to those seen with phenytoin, phenobarbital and carbamazepine. Whether there is cross-reactivity among lamotrigine and the other anticonvulsants is not known. Lamotrigine reactions may occur more often in those who are on concurrent valproic acid.

Sulphonamide antibiotics and other aromatic amines [6,7]

The sulphonamide antibiotics such as sulphamethoxazole and sulphadiazine are relatively common causes of HSR. The reaction is not based on the sulphur moiety, but on the aromatic amine end of the molecule. Because of that, there is a concern over cross-reactivity to other aromatic amine drugs. These include procainamide, dapsone and acebutolol. Patients can probably use other sulphonamide drugs that are not antibiotics, i.e. sulphonylureas, but must avoid sulphonamide antibiotics in the future.

Minocycline is a drug that is recognized as a cause of HSR [8,9]. Patients have developed reactions 3–4 weeks into therapy with a rash, fever, hepatitis, and so on, similar to the syndrome described above. Cross-reactivity with minocycline and other antibiotics of that class is not clear. There are structural differences in minocycline that may make it more likely to be a cause of HSR and it may make it unique within that class.

Many drugs can cause HSR but these reactions may be missed or misinterpreted because the drugs are used less often than anticonvulsants or sulphonamide antibiotics. Examples are nitrofurantoin, metronidazole and allopurinol [10].

Azathioprine presents as a different syndrome, but it is important to recognize it as a hypersensitivity reaction. Within 1–2 weeks of the start of azathioprine therapy, patients will develop fever, swelling of the face and diarrhoea. The reaction may appear to be minor, but troubling enough for the patient to notify the doctor. On second exposure to azathioprine, patients have gone into shock and this can be potentially lethal. The risk of azathioprine shock is to be recognized and treated with respect [11].

Pathogenesis

The pathogenesis of HSR is not known, but there are clearly pharmacological and immunological steps that are under genetic control [12]. A pharmacological defect results in an imbalance in the clearance of toxic, reactive metabolites of the parent compound. Once the drug is absorbed, reactive metabolites are formed through oxidative metabolism from numerous pathways such as cytochromes P-450 in the liver, myeloperoxidases in white cells, prostaglandin synthetase and other enzymes in the skin and thyroid peroxidases in the thyroid gland.

Studies have used the lymphocyte toxicity assay in which reactive metabolites of the drug are generated *in vitro* by using P-450 sources from mice [1,6,7]. The reactive metabolites are more toxic to the cells of patients than they are to control cells. Detoxification pathways in lymphocytes include glutathione transferases and epoxide hydrolases. The best evidence would suggest that glutathione pathways are involved for sulphonamides and the epoxide hydrolase pathway is involved for anticonvulsants, but this is not proven and is only surmised from *in vitro* studies. It is clear that the defect is inherited and that siblings of patients who have had reactions are at very high risk of having a reaction if exposed to the same drug.

The exact nature of the metabolites is not always known, but work has shown that the sulphonamide metabolite is first a hydroxylamine and, ultimately, a nitroso compound that is very toxic to cells and will react with intracellular proteins and cause direct toxicity to the cell or act as a hapten and elicit an immune response. Metabolites bind to the enzymes that created them and patients have been seen who have antibodies to cytochrome P-450 enzymes. Thyroiditis probably develops in the same way. Patients will metabolize either the sulphonamide or anticonvulsant to reactive metabolite in their thyroid, the metabolite–peroxidase complex is immunogenic, and thyroid peroxidase antibodies are generated. These antibodies are identical to the antimicrosomal antibodies that are seen in the serum of patients with acute lymphocytic thyroiditis [4].

Sulphonamides have other pharmacogenetic aspects. The normal clearance mechanism for sulphonamides in the body is through N-acetylation. North American and European white and black populations are roughly equally divided into slow acetylators (poor metabolizers) or fast acetylators (extensive metabolizers) of sulphonamides. Work has shown that the predominance of

patients who have hypersensitivity reactions are slow acetylators, suggesting that more parent compound is available for oxidative metabolism [13]. An alternate, and probably more likely interpretation of the data, is that patients who are fast acetylators are protected from developing this reaction, even if they have a pharmacogenetic defect in detoxification. There is much work that needs to be done in this area and there may be differences in the two major N-acetyl transferase genes that determine which tissues are involved and which patients have reactions.

For the aromatic anticonvulsants (phenytoin, phenobarbital, carbamazepine), arene oxides have been suspected as the reactive metabolite, but this has never been proven and a defect in epoxide hydrolases is the putative defect.

Management

After HSR has been recognized by the presence of fever, rash and lymphadenopathy on physical examination, there are a minimum of tests that will help to evaluate internal organ involvement which may be asymptomatic: liver transaminases, complete blood count and blood smear examination, urinalysis and serum creatinine. If there are any respiratory symptoms, a chest X-ray should follow. Further testing is guided by history and physical examination. And, if the rash has a blistering or pustular eruption, a biopsy would be helpful.

Patients should be followed closely during this time with follow-up tests in 1 week if there are no abnormalities.

The role of corticosteroids in therapy is still a debatable issue. In acute, drug-induced renal failure, it appears that oral corticosteroids are helpful to prevent dialysis or reduce the amount of time on dialysis. The authors recommend corticosteroids in this situation. If prednisone at a dose of 1–2 mg/k is used, it will often ameliorate symptoms but will need to be used on a continuous basis for up to 2–3 months. It is often best to follow patients and treat them symptomatically, and avoid corticosteroids. In patients who have rapidly advancing TEN and possible internal organ involvement (e.g. respiratory distress syndrome) as part of HSR, the authors have found that pulse methoprednisolone at a dose of 1 g/day, for 3 days, is extremely useful in controlling pain and stopping progression of the disease. While this requires close monitoring for infection and may require prophylactic antibiotics, it can be life-saving. Low-dose corticosteroids for TEN are absolutely contraindicated and will probably increase the risk of side-effects without providing help. Intravenous immunoglobulin (0.75 g/kgld × 4 d) has shown excellent results and is our current treatment for TEN [14].

Patients and their families are informed that the patient should avoid drugs in the same chemical class. Specifically, if they reacted to phenytoin, phenobarbital or carbamazepine, they are told that 75% of patients will react to all of these drugs and they should be avoided. Other anticonvulsants can be used, but most patients will want to be monitored closely. Patients who react to sulphonamide antibiotics should be warned against other sulphonamide antibiotics, as well as dapsone, procainamide and other drugs that may have an aromatic amine structure.

Siblings will be at increased risk compared to the general population and this risk may be as high as 1 in 4 of having a hypersensitivity reaction. This information needs to be transmitted to all siblings of the patient.

At 3 weeks after the initiation of the reaction, patients are assessed for recurrence. Patients are seen again in 3 months for follow-up with specific attention paid to thyroid function. More complex cases or patients who have been started on prednisone will need to be followed much more closely.

Futher research

Ultimately, identification of the genetic defects that lead to drug reactions will occur. This will allow for the screening of populations before they receive the drugs that cause such severe toxicity.

REFERENCES

1 Shear NH, Spielberg SP. Anticonvulsant hypersensitivity syndrome: *in vitro* assessment of risk. *J Clin Invest* 1988; 82: 1826–32.
2 Roujeau JC, Bioulac-Sage P, Bourseau C *et al*. Acute generalized exanthematous pustulosis. *Arch Dermatol* 1991; 127: 1333–8.
3 Bastuji-Garin S, Rzany B, Stern RS *et al*. Clinical classification of cases of toxic epidermal necrolysis, Stevens–Johnson syndrome and erythema multiforme. *Arch Dermalol* 1993; 129: 892–6.
4 Gupta A, Eggo MC, Uetrecht JP *et al*. Drug-Induced hypothyroidism: the thyroid as a target organ in hypersensitivity reactions to anticonvulsants and sulfonamides. *Clin Pharmacol Ther* 1992; 51: 56–67.
5 Chang DKM, Shear NH. Cutaneous reactions to anticonvulsants. *Semin Neurol* 1992; 12: 329–37.
6 Shear NH, Spielberg SP, Grant DM, Tang BK, Kalow W. Differences in metabolism of sulfonamides predisposing to idiosyncratic toxicity. *Ann Intern Med* 1986; 105: 179–84.
7 Rieder MJ, Uetrecht JP, Shear NH *et al*. Diagnosis of sulfonamide hypersensitivity reactions by *in vitro* rechallenge with hydroxylamine metabolites. *Ann Intern Med* 1989; 110: 286–9.
8 Gough A, Chapman S, Wagstaff K, Emery P, Elias E. Minocycline-induced autoimmune hepatitis and systemic lupus erythematosus-like syndrome. *Br Med J* 1996; 312: 169–72.
9 Knowles SR, Shapiro L, Shear NH. Serious adverse reactions induced by minocycline: report of 13 cases and review of the literature. *Arch Dermatol* 1996; 132:934–9.
10 Knowles S, Choudhury T, Shear NH. Metronidazole hypersensitivity. *Ann Pharmacother* 1994; 28: 325–6.
11 Knowles SR, Gupta AK, Shear NH, Sauder DN. Azathioprine hypersensitivity-like reactions: a case report and a review of the literature. *Clin Exp Dermatol* 1995; 20: 353–6.
12 Park BK, Tirmohamed M, Kitteringham NR. The role of cytochrome P450 enzymes in hepatic and extra hepatic human drug toxicity. *Pharmaco Ther* 1995; 18: 385–424.
13 Rieder MJ, Shear NH, Kanee A *et al*. Prominence of slow acetylator phenotype among patients with sulfonamide hypersensitivity reactions. *Clin Pharmacol Ther* 1991; 49: 13–17.
14 Viard I, Wehrli P, Bullani R, *et al*. Inhibition of toxic epidermal necrolysis by blockards of CD95 with human intravenous immunoglobulin. *Science* 1998; 282: 490–3.

Pigmentary disturbances

More generalized pigmentary disturbances than those seen with FDE can occur in association with the administration of a variety of drugs. Many of these pigmentary disturbances tend to be more pronounced in sun-exposed areas, suggesting that photochemical changes may be responsible. Chronic therapy and inflammation are also risk factors for some drug-induced pigmentation.

Minocycline, a tetracycline antibiotic is widely prescribed for acne because of its safety and efficacy. Minocycline among the tetracyclines is noted for its ability to cause grey pigmentation most apparent in areas of chronic inflammation and brown discoloration in a generalized distribution with accentuation in sun-exposed areas [1]. Mucus membranes and acral areas may be involved. A recent study comparing the side-effect profile of minocycline at doses of 100 mg, 100/200 mg on alternate days and 200 mg daily revealed an incidence of side-effects of 2%. The pigmentary disturbance was the only side-effect that was clearly dose related with a 10-fold increase in pigmentation associated with higher doses [2].

Histology and electron microscopy suggest haemosiderin or a pigment with haemosiderin staining properties is responsible for the blue–grey discoloration found in sites of cutaneous inflammation. Increased melanin in the basal layer and dermal melanophages may correlate with the muddy-brown discoloration [3].

REFERENCES

1 Basler RS. Minocycline-related hyperpigmentation. *Arch Dermatol* 1985; 121: 606–8.
2 Goulden V, Glass D, Cunliffe WJ. Safety of long-term high-dose minocycline in the treatment of acne. *Br J Dermatol* 1996; 134: 693–5.
3 Fenske N, Millns J, Greer K. Minocycline-induced pigmentation at sites of cutaneous inflammation. *J Am Med Assoc* 1980; 244: 1103–6.

Serum sickness-like reactions

SSLRs are defined by the presence of fever, rash (usually urticarial), arthralgia and lymphadenopathy 1–3 weeks after drug ingestion. In contrast to true serum sickness, immune complexes, hypocomplementaemia, vasculitis and renal lesions are absent [1]. Most cases have occurred after repeated exposures to the suspect drug. No mortality or renal failure attributable to SSLRs are reported.

Epidemiological studies in children have suggested that the risk of SSLRs is greater with cefaclor as compared to other antibiotic therapy, including other cephalosporins. A retrospective cohort study estimated the risk of SSLR in children after antibiotic exposure by review of the computerized outpatient records of the Harvard Community Health Plan [2]. The relative risk of SSLRs for cefaclor versus amoxicillin was 19:1 and for sulphonamides versus amoxicillin, it was 12:1. Using the database of the World Health Organization Collaborating Center for International Drug Monitoring, there were 722 reports of SSLRs to cefaclor compared to 34 for amoxicillin and 12 for cephalexin [3]. Therefore, according to prospective and retrospective data, the estimated pooled incidence of cefaclor related SSLR varies from 0.02 to 0.2% per drug course in paediatric patients.

While the pathogenesis is unknown, Kearns *et al.* have postulated that in genetically susceptible hosts, a reactive cefaclor metabolite is generated during its metabolism that may bind with tissue proteins and elicit an inflammatory response manifesting as a SSLR [4].

Treatment is symptomatic with antihistamines and topical antipruritics. The culprit drug should be discontinued. More severe symptoms such as arthralgia/arthritis may benefit from a short course of oral corticosteroids. Patients are advised to avoid the specific drug in the future. The cefaclor SSLR appears to be specific for this cephalosporin [5].

REFERENCES

1 Hebert A, Sigam E, Levy M. Serum sickness-like reactions from cefaclor in children. *J Am Acad Dermatol* 1991; 25: 805–8.
2 Heckbert S, Stryker W, Coltin K, Manson J, Platt R. Serum sickness in children after antibiotic exposure: estimates of occurrence and morbidity in a Health Maintenance Organization population. *Am J Epidemiol* 1990; 132: 336–42.
3 Stricker BH, Tijssen JG. Serum sickness-like reactions to cefaclor. *J Clin Epidemiol* 1992; 45: 1177–84.
4 Kearns G, Wheeler J, Childress S, Letzig L. Serum sickness-like reactions to cefaclor: role of hepatic metabolism and individual susceptibility. *J Pediatr* 1994; 125: 805–11.
5 Lowery N, Kearns G, Young R, Wheeler JG. Serum sickness-like reactions associated with cefprozil therapy. *J Pediatr* 1994; 125: 325–8.

27.3 Poisoning and Paediatric Skin

GIUSEPPE MICALI AND DENNIS P. WEST

Percutaneous route of poisoning
Fundamentals of percutaneous absorption
Percutaneous absorption and systemic toxicity

Drugs

Chemicals

Cutaneous symptoms following inhalation, ingestion or injection of some toxicants

Poisoning can be classified according to the type of toxicity produced. Drugs may have a direct toxic effect: they are inherently toxic at some doses without being metabolically altered or chemically combined with other substances. Some drugs may demonstrate toxicity through interference with metabolic processes. Other drugs may be hazardous after conversion to a toxic metabolite [1].

Poisoning is usually associated with acute exposure to a toxic agent. Chronic poisoning is described as toxicity produced over a prolonged period of time; it usually relates to accumulation of a toxic agent in the host, with resulting damage to affected tissues and organ systems [1]. Fatal or near-fatal effects have resulted from accidental as well as intentional ingestion, inhalation, injection or skin exposure to a toxic agent.

Systemic poisoning from percutaneous absorption of certain substances (i.e. lead, mercury) is well known [2] and may also produce fatal or near-fatal effects without cutaneous symptoms [3,4]. Alternatively, systemic poisoning by ingestion, inhalation or injection may produce cutaneous signs. For substances or drugs causing cytotoxic reactions through an immunological mechanism see Chapter 27.2.

Any given toxic agent will pass through one or more portals of entry, although at possibly different rates. The most frequent modes of entry are percutaneous, gastrointestinal and respiratory routes [1].

In general, the respiratory route provides the most rapid rate of entry and the percutaneous route the least rapid, although overall entry depends both on the amount of toxic agent present and saturability of the epithelium involved [1].

Route of entry may be either of minor consideration or highly significant depending on the poison and whether it is a liquid, solid or gas [5]. The circulatory system typically offers an excellent carrier system for a poison because it can accommodate both water-soluble as well as lipid-soluble compounds via its aqueous component or by its protein composition. Blood proteins may serve to bind a toxicant for release at a tissue remote from the site of entry. Such transport may carry the poison to a site of toxic action, a site of metabolism, a site of storage or to an organ of elimination. All of these events may occur simultaneously, and the resulting dynamic flux makes the study of poisoning quite complex [1].

REFERENCES

1 Guthrie FA, Hodgson E. Absorption and distribution of toxicants. In: Hodgson E, Levi PE, eds. *Modern Toxicology*. New York: Elsevier, 1987.
2 Vale JA, Meredith TJ. Poisoning. In: Barltrop D, Brueton MJ, eds. *Pediatric Therapeutics. Principles and Practice*. Oxford: Butterworth-Heinemann, 1990.
3 Emmett EA. Toxic response of the skin. In: Amdur MO, Doull J, Klaassen KD, eds. *Toxicology. The Basic Science of Poison*, 4th edn. New York: Pergamon Press, 1991.
4 Leikin JB, Paloucek FP. *Poisoning and Toxicology Handbook*. Hudson: Levi-Comp, 1995.
5 Rosenstock L, Culle MR. *Textbook of Clinical, Occupational and Environmental Medicine*. Philadelphia: WB Saunders, 1994.

Percutaneous route of poisoning

The skin is a membrane that is relatively impermeable to most ions as well as aqueous solutions. However, it is permeable to a large number of toxicants in the solid, liquid or gaseous phases. The skin not only serves as a passive barrier to diffusion but also plays a role in the biotransformation of topically applied substances before they enter the systemic circulation. The epidermis accounts for a major portion of biochemical transformation within skin, although total metabolic activity within skin is relatively low compared to some other organs [1].

The full-term infant has a well-developed epidermis which, similarly to adults, possesses excellent barrier properties. By contrast, the infant who is born prematurely, particularly before 22 weeks of gestation, has a thin epidermis with a poorly developed stratum corneum (SC). Although rapid postnatal maturation of the epidermis occurs over the first 2–3 weeks of age [2] the preterm infant's skin is a poor barrier in this early neonatal period [3] and this may result in increased absorption through the percutaneous route.

Moreover, as the ratio of surface area to body weight in the newborn is approximately three times that of the adult, given an equal area of application of a drug to the skin of the newborn and adult, the proportion absorbed per kilogram of body weight is much more in the infant [4].

REFERENCES

1 Riviere JE. Predicting percutaneous absorption. *Acta Pharm Nord* 1992; 4: 119–20.
2 Evans NJ, Rutter N. Development of the epidermis in the newborn. *Biol Neonate* 1986; 49: 74–80.
3 Harpin VA, Rutter N. Barrier properties of the newborn infant's skin. *J Pediatr* 1983; 102: 419–25.
4 Freeman S, Maibach HI. Systemic toxicity in man secondary to percutaneous absorption. In: Marks R, Plewig G, eds. *The Environmental Threat to the Skin.* London: Martin Dunitz, 1992.

Fundamentals of percutaneous absorption

For percutaneous absorption to occur, a topically administered drug must diffuse through the SC and be absorbed into the inner epidermis and dermis. The drug must be in solution and penetrate readily through the vehicle and SC. Many drugs for topical use on the skin are capable of producing systemic side-effects, the occurrence and severity of which depend largely on the following factors: (a) physicochemical properties of the drug, such as molecular weight and size, water and lipid solubility; (b) chemical and physical properties of the vehicle; (c) drug concentration in the vehicle; (d) thickness of the SC; and (e) temperature, humidity, occlusion and presence of skin diseases or damage [1–3] (see Chapter 27.1).

REFERENCES

1 Micali G, Distefano G. Percutaneous absorption in neonates: a review. *G Int Dermatol Pediatr (Italy)* 1989; 1: 31–8.
2 Rasmussen JE. Percutaneous absorption in children. In: Dobson RL, ed. *Year Book of Dermatology.* Chicago: Year Book Medical, 1979.
3 Ghadially R, Shear NH. Topical therapy and percutaneous absorption. In: Yaffe SJ, Aranda JV, eds. *Pediatric Pharmacology. Therapeutic Principles in Practice,* 2nd edn. Philadelphia: WB Saunders, 1992.

Percutaneous absorption and systemic toxicity

Several drugs and chemicals have been reported as the cause of systemic toxicity by percutaneous absorption in newborns and infants [1]. The ability of a substance to cause systemic toxicity by percutaneous absorption depends on its capability for penetration of the epidermis with some entry by way of follicular and sweat duct routes and subsequently entry into the systemic circula-

Table 27.3.1 Examples of compounds reported to produce systemic toxicity after percutaneous absorption in paediatric patients

Drugs	
Adrenaline	Malathion
Benzocaine	Mercurials
Boric acid	Methanol
Camphor	Neomycin
Castellani's solution	Oestrogens
Chlorhexidine	Phenol
Cocaine	*Podophyllum* resin
Corticosteroids	Promethazine
Diethyltoluamide	Resorcinol
Diphenhydramine	Salicylic acid
Diphenylpyraline	Silver nitrate
Ethanol	Tars
Hexachlorophene	Warfarin
Iodine	*Chemicals*
Isopropanol	Aniline dye
Lidocaine	Carbon tetrachloride
Lindane	Naphthalene
Mafenide	Paraquat

tion from the dermis. There are a number of toxicants, especially lipophilic substances, such as organophosphate insecticides and polychlorinated biphenyls, that penetrate the skin quite readily [2,3].

Systemic toxicity via percutaneous absorption may result either from unintended absorption of compounds used for the treatment of a dermatological disorder as well as from accidental absorption of compounds used for non-dermatological purposes [4–6] (Table 27.3.1).

REFERENCES

1 West DP, Worobec S, Solomon LM. Pharmacology and toxicity of infant skin. *J Invest Dermatol* 1981; 76: 147–50.
2 Emmett EA. Toxic responses of the skin. In: Amdur MO, Doull J, Klaassen CD, eds. *Casarett and Doull's Toxicology. The Basic Science of Poisons,* 4th edn. New York: Pergamon Press, 1991.
3 Stoughton RB. Percutaneous absorption of drugs. *Ann Rev Pharmacol Toxicol* 1989; 29: 55–69.
4 Litovitz TL, Felberg L, Soloway RA, Ford M, Geller R. 1994 annual report of the American Association of Poisoning Control Centers Toxic Exposure Surveillance System. *Am J Emerg Med* 1995; 13: 551–97.
5 Knight M. Adverse drug reactions in neonates. *J Clin Pharmacol* 1996; 34: 128–35.
6 Malloy-McDonald MB. Skin care for high-risk neonates. *J Wound Ostomy Cont Nurs* 1995; 22: 177–82.

Drugs

Adrenaline

Adrenaline (1:1000, 0.1 ml) applied locally to a haemorrhaging circumcision in a 2-day-old infant produced local and systemic effects. The infant became tachycardic and had local pallor of the penis and base of the shaft. He also had perioral pallor and acrocyanosis [1].

REFERENCE

1 Denton J, Schreiner RL, Pearson J. Circumcision complication. Reaction to treatment of local hemorrhage with topical epinephrine in high concentration. *Clin Pediatr* 1978; 17: 285–6.

Benzocaine

Topical application of benzocaine to both the skin and mucous membranes may cause methaemoglobinaemia [1–5]. A majority of cases are infants.

REFERENCES

1 Rodriguez LF, Smolik LM, Zbehlik AJ. Benzocaine-induced methemoglobinemia: report of a severe reaction and review of the literature. *Ann Pharmacother* 1994; 28: 643–9.
2 Eldadah M, Fitzgerald M. Methemoglobinemia due to skin application of benzocaine. *Clin Pediatr* 1993; 32: 687–8.
3 Olson ML, McEvoy GK. Methemoglobinemia induced by local anesthetics. *Am J Hosp Pharm* 1981; 38: 89–93.
4 Steinberg JB, Zepernick RGL. Methemoglobinemia during anesthesia. *J Pediatr* 1962; 61: 885–6.
5 Haggerty RJ. Blue baby due to methemoglobinemia. *N Engl J Med* 1962; 267: 1303.

Boric acid

Boric acid may be present in talcum powders, ointments and solutions in 5–10% concentrations. There are numerous reports of boric acid toxicity in premature or newborn infants after topical application of talcum powders and solutions in the treatment of diaper dermatitis or burns [1–5]. Usually, the patients developed nausea, vomiting, diarrhoea, erythrodermic rash, central nervous system (CNS) irritability and in severe cases renal failure and shock, sometimes leading to death [4–8]. Extensive desquamation occurred 1–2 days after the onset of rash. Although concentrated boric acid is not commonly available for topical application today, caution is in order because the chemical itself is still readily available [9].

REFERENCES

1 Skipworth GB, Goldstain N, McBride WP. Boric acid intoxication from 'medicated talcum powder'. *Arch Dermatol* 1967; 95: 83–6.
2 Baker DH, Wilson RE. The lethality of boric acid in the treatment of burns. *J Am Med Assoc* 1963; 186: 1169–70.
3 Goldbloom RB, Goldbloom A. Boric acid poisoning—report of four cases and a review of 109 cases from the world literature. *J Pediatr* 1953; 43: 631–43.
4 Ducey J, Williams DB. Transcutaneous absorption of boric acid. *J Pediatr* 1953; 43: 644–51.
5 Brooke C, Boggs T. Boric-acid poisoning: report of a case and review of the literature. *Am J Dis Child* 1951; 82: 465–72.
6 Rubenstein AD, Musher DM. Epidemic boric acid poisoning simulating staphilococcal toxic epidermal necrolysis of the newborn infant: Ritter's disease. *J Pediatr* 1970; 77: 884–7.
7 Fisher R, Freimuth HC, O'Conner KAO. Boron absorption from borated talc. *J Am Med Assoc* 1995; 157: 503–5.
8 Valdes-Dapena MA, Arey JB. Boric acid poisoning. Three fatal cases with pancreatic inclusions and a review of the literature. *J Pediatr* 1962; 61: 531–46.
9 Siegel E, Wason S. Boric acid toxicity. *Pediatr Clin N Am* 1986; 33: 363–7.

Camphor

Topical camphor is most commonly used as an antiseptic and rubefacient. In remedies for the common cold, it is often used by application to the chest or via a vaporizer. It has also been used as a topical analgesic for herpes simplex [1].

Although the majority of reported cases are due to oral ingestion, some case reports in infants have described systemic toxicity following topical application of a camphorated ointment [2–5]. An unusual case is that of a 7-year-old white male who had normal growth and development until the age of 15 months, when he developed serious alteration in cerebral function after skin exposure by crawling through spirits-of-camphor spilled by a sibling [2]. One year later, a brief major motor seizure occurred after inhalation of a camphorated vaporizer preparation. When considering the risks versus benefits, some authors emphasize that there is essentially no rationale for the continued use of topical camphor products in children [3,5].

REFERENCES

1 Siegel E, Wason S. Camphor toxicity. *Pediatr Clin N Am* 1986; 33: 375–80.
2 Skoglund RR, Ware LL, Schanberger JE. Prolonged seizures due to contact and inhalation exposure to camphor. A case report. *Clin Pediatr* 1977; 16: 901–2.
3 Calvelli MM, Pesenti P, Ronconi GF. Poisoning caused by the cutaneous application of camphorated balsam ointment in a nursing infant. *Pediatr Med Chir* 1987; 9: 513–14.
4 Joly C, Bouillie C, Hummel M. Acute poisoning by camphor administered externally in an infant. *Ann Pediatr* 1980; 27: 395–6.
5 Dupeyron JP, Quattrocchi F, Castaing H, Fabiani P. Acute poisoning of an infant by cutaneous application of a local counterirritant and pulmonary antiseptic salve. *J Eur Toxicol* 1976; 9: 313–20.

Castellani's solution

Castellani's solution (or paint) has been used for the local treatment of fungal skin infections. Its ingredients include boric acid, fuchsin, resorcinol, water, phenol, acetone and ethanol. The application of Castellani's solution to napkin dermatitis and other areas, where absorption is enhanced, may cause serious complications as reported in a 6-month-old boy who became cyanotic and methaemoglobinaemic after two applications of Castellani's solution to the napkin area [1]. Another case is that of a 6-week-old infant who, some hours after the application of Castellani's paint to the entire body surface except the face for the treatment of a severe seborrhoeic eczema, became drowsy and had shallow breathing and blue urine [2]. Another 16 infants with seborrhoeic eczema were painted twice daily for 48 h in the napkin area and skin folds, and phenol was detected in the urine of four patients [2].

REFERENCES

1 Lundell E, Nordman R. A case of infantile poisoning by topical application of Castellani's solution. *Ann Clin Res* 1973; 5: 404–6.
2 Rogers SCF, Burrows D, Neill D. Percutaneous absorption of phenol and methyl alcohol in Magenta Paint BPC. *Br J Dermatol* 1978; 98: 559–60.

Chlorhexidine

Chlorhexidine, an antimicrobial skin cleanser, has been detected in low levels in the serum of preterm and term neonates with intact skin, after standard bathing. Although no clinical toxic effects were documented, there were more positive results in preterm babies [1].

REFERENCE

1 Cowen J, Ellis SH, McAinsh J. Absorption of chlorhexidine from the intact skin of newborn infants. *Arch Dis Child* 1979; 54: 379–83.

Cocaine

There are reports of hypertension and seizures after application of a solution of tetracaine 0.5%, adrenaline 0.05% and cocaine 11.8% (TAC) to burns or mucous membranes of children, raising concern for potential toxicity during routine use [1–3]. Documentation of cocaine serum levels in 75% of 77 children 15 min after application of TAC has raised additional concerns [4]. There is a report in the literature of a 7-month-old child who died after 10 ml of TAC was applied to a lip laceration [5].

REFERENCES

1 Bonadio WA. TAC; a review. *Pediatr Emerg Care* 1989; 5: 128–30.
2 Wehner D, Hamilton GC. Seizures following topical application of local anesthetics to burn patients. *Ann Emerg Med* 1984; 13: 456–8.
3 Daya MR, Burton BT, Schleiss MR *et al.* Recurrent seizure following mucosal application of TAC. *Ann Emerg Med* 1988; 17: 646–8.
4 Terndrup TE, Walls HC, Mariani PJ, Gavula DP, Madden CM, Cantor RM. Plasma cocaine and tetracaine levels following application of topical anesthesia in children. *Ann Emerg Med* 1992; 21: 162–6.
5 Dailey RH. Fatality secondary to misuse of TAC solution. *Ann Emerg Med* 1988; 17: 159–60.

Corticosteroids

Systemic effects resulting from percutaneous absorption of steroids have been well documented in children. Major risk factors include occlusion and use of high or very high potency steroids [1,2].

Chronic suppression of adrenal function and impairment of growth are significant risk factors in infants and children treated with high potency topical corticosteroids [1,2].

REFERENCES

1 Munro DD. The effect of percutaneously absorbed steroids in hypothalamic–pituitary–adrenal function after intensive use in patients. *Br J Dermatol* 1976; 94(S): 67–76.
2 Borzyskowski M, Grant DB, Wells RS. Cushing's syndrome induced by topical steroids used for the treatment of non-bullous ichthyosiform erythroderma. *Clin Exp Dermatol* 1976; 1: 337–42.

Diethyltoluamide

Diethyltoluamide (DEET) has been used as an insect repellent for several decades. Although it has an overall low incidence of toxic effects [1], use of high concentrations or prolonged use in children is discouraged because of reports of toxic encephalopathy [2–7].

Cases have been reported where major motor seizure activity occurred following brief cutaneous exposure to DEET [8,9].

REFERENCES

1 Osimitz TG, Grothaus RH. The present safety assessment of deet. *J Am Mosquito Control Assoc* 1995; 11: 274–8.
2 Edwards DL, Johnson CE. Insect-repellent-induced toxic encephalopathy in a child. *Clin Pharm* 1987; 6: 496–8.
3 Grybowksy J, Weinstein D, Ordway NK. Toxic encephalopathy apparently related to the use of an insect repellent. *N Engl J Med* 1961; 264: 289–91.
4 Heick HMC, Shipman RT, Norman MG *et al.* Reye-like syndrome associated with use of insect repellent in a presumed heterozygote for ornithine carbamoyl transferase deficiency. *J Pediatr* 1980; 97: 471–3.
5 de Garbino JP, Laborde A. Toxicity of an insect repellent: *N-N*-diethyltoluamide. *Vet Hum Toxicol* 1983; 25: 422–3.
6 Zadicoff CM. Toxic encephalopathy associated with use of insect repellent. *J Pediatr* 1979; 95: 140–2.
7 Orasky S, Roseman B, Fish D *et al.* Seizures temporally associated with use of DEET insect repellent. New York and Connecticut. *MMWR* 1989; 38: 678–80.
8 Roland EH, Jan JE, Rigg JM. Toxic encephalopathy in a child after brief exposure to insect repellents. *Canad Med Assoc J* 1985; 132: 155–6.
9 Lipscomb JW, Kramer JE, Leikin JB. Seizure following brief exposure to the insect repellent *N,N*-diethyl-*m*-toluamide. *Ann Emerg Med* 1992; 21: 315–17.

Diphenhydramine

Diphenhydramine hydrochloride toxicity has been frequently described in children [1–5] after topical application of lotions and sprays for treatment of severe itching [1].

REFERENCES

1 Chan CY, Wallander KA. Diphenhydramine toxicity in three children with varicella-zoster infection. *Drug Intell Clin Pharm* 1991; 25: 130–2.
2 Bernhardt DT. Topical diphenhydramine toxicity. *Wisc Med J* 1991; 90: 469–71.
3 Reilly JF Jr, Weisse ME. Topically induced diphenhydramine toxicity. *J Emerg Med* 1990; 8: 59–61.
4 Huston RL, Cypcar D, Cheng GS, Foulds DM. Toxicity from topical administration of diphenhydramine in children. *Clin Pediatr* 1990; 29: 542–5.
5 Patranella P. Diphenhydramine toxicity due to topical application of Caladryl. *Clin Pediatr* 1986; 25: 163.

Diphenylpyraline

Diphenylpyraline hydrochloride has been used topically in Germany for the treatment of eczematous and other itching dermatoses. Its use caused symptomatic psychosis in 12 patients, nine of whom were children. The amount of active drug applied ranged from 225 to 1350 mg. Symptoms included psychomotor restlessness, disorientation, optic and acoustic hallucinations, all of which disappeared within 4 days after discontinuation of the offending agent [1].

REFERENCE

1 Camman R, Hennecke H, Beier R. Symptomatische Psychosen nack Kolton-Gelee-Applikation. *Psychiat Neurol Med Psycol* 1971; 23: 426–31.

Ethanol

Ethanol is a commonly used topical antiseptic in newborn nurseries for numerous procedures such as venepuncture and arterial cannulation. It primarily evaporates from the surface of the skin, but some degree of percutaneous absorption is known to occur.

Twenty-eight children of both genders ranging in age from 3 months to 1 year, presented with alcohol intoxication from percutaneous absorption [1]. The poisoning occurred in Argentina where it was a popular procedure to apply alcohol-soaked cloths to the abdomens of babies as a home remedy for the treatment of disturbances of the gastrointestinal tract such as cramps, pain, vomiting and diarrhoea, or because of crying, excitability and irritability. Alcohol-soaked cloths had been applied on the babies' abdomen under rubber pants, and the number of applications varied from one to three; it was estimated that each application contained approximately 40 ml ethanol. Medical consultation took place from 1 to 23 h after application. Alcoholic breath and abdominal erythema were valuable clues to the diagnosis. All 28 children showed some degree of CNS depression, 24 showed miosis, 15 hypoglycaemia, five convulsions, five respiratory depression and two died. Eleven children had blood alcohol levels of 0.6–1.49 g%. Of the two who died, one was autopsied: the findings were consistent with ethyl alcohol intoxication.

Other reported cases of alcohol intoxication from percutaneous absorption include a preterm infant treated with local application of alcohol-soaked compresses on the legs to relieve hypodermic needle-induced haematomas [2].

A 2-year-old child treated with alcohol-soaked bandages applied to damaged skin [3] and a 1-month-old child who was found to be intoxicated from ethanol-soaked gauze pads which had been applied to the umbilical stump and contiguous skin over several days for the purpose of promoting umbilical cord detachment [4] have been recorded.

REFERENCES

1 Gimenez ER, Vallejo NE, Roy E et al. Percutaneous alcohol intoxication. *Clin Toxicol* 1968; 1: 39.
2 Castot A, Garnier R, Lanfranchi C et al. Effects systemiques indesiderables des medicaments appliqué sur la peau, chez l'enfant. A propos de quelques observations. *Therapie* 1980; 35: 423–32.
3 Puschel K. Percutaneous alcohol intoxication. *Eur J Pediatr* 1981; 136: 317–18.
4 Dalt LD, Dall'Amico R, Laverda AM, Chemollo C, Chianetti L. Percutaneous ethyl alcohol intoxication in a 1-month old infant. *Pediatr Emerg Care* 1991; 7: 343–4.

Hexachlorophene

Hexachlorophene was widely used in nurseries for the prevention of *Staphylococcus aureus* infection. In 1972 in France, as a result of the accidental addition of 6.3% of hexachlorophene to batches of baby talcum powder, 204 babies fell ill and 36 died from respiratory arrest [1]. Several other cases of hexachlorophene myelinopathy caused by percutaneous absorption in premature infants have been reported [2–8].

Among affected infants, common findings were the presence of skin rash or wounds, prematurity with low birth weight and repeated exposure to hexachlorophene. Factors contributing to hexachlorophene toxicity in infants include multiple exposures to the drug, increased drug concentration, absence of adequate rinsing, presence of large areas of abraded skin, hepatic, biliary or renal disease and low birth weight. Ultraviolet (UV) lights help to dechlorinate (detoxify) hexachlorophene and exert a protective effect. Although rarely used now, and not recommended, general suggestions for use of hexachlorophene have included: limit exposure to one or two baths with accurate thorough rinsing; and do not use in infants under 1200 g or under 35 weeks of age or on large areas of abraded skin, with hepatic dysfunction [9,10].

REFERENCES

1 Martin-Bouyer G, Lebreton R, Toga M et al. Outbreak of accidental hexachlorophene poisoning in France. *Lancet* 1982; i: 91–5.
2 Chilcote R, Curley A, Loughlin HH, Jupin JA. Hexachlorophene storage in a burn patient associated with encephalopathy. *Pediatrics* 1977; 59: 457–9.
3 Larregue M, Laidet B, Ramdene P, Djeridi A. Caustic diaper dermatitis and encephalitis secondary to the application of talcum contaminated with hexachlorophene. *Ann Dermatol Vénéréol* 1984; 111: 789–97.
4 Marquardt ED. Hexachlorophene toxicity in a pediatric burn patient. *Drug Intell Clin Pharm* 1986; 20: 624.
5 Shuman RM, Leech RW, Albord EC. Neurotoxicity of hexachlorophene in humans. II. A clinicopathological study of 46 premature infants. *Arch Neurol* 1975; 32: 320–5.
6 Goutieres F, Arcardi J. Accidental percutaneous hexachlorophene intoxication in children. *Br Med J* 1977; 2: 663–5.
7 Curley A, Hawk RE, Kimbrough RD et al. Dermal absorption of hexachlorophane in infants. *Lancet* 1971; ii: 296–7.
8 Powell H, Swarmer O, Gluck L et al. Hexachlorophene myelinopathy in premature infants. *J Pediatr* 1973; 82: 976–81.

9 Menni S, Piccinno R. Cloro e cute infantile. *G Ital Dermatol Venereol* 1994; 129: 471–6.
10 Tryala EE, Hillman LS, Hillman RE *et al*. Clinical pharmacology of hexachlorophene in newborn infants. *J Pediatr* 1977; 91: 481–6.

Iodine

Iodine has been reported to be absorbed percutaneously [1]. Twenty-one neonates admitted to an intensive care unit repeatedly received skin preparation with iodine antiseptic, and all showed significantly high levels of TSH and low free triiodothyronine (T3). Urinary iodine was also significantly increased [2]. Povidone iodine is a water-soluble iodine complex which retains the broad-range microbicidal activity of iodine but minimizes the undesirable effects of iodine tincture. However, toxicity may still occur with topical povidone iodine, primarily when it is used on large areas of burned skin or on neonates [3].

REFERENCES

1 Chabrolle JP, Rossier A. Goitre and hypothyroidism in the newborn after cutaneous absorption of iodine. *Arch Dis Child* 1978; 53: 495–8.
2 Vilain E, Bompard Y, Clement K, Laplanche S, de Kermadec S, Aufrant C. Brief antiseptic application of iodine in neonatal intensive care units: effects on thyroid function. *Arch Pediatr* 1994; 1: 795–800.
3 Mofenson HC, Caraccio TR, Greensher J. Iodine. In: Haddad LM, Winchester JF, eds. *Poisoning and Drug Overdose*. Philadelphia: WB Saunders, 1983.

Isopropanol

After preoperative skin disinfection in paediatric surgery, 26 children had detectable serum levels of isopropanol [1].

REFERENCE

1 Wittmann S, Gilg T, Dietz HG, Grantzow R, Peschel O, von Meyer L. Isopropanol and acetone level in serum after preoperative surface disinfectant with antiseptics containing isopropanol. *Blutalkohol* 1992; 29: 326–35.

Lidocaine

Lidocaine hydrochloride is widely used for both topical and local injection anaesthesia. Serum lidocaine concentrations higher than 6 µg/ml have been associated with toxicity [1]. Clinical signs include those of CNS stimulation followed by depression and subsequent inhibition of cardiovascular function. Systemic toxicity from viscous lidocaine applied to the oral cavity in two children has been reported [2,3]. In one, the mother had been applying lidocaine hydrochloride 2% solution to the infant's gums with her finger five to six times daily for 1 week; the child experienced two generalized seizures within 1 h. The other child had a seizure after having received 227.8 mg/kg oral viscous lidocaine for stomatitis herpetica over a 24-h period. In this case, however, ingestion and absorption from the gastrointestinal tract may have contributed to the clinical picture. It has been suggested that for paediatric patients viscous lidocaine should be applied with an oral swab to individual lesions, thus limiting oral ingestion and buccal absorption by decreasing the surface area exposed to lidocaine [2].

REFERENCES

1 Selden R, Sasahara AA. Central nervous system toxicity induced by lidocaine. *J Am Med Assoc* 1967; 202: 908–9.
2 Giard MJ, Uden DL, Whitelock DJ *et al*. Seizures induced by oral viscous lidocaine. *Clin Pharm* 1983; 2: 110.
3 Mofenson HC, Caraccio TR, Miller H *et al*. Lidocaine toxicity from topical mucosal application. *Clin Pediatr* 1983; 22: 190–2.

Lindane

Lindane, a chlorinated hydrocarbon, is the γ-isomer of benzene hexachloride. Topical 1% lotion used for the treatment of scabies may cause significant CNS toxicity in infants [1–6].

A premature, malnourished infant had one application of lindane over most of the skin surface with subsequent soap and water bath after 24 h. Two days later the infant showed a marked mental and motor deficit. A serum lindane level 46 h after application was 0.10 µg/ml (0.005 µg/ml is the reported mean level after treatment in infants and children according to one group) [3]. Risk of toxicity appears minimized when lindane is used with precautions [7].

REFERENCES

1 Boffa MJ, Brough PA, Ead RD. Lindane neurotoxicity. *Br J Dermatol* 1995; 133: 1013.
2 Matsuoka LY. Convulsions following application of gamma benzene hexachloride. *J Am Acad Dermatol* 1981; 5: 98–9.
3 Pramanik AK, Hansen RC. Transcutaneous gamma benzene hexachloride absorption and toxicity in infants and children. *Arch Dermatol* 1979; 115: 1224–5.
4 Lee B, Groth P. Scabies: transcutaneous poisoning during treatment. *Pediatrics* 1977; 59: 643.
5 Ginsburg CM, Lowry W, Reisch JS. Absorption of lindane (gamma benzene hexachloride) in infants and children. *J Pediatr* 1977; 91: 998–1000.
6 USFDA. Gamma benzene hexachloride (Kwell) and other products alert. *FDA Drug Bull* 1976; 6: 28.
7 Solomon LM, Fahrner L, West DP. Gamma benzene hexachloride toxicity. A review. *Arch Dermatol* 1977; 113: 353–7.

Mafenide

Mafenide is a topical sulphonamide which has been used for the treatment of burns. Methaemoglobinaemia caused by percutaneous absorption of mafenide acetate has been reported in two children [1].

REFERENCE

1 Ohlgisser M, Adler MN, Ben-Dov B *et al*. Methemoglobinaemia induced by mafenide acetate in children. A report of two cases. *Br J Anaesth* 1978; 50: 299–301.

Malathion

Four children developed systemic toxicity including hyperglycaemia, following hair washing with a solution containing 50% malathion in xylene, for the purpose of louse control [1]. A single application of 0.5% malathion represents a relatively safe approach that has been employed for the treatment of lice, although the use of the compound in the environment as a pesticide should be guarded [1,2].

REFERENCES

1 Ramu A, Slonim EA, London M *et al.* Hyperglycemia in acute malathion poisoning. *Isr J Med Sci* 1973; 9: 631–4.
2 Marty MA, Dawson SV, Bradman MA, Harnly ME, Dibartolomeis MJ. Assessment of exposure to malathion and malaoxon due to aerial application over urban areas of Southern California. *J Expo Anal Environ Epidemiol* 1994; 4: 65–81.

Mercurials

With a few exceptions, the use of mercurial compounds in medicine is uncommon. However, attention should be paid to the possibility of mercurial poisoning, as various forms of mercury are still present in numerous products, and in various countries, even in over-the-counter remedies, and sometimes without identification on the label.

Although there are considerable differences between various mercurials regarding rate of absorption through skin, all mercurial preparations are potentially hazardous and may cause intoxication [1]. Mercury is readily absorbed through intact skin; absorption of ammoniated mercury chloride in psoriatic patients has been demonstrated [2]. There have been some cases [3–5] of children who died following treatment of an omphalocele with topical merbromin (an organic mercurial antiseptic). Poisoning of a nursing infant has followed the use of perchloride of mercury lotion for cracked nipples [6].

Systemic absorption has been also observed following application to the oral mucosa of phenylmercury borate-containing mouthwashes causing acrodynia in small children [7].

REFERENCES

1 Gotelli CA, Astolfi E, Cox C, Cernichiari E, Clarkson TW. Early biochemical effects of an organic mercury fungicide on infants: 'dose makes the poison'. *Science* 1985; 227: 638–40.
2 Bork K, Morsches B, Holzmann H. Zum problem der Quecksilber-Resorption aus weisser Prazipatatsalbe. *Arch Dermatol Forsch* 1973; 248: 137–43.
3 Stanley-Brown EG, Frank JE. Mercury poisoning from application to omphalocele. *J Am Med Assoc* 1971; 216: 2144–5.
4 Clark JA, Kasselberg AG, Glick AD *et al.* Mercury poisoning from merbromin (mercurochrome) therapy of omphalocele. *Clin Pediatr* 1982; 21: 445–7.
5 Yeh TF, Pildes RS, Firor HV. Mercury poisoning from mercurochrome therapy of an infected omphalocele. *Clin Toxicol* 1978; 13: 463–7.
6 Hunt GM. Mercury poisoning in infancy. *Br Med J* 1966; i: 1482.
7 Bork K. *Cutaneous Side Effects of Drugs.* Philadelphia: WB Saunders, 1988.

Methanol

Methanol poisoning may occur from skin absorption or inhalation [1]. An 8-month-old child died from methanol toxicity after application of olive oil and warm methanol compresses on the chest for the treatment of a common cold [2]. Other reported cases include a 27-week gestational age infant who developed extensive haemorrhagic skin necrosis on the back and buttocks after cleaning the skin site for umbilical arterial catheterization with methylated spirits [3]. Systemic toxicity consisting of profound metabolic acidosis and high formate serum levels have been reported following cutaneous burns [4,5]. These reports include a 15-year-old female presenting with minor degree burns but with severe systemic signs of toxicity and a 3-year-old female burned by formic acid while playing near a leather-tanning room. Formic acid, or formate, is a strong corrosive agent used in industry and agriculture. It is well known as the toxic metabolite produced in methanol poisoning [4].

REFERENCES

1 Litovitz T. The alcohols: ethanol, methanol, isopropanol, ethylene glycol. *Pediatr Clin N Am* 1986; 33: 311–23.
2 Kahn A, Blum D. Methyl alcohol poisoning in an 8-month-old boy: an unusual route of intoxication. *J Pediatr* 1979; 94: 841–3.
3 Harpin VA, Rutter N. Percutaneous alcohol absorption and skin necrosis in a preterm infant. *Arch Dis Child* 1982; 57: 477–9.
4 Sigurdsson J, Bjornsson A, Gudmundsson ST. Formic acid burn—local and systemic effects. Report of a case. *Burns Incl Therm Inj* 1983; 9: 358–61.
5 Chan TC, Williams SR, Clark RF. Formic acid skin burns resulting in systemic toxicity. *Ann Emerg Med* 1995; 26: 383–6.

Neomycin

A triple antibiotic spray containing neomycin has been implicated in percutaneous toxicity. A 26-week gestational age infant received chronic local triple antibiotic therapy and developed a severe nerve deafness. The phenomenon was secondary to percutaneous absorption of neomycin, a well-known ototoxic agent [1].

Absorption of neomycin may be increased if associated with dimethylsulphoxide. In a young girl with chronic dermatomyositis, approximately 30% of the body surface was treated with an ointment containing 1% neomycin and 11% dimethylsulphoxide for a 2-month period. Vertigo, nystagmus and complete loss of hearing occurred [2].

REFERENCES

1 Morrel P, Hey E, Mackee IW *et al.* Deafness in preterm baby associated with topical antibiotic spray containing neomycin. *Lancet* 1985; i: 1167–8.
2 Herd JK, Cramer A, Hoak FC *et al.* Ototoxicity of topical neomycin augmented by dimethyl sulfoxide. *Pediatrics* 1967; 40: 905–7.

Oestrogens

Topical application of oestrogen-containing preparations may lead to absorption of these hormones with systemic oestrogen effects. Pseudoprecocious puberty in female infants and feminization in males resulted from 2–10 daily topical applications of a topical ointment containing oestrogens for a period of 2–18 months in the treatment or prevention of ammoniacal dermatitis [1]. These agents produced not only local effects (pigmentation and pubic hair), but also distant effects such as areolar pigmentation and mammary enlargement or gynaecomastia. Female infants developed vaginal discharge and bleeding.

REFERENCE

1 Beas F, Vargas L, Spada RP *et al.* Pseudoprecocious puberty in infants caused by a dermal ointment containing estrogens. *J Pediatr* 1969; 75: 127–30.

Phenols

Phenol can be applied as a local anaesthetic (0.5–2.0%) or as one component of multi-ingredient antifungals, such as Castellani's paint (4.4% phenol). Moderate to severe toxicity has been reported after the application of 2–4% phenol solutions in infants [1]. Use of a 2% phenol solution on an umbilical stump in a 1-day-old child produced circulatory collapse and death within 11 h [2]. Another child similarly treated developed severe methaemoglobinaemia that required exchange blood transfusions [2].

An outbreak of illness occurred among 29 infants in a newborn nursery and was characterized by sweating, fever, tachycardia, tachypnoea, hepatomegaly and acidosis. Nine infants became seriously ill and two died. An epidemiological study revealed that illness was caused by percutaneous absorption of pentachlorphenol, which was used for terminal rinse of the napkins as an antimicrobial neutralizing agent [3].

Cresol and chlorocresol are phenolic compounds which are caustic and exert their toxic effect directly on cells by denaturation and precipitation of proteins. There is an impressive report in the literature of a 12-month-old child who died apparently from absorption of a cresol-containing household remedy after the fluid had been spilled on his head [4].

REFERENCES

1 Thiemes C, Haley T. *Clinical Toxicology*, 3rd edn. Philadelphia: Lea & Febiger, 1972.
2 Von Hinkel GK, Kitzell HW. Phenolvergifungen bei neugeborenen durch kutane resorption. *Dtsch Gesundh-Wes* 1968; 23: 240.
3 Armstrong RW, Eichner ER, Klein DE *et al.* Pentachlorophenol poisoning in a nursery for newborn infants. Epidemiologic and toxicologic studies. *J Pediatr* 1969; 75: 317–24.
4 Green MA. A household remedy misused—fatal cresol poisoning following cutaneous absorption (a case report). *Med Sci Law* 1975; 15: 65–6.

Podophyllum resin

Podophyllum resin is a powerful skin irritant widely used in the local treatment of condyloma acuminatum. Absorption of the resin may lead to severe toxicity. A 19-year-old girl who developed weakness of the legs 2 days after a single application of 25% *Podophyllum* solution has been reported [1]. Another case includes an 18-year-old girl who became comatose about 24 h after the application of 25% *Podophyllum* ointment to vulvar warts. She died after 8 days [2].

REFERENCES

1 Grabbe W. Gefahren bei der Behandlung spitzer kondylome mit podophyllin bei geichzeitiger neosalvarsan-therapie. *Hautarz* 1951; 2: 325–6.
2 Ward JW, Clifford WS, Monaco AR *et al.* Fatal systemic poisoning following podophyllin treatment of condyloma acuminatum. *South Med J* 1954; 47: 1204.

Promethazine

Promethazine 2% cream applied to the skin of a 16-month-old male weighing 11.5 kg and suffering from generalized eczema, caused the child to fall asleep; he woke a few hours later with abnormal behaviour, loss of balance, inability to focus, irritability, drowsiness and failure to recognize his mother. One day later all symptoms had spontaneously disappeared. Known symptoms of promethazine toxicity include disorientation, hallucinations, hyperactivity, convulsions and coma [1].

REFERENCE

1 Bloch R, Beysovec L. Promethazine toxicity through percutaneous absorption. *In Contin Prac* 1982; 9: 28.

Resorcinol

Resorcinol is used for its keratolytic properties and is also a constituent of Castellani's solution [1]. Five deaths occurred in seven cases of acute poisoning in babies as a consequence of topical resorcinol application, in some instances to limited areas [2]. Other reported cases include an infant treated with 12.5% resorcinol ointment applied to the napkin area causing cyanosis, a maculopapular skin eruption, haemolytic anaemia and haemoglobinaemia.

REFERENCES

1 Freeman S, Maibach HI. Systemic toxicity in man secondary to percutaneous absorption. In: Marks R, Plewig G, eds. *The Environmental Threat to the Skin*. London: Martin Dunitz, 1992.
2 Cunningham AA. Resorcin poisoning. *Arch Dis Child* 1956; 31: 173–6.

Salicylic acid and salicylates

Salicylate poisoning in small children is often more serious than in older people because they are more likely to develop metabolic acidosis [1].

Although ingestion of aspirin tablets is the most frequent cause of salicylate poisoning, percutaneous absorption of sufficient amounts of salicylic acid or methylsalicylate also results in toxicity [2,3].

Ten fatal cases of percutaneous salicylate intoxication have been reported in children under 3 years of age [4]. Symptoms were those of salicylism.

A case of a 3-month-old infant with lamellar ichthyosis who developed severe salicylate intoxication after the application of a 4% salicylic acid ointment has been reported [5]. Salicylate intoxication may also occur inadvertently by application of salicylate-containing teething gels to the gums [6].

REFERENCES

1 Proudfoot AT. Toxicity of salicylate. *Am J Med* 1983; 75: 99–103.
2 Weigert SR, Gorisch V, Kluge C. Percutaneous salicylic acid poisoning in infancy. *Zeitschr Arztli Fortbild* 1983; 72: 427–32.
3 Lucas D. Salicylic acid poisoning in infancy. *Archiv Kinderheilk* 1971; 82: 168–74.
4 Van Weiss JF, Lever WF. Percutaneous salicylic acid intoxication in psoriasis. *Arch Dermatol* 1964; 90: 614–19.
5 El Assan Mohammed Abdel-Magid, Fathel-Rahman El Awad Ahmed. Salicylate intoxication in an infant with ichthyosis transmitted through skin ointment—a case report. *Pediatrics* 1994; 94: 939–40.
6 Paynter AS, Alexander FW. Salicylate intoxication caused by teething ointment. *Lancet* 1979; ii: 1132.

Silver nitrate

Fatal methaemoglobinaemia has been described in two children suffering from burns involving 70–80% of the body surface who were treated with silver nitrate solution [1,2].

In children, another important complication of the use of topical silver nitrate is electrolyte imbalance.

REFERENCES

1 Ternberg JL, Luce E. Methemoglobinemia: a complication of the silver nitrate treatment of burns. *Surgery* 1968; 63: 328–30.
2 Cushing AH, Smith S. Methemoglobinemia with silver nitrate therapy of a burn; report of a case. *J Pediatr* 1969; 74: 613–15.

Tars

A case of methaemoglobinaemia has been reported in a 3-month-old infant with severe atopic eczema following a 5-day application of an ointment containing 2.5% crude coal tar and 5% benzocaine to about half the body surface [1]. Benzocaine has not been attributed to causing methaemoglobinaemia. On the fifth day the infant suddenly became critically ill, cyanotic and anoxic; death appeared imminent.

REFERENCE

1 Goluboff N, MacFadyen DJ. Methemoglobinemia in an infant associated with application of a tar-benzocaine ointment. *J Pediatr* 1955; 47: 222–6.

Warfarin

The risk of transdermal toxicity by warfarin in infants has rarely been reported [1,2].

In Vietnam, the application of a talcum powder contaminated with warfarin in 741 infants caused an epidemic of haemorrhagic disease which was fatal for 177 babies [3].

REFERENCES

1 Green P. Haemorrhagic diathesis attributed to 'warfarin' poisoning. *Canad Med Assoc J* 1955; 72: 769–70.
2 Fristedt B, Sterner N. Warfarin intoxication from percutaneous absorption. *Arch Environ Health* 1965; 11: 205–8.
3 Martin-Bouyer G, Linh PD, Tuan LC *et al.* Epidemic of haemorrhagic disease in Vietnamese infants caused by warfarin-contaminated talcs. *Lancet* 1983; i: 230–2.

Chemicals

Aniline dye

Percutaneous toxicities have been reported with aniline dye used to mark new napkins. Cyanosis in infants of 3–64 days of age was attributed to absorption of aniline dye from the buttock area [1].

REFERENCE

1 Kagan BM, Mirman B, Kalvin J *et al.* Cyanosis in premature infants due to aniline dye intoxication. *J Pediatr* 1949; 34: 574–8.

Carbon tetrachloride

Fatal poisoning has occurred in a child after too liberal use of this solvent to remove adhesive plasters [1].

REFERENCE

1 Breathnach SM. Drug reactions. In: Champion RH, Burton JL, Burns JL, Breathnach SM, eds. *Textbook of Dermatology*, Vol. 4, 6th edn. Oxford: Blackwell Science, 1998.

Naphthalene

Naphthalene is commonly found in moth repellent products such as mothballs, flakes and crystals in 100% concentration. It is well absorbed following oral, dermal and inhalation exposure.

Cases of severe toxicity and death by dermal exposure to naphthalene have been documented in infants [1,2]. A tragic case is that of a 6-day-old female exposed for 3 days to napkins and blankets that had been stored in naphthalene and subsequently rinsed in water. Naphthalene's insolubility probably minimized its removal by water. Daily baby oil rubdowns may have facilitated the dermal absorption of naphthalene. After 2 days jaundice, cyanosis and a loud flow murmur developed. She died after 4 days. Postmortem examination showed extramedullary haemopoiesis in the heart, liver, spleen and adrenals. There were gross and microscopically evident haemoglobin deposits in the renal tubules [3].

In those reports involving inhalation and dermal absorption, it is not clear whether one route exclusively contributed to the development of toxicity [3].

REFERENCES

1 Dawson JP, Thayer WW, Desforges JF. Acute hemolytic anemia in the newborn infant due to naphthalene poisoning. Report of two cases with investigation into the mechanism of the disease. *Blood* 1958; 13: 1113–25.
2 Schafer WB. Acute hemolytic anemia related to naphthalene. Report of a case in a newborn infant. *Pediatrics* 1951; 7: 172–4.
3 Siegel E, Wason S. Mothball toxicity. *Pediatr Clin N Am* 1986; 33: 369–74.

Paraquat

Paraquat is a defoliant and contact herbicide. If ingested, paraquat poisoning is, in the majority of cases, lethal. Systemic toxicity from percutaneous absorption has also been described in adults, but rarely in children [1]. It may be seen also in adolescents as an occupational illness [2]. Symptoms of toxicity from cutaneous exposure to highly concentrated material include skin necrosis as well as CNS and pulmonary symptoms.

REFERENCES

1 Roth B, Bulla M, von Lilien T, Statz A, Okonek S. Clinical findings and treatment of paraquat poisoning in childhood. *Mon Kinder* 1983; 131: 458–63.
2 Weinbaum Z, Samuels SJ, Schenker MB. Risk factors for occupational illnesses associated with the use of paraquat (1,1'-dimethyl-4,4'-bipyridylium dichloride) in California. *Arch Environ Health* 1995; 50: 341–8.

Cutaneous symptoms following inhalation, ingestion or injection of some toxicants

Systemic poisoning by ingestion, inhalation or injection of some toxicants may produce cutaneous symptoms. However, reports in infants are scarce.

After an accident in 1976 in a chemical plant in Seveso, Italy, 2,3,7,8-tetrachlorodibenzo-*p*-dioxin (TCDD) spread over a populated area. Children, as well as adults, were affected and the contamination took place not only through direct exposure but also through inhalation and ingestion of contaminated foods such as fruits and vegetables.

Cutaneous manifestations were recognized as early and late lesions. Early lesions appeared within a few hours, or a few days, after the accident and were ascribed to direct cutaneous exposure to the toxic cloud or to contaminated soil. Late lesions were represented by an acneiform eruption (chloracne) appearing some 30–60 days after the accident and considered to result both from direct exposure to TCDD as well as from inhalation and ingestion of contaminated foods. Most of the patients were children aged 2–10 years and adolescents. The eruption was characterized by comedo-like and cystic lesions; the malar area was most frequently affected, while the centrofacial region was constantly spared as reported in other chloracne cases [1,2].

Severe cutaneous manifestations were detected in eight children, all of whom had shown early lesions. All of them showed diffuse follicular hyperkeratosis associated with comedones on the limbs. In three of these patients granuloma annulare or erythema elevatum diutinum like lesions occurred on the palms, and two sisters had comedones and cysts of the axillae. The only sequelae at follow-up were atrophic cicatricial skin changes [3–5].

In 1987, a family of nine (father, mother and seven children: 12-, 8- and 4-year-old boys; 11-, 9- and 3-year-old girls; and a 2-month-old infant), was intoxicated by a chlorinated hydrocarbon mixture [6]. The product was introduced into the home in the form of an edible oil, which had been stored in a plastic container where, presumably, it had become contaminated with hexachlorobenzene, pentachlorophenol and a mixture of chlorinated dibenzo-*p*-dioxins and chlorinated dibenzofurans.

The cutaneous manifestations in the father and the four eldest children were comedones, papules, cysts and milia on the forehead, cheeks, neck, thorax, shoulders, back, buttocks, abdomen and genitals; and in two girls on the earlobes. The father and the two eldest sons also had hypertrichosis, hyperpigmentation of the skin, follicular hyperkeratosis and increased cutaneous fragility. The mother and the three youngest children, including the newborn baby, only had discrete papules on the cheeks. Cutaneous lesions were preceded by systemic symptoms.

Ingestion of hexachlorobenzene (a chlorinated hydrocarbon different from that of lindane), a fungicide added to wheat seedlings, was the cause of porphyria involving more than 4000 people in Turkey from 1956 to 1961 [7]. Initial symptoms mentioned by most subjects were weakness, loss of appetite, photosensitivity and development of erythema, which occurred principally on the sun-exposed areas of skin, but was often generalized with accompanying pruritus. Hyperpigmentation was maximum in exposed areas of skin, but in many subjects the entire skin became darker. Hypertrichosis occurred principally on the forehead, cheeks, arms and legs, and was sufficiently distinctive in the age group of 5–15 years

Table 27.3.2 Examples of chemotherapy drugs used in children that are known to cause cutaneous changes through cytotoxic effects

Actinomycin D
Adriamycin
Bleomycin
Cyclophosphamide
Cytarabine
Dactinomycin
Daunomycin
Decarbazine
Fluorouracil
Methotrexate
Nitrosoureas

for the children to be described by some as 'monkey children'.

Development of bullae, often up to 5 cm in size, occurred frequently, healing with severe mutilating scars. During the early period of active porphyria, affected people were irritable, with colic, loss of appetite, weakness and red or brown urine (porphyrinuria). Most patients were between the ages of 6 and 15 years. In some villages almost all of the children under the age of 2 years, who were breast-fed by mothers who had eaten the contaminated wheat, died of the condition known as pembe yara, which included symptoms of weakness, convulsions and localized cutaneous annular erythema.

Thallium poisoning following ingestion may produce serious symptoms. Hair loss is consistently present [8–11].

Two children developed skin bullae after accidental ingestion of kerosene [12].

In some countries, children with typical palmoplantar keratoderma as a result of endemic arsenic poisoning of drinking water, may still be recognized [13].

In children as well as in adults, systemic administration of some cancer chemotherapy drugs may produce changes in the skin and its appendages. Changes are mostly due to the cytotoxic effects caused by interference with critical intracellular processes, including nucleic acid formation and ribosomal function. Cytotoxic reactions, disorders of pigmentation, exathematous and follicular rashes, are among skin complications induced by chemotherapy [14–17] (Table 27.3.2).

REFERENCES

1 Tindall JP. Chloracne and chloracnegens. *J Am Acad Dermatol* 1985; 13: 539–58.
2 Taylor JS. Environmental chloracne: update and overview. *Ann NY Acad Sci* 1979; 320: 295–307.
3 Caputo R, Monti M, Ermacora E *et al.* Cutaneous manifestations of tetra-chlorobenzo-*p*-dioxin in children and adolescents. Follow-up 10 years after the Seveso, Italy, accident. *J Am Acad Dermatol* 1988; 19: 812–19.
4 Caputo R. Cutaneous manifestations of tetrachlorobenzo-*p*-dioxin in children and adolescents. In: Marks R, Plewig G, eds. *The Environmental Threat to the Skin*. London: Martin Dunitz, 1992.
5 Moccarelli P, Marocchi A, Brambilla P. Clinical laboratory manifestations of exposure to dioxin in children. A 6-year study effects of an environmental disaster near Seveso, Italy. *J Am Med Assoc* 1986; 256: 2687–95.
6 Rodriguez-Pichardo A, Camacho F. Chloracne as a consequence of a family accident with chlorinated dioxins. *J Am Acad Dermatol* 1990; 22: 1121.
7 Cripps DJ, Gocmen A, Peters HA. Porfiria turcica. Twenty years after hexachlorobenzene intoxication. *Arch Dermatol* 1980; 116: 46–50.
8 Prick JJC, Smitt WGS, Muller L. *Thallium Poisoning*. Amsterdam: Elsevier, 1955.
9 Heyl T, Barlow RJ. Thallium poisoning: a dermatological perspective. *Br J Dermatol* 1989; 121: 787–92.
10 Grossman H. Thallotoxicosis. *Pediatrics* 1955; 16: 865–72.
11 Niehues R, Horstkotte, Klein RM *et al.* Repeated ingestion with suicidal intent of potentially lethal amounts of thallium. *Dtsch Med Wochenschr* 1995; 120: 403–8.
12 Annobil SH. Skin bullae following kerosene poisoning. *Ann Trop Paediatr* 1988; 8: 45–7.
13 Foy HM, Tarmapai S, Eamchan P, Metdilogkul O. Chronic arsenic poisoning from well water from a mining area in Thailand. *Asia-Pac J Pub Health* 1992–93; 6: 150–2.
14 Nixon DW, Pirozzi, D, York RM *et al.* Dermatologic changes after systemic cancer therapy. *Cutis* 1981; 27: 181–94.
15 Adrian RM, Hood AF, Skarin AT. Mucocutaneous reactions to antineoplastic agents. *CA Cancer J Clin* 1980; 30: 143–57.
16 Levine N, Greenwald ES. Mucocutaneous side effects of cancer chemotherapy. *Cancer Treat Rev* 1978; 5: 67–84.
17 Kanwar VS, Gajjar A, Ribeiro RC, Bowman L, Parham DM, Jenkins JJ III. Unusual cutaneous toxicity following treatment with dactinomycin: a report of two cases. *Med Pediatr Oncol* 1995; 24: 329–33.

Acknowledgements

We wish to acknowledge Maria Letizia Musumeci MD, from Clinica Dermatologica, Universita di Catania, Italia, for her assistance in this chapter.

Section 28
Paediatric Dermatological Surgery and Laser Therapy

28.1

Basic Skin Surgery Techniques

MARY MALONEY

Basic cutaneous surgery is important in the paediatric population. There are a multitude of biopsy and surgical treatment techniques that can and should be performed in the office, both to provide cost-effective medical care, as well as to decrease the anxiety and trauma of an operative procedure. Proficiency in these techniques allows the attending doctor to perform in a confident and rapid fashion, two very important features when dealing with the paediatric population. This chapter reviews in-office surgical procedures, as well as the indications for such procedures and the possible complications.

Local anaesthesia

The use of local anaesthesia for surgical procedures avoids the small but real risks of morbidity and mortality associated with general anaesthesia. Local anaesthesia must have a reasonably rapid onset of action, be effective and have a long enough duration of activity to allow for completion of the procedure at hand. Local anaesthetics include topical as well as local injectable anaesthetics.

Topical anaesthesia does not provide deep anaesthesia but may be very useful for superficial procedures. It will also provide anaesthesia prior to injectable local anaesthesia or other needle sticks.

Topical anaesthesia, as initially developed with lidocaine cream, was poorly effective, with limited penetration of intact skin and a very limited duration of anaesthesia.

The development of a 'eutectic mixture' in 1985 by Broberg and Evers essentially revolutionized topical anaesthesia [1]. EMLA, an acronym for eutectic mixture of local anaesthetics, contains lidocaine (25 mg/l) and prilocaine (25 mg/l). Such high concentrations of the anaesthetics are necessary for absorption and penetration. Maximal analgesia is obtained in 1–2 h when applied under occlusion with plastic wrap [2], and persists for 1–2 h [2,3].

Topical amethocaine 4% gel (Ametop) is a newer product which has the advantages of only needing 30–45 min contact prior to the procedure and the anaesthesia remaining effective for 4–6 h. It may not be available worldwide.

EMLA cream or Ametop provide good analgesia for a wide variety of minor procedures including pulsed dye laser, curettage of molluscum, venepuncture, shave biopsies and other superficial procedures. However, the depth of anaesthesia is to a maximum of 5 mm and so deep biopsies will still produce pain [2]. In these instances, injectable anaesthesia is required.

Injectable anaesthetics

Local injectable anaesthetics must produce anaesthesia relatively rapidly. The duration of the anaesthetic must be tailored to the length of the procedure (Table 28.1.1). It is important to minimize the discomfort of the injection of a local anaesthetic, especially in a paediatric population. It should also be relatively free from toxic effects and should be non-sensitizing. There are a number of local anaesthetics that meet these requirements [4,5]. The commonly used local anaesthetics all fall into two groups: the amide and the ester groups. Local injectable anaesthetics are composed of an aromatic ring portion, which accounts for the lipid solubility of the anaesthetic, and an amide portion, which accounts for the water solubility. These are linked by an intermediate chain which contains either an amide or an ester. It is this linkage area which classifies the anaesthetic.

The ester group which includes cocaine, procaine and tetracaine was the first developed local anaesthetic. This ester group produced a number of sensitizations with both type 1 and 4 allergic reactions. Development of the

Table 28.1.1 Local anaesthetic properties

Anaesthetic	pKa (25°C)	Site of metabolism	Max duration (min) Plain	With Epinephrine
Amide				
lignocaine	7.91	Liver	120	400
mepivocaine	7.76	Liver	120	400
bupivacaine	8.16	Liver	240	480
etidocaine	7.74	Liver	200	360
prilocaine	7.9	Liver	120	400
Ester				
procaine	9.05	Plasma	30–50	90
chloroprocaine	8.97	Plasma	60	—
tetracaine	8.46	Plasma	175	—

amide group significantly reduced sensitization and has become the anaesthetic agent of choice in most instances. This group includes lignocaine (lidocaine) mepivacaine, bupivacaine, prilocaine and etidocaine. Parabens are added to the anaesthetic solutions to act as a preservative. Adrenaline (epinephrine) is frequently added to local anaesthetic solutions. Adrenaline causes vasoconstriction in the area and will therefore decrease bleeding during the procedure. It provides a less bloody field for the surgical procedure.

Adrenaline also slows absorption of the local anaesthetic, prolonging the duration of anaesthesia and decreasing the rate of systemic absorption. With this decreased rate of absorption, a larger total volume of anaesthesia may be used safely. However, there is a risk of vasoconstriction when it is used around the digits. If both digital arteries are constricted, the digit can undergo necrosis. This is most commonly seen in patients who have peripheral vascular disease, but as a standard of care, most doctors avoid the use of adrenaline in any patient population around the digits.

To stabilize adrenaline, the solution must be acidic. This lower pH makes the anaesthetic significantly more painful at the time of injection. It has been found that warming the solution to 37°C and the addition of sodium bicarbonate to the vial before the anaesthetic is used does not affect the stability of the solution and significantly decreases the pain at injection [6,7].

Standard anaesthetic solutions containing adrenaline usually contain a concentration of adrenaline of 1:100000. However, the vasoconstrictive effect will be seen at 1:200000 and even to 1:400000, and may be diluted to these concentrations easily.

Adverse reactions may be divided into allergic and toxic reactions. Allergic reactions with the amide group of local anaesthetics are rare. Less than 1% of reactions to local anaesthetics are allergic in nature. These include immunoglobulin E (IgE)-mediated (anaphylactic) reac-

tions and delayed hypersensitivity [8]. Occasionally these reactions may be traced to the paraben preservative in the solution, rather than the lignocaine itself.

Toxic reactions are dose-related phenomena. 'Safe' amounts of local anaesthetic are usually calculated on the standard 70-kg man. As an example, toxicity may be seen above 3mg/kg of 1% lignocaine solution. The slowed systemic absorption allows a maximum dose of 7mg/kg when adrenaline is added to the solution. Children require less anaesthetic to reach toxicity [5]. Toxic levels may result from inadvertent intravascular injection, excessive amount of locally injected anaesthetic, or impaired hepatic function decreasing the metabolism of the injected amide anaesthetic. Toxic effects are largely seen in the central nervous system (CNS) and cardiovascular systems and will include light-headedness, disorientation, irritability or restlessness, slurred speech, nystagmus and muscle twitching. In the late stages, convulsions may occur, as well as respiratory depression and eventually death. The cardiovascular effects will include a fall in blood pressure (as these agents are vasodilators), arrhythmias and cardiovascular collapse. If early signs of toxicity appear, the surgery should be concluded, supportive measures instituted and the patient carefully monitored.

Other local anaesthetic agents that have been documented are 1% diphenhydramine [9,10] and sodium chloride [11], neither of which are used in routine clinical practice.

Biopsy techniques

There are three distinct biopsy techniques, each with their own indications and limitations [12]. It is important to evaluate carefully the lesion in question and determine the technique that will accomplish that goal.

Before either a biopsy or excisional surgery is performed, the skin needs to be prepared to decrease the bacterial 'load'. Such treatment does not sterilize the skin, but decreases the risk of postoperative infection [13–15]. Table 28.1.2 lists the available agents used for this purpose in the USA.

The shave biopsy is the most superficial type, and its advantage is that it will leave the least scar of any of the techniques. It is especially suited for removal of relatively superficial lesions and will remove them easily and in most cases completely. For processes with deeper components, this technique may provide incomplete removal or an inadequate tissue sample for the histopathologist. In the instance of benign tumours, the advantages may outweigh the disadvantages. However, for diagnostic biopsies of inflammatory conditions, this method is clearly inadequate.

The punch biopsy has the advantage of obtaining deeper elements of tissue for histopathological evalua-

Table 28.1.2 Skin preparation solutions

	Spectrum of activity	Onset	Sustained activity	Comments
Alcohol (70%)	Gram-positive	Fast	None	No activity against spores, fungi, viruses; 75% bacterial reduction with wipe
Iodophor (Betadine)	Gram-positive Gram-negative	Moderate	1 h	Activity enhanced if not removed
Chlorhexidine (Hibiclens hibitane)	Gram-positive Gram-negative	Fast	Hours	Eye irritant
Hexachlorophene (Phisohex)	Gram-positive	Slow	Hours	Not sporicidal

tion. It will provide a more complete sampling of a disorder that has such a deep component. It may also act as a punch excision of small lesions that need to be completely removed. In such an instance, the size of the punch should be chosen so as to completely encompass the lesion and include a small margin of normal appearing epidermis. Punches come in a variety of sizes, as small as 2 mm and extending to 2 cm in size. There are several types to be chosen, including machine held, hand held and disposable. It is the operator's choice which size and style to use.

The disadvantage of the punch biopsy/excision is that it will leave a more discernible mark or scar. In noncosmetic areas, the resulting scar is usually insignificant. However, care must be taken in more cosmetic areas to place the biopsy in the least visible area and frequently to close the defect with one or two fine sutures. If suturing is to be performed, it is usually helpful to stretch the tissue at 90° angle from the proposed line of closure to create a partially elliptical defect which will close more easily.

The third form of biopsy is an incisional or excisional biopsy, which represents an elliptical or fusiform excision. If this biopsy is to include the entire lesion, it will be an ellipse around the lesion in question extended down to the subcutaneous tissue. An incisional biopsy will include representative tissue from the lesion, and again extend down to at least the subcutaneous tissue. At this point, the wound will be closed usually with an initial layer of dermal absorbable sutures followed by a layered epidermal closure of sutures, staples or adhesive strips, depending upon the location and the tension on the wound. This type of biopsy allows the best representative sampling or the entire lesion for evaluation histopathologically. However, it will clearly cause the most scarring, as in most instances it will result in the largest defect and the most noticeable scar.

Excision

There are a multitude of indications for an excision to be performed in any patient population. These range from a small benign lesion being removed for cosmetic reasons to a cutaneous malignancy. Whenever a lesion is to be removed, it is important that both the doctor and the parent understand the reason for removal, the proposed method of removal, alternatives to surgical removal and reasonable expectations regarding resulting scarring. These areas make up the basis of informed consent and must not be ignored in any patient population. No surgery should be embarked upon without consent from the legal guardian or the patient if they have reached the age of legal consent. This is important not only for medicolegal reasons, but also to be certain that goals and expectations are clearly laid out and agreed to by both the doctor and the patient before a procedure is undertaken.

The method of surgical excision will depend on the location, normal skin lines and the required margin around the lesion to be excised. In an area where the normal lines of tension cannot be fully predicted, a circular excision may be the best approach. The defect can then be undermined, which will almost invariably clearly define the optimal closure line. Closure can then be completed by the removal of standing cones or the planning of M-plasties, depending on the location and nature of the tissue. In other areas, an ellipse or a fusiform excision can be easily planned to follow existing contours.

The actual technique of a surgical excision requires simple self-confidence in the knowledge of the technique and the ability to perform this. The scalpel should be held comfortably and a firm excision undertaken to cut smoothly into the dermis, taking care not to make too many repeated superficial cuts to attain the same end. The repeated tracing of the incision tends to cause 'stair-stepping' of the tissue (Fig. 28.1.1) and therefore an irregular wound to reapproximate. Cross-hatching and nicking of the wound edge should similarly be avoided (Fig. 28.1.2). In most instances, the excision is extended to the subcutaneous fat and removed at that level either by scissors or sharp scalpel dissection. Care should be taken to make the depth of the wound uniform, avoiding the tendency of producing a deeper wound at one end. The specimen

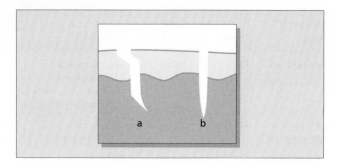

Fig. 28.1.1 (a) Stair-stepping of an incision caused by multiple, repeated and shallow passes along an incision line. (b) The correct 90° incision from a single firm stroke of the scalpel.

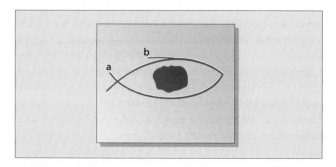

Fig. 28.1.2 (a) Cross-hatching caused by extension of the incision beyond the distal point. (b) Nicking of the wound margin caused by a slip of the scalpel as it passes along the planned incision line.

should be immediately handed off the surgical field to an assistant so that it does not become lost or desiccated during the remainder of the procedure. Haemostasis should then be obtained immediately. It is important to take care to produce a dry field without indiscriminate desiccation of surrounding tissue.

Undermining of the wound margins will free the skin from the underlying tissues and allow it to close more smoothly and easily with less tension. The plane of undermining varies, depending on the body location. In most locations, one undermines at the level of the superior subcutaneous fat. It is important to be careful when undermining not to damage deep or surrounding structures and not to crush the overlying epidermis as it is everted during the undermining procedure. Undermining should take place with a spreading motion of the scissors rather than snipping. This will prevent damage to surrounding blood vessels and nerves. On rare occasions it is necessary to undermine sharply with either scissors or a scalpel blade. This most frequently occurs when there have been previous surgical procedures in the area and there is dense scarring. Before initiating closure, the wound edges need to be everted, bleeding sites identified and then appropriately cauterized. The remainder of the wound, should then be inspected for bleeding or oozing so as to prevent formation of a haematoma.

For wounds under even mild tension, closure is begun with buried sutures closing the deep portion of the wound. These sutures will resorb slowly and provide the wound with more long-lasting support, even after cutaneous sutures have been removed. These sutures will also obliterate dead space at the deep margin and therefore decrease the possibility of a haematoma or seroma.

There are a number of techniques for closure of the epidermis, and it is important to select carefully the most appropriate closure method dependent on the location of the wound, tension and the possible tension created by a moving body part. Choices include the following methods.

The adhesive strip has been used for several years, first as a 'butterfly' adhesive and now being known as an adhesive closure material. This may be used when buried sutures have removed all evidence of tension and there is good epidermal apposition. There should be no possibility of extensive movement, and so this type of closure would not be the closure of choice on the trunk, extremities or moving jawline. It would also not be applicable where hair would interfere with the adherence of these strips to the skin. This would include the beard area, the scalp and any other location in a patient with excessive body hair. It is important to note that rapidly growing hair such as found in the beard area will interfere with skin adhesion. Application of a gum or glue such as benzoin or mastisol greatly increases the adherence of the adhesive strip and increases the tension that the strip will bear [16].

Suturing the wound is most commonly achieved with a synthetic non-absorbable suture alone or absorbable buried sutures followed by a non-absorbable suture. The surgeon should choose the smallest size of suture applicable.

The absorbable buried suture will relieve tension and may provide wound security after the cutaneous sutures have been removed. These sutures should be placed so that the knot is 'buried' (Fig. 28.1.3). This prevents the knots from causing a firm nodule along the suture line or from actually extruding through the incision. Buried sutures can work to the surface late in the course of wound healing. The risk of suture 'spitting' must be weighed against the benefit of improved wound security. In most instances this will depend on wound tension; the greater the tension, the more beneficial the buried absorbable suture.

Choice of the non-absorbable cutaneous suture depends on wound tension and location (Table 28.1.3). Options include a braided synthetic suture, which is easy to handle; a monofilament synthetic suture, which is especially useful in a contaminated wound; and a non-synthetic suture such as silk. In children it may be useful to use a rapid absorbing gut suture or a similar absorbable suture. These sutures should fall out on their own, ending the necessity of suture removal.

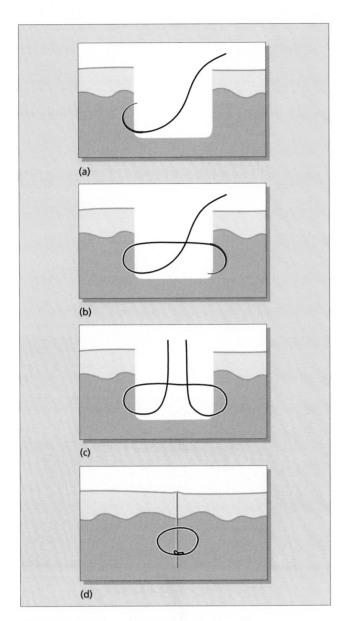

(a)

(b)

(c)

(d)

Fig. 28.1.3 Schematic of the intradermal buried suture. (a) The needle starts from deep to more superficial on one margin. (b) The needle then passes from superficial to deep on the opposite margin. (c) Stitch in place before tying. (d) The tied suture approximating the wound with the knot buried.

The method of placing sutures is also a very important choice for the surgeon. Choices include a simple uninterrupted suture, mattress suture, running or running locked suture, and a running subcuticular suture. Each will be discussed in detail.

The simple interrupted suture is the basis of all cutaneous sutures. The needle should enter the skin at a 90 degree angle and have a somewhat flask-like course through the deeper tissue, as illustrated in Fig. 28.1.4a. This causes slight wound eversion, which will prevent any depression of the final incision line. Incorrect suture (as demonstrated in Fig. 28.1.4b) is a simple flat semi-circle motion, which can accentuate inversion of the wound and lead to a less cosmetically acceptable scar. Care must be taken to have the suture enter and exit the wound at the same distance from the wound edge and to extend to the same depth on both sides of the incision. Careful attention to this will prevent an uneven wound (Fig. 28.1.4c).

The vertical mattress suture (Fig. 28.1.5a–d) is a suture designed to add strength to a wound closure, carrying more tension. It can also obliterate dead space with the depth of the second pass. Lastly, this suture helps to evert the epidermal wound margin, thus producing a more cosmetically acceptable scar. It is not uncommon to use this suture at intervals in a wound even if that wound is not under significant tension. Again, such an intermittent use of the suture will help with wound eversion.

The horizontal mattress suture (Fig. 28.1.6a–d) is designed principally to relieve tension along the wound margins. The suture may be placed initially to relieve tension while the remainder of the wound is sutured. The suture can then be removed when tension is shared more evenly along the entire wound, or in some cases may be left in place for 24–48 h.

Continuous running suture (Fig. 28.1.7a–d) is a simple continuous suture that can be used on wounds with little or no tension. It is a rapid suture to place and can give a good cosmetic result. The one disadvantage of this suture is that if a haematoma or seroma develops, one is unable to remove just a single suture to drain the collection of fluid.

The running intradermal suture is the most cosmetic of all sutures. The suture is only visible at the two ends of the

Table 28.1.3 Non-absorbable sutures. Adapted from Maloney [17]

Filament	Type	Knot security	Strength	Reactivity
Silk	Braided	4+	1+	High
Nylon	Braided	2+	3+	Low
	Monofilament	3+	3+	Low
Polyester	Braided	4+	4+	Low
Polypropylene	Monofilament	1+	1+	Low
Polybutester	Monofilament	2+	2+	Lowest
Absorbable sutures that may be used for cutaneous closure				
Fast absorbing plain gut	Monofilament	1+	2+	High
Polyglactin 910	Braided	3+	4+	Low

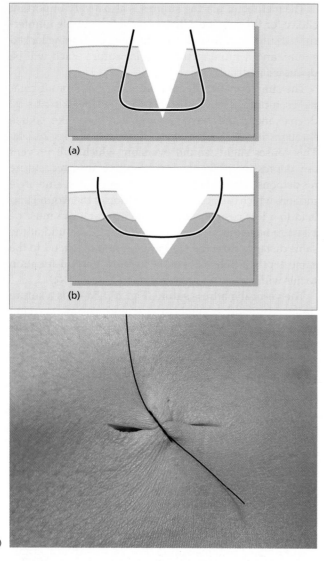

Fig. 28.1.4 (a) The correct flask-shaped placement of the interrupted cutaneous suture. (b) The incorrect method of an interrupted suture, placed in a flat semi-circular motion, creating a circular suture that can accentuate inversion of a wound. (c) Inversion of the wound caused by an incorrectly placed interrupted suture.

incision (Fig. 28.1.8a–e), and the suture is placed by intra-dermal bites along the entire wound length. This suture leaves no suture tracking but can be used only on wounds that have little or no tension. There is again the risk of having to remove the entire length of suture if any under-lying complication develops.

There is no correct number of sutures to be placed in closing a particular wound. The wound should be closed in a fashion such that there is no 'gaping' of any portion on the wound and that the epidermis is nicely approximated. Enough sutures need to be placed to share the full tension of the wound, avoiding any single suture carrying the majority of wound tension.

Staples are made of stainless steel and therefore are very

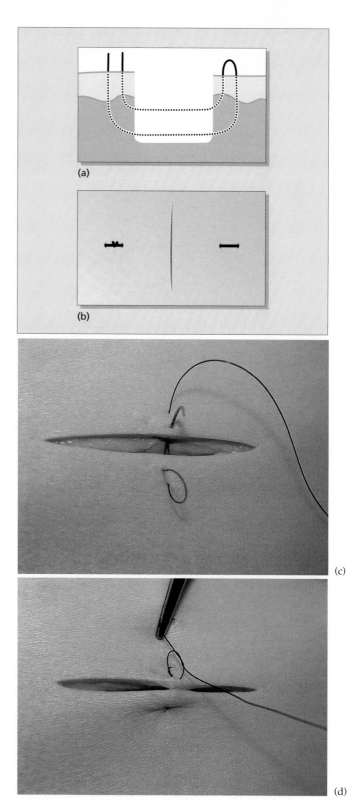

Fig. 28.1.5 The vertical mattress suture. (a) The path of the suture. (b) The appearance schematically of the tied suture with the suture line lying vertical to the incision line. (c) Placement of the vertical mattress suture. (d) Tying the vertical mattress suture, creating wound eversion.

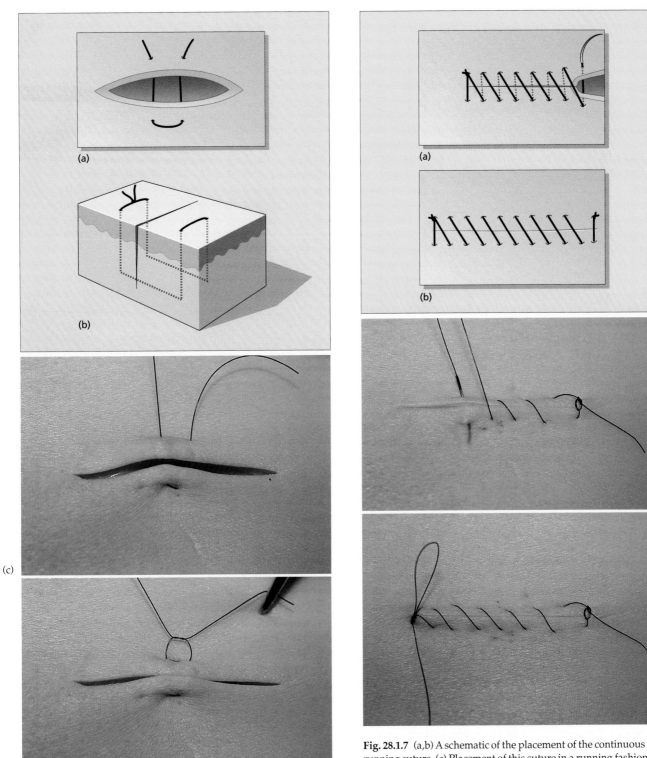

Fig. 28.1.6 The horizontal mattress suture. (a) Schematic of the placement. (b) A schematic showing the patch of the suture in the dermis. This shows the nature of the suture line lying on the surface being horizontal with the incision line. (c) Placement of the suture. (d) Tying of the suture showing the resulting wound eversion.

Fig. 28.1.7 (a,b) A schematic of the placement of the continuous running suture. (c) Placement of this suture in a running fashion. (d) Appearance of the suture when fully placed.

non-reactive. They are easy and rapid to place, but one may sacrifice careful wound opposition as staple placement is not quite as fine a technique. However, staples will hold under moderate tension.

Tissue adhesives (cyanoacrylates) have been developed

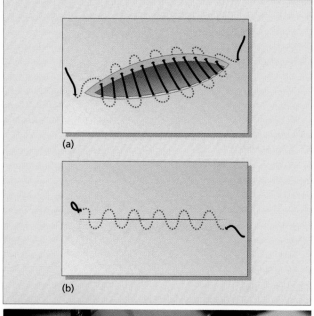

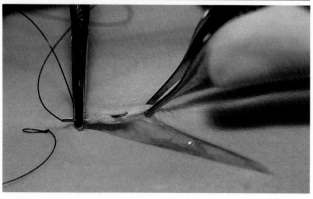

(c)

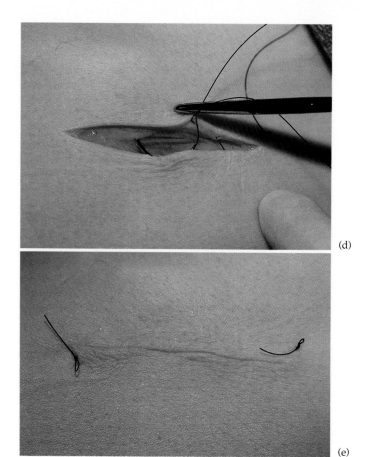

(d)

(e)

Fig. 28.1.8 (a,b) A schematic of the placement of the running intradermal suture. (c,d) Actual placement of the suture. (e) Appearance of the suture line when the suture has been placed and tied.

and have proven very effective in wounds that are not under tension. They are especially useful in the pediatric population as there is no need for bulky dressings or suture removal. At this time they remain expensive, but are easy to apply. Further work is sure to provide stronger adhesive properties for wounds under some tension, and the cost should diminish over time.

Closure of wounds of unequal length

In many instances, wounds will be created that are of unequal length. This may be the result of the lesion to be excised or of the anatomical location. There are two basic ways to approach this problem. The first approach is to sew the wounds together by the rule of halves. The initial suture is placed in the centre of the wound and the remaining distances are continually halved by suture placement (Fig. 28.1.8a,b). This method essentially shares the excess length of one side of the wound over the entire length of the closure, ending with a cosmetic closure with no evidence of the unequal sides.

The second method involves shortening of the longer

side by the removal of what is known as a Burow's or von Burow's triangle. This triangle of skin is removed as shown in Fig. 28.1.9a and c, and that defect is then closed. This shortens the long side of the wound, thereby making the sides equal in length. This defect is then sutured in a standard fashion. The benefit of this method is that the excess skin can be removed at any point along the long side. It can thereby be placed in the most cosmetic site depending on the location of the wound and the long side of the wound.

Either of the above are correct repairs of this problem. The use will depend on the clinical setting and the location of the wound. When a von Burow's triangle can be removed in a cosmetic area, such as into the hairline or into a fold, this may be the method of choice. The rule of sewing by halves may be the choice in other locations.

Standing cone (dog-ear) repair

Wounds that have been created that do not meet the 30

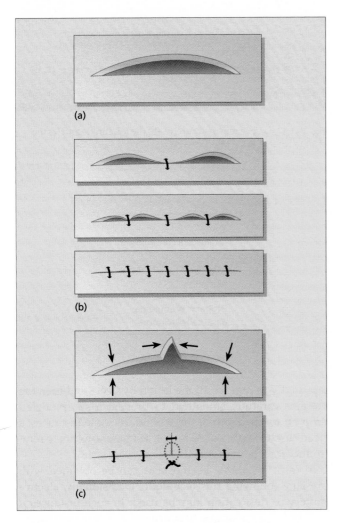

Fig. 28.1.9 (a) Depicts a wound of unequal length. (b) Shows closure of this wound by the rule of halves. The wound length is continually halved with simple interrupted sutures, sharing the excess tissue along one margin. (c) Correction of the unequal length by the placement of a von Burow's triangle which may be placed at any point along the long margin of the wound.

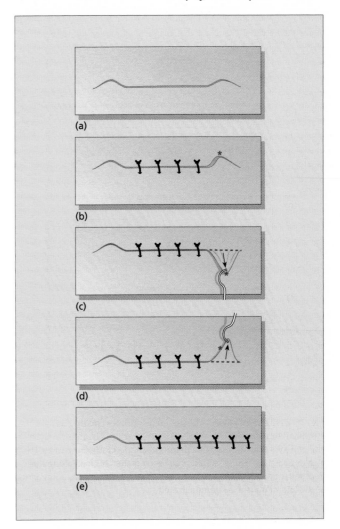

Fig. 28.1.10 Dog-ear correction. (a) The appearance of redundant tissue at the ends of the wound. (b) The cone of tissue to be removed is identified with its central focal point. (c) Tissue is pulled to one side and an incision made along the dotted line. (d) The redundant skin is then pulled in the other direction and again removed along the dotted line. (e) The wound is then lengthened and the length of this wound is sutured with simple interrupted sutures.

degree angle rule of the standard ellipse may close with puckering at one or both distal ends of the incision. Similarly, excisions that are planned in a circular fashion and then closed in a side-to-side fashion will by definition have these standing cones or puckers at the ends of the incision. One simple method of minimizing these is to undermine the entire wound including the ends of the ellipse to free the tissue to allow it to slide easily and to close smoothly. When this undermining technique does not provide a resolution, they will need to be repaired or removed. The standard method of repair is the length-extension technique, which simply removes the triangular shaped standing cone and then continues the final repair with a somewhat extended length of the wound [18] (Fig. 28.1.10). This redundant skin can be removed at various angles depending on the location and how this will fit with the normal body contours. There are other methods of repair of the standing cone that are beyond the scope of this chapter.

M-plasty

An M-plasty is an M-shaped modification of one end of an elliptical excision. This M-shaped modification (Fig. 28.1.11) may shorten a wound, spare further tissue or actually be another form of dog-ear repair. The M-plasty is designed by initially marking the geometric design before surgery is begun, as even anaesthesia can distort these lines. The closure then proceeds with the only addition being what is called a tip stitch to keep the tip of the M in

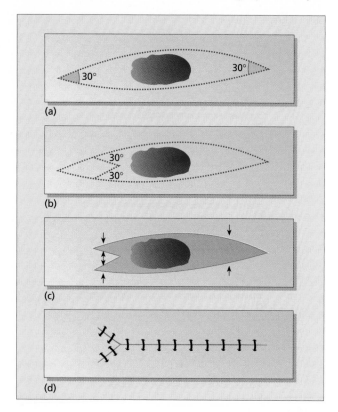

(a)

(b)

(c)

(d)

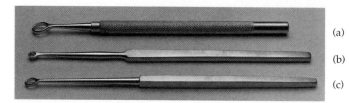

(a)

(b)

(c)

Fig. 28.1.12 (a) The rein oval curette, (b) the fox curette and (c) the cannon curette. From Maloney [17].

Table 28.1.4 Lesions amenable to curettage

Warts
Molluscum contagiosum
Milia
Sebaceous hyperplasia
Epidermal cysts
Vellus hair cysts
Pyogenic granuloma
Basal cell carcinoma

Fig. 28.1.11 The M-plasty is designed by initially creating an elliptical excision with 30° angles at each margin. The margin to be shortened is then divided in a diamond-shaped fashion creating two angles of 30° as demonstrated. The lesion is then excised along this geometric pattern and the wound is sutured, creating two short arms at the lateral margin as demonstrated.

place during initial healing. This geometric design is most useful to prevent wounds extending into sensitive cosmetic areas or abutting lip or eyelid tissue.

Curettage

The curette for use in the skin was developed in the late 1800s and may be an under-utilized instrument and technique. The sharp cutting edge portion of the curette is unique in its ability to remove superficial and/or friable tissue while little damaging normal epidermis. However, this instrument is not useful in dealing with fibrotic lesions or lesions imbedded in scar. A curette is an important instrument and technique in the paediatric population.

The curette should be firmly grasped with the exact location frequently determined by the shape and contour of the curette chosen (Fig. 28.1.12). There are many curettes with different grips and the surgeon should choose one that fits the size of their hand most comfortably. The curette is then firmly and sharply pulled over the lesion to remove it from the normal surrounding skin. If there is depth to the lesion, the curette needs to be used

repeatedly to remove all the lesion by 'feel', and then the margins carefully smoothed to prevent a sharp-angled drop off to the depth of the wound. In some instances, a clean curette may be used for the last pass so as not to reintroduce infectious materials such as wart virus.

In most instances, haemostasis can be obtained with pressure following this technique. Occasionally, electrocautery or desiccation may be used. In such instances it may be used for simple haemostasis or to further help in the destruction of the lesion. This may be the case in skin tumours or in the treatment of wart virus. Curettes may also be used to remove the sac lining of an epidermal inclusion cyst (Table 28.1.4).

Cryosurgery

Modern cryosurgery was first begun in the mid-1800s by James Arnot, who used a blind solution that would approach −24 degrees. Pusey in the early 1900s made the technique easily clinically applicable with the use of carbon dioxide (CO_2) sticks. From that point, other gases were used, with the most common including a solid CO_2 'slush', liquid nitrous oxide, and finally, liquid nitrogen. Solid CO_2 cryo agent is held in direct contact with the lesion to be treated while the other agents in a liquid form may be applied by a cotton swab or by a cryosurgical spray unit. Liquid nitrogen is by far the most commonly used agent.

Cryosurgery is based on controlled cell death through freezing. The cryo agent is applied to the lesion and there are cellular changes which occur in a rapid fashion. Cell death of treated cells usually occurs within several days, and inflammatory response develops in and around the

Table 28.1.5 Common skin conditions treated by cryosurgery

Warts
Molluscum contagiosum
Pyogenic granuloma
Acne cysts
Bowen's disease

Table 28.1.6 Lesions amenable to electrosurgery

Warts
Skin tags
Telangiectases
Pyogenic granuloma
Hair removal (electrolysis)

treated area. The deeper or thicker the lesion to be treated, the longer the freeze time required and the greater amount of resulting tissue necrosis. Superficial lesions treated in this fashion usually heal with essentially no resulting scarring. The greater the depth and tissue loss, the more probable that small amounts of scarring will develop as an end result of the treatment [19].

Other possible side-effects include a tingling or burning discomfort which may last several hours; oedema, especially in areas of lax tissue; blisters, either fluid-filled or haemorrhagic blisters; and postinflammatory hyper- or hypopigmentation. More severe side-effects can include paraesthesias when a large sensory nerve trunk is damaged, hair loss, hypertrophic scarring or a through-and-through defect on a structure such as an ear or nasal ala [20]. The risk of complication increases with the intensity of the freeze. Cryotherapy has been used to treat a large number of lesions, both benign and malignant. Dermatology will continue to rely on this cost-effective treatment for many conditions. Table 28.1.5 lists the common conditions treated with cryotherapy.

Electrosurgery

Electrical currents have been used in the treatment of dermatological conditions for many years. There are several distinct types of electrosurgery, each with their own uses [21–23]. Electrolysis is achieved by chemical reaction at the tip of the electrode and requires direct current to cause this chemical reaction. Electrocautery uses the resistance of the tip to generate heat which is then transferred to the surgical site. No electricity passes through the patient. The cautery tip is simply a heated tip much like a branding iron or hot poker. High frequency electrosurgery uses a bipolar machine with the passage of current through the patient, requiring the patient to be grounded to prevent sparking or burning from passage of the electricity. Electrofulguration occurs when there is a spark between the instrument tip and the area to be treated, the tip not being in direct contact with the skin. Electrodesiccation occurs when the tip is in direct contact with the area to be treated and no sparking occurs.

Electrodesiccation remains the mainstay of haemostasis during surgical procedures. Cautery may be used in some patients with unprotected pacemakers. Other uses are listed in Table 28.1.6. At the basis of the use of electric current is that such current will cause cellular desiccation and death. There will also be thrombosis of small blood vessels with actual destruction of the vessel itself. Because it cauterizes as it works, there will be little or no bleeding, making it a bloodless type of surgery.

One of the risks of electrosurgery is that it is relatively uncontrolled, and there may be tissue damage beyond the clinical lesion. With care, this damage may be minimized. There will be an inflammatory infiltrate called to the area of injury. The more tissue injury that occurs, the greater the chance of resulting scarring. Electrosurgery can damage or destroy adnexal structures, therefore leaving resulting scars devoid of follicles or other adnexal structures.

Other surgical procedures

Skin resurfacing

Skin resurfacing has been used to improve scars as a result of surgical procedures or other scarring processes. Resurfacing techniques have on occasion been used to remove imbedded foreign material as a result of trauma such as road burns or powder burns. Such resurfacing has been done with dermabrasion techniques [24–26] with either diamond-studded wheels and fraizes or wire brushes. They spin at 20 000–30 000 revolutions/min and will remove the dermis and papillary dermis and in some instances extend into the deeper dermis. Abrasions that are extended too deeply may cause scarring or an unsightly scar. Dermabrasions that are too superficial will produce no significant improvement of the underlying condition. Dermabrasion is frequently used for scar revision, acne scarring and a large number of other benign but superficial lesions.

The improved pulsing of the CO_2 laser with shorter pulse durations has allowed the development of resurfacing by such CO_2 lasers. This technique is bloodless and will grow in application [27–31].

Hair transplantation

Hair transplantation, while commonly thought of as useful in balding men, may be important in children who have had traumatic or congenital hair loss. Hair transplantation may be achieved by the movement of hair-bearing skin into an area of alopecia, scalp reduction which entails the removal of the alopecic area with primary closure, punch grafting and micrografting which moves single hairs to create a more normal hairline. All of these techniques have a place in dermatological surgery and may occasionally be useful in the paediatric population.

Mohs micrographic surgery

Mohs micrographic surgery was developed as a method of removing cutaneous malignancies [32]. This method includes the careful removal of a narrow margin of epidermis around the cutaneous tumour. The tissue removed is then carefully mapped and marked, and horizontal frozen sections are prepared. In this way, the entire epidermal and deep margins are viewed histopathologically and small foci of tumour can be carefully traced. This method gives the highest cure rates for cutaneous tumours as well as conserving tissue in cosmetically important areas. While this is used most commonly in the older population when tumours are most common, it has been very useful in a few instances in the paediatric population [33]. This technique has been used for children with basal cell naevus syndrome, with invasive tumours where both a high cure rate and tumour preservation are important, and in children with dermatofibrosarcoma protuberans, a fibrotic tumour that is difficult to eradicate with conventional excision.

Wound management

The biology of wound healing is beyond the limitations of this chapter. There are many reviews which cover this topic well [34–39]. However, wound management is important for the creation of an optimal environment for wound healing. It is clear that a moist environment maximizes both granulation of a wound and epidermal migration. There are a variety of approaches to wound management that range from simple to complicated.

Wound care should first include a daily cleaning of the wound with sterile saline, soap and water, or half strength hydrogen peroxide (1.5%). Cleaning with such materials will provide gentle mechanical debridement for any accumulating debris or crust which can act as a medium for colonization with bacteria. Once this has been removed, an ointment should be applied, e.g. bacitracin, polysporin, garamycin, silvadene or even petrolatum. It has clearly been shown that this will speed wound healing. The addition of antibiotic does not seem to play a significant role in this wound-healing effect. Several studies have shown that application of the base of the named ointments were as effective in promoting healing as the ointment itself.

A dressing needs to be firmly held in place with tape or with a soft 'wrap around' gauze. A circular 'wrap around' on the extremity or digit must be applied carefully to avoid excessive constriction of the tissues, thereby causing distal oedema or hypoxia [40].

There are a wide variety of newer dressings which may be placed directly over a wound, replacing the ointment application and bandaging process [41–43]. Such dressings maintain a moist milieu and may be left in place longer than 24 h, decreasing the need for as frequent dressing changes. They are far more expensive than the ointment and dressing as listed above, but in some instances will be a significant benefit.

Complications

Surgical procedures should not be undertaken unless the potential complications of that procedure are fully understood. Anticipation of a complication may prevent its occurrence, while recognition of a complication is mandatory for appropriate therapy. A range of complications are discussed here.

Bleeding [44,45]

Interference with normal clot formation may occur at various points along the clotting pathway. Full discussion is beyond the scope of this chapter. Interference with haemostasis may be caused by an acquired or congenital defect in the clotting cascade, thrombocytopenia, platelet dysfunction or drugs.

Inherited disorders of clotting defects are frequently well identified before a surgical procedure is planned. In these instances, management of the problem will be best obtained by replacement of the missing factor. However, in some instances, a clotting disorder will not be suspected until the patient has a surgical or dental procedure. In these instances, it is possible for the dermatology surgeon to be the first to recognize excessive intraoperative bleeding.

Platelets initiate the clotting cascade. Their absence or dysfunction will therefore lead to an intraoperative bleeding problem. Thrombocytopenia may be caused by impaired production, excessive destruction, disseminated intravascular coagulation or abnormal sequestration in the spleen or haemangioma. Surgery can be safely performed with attention to intraoperative haemostasis when platelet counts are above 50 000. Below that number, surgery may be performed, but care must be taken and platelet transfusion should be available if required.

Non-functioning platelets are the more common defect seen. Non-functioning platelets are almost always the result of medication, most commonly aspirin. Aspirin irreversibly inactivates phospholipase and this in turn inactivates the platelet for its circulating life. Non-steroidal anti-inflammatory drugs (NSAIDs) similarly inhibit platelet function; however, the NSAID effects are reversible [46]. Aspirin is not commonly used in the younger paediatric population, but may be used for specific indications, or in the older paediatric population.

NSAIDs are being used more frequently in the entire paediatric population.

Other drugs causing bleeding are typically heparin or coumadin. These drugs affect clot formation during the later phase of clot stabilization. Therefore one would expect to see bleeding 2–3 days postoperatively, and, in most instances, there is no increased intraoperative bleeding. Cutaneous surgery can be safely performed with any of the anticoagulative drugs, but knowledge of these drugs is imperative to minimize the risks of bleeding [46,47].

The complications resulting from ineffective haemostasis include acute intraoperative bleeding, immediate postoperative bleeding and late postoperative bleeding.

Acute bleeding is most usually caused by interrupting an artery. A transected artery will tend to retract, and the bleeding ends are usually easily found. Small diameter vessels may be cauterized, whereas larger vessels may require tying off with an absorbable suture. Occasionally, vessels are unroofed without being fully transected; these arteries bleed copiously and will not be effectively treated with cautery. The surgeon must complete the transection and then deal with the bleeding artery appropriately.

The other common bleeding problem is the excessive oozing related to aspirin use. In these instances, wounds bleed briskly, but no single bleeding site can be identified. Meticulous haemostasis must be obtained with an electrocoagulating device to obtain a dry field. Early postoperative bleeding is frequently the result of a small arterial bleeder overlooked because of vasoconstriction due to the epinephrine in the local anaesthetic. As the epinephrine effect wears off, the vessel may actively bleed, resulting in an acute haematoma. Other causes of bleeding at this time include excessive vasodilation usually caused by exercising or local trauma. Such bleeding may be controlled with 10–15 min of direct pressure, but may require the wound to be opened and the bleeder identified and treated appropriately.

Late postoperative bleeding may be the result of trauma or any defect causing interference with maceration of the clot. Late bleeding usually causes a slowly developing haematoma or a far-reaching ecchymosis. If identified early, the wound may be opened and the bleeding site identified. However, in some instances, the patient does not recognize the occurrence of this complication, and an organized haematoma may be identified at the time of suture removal. Such an organized haematoma may require removal or can be treated with warm compresses and massage, which will heal with time.

Seromas may develop in any wound irrespective of a bleeding problem. They are most common in wounds where the dead space is not obliterated and can act as either a culture media or a mechanical interference with wound healing. The seromas can be evacuated through a large-bore needle and do not usually require opening of the entire wound.

Allergic reactions

Allergic reactions can be divided into type I and IV. Type I reactions are extremely uncommon in dermatological surgery. The most likely cause of type I reaction in this setting would be injected anaesthetics. As discussed above, the ester family of anaesthetics (including procaine) is the more likely of the anaesthetics to cause this kind of reaction. A few cases of allergic reaction have been reported to the amide type of anaesthetics. There has also been a single case report of an anaphylactic reaction to chlorhexidine gluconate when it was applied mucosally [48].

The vast majority of allergic reactions include type IV contact sensitivity to topical agents. Such agents include povidone-iodine, chlorhexidine gluconate, amide anaesthetics, adhesive tapes and topical antibiotics. Topical antibiotics are probably the most common offender producing contact allergy. Of these, neomycin causes sensitization in as many as 8% of patients, and, interestingly, neomycin and bacitracin sensitivity may well develop in the same patient. This is a phenomenon of cosensitization rather than cross-sensitization [49].

A contact sensitization or contact allergy may be confused with an early wound infection. Points to differentiate include early vesiculation and a geometric pattern of reaction that are both seen with contact sensitivity. In most instances of contact sensitivity to a topical antibiotic, the reaction will include the suture line itself and again move outwards in a geometric pattern. Interestingly, patients frequently increase their application, subsequently involving larger and larger areas of dermatitis. Appropriate treatment of contact allergy is important to appropriate wound healing. Secondary infection is not uncommon when contact allergy occurs. Treatment may include oral antibiotics as well as the appropriate topical steroid. Wound healing will be slowed in such cases and suture removal may therefore need to be delayed.

Wound infection

Wound infection rates will vary according to the patient population, and the preoperative risk for infection [50]. The infection rate in patients with coexisting dermatitis is frequently higher than in people with an otherwise normal epidermal barrier. Generally, wound infections occur in approximately 3% of cutaneous surgical procedures [51]. With development or increasing erythema, warmth and tenderness, a wound infection should be suspected. If pus is available for culture, a Gram stain and culture should be performed, especially in an immunocompromised host or patient where unusual infections might occur. If no material is available, treatment with antibiotics for the presumed organism (*Staphylococcus aureus*) is prudent. Wound infection around the ear may involve *Pseudomonas* organisms and can go on to develop into what is known as malignant external otitis. Such infection is serious and will require intravenous antibiotics and frequently hospitalization.

Wound dehiscence

Wound dehiscence may be the result of one of several factors. It can be the result of excessive tension on a sutured wound, infection, haematoma or seroma, or trauma to or excessive movement of the surgical site. The wound may open completely with resulting bleeding or it may separate at just a portion of the incision line, separating only 1–3 mm wide. The cause of dehiscence should be sought so that an unsuspected haematoma or infection will be recognized.

Management of the open wound depends on the size of the dehiscence, its location and the patient. The wound that has only opened 1–2 mm will easily heal by second intention and in most instances leaves a completely acceptable cosmetic result. If the wound is opened more fully and the patient notifies the doctor immediately, the wound can be cleaned and simply resutured. If there has been a time delay of over 24 h or if there is any sign of infection, the wound should be allowed to heal by second intention and then managed further for the ultimate cosmetic effect following full healing. It has been found that even large wounds that have dehisced have healed with an amazingly good cosmetic result without resuturing. However, if the resulting scar is depressed or noticeable, the area can be re-excised and resutured with careful attention to immobilizing the wound and providing prolonged support even after the sutures have been removed with agents such as Steri-strips or adhesive strips.

Wound necrosis is frequently due to other complications such as undue wound tension, a compromised blood supply, a haematoma or infection. Whatever the cause, the tissue loss should be identified and any wound infection (either primary or secondary to tissue loss) should be treated. Seromas or haematomas should similarly be evacuated. Completely devitalized tissue should be debrided to speed healing, but one must be very careful not to remove still vital tissue. When tissue necrosis occurs, it is most prudent to allow the defect to heal by second intention, although in rare instances, the area can be excised and reclosed with a side-to-side closure, a flap or a graft.

Scarring

There are several complications that may occur in the final scarring event. There may be postinflammatory hyper- or hypopigmentation and this should be managed conserva-

tively. In most instances, this discoloration will resolve spontaneously over months.

Hypertrophic or keloidal scarring is more difficult to manage. Hypertrophic scarring will include scars that are thickened but do not extend beyond the area of surgical trauma. Keloids are the result of uncontrolled scar formation that extend far beyond the site of surgical trauma. Hypertrophic scars are more easily managed with high potency topical steroids, steroid injection into the wound itself, massage and time. These scars frequently occur in certain body locations, such as the chest and back, and on areas with frequent movement. The scars may also result from thermal injury, such as burn scars.

In an effort to diminish the risk of keloid formation, buried sutures as a source of foreign body tissue reaction can be avoided, cautery can be minimized and nonreactive sutures can be used. In a known keloid former, interlesional steroid injections may be given at the time of surgery in an attempt to decrease the risk of keloid formation. When this is done, wound healing may occur more slowly and it may be prudent to support the wound for a longer time period. This would include leaving cutaneous sutures in for several days longer than the norm, and then supporting the wound with adhesive strips for several weeks postoperatively.

Treatment of a formed keloid includes topical high-potency steroids, injectable steroids, silicone gel sheeting [52], laser therapy (CO_2 [53] and pulsed dye laser [54]) and occasionally judicial scar revision. Keloids and hypertrophic scarring are discussed in more detail in Chapter 28.3.

REFERENCES

1 Evers H, von Dardel O, Juhlin L *et al.* Dermal effects of compositions based on eutectic mixture of lignocaine and prilocaine (EMLA). *Br J Anaesth* 1985; 57: 997–1005.
2 de Ward-van der Spek FB, van den Berg GM, Oranje AP. EMLA cream: an improved local anesthetic. Review of current literature. *Pediatr Dermatol* 1992; 9: 126–31.
3 Nielsen JC, Arendt-Nielsen L, Bjerring P, Svensson P. The analgesic effect of EMLA cream on facial skin. *Acta Derm Venereol (Stockh)* 1992; 72: 281–4.
4 Skidmore RA, Patterson JD, Tomsick RS. Local anesthetics. *Dermatol Surg* 1996; 22: 511–22.
5 Auletta MJ. Local anesthesia for dermatologic surgery. *Semin Dermatol* 1994; 13: 35–42.
6 Larson PO, Ragi G, Swandby M, Darcey B, Polzin G, Carey P. Stability of buffered lidocaine and epinephrine used for local anesthesia. *J Dermatol Surg Oncol* 1991; 17: 411–14.
7 Stewart JH, Cole GW, Klein JA. Neutralized lidocaine with epinephrine for local anesthesia. *J Dermatol Surg Oncol* 1989; 15: 1081–3.
8 Glinert RJ, Zachary CB. Anesthetic allergy. *J Dermatol Surg Oncol* 1991; 17: 491–6.
9 Dire DJ, Hogan DE. Double-blinded comparison of diphenhydramine versus lidocaine as a local anesthetic. *Ann Emerg Med* 1993; 22: 1419–22.
10 Green SM, Rothrock SG, Gorchynski J. Validation of diphenhydramine as a dermal local anesthetic. *Ann Emerg Med* 1994; 23: 1284–9.
11 Skidmore RA, Patterson JD, Tomsick RS. Local anaesthetics. *Dermatol Surg* 1996; 22: 511–22.
12 Winkelmann RK. Skin biopsy. In: Epstein E, Epstein E, eds. Lea & Febiger, 1979: 95–101.

13 Sebben JE. Sterile technique and the prevention of wound infection in office surgery. Part II. *Dermatol Surg Oncol* 1989; 15: 38–48.

14 Maki DG, Ringer M, Alvarado CJ. Prospective randomised trial of povidone-iodine, alcohol, and chlorhexidine for prevention of infection associated with central venous and arterial catheters. *Lancet* 1991; 338: 339–43.

15 Roth RR, James WD. Microbiology of the skin: resident flora, ecology, infection. *J Am Acad Dermatol* 1989; 20: 367–90.

16 Moy RL, Quan MB. An evaluation of wound closure tapes. *J Dermatol Surg Oncol* 1990; 16: 721–3.

17 Maloney ME. *Suture Selection in the Dermatologic Surgical Suite*. Edinburgh: Churchill Livingstone, 1991: 42–7.

18 Dzubow LM. The dynamics of dog-ear formation and correction. *J Dermatol Surg Oncol* 1985; 11: 722–8.

19 Pusey W. The use of carbon dioxide in the treatment of nevi and other lesions of the skin. *J Am Med Assoc* 1907; 49: 1354–6.

20 Kuflik EG. Cryosurgery updated. *J Am Acad Dermatol* 1994; 31: 925–44.

21 Blankenship ML. Physical modalities. Electrosurgery, electrocautery and electrolysis. *Int Soc Trop Dermatol* 1979; 18: 443–52.

22 Sebben JE. The status of electrosurgery in dermatologic practice. *J Am Acad Dermatol* 1988; 19: 542–9.

23 Sebben JE. Electrodes for high-frequency electrosurgery. *J Dermatol Surg Oncol* 1989; 15: 805–10.

24 Roenigk HH Jr. Dermabrasion: state of the art. *J Dermatol Surg Oncol* 1985; 11: 306–14.

25 Harmon CB, Zelickson BD, Roenigk RK *et al.* Dermabrasive scar revision. Immunohistochemical and ultrastructural evaluation. *Dermatol Surg* 1995; 21: 503–8.

26 Yarborough J. Dermabrasive surgery. *Clin Dermatol* 1987; 5: 75.

27 Chernoff WG, Schoenrock LD, Cramer H, Wand J. Cutaneous laser resurfacing. *Int J Aesthetic Restor Surg* 1995; 3: 57–68.

28 David LM, Sarne AJ, Unger WP. Rapid laser scanning for facial resurfacing. *Dermatol Surg* 1995; 21: 1031–3.

29 Lowe NJ, Lask G, Griffin ME, Maxwell A, Lowe P. Skin resurfacing with the ultrapulse carbon dioxide laser. *Dermatol Surg* 1995; 21: 1025–9.

30 Lowe NJ, Lask G, Griffin H. Oaser skin resurfacing. *Dermatol Surg* 1995; 221: 1017–19.

31 Ho C, Gguyen Q, Lowe NJ, Griffin ME, Lask G. Laser resurfacing in pigmented skin. *Dermatol Surg* 1995; 21: 1035–7.

32 Telfer NR. Mohs micrographic surgery for nonmelanoma skin cancer. *Clin Dermatol* 1995; 13: 593–600.

33 Dinehart SM, Dodge R, Stanley W, Franks HH, Pollack SV. Basal cell carcinoma treated with Mohs surgery. A comparison of 54 younger patients with 1050 older patients. *J Dermatol Surg Oncol* 1992; 18: 560–6.

34 Clark RAF. Basics of cutaneous wound repair. *J Dermatol Surg Oncol* 1993; 19: 693–706.

35 Kirsner RS, Eaglstein WH. The wound healing process. *Dermatol Clin* 1993; 11: 629–39.

36 Clark RAF. Biology of dermal wound repair. *Dermatol Clin* 1993; 11: 647–66.

37 Mertz PM, Ovington LG. Wound healing microbiology. *Dermatol Clin* 1993; 11: 739–47.

38 Thompson WM. Regulation of cutaneous wound healing by growth factors and the microenvironment. *Cutaneous Wound Healing* 1991; 6: 604–11.

39 Galanga V. Growth factors and wound healing. *J Dermatol Surg Oncol* 1993; 19: 711–14.

40 Giandoni MB, Vinson RP, Grabski WJ. Ischemic complications of tubular gauze dressings. *Dermatol Surg* 1995; 21: 716–18.

41 Hutchinson JJ, McGuckin M. Occlusive dressings: a microbiologic and clinical review. *Am J Infect Control* 18: 257–68.

42 Phillips TJ, Palko MJ, Bhawan J. Histologic evaluation of chronic human wounds treated with hydrocolloid and nonhydrocolloid dressings. *J Am Acad Dermatol* 1994; 30: 61–34.

43 Kannon GA, Garrett AB. Moist wound healing with occlusive dressings. A clinical review. *Dermatol Surg* 1995; 21: 583–90.

44 Salasche SJ. Acute surgical complications: cause, prevention, and treatment. *J Am Acad Dermatol* 1986; 15: 1163–85.

45 Maloney ME. Management of surgical complications and suboptimal results. In: Wheeland RG, ed. *Cutaneous Surgery*. Philadelphia: WB Saunders, 1994: 921–34.

46 Lawrence C, Sakuntabhai A, Tiling-Grosse S. Effect of aspirin and non-steroidal anti-inflammatory drug therapy on bleeding complications in dermatologic surgical patients. *J Am Acad Dermatol* 1994; 31: 988–92.

47 Otley CC, Fewkes JL, Frank W, Olbricht SM. Complications of cutaneous surgery in patients who are taking warfarin, aspirin, or non-steroidal anti-inflammatory drugs. *Arch Dermatol* 1996; 132: 161–6.

48 Okano M, Nomura M, Hata S *et al.* Anaphylactic symptoms due to chlorhexidine gluconate. *Arch Dermatol* 1989; 125: 50–2.

49 Gette MT, Marks JG, Maloney ME. Frequency of postoperative allergic contact dermatitis to topical antibiotics. *Arch Dermatol* 1992; 128: 356–67.

50 Nichols RL. Surgical wound infection. *Am J Med* 1991; 91: 545–645.

51 Futoryan T, Grande D. Postoperative wound infection rates in dermatologic surgery. *Dermatol Surg* 1995; 21: 509–14.

52 Fulton JE Jr. Silicone gel sheeting for the prevention and management of evolving hypertrophic and keloid scars. *Dermatol Surg* 1995; 21: 947–51.

53 Spicer MS, Goldberg DJ. Lasers in dermatology. *J Am Acad Dermatol* 1996; 34: 1–25.

54 Alster TS. Improvement of erythematous and hypertrophic scars by the 585-nm flashlamp-pumped pulsed dye laser. *Ann Plast Surg* 1994; 32: 186–90.

28.2 Treatment of Giant Congenital Melanocytic Naevi

LINDA E. DE RAEVE

Congenital melanocytic naevi (CMN) are common lesions found in about 1% of newborns. They represent a special group of melanocytic lesions because of the potential for development of malignant melanoma [1–3].

CMN are usually classified by their size [2]. Small congenital melanocytic naevi (SCMN) are defined as those measuring less than 1.5 cm in their largest diameter, medium-sized lesions (MCMN) are 1.5–20 cm in their largest diameter and giant congenital melanocytic naevi (GCMN) are 20 cm or more. Another more useful functional definition defines small naevi as those amenable to simple excision and primary closure, and giant naevi as lesions that cannot be easily excised and closed in one surgical stage [4,5].

The sizes of the lesions have different implications for diagnosis, treatment and prognosis. GCMN often cover a large portion of the body surface such as the back or the extremity. Such naevi are often descriptively called coat-sleeve, cape-like, bathing trunk or giant hairy naevi. They are unevenly pigmented, have an irregular surface and over 95% have a component consisting of large coarse terminal hairs. In some cases, GCMN situated on the head or neck are associated with leptomeningeal melanocytosis, the so-called neurocutaneous melanosis [6]. GCMN situated in the lumbosacral area may be associated with meningomyelocele or spina bifida. In children with GCMN overlying the head or midline posterior spine it is appropriate to evaluate the child for underlying abnormalities by magnetic resonance imaging (MRI), since the presence of this condition may influence subsequent management decisions.

REFERENCES

1 Arons MS, Hurwitz S. Congenital nevocellular nevus. Review of treatment controversy. *Plast Reconstr Surg* 1983; 72: 355–65.
2 Kaplan EN. The risk of malignancy in large congenital nevi. *Plast Reconstr Surg* 1974; 53: 421–8.
3 Lorentzen M, Pers M, Bretteville-Jensen G. The incidence of malignant transformation in giant pigmented nevi. *Scand J Plast Reconstr Surg* 1977; 11: 163–7.
4 Pack GT, Davis J. Nevus giganticus pigmentosus with malignant transformation. *Surgery* 1961; 49: 347–54.
5 Lanier VC, Pickrell KL, Georgiade NC. Congenital giant naevi: clinical and pathological considerations. *Plast Reconstr Surg* 1976; 58: 48–54.
6 Kadonaga JN, Frieden IJ. Neurocutaneous melanosis: definition and review of the literature. *J Am Acad Dermatol* 1991; 24: 747–55.

Management

The approach to the management of CMN is one of the most debated subjects in paediatric dermatology [1]. In recent years this approach has been considerably changed by more accurate information on evaluation of the risk of malignancy occurring in these naevi [2] and by the development of new surgical techniques.

With regard to SCMN the risk of malignant change has been estimated to be 2.6–4.9% [3,4]. The risk of malignant change in MCMN has not yet been quantified [5]. The incidence of malignant melanoma in GCMN has first been reported to vary from 1.8 to 42% [6]. Part of the discrepancy among figures in these reports results from the large variability in the criteria defining GCMN. There is also biased reporting and the lack of adequate prospective data.

The lifetime risk of malignant melanoma arising in GCMN has been estimated by Rhodes *et al.* to be about 6.3% [7]. In GCMN 60% of melanomas develop within the first decade, 10% within the second decade and 30% later in life. As malignancy risk is substantially increased (17-fold relative risk as compared to the general population) and as these changes mostly occur prior to puberty, most authorities now agree that GCMN should be removed whenever and as early as technically possible [7–9].

Besides these considerations on malignancy risk, the management of GCMN is also influenced by aesthetic considerations. These GCMN have considerable consequences for both patients and family. As they often cover extensive areas of the body, they can be an aesthetic tragedy and contribute to severe psychological sequelae, which should not be underestimated.

Management of GCMN thus presents a tremendous challenge to those caring for these patients. The choice of surgical methods must take into consideration the importance of the cosmetic appearance, the reduction of malignancy risk and the maintenance of normal function [9–11]. In order to reduce the risk of malignancy a complete excision is preferred, whenever such surgery is feasible and practical. However, surgical excision too early in life is often not practical because of the cosmetic and functional disability caused by extensive surgery. Excision of giant lesions mostly requires multiple procedures: this increases the number of blood transfusions and the risks of general anaesthesia [12]. Serial excisions with primary wound closing are sometimes not possible due to the localization of the naevus. An alternative to excision is skin grafting or skin flaps. Split-skin grafting, however, can be limited by donor sites and in general the cosmetic results with skin grafts are poor. Great strides have been made in excisional surgery with the use of tissue expanders; however, all of the tumour cannot always be removed easily and complete removal may be incompatible with acceptable cosmetic results [13]. Another possibility offered for these patients is the use of cultured epithelial autografts or allografts [14].

Dermabrasion

A treatment that has been used by several authors for GCMN is dermabrasion. The fact that pigmented melanocytes can be removed by dermabrasion in the neonate was discovered by accident by Johnson in 1977 [15]: a newborn with a large pigmented naevus of the forehead and scalp had part of the lesion scuffed by obstetrical forceps during delivery. Ten days later epithelialization was complete without pigmentation. Based on this, Johnson described how he dermabraded three other pigmented naevi and suggested that reducing the total number of melanocytes to a minimum early in life might well have prophylactic value to malignant change. However, in two lesions dermabraded at 11 and 17 months pigmentation returned. Miller and Becker in 1979 reported on two GCMN cases similarly treated at age 4 weeks, 7 weeks and 9 weeks [16]. The first dermabrasion, 4 weeks after birth, had the best cosmetic results and the least amount of residual naevus.

These reports that better cosmetic results can be achieved by early rather than by later dermabrasion have led authors to postulate that naevus cells at birth are located predominantly in the superficial papillary dermis and that they only later migrate into the deeper dermis [15–17]. This theory however is not generally accepted, as skin biopsies of GCMN taken shortly after birth compared to those taken later have not substantiated this hypothesis. Walton *et al.* [9] studied the depth of penetration of naevus cells in SCMN: they concluded that SCMN have a variable pattern of histological appearance with naevus cells at varying levels throughout the dermis with naevus cells only in the upper dermis in 63% and in the upper and deep dermis as well as the subcutis in 37%. Zitelli *et al.* [18] studied larger CMN. They showed that in GCMN naevus cells already occupy the entire dermis and often deeper structures in the neonatal period and that the depth of

invasion of CMN does not change with time; postdermabrasion biopsies still showed the presence of naevus cells in the deep dermis and subcutis. Based on this published information it is clear that there are various subsets of histological patterns of CMN and these patterns do not appear to change remarkably during the first years of life [19]. Whether or not dermabrasion alters the risk of malignant change is not known, but it may improve the cosmetic appearance. However, there is a tendency for most naevi so treated to repigment.

Curettage in the neonatal period

Moss in 1987 described a new approach to the treatment of GCMN, using a curette to remove naevus cells in the first weeks of life [20]. This treatment is based on the observation that there appears to be in these GCMN in the first weeks of life a cleavage plane between the upper dermis containing most of the pigmented naevus cells and the lower dermis. He obtained encouraging cosmetic results and recommended this technique as an atraumatic method for removing the upper dermis with most of the pigmented naevus cells. The author has used this technique for the treatment of newborns with GCMN in the first few weeks of life during the past 10 years. Under general anaesthesia the GCMN is scraped with a sharp curette from the centre to the periphery of the naevus. In the first 2 weeks of life this curettage is easy to perform and the cleavage plane described above easily found. The only area where it is more difficult is at the junction of the naevus with the normal skin. The earlier the curettage is performed, the easier it is to find the cleavage plane. Later it becomes progressively more difficult to find. The advantage of curettage over dermabrasion is the ability to discern the level of destruction within the dermis when the operation is performed before 2 weeks of age, and this separation level seems to be the correct level in terms of cosmetic results. Dermabrasion is inaccurate in that if it is performed too superficially it can result in return of the naevus while if performed too deeply hypertrophic scarring or changes in pigmentation may occur.

Another advantage of the curettage procedure is that it is a relatively atraumatic procedure with minimal blood loss and a one-stage procedure well tolerated by the infant. Healing takes place rapidly with minimal scarring and cosmetic results are favourable [21]. In order to evaluate whether or not this procedure alters the risk of malignant change, these GCMN were examined histologically before and after curettage.

The histological features of the naevi prior to curettage showed that the upper dermis was entirely occupied by heavily pigmented naevus cells, while the lower dermis contained a less dense, diffuse infiltration of nonpigmented naevus cells. The curetted material consisted

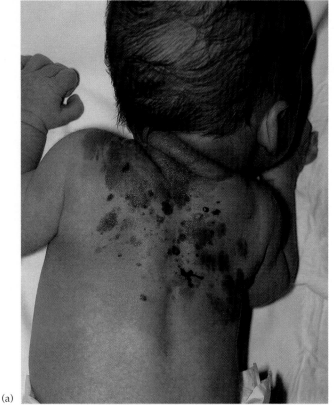

(a)

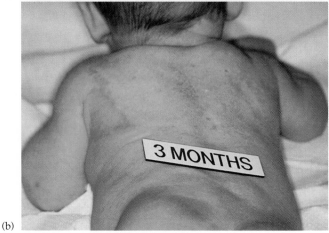

(b)

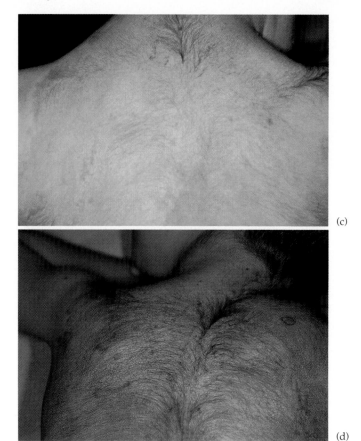

(c)

(d)

Fig. 28.2.1 (a) GCMN on the back of a newborn just prior to curettage. (b) Three months follow-up. (c) Two years follow-up. (d) Four years follow-up. Reproduced with permission from the *Archives of Dermatology*.

of epidermis with underlying upper dermis, as described by Moss [20].

Histological findings prior to curettage have already shown deep dermal involvement in the neonatal period but two populations of naevus cells have been identified: the superficially located heavily pigmented naevus cells and the deeper dermal non-pigmented naevus cells. Positive HMB-45 staining of the superficially located dermal pigmented naevus cells and negative staining of the deeper dermal non-pigmented naevus cells in these GCMN demonstrates that the biological behaviour of these two populations of naevus cells seems to be different, as they are different in their expression of melanocytic

antigen [21]. The significance of these findings awaits further study [22,23]. Follow-up biopsies after curettage showed that the entire upper dermis was composed of a dense connective tissue with some degree of sclerosis, but the heavily pigmented naevus cells were no longer seen; HMB-45 staining was negative. The deeper dermis still contained a diffuse infiltration of non-pigmented naevus cells as observed prior to curettage, but no pigmented naevus cells and there was no immunoreactivity for HMB-45.

Curettage will thus not eliminate the naevus cells in the deeper dermis but it seems reasonable to assume that early removal of an important number of pigmented

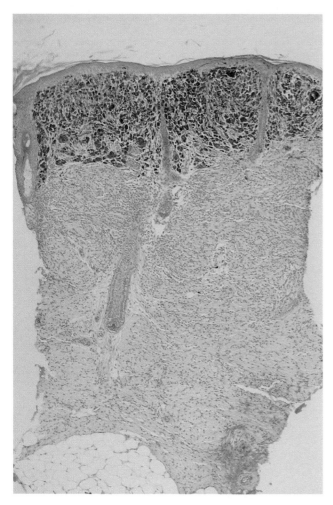

Fig. 28.2.2 Histological section prior to curettage: the upper dermis is occupied by heavily pigmented naevus cells; the lower dermis contains non-pigmented naevus cells. (Haematoxylin and eosin.) Reproduced with permission from the *Archives of Dermatology.*

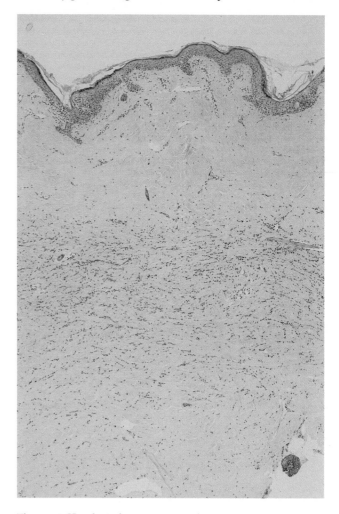

Fig. 28.2.3 Histological section 4 years after curettage: dense connective tissue with sclerosis and no pigmented naevus cells in upper dermis. (Haematoxylin and eosin.) Reproduced with permission from the *Archives of Dermatology.*

naevus cells will minimize the risks of malignancy. Certainly the deeper naevus cells which remain after the debulking procedure can give rise to melanoma [24], and there is concern that the scar tissue induced by this procedure may mask the ability to detect malignant growth to the deeper component. Only long-term follow-up on a large number of treated patients will answer some of these critical questions. The cosmetic improvement, however, is impressive and may spare a child with a GCMN from another treatment method with less acceptable aesthetic and functional results.

REFERENCES

1 Alper JC. Congenital naevi: the controversy rages on. *Arch Dermatol* 1985; 121: 734–5.

2 Rhodes AR. Pigmented birthmarks and precursor melanocytic lesions of cutaneous melanoma identifiable in childhood. *Pediatr Clin N Am* 1983; 30: 435–63.

3 Rhodes AR, Melski JW. Small congenital nevocellular nevi and the risk of cutaneous melanoma. *J Pediatr* 1982; 100: 219–24.

4 Rhodes AR, Sober AJ, Day CL *et al.* The malignant potential of small congenital nevocellular nevi. *J Am Acad Dermatol* 1982; 6: 230–41.

5 De Raeve L, Danau W, De Backer A, Otten J. Prepubertal melanoma in a medium-sized congenital naevus. *Eur J Pediatr* 1993; 152: 734–6.

6 Hurwitz S. Pigmented nevi. *Semin Dermatol* 1988; 7: 17–25.

7 Rhodes AR, Wood WC, Sober AJ, Mihm MC. Non-epidermal origin of malignant melanoma associated with a giant congenital nevocellular nevus. *Plast Reconstr Surg* 1981; 67: 782–90.

8 Quaba AA, Wallace AE. The incidence of malignant melanoma (0–15 years of age) arising in 'large' congenital naevocellular naevi. *Plast Reconstr Surg* 1986; 78: 174–9.

9 Walton RG, Jacobs AH, Cox AJ. Pigmented lesions in newborn infants. *Br J Dermatol* 1976; 95: 389–96.

10 Kopf AW, Bart RS, Hennessy P. Congenital nevocytic naevi and malignant melanomas. *J Am Acad Dermatol* 1979; 1: 123–30.

11 Lorentzen M, Pers M, Bretteville-Jensen G. The incidence of malignant transformation in giant pigmented nevi. *Scand J Plast Surg* 1977; 11: 163–7.

12 Brackman ME, Kopf AW. Iatrogenic effects of general anesthesia in children. Considerations in treating large congenital nevocytic nevi. *J Derm Surg Oncol* 1986; 12: 363–7.

13 Bauer BS, Johnson PE, Lovato G. Applications of soft tissue expansion in children. *Pediatr Dermatol* 1986; 3: 281–90.

14 Gallico GG, O'Connor NE, Compton CC, Remensnijder JP, Rehinde O, Green H. Cultured epithelial autografts for giant congenital nevi. *Plast Reconstr Surg* 1989; 84: 1–9.

15 Johnson HA. Permanent removal of pigmentation from giant hairy naevi by dermabrasion in early life. *Br J Plast Surg* 1977; 30: 321–3.

16 Miller CJ, Becker DW. Removing pigmentation by dermabrading naevi in infancy. *Br J Plast Surg* 1979; 32: 124–6.

17 Chait LA, White B, Skudowitz RB. The treatment of giant hairy naevi by dermabrasion in the first few weeks of life. *S Afr Med J* 1981; 20: 593–4.

18 Zitelli JA, Grant MG, Abell E, Boyd JB. Histologic patterns of congenital nevocytic nevi and implications for treatment. *J Am Acad Dermatol* 1984; 11: 402–9.

19 Nickoloff BJ, Walton R, Pregerson-Rodan K, Jacobs AH, Cox AJ. Immunohistologic patterns of congenital nevocellular nevi. *Arch Dermatol* 1986; 122: 1263–8.

20 Moss ALH. Congenital 'giant' naevus: a preliminary report of a new surgical approach. *Br J Plast Surg* 1987; 40: 410–19.

21 De Raeve LE, De Coninck AL, Dierickx PR, Roseeuw DI. Neonatal curettage of giant congenital melanocytic naevi. *Arch Dermatol* 1996; 132: 20–2.

22 Gown AM, Vogel AM, Hoak D, Gough F, McNutt MA. Monoclonal antibodies specific for melanocytic tumors distinguish subpopulations of melanocytes. *Am J Pathol* 1986; 123: 195–203.

23 Skelton III HG, Smith KJ, Barrette TL, Lupton GP, Graham JH. HMB-45 staining in benign and malignant melanocytic lesions. A reflection of cellular activation. *AM J Dermatopathol* 1991; 13: 543–50.

24 Swerdlow AJ, English JSC, Qiao Z. The risk of melanoma in patients with congenital naevi: a cohort study. *J Am Acad Dermatol* 1995; 32: 595–9.

28.3 More Complex Skin Surgery

PAUL J. SMITH AND LOSHAN KANGESU

For many years plastic surgeons have concentrated on perfecting techniques related to reconstructive and cosmetic work. Simple wound closure must be undertaken so well that the surgeon doubts, upon completion of the deep sutures, whether or not any cutaneous sutures are necessary. Unless, with each wound closure this doubt arises, then wound closure has been technically inadequate. These are the standards that should be set in surgery. Only concentration on basic principles can lead to sound surgical practice. This chapter discusses basic surgical principles and plastic surgical techniques.

Wound healing

Wound healing has been studied extensively in skin and there is a distinction between primary healing that occurs in the incised wound where the skin edges are in close apposition, and secondary healing where the edges are far apart. During wound healing there is interaction of cellular and extracellular events such as cell migration, proliferation and differentiation. There is also synthesis and remodelling of extracellular matrix culminating finally in tissue repair with scar formation. Three phases of wound healing are recognized: (a) the period of haematoma formation, inflammation and removal of foreign material; (b) the phase of granulation tissue growth and epithelial migration; and (c) the phase of connective tissue remodelling, wound contraction and scar formation. These phases overlap and occur in both primary and secondary healing but to differing extents. In secondary healing the entire process is prolonged, but particularly the second and third phases with reliance on the wound reducing in size. The latter is due to both wound contraction which is thought to be mediated by myofibroblasts and cicatrization (or contracture), which is due to fibrosis. Although the processes causing the wound to shrink in size are useful to the wounded animal, they can be disastrous to the surgical wound because they may produce deformity. The surgeon aims to achieve primary healing and prevent secondary wound healing by direct suture of skin edges and also by use of skin flaps and grafts.

The tensile strength of a wound is a measure of its load capacity per unit area. Collagen fibres are largely responsible for the tensile strength of wounds and the rate of healing varies between species and individuals, as well as between different tissues in the same individual. All wounds gain strength at approximately the same rate during the first 14–21 days. Animal experiments have shown in the rat that the tensile strength of the wound at 7 days is 40%, at 14 days 80% and 10 months before it reaches its maximum. Even so, wound tensile strength only reaches about 80% of that in normal skin [1].

REFERENCE

1 Levenson SM, Geever EF, Crowley LV, Oatesif SD, Berard CW, Rosen H. The healing of rat skin wounds. *Ann Surg* 1965; 161: 293–308.

Methods of wound cover

The surgeon has a choice of methods of wound cover, but a successful outcome in terms of subsequent scarring and cosmetic result are dependent on the adherence to basic plastic surgical principles. These involve correct planning, accurate approximation of skin edges, measures to minimize wound haematoma, minimal handling of the skin edges, avoidance of excess tension on the skin edge and prevention of unnecessary wound contamination. Factors beyond the surgeon's control that may cause a poor scar are the age of the patient, the site and also direction of the wound. In general, apart from scars in infants (1–3 months) which often heal as fine lines, children's scars remain erythematous and harder for a longer duration than in adults and in addition children are more prone to developing hypertrophic and even keloid scars (see below).

The size of the anticipated skin defect influences the surgeon's choice of wound cover. Obviously, small wounds are closed directly. Conversely, larger defects will require skin flaps and skin grafts. Where it is possible to delay the excision of a lesion, techniques such as serial excision and tissue expansion may be employed.

Direct closure

The vast majority of skin lesions are suitable for excision and direct closure. In general, lesions are excised as an ellipse. The skin of infants and smaller children is very elastic and padded by a type of adipose tissue commonly called 'baby fat' which maintains the skin at maximal distension. One consequence of this is that wounds that one may not expect to close directly in older children and adults can be approximated with comparative ease in infants.

When planning elliptical incisions one is generally taught that the length of the ellipse will be equal to three times the diameter of the lesion and this is a useful guide when explaining the procedure to patients. However, in reality one can make the limbs of the ellipse shorter thus decreasing the length of the final scar. The longitudinal axis of the ellipse should be designed to lie along or parallel to a line of skin tension. The existence of lines of tension in the skin was first noted by Dupuytren in 1832 [1] and subsequently investigated by Karl Langer [2], Professor of Anatomy at Joseph's Academy in Vienna. The work was presented in the second of four papers in 1861 [2]. Although some of Langer's lines run across natural creases, they form the basis of our understanding of lines of skin tension which have attracted numerous descriptive terms as listed by Borges [3]. A scar is less conspicuous if it lies along or parallel to a line of skin tension. In the face

these lines correspond to wrinkle lines in elderly people where they are also known as lines of facial expression. In the neck these lines correspond with the lines of dependency where the effects of gravity produce horizontal creases. Lines of skin tension also lie horizontally in flexion creases and in the limbs: where it is difficult to choose the correct line it is preferable to follow the line that falls when the limb is in the relaxed position. In the child's face it is often difficult to plan the direction of excision due to their stretched skin and absence of facial lines. In this instance the excision should be planned so that the scar will eventually lie in a line of facial expression (Fig. 28.3.1). Another principle in planning surgical wounds on the face is the appreciation of cosmetic units (Fig. 28.3.2) and the placement of scars at the junction of these units. Furthermore, if possible, scars can be hidden in the hair-bearing skin of the scalp or eyebrow. In this instance the skin should not be cut perpendicular to the surface as is the normal teaching, but parallel to the direction of the hair follicles to prevent their disruption and subsequent local balding. The sex of the child is important when planning excisions within the hair scalp due to the chance of subsequent balding in boys [4].

REFERENCES

1 Dupuytren G. *Leçons Orales de Clinique Chirurgicale Faites à l'Hôtel-Dieu de Paris*. Paris: Baillière, 1832–4.
2 Langer K. Zur Anatomie und Physiologie der Haut. *Sitzungsb Acad Wissensch* 1861; 45: 223. [On the anatomy and physiology of the skin (trans. T. Gibson). *Br J Plast Surg* 1978; 31: 3–8, 93–106, 185–99, 273–8.]
3 Borges AF. *Elective Incisions and Scar Revision*. Boston: Little, Brown, 1973.
4 McGregor IA. *Fundamental Techniques of Plastic Surgery*, 8th edn. Edinburgh: Churchill Livingstone, 1989.

Skin graft

Skin grafts offer the simplest method of covering defects that are too large for direct closure. Skin grafts are sheets of skin that are completely detached from their source of origin so rendering them avascular. Following transfer to a recipient site, their survival depends on acquiring a new blood supply from the wound bed.

Skin grafts contain epidermis and variable amounts of dermis. If the entire thickness of dermis is included, they are described as full-thickness grafts, whereas if there is a variable amount of dermis, they are called split-thickness grafts (Fig. 28.3.3). The history of skin grafting dates back to pre-Christian times in India but the skill became lost until rediscovery in the 19th century. In 1804, Baronio of Italy carried out a successful autograft on sheep and in 1817, Sir Astley Cooper in London grafted a full-thickness piece of skin from an amputated thumb onto the stump [1,2]. In 1823, Bünger first applied a skin graft from the thigh to the nose [3]. Early skin

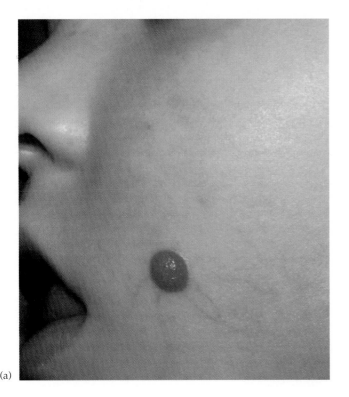

(a)

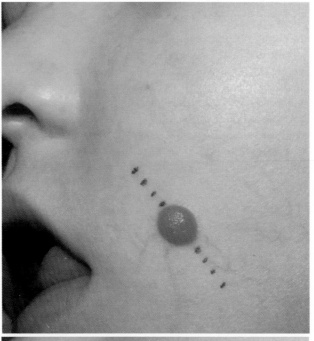

(b)

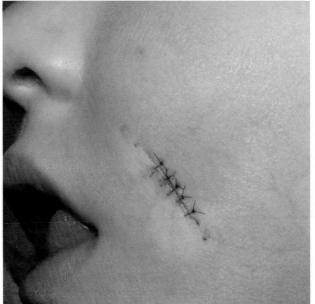

(c)

Fig. 28.3.1 Excision of Spitz naevus on a 3-year-old girl. (a) The lines of skin tension are not obvious on the stretched skin of a child. (b) Therefore the excision should be planned so that the scar falls in a future skin crease. (c) The sutured wound after excision of the naevus as a short ellipse.

grafts were exceptionally thin and had little more than epidermis alone [4–6], but it was the true split-thickness skin graft [7] that allowed larger wounds to be resurfaced. In the 1870s Lawson [8], Le Fort and Wolfe all used full-thickness skin grafts to treat ectropion, but it is Wolfe, an Austrian ophthalmologist who later settled in Melbourne, Australia, with whom they are most commonly associated [9].

Differences between split-thickness and full-thickness skin grafts

There are important differences between split-thickness and full-thickness grafts that are relevant when planning surgery. Split-thickness grafts are preferable when larger areas require cover. The donor sites heal in 10–14 days by epidermal migration from the wound edge and from foci of epidermal cells in the cut ends of skin appendages. The maximum size of full-thickness grafts is often limited by the ability to obtain primary closure of the donor site.

Split-thickness skin grafts are thinner and have lower metabolic requirements than full-thickness grafts, and therefore they exhibit better take and are preferable if the wound bed is not well vascularized. Split-skin grafts contract more than full-thickness skin grafts and in general produce a less favourable cosmetic result because they are less able to correct a greater contour defect, exhibit poorer texture, have unpredictable pigmentation (either hypo- or hyperpigmentation), lower durability and also

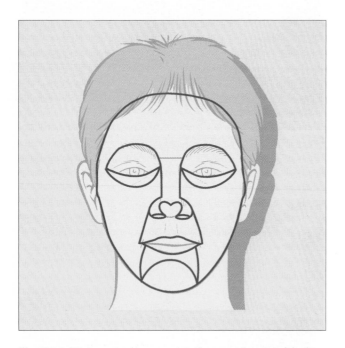

Fig. 28.3.2 It is important to appreciate the cosmetic units of the face. Scars are less conspicuous if they lie along the border of adjacent cosmetic units.

a more visible donor site. Furthermore, split-thickness grafts in children fail to grow with the child unlike full-thickness grafts. Hence children with split-skin grafts overlying joints often require scar release as they grow. Finally, the skin adnexae are preserved in full-thickness skin grafts, whereas split-skin grafts are hairless and require long-term use of emollients to prevent drying of their surface.

Split-skin graft storage

Split-skin grafts can be stored wrapped in saline soaked gauze at 4°C for up to 3 weeks. Studies on keratinocyte viability of stored skin have shown that cell viability falls significantly after 10 days in skin stored with saline, but longer preservation is possible if the skin is stored in nutrient tissue culture medium [10]. Split-thickness skin can also be cryopreserved for long-term storage in skin banks for use as a dressing material for patients with massive burns [11]. Non-viable skin that is preserved in glycerol or lyophilized can also be used as a temporary dressing.

Donor sites

Split-thickness skin donor sites usually heal well with minimal scarring, but there is always the risk of hypertrophic scarring in children (Fig. 28.3.4). The most common donor site for split-thickness skin grafts is the thigh, but if only a small graft is required in children the buttock is a good site as the scar can be hidden. The donor sites for full-thickness skin grafts are more specific. For grafts to the face in children, the best colour match is obtained from postauricular skin. In adults the upper eyelid, preauricular area and supraclavicular fossa are also useful sites, but there is insufficient skin laxity at these sites in children. Larger grafts in children are usually taken from the groin crease. The graft should be taken as

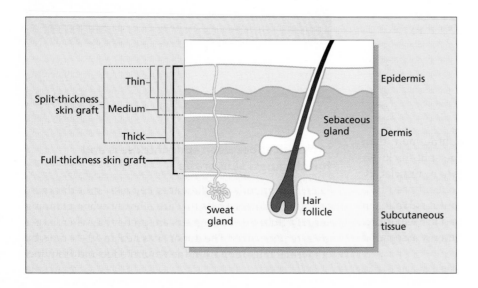

Fig. 28.3.3 Diagram of skin illustrating the relative thickness of thin and thick split-thickness skin grafts and also full-thickness skin grafts.

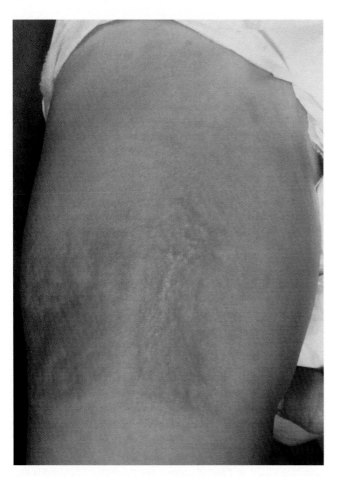

Fig. 28.3.4 Split-thickness skin graft donor site that had become hypertrophic on a 20-month-old girl, 1 year postoperatively. The scar improved with time.

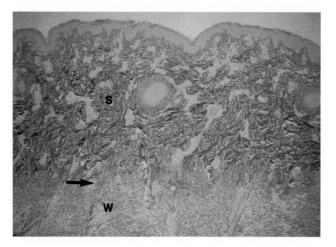

Fig. 28.3.5 Histology section of split-skin grafted area at 3 weeks showing the scar interface (arrow) between the skin graft (S) and the wound bed (W). (Elastic van Gieson, ×100.)

lateral as possible and always lateral to the femoral artery to minimize the chance of transferring skin that will be hairy postpuberty.

Biology of skin grafts

When a skin graft is harvested it is very pale and on grafts that are kept exposed a pink hue is visible after 8–12 hs. At 2–4 days if grafts are successful, they are bright pink and distended. Some grafts have a bluish tint at this time probably because the arterial inflow precedes the development of the venous outflow. These observations have attracted much interest, but there is still no unifying agreement about the microscopic events. When a graft is applied to a wound bed, it adheres by a fibrin bond and graft survival is explained by two separate phases. First, there is the phase of serum imbibition during which grafts are nourished by diffusion of metabolites to and from the wound bed across a thin film of serum. During this period grafts gain weight and cell survival is probably dependent on anaerobic pathways [12]. After day 2, graft survival is

maintained by capillary ingrowth from the wound bed accounting for the bright pink colour of grafts. There is disagreement about whether new blood vessels from the wound bed link directly with the cut vessel on the graft, a process termed capillary inosculation [6,13] or if the capillaries growing from the wound bed forge new pathways into the grafts [14]. Lymphatic growth occurs after 7 days.

The delicate bond between graft and wound bed is susceptible to damage from shear forces in the first week and therefore grafts need protection from movement for the first 2 weeks. Grafts become firmly attached to the wound bed by the ingrowth of connective tissue that forms a scar interface with the grafts (Fig. 28.3.5) and the cellular events resemble those in classical primary healing of opposed skin edges. Graft contracture occurs at this plane and becomes progressive for 3–4 months. Hence when grafts are used to release contractures across flexure creases, the joint should be splinted for that time. It is not known why full-thickness grafts contract less than split-thickness grafts, but the ratio of reticular to papillary dermis appears to be important. This is evident from the observation that a split-skin graft will contract more than a full-thickness skin graft even when both are of the same thickness.

Nerves grow into grafts both from the surrounding wound edge and the wound bed [15] (Fig. 28.3.6). Again there is debate as to whether nerves follow the neurolemmal sheaths of nerves transferred with the graft [16], or whether they make new pathways [17]. In patients, sensations of pain, light touch and temperature return in that order. However, sensation will never be equal to normal skin as specialized nerve endings such as Merkel cells and Meissner's corpuscles appear to degenerate [17,18] and so sensation is mediated directly from bare nerve endings. The release of neurotrophic factors such as nerve growth

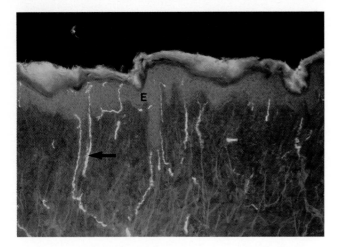

Fig. 28.3.6 Immunohistochemical stain of section of split-skin graft at 6 weeks showing nerve fibres (arrow) that have grown from the wound bed. Some fibres are within the epidermis (E). (Protein gene product 9.5, a pan-neural marker, ×200.)

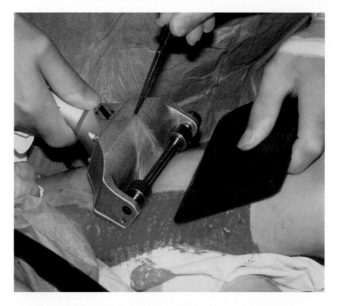

Fig. 28.3.7 The use of a power dermatome to excise split-thickness skin from the thigh of a child with burn injury.

factor (NGF) from target cells within a graft may influence the quality of reinnervation [19]. Previous studies have suggested that within skin grafts, skin appendages such as hair follicles and sebaceous glands may be a focus of neurotropism. Full-thickness skin grafts, acquire a better sensation than split-thickness skin grafts [18] possibly because of a greater number of target organs.

Surgical technique

With an understanding of the biology of skin graft survival, it is now possible to appreciate four factors essential to achieve satisfactory skin graft take.
1 Selection of a vascularized wound bed.
2 Avoidance of haematoma or seroma.
3 Perfect graft immobility on the wound bed.
4 Minimizing microbial contamination.
It is essential to apply skin grafts on to a vascularized wound bed. Exposed bone and tendons cannot support overlying grafts, but grafts will grow on periosteum and paratenon. By the same token, necrotic debris (slough) must be removed prior to grafting. Haematomas beneath the grafts are the commonest cause of graft failure as they are a barrier to the revascularization process and it is essential to secure haemostasis on the wound bed before applying the graft. Perforations in the graft may allow small amounts of blood and seroma to drain out. Grafts must be held on the wound bed without any movement for at least 7 days to avoid damage to new vessel growth. Tie over dressings are one way of preventing this movement. Grafts become stable only after 14 days and so if grafts are across joints or directly on muscle, limb splints should be worn for the period. Sometimes dressings can be harmful as they create shear forces between the graft and the wound bed. In such situations, as with grafts on the shoul-

der or parts of the lower leg, it is often better to expose grafts. Excess pressure (over 30 mmHg) from dressings should be avoided to prevent pressure necrosis of grafts.

Grafts are always contaminated by skin flora and there is a tendency to overstate the importance of infection as a cause of graft failure as this overlooks other reasons. In practice only a few bacteria are harmful. *Streptococcus pyogenes* (Lancefield group A) is very harmful to grafts because it produces streptokinase that breaks down the fibrin bond between grafts and the wound bed. *Pseudomonas aeruginosa* is of moderate harm to skin grafts especially in burn patients where it is a common contaminant. Thus any wound that is more than a few days old should have its bacterial status assessed prior to grafting. The presence of *S. pyogenes* is a contraindication to grafting and surgery should be postponed until the bacteria is eradicated with systemic antibiotics.

Full-thickness grafts are excised with a scalpel blade. Subcutaneous fat is meticulously removed with scissors to promote maximum contact between the skin and the wound bed. Split-thickness skin grafts can be taken with a hand-held Watson knife (or other modification of the Humby knife) or with a powered dermatome (Fig. 28.3.7). Some experience is required to cut the correct thickness of skin grafts (0.3–0.35 mm). Grafts that are too thin are unstable, and significant morbidity is caused from grafts that are too thick because of poor take of the graft and delayed healing of the donor site also leads to hypertrophic scarring. Numerous dressings have been used for donor sites (summarized by Feldman [20]), but paraffin gauze remains the most common in use. Semi-occlusive dressings (Opsite) have been shown to enhance donor site healing and are good for small wounds. However, the

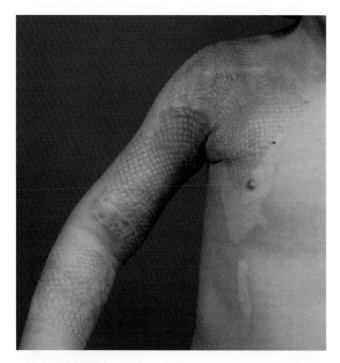

Fig. 28.3.8 Although meshing is sometimes a necessity especially in burn surgery, the cosmetic result may be very unsatisfactory due to persistence of the mesh pattern.

fluid collection beneath the dressing is a potential nidus for infection and regular wound checks with aspiration of the fluid is required. Calcium alginate dressings (Kaltostat) also promote wound healing, and when impregnated with bupivacaine provide good postoperative analgesia [21]. Donor site dressings should be left intact until they separate spontaneously once the wound has healed after 10–14 days.

Skin graft expansion

If split-skin graft donor sites are limited, as is often the case in burns, the sheets of split-thickness skin can be meshed so that they can cover a larger area [22]. During healing epidermal cells migrate to fill the interstices of the mesh. However, mesh grafts give a poor cosmetic result as the mesh pattern often persists (Fig. 28.3.8). Another way of expanding skin is the so-called Chinese method where the split-thickness skin is finely diced and then spread over a large area [23]. Although wound cover is achieved, the new skin is very fragile because of the lack of dermal support, akin to problems with cultured keratinocyte grafts (see below).

REFERENCES

1 Davis JS. Story of plastic surgery. *Ann Surg* 1941; 113: 651–56.
2 Hauben DJ, Baruchin A, Mahler A. On the history of the free skin graft. *Ann Plast Surg* 1982; 9: 242–5.

3 Bünger C. Gelungener versuch einer Nasenbildung aus einem völlig getrennten Haustück dem biene. *Jahresber Chir Augen-Heilk* 1822; 4: 569–82.
4 Réverdin JL. Greffe épidermique-expérience faite dans le service de M le Docteur Guyon, a l'Hôpital Necker. *Bull Imp Soc Chir Paris* 1869; 10: 511–15. [Trans. Ivy RH, in: McDowell F, ed. *Silvergirl's Surgery: Plastic Surgery*. Austin, Texas: Silvergirl, 1987: 3–5.
5 Ollier LXEL. Greffes cutanées ou autoplastiques. *Bull Acad Med Paris*, 1872; 1(2 Série): 243–50. [Trans. Ivy RH, in: McDowell F, ed. *Silvergirl's Surgery: Plastic Surgery*. Austin, Texas: Silvergirl, 1987: 10–11.]
6 Thiersch C. Uber die feineren anatomischen Varänderunger bei Aufheilung von Haut auf Granulationen. *Verhandlung Deutsch Gesellsch Chir Berlin* 1874; 3: 69–75. [Trans. May H, May H, in: McDowell F, ed. *Silvergirl's Surgery: Plastic Surgery*. Austin, Texas: Silvergirl, 1987: 12–13.]
7 Blair VP, Brown J. The use and uses of large split skin grafts of intermediate thickness. *Surg Gynaecol Obstet* 1929; 49: 82–97.
8 Lawson G. On the transplantation of portions of skin for the closure of large granulating surfaces. *Trans Clin Soc London* 1871; 4: 49–53.
9 Kelton PL. Skin grafts. *Select Read Plast Surg* 1992; 7: 1–25.
10 Fahmy FS, Navsaria HA, Frame JD, Jones CR, Leigh IM. Skin graft storage and keratinocyte viability. *Br J Plast Surg* 1993; 46: 292–5.
11 Athreya BH, Grimes EL, Lehr Greene AE, Coriell LL. Differential susceptibility of epithelial cells and fibroblasts of human skin to freeze injury. *Cryobiology* 1969; 5: 262–9.
12 Hübscher C. Beiträge zue Hautverpflanzung nach Thiersch. *Beitr Klin Chir* 1888; 4: 395.
13 Peer LA, Walker JC. The behaviour of autogenous human tissue grafts. Part 1. *Plast Reconstr Surg* 1951; 7: 6 (part 2 p. 73).
14 Converse JM, Rapaport FT. The vascularisation of skin autografts and homografts: an experimental study in man. *Ann Surg* 1956; 143: 306–15.
15 Pontén B. Grafted skin: observations on innervation and other qualities. *Acta Chir Scand* 1960; (suppl 257): 11–78.
16 Fitzgerald MJT, Martin F, Paletta FX. Innervation of skin grafts. *Surg Gynaecol Obstet* 1969; 124: 808–12.
17 Waris T. Innervation of scar tissue in the skin of the rat. *Scand J Plast Reconstr Surg* 1978; 12: 173–80.
18 Waris T, Rechardt L, Kyösola K. Reinnervation of human skin grafts: a histochemical study. *Plast Reconstr Surg* 1983; 72: 439–45.
19 Seckel BR. Enhancement of peripheral nerve regeneration. *Muscle Nerve* 1990; 13: 785–800.
20 Feldman DL. Which dressing for split-thickness skin graft donor sites? *Ann Plast Surg* 1991; 27: 288.
21 Butler PEM, Eadie PA, Lawlor D, Edwards G, McHugh M. Bupivacaine and Kaltostat reduces post-operative donor site pain. *Br J Plast Surg* 1993; 46: 523–4.
22 Tanner JC, Vanderput J, Olley JF. The mesh skin graft. *Plast Reconstr Surg* 1964; 34: 287–92.
23 Zhang M-L, Wang C-Y, Chang Z-D, Cao D-X, Han X. Microskin grafting II. Clinical report. *Burns* 1986; 12: 544–8.

Skin grafting for epidermolysis bullosa

Epidermolysis bullosa comprises a group of hereditary blistering disorders that involve skin, oral and other mucosae (see Chapter 19.4). Surgery becomes appropriate when dealing with dystrophic epidermolysis bullosa. In this, blisters appear at birth or soon after; they may appear spontaneously and once they burst leave a raw and painful area. Healing occurs by scar formation which may lead to severe contractures. Hands become severely deformed and there is fusion of the digits which are held flexed within an epidermal cocoon. The thumb becomes adducted. In severely affected hands, the digits are entirely encased and flexed within an epidermal cocoon creating a pseudosyndactyly and are unable to participate in any precision work. The general condition of the patient is such that they are difficult to anaesthetize with oral blistering and scarring impairing opening the mouth, carious

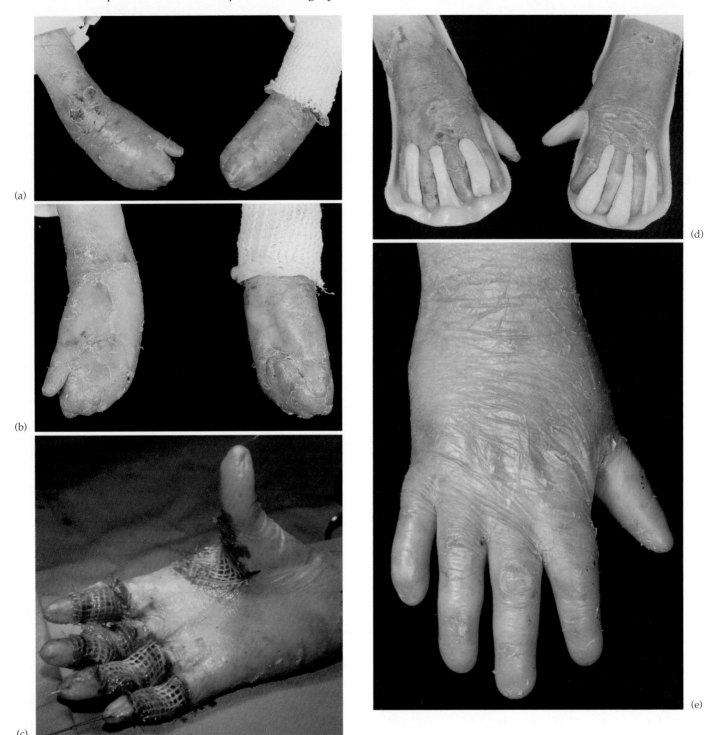

(a)

(b)

(c)

(d)

(e)

Fig. 28.3.9 Sequence showing surgery with skin grafting for hand deformity in dystrophic epidermolysis bullosa in a 5-year-old boy. (a,b) Preoperative views showing adduction of both thumbs with flexion contractures and pseudosyndactyly of fingers. (c) Position of hand at the end of surgery. The contractures have been released and split-thickness skin grafts have been applied to the raw areas. Paraffin gauze covers the grafts. (d) Splinting of the hands in the postoperative period is essential to prevent recurrence of the deformity. (e,f) Early postoperative result.

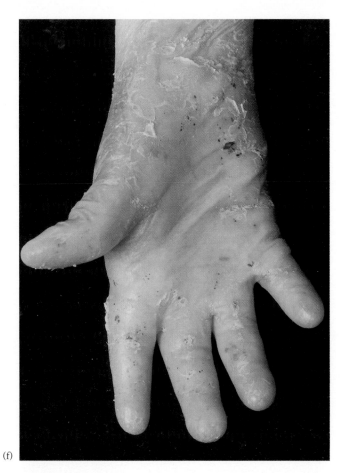

(f)

Fig. 28.3.9 *Continued.*

teeth, laryngeal involvement and dysphagia. Conjunctival and corneal erosions occur but these children now tend to survive into adult life due to improved standards of care and with this survival there is the necessity to return their hands to a functional state.

Surgery is undertaken essentially to separate the digits and to release joint contractures [1]. Skin grafting is required to cover the volar defects following contracture release but is not required following the release of pseudosyndactyly. Upon completion of the grafting, very careful postoperative immobilization and immediate splintage, with the splints being made in theatre, is essential for a satisfactory outcome. The aim of surgery is to return the hand to a functional state. It is maintained in that functional state by appropriate splintage using modern soft light-weight appliances [2]. An example of what can be achieved using surgery is shown in Fig. 28.3.9.

REFERENCES

1 Terrill PJ, Mayou BJ, Pemberton J. Experience in the surgical management of the hand in dystrophic epidermolysis bullosa. *Br J Plast Surg* 1992; 45: 435–42.
2 Mullett FLH, Smith PJ. Hand splintage following surgery for dystrophic epidermolysis bullosa. *Br J Plast Surg* 1993; 46: 192–3.

Skin flaps

As opposed to skin grafts which are avascular at the time of transplantation, skin flaps are vascularized segments of tissue that are transferred from one site to another. In comparison with skin grafts, local skin flaps provide similar tissue, and resurface defects without leaving a contour defect thus giving a better aesthetic result. In addition, skin flaps can resurface exposed bone or tendons and are also preferable to grafts for cover of vital structures such as major nerves and blood vessels. Furthermore, sensation on skin flaps is better than on skin grafts [1].

One of the major advances in plastic surgery in the past two decades has been the increased understanding of the skin blood supply. Although the subject was studied by Manchot in the 19th century [2] and more recently Salmon [3] the subject gained interest in the English literature only after the 1970s [4]. Recent significant contributions have been from Cormack and Lamberty [5] and Taylor *et al.* [6].

The immediate blood supply to the skin is from the subdermal plexus which is fed by one of three systems: (a) perforators from the underlying muscle; (b) perforators from the underlying deep fascia; and (c) a direct cutaneous system. Skin flaps are described as random or axial pattern depending on the blood supply [4,7]. In random pattern flaps the subdermal plexus is fed by perforators from the underlying muscle or fascia. Axial pattern flaps have a direct cutaneous supply that extends to the entire length of the flap. Skin flaps are also classified by their proximity to the defect. Local flaps arise from the immediate vicinity of the defect, whereas distant flaps arise from an adjacent region of the body. Free flaps are flaps that are transported from one part of the body with their blood supply identified and then reanastomosed using microsurgical techniques to blood vessels at the recipient site. Skin flaps can also be transferred together with their underlying fascia, muscle or even bone and are described respectively by the terms fasciocutaneous, musculocutaneous and osseocutaneous flaps. The rest of this discussion will be confined to the use of local skin flaps with a random blood supply for the coverage of small defects.

The following are examples of local skin flaps that are often used in various parts of the body when direct closure is not possible or when direct closure would cause undue distortion of the local tissue.

Advancement flaps: rectangular and V–Y

In these flaps tissue proximal to the defect is advanced forwards. In the rectangular advancement flap it is often necessary to excise small triangles adjacent to the base of the flap (Burow's triangle) to facilitate advancement (Fig. 28.3.10). The V–Y island flap, so-called because a

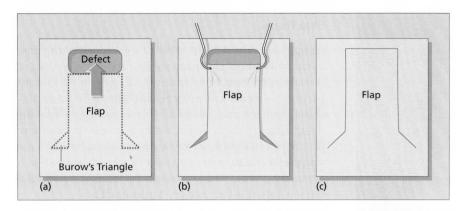

Fig. 28.3.10 Rectangular advancement flap. (a–c) In order to cover the defect a rectangular shaped local skin flap is advanced forwards. Advancement of the flap is aided by excising (von Burow's) triangles of skin at the base of the flap.

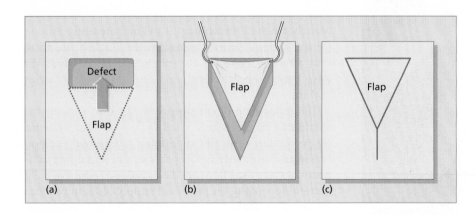

Fig. 28.3.11 V–Y advancement flaps. (a) Although the defect is similar in shape to that in Fig. 28.3.10, a V-shaped incision is made in adjacent skin to create a triangular island of skin. The viability of the skin is maintained by an intact vascular supply on its deep surface. (b) The flap is advanced into the defect and the entire wound is closed as a Y.

V-shaped incision is made but final closure is in the shape of a Y, is a more straightforward procedure (Figs 28.3.11, 28.3.12).

Pivot flaps: transposition and rotation

These flaps have in common a pivot point and an arc through which the flap is rotated. The radius of the arc is the line of greatest tension of the flap and its realization is important to the planning of these flaps. In transposition flaps, a rectangular or square area of skin and subcutaneous tissue adjacent to the defect is moved to cover the defect (Fig. 28.3.13). In rotation flaps, a semicircular area of skin and subcutaneous tissue adjacent to the defect is rotated to fill the defect. In the planning of rotation flaps the defect has to be first triangulated and so a small amount of normal skin has to be excised together with the lesion. The triangle will have two equal sides and one shorter side. The tissue movement is based on the arc of a semicircle the circumference of which may need to be eight times the length of the short side of the triangle (Fig. 28.3.14). A releasing back cut may be necessary to facilitate flap movement. The secondary defect may be closed directly or require a split-skin graft.

Rhomboid flap

This is a type of local transposition flap that was originally described by Limberg in 1946 in Russian and subsequently in English in 1966 [8]. The defect is made into a rhomboid shape and then a transposition flap from any one of the four sides of the rhomboid can be used to fill the defect. The secondary defect from where the flap arose is closed directly giving this flap the unique property of a moving pivot point (Fig. 28.3.15). There have been some modifications of Limberg's original description including that suggested by Quaba and Sommerlad [9] which allows for ease of flap design.

REFERENCES

1 Santoni-Rugiu P. An experimental study on the reinnervation of free skin grafts and pedicle flaps. *Plast Reconstr Surg* 1996; 38: 98–104.
2 Manchot C. *Die Hautarterien des Menschlichen Körpers*. Leipzig: FCW Vogel, 1889. [Trans. Ristic J, Morain WD. *The Cutaneous Arteries of the Human Body*. New York: Springer-Verlag, 1983].
3 Salmon M. *Les Artères de la Peau*. Paris: Masson, 1936.
4 McGregor IA, Morgan G. Axial and random pattern flaps. *Br J Plast Surg* 1973; 26: 202–13.
5 Cormack GC, Lamberty BGH. *The Arterial Anatomy of Skin Flaps*. Edinburgh: Churchill Livingstone, 1987.
6 Taylor IG, Palmer JH, McManamny D. The vascular territories of the body (angiosomes) and their clinical application. In: McCarthy JG, ed. *Plastic Surgery*, Philadelphia: WB Saunders, 1990.

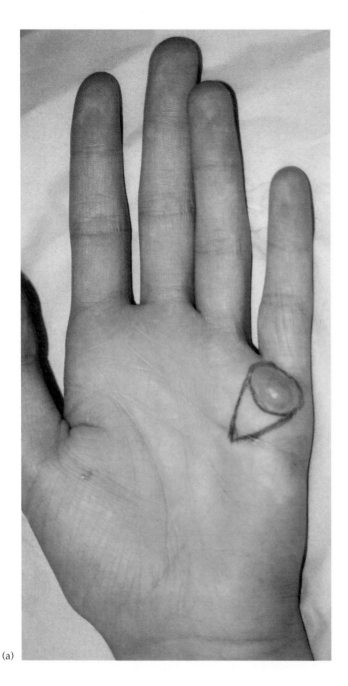

(a)

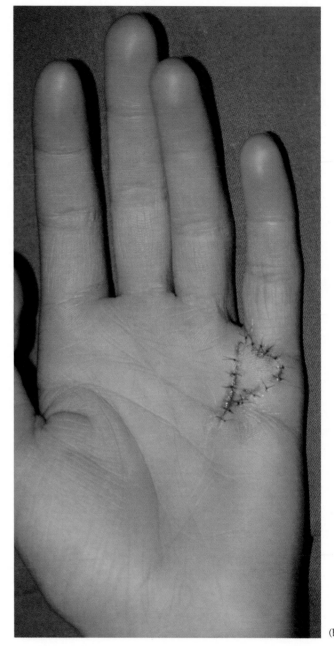

(b)

Fig. 28.3.12 (a) A subcutaneous lesion was excised from the hand of this 15-year-old boy and the defect was closed (b) with V–Y advancement flap as illustrated in Fig. 28.3.11.

7 Smith PJ. The vascular basis of axial pattern flaps. *Br J Plast Surg* 1973; 26: 150–7.
8 Limberg AA. Design of local flaps. In: Gibson T, ed. *Modern Trends in Plastic Surgery*, 2nd edn. London: Butterworths, 1966.
9 Quaba AA, Sommerlad BC. A square peg in a round hole: a modified rhomboid flap and its clinical application. *Br J Plast Surg* 1987; 40: 163–70.

Covering large defects

Serial excision

On occasions when a large benign lesion has to be excised, it may be possible to excise it in two or more stages (Fig. 28.3.16). This technique utilizes the ability of the surrounding skin to 'expand' over time. In each stage of the serial excision the maximum amount of the lesion is excised that will allow the wound to be closed comfortably without undue tension. If a wound is closed with excessive tension the scar will stretch sometimes to a

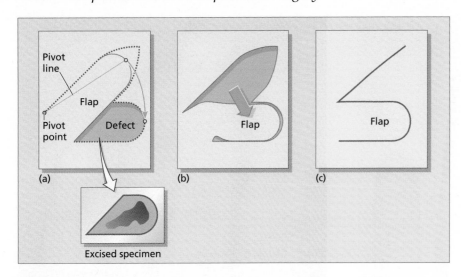

(a)

Excised specimen

(b)

(c)

Fig. 28.3.13 Transposition flap. (a,b) The defect is resurfaced by transposing adjacent skin. Careful planning is required to ensure that the tip of the flap will reach the full extent of the defect by measuring from the pivot point. (c) In this diagram the resulting secondary defect is directly closed, but may require a skin graft.

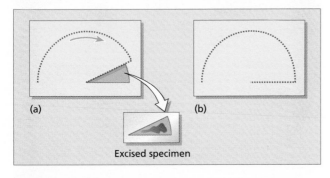

(a)

(b)

Excised specimen

Fig. 28.3.14 Rotation flaps. (a,b) In this instance the defect which is triangular in shape is filled by rotating a semicircular piece of skin. The flaps need to be large, often eight times the circumference of the defect. Also note that the radius of the flap is longer than that of the defect.

width resembling the size of the original lesion. These staged excisions are planned so that the vertical length of the scar barely exceeds the longest diameter of the lesion. In all but the final stage the excisions are intralesional as are the suture holes. Although individual patient variations exists, often it is possible to plan subsequent stages of excisions after a minimum of 3 months.

Tissue expansion

Since the 1980s tissue expansion has provided an important addition to the plastic surgeon's repertoire. Skin expansion is seen physiologically in the gravid abdominal skin and has been used for reasons of beauty or tradition by various races—such as the Hottentots who stretch their labia and the women of Chad who stretch their lips.

Tissue expansion as currently practised was first described by Radovan in 1976 (subsequently published in

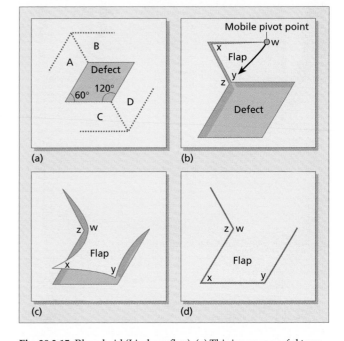

(a)

(b)

(c)

(d)

Fig. 28.3.15 Rhomboid (Limberg flap). (a) This is a very useful type of transposition flap that is designed by making the defect into the shape of a rhomboid. Thereafter any one of four transposition flaps (A, B, C or D) can be raised to cover the defect. The remaining illustration show the effect of creating flap B. (b,c) The pivot point is W. Direct closure of the secondary donor defect approximates Z to W (d), in effect moving the pivot point so that the tip of the flap (XY) reaches the far edge of the defect.

1982 [1]), involved the subcutaneous insertion of a silicon bag which was inflated with saline over a period of weeks thus causing stretching of the overlying skin. The expanded skin can then be used as an advancement or transposition flap to cover any adjacent skin defect.

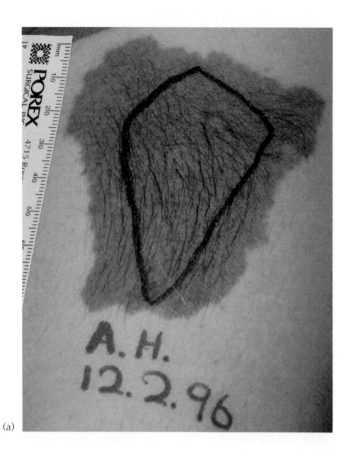

(a)

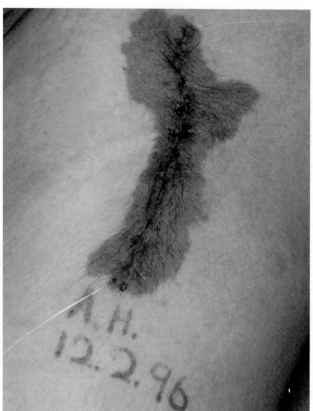

(b)

Fig. 28.3.16 First stage of serial excision of scar. (a) This 12-year-old girl had a large pigmented congenital naevus on her left arm. The planned area of excision is marked. (b) Following the first-stage excision, note that the suture marks are intralesional. A further stage of excision is planned to remove the remnant lesion.

Valuable experimental data was provided by Austad *et al.* [2] in the early 1980s who also introduced a self-expanding prosthesis which contained a hyperosmotic substance that drew in surrounding tissue water by osmosis. The permeability of the wall of the prosthesis and the osmolarity of its contents dictated the rate of expansion. Experimental data largely from animal studies has shown that the thickness of the epidermis remains unchanged by tissue expansion, although there is increased mitotic activity during expansion. Electron micrograph studies have shown that the undulations of the dermal and epidermal junction are unfolded during expansion and there is a reduction in intercellular distance in the epidermis. The skin appendages are compressed during expansion but do not degenerate. There is some evidence of increased melanocytic activity and this has been used to explain the hyperpigmentation of the expanded area

that sometimes occurs and which reverses at the end of expansion. The dermis is affected quite significantly and thins during expansion and a fibrous capsule forms around the prosthesis. There is also atrophy of fat. Nerves are largely unaffected and seem to stretch although at certain sites such as the forehead, distortion can cause considerable pain. Interestingly, there is increased angiogenesis in the expanded skin much akin to processes occurring in vascular surgical delay thus allowing long transposition flaps of expanded skin to be designed. When muscle either overlying or beneath the prosthesis is examined there are features of atrophy but muscle function remains unchanged.

The physical properties of skin depend mainly on the patterns of the fibrous weave of the dermis. These properties can be divided into four groups: (a) skin tension, which if excessive in sutured wounds leads to hypertrophic or stretched scars; (b) skin extensibility, that allows for movement across joints and closure of simple skin defects and is maximal in infancy but with age gives way to skin laxity; (c) directional variations, that give rise to Langer's lines; and (d) viscoelastic properties which are creep and stress relaxation. Creep occurs in the first few minutes when a constant force is applied to skin causing it

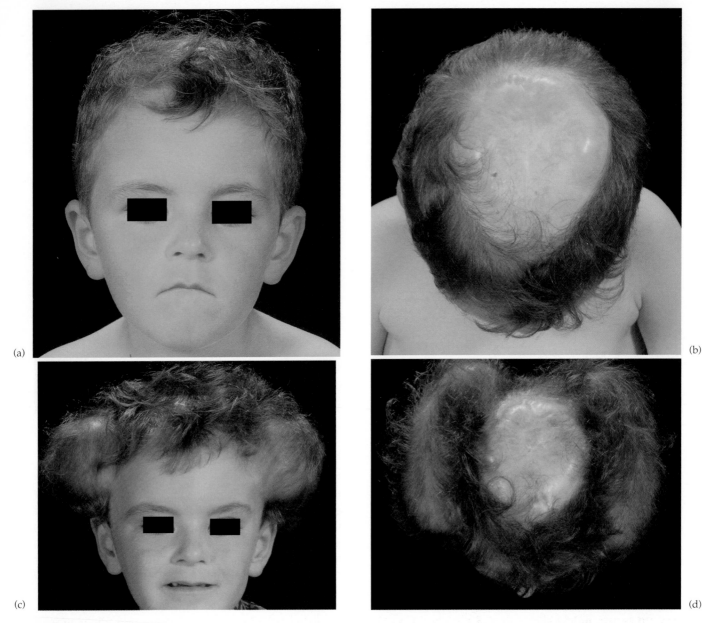

(a)

(b)

(c)

(d)

Fig. 28.3.17 Use of tissue expansion to resurface scarring alopecia. (a,b) Preoperative appearance. (c,d) Following insertion and inflation of expanders. The extra hair-bearing skin can now be used to cover the defect. (e,f) Postoperative appearance 1 year after surgery. *Continued opposite.*

to stretch. It is clinically important when it is utilized to close defects that appear initially just too large for primary closure. Skin can be load cycled, that is, repeated attempts at stretching will increase the stretch. The phenomenon is thought to be due to the realignment of dermal fibres and displacement of tissue fluid and ground substance from the dermis. Stress relaxation is the corollary of creep and is the measured force when skin is stretched at a constant distance. Within a few minutes, the measured stress declines as the skin stretches. Stress relaxation explains

why a flap that appears too tight immediately after the operation, may look satisfactory later on.

Gibson summarized the three ways in which skin can be stretched: (a) extensibility; (b) by mechanical creep; and (c) biological creep which is what occurs in the gravid abdominal wall and during tissue expansion [3]. The term 'biological' is misleading as a significant contribution to the expansion is from the mechanical effect of the expander to both the overlying and surrounding skin and soft tissue which is recruited into the area.

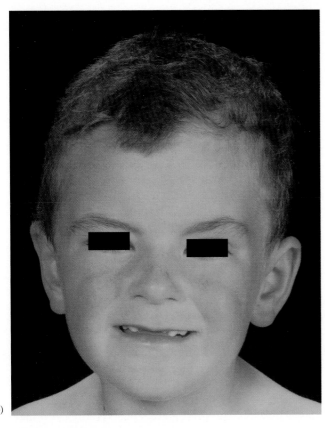
(e)

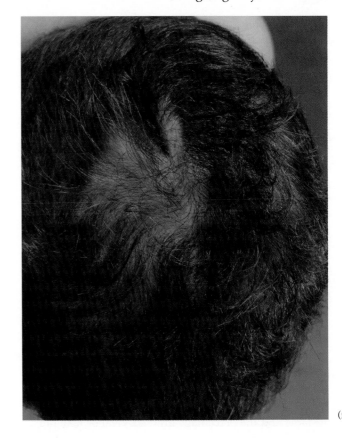
(f)

Fig. 28.3.17 *Continued.*

Tissue expansion has been used most successfully in the scalp and for breast reconstruction. Complications are higher when used in limbs, but even here when patient selection is appropriate the risks are acceptable. Careful planning is required for a successful outcome. As a rule, expanders are placed beneath the galea in the scalp, beneath muscle in breast reconstruction and beneath the skin, but not in a subfascial plane, in the limbs. The selection of implant requires some experience but a useful guide has been provided by Joss *et al.* [4], who explained that the length of the expander should correspond to the length of the defect but the width should be twice the width of the defect.

In children, tissue expansion is often used in the scalp for reconstruction following excision of giant pigmented naevi, aplasia cutis and of postburn alopecia (Fig. 28.3.17). Expanders are placed in the surrounding skin through radial or V-shaped incisions [5] and in general children tolerate the expanders very well. Complications from the use of the expanders include infection, extrusion and failure to cover the required defect which is most often due to poor planning.

REFERENCES

1 Radovan C. Breast reconstruction after mastectomy using the temporary expander. *Plast Reconstr Surg* 1982; 69: 195–208.
2 Austad ED, Pasyk KA, McClatchey KD, Cherry GW. Histomorphologic evaluation of guinea pig skin and soft tissue after controlled tissue expansion. *Plast Reconstr Surg* 1982; 70: 704–10.
3 Gibson T, Kenedi RM. Biochemical properties of skin. *Surg Clin North Am* 1967; 47: 279–94.
4 Joss GS, Zoltie N, Chapman P. Tissue expansion technique and the transposition flap. *Br J Plast Surg* 1990; 43: 328–33.
5 Matton GE, Tonnard PL, Monstrey SJ, van Landuyt SH. A universal incision for tissue expander insertion. *Br J Plast Surg* 1995; 48: 172–6.

Cultured keratinocytes

Rhinewald and Green [1] showed that keratinocytes, the cells that make up 90% of the epidermis can be grown *in vitro*. They achieved a massive expansion in cell number by optimizing the culture medium to produce a rapid rate of cell division and by the technique of repeated subculturing. Starting with a $3\,cm^2$ piece of skin, the area of potential epidermis can be expanded more than 5000-fold within 3–4 weeks, yielding sufficient keratinocytes to cover nearly the entire body surface of an adult human ($1.7\,m^2$) [2].

The first clinical trials with keratinocytes were on two children with severe burn injuries, one had a 40% and the other 80% body surface area (BSA) burn. Cultured autologous keratinocytes were used to provide part of the wound cover. On freshly excised wounds over 50% of grafts showed initial take [3]. In the following decade numerous clinical reports of cultured keratinocytes on burn patients were published from around the world. Cultured autologous keratinocytes have also been used in children following the excision of giant pigmented naevi [4], in those with epidermolysis bullosa [5] and following the division of Siamese twins [6].

There was optimism that allogeneic cultured keratinocytes may provide an off-the-shelf wound cover in burn care [7] since Langerhans' cells, which contribute to immune surveillance, do not survive in culture. Furthermore, cultured keratinocytes have reduced expression of HLA class I antigens [8]. Unfortunately, in patients, it appears that allogeneic keratinocytes do not survive long term [9], but the mechanism for this failure is unclear. Although animal studies have shown immune rejection of allogeneic cultured keratinocytes [10] there is no convincing data to show rejection in humans.

The wealth of clinical reports on cultured keratinocytes have highlighted the fact that grafted areas are often unstable and the percentage graft survival or take rate is also variable. It appears that the nature of the wound bed on which the keratinocytes are applied is critical to their initial survival and mechanical durability of the new epidermis. If the keratinocytes are applied to a chronic granulating wound cell survival is poor and any resulting epidermis is fragile, easily abraded and prone to blistering. However, it has been shown both experimentally [11] and in burn patients that if a dermal wound bed is created keratinocyte survival is high and the grafted area is durable. Cuono *et al.* [12] showed that on burn patients it was possible to create a dermal wound bed using allografted skin. The epidermis is known to be more immunogeneic than dermis and in patients with major burns who are partly immunocompromised from their injury, the allografted dermis becomes permanently engrafted. The technique thus involves application of allografted skin onto a debrided wound bed. After a few weeks once the dermis has engrafted, the allografted epidermis is removed by shaving or dermabrasion and then cultured autologous keratinocytes are grafted on to the dermal wound bed. This method has been adopted worldwide in the treatment of burns and although the publication of large clinical trials is awaited the results appear promising with over 60% of the grafted area showing successful epidermal cover.

At the time of grafting, the sheets of cultured keratinocytes are approximately six cells thick and initially transparent (Fig. 28.3.18). However, as the cells grow and become stratified, a cornified layer develops and the surface becomes opaque. Histologically, the epidermis is initially acanthotic and the dermoepidermal junction is flat for several months without rete ridges. If there is a dermal wound bed, epidermal maturation is faster. Eventually there is mesenchymal remodelling beneath the epidermis with formation of a new dermis that even becomes innervated [13,14].

In summary, cultured keratinocytes are still not in routine clinical use worldwide but the topic has given rise to several avenues of research. These include attempts to develop synthetic dermal substitutes, as the use of cadaveric allograft skin to provide a dermal wound bed has potential risks of transmitting infections such as the human immunodeficiency virus (HIV). Another problem with autologous keratinocytes is the 3–4 week delay required to produce sheets of cells and other workers are trying to develop alternative delivery systems whereby subconfluent cells are grafted on to wounds after only 1–2 weeks in culture [15,16]. Finally, since the Rhinewald and Green technique to produce sheets of cultured autologous keratinocytes is still under patent, they are very expensive to purchase. A 25 cm² graft begins at US$350 (approximately £233) (Biosurface Technology, now Genzyme, Cambridge, Massachusetts). Cultured autologous keratinocytes may play a valuable role particularly in burn management in the future, but their present use should be confined to clinical trials.

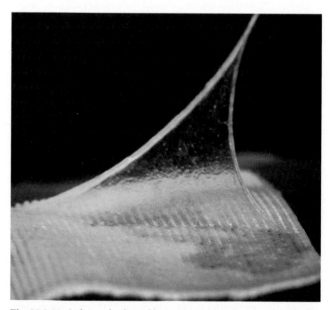

Fig. 28.3.18 A sheet of cultured keratinocytes at the time of grafting. It is six to eight cells thick and although transparent will become opaque with the formation of a differentiated epidermis.

REFERENCES

1 Rheinwald JG, Green H. Serial cultivation of strains of human epidermal keratinocytes: the formation of keratinizing colonies from single cells. *Cell* 1975; 6: 331–44.

2 Green H. Cultured cells for the treatment of disease. *Sci Am* 1991; 265: 64–70.

3 O'Connor NE, Mulliken JB, Banks-Schlegel S *et al*. Grafting of burns with cultured epithelium prepared from autologous epidermal cells. *Lancet* 1981; i: 75–8.

4 Gallico GG, O'Connor NE, Compton CC, Remensnyder JP, Kehinde O, Green H. Cultured epithelial autografts for giant congenital naevi. *Plast Reconstr Surg* 1989; 84: 1–9.

5 Carter DM, Lin AN, Varghese MC *et al*. Treatment of junctional epidermolysis bullosa with epidermal autografts. *J Am Acad Dermatol* 1987; 172: 246–50.

6 Higgins CR, Navsaria HA, Stringer M, Spitz L, Leigh IM. Use of two-stage keratinocyte dermal grafting to treat the separation site in conjoined twins. *J Roy Soc Med* 1994; 87: 108–9.

7 Hefton JM, Amberson JB, Biozes DG, Weksler ME. Loss of HLA-DR expression by human epidermal cells after growth in culture. *J Invest Dermatol* 1984; 83: 48–50.

8 Nanchahal J, Otto WR, Dover R, Dhital SK. Cultured composite skin grafts: biological skin equivalents permitting massive expansion. *Lancet* 1989; ii: 191–2.

9 Brain A, Purkis P, Coates P *et al*. Survival of cultured allogeneic keratinocytes transplanted to deep dermal bed assessed with probe specific for Y chromosome. *Br Med J* 1989; 298: 917–19.

10 Carver N, Navsaria HA, Green CJ, Leigh IM. Acute rejection of cultured keratinocyte allografts in nonimmunosuppressed pigs. *Transplantation* 1991; 52: 918–21.

11 Kangesu T, Navsaria HA, Manek S *et al*. Kerato-dermal grafts: the importance of dermis for the *in-vivo* growth of cultured keratinocytes. *Br J Plast Surg* 1993; 46: 401–9.

12 Cuono C, Langdon R, McGuire J. Use of cultured epidermal autografts and dermal allografts as skin replacement after burn injury. *Lancet* 1986; i: 1123–4.

13 Compton CC, Gill JM, Brafford DA *et al*. Skin regenerated from cultured epithelial autografts on full-thickness burn wounds from 6 days to 5 years after grafting. *Lab Invest* 1989; 60: 600–12.

14 Kangesu T, Manek S, Terenghi S *et al*. Nerve and blood vessel growth in cultured keratinocyte grafts. *Plast Reconstr Surg* 1998; 101: 1029–38.

15 Kaiser HW, Stark GB, Kopp J *et al*. Cultured autologous keratinocytes in fibrin glue suspension, exclusively and combined with STS-allograft: preliminary clinical and histopathological report of a new technique. *Burns* 1994; 20: 23–9.

16 Barlow YM, Burt AM, Clarke JA *et al*. The use of a polymeric film for the culture and transfer of sub-confluent autologous keratinocytes to patients. *J Tissue Viabil* 1992; 2: 33–6.

Hypertrophic and keloid scars

Clinical features

Although one hopes that all scars heal perfectly as thin lines, often this is not the case. In children in particular, there is a significant risk of hypertrophic and even keloid scar formation. There are many similarities between both hypertrophic and keloid scars and they are indistinguishable histologically. In both the pathology is within the dermis where there is dense hyalinized fibrous tissue with excess collagen deposition that is organized as discrete nodules. Frequently the rete pegs in the papillary dermis of the lesions are obliterated. Unlike normal dermis where collagen is arranged in discrete fascicles separated by interstitial space, the collagen nodules in keloids and hypertrophic scars appear avascular and are

arranged in a haphazard manner. Keloid nodules are thought to have a glassy appearance compared with hypertrophic scars.

The distinction between keloid and hypertrophic scars is a clinical one and it is incorrect to think of them as the same phenomenon that is qualitatively similar but quantitatively different. Keloid scars (Fig. 28.3.19) are most likely in patients of African origin but also in Chinese and Celts. In addition, there may be a familial predilection. They can occur at any age but are most prevalent in patients between 10 and 30 years of age [1]. They are rare in very young children [2] and the elderly. Keloids develop a few months after the wound repair, and occur most commonly on the lower face, neck, ear lobes, presternal area and back. Their characteristic feature is that they outgrow the boundaries of the original scar invading surrounding normal tissue. They rarely subside and treatment is largely unsuccessful.

Hypertrophic scars are less associated with racial origin and have lower familial tendency. They can occur at any age, but are most frequent below the age of 20 years. Hypertrophic scars develop a few weeks after injury and are prevalent on scars across flexor surfaces (Fig. 28.3.20). Hypertrophic scars stay within the boundaries of the original scar and subside over a 2–3 year period. Patients are troubled by the appearance of the scar, persistent itching and contracture.

Aetiology

Clues to the aetiology of both hypertrophic and keloid scars lie in some clinical observations. Both types of scars are common in some areas such as the sternum and shoul-

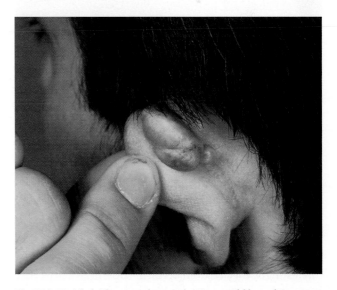

Fig. 28.3.19 A keloid scar on the ear of a 10-year-old boy after surgery for correction of prominent ears.

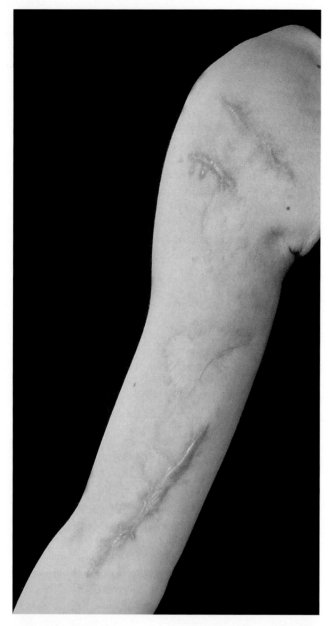

Fig. 28.3.20 Hypertrophic scars on the flexure aspect of this 12-year-old girl. She had hypertrophic burn scars that were revised when the scars were thought to be inactive, but the new wounds also became hypertrophic.

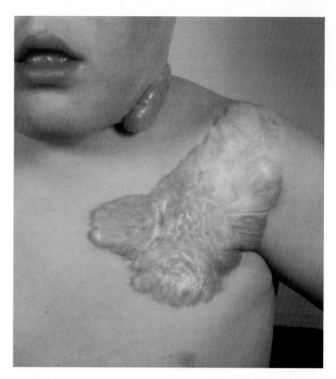

Fig. 28.3.21 Severe hypertrophic scars are common following burns as on this 3-year-old boy who sustained deep partial-thickness burns. The scars can mimic keloids but do not extend beyond the boundary of the original wound.

ders. Hypertrophic scars often occur where the axis of the wound crosses natural lines of skin tension rather than parallel to them. This gave rise to the theory that abnormal mechanical stresses are an important trigger of hypertrophic scarring. Hypertrophic scars are very common following a burn injury, particularly in children (Fig. 28.3.21). Interestingly, they seldom occur in superficial burns that have healed quickly, but are likely to form at sites where the burn injury was deeper and the wound slow to heal. Similarly, parts of wounds that dehisced and became infected are also more likely to become hypertrophic than areas of uneventful primary healing.

Other theories for the aetiology of hypertrophic and keloid scars include the suggestion that there were abnormalities of the immune system, but Cohen *et al.* [3] were unable to show any derangement of local or systemic immune factors. Tissue culture and biochemical studies have confirmed the increased production of collagen in keloid scars. Furthermore, fibroblasts that have been isolated from keloid scars continue to overproduce collagen when in culture. Hence it appears that once the fibroblasts have been stimulated to behave abnormally, they continue to do so even when removed from the abnormal environment [4]. Specific collagen studies have shown that the overproduction is mainly of collagen type I and not type III that is seen in wound healing. One popular concept is that hypoxia may stimulate or be responsible for the propagation of hypertrophic and keloid scars. Kischer *et al.* [5], observed increased occlusion of the microcirculation within lesions due to endothelial cell proliferation. It was hypothesized that perivascular myofibroblast contraction may contribute to microvascular occlusion. The resulting hypoxia could stimulate endothelial hyperplasia causing further hypoxia which eventually would lead to excess collagen production.

The symptoms of severe itching in hypertrophic scars

has attracted some interest and a high concentration of neuropeptides has been shown in hypertrophic scars when compared with normal skin [6]. These nerves may be responsible for the itching, but since some neuropeptides are trophic agents it has even been suggested that they may stimulate growth of the abnormal scars.

Treatment

Hypertrophic scars by their nature will regress with time. However, at the earliest suggestion that a scar may become hypertrophic, it is advisable to institute preventive measures. The mainstay of management is the use of pressure garments [7]. Quinn [8] introduced the use of silicone gel for hypertrophic and keloid scars. To be effective silicone gel needs to be applied for at least 12 h/day. As a practical guide, as soon as a wound is seen to be hypertrophic and in all healed burn wounds, the authors would advocate use of pressure garments (Fig. 28.3.22) in conjunction with silicone gel which can be worn inside the garment for a minimum period of 6 months. Children cope very well with this regime, but occasionally some develop an atopic sensitivity to silicone gel.

Intralesional steroid injections can be used for hypertrophic scars but surgery is not advised in the active phase when scars are red and itchy. Thereafter options for surgical treatment include excision and direct closure but this may result in scar recurrence. Alternatives are the use of Z-plasty techniques to realign the direction of the scars to lie parallel with the lines of skin tension, or to introduce local unaffected flaps to relieve tension and break up the scar.

Treatment of keloid scars is frustrating. Surgical excision alone is unlikely to be successful, and the lesions are likely to recur and may be larger than their original size. Intralesional excision is thought to be less harmful as it does not damage normal tissue. Intralesional steroid injections can in many instances decrease the size of keloids. It is the authors' practice to use intralesional injections of triamcinolone 10 mg/ml (maximum 1 ml), at 6-week intervals. A minimum of three injections is necessary before the benefit of the treatment can be assessed. In young children this may necessitate a general anaesthetic in order to give the injections. If steroid injections are unsuccessful, the next option would be to combine intralesional surgical excision with postoperative steroid injections. Complications of steroid injections such as local fat atrophy and depigmentation are due to extravasation into normal tissue.

Many workers have used radiotherapy following excision of keloids, but the authors do not recommend their use in children due to the risk of future malignancy. However, patients are often willing to take that risk, such is the social stigma from keloids. A summary of various regimes of surgery, radiotherapy and steroids in the treatment of keloids was published by Lawrence [9]. Although quantitative comparison of publised data is not possible due to numerous variations in patient cohort and treatment protocols, it nevertheless provides an impression of treatment efficacy. Analysis showed that steroid injections alone had a mean success rate of 66%. Surgery alone had a mean success rate of 28%, that increased to 52% when combined with postoperative steroid injections and 75% with radiotherapy.

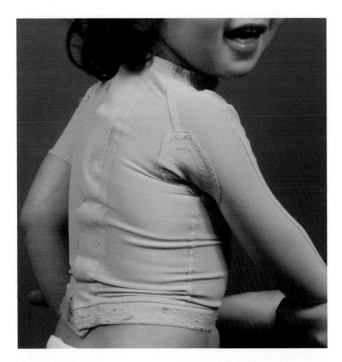

Fig. 28.3.22 Pressure garments, sometimes with silicone gel applied directly on the scar form the mainstay of treating hypertrophic scars in burns. They need to be worn for at least 6 months and usually for 2–3 years.

REFERENCES

1 Ketchum LD, Cohen IK, Masters FW. Hypertrophic scars and keloids: a collective review. *Plast Reconstr Surg* 1974; 53: 140–54.

2 Moustafa MFH, Abdel-Fattah AFMA. Keloids of the earlobe in Egypt. Their rarity in childhood and their treatment. *Br J Plast Surg* 1976; 29: 59–60.

3 Cohen IK, McCoy BJ, Mohanakumar T, Diegelmann RF. Immunoglobulin, complement, and histocompatibility antigen studies in keloid patients. *Plast Reconstr Surg* 1979; 63: 689–95.

4 Cohen IK, Keiser HR. Collagen synthesis in keloid and hypertrophic scar following intralesional use of triamcinolone. *Surg Forum* 1972; 23: 509–10.

5 Kischer CW, Theis C, Chavapil M. Perivascular myofibroblasts and microvascular occlusion in hypertrophic scars and keloids. *Human Pathol* 1982; 13: 819–24.

6 Crowe R, Parkhouse N, McGrouther DA, Burnstock G. Neuropeptide containing nerves in painful hypertrophic scar tissue. *Br J Dermatol* 1994; 130: 444–52.

7 Larson DL. Contracture and scar formation in the burn patient. *Clin Plast Surg* 1974; 1: 653–6.

8 Quinn KJ. Silicone gel in scar treatment. *Burns* 1987; 13: S33–40.

9 Lawrence WT. In search of the optimal treatment of keloids: report of a series and review of the literature. *Ann Plast Surg* 1991; 27: 164–78.

Scar revision

There should be little reason for scar revision following elective surgery. Local skin flaps may be bulky initially, but the vast majority settle down with time. The majority of patients who request scar revision are those with wounds that were the result of trauma, or those that have contracted unexpectedly or become hypertrophic. Scars are unsightly if they are tethered to the underlying muscle or fascia, contracted, raised or widened. Circular scars contract to produce a pin-cushion effect of the normal tissue within the scar.

It is essential to allow scars to mature before attempting revision, which means waiting for the itching and redness to resolve. It is the authors' practice to wait for a minimum of 1 year in adults and 2 years in children before considering revision. In that time, scar remodelling and softening may be adequate to even avoid further surgery. In children of early teenage it may be worthwhile waiting until they are 17 or 18 to reduce the risk of hypertrophic scar formation. Prior to surgery, it must be stressed to the patient or parent that the original deformity may recur or even be worse. It is also important to pin-point the exact feature of the scar that the patient dislikes and avoid excessive corrective surgery.

Surgery for scar revision is one of the most challenging in plastic surgery. Much scar revision involves excision of the scar with untethering of the local tissue, and then reapproximation of appropriate tissue layers. Sometimes, the scar can be de-epithelialized and buried subcutaneously to provide a firm anchor to the repair and correct a sunken contour deformity. If a scar is unsightly because it lies across a natural line of skin tension, then attempts can be made to realign the scar with the techniques of Z-plasty (Fig. 28.3.23) or W-plasty (Fig. 28.3.24). The details are quite complex and outside the limits of this text [1–3], but in principle if a straight scar is up to 35° across a line of skin tension, a Z-plasty is chosen. If the angle is between 35 and 90°, a W-plasty is performed with multiple small flaps with acute angles.

REFERENCES

1 Borges AF. Improvement in anti-tension-line scars by the W-plasty operation. *Br J Plast Surg* 1959; 12: 29–33.
2 McGregor IA. The theoretical basis of the Z-plasty. *Br J Plast Surg* 1957; 9: 256.
3 McGregor IA. *Fundamental Techniques of Plastic Surgery*, 8th edn. Edinburgh: Churchill Livingstone, 1989.

Management of the burn wound

Each year in the UK, there are an estimated 600 deaths and over 10 000 hospital admissions from burn injuries [1]. In the USA, it is estimated that each year there are approximately 2 million burn injuries that require medical attention. These account for more than 500 000 hospital emergency department admissions and 70 000 inpatient admissions [2]. Approximately 50% of admissions to burns units in the UK are children, the vast majority of

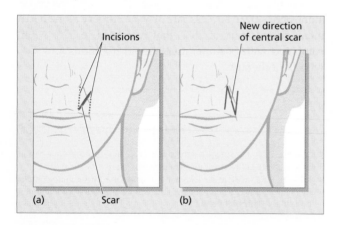

Fig. 28.3.23 A Z-plasty can also be used to change the direction of a scar so that it falls into a line of natural skin tension. (a) The scar initially passes across the line of relaxed skin tension which is along the nasolabial groove. Thus it would be very noticeable during normal facial expressions. (b) After excision of the scar and transposition of the flaps, the central limb of the scar is along the nasolabial groove. The price is two further scars from the lateral limbs of the Z-plasty. However, with good planning these will also fall in or close to lines of relaxed skin tension and the final scar be less noticeable than the original.

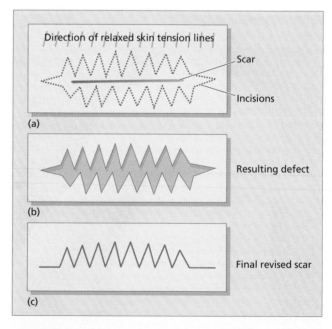

Fig. 28.3.24 A W-plasty is an alternative to a Z-plasty and is indicated when the angle between the scar and relaxed skin tension lines is between 35 and 90°. (a) The scar is excised with a running W incision. Closure of the resultant defect (b) produces a zig-zag scar where each limb of the scar is close in alignment with the skin tension lines.

whom are children between the age of 1 and 3 years who have sustained scalds from domestic accidents.

Thermal injuries can result from a wide range of temperatures, varying from frostbite at the lowest end of the spectrum to electrical burns at the highest. The severity of the injury depends on the aetiology, size and depth of the wound. Apart from the local tissue damage to the integument, there are diverse systemic effects which cause major burn injuries to be classified amongst the most severe forms of traumatic injury [3].

The depth of local burn injury is classified as (a) superficial partial-thickness (Fig. 28.3.25); (b) deep partial-thickness (Fig. 28.13.26); and (c) full-thickness (Fig. 28.3.27), in relation to the anatomy of the skin. In superficial partial-thickness burns, only the epidermis is involved with minimal damage to the underlying dermis. Such wounds heal spontaneously with epithelialization occurring from the epidermal lining of skin appendages as well as from the unburned skin edge. In deep partial-thickness burns, the injury extends into the dermis and in full-thickness burns, damage includes the complete thickness of epidermis and dermis. If these wounds only involve a small area, they could also heal spontaneously by a combination of epidermalization and wound contraction; but in practice, in view of the cosmetic and functional deformities that arise from contraction, and also because healing would be a slow process, many deep partial-thickness wounds are treated surgically. Deep partial-thickness injuries are usually debrided by early tangential excision, where the burned area is progressively shaved until healthy dermis is reached [4]. For full-thickness injuries,

complete excision of the skin may require excision down to fat or the fascial plane. After debridement, wounds are routinely resurfaced with autologous skin grafts. Early surgery correlates well with decreased mortality [5] and an improved cosmetic appearance due to a reduced incidence of hypertrophic scarring in grafted areas [6].

There are an array of dressing materials for burn wounds due to aggressive marketing tactics. In principle, a superficial wound can be dressed with a non-adherent material the cheapest of which is paraffin gauze. The authors' initial experience with a silicone-backed dressing (Mepitel) has been promising particularly in children as the material does not adhere to the wound, making dressing changes more tolerable. Semi-permeable occlusive materials (Opsite) can also be used, but dressings must be inspected regularly to aspirate excessive serous collections, and these dressings should be discontinued at the first sign of infection as they otherwise create an ideal environment for bacterial growth. Use of a topical bacteriostatic agents such as the sulphonamide in silver sulpha-

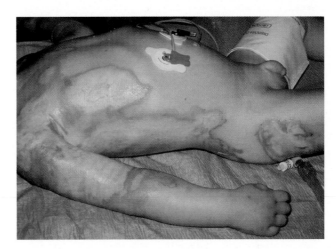

Fig. 28.3.26 A 1-year-old child with mixed depth burns. The injury on the right arm is of deep partial-thickness.

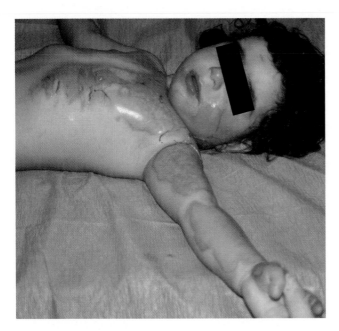

Fig. 28.3.25 A 11-month-old boy with superficial partial-thickness burns from a scald.

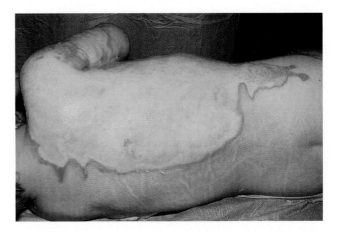

Fig. 28.3.27 A 2-year-old child with mostly full-thickness burns.

diazine (Flamazine) is also appropriate to decrease the risk of bacterial contamination, but the doctor must be sure that the wound is superficial because the white staining of the wound by Flamazine makes subsequent assessment of burn depth more difficult. Small deep partial-thickness wounds that are treated conservatively can be dressed with Flamazine. Wounds that are destined for early surgery are best dressed with paraffin gauze as it is cheap and will not stain the tissue.

REFERENCES

1 Muir IFK, Barclay TLK, Settle JAD. *Burns and their Management*, 3rd edn. London: Butterworths, 1987.

2 American Burn Association. Appendix B to hospital resources document: guidelines for service standards and severity classifications in the treatment of burn injury. *Am Coll Surg Bull* 1984; 69: 24–8.

3 Robson MC, Smith DJ. Thermal injuries. In: Jurkiewicz MJ, Krizek TJ, Mathes SJ, Ariyan S, eds. *Plastic Surgery: Principles and Practice*, vol. 2. St Louis: CV Mosby, 1990: 1355–410.

4 Janzekovic A. A new concept in the early excision and immediate grafting of burns. *J Trauma* 1970; 10: 1103–8.

5 Scott-Conner CEH, Meydrech E, Wheeler WE, Cil JA. Quantitation of rate of wound closure and the prediction of death following major burns. *Burns* 1988; 14: 373–8.

6 McDonald S, Deitch EA. Hypertrophic skin grafts in burn patients: a prospective analysis of variables. *J Trauma* 1987; 27: 147–50.

Conclusion

It is easy to see that in the simple matter of dealing with wounds, scars and their subsequent care, a knowledge of the basic scientific aspects of wound healing and the natural history of scar formation is essential. On being presented with a patient who asks whether scar revision can be undertaken, the experienced plastic surgeon will determine the mechanism of injury, the initial treatment, the expertise of the initial surgeon, the technical correctness of the operation, the time elapsed since the injury, whether primary healing occurred or if infection or dehiscence led to secondary intention healing, the direction of the scar, the skin type of the patient and the expectations of the patient and family. Assessment of these issues will help in the decision over whether or not revision is indicated. If so, a decision then needs to be made over whether a simple direct excision or reorientation of the scar by either Z-plasty or W-plasty will suffice. The surgeon then must determine how technically the wound should be closed. It is too often assumed that surgery is about the last decision only, the technical one. It is not, it is a matter of judgement.

Acknowledgements

The authors would like to thank the following consultant plastic surgeons for giving their permisssion to allow us to use photographs of their patients: Roy Sanders (Figs. 28.3.1, 28.3.16), Chris C. Walker (Figs. 28.3.4, 28.3.8, 28.3.22), Jim Frame (Figs. 28.3.7, 28.3.25, 28.3.26, 28.3.27), David Elliot (Fig. 28.3.12), Barry Jones (Fig. 28.3.17) and Brian Morgan (Fig. 28.3.20).

28.4 Lasers for Vascular and Pigmented Lesions

MOISE L. LEVY

Vasculur lesions
Argon laser
Argon-pumped tunable dye laser
Flashlamp excited dye laser
Copper vapour laser

Pigmented lesions
Benign cutaneous pigmented lesions

Special considerations

Vascular lesions

A wide variety of cutaneous vascular disease can be seen in any paediatric dermatology practice. Patients seeking treatment of such disease are usually those with port-wine stains. Additionally, however, patients (and parents of patients) may seek consultation regarding available treatment for haemangiomas, telangiectasias, capillary ectasias or spider angiomas and pyogenic granulomas. Angiofibromas may also be considered. Lasers have been utilized for treatment of vascular skin disease since the 1960s. Initially, the ruby laser was utilized for this indication, but was found to produce non-specific thermal damage to affected tissues. Scarring and skin dyspigmentation of treated skin resulted. Subsequently, a variety of different lasers have evolved which allow more selective targeting of tissues resulting in significantly less thermal damage to uninvolved tissues.

Argon laser

Argon lasers release a blue–green continuous beam of light with wavelengths between 488 and 514nm [1]. Argon light is absorbed by both oxyhaemoglobin and melanin. Because of the relatively non-specific absorption of this light by vascular structures, the initial popularity of argon lasers for the treatment of vascular lesions has faded. Significant thermal destruction of the epidermis and dermal structures limited the use of the argon laser for the treatment of vascular lesions, particularly in children [2]. Textural changes of the skin, as well as dyspigmentation has been reported in 20–30% of patients who have undergone such treatment [3].

In an attempt to overcome such difficulties, a variety of approaches to minimize significant thermal destruction of uninvolved tissues have been devised. A very tedious and time-consuming method utilizing magnification of affected vessels and tracing of involved areas does seem to minimize the ill effects of the poorly selective absorption of this continuous wave laser energy. Other than port-wine stains, a wide variety of vascular lesions including telangiectasias, macular stains and angiofibromas have been successfully treated with this laser modality.

Argon-pumped tunable dye laser

The argon-pumped tunable dye laser is a continuous wave laser which can be truly 'tuned' to a variety of wavelengths from, blue to green to yellow, depending on the target desired for such treatment [4]. When treating vascular lesions, wavelengths in the yellow band are most appropriate owing to the fact that haemoglobin maximally absorbs light at 577nm. The argon-pumped tunable dye laser can be tuned to emit light both at 577nm as well as 585nm which has been proven to yield improved clearing of vascular lesions owing to its deeper penetration within the dermis.

Due to the continuous nature of energy production by such equipment, side-effects such as textural skin change or dyspigmentation seen with the argon (or other continuous wave lasers) can still be seen. One group found that areas measuring 8–10cm can be treated in approximately 1h with sessions being repeated on a monthly basis until an entire port-wine stain, for example, is covered [2]. Utilizing 0.08W of power with increments up to 0.8W, such treatments are administered at 4–6-week intervals. Of patients treated with this method 40% were reported to have 80–100% clearing of port-wine stains. The average age of patients in this group was 8 years old. Most individuals utilizing the argon-pumped dye laser for treatment of vascular lesions will utilize either the very tedious method of tracing individual vessels guided by suitable magnification over very extended periods of time (as outlined above) or robotic scanners such as the Hexascan. Utilizing the Hexascan, pulses of energy measuring 1mm can be delivered in a manner to dissipate more effectively

1809

the accumulation of thermal energy at a given treatment site which can occur utilizing only continuous wave lasers. The Hexascan allows for the arrangement of energy pulses into hexagonal grids measuring from 3 to 13 mm [4]. The pulses of energy are delivered at 50 ms intervals to minimize thermal injury. While 577–585 nm is most often used for vascular lesions, one author utilizes green light at 514 nm for individuals with a light complexion and 'large or recurrent lesions'. When compared to the flashlamp excited dye lasers (FEDL) utilizing either 577 or 585 nm wavelength, this technology has proven to be roughly equivalent in its use for treatment of port-wine stains [5]. Undesirable side-effects such as dyspigmentation, textural change or hypertrophic scarring were infrequent with either technology based on one investigation. Overall, however, the argon-pumped dye laser seemed to produce slightly less clearing at the 6-week interval chosen for investigation in this study and slightly greater amounts of dyspigmentation. A benefit to the argon-pumped dye laser when compared to the FEDL is the lack of significant purpura which is prominent after treatment with the FEDL. Lesions which can be treated by the argon-pumped dye laser include the spectrum of vascular and macular pigmented lesions.

Flashlamp excited dye laser

Utilizing a technique known as selective photothermolysis, the principle of restricting desired thermal damage to selected pigmented targets, a variety of lasers, (including vascular lesion lasers) have proven to be extremely useful in the treatment of vascular and pigmented lesions [6]. Vascular lesions such as port-wine stains, haemangiomas, telangiectasia and angiofibromas, among others can be effectively treated with the FEDL. Initial clinical trials utilizing this equipment employed light produced at 577 nm coincident with one of the maximum absorption peaks for oxyhaemoglobin [7]. Subsequent investigations discovered that deeper penetration within the dermis to approximately 1.2 mm could be obtained utilizing light produced at 585 nm [8]. Additionally, less light was absorbed by melanin while conserving very high amounts of absorption of this energy by the targeted oxyhaemoglobin. The laser energy is delivered at 450 ms which is within the estimated thermal relaxation time for cutaneous vessels measuring 10–40 μm. The purpura seen clinically after treatment with these lasers is consistent with a mild superficial haemorrhage due to vaporization of the targeted vessels [6]. Only minimal perivascular tissue damage is seen with such technology.

Such energy can be delivered through a variety of spot sizes, now up to 10 mm. The response to therapy of port-wine stains to treatment with the FEDL has been thoroughly investigated. Overall, most patients can expect significant improvement (lightening) of their lesions after

multiple treatment sessions. One group has found approximately 75% improvement in facial port-wine stains in children after five to seven treatments [9]. This is consistent with the author's experience, while others have cited more favourable results [10,11]. Variables do exist which must be kept in mind when considering treatment of port-wine stains. The size of port-wine stains was considered to be a useful indicator of treatment outcome by Morelli *et al.* [12]. Lesions less than 20 cm² (15 of 47 patients) cleared completely in their series of 83 children while only three of 36 patients with lesions larger than 20 cm² showed the same result. These results were cited irrespective of the site of the lesion being treated.

In general, when treatment can begin during infancy or early childhood overall results seem to be better. The central portion of the face and lower extremities clear less readily in the same period of time required to achieve improvement of a given lesion over the periorbital, temporal or malar areas of the face, the neck, trunk or upper extremities (Fig. 28.4.1). Lighter port-wine stains respond better with this modality than the nodular and darker lesions seen in older patients. This point is a source of some debate in the literature. Orren *et al.* found that age had no relation to ultimate outcome of therapy [13]. More recently, van der Horst *et al.* [14] prospectively evaluated a group of 100 patients, both paediatric and adult. An average of five treatments was chosen for evaluation purposes and no benefit for treatment of port-wine stains in early childhood was found [14]. Finally, another group concluded, after reviewing their extensive experience with a group of 640 patients who were treated with FEDL, that older patients responded better than younger patients [15]. This same group also found no correlation between colour of the vascular malformation and its ultimate response to laser treatment. Morelli's group, however, felt strongly that patients beginning therapy when younger than 1 year old had markedly improved clearing [16].

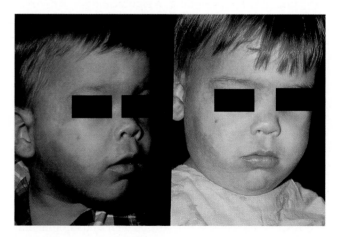

Fig. 28.4.1 The lightening of a port-wine stain (left) before and (right) after three treatments with the FEDL.

When preparing patients or families for such treatment, they must be carefully counselled regarding the length of treatment generally required as well as being given an honest appraisal of the expected results. While this author concurs that most patients achieve maximum clearing with the use of the traditional FEDL (577 or 585 nm) after five to seven treatments as cited by others [9,13], some patients do seem to benefit from more treatment sessions [6]. The possibility of darkening, and possibly hypertrophic changes of treated areas years after treatment should be discussed. Such changes, seen in many non-treated port-wine stains, remain possible since most lesions cannot be totally cleared.

The treatment is not painless and provisions for the use of distraction methods (e.g. child life workers, who are trained in child development and assist with distraction methods during painful procedures), as well as the potential need for local or general anaesthesia must be discussed. Pain control is reviewed in Chapter 28.5. Utilizing 'test patches' (Fig. 28.4.2) or a few pulses of energy delivered to a given lesion with 0.25–0.5 J/cm^2 increments can be a useful part of the initial treatment session particularly in patients with darker skin who will be at a greater risk for dyspigmentation or when treating areas such as eyelids or the neck. The latter areas are more subject to scarring. Initial power settings for the treatment of port-wine stains can be between 5.5 and 6.25 J/cm^2. Telangiectasias may require higher initial power settings. Care must be exercised regarding areas more prone to scarring such as the eyelids or neck. Between 0.25 and 0.50 J/cm^2 less of those power densities selected for use elsewhere may be appropriate. Eye protection must be utilized when treating around the eyes. Eyeglasses specific for the wavelength used, gauze or sterile corneal protectors must be applied in such instances. Haemangiomas may also respond well to treatment with this modality when therapy is delivered either early or late in the growth of such lesions. Utilizing power densities between 6 and 9 J/cm^2 with 5 mm spot sizes and treating at 4–8-week intervals for a total of two to three sessions, improvement (but not complete resolution) can be expected [17,18]. Larger spot sizes (e.g. 7 or 10 mm) are appropriate for larger lesions but are used at lower power densities. The special clinical situation of ulcerated haemangiomas deserves mention. Morelli *et al.* have reported excellent results using the FEDL (6.0–6.5 J/cm^2, 5 mm spot size) [19]. Others have cited similar results using different treatment parameters [20]. Children have significant associated discomfort when these lesions occur in the perineal region. Pain was relieved after one session according to these authors, with one to three sessions given at 2–4-week intervals resulting in healing of the ulcerations (Fig. 28.4.3).

Adverse effects in patients treated with FEDL are unusual. One group found atrophic scarring to occur in 0.1%, hyperpigmentation in 1.0%, transient hypopigmentation 1.4% and a mild dermatitis in 0.04% of treated

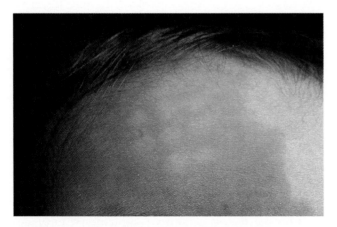

Fig. 28.4.2 Initial small test area showing a good response to the FEDL. Courtesy of Dr J. Harper.

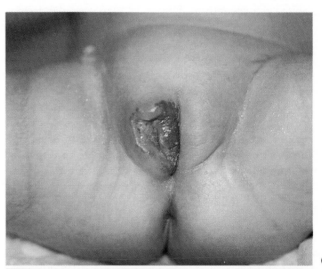

(a)

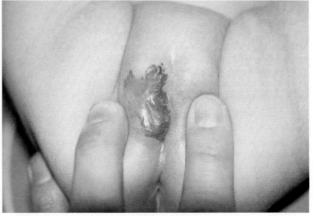

(b)

Fig. 28.4.3 (a) Ulcerated haemangioma on the labia majora of an infant. This lesion was complicated by bleeding and extreme pain unresponsive to medical therapies. (b) One month after a single treatment with the 585 nm FEDL, the ulceration illustrated in (a) has resolved. Pain relief was evident 2–3 days after the laser treatment.

patients [21,22]. A review of 701 patients found hyperpigmentation occurring in 9% of the patients [22]. This, however, generally resolved within 1 year. Atrophic scarring occurred in 4% of the patients with hypertrophic scarring being seen in less than 1% of patients. The former tended to occur more commonly in the younger patients.

Finally, longer pulse duration (1500 ms) and wavelength (595 or 600 nm) FEDL are now available for treating such vascular malformations. Preliminary indications from the author's use of this equipment suggest more clearing of lesions previously treated multiple times with the 585 nm/450 ms FEDL. These lasers may prove to be of use particularly for those patients whose results have 'plateaued' after a series of treatments with the 585 nm/450 ms FEDL.

Copper vapour laser

Copper lasers can be 'tuned' to emit light at the green wavelength for treating pigmented lesions or to the yellow wavelength at 578 nm to treat vascular lesions [1,16]. This laser produces energy with an extremely short pulse duration of 20 ns at a very high frequency. While technically a pulsed laser, this laser functions more like a continuous wave laser owing to the short pulse duration and high frequency of energy production. Side-effects, therefore, are more similar to those seen after treatment with the argon or argon-pumped dye lasers. The copper vapour lasers have proven to be more useful than FEDL for the treatment of nodular vascular lesions such as 'mature' port-wine stains or angiokeratomas. Postoperatively, patients do not experience the purpura seen after treatment with the FEDL, but will have eschar formation over the treated sites. Small spot sizes (100 to 200μ) and an average power of 200 W will generally prove to be appropriate for clinical use.

REFERENCES

1 Wheeland RG. Clinical uses of lasers in dermatology. *Lasers Surg Med* 1994; 16: 2–23.
2 Scheibner A, Wheeland RG. Use of the argon-pumped tunable dye laser for port-wine stains in children. *Dermatol Surg Oncol* 1991; 17: 735–9.
3 Spicer MS, Goldberg DJ. Lasers in dermatology. *J Am Acad Dermatol* 1996; 34: 1–25.
4 Apfelberg DB. Argon-pumped tunable dye laser. *Ann Plast Surg* 1994; 32: 394–400.
5 Dover JS, Geronemus R, Stern RS *et al.* Dye laser treatment of port-wine stains: comparison of the continuous-wave dye laser with a robotized scanning device and the pulsed dye laser. *J Am Acad Dermatol* 1994; 32: 237–40.
6 Anderson RR, Parrish JA. Selective photothermolysis: precise microsurgery by selective absorption of pulsed radiation. *Science* 1983; 220: 524–7.
7 Morelli JG, Tan OT, Garden J *et al.* Tunable dye laser (577 nm) treatment of port wine stains. *Lasers Surg Med* 1986; 6: 94–9.
8 Tan OT, Morrison P, Kurban AK. 585 nm for treatment of port-wine stains. *Plast Reconstr Surg* 1990; 86: 1112–17.
9 Goldman MP, Fitzpatrick RE, Ruiz-Esparza J. Treatment of port-wine stains (capillary malformation) with the flashlamp-pumped pulsed dye laser. *J Pediatr* 1993; 122: 71–7.
10 Tan OT, Sherwood K, Gilchrest BA. Treatment of children with port-wine stains using the flashlamp-pulsed tunable dye laser. *N Engl J Med* 1989; 320: 416–21.
11 Reyes BA, Geronemus R. Treatment of port-wine stains during childhood with flashlamp-pumped pulsed dye laser. *J Am Acad Dermatol* 1990; 23: 1142–8.
12 Morelli JG, Weston WL, Huff JC *et al.* Initial lesion size as a predictive factor in determining the response of port-wine stains in children treated with the pulsed dye laser. *Arch Pediatr Adolesc Med* 1995; 149: 1142–4.
13 Orren SS, Waner M, Flock S *et al.* Port-wine stains—an assessment of 5 years of treatment. *Arch Otolaryngol Head Neck Surg* 1996; 122: 1174–9.
14 van der Horst CMAM, Koster PHL, de Borgie CAJM *et al.* Effect of timing of treatment of port-wine stains with the flash-lamp-pumped pulsed-dye laser. *N Engl J Med* 1998; 338: 1028–33.
15 Kutugampola GA, Lamigan SW. Five years' experience of treating port-wine stains with the flashlamp-pumped pulsed dye laser. *Br J Dermatol* 1997; 137: 750–4.
16 Kauvar ANB, Geronemus RG. Repetitive pulsed dye laser treatments improve persistent port-wine stains. *Dermatol Surg* 1995; 21: 515–21.
17 Barlow RJ, Walker NPJ, Markey AC. Treatment of proliferative haemangiomas with the 585 nm pulsed dye laser. *Br J Dermatol* 1996; 134: 700–4.
18 Landthaler M, Hohenleutner U, El-Raheem T. Laser therapy in childhood haemangiomas. *Br J Dermatol* 1995; 133: 275–81.
19 Morelli JG, Tan OT, Weston WL. Treatment of ulcerated hemangiomas with the pulsed tunable dye laser. *Am J Dis Child* 1991; 145: 1062–4.
20 Lacour M, Syed S, Linward J *et al.* Role of the pulsed dye laser in the management of ulcerated capillary haemangiomas. *Arch Dis Child* 1996; 74: 161–3.
21 Waner M, Dinehart S. Lasers in facial plastic and reconstructive surgery. In: Davis RK, ed. *Lasers in Otolaryngology: Head and Neck Surgery*. New York: WB Saunders, 1990: 156–91.
22 Seukeran DC, Collins P, Sheehan-Dare RA. Adverse reactions following pulsed tunable dye laser treatment of port-wine stains in 701 patients. *Br J Dermatol* 1997; 136: 725–9.

Pigmented lesions

Benign cutaneous pigmented lesions

Dermatologists and plastic surgeons have utilized a variety of methods for treating benign pigmented lesions of the skin such as cryotherapy, tattoo, chemical peels and others. Utilizing a variety of lasers will allow targeting of light at epidermal or dermal depths should allow effective clearing of a variety of such lesions. Lentigines, café-au-lait macules, ephelides, melanocytic and Becker's naevi, naevus of Ota and even melasma and postinflammatory hyperpigmentation have been managed with variable success with a variety of laser modalities [1].

Argon laser

Utilizing the blue–green wavelength of light at 514 nm produced by the argon laser, a variety of pigmented lesions have been successfully treated. Examples include naevi, café-au-lait macules and naevus of Ota. Because of the non-selective absorption by tissues treated with the argon laser, dyspigmentation and textural skin changes seen have relegated this equipment to a position well behind more pigment-specific lasers in the treatment of such lesions. Spot sizes of 0.2–1 mm with 0.5–1.5 W and 1–2 s pulses can be used.

Copper vapour laser

Copper vapour lasers, when utilizing the 511 nm green band, have proven to be useful in the treatment of a variety of benign pigmented lesions. Specifically, ephelides and lentigines have been successfully treated. Additionally, benign melanocytic naevi and even some cases of postinflammatory hyperpigmentation have been successfully managed with such equipment.

Pulsed pigmented dye laser

Pulsed dye lasers with wavelengths of 504–510 nm (green light) have been shown to modify successfully the appearance of a variety of benign pigmented skin lesions. Generally, patients require between two and five treatments given at 6–12-week intervals [2]. The success of the pulsed dye lasers for the treatment of pigmented lesions has been attributed to their ability to minimize damage to the basement membrane lowering the risks of pigmentary incontinence and postinflammatory hyperpigmentation from such therapy. The principle of selective photothermolysis, as described for vascular lesions above, explains the utility of such equipment. Using a pigmented lesion dye laser (504 nm) at 2.0–3.5 J/cm² macular areas of hypermelanosis were successfully cleared after an average of two to four sessions (Fig. 28.4.4). While initial investigations did not demonstrate recurrence of some pigmented lesions such as café-au-lait macules, with longer follow-up periods these lesions, in certain individuals, have been found to slowly repigment approximately 1 year after treatment [3].

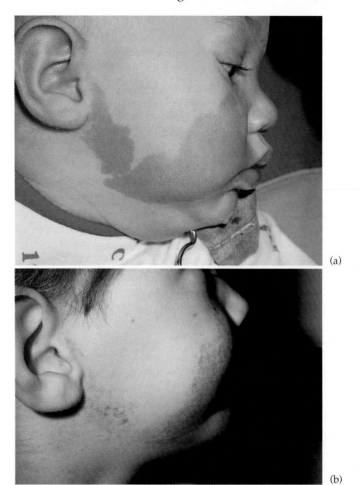

(a)

(b)

Fig. 28.4.4 Large café-au-lait macule (a) before and (b) after two complete and three partial treatments with the pulsed pigment dye laser. Courtesy of Dr Ilona Frieden.

Q-switched yttrium–aluminium–garnet

The Q-switched neodymium : yttrium–aluminium–garnet (Nd : YAG) laser utilizes the property of selective photothermolysis delivering very high energy densities with short pulsed intervals. When the frequency of the energy being delivered is doubled, green light delivered at 532 nm is produced [1]. At this wavelength, relatively superficial (epidermal) pigmentation can be effectively treated. Representative lesions would include lentigines, café-au-lait macules or ephelides. Without frequency-doubling, the Q-switched Nd : YAG laser produces energy in the near infrared range at 1064 nm. The Q-switch is a shutter device which allows very short high-dose energy bursts of light to be emitted [3]. At this wavelength, deeper melanocytic lesions such as the naevus of Ota can be treated [4]. After treatment, which is done under local or general anaesthesia, minor crusting of the skin is seen. Treatments are administered every 3–6 months. Patients generally require three to five treatments with the usual complications seen with laser therapy occurring in some instances. Mechanistically, the light is absorbed by

pigment particles which vaporize and fragment. The pigment is then phagocytozed and cleared. Power densities between 4.5 and 5 J/cm² at 1064 nm wavelength, with 3 mm spot size and 5 Hz are useful to treat naevus of Ota. Moisturizing ointments or gels are generally sufficient for postoperative management, although non-adherent dressings may hasten healing and will minimize patient discomfort.

Q-switched ruby laser

Utilizing the red light (694 nm) produced by the Q-switched ruby laser, a variety of epidermal or dermal melanocytic lesions have been successfully managed [5–7]. With the short pulse duration (20–40 ns) and high peak energy produced by such lasers, advantage can be taken of the wide absorption spectrum of melanin with the ruby laser. As with many of the other lasers, the sensation during treatment is similar to that of a small elastic band snapping on the skin. Many patients require either no anaesthesia or only minimal local anaesthetic.

Immediately after treatment, mild petechiae or purpura can be seen at the treatment site in addition to a whitening of the treated area. Occasionally, small erosions can be seen at treatment sites but no significant amount of exudate or bleeding is seen. Mild oedema occurs followed by an erythematous response lasting 7–10 days. Patients with darker skin such as types IV or V are at risk for hypopigmentation which is seen to resolve generally over many months. Test patches should be utilized in such cases, if not with all patients. Regardless of the lesion being treated, histological changes subsequent to treatment of pigmented lesions with the ruby laser demonstrate vacuolization of melanocytes and keratinocytes [5]. Rupture of melanosomes is also seen. No damage to the appendages has been consistently documented and no gross evidence of fibrosis is seen months after treatment. A wide variety of pigmented lesions including lentigines, café-au-lait macules, naevus of Ota and melanocytic naevi have been successfully treated. Small macular lesions can be well managed with one or two treatments, although lesions such as café-au-lait macules have been seen to recur slowly approximately 1 year after the initial treatment. Up to five treatment sessions have been found to be necessary for removal of naevus of Ota. One study cited a 3-year follow-up after treatment of a group of 114 patients with naevus of Ota [8]. No recurrence was noted during that interval. Even greater numbers of treatment sessions have been required to achieve significant clearing of pigment from naevocellular naevi [9]. There is controversy regarding the advisability of treating congenital or acquired naevi with any laser. Such a decision must be guided in individual cases after careful discussion with patients or parents and prior skin biopsy.

Alexandrite laser

The Alexandrite laser is another Q-switched laser producing energy at 755 nm. The long wavelength allows for more effective treatment of pigmented lesions with deeper dermal involvement [1]. The utility of this laser modality is probably similar to the ruby laser.

Other clinical indications for laser treatment

While multiple other clinical conditions are currently being explored for their suitability for treatment with laser technology, in the paediatric and adolescent patient indications are generally more focused. Erythematous and hypertrophic scars represent a clinical problem seen frequently in paediatric and adolescent patients, whether as a postoperative complication or subsequent to rapid growth during puberty [10]. Erythematous scars after

treatment of severe acne are another potential indication for laser treatment. The FEDL at a wavelength of 585 nm has been successfully applied to the treatment of such clinical problems [11]. Generally, patients with lighter skin colours (e.g. types I, II or III) seem to be the best candidates for treatment with this modality. Power densities between 6.5 and 6.75 J/cm^2 were used without overlapping pulses. One or two treatment sessions at 6–8-week intervals with this equipment has proved to be a useful treatment modality.

Improvement in the erythema, skin texture and elevation, and patient complaints of pruritus, have all been seen to respond. The author has seen great improvement in the erythema of such lesions after treatment with flashlamp pulsed dye vascular lesion lasers while softening and flattening of hypertrophic scars have responded less well. The mechanism for efficacy of FEDL treatment of scars is generally unknown. While the erythema may certainly represent the vasculature within these lesions (and therefore a target upon which the light will act), the effect of this treatment on the supporting tissues is difficult to explain. Histopathology of treated areas has shown normal number and appearance of dermal fibroblasts with a more loose appearing collagen structure overall. Interestingly, mast cells have been found to be present in increased numbers of laser-treated scars when compared to controlled lesions.

Similarly striae have been found to respond well to treatment with the (vascular) FEDL. Using the 10 mm spot size at a power density of 3 J/cm^2 or 7 mm with a power density of 4 J/cm^2 results in clinical and histopathological improvement at 8 weeks after treatment [11]. Striae with significant erythema represent the best lesions for such therapy.

Angiofibromas, which can represent a significant cosmetic concern for some patients, can also be successfully modified with either the argon or (vascular) FEDL [12]. Again, those lesions with a significant vascular component respond best to such therapy. The author has found great results from treatment of such lesions after one to three treatment sessions given 1–3 months apart. Smaller papules tend to respond best.

Verrucae, unresponsive or partially responsive to routine medical intervention, may be candidates. Paring of such lesions followed by double or triple pulsing with 8.0–8.5 J/cm^2 (or more) can be considered. Treatments should be repeated at monthly intervals. Response should be evident after two or three sessions. Subsequent treatments are guided by the clinical response. Due to the higher power densities used, appropriate smoke evacuators and masks should be used due to the plume generated. An alternative is to treat the warts through a clear gel dressing. Such treatment is very uncomfortable making suitable anaesthesia or analgesia necessary for most patients.

REFERENCES

1 Wheeland RG. Clinical uses of lasers in dermatology. *Lasers Surg Med* 1994; 16: 2–23.

2 Tan OT, Morelli JG, Kurban AK. Pulsed dye laser treatment of benign cutaneous pigmented lesions. *Lasers Surg Med* 1992; 12: 538–42.

3 Spicer MS, Goldberg DJ. Lasers in dermatology. *J Am Acad Dermatol* 1996; 34: 1–25.

4 Apfelberg DB. Argon and Q-switched yttrium–aluminum–garnet laser treatment of nevus of Ota. *Ann Plast Surg* 1995; 35: 150–3.

5 Taylor CR, Anderson RR. Treatment of benign pigmented epidermal lesions by Q-switched ruby laser. *Int J Dermatol* 1993; 32: 908–12.

6 DePadova-Elder SM, Milgraum SS. Q-switched ruby laser treatment of labial lentigines in Peutz–Jeghers syndrome. *J Dermatol Surg Oncol* 1994; 20: 830–2.

7 Chang CJ, Nelson JS. Q-switched ruby laser treatment of mucocutaneous melanosis associated with Peutz–Jeghers syndrome. *Ann Plast Surg* 1996; 36: 394–7.

8 Watanabe S, Takahashi H. Treatment of nevus of Ota with the Q-switched ruby laser. *N Engl J Med* 1994; 331: 1745–50.

9 Waldorf HA, Kauvar ANB, Geronemus RG. Treatment of small and medium congenital nevi with the Q-switched ruby laser. *Arch Dermatol* 1996; 132: 301–4.

10 Alster TS. Improvement of erythematous and hypertrophic scars by the 585-nm flashlamp-pumped pulsed dye laser. *Ann Plast Surg* 1994; 32: 186–90.

11 McDaniel DH, Ash K, Zukowski M. Treatment of stretch marks with the 585-nm flashlamp-pumped pulsed dye laser. *Dermatol Surg* 1996; 22: 332–7.

12 Boixeda P, Sanchez-Miralles E, Azana JM *et al.* CO_2 argon, and pulsed dye laser treatment of angiofibromas. *J Dermatol Surg Oncol* 1994; 20: 808–12.

Special considerations

Safety issues are of paramount importance when using lasers of any type. All personnel, including doctors, nurses and any technical personnel, must be well versed regarding all applicable laser safety regulations. Local rules and regulations relative to laser use exist in most areas. Basic laser physics and principles of use are covered by most courses dealing with the use of lasers in dermatology and plastic surgery. Safety eyewear particular for the type of equipment being used must be employed by all individuals present during a given procedure. Such eyewear should be placed on the door of the treatment suite for individuals who might enter during a treatment. Laser warning signs should also be posted on the outside door(s). Protection of the patient's eyes must also be kept in mind, e.g. taping eyelids shut while under anaesthesia, application of gauze pads or direct application of opaque corneal occluders. Laser operators must be careful to ensure that corneal occluders, when employed, are made of materials which will not be absorbed by the type of laser energy being used.

While the treatment of many types of vascular or pigmented lesions in childhood may be driven by the concern for the psychological impact of such lesions, the treatment itself may be fraught with such obstacles. Laser treatment with most vascular or pigmented lesion lasers is not painless. In most cases, however, the sensation is generally described as being similar to a mild pin-prick, a spark or a mild to moderate pop with an elastic band. Very small lesions can often be effectively treated with either no local

anaesthesia or with the application of eutectic mixture of local anaesthetics (EMLA) [1]. When treating large areas, particularly over the head and neck region, some degree of analgesia, sedation or anaesthesia can be considered appropriate. In either case, the use of careful, though direct, counselling of patients (when feasible) and their parents regarding the expectations of treatment and how a given treatment can be accomplished is essential. In the author's institution, child-life workers or play therapists are widely used as aides to the treatment of localized lesions on most children. Frank discussions with families and their children regarding the use of pain control measures are as much a part of the treatment as the discussion of the treatment itself. For those families wary of utilizing medication for pain control, counselling regarding the option of waiting until a time at which the child can make his or her own decision regarding how to pursue such therapy should be made. Local anaesthesia can often be effectively delivered by nerve blocks or regional/field blocks. To ease the discomfort of needle-sticks or chilling of the skin, application of EMLA may be of use. Other topical anaesthetic options exist.

Amethocaine gel has been studied under a controlled setting of laser treatments to EMLA and was felt to be more effective in pain reduction [2]. Amethocaine 4% gel (Ametop) is now the preferred option in some centres; compared to EMLA, it acts more rapidly (within 30 min), provides longer postoperative anaesthesia and causes vasodilation which is advantageous for laser treatment. However, it can cause an allergic reaction in some patients.

Iontophoresis of lidocaine with epinephrine has been used without any consequence on the clinical response to treatment [3].

The use of oral medications, such as midazolam (0.5–0.75 mg/kg per dose) or diazepam (0.2–0.3 mg/kg per dose) are useful as sedatives, but provide no analgesia. The use of such medications, as with any form of conscious sedation, must be administered together with appropriate monitoring of vital signs [4].

When these measures prove to be insufficient to achieve treatment of a particular lesion in a child, consideration should be given to the use of general anaesthesia. This requires the expertise of a trained anaesthetist. For large lesions, the use of general anaesthesia will allow for the treatment of an entire lesion rather than treating small sections over a very extended period of time. This is an important consideration when considering the need for multiple treatments of most vascular and some pigmented lesions. Such pain management can be accomplished safely [5]. The risk of a catastrophic complication (e.g. death, disability) from general anaesthesia has been estimated to be 1 in 20 000 to 1 in 40 000 [6], although this is variable worldwide and in many university centres the risk would be much lower.

Physicians must keep in mind that laser treatment of vascular and pigmented lesions requires multiple sessions and that the psychological well-being of the child during treatment is very dependent upon his or her level of comfort during those treatments.

Concern regarding the flammability of tissues (other than those being targeted for treatment with a given laser) or objects in the vicinity of a lesion being treated is also of importance. Argon lasers which generate blue–green light are associated with significant absorption by melanin. In the presence of high concentrations of supplemental oxygen, a small flash seen at the skin surface may result in combustion of flammable targets without appropriate precautions. The use of the FEDL is not without similar risk during its use [7]. While gauze, light coloured hair and clear plastic masks or tubing cannot be ignited by direct exposure to the light from these (vascular FEDL) lasers, any small flash in the presence of high concentrations of supplemental oxygen can be quite dangerous. Care must also be exercised with any laser with regard to cleaning agents applied to the skin surface prior to treatment. Alcohol, if used at all to prepare skin surfaces for treatment, must be allowed to dry completely before beginning treatment. Dark hair is quite flammable with the use of the vascular or pigmented lesion lasers. Moistening of hair with water in the vicinity of the treatment site is helpful to diminish this potential hazard.

REFERENCES

1 Tan OT, Stafford TJ. EMLA for laser treatment of port-wine stains in children. *Lasers Surg Med* 1992; 12: 543–8.

2 McCafferty DF, Woolfson AD, Handley J *et al*. Effect of percutaneous local anaesthetic on pain reduction during pulse dye laser treatment of port-wine stains. *Br J Anaesth* 1997; 78: 286.

3 Nunez M, Miralles ES, Boixeda P *et al*. Iontophoresis for anesthesia during pulsed dye laser treatment of port-wine stains. *Pediatr Dermatol* 1997; 14: 397–400.

4 American Academy of Pediatrics Committee on Drugs. Guidelines for monitoring and management of pediatric patients during and after sedation for diagnostic and therapeutic procedures. *Pediatrics* 1992; 89: 1110–15.

5 Grevelink JM, White VR, Bonoan R *et al*. Pulsed dye laser treatment in children and the use of anesthesia. *J Am Acad Dermatol* 1997; 37: 75–81.

6 Cohen MM, Cameron CB, Duncan PG. Pediatric anesthesia morbidity and mortality in the perioperative period. *Anesth Analg* 1990; 70: 160–7.

7 Epstein RH, Brummett Jr RR, Lask GP. Incendiary potential of the flash-lamp pumped 585-nm tunable dye laser. *Anesth Analg* 1990; 71: 171–5.

28.5   Sedation and Anaesthesia

LAWRENCE F. EICHENFIELD

Pain perception

Local anaesthetics

Techniques to decrease the pain of injection

Topical anaesthetics

Perioperative analgesics

Sedation

Pharmacological agents

Other techniques: anxiety alleviation, reassurance and rewards

Painful cutaneous procedures in children may be made less so by a knowledge of sedatives, analgesics, topical, intralesional and general anaesthetics.

Pain perception

Children of all ages, including infants, perceive pain. Multiple factors influence a child's perception of pain during a surgical procedure. These include the type of painful stimulus, fear and anxiety, and the child's personal history of medical or painful events [1]. Children have various states of cognitive development, cultural backgrounds, personality traits, emotional states and past experiences, which may influence pain. Anxiety may also be affected by the physical location of a procedure (clinic, office, hospital, etc.), the approach and demeanour of the doctor and health-care staff, and the dynamic between the child and family members. Age is a significant variable in the perception of pain, and historically of the doctor's misperception of the absence of pain.

It was previously common for doctors to not use anaesthetics for procedures in infants, believing that infants do not feel pain and have no memory of it. This was based upon assumptions that complete myelinization is necessary for nerve tract function and pain perception. It has now been clearly established that newborns and premature infants have fully developed physiological responses to pain, with intact neural circuitry and significant hormonal and metabolic response to painful stimuli, that is suppressed with anesthesia [2,3]. Younger children may have lower pain thresholds, and may not tolerate procedures as well as older children. Partially, this is due to the inability of very young children to understand fully the procedure, and the inability of children to disassociate their feelings from their actions. Definitions relevant to sedation and anaesthesia are listed below.

Analgesia: analgesia is defined as the relief of the perception of pain without intentional production of a sedated state. Altered mental status may be a secondary effect of medications administered for this purpose.

Anxiety alleviation: anxiety alleviation is a state in which there is no change in a patient's level of awareness, only a decrease of apprehension for the situation.

Conscious sedation: conscious sedation is a medically controlled state of depressed consciousness that (a) allows protective reflexes to be maintained; (b) retains the patient's ability to maintain a patent airway independently and continuously; and (c) permits appropriate response by the patient to physical stimulation or verbal command, e.g. 'open your eyes'.

Deep sedation: deep sedation is a medically controlled state of depressed consciousness or unconsciousness from which the patient is not easily aroused. It may be accompanied by a partial or complete loss of protective reflexes and includes the inability to maintain a patent airway independently and respond purposefully to physical stimulation or verbal command.

General anaesthesia: general anaesthesia is a medically controlled state of unconsciousness accompanied by a loss of protective reflexes, including the inability to maintain a patent airway independently and respond purposefully to physical stimulation or verbal command.

REFERENCES

1 Cunningham BB, Eichenfield LF. Decreasing the pain of procedures in children. *Curr Prob Derm* 1999; ii: 1–36.
2 Anand KJS, Hickey PR. Pain and its effects in the human neonate and fetus. *N Engl J Med* 1987; 317: 1321.
3 Walco GA, Cassidy RC, Schechter NL. Pain, hurt, and harm. The ethics of pain control in infants and children. *N Engl J Med* 1994; 331: 541–4.

Local anaesthetics

History

The first topical anaesthetic was probably cocaine, the numbing qualities of which were noted in Peru some centuries ago. The first description of its medical use was in 1884 by Carl Koller, as a topical ophthalmic anaesthetic [1]. The first synthetic anaesthetic was the ester procaine, developed in 1905. Lignocaine, the first synthetic amide anaesthetic, was created in 1943 [2].

Mechanism

Pain sensation is mediated through unmyelinated C fibres and myelinated Aδ fibres. Local anaesthetics interfere with the generation of the membrane action potential by impeding the inward flux of sodium, blocking the transmission of the painful stimulus. Local anaesthetics are generally esters or amides. Esters include cocaine, chloroprocaine (Nesacaine), procaine (Novocain), tetracaine (Pontocaine) and benzocaine. Amides include lignocaine (Xylocaine), bupivicaine (Marcain), priocaine (Citanest), mepivicaine (Carbocaine) and etidocaine (Duranest). Variations in properties affecting lipophilicity, pKa and protein binding influence potency, speed of onset, duration as well as potential toxicity [3]. Esters have a higher tendency to cause allergic reactions than the amides.

Lignocaine is usually administered as a 0.5–2% (5–20 mg/ml) solution, with 1% solution standardly used in paediatric patients. The maximum suggested dose is 5 mg/kg, or a maximum volume of 0.5 ml of 1% lignocaine per kilogram of body weight. The addition of adrenaline counteracts the natural vasodilatory effect of lignocaine, decreasing the rate of absorption, increasing duration of action and decreasing systemic toxicity per dose. The suggested maximum dose of lignocaine 1% plus adrenaline is 7 mg/kg, equivalent to a maximum volume of 0.7 ml per kilogram of body weight. (Note that for an average newborn of 4 kg, the maximum volume is only 2.8 ml.) Lignocaine with adrenaline is not advised for use in procedures involving distal digits, penis or pinna of the ear, due to the risk of vasoconstriction of distal end arteries and cutaneous necrosis.

A disadvantage of lignocaine as a local anaesthetic is the pain associated with its injection. The addition of a 1:10 ratio of 8.4% sodium bicarbonate (1 mmol/ml) to 1% lignocaine (with or without adrenaline) has been shown to decrease pain without significant alteration of onset, extent or duration of anaesthesia [4]. Elevation of the pH of the mixture, as well as faster nerve penetration due to an increase in the uncharged form, may explain the reduction in pain. Lignocaine is more soluble and has a longer shelf-life at acid pH. After the addition of bicarbonate as a buffer, the mixture should be refrigerated, as lignocaine activity drops to 66% of the initial concentration after 4 weeks at room temperature. Refrigeration at a temperature of 0–4°C maintains lignocaine at 90% of its initial concentration [5]. The average duration of anaesthesia with plain lignocaine is 40–60 min, and is slightly decreased to 30 min with the addition of bicarbonate [6]. For extended procedures the addition of lignocaine with adrenaline is recommended. Several studies have shown that buffered lignocaine has enhanced antimicrobial activity *in vitro*. It is unknown if this effect decreases the incidence of postoperative wound infections. Mepivacaine may also be buffered at a ratio of 1:10, and 0.5% bupivicaine with 1:100–1:200 of 8.4% sodium bicarbonate.

Adverse effects

Allergic reactions to esters are related to their metabolism to paraminobenzoic acid, a powerful allergen, limiting their usefulness. True allergic reactions to lignocaine and other amides are rare, comprising less than 1% of adverse reactions [7]. Central nervous system (CNS) toxicity includes symptoms of drowsiness, numbness of the lips and tongue, nausea and vomiting, metallic taste sensation and, at increasing blood levels, diplopia, nystagmus, tremors, seizures, apnoea and coma. Cardiovascular toxicity is generally noted after CNS symptomatology develops [8]. Effects include prolonged electrocardiographic intervals, bradycardia, hypotension, decreased myocardial contractility and cardiac arrest. Local toxicity to lignocaine and other local amide anaesthetics includes pain, haematoma or ecchymosis, infection, cutaneous necrosis and nerve damage. There are alternatives to local anaesthetics, including normal saline with 0.9% benzyl alcohol, which is reported to give immediate anaesthesia lasting several minutes with little pain on injection.

REFERENCES

1 Calverley RK, Scheller MS. Anesthesia as a specialty: past, present and future. In: Barash PG, Cullen BF, Stoelting RK, eds. *Clinical Anesthesia*, 2nd edn. Philadelphia: JB Lippincott, 1992: 3–33.
2 Grekin RC, Auletta MJ. Local anesthesia in dermatology surgery. *J Am Acad Dermatol* 1988; 19: 599–614.
3 Norris RL. Local anesthetics. *Emerg Med Clin N Am* 1992; 10: 707–18.
4 Christoph RA, Buchanan L, Begalid K, Schwartz S. Pain reduction in local anesthetic administration through pH buffering. *Ann Emerg Med* 1988; 17: 117–20.
5 Larson PO, Gangaram R, Swandby M, Darcey B, Pozin G, Carey P. Stability of buffered lidocaine and epinephrine used for local anesthesia. *J Dermatol Surg Oncol* 1991; 17: 411–14.
6 Holmes SG. Choosing a local anesthetic. *Dermatol Clin* 1994; 12: 817–23.
7 Norris RL. Local anesthetics. *Emerg Med Clin N Am* 1992; 10: 707–18.
8 Grekin RC, Auletta MJ. Local anesthesia in dermatology surgery. *J Am Acad Dermatol* 1988; 19: 599–614.

Techniques to decrease the pain of injection

There are several techniques that may be employed to decrease the pain of lignocaine infiltration [1]. Small gauge needles 2.5 cm in length (generally 30 gauge) are sharp and will penetrate tissue easily, and allow extension of anaesthetic into an area of several centimetres without repuncture of the surface. Counterstimulation techniques, such as pinching or rubbing of the injection site prior to infiltration may distract the patient from the pain of the injection. Topical application of ice, or freezing of the skin with ethyl chloride, warming of anaesthetic to body temperature and slow injection of fluid may also minimize injection pain.

Topical anaesthetics

Eutectic mixture of local anaesthetics

Eutectic mixture of local anaesthetics (EMLA) is 2.5% lignocaine and 2.5% prilocaine in an oil-in-water emulsion, that induces topical anaesthesia of intact skin. EMLA melts at a lower temperature than lignocaine or prilocaine alone, resulting in a stable solution at room temperature. It has been shown to be efficacious in hundreds of reports for needle-sticks, venepuncture, intravenous catheterization, lumbar puncture, debridement of ulcers, treatment of molluscum contagiosum, laser treatment of skin and genital mucosa, and other superficial skin surgery [2,3]. EMLA alone does not appear to provide sufficient analgesia for deep biopsies or scalpel excision of skin. Standard usage requires placement of the product on the skin surface with occlusive wrap, such as Tegaderm or cellophane wrap, for 60–120 min. Patch preparations of 5% EMLA may allow easier application with equivalent efficacy [4]. The standard dosing regime is 1–2 g of EMLA per square centimetre, with a maximum recommended dose of 10 g per application. The depth and degree of analgesia is related to the duration of application (Table 28.5.1). The maximal depth of analgesia is 5 mm. Mucous membranes, genital skin and diseased skin absorb more

rapidly, allowing for shorter application times (5–40 min) in these areas.

Reported local side-effects include transient blanching, erythema, oedema, eye irritation, dermatitis and purpura. Methaemoglobinaemia has been reported in neonates under 3 months of age, and is due to deficient enzyme methaemoglobin reductase in the neonate and a prilocaine-induced methaemoglobin stress [5]. Use of medications by infants associated with methaemoglobinaemia (including sulphonamides, acetaminophen, dapsone, benzocaine, phenytoin and phenobarbital) may increase the risk of EMLA-associated methaemoglobinaemia, as stated in the prescribing information. The incidence of adverse effect is very low with proper use.

Other topical anaesthetics

Lignocaine cream 30–40% in emollient base may be equal to EMLA or slightly less efficacious at inducing local anaesthesia. It requires prolonged application time under occlusion. Commercial preparations are not available, and there is more limited medical literature discussing its use in children as compared to prilocaine/lignocaine (EMLA cream). Liposomal lidocaine preparations (4% and 5%) utilize liposome technology to allow rapid cutaneous penetration and anaesthesia.

Tetracaine–adrenaline–cocaine

A solution containing 5.9–11.8% cocaine, 1:1000 to 1:4000 adrenaline and 0.25–2.0% tetracaine (TAC) has been used for lacerated skin. The agent is not considered useful for intact skin and problems with toxicity, including seizures and death, limit its use for dermatological procedures. It should not be used near mucus membranes where rapid absorption can occur.

Amethocaine gel

Amethocaine 4.0% gel appears to have very rapid onset and perhaps a longer duration of cutaneous anaesthesia than EMLA cream. Amethocaine is lipid soluble, with a high affinity for neural tissue [6].

Iontophoresis devices

Iontophoresis devices have been advocated for needleless delivery of lignocaine to skin. A low level current is applied to the skin under lignocaine solution or an impregnated patch, allowing cutaneous absorption of the charged agent. Improved deep sensory blockade and more rapid onset than EMLA are advantages. Disadvantages include the cost of the iontophoresis device and mild discomfort during the application of the electrical current.

Table 28.5.1 EMLA: pain and sensory blockage after 2 g/cm² to dorsal hand. Adapted from Arendt-Nielsen [7]

Application time (mins)	Time of onset of pain block after cream removal	Duration of pain blockade	Total sensory blockade reached
15		0	No
30	30	60	No
60	15	75	No
80	0	100	Yes
100–120	0	120–140	Yes

Topical anaesthesia for mucosal surfaces

Topical Cetacaine, benzocaine and viscous lignocaine are effective topical agents for mucosal surfaces. They are useful to decrease the pain of intralesional lignocaine injection, while insufficient alone for scalpel surgery. Anaesthetic effect is almost immediate upon application of solution or gel. While benzocaine is a known sensitizer of contact dermatitis, it is uncommon when used preoperatively, presumably due to lack of repeated exposure.

REFERENCES

1 Eichenfield LF, Weilepp A. Pain control in pediatric procedures. *Curr Opin Dermatol* 1997; 4: 151–61.
2 Garjraj NM, Pennant JH, Watcha MR. Eutectic mixture of local anesthetics (EMLA). *Anesth Analg* 1994; 78: 574–83.
3 Stewart JH, Cole GW, Klein JA. Neutralized lidocaine with epinephrine for local anesthesia. *J Dermatol Surg Oncol* 1989; 15: 1081–3.
4 Chang PC, O'Connor G, Rogers PJC *et al.* A multicentre randomized study of single-unit dose package of EMLA patch vs. EMLA cream 5% for venepuncture in children. *Canad J Anesth* 1994; 41: 59–63.
5 Jakobson B, Nilsson A. Methaemoglobinemia in children treated with prilocain-lidocaine cream and trimethoprim-suphamethoxazole. A case report. *Acta Anaesth Scan* 1985: 453–5.
6 Lawson RA, Smart NG, Gudteonac AC *et al.* Evaluation of an amethocaine gel preparation for percutaneous analgesia before venous canulation in children. *Br J Anesth* 1995; 75: 282–5.
7 Arendt-Nielsen L, Bjerring P. Laser-induced pain for evaluation of local analgesia: a comparison of topical application (EMLA) and local injection (lidocaine). *Anesth Analg* 1988; 67(2): 115–23.

Perioperative analgesics

The use of medications to alleviate postprocedure pain and discomfort has been a standard practice in paediatric dermatology. Preoperative and perioperative pain relief may benefit the patient by decreasing postoperative pain, decreasing medication requirements postoperatively and possibly by mediating the body's inflammatory response.

Preoperative medications also decrease the pain and discomfort of procedures generally performed without local regional anaesthesia (such as cryotherapy), as well as that of local/regional anaesthesia administration. The use of preoperative acetaminophen (15 mg/kg orally or per rectum) or acetaminophen with codeine suspension (0.4 cm³/kg, equivalent to 0.96 mg/kg of 2.4 mg/cm³ codeine with acetaminophen) may be quite useful for perioperative pain. An added benefit of codeine is its mild to moderate sedative effect, useful in young children. If utilizing concurrent sedative agents (diazepam, midazolam, chloral hydrate), doctors should be aware of the risk of respiratory depression with opiate and opiate-like agents. Non-steroidal anti-inflammatory agents such as ibuprofen and ketorolac (Tordal) may also be used perioperatively, although effects on coagulation and haemostasis should be considered.

Sedation

The goal of sedation is to guard the safety and welfare of patients, minimize physical discomfort or pain, minimize negative psychological responses to treatment by providing analgesia, control behaviour, maximize the potential for amnesia and to return patients to a state in which they are safe to discharge, as determined by recognized criteria. Sedatives and general anaesthesia may be appropriate for diagnostic and therapeutic procedures in children. Sedation should be considered as a continuum within which a patient may change state from light sedation to deep sedation to obtundation. As such, the risks and benefits of specific agents and analysis of the health of the patient, adequacy of the facilities, equipment, staff education and monitoring must be considered.

Doctors should be aware of national and regional guidelines such as those in the USA of the American Academy of Pediatrics and the American Academy of Dermatology, for use of sedation in the office and hospital setting in children that may dictate appropriate monitoring, equipment, sedation protocols and staff training [1,2]. In general, deep sedation and general anaesthesia for dermatological procedures in children are most safely performed with the assistance of an anaesthesiologist. Conscious and deep sedation may be safely performed in an ambulatory setting if the facility and staff are appropriately equipped and trained. Selecting an appropriate sedative technique requires preoperative assessment of the child's medical status, the painfulness of the procedure, the duration of the procedure, the need or absence of need for the child to be motionless, the expertise of the practitioner in performing the sedation, the facility resources for monitoring the patient and responding to adverse events, and knowledge of minimal levels of monitoring and personnel appropriate for the level of sedation used [3]. Preoperative assessment must include the general health of the child, with an awareness that underlying systemic diseases may greatly increase the risk of adverse occurrence with sedative medications. As protective airway reflexes may be compromised to varying degrees depending upon sedative agents, dose and baseline medical state, nil by mouth status should be assured for elective sedative procedures. Monitoring may include the use of a pulse oximeter, which continuously measures heart rate and arterial oxygen saturation using a spectrophotometric technique.

Pharmacological agents

There is a broad array of medications used as sedative, hypnotic, analgesic and anaesthetic agents. Analgesia refers to the relief of pain, amnesia to lack of memory, hypnosis to lack of consciousness and sedation to a change in consciousness. Anxiolytic effects may decrease anxiety without specific analgesic effects. Local, topical or regional anaesthesia, with conscious sedation medication inducing amnesia, may produce the desired effect of a painless or minimally painful experience not remembered by the patient.

Benzodiazepines

Benzodiazepines are sedative/hypnotic agents with potent antianxiety effects. While having no analgesic effect, they are used for their hypnotic and amnesic effect with relatively little cardiovascular or respiratory depression at recommended dosages as compared to barbiturates. Diazepam (Valium) may be given orally, sublingually, rectally, intravenously and intramuscularly, though the intramuscular route is not suggested. Dosages vary by route of administration (0.05–0.2 mg/kg intramuscular or intravenous, 0.2–0.4 mg/kg orally or per rectum; 10 mg maximum dose). The degree of sedation may be influenced by dosage, and concurrent use of narcotics. Onset of action is 30–60 min, and duration is 3 or more hours. Prolonged sedation is not uncommon.

Midazolam (Versed, Roche Laboratories) is a short-acting benzodiazepine that is useful for preoperative or operative sedation in children. The medication is a very rapid acting agent of short duration, with an excellent safety profile. Onset of action is more rapid than diazepam, with shorter duration of action. Route of administration includes intravenous, oral, intranasal, intramuscular and rectal. Required dosages vary greatly by route; intravenous dosing is 0.05 mg/kg intravenously, titrated up to 0.1 mg/kg/dose up to a maximum of 7.5 mg. Intranasal and oral routes require higher dosing due to variable absorption: nasal dosing 0.2–0.5 mg/kg; and oral dosing 0.5–0.7 mg/kg up to 20 mg. Midazolam has potent anxiolytic effects, but is without analgesic properties. Amnesic effect is profound, making the agent useful for repetitive procedures (e.g. pulsed dye laser treatments). The addition of an analgesic agent, such as acetaminophen/codeine, or fentanyl may be reasonable, though the combination increases the risks of respiratory depression [4]. Pulsed oximetry monitoring is recommended, as higher doses of midazolam are associated with transient drops in transcutaneous oxygen saturation. Flumazenil is a specific antagonist for benzodiazepines, and may reverse the depressant effects in a dose-dependent fashion.

Barbiturates

Barbiturates are potent sedative/hypnotic agents with amnesic, but no analgesic effects. These medications are non-specific CNS depressants, with more profound respiratory and cardiovascular depressant effects than benzo-

diazepines. Pentobarbital (Nembutal) may be used orally, or less commonly by rectum or intramuscular injection (1.5–6 mg/kg, maximum dose 100 mg) with a 30-min onset of action and a duration of several hours. Barbiturates have no analgesic effect, and may lower the pain threshold, rendering them unreliable as sedatives without local or systemic analgesia for painful procedures. Their use in paediatric procedures has decreased greatly due to the better safety/toxicity profile of benzodiazepines.

Ketamine

Ketamine hydrochloride is an anaesthetic agent that may be given by the intramuscular or intravenous route. It produces profound amnesia and sedation with a 'trance-like' state. Onset is rapid: 1 min for the intravenous route (0.5 mg with infusion of 0.01–0.2 mg/kg/min) and 5 min for the intramuscular route (0.5–1 mg/kg), and sedation duration is quite variable lasting hours in some individuals [5]. Oral ketamine has been used at doses of 1 mg/kg with sedation 30–45 min postadministration. Postprocedure nausea and prolonged unarousability are problems with its use. Ketamine may cause unpleasant dreams and emersion reactions. There is significant risk of vomiting, aspiration and laryngospasm, as well as elevation of intracranial pressure and blood pressure. Monitoring of vital signs, oxygenation and blood pressure is mandatory.

Opiates

Opiates and synthetic opiates are primarily used for analgesia, often as an adjunct to sedative/hypnotic agents. Morphine, meperidine (Demerol) and fentanyl are potent pain relievers. However, systemic use in conjunction with sedative/hypnotic agents may yield inconsistent circulatory and respiratory depression, nausea and vomiting. Fentanyl, a synthetic opioid agonist, has rapid onset and relatively short duration when given intravenously (1–3 μg/kg), allowing titration of medication for pain relief with less risk of prolonged depressive effects and hypotension. Fentanyl lozenges have been utilized for paediatric procedures, though respiratory depression and emesis have been observed with their use [6,7]. Codeine may be useful perioperatively and postoperatively for procedural related pain (see above). If utilizing concurrent sedative agents (diazepam, midazolam, chloral hydrate), doctors should be aware of the risk of respiratory depression with opiate and opiate-like agents.

Chloral hydrate

Chloral hydrate is a sedative/hypnotic agent that has

been used in children for several decades. Doses of 25–50 mg/kg (up to 100 mg/kg) are administered orally and induce sleep lasting 3–6 h, with amnesiac effect. Chloral hydrate has a slow onset and long duration of action. It is classified as a conscious sedation medication and requires prolonged monitoring both during and at the conclusion of a procedure. It lacks analgesic properties, and is not suitable for use as a sole agent for painful procedures. Several deaths have been reported from chloral hydrate use, most commonly from overdosage or its use in children with underlying cardiac or systemic disease. It has been reported to cause liver tumours, but there is no evidence that children receiving sedative dosages are at risk for this [8].

Demerol—promethazine—thorazine

A sedative that was previously commonly used is the combination of intramuscular meperidine (Demerol), promethazine (Phenergan) and chlorpromazine (Thorazine), known as DPT. This mixture has potent analgesic and sedative qualities, but has unpredictable efficacy and side-effects. There is a trend towards decreased use of DPT because of its long duration of action and side-effects including respiratory depression and seizures. A recent statement of the American Academy of Pediatrics concludes that 'neither the combination itself nor its dosages are based on sound pharmacological data. There is a high rate of therapeutic failure, as well as a high rate of serious adverse reactions, including respiratory depression and death associated with its use' [9].

Propofol

Propofol is an intravenous anaesthetic which provides rapid onset of an unconscious sedation. Propofol is an aqueous formulation that appears milky in colour. The agent has almost immediate onset of sedation after bolus dosing (0.4–1.0 mg/kg followed by continuous infusion of 30–50 μg/k/min). Propofol has relatively limited haemodynamic instability and short duration of action, allowing a 'clean head wake-up' with little nausea or hangover effect commonly reported with traditional gas anaesthetic agents. Antiemetic properties have also been observed. The agent is safe for outpatient surgery even in children under 2 years of age, and has no known cumulative hazardous physical effects. Propofol does not have profound analgesic qualities and concurrent analgesics for painful procedures are appropriate. In a study of propofol for pulsed dye laser treatments in 48 paediatric outpatients, 62% were calm and pain-free upon awakening. The mean recovery time was 25 min, and none of the patients experienced emesis [10]. Respiratory depression is dose dependent, and hypoxia and apnoea are not uncommon, thus limiting its use to individuals and facilities proficient in critical airway and ventilatory management.

Nitrous oxide

Nitrous oxide (N_2O) is a gas anaesthetic that has analgesic effects and rapidly induces a sedated, disassociative state with a euphoric feeling and profound amnesic effect. When used alone at 35–50% concentrations N_2O has analgesic effects with minimal respiratory and cardiovascular effects [11,12]. It is commonly administered with other agents to achieve general anaesthesia. There is an extensive history of its use for paediatric procedures. N_2O use requires extensive training and/or credentialing of personnel, a fail-safe system for oxygen/gas delivery to prevent anoxia, a scavenger device to eliminate gas traces and continuous oximetry monitoring. Concerns have been raised about possible teratogenicity and spontaneous abortions from N_2O gas [13].

General gas anaesthesia

The use of general gas anaesthesia is appropriate for painful surgical procedures in children which are necessary and which cannot be safely or effectively performed awake or with the use of local anaesthetics and sedative/hypnotic agents. The decision to utilize general anaesthesia is individualized, dependent upon the age of the patient, the underlying health of the patient, the extent of the procedure planned, the location of surgical procedure, the need for a motionless patient and the medical and personnel resources available to induce and administer anaesthetic agents appropriately, and monitor and assure safe postoperative recovery. A variety of anaesthetic gases are commonly used, including halothane, isoflurane, sevofluorane and N_2O. The risks of general anaesthesia are dependent upon a variety of factors including the age of the patient and underlying systemic conditions [14]. Its use should be restricted to anaesthesiologists and other health professionals trained and accredited in its use.

Laryngeal masks

Induction of anaesthesia with inhalational gases (halothane, isoflurane, sevoflurane) is done with mask inhalation, followed by endotracheal visualization and intubation. Laryngeal masks are devices that allow placement of a hypopharyngeal airway, without the need for visualization or intubation of the trachea. After initial face mask induction of anaesthesia, the device, a deflated 'mask-on-a-stick' is placed in the mouth and pushed towards below the epiglottis superior to the vocal cords. Air is then inserted via a syringe (similar to a Foley catheter) and the breathing loop is connected to the exposed end. This device has gained widespread acceptance for paediatric surgical cases where there is no 'critical airway', and has been used successfully for dermatological and laser surgery in children [15].

REFERENCES

1 American Academy of Pediatrics. Guidelines for monitoring and management of pediatric patients during and after sedation for diagnostic and therapeutic procedures. *Pediatrics* 1992; 89: 1110–15.

2 Committee on Guidelines of Care, Task Force on Office Surgical Facilities. Part I. Guidelines of care for office surgical facilities. *J Am Acad Dermatol* 1992; 26: 763–5.

3 Litman RS. Recent trends in the management of pain during medical procedures in children. *Pediatr Ann* 1995; 24: 158–63.

4 Yaster M, Nichols DG, Desphande JK, Wetzel RC. Midazolam-fentanyl intravenous sedation in children: case report of respiratory arrest. *Pediatrics* 1990; 86: 463–7.

5 Green SM, Nakamura R, Johnson NE. Ketamine sedation for pediatric procedures. Part 1. A prospective series. *Ann Emerg Med* 1990; 19: 1024–32.

6 Litman RS. Recent trends in the management of pain during medical procedures in children. *Pediatr Ann* 1995; 24: 158–63.

7 Ashburn MA, Streisand JB, Tarver SD *et al.* Oral transmucosal fentanyl citrate for premedication in paediatric outpatients. *Canad J Anaesth* 1990; 37: 857–66.

8 American Academy of Pediatrics Committee on Drugs and Committee on Environmental Health. Use of chloral hydrate for sedation in children. *Pediatrics* 1993; 94: 471–3.

9 American Academy of Pediatrics Committee on Drugs. Reappraisal of lytic cocktail/Demoral, Phenergan, and Thorazine (DPT) for the sedation of children. *Pediatrics* 1995; 95: 598–602.

10 Vischoff D, Charest J. Propofol for pulsed dye laser treatments in pediatric outpatients. *Canad J Anesth* 1994; 41: 728–32.

11 American Academy of Pediatrics. Guidelines for monitoring and management of pediatric patients during and after sedation for diagnostic and therapeutic procedures. *Pediatrics* 1992; 89: 1110–15.

12 Litman RS, Berkowitz RJ, Ward DS. Levels of consciousness and ventilatory parameters in young children during sedation with oral midazolam and nitrous oxide. *Arch Pediatr Adoles Med* 1996; 150: 671–5 (see comments).

13 Rowland AS, Baird DD, Weinberg CR, Shore DL, Shy CM, Wilcox AJ. Reduced fertility among women employed as dental assistants exposed to high levels of nitrous oxide. *N Engl J Med* 1992; 327: 993–7.

14 Cohen MM, Cameron CB, Duncan PG. Pediatric anesthesia morbidity and mortality in the perioperative period. *Anesth Analg* 1990; 70: 160–7.

15 Epstein RH, Halmi BH. Oxygen leakage around the laryngeal mask airway during laser treatment of port-wine stains in children. *Anesth Analg* 1994; 78: 486–9.

Other techniques: anxiety alleviation, reassurance and rewards

Hypnosis

Hypnosis may be effective in decreasing pain and anxiety of surgical procedures in children. A variety of techniques are used such as visual imagery for distraction and reducing awareness and perception of pain. Hypnosis has been useful for chronic pain treatment as well as for acute management of painful injuries and procedures.

Other techniques

These include the use of illustrated procedure books, use of dolls to display the planned procedure, concealment of the needle, draping of the surgical tray and constructing a curtain which obscures the procedure from the patient's field of view. For infants, cuddling, swaddling, using a pacifier or feeding a mixture of sucrose and water may soothe the child. Distraction techniques involving visual imagery or deep breathing may be useful. In the older child, singing, storytelling and lively background music may be helpful [1,2]. Parents should be strongly discouraged from threatening to punish a child for not cooperating. The parent should be the key emotional support for the child during the procedure and should have both hands free and full attention focused on soothing the child. The doctor should have adequate assistance in restricting the child and should not ask the parents to fulfil this role. The use of positive reinforcement and rewards is another key tool. Gifts of stickers, trinkets and sweets ensure that the child leaves feeling he or she has done a great job, regardless of how difficult the procedure has been.

REFERENCES

1 Rothman KF. Pain management for dermatologic procedures in children. *Adv Dermatol* 1995; 10: 287–308.

2 Eichenfield LF, Weilepp A. Pain control in pediatric procedures. *Curr Opin Dermat* 1997; 4: 157–61.

Section 29
Miscellaneous Disorders

29.1   Alopecia Areata

YVES DE PROST AND CHRISTINE BODEMER

Definition

Alopecia areata (AA) is a non-scarring, recurrent, hair disease which can potentially cause hair loss in any hair-bearing area.

History

In earlier years all hair disorders were called tinea. Now this term is almost only limited to fungus infections [1]. The psychological aspects of hair are very important. Although hair has no vital function, the classic tale of Samson and Delilah in the Old Testament underlines its enormous significance. Julius Caesar designates his nickname to 'caesaries' that means thick healthy hair. It symbolizes royal dignity [2]. Hair loss has always been very distressing for young and old people [2–4].

REFERENCES

1 Lachapelle J-M, Tennstedt D, DeGreef H *et al*. *Two Centuries of Dermatology: Jean Louis Alibert*. Belgium: Glaxo, 1992 (in Flemish).
2 Berg C. *The Unconscious Significance of Hair*. London: George Allen & Unwin, 1951.
3 Peereboom-Wynia JDR. *Hair-root characteristics of the human scalp hair in health and disease*. Thesis, Erasmus University, Rotterdam, 1982.
4 Stroud JD. Hairloss in children. *Pediatr Clin N Am* 1983; 30: 641–57.

Aetiology

Epidemiology

Alopecia is relatively frequent, with a prevalence of about 2% [1]. The first manifestations generally occur during childhood, usually after the age of 5 years. In 63% of adults with alopecia, onset occurs before the age of 20 years [2]. A family history of alopecia is found in 5–25% of cases.

Associated conditions

A history of allergy is found in 10–30% of cases, but this association is unexplained [3]. Thyroid disorders were found in 59 of the 736 patients described by Muller and Winkelman, with goitre, hypothyroidism, exophthalmia, Hashimoto's disease and hyperthyroidism being recorded [4]. However, thyroid disease is infrequent relative to antithyroid antibodies, which can be present at high titres [5]. Alopecia can be associated with auto-immune diseases, especially Hashimoto's disease. All patients presenting with alopecia should undergo ultra-sensitive thyroid-stimulating hormone (TSH) assay and possibly tests for antithyroid antibodies. Other associated autoimmune diseases include Addison's disease, lupus erythematosus, myasthenia, thymoma, the polyglandular autoimmune syndrome and vitiligo. Between 1.3 and 9% of patients with Down's syndrome have alopecia [6]. This association is unclear, but there is abnormal T-mediated immune responses in Down's syndrome [6].

Pathogenesis

AA is generally believed to be an autoimmune disease, but there is no concrete evidence of a primary autoimmune mechanism. New technologies applicable to the hair follicle (hair follicle culture, single-hair reverse transcriptase–polymerase chain reaction (PCR), animal models) provide insight into the complex and intricate underlying immunological, genetic and biological mechanisms.

Without any doubt several pathophysiological mechanisms are recognized. Immunological factors include autoimmune phenomena that probably trigger cytokine secretion in the hair follicle, and also lymphocytotoxicity phenomena. The role of cytokines such as interleukin 10 (IL-10) has also been reported [7]. However, these immunological phenomena are probably secondary, and the initial event is unknown. Recent work has pointed to the involvement of certain viruses, particularly cytomegalovirus [8].

Immunological hypothesis

Role of T lymphocytes. Immunohistochemical studies have shown peri- and intrafollicular responses suggesting immune attack against a hair follicle (HF) antigen. AA is characterized microscopically by a perifollicular lymphocytic infiltrate composed mainly of CD4+ cells, together with expression of HLA-DR antigens and intercellular adhesion molecule type 1 (ICAM-1) on the follicular epithelium [9–11]. Autoreactive T lymphocytes (cells proliferating to irradiated autologous peripheral blood mononuclear cells in the absence of exogenous antigen) were found in larger numbers in scalp biopsy specimens than in peripheral blood [12]. Absolute numbers of peripheral blood mononuclear cells and their phenotype ratios vary between reports [13–15].

Strong indirect evidence of an important role for T cells in the pathogenesis of AA is provided by the clinical efficacy of immunosuppressive agents such as corticosteroids and cyclosporin.

One animal model of AA is the DEBR rat, which displays perifollicular and intrabulbar infiltration of hair follicles by T cells, and hairs in a state of dystrophic anagen [16]. Another model is the ageing C3H/HEJ mouse, which develops non-scarring alopecia on the abdomen, with histologically an anagen follicle infiltrated and surrounded by T cells [17]. T cells apparently interact with hair follicle cells, either by direct contact and cytotoxicity, or indirectly via lymphokines. Happle and Hoffmann provided evidence that cytokines participate in the pathogenesis of AA [18]. They used semiquantitative reverse transcriptase PCR on RNA extracted from scalp biopsies before and after successful treatment with diphenylcycloproperone (DCP). Before treatment they detected increased intralesional levels of interferon-γ (IFN-γ) and IL-1β transcripts, corresponding to the T-helper (Th-1) cytokine pattern. IFN-γ is involved in adhesion molecule expression on hair follicles, and these results might explain the aberrant expression of ICAM-1 and HLA-DR on affected hair follicle keratinocytes. Furthermore, IL-1β has been shown to inhibit hair growth *in vitro* and might be one of the factors triggering hair growth arrest *in vivo* [19]. Steady-state IL-10 RNA levels were found to be increased after successful DCP treatment, suggesting a substantial role for IL-10. IL-10 can inhibit Th-1 cytokine production and reduce expression of ICAM-1 and HLA-DR molecules on hair follicles [20].

Role of keratinocytes and melanocytes. Follicular keratinocytes appear to play a crucial part in the pathogenesis of AA. Keratinocytes produce proinflammatory cytokines (IL-1β, IL-8 and tumour necrosis factor α (TNF-α)), together with other T-cell chemotactic factors, under the influence of external and internal stimuli. T cells attracted to follicular keratinocytes may interact with them and release additional cytokines. However, no such external or internal keratinocyte stimuli have so far been identified. Increased HLA expression by hair-matrix keratinocytes appears to be a relatively late event and may result from cytokine release by infiltrating immune cells. Several authors have focused on the recent identification of antigens expressed on normal hair follicles but not on

adjacent epidermis and dermis. Most of these antigens are autoantigens, reacting with antibodies present in the donor's serum [21]. Some such autoantibodies appear to be more frequent and present at higher titres in patients with AA [22]. The potential pathogenic role of such autoantibodies is unclear. They could be responsible for selective damage to hair follicles, but also reflect a secondary immune response to isolated cells from damaged follicles that find their way into the systemic circulation. Chronic progressive disease requires the persistence of the antigen, HLA class II molecule expression, and the persistence of inflammatory T cells. The distinction between T cells specific for autoantigens and viruses is difficult to make, and the possible involvement of persistent viral infections requires further study. AA autoantibodies are also directed against the melanocytes in hair follicles [23]. Clinical, morphological and functional evidence indicates a role for melanocytes with frequent sparing of non-pigmented hairs, regrowing of initially white hairs, unusual outer root sheath distribution of hair bulb melanocytes, abnormal melanosomes in affected melanocytes in the hair follicle, decreased numbers of melanocytes and melanosomes, decreased melanization and poorly developed dendritic processes in biopsies of regrowing white hair.

Biological hypothesis: dermal papilla dysfunction

The dermal papilla plays an important regulatory role in hair follicle function [24]. Transplanted papillae placed in the proximity of follicular epithelium induces follicular development and hair shaft formation in animals [25]. The dermal papilla could be an important target in AA, with lymphocytic infiltrates around follicles, loss of the normal regular arrangement of dermal papilla cells in apparently unaffected scalp areas [26], degenerative changes in involved scalp dermal papilla cells, apoptosis of dermal papilla cells [27] and release of soluble factors that stimulate lymphocyte proliferation by cultured dermal papilla cells [28].

Genetic hypothesis

A family history is reported in 10–47% of cases, and there have been occasional reports of simultaneous onset in identical twins [29]. The likely mode of inheritance is autosomal dominant with variable penetrance [30]. A correlation has been found between certain HLA markers and AA. In particular DR4 and DR5 are more frequent in unrelated AA patients than in controls [31]. Predisposition to autoimmunity is also associated with certain HLA alleles. However, environmental factors (e.g. microorganisms) may be relevant in individuals with a genetic susceptibility. Antigen presentation is governed by interactions between cells bearing HLA molecules and the

T-cell receptor, and susceptibility genes are likely to involve these particular molecules. Other genes are probably needed for disease onset, and yet others for persistence or regression. Cork *et al.* recently showed an association between an allele of the IL-1 receptor antagonist gene and the clinical severity of AA [32]. Other genes such as those encoding T-cell receptor chains and cytokines remain to be investigated.

Psychological hypothesis

Psychiatric studies of AA have given conflicting results [2,33–35]. It has been suggested that psychiatric diagnoses are more prevalent in AA patients, with high lifetime prevalence rates of depression (39%) and generalized anxiety disorders (39%) [36].

REFERENCES

1 Gollnick H, Orfanos CE. Alopecia areata pathogenesis and clinical picture. In: Orfanos CE, Happle R, eds. *Hair and Hair Diseases*. Berlin: Springer-Verlag, 1990: 529–69.
2 Safari K. Prevalence of alopecia areata in the First National Health and Nutrition Examination Survey (letter). *Arch Dermatol* 1992; 128: 702.
3 De Weert J, Temmermann L, Kint A. Alopecia areata: a clinical study. *Dermatologica* 1984; 168: 224–9.
4 Muller SA, Winkelman RK. Alopecia areata. *Arch Dermatol* 1963; 88: 290–7.
5 Friedman PS. Alopecia areata an autoimmunity. *Br J Dermatol* 1981; 105: 153–7.
6 Wunderlich C, Braun-Falco O. Mongolismus and alopecia areata. *Med Welt* 1965; 10: 477–81.
7 Hoffman R, Eicheler W, Huth A, Wenzel E, Happle R. Serum interleukin-10 levels in patients with alopecia areata undergoing topical immunotherapy. *Eur J Dermatol* 1995; 5: 267–9.
8 Skinner RB, Light WH, Leonardi C, Bale GF, Rosenberg W. A molecular approach to alopecia areata. *J Invest Dermatol* 1995; 104: 35–45.
9 Messenger AG, Bleehen SS. Expression of HLA-DR by anagen hair follicles in alopecia areata. *J Invest Dermatol* 1978; 85: 569–72.
10 Perret C, Weisner Menzel L, Happle R. Immunohistochemical analysis of T cell subsets in the peribulbar and intrabulbar infiltrates of alopecia areata. *Acta Derm Venereol* 1984; 64: 26–30.
11 Nickoloff BJ, Griffiths CEM. Aberrant intercellular adhesion molecule-1 (ICAM-1) expression by hair-follicle epithelial cells and endothelial leukocyte adhesion molecule-1 (ELAM-1) by vascular cells are important adhesion-molecule alterations in alopecia areata. *J Invest Dermatol* 1991; 96(suppl): 91S–2S.
12 Kalish R, Johnson K, Hordinsky M. Alopecia areata. Autoreactive T cells are variably enriched in scalp lesions relative to peripheral blood. *Arch Dermatol* 1992; 128: 1072–7.
13 Galbraight GMP *et al.* Increased ratio of helper to suppressor T-cells in alopecia areata. *Br J Dermatol* 1984; 110: 171–5.
14 Valsecchi R, Bon Tempelli M, Vicari O. Peripheral T-cell subsets in patients with alopecia areata in different clinical phases. *Dermatologica* 1985; 171: 170–4.
15 Bystryn JC, Tamesis J. Immunological aspects of hair loss. *J Invest Dermatol* 1991; 96: 88S.
16 Oliver RF *et al.* The DEBR rat model for alopecia areata. *J Invest Dermatol* 1991; 96: 97S.
17 Sundberg JP, King LP. An alopecia areata-like disease in C3M/MEJ mice. *Clin Res* 1992; 40: 781A (abstract).
18 Happle R, Hoffmann R. Cytokine patterns in alopecia areata before and after topical immunotherapy. *J Invest Dermatol* 1995; 104 (suppl): 14S–15S.
19 Harmon CS, Nevins TD. IL-1a inhibits human hair follicle growth and hair fiber production in whole-organ cultures. *Lymphok Cytokin Res* 1993; 12: 197–203.
20 de Waal Malefyt R, Abrams J, Bennet B, Figdor C, Vries JE. Interleukin 10 inhibits cytokines synthesis by human monocytes: an autoregulatory role of IL-10 produced by monocytes. *J Exp Med* 1991; 174: 1209–20.
21 Tobin DJ, Orentreich N, Bystryn JC. Autoantibodies to hair follicles in normal individuals. *Arch Dermatol* 1994; 130: 395–7.
22 Tobin DJ, Orentreich N, Fenton DA, Bystryn JC. Antibodies to hair follicles in alopecia areata. *J Invest Dermatol* 1994; 102: 721–4.
23 Tobin DJ, Bystryn JC. Immunity to hair follicles in alopecia areata. *J Invest Dermatol* 1995; 104 (suppl): 13S–14S.
24 Johnson WC, Helwig EB. Histochemistry of the acid mucopolysaccharides of skin in normal and in certain pathologic conditions. *Am J Clin Pathol* 1963; 40: 123–31.
25 Oliver RF. The experimental induction of whisker growth in the hooded rat by implantation of dermal papillae. *J Embryol Exp Morphol* 1967; 18: 43–51.
26 McDonald HSP, Nutbrown M, Pepall L, Thornton MJ, Randall VA, Cunliffe WJ. Immunohistologic and ultrastructural comparison of the dermal papilla and hair follicle bulb from 'active' and 'normal' areas of alopecia areata. *J Invest Dermatol* 1991; 96: 673–81.
27 Norris DA, Duke R, Whang K, Middleton M. Immunologic cytotoxicity in alopecia areata: apoptosis of dermal papilla cells in alopecia areata. *J Invest Dermatol* 1995; 104(suppl): 8S–9S.
28 McDonagh AJG, Elliot KR, Messenger AG. Cytokines and dermal papilla function in alopecia areata. *J Invest Dermatol* 1995; 104(S): 9S–10S.
29 Hendren OS. Identical alopecia areata in identical twins. *Arch Dermatol* 1949; 60: 793–5.
30 Sauder DN. Alopecia areata: an inherited autoimmune disease. In: Brown AC, Crounse RG, eds. *Hair, Trace Elements and Human Illness*. New York: Praeger, 1980: 343–7.
31 Duvic M, Hordinsky MK, Fiedler VC, O'Brien WR. HLA-D locus associations in alopecia areata. *Arch Dermatol* 1991; 127: 64.
32 Cork MJ, Tarlow JK, Clay FE *et al.* An allele of the interleukin-1 receptor antagonist as a genetic severity factor in alopecia areata. *J Invest Dermatol* 1995; 104(suppl): 15S–16S.
33 Van Moffaert M. Psychosomatics of alopecia. *Dermatologica* 1985; 171: 501.
34 Koo J, Shellow WV, Hallman CP, Edwards JE. Alopecia areata and increased prevalence of psychiatric disorders. *Int J Dermatol* 1994; 33: 849–50.
35 Colon EA *et al.* Lifetime prevalence of psychiatric disorders in patients with alopecia areata. *Compr Psychiatr* 1991; 32: 245–51.

Pathology

Alopecia areata shows patchy or (in the most extreme situations) total premature conversions of the hair follicles from the anagen phase into the catagen–telogen phase. Subsequently this process leads to acute or subacute shedding of hairs [1–3]. In the early stage there is a lymphocytic infiltrate around the anagen hair bulb and hair sheath. A lymphocytic vasculitis including plasma cells, mast cells and eosinophils may be observed [3]. Perret *et al.* found that the majority of the lymphocytes are of the T-helper class (CD4) [4]. In the late stage the infiltrate has been diminished and a perifollicular fibrosis has developed. Telogen hairs are present high in the dermis, have a rudimentary hair bulb and a thickened fibrous tissue sheath [1].

REFERENCES

1 McKee PH. *Pathology of the Skin*, 2nd edn. London: Mosby-Wolfe, 1996.
2 Nelson DA, Spielvogel RI. Alopecia areata. *Int J Dermatol* 1985; 24: 26–34.
3 Bergfield WF. Alopecia: histologic changes. *Adv Dermatol* 1989; 4: 310–22.
4 Perret C, Wiesner-Menzel L, Happle R. Immunohistochemical analysis of T-cell subsets in the peribulbar and intrabulbar infiltrates of alopecia areata. *Acta Derm Venereol* 1984; 64: 26–30.

Clinical features

The most common form in children is patchy alopecia [1,2]. Hair loss is generally well circumscribed, and the scalp usually has a normal appearance (Fig. 29.1.1). The hair loss is discovered by the mother when washing the child's hair or, occasionally, by the hairdresser. The edges of the area of alopecia can show dystrophic hairs known as exclamation mark hairs. These hairs, which are a few millimetres long, are broader at the end than at the scalp level [2]. The course is unpredictable, with spontaneous regrowth in some cases, occasionally with a few white hairs and the appearance of other patches in other cases. If AA predominates in the occipital region, behind the ears, creating a ring of hair loss, it is called 'ophiasis'. This aspect, rarer in children than in adults, generally carries a poor prognosis [3].

AA totalis (AAT) is a loss of all scalp hair, often the eyebrows and eyelashes being preserved (Fig. 29.1.2). It can be created by extension and coalescence of patchy alopecia, or occur within a short space of time. Onset is accompanied by pruritus and sometimes mild erythema.

Alopecia universalis is the most severe stage, with loss of all scalp hair, the eyebrows, eyelashes and body hair. Fortunately it is rare in children but can occur at all ages, even in neonates.

In all these forms the general physical paediatric examination reveals no abnormalities. Nail involvement, usually in the form of pitting, which can affect all the nails, is observed in 7–66% of cases [4]. Nail dystrophy varies in severity to the degree of hair loss [3] and can precede or follow remission of AA.

Prognosis

The onset of alopecia is generally gradual. In certain well-documented cases alopecia occurs after a life event such as an accident or loss of a close relative or friend [5]. Immunological modifications triggered by stress are now a major focus of study and also occur in other autoimmune conditions. However, the importance of this phenomenon has been exaggerated and it must be borne in mind that most children with alopecia have no history of mental trauma. In contrast, severe chronic alopecia can have a major psychological impact and requires appropriate counselling [6].

The outcome of alopecia is unpredictable. The prognosis is usually very good for small patchy forms, i.e. the majority of cases in children, with spontaneous regrowth within weeks or months. Large patchy forms have a tendency to be chronic, as do mainly ophiasic forms and both AAT and alopecia universalis. The most frequently cited factors of poor prognosis are a personal history of allergy, a family history of alopecia and long-standing alopecia [3].

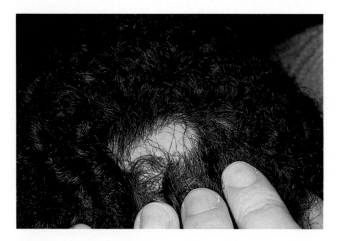

Fig. 29.1.1 A localized area of AA.

Differential diagnosis

The differential diagnosis includes tinea capitis (ringworm), trichotillomania (hair pulling tic) and traction alopecia [3,7].

REFERENCES

1 Price VH. Alopecia areata: clinical aspects. *J Invest Dermatol* 1991; 96: 64–8.
2 Peereboom-Wynia JDR, Koerten HK, van Joost T *et al.* Scanning electron microscopy comparing exclamation mark hairs in alopecia areata with normal hair fibres mechanically broken by traction. *Clin Exp Dermatol* 1989; 14: 47–52.
3 de Waard-van der Spek FB. Oranje AP, De Raeymacker DMJ *et al.* Juvenile versus maturity-onset alopecia areata: a comparative retrospective clinical study. *Clin Exp Dermatol* 1989; 14: 429–33.
4 Baran R, Dawber RPR. *Diseases of Nails and Their Management.* Oxford: Blackwell Science 1984: 192–5.
5 Colon EA *et al.* Lifetime prevalence of psychiatric disorders in patients with alopecia areata. *Compr Psychiatr* 1991; 32: 245–51.

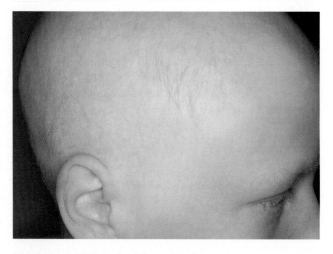

Fig. 29.1.2 AAT: alopecia of the total scalp.

6 de Waard-van der Spek FB, Oranje AP, de Roeymaeker DM, Peereboom-Wynia JDR. Juvenile versus maturity-onset alopecia areata—a comparitive retrospective clinical study. *Clin Exp Dermatol* 1989; 14: 429–33.
7 Oranje AP, Peereboom-Wynia JDR, De Raeymaecker DMJ. Trichotillomania in childhood. *J Am Acad Dermatol* 1986; 15: 614–19.

Treatment

Treatment is very disappointing. The existence of an abundance of therapeutic modalities reflects the lack of any safe and consistently effective approach. None of the methods proposed shows more than 30% efficacy in severe alopecia. Several general rules need to be underlined before each approach is discussed in detail.

1 When a given method fails in a patient, other methods should be tried.

2 A long period (between 3 and 6 months) usually elapses before regrowth—this is the minimum treatment period before an approach can be considered to have failed.

3 Spontaneous regrowth frequently occurs in patchy AA. Therapeutic trials must therefore be placebo-controlled and double-blind, preferably with parallel treatment groups.

Alopecia is not associated with systemic involvement, and treatment should be free of major adverse effects. In children it is important to consider whether the treatment is worse than the disease. A restrictive approach should be kept in mind.

Classical local treatments

The aim of these treatments is to induce scalp irritation with substances such a phenol, benzoyl-benzoate, *Croton* oil, coal tar and acetic acid, or mechanical means such as cryotherapy. Such treatments have not been tested in comparative trials.

Topical corticosteroids

These agents are mainly used in patchy AA, and the results are highly variable. They must not be used for more than 2 months in case of failure, given the risk of scalp atrophy. Intralesional steroids should be avoided as they give inconsistent and short-lived results, and can also cause skin atrophy. They should never be used to treat alopecia of the eyebrows, as there is a risk of amaurosis due to crystal embolism of the ophthalmic artery.

Anthralin

This approach was first used by Schmoeckel, and later by Fiedler-Weiss and Buys, for the treatment of patchy AA [1]. Fiedler-Weiss obtained good results in 17 out of 66 patients with patchy AA, 25% of whom were treated with 0.5% anthraline for 6 months then a 1% preparation for the following 6 months [1]. The results were durable in 12 patients. The time required for regrowth was 11 weeks, and a cosmetically acceptable result was obtained after 6 months.

Treatment with contact allergens

The principle of this type of treatment is to create antigenic competition by provoking contact eczema on the scalp. The first step is sensitization by means of a patch test on the forearm or scalp, and then application of increasing concentrations of the allergen after 15 days. The aim is to obtain frank contact eczema, without creating too much discomfort for the patient. The mechanism of action forwarded by Happle involves antigenic competition with putative hair follicle antigens [2,3]. The perifollicular infiltrate is amplified by dinitrochlorobenzene (DNCB) application, with a particularly marked increase in the number of suppressor T lymphocytes that have a local immunoregulatory effect. Therapeutic efficacy is obtained in 25–70% of cases according to the series and the precise endpoint. If aesthetically acceptable regrowth is used as the endpoint, the treatment is effective in about 30% of cases. The authors have treated 42 alopecia patients with local DNCB applications [4]. Seven patients showed widespread scalp hair growth that persisted for at least 6 months after 3–15 months of treatment. The mean time to regrowth was 5.5 weeks. Seventeen patients had poor results; the regrowth only involved about 50% of the entire hairless surface, while five showed only downy regrowth. Treatment failed in 18 cases. Since DNCB is thought to be a potentially mutagenic agent, the use of two other allergens, dibutylester squaric acid and diphencyprone (DPCP) is preferred [5,6]. The results are similar to those obtained with DNCB, but DPCP gives rise to more frequent and serious contact reactions. In summary, treatment with contact allergens has to be proven effective, but the patients, their friends and family, and the doctors and pharmacists who use the technique, may all suffer from side-effects. The potential benefits of this approach for children must be carefully balanced. A recent study assessed the efficacy of DPCP treatment in children with severe AAT and alopecia areata localis (AAL) showing no spontaneous remission [7].

Photochemotherapy

This technique was first used by Rollier and Warcewski in 1974. Later studies confirmed that good results can be obtained in 30–70% of cases [8]. This treatment can only be offered to children over 12 who are refractory to other treatments and have severe forms of AA. There are several photochemotherapy methods. In the first, following local application of a solution of meladinin, only the scalp is irradiated. Alternatively, oral administration of psoralens is followed by irradiation of either the scalp or the whole body. The treatment regime is usually three irradiations per week at doses that are increased gradually up to 8 J/cm^2. If the treatment is successful, regrowth is obtained between the 50th and 80th session. Claudy and Gagnaire consider it best to use systemic psoralens and full-body irradiation [8]. The main problem with photochemotherapy is that patients relapse when the sessions are tapered [9]. The method probably corrects the immune dysregulation, as in psoriasis. Studies of a mouse model have shown that ultraviolet A irradiation of the skin reduces the number of T-helper lymphocytes and Langerhans' cells, and increases that of T-suppressor cells.

Inosiplex

This agent has immunomodulating properties *in vitro* that mainly consist of stimulating T lymphocyte and phagocyte functions. However, its effect *in vivo* remains to be established. Galbraith and Fudenberg have obtained good results, particularly when administered continuously at high doses, i.e. 50 mg/kg/day, or one 500-mg tablet per 10 kg of body weight [10]. Treatment must last at least 6 months. Galbraith *et al.* obtained 11 good results in a series of 25 patients, although good result was not clearly defined. The perifollicular lymphocyte infiltrate was attenuated in patients who responded [11]. This treatment has the advantage of being simple, acceptable for children and relatively non-toxic, but its efficacy, which is probably low, needs to be confirmed in other studies. It should only be tried in AAT and alopecia universalis.

Minoxidil

Minoxidil is currently in vogue, but its mechanism of action remains to be identified. Its trichogenic action is a well-known side-effect of systemic treatment of hypertension. Minoxidil has a local vasodilatory effect and directly stimulates the mitotic activity of hair follicles and keratinocytes. Fiedler-Weiss *et al.* treated 48 alopecia patients with a 1% solution of minoxidil twice daily under an occlusive dressing [12]. Terminal hairs regrew in 25 cases but acceptable aesthetic results were only obtained in 11, and were durable in only one-third of these patients. Fenton obtained regrowth in 16 out of 30 patients with a 1% solution [13]. The authors' results have been less encouraging [14]. Using a 4% solution the authors only observed full regrowth in one out of 25 patients with AA [14]. Fiedler-Weiss *et al.* obtained slightly better results with a 5% solution, but had problems with crystal formation at this concentration.

Cyclosporin

Patients treated with this powerful immunosuppressive agent can develop hypertrichosis. Gilhar has shown that cyclosporin stimulates hair regrowth on human skin grafts in nude mice [15]. The severity of side-effects (nephrotoxicity, hypertension and lymphoma) rules out the use of oral cyclosporin in children with AA [16]. The authors used it topically in a placebo-controlled trial involving 43 patients with severe AA [16]. Terminal hairs, generally in small tufts 0.5–2 cm in diameter, grew in seven patients, between the second and sixth month of treatment. Complete regrowth never occurred. Cyclosporin was thus more effective than the placebo, but regrowth was weak, took a long time to appear and was always incomplete. Other teams have reported no benefit [17].

FK-506

One promising agent for the treatment of AA is FK-506, another immunosuppressive agent that stimulates hair growth in CD-1 mice when applied to the skin [18].

REFERENCES

1 Fiedler-Weiss VC, Buys CM. Evaluation of anthralin in the treatment of alopecia areata. *Arch Dermatol* 1987; 123: 1491–5.
2 Happle R. Antigenic competition as a therapeutic concept for alopecia areata. *Arch Dermatol Res* 1980; 267: 109–14.
3 Van der Steen PHM, Happle R. Immunological treatment of alopecia areata including the use of diphencyprone. *J Dermatol Treat* 1992; 3: 35–40.
4 De Prost Y, Paquez F, Touraine R. Dinitrochlorobenzene treatment of alopecia areata. *Arch Derm* 1982; 118: 542–5.
5 Happle R, Hausen BM, Wiesner Menkel L. Diphencyprone in the treatment of alopecia areata. *Acta Derm Venereol* 1983; 63: 49–52.
6 Orecchia G, Malagoli P. Topical immunotherapy in children with alopecia areata. *J Invest Dermatol* 1995; 104: 35–6S.
7 Schuttelaar M-LA, Plinck EB, Peereboom-Wynia JDR, Vuzevski VD, Mulder PGH, Oranje AP. Alopecia areata in children: treatment with diphencyprone. *Br J Dermatol* 1996; 135: 585–8.
8 Claudy AL, Gagnaire D. PUVA treatment for alopecia areata. *Arch Dermatol* 1983; 119: 975–8.
9 Healy E, Rogers S. PUVA treatment for alopecia areata does it work? A retrospective review of 102 cases. *Br J Dermatol* 1993; 129: 42–4.
10 Galbraith GM, Thiers BH, Fundenberg HH. An open label trial of immunomodulation therapy with Inosiplex (isprinosine) in patients with alopecia totalis and cell-mediated immunodeficiency. *J Acad Dermatol* 1984; 11: 224–30.
11 Galbraith GMR, Thiers BH, Jensen J, Hoehler F. A randomized double-blind study of Inosiplex (isoprinosine) therapy in patients with alopecia areata totalis. *J Am Acad Dermatol* 1987; 16: 977–83.
12 Fiedler-Weiss VC, West DP, Fu JP. Alopecia areata treated with topical minoxidil. *Arch Dermatol* 1984; 120: 457–63.
13 Fenton DA, Wilkinson JD. Topical minoxidil in the treatment of alopecia areata. *Br Med J* 1983; 287: 1075–7.
14 De Prost Y, Paquez F, Baspeyras M, Touraine R. Traitement de pelades sävâres par applications locales de Minoxidil. *Ann Dermatol Vénéréol* 1984; 11: 613–14.
15 Gilhar A, Pillar T, Etzioni A. Topical cyclosporine A in alopecia areata. *Acta Derm Venereol (Stockh)* 1989; 69: 803–4.
16 De Prost Y, Teillac D, Paquez F. Placebo-controlled trial of topical cyclosporin in severe alopecia areata. *Lancet* 1986; ii: 803–4.
17 Rongioletti F, Guarrera M, Tosti A, Guerra L, Pigatto P. Topical cyclosporin A fails to improve alopecia areata: a double blind study. *J Dermatol Treat* 1992; 3: 13–14.
18 Yamamoto S, Jiang H, Kato R. Stimulation of hair growth by topical application of FK506, a potent immunosuppressive agent. *J Invest Dermatol* 1994; 102: 160–4.

29.2 Granuloma Annulare

CAMERON KENNEDY

Definition

Granuloma annulare is an inflammatory disorder of the dermis and/or subcutis characterized by degeneration of connective tissue and a surrounding predominantly of histiocytic infiltrate. Almost always there is healing without scarring.

History

The term granuloma annulare was introduced by Radcliff-Crocker in 1902 [1] but probably the first clinical description was by Colcott-Fox in 1895 [2] of a 'ringed eruption on the fingers' of an 11-year-old girl. From these early reports onwards, granuloma annulare has been described in patients of all ages. Only occasionally are paediatric cases identified as such, and most experimental work has been on adults.

Early authors considered the underlying cause to be tuberculosis [3,4], but as the incidence of this disease fell, reported cases of granuloma annulare were increasingly not associated with tuberculosis [5]. From the 1960s, other disease associations have been investigated, notably abnormal glucose tolerance and overt diabetes [6,7,8,9], but in most patients, perhaps particularly in children, granuloma annulare occurs without relationship to other diseases.

The 1950–60 period saw the recognition of the subcutaneous form of granuloma annulare, a variant rarely found outside the paediatric age group, and its distinction from nodules associated with rheumatoid arthritis and rheumatic fever [10,11,12,13].

Aetiology

In most cases granuloma annulare occurs for no apparent reason.

Familial incidence

Overall there is no convincing evidence that genetic factors are important, although granuloma annulare has been reported in mother and child, twins, siblings and successive generations [14,5,15,16,17,18,19].

Triggering factors

Occasionally, the onset has been associated with a triggering factor. Subcutaneous granuloma annulare in children has been recorded to follow non-specific trauma in up to 25% [10] and it is possible that trivial injuries have a role with dermal granuloma annulare on the hands and feet. Other triggers include insect bite [20,21,22], octopus bite [23], tuberculin test [24], sun exposure [25,26,27], psoralens and ultraviolet A (PUVA) [28], ultraviolet B (UVB) [29] and occupational contact with corticosteroid powder [30]. Granuloma annulare has been recorded localizing to scars from herpes zoster [31,32], in association with viral warts [33] and possibly *Borrelia burgdorferi* infection [34]. Within a controlled study there was no evidence for this association [35].

Human leucocyte antigen (HLA) associations

HLA associations have been seen in some populations. In Denmark an association was reported for localized granuloma annulare and HLA-B8 [36]. A study from Israel mainly of Ashkenazi Jews, showed that 95% of cases of generalized granuloma annulare had the HLA-B35 compared with 35% of controls and there was also a significant association with HLA-A31; these associations were not found in the localized granuloma annulare population [37]. The Israeli group did not confirm the HLA-B8 findings from Denmark, illustrating that HLA genes are population specific. A group in Belfast reported on 59 cases of localized granuloma annulare and found increases in HLA-A29, HLA-B14 and HLA-B15 [38].

Association with diabetes mellitus

From a recognition of the pathological similarities between granuloma annulare and necrobiosis lipoidica diabeticorum, a link between granuloma annulare and diabetes mellitus has long been suspected [6], but remains controversial [39,40]. Also, overt diabetes does not seem unduly prevalent in the granuloma annulare population [5]. Difficulties with interpreting the literature include a failure to define cases as localized or generalized granuloma annulare, selectivity, different methods for assessing carbohydrate intolerance, lack of control in some series and few of these studies include any or significant numbers of children.

Haim *et al.* [1973] [41] reported on 52 cases of granuloma annulare, 39 of which were localized granuloma annulare (eight of whom were under the age of 20 years), and 13 cases of generalized granuloma annulare (none under the age of 20 years) and found significant carbohydrate intolerance only in the generalized granuloma annulare group.

Mobacken *et al.* also showed an association between generalized granuloma annulare and insulin-dependent diabetes mellitus in adults, but not localized granuloma annulare [8,42]. Uncontrolled studies [43,9,36,44] have shown similar results.

In the largest of these series, Dabski and Winkelmann [44] found that 20% of 100 cases of generalized granuloma annulare were diabetic, but this series included only six patients under the age of 20 years. A more recent small series of generalized granuloma annulare in adults showed no association with diabetes [40].

Although most of the literature examining a relationship between localized granuloma annulare and diabetes mellitus has not found a relationship, in a retrospective study of 557 cases, 300 of whom were under the age of 24 years at diagnosis, insulin-dependent diabetes mellitus was found in 10 of the 300, significantly more than would have been predicted from population statistics [45].

Some further light is shed on granuloma annulare as a prediabetic state in a controlled study on 14 patients (mean age 37 years) in whom those with overt diabetes were excluded, with various types of granuloma annulare; there was evidence for both impaired carbohydrate tolerance and insulin resistance [46].

There have been some individual case reports in which there is a noteworthy relationship between granuloma annulare and diabetes in childhood [47], and occasionally granuloma annulare and necrobiosis lipoidica occurring in the same patient [48].

In conclusion, a large prospective controlled study of well-defined granuloma annulare patients whose disease begins in childhood is needed to assess the connection between granuloma annulare and insulin-dependent diabetes mellitus. Meanwhile, a simple history and urinalysis for sugar are appropriate investigations for the paediatric case and more complex procedures are unnecessary.

Association with other diseases

Granuloma annulare has also been associated with Hodgkin's disease [49], other lymphomas [50], chronic Epstein–Barr virus infection [51], human immunodeficiency virus [52,29], following bone marrow transplantation [53] and with antithyroid antibodies [25], but these have all been in adult patients and the association could be fortuitous.

Pathogenesis

Although connective tissue degeneration and surrounding granuloma formation are the defining histological events in granuloma annulare, vascular changes and the presence of lymphocytes and neutrophils have prompted speculation over the initial process in the genesis of the skin lesions.

Dahl *et al.* [1977] [54] found evidence of small vessel vasculitis with variable degrees of endothelial swelling and necrosis in 35 of 38 cases of granuloma annulare, together with extravasation of fibrin in necrobiotic areas, and in some there was deposition of immunoglobulin M (IgM) and complement C3 in the vessel walls and at the epidermal junction. Neutrophils and nuclear dust were seen, but were not a prominent feature. In a later study [55] immune reactants were infrequent and inconstant. In a study of 10 lesions reported by patients to be less than a week old, Bergmann *et al.* [1993] [56] confirmed the presence of neutrophils and nuclear dust, but found frank vasculitis in only one lesion, and there was no evidence of deposition of immune reactants.

There may, however, be an excess of circulating immune complexes in granuloma annulare patients. In one series of patients with localized granuloma annulare, immune complexes were detected by the Raji cell technique in 18 of 30 patients but in only four of 90 controls [57]. If immune complexes are relevant, it is unlikely that autoantibodies to collagen are involved [58].

Although an early study found evidence for defective neutrophil function *in vivo* in granuloma annulare patients [59], neither leucocytes, plasma nor serum can replicate this phenomenon [60,61,62].

Increased circulating factor VIII-related antigen has been associated with both vasculitis and angiopathy, including that occurring in diabetics, and an increased level was reported in patients with necrobiosis lipoidica and generalized but not localized granuloma annulare [63].

Vascular occlusion in granuloma annulare may also be contributed to by decreased tissue fibrinolytic activity [64] and increased circulating fibronectin [65].

Cellular immune mechanisms

The presence of lymphocytes with histiocytes in the cellular infiltrate in granuloma annulare would suggest that delayed hypersensitivity contributes to the pathogenesis. Lymphocyte accumulation has been described as an early event [66]. Most of these lymphocytes are activated T cells, the majority being T-helper cells [67,68]. Cells with the immunophenotype of Langerhans' cells are increased in the dermal infiltrate and in the overlying epidermis [68]. There is some evidence for circulating cytokine excess, e.g. leucocyte inhibitory factor [69] and macrophage inhibitory factor [70], although neither were detected in another study [60]. There are interleukin 2 positive cells in the infiltrates [68].

Although these studies indicate that T lymphocytes have an important role, it is far from clear whether they are the initial event, nor is the relationship to neutrophil activity in the lesions apparent.

Pathology

Routine histology

As with the clinical manifestations, there is a range of histopathological appearances in granuloma annulare. In all cases there is at least some degree of a process called 'necrobiosis'. This consists of degeneration of dermal and/or subcutaneous connective tissue, seen as blurring and loss of definition of the collagen bundles, often with separation of them, reduced numbers of fibroblast nuclei, altered staining (usually basophilia) and a surrounding lymphohistiocytic granulomatous reaction. The standard interpretation has been that there is degeneration of collagen fibres, but recent work suggests that the primary event in the connective tissue is a loss of elastic fibres [71]. The foci of connective tissue degeneration usually stain for mucin and fibrin, and with appropriate processing lipid microdroplets may be seen. Elastic fibres are absent or abnormal. The diagnosis is usually best made under low power. Three major patterns of inflammatory infiltrate have been described: interstitial histiocytic, palisading granulomatous and sarcoidal [70], although mixtures of these patterns are common in a single lesion [71]. At the periphery of each of these patterns the vessels are surrounded by mononuclear cell infiltrates.

Histiocytic pattern. The most common appearance in papules and plaques of granuloma annulare, especially the generalized form, is a diffuse infiltration of histiocytes between the collagen bundles in the mid and upper dermis. Foci of necrobiotic change may be insignificant on haematoxylin and eosin stained sections, but often more apparent when mucin stains such as colloidal iron and alcian blue are used.

Palisading granuloma. The best known pattern is the palisading granuloma, in which areas of necrobiosis are surrounded by lymphocytes and histiocytes, then a peripheral rim of histiocytes whose long axes are arranged radially, and variable numbers of giant cells are present (Fig. 29.2.1). Eosinophils do occur, but plasma cells are rare [72]. The dermis between necrobiotic granulomas is relatively normal. This pattern is particularly common in localized granuloma annulare.

Sarcoidal. An uncommon pattern, seen in about 3% of cases [70] although relatively more common in localized than generalized granuloma annulare [71] is the formation of epithelioid nodules (Fig. 29.2.2). There is usually some degree of the infiltrative change beyond such nodules. If present, eosinophils and central mucin can be helpful in distinguishing this pattern from sarcoidosis.

Subcutaneous granuloma annulare. In subcutaneous granuloma annulare the areas of necrobiosis tend to be larger and may extend through the fat, and rarely into underlying structures such as muscle [73].

Vasculitis and vascular occlusion. Vasculitis with endothelial swelling, necrosis of the vessel wall, neutrophil debris and even occlusion is sometimes seen [54], perhaps more with the palisading granuloma pattern [70], but is not necessarily the earliest event and neutrophils may be present without vasculitis [56]. Deposition of amorphous material in the basement membrane region of capillaries is also seen, especially in generalized granuloma annulare, reminiscent of diabetic microangiopathy [71].

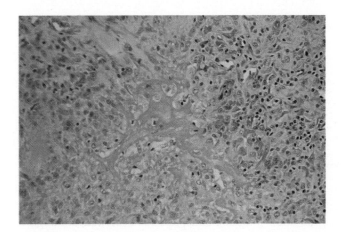

Fig. 29.2.1 Dermal granuloma annulare. Granulomatous reaction around eosinophilic necrobiotic connective tissue. Courtesy of Professor J.W.B. Bradfield, Bristol Royal Infirmary.

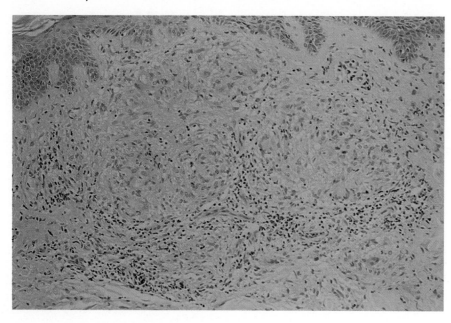

Fig. 29.2.2 Dermal granuloma annulare. Sarcoid-like accumulation of epithelioid cells with peripheral lymphocytes. Courtesy of Professor J.W.B. Bradfield, Bristol Royal Infirmary.

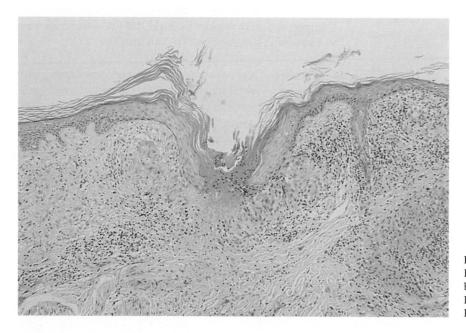

Fig. 29.2.3 Perforating granuloma annulare. Extrusion of necrobiotic material through a breach in the epidermis. Courtesy of Professor J.W.B. Bradfield, Bristol Royal Infirmary.

Elastic tissue. Elastic tissue is reduced or absent in the necrobiotic areas, particularly in generalized granuloma annulare [74] and phagocytosed elastotic material can often be seen in individual histiocytes [75]. These changes can also occur in subcutaneous nodular granuloma annulare.

Epidermal and follicular perforation. In most cases of granuloma annulare the epidermis is normal, although it may be thinned, particularly in the papular umbilicated type [76]. However, in perforating granuloma annulare an underlying necrobiotic granuloma communicates to the surface through an epidermal defect [77] (Fig. 29.2.3). There is usually some epidermal hyperplasia at the edge of the perforation. A variant of this process is transfollicular perforation [78].

Histochemistry. The mucin in granuloma annulare is colloidal iron positive, hyaluronidase labile, alcian blue positive at pH 3.0 but negative at pH 0.4 and toluidine blue positive at pH 3.0 but not at pH 2.0. Abundant hydrolase and esterase activity is found, typical of a histiocytic infiltrate. Perhaps distinctive for granuloma annulare is possible staining for lysozyme, compared with necrobiosis lipoidica and rheumatoid nodule which are negative [79]. There is evidence of both increased collagen production [80,81] and collagenase [82].

Immunocytochemistry. Necrobiotic areas are rich in fibrin. Immunoglobulin and C3 are sometimes but not regularly seen in vessel walls [54,70,83]. Immunoperoxidase techniques have shown activated T lymphocytes with an excess of helper/inducer cells and CD-1 positive dendritic cells, i.e. Langerhans' cell phenotype, in the perivascular and granulomatous infiltrates [68]. Interleukin 2 positive cells and interleukin 2 receptor positive cells were also increased, as occurs in cell-mediated responses [68]. The histiocytes may be a locally derived, immunocytochemically distinct population [84].

Electron microscopy. The ultrastructural details of collagen and elastic tissue degeneration, fibrin accumulation and multilayered basal lamina thickening around capillaries have been described [70,71,85].

Clinical features

Prevalence

Point prevalence in the community has never been determined. It has been stated that 0.1–0.4% of new patients (all ages) attending dermatologists have granuloma annulare [39]. Granuloma annulare can occur at any age, but overall is commonest in children and young adults [5]. Some clinical subtypes are, however, almost always reported in children: the subcutaneous 'pseudorheumatoid nodule' and the papular umbilicated type [76]. Generalized granuloma annulare occurs in children [86] but in a series of 100 cases, only 8% were under the age of 20 years [44]. The reported female predominance for generalized granuloma annulare [44] probably does not apply in the paediatric age range.

Familial cases have been recorded (see above).

The uncommon variety, perforated granuloma annulare, may be more common in Hawaii than elsewhere [87] but there are no other reports to suggest geographical or racial basis for differences in prevalence.

Seasonal fluctuation in granuloma annulare has been described, with lesions appearing on the elbows in spring and subsiding in October [88] but such changes have not been described in other patients.

Localized granuloma annulare

This is the commonest form in children. Lesions are single or a few in number. The most easily recognizable pattern is a ring composed of smooth, firm papules, often coalescent with each other (Figs 29.2.4, 29.2.5). Papules may be skin coloured, red, violaceous or paler than surrounding

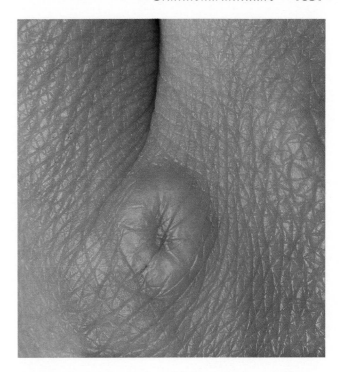

Fig. 29.2.4 Smooth annular dermal plaque on the dorsum of the hand.

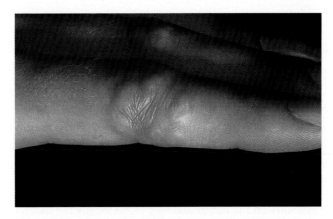

Fig. 29.2.5 Ring of dermal papules on the side of the finger.

normal skin, and can be made more visible by stretching the skin between the finger and thumb.

Isolated papules as well as ring-shaped configuration may be present, and sometimes the subcutaneous form (see below) may coexist. The rings gradually enlarge but are usually less than 5 cm across. They may be multiple. Sometimes the papular component is not evident, the lesions presenting as purplish rings (Fig. 29.2.6). Rarely, they may be notably inflammatory and oedematous [16].

The skin surface is usually normal over localized granuloma annulare, although on exposed sites the stratum corneum can have a compacted shiny appearance.

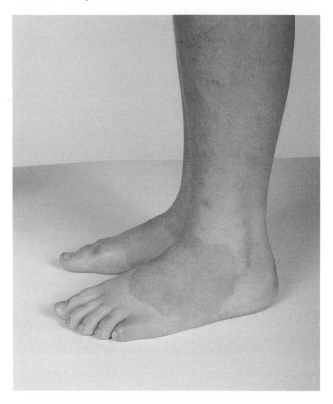

Fig. 29.2.6 Purple patch of granuloma annulare on dorsum of the foot.

The commonest sites are the backs of the hands, fingers, tops of the feet, legs and forearms [5], although granuloma annulare has been reported on almost all body sites including the ear [89] and the eyelid [90].

Granuloma annulare has been recorded on the buccal mucous membrane [91] but this isolated report was in an adult with acquired immune deficiency syndrome (AIDS).

Lesions are usually asymptomatic, but can be painful, especially on the hands and feet. Occasionally the lesions itch.

Linear granuloma annulare. Linear arrays of granuloma annulare papules have been described on the finger [92] and trunk [93] in adults but not as yet in children.

Generalized granuloma annulare

The individual lesion in generalized granuloma annulare is usually a small skin-coloured papule, although macules and nodules can occur, and the colour may be erythematous, yellowish or violaceous. There is no surface change. The distinctive annular configuration of lesions is only seen in about two-thirds of cases [44]. Sometimes lesions aggregate into reticulate and circinate patterns. Lesions are widespread, symmetrical and when non-annular tend to favour the trunk more than the limbs. In some cases the disease occurs mainly on sun-exposed sites. The eruption may be disfiguring but is otherwise usually asymptomatic.

It is impossible to say from the literature whether generalized granuloma annulare in children is significantly associated with diabetes and hyperlipidaemia as it may be in adults [44,94].

Subcutaneous granuloma annulare

This variant of granuloma annulare has been described under several synonyms including benign rheumatoid nodule, pseudorheumatoid nodule, isolated subcutaneous nodule, subcutaneous palisading granuloma and palisading granuloma nodosum [95]. It most commonly occurs in younger children, and is rare beyond the second decade.

The lesion usually presents as a nodule or mass, which may be rapidly growing at presentation. It may

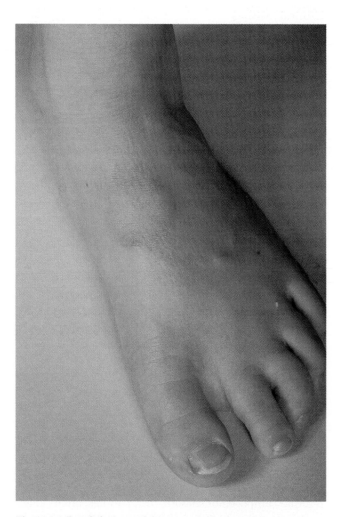

Fig. 29.2.7 Purplish ring and deeper nodules: dermal and subcutaneous granuloma annulare.

be mobile, but often appears to be fixed to underlying periosteum or muscle. Lesions are frequently multiple. The characteristic sites are the lower limb, especially the foot (Fig. 29.2.7) and pretibial area, hands, forearms and scalp [96,97]. At the latter site the occiput is a common location [73]. The buttock and eyebrow [98] are occasional sites.

Lesions are usually asymptomatic.

Typical localized granuloma annulare can occur elsewhere: in 25% in one series of 54 cases [10]. In most cases, subcutaneous granuloma annulare in children is not associated with any systemic disease [73,96,95,97] although with long-term follow-up small numbers of children do develop rheumatoid factor and even rheumatoid arthritis [99,100]. Whether these few cases are intrinsically different from the majority, in whom there is no systemic disease remains to be established.

Perforating granuloma annulare and papular umbilicated granuloma annulare

There is probably a spectrum of change variously reported as perforating granuloma annulare [77] and papular umbilicated granuloma annulare [76], in which a breach in the epidermis with transepidermal elimination of necrobiotic connective tissue is sometimes but not always seen.

Lucky *et al.* [76] reported four cases of an eruption of asymptomatic papules symmetrically located on the dorsa of the hands and fingers in four boys. The papules were 1–4 mm diameter, smooth, flesh-coloured to hypopigmented, usually flat topped, but some with central depressions (Fig. 29.2.8). There were occasional typical localized granuloma annulare lesions. The histology of these cases showed no true perforation, although some of the other features associated with perforating granuloma annulare were minimally present.

In cases described as perforating granuloma annulare, umbilication of the papules is a feature, the depressed centre sometimes being associated with discharge of viscous or creamy material, or with scale or crust [101,77]. The localized form is typically over the backs of the hands and sides of the fingers and the condition can be generalized [39]. When widespread, the arms and legs are frequently involved [87]. The incidence of widespread perforating granuloma annulare may be higher in Hawaii than elsewhere.

Prognosis

Granuloma annulare is ultimately a self-limiting condition, and only very rarely has it been associated with tissue destruction and scarring [44]. Localized granuloma annulare can last from months to more than 20 years, although it has been stated that 50% clear spontaneously in 2 years [39]. About 40% of all cases, children and adults, may get recurrent eruptions, usually at the same sites, but these tend to resolve more quickly than primary lesions [5].

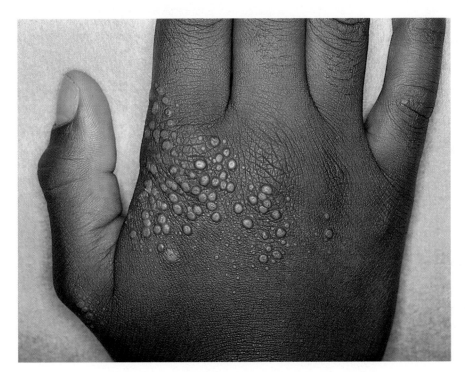

Fig. 29.2.8 Discrete dermal papules, many are umbilicated. Courtesy of Dr Anne W. Lucky, and the *Archives of Dermatology*.

Table 29.2.1 Treatment—localized lesions of granuloma annulare

Treatment	Children included	Nos	Comment	References
Local corticosteroid				
flurandrenolide tape	—	—	Convenient; no reported trials	—
triamcinolone by jet injector	Yes	25	17 cleared (68%) 12/27 saline controls cleared (44%)	[105]
clobetasol propionate under hydrocolloid occlusion	No	3	1 cleared, 2 improved	[106]
Cryotherapy	Yes	31	25 cleared; nitrous oxide preferred	[107]
Scarification	No	2	Improved, over 5 months	[108]
Intralesional interferon β1	No	4	Improved	[109]

Table 29.2.2 Treatment—generalized lesions of granuloma annulare (GA) (and some localized lesions or LGA)

Treatment	Type GA	Children included	Nos	Comment	References
Antimalarials	GGA	All	6	Cleared after 4 weeks	[110]
Dapsone	GGA	No	10	4 cleared	
	LGA	Yes (1)	6	2 cleared (all but 1 needed maintenance)	[111]
	GGA	Yes (1)	6	6 cleared	[112]
Isotretinoin	GGA	No	1	Nearly cleared	[113]
	GGA	No	5	Cleared/nearly cleared	[114]
	GGA	No	1	Nearly cleared	[115]
Etretinate	GGA	No	1	Nearly cleared	[116]
Pentoxifylline	GGA	No	1	Nearly cleared	[117]
Niacinamide	GGA	No	1	Nearly cleared	[118]
Potassium Iodide	GGA	No	4	Improved	[119]
Photochemotherapy (PUVA)	GGA	No	5	5 cleared; maintenance required	[120]
	GGA	No	3	3 cleared; new lesions after stopping	[121]
Cyclosporin	LGA	No	1	Improved	[122]
	GGA	No	1	Improved	
	GGA	No	1	Cleared	[123]
Chlorambucil	GGA	No	6	1 cleared 4 improved	[124]

Generalized granuloma annulare lasts on average 3–4 years but can last a decade or more [44]. Subcutaneous granuloma annulare lesions also tend to last months to several years, all resolving by the second decade [96].

Differential diagnosis

Clinical appearances and a characteristic location will enable a diagnosis to be made in most cases of typical localized granuloma annulare. Occasionally ring-shaped arrays of warts can be confused, but the surface is verrucous. Knuckle pads are flesh-coloured thickenings confined to knuckles. Tinea corporis will have a scaly periphery, and confirmation is easily made by microscopy and culture. Other asymmetrical or localized annular disorders that may occasionally mimic granuloma annulare include lichen planus, erythema annulare centrifugum, secondary syphilis [102], sarcoidosis and erythema elevatum diutinum. When in the form of plaques, granuloma annulare may be mimicked by follicular mucinosis, non-X histiocytosis, juvenile xanthogranuloma and xanthomas.

The differential diagnosis of generalized granuloma annulare includes lichen scrofulosorum, lichen nitidus, sarcoidosis, non-X histiocytosis, eruptive xanthoma, secondary syphilis, lipoid proteinosis and lymphoma. In adults an additional consideration is the papular eruption of HIV [103] and this may also be true for children although it does not seem to have been documented yet.

The differential diagnosis of generalized perforating granuloma annulare includes perforating collagenosis, molluscum contagiosum and lichen nitidus; sarcoidosis can resemble the papular umbilicated variant on the backs of the hands.

Prior to biopsy, there is a wide differential diagnosis for subcutaneous granuloma annulare including tumours, cysts, deep-seated infections, panniculitis, and so on. Radiological techniques, especially MRI, can be helpful in some cases [104]. After biopsy, the nodules of juvenile rheumatoid nodule, lupus erythematosus, scleroderma, rheumatic fever and sarcoidosis may occasionally need to be excluded.

On histological grounds, granuloma annulare can sometimes be confused with necrobiosis lipoidica, as well as rheumatoid nodule [125]. These conditions can on occasions coexist in the same patient [126,48].

Treatment

Most cases of granuloma annulare in childhood are asymptomatic. Explanations should be given about the harmless nature of the disorder and the ultimate resolution without scarring. Treatment may be justified if lesions are painful or tender, e.g. over the backs of hands or on the feet, and for disfigurement.

Hardly any of the many treatments recorded as successful in the literature have been subjected to comparison with placebo or other treatments, and numbers treated in any given series are small or anecdotal. Furthermore, few trials include children.

For localized lesions, a corticosteroid by intralesional injection or under occlusion will usually be the treatment of choice.

For completeness, most treatments for granuloma annulare recorded since the 1970s are shown in Tables 29.2.1 and 29.2.2.

REFERENCES

1 Radcliff-Crocker H. Granuloma annulare. *Br J Dermatol* 1902; 14: 1–9.
2 Colcott-Fox T. Ringed eruption of the fingers. *Br J Dermatol* 1895; 7: 91–5.
3 Graham-Little E. Granuloma annulare. *Br J Dermatol* 1908; 20: 213–57.
4 Halliwell EO, Ingram JT. Granuloma annulare. *Br J Dermatol* 1935; 47: 319–40.
5 Wells RS, Smith MA. The natural history of granuloma annulare. *Br J Dermatol* 1963; 75: 199–205.
6 Rhodes EL, Hill DM, Ames AC, Tourle CA, Taylor CG. Granuloma annulare: prednisone glycosuria tests in a non-diabetic group. *Br J Dermatol* 1966; 78: 532–5.
7 Haim S, Friedman-Birnbaum R, Shafrir A. Generalized granuloma annulare: relationship to diabetes mellitus as revealed in eight cases. *Br J Dermatol* 1970; 83: 302.
8 Mobacken H, Gisslen H, Johannisson G. Cortisone-glucose tolerance test in a non-diabetic group. *Acta Derm Venereol (Stockh)* 1970; 50: 440–4.
9 Hammond R, Dyess K, Castro A. Insulin production and glucose tolerance in patients with granuloma annulare. *Br J Dermatol* 1972; 87: 540–7.
10 Draheim JH. A clinicopathologic analysis of 'rheumatoid' nodules occurring in 54 children. *Am J Pathol* 1959; 35: 678.
11 Lowney ED, Simons HM. 'Rheumatoid' nodules of the skin. *Arch Dermatol* 1963; 88: 853–8.
12 Rubin M, Lynch FW. Subcutaneous granuloma annulare. *Arch Dermatol* 1966; 93: 416–20.
13 Burrington JD. 'Pseudorheumatoid' nodules in children: report of 10 cases. *J Pediatr* 1970: 45: 473–8.
14 Spitzer VR. Granuloma annulare familiare. *Dermatologica* 1961; 123: 38–41.
15 Arner S, Aspegren N. Familial granuloma annulare. *Acta Derm Venereol* 1968; 48: 253–4.
16 Burnett JW, Wood C, Sina B, Dilaimy M. Inflammatory granuloma annulare. *Cutis* 1986; 37: 267–8.
17 Goolamali SK, Stevenson CJ. Granuloma annulare in identical twins. *Br J Dermatol* 1972; 86: 636.
18 Bowen JR. Subcutaneous granuloma annulare in identical twins. *Del Med J* 1982; 54: 509–12.
19 Abrusci V, Weiss E, Planas G. Familial generalized perforating granuloma annulare. *Int J Dermatol* 1988; 27: 126–7.
20 Curwen W. Granuloma annulare, multiple, suggesting an unusual insect-bite reaction. *Arch Dermatol* 1963; 88: 355.
21 Moyer DG. Papular granuloma annulare. *Arch Dermatol* 1964; 89: 41–5.
22 Takigawa M, Aoshima T. Generalized granuloma annulare in a 15-month infant. *Dermatologica* 1976; 153: 202–5.
23 Fulghum D. Octopus bite resulting in granuloma annulare. *South Med J* 1986; 79: 1434.
24 Beer WE, Jones EW. Granuloma annulare following tuberculin heaf tests. *Trans Rep St John's Hosp Dermatol Soc London* 1966; 52: 68–70.
25 Gross PR, Shelley WB. The association of generalized granuloma annulare with antithyroid antibodies. *Acta Derm Venereol (Stockh)* 1971; 51: 59–62.
26 Leppard B, Black MM. Disseminated granuloma annulare. *Trans Rep St John's Hosp Dermatol Soc London* 1972; 58: 186–90.
27 Reinhard M, Undeutsch W, Lampe P. Das atypische granuloma annulare. *Arch Dermatol Forsch* 1971; 240; 79–94.
28 Dorval JC, Leroy JP, Masse R. Granulomes annulaires dissemines pares puvatherpaie. *Ann Dermatol Vénéréol (Paris)* 1979; 106: 79–80.
29 Cohen PR, Grossman ME, Silvers DN, DeLeo VA. Human immunodeficiency virus-associated granuloma annulare. *Int J STD AIDS* 1991; 2: 168–71.
30 Morelli M, Fumagalli M, Altomare GF, Pigatto PD. Contact granuloma annulare. *Contact Derm* 1988; 18: 317–18.
31 Friedman SJ, Fox BJ, Albert HL. Granuloma annulare arising in herpes zoster scars. *J Am Acad Dermatol* 1986; 14: 764–70.
32 Krahl D, Hartschub W, Tilgen W. Granuloma annulare perforans in herpes zoster scars. *J Am Acad Dermatol* 1993; 29: 859–62.
33 Ward WH. Warts and granuloma annulare. *Br Med J* 1956; 2: 1484.
34 Berger BW. Dermatologic manifestations of Lyme disease. *Rev Infect Dis* 1989; 11 (suppl).
35 Halkier-Sorensen L, Kragballe K, Hansen K. Antibodies to the *Borrelia burgdorferi* flagellum in patients with scleroderma, granuloma annulare and porphyria cutanea tarda. *Acta Derm Venereol (Stockh)* 1989; 69; 116–19.
36 Andersen BL, Verdich J. Granuloma annulare and diabetes mellitus. *Clin Exp Dermatol* 1979; 4: 31–7.
37 Friedman-Birnbaum R, Gideoni O, Bergman R, Pollack S. A study of HLA antigen association in localized and generalized granuloma annulare. *Br J Dermatol* 1986; 115: 329–33.
38 Middleton D, Allen GE. HLA antigen frequency in granuloma annulare. *Br J Dermatol* 1984; 110: 57–9.
39 Muhlbauer JE. Granuloma annulare. *J Am Acad Dermatol* 1980; 3: 217–30.
40 Gannon TF, Lynch PJ. Absence of carbohydrate intolerance in granuloma annulare. *J Am Acad Dermatol* 1994; 30: 662–3.
41 Haims S, Friedman-Birnbaum R, Haim N, Shafrir A, Ravina A. Carbohydrate tolerance in patients with granuloma annulare. *Br J Dermatol* 1973; 88: 447.
42 Blohme G, Mobacken H, Waldenstrom J. Early insulin response to glucose injection intravenously in patients with localised granuloma annulare. *Acta Derm Venereol (Stockh)* 1974; 54: 259–63.
43 Romaine R, Rudner EJ, Altman J. Papular granuloma annulare and diabetes mellitus. *Arch Dermatol* 1968; 98: 152–4.
44 Dabski K, Winkelmann RK. Generalized granuloma annulare: clinical and laboratory findings in 100 patients. *J Am Acad Dermatol* 1989; 20: 39–47.
45 Muhlemann MF, Williams DRR. Localized granuloma annulare is asso-

ciated with insulin-dependent diabetes mellitus. *Br J Dermatol* 1984; 111: 325–9.

46 Kidd GS, Graff GE, Davies BE, McDermott MT, Aeling JL, Hofeldt FD. Glucose tolerance in granuloma annulare. *Diabetes Care* 1985; 8: 380–4.

47 Goldin D, Rook A, Gairdner D. Granuloma annulare in Mauriac's syndrome. *Br J Dermatol* 1975; 93: 31.

48 Schwartz ME. Necrobiosis lipoidica and granuloma annulare. *Arch Dermatol* 1982; 118: 192–3.

49 Schwartz RA, Hansen RC, Lynch PJ. Hodgkin's disease and granuloma annulare. *Arch Dermatol* 1981; 117: 185–6.

50 Barksdale SK, Perniciaro C, Halling KC, Strickler JG. Granuloma annulare in patients with malignant lymphoma: clinicopathologic study of 13 new cases. *J Am Acad Dermatol* 1994; 31: 42–8.

51 Spencer SA, Fenske NA, Espinoza CG, Hamill JR, Cohen LE, Espinoza LR. Granuloma annulare-like eruption due to chronic Epstein–Barr virus infection. *Arch Dermatol* 1988; 124: 250–5.

52 Ghadially R, Sibbald RG, Walter JB, Haberman HF. Granuloma annulare in patients with human immunodeficiency virus infections. *J Am Acad Dermatol* 1989; 20: 232–5.

53 Nevo S, Drakos P, Goldenhersh MA *et al.* Generalized granuloma annulare post autologous bone marrow transplantation in a Hodgkin's disease patient. *Bone Marrow Trans* 1994; 14: 631–3.

54 Dahl MV, Ullman S, Goltz RW. Vasculitis in granuloma annulare. *Arch Dermatol* 1977; 113: 463.

55 Thyresson HN, Doyle JA, Winkelmann RK. Granuloma annulare: histopathologic and direct immunofluorescent study. *Acta Derm Venereol (Stockh)* 1980; 60: 261–3.

56 Bergman R, Pam Z, Lichtig C, Reiter I, Friedman-Birnbaum R. Localized granuloma annulare. *Am J Dermatopathol* 1993; 15: 544–8.

57 Peserico A, Ossi E, Salvador L *et al.* Circulating immune complexes in granuloma annulare. *Arch Dermatol* 1988; 280: 325–6.

58 Evans CD, Pereira RS, Yuen CT, Holden CA. Anti-collagen antibodies in granuloma annulare and necrobiosis lipoidica. *Clin Exp Dermatol* 1988; 13: 252–4.

59 Gange RW, Black MM, Carrington P. Defective neutrophil migration in granuloma annulare, necrobiosis lipoidica, and sarcoidosis. *Arch Dermatol* 1979; 115: 32.

60 Cherney KJ, Lindroos WE, Goltz RW, Dahl MV. Leukocyte function in granuloma annulare. *Br J Dermatol* 1979; 101: 23–31.

62 Friedman-Birnbaum R, Bergman R, Obedeanu N, Meshulam T, Merzbach D. Neutrophil migration in granuloma annulare: comparative study between localized and generalized types and between active and regressive states. *J Dermatol* 1985; 12: 455–8.

62 Majewski BBJ, Rhodes EL, Watson B. Neutrophil mobility in granuloma annulare and necrobiosis lipoidica. *Clin Exp Dermatol* 1981; 6: 583–90.

63 Majewski BBJ, Koh MS, Barter S, Rhodes EL. Increased factor VIII-related antigen in necrobiosis lipoidica and widespread granuloma annulare without associated diabetes. *Br J Dermatol* 1982; 107: 641–5.

64 Misch KJ, Yuen CT, Rhodes EL. Decreased tissue fibrinolytic activity in granuloma annulare. *Clin Exp Dermatol* 1987; 12: 437–9.

65 Koh MS, Majewski BBJ, Barter S, Rhodes EL. Increased plasma fibronectin in diabetes mellitus, necrobiosis lipoidica and widespread granuloma annulare. *Clin Exp Dermatol* 1984; 9: 293–7.

66 Charles CR, Cooper PH, Helwing EB. The fine structure of granuloma annulare. *Lab Invest* 1977; 36: 444–51.

67 Buechner SA, Winkelmann RK, Banks PM. Identification of T-cell subpopulations in granuloma annulare. *Arch Dermatol* 1983; 119: 125–8.

68 Modlin RL, Horwitz DA, Jordan RR, Gebhard JF, Taylor CR, Rea TH. Immunopathologic demonstration of T lymphocyte subpopulations and interleukin 2 in granuloma annulare. *Pediatr Dermatol* 1984; 2: 26–32.

69 Friedman-Birnbaum R, Gilhar A, Haim S, Golan DT. Leucocyte inhibitory factor (LIF) in granuloma annulare: a comparative study between the generalized and localized types. *Acta Derm Venereol* 1983; 63: 242–3.

70 Umbert P, Winkelmann RK. Histologic, ultrastructural, and histochemical studies of granuloma annulare. *Arch Dermatol* 1977; 113: 1681–6.

71 Hanna WM, Moreno-Merlo F, Andsighetti L. Granuloma annulare: an elastic tissue disease? Case report and literature review. *Ultrastruct Pathol* 1999; 23: 33–8.

71 Friedman-Birnbaum R, Weltfriend S, Munichor M, Lichtig C. A comparative histopathologic study of generalized and localized granuloma annulare. *Am J Dermatopathol* 1989; 11: 144–8.

72 Silverman RA, Rabinowitz AD. Eosinophils in the cellular infiltrate of granuloma annulare. *J Cutan Pathol* 1985; 12: 13–17.

73 Kossard S, Goellner JR, Su WPD. Subcutaneous necrobiotic granulomas of the scalp. *J Am Acad Dermatol* 1980; 3: 180–5.

74 Friedman-Birnbaum R, Weltfriend S, Kerner H, Lichtig C. Elastic tissue changes in generalized granuloma annulare. *Am J Dermatopathol* 1989; 11: 429–33.

75 Burket JM, Zelickson AS. Intracellular elastin in generalized granuloma annulare. *J Am Acad Dermatol* 1986; 14: 975–81.

76 Lucky AW, Prose NS, Bove K, White WL, Jorizzo JL. Papular umbilicated granuloma annulare. *Arch Dermatol* 1992; 128: 1375–8.

77 Owens DW, Freeman RG. Perforating granuloma annulare. *Arch Dermatol* 1971; 103: 64–7.

78 Bardach HG. Granuloma annulare with follicular perforation. *Dermatologica* 1982; 165: 47–53.

79 Padilla RS, Mukai K, Dahl MV, Burgdorf WH, Rosai J. Differential staining pattern of lysozyme in palisading granulomas: an immunoperoxidase study. *J Am Acad Dermatol* 1983; 8: 634–8.

80 Oikarinen A, Kinnunen T, Kallioinen M. Biochemical and immunohistochemical comparison of collagen in granuloma annulare and skin sarcoidosis. *Acta Derm Venereol (Stockh)* 1989; 69: 277–83.

81 Kallioinen M, Sandberg M, Kinnunen T, Oikarinen A. Collagen synthesis in granuloma annulare. *J Invest Dermatol* 1992; 98: 463–8.

82 Saarialho-Kere UK, Chang ES, Welgus HG, Parks WC. Expression of interstitial collagenase, 92-kDa gelatinase, and tissue inhibitor of metalloproteinases-1 in granuloma annulare and necrobiosis lipoidica diabeticorum. *J Invest Dermatol* 1993; 100: 335–42.

83 Nieboer C, Kalsbeek GL. Direct immunofluorescence studies in granuloma annulare, necrobiosis lipoidica and granulomatosis disciformis Miescher. *Dermatologica* 1979; 158: 427–32.

84 Mullans E, Helm KF. Granuloma annulare: an immunohistochemical study. *J Cutan Pathol* 1994; 21: 135–9.

85 Friedman-Birnbaum R, Ludatscher RM. Comparative ultrastructural study of generalized and localized granuloma annulare. *Am J Dermatopathol* 1986; 8: 302–8.

86 Dicken CH, Carrington SG, Winkelmann RK, Rochester MD. Generalized granuloma annulare. *Arch Dermatol* 1969; 99: 556–63.

87 Samlaska CP, Sandberg GD, Maggio KL, Sakas EL. Generalized perforating granuloma annulare. *J Am Acad Dermatol* 1992; 27: 319–22.

88 McLelland J, Young S, Marks JM, Lawrence CM. Seasonally recurrent granuloma annulare of the elbows. *Clin Exp Dermatol* 1991; 16: 129–30.

89 Mills A, Chetty R. Auricular granuloma annulare. *Am J Dermatopathol* 1992; 14: 431–3.

90 Wojno T, Tenzle RR, Thomas M. Granuloma annulare of the eyelid. *Ann Ophthalmol* 1985; 17: 73–5.

91 Green TL, Hikado M, Greenspan D. Granuloma annulare of the buccal mucosa in association with AIDS. *Oral Surg Oral Med Oral Pathol* 1989; 67: 319–21.

92 McDow RA, Fields JP. Linear granuloma annulare of the finger. *Cutis* 1987; 39; 43–4.

93 Harpster EF, Mauro T, Barr RJ. Linear granuloma annulare. *J Am Acad Dermatol* 1989; 21: 1138–41.

94 Friedman-Birnbaum R. Generalized and localized granuloma annulare. *Int J Dermatol* 1986; 25: 364.

95 Davids JR, Kolman BH, Billman GF, Krous HF. Subcutaneous granuloma annulare: recognition and treatment. *J Pediatr Orthop* 1993; 13; 582–6.

96 Minifee PK, Buchino JJ. Subcutaneous palisading granulomas (benign rheumatoid nodules) in children. *J Pediatr Surg* 1986; 21: 1078–80.

97 Evans MJ, Blessing K, Gray ES. Pseudorheumatoid nodule (deep granuloma annulare) of childhood: clinicopathologic features of 20 patients. *Pediatr Dermatol* 1994; 11: 6–9.

98 Ferry AP. Subcutaneous granuloma annulare ('pseudorheumatoid nodule') of the eyebrow. *J Pediatr Ophthalmol* 1977; 14: 154–7.

99 Berardinelli JL, Hyman CJ, Campbell EE, Fireman P. Presence of rheumatoid factor in 10 children with isolated rheumatoid-like nodules. *J Pediatr* 1972; 81: 751–7.

100 Moore TL, Dorner RW, Zuckner J. Complement fixing hidden rheumatoid factor in children with benign rheumatoid nodules. *Arthritis Rheum* 1978; 21: 930–4.

101 Calnan CD. Granuloma annulare. *Br J Dermatol* 1954; 66: 254.

102 Jain HC, Fisher BK. Annular syphilid mimicking granuloma annulare. *Int J Dermatol* 1988; 27: 340–1.

103 Smith KJ, James WD, Barrett TL, Lupton GP. Papular eruption of human immunodeficiency virus disease. *Am J Dermatopathol* 1991; 13: 445–51.

104 Chung S, Frush DP, Prose NS *et al*. Subcutaneous granuloma annulare: MR imaging features in six children and literature review. *Radiol* 1999; 210: 845–9.

105 Sparrow G, Abell E. Granuloma annulare and necrobiosis lipoidica treated by jet injector. *Br J Dermatol* 1975; 93: 85–9.

106 Volden G. Successful treatment of chronic skin diseases with clobetasol propionate and a hydrocolloid occlusive dressing. *Acta Derm Venereol (Stockh)* 1992; 72: 69–71.

107 Blume-Peytavi U, Zouboulis CC, Jacobi H, Scholz A, Bisson S, Orfanos CE. Successful outcome of cryosurgery in patients with granuloma annulare. *Br J Dermatol* 1994; 130: 494–7.

108 Wilkin JK, DuComb D, Castrow FF. Scarification treatment of granuloma annulare. *Arch Dermatol* 1982; 118: 68.

109 Baba T, Hoshion M, Uyeno K. Resolution of cutaneous lesions of granuloma annulare by intralesional injection of human fibroblast interferon. *Arch Dermatol* 1988; 124: 1015–16.

110 Simon M, von den Driesch P. Antimalarials for control of disseminated granuloma annulare in children. *J Am Acad Dermatol* 1994; 31: 1064–5.

111 Steiner A, Pehamberger H, Wolff K. Sulfone treatment of granuloma annulare. *J Am Acad Dermatol* 1985; 13: 1004–8.

112 Czarnecki DB, Gin D. The response of generalized granuloma annulare to dapsone. *Acta Derm Venereol* 1986; 66: 82–4.

113 Schleicher SM, Milstein HJ. Resolution of disseminated granuloma annulare following isotretinoin therapy. *Cutis* 1985; 36; 147–8.

114 Schleicher SM, Milstein HJ, Lim SJM. Resolution of disseminated granuloma annulare with isotretinoin. *Int J Dermatol* 1992; 31: 371–2.

115 Ratnavel RC, Norris PG. Perforating granuloma annulare: response to treatment with isotretinoin. *J Am Acad Dermatol* 1995; 32: 126–7.

116 Botella-Estrada R, Guillen C, Sanmartin O, Aliaga A. Disseminated granuloma annulare: resolution with etretinate therapy. *J Am Acad Dermatol* 1992; 26: 777–8.

117 Rubel DM, Wood G, Rosen R, Jopp-McKay A. Generalised granuloma annulare successfully treated with pentoxifylline. *Australas J Dermatol* 1993; 34: 103–8.

118 Ma A, Medenica M. Response of generalized granuloma annulare to high-dose niacinamide. *Arch Dermatol* 1983; 119: 836–9.

119 Gressel M, Graves K, Kalivas J. Treatment of disseminated granuloma annulare with potassium iodide. *Arch Dermatol* 1979; 115: 639–40.

120 Kerker BJ, Huang CP, Morison WL. Photochemotherapy of generalized granuloma annulare. *Arch Dermatol* 1990; 126: 359–61.

121 Hindson TC, Spiro JG, Cochrane H. PUVA therapy of diffuse granuloma annulare. *Clin Exp Dermatol* 1988; 13: 26–7.

122 Gupta AK, Ellis CN, Nickoloff BJ *et al*. Oral cyclosporine in the treatment of inflammatory and non-inflammatory dermatoses. *Arch Dermatol* 1990; 126: 339–50.

123 Filotico R, Vena GA, Coviello C, Angelini G. Cyclosporine in the treatment of generalized granuloma annulare. *J Am Acad Dermatol* 1994; 30: 487–8.

124 Kossard S, Winkelmann RK. Low-dose chlorambucil in the treatment of generalized granuloma annulare. *Dermatologica* 1979; 158: 443–50.

125 Patterson JW. Rheumatoid nodule and subcutaneous granuloma annulare. *Am J Dermatopathol* 1988; 10: 1–8.

126 Jorizzo JL, Olansky AJ, Stanley RJ. Superficial ulcerating necrobiosis in rheumatoid arthritis. *Arch Dermatol* 1982; 118: 255.

29.3 Knuckle Pads

ELAINE C. SIEGFRIED

Definition

Knuckle pads are defined by their clinical appearance. They are easily recognized, firm, well-defined thickenings of the skin that develop over the extensor aspects of any digital joint. The term 'knuckle pads' has been accepted for this condition, but synonyms include Garrod's nodes, helodermia, subcutaneous fibroma, keratosis, supracapitularis, discrete keratodermas, tylositas articuli and the French term coussinets des phalanges [1]. Age of onset, familial occurrence and associated abnormalities further subdivide knuckle pads into distinct categories.

History

Knuckle pads were recorded in painting and sculpture in ancient Greece and during the Renaissance, including a prominent lesion on the right thumb of Michelangelo's *David* [2]. This condition was first described in the medical literature by Garrod in 1893. Since that time, little insight has been gained into the pathophysiology of the disorder.

Aetiology

Reported cases of knuckle pads fall into three categories: idiopathic, familial and those associated with other fibrosing conditions [2–4]. Idiopathic and familial knuckle pads occur in childhood; onset is in adulthood for those with associated fibrosing diseases.

Clinicians frequently suspect repetitive trauma as the cause of knuckle pads; some authors refer to these as 'false' knuckle pads [5]. Examples are 'chewing pads', caused by a tic-like habit of chewing the dorsal aspects of the middle phalangeal joints [5], or knuckle pads related to occupational exposure [3,6]. A medical history and consistent distribution of lesions will usually support a suspicion of trauma. Knuckle pads have not been described as a common sign of compulsive habits or obsessional concerns [7]. In children, knuckle pads are most often sporadic and idiopathic [2,3].

Knuckle pads have been reported as an autosomal dominantly inherited condition [3,4]. The familial form can be isolated, or linked to other anomalies. Associated abnormalities limited to skin are palmoplantar keratoderma with or without ichthyosis vulgaris. Bart–Pumphry syndrome includes palmoplantar keratoderma, leuconychia, syndactyly and hearing loss (either sensorineural or mixed conductive and sensorineural). 'Breast cysts and cyst-like skin lesions' also occurred in one affected family [8], and amyotrophy in another [9]. Molecular analyses have not been done for this syndrome.

Knuckle pads in association with other fibrosing diseases occur in adulthood. This spectrum of abnormalities has been referred to as Touraine's polyfibromatosis. It can occur as a sporadic or familial condition, and includes Dupuytren's contracture (palmar fibromatosis), Peyronie's disease (penile fibromatosis), plantar nodules and aponeurotic fibrosis [8,10,11].

Pathology

Two different histological patterns of knuckle pads have been described, notably changes within the epidermis versus more prominent dermal pathology [3]. Conspicuous epidermal changes are more often seen in idiopathic knuckle pads of childhood. Skin biopsy specimens feature regular acanthosis and marked compact hyperkeratosis (Fig. 29.3.1). The histological features seen with Touraine's polyfibromatosis have been described as 'true fibroma', with proliferation of dermal fibroblasts and thickened, irregular collagen bundles under a hyperkeratotic epidermis [2,3,8]. Histological features have not been specifically described for autosomal dominant knuckle pads or the associated palmoplantar keratoderma [8].

Clinical features

The onset of knuckle pads is generally inconspicuous, occurring over a period of months or years. Idiopathic knuckle pads of childhood are most often reported in adolescence; onset may be earlier for familial forms. Knuckle pads are most commonly described over the dorsa of the proximal interphalangeal joints, but can occur over the dorsal aspects of any joints of the hands and feet [2]. The

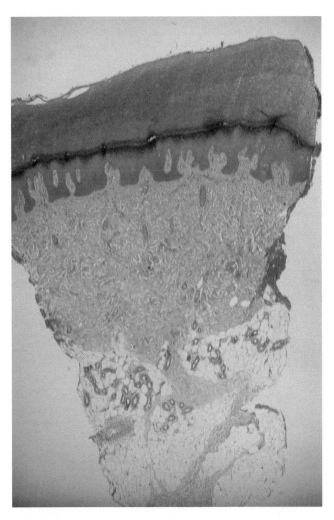

Fig. 29.3.1 This biopsy specimen was taken from the 14-year-old girl whose hand is pictured in Fig. 29.3.2. It reveals the typical histological features of idiopathic knuckle pads of childhood: regular acanthosis and marked compact hyperkeratosis (10× magnification).

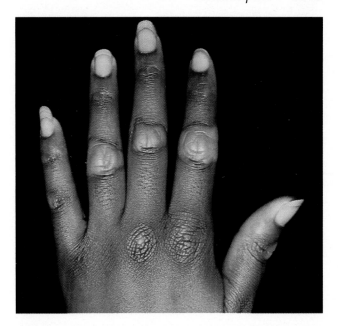

Fig. 29.3.2 This 14-year-old girl has idiopathic knuckle pads of childhood. Note the prominent hypopigmentation typically seen in dark-skinned patients.

Differential diagnosis

Knuckle pads should be distinguished from other cutaneous disorders, especially those with more ominous associations [3]. A medical history, physical examination and skin biopsy are usually sufficient to make the correct diagnosis. In children, the differential diagnosis includes: callosities, hypertrophic scars, deep granuloma annulare, rheumatoid nodules, Gottren's papules, the cutaneous lesions of Farber's disease (lipogranulomatosis) and the scar-like changes that can be seen with erythropoietic protoporphyria, epidermolysis bullosa acquisita or dystrophic forms of hereditary epidermolysis bullosa [3,13].

Treatment

For conditions with no uniformly successful therapy, the benefits of treatment must outweigh the risks. In addition, a period of watchful waiting is reasonable for conditions that may show spontaneous improvement. People with knuckle pads should be alerted to the possible exacerbating role of trauma, and the potential benefit of protective measures. Motivated patients may choose from a variety of more proactive therapeutic options. Those with primarily epidermal lesions may benefit from the use of topical keratolytic agents such as α-hydroxy acids, salicylic acid or urea, with or without occlusion. Topical calcipotriol has been used with success in some forms of ichthyosis, and may be considered [14,15]. Knuckle pads that exhibit primarily dermal pathology may respond to corticosteroids; intralesional steroids are appropriate only for assenting

lesions are flat or convex with a slightly rough surface. They may have prominent pigment change in people with darker type IV or V skin (Fig. 29.3.2). A possibly related, idiopathic variant has been described that involves lateral, rather than dorsal aspects of the proximal interphalangeal joints, dubbed 'pachydermodactyly' [12]. People with the familial form may also have thickened plaques over the knees and elbows [3]. Knuckle pads are usually asymptomatic, but can be disfiguring.

Prognosis

There is no uniformly successful treatment for knuckle pads. Lesions usually persist for several years, or remain indefinitely, but spontaneous resolution has been reported [3].

patients, generally adolescents or older. Potent topical steroids under occlusion are easier to administer, but their use must be carefully monitored. Silicone gel dressings have been successfully used to shrink hypertrophic scars and keloids, and are another safe, painless therapeutic option [16,17].

REFERENCES

1 Mackey SL, Cobb MW. Knuckle pads. *Cutis* 1994; 54: 159–60.
2 Nahass GT, Goldstein BA, Zhu W, Serfling U, Penneys NS, Leonardi CL. Comparison of Tzanck smear, viral culture, and DNA diagnostic methods in detection of herpes simplex and varicella-zoster infection. *J Am Med Assoc* 1992; 268: 2541–4.
3 Paller AS, Herbert AA. Knuckle pads in children. *Am J Dis Child* 1986; 140: 915–17.
4 Kodama BF, Gentry RH, Fitzpatrick JE. Papules and plaques over the joint spaces. *Arch Dermatol* 1993; 129: 1044–7.
5 Meigel WN, Plewig G. Chewing pads, a variant of knuckle pads. *Hautarzt* 1976; 27: 391–5 (in German).
6 Richards TB, Gamble JF, Castellan RM, Mathias CG. Knuckle pads in live-chicken hangers. *Contact Derm* 1987; 17: 13–16.
7 Stein DJ, Hollander E. Dermatology and conditions related to obsessive–compulsive disorder. *J Am Acad Dermatol* 1992; 26: 237–42.
8 Ramer JC, Vasily DB, Ladda RL. Familial leuconychia, knuckle pads, hearing loss, and palmoplantar hyperkeratosis: an additional family with Bart–Pumphrey syndrome. *J Med Genet* 1994; 31: 68–71.
9 Jacyk WK, Bill PL. Palmoplantar keratoderma with amyotrophy. *Dermatologica* 1988; 176: 251–6.
10 Wooldridge WE. Four related fibrosing diseases. When you find one, look for another. *Postgrad Med* 1988; 84: 269–71.
11 Gonzalez SM, Gonzalez RI. Dupuytren's disease. *Western J Med* 1990; 152: 430–3.
12 Perez B, Gomez MI, Sanchez E, Munoz E, Ledo A. Pachydermodactyly: a case report. *J Dermatol* 1995; 22: 43–5.
13 Amirhakimi GH, Haghighi P, Ghalambor MA, Honari S. Familial lipogranulomatosis (Farber's disease). *Clin Genet* 1976; 9: 625–30.
14 Delfino M, Fabbrocini G, Sammarco EM, Santoianni P. Efficacy of calcipotriol versus lactic acid cream in the treatment of lamellar and X-linked ichthyoses. *J Dermatol Treat* 1994; 5: 151–2.
15 Russell S, Young MJ. Hypercalcemia during treatment of psoriasis with calcipotriol. *Br J Dermatol* 1994; 130: 795–6.
16 Dockery GL, Nilson RZ. Treatment of hypertrophic and keloid scars with silastic gel sheeting. *J Foot Ankle Surg* 1994; 33: 110–19.
17 Rusciani L, Rossi G, Bono R. Use of cryotherapy in the treatment of keloids. *J Dermatol Surg Oncol* 1993; 19: 529–34.

29.4 Striae

FREDERIC CAMBAZARD AND JEAN-LOÏC MICHEL

Definition

Striae are well-defined linear atrophic skin lesions secondary to connective tissue alterations. They are most often located on the hips or breasts and appear during puberty or pregnancy [1].

History

Cutaneous striae were first described by Roederer in 1773. They are common, benign, asymptomatic skin manifestations with principally an aesthetic consequence. Many groups have been defined, based on clinical manifestations (striae albae, atrophicae, distensae, rubrae, lineae or atrophia lineares—striata, or atrophoderma striatum, or lineae atrophicae—distensae) or on aetiological factors (striae adolescentium, gravidarum) [2]. The first histological descriptions of striae were made by Troisier and Ménétrier in 1889 and later by Unna in 1894. Striae were described by Cushing in his first description of Cushing's syndrome. He pointed out the action of steroid hormones in the pathogenesis of striae [3].

Aetiology

Striae are due to a breaking of dermal connective tissue, with initially an inflammatory reaction. This break may be secondary to biochemical or mechanical factors, although a genetic predisposition also plays an important role [4]. Steroid hormones and skin distension are the main aetiological factors [1].

Sex

Striae are found in more than 40% of the population. Sometimes very discrete, they are often unrecognized. Striae are more often found in women (60–80%) [2,5] than in men (10–30%) [5,6]. Pregnancy explains this difference, but also physiological hormones [7]. Striae are twice as frequent in girls than in boys [8,9].

Ethnic background

Striae are more frequent in Caucasian and red-haired individuals than in those with dark-skin, being rare in Asian or black people.

Age

Striae develop usually between 5 and 49 years of age [10–12]. They do not occur in the elderly. Striae are seen in young adolescents, but their frequency increases with age in particular at the beginning of adulthood. While only 8% of adolescents of both sexes have striae, they are present in up to 80% of women between 22 and 41 years of age [2]. In childhood striae are commonly due to steroid therapy [13,14]. Steroid therapy induces more striae during puberty than would normally be expected. Pathological states, such as ascites or pleural-pulmonary lesions, lead to more striae in younger patients than in adults [15].

Puberty

Puberty and accelerated growth are the main physiological factors. In adolescents, striae appear when the secondary sexual characteristics develop [9]. Striae can be observed in girls at 9 or 10 years of age. So in girls they can be present before menarche and before the development of axillary hair. In prepubertal boys, striae rarely occur. Most often in boys, striae appear after the development of pubic hair. In male adolescents between 14 and 20 years of age, striae are mainly located on the hips. However, in girls (between 12 and 16 years of age) striae are present on the breasts, hips or thighs [9].

No direct relationship with obesity or rapid body growth exists [6]. Striae do correlate with severity of acne vulgaris. Acne develops in 47% of adolescents with striae and in only 9% in adolescents without striae [9].

Pregnancy [16,17]

Striae formation during pregnancy confirms the pathogenesis of these skin lesions. More than 90% of females have striae during pregnancy, mainly during the last trimester. In this period, the level of corticosteroids rises, especially after the seventh month of gestation. There is also a relationship between striae and facial acne during pregnancy.

Striae are not dependent solely on the increase of the abdominal girth. Striae largely depend on the patient's individual condition with a familial predisposition. Women with a greater weight gain, primigravida and younger pregnant women are more prone to striae than others. The pre-existence of acne or striae during adolescence are predictive signs of developing lesions during pregnancy. Striae are rarer in older primigravidas than in younger mothers. In multigravidas, new striae are less numerous in already involved areas, but may occur in new anatomical sites and the number of striae increases with the number of pregnancies.

Corticosteroids

The role of corticosteroids in striae formation during puberty or pregnancy is confirmed by the relation between the daily urinary excretion of 17 ketosteroids and striae [18].

The role of steroids as an intrinsic aetiological factor is observed in Cushing's syndrome [3]. Striae are side-effects of systemic treatment with corticosteroids, or adrenocorticotrophic hormone (ACTH), particularly during adolescence. Dexamethasone given in adolescence for congenital adrenal hyperplasia may induce striae [19,20]. The relationship between the topical use of corticosteroids and the local development of striae is also well known [21–25] in particular during puberty. Then striae appear within a few weeks to 3 months [10,12–14,26–31]. Striae are seen in unusual places, such as the face [32], axillae [33] and limbs [32,34]. Pre-existing striae will become bigger. Sometimes striae occur in areas distant from the topical site of application. Complications such as ulceration [32] or skin rupture may occur with protrusion of adipose tissue [35] or peritoneous fistula [36] during steroid therapy. Striae are more frequently caused by external application of creams or ointments than by injections. Injections more often cause cutaneous atrophy. Potent corticosteroids are more likely to produce striae. Long-term treatment, occlusion with plastic film, application in thin and deep cutaneous folds or on a pre-existing pathological skin that increase steroid cutaneous absorption, favour the development of striae [34]. Anabolic steroids may also induce striae [37].

Mechanical factors

Increase in skin tension is another pathogenic factor in striae formation [38]. Skin distension may be slow and progressive (with a smaller probability of the development of striae) [15] or more suddenly as in a growth spurt during puberty or in pregnancy. In pregnancy, striae occur first on the abdomen and thighs and then on the breasts [16]. The size of the breast is less important than the stretching of the skin during pregnancy. Striae appear more readily on the hips than on the abdomen. Biochemical properties show an increased skin extensibility in women [39] (compared to men) which decreases after the age of 20 years [7].

Exaggerated muscular activities, such as lifting of weights or other sports (such as seen in basketball or football players) can induce striae [40]. The regular practice of sport or physical exercise rarely induces striae. More unusual mechanical causes such as oedema, ascites, subcutaneous tumours or incorrect posture may favour striae formation.

Obesity acts on striae only in puberty [9] or with steroid involvement [41,42] and striae are absent in markedly obese preadolescent boys and girls. Obese patients who have abdominal striae have a urinary level of 17 ketosteroids twice that found in normal individuals [41]. In obese individuals, striae often appear in other less frequent areas, such as the arms, forearms, abdomen and groin. No relationship was found between striae and diabetes or glucose tolerance.

Other aetiological factors [2]

Striae may also occur with low-calorie and low-protein diets (intense slimming diets, undernourished refugees), caused by deficient synthesis of the connective tissue. In chronic infectious and consumptive diseases, such as tuberculosis, typhoid fever, typhus, tonsillitis, meningitis, scarlet fever, Hodgkin's disease and others, striae develop due to the same cause. In these circumstances, higher steroid secretion is observed and considered as the main factor. Other contributive factors are weight variations, cachexia, higher circulating levels of sexual hormones in chronic liver diseases and sometimes bacteriological toxins.

Pathogenesis

Striae are the result of breaks in the connective tissue. This mechanical factor is underlined by the involved sites and direction of the striae in the tension lines of the skin. Often striae appear at sites with a large concentration of adipose cells that diminish the union between the skin and the surrounding tissues. Striae never occur on the hands or feet, face or extensor surfaces of the limbs. In these areas, deep dermis is filled by dense bundles of collagen, diminishing skin mobility and increasing skin resistance. The relationship between striae and adipose tissue explain the greater incidence in females, the different topography in males and females and the absence of striae during childhood. Collagen fibres are implicated in the development of striae. The intensity of the cross-linking of peptide chains of collagen, which increases with age, augment the cutaneous resistance to damage [15]. The lack of cross-linking causes excessive elasticity and facilitates the rupture of fibres if the traction is too intensive.

Striae may be a consequence of local trauma, repeated cutaneous incision [43,44] and localized cutaneous stretching. Mechanical factors are not sufficient by themselves to explain striae. This is illustrated with skin expanders [45]. These silastic subcutaneous envelopes are filled with increasing amounts of fluid to expand the skin. This therapeutic manoeuvre lasts several weeks. Striae almost never develop [46]. The genetic constitution of connective tissue also interferes with the development of striae [47]. Individual susceptibility is of some influence. Some children are more predisposed to develop striae and their constitutional alteration may not be clinically detectable. Striae have been described in a prepubertal girl in association with anetoderma and pilomatricoma [48]. Striae are included in well-defined genetic diseases, such as Marfan's syndrome [49–56], pseudoxanthoma elasticum [57] or Buschke–Ollendorff syndrome. However, in some diseases such as in Ehlers–Danlos syndrome, striae are rare even during pregnancy, because cutaneous extensibility limits any destruction of connective tissue.

Major intrinsic factors for striae development are adrenal activity or steroid treatment. Steroids induce atrophy of the epidermis and dermis, reduce fibroblasts, adipose tissue and skin appendages [21]. They alter the synthesis of fibroblasts, the collagen fibres and ground substance formation. They increase synthesis of non-sulphated glycosaminoglycans reducing the cohesion of collagen fibrils and with their catabolic action, collagen type I disappears, leaving only type III.

Pathology

Histopathological findings are sometimes contradictory, depending on the different staining techniques and the evolution of the striae. Many authors believe that striae are a type of skin scar representing the healed stage of earlier disintegration of connective tissue [58–60].

The epidermis is still normal in the early stages, and later atrophic. The stratum granulosum may disappear. The rete ridges are shortened with a straightened dermoepidermal junction. Melanin is absent but increased in the surrounding basal layer. Keratinocytes cultured from striae have a lower survival rate [61].

The dermis is thinned by up to 50% or even absent, with alterations of elastic and collagen fibres. Sometimes electron microscopy shows no abnormalities [58]. Coarse, thin, curly and clustered elastic fibres are observed in the borders of the striae. Alterations begin in the deep dermis. In older lesions, elastic fibres may be totally absent [13], or may have a normal structure [58], or may be immature

with an insufficient protein matrix. They appear thinned and agglomerated in a linear arrangement with scanning microscopy. There is also neosynthesis of new elastic fibres in later lesions [52,58,62,63].

The collagen fibres are also altered with dense groups of straight fine bundles of collagen arranged in a parallel disposition to the epidermis [58]. Fibrils with a thinner diameter [59] than normal fibrils have a perpendicular disposition to the direction of the stria [64] and collagen bundles may be stretched or fragmented [59,60].

The fibroblasts are often quiescent [59]. Ground substance is abundant with vascular ectasia, haemorrhage and a perivascular cellular infiltrate with lymphocytes, monocytes, macrophages and occasionally increased mast cells [65]. Arterioles and venules are arranged in parallel to the collagen fibres.

Hair follicles, sweat and sebaceous glands may be deformed or destroyed. Connective tissue alterations may extend to normal skin around the striae from 0.5 to 3 cm with a sharp demarcation from normal skin. This may be caused by inflammation and degranulation of mast cells, leading to regeneration of elastic and collagen fibres, directed to the mechanical force [38,58,60].

Clinical features

Striae are well-defined atrophic skin lesions. The lesions are often inflammatory at the beginning (Fig. 29.4.1). They form linear, papular, smooth, red or purple, sometimes pruritic or sensitive, well-demarcated skin lesions. Exceptionally, lesions may be ecchymotic. During steroid therapy, striae are more red and larger (Fig. 29.4.2). This inflammatory phase is sometimes not observed. It usually lasts from a few months to 1 or 2 years. Then the red coloration disappears and hypertrophic striae evolve to a plane and later depressed skin lesion [66]. This 'scarring' process leads to a pearly white, rarely pigmented lesion

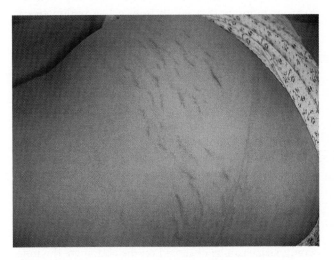

Fig. 29.4.1 Typical early red striae during puberty.

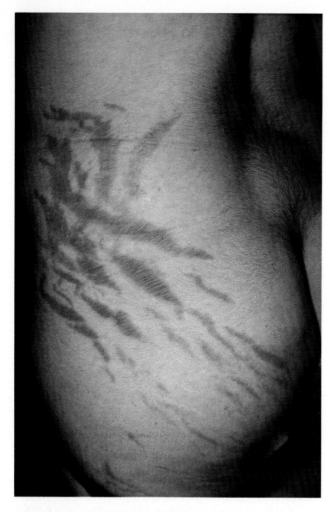

Fig. 29.4.2 Large and red striae during systemic steroid therapy.

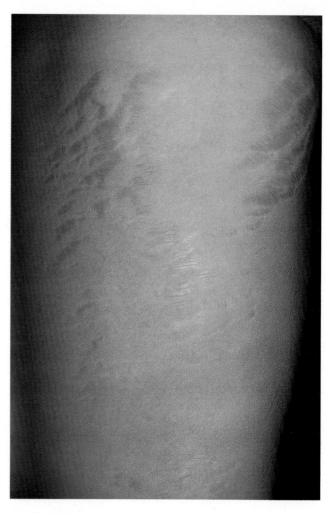

Fig. 29.4.3 White striae atrophica.

with a soft surface and small wrinkles across to the axis of the stria [67] (Fig. 29.4.3). On the striae hairs are atrophic and there is no sebum secretion.

The length of each stria varies from a few millimetres to 20 cm or more, with a width from a few millimetres to a few centimetres. Striae are multiple, linear, sometimes undulated, rarely circular, grouped with a parallel disposition in the same body place. They occur symmetrically in some specific anatomical areas. Striae follow Langer's lines that form the cleavage lines of the skin: they are perpendicular to the axes of skin tension [38]. Involved areas are always the same: hips (transverse direction); buttocks (striae oblique from the external superior quadrant to the inferior internal quadrant); lumbosacral region (transverse direction); breasts (with a radiated disposition from the nipple); and shoulders (oblique direction). In women, striae are found on the hips, abdomen and breasts, while in men they predominate on the lumbosacral area (52%), the outer side of thighs and the hips (29%). Less commonly, striae can be observed on the abdomen, the inner side of the thighs or very rarely on the neck, axillae or

limbs [68]. On the abdomen, vertical striae, and around the navel concentric striae, are observed. On the limbs, striae are transverse during longitudinal growth and longitudinal if growth is circumferential. If caused by systemic steroid therapy, striae are predominately on the abdomen and hips.

Prognosis

Striae always tend to improve with time, as they become narrower and far less obvious. Even if they persist throughout life they become much more discrete. Unusual complications include acute oedema [69] (during ascites), ulceration [32], skin rupture with protrusion of adipose tissue [35] and peritoneal fistula [36], but always secondary to treatment with systemic or topical steroids [32,36] or etretinate [35], in addition to mechanical factors on pre-existing striae.

Dermatoses such as bullous impetigo, psoriasis or other inflammatory skin diseases can begin inside the striae. This phenomenon has also been observed in pruritic urticarial papules and plaques in pregnancy. A possible explanation may be a more sensitive and less resistant skin [70–72].

Differential diagnosis

Striae usually do not mimic other skin diseases. However, striae are sometimes unusual and atypical, red and papular, but their disposition and context of occurrence make the diagnosis simple. In older lesions, linear scars must be differentiated from striae for sometimes legal reasons [73]. However, scars do not have the same distribution, and are associated with the notion of pre-existing trauma. Scars are also firm and not soft as are striae.

Linear focal elastosis is an entity described in 1989 by Burket *et al.* [74] that looks like dorsolumbar striae [75–79]. However, this disease occurs in elderly white men and the lesions are raised and yellow, without any of the usual aetiological factors of striae. Histological findings are completely different and include a thickened dermis with basophilic and fragmented elastic fibres and normal collagen fibres. An exceptional case of linear focal elastosis was described in a young black man who had been aware of these lesions since early childhood [80].

Primary or secondary anetoderma and skin lesions of pseudoxanthoma elasticum do not have the same clinical manifestations.

In extreme cases, Cushing's syndrome must be considered, but this is rarely the cause.

Treatment and prognosis

Multiple topical treatments have been proposed to prevent or cure striae [81], but their effects are difficult to prove, because such skin lesions also spontaneously improve. Aetiological factors should be eliminated such as Cushing's syndrome and iatrogenic effects of topical steroids (especially during puberty). Topical treatments that have been tried, are hydroxyproline precursors, collagen derivates, vitamin E and others. Topical tretinoin has been used with a significant improvement in 15 of 16 patients who completed the study, but local tolerance was often difficult [82]. There is no proved effective measure to prevent or cure striae. Aesthetic aspects of striae spontaneously improve after a few years. Therefore, in most cases the prognosis is good.

REFERENCES

1 Moretti G, Rebora AA, Guarrera M. Striae distensae: how and why they are formed. In: Moretti G, Rebora AA, eds. *Striae Distensae*. Milan: Brocades, 1976: 9.
2 Bittencourt-Sampaio S. *Striae Atrophicae*. Rio de Janeiro: ZMF Editora, 1995.
3 Cushing H. The basophil adenomas of the pituitary body and their clinical manifestations. *Johns Hopkins Hosp Bull* 1932; 1: 137–95.
4 De Lacharriere O. Vergetures. *Encyl Med Chir (Paris, France) Dermatologie* 12640 A⁴⁰, 7, 1988.
5 Bismark HD. Zur Konstitutionellen Bedeutung der striae cutis atrophicae. *Med Klin* 1967; 62: 51–3.
6 Elton RF, Pinkus H. Striae in normal men. *Arch Dermatol* 1966; 94: 33–4.
7 Berardesca E, Gabba P, Farinelli N, Borroni G, Rabbiosi G. Skin extensibility time in women. Changes in relation to sex hormones. *Acta Derm Venereol* 1989; 69: 431–3.
8 Larsson PA, Liden S. Prevalence of skin diseases among adolescents 12–16 years of age. *Acta Derm Venereol* 1980; 60: 415–23.
9 Sisson WR. Colored striae in adolescent children. *J Pediatr* 1954; 45: 520–30.
10 Meara RH. Atrophic striae following topical fluocinolone therapy. *Br J Dermatol* 1964; 76: 481–2.
11 Behl PN, Sehgal VK, Sood NK. Striae atrophicae: a clinicopathological study. *Int J Dermatol Venereol Lepro* 1974; 40: 236–9.
12 Gschwandtner WR. Striae cutis atrophicae nach lokalbehandlung mit corticosteroiden. *Hautarzt* 1973; 24: 70–3.
13 Chernosky ME, Knox JM. Atrophic striae after occlusive corticosteroid therapy. *Arch Dermatol* 1964; 90: 15–19.
14 Grupper C, Segal M. Vergetures purpuriques après corticothérapie locale sous traitement occlusif. *Bull Soc Fr Dermatol Syph* 1964; 71: 479–82.
15 Shuster S. The cause of striae distensae. *Acta Dermatol Venereol (Stockh)* 1979; 59 (suppl 85): 161–9.
16 Esteve E, Saudeau L, Pierre F, Barruet K, Vaillant L, Lorette G. Signes cutanés physiologiques au cours de la grossesse normale: étude de 60 femmes enceintes. *Ann Derm Venereol* 1994; 121: 227–31.
17 Marin AG, Leal-Khouri S. Physiologic skin changes associated with pregnancy. *Int J Dermatol* 1992; 31: 375–8.
18 Shirai Y. Studies on striae cutis of puberty. *Hiroshima J Med Sci* 1959; 8: 215–22.
19 Gardner LI, Morillo E. Striae as complication of one dose dexamethasone therapy of virilizing adrenal hyperplasia. *Pediatr Res* 1980; 14: 478 (abstract).
20 Guest G, Rappaport R, Philippe F, Thibaud E. Survenue de vergetures graves chez des adolescents atteints d'hyperplasie surrénale congénitale par defaut de 21-hydroxylation et traités par la dexaméthasone. *Arch Fr Pediatr* 1983; 40: 453–6.
21 Calnan CD. Use and abuse of topical steroids. *Dermatologica* 1976; 152 (suppl 1): 247–51.
22 Morman MR. Possible side effects of topical steroids. *Am Fam Phys* 1981; 23: 171–4.
23 Harris DWS, Hunter JAA. The use and abuse of 0.05 per cent clobetasol propionate in dermatology. *Dermatol Clin* 1988; 6: 643–7.
24 Goa KL. Clinical pharmacology and pharmacokinetic properties of topically applied corticosteroids. A review. *Drugs* 1988; 36 (suppl 5): 51–61.
25 Mills CM, Marks R. Side effects of topical glucocorticoids. *Curr Prob Dermatol* 1993; 21: 122–31.
26 Bazex A, Salvador R, Dupre A, Parant M, Christol B. Vergetures pourpres transversales de la face antérieure des cuisses chez un psoriasique traité, par corticoides sous pansement occlusif. *Bull Soc Fr Dermatol Syph* 1964; 71: 197–8.
27 Adam JE, Craig C. Striae and their relation to topical steroid therapy. *Canad Med Assoc J* 1965; 92: 289–91.
28 Bureau Y, Barriére H, Litoux P, Bureau B. Vergetures pourpres secondaires à l'application prolongée et étendue d'une créme aux corticoides. *Bull Soc Fr Dermatol Syph* 1967; 74: 498–501.
29 Michel PJ, Cretin J, Campagni JP. Un cas de vergetures de la partie supéro-interne des deux cuisses après corticothérapie locale prolongée. *Bull Soc Fr Dermatol Syph* 1969; 76: 899.
30 Depaoli M. Strie atrophiche cutanee da corticoterapia locale. *Minerva Med* 1970; 61: 2773–7.
31 Barkey WF. Striae and persistent tinea corporis related to prolonged use of betamethasone dipropionate 0.05% cream/clotrimazole 1% cream (Lotrisone cream). *J Am Acad Dermatol* 1987; 17: 518–19.
32 Stroud JD, Van Dersal JV. Striae. *Arch Dermatol* 1971; 103: 103–4.
33 Sörensen GW, Odom RB. Axillary and inguinal striae induced by systemic absorption of a topical corticosteroid. *Cutis* 1976; 17: 355–7.
34 Resina O, Gago IS, Montes B, Castro R. Estrias atroficas. *Acta Dermo Sif* 1975; 66: 293–304.
35 Bordier C, Flechet ML, Thomine E, Lauret P. Rupture de vergetures au cours d'un psoriasis pustuleux traité, par étrétinate (Tigason). *Ann Dermatol Vénéréol* 1984; 111: 929–31.
36 Lawrence SH, Salkin D, Schwartz JA, Fortner HC. Rupture of abdominal wall through stria distensa during cortisone therapy. *J Am Med Assoc* 1953; 152: 1526–7.

37 Scott MJ, Scott AM. Effects of anabolic-androgenic steroids on the pilosebaceous unit. *Cutis* 1992; 50: 113–16.

38 Agache P, Ovide MT, Kienzler JL, Laurent R. Mechanical factors in striae distensae. In: Moretti G, Rebora AA, eds. *Striae Distensae*. Milan: Brocades, 1976: 87.

39 Pierard GE, Lapiére CM. Physiopathological variations in the mechanical properties of skin. *Arch Dermatol Res* 1977; 260: 231–9.

40 Levine N. Dermatologic aspects of sports medicine. *J Am Acad Dermatol* 1980; 3: 415–24.

41 Simkin B, Arce R. Steroid excretion in obese patients with colored abdominal stria. *N Engl J Med* 1962; 266: 1031–5.

42 Gogate AN, Prunty FTG. Adrenal cortical function in 'obesity with pink stria' in the young adults. *J Clin Endocrinol Metab* 1963; 23: 747–51.

43 Okamoto J, Onizuka T. Skin striae due to serial excisions of scar. *Jpn J Plast Surg* 1977; 20: 129–33.

44 Ono T, Matsunaga W, Yoshimura K. Striae distensae after tension-requiring skin sutures. *J Dermatol* 1991; 18: 47–51.

45 Marcus J, Horan DB, Robinson JK. Tissue expansion: past, present and future. *J Am Acad Dermatol* 1990; 23: 813–25.

46 Antonyshyn O, Gruss JS, Mackinnon SE, Zuker R. Complications of soft tissue expansion. *Br J Plast Surg* 1988; 41: 239–50.

47 Pottkotter L, Pyeritz RE, Glesby MJ. Striae and systemic abnormalities of connective tissue. *J Am Med Assoc* 1989; 262: 3132.

48 Jones CC, Tschen JA. Anetodermic cutaneous changes overlying pilomatricomas. *J Am Acad Dermatol* 1991; 25: 1072–6.

49 Loveman AB, Gordon AM, Fliegelman MT. Marfan's syndrome. Some cutaneous aspects. *Arch Dermatol* 1963; 87: 428–35.

50 Morita H. A case report of Marfan's syndrome with striae atrophicae. *Jap J Dermatol* 1964; 74: 107.

51 Moretti G, Le Coulant P, Staeffen J, Catanzano G, Brouset A. La peau dans le syndrome de Marfan. *Presse Med* 1964; 72: 2985–90.

52 Pinkus H, Keech MK, Mehregan AH. Histopathology of striae distensae with special reference to striae and wound healing in the Marfan syndrome. *J Invest Dermatol* 1966; 46: 283–92.

53 Cohen PR, Schneiderman P. Clinical manifestations of the Marfan syndrome. *Int J Dermatol* 1989; 28: 291–9.

54 Cabré J, Gonzalez JA, Lacombe JAS, Vidal J. Manifestaciones cutaneas del sindrome de Marfan. *Actas Dermo Sif* 1973; 64: 9–10.

55 Glesby MJ, Pyeritz RE. Association of mitral valve prolapse and systemic abnormalities of connective tissue. A phenotypic continuum. *J Am Med Assoc* 1989; 262: 523–8.

56 Herman KL, Salman K, Rose LI. White forelock in Marfan's syndrome: an unusual association with review of the literature. *Cutis* 1991; 48: 82–4.

57 Viljoen DL, Beatty S, Beighton P. The obstetric and gynaecological implications of pseudoxanthoma elasticum. *Br J Obstet Gynecol* 1987; 94: 884–8.

58 Zheng P, Lavker RM, Kligman AM. Anatomy of striae. *Br J Dermatol* 1985; 112: 185–93.

59 Pieraggi MT, Julian M, Delmas M, Bouissou H. Striae: morphological aspects of connective tissue. *Virch Arch Pathol Anat* 1982; 396: 279–89.

60 Arem AJ, Kischer CW. Analysis of striae. *Plast Reconstr Surg* 1980; 65: 22–9.

61 Klehr N. Striae cutis atrophicae: morphokinetic examination in vitro. *Acta Derm Venereol* 1979; 59: 105–8.

62 Breathnach AS. Ultrastructure of epidermis and dermis in striae atrophicae. In: Moretti G, Rebora AA, eds. *Striae Distensae*. Milan: Brocades, 1976: 35.

63 Tsuji T, Sawabe M. Elastic fibers in striae distensae. *J Cutan Pathol* 1988; 15: 215–22.

64 De Pasquale V, Franchi M, Govoni P *et al*. Striae albae: a morphological study on the human skin. *Basic Appl Histochem* 1987; 31: 475–86.

65 Sheu HM, Yu HS, Chang CH. Mast cell degranulation and elastolysis in the early stage of striae distensae. *J Cutan Pathol* 1991; 18: 410–16.

66 Nigam PK. Striae cutis distensae. *Int J Dermatol* 1989; 28: 426–8.

67 Tsuji T, Sawabe M. Hyperpigmentation in striae distensae after bleomycin treatment. *J Am Acad Dermatol* 1993; 28: 503–5.

68 Basak P, Dhar S, Kanwar AJ. Involvement of the legs in idiopathic striae distensae. A case report. *Indian J Dermatol* 1989; 34: 21–2.

69 Peterson JL, McMarlin SL, Read SI. Edematous striae distensae. *Arch Dermatol* 1984; 120: 1097–8.

70 Bronstein SW, Bickers DR, Lamkin BC. Bullous dermatosis caused by *Staphylococcus aureus* in locus minoris resistentiae. *J Am Acad Dermatol* 1984; 10: 259–63.

71 Zeulke R, Rapini R, Puhl S, Ray T. Dermatitis in locus minoris resistentiae. *J Am Acad Dermatol* 1982; 6: 1010–13.

72 Ford MJ, Gammon WR, Kilpatrick TM. Pustular eruption of the striae in a primigravida. *Cutis* 1992; 50: 225–8.

73 Davies H. Adolescent lumbar striae mistaken for non-accident injury. *Police Surg* 1985; 27: 72–6.

74 Burket JM, Zelickson AS, Padilla RS. Linear focal elastosis (elastotic striae). *J Am Acad Dermatol* 1989; 20: 633–6.

75 Linn HW. Transverse striae atrophicae of the back. *Aust J Dermatol* 1968; 9: 352–3.

76 Carr RD, Hamilton JF. Transverse striae of the back. *Arch Dermatol* 1969; 99: 26–30.

77 Schnitzler L, Paumard M. Stries dorso-lombaires des sujets jeunes, a type de vergetures. *Bull Soc Fr Dermatol Syph* 1971; 78: 253–5.

78 Cabré J. Estrias atroficas dorso-lumbares en un adolescente. *Actas Dermo Sif* 1973; 64: 537–42.

79 McKusick VA. Transverse striae distensae in the lumbar area in father and two sons. *Birth Defects* 1971; 7: 260–1.

80 Moiin A, Hashimoto K. Linear focal elastosis in a young black man: a new presentation. *J Am Acad Dermatol* 1994; 30: 874–7.

81 Mallol J, Belda MA, Costa D, Noval A, Sola M. Prophylaxis of striae gravidarum with a topical formulation. A double blind trial. *Int J Cosmet Sci* 1991; 13: 51–7.

82 Elson ML. Treatment of striae distensae with topical tretinoin. *J Dermatol Surg Oncol* 1990; 16: 267–70.

Hyperhidrosis

CHANTAL DANGOISSE AND MICHELINE SONG

Definition

Hyperhidrosis is a common and distressing clinical condition, characterized by an excessive production of sweat by the eccrine sweat glands.

Aetiology [1–3]

The eccrine sweat glands are distributed over the whole skin surface, excluding the mucosae. Their number is estimated at 2–5 million [4]. The density of eccrine glands varies according to site; they are most numerous on the palms, soles, forehead and in the axillae [5]. Eccrine glands are composed of simple tubular ducts which descend the epidermis to the mid and deep dermis, and to the hypodermis, where they coil in a nest-like arrangement (Fig. 29.5.1). The components of the eccrine glands are the sweat pore on the skin surface, a wavy ascending transdermal and transepidermal duct and the secretory coil in the lower dermis, with its rich vascular supply and innervation (Fig. 29.5.2). The duct consists of several layers of cuboidal cells which are metabolically active. The secretory coil is composed of two types of cells: large clear cells which are secretory and small dark cells of unknown function. The clear cells are surrounded by myoepithelial cells, smooth muscle-like cells whose contraction causes the expulsion of the sweat. These cells also provide resistance to the important osmotic gradient at this level.

Each gland receives a unique arteriole which divides into two to four branches and gives rise to numerous capillaries (around 1500 per gland) surrounding the secretory coil. The glands also receive rich innervation from sympathetic postganglionic cholinergic nerves, which consist of non-myelinated class C nerve fibres. The fibres are derived from the premotor area of the cortex and act as a relay in the anterior hypothalamus, bulb and spinal cord before arriving at the eccrine glands [6]. Acetylcholine is the main neurotransmitter.

The role of the eccrine sweat gland is to generate sweat from plasma. A nervous or pharmacological stimulus induces secretion of acetylcholine around the clear cells. As a consequence, there is a change in the permeability of the cellular membrane, with passive redistribution of potassium ions, an increase in intracytoplasmic sodium and active secretion of sodium in the intercellular canaliculi. In addition, the work of Sato showed that calcium flux plays a central and essential part in the stimulation of active sweat secretion [1]. The sweat duct also has intense metabolic activity and the capacity of reabsorbing sodium ions.

The secretion of eccrine sweat glands is intermittent. Under basal conditions, only water (as vapour) is emitted, corresponding to the insensible perspiration or transepidermal water loss which is independent of nervous control. Real sweat is produced when the eccrine sweat gland is stimulated by various stimuli.

Mental stimuli

Mental stimuli originates in the corticosuperior centres. They induce sweating on the forehead, palms and soles without any vasodilatation. Emotional sweating is induced by fear, anxiety and embarrassment.

Hypothalamic stimuli

Central stimuli occurring in the hypothalamus where the heat-regulating centre is situated, induce generalized hyperhidrosis, except of the palms and soles. Anoxia, hypoglycaemia and increase in blood temperature represent central stimuli. The heat-regulating centre is activated by changes in the temperature of the perfusing blood, hormones, circulatory changes, as well as by axon and spinal reflexes.

Gustatory stimuli

Gustatory sweating occurs in many normal individuals on the lips, face and nose after eating, especially when the food is hot and spicy. The central connections of this reflex are not fully known.

The major function of the eccrine sweat gland is thermal regulation. The preoptic hypothalamic area plays an essential part in the regulation of body temperature. The elevation of hypothalamic temperature, associated with

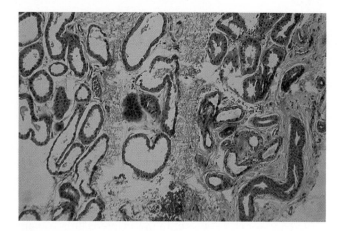

Fig. 29.5.1 Eccrine sweat glands in the mid dermis.

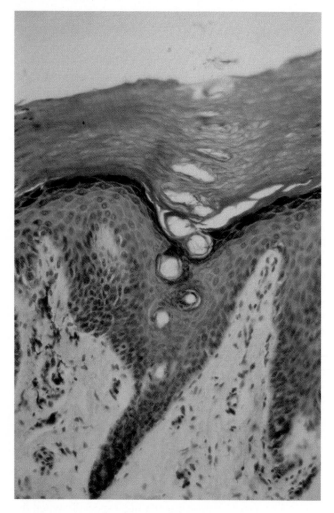

Fig. 29.5.2 Wavy transepidermal eccrine duct.

an increase in body temperature, provides the strongest stimulus for thermoregulatory sweat excretion. Thus, generalized hyperhidrosis is a physiological process which occurs during vigorous physical exercise, in obese individuals, and when the environmental temperature is high. Although sweat glands are morphologically normal at birth, they are functionally inadequate because of their immature innervation. The result is lower transepidermal water loss and difficulties in thermoregulation. Sweat glands may not become fully functional until the age of 2 years [7].

REFERENCES

1 Sato K. The physiology, pharmacology and biochemistry of the eccrine sweat glands. *Rev Physiol Biochem Pharmacol* 1977; 79: 51–131.
2 Sato K. The physiology and pharmacology of the eccrine sweat gland. In: Goldsmith LA, Sterner JH, eds. *Biochemistry and Physiology of the Skin.* London: Oxford University Press, 1983: 596–641.
3 Sato K, Sato F. Individual variations in structure and function of human eccrine sweat gland. *Am J Physiol* 1983; 245: 203–8.
4 Szabo G. The number of eccrine sweat glands in human skin. In: Montagna W, Ellis R, Silver A, eds. *Advances in Biology of Skin*, vol. 3. New York: Pergamon, 1962: 1–4.
5 Randall WC. Quantitation and regional distribution of sweat glands in man. *J Clin Invest* 1946; 25: 761–7.
6 Uno H. Sympathetic innervation of the sweat glands and piloerector muscle of macaques and human beings. *J Invest Dermatol* 1977; 69: 112–20.
7 Green M. Comparison of adult and neonatal skin eccrine sweating. In: Maibach H, Boisits EK, eds. *Neonatal Skin. Structure and Function.* New York: Marcel Dekker, 1982: 35–63.

Clinical features

Hyperhidrosis may be classified as primary (idiopathic) or secondary. Primary hyperhidrosis is diagnosed by elimination of all other possible causes.

Secondary hyperhidrosis

Secondary hyperhidrosis may be further subdivided into generalized and localized forms.

Generalized hyperhidrosis. Abnormal stimulation of the sweat regulation centre, or of the sympathetic pathway between the hypothalamus and the nerve endings, can cause generalized sweating. Neurological causes include brain tumour, hypothalamic lesions, encephalitis and cerebral anoxia. Increased catecholamine production due to shock, hypoglycaemia, Cushing's syndrome and varied emotional stimuli can also cause generalized hyperhidrosis [1,2].

Generalized sweating of unknown mechanism is associated with endocrinological disorders, such as diabetes mellitus, hyperthyroidism and hyperpituitarism, and as a side-effect of antidepressants. A rise in body temperature and as a consequence a rise in the temperature of the blood, the hypothalamus induces sweating. Generalized sweating accompanies fever and many infectious processes including chronic infection such as tuberculosis, malaria and brucellosis.

Instability of the sweat-regulating centre is also described in alcoholic intoxication, neonatal heroine withdrawal syndrome [3], salicylism, Hodgkin's disease and after vomiting. Infants with familial dysautonomia [4] suffer from hyperhidrosis. Children with oesophageal atresia and choanal atresia develop episodes of glossoptosis apnoea, associated with many clinical manifestations of dysautonomia, including hyperhidrosis [5]. Neonates at risk of sudden death frequently have excessive sweating during sleeping or feeding [3,5,6].

Localized hyperhidrosis. Lesions affecting any part of the sympathetic pathway from the cerebral cortex to the peripheral nerves may result in segmental and often asymmetrical sweating. These causes include brain tumours and abscesses, lesions of the spinal cord, subclavian aneurysm, cervical rib, osteoma of the vertebra, trauma of peripheral nerves and sympathectomy [1,2,7,8].

Compensatory hyperhidrosis can also be the first sign of Ross's syndrome. In this disorder, hyperhidrosis is due to selective degeneration of the sympathetic pathways. It is characterized by widespread hypohidrosis, tonic pupil and loss of reflexes [1].

Gustatory sweating stimulated by taste or even chewing occurs secondary to peripheral neuropathy in diabetes mellitus, and due to outer parotid gland damage [9,10]. Gustatory hyperhidrosis of the malar region is termed Frey's syndrome [11].

Palmoplantar hyperhidrosis is associated with endocrinological disorders, such as hyperthyroidism, and acromegaly and has been reported in association with certain drugs. Sticky skin was reported during treatment with etretinate and acitretin [12,13].

Severe localized hyperhidrosis may be associated with a glomus tumour [14]. Sweat eccrine gland hamartomas are extremely rare. These lesions are characterized by increased sweat secretion in limited areas. A hyperplasia of normal, mature eccrine secretory coils and/or increase in the number and size of glands may be observed; the diagnosis is established by biopsy [15]. Some sweat eccrine gland hamartomas are caused by increased local sensitivity of the sweat glands to neurotransmitters. In this case, histological examination is normal and pharmacological tests show an exaggerated response to acetylcholine [16].

Other organoid hamartomas have been reported to cause localized hyperhidrosis. These include eccrine-pilar angiomatous hamartoma, seborrhoeic naevus et sudoriferis and the blue rubber bleb naevus syndrome [17–20].

Granulosis rubra nasi, described by Jadassohn in 1901, is a rare childhood cause of localized hyperhidrosis (Fig. 29.5.3) [21]. The pathogenesis is unknown. This inherited disorder occurs only in children, and begins to resolve at puberty. Diffuse erythema and persistent hyperhidrosis of the nose is followed by the development of red macules and papules, and occasionally vesicles. This disorder is usually associated with hyperhidrosis of the palms and soles.

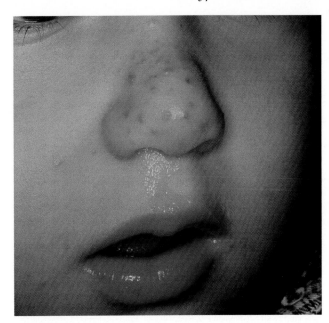

Fig. 29.5.3 Granulosis rubra nasi. Courtesy of Professor Yves de Prost.

Primary (idiopathic) hyperhidrosis

Primary idiopathic hyperhidrosis is diagnosed when underlying conditions have been ruled out. Primary hyperhidrosis is usually restricted to the palms and soles, but sometimes involves the axillae. Palms are also frequently diffusely red and cold, a presumed sign of autonomic hypersensitivity. One study estimated the prevalence in Israeli children at between 0.6 and 1% [22]. Primary hyperhidrosis is most common in childhood and adolescence, and appears to improve thereafter with age. Several authors have reported the occurrence of this disorder in neonates [23–25]. The cause of this condition is unknown. Anatomically and functionally, the sympathetic chain, sweat glands and sweat content are normal. The sweating is aggravated by emotional stress and during sleep. Several authors have suggested that emotional hyperhidrosis may be familial [26–28]. The condition is socially distressing, disrupts school routines and recreational activities and may precipitate significant psychological difficulty. Complications of palmoplantar hyperhidrosis are dyshidrosis, contact dermatitis and maceration leading to intertrigo. Pitted keratolysis and bromhidrosis also occur. Primary hyperhidrosis tends to aggravate juvenile plantar dermatosis and Weber–Cockayne epidermolysis bullosa.

REFERENCES

1 Champion RH. Hyperhidrosis. In: Champion RH, Burton JL, Burns JL, Breathnach SM, eds. *Textbook of Dermatology* Vol. 3, 6th edn. Oxford: Blackwell Science, 1998: 1991–5.
2 Sato K. Disorders of the eccrine sweat gland. In: Fitzpatrick TB, Eisen AZ,

Wolff K, Freedberg IM, Frank Austen K, eds. *Dermatology in General Medicine*. New York: McGraw-Hill, 1993: 740–53.

3 Green M. Comparison of adult and neonatal skin eccrine sweating. In: Maibach H, Boiisits EK, eds. *Neonatal Skin. Structure and Function*. New York: Marcel Dekker, 1982: 35–63.

4 Axelrod FB, Porges RF, Sein ME. Neonatal recognition of familial dysautonomia. *J Pediatr* 1987; 110: 946–8.

5 Cozzi F, Myers NA, Madonna L *et al*. Esophageal atresia, choanal atresia and dysautonomia. *J Pediatr Surg* 1991; 26: 548–52.

6 Southall DP. Role of apnea in the sudden infant death syndrome: a personal view. *Pediatrics* 1988; 81: 73–84.

7 Kewalramani LS. Autonomic dysreflexia in traumatic myelopathy. *Am J Phys Med* 1980; 59: 1–21.

8 Pool JL. Unilateral thoracic hyperhidrosis caused by osteoma of the tenth dorsal vertebra. *J Neurosurg* 1956; 13: 111–15.

9 Watkins PJ. Facial sweating after food: a new sign of diabetic autonomic neuropathy. *Br Med J* 1973; 1: 583–7.

10 Stuart DD. Diabetic gustatory sweating. *Ann Int Med* 1978; 89: 223–4.

11 Harrison K, Donaldson I. Frey's syndrome. *J Roy Soc Med* 1979; 72: 503–8.

12 Penneys NS, Hernandez D. A sticky problem with etretinate. *N Engl J Med* 1991; 327: 521.

13 Pilkington T, Brogden RN. Acitretin: a review of its pharmacology and therapeutic use. *Drugs* 1992; 43: 597–627.

14 Cooke SAR. Misleading features in the clinical diagnosis of the peripheral glomus tumour. *Br J Surg* 1971; 58: 602–6.

15 Chan P, Kao GF, Pierson DL, Rodman OG. Episodic hyperhydrosis on the dorsum of the hands. *J Am Acad Dermatol* 1985; 12: 937–42.

16 Lorette G, Rouesnel S, Grangeponte MC, Goergesco G, Vaillant L. Idiopathic localized paroxysmal hyperhidrosis. Free comunication 07 in the 7th International Congress of Pediatric Dermatology. Buenos Aires, Argentina, 1994.

17 Zeller DJ, Goldman RL. Eccrine pilar angiomatous hamartoma: report of a unique case. *Dermatologica* 1971; 143: 100–4.

18 Smith VC, Montesinos E, Revert A *et al*. Eccrine angiomatous hamartoma: report of three patients. *Pediatr Dermatol* 1996; 13: 139–42.

19 Arnold HL Jr. Nevus seborrheicus et sudoriferus: a unilateral linear physiologic anomaly. *Arch Dermatol Syph* 1945; 51: 370–2.

20 Fine RM, Derbes VJ, Clark WH. Blue rubber bleb nevus. *Arch Dermatol* 1961; 84: 802–5.

21 Aram H, Mohaghegi AP. Granulosis rubra nasi. *Cutis* 1972; 10: 463–4.

22 Adar R, Kurchin A, Zweig A, Mozes M. Palmar hyperhidrosis and its surgical treatment. *Ann Surg* 1977; 186: 34–41.

23 O'Donoghue G, Finn D, Brady MP. Palmar primary hyperhidrosis in children. *J Pediatr Surg* 1980; 15: 172–4.

24 Verbov J, Baxter J. Onset of palmar sweating in newborn infants. *Br J Dermatol* 1974; 90: 269–76.

25 Millar AJW, Steiner Z, Rode H, Cywes S. Transaxillary transpleural sympathectomy for palmar hyperhidrosis in children. A 3 to 7 years follow-up of 9 cases. *Eur J Pediatr Surg* 1994; 4: 3–6.

26 Cloward RB. Hyperhidrosis. *J Neurosurg* 1969; 30: 545–51.

27 Shih CJ, Wang YC. Thoracic sympathectomy for palmar hyperhidrosis. *Surg Neurol* 1978; 10: 291–6.

28 James WD, Schoomaker EB, Rodman OG. Emotional eccrine sweating. A heritable disorder. *Arch Dermatol* 1987; 123: 925–9.

Differential diagnosis

In children, hereditary conditions causing hyperhidrosis must be excluded. These include Böök's syndrome, Charcot–Marie–Tooth syndrome, the nail–patella syndrome, pachydermoperiostosis, dyskeratosis congenita, Weaver's syndrome and Papillon–Lefèvre syndrome [1–6].

Treatment

The initial treatment of primary hyperhidrosis consists of conservative and simple measures. When conservative measures fail, and the disorder is severe or disabling, surgery should be considered.

Topical treatment

Removing the sweat by washing or by absorption can improve comfort. The use of cotton clothes and absorbing powders is helpful. A number of topical medications [7–9] denature keratin and cause temporary mechanical blockage of the eccrine sweat glands ducts at different levels. These include tanning agents, such as trichloracetic acid, tannic acid (2–5% solution), and aldehydes, such as formaldehyde (5–20% solution) and glutaraldehyde (10% solution). Side-effects such as allergic contact dermatitis and staining limit their use, and these agents are essentially only suitable for the feet.

Metal salts (aluminium, gallium and vanadium) in high concentrations are particularly effective in axillary hyperhidrosis [10]. These agents are less effective in palmoplantar hyperhidrosis. Zirconium salts may cause granulomas and are therefore no longer used [9].

The most useful topical preparation is 20% aluminium chloride hexahydrate in alcohol [11–13], applied nightly for two or more nights. An irritant dermatitis is an occasional side-effect.

Topically applied anticholinergic drugs (with occlusion) can inhibit sweating for hours or days, but systemic effects due to absorption restrict the use of this treatment.

Iontophoresis [14–17] is one of the most effective treatments for palmoplantar hyperhidrosis. It has been postulated that passing a direct current through the skin leads to hyperkeratinization and subsequent obstruction of the eccrine sweat gland unit [18]. However, several investigators have disputed this theory and believe that the actual mechanism of action remains unknown [15,19,20]. Currently, tap water, because it is effective and safe, is the most commonly used conducting medium [21]. Solutions of anticholinergic drugs such as poldine methylsulphate, glycopyrrhonium bromide and atropine were shown to have a longer lasting effect than water [22]. However, the frequent side-effects of systemic anticholinergic blockade has prevented this therapy from gaining wide acceptance. A portable delivery system is available for home treatment [23]. Repeated daily baths with an amperage of 15–20 mA will improve hyperhidrosis in 70–88% of patients. Since complete inhibition of hyperhidrosis lasts only for 1–2 weeks, maintenance treatment is required [17]. Side-effects are minimal (intermittent tingling sensation, scaling secondary to irritation), and are prevented by avoiding high current densities [17].

Systemic treatment

Most systemic therapies result in an unsatisfactory outcome or unacceptable side-effects, and are therefore disappointing. These treatments should therefore be avoided in children, or attempted only when traditional topical therapies have failed.

Anticholinergic drugs. Anticholinergic drugs such as atropine (0.01 mg/kg every 4 or 6 h) and probanthine (1.5 mg/kg/day) cause pharmacological blockade of sweat gland neurotransmitters. However, side-effects include dryness of the mouth, blurred vision, glaucoma and even convulsions.

Ganglion-blocking drugs. Ganglion-blocking drugs [9] have significant side-effects, including hypotension.

Sedatives. Sedatives and tranquillizers cause significant side-effects and give only partial relief, but these agents can be helpful in cases with a significant emotional component. Tricyclic antidepressants may also be used [24].

Inhibition of sympathetic stimulation. Central inhibitors of the sympathetic nervous system such as clonidine [25] are somewhat hopeful. Kuritzky *et al.* reported that clonidine provided relief in two adult cases of localized paroxysmal hyperhidrosis [26]. In practice, clonidine appears actually to be disappointing.

Other drugs. Calcium channel blocking agents may prevent the essential initial step of calcium influx into the eccrine secretory cells. Side-effects are minimal [27]. The effectiveness of prostaglandin inhibitors has not been thoroughly evaluated in the treatment of hyperhidrosis [28].

Surgical treatment

When conservative measures fail to control severe cases, surgery is the treatment of choice. Since this condition is not life-threatening, surgical treatment carries a low risk of morbidity and of unpleasant side-effects.

The surgical removal of the axillary sweat gland field, using a diamond-shaped excision technique, generally gives good results [29] but it may result in disfiguring scarring.

Sectioning the sympathetic nerve supply is the alternative surgical approach [30,31]. Because of a high morbidity and complication rate, the surgical transthoracic technique should be avoided. Several studies have resulted in increased interest in a thoracoscopic approach to the thoracic chain. The thoracoscopic technique has simplified the operation and significantly improved results [32–37]. Under general anaesthesia, after induction of a pneumothorax, resection or destruction by electrocautery of the upper thoracic sympathetic ganglia (T2 and T3) is performed. The bilateral procedure takes an experienced operator less than 20 min, and patients can leave the hos-

pital within 24–48 h. There are no appreciable technical difficulties in the treatment of paediatric patients [36–38]. The results are impressive, with immediate relief of symptoms in more than 90% of cases [36,37]. In the treatment of children, several centres report a success rate of 98% and a long-term recurrence rate of only 1–2% [9,31,37,38].

The complications are as follows.

1 Pneumothorax (less than 1%) [31,36,37].

2 Horner's syndrome (0–3%) [37].

3 Compensatory hyperhidrosis (incidence 31–46%) [31–33,39]. Increased perspiration after sympathectomy may affect the axillae, feet or trunk. The more extensive the resection of the sympathetic chain, the higher the risk of compensatory hyperhidrosis [38]. This side-effect prevents the treatment of all four limbs because of the risk of severely imbalanced thermal regulation. The mechanism of compensatory hyperhidrosis is unknown. The patient should be warned about this quite common side-effect.

4 Gustatory symptoms [40], attributed to sprouting of vagal fibres into the severed sympathetic chain, can occur.

5 Late recurrences of sweating [41], due to regeneration of sympathetic fibres or reinnervation through alternative pathways, can unfortunately occur. Excessive sweating can return, even after a number of years.

Based on long-term follow-up, thoracoscopic sympathectomy has a low operative morbidity and a high success rate [37]. When medical therapy has failed, this minimally invasive and relatively safe method of treating hyperhidrosis should be offered to children with severe hyperhidrosis [36–38,42].

REFERENCES

1 Böök JA. Clinical and genetical studies of hypodontia: premolar aplasia, hyperhidrosis and canities prematura: a new hereditary syndrome in man. *Am J Hum Genet* 1950; 2: 240–3.

2 Pechman KJ, Bergfeld WF. Palmar-plantar hyperhidrosis occurring in a kindred with nail–patella syndrome. *J Am Acad Dermatol* 1980; 3: 627–32.

3 James WD, Schoomaker EB, Rodman OG, Emotional eccrine sweating. A heritable disorder. *Arch Dermatol* 1987; 123: 925–9.

4 Gomez Rodrigues N, Atanes Sandoval A, Grana Gil J, Aspe de la Iglesia B, Sato Crespo JM, Comesana-Castro ML. Paquidermoperiostosis (osteo-artropatia hypertrofica primaria). *Ann Med Int* 1990; 7: 80–2.

5 Dumic M, Vukovic J, Cvitkovic M, Medica I. Twins and their mildly affected mother with Weaver syndrome. *Clin Genet* 1993; 44: 338–40.

6 Haneke E. The Papillon–Lefèvre syndrome: keratosis palmoplantaris with periodontopathy. *Hum Genet* 1979; 51: 1–35.

7 Shelley WB, Hurley HJ. Studies on topical antiperspirant control of axillary hyperhidrosis. *Acta Derm Venereol (Stockh)* 1975; 55: 241–60.

8 Grise K. Treatment of hyperhidrosis. *Clin Exp Dermatol* 1982; 7: 183–8.

9 Lambert D, Collet E, Lacroix M. Hyperhidrose et dysidrose palmaire. *J Eur Echange Cosmét Dermatol (Paris)* 1995.

10 Hölzle E, Kligman AM. Mechanism of antiperspirant action of aluminium salts. *J Soc Cosmet Chem* 1979; 30: 279–95.

11 Brandrup F, Larsen PO. Axillary hyperhidrosis: local treatment with aluminium chloride hexahydrate 25% in absolute ethanol. *Acta Derm Venereol (Stockh)* 1978; 58: 461–5.

12 Scholes KT, Crow KD, Ellis JP et al. Axillary hyperhidrosis treated with alcoholic solution of aluminium chloride hexahydrate. *Br Med J* 1978; 2: 84–5.

13 Goh CL. Aluminium chloride hexahydrate versus palmar hyperhidrosis. Evaporimeter assessment. *Int J Dermatol* 1990; 29: 368–70.

14 Levit F. Simple device for the treatment of hyperhidrosis by iontophoresis. *Arch Dermatol* 1968; 98: 505–7.

15 Hölzle E, Ruzicka T. Treatment of hyperhidrosis by a battery-operated iontophoretic device. *Dermatologica* 1986; 172: 41–7.

16 Sloan JB, Soltani K. Iontophoresis in dermatology. A review. *J Am Acad Dermatol* 1986; 15: 671–84.

17 Hölzle E, Alberti N. Long-term efficacy and side effects of tap water iontophoresis of palmoplantar hyperhidrosis—the usefulness of home therapy. *Dermatologica* 1987; 175: 126–35.

18 Dobson RL, Lobitz WC. Some histochemical observations on the human eccrine sweat glands. *Arch Dermatol* 1957; 75: 653–66.

19 Hill AC, Baker GF, Janssen GT. Mechanism of action of iontophoresis in the treatment of palmar hyperhidrosis. *Cutis* 1981; 28: 69–72.

20 Stolman LP. Treatment of excess sweating of the palms by iontophoresis. *Arch Dermatol* 1987; 123: 893–6.

21 Shrivastava SN, Singh G. Tap water iontophoresis for palmar hyperhidrosis. *Br J Dermatol* 1977; 96: 189–95.

22 Abell E, Morgan K. The treatment of idiopathic hyperhidrosis by glucopyrronium bromide and tap water iontophoresis. *Br J Dermatol* 1974; 91: 87–91.

23 Akins DL, Meisenheimer JL, Dobson RL. Efficacy of the Drionic Unit in the treatment of hyperhidrosis. *J Am Acad Dermatol* 1987; 16: 828–32.

24 Cohen JB, Wilcox C. A comparison of fluoxepine, imipramine and placebo in patients with major depressive disorders. *J Clin Psychiatr* 1985; 46: 26–31.

25 Sandyk R, Gilman MA, Iacono RP, Bamford CR. Clonidine in neuropsychiatric disorders: a review. *Int J Neurosci* 1987; 35: 205–15.

26 Kuritzky A, Hering R, Goldhammer G, Bechar M. Clonidine treatment in paroxysmal localized hyperhidrosis. *Arch Neurol* 1984; 41: 1210–11.

27 Braunwald E. Mechanism of action of calcium-channel blocking agents. *N Engl J Med* 1982; 307: 1618–27.

28 Tkach JR. Indomethacin treatment of generalized hyperhidrosis. *J Am Acad Dermatol* 1982; 6: 545–6.

29 Skoog T, Thyresson N. Hyperhidrosis of the axillae. A method of surgical treatment. *Acta Chir Scand* 1962; 124: 531–8.

30 Kotzareff A. Résection partielle du tronc sympathique cervical droit pour hyperhydrose unilatérale. *Rev Med Suisse Romande* 1920; 40: 111–13.

31 Loew NW, Ellis H. Transthoracic sympathectomy for palmar hyperhidrosis in children under 16 years of age. *Ann Roy Coll Surg Engl* 1989; 71: 70–1.

32 Kux M. Thoracic endoscopic sympathectomy in palmar and axillary hyperhidrosis. *Arch Surg* 1978; 113: 264–6.

33 Byrne J, Walsh T, Hederman WP. Endoscopic transthoracic electrocautery of the sympathetic chain for palmar and axillary hyperhidrosis. *Br J Surg* 1990; 77: 1046–9.

34 Edmonson RA, Banerjee AK, Rennie JA. Endoscopic transthoracic sympathectomy in the treatment of hyperhidrosis. *Ann Surg* 1992; 215: 289–93.

35 Claes G, Göthberg G, Drott C. Endoscopic electrocautery of the thoracic sympathetic chain—a minimal invasive method to treat palmar hyperhidrosis. *Scand J Plast Reconstr Hand Surg* 1993; 27: 29–33.

36 Claes G, Drott C. Hyperhidrosis. *Lancet* 1994; 343: 247–8.

37 Drott C, Göthberg G, Claes G. Endoscopic transthoracic sympathectomy: an efficient and safe method for the treatment of hyperhidrosis. *J Am Acad Dermatol* 1995; 33: 78–81.

38 Hehir DJ, Brady MP. Long-term results of limited thoracic sympathectomy for palmar hyperhidrosis. *J Pediatr Surg* 1993; 28: 909–11.

39 Shelley WB, Florence R. Compensatory hyperhidrosis after sympathectomy. *N Engl J Med* 1960; 263: 1056–8.

40 Bloor K. Gustatory sweating and other responses after cervico-thoracic sympathectomy. *Brain* 1969; 92: 137–46.

41 Beatty RA. The use of clip-suture in thoracic sympathectomy. *J Neurosurg* 1994; 81: 482.

42 Millar AJW, Steiner Z, Rode H *et al.* Transaxillary transpleural sympathectomy for palmar hyperhydrosis in children. A 3 to 7 years follow-up of nine cases. *Eur J Pediatr Surg* 1994; 4: 3–6.

29.6 Pigmented Purpuras

LINDA G. RABINOWITZ

Schamberg's disease

Lichen aureus

Purpura annularis telangiectodes

Pigmented purpuric lichenoid dermatosis of Gougerot and Blum

Eczematid-like purpura of Doucas and Kapetanakis
(itching purpura)

The pigmented purpuras, also known in the literature as purpura simplex and purpura pigmentosa chronica, refer to a group of benign conditions that are similar in clinical and histological appearance. In addition to having comparable morphology, these disorders exhibit a distribution of lesions that is remarkably alike. The aetiologies of these entities are poorly understood. Each is considered to be a capillaritis (inflammation of superficial dermal blood vessels) associated with leakage of blood into the surrounding dermis and the presence of haemosiderin-laden macrophages.

Five dermatoses are included under the umbrella of pigmented purpuras. These include Schamberg's disease (progressive pigmented purpuric dermatosis), pigmented purpuric lichenoid dermatosis (PPLD) of Gougerot and Blum, purpura annularis telangiectodes (Majocchi's disease), lichen aureus and eczematid-like purpura of Doucas and Kapetanakis (itching purpura).

Many clinicians view these entities as variants of a single disorder and believe they should be lumped together and not separated [1,2]. Others prefer to consider these as distinct conditions, since subtle differences exist. Ratnam *et al.* [2] favour the inclusive term purpura simplex because of the clinical and histological similarities. These authors studied 174 cases of pigmented purpura in order to identify specific and general features of the five different clinical subtypes. Of the 174 patients, 46% were diagnosed as having Schamberg's disease. Lichen aureus was present in 11% and itching purpura in 10% of patients. Majocchi's disease (6%) and PPLD of Gougerot and Blum (5%) were the least frequently observed variants. A number of cases was unclassified (20%). Although most reports indicate a male preponderance, this study noted a slightly higher incidence of pigmented purpura in females. The mean age at diagnosis was 54 years. Approximately 14% of cases were related to administration of medications, including non-steroidal anti-inflammatory agents, diuretics, meprobamate, ampicillin and zomepirac sodium. At least one case in each subtype was caused by a drug reaction. All patients had clearing of skin lesions within a few months after the triggering medication was discontinued. With regard to clinical presentation, 57% of patients had the eruption confined to the lower limbs. A generalized distribution was noted in 28% of cases. Itching was mild or absent in 85% of affected patients. Two-thirds of all individuals had improvement or clearing of their condition without treatment. Those with Schamberg's disease and PPLD of Gougerot and Blum had the most persistent and chronic courses [2].

Generally, the pigmented purpuras occur most frequently on the legs of middle-aged adults, but they do occur in older and younger patients and can appear at sites other than the lower extremities, such as the arms or trunk. The differential diagnosis is similar for each of the clinical subtypes. Haematological abnormalities, fixed or other drug eruptions, bruising, Kaposi's sarcoma and leucocytoclastic vasculitis may simulate the pigmented purpuras. There is no single satisfactory treatment for this group of disorders, but some patients benefit from topical corticosteroids or psoralens and ultraviolet A light (PUVA). Ascorbic acid and non-steroidal anti-inflammatory agents have not been proven to be effective treatments [3].

Schamberg's disease

Definition

Schamberg's disease, also known as progressive pigmented purpura and progressive pigmentary dermatosis, is a benign, chronic condition characterized by petechiae and hyperpigmented macules that occur predominantly on the lower extremities. Although it is most commonly seen in adults, this condition may affect individuals during late childhood and adolescence.

History

Progressive pigmentary dermatosis was initially described by Schamberg in 1901 [4]. His patient was a 15-year-old boy who was noted to have peculiar red–brown patches on his lower legs at the age of 11 years. He identified pinhead-sized reddish-brown puncta or 'cayenne pepper' spots at the borders of the patches. Although Schamberg did not describe pigment deposition in his patient, Kingery, in 1918, reported the presence of haemosiderin deposits. Kingery theorized that the haemosiderin was due to leakage of blood from cutaneous capillaries [5].

Aetiology

The precise aetiology of this disorder has not been determined, but a hypersensitivity reaction is believed to be the underlying pathogenetic mechanism. Immune complex deposition has been identified in papillary blood vessels, suggesting a type III reaction [6]. Langerhans' cell-mediated injury may also be involved in the process, resulting in capillary leakage [7]. Immunohistological analysis of the infiltrate and lesional keratinocytes demonstrates some features of delayed-type cellular reactions [8]. Several factors responsible for this disorder have been suggested in the literature. Acetaminophen, aspirin, thiamine, carbromal and meprobamate have been reported to trigger and maintain these skin lesions [9,10]. Chronic irritation and local contact allergens may induce capillaritis. Whatever the pathogenetic mechanism, the result appears to be dilation and increased fragility of superficial dermal capillaries with resultant extravasation of red blood cells. Macrophages engulf the erythrocytes and result in haemosiderin deposition, responsible for the clinically apparent reddish-brown hyperpigmentation. Gravity-dependent sites have increased intravascular pressure, and this may explain why lower limbs are primarily affected.

Detailed analysis of cell adhesion molecule (CAM) modulation has been performed and findings demonstrate characteristic modifications in the expression of CAMs in the pigmented purpuras. Studies indicate the involvement of the epidermis in this disorder. This modulation shows close parallels to those reported for chronic delayed-type immune reactions of the skin [11]. The T cells in pigmented purpura are activated by an antigenic stimulus and may use cellular adhesion to local tissue cells such as endothelial cells, fibroblasts and keratinocytes. Adhesion to blood vessels and Langerhans' cells is also possible. Involvement of the epidermis is always present, demonstrated by epidermotropic T cells and upregulation of adhesion molecules on keratinocytes. Researchers speculate that pigmented purpuras are related to cytokine-mediated immunity and depend on a delayed-type hypersensitivity reaction. The pattern of CAM expression suggests an active role of T lymphocytes [11,12].

Pathology

All of the pigmented purpuras are characterized histologically by a lymphohistiocytic perivascular infiltrate in the papillary dermis. Early lesions may demonstrate endothelial cell swelling. Older lesions have dilated capillaries, proliferation of the endothelium, haemosiderin-laden macrophages and a less pronounced inflammatory infiltrate. Variable erythrocyte extravasation is present in all subtypes of pigmented purpura [1]. Epidermal spongiosis and patchy parakeratosis are seen in some of the subtypes, including PPLD of Gougerot and Blum as well as eczematid-like purpura of Doucas and Kapetanakis. The epidermis is normal in lichen aureus. The histological differential diagnosis includes stasis dermatitis which has similar findings but this process extends deeper into the dermis and the epidermal changes are more marked. There is also dermal fibrosis in stasis dermatitis. The lymphocytes in the perivascular infiltrate are often adjacent to macrophages and Langerhans' cells suggesting antigen transfer to T lymphocytes, characteristic of delayed hypersensitivity reactions [1].

Clinical features

Children, adolescents and adults are affected by this disorder which is more common in males. The cutaneous lesions of Schamberg's disease are reddish-brown hyperpigmented macules (Fig. 29.6.1) that, upon close inspection, contain sprinkles of petechiae (often referred to as 'cayenne pepper'). Lesion size and shape are variable. The macules may enlarge and become coalescent. Petechiae are typically located at the periphery of the brown macules but may be noted throughout the lesions (Fig. 29.6.2). In addition, fine telangiectases may occasionally be noted at the periphery of lesions. Older lesions tend to be darker brown in colour and may have atrophic centres. The lower limbs are most commonly involved; however, lesions may appear on the trunk and upper extremities. Typically, the distribution is bilaterally symmetrical; however, a unilateral presentation has been reported to occur [13,14]. The lesions develop slowly and are usually asymptomatic but may be pruritic. Laboratory evaluation, including platelet number and function, is normal. Occasionally, peripheral eosinophilia may be present [15]. Results of laboratory testing, including platelet counts, bleeding time and prothrombin time/partial thromboplastin times are normal.

Prognosis

Although this disorder is not associated with systemic disease, it is a distressing condition because of the cosmet-

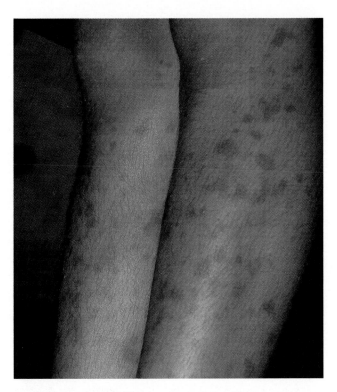

Fig. 29.6.1 Hyperpigmented macules distributed over the lower extremities in a young girl with Schamberg's disease.

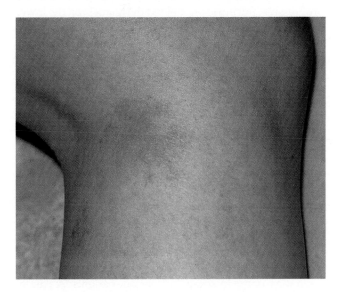

Fig. 29.6.2 Petechiae are present at the periphery of the hyperpigmented macules in Schamberg's disease.

ically disfiguring nature of the eruption. Schamberg's disease has a chronic course marked by phases of resolution and recurrence. It is notoriously resistant to treatment. Lesions may clear within a few months or may persist for as long as 40 years.

Differential diagnosis

Progressive pigmented purpura may be thought to be purpura or ecchymoses. Platelet disorders (decrease in number or function), coagulopathies, vasculitis, Henoch–Schönlein purpura, cryoglobulinaemia and drug eruptions are included in the differential diagnosis. The lesions in Schamberg's disease are macular and never palpable, in contrast to those seen in leucocytoclastic vasculitis. Chronic hyperpigmentation is not a typical feature of Henoch–Schönlein purpura. Referrals to haematologists or rheumatologists are not necessary.

Treatment

Unfortunately, there is no highly effective treatment for this condition. Time, patience, education and reassurance are the keys to management. Psoralens ultraviolet A (PUVA) has been shown to be effective in some cases [16]. This may be related to the role of Langerhans' cells. Therapies that have been recommended but with variable success include ascorbic acid, antihistamines, topical and systemic corticosteroids and support stockings. Although systemic corticosteroids may be the most effective of all therapies, the disease tends to recur when the medication is discontinued. Additionally, it is questionable whether systemic corticosteroids should be prescribed for a chronic benign condition [17].

Lichen aureus

Definition

Lichen aureus, also termed lichen purpuricus, is a benign pigmented purpura that differs clinically and histologically from the other subtypes in this group. Clinically, lesions are grouped lichenoid papules that have a distinct golden or rust colour. Histologically, epidermal changes are lacking. This entity, although distinctive, is quite rare.

History

In 1958, Marten reported the first case of lichen aureus, using the term lichen purpuricus. In 1960, Calnan introduced the term lichen aureus, highlighting the golden colour of the lesions [18].

Aetiology

The aetiology of lichen aureus is not known. Capillary fragility is thought to be a factor, but precise pathophysiological mechanisms are unclear. Sporadic cases implicate asymptomatic infections and drugs as possible aetiologies [18]. Although it has been hypothesized that venous insufficiency may be a precipitating factor [19], none of the paediatric cases reported has been associated with deep venous insufficiency [18].

Pathology

The histopathological findings are similar to those seen in Schamberg's disease, with the exception that lichen aureus features a normal epidermis. The papillary dermis contains a lymphohistiocytic perivascular infiltrate and a few extravasated red blood cells. The endothelial cells of the capillaries in the papillary dermis appear swollen. Haemosiderin is found in varying amounts. Lichen aureus differs histologically from the other pigmented purpuras by the presence of a dense band-like infiltrate of histiocytes and lymphocytes in the papillary dermis that is separated from the epidermis by a zone of normal collagen (Grenz zone). In early lesions the infiltrate is patchy, whereas in the late stages it changes into a band-like pattern. Direct immunofluorescence studies have not revealed significant abnormalities [18].

Clinical features

Of 104 reported cases of lichen aureus, children represent 17% of the total number of cases [18]. The lesions of lichen aureus may arise suddenly at any site but are most common on the lower extremities. Occurrence on the arm and finger has been reported [3]. As with Schamberg's disease, lichen aureus is either asymptomatic or mildly pruritic. The typical lesions are localized and are comprised of grouped lichenoid papules, each measuring a few millimetres, that have a golden, copper or rust colour. There may be a petechial component, giving a purplish hue. Lesions may be isolated or may coalesce into plaques that range in size from 1 to 20 cm. The sharply demarcated plaques may be solitary or multiple, but are usually unilateral [20]. A zosteriform pattern has been reported rarely [21]. Despite the petechial component, there are no haematological abnormalities. Platelet number and function, prothrombin time, bleeding time and haemoglobin levels are all normal.

Prognosis

The plaques of lichen aureus can be persistent and sometimes permanent. The condition may regress within a period ranging from 6 months to 18 years. In five of eight paediatric patients, it resolved in 2–4 years [18].

Differential diagnosis

Lichen aureus must be differentiated from other conditions that have a golden to rust-coloured appearance. Clinically and histologically, the condition most closely resembling lichen aureus is PPLD of Gougerot and Blum. Other conditions in the differential diagnosis include Schamberg's disease, Majocchi's disease and fixed drug eruptions. Lichen aureus is often confused with bruising

because of the golden colour. Unlike a bruise, the colour of lichen aureus remains unchanged, and only rarely is there a history of preceding trauma [22].

Treatment

Treatment of lichen aureus is often unsatisfactory. Topical corticosteroids may result in flattening of the papular component as well as some fading of the dyspigmentation. Occasionally, potent topical corticosteroids will result in dramatic and rapid resolution of the lesions [23].

Purpura annularis telangiectodes

Definition

Purpura annularis telangiectodes, also referred to as Majocchi's purpura or Majocchi's disease, is a pigmented purpura that features annular and telangiectatic lesions. It is a rare dermatosis that may be seen in adolescents and young adults. It is the only subtype that has a female predominance. Familial occurrence has been reported [24].

History

In 1896, Majocchi, an Italian dermatologist, described a progressive, purpuric pigmented dermatosis on the lower limbs of a 21-year-old male. The primary lesions were macular rings which consisted of pigmented purpura and punctate red dots [25]. The centres were depigmented and atrophic. MacKee reported the first case in the American literature in 1915 [3].

Clinical features

Majocchi's disease is characterized by annular lesions with peripheral telangiectases. There are three stages: (a) telangiectatic; (b) haemorrhagic and pigmentary; and (c) atrophic. The telangiectatic stage demonstrates a rose-coloured macule with dilated capillaries. Erythematous, follicular puncta that enlarge into annular lesions are typical of the second stage, as are yellowish brown centres as the lesions expand into rings. The atrophic, and final, stage may occur in some, but not all, patients. A patient may have lesions in different stages at the same point in time. The eruption is usually bilateral and symmetrical and develops on the legs in most cases. The arms and trunk may be involved. The ringed lesions may be few in number or numerous and can range in size from 1 to 3 cm. They are either only mildly pruritic or asymptomatic.

Prognosis

The course is chronic and is characterized by recurrences and remissions over a period of months to years. Individual lesions may remain unchanged or may gradually extend centrifugally.

Treatment

Topical corticosteroids might be helpful, as with the other pigmented purpuras.

Pigmented purpuric lichenoid dermatosis of Gougerot and Blum

Definition

PPLD of Gougerot and Blum is also referred to as lichenoid purpura and purpuric pigmented lichenoid dermatitis. Lichenoid papules are present in addition to the purpura seen in Schamberg's disease.

History

The first case of pigmented purpuric lichenoid dermatosis was reported by Gougerot and Blum in 1925 [26]. This rare disorder features orange–red lichenoid papules on the legs.

Clinical features

Because PPLD of Gougerot and Blum occurs primarily in men aged between 40 and 60 years and is extremely rare in the paediatric age group, detailed discussion in this text is limited.

Eczematid-like purpura of Doucas and Kapetanakis (itching purpura)

Definition

This pigmented purpura, also of unknown aetiology, is very similar to Schamberg's disease, but it is distinguished by intense itching.

History

Doucas and Kapetanakis described this entity in 1953 as a recurrent, purpuric eruption that commenced on the legs and resulted in haemosiderin deposition [27]. Loewenthal emphasized the intense pruritus associated with this condition [28].

Pathology

Histopathological findings are similar to those of the other pigmented purpuras. There are variable epidermal changes, including spongiosis.

Clinical features

The cutaneous lesions characteristic of this disorder are similar to those seen in Schamberg's disease, but extremely pruritic reddish papules and mild scaling are also present. Middle-aged men are most frequently affected, and the condition is rare during childhood. There appears to be a seasonal relationship, with most cases occurring during the spring and summer months [29].

Prognosis

After a course of months to years, the lesions resolve spontaneously. The duration of the condition tends to be shorter than that of Schamberg's disease.

Differential diagnosis

Eczematid-like purpura of Doucas and Kapetanakis is similar to Schamberg's disease, but the latter entity is more persistent, much less pruritic and more common in children. The distinction between these two disorders is otherwise ill-defined.

Treatment

Management includes measures to control the intense pruritus. Topical corticosteroids and antihistamines may be beneficial.

REFERENCES

1 Lever WF, Schaumburg-Lever G, eds. *Histopathology of the Skin*, 7th edn. Philadelphia: JB Lippincott, 1990: 192–3.
2 Ratnam KV, Su WPD, Peters MS. Purpura simplex (inflammatory purpura without vasculitis): a clinicopathologic study of 174 cases. *J Am Acad Dermatol* 1991; 25: 642–7.
3 Newton RC, Raimer SS. Pigmented purpuric eruptions. *Dermatol Clin N Am* 1985; 3: 165–9.
4 Schamberg JF. A peculiar progressive pigmentary disease of the skin. *Br J Dermatol* 1901; 13: 1–5.
5 Kingery LB. Schamberg's progressive pigmentary dermatosis: report of a case with histologic study. *J Cutan Dis* 1918; 36: 166–72.
6 Iwatsuki K, Aoshima T, Tagami H. Immunofluorescence study in purpura pigmentosa chronica. *Acta Derm Venereol* 1980; 60: 341–70.
7 Aiba S, Tagami H. Immunohistologic studies in Schamberg's disease: evidence for cellular immune reaction in lesional skin. *Arch Dermatol* 1988; 124: 1058–62.
8 Simon M Jr, Heese A, Gotz A. Immunopathological investigations in purpura pigmentosa chronica. *Acta Derm Venereol* 1989; 69: 101–4.
9 Abeck D, Gross GE, Kuwert C *et al.* Acetaminophen-induced progressive pigmentary purpura (Schamberg's disease). *J Am Acad Dermatol* 1992; 27: 123–4.
10 Draelos ZK, Hansen RC. Schamberg's purpura in children: case study and literature review. *Clin Pediatr* 1987; 26: 659–61.
11 von den Driesch P, Simon M. Cellular adhesion antigen modulation in purpura pigmentosa chronica. *J Am Acad Dermatol* 1994; 30: 193–200.
12 Burrows NP, Jones RR. Cell adhesion molecule expression in capillaritis. *J Am Acad Dermatol* 1994; 31: 826 (letter).
13 Hersh CS, Shwayder TA. Unilateral progressive pigmentary purpura (Schamberg's disease) in a 15-year-old boy. *J Am Acad Dermatol* 1991; 24: 651.

14 Friedman SA, Byrd RC. Schamberg's disease: report of a case. *J Am Osteop Assoc* 1987; 87: 140–1.

15 Carpentieri U, Gustavson LP, Grim CB *et al.* Purpura and Schamberg's disease. *Southern Med J* 1978; 71: 1168–70.

16 Simon M Jr, Hunyadi J. PUVA-Therapie der Ekzematidartigen Purpura. *Aktuel Dermatol* 1986; 12: 100–2.

17 Sherertz EF. Pigmented purpuric eruptions. *Semin Thromb Hemost* 1984; 10: 190–5.

18 Gelmetti C, Cerri D, Grimalt R. Lichen aureus in childhood. *Pediatr Dermatol* 1991; 8: 280–3.

19 Shelley WB, Swaminathan R, Shelley ED. Lichen aureus: a hemosiderin tattoo associated with perforator vein incompetence. *J Am Acad Dermatol* 1984; 11: 260–4.

20 Khana M, Levy A, Shewach-Millett M *et al.* Lichen aureus occurring in childhood. *Int J Dermatol* 1985; 10: 666–7.

21 Braun-Falco O, Abeck O, Betke M *et al.* Lichen aureus zosteriformis. *Hautarzt* 1989; 40: 373–5.

22 Ruiz-Esmenjaud J, Dahl MV. Segmental lichen aureus: onset associated with trauma and puberty. *Arch Dermatol* 1988; 124: 1572–4.

23 Rudolph RI. Lichen aureus. *J Am Acad Dermatol* 1983; 8: 722–4.

24 Dowd PM, Champion RH. Pupura. In: Champion RH, Burton JL, Burns DA, Breathnach SM, eds. *Textbook of Dermatology*, 6th edn. Oxford: Blackwell Science, 1998: 2141–54.

25 Majocchi D. Sopra una dermatosi telangiectode non ancora descritla: purpura annularis. *Ital Mal Ven* 1896; 31: 263–4.

26 Gougerot H, Blum P. Purpura angioscléreux prurigineous avec elements lichenoides. *Bull Soc Fr Derm Syph* 1925; 32: 161–3.

27 Doucas C, Kapetanakis J. Eczematid-like purpura. *Dermatologica* 1953; 106: 86–95.

28 Loewenthal LA. Itching purpura. *Br J Dermatol* 1954; 66: 95–103.

29 Mosto SJ, Casala AM. Disseminated pruriginous angiodermatitis (itching purpura). *Arch Dermatol* 1965; 91: 351–6.

29.7 Hypereosinophilic Disorders

NERYS ROBERTS, RICHARD J. ANTAYA AND RICHARD STAUGHTON

Eosinophils have been easily recognizable in tissues for over a century, because of the characteristic staining of their granules with eosin on haematoxylin, yet their precise role in health and disease is only gradually being elucidated. Eosinophils increase vascular permeability leading to oedema, stimulate fibrous tissue deposition and contribute to the formation of bullae and chronic inflammation.

In the clinical setting, circulating eosinophilia most often, in the West, signals an atopic condition (eczema, asthma, hay fever) or other allergic state (e.g. drug reaction); in the East or Africa, an underlying internal parasitosis is the cause until proven otherwise. International air travel can thus spring occasional clinical surprises.

Congenital eosinophilia

In the newborn, the blood eosinophil count is $<0.7\times10^9/l$, although counts of $1–2\times10^9/l$ are seen occasionally in otherwise normal infants [1,2]. Cord blood contains more eosinophils and precursor cells than adult peripheral blood.

Congenital eosinophilia following intrauterine blood transfusions, with exchange transfusions is not uncommon, and occurred in 60% of neonates in one series [3]. This is thought to be the result of a hypersensitivity reaction since it can be associated with a rash, thrombocytopenia and lymphopenia.

Familial or hereditary eosinophilia was described with multiple family members with eosinophilia, but initial reports were not followed by other familial cases, so that it is difficult to be certain if this is a distinct entity.

In Down's syndrome, eosinophil numbers are normal, but there is a higher percentage of eosinophils with multilobed nuclei in the bone marrow.

Neonatal eosinophilia

In neonates, tissue eosinophilia is seen in erythema toxicum neonatorum, infantile acropustulosis and transient neonatal pustular melanosis.

Peripheral blood eosinophilia may be a feature of incontinentia pigmenti, but marked peripheral blood eosinophilia in a baby with erythroderma should arouse suspicion of an immunodeficiency, especially Omenn's syndrome.

Infantile eosinophilia

Very marked peripheral blood eosinophilia in infants must be taken seriously, as it may herald either idiopathic hypereosinophilic syndrome (HES) or leukaemia. A high to moderate eosinophilia is a feature of eosinophilic pustular folliculitis. Eosinophilia is common in atopic dermatitis, where tissue eosinophilia is characteristic. Tissue eosinophilia may also be a feature of Langerhans' cell histiocytosis.

Eosinophilia in older children

Marked eosinophilia is seen in idiopathic HES and in Kimura's disease/angiolymphoid hyperplasia with eosinophilia which is detailed in a separate section (see Chapter 29.8).

Moderate peripheral blood eosinophilia is a feature of Wells' syndrome, eosinophilic fasciitis and Ofuji's syndrome. Clearly the possibility of parasitic infection must be considered.

Tissue eosinophilia is a feature of numerous dermatoses discussed elsewhere. A low molecular weight chemotactic factor for eosinophils has been found in the skin of patients with bullous pemphigoid, atopic eczema, drug reaction and contact sensitivity [4]. Other dermatoses include scabies, urticaria, polyarteritis nodosa, Churg–Strauss syndrome, systemic sclerosis, dermatitis herpetiformis and pemphigus.

REFERENCES

1 Lawrence R Jr, Church JA, Richards W, Lipsey AI. Eosinophilia in the hospitalized neonate. *Ann Allergy* 1980; 44: 349–52.
2 Kien CL, Chusid MJ. Eosinophilia in children receiving parenteral nutrition support. *JPEN* 1979; 3: 468–9.
3 Chudwin DS, Ammann AJ, Wara DW, Cowan MJ, Phibbs RH. Posttransfusion syndrome: rash, eosinophilia, and thrombocytopenia following intrauterine and exchange transfusions. *Am J Dis Child* 1982; 136: 612–14.
4 Dierksmeier U, Frosch PJ, Czarnetzki BM. Eosinophil chemotactic factor (ECF) in blister fluid of dermatological diseases. *Br J Dermatol* 1980; 102: 43–8.

Eosinophilic pustular folliculitis in infancy and childhood

SYN. OFUJI'S DISEASE

Definition

Eosinophilic pustular folliculitis is an uncommon disorder first described in adults by Ofuji *et al.* in 1970 [1]. There have been only a few reports of this entity in children. In 1984 Lucky *et al.* [2] described a variant in infants that has its own set of characteristics which distinguish it from the adult and childhood forms. There is debate over whether the infantile form is truly a variant of the adult form or a completely separate disorder [2–5]; and the name *eosinophilic pustulosis of the scalp* has been proposed for infants in whom the scalp is primarily affected. The described form seen in adult patients with human immunodeficiency virus (HIV) infection has not been observed in infancy or childhood [6].

Aetiology and pathogenesis

The origin of this dermatosis is unknown. Currently many theories exist, particularly for the classic adult form, none of which have been validated. Most theories evoke immunological mechanisms in the initiation of lesions [7]. An eosinophil chemotactic factor has been identified in the stratum corneum of an adult patient with eosinophilic pustular folliculitis, and because of the clinical response of some patients to indomethacin, a cyclo-oxygenase inhibitor; it has been suggested that this chemotactic factor may be a metabolite in the cyclo-oxygenase pathway [8,9].

An exaggerated response to skin saprophytes or dermatophytes, or autoantibodies directed against the intercellular substance of the lower epidermis [10] or the cytoplasm of basal cells of the epidermis and the outer sheath of hair follicles [11], have also been proposed

aetiologies in adult eosinophilic pustular folliculitis. Sebaceous gland activity has been postulated to be an aetiological factor, especially for the classical and HIV-related forms [12]; however, it is presumed that this is probably not so for the paediatric variants [13].

Boone *et al.* described three children, two with childhood onset and one with onset in infancy, who tested positive with immunoglobulin E (IgE) radioallergosorbent testing to the dust mite *Dermatophagoides pteronyssinus* (DPT), suggesting a hypersensitivity reaction in the pathogenesis of eosinophilic pustular folliculitis. Two of the three patients had neither personal nor family history of atopy [13].

Eosinophilic pustular folliculitis shares some histopathological characteristics with erythema toxicum neonatorum and some hypothesize it may represent a more persistent form [6].

Pathology

Histopathology of the infantile scalp lesion displays a moderate to dense perifollicular and periappendageal inflammatory infiltrate in the upper and mid dermis composed predominantly of eosinophils together with neutrophils and mononuclear cells. The infiltrate may extend to the deep dermis [14,15] and panniculus [3,6]. Most cases demonstrate interstitial eosinophilic flame figures between collagen bundles, representing degranulated eosinophils [3,16]. Eosinophil, neutrophil and mononuclear cell exocytosis into the pilosebaceous unit, with spongiosis, subsequent abscess formation and ultimate destruction of the hair follicle is frequently demonstrated in the adult and older paediatric cases; while most, but not all, of the infantile cases present with simply perifollicular mixed, but predominantly eosinophilic, inflammation [7]. Sebaceous glands may be infiltrated, and with follicular involvement, the infundibulum is most affected [15]. The epidermis may also exhibit exocytosis, spongiosis and occasionally eosinophilic subcorneal pustules, parakeratosis or crust [3]. The scalp is the preferred biopsy site in infants, as it is invariably affected in this age group and consistently yields a specific histological picture [6,15].

Clinical features and prognosis

Eosinophilic pustular folliculitis (Fig. 29.7.1a–d) is characterized by recurrent crops of pruritic annular or polycyclic plaques, composed of coalescing, sterile papulopustules on the seborrhoeic areas of the face, trunk and extremities. There is a tendency for central healing with peripheral extension. Scalp involvement is present in only 6% of adult patients [17]. This classical form has been reported in children [13,18–20] and adolescents rarely.

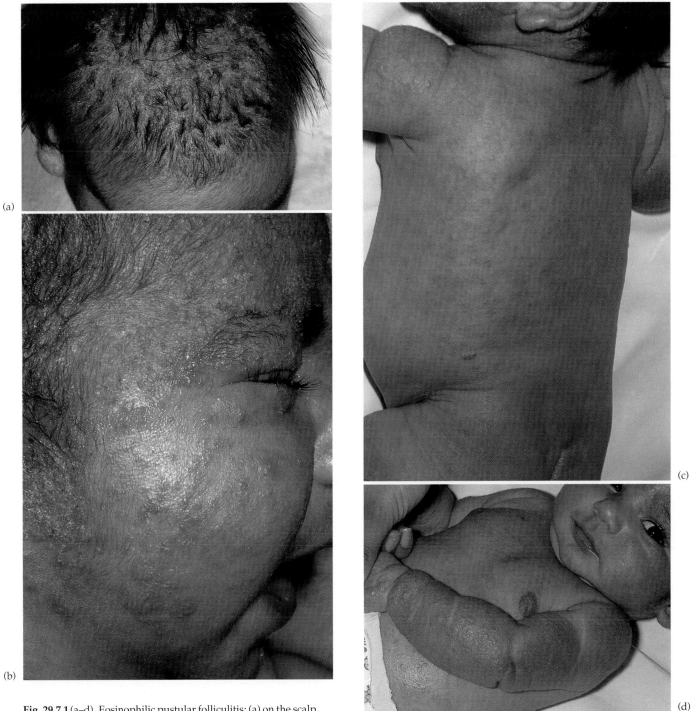

Fig. 29.7.1 (a–d) Eosinophilic pustular folliculitis; (a) on the scalp, (b) face, (c) trunk and (d) limbs. Note the sparing of the skin creases.

Eosinophilic pustular folliculitis in infancy appears to be a variant of this disorder which principally involves the scalp [14]. These lesions, similar to those in the adult form, occur as grouped, pruritic firm papules (occasionally vesicles) which evolve into follicular pustules, measuring pinpoint to 3 mm, on an erythematous base. The lesions can present as a solitary plaque as small or as scattered pus-

tules throughout the scalp [7]. Unlike the adult and childhood forms, annular or serpiginous plaques are not observed in infants and small children. They resolve spontaneously without scarring [17] after evolving through a yellow, crusted phase in approximately 5–10 days, often leaving a 3–4 mm hyperpigmented macule [16]. New crops of lesions appear approximately every 2–8 weeks

[12]. Whereas the majority of infants commonly have involvement of the scalp, the extremities, hands, feet and trunk. The face [3,6,15], groin [5] and genitals [3] may rarely be affected. In the infantile variant age of onset is greatest in the first 6 months of life, with approximately one-quarter presenting at or just after birth. Spontaneous resolution is mostly between 4 and 36 months. It appears that the earlier the disorder appears, the less chronic it becomes. Although there does not seem to be a familial predisposition, eosinophilic pustular folliculitis has been reported in two brothers, born at different times, both with onset in the neonatal period [14].

In all age groups there is peripheral eosinophilia and leucocytosis associated with exacerbations and an absence of systemic symptoms. Both classical and infantile forms exhibit a strong male predominance; however, in the 4–9 year age group, which by far represents the smallest cohort, females have been reported more often. The clinical characteristics of eosinophilic pustular folliculitis in this age group falls between the other groups in that scalp involvement is unusual, seborrhoeic areas are less involved than the classical form and there are less annular and more diffuse lesions as seen in the infantile form [18].

A Wright's stained smear of pustular contents demonstrating abundant eosinophils may be helpful in making the diagnosis. The diagnosis is based on the clinical presentation, associated haematological abnormalities and histological evidence of eosinophilic folliculitis.

Differential diagnosis

The differential diagnosis for eosinophilic pustular folliculitis in infancy should include most pustular eruptions in infancy in particular: scalp pyoderma or infectious folliculitis caused by *Staphylococcus aureus*; scabies; erythema toxicum neonatorum; herpes simplex infection; infantile acropustulosis; Langerhans' cell histiocytosis; and incontinentia pigmenti.

When eosinophilic pustular folliculitis presents in older children the differential diagnosis should include: fungal, parasitic and herpetic infections; eosinophilic cellulitis; insect bites; eczema; and impetigo.

Treatment

Because of the rarity of this disorder, there have been no controlled clinical trials for the treatment of eosinophilic pustular folliculitis in adults or children. In addition, its recurrent and self-limited features, especially in infants, make evaluation of anecdotal treatments difficult. Antihistamines are indicated for associated pruritis and there may be a role for the newer eosinophil antimigration drugs like cetirizine dihydrochloride [21]. While not consistently effective, most have found mid to high potency topical steroids to reduce pruritis and hasten involution of the lesions in infants [2,6,15], with response usually within 1–2 days of application. Dapsone at a dose of 2 mg/kg/day was effective in one infant who was unresponsive to topical steroids; however, it was discontinued secondary to haematological side-effects. The eruption recurred after the dapsone was stopped [14]. Neither oral erythromycin nor cephalexin produces any apparent change in the course of this disease [6].

In adults treatment options including topical steroids, non-steroidal anti-inflammatory drugs, such as indomethacin, and isotretinoin [7] have been used with some success. In the acquired immunodeficiency syndrome (AIDS)-associated variety psoralens and ultraviolet A (PUVA) [15] and oral metronidazole [22] have been reported to be efficacious.

REFERENCES

1 Ofuji S, Ogino A, Horio T *et al.* Eosinopilic pustular folliculitis. *Acta Derm Venereol* 1970; 50: 195–203.
2 Lucky A, Esterly NB, Heskel N, Krafchik BR, Solomon LM. Eosinophilic pustular folliculitis in infancy. *Pediatr Dermatol* 1984; 1: 202–6.
3 Taieb A, Bassan-Andrieu L, Maleville J. Eosinophilic pustulosis of the scalp in childhood. *J Am Acad Dermatol* 1992; 27: 55–60.
4 Taieb A. Infantile eosinophilic pustular 'folliculitis' in infancy: a nonfollicular disease. *Pediatr Dermatol* 1994; 11: 186 (letter).
5 Larralde M, Morales S, Santo Munoz A, Lamas F, Schroh R, Corbella C. Eosinophilic pustules folliculitis in infancy: report of two new cases. *Paed Dermatol* 1999; 16(2): 118–20.
6 Duarte AM, Rramer J, Yusk JW, Paller A, Schachner LA. Eosinophilic pustular folliculitis in infancy and childhood. *Am J Dis Child* 1993; 147: 197–200.
7 Otley CC, Avram MR, Johnson RA. Isotretinoin treatment of human immunodeficiency virus associated eosinophilic folliculitis. *Arch Dermatol* 1995; 2131: 1047–50.
8 Takematsu H, Tagami H. Eosinophilic pustular folliculitis: studies on possible chemotactic factors involved in the formation of pustules. *Br J Dermatol* 1986; 114: 209–15.
9 Miyauchi T, Fujigaki H, Uehara N, Hayashi S, Hironaga M. Effect of indomethacin on eosinophilic folliculitis. *Acta Dermatol (Kyoto)* 1985; 80: 9–13.
10 Vakilzadeh F, Suter L, Knop J, Macher E. Eosinophilic pustulosis with pemphigus-like antibody. *Dermatologica* 1981; 162: 265–72.
11 Nunzi E, Parodi A, Rebora A. Ofuji's disease: high circulating titers of IgG and IgM directed to the basal cell cytoplasm. *J Am Acad Dermatol* 1985; 12: 268–73.
12 Fearfield LA, Rowe A, Francis N, Bunker CB, Staughton RCD. Itchy folliculitis and human immunodeficiency virus infection L clinicopathological and immunological features, pathogenesis and treatment. *Brit J Dermatol* 1999; 141: 3–11.
13 Boone M, Dangoisse C, Andre J, Sass U, Song M, Ledoux M. Eosinophilic pustular folliculitis in three atopic children with hypersensitivity to *Dermatophagoides pteronyssinus*. *Dermatology* 1995; 190: 164–8.
14 Dupond AS, Aubin F, Bourezane Y, Faivre B, Van Landuyt H, Humbert PH. Eosinophilic pustular folliculitis in infancy: report of two affected brothers. *Br J Dermatol* 1995; 132: 296–9.
15 Giard F, Marcoux D, McCuaig C, Powell J, Russo P. Eosinophilic pustular folliculitis (Ofuji disease) in childhood: a review of four cases. *Pediatr Dermatol* 1991; 8: 189–93.
16 Onorato J, Heilman ER, Laude TA. Pruritic pustular eruption in an infant (clinical conference). *Pediatr Dermatol* 1994; 10: 292–4.
17 Garcia-Patos V, Pujol RM, de Moragas JM. Infantile eosinophilic pustular folliculitis. *Dermatology* 1994; 189: 133–8.
18 Dekio S, Jidoi J, Kawasaki Y. Eosinophil-infiltrating folliculitis in childhood—report of a case. *J Dermatol* 1989; 16: 388–91.

19 Takematsu H, Nakamura K, Igarashi M, Tagami H. Eosinophilic pustular folliculitis—report of two cases with a review of the Japanese literature. *Arch Dermatol* 1985; 121: 917–20.

20 De Dulanto F, Armijo M, Diaz L *et al.* Folicilitis pustulosa eosinofilica (sindrome de Ofuji). *Med Cutan ILA* 1977; 5: 323–30.

21 Fadel R, Herpin-Richard N, Rihoux JP, Henocq E. Inhibitory effect of cetirizine on eosinophil migration *in vivo. Clin Allergy* 1987; 17: 373–9.

22 Smith RJ, Skelton HG, Yeager J, Ruiz N, Wagner KF. Metronidazole for eosinophilic pustular folliculitis in human immunodeficiency virus type 1-positive patients *Arch Dermatol* 1995; 131: 1089–91 (letter).

The idiopathic hypereosinophilic syndrome

Definition

This term idiopathic HES is used to describe patients with a persistent, non-malignant eosinophilia of more than 1.5×10^9/l with evidence of organ damage.

Aetiology and pathogenesis

It is still not clear whether eosinophils or their precursors themselves are abnormal in HES, or whether there is a problem in the regulatory mechanism of eosinophil production. The striking male preponderance (9:1) also remains unexplained. The mean age at onset is 37 years and the disorder is distinctly rare in childhood. Eighteen cases of childhood hypereosinophilia of unknown cause were recorded to 1987, five of whom died of a leukaemic process, and the others probably had HES.

Clinical features

Presentation may be with an asymptomatic eosinophilia in as many as 10% of cases, but angio-oedema or muscle pains was the presenting feature in 14% of the National Institutes of Health (NIH) series [1], whilst a rash of fever was the main problem in another 12%. Tiredness, excessive sweating, cough, breathlessness and retinal lesions are other common presentations.

The skin is involved in 70% of cases and retinal lesions (90%), endomyocardial fibrosis (80%), thromboembolic disease (80%), lymphatic and spleen involvement (60%) and central nervous system involvement (50%) are seen in over half of the cases, whilst respiratory tract involvement occurs in about 40%.

The skin lesions of HES are varied. Urticaria, angio-oedema and erythematous pruritic papulonodular lesions are well documented. Eczematous changes can be seen, but there are no distinguishing features from other types of eczema. Immediate pressure urticaria has been observed in some patients. Dermographism may be marked, although this does not correlate with other features of the disease. Cutaneous ulceration, the result of dermal arteri-

ole thrombosis, is also well documented, and three cases who were later found to have lymphomatoid papulosis have been reported [2]. It was postulated that the abnormal lymphocytes may have induced the eosinophilia.

Differential diagnosis

The diagnosis rests on the exclusion of other possible causes of eosinophilia such as parasitic infection, tumours and hypersensitivity (although these sometimes only become apparent at a later date). The importance of recognizing HES as an entity is that it is now established that patients with a persistent eosinophilia of this degree can develop a series of problems related to eosinophil toxicity.

Treatment

The response to corticosteroids is variable, and it has been suggested that dapsone may be the drug of choice. Disodium cromoglycate was helpful in one patient, but topical steroids are generally ineffective. More recently, bone marrow transplantation and interferon-α have been used with benefit.

REFERENCES

1 Fauci AS, Harley JB, Roberts WC, Ferrans VJ, Gralnick HR, Bjornson BH. NIH conference: the idiopathic hyper eosinophilic syndrome: clinical, pathophysiologic, and therapeutic considerations. *Ann Intern Med* 1982; 97: 78–92.

2 Whittaker SJ, Russell-Jones R, Spry CJ. Lymphomatoid papulosis and its relationship to 'idiopathic' hypereosinophilic syndrome. *J Am Acad Dermatol* 1988; 18: 339–44.

Eosinophilic cellulitis (Wells' syndrome)

Definition

This syndrome was first described by Wells in 1971 [1] as 'a changing symptom complex with a phase of the disease characterised by episodes of acute eosinophilic cellulitis followed by granulomatous dermatitis with its distinctive histopathology'.

Aetiology

This is a rare condition, with less than 25 reported cases in the literature, with eight paediatric cases. There is no sex preference. It is postulated that different triggers such as insect bites, fungal infection, drug eruptions (especially antibiotics, cholesterol-lowering drugs and local anaesthetics) or surgery may induce a hypersensitivity reaction with eosinophil-induced cytotoxicity of collagen and histiocytic phagocytosis as a response to the damage.

Pathology

Where there is blistering, it is subepidermal and crowded with eosinophils. There is marked dermal oedema and infiltration with eosinophils and phagocytic histiocytes together with scattered 'flame figures' in the mid to deep dermis, which consist of a core of collagen and eosinophilic debris which is surrounded by eosinophils, palisading histiocytes and in established lesions foreign body type giant cells. The collagen appears displaced rather than destroyed. Extracellular eosinophil granules may be seen free in the dermis, within phagocytes and in the flame figures. Major basic protein (MBP) is abundant within the eosinophils and in the flame figures [2]. Eosinophils and other cells can be seen transiting through oedematous small venules, but there is no structural vasculitis.

In cases subjected to direct immunofluorescence (IMF) perivascular C3, IgM and IgA have been observed. Dermal fibrin may also stain positively.

Electron microscopy reveals eosinophil granule coating collagen fibres in the flame figures.

Clinical features

Patients are generally well, but may be febrile and occasionally there is general malaise. Presentation can be abrupt, especially in severe cases with single or multiple itchy lesions which can spread rapidly and evolve over a few weeks, and often recur over many months. Lesions begin as red plaques, which clinically resemble urticaria and cellulitis, often with some blistering, haemorrhagic in some cases. The lesions can extend rapidly, often with a blue central discoloration and peripheral red rim, and are sometimes painful at the outset. The skin is not generally hot to the touch. Lesions undergo gradual resolution over about 4–8 weeks and often develop a greenish hue and firm induration before resolving without scarring, although postinflammatory hyperpigmentation is common. Any site can be involved. Mucosal involvement with tongue swelling (one case) and throat swelling (one case) were a feature in Wells' original cases.

Milder cases have multiple annular or circinate erythematous plaques with infiltrated borders persisting and recurring over a few years. Erythematous papulonodular lesions with a faint punctate erythema at another skin site were noted in one patient, and in another scaling (mycology negative) of the feet was associated with scaly, itchy annular lesions resembling granuloma annulare which showed the histology of eosinophilic cellulitis.

Wells and Smith described two paediatric cases [3].Both patients had been given penicillin prior to their illness. An 11-year-old boy with an intermittent fever and widespread urticarial lesions, some with blisters, which developed into erythematous plaques associated with a polymorphonu-clear leucocytosis. He had received a course of penicillin prior to his eruption, when he had mumps. A 12-year-old boy developed widespread itchy infiltrated lesions on the trunk and thighs which persisted for many weeks, following a course of penicillin for an erysipelas-like rash on his ankle. He had a leucocytosis with up to 44% eosinophils. Biopsies from both boys showed typical histological features, and both had recurrent attacks over a 3-year period, which were only partially controlled with systemic corticosteroid therapy.

Lindskov *et al.* described four cases in children [4]. A 4-year-old girl presented with a 1-month history of an itchy, reddish brown granulomatous infiltration of the left arm, with severe blistering and a few papulovesicular lesions at other sites. She had three episodes lasting 3 weeks to 2 months. There was a partial response to prednisolone. A 5-year-old girl developed multiple yellow–green and purple lesions with marked blistering on her limbs and tender subcutaneous nodules on the scalp. She had a low grade fever and diffuse pains with some stiffness. A 20-month-old boy presented with generalized, pruritic, herpetiform papulovesicles which had a tendency to coalesce and persisted for 2 months, and subsequent outbreaks occurred over 2 years. A 9-year-old boy had three episodes of fever and an acute widespread, vesiculopapular eruption, lasting for 2 weeks each, over 2 years. Biopsies from all four patients showed the characteristic features of eosinophilic cellulitis. In addition, in the patient with scalp nodules, there were extensive subcutaneous necrotizing granulomas surrounded by a rim of histiocytes and a massive diffuse infiltration of partially ruptured eosinophilic cells and granules.

Differential diagnosis

Tissue biopsy is the diagnostic investigation. Peripheral blood eosinophilia is a feature, but is not usually sufficiently severe or persistent to cause confusion with HES. Furthermore, the lack of multisystemic involvement and the presence of flame figures (which are not seen in the cutaneous lesions of HES although perivascular eosinophil and monocyte infiltration can be marked) help to differentiate these conditions.

Serological tests for *Toxocara* should be carried out to exclude *Toxocara* infection. Heiner and Kevy [5] described a child with itchy papular erythema due to *Toxocara canis* larva migrans infection, and the biopsy showed dermal infiltration of eosinophils and histiocytes with areas of 'fibrinoid degeneration of collagen'. Rook and Staughton [6] similarly observed perivascular and fat infiltration by eosinophils and histiocytes in an adult patient with toxocariasis and infiltrated skin lesions.

The resolving lesions may resemble morphoea.

The Churg–Strauss syndrome is differentiated clinically by the lack of systemic upset and the favourable outcome, and histologically by the presence of a true vasculitis. Clinically the lesions tend to be purpuric, with tender subcutaneous nodules and cutaneous infarcts rather than urticarial/cellulitic lesions.

Treatment

Often no treatment is necessary, low dose corticosteroids are helpful if needed.

REFERENCES

1 Wells GC. Recurrent granulomatous dermatitis with eosinophilia. *Trans St John's Hosp Dermatol Soc* 1971; 57: 46–56.
2 Peters MS, Schroeter AL, Gleich GJ. Immunofluorescence identification of eosinophil granule major basic protein in the flame figures of Well's syndrome. *Br J Dermatol* 1983; 109: 141–8.
3 Wells GC, Smith NP. Eosinophilic cellulitis. *Br J Dermatol* 1979; 100: 101–9.
4 Lindskov R, Illum N, Weismann K, Thomsen OF. Eosinophilic cellulitis: five cases. *Acta Derm Venereol* 1988; 68: 325–30.
5 Heiner DC, Kevy SV. Visceral larva migrans. Report of syndrome in three siblings. *New Eng J Med* 1956; 254: 629.
6 Rook AJ, Staughton RCD. Cutaneous manifestations of toxocariasis. *Dermatologica* 1972; 144: 129.

Eosinophilic fasciitis

Aetiology and pathogenesis

Also known as Shulman's syndrome, eosinophilic fasciitis appears to be a distinct entity, although it may be an early phase of systemic sclerosis or a variant of linear scleroderma. It can occur in association with other connective tissue disorders. Preceding trauma or strenuous exertion have been implicated in some cases. There is a male preponderance in both children and adults. Over a hundred cases have now been reported, the youngest being only 2 years old.

An eosinophil chemotactic activity has been detected in the sera of patients with eosinophilic fasciitis [1]

Pathology

There is dermal sclerosis with inflammation and fibrosis of the fat and deep fascia. The fascia becomes thickened, with collagen hypertrophy and infiltration by lymphocytes, plasma cells, histiocytes and eosinophils. Lack of new collagen deposition in early lesions distinguishes this from scleroderma. IMF demonstrates IgG and C3 in the deep fascia. The serum of these patients contains a serum factor which suppresses *in vitro* myeloid and erythrocyte precursors.

Clinical features

Painful swelling of the distal part of the limbs, progressing to indurated lesions which limit movement of the hands and feet, is the usual presentation, although occasionally the face or abdomen has been affected. There may be superficial blistering and haemorrhage. Polyarthritis is rarely associated, and subsequent development of aplastic anaemia is reported more commonly than by chance. Raynaud's phenomenon and nail-fold capillary defects are not usually a feature.

Peripheral blood eosinophilia, up to 30%, is observed in the majority (about 70% of cases) but it is transient. The sedimentation rate is raised, and there is hypergammaglobulinaemia. Bone marrow biopsy may reveal plasmacytosis and eosinophilia, and rarely aplastic anaemia and thrombocytopenia occur. Serum aldolase may be elevated, but creative phosphokinase is normal. A deep biopsy including muscle fascia is necessary for diagnosis.

Treatment

Corticosteroid therapy is effective, but spontaneous resolution can occur.

REFERENCE

1 Wasserman SI, Seibold JR, Medsger TA Jr, Rodman GP. Serum eosinophilotactic activity in eosinophilic fasciitis. *Arthritis Rheum* 1982; 25: 1352–6.

29.8 Angiolymphoid Hyperplasia with Eosinophilia

LINDA G. RABINOWITZ

Definition

Angiolymphoid hyperplasia with eosinophilia (ALHE) is a rare condition that is considered to be either a benign vascular neoplasm or an inflammatory process of the skin. It represents a distinct disease process, probably unrelated to Kimura's disease, and is characterized by nodules that are located in the dermis as well as the subcutaneous tissues. Similar cases have been reported under a variety of names including atypical pyogenic granuloma, pseudopyogenic granuloma, histiocytoid haemangioma, epithelioid haemangioma and inflammatory angiomatous nodules. There is a broad spectrum of clinical and histological presentations.

History

In 1948, Kimura initially described subcutaneous nodules that were similar to those seen in ALHE. They were reported to be 'eosinophilic lymph folliculosis' of the skin [1]. In 1969, Wells and Whimster identified these subcutaneous nodules as subcutaneous ALHE [2]. Subsequently, the dermal nodules were reported as pseudogranuloma pyogenicum or atypical pyogenic granulomas. It later became apparent that these intradermal and subcutaneous lesions shared the same disease process [1]. In 1979, Rosai *et al.* suggested that the term histiocytoid haemangioma be used, since it was believed that the primary event was vascular proliferation, a feature typical of haemangiomas [3]. Nevertheless, the use of multiple terms for this entity has added to the semantic confusion in the literature.

Aetiology

Although the pathogenesis of ALHE is not entirely clear, the disorder is distinguished by proliferation of endothelial cells and an accompanying inflammatory reaction. It has been debated whether the lesions represent true vascular neoplasms or reactive healing phenomena. A small percentage of patients have a history of previous trauma to the skin at the site affected by ALHE [4].

Pathology

Histopathological evaluation reveals two essential findings in these lesions. The first is anomalous vascular hyperplasia which features irregularly shaped capillaries that have swollen pleomorphic 'histiocytoid' endothelial cells protruding into the lumina. This has been described as a 'hobnail' appearance [4]. The endothelial cell layer may be two or three cells thick. The blood vessels are thick walled, and arteriovenous shunts may be present. The second essential finding is an inflammatory infiltrate containing germinal centres and lymphocytes, histiocytes and eosinophils. There is variability in the intensity of this mixed cellular infiltrate which is found in the dermis and/or subcutaneous tissues. Although eosinophils are usually prominent in the infiltrate, they may be absent or few in number. Direct immunofluorescence staining reveals immunoglobulin A (IgA), IgM and C3 deposition around blood vessels, suggesting an immunological phenomenon [5].

Clinical features

ALHE is a rare disorder characterized by solitary or multiple dermal or subcutaneous papules and nodules that are usually located on the head and neck of young adults. There is a slight female predominance, and the median age of onset is 32 years. There is a low incidence in African-Americans [4].

Clinically, there are dome-shaped papules, nodules or plaques which range in colour from pink to red–brown and have a predilection for the scalp, forehead and sites in and around the ears. Other less common sites of involvement include the palm, genitalia and oral mucosae. Some of the dermal papules or nodules may have overlying superficial erosions and crusting. Subcutaneous lesions typically lack distinguishing surface changes. Symptoms might include pruritus or pain, and lesion tenderness is present in almost one-third of patients. Each dermal nodule typically measures 1–2 cm. Subcutaneous lesions may be as large as 5–10 cm. Some nodules have palpable pulsations, and spontaneous bleeding has been reported to occur. Peripheral blood eosinophilia is not always present.

Prognosis

The clinical course of ALHE is protracted, and lesions may increase in number over time and persist indefinitely. Spontaneous resolution is exceedingly rare, but has been reported to occur [4]. Recurrences are seen in some cases. No serious sequelae have been associated with ALHE.

Differential diagnosis

Lesions of ALHE may be confused with haemangiomas, pyogenic granulomas and, possibly, inflamed epidermal cysts. The clinical differential diagnosis includes all vascular neoplasms, bacillary angiomatosis, verruga peruana, Kaposi's sarcoma, granuloma faciale and metastatic tumours. Establishing the diagnosis of ALHE prior to obtaining skin biopsy results is unlikely because of the non-specific clinical morphology. The histological differential diagnosis includes angiosarcoma, but this disorder is seen most frequently in older adults and biopsy specimen findings reveal large endothelial cells and immature blood vessels. ALHE, in contrast to angiosarcoma, is often dominated by tissue eosinophilia. Other entities that should be distinguished from ALHE are spindle cell haemangioendothelioma, intravascular papillary endothelial hyperplasia, persistent arthropod reaction and pseudolymphomas.

Although the relationship of Kimura's disease to ALHE has been unclear, it is now generally accepted that these are separate entities [6,7]. Unlike ALHE, Kimura's disease typically affects young Asian males. In addition, these children almost always have contiguous lymphadenopathy, a clinical finding not seen in patients with ALHE. Lesions usually arise in the subcutaneous tissue, are larger than those seen in ALHE, and may not be limited to the head/neck area. The skin overlying the nodules is normal.

Peripheral eosinophilia is seen in virtually all cases, whereas this feature is variably present in patients with ALHE. Kimura's disease does not exhibit the distinctive endothelial cells (hobnailing) typical of ALHE. However, there are huge numbers of eosinophils in the cellular infiltrates, and eosinophilic microabscesses may be noted.

Treatment

Generally, nodules of ALHE are removed surgically. Some patients have been treated with topical, intralesional or systemic corticosteroids with variable success. Systemic vinblastine has been reported to be beneficial in isolated reports. Pentoxifylline has been useful in at least one patient [8,9].

REFERENCES

1 Lever W, Schaumburg-Lever G. *Histopathology of the Skin*, 7th edn. Philadelphia: JB Lippincott, 1990: 714–15.
2 Wells GC, Whimster IW. Subcutaneous angiolymphoid hyperplasia with eosinophilia. *Br J Dermatol* 1969; 81: 1–15.
3 Rosai J, Gold J, Landy R. The histiocytoid hemangiomas: a unifying concept embracing several previously described entities of skin, soft tissue, large vessels, bone, and heart. *Hum Pathol* 1979; 10: 707–30.
4 Olsen TG, Helwig EB. Angiolymphoid hyperplasia with eosinophilia. *J Am Acad Dermatol* 1985; 12: 781–96.
5 Grimwood R, Swinehart JM, Aeling JL. Angiolymphoid hyperplasia with eosinophilia. *Arch Dermatol* 1979; 115: 205–7.
6 Helander SD, Peters MS, Kuo TT, Su WP. Kimura's disease and angiolymphoid hyperplasia with eosinophilia: new observations from immunohistochemical studies of lymphocyte markers, endothelial antigens, and granulocyte proteins. *J Cutan Pathol* 1995; 22: 319–26.
7 Chun SI, Ji HG. Kimura's disease and angiolymphoid hyperplasia with eosinophilia: clinical and histopathologic differences. *J Am Acad Dermatol* 1992; 27: 954–8.
8 Person JR. Angiolymphoid hyperplasia with eosinophilia may respond to pentoxifylline. *J Am Acad Dermatol* 1994; 31: 117–18.
9 Cheney ML, Googe P, Bhatt S, Hibberd PL. Angiolymphoid hyperplasia with eosinophilia (histiocytoid hemangioma): evaluation of treatment options. *Ann Otol Rhinol Laryngol* 1993; 102: 303–8.

Amyloidosis

TERI A. KAHN

Definition

Amyloidosis, also known as the β-fibrilloses, comprises a diverse group of disease processes that result in the extracellular deposition of β-pleated protein-derived fibrils in various tissues [1–3]. The most common forms of amyloidosis consist of one of three major types of proteins within the fibrils: amyloid light chain (AL) protein, amyloid A (AA) protein or keratinocyte-derived amyloid (K amyloid) [1,2,4]. The quantity and site of amyloid deposition determine whether there is associated clinical disease or merely an incidental histological finding. Disease classification may be based on the location of the amyloid deposits (systemic versus localized), and by whether the amyloid deposition is a primary or secondary disease process (Table 29.9.1). In this chapter, the emphasis will be on cutaneous disease presentations of amyloidosis which affect children. Overall, cutaneous amyloidosis is extremely rare in children, and the most likely types of primary localized cutaneous amyloidosis (PLCA) to occur in this age group are lichen or macular amyloidosis. The systemic forms in children, which are even more uncommon, are usually familial and will be reviewed briefly.

History

The first probable case of systemic amyloidosis was described by Fontanus (Fonteyn) in 1639, but Rokitansky is credited with identifying a lardaceous or waxy amyloid-like degradation in tissue in association with tuberculosis, syphilis and rickets more than 50 years ago [5]. During that time, Schleiden coined the term 'amyloid' to describe a constituent of plants [5], and Virchow used the term 'amyloid change' (cellulose-like) in 1854, when he observed the similar reactions of amyloid and cellulose polysaccharide to iodine and sulphuric acid [6]. Guttman in 1928 reported the first case of primary localized cutaneous amyloidosis, and Freudenthal introduced the term 'lichen amyloidosis' in 1930 [6].

Special stains have been used to identify amyloid since 1875 [5]. In 1930, Freudenthal implicated keratinocytes in the causation of lichen amyloidosis. Glenner and Page described the AL protein in 1971 [7], and Hashimoto and Kumakiri further elucidated the role of keratinocytes in cutaneous amyloid production in 1979 [4].

Aetiology

Ultrastructurally, amyloid is composed of straight, non-branching fibrils 7.5–10.0 nm in diameter, arranged haphazardly in a 'felt-like' array [1–3,5]. The fibrils are arranged in an antiparallel (β-pleated) configuration which is responsible for the affinity of amyloid to cotton dyes (e.g. Congo red) [1–3,5]. Several sources of amyloid-fibrillar proteins have been identified. Plasma cells secrete AL protein from intact immunoglobulin G (IgG) light chains (primarily lamda) in three main disease states (immunocytic amyloidoses): primary systemic amyloidosis, amyloidosis associated with plasma cell dyscrasias (in particular, multiple myeloma) and localized nodular (tumefactive) amyloidosis of the skin or other organs [1,3,7]. Serum amyloid A (SAA) protein is a normal serum protein synthesized by the liver in association with serum high-density lipoprotein (HDL), and it behaves as an acute phase reactant. During inflammatory states, macrophages phagocytose SAA and transform SAA into AA protein [1]. AA is present in both reactive (secondary) systemic amyloidosis and systemic heredofamilial amyloidosis [1]. Damaged and degenerating keratinocytes (e.g. due to psoralens and ultraviolet A) [8] are the source of Keratinoid amyloid, which is the principal amyloid protein in PLCA [4,9]. Transthyretin, a type of prealbumin, is the source of amyloid in some of the heredofamilial neurotropic amyloidoses [10].

Cutaneous amyloidosis in children may be due to genetic or environmental factors. Familial cutaneous lichen amyloidosis is autosomal dominant [11–15]. A form of lichen amyloidosis occurs in association with Sipple syndrome (multiple endocrine neoplasia (MEN) type 2A) [16–18], and a mutation of the RET proto-oncogene on chromosome 10 is believed to be responsible for this constellation of findings [19]. However, patients with familial cutaneous lichen amyloidosis do not have this gene mutation and therefore do not appear to be at risk for developing Sipple syndrome [20]. The genetic defect in

Table 29.9.1 Classification of amyloidoses

Type of amyloidosis	Origin of amyloid	Distribution of amyloid in tissue
Cutaneous amyloidosis		
PLCA	Keratinocytes	Papillary dermis
lichenoid		
macular		
biphasic		
bullous		
poikiloderma-like		
Nodular	Immunoglobulin AL protein	Papillary, reticular dermis, subcutaneous fat, eccrine glands and blood vessels
Secondary	Keratinocytes	Adjacent tissue
tumour associated		
Systemic amyloidosis		
Primary	Immunoglobulin AL protein	Dermis, vessel walls, subcutaneous fat, eccrine glands and mesenchymal tissues
Secondary		
JRA, Hodgkin's lymphoma, tuberculosis	SAA protein → AA protein	Subcutaneous fat, vessel walls, eccrine glands, parenchymal organs
Heredofamilial		
familial Mediterranean fever	SAA protein → AA protein	
Muckle–Wells syndrome	SAA protein → AA protein	
neurotropic	Transthyretin (prealbumin)	

JRA, juvenile rheumatoid arthritis; PCLA, primary localized cutaneous amyloidosis.

Partington's syndrome (X-linked cutaneous amyloidosis) has been localized to Xp22–p21 [21]. Macular amyloidosis is frequently an early form of lichen amyloidosis, but it may also occur due to friction from nylon brushes, back scratchers or sharp fingernails [22,23].

Pathology

Although amyloid is derived from many different sources, the different forms of amyloid are morphologically the same on histological sections [1–3,5,6]. In haematoxylin and eosin stain, amyloid appears as amorphous, eosinophilic extracellular aggregates, without accompanying inflammation [1–3,5,6]. Special stains are helpful when minimal amounts of amyloid are present. Amyloid stains metachromatically with toluidine blue, crystal violet or methyl violet [1–3,5,6,24]. Congo red and other cotton dyes produce an apple-green birefringence in polarized light and are the most specific stains for the detection of amyloid. With thioflavine T, fluorescent microscopy reveals a yellow–green fluorescence [1–3,5,6]. Under the electron microscope, amyloid deposits are seen as straight, non-branching fibrils 7.5–10.0 nm in diameter, arranged in a 'felt-like' array [1–3,5,6]. The fibril is composed of two twisted β-pleated sheet micelles helically arranged in antiparallel conformation, as seen by X-ray crystallography [1–3,5,6].

Clinical features

Cutaneous amyloidoses (Table 29.9.2)

Primary localized cutaneous amyloidosis (PCLA). Lichen amyloidosis is the most common form of PLCA. Its peak incidence is between 40 and 60 years, although in children it usually occurs in adolescence [12–14]. It is most prevalent in Chinese people residing in Taiwan, Singapore and Indonesia [12–14]. Lichen amyloidosis presents with intensely pruritic flesh-coloured, grey or yellowish-brown papules ranging in size from 1 to 10 mm. They are most commonly located on the pretibial surfaces but may also occur on the extensor surfaces of the forearms, the trunk, shoulders and sacrum (Fig. 29.9.1).

Macular amyloidosis occurs more commonly in children than lichen amyloidosis [25]. It is seen more frequently in people of Latin American, Asian or Middle Eastern origin [22–25]. Typically occurring during adolescence, the macular form presents as poorly delineated hyperpigmented patches or as a linear rippling of the skin by moderately pruritic, closely aggregated greyish-brown macules. This presentation most commonly involves the lower extremities but may also involve the mid-back or arms (Fig. 29.9.2). Rubbing the affected area with a nylon brush or back scratcher may lead to the macular form known as 'friction amyloidosis' [22,23].

Diffuse biphasic amyloidosis is the existence of both macular and lichen amyloidosis in the same patient. Rubbing and scratching may transform the macular to the

Table 29.9.2 Cutaneous amyloidosis in children

PLCA
Major types
  lichenoid
     sporadic
     FPCA late stage
  macular:
     sporadic ('friction' amyloidosis)
     FPCA early stage
  biphasic
     sporadic
     FPCA early stage
Less common types
  FPCA associated with Sipple syndrome
  poikiloderma-like
  bullous
  genodermatoses-associated macular variant

Secondary cutaneous amyloidoses
Skin-tumour associated

FPCA, familial primary cutaneous amyloidosis.

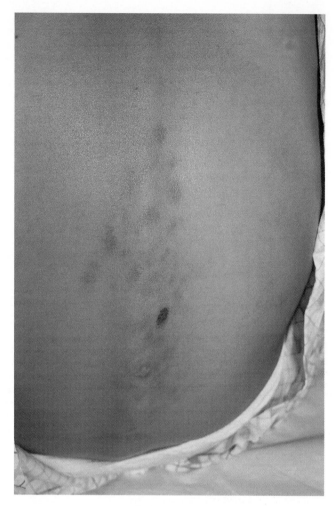

Fig. 29.9.2 Macular amyloidosis. Hyperpigmented patches with superficial erosion in a 12-year-old girl.

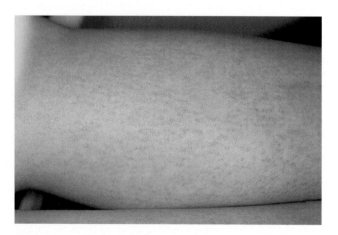

Fig. 29.9.1 Lichen amyloidosis: flesh-coloured papules on the lower legs of a 17-year-old girl.

lichenoid form, and intralesional steroids may transform the lichenoid to the macular form [3–5,22,23].

Familial primary cutaneous amyloidosis (FPCA) is an autosomal dominant disorder with incomplete penetrance [11–15]. The onset is during puberty as either the macular or biphasic form of amyloidosis, and it progresses with age into the lichenoid form [11–15]. The most common locations are the interscapular and pretibial areas, and the intensity of the pruritus is much greater than the clinical appearance [14].

In all of the sporadic and familial forms of lichenoid, macular or biphasic forms of amyloidosis, there is no risk for developing systemic amyloidosis [3,5,6]. However, there is one form of familial primary cutaneous amyloidosis where the cutaneous lesions may signal the risk for developing Sipple syndrome, or multiple endocrine neoplasia 2A (MEN 2A) [16–18]. Sipple syndrome is an autosomal dominant disorder associated with the triad of parathyroid hyperplasia, phaeochromocytoma and

medullary carcinoma of the thyroid. In some kindreds, cutaneous lichen or biphasic amyloidosis presents as an intensely pruritic plaque involving the interscapular area [16–18]. The cutaneous amyloidosis usually occurs in childhood or adolescence and frequently precedes the development of the neoplasms [16–18]. Therefore, young patients presenting with interscapular amyloidosis should be evaluated for the risk of developing MEN 2A, including the presence of the mutation for the RET proto-oncogene on chromosome 10 [20]. PLCA was also reported to occur in a family with medullary thyroid carcinoma, without other endocrinopathies [26].

Poikiloderma-like cutaneous amyloidosis is an extremely rare autosomal dominant disorder associated with poikiloderma, lichen amyloid papules, short stature and photosensitivity. The skin lesions appear early in life, and palmoplantar keratosis and blister formation may rarely occur. Amyloid deposition is present in both the poikilodermatous and the lichenoid lesions [23,27].

A single report of bullous amyloidosis describes bullous lesions around joints in adolescents, with onset of disease between 10 and 13 years of age. Biopsy confirmed the presence of amyloid within the bullae [28]. Nodular, anosacral and vitiliginous amyloidoses have not been reported to occur in children.

Genodermatosis-associated amyloidosis comprises several syndromes that have asymptomatic macular amyloid within cutaneous hyperpigmentation. Partington's syndrome, or X-linked reticulate pigmentary disorder with systemic manifestations, was formerly known as X-linked cutaneous amyloidosis [29]. Partington originally reported a family where the affected males had generalized and reticulated 'muddy' brown pigmentation, with xerosis and hypopigmentation on the torso and proximal extremities. These male infants had severe systemic involvement, including ulcerative colitis, failure to thrive, photophobia with corneal dystrophy, unruly hair, recurrent pneumonia and chronic pulmonary disease that led to premature death. The females only had macular naevoid hyperpigmentation along Blaschko's lines without systemic disease. Amyloid deposits were present in the pigmented skin of both sexes [29]. A 10-year follow-up study revealed that the amyloid deposits were not a consistent finding [30], and other reports have since confirmed that amyloid was not always found in identical clinical presentations, leading to the change in the name of the syndrome [31,32]. Other genodermatoses associated with asymptomatic macular amyloid include pachyonychia congenita (Tidman–Wells–MacDonald variant) [33], epidermolysis bullosa (Weber–Cockayne type) [34], dyskeratosis congenita [35] and the Nageli–Franceschetti–Jadassohn syndrome [36].

Secondary cutaneous amyloidosis. Skin tumour-associated amyloidosis is the asymptomatic deposition of amyloidosis within and around tumours. In the paediatric population, these would include pilomatrixomas, porokeratosis of Mibelli and melanocytic naevi [3].

Systemic amyloidosis. Primary systemic or immunocytic amyloidosis is extremely rare in childhood [25,37]. Infiltration of amyloid in the tongue leads to macroglossia, and amyloid deposition within the blood vessel walls leads to 'pinch purpura' and purpura after the Valsalva manoeuvre. Waxy, smooth, shiny asymptomatic amber or yellow papules may occur in flexural areas, or on the central part of the face, lips and oral mucosa. A leonine facies may occur as well as sclerodermatous-type changes on the hands [3]. Rectal biopsy is often diagnostic for amyloidosis [3].

Reactive or secondary systemic amyloidosis is associated with chronic inflammatory diseases. These include juvenile rheumatoid arthritis, Hodgkin's disease and tuberculosis [38–40]. The amyloid deposits involve mainly the kidneys, spleen, liver and heart, and skin findings are rare. Recessive dystrophic epidermolysis bullosa has been reported in association with systemic amyloidosis involving the heart, stomach, kidneys and thyroid gland [41].

Heredofamiliar syndromes include several entities with systemic amyloidosis and other distinctive cutaneous findings that are not cutaneous amyloid. Familial Mediterranean fever (recurrent hereditary polyserositis) is an autosomal recessive disorder of febrile episodes associated with transient symptoms most commonly localized to serosal surfaces. Amyloid nephropathy occurs in childhood and can result in death from renal failure. [38,39,42]. Cutaneous changes include an erysipelas-like erythema around the ankles or dorsae of the feet, and over the extensor surfaces of the legs. Biopsy reveals vasculitis, and this rash is highly specific for familial Mediterranean fever. Other cutaneous findings include Henoch–Schönlein purpura, urticaria and a unilateral, painful, red, swollen scrotum associated with fever, leucocytosis and elevated erythrocyte sedimentation rate which spontaneously resolves within 24–72 h. Erythema nodosum-like lesions may occur in adult patients with familial Mediterranean fever [42].

Muckle–Wells syndrome is an autosomal dominant disorder associated with recurrent attacks of urticaria and flu-like symptoms present during adolescence, followed by progressive deafness and amyloid nephropathy [43].

Neurotropic amyloidoses are autosomal dominant disorders associated with amyloid neuropathy affecting Portuguese, Swedish and Finnish families [10,40,44]. Patients have the constellation of painless ulcers with eventual loss of digits, carpal tunnel syndrome, malabsorption, vitreous opacities and cardiac involvement. The neuropathy may occur in adolescence, but the other skin changes, including hyperpigmented atrophic scars, hypotrichosis blisters and sclerodermatous changes do not appear until adulthood [10,25,40,44].

Prognosis

The localized cutaneous forms of amyloidosis persist unchanged or may slowly progress. In systemic amyloidosis, mortality is related to visceral involvement and is especially high with renal or cardiac amyloidosis.

Differential diagnosis

Lichen amyloidosis may be confused with lichen simplex chronicus, pretibial myxoedema, confluent and reticulated papillomatosis of Gougerot and Carteaud, lichen myxoedematosus, colloid milium, stasis dermatitis and lichen planus [23,25]. Macular amyloidosis may resemble stasis dermatitis, postinflammatory hyperpigmentation, pigmented purpuric dermatoses, pityriasis versicolor, erythema dyschromicum perstans, and hyperpigmentation due to endocrine disorders, drugs or heavy metals [45]. Poikiloderma-like cutaneous amyloidosis must be differentiated from Rothmund–Thomson syndrome, and

Partington's syndrome can clinically resemble incontinentia pigmenti. Histopathology and special stains are so specific and distinctive that they can easily confirm the diagnosis of amyloidosis.

Treatment

Treatment is not totally satisfactory for localized cutaneous amyloidosis. Topical and intralesional corticosteroids offer some relief from the pruritus, often in conjunction with oral antihistamines [3,6,23–25]. Cryosurgery has limited success, but dermabrasion may be helpful for some patients [46]. Etretinate may be effective for some patients with lichen amyloidosis [47] but is not recommended for female patients until after child-bearing age.

Treatment for systemic amyloidosis is disease-specific. Primary systemic amyloidosis is somewhat responsive to melphalan, prednisone and peritoneal dialysis [2,3]. Secondary systemic amyloidosis requires treatment of the underlying disease as well as cytotoxic or supportive care for the systemic amyloidosis. For familial Mediterranean fever, colchicine is a successful treatment for the renal amyloidosis [48].

REFERENCES

1 Glenner GG. Amyloid deposits and amyloidosis. The beta-fibrilloses. Part 1. *N Engl J Med* 1980; 302: 1283–92.
2 Glenner GG. Amyloid deposits and amyloidosis. The beta-fibrilloses. Part 2. *N Engl J Med* 1980; 302: 1333–43.
3 Breathnach SM. Amyloid and amyloidosis. *J Am Acad Dermatol* 1988; 18: 1–16.
4 Kumakiri M, Hashimoto K. Histogenesis of primary localized cutaneous amyloidosis: sequential change of epidermal keratinocytes to amyloid via filamentous degeneration. *J Invest Dermatol* 1979; 73: 150–62.
5 Kyle RA. Amyloidosis. Part 1. *Int J Dermatol* 1980; 19: 537–9.
6 Wong C-K. History and modern concepts. *Clin Derm* 1990; 8: 1–6.
7 Glenner GG, Terry W, Harada M, Isersky C, Page D. Amyloid fibril proteins: proof of homology with immunoglobulin light chains by sequence analyses. *Science* 1971; 172: 1150–1.
8 Hashimoto K, Kumakiri M. Colloid-amyloid bodies in PUVA-treated human psoriatic patients. *J Invest Dermatol* 1979; 72: 70–80.
9 Hashimoto K. Progress in cutaneous amyloidosis. *J Invest Dermatol* 1984; 82: 1–3.
10 Benson MD. Inherited amyloidosis. *J Med Genet* 1991; 28: 73–8.
11 Sagher F, Shanon J. Amyloidosis cutis: familial occurrence in three generations. *Arch Derm* 1963; 87: 171–5.
12 Rajagopalan K, Tay CH. Familial lichen amyloidosis. Report of 19 cases in four generations of a Chinese family in Malaysia. *Br J Derm* 1972; 87: 123–9.
13 Ozaka M. Familial lichen amyloidosis. *Int J Dermatol* 1984; 23: 190–3.
14 Newton JA, Jagjivan A, Bhogal B, McKee PH, McGibbon DH. Familial primary cutaneous amyloidosis. *Br J Derm* 1985; 112: 201–8.
15 De Pietro WP. Primary familial cutaneous amyloidosis: a study of HLA antigens in a Puerto Rican family. *Arch Derm* 1981; 117: 639–42.
16 Gagel RF, Levy ML, Donovan DT, Alford BR, Wheeler T, Tshen JA. Multiple endocrine neoplasia type 2A associated with cutaneous lichen amyloidosis. *Ann Int Med* 1989; 111: 802–6.
17 Kousseff BG, Espinoza C, Zamore GA. Sipple syndrome with lichen amyloidosis as a paracrinopathy: pleiotropy, heterogeneity, or a contiguous gene? *J Am Acad Dermatol* 1991; 25: 651–7.
18 Robinson MF, Furst EJ, Nunziata V *et al.* Characterization of the clinical features of five families with hereditary primary cutaneous lichen amyloidosis

and multiple endocrine neoplasia type 2. *Henry Ford Hosp Med J* 1992; 40: 249–52.
19 Mulligan LM, Kwok JBJ, Healey CS *et al.* Germ-line mutations of the RET proto-oncogene in multiple endocrine neoplasia type 2A. *Nature* 1993; 363: 458–60.
20 Hofstra RMW, Sijmons RH, Stelwagen T *et al.* RET mutation screening in familial cutaneous lichen amyloidosis and in skin amyloidosis associated with multiple endocrine neoplasia. *J Invest Dermatol* 1996; 107: 215–18.
21 Gedeon AK, Mulley JC, Kozman H, Donnelly A, Partington MW. Localization of the gene for X-linked reticulate pigmentary disorder with systemic manifestations (PDR), previously known as X-linked cutaneous amyloidosis. *Am J Med Genet* 1994; 52: 75–8.
22 Wong C-K, Lin C-S. Friction amyloidosis. *Int J Dermatol* 1988; 27: 302–7.
23 Wang W-J. Clinical features of cutaneous amyloidoses. *Clin Derm* 1990; 8: 13–19.
24 Wong C-K. Cutaneous amyloidoses. *Int J Dermatol* 1987; 26: 273–7.
25 Mallory SB. Infiltrative diseases. In: Schachner LA, Hanson RC, eds. *Pediatric Dermatology*, vol. 2. New York: Churchill Livingstone, 1988: 859–61.
26 Ferrer JP, Halperin I, Conget I, Alsina M, Martinez-Osaba MJ. Primary localized cutaneous amyloidosis and familial medullary thyroid carcinoma. *Clin Endocrinol* 1991; 34: 435–9.
27 Ogino A, Tanaca S. Poikiloderma-like cutaneous amyloidosis. *Dermatologica* 1977; 155: 301–9.
28 DeSouza AR. Amiloidose cutanea bullosa familial. Observacao de 4 casos. *Rev Hosp Clin Fac Med S Paulo* 1963; 18: 413–17.
29 Partington MW, Marriott PJ, Prentice RS, Cavaglia A, Simpson NE. Familial cutaneous amyloidosis with systemic manifestations in males. *Am J Med Genet* 1981; 10: 65–75.
30 Partington MW, Prentice RS. X-Linked cutaneous amyloidosis: further clinical and pathological observations. *Am J Med Genet* 1989; 32: 115–19.
31 Ades LC, Rogers M, Sillence DO. An X-linked reticulate pigmentary disorder with systemic manifestations: report of a second family. *Pediatr Dermatol* 1993; 10: 344–51.
32 Salmon JK, Frieden IJ. Congenital and genetic disorders of hyperpigmentation. *Curr Prob Dermatol* 1995; 7: 182–3.
33 Tidman MJ, Wells RS, Macdonald DM. Pachyonychia congenita with cutaneous amyloidosis and hyperpigmentation: a distinct variant. *J Am Acad Dermatol* 1987; 16: 935–40.
34 Kantor GR, Kasick JM, Bergfeld WF, McMahon JT, Krebs JA. Epidermolysis bullosa of the Weber–Cockayne type with macular amyloidosis. *Cleve Clin Q* 1985; 52: 425–8.
35 Llistosella E, Moreno A, deMoragas JM. Dyskeratosis congenita with macular cutaneous amyloid deposits. *Arch Dermatol* 1984; 120: 1381–2.
36 Frenk E, Mevorah B, Hohl D. The Nageli–Franceschetti–Jadassohn syndrome: a hereditary ectodermal defect leading to colloid-amyloid formation in the dermis. *Dermatology* 1993; 187: 169–73.
37 Pick AI, Versano I, Schreibman S, Ben-Bassat M, Shoenfeld Y. Agammaglobulinemia, plasma cell dyscrasia, and amyloidosis in a 12-year-old child. *Am J Dis Child* 1977; 131: 682–6.
38 Woo P. Amyloidosis in pediatric rheumatic diseases. *J Rheum* 1992; 19: 10–16.
39 Woo P. Amyloidosis in children. *Ballière's Clin Rheumatol* 1994; 8: 691–97.
40 Kyle RA. Amyloidosis. Part 3. *Int J Dermatol* 1981; 20: 75–80.
41 Yi S, Naito K, Nogami R, Maekawawa Y, Arao T. Complicating systemic amyloidosis in dystrophic epidermolysis bullosa, recessive type. *Pathology* 1988; 20: 184–7.
42 Gedalia A, Adar A, Gorodischer R. Familial Mediterranean fever in children. *J Rheum* 1992; 19: 1–9.
43 Muckle TJ. The Muckle–Wells syndrome. *Br J Dermatol* 1979; 100: 87–92.
44 Meretoja J. Familial systemic paramyloidosis with lattice dystrophy of the cornea, progressive cranial neuropathy, skin changes and various internal symptoms: a previously unrecognized heritable syndrome. *Ann Clin Res* 1969; 1: 314–24.
45 Wang C-K, Lee JY-Y. Macular amyloidosis with widespread diffuse pigmentation. *Br J Dermatol* 1996; 135: 135–8.
46 Wong C-K, Li W-M. Dermabrasion for lichen amyloidosus. *Arch Dermatol* 1982; 118: 302–4.
47 Helander I, Hopsu-Havu VK. Treatment of lichen amyloidosus by etretinate. *Clin Exp Dermatol* 1986; 11: 574–7.
48 Zemer D, Pras M, Sohar E, Modan M, Cabili S, Gafni J. Colchicine in the prevention and treatment of the amyloidosis of familial Mediterranean fever. *N Engl J Med* 1986; 314: 1001–5.

Carotenaemia

PETER T. CLAYTON

Definition

Carotenaemia is a condition in which the plasma concentration of carotenoids (principally β-carotene) is elevated producing a yellowish discoloration of the skin (xanthodermia). Carotenoids are pigments which are synthesized by plants and which are present in foods such as carrots and all green vegetables. They are generally C_{40} tetraterpenoids formed from eight isoprenoid units joined so that the configuration is reversed in the centre [1]. The most abundant carotenoid in the diet is β-carotene the structure of which is shown in Fig. 29.10.1. Carotenoids are an important source of vitamin A. Normal plasma concentrations of β-carotene and vitamin A in children are given in Table 29.10.1 [2].

History

Prior to the 20th century there were occasional observations on 'aurantiasis' and 'carotenosis cutis' as forms of xanthodermia which were different from jaundice. In 1926 Greene and Blackford showed that it was possible to distinguish carotenaemia from jaundice by shaking serum with equal volumes of petroleum ether and absolute alcohol. Carotene colours the upper petroleum ether layer whereas bile pigments are found in the middle alcohol layer [3]. The food rationing of World War II provided the background to a series of observations on dietary carotenaemia. In the UK there was a successful campaign promoting the consumption of root vegetables (particularly carrots and swedes) and in 1941, Almond and Logan described four housewives who developed orange pigmentation of their palms and nasolabial folds following the ingestion of 2.7 kg of carrots weekly for 7 months. One of the four women was breast-feeding an infant and this infant also developed pigmentation which disappeared following a change to bottle feeding [4]. In 1958, Lord Cohen of Birkenhead reported 50 cases of xanthodermia diagnosed in the war years in the UK and associated with a raw carrot intake of 1.8–3.6 kg daily. Xanthodermia appeared after 6–8 months but if carrots were omitted from the diet the yellowish tinge faded in 2–6 weeks. Lord Cohen also described carotenaemia in hyperlipidaemic

states (including diabetes mellitus, the nephrotic syndrome and myxoedema). He was the first to describe a case of carotenaemia with low plasma vitamin A concentration and postulate that this was due to an inborn error in the conversion of β-carotene to vitamin A [5].

Aetiology and/or pathogenesis

A normal intake of β-carotene is 900–1200 μg/day. Ingested carotene is largely converted to vitamin A (retinol) in the intestinal mucosa by β-carotene 15,15'-oxygenase and retinaldehyde reductase (Fig. 29.10.1). A small proportion is absorbed unchanged. The absorption of β-carotene is increased in subjects taking a high-fat diet. The highly lipid-soluble pigment is present in the lipoprotein fractions of plasma (particularly low-density lipoprotein or LDL) and there is a close correlation between serum lipoprotein levels and serum β-carotene concentration [6]. Carotenaemia or hypercarotenaemia can therefore arise either as a result of excessive ingestion of β-carotene or as a result of defective conversion to vitamin A (metabolic carotenaemia) or as a result of hyperlipidaemia.

Excessive ingestion of carotene

Foods with a high content of β-carotene [7] are listed in Table 29.10.2. Ingestion of large amounts of any of these carotene-rich foods could give rise to carotenaemia. It is important to remember that β-carotene is also used as a food additive; its presence is usually declared on the package (as β-carotene or E160). Prince and Frisoli [8] have studied the accumulation of β-carotene in the plasma and skin in adult volunteers given a large daily dose of the pigment. The plasma concentration rises to a plateau over 9–10 days. Accumulation in the skin takes a further 2 weeks. On cessation of administration plasma carotene concentrations decay with a half-life of around 15 days [8].

Hyperlipidaemia

The concentration of β-carotene in the blood rises when the lipoprotein concentrations rise. The conditions which have been documented as giving rise to carotenaemia

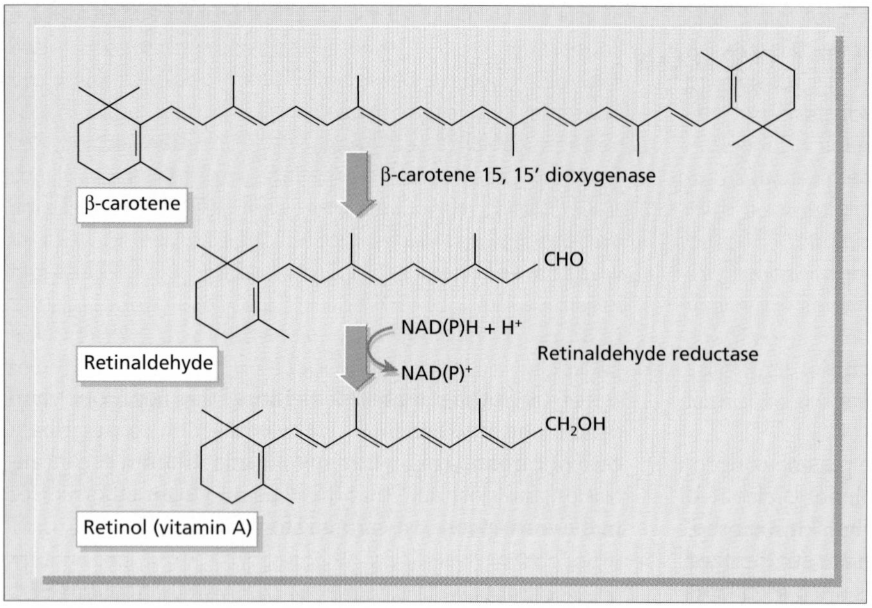

β-carotene

β-carotene 15, 15′ dioxygenase

CHO

Retinaldehyde

NAD(P)H + H$^+$

NAD(P)$^+$

Retinaldehyde reductase

CH$_2$OH

Retinol (vitamin A)

Fig. 29.10.1 Metabolism of β-carotene to vitamin A. β-Carotene 15,15′-dioxygenase is located in the intestinal mucosa.

Table 29.10.1 Normal ranges for serum concentrations of β-carotene and vitamin A in children (0.025–0.975 fractiles). To convert μmol/l to μg/l multiply by 537 for β-carotene and 286 for vitamin A (retinol). Data from Malvy *et al.* [2]

Analyte	Serum concentration	
	μmol/l	μg/l
β-carotene	0.56–2.85	300–1530
Vitamin A	0.67–2.39	182–683

include diabetes mellitus (which usually gives rise to increased plasma very low-density lipoprotein or VLDL) hypothyroidism (increased LDL) and the nephrotic syndrome (increased LDL and VLDL) [5]. Other causes of hyperlipoproteinaemia in childhood include obstructive jaundice, hepatic glycogenoses, renal dialysis, acute porphyria, cholesterol ester storage disease and the primary hyperlipidaemias [9]. It has also been reported in some patients with anorexia nervosa [10]. The mechanisms responsible for the hyperlipidaemia in these conditions are beyond the scope of this chapter. In hyperthyroidism the conversion of β-carotene to vitamin A is reduced so that this is an additional mechanism for the carotenaemia.

Metabolic carotenaemia

The inborn error(s) of β-carotene metabolism are at present ill-defined. The combination of an elevated serum carotene concentration and low serum vitamin A suggests that the defect is in one of the enzymes responsible for converting carotene to vitamin A. Bloomstrand and Werner [11] fed labelled carotene to one patient with meta-

bolic carotenaemia and to healthy volunteers. The patient failed to convert carotene to vitamin A and the authors suggested that the defect was in the mucosal β-carotene 15,15′-dioxygenase [11]. Attard-Montalto *et al.* [12] described a 5-year-old girl with xanthodermia, elevated serum β-carotene and low serum vitamin A. The serum concentration of retinol-binding protein (RBP) was at the low end of the normal range. Vitamin A supplements failed to correct the low serum vitamin A concentration. The authors proposed that the primary defect was in the RBP: deficiency of RBP was responsible for defective transport of vitamin A out of intestinal mucosal cells and hepatocytes. Accumulation of vitamin A within these cells was responsible for defective conversion of β-carotene to vitamin A [12]. No direct proof for this hypothesis has been obtained.

Pathology

When the concentration of β-carotene in the blood is high, it accumulates both in the epidermis and in the subcutaneous fat. Here it absorbs light with absorption maxima at 475, 490 and 510 nm, producing the orange–yellow discoloration [8]. There is no strong evidence that elevated concentrations of β-carotene have any adverse effects in the skin or in other tissues in which it accumulates. Shoenfeld *et al.* in 1982 described a single patient, aged 21, who had mild neutropenia and gingival and buccal erosions while she was taking a high carotene diet. The neutropenia resolved on a low carotene diet and returned when ingestion of large amounts of carrot juice was resumed [13]. Kaspar *et al.* in 1991 reported two children with dietary carotenaemia and raised transaminases which fell when the dietary carotene intake was normalized [14].

Table 29.10.2 Carotene content of foods

Moderate (50–250 µg/100 g)	High (300–600 µg/100 g)	Very high (>600 µg/100 g)
Vegetables		
Aubergine	Asparagus	Cabbage (savoy)
Baked beans	Broccoli	Carrots
Broad beans	Brussels sprouts	Chilli (red)
Cauliflower	Courgette	Cress
Celery	Green beans	Curly kale
Fennel	French beans	Mange-tout
Marrow	Leeks	Peppers (red)
Peas (sugarsnap)	Peas (tinned/frozen/fresh)	Parsley
Peppers (green/yellow)	Petit pois	Pumpkin
Runner beans	Squash (acorn)	Spinach
Swede		Spring greens
Sweetcorn		Squash (butternut)
Sweet potato (white flesh)		Sweet potato (orange flesh)
		Tomato (fresh/tinned)*
		Tomato purée*
		Watercress
		Yam (yellow flesh)
Fruit		
Apricot (canned in syrup)	Peach (dried)	Apricot (dried)
Banana	Plum	Melon (canteloupe, flesh)
Blackberry		Watermelon*
Blackcurrant		
Orange		

*Major carotenoid is lycopene.

However, it is by no means certain that liver damage was caused by high tissue concentrations of β-carotene and, in most cases of dietary carotenaemia, transaminases are normal (see below). Nishimura [15] in 1993 compared the serum carotene levels in 82 patients with 'biliary dyskinesia' with 27 control subjects. The patients with abnormal gallbladder contraction rates had a higher incidence of serum carotene levels (>5.6 µmol/l) than the controls. The carotenaemic patients were diagnosed as having metabolic or hyperlipidaemic carotenaemia. Nishimura suggested that there was a close relationship between metabolic carotenaemia and biliary dyskinesia [15]. These findings have not yet been confirmed by other investigators.

It is possible that high skin and tissue concentrations of β-carotene are in fact beneficial. Carotenoids are believed to protect cells against the harmful effects of free radicals. Someya *et al.* [16] have shown that, in the guinea pig, carotene supplementation prevents the skin lipid peroxidation caused by ultraviolet irradiation [16]. It has been postulated that the free radical scavenging activity of carotenoids may help to prevent atherosclerosis and cancer. Individuals with blood β-carotene levels towards the upper limit of the normal range have a lower incidence of cancer and heart disease than those with lower β-carotene levels. Conversely, two studies have shown that supplementation with β-carotene does not prevent cancer and heart disease in well-nourished individuals and, indeed, in high-risk groups (smokers and people exposed to asbestos) the morbidity and mortality appeared to be increased by supplementation. However, there were no excess cases of death and disease in those who attained the highest blood β-carotene levels during supplementation [17].

Dietary carotenaemia (and some cases of hyperlipidaemia) give rise to mildly elevated plasma concentrations of vitamin A. The hypervitaminosis A is never sufficient to cause signs of intoxication; liver function tests are normal [18]. Metabolic carotenaemia may produce low plasma vitamin A concentrations. In such individuals it may be possible to show defective dark adaptation on careful visual testing [5]. In theory, prolonged systemic vitamin A deficiency might lead to more significant ocular problems. Xerosis, swelling and destruction of the cornea could occur and the retinal defect could progress to night blindness. In the skin, hyperkeratosis could also occur and there may be increased susceptibility to infection. To date these problems have never been documented but that may be because metabolic carotenaemia has not been described in children from developing countries. It is important to remember that such children may already be prediposed to vitamin A deficiency by their poor dietary intake of vitamin A [19].

Clinical features

Carotenaemia produces a yellow–orange pigmentation of the skin which is usually most obvious on the palms, soles and nasolabial folds and is absent from the sclerae (Fig. 29.10.2). The urine and stools have a normal colour.

Excessive ingestion

A careful dietary history should be taken. Carotenaemia has been documented in the first year of life in breast-fed infants whose mothers ingest over 1.5 kg of carrots per week or more than 10 tangerines per day [20]. Carotenaemia has also been documented in infants whose

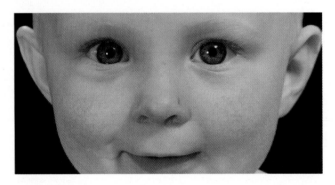

Fig. 29.10.2 Facies of an infant with metabolic carotenaemia. In this case the pigmentation was most obvious in the skin of the tip of the nose, the cheeks and the pinnae. Note the absence of pigmentation in the sclerae.

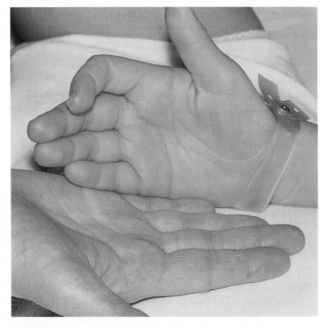

Fig. 29.10.3 Comparison of the skin colour of the palm of a child with carotenaemia (upper) and a normal palm (lower).

parents were strict vegetarians and believed that carrot juice was better for their infant than milk. Such infants may also show evidence of failure to thrive. Carotenaemia may also occur in infants who are difficult to wean onto a balanced range of solids and show a marked preference for pureed carrots and green vegetables. It has been diagnosed in infants who have ingested two to four tangerines per day for 4 weeks. Older children may select a vegetarian diet with a high content of β-carotene and the clinician should consider the possibility that this is part of the anorexia nervosa syndrome [21]. Dietary carotenaemia has also been recorded in areas of West Africa where red palm oil (which has a high carotene content) is used for cooking. Finally, it should be recalled that β-carotene has been used for treatment of photodermatoses such as porphyria and so a careful drug history must be taken. Laboratory investigations reveal an elevated plasma β-carotene concentration and a slightly elevated plasma vitamin A concentration.

Hyperlipidaemias

A full medical history and examination (including urinalysis) should be undertaken. Weight loss could be the result of diabetes or anorexia nervosa. A history of polyuria and polydipsia points strongly to diabetes which can be confirmed by testing the urine for sugar. A history of lethargy, developmental delay, constipation and poor linear growth should trigger a search for features of hypothyroidism such as the coarse facies, large tongue, umbilical hernia and bradycardia. A history of periorbital swelling should lead to a general search for oedema and ascites, and the urine should be checked for the heavy proteinuria that is characteristic of the nephrotic syndrome. Symptoms suggestive of fasting hypoglycaemia (pallor, sweating, jitteriness, loss of consciousness, convulsions) and poor linear growth are suggestive of one of the hepatic glycogenoses and such a diagnosis will usually be obvious from massive hepatomegaly. The hyperlipidaemia of cholestasis and of homozygous familial hypercholesterolaemia may be associated with the presence of cutaneous xanthomas.

Investigations will be directed by the clinical findings but may include β-carotene, vitamin A, cholesterol, triglycerides, blood glucose, glycosylated haemoglobin, thyroid function tests, liver function tests, plasma albumin and renal function tests.

Inborn error(s) of carotene metabolism

The pigmentation is identical to that produced by excessive ingestion of carotene. The age of presentation ranges from 6 months to 24 years. The β-carotene intake is normal or low; some of the older patients have shown an aversion to β-carotene and have adopted a low carotene diet [22].

Some parents of affected infants and toddlers have described loose stools regularly induced by ingestion of carotene-containing foods. There may be a family history of other affected individuals. The plasma concentration of β-carotene is elevated (5–22 μmol/l) and the plasma concentration of vitamin A may be normal or low.

Prognosis

There are no proven adverse effects of dietary carotenaemia. The skin pigmentation can be eliminated by reducing the excessive carotene intake. In the occasional case in which there has been neutropenia or transaminaemia these have also resolved. In children who have carotenaemia associated with hyperlipidaemia, discussion of the prognosis should focus on the cause of the hyperlipidaemia. Metabolic carotenaemia is a benign condition. Parents can be advised that any symptoms associated with ingestion of β-carotene will resolve when a low carotene diet is instituted. Any potential effects of vitamin A deficiency can be avoided by a vitamin A supplement.

Differential diagnosis

Yellowish pigmentation of the skin (xanthodermia) is most commonly due to jaundice. It is occasionally seen when substances such as picric acid, saffron and mepacrine are ingested and stain the skin. In all these conditions, unlike in carotenaemia, the sclerae are also pigmented. The diagnosis of carotenaemia and its cause can often be elucidated from the history and examination (as indicated above) but differential diagnosis is aided by measurements of plasma concentrations of β-carotene, vitamin A and lipids (Table 29.10.3).

Treatment

Excessive ingestion of β-carotene should be managed by first reassuring the parents and the referring doctor that the child does not have jaundice or any other significant medical problem. General dietary advice should be given to ensure that the child will in future receive a balanced diet and the parents can also be told how they can eliminate the cutaneous pigmentation by cutting down the child's excessive intake of β-carotene.

Children with hyperlipidaemia should be treated on the basis of the underlying cause. Parents of children with metabolic carotenaemia should be reassured that it is a benign condition but that the pigmentation can be reduced or eliminated by the use of a low carotene diet. This involves avoidance or restriction of certain vegetables and fruit and avoidance of foods which contain E160 carotenoid additives. The fruit and vegetables in Table 29.10.2 which have a very high carotene content should be avoided altogether. Those with a high content should be restricted to a maximum of one portion per week but those with a moderate content can be allowed two portions daily. Children with metabolic carotenaemia should avoid carrot juice, apricot juice, mango juice, tomato juice and any squash or carbonated drinks with added β-carotene. Meat, fish eggs and poultry can be used freely in the diet but ox liver should be avoided. Chilli, paprika, cayenne pepper and curry powder have a high β-carotene content and should be omitted from the diet. Foods with a high content of cow's milk fat should also be avoided as should butter and margarine (except for products with no added β-carotene). Flour, bread, pasta and breakfast cereals can be taken freely. Cakes and biscuits which are made with butter or margarine should be avoided but those made with vegetable oil as the fat source can be used in the diet. Yellow-coloured sweets, desserts, preserves and so on should be checked for added β-carotene (e.g. high content in lemon curd). If children with metabolic carotenaemia have a low plasma vitamin A concentration this can usually be corrected by an oral vitamin A supplement (2500 units/day).

Acknowledgements

I am grateful to Marjorie Dixon, Chief Dietitian at the Great Ormond Street Hospital for valuable advice on the low carotene diet.

Table 29.10.3 Differential diagnosis of carotenaemia

Cause	Plasma carotene	Plasma vitamin A	Plasma cholesterol and/or triglycerides
Dietary carotenaemia	↑	↑	N
Metabolic carotenameia	↑	N/↓	N
Hyperlipidaemia	↑	N/↑	↑

N, normal.

REFERENCES

1 Furr HC. Carotenoids. In: Macrae R, Robinson RK, Sadler MJ, eds. *Encyclopaedia of Food Science, Food Technology and Nutrition*. London: Academic Press 1993: 707–18.

2 Malvy DJ, Burtschy B, Dostalova L, Amedee-Manesme O. Serum retinol, β-carotene, α-tocopherol and cholesterol in healthy French children. *Int J Epidemiol* 1993; 22: 237–46.

3 Greene CH, Blackford L. Carotenemia. *M Clin N Am* 1926; 10: 733–44.

4 Almond S, Logan RFL. Carotinaemia. *Br Med J* 1942; ii: 239–41.

5 Cohen L. Observations on carotenaemia. *Ann Intern Med* 1958; 48: 219–27.

6 Traber MG, Diamond SR, Lane JC, Brody RI, Kayden HJ. β-Carotene transport in human lipoproteins. Comparisons with α-tocopherol. *Lipids* 1994; 29: 665–9.

7 Holland B, Welch AA, Unwin ID, Buss DH, Paul AA, Southgate DAT. *McCance and Widdowson's The Composition of Foods*, 5th edn. London: Royal Society of Chemistry, Ministry of Agriculture, Food and Fisheries, Her Majesty's Stationery Office, 1991.

8 Prince MR, Frisoli JK. Beta-carotene accumulation in serum and skin. *Am J Clin Nutr* 1993; 57: 175–81.

9 Lloyd JK. Plasma lipid disorders. In: Clayton BE, Round JM, eds. *Chemical Pathology and the Sick Child*. Oxford: Blackwell Scientific Publications, 1984.

10 Mordasini R, Klose G, Greten H. Secondary type II hyperlipoproteinemia in patients with anorexia nervosa. *Metabolism* 1978; 27: 71–9.

11 Bloomstrand R, Werner B. Studies on the intestinal absorption of radioactive beta-carotene and vitamin A in man. Conversion of beta-carotene into vitamin A. *Scand J Clin Lab Invest* 1967; 19: 339–45.

12 Attard-Montalto S, Evans N, Sherwood RA. Carotenaemia with low vitamin A levels and low retinol-binding protein. *J Inherit Metab Dis* 1992; 15: 929–30.

13 Shoenfeld Y, Shaklai M, Ben-Baruch N, Hirschorn M, Pinkhas J. Neutropenia induced by hypercarotenaemia. *Lancet* 1982; i: 1245.

14 Kaspar P, Polsky A, Kudlova E, Novakova V. Carotenemia. *Cesk-Pediatr* 1991; 46: 275–7.

15 Nishimura T. A correlation between carotenemia and biliary dyskinesia. *J Dermatol* 1993; 20: 287–92.

16 Someya K, Totsuka Y, Murakoshi M, Kitano H, Miyazawa T. The antioxidant effect of palm fruit carotene on skin lipid peroxidation in guinea pigs estimated by the chemiluminescence–HPLC method. *J Nutr Sci Vitaminol Tokyo* 1994; 40: 315–24.

17 Rowe PM. Beta-carotene takes a collective beating. *Lancet* 1996; 347: 249.

18 Pollitt N. β-carotene and the photodermatoses. *Br J Dermatol* 1975; 93: 721–4.

19 Favaro RM, de-Souza NV, Batistal SM, Ferriani MG, Desai ID, Dutra-de-Oliviera JE. Vitamin A status of young children in southern Brazil. *Am J Clin Nutr* 1986; 43: 852–8.

20 Honda T. In: Jelliffe EFP, Jelliffe DB, eds. *Adverse Effects of Foods*. New York: Plenum Press, 1982: 389–96.

21 Bilimoria S, Keczkes K, Williamson D, Rowell NR. Hypercarotenaemia in weight watchers. *Clin Exp Dermatol* 1979; 4: 331–5.

22 Monk B. Carotenaemia. *Int J Dermatol* 1983; 22: 376–7.

Index

Page numbers in *italic* refer to figures. Alphabetical order is word-by-word.

in pityriasis rubra pilaris 664
in herpes simplex virus infection 321–2
in HPV infection 309
in Jessner's lymphocytic infiltrate 816
in leishmaniasis 516
in leprosy 537–8
in lichen planus 678–9
in polymorphic light eruption 895
in sarcoidosis 1549
in toxic shock syndrome 379
T-cell receptor and atopic disease 174
Tabanus 551, 552
tabby mouse 1164–5
tache noir 441
tachycardia in hyperthyroidism 1627
tacrolimus
    in alopecia areata 1832
    in atopic dermatitis 184, 228
    in GVHD 1707
talcum powder 156
talipes in pigmentary mosaicism 1245
tanapoxviruses 352, *353*, 360–1
tanning beds 923
tar preparations 1737
    in atopic dermatitis 184, 222
    in napkin dermatitis 156
    poisoning 1761
    in psoriasis 662
    in seborrhoeic dermatitis of adolescence
        276
target lesion 573, 628, 629–30
tartrazine 232, 591
TAT gene 1137
tattooing in vitiligo 888
taurodontia 1173
Tay–Sach's disease 1200
Tay's syndrome *see* trichothiodystrophy
TDT test 171
tea tree 300
Tedania ignis 580
teeth
    in Cockayne's syndrome 1333
    in dyskeratosis congenita 1346
    in dystrophic epidermolysis bullosa 1084,
        1093–4
    in EDS 1270
    in EEC syndrome 1181
    effects of thumb/finger-sucking 1721
    in Gorlin syndrome 1251
    grinding 1721
    in Hay–Wells syndrome 1178
    in hidrotic ectodermal dysplasia 1170
    Hutchinson's 1514
    in incontinentia pigmenti 1240–1
    in junctional epidermolysis bullosa 1095
    in Langerhans' cell histiocytosis 1419
    mulberry molars 1514
    in Naegeli–Franceschetti–Jadassohn
        syndrome 1185
    natal 1307
    in oculodentodigital dysplasia 1184
    in pigmentary mosaicism 1245
    pigmentation/discoloration 1450
    in Rapp–Hodgkin syndrome 1175, *1176*
    in Rothmund–Thomson syndrome 1342
    in Schöpf–Schultz–Passarge syndrome
        1183
    in tooth and nail syndrome 1172
    in trichodentosseous syndrome 1173
    in trichothiodystrophy 1338
    in X-linked hypohidrotic ectodermal
        dysplasia 1165, *1166*
Tegenaria agrestis 574

telangiectasia
    in dermatomyositis 1675
    differential diagnosis 114, 992
    generalized essential 992
    hereditary benign 992
    hereditary haemorrhagic
        (Rendu–Osler–Weber disease) 992,
        994, 1450
    localized 992
    syndromic 992–4
    treatment 991, 1809, 1810, 1811
    unilateral naevoid 992, *1052*
    see also ataxia telangiectasia
telangiectasia macularis eruptiva perstans
    600, *601*, 605, 607, 992
temper tantrums 1533
temperature
    regulation 1853–4
    role in napkin dermatitis 141
TEN *see* toxic epidermal necrolysis
tenascin in hair follicle development 32–3,
    35
tenosynovitis in gonorrhoea 1519
tensioactive agents 50
terbinafine 1741
    adverse effects 1746
    in black piedra 469
    in candidiasis 465
    in dermatophytoses 458–9
    in sporotrichosis 486
    topical 1738
terconazole 458
terfenadine 1740
    in atopic dermatitis 190
    in hypersensitivity to plants and plant
        products 298
testes
    maldescent, and X-linked recessive
        ichthyosis 1104
    oestrogen-producing tumours 1636, 1637
    pain, in Henoch–Schönlein purpura 1566
testicular feminization syndrome 1065,
    1636–7
testitoxicosis 1632
testolactone 1634
testosterone
    and acne 643, 1744
    free plasma 1635
tetracaine 1767, 1818, 1819
tetracyclines
    adverse effects 648, 1740
        dyschromatosis 870
        fixed drug eruptions 1746
        hyperpigmentation 857–8
        lichenoid drug eruption *686*
        phototoxicity 918
        urticaria 590
    in *Chlamydia* infection 1525
    in dystrophic epidermolysis bullosa
        1088
    in perioral dermatitis 264
    in recurrent aphthous stomatitis 1437
    in rickettsial infections 441, 442–3, 444,
        445, 446
    and Stevens–Johnson syndrome 632
    and toxic epidermal necrolysis 635
tetrahydrobiopterin 882
tetrasomy 22p 1061
TEWL *see* transepidermal water loss
TGase *see* transglutaminase
thalidomide
    in actinic prurigo 900
    in Behçet's disease 1608–9

in GVHD 1707
    in Jessner's lymphocytic infiltrate 817
    in Langerhans' cell histiocytosis 1424
    in leprosy 545
    in lupus panniculitis 626
thallium poisoning 1478, 1763
thelarche 1631, 1632
    premature 1632, *1633*
theophylline 45
    in atopic dermatitis 190
    transdermal therapeutic delivery systems
        1734
therapeutic principles 1731–42
thiabendazole 477, 530
thiazides *686*
Thibierge–Weissenbach syndrome 785
thimble jellyfish 578
thimerasol (thiomersal) 288, 290
thioredoxin reductase 882
thiurams 290, *293*
threadworms 1504–5, 1520, 1538
3A syndrome 1630
thrombocytopenia
    in Fanconi's syndrome 1348, 1349
    in Kasabach–Merritt syndrome 1015
    in NLE 113
    transient 66
    in Wiskott–Aldrich syndrome 1697, 1698
thrombocytopenic purpura 1450, 1579
thrombocytosis in Kawasaki's disease 1619
thrombomodulin in purpura fulminans
    1577
thrombophlebitis 624, 1608
thrombosis in purpura fulminans 1579–80
thrush *see* candidiasis
thumb
    anomalies in Gorlin syndrome 1253
    duplication 1498
    sucking 1719, 1720, 1721, 1728
thumb sign in Marfans's syndrome 1290,
    1291
thymidine kinase 326
thymoma 881
thymopentin in atopic dermatitis 226
thymus
    in ataxia telangiectasia 1680
    hypoplasia with bullous pemphigoid 744
thyroid
    in Cowden's syndrome 1354
    function disorders 1623–7, 1827
    lingual 1456, 1623
    papillary carcinoma 82
thyroiditis
    autoimmune 1625
    Hashimoto's 1623, 1626, 1627
    in hypersensitivity syndrome reaction
        1749
    and ILVEN 962
thyrotropin in hypothyroidism 1625
thyroxine replacement therapy 1625
tibia, sabre 433, *434*, 1514
ticks 421, 422, 438
TIMP-1 997, 998
tin-protoporphyrin 919
tinea capitis 450–1, *453*
    aetiology 448–9
    carriage of spores 449
    differential diagnosis 457
    ectothrix infections 451, *452*
    endothrix infections 451–2
    in HIV infection 363, *364*
    treatment 458–9
tinea corporis 452–3